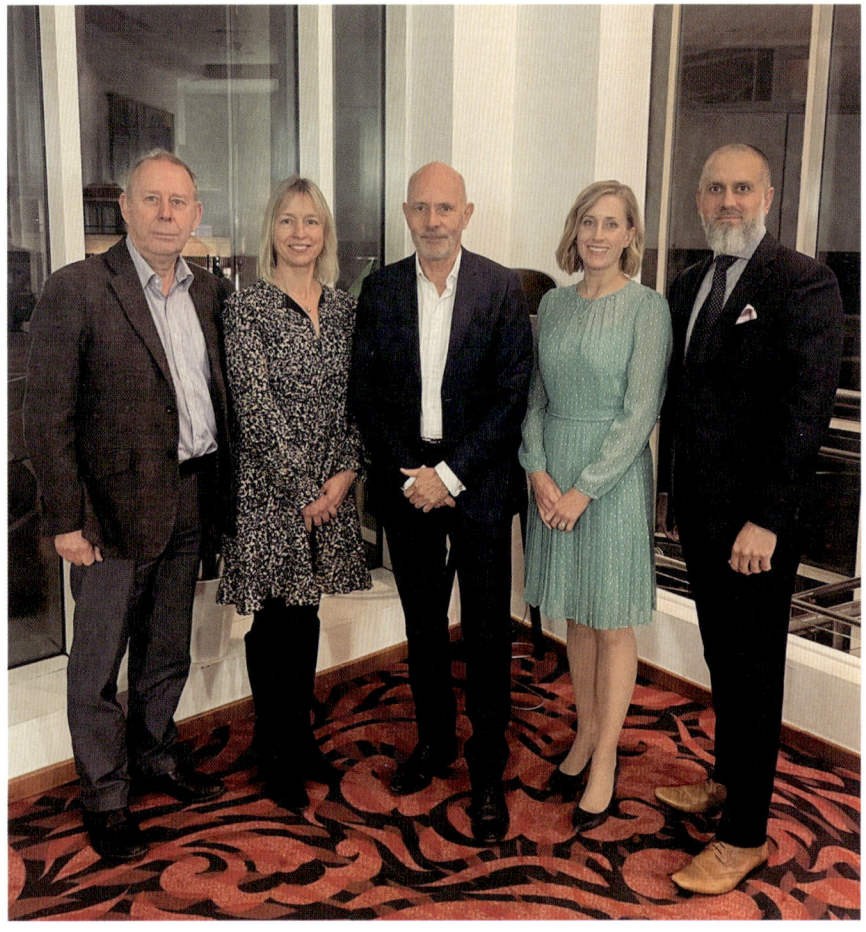

The Editors
From left to right: Jonathan Barker, Tanya Bleiker, Christopher Griffiths,
Rosalind Simpson, Walayat Hussain

Rook's
Textbook of
Dermatology

TENTH EDITION

EDITED BY

Christopher Griffiths OBE, MD, FMedSci

Emeritus Professor of Dermatology
The University of Manchester
Manchester, UK

Adjunct Professor & Consultant Dermatologist
King's College London
London, UK

Jonathan Barker MD, FRCP

Professor of Medical Dermatology
St John's Institute of Dermatology
Faculty of Life Sciences and Medicine
King's College London
London, UK

Tanya Bleiker FRCP

Consultant Dermatologist
University Hospitals of Derby and Burton NHS Foundation Trust
Derby, UK

Walayat Hussain FRACP

Consultant Dermatological & Mohs Micrographic Surgeon
Dermatology Surgical & Laser Unit
Chapel Allerton Hospital
Leeds, UK

Rosalind Simpson MRCP, PhD

Associate Professor and Consultant Dermatologist
Centre of Evidence Based Dermatology
University of Nottingham
Nottingham, UK

IN FOUR VOLUMES

VOLUME 2

WILEY Blackwell

Registered Office(s)
John Wiley & Sons, Inc., 111 River Street, Hoboken, NJ 07030, USA
John Wiley & Sons Ltd, The Atrium, Southern Gate, Chichester, West Sussex, PO19 8SQ, UK

Editorial Office(s)
9600 Garsington Road, Oxford, OX4 2DQ, UK
The Atrium, Southern Gate, Chichester, West Sussex, PO19 8SQ, UK

For details of our global editorial offices, customer services, and more information about Wiley products visit us at www.wiley.com.

Wiley also publishes its books in a variety of electronic formats and by print-on-demand. Some content that appears in standard print versions of this book may not be available in other formats.

Library of Congress Cataloging-in-Publication Data has been applied for.

Set ISBN (4 Volumes): 9781119709213

Cover Design: Wiley
Cover Image: © khamkula/Adobe Stock

Set in 9.5/12pt, Palatino LT Std by Straive, Chennai, India

Printed in Great Britain by Bell & Bain Ltd, Glasgow

10 9 8 7 6 5 4 3 2 1

Contents

PART 4
Inflammatory Dermatoses

CHAPTER 35

Psoriasis and Related Disorders

Brian Kirby[1] *and A. David Burden*[2]

[1] St Vincent's University Hospital and Charles Institute, University College Dublin, Dublin, Ireland
[2] Institute of Infection and Immunity, University of Glasgow, Glasgow, UK

PART 4: INFLAMMATORY DERMATOSES

Definition

Psoriasis comprises a family of common, immune-mediated and often genetically determined, inflammatory skin diseases, recognised by its distinctive clinical appearances, and associated with diseases in other organs, in particular psoriatic arthritis. There is a fundamental classification into plaque forms of the disease and pustular forms, which may co-exist. Chronic plaque psoriasis (psoriasis vulgaris) is the commoner form and is characterised by red, scaly, sharply demarcated plaques of variable extent and severity. Pustular psoriasis is characterised by the presence of sterile pustules and is distinct from psoriasis vulgaris in its genetic susceptibility, pathogenesis, clinical features and response to treatment.

Pending a full aetiological and molecular classification, Box 35.1 provides a provisional working classification.

This chapter is divided into three sections: plaque psoriasis, pustular psoriasis and psoriatic arthritis.

CHRONIC PLAQUE PSORIASIS (PSORIASIS VULGARIS)

Epidemiology

Incidence and prevalence

Psoriasis is estimated to affect at least 60 million people worldwide [1]. The point prevalence rises during childhood and affects approximately 1–3% of the adult population [1,2], with wide geographic variation, and some evidence for an increasing prevalence in all

Rook's Textbook of Dermatology, Tenth Edition. Edited by Christopher Griffiths, Jonathan Barker, Tanya Bleiker, Walayat Hussain and Rosalind Simpson.

age groups [3]. The annual incidence in adults has been reported as between 0.03% and 0.32% [1]. These figures relate primarily to plaque psoriasis, which accounts for 90% of all cases. The epidemiology of disease variants is less well described.

Ethnicity

Psoriasis appears to be more common in high income populations [1]. It is rare in American Indians [4] and in sub-Saharan Africa [5]. In the USA, the standardised incidence rate is higher in white people than in Hispanic/Latino and African American people [6].

Box 35.1 Provisional working classification of psoriasis

Clinical forms of psoriasis (based on morphology or natural history)
- Plaque psoriasis (psoriasis vulgaris)
- Acute guttate psoriasis
- 'Unstable' psoriasis
- Erythrodermic psoriasis
- Pustular psoriasis
- Atypical forms of psoriasis

Other specified forms of psoriasis (based on age or precipitants)
- Linear and segmental psoriasis
- Psoriasis in childhood and old age
- Photoaggravated psoriasis
- Drug-induced or exacerbated psoriasis
- HIV-induced or exacerbated psoriasis

Psoriasis affecting specific sites
- Scalp psoriasis
- Follicular psoriasis
- Seborrhoeic psoriasis (sebopsoriasis)
- Flexural psoriasis (inverse psoriasis)
- Genital psoriasis
- Non-pustular palmoplantar psoriasis
- Nail psoriasis
- Mucosal lesions
- Ocular lesions

Age at onset

There are two peak ages of incidence, the first occurring between 16 and 22 years and the second between 57 and 62 years of age. This underlies the concept of type I and type II psoriasis [7]. In 35% of patients, disease onset is before the age of 20 years and 58% before age 30 years. In a UK study, the mean age of onset was 33 years with the mode in the second decade. In 75% of patients, the disease onset was before 46 years of age [8].

Sex

Some studies have reported an earlier age of onset in girls, although psoriasis affects adult women and men with equal frequency [9,10]. Studies assessing the use of systemic and biological treatment in cohorts of patients with severe disease consistently report that men are about twice as likely to receive systemic treatment as women, suggesting that men may have more severe disease [11,12].

Pathophysiology

Genetics

There is overwhelming evidence of an important genetic component to the aetiology of psoriasis. Lomholt's classical epidemiological survey of psoriasis in the Faroe Islands, in which he examined more than 10 000 inhabitants, made the key observation that the prevalence of psoriasis was greater among relatives of those affected than controls [2]. Based on population data, lifetime risks of psoriasis are 4%, 28% and 65% if neither, one or both parents are affected [13]. A bimodal peak in the age at disease onset curve has been used as evidence for two pathogenetically distinct types of psoriasis (type I psoriasis of early-onset, hereditable, strongly HLA-C:06:02 associated and more severe, type II of late-onset, sporadic, HLA-C:06:02 unrelated, and generally milder) [7], although the genetic epidemiology is more complex than this [14]. Support for population studies comes from the analysis of family pedigrees in which psoriasis appears in multiple generations [15]. The pattern of inheritance may be autosomal dominant with reduced penetrance, or consistent with a recessive model. Most authorities regard the data as suggesting polygenic or multifactorial inheritance.

The most robust data supporting a genetic basis to psoriasis come from studies examining concordance for the disease in twins. Examination of individuals in twin registries has shown concordance for psoriasis almost three times more frequently in monozygotic twins than dizygotic twins, giving estimates of heritability from 60% to 90% [16,17,18,19]. When monozygotic twins are concordant for psoriasis, the age of onset, distribution of the disease and severity are similar, suggesting that genetic factors play a role in these parameters. Based on the variable extent and pattern in which it is inherited, it is suggested that psoriasis represents a spectrum of genetic diseases. At one end are rare families in which changes in a single gene may be sufficient to cause the disease. At the opposite end of the spectrum is the more common form in which a family history may be lacking. In these individuals, it is likely that changes in multiple genes, interacting both with each other and the environment, are required for disease expression [20].

All the above investigations have studied chronic plaque psoriasis. Guttate psoriasis is almost invariably *HLA-C:06:02* associated [21,22] and thought to be closely linked pathogenically to early-onset plaque psoriasis. Late-onset plaque psoriasis shares many susceptibility loci with early-onset disease, and may have additional specific susceptibility genes, e.g. *IL1B* [23]. The genetics of pustular psoriasis is discussed later. Little is known about the genetic epidemiology of other forms of psoriasis.

Molecular genetics

Classical genome-wide linkage analysis in pedigrees multiply affected by psoriasis has identified nine chromosomal regions with evidence for linkage (*PSORS1–PSORS9*) [24]. By far the major psoriasis genetic determinant is *PSORS1*, located within the major histocompatibility complex (MHC) on chromosome 6p, spanning an approximately 150-kb segment within the class I region [25,26]. Identification of the causative gene at this locus is hampered by the extensive linkage disequilibrium observed within the MHC. The consensus major risk allele at this site is *HLA-C:06:02*, and there may be additional independent associations within the MHC,

Table 35.1 Psoriasis susceptibility genes identified by GWAS and their pathway.

Type 1 interferon signalling	NFκB signalling	Antigen presentation	IL-23/ IL-17 axis	Epidermal barrier function
IFIH1/MDA5	CARD14	HLA-C	IL23A	CDSN
ZNF313/RNF114	REL	ERAP1	IL12B	LCE3B/LCE3C
DDX58	TNIP1		IL23R	KLF4
EXOC2	TRAF3IP2 (Act1)		SOCS1	
ELMO1	TNFAIP3		TYK2	
TYK2	NFKBIA		TNFSF15	
	NFKBIZ		PTPN2	
	IKBKE		STAT3	
	CARM1		IRF4	

for instance with *MICA* and *CDSN* [27,28]. Phenotypic variants of psoriasis are genetically heterogeneous at the level of *PSORS1*. Thus, guttate psoriasis is strongly associated with *PSORS1* [22], whereas late-onset plaque psoriasis is not [29].

Of particular interest is *PSORS2*, a replicated locus first mapped to chromosome 17q in 1994 [25] and identified as the gene *CARD14* by exome sequencing in 2012 [30,31]. Heterozygous gain-of-function mutations in *CARD14* mediate nuclear factor kappa light chain enhancer of activated B-cell (NFκB) signal transduction in affected keratinocytes leading to enhanced production of pro-inflammatory cytokines.

The availability of large, well-characterised cohorts of plaque psoriasis patients together with advances in high-throughput genotyping have combined to permit disease case–control association studies producing robust replicated data on associated disease susceptibility genes. Genome-wide association studies (GWAS) [32,33,**34**,35,36,**37**], meta-analyses of GWAS and genome-wide imputation along with exome chip analysis provide evidence for over 65 susceptibility loci in white populations [38,39]. Candidate genes at these loci tend to cluster in a limited number of biological pathways, primarily involved in innate and adaptive immunity (Table 35.1). The relative risk attributed to individual polymorphisms in known genes is low, but there is also evidence of additive association between genes (epistasis), for instance between *HLA-C* and *ERAP1* [37]. It is currently estimated that about 25% of the heritability of psoriasis can be explained by known susceptibility loci [38]. The genetic contribution to disease course and severity, and of co-morbidities (psoriatic arthritis, obesity), is being explored [20]. As the genetic architecture of psoriasis becomes more fully understood, investigation of gene–environment interactions may suggest interventions that prevent or modify the natural history of the disease.

The impact on the management of psoriasis of translating genetic information into the clinic is yet to be fully realised. Currently, too small a proportion of the heritability is accounted for by known loci for genotyping to contribute to the diagnosis, although rare genetic mutations of major effect (e.g. in *CARD14* or *IL36RN*) may be useful in subclassifying psoriatic diseases. The most immediate consequence of a greater understanding of the genetic basis of psoriasis has been in the identification of therapeutic targets (interleukin [IL]-23, IL-17, Tyk2), and the selection and monitoring of individual treatments. As more selective treatments emerge, the likelihood of a differential responsiveness to treatment between

patients depending on genotype will increase. For instance, there is evidence that patients who have the *HLA-C* risk allele may respond better to ustekinumab [40] and that those who are *HLA-C:06:02* negative and have psoriatic arthritis are more likely to respond to adalimumab [41].

Environmental factors

Disease concordance rates in twin studies do not reach 100% even when older identical twins are examined, indicating that the environment plays a role in disease expression. Some of the known triggers and exacerbating factors described below are also complications of psoriasis and its treatment, for instance psychological distress, and in an individual patient it can be difficult to know the direction of causality.

Infection

An association between tonsillitis and psoriasis was first noted over 100 years ago [42]. It is now well recognised that psoriasis can be triggered by streptococcal infection, particularly guttate psoriasis but also psoriasis vulgaris [**43**]. Oligoclonal expansion of T cells occurs in the tonsils in response to streptococcal colonisation, and the same T-cell repertoire may be found in the peripheral blood and skin of patients with guttate psoriasis [**44**,45]. It has been proposed that psoriasis is an autoimmune disease that is fuelled by persistent intracellular streptococcal infection [45]. Streptococci are facultative intracellular bacteria and are not eliminated by standard antibiotic therapy, which may explain the lack of efficacy of antibiotics in treating guttate psoriasis [46].

Tonsillectomy appears to be effective in some patients. Of 29 patients with plaque psoriasis exacerbated by sore throats, 13/15 randomised to tonsillectomy showed significant improvement in psoriasis over 2 years compared with none in the control group [47,48]. The tonsillectomy group was also found to have reductions in skin homing T cells compared with controls [47]. In a subsequent study, the benefit of tonsillectomy was found to be greatest in the those who were HLA-C:06:02 homozygotes [49].

Respiratory viral infections have also been shown to exacerbate psoriasis [50]. Covid-19 infection is associated with exacerbation of psoriasis in up to 25% of patients [51].

The role of HIV infection in the exacerbation of psoriasis is discussed later.

Medications

Many drugs have been reported to trigger the onset and/or exacerbation of psoriasis [52,**53**]. The most important medications that may trigger or exacerbate psoriasis in current clinical practice are lithium salts, synthetic antimalarials [54] and TNF-α inhibitors [**55**]. Interferon-α was a potent inducer of psoriasis when it was used as a treatment for hepatitis C infection [56]. Beta-blockers, calcium channel blockers, angiotensin-converting enzyme inhibitors and non-steroidal anti-inflammatory drugs have been implicated in small case series or population-based case–controlled studies [57,58]. Given the known co-morbidities of psoriasis, these drugs are widely prescribed in patients with psoriasis and yet, in most, do not appear to have a major detrimental effect.

Although psoriasis may respond to oral corticosteroids, both tachyphylaxis and rebound phenomena may occur. Withdrawal of corticosteroids may lead to rebound of the disease and the development of unstable psoriasis – withdrawal should be by steady dose reduction rather than abrupt termination [59].

Alcohol misuse

There is good evidence that excessive alcohol consumption is associated with moderate to severe psoriasis [60–63]. One Finnish study of over 5000 patients reported an excess mortality from alcohol-related causes in patients with psoriasis who had been admitted to hospital for treatment of their disease. The standard mortality ratios for alcohol-related deaths were 4.46 (95% CI 3.60–5.45) for men and 5.60 (95% CI 2.98–8.65) for women [64]. Psoriasis appears to be more prevalent in patients with alcoholic liver disease and patients undergoing outpatient treatment for alcohol dependence [65]. Alcohol misuse, as measured by anonymous questionnaires, is present in about 30% of patients with moderate to severe disease [66,67]. Alcohol misuse is associated with more severe skin disease, increased levels of anxiety and depression, and contributes to increased cardiovascular risk [68]. Screening for alcohol misuse should be considered in those with more severe disease [67]. There is a close relationship between alcohol misuse and cigarette smoking [60–62].

Cigarette smoking

Cigarette smoking is increased among patients with plaque psoriasis compared with the normal population [69]. The odds ratio of ever having been a smoker in psoriasis compared with the general population is 1.84 (95% CI 1.4–2.3) [70]. Patients who smoke are at increased risk of developing psoriasis, of having more severe disease and of a poorer response to biologic treatments [71]. Smoking has multiple immunological and pro-inflammatory effects that may contribute to the initiation and persistence of psoriasis [72]. There is a particularly strong association between cigarette smoking and palmoplantar pustulosis. The effect of smoking cessation on the activity of psoriasis and response to treatment has not been established.

Psychological distress

There is a complex relationship between psoriasis and psychological distress. In different studies between 31% and 88% of patients with psoriasis report that psychological distress triggers or exacerbates their disease [73]. The mechanisms that mediate this effect are not fully understood, but may include interactions between the peripheral nervous system, immune pathways and the hypothalamic–pituitary–adrenal axis [74]. Neurotransmitters have immunomodulatory properties and may play a role in the maintenance of plaques [75]. For instance, in imiquimod-induced psoriasiform inflammation in a murine model, pharmacological ablation of a subset of cutaneous nociceptive neurons caused a reduction in IL-23 production from dermal dendritic cells, with a consequent reduction in IL-23 dependent cytokines from Th17 cells and reduced inflammation [76]. Acute experimental psychological stress can affect Langerhans cell function [77], skin barrier function [78] and hypocortisolaemic responses in patients with psoriasis compared with healthy controls [79]. High worry levels are associated with a decreased response to PUVA [80].

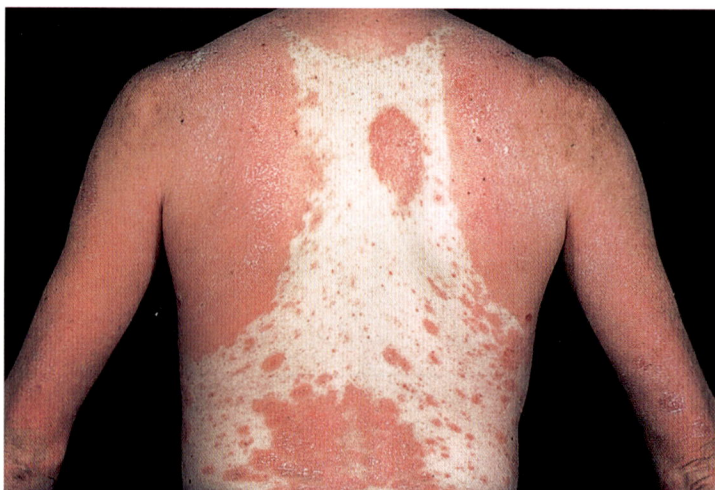

Figure 35.1 Although sunlight is generally beneficial, psoriasis may be provoked by sunlight in a minority. Courtesy of St John's Institute of Dermatology, London, UK.

The question arises whether interventions that focus on psychological distress can improve the physical disease. Several small studies have demonstrated increased efficacy of UVB and PUVA when supplemented with stress-reducing psychological interventions [81]. Various forms of cognitive-behavioural therapy (one to one, group and online) have been shown to reduce distress in patients with psoriasis, and in some studies have also improved health-related quality of life, and the activity of psoriasis as measured by PASI [82,83]. These studies provide some evidence that there is a causal association between psychological distress and the clinical activity of psoriasis.

Sunlight

Although sunlight is generally beneficial, psoriasis may be provoked by sunlight (Figure 35.1) and cause summer exacerbations in exposed skin in 5–20% of patients. Some of these patients gave a history of polymorphic light eruption (PLE) with psoriasis appearing as a Koebner phenomenon within PLE lesions [84]. In a study of 20 British patients, severely photosensitive psoriasis was found in younger patients, affecting women almost exclusively [85]. Although monochromator testing is generally normal, psoriasis may be induced by low-dose broadband UVA directly, without koebnerisation. Photochemotherapy can be helpful in these patients [86].

Physical trauma

Psoriasis can occur in sites of cutaneous trauma and old scars – the Koebner phenomenon, which was first described by Heinrich Koebner in 1877. The mechanisms are analogous to accelerated wound healing and it is proposed that trauma can initiate innate immune activation, keratinocyte hyperproliferation and angiogenesis. Up to 25% of patients report the development of psoriasis in sites of skin trauma [87] and this is more frequent in patients who are *HLA-C:06:02* positive [88].

Pathogenic mechanisms

Progress in the understanding of the pathogenesis of plaque psoriasis in recent years has proceeded in tandem with a greater understanding of innate and adaptive immunity [89]. It has facilitated the development of targeted biologic and small molecule treatments and has itself been informed by the effectiveness of these treatments [90]. There is a complex network of inflammation in psoriasis plaques, involving many cell types and inflammatory mediators (interferons, cytokines and chemokines) with the potential to generate self-amplifying loops, moderated by susceptibility gene variants and environmental triggers.

Plaques of psoriasis represent hyperproliferation and activation of keratinocytes and endothelial cells, which are in turn caused by the infiltration of inflammatory and immune cells including neutrophils, dendritic cells, mast cells, T lymphocytes, innate lymphoid cells, natural killer cells (NK cells), and NK T cells. The pattern of inflammation is mixed, having features of both autoinflammation and adaptive immunity. A bimodal pattern has been proposed in which innate immunity and autoinflammation dominate in early and unstable lesions, and T-cell adaptive immunity in established chronic plaques [91]. The Th17 cell and the IL-23/IL-17 axis are involved in the interplay of innate and adaptive immunity and have emerged as central to the pathogenesis of plaque psoriasis, with evidence coming from genetics, immunology and the high efficacy of treatments targeting this pathway [92].

The recruitment of neutrophils and plasmacytoid dendritic cells (pDCs) are early events in the development of plaques of psoriasis [93]. Activated neutrophils release neutrophil extracellular traps (NETs), web-like structures of DNA, RNA, enzymes and antimicrobial peptides (AMPs) such as LL37 (derived from the AMP cathelicidin). Self-DNA in complex with LL37 in NETs or from keratinocytes can bind TLR9 in pDCs and induce the production of interferon-α [94,95,96]. NETs also activate monocytes to produce Th17-polarising cytokines, which induce memory T-cells with a Th17 phenotype. In patients with psoriasis who carry the risk allele at TRAF3IP2, the encoded D10N variant of Act1 promotes unrepressed STAT3-mediated IL-17A production, contributing to the elevated IL-17A seen in psoriasis plaques [97]. IL-17A is also released by innate immune cells including mast cells and innate lymphoid cells [98].

In established plaques, myeloid dendritic cells direct the inflammatory cascade by producing IL-12 which activates Th1 cells, and IL-23 which maintains the activation of Th17 cells [99]. In psoriasis, regulatory T-cell function is impaired, which disturbs the balance of Th1 and Th17 cells [100]. Some T-cell clones in psoriasis plaques recognise T-cell auto-antigens, including ADAMTSL5 secreted by melanocytes, in an HLA-C:06:02 restricted manner [101]. The extent to which Th17 cell autoimmunity is primary or secondary in the pathogenesis psoriasis is unclear [102]. T-cell cytokines including IL-17A and IL-17F co ntribute to driving keratinocyte proliferation and the activation of keratinocytes to produce further pro-inflammatory cytokines (IL-1, IL-6, TNF-α, IL-36), chemokines (CXCL10, CCL20, IL-8) and AMPs, which can set up self-perpetuating autocrine inflammatory loops. Key pro-inflammatory cytokines involved in the inflammatory network in psoriasis act through a limited set of intracellular signalling and transcription pathways, in particular JAK-STAT signalling in the case of interferon α, interferon γ, interleukin 12, interleukin 23 and

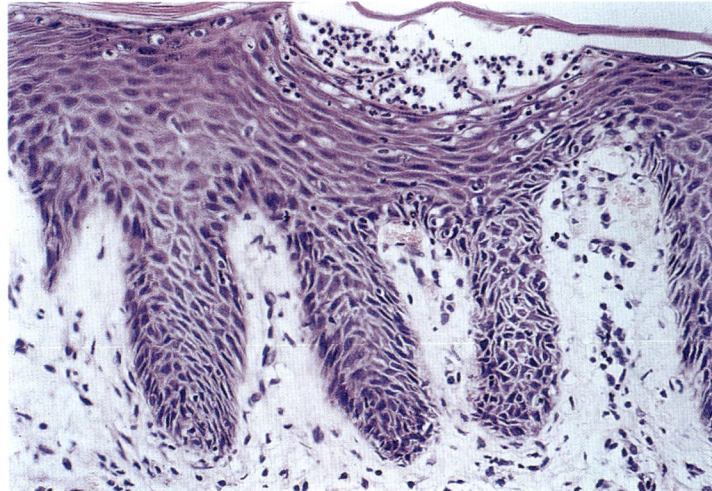

Figure 35.2 Psoriasis: intraepidermal spongiform pustule (of Kogoj). H&E, ×100. Courtesy of St John's Institute of Dermatology, London, UK.

NFκB in the case of TNF-α, which present therapeutic targets for small molecule inhibitors [103]. When plaques of psoriasis resolve, oligoclonal populations of resident memory T cells that produce IL-17A persist at the site of previous inflammation at a higher frequency than in non-lesional skin, which may account for the tendency for plaques to recur in the same anatomical location [104].

Histopathology
Early changes
Vasodilatation, papillary oedema and leukocyte infiltration appear to precede epidermal changes in early developing lesions [105]. Compact hyperkeratosis, disappearance of the granular layer and epidermal hyperplasia follow. Mitotic figures in keratinocytes and leukocytic infiltration in spongiotic foci are seen in the lower half of the epidermis. Scattered mounds of parakeratosis set in a predominantly orthokeratotic stratum corneum appear, with or without neutrophils (Figure 35.2). Epidermal hyperplasia with rete ridges of even length and prominently dilated, tortuous papillary capillaries associated with mixed mononuclear and neutrophil infiltrates are seen [106].

Changes in fully developed plaques
There is parakeratosis associated with focal orthokeratosis, near absence of the granular layer, hyperplasia with elongation of rete ridges and supra-papillary epidermal thinning [107] (Figure 35.3). The rete ridges are often clubbed, branched or fused at their bases, with mononuclear leukocyte infiltrates in the lower half of the epidermis. Neutrophils may sometimes be seen in the stratum corneum (Munro microabscesses) (Figure 35.4). Dilated, tortuous, papillary blood vessels almost touch the undersurface of the thinning supra-papillary epidermis and are surrounded by a mixed mononuclear and neutrophil infiltrate, as well as extravasated erythrocytes. Invasion of the epidermis with leukocytes takes place particularly in the supra-papillary region [106,108]. Necrotic keratinocytes may be seen in the upper and mid epidermis [109].

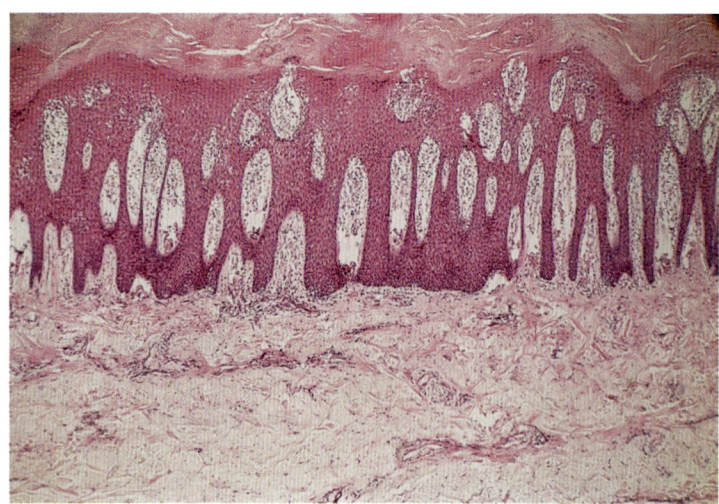

Figure 35.3 Psoriasis irregular epidermal hyperplasia with suprapapillary thinning. H&E, ×50. Courtesy of St John's Institute of Dermatology, London, UK.

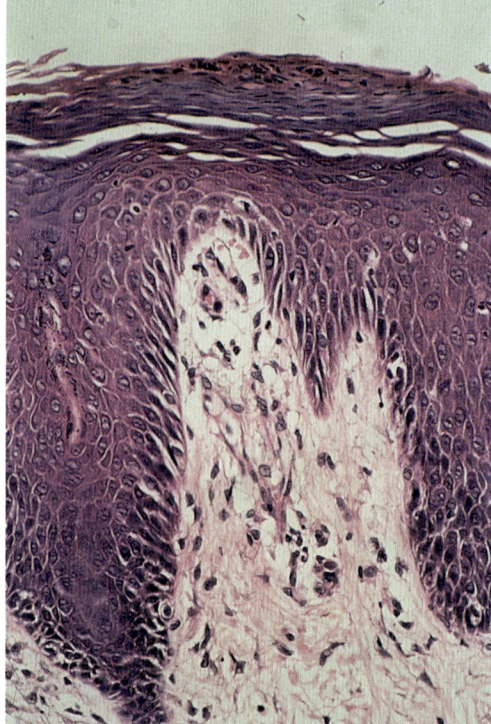

Figure 35.4 Psoriasis: Munro microabscess formation in lesional stratum corneum. H&E, ×200. Courtesy of St John's Institute of Dermatology, London, UK.

Clinical features

History

Pruritus is often the dominant symptom and, although not as severe as in atopic eczema [110,111], is experienced by the majority of patients and contributes to the impairment in quality of life, partly through disturbed sleep [112–115]. Skin tightness and burning are frequent in unstable, erythrodermic or pustular psoriasis and pain may be experienced in areas of fissure formation, particularly in palmoplantar or flexural disease [116]. Shedding of scale can be a significant symptom, for instance in scalp psoriasis, and contributes to feelings of embarrassment. The impact of the disease and its symptoms on patients' relationships, activities and occupation can be severe and its assessment may be assisted by patient completed questionnaires.

The first manifestation of psoriasis may develop at any age and in general those with earlier onset disease are more likely to have a family history of psoriasis. The course of the disease including the frequency of relapses and remissions varies greatly between individuals. Exacerbating factors should be enquired after and responses to previous treatments noted. It is important to ask concerning the involvement by psoriasis of specific sites that may not be volunteered by the patient, for instance the ano-genital region [117]. A detailed medical history should be taken including an enquiry into symptoms of common co-morbidities, particularly of articular symptoms.

Presentation

Chronic plaque psoriasis is the most common type of psoriasis, accounting for about 80–90% of all cases [118]. It presents as a papulo-squamous rash, and the diagnosis is based on the characteristics of individual lesions and their distribution on the skin. Typical lesions are red scaly plaques, which are remarkably well demarcated from unaffected skin, with sharply delineated edges (Figure 35.5). Plaques may be encircled by a clear peripheral zone, the halo or ring of Woronoff (Figure 35.6) [119]. There may be any number of lesions or only a single one. When multiple, lesions are usually monomorphic and distributed relatively symmetrically over the scalp, trunk and extensor surfaces of the limbs. They vary in diameter from one to several centimetres and are oval or irregular in shape. Large plaques may form by coalescence of smaller plaques and are commonly seen on the legs and sacral region. Involuting lesions may clear from the centre initially, producing annular or arcuate shapes. Postinflammatory hyperpigmentation or hypopigmentation are common [120], particularly in patients with skin of colour [121]. Linear and geometric configurations may arise at the sites of trauma as an isomorphic (Koebner) phenomenon (Figure 35.7).

Most psoriasis lesions are surmounted by silvery white scales, which vary considerably in thickness (Figure 35.8). The amount of scaling may be minimal in partially treated disease, and in the flexures. When scaling is not evident it can often be induced by light scratching, a useful sign in diagnostically uncertain lesions. The successive removal of scales usually reveals an underlying smooth, glossy red membrane with small bleeding points where the thin supra-papillary epidermis has been torn off (Auspitz sign) (Figure 35.9). The epidermal thickening characteristic of the psoriasis process causes the lesions to be raised from the adjoining skin and easily palpable. There is evidence that the thickness of untreated plaques varies between patients but is relatively constant in an individual and may predict response to treatment [122].

These diagnostic features may not all be present at the same time or in every case and are sometimes obscured or evanescent. The variety of morphologies of chronic plaque psoriasis has led some authors to attempt a sub-classification according to phenotype and to speculate that it may in fact be several distinct disease entities [122,**123**,124].

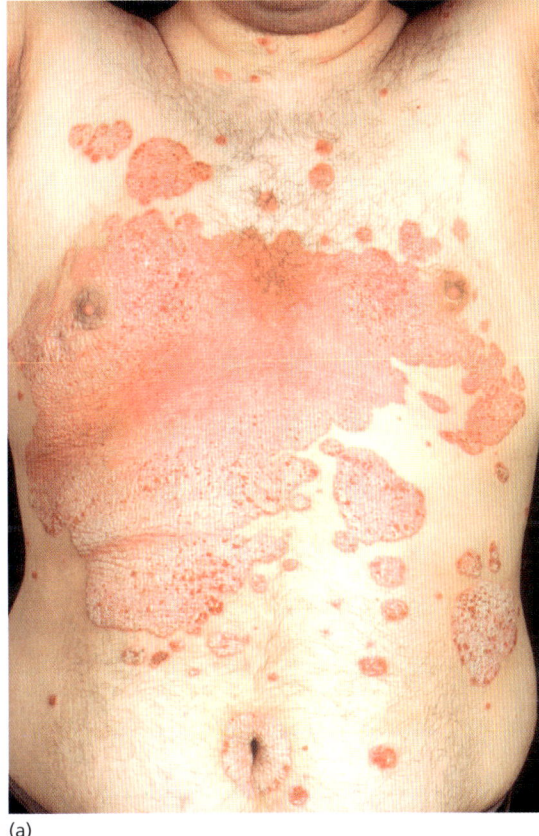

(a)

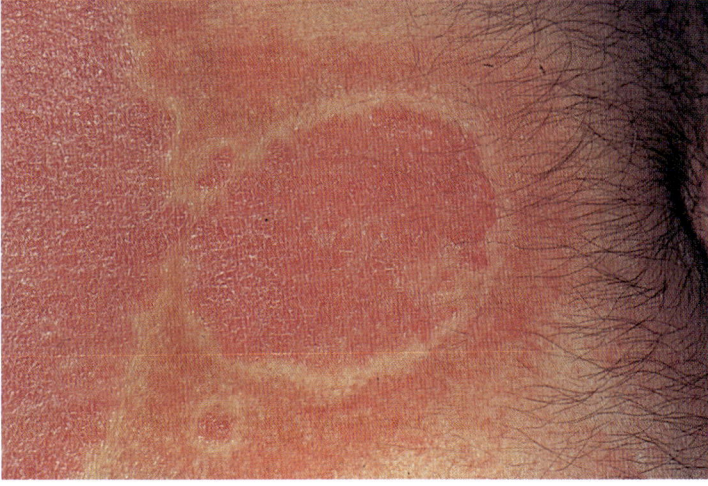

(a)

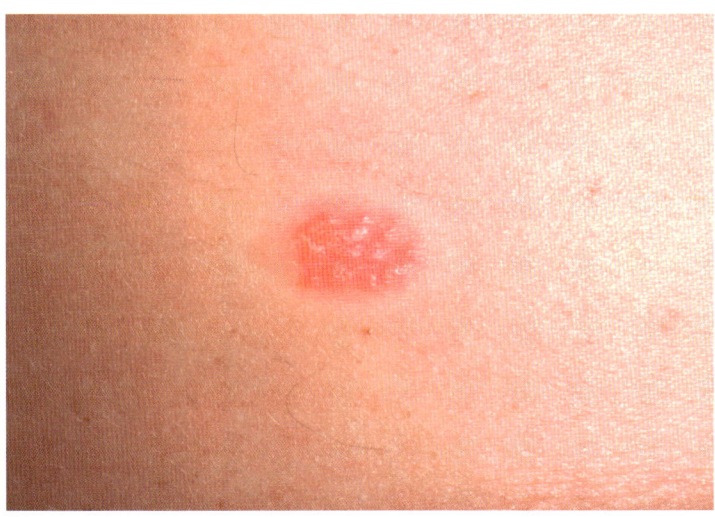

(b)

Figure 35.6 (a,b) Plaques may be encircled by a clear peripheral zone, the halo or ring of Woronoff.

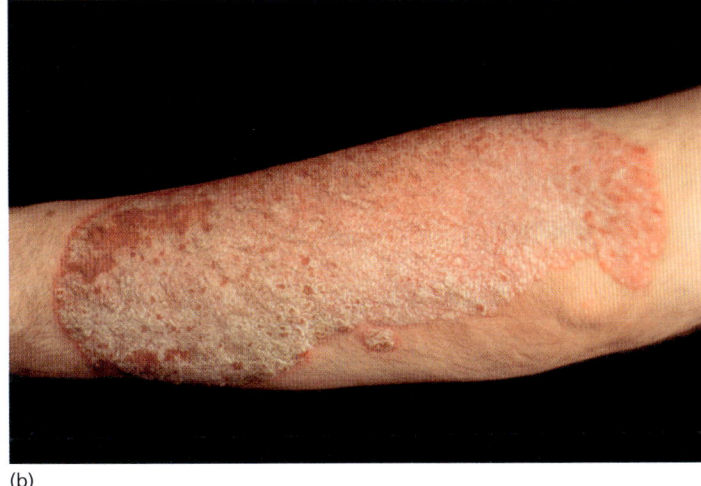

(b)

Figure 35.5 (a,b) Psoriasis is characterized by well-demarcated red scaly plaques.

Psoriasis affecting specific sites

Scalp psoriasis

The scalp is one of the most common areas to be affected by plaque psoriasis and often the site first affected. The whole scalp may be diffusely involved or multiple discrete plaques of varying size may be seen [125]. Very thick plaques can develop, especially at the occiput. Plaques tend to be restricted to hair-bearing areas, extending a short distance beyond the hairline and around the ears.

The rate of hair growth is normal [126] and common scalp psoriasis is not a frequent cause of alopecia, although it may occur [127]. Erythrodermic psoriasis may be associated with severe hair loss,

as may vigorous local treatment. A morphological entity consisting of plaques of asbestos-like scaling, firmly adherent to the scalp and associated hair, has been termed pityriasis (tinea) amiantacea [128] (Figure 35.10). It is most common in children and young adults, and is best regarded as a non-specific reaction pattern, which may be seen in other scaling scalp conditions. It may be an early manifestation occurring before the other signs of psoriasis. Hair loss, sometimes cicatricial, may be seen in pityriasis amiantacea.

Follicular psoriasis

Psoriasis affecting hair follicles on the trunk and limbs – follicular psoriasis (Figure 35.11) – may occur as an isolated phenomenon, or in association with plaque psoriasis [129]. The lesions are smaller than the typical lesions of guttate psoriasis and may be either grouped or diffuse [130,131]. In children it may be confused with pityriasis rubra pilaris (PRP).

Seborrhoeic psoriasis (sebopsoriasis)

Plaques of thin, sharply demarcated erythema with variable scale may occur in the typical distribution of seborrhoeic dermatitis,

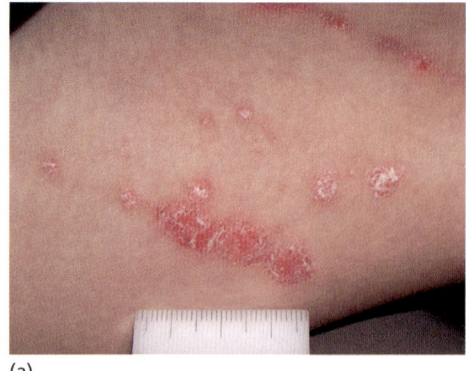

(a)

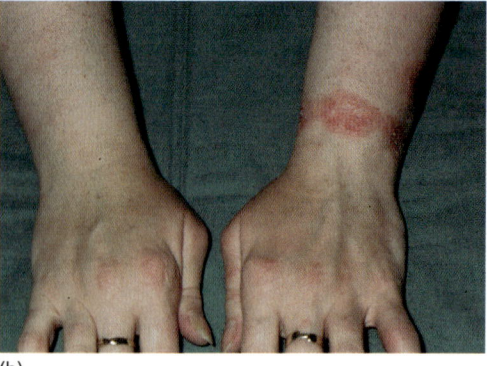

(b)

Figure 35.7 (a) Koebner phenomenon. Psoriasis appearing in the line of a scratch. (b) Psoriasis provoked by the friction of wearing a watch.

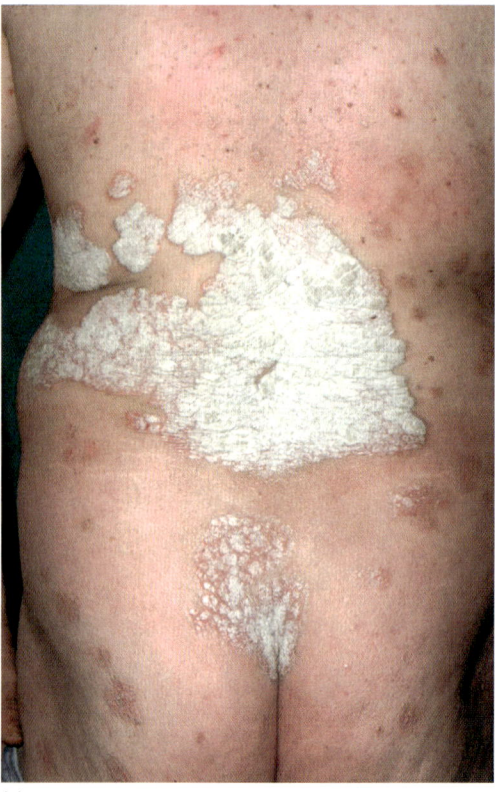

(a)

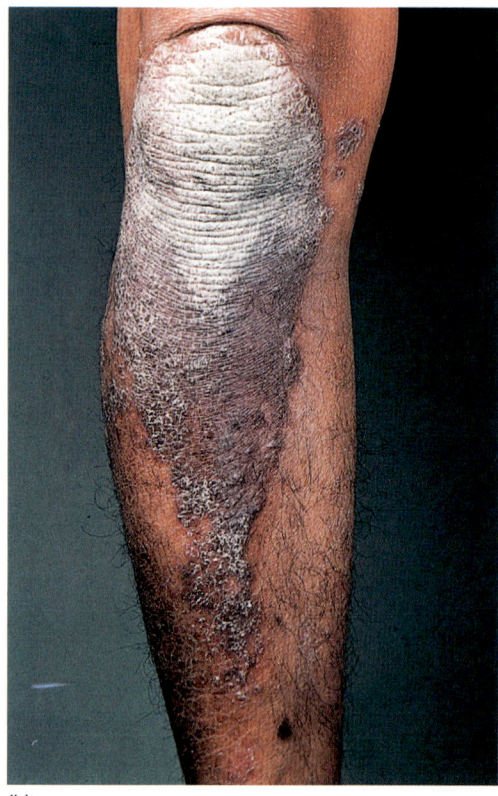

(b)

Figure 35.8 (a) Most plaques of psoriasis are surmounted by silvery white scaling, which varies considerably in thickness. (b) In dark-skinned races, the quality of the colour is lost. Courtesy of St John's Institute of Dermatology, London, UK.

involving paranasal areas, external ears, medial eyebrows, hairline, pre-sternal and inter-scapular chest wall [**123**]. These may occur in individuals with plaque psoriasis elsewhere. When it arises as an isolated phenomenon, it is difficult to distinguish from seborrhoeic dermatitis, and may represent a koebnerisation of psoriasis within this entity. Involvement of the face other than in a seborrhoeic distribution is uncommon in adults, and when it occurs is often an indication of widespread psoriasis elsewhere on the skin [132,133].

Flexural psoriasis (inverse psoriasis)

Psoriasis involving the inguinal creases, axillae, submammary folds (Figure 35.12), gluteal cleft, umbilicus (Figure 35.13) and other body folds is more common in older adults and is associated with obesity [134]. Flexural involvement is often seen in individuals with

plaque psoriasis elsewhere on the skin. Less frequently, lesions are confined to flexural sites, and sometimes referred to as inverse psoriasis [135]. Inverse psoriasis may occur as a primary disorder or as a Koebner phenomenon on top of infective or seborrhoeic intertriginous dermatoses. Failure to respond to antibacterial or antifungal preparations should arouse suspicion.

Flexural plaques are thin, scaling is greatly reduced or absent, and a confident diagnosis may therefore be difficult. The surface has a glazed hue and fissuring at the depth of the skin fold is common, especially in the gluteal cleft. The edges of the lesions are usually well defined, unless secondary infection or medicament dermatitis, both quite common events, have occurred. Involvement of the napkin area (psoriatic napkin eruption) may be the first presentation of psoriasis in infancy [136].

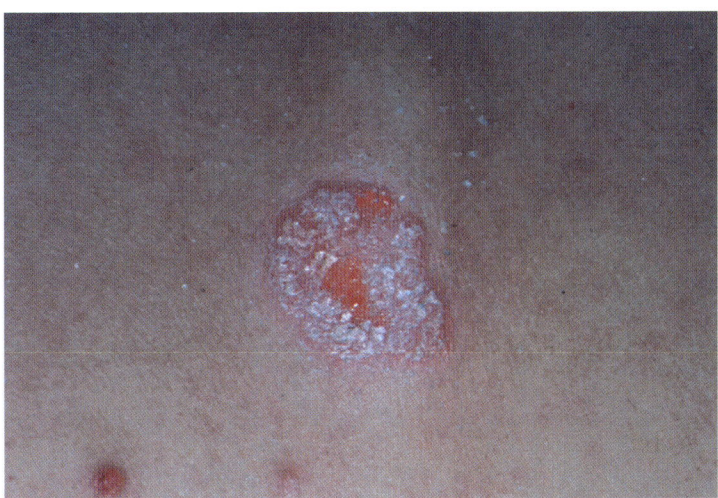

Figure 35.9 Auspitz sign: removal of the thinned suprapapillary epidermis by gentle scraping reveals vascular bleeding points. Courtesy of St John's Institute of Dermatology, London, UK.

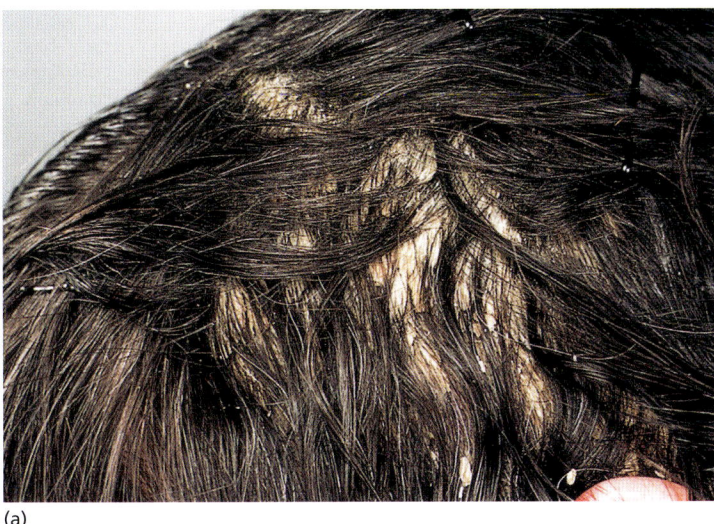

(a)

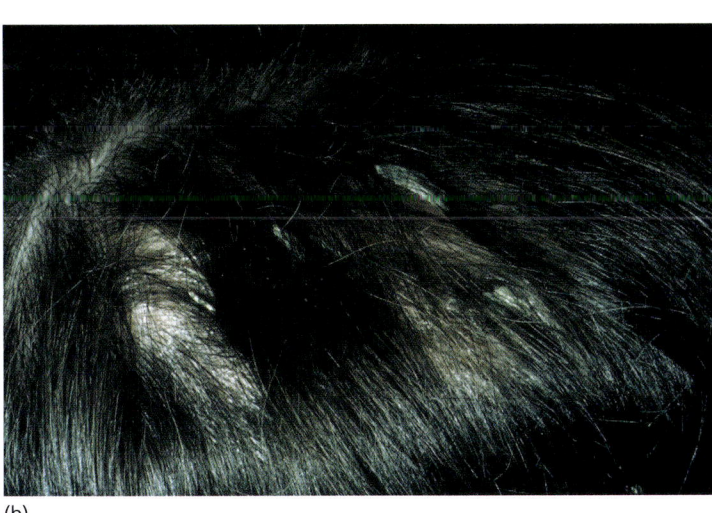

(b)

Figure 35.10 (a) The disease often first appears in the scalp, where it may present as pityriasis amiantacea. (b) Pityriasis amiantacea in psoriasis. Courtesy of St John's Institute of Dermatology, London, UK.

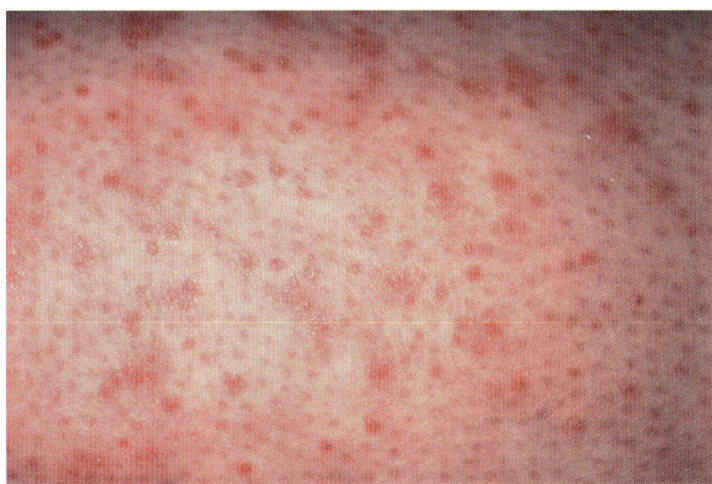

Figure 35.11 Psoriasis around hair follicle openings (follicular psoriasis).

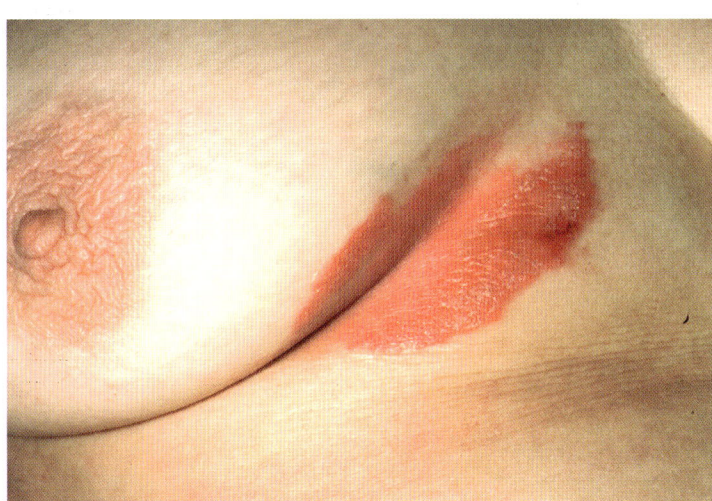

Figure 35.12 Submammary flexural psoriasis.

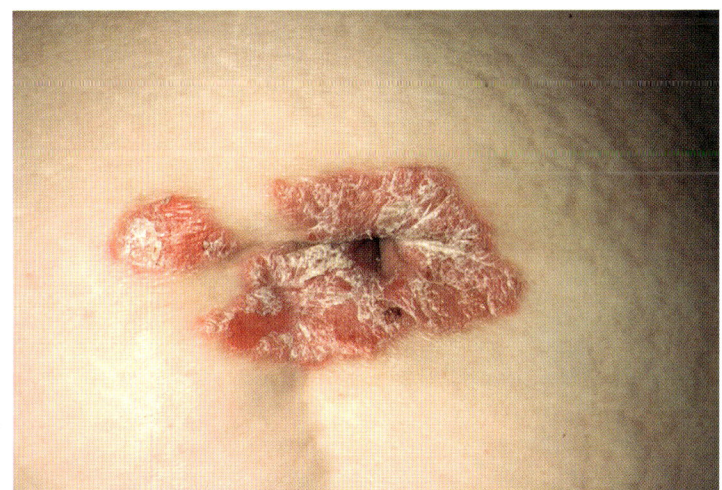

Figure 35.13 Flexural psoriasis affecting the umbilicus.

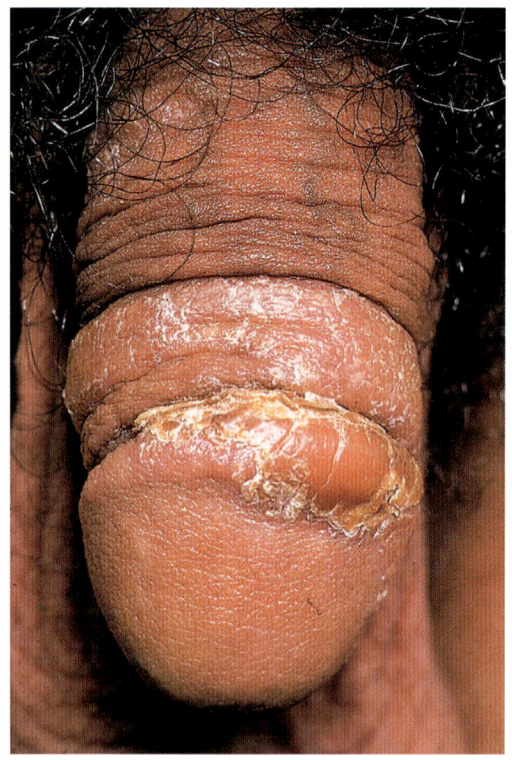

(a)

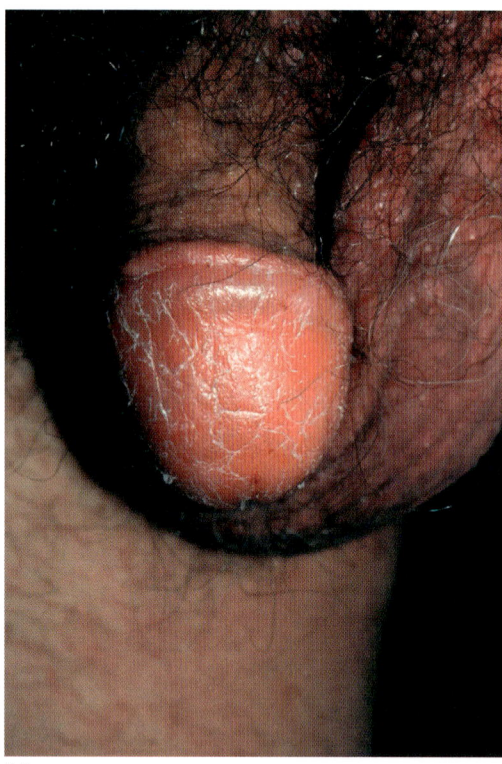

(b)

Figure 35.14 (a) Penile psoriasis in a circumcised man. Courtesy of St John's Institute of Dermatology, London, UK. (b) Penile psoriasis in a circumcised man retaining its typical psoriatic morphology.

Genital psoriasis

Genital skin can be considered a type of flexural skin, and there are similarities between psoriasis as it affects flexural and genital sites. The genital skin is often involved in individuals with inverse psoriasis, less frequently in those with plaque psoriasis and may be the only manifestation of psoriasis [137]. It has been shown to cause particular problems with sexual function [117,138–140].

Skin of the scrotum and penile shaft may be affected by psoriasis, but the glans penis is the most frequently affected part. In circumcised men, lesions on the glans are similar in appearance to plaques at other sites. In the uncircumcised, the plaques may lack scale but the colour and well-defined edge are usually distinctive (Figure 35.14). Where confirmatory signs elsewhere are absent, a diagnostic biopsy may be necessary as it may resemble erythroplasia or plasma cell balanitis.

Patients with vulval involvement often complain of marked pruritus. The most common vulval presentation is a symmetrical, red, non-scaly, well-demarcated thin plaque affecting the labia majora. Psoriasis is among the commoner causes of chronic vulvitis in children, and among adults should be considered in the differential diagnosis of chronic erythematous vulvitis without vaginitis [141].

Non-pustular palmoplantar psoriasis

On the palms and soles (Figure 35.15), psoriasis may present as typical scaly patches on which a fine silvery scale can be evoked by scratching, as less well-defined plaques resembling lichen simplex or hyperkeratotic eczema. Mixed forms occasionally occur [142]. It is often difficult to distinguish between psoriasis and eczema, with which it may sometimes appear to alternate. A sharply defined edge at the wrist, forearm or palm (Figure 35.16) and absence of vesiculation are helpful. On the dorsal surface, the knuckles frequently show a dull-red thickening of the skin. Elsewhere on the hands and feet, psoriasis retains its typical character. There may be a relationship to trauma or occupational irritants [143].

Nail psoriasis

The nails grow more quickly in patients with psoriasis [144]. Nail dystrophy may be seen in association with all types of psoriasis or occasionally as an isolated feature. Estimates of its incidence vary considerably. Minor degrees of involvement (e.g. pitting) are difficult to define clinically but abnormalities of the nail unit have been detected by ultrasonography in up to 73% of patients with plaque psoriasis [145]. On clinical examination, nail changes are present in about 40% of cases at any point in time [146] and the lifetime prevalence is 80–90% [147]. Nail psoriasis is characterised by hyperkeratosis of the nail matrix and often the nail plate. In one reported case series, parakeratosis was present in 78% of cases and unlike plaque psoriasis hypergranulosis is a common feature. Neutrophilic infiltration of the nail bed is present in 63% of patients [148].

Nail psoriasis is associated with more extensive psoriasis, longer disease duration, family history of psoriasis and the presence of psoriatic arthritis. In one German study, psoriatic arthritis was present in more than twice as many psoriasis patients with nail disease [146].

Psoriasis may affect any part of the nail unit, including the nail matrix, nail bed and hyponychium. Nail matrix disease presents with pits, ridges and grooves of the nail plate. Pitting (Figure 35.17) is the most frequent change seen in fingernails, individual pits

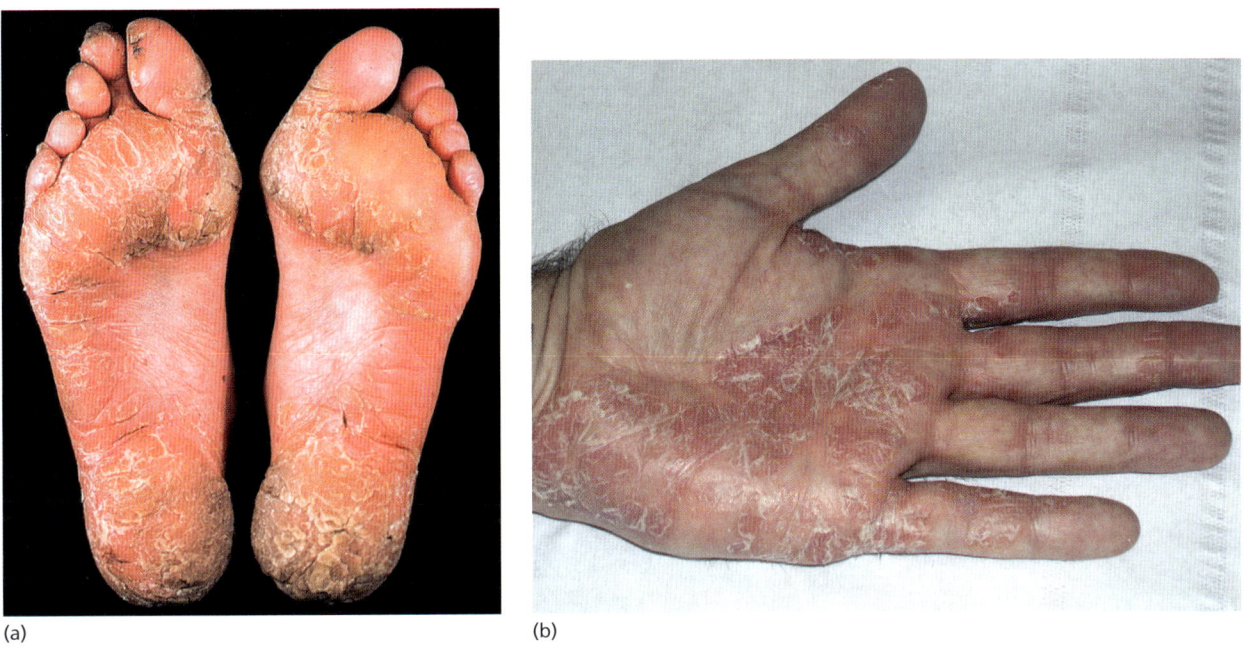

(a)   (b)

Figure 35.15 (a) On the palms and soles, psoriasis may present as typical scaly plaques. Courtesy of St John's Institute of Dermatology, London, UK. (b) Typical psoriatic plaques on the palm.

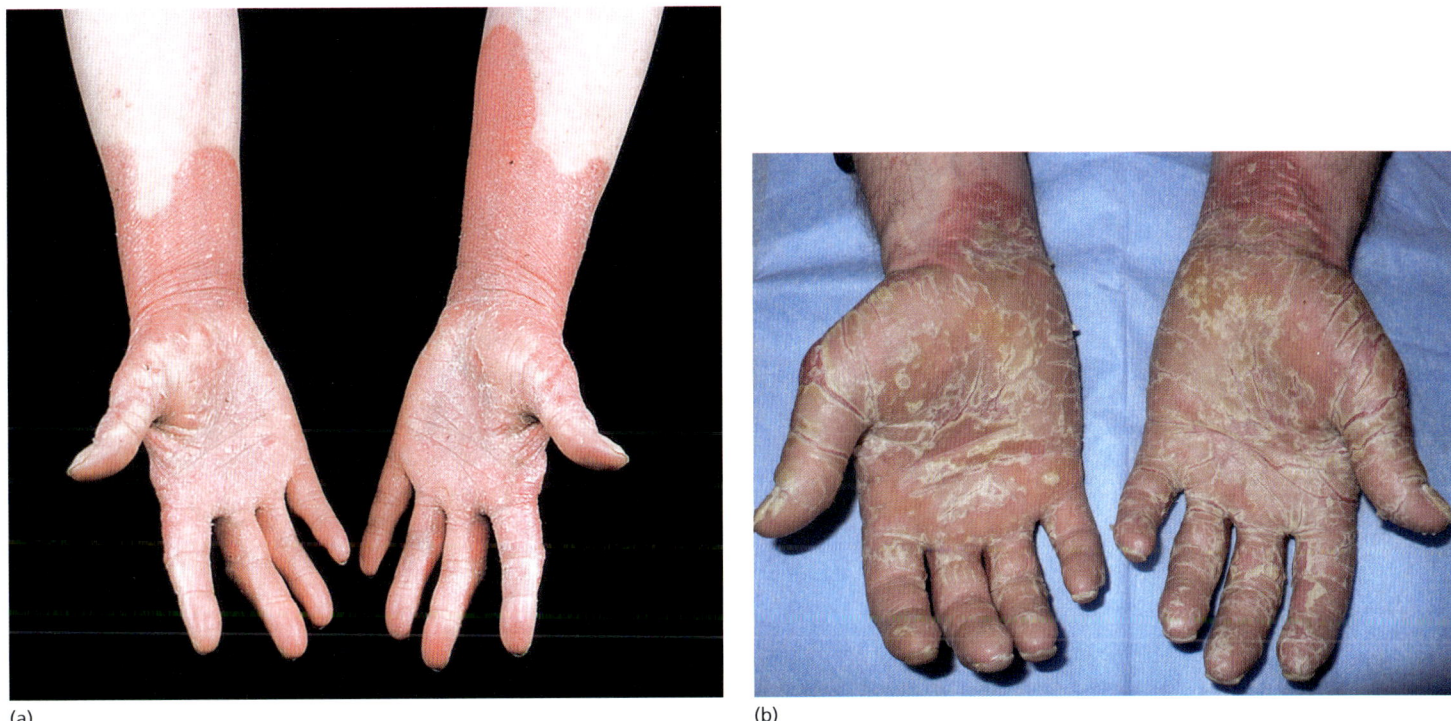

(a)   (b)

Figure 35.16 (a) A sharply defined edge at the wrist or forearm and absence of vesiculation are helpful diagnostic features. Courtesy of St John's Institute of Dermatology, London, UK. (b) Severe confluent palmar psoriasis.

being uniform in size at about 1 mm diameter and sometimes arranged longitudinally. Nail bed disease can be seen as subungual 'oil drops' that are highly specific for psoriasis (Figure 35.18) [149]. Nail bed disease also causes subungual hyperkeratosis, splinter haemorrhages and distal onycholysis (Figure 35.19). It can be difficult to distinguish clinically between toenail bed psoriasis and onychomycosis, which quite often coexists [150,151].

Mucosal lesions

Whether psoriasis affects the oral mucosa is a matter of controversy [152]. True mucosal involvement appears to be rare. Geographic tongue (benign migratory glossitis) (Figure 35.20) and fissured tongue are both more frequent among patients with psoriasis than healthy controls [153–155]. The association of both psoriasis and geographic tongue with *HLA-C:06:02* provides further evidence that

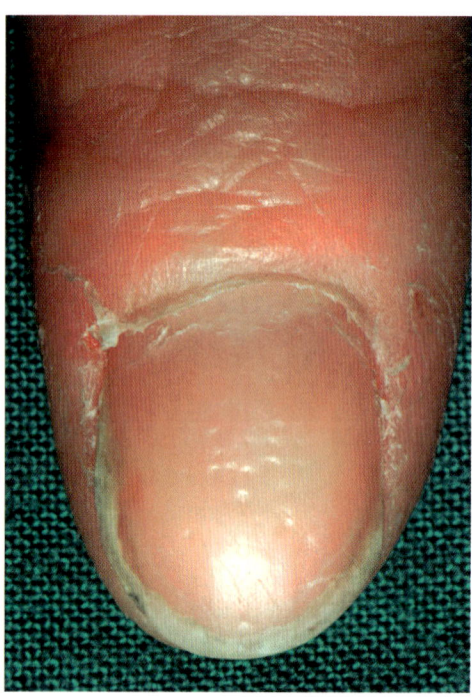

Figure 35.17 Psoriatic nail pitting.

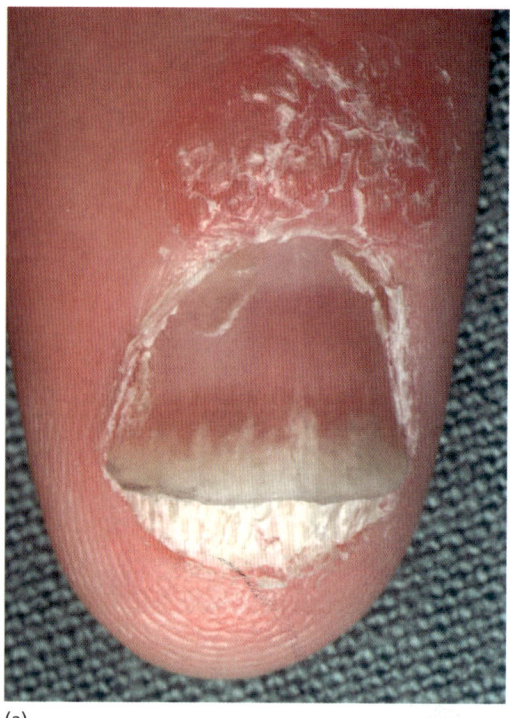

(a)

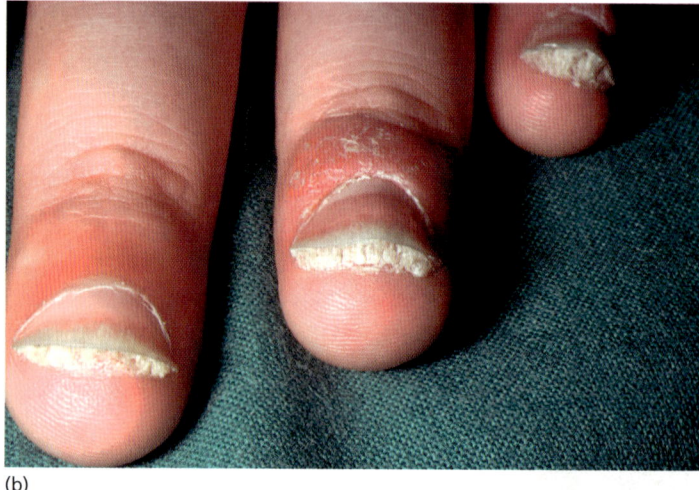

(b)

Figure 35.19 (a) Psoriatic subungual hyperkeratosis with distal onycholysis. (b) Marked psoriatic subungual hyperkeratosis.

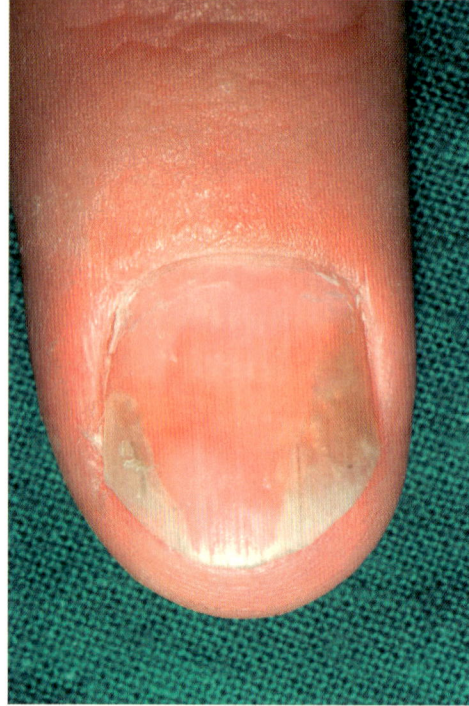

Figure 35.18 Salmon patches ('oil drops'), with distal onycholysis.

the two disorders are related [156], but whether geographic tongue is an oral manifestation of psoriasis *per se* remains to be established.

Ocular lesions

Psoriasis may affect ocular structures directly, or by associated immunological phenomena. Direct involvement of the eyelids or eyelid margins may cause blepharitis and its consequences, which are the most frequent ocular complications of psoriasis

[157]. A chronic non-specific conjunctivitis has also been reported to be common in psoriasis, and xerosis may also be seen [158]. Keratitis is rare. Uveitis is an important immunologically mediated complication and has been found to be associated with more extensive psoriasis [159]. It is more strongly associated with psoriatic arthritis [160].

Clinical variants (based on morphology or natural history)

Acute guttate psoriasis

This describes the sudden onset of a shower of small lesions (Latin plural *Guttae* meaning drops), appearing diffusely over the body (Figure 35.21). It should be distinguished from small plaque psoriasis and follicular psoriasis, which follow a more chronic

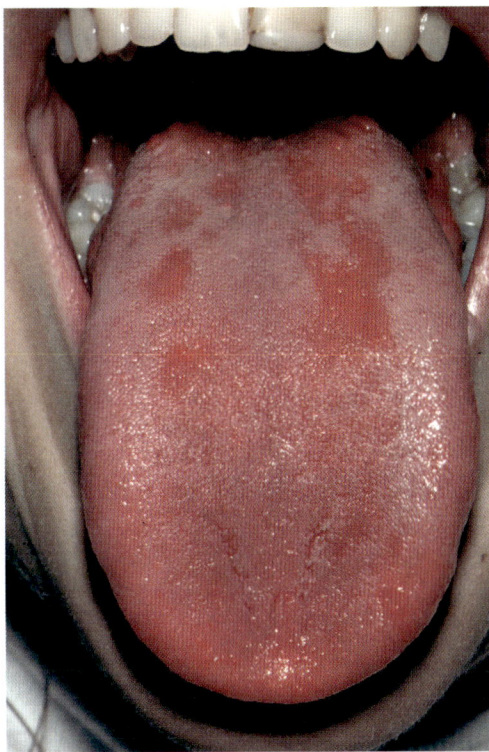

Figure 35.20 Geographic tongue in a patient with psoriasis

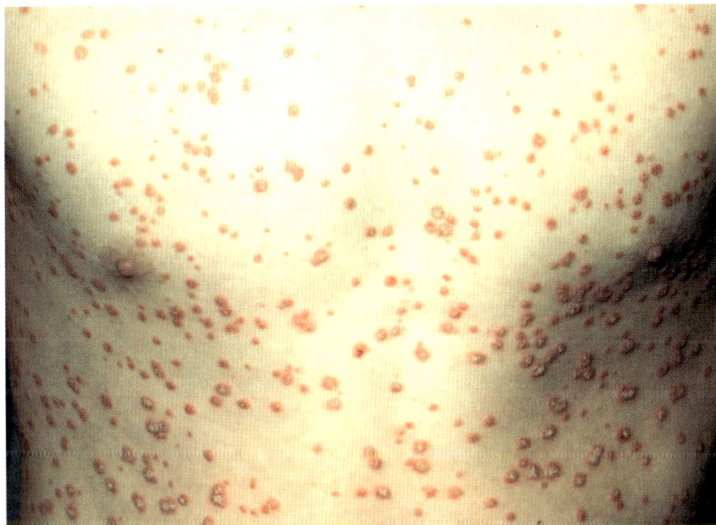

Figure 35.21 Extensive lesions of guttate psoriasis in a young man.

slightly oval. They are scattered more or less evenly over the body, particularly on the trunk and proximal part of the limbs, rarely on the soles but not infrequently on the face, ears and scalp. Lesions on the face are often sparse, difficult to see and disappear quickly. Although guttate lesions are normally profuse, there are occasionally no more than half a dozen present on the body, and in the early stages the colour is not specific. The diagnosis is made chiefly from the nature of the scaling, the general distribution and evidence for preceding infection. Lesions usually resolve over about 3 months. A significant minority of patients with acute guttate psoriasis subsequently develop plaque psoriasis [163].

'Unstable' psoriasis (syn. active psoriasis, eruptive inflammatory psoriasis)

In contrast to the lesions in plaque psoriasis, which are static for prolonged periods, in some individuals and in some phases of the disease there is more marked activity in the form of enlargement of plaques that can become more intensely red (Figure 35.22), and the development of many new smaller plaques. Patients may complain of more pain or pruritus within the plaques. The Koebner phenomenon is thought to be more frequent in this phase of the disease [122]. The immediate outcome is unpredictable; the lesions may return to the inactive state, or progress to localised pustulation or erythrodermic psoriasis. Patients may develop unstable phases repeatedly, settling back again into the stable forms of the disease. Recognised precipitants include withdrawal of systemic or potent topical corticosteroids, treatment with irritants such as tar or dithranol, acute infection and severe emotional distress. Serum levels of IL-17 and the IL-1 receptor antagonist are higher in patients during the unstable phase of the disease [164].

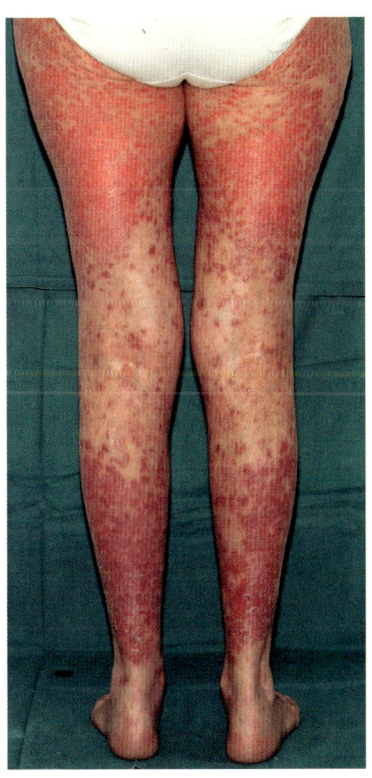

Figure 35.22 Extensive tender fiery red plaques of unstable psoriasis.

course. In one series, 12% of all affected psoriasis patients had experienced acute guttate psoriasis [161]. It is more common in children and young adults in whom it may be the first presentation of psoriasis. It frequently follows several weeks after pharyngitis caused by group A streptococci, serological evidence for which can be found in about 60% of individuals [161]. A guttate flare may also occur in adults with plaque psoriasis and in this context is more common in patients whose psoriasis had its onset in childhood [162].

In the early stages of acute guttate psoriasis there may be little scaling. The lesions are from 2 or 3 mm to 1 cm in diameter, round or

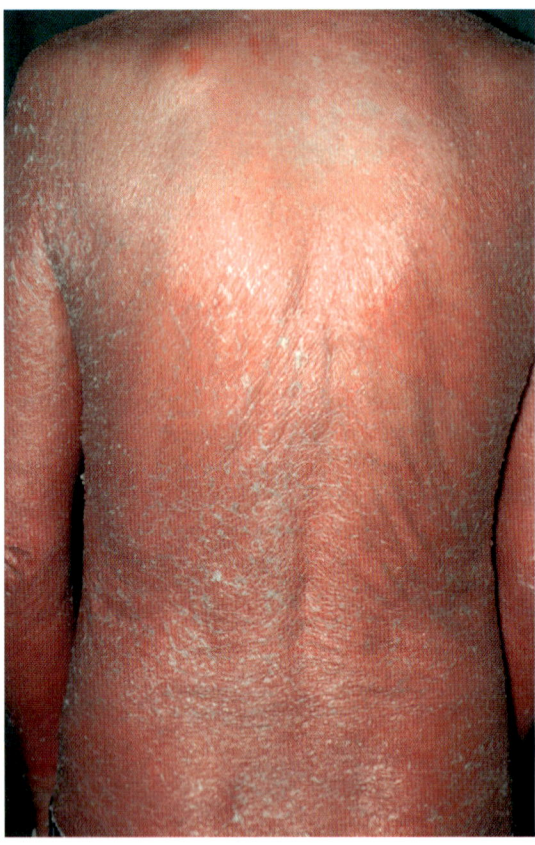

Figure 35.23 Erythrodermic psoriasis in an older man.

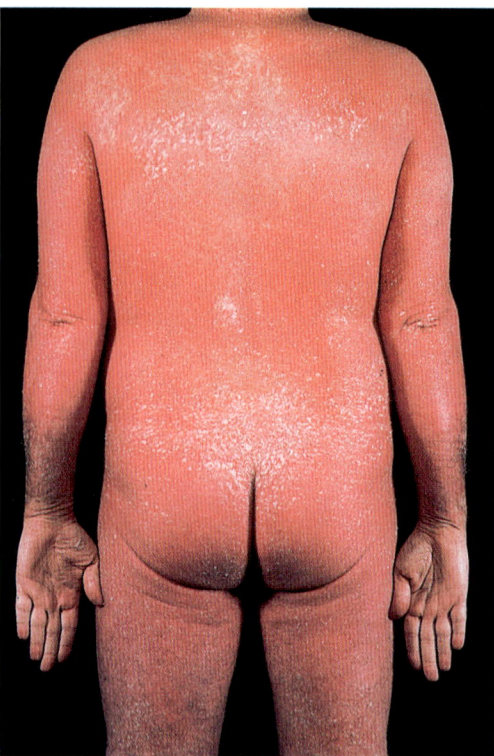

Figure 35.24 Acute unstable erythrodermic psoriasis. Courtesy of St John's Institute of Dermatology, London, UK.

Erythrodermic psoriasis

Erythrodermic psoriasis, in which most or all of the body surface is affected by psoriasis, is uncommon, occurring in 1–2% of patients [165,166]. Psoriasis has been found to be the underlying cause in about 25% of cases of erythroderma [166]. Erythroderma in psoriasis may be chronic, due to the gradual extension of plaque psoriasis (Figure 35.23), or acute as part of the spectrum of 'unstable' psoriasis (Figure 35.24). In the chronic form, the individual may be systemically well, the clinical characteristics of psoriasis are retained and there are usually some areas of uninvolved skin. Mild topical treatments are well tolerated and the overall prognosis is good.

The acute form is often precipitated by environmental or therapeutic triggers including systemic illness, alcohol excess, antimalarials, irritating topical treatments, ultraviolet radiation or by withdrawal of systemic treatments including corticosteroids, ciclosporin, methotrexate or TNF inhibitors. The patient may be febrile and systemically ill. Dependent oedema is common. Itching is often severe. The entire skin may be affected and the clinical characteristics of psoriasis are often lost. There may be clinical overlap with generalised pustular psoriasis. Untreated, the course is prolonged, relapses are frequent and there is an appreciable mortality. Complications are those of skin failure, including sepsis, hypothermia or hyperthermia, hypoalbuminaemia, anaemia, dehydration and high output cardiac failure [167].

Pustular psoriasis

See later.

Atypical forms of psoriasis

In a disease as common and variable as psoriasis, atypical forms are frequent. Many unusual localisations have been recorded, including digital and interdigital forms. Verrucous lesions particularly affect the legs. Rupioid, elephantine and ostraceous psoriasis are terms sometimes used to describe plaques associated with gross hyperkeratosis. Rupioid psoriasis refers to limpet-like cone-shaped lesions. The term elephantine psoriasis might be used to describe unusual but very persistent, thickly scaled, large plaques that sometimes occur on the back, limbs, hips or elsewhere (Figure 35.25) [168]. Ostraceous psoriasis, an infrequently used term, refers to a ring-like hyperkeratotic lesion with a concave surface, resembling an oyster shell [169].

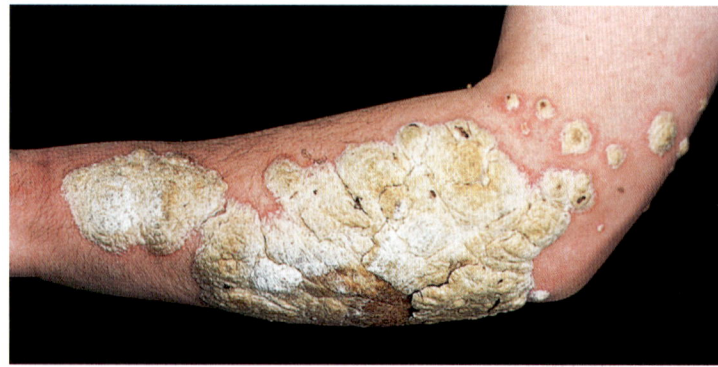

Figure 35.25 Elephantine psoriasis: large plaques with gross hyperkeratosis. Courtesy of St John's Institute of Dermatology, London, UK.

Other specified forms of psoriasis (based on age, precipitants)

Linear and segmental psoriasis

True linear or segmental psoriasis, in which lesions are unilateral or Blaschko-linear, is extremely rare (Figure 35.26) [170]. It has been called isolated linear psoriasis when it occurs alone, or superimposed linear psoriasis when, as occurs more frequently, it arises in association with non-segmental plaque psoriasis (Figure 35.27) [171]. The segmental lesions tend to arise at a young age, and are often more severe and treatment refractory than the associated non-segmental disease [172,173]. Segmental manifestations are thought to represent genetic mosaicism arising by postzygotic loss of heterozygosity or a postzygotic new mutation at a psoriasis susceptibility locus [171].

This phenomenon should not be confused with inflammatory linear verrucous epidermal naevus, or a Koebner response of psoriasis on verrucous epidermal naevus of the non-inflammatory type or at the site of prior herpes zoster.

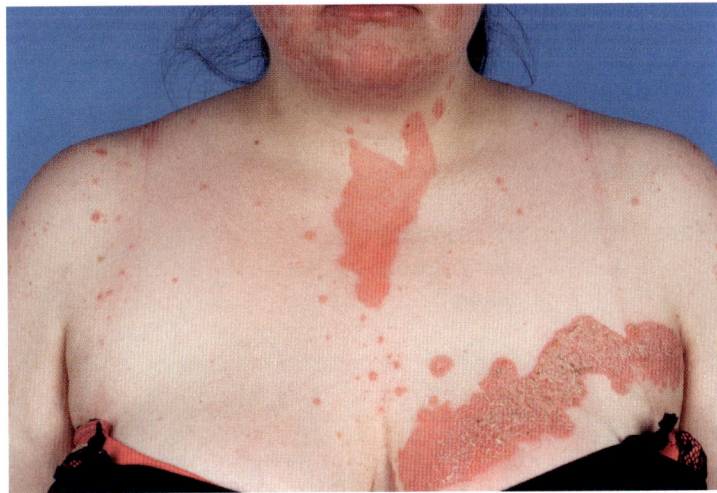

Figure 35.26 Segmental psoriasis.

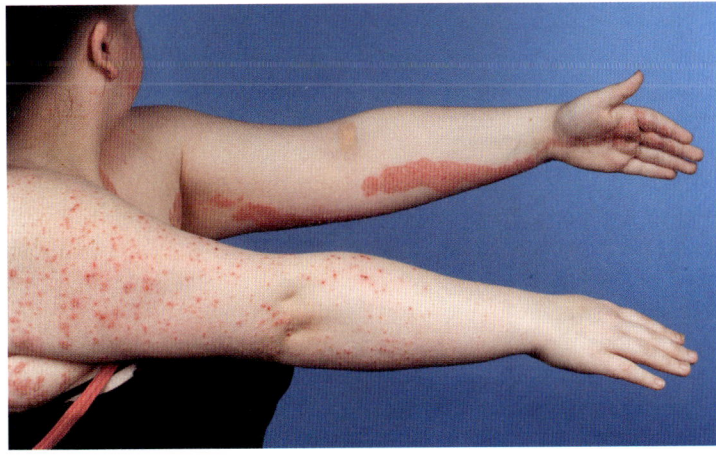

Figure 35.27 Linear psoriasis on the left upper limb associated with guttate psoriasis on the right upper limb.

Psoriasis in childhood and old age

Psoriasis is common in children with a cumulative prevalence up to 18 years of 0.71% [174]. Congenital psoriasis is very rare. In some series girls outnumber boys [174,175]. Psoriasis in children is significantly associated with several co-morbidities including obesity and diabetes [174,176]. There is no evidence that onset of psoriasis in childhood predicts severe disease in adult life [162].

All of the clinical variants of psoriasis described in adults are recognised in childhood but with a different frequency according to the age group. Establishing the diagnosis in infancy can be challenging because of limited involvement or an atypical appearance. The napkin area is frequently the first site affected; under the age of 2 years, napkin psoriasis with or without disseminated lesions is the most frequent form, presenting with well-defined erythema devoid of scale [135]. At this site, psoriasis must be differentiated from irritant contact dermatitis and seborrhoeic dermatitis. Napkin seborrhoeic dermatitis is a particular diagnostic problem as a significant proportion of affected children develop plaque psoriasis in adulthood [177].

Guttate psoriasis is more frequent in children than adults, particularly under the age of 12 years [177]. In older children, plaque psoriasis is the most frequent presentation, and the face and anogenital sites appear to be affected more frequently than in adults [135,178]. The disease often first appears in the scalp, where it may present as pityriasis amiantacea. Apart from the common forms, several other patterns of psoriasis occur in childhood. Interdigital tinea is uncommon in children and a toe cleft intertrigo may be psoriatic. Other flexural forms also occur. The disease may mimic chronic blepharitis, usually unilaterally, with a small plaque of psoriasis on one eyelid extending to the lid margin, or on the cheek at the angle of the mouth. Erythrodermic and pustular variants of psoriasis are rare in childhood. Pustular psoriasis may be the first presentation of psoriasis and tends to follow a benign course. Although localised pustular psoriasis is extremely rare in children, parakeratosis pustulosa (an indolent and recurrent scaling pustular acrodermatitis, sometimes around the nail of only one digit) often proves to be psoriatic [179]. Psoriatic arthritis is relatively uncommon in childhood.

In older age groups, psoriasis that starts for the first time after the age of 65 years tends to be less extensive than early-onset disease [180]. There is less often a family history of psoriasis. Plaque psoriasis with prominent scalp involvement is the commonest phenotype. Inverse psoriasis and erythrodermic psoriasis may be more common than in early-onset disease [133,181,182], whereas guttate and generalised pustular psoriasis are rare [178].

Drug-induced or exacerbated psoriasis

See later.

Photoaggravated psoriasis

See later.

HIV-induced or exacerbated psoriasis

The association between severe psoriasis, psoriatic arthritis and HIV infection is well recognised. Psoriasis may be the first presentation of HIV infection, as may the deterioration in previously stable disease. Plaque psoriasis is the most frequent phenotype, with a predilection for the scalp and palmoplantar skin [183]. Sebopsoriasis, rupioid psoriasis and erythrodermic psoriasis are also common, as are mixed patterns [184]. Psoriasis tends to be more prevalent in the later stages of HIV-related immunodysfunction, but may occur earlier. The mechanisms of worsening of psoriasis in HIV infection are unclear and represents a paradox, given that T cells are the major target of HIV. Suggested explanations include HIV-induced reduction in regulatory T cells, an increased number of memory CD8+ T cells, effects of HIV on dendritic cell populations, HIV proteins acting as superantigens, or shared genetic variants between psoriasis and HIV responder status [185]. One suggestion is that HIV affects peripheral blood Th cells and affects to a lesser degree cutaneous resident memory T cells which are pathogenic in psoriasis [186]. Psoriasis tends to improve with a reduced viral load, especially on treatment with antiretroviral therapy [187].

Differential diagnosis

The clinical characteristics already described are usually sufficient to enable the diagnosis to be made, but doubt may arise in atypical cases, in particular sites, and when psoriasis is complicated by or alternates with other diseases. The diseases that need to be distinguished from psoriasis vary depending on the clinical variant of psoriasis and the site affected (Table 35.2).

In seborrhoeic dermatitis, the lesions are lighter in colour, less well defined and covered with a dull or branny scale. Eczema at times develops a psoriasiform appearance, especially on the legs. Hyperkeratotic eczema of the palms is a common cause of misdiagnosis. Colour, scratch-evoked scaling and well-defined margins are suggestive of psoriasis, and nail changes may be diagnostic. Lichen planus can give rise to difficulty when the two diseases coexist, especially when present as hypertrophic lesions on the legs, as penile lesions and on the palms. The violaceous colour, Wickham's striae and the presence of oral changes are usually decisive. Chronic hand or foot eczema can be difficult to differentiate from palmar or plantar psoriasis, and the presence of exudate or microvesicles should be sought to support the former diagnosis. Lichen simplex can resemble psoriasis closely, particularly on the scalp and near the elbow. The intensified skin markings, rather ill-defined edge and

the marked itching are characteristic, and the point of the elbow tends to be avoided. Pityriasis lichenoides chronica can closely resemble guttate psoriasis, but the lesions are usually less evenly scattered, have a brownish red or orange-brown colour and are capped by a 'mica-like' scale. Candidiasis shows a glistening deep red colour suggestive of psoriasis, particularly in the flexures, but scaling tends to be confined to the edge, and small satellite pustules and papules are usually evident outside the main area. Tinea cruris has a well-defined, often polycyclic edge, but *Trichophyton rubrum* infections, especially of the palm, may cause difficulty. If corticosteroids have been applied, scaling may be absent and the diagnosis must be made by mycological examination of skin scrapings.

Less common causes of confusion are PRP and secondary syphilis. The resemblance to PRP may be close, especially in the erythrodermic phase. In PRP dark red follicular lesions are apparent, and the acquired palmar and plantar keratoderma has a yellow-orange tinge. The psoriasiform lesions of syphilis may cause difficulty to the inexperienced; condylomas, mucosal lesions and other signs of the disease are usually found, if sought. Porokeratosis of Mibelli on the palms and soles, patches of Bowen and Paget disease and penile erythroplasia may resemble psoriasis, but the lesions are often solitary. Mycosis fungoides can clinically also appear similar to psoriasis. In atypical psoriasis that does not respond to conventional therapy, this diagnosis should be considered and appropriate investigations performed. The coexistence of two inflammatory diseases should also be considered – for example, allergic contact dermatitis in the context of psoriasis.

Classification of severity

Aspects of the severity of psoriasis include the extent and severity of the inflammation at a particular time point, cumulative activity of psoriasis over time, the involvement of areas of skin that may cause specific problems (for instance, face, hands or genital skin), the presence or absence of co-morbid conditions, the impact of the disease on an individual's quality of life, and the responsiveness of the affected skin to treatments. Psoriasis varies in its severity between patients, and over time. Instruments to measure various elements of the severity of psoriasis have been developed for research, including drug development, and for clinical practice, including treatment selection and determining the response to treatment (see later) [188,189].

The Psoriasis Area and Severity Index (PASI) has been widely used in clinical trials and adopted in clinical practice, and its use in a specialist setting as both a severity score and an outcome measure has been endorsed in several European clinical practice guidelines and systematic literature reviews [190]. The PASI was initially developed in 1978 as an outcome measure in a clinical trial of etretinate in psoriasis and has since been partially validated [191]. Affected body surface area (BSA) is estimated for the head and neck, trunk, upper limbs and buttocks separately with a correction factor to allow for the differing surface areas of these four regions. Erythema, scaling and induration are graded in each region and a combined score ranging from 0 to 72 calculated as in Table 35.3. PASI is not appropriate in forms of psoriasis other than plaque disease, e.g. guttate or pustular psoriasis, when a record of percentage BSA affected may be preferred. PASI has been criticised as non-linear with a low response distribution, resulting in a lack

Table 35.2 The diseases that need to be distinguished from psoriasis vary depending on the clinical variant of psoriasis and the site affected.

Chronic plaque psoriasis	Guttate psoriasis	Flexural psoriasis	Erythrodermic psoriasis
Lichen simplex	Pityriasis rosea	Seborrhoeic dermatitis	Drug induced
Discoid eczema	Lichen planus	Candidiasis	Eczema
Lichen planus	Pityriasis lichenoides chronica	Tinea cruris	Cutaneous T-cell lymphoma/Sézary syndrome
Pityriasis rubra pilaris	Secondary syphilis	Bacterial intertrigo	Pityriasis rubra pilaris
Bowen disease		Allergic contact dermatitis	
Tinea corporis		Hailey–Hailey disease	
Cutaneous lupus		Langerhans cell histiocytosis	
Mycosis fungoides			

Table 35.3 Erythema, scaling and induration are graded in each region and a combined score ranging from 0 to 72 calculated as Psoriasis Area Severity Index (PASI).

	Thickness 0–4	Scaling 0–4	Erythema 0–4	× Area 0–6	Total
Head	a	b	c	d (a + b + c)	× 0.1 = A
Upper limbs	e	f	g	h (e + f + g)	× 0.2 = B
Trunk	i	j	k	l (i + j + k)	× 0.3 = C
Lower limbs	m	n	o	p (m + n + o)	× 0.4 = D
					PASI = A + B
					+ C + D
Severity	0 = none 1 = mild 2 = moderate 3 = severe 4 = very severe	Area 0 = no involvement 1 = 0 <10% 2 = 10 <30% 3 = 30 <50% 4 = 50 <70% 5 = 70 <90% 6 = 90 <100%		Axillae = upper limb Neck/buttocks = trunk Genito-femoral = lower limb	

of sensitivity to change in milder psoriasis [192,193], and because it is complicated to calculate. The static Physician Global Assessment (sPGA) may be more appropriate in a non-specialist environment [193]. This is an assessment of the average erythema, scaling and induration of all psoriasis lesions on a 5-, 6- or 7-point rating ranging from 'clear' to 'very severe', without assessment of affected BSA. Although not well standardised, it is straightforward to use and easy to understand [194].

The impact of psoriasis on the individual can be measured using health-related quality of life (HRQoL) instruments [195]. The most frequently used measure of HRQoL has been the skin-specific tool the Dermatology Life Quality Index (DLQI), which is simple to administer, validated and useful in clinical trials and in clinical practice [**196**]. This 10-point questionnaire generates a score from 0 to 30, and scores of greater than 10 have been shown to reflect a very large effect on a patient's life [197]. The DLQI has been criticised for being influenced by the patient's age and gender, and as being relatively insensitive to the effects of psoriasis on mood, stress, sleep, fatigue and addictive behaviours [198,199]. More recently developed scores include Skindex-17, and in clinical trials, generic quality of life instruments such as the 36-item Short Form Health Survey (SF-36) and EQ-5D are also often used [200]. Quality of life scores (e.g. DLQI) correlate only moderately with psoriasis severity scores (e.g. PASI), because they measure different aspects of the disease [188]. Psoriasis on the face, hands or genitals may have a disproportionate effect on quality of life resulting in a high HRQoL score with a relatively low PASI. Alternatively, a mismatch between a low PASI and significantly impaired HRQoL score can suggest co-morbid depression, and psychological support should be considered under these circumstances [201].

The severity of psoriasis is continuously distributed and, although attempts have been made to categorise psoriasis as mild, moderate or severe, the thresholds are arbitrary and not standardised. Severe psoriasis has been variously defined as a PASI >12 [202], as a PASI ≥10 with a DLQI ≥10 [203] or a score of 10 or more in either the PASI or DLQI or BSA >10% [**204**]. A recent consensus statement from the International Psoriasis Council rejected the notion of mild,

moderate or severe psoriasis, in favour of a classification into two groups, candidates for topical treatment or candidates for systemic treatment, the latter group characterised by either an affected BSA of ≥10%, or the involvement of high impact sites, or failure of topical treatment [205].

Complications and co-morbidities

Patients with psoriasis, particularly those with more severe disease, experience increased morbidity and mortality from a range of systemic diseases affecting most major organ systems, [**206**,207,208] (Box 35.2). Patterns of disease association are recognised, but the direction of causality is complex. Mendelian randomisation studies suggest that smoking, obesity and cardiovascular disease are causal for psoriasis [209]. Mechanisms may include shared genetic susceptibility or pathomechanisms, systemic effects of inflammation, effects of treatments for psoriasis on other systems or vice versa, and the consequences of behavioural responses to living with chronic disease. There is also some evidence of under-representation of several diseases in the psoriasis population, for instance cutaneous infections in early-onset psoriasis [7].

Box 35.2 Co-morbidities of psoriasis vulgaris

Immune-mediated inflammatory diseases
- Psoriatic arthritis
- Crohn's disease
- Ulcerative colitis
- Coeliac disease
- Uveitis

Infections

Cancer
- Non-melanoma skin cancer
- Lymphoma

Metabolic syndrome
- Obesity
- Hyperlipidaemia
- Hypertension
- Diabetes

Cardiovascular disease
- Myocardial infarction
- Stroke
- Peripheral vascular disease
- Atrial fibrillation
- Venous thromboembolism

Hepatobiliary
- Non-alcoholic fatty liver disease
- Alcoholic liver disease

Psychiatric/psychological
- Anxiety
- Depression

Miscellaneous
- Gout
- Amyloidosis

Immune-mediated inflammatory diseases

Psoriatic arthritis is the most frequent inflammatory disease associated with psoriasis (see later). Inflammatory bowel disease (IBD) is also more frequently observed, an observation that has led to considerable advances in our understanding of shared genetic mechanisms particularly with respect to innate immunity and key T-cell differentiation pathways. In a recent meta-analysis, the prevalence of Crohn disease and ulcerative colitis in psoriasis was 0.7% (95% CI 0.2–1.3%) and 0.5% (95% CI 0.3–0.8%), respectively. The prevalence of psoriasis in Crohn disease was 3.6% (95% CI 3.1–4.6%) and in ulcerative colitis 2.8% (95% CI 2.0–3.8%). The presence of Crohn disease or ulcerative colitis was significantly associated with psoriasis, with an odds ratio of 2.0 (95% CI 1.4–2.9) and an odds ratio of 1.5 (95% CI 1.2–2.0), respectively [210]. The incidence and prevalence of uveitis is also increased in psoriasis (risk ratio 1.29, 95% CI 1.10–1.51), and the risk may be greater in those who also have psoriatic arthritis [211].

There are reports of an association between psoriasis and coeliac disease. In a meta-analysis of published cohorts in 2020, odds ratios of 2.16 (95% CI 1.74–2.69) for coeliac disease in patients with psoriasis and 1.8 (95% CI 1.36–2.38) for psoriasis in patients with coeliac disease were calculated [212]. There may be an increased risk of several end-organ specific autoimmune diseases including alopecia areata, vitiligo, pemphigus and urticaria, particularly in psoriatic arthritis [213,214].

Infection

It has long been known that patients with psoriasis may carry staphylococci on their plaques [215] and using modern culture-independent molecular techniques the microbiota of psoriasis plaques has been shown to differ from uninvolved skin and from the skin of unaffected individuals [216,217]. Despite this, clinical infection of psoriasis lesions is rare. Occasionally, flexural psoriasis becomes clinically infected, especially if fissuring occurs (e.g. in the natal cleft). The relative resistance of psoriasis skin to infection may relate to the overexpression of antimicrobial peptides (cathelicidins and β-defensins) [218]. Retrospective reports suggest that psoriasis may be a risk factor for infection in joint replacement surgery [219] leading orthopaedic surgeons to defer elective surgery in those with psoriasis plaques until these have been adequately treated.

In addition to the known effect of streptococcal infection in triggering disease, patients with psoriasis have been shown in a prospective study to be 10 times more likely to develop pharyngitis than household controls, and streptococci are more likely to be isolated in association with a sore throat than controls [**220**]. There is also evidence for an increase in risk of respiratory and abdominal infections resulting in hospital admission [221]. This effect is independent of systemic treatment [221], but the risk appears to be greater in those receiving immunosuppressive treatment [222].

Cancer

There are reports of an association between various cancers and psoriasis, although some of the studies are of low methodological quality with insufficient accounting for potential confounding variables (for instance smoking, alcohol consumption and obesity) [223,224]. The extent to which these effects may relate to psoriasis per se, treatment or disease severity or treatment is not apparent.

The strongest association is with non-melanoma skin cancer, the incidence of which is raised in patients with psoriasis compared with the general population (risk ratio 1.72, 95% CI 1.46–2.02) [225]. High-dose PUVA is known to increase the risk of cutaneous squamous cell carcinoma and basal cell carcinoma [226], and this may be compounded by treatment with ciclosporin [227], and possibly high-dose UVB [228]. There does not appear to be an increased risk with TNF inhibitors [229].

There is evidence for a modestly increased risk in psoriasis of systemic lymphoma, particularly Hodgkin lymphoma (risk ratio 1.40, 95% CI 1.24–1.57) [223,230]. Although rare, this association creates significant challenges for psoriasis treatment. A possible association between psoriasis and cancer in other organs including the renal tract, pancreas and colon, remains uncertain [223,224,231,232].

Metabolic syndrome and its components (hypertension, hyperlipidaemia, obesity, diabetes)

The metabolic syndrome (truncal obesity, hyperlipidaemia, hypertension and insulin resistance) is increasing in prevalence in the general population. There are complex interrelationships between metabolic syndrome and chronic inflammation. In a representative sample of the UK population in 2012, the prevalence of metabolic syndrome was found to be significantly elevated in patients with psoriasis at 34% compared with 26% of the unaffected population (odds ratio 1.50, 95% CI 1.40–1.61) [**233**]. Similar results have been published in a meta-analysis of observational studies [**234**]. The risk is highest in those with more extensive disease. Psoriasis has been shown in many population-based epidemiological studies to be statistically associated with arterial hypertension [235], hyperlipidaemia [236], type 2 diabetes [237,**238**] and obesity [239,240].

The strongest of these associations is with obesity [**233**], which can be seen in childhood psoriasis, and tends to predate the onset of psoriasis [176]. Obesity in adults appears to be a risk factor for the development of psoriasis [209,241,242]. Patients who are obese have more severe psoriasis than patients with a normal body weight [176,243]. Obesity may decrease treatment responsiveness and appears to be one of the main reasons for the development of premature cardiovascular disease [244,245]. Weight loss in obese patients with psoriasis, either by low-energy diet or bariatric surgery, improves quality of life and psoriasis severity [**246**,247]. In a randomised trial in overweight or obese patients receiving systemic treatment, an intervention group who received a supervised calorie restricted diet with a programme of aerobic exercise for 20 weeks had a significantly greater improvement in PASI compared with a group randomised to non-intervention [248]. In an open label study of a very low calorie ketogenic diet in 37 patients with overweight or obese patients with stable plaque psoriasis, a mean weight reduction of 10.6 kg was associated with PASI75 rate of 65% [249].

In relation to the components of the metabolic syndrome, there is evidence of under-treatment, and lack of physician awareness, in comparison to other chronic inflammatory diseases such as rheumatoid arthritis [250]. In a Danish nationwide registry of psoriasis patients, 28% of those with hypertension were not prescribed treatment [251].

Cardiovascular disease

Patients with severe psoriasis die at a younger age than unaffected people and cardiovascular disease accounts for the majority of this excess mortality [206]. Psoriasis significantly increases the risk of stroke (risk ratio 1.21, 95% CI 1.04–1.4) and myocardial infarction (risk ratio 1.22, 95% CI 1.05–1.42) separately [252]. The risk appears to be greatest in younger patients with more severe disease or with psoriatic arthritis [253]. There is also an increased risk of peripheral vascular disease, atrial fibrillation and of venous thromboembolism [254–256].

Much of the increased vascular risk probably relates to behaviours (such as cigarette smoking, which is more frequent among those with psoriasis) and traditional cardiovascular risk factors such as the components of the metabolic syndrome. The extent to which psoriasis contributes independently and in addition to these conventional risk factors is controversial, but some epidemiological studies have demonstrated an increased vascular risk after correcting for many known risk factors [257,258]. Systemic inflammation in psoriasis has been associated with visceral adiposity and coronary artery disease [259].

Hepatobiliary disease

Death rates due to liver disease have been reported to be significantly elevated in patients with severe psoriasis [260]. Non-alcoholic fatty liver disease is the most frequently identified liver pathology, present in up to 50% of patients with psoriasis [261–263]. It is associated with obesity, metabolic syndrome and more severe psoriasis. In a recent UK study of 400 adults with severe psoriasis investigated by transient elastography, 14.1% (95% CI 10.4–17.9%) were found to have advanced liver fibrosis [264].

Alcoholic liver disease is also common [65]. Neutrophilic cholangitis is a recognised cause of liver dysfunction in patients with generalised pustular psoriasis and occasionally plaque psoriasis [265].

Psychological and psychiatric morbidity

Psoriasis is associated with significant psychological consequences, including dysfunctional thought, pathological worrying, fear of stigmatisation, alexithymia, effects on self-image, personality and temperament [266,267–270]. Excessive alcohol consumption has been found significantly more commonly in men with severe psoriasis than in other groups with the disease and could be a consequence of stress caused by severe skin disease [271].

Psoriasis is also associated with a significant psychiatric morbidity, including an increased prevalence of depression, anxiety and bipolar disorder [272]. In a study utilising the Clinical Practice Research Database, the hazard ratios for a diagnosis of anxiety, depression or suicidality corrected for age and gender were 1.39, 1.31 and 1.44, respectively. The risk of depression in those with severe psoriasis is higher still [273,274]. In a meta-analysis, 28% of patients in tertiary care had depressive symptoms and up to 19% a diagnosis of clinical depression [275].

Miscellaneous

Psoriasis is associated with an increased risk of hyper-uricaemia and gout [276,277]. Several epidemiological studies have reported an increased risk of asthma, obstructive sleep apnoea and chronic obstructive pulmonary disease independently of smoking [278–281]. There are rare reports of acute respiratory distress syndrome complicating erythrodermic or generalised pustular psoriasis [282]. Renal involvement due to psoriasis is rare: secondary amyloidosis has occasionally been reported, as have instances of immunoglobulin A nephropathy [283]. There are conflicting reports of the frequency of cognitive impairment and dementia in psoriasis [284–287].

Pregnancy outcomes in patients with mild psoriasis appear to be unaffected, but in severe disease a higher prevalence of adverse outcomes including spontaneous abortion, gestational diabetes, pre-eclampsia, pre-term birth and low birth weight have been suggested although these findings are not consistent between studies in different populations [288,289,290,291]. Fertility does not appear to be negatively affected [292].

Disease course and prognosis

In many instances, plaque psoriasis is persistent, changing little over years. In other individuals, the disease is less stable with considerable variation in the extent and degree of inflammation, sometimes in relation to environmental triggers such as infections, alcohol consumption, emotional distress or climate. A deterioration in the symptoms and extent of psoriasis in the winter months is common, with a tendency for it to be milder in the autumn [293]. In the few longitudinal studies that have been reported, spontaneous remission occurs in between a third and a half of patients, and has been described for as long as 54 years [2,10]. The cause of these spontaneous remissions is unknown. Psoriasis can be maintained in prolonged remission using systemic or biological treatment, but untreated, relapse is the rule. The time to relapse after treatment varies enormously between individuals and between therapeutic modalities.

Acute guttate attacks carry a better prognosis than those of a slower onset and have longer remissions after treatment [294]. Few studies have assessed the long-term prognosis for first episodes of guttate psoriasis. In one study, only five of 15 patients followed up 10 years after an initial episode of guttate psoriasis had developed plaque disease [295]. At the other extreme, erythrodermic and pustular forms carry an appreciable mortality and arthropathic forms a considerable morbidity. Severe plaque psoriasis shortens life expectancy by an average of 4–6 years [206,296].

Investigations

The diagnosis of psoriasis is usually apparent on clinical examination and there is no reliable diagnostic test. A biopsy of lesional skin may occasionally be helpful in atypical cases to exclude other pathologies. There is no constantly present laboratory abnormality in uncomplicated psoriasis. High sensitivity C-reactive protein may be mildly elevated, with higher levels seen in psoriatic arthritis and especially in generalised pustular psoriasis [297]. Identification of biomarkers in the skin or peripheral blood of disease severity, natural history, risk of co-morbidities, and response to treatment is a focus of research in stratified medicine [298–301]. Screening for known co-morbidities should also be undertaken which will include assessments for psoriatic arthritis, metabolic syndrome and depression. Investigations appropriate for initiating or monitoring of systemic and biological treatments may be required.

Management

General

Every patient with psoriasis presents an individual problem. Treatment depends upon many variables including age, gender, occupation, personality, general health and resources, as well as the type, extent, site, duration and natural history of the disease. Extensive psoriasis may be ignored by the phlegmatic, yet minor lesions on exposed areas can be ruinous for others. Treatment should be appropriate to disease severity and importance in that individual. It should not be more unpleasant, intolerable or dangerous than the disease itself. Reassurance and emotional support are invaluable, stressing the non-contagious and benign nature of psoriasis, and the availability of a wide range of effective treatments.

The importance of talking to patients, trying to allay their concerns, coupled with advice on how to handle negative beliefs about their disease cannot be overestimated.

Attention to the patient's general, physical and psychological health is always worthwhile. Known co-morbidities, for instance psoriatic arthritis and cardiovascular disease, should be actively looked for and treated. Lifestyle and behaviours that contribute to general health and treatment responsiveness such as weight management and smoking cessation should be addressed.

The disease remains incurable and there is no current evidence that treatment alters its natural history. This is, however, an area of active research. Trials are ongoing to assess whether early effective intervention may alter the course of the disease and prevent associated co-morbidities such as psoriatic arthritis, cardiovascular disease and psychological distress [1,2]. The patient should be encouraged to consider realistic targets for treatment, which may be subjective, or utilise a numerical scoring system such as DLQI. For physicians, response to treatment should be recorded objectively using appropriate severity scores such as PASI and PGA. It is useful to consider treatment in two phases: induction and subsequent maintenance of remission. In inducing remission, 75% reduction in PASI from baseline (PASI 75) has been widely adopted as a minimum response criterion for severe plaque psoriasis in clinical trials. With the availability of higher efficacy treatments, this standard has changed to PASI 90, or perhaps preferably a low absolute PASI (e.g. PASI <2) and/or a low absolute DLQI [3]. However, the physician must take a long-term view, and long-term safe control of psoriasis is equally important. The cost of treatment is a significant consideration in planning a treatment strategy. The management of psoriasis is a rapidly developing and increasingly specialised therapeutic area and up-to-date local and national guidelines should be consulted.

Topical treatment

Topical therapies are the mainstay of treatment for psoriasis of limited extent. Patients with more extensive psoriasis also often use topical therapies, at least for selected body areas. The main groups of topical therapies are emollients, corticosteroids, vitamin D and its analogues, coal tar and dithranol (Table 35.4). As well as differences

Table 35.4 Properties of topical treatments.

Treatment	Relative short-term efficacy	Suitability for inducing clearance	Suitability for maintenance of clearance	Patient acceptability
Topical corticosteroids	√ √ √ √	√ √ √	√	√ √
Vitamin D analogues	√ √ √	√ √ √	√ √ √	√ √
Out-patient dithranol	√ √	√ √	–	–
Coal tar	√ √	√	√	–

in efficacy and side effects, some of these preparations are easier to use than others for different patterns of psoriasis. There is a need for more effective and better tolerated treatments for patients who fail to respond to first line topical treatment.

There are several topical therapies in development and have undergone phase II and III trials.

Topical corticosteroids

Topically applied corticosteroids are of established value in psoriasis [4,5]. Potent and very potent topical corticosteroids are the most effective topical monotherapies for outpatient use and are recommended by the National Institute for Health and Care Excellence (NICE) as first line topical treatment on cost-effectiveness grounds [6]. Mild to moderate potency corticosteroids are the treatment of choice on the face and neck, flexures and genitalia. Potent and very potent corticosteroids are suitable for scalp psoriasis [5] and plaque psoriasis at sites of thick skin such as the palms and soles. Newer formulations of corticosteroids, particularly foams, are easier to apply than traditional creams or ointments and can be used for scalp, truncal or limb psoriasis. Intralesional corticosteroid infiltrated intradermally into localised lesions of psoriasis by needle injection may be a valuable technique in small resistant plaques, for instance on the backs of the hands and knuckles. The effect may be long lasting in some patients [7].

Topical corticosteroids are associated with a lower incidence of short-term local adverse events than other topical treatments [4]. They generally lack irritancy, do not stain skin or clothing and have the merits of ease of application. They are frequently combined with other topical agents to counteract irritancy. The combination of a potent topical corticosteroid with calcipotriol provides the most effective strategy for topical treatment of limited plaque psoriasis over a short period of time [4,5]. The potential side effects of topical corticosteroids are well known and include cutaneous atrophy (Figure 35.28), tachyphylaxis, rebound flare and systemic absorption, although there is a lack of data about the magnitude of these risks [4]. It is prudent to limit the use of potent topical corticosteroids to stable plaque psoriasis affecting limited areas, as long-term use may exacerbate the disease. Potent topical corticosteroids tend not to induce a lasting remission, unlike tar or dithranol which have the potential to do so.

Vitamin D analogues

The naturally occurring active metabolite of vitamin D_3, 1,25-dihydroxyvitamin D_3 (calcitriol) [8] and synthetic analogues calcipotriol [2–4] and 1,24-dihydroxyvitamin D_3 (tacalcitol) [9,10]

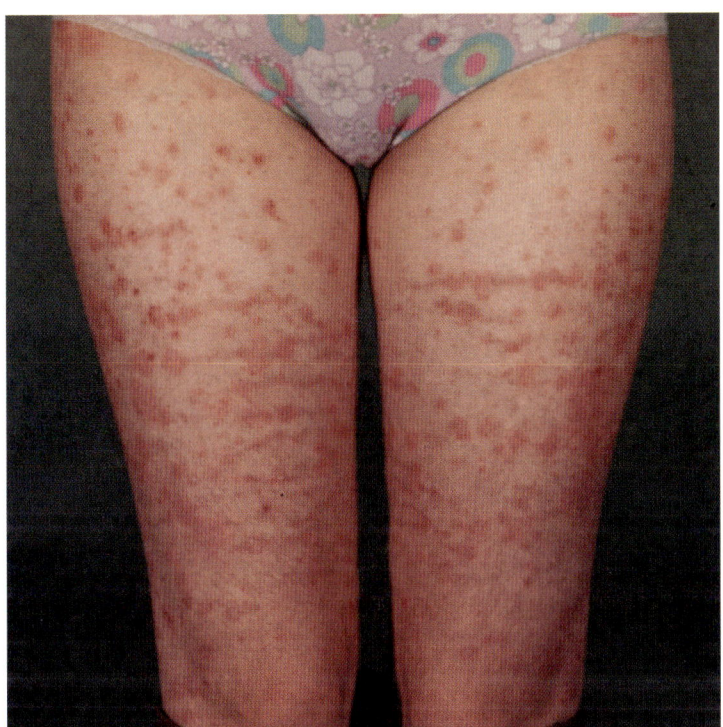

Figure 35.28 Striae induced by potent topical corticosteroids in psoriasis.

have all been shown to be effective when applied topically in psoriasis. The mechanism of action of these agents is via vitamin D receptor-mediated effects on the proliferation and differentiation of epidermal keratinocytes [8,11] and on immunocytes [12]. Topical formulations of calcipotriol and other vitamin D analogues are widely prescribed therapies for plaque psoriasis. Systematic reviews of calcipotriol attest to its equivalence or superiority to other available topical therapies apart from potent topical corticosteroids [4,13]. The most widely prescribed analogue in current use, calcipotriol (50 μg/g) ointment, has been reported to be at least as effective as 0.1% betamethasone valerate ointment [14,15] and more effective than short-contact dithranol therapy [16] in plaque psoriasis. Calcipotriol (50 μg/g) ointment has also been shown to be effective and safe in children when administered in amounts up to 45 g/week/m² [17]. Side effects of calcipotriol include local irritation, which may affect up to 20% of patients, and can be particularly troublesome on the face. Vitamin D and its analogues all have the potential to affect systemic calcium homeostasis with hypercalciuria and hypercalcaemia [18]. It is prudent to restrict the amount of calcipotriol (50 μg/g) ointment to fewer than 100 g or 50 g/m² per week, and to monitor serum and urinary calcium levels should these doses be exceeded.

Combining calcipotriol monotherapy applied in the morning with a potent topical corticosteroid such as halobetasol ointment applied in the evening for 2 weeks was superior to either drug used twice daily [19]. Based on this observation, a stable ointment formulation of calcipotriol 50 μg/g and betamethasone dipropionate 0.5 mg/g has been licensed for therapy. This combination shows superior efficacy to either calcipotriol or betamethasone alone with better clearance and faster onset of action [20]. The introduction of a gel and foam formulation of the combination product has improved

tolerability in managing scalp psoriasis and is also useful for plaque psoriasis at other sites [21,22].

Long-term treatment of plaque psoriasis with calcitriol (3 μg/g) ointment confirmed shorter term efficacy studies [8]. No statistically significant changes in serum or urinary calcium levels have been found, even in patients using large quantities to treat up to 35% of the BSA for 3 months [23].

Tacalcitol 4 μg/g ointment applied once daily is effective for the treatment of plaque psoriasis but is probably less effective than calcipotriol 50 μg/g ointment [4].

Calcipotriol and tacalcitol have been combined with other therapies. Calcipotriol ointment enhances the efficacy of PUVA and UVB phototherapy [24,25]. Tacalcitol ointment when combined with PUVA is UVA sparing [26] and calcitriol is UVB sparing in combination [27]. Calcipotriol 50 μg/g ointment used in combination with methotrexate may enable lower cumulative doses of methotrexate to be used [28].

Dithranol

Dithranol is a synthetic derivative of chrysarobin, which was originally extracted from the bark of the araroba tree. The use of dithranol for the treatment of psoriasis was first described by Unna in 1916 [29] and its use became widespread following the discovery that its stability can be increased by combination with salicylic acid. The mechanism of action of dithranol may relate to its antiproliferative and pro-apoptotic effects on keratinocytes [30–32]. It also reduces neutrophil and lymphocyte migration [33,34].

Dithranol therapy for psoriasis was formalised in the Ingram regimen; in-patients were treated with a tar bath, suberythemogenic UVB and then dithranol in Lassar's paste applied to plaques, starting at a concentration of 0.05–0.1% and increased cautiously to reduce irritation up to a maximum concentration of 4% [35,36]. The stiff paste prevented spread onto perilesional skin, which can become irritated by dithranol. Clearance rates with the Ingram regimen were reported at over 95% with remission times of 6 months or longer [36,37]. Clearance rates and remission times were similar to PUVA in a randomised controlled trial of 224 patients [38]. In the 1980s, the recognition that dithranol could penetrate the epidermis in 100 minutes led to the concept of short-contact dithranol. This, in conjunction with increased financial pressure on in-patient dermatology beds, led to the development of day care centres for psoriasis therapy. Out-patient short-contact dithranol is less effective [39] but more cost-effective than in-patient therapy [40]. It has a similar efficacy to topical vitamin D analogues in head-to-head trials [41]. Dithranol produces brown staining of the skin which resolves about 2 weeks after therapy is completed. It is not generally useful for facial or flexural psoriasis due to significant irritation. Despite these modifications, the use of dithranol as an out-patient therapy for psoriasis has declined.

Coal tar

Coal tar is the by-product of coal distillation and contains over 100 000 individual compounds, predominantly hydrocarbons. Coal tar was pioneered for the treatment of psoriasis by Goeckerman in the 1920s, applied on an in-patient basis for 24 h in combination with suberythemogenic doses of UVB [42]. In a day care setting, modified Goeckerman regimens cleared over 90% of patients with an average duration of remission of 8 months [43]. The mode of action of topical tar therapy is incompletely understood but clearance of psoriasis with the Goeckerman regimen is associated with decreased serum levels of inflammatory cytokines [44].

The efficacy of the modified Goeckerman regimen using coal tar applied for 5 h/day in combination with narrow-band UVB in patients with moderate to severe psoriasis has been confirmed in a Taiwanese study. After 4–6 weeks of therapy, the mean PASI reduced from 27.1 to 6.9. There were significant improvements in anxiety, depression and quality of life scores and the mean remission time (i.e. maintenance of PASI-75) was 22 months [45]. There are a number of reports of the success of modified Goeckerman regimens in patients whose psoriasis is refractory to biologic therapy [46,47]. The use of topical tar therapies in an in-patient setting and day care setting has reduced considerably in recent years, due to a reduction in dermatology in-patient beds and the inconvenience for patients of attending day care centres. Nonetheless, despite the advances in psoriasis therapies, the efficacy and safety of the Goeckerman regimen remains impressive [48].

The use of coal tar outside of the setting of day care and in-patient treatment has had less impressive results. There are a small number of randomised controlled trials assessing the efficacy of new formulations of coal tar. In mild to moderate disease, a 1% coal tar solution is similar in efficacy to calcipotriol cream and 5% coal tar cream [49,50]. In the short term, coal tar may cause folliculitis and contact allergy has been reported occasionally [51].

Topical calcineurin inhibitors

The topical calcineurin inhibitors tacrolimus and pimecrolimus were initially developed for the treatment of atopic eczema in childhood. Both preparations have been shown to be effective for psoriasis affecting the face, neck, flexures and genitalia [52,53]. Their advantage is that unlike topical corticosteroids they are not absorbed systemically and do not produce skin atrophy, making them more suitable for long-term use.

Novel topical agents

Tapinarof is a novel topical agent that is undergoing phase III clinical trials. It binds to the intracellular arylhydrocarbon receptor which results in downregulation of inflammatory cytokines including IL-17A and F. In two phase III randomised controlled studies, patients with moderate disease (PASI 8.7–9.1) were treated with taparinof 1% cream once daily for 12 weeks compared with placebo. The primary end-point of PGA 0/1 (clear or almost clear) was achieved by 35.4–40.2% of taparinof treated patients compared with 6–6.3% of patients treated with placebo cream. Between 36.1% and 47.6% of patients achieved PASI-75 [54]. It is well tolerated although a small number of patients develop folliculitis. Taparinof was approved for use in the treatment of psoriasis by the US Food and Drug Administration in 2022.

Roflumilast is a topical PDE4 inhibitor with a similar mechanism of action to apremilast. In a phase IIb study, topical roflumilast 0.3% cream was compared with 0.15% cream and placebo vehicle in patients with mild to moderate psoriasis. At week 6, an IGA score of clear or almost clear was achieved in 28% of the roflumilast 0.3% cream group, 23% in the 0.15% cream group and in 8% of the vehicle group. The treatment was well tolerated and was especially effective in intertriginous areas [54]. These findings were replicated in two larger phase III studies. At week 8, an IGA of 0/1 was achieved in 37.5–42.4% of patients using roflumilast compared with 6.1–6.9% of placebo patients [55]. Roflumilast is licensed for the treatment of psoriasis in the USA.

Phototherapy
Narrow-band UVB

Phototherapy with narrow-band UVB (NB-UVB) is recommended for patients with moderate to severe psoriasis [1]. Broadband UVB sources (290–320 nm) were used for nearly 100 years as part of the Goeckerman and Ingram regimens. The recognition that the optimal wavelength for treating psoriasis was approximately 312 nm [2] led to the development of TL-01 bulbs that produced wavelengths 311–313 nm: NB-UVB. NB-UVB evolved rapidly in the mid-1990s replacing broadband UVB therapy, as it is more effective and better tolerated [3,**4**].

UVB exerts pleiotropic effects on the skin and the mechanism of action of NB-UVB remains incompletely understood. NB-UVB causes cutaneous immunomodulation partly by increasing vitamin D [5] and similarly to PUVA induces apoptosis of T cells [6,7]. It also reduces epidermal hyperproliferation [8]. Studies also indicate that induction of keratinocyte apoptosis is involved in remodelling and resolution of hyperplastic psoriatic epidermis in response to NB-UVB [9,**10**]. NB-UVB may also reduce systemic inflammation in psoriasis as measured by C-reactive protein and cytokine levels in peripheral blood [**11**]. Nonetheless it is a non-immunosuppressant therapy and is also safe in the periconceptual period and at all stages of pregnancy.

The efficacy of NB-UVB is comparable to PUVA with clearance rates (<1% BSA) of over 90%, and average remission time of 16 weeks [**12**]. NB-UVB has been combined with numerous therapies with apparent success, including methotrexate, acitretin, fumaric acid esters (FAEs) and biologic therapies. NB-UVB should be avoided in patients who are taking ciclosporin due to concerns regarding accelerated cutaneous carcinogenesis [13]. Several factors determine treatment outcomes with NB-UVB. Psoriasis severity, BMI, smoking status, impairment of quality of life among others appear to predict outcomes and remission times in psoriasis patients treated with NB-UVB [5,13].

UVB erythema is maximal at 48–72 h and this fact coupled with the dose–response curve for NB-UVB suggests that treatment should be given three times weekly. Thrice-weekly NB-UVB has been shown to clear psoriasis more quickly than twice-weekly NB-UVB [14]. The British Photodermatology Group has published guidelines on dosing regimens for NB-UVB [13]. The initial dose is based on skin phototesting and the determination of the minimal erythemal dose (MED) or on skin phototype. Patients' estimation of their skin phototype may be inaccurate so MED phototesting is preferred.

NB-UVB can cause erythema and pruritus in the acute setting and, rarely, blisters can develop in the resolving plaques [15]. The cutaneous carcinogenic potential is unknown, but animal studies suggest that NB-UVB may be less carcinogenic than PUVA, leading some authors to suggest that it can be used in patients who have reached the maximum number of lifetime PUVA treatments [13]. Due to concerns regarding an increased risk of cutaneous squamous cell carcinoma (SCC), the scrotum and genital skin should be protected from irradiation. Longitudinal prospective studies are needed to establish the long-term side effects of NB-UVB.

NB-UVB is a highly effective, cost-effective remission-inducing therapy in psoriasis with a long safety record [16]. It should continue to play a significant role in psoriasis management. Regular attendance at hospital phototherapy departments is required and limits the utility of phototherapy for some patients.

PUVA photochemotherapy

PUVA is the acronym used for the combination of psoralens and long-wave ultraviolet radiation (UVA 320–400 nm). Psoralens bind to DNA and when activated by UVA cause permanent DNA damage with resulting cell death [1]. This reduces keratinocyte hyperproliferation, decreases antigen-presenting cells in the dermis, reduces angiogenesis, causes T-cell apoptosis with associated clearance and remission of psoriasis [2–4]. The psoralens that are commonly used are 8-methoxypsoralen (8-MOP), 5-methoxypsoralen (5-MOP) and trioxypsoralen (T-MOP). Psoralens are used either topically or orally in combination with UVA. Small studies comparing topical bath PUVA to oral systemic PUVA have reported similar efficacy rates although bath PUVA is more time-consuming and resource intensive. Bath PUVA is not associated with nausea and obviates the need to wear UVA protective spectacles on treatment days.

Oral PUVA therapy is given in dermatology centres according to dosing protocols. 8-MOP is usually given at a dose of 0.6 mg/kg 2 h before UVA therapy although it may be dosed according to the BSA. As the skin reacts to PUVA by developing pigmentation and epidermal hyperplasia, increasing doses are required as courses progress. PUVA is usually given as a twice-weekly treatment and the average number of treatments to clearance is 18. Twice-weekly PUVA is as effective as three-times-weekly PUVA. The initial dose of UVA is calculated as 70% of the minimal phototoxic dose and 20% increments are given until erythema occurs. The scrotum and genital skin are more sensitive to the development of PUVA-induced skin cancers and should be protected from irradiation.

This modality is highly efficacious in treating psoriasis with reported clearance rates of over 90% [5,6,7,8]. When PASI-75 results are reported using conservative analyses such as intention-to-treat, PUVA still compares favourably to systemic and biologic agents [9]. The average duration of remission (the time taken for 50% of a patient's psoriasis to return) is approximately 6 months. Guidelines on the use of PUVA for psoriasis have been published [10].

PUVA can cause both acute and chronic side effects; these include erythema, maximal at 72–96 h, and blistering that is usually dose and skin phototype dependent. PUVA may also cause neurogenic pruritus (PUVA itch), commoner in fairer skin types and usually dose related [11]. Patients describe a crawling under the skin that affects both psoriasis and clinically normal skin. If treatment continues, PUVA itch usually persists. PUVA is associated with an increased incidence of non-melanoma skin cancer [12,**13**,14]. This is true for both basal cell carcinoma and SCC although the incidence of SCC is increased more dramatically. The risk of SCC increases with the cumulative number of treatments, the total dose of UVA and in fairer skin types. Immunosuppression with ciclosporin also appears to increase this risk. The relative risk of cutaneous SCC

starts to increase after 250 treatments in a lifetime. The British Photodermatology Group therefore recommends that a patient does not receive more than 200 treatments of PUVA [10]. One study has reported an increased risk of malignant melanoma associated with high-dose PUVA (>400 treatments) but this finding has not been replicated [15]. Due to the observed increased incidence in SCC, several studies have attempted to make PUVA regimens more efficient. PUVA may be combined effectively with oral retinoids, so-called Re-PUVA. This allows an overall dose reduction in UVA but remission times are typically shorter [16].

PUVA has been associated with cataract formation in mice but to date the relative risk of cataracts is the same in patients who have received PUVA compared with the background population. Nonetheless, it is still recommended that patients wear UVA protecting plastic-lensed glasses on treatment days. Psoralens are teratogenic and patients should be advised about this risk even in patients undergoing topical or bath PUVA. The use of PUVA is declining due to lack of access in many centres in the UK and Ireland and has been largely replaced with NB-UVB. It offers superb efficacy combined with a known toxicity profile. It is also a cost-effective therapy for severe disease and is non-immunosuppressive.

Systemic therapy

The initiation of systemic therapy is a shared decision between patient and clinician, after consideration of the risk–benefit profiles of the available treatments. In general, systemic treatment is used for more extensive disease that is not responsive to topical therapy or phototherapy. However, the impact of disease may be sufficient that a patient in conjunction with their dermatologist would opt for earlier systemic treatment. Logistical factors may also play a part (e.g. ability to attend for regular phototherapy). The main systemic treatments in current clinical practice are methotrexate, ciclosporin, acitretin, dimethyl fumarate (DMF) and apremilast (Table 35.5). The choice of the most suitable agent in an individual depends on many variables including the person's age and plans for conception, the presence of psoriatic arthritis or other co-morbidities and the pattern of activity (including high-impact sites) and current severity of their psoriasis.

Methotrexate

The successful use of aminopterin therapy for psoriasis was first described in 1951 [1]. It was soon replaced by methotrexate, which is a more stable folate antagonist that inhibits DNA synthesis by dihydrofolate reductase inhibition [1]. Although initially thought to inhibit keratinocyte hyperproliferation, it appears to inhibit lymphocyte proliferation and probably acts via this mechanism in psoriasis and psoriatic arthritis. Methotrexate is given orally at doses rising to a maximum of 25 mg weekly, and also by subcutaneous or intramuscular injection [2]. Subcutaneous weekly methotrexate is used widely in the treatment of inflammatory arthritis and more recently in psoriasis [3]. It has been suggested that this method increases the bioavailability of methotrexate and may reduce side effects [4]. Lower doses of methotrexate may be effective, particularly in the elderly, which may relate to reduced renal excretion in this age group. Methotrexate is metabolised in the liver and significant enterohepatic circulation occurs but is mainly excreted via the kidneys. The modern use of methotrexate

Table 35.5 Properties of systemic treatments.

Treatment	Relative efficacy in psoriasis	Suitability for inducing clearance	Suitability for maintenance of remission	Patient acceptability	Relative efficacy in psoriatic arthritis
Phototherapy	√ √ √	√ √ √	–	√ √	–
Methotrexate	√ √	√ √	√ √	√ √	√ √
Ciclosporin	√ √ √	√ √ √	√	√ √ √	√
Acitretin	√	√	√ √	√	–
Fumaric acid esters	√ √	√ √	√ √	√	–
Hydroxycarbamide	√	√	√ √	√ √	–

for psoriasis is supplemented by folic acid. There is a wide variety in the dosing regimens of folic acid used [5,6].

Methotrexate is often used as the first systemic agent in plaque psoriasis, particularly if there is concomitant psoriatic arthritis. Methotrexate is by a considerable margin the least expensive systemic therapy for psoriasis. The British National Formulary NHS indicative price is £10 per month for 15 mg orally per week and for subcutaneous methotrexate is between £13.77 and £14.85 for a 25 mg injection.

Early uncontrolled series of the efficacy of methotrexate in psoriasis reported clearance rates of up to 80% of patients with moderate to severe psoriasis [7]. More recent placebo-controlled and active comparator studies have revealed a lower efficacy. In small studies comparing methotrexate with ciclosporin, the efficacy of methotrexate 15 mg/week was found to be similar to ciclosporin 3 mg/kg/day at 16 weeks [8] whereas methotrexate 7.5 mg/week, increasing to 15 mg/week if necessary, was found to be inferior to ciclosporin 3 mg/kg/day increasing to 5 mg/kg/day at 12 weeks [9]. Methotrexate has also been used as an active comparator in clinical trials for the development of the biologic agents adalimumab and briakinumab [10,11]. PASI-75 was achieved at week 16 in 35.5% of patients receiving methotrexate 7.5 mg orally increasing as tolerated and needed up to 25 mg/week, as against a PASI-75 rate in the placebo arm of 18.9% [10]. In the second study using a similar methotrexate dosing strategy, PASI-75 was seen at week 24 in 39.9% of the methotrexate arm (no placebo arm) [11]. Registry data supports increased efficacy of adalimumab compared with methotrexate [12]. Methotrexate can take up to 6 months to achieve maximum efficacy although improvement can be seen after about 2 months therapy. Subcutaneous methotrexate has been evaluated in a randomised controlled trial for psoriasis. At week 16, PASI-75 was achieved in 41% of patients compared with 10% in the placebo group [3].

In those patients in whom methotrexate is effective, long-term studies have reported both long-term safety and efficacy with some studies reporting favourable outcomes in patients treated for 20 years or more [13]. Prospective studies have reported a mean drug survival of between 7.7 and 22.3 months [14].

Methotrexate therapy for psoriasis can cause a myriad of side effects including infections, nausea, bone marrow suppression, mucositis and hepatotoxicity. In the largest registry data, the reported risk of serious infection is 14.18 per 1000 patient years. The majority of these are lower respiratory tract infections and soft-tissue infections. In several registries, this is similar to the infection rates reported with TNF-inhibitors and ustekinumab [15].

Low-dose once-weekly methotrexate (up to 25 mg weekly) for psoriasis is associated with hepatic fibrosis in a minority of patients [16]. A systematic review assessing hepatotoxicity from methotrexate in psoriasis patients revealed that hepatic fibrosis was increased with a risk difference compared with controls of 0.22 (95% CI 0.04–0.41). There was no association between the cumulative methotrexate dose and the development of liver fibrosis. The review commented that the quality of the evidence on this topic was poor [17]. Methotrexate hepatotoxicity nonetheless appears to be commoner in psoriasis patients than in those with rheumatoid arthritis [18]. This may be due to increased risk factors for liver injury among psoriasis patients such as obesity, alcohol misuse and diabetes and the fact that higher therapeutic doses are generally used when treating psoriasis compared with rheumatoid arthritis [18]. Standard liver function tests are considered insufficient to monitor patients for the development of hepatic fibrosis. In a significant minority of patients, liver fibrosis can occur with normal liver enzymes. In the past, liver biopsies have been recommended in order to detect occult fibrosis but the use of the serum aminoterminal peptide of pro-collagen III (PIIINP) as a biomarker of fibrosis has reduced the need for routine liver biopsies in these patients [19]. Although, to date, the level of evidence in psoriasis patients is limited [17], the use of PIIINP is recommended in guidelines [3]. The detection and monitoring of hepatic fibrosis is aided by the use of transient elastography, which is now in routine clinical use in many centres [20]. Other non-invasive tools such as FIB-4 for detecting hepatic fibrosis have been reported [21]. Some studies in rheumatoid arthritis suggest that the use of concomitant folic acid may reduce abnormalities in liver enzymes [22]. There are no long-term studies assessing the use of concomitant folic acid with methotrexate therapy in psoriasis patients in terms of reducing hepatic fibrosis. Pulmonary fibrosis has only been reported rarely in psoriasis patients treated with methotrexate [23]. This contrasts with rheumatoid arthritis where pulmonary fibrosis induced by methotrexate is a significant concern. However, guidelines do recommend a chest X-ray prior to starting methotrexate therapy. This is to screen for pre-existing pulmonary pathology that may be exacerbated by methotrexate [2].

Methotrexate is teratogenic and it is advised that women of child-bearing age use adequate contraception during methotrexate therapy and for 6 months after methotrexate cessation. It is also recommended that men do not father children while taking methotrexate and for 6 months after cessation of therapy.

Methotrexate is a cost-effective, safe treatment for psoriasis, but it requires a persistent attitude from both patient and physician. The superior efficacy of biologic therapies and decreased monitoring required may make these drugs more attractive to prescribe. Nonetheless a significant number of patients will achieve excellent, long-term control of their disease with methotrexate therapy and the treatment of psoriasis demands a long-term perspective.

Methotrexate is often used and licensed for the use in combination with biologic treatments for the treatment of psoriatic arthritis. This has been studied less often in psoriasis. In a randomised controlled trial, methotrexate in combination with etanercept was more effective than etanercept monotherapy [24]. Methotrexate therapy in combination with infliximab is a recommended approach as it may reduce the immunogenicity of infliximab although this has not been studied in randomised controlled trials. The use of combination therapies probably increases the risk of serious infection and for most psoriasis patients is not needed for control of the disease. The question of whether concomitant methotrexate therapy increases drug survival is one that needs to be addressed in prospective studies. It is established practice to use methotrexate in conjunction with adalimumab for the treatment of rheumatoid arthritis. This is based on studies that report increased adalimumab drug levels and decreased anti-drug antibody formation in rheumatoid arthritis and ankylosing spondylitis patients treated with methotrexate and adalimumab compared with adalimumab alone [25,26]. One study in psoriasis has suggested that the combination of methotrexate and adalimumab is more effective compared with adalimumab alone after 1 year but the 3-year follow-up report of this study did not report any statistically significant differences in terms of efficacy and drug survival [27,28].

Ciclosporin

Ciclosporin was reported as being effective for psoriasis in 1979 following a serendipitous observation in patients with psoriatic arthritis who received the treatment as part of a pilot study in inflammatory arthritis [29]. Ciclosporin works by inhibiting IL-2 production by lymphocytes via calcineurin inhibition. This results in the reduction of NFκB and multiple cytokines including IL-2, TNF-α and IL-8. The observation that ciclosporin was effective in psoriasis reinforced a change in thinking about the psoriasis pathogenesis paradigm [30]. Prior to this, psoriasis was considered to be primarily a disease of keratinocyte hyperproliferation with secondary inflammation. The efficacy of ciclosporin confirmed the primacy of immunological abnormalities and led to a large body of research suggesting that psoriasis is an immune-mediated disease. Calcineurin is also expressed in epidermal keratinocytes and other cell types in skin so that inhibition of nuclear factor of activated T-cell (NFAT) signalling in both the acquired and innate immune system may be important to its therapeutic efficacy.

Double-blind placebo-controlled trials confirmed early observations of efficacy and suggest a maximum dose of 5 mg/kg/day [31,**32**]. Ciclosporin 5 mg/kg/day is more effective than 2.5 mg/kg/day [33]. Over 80% of patients achieved PASI-75 at week 16 [33].

There are two randomised controlled trials of ciclosporin compared with methotrexate therapy. In a study of 88 patients randomised to either ciclosporin 2.5–5 mg/kg/day or methotrexate 15–22.5 mg weekly, there were similar responses in both groups. Thirty-three per cent of patients in the ciclosporin group achieved complete remission and 71% partial remission. In the methotrexate

group, 40% and 60% achieved complete and partial remission, respectively [8]. In a similar comparative study, Flystrom reported greater efficacy of ciclosporin (PASI-75 achieved in 58%) compared with methotrexate in a study of 84 patients [9].

The long-term use of ciclosporin is associated with significant side effects. The major issues relate to renal impairment, hypertension and possible increased risk of malignancies [34].

As a consequence, ciclosporin is not recommended for maintenance treatment of psoriasis. [35]. It is used predominantly for the induction of remission when a swift response is required. It is also a safe treatment throughout all stages of pregnancy with appropriate monitoring for hypertension and renal impairment. Transition to another therapy with a more favourable side-effect profile is then recommended for long-term disease control.

Acitretin

Acitretin is a metabolite of etretinate, which was the first retinoid used in the treatment of psoriasis. Etretinate has a narrow therapeutic window and a long half-life and its use has been superseded by acitretin. Acitretin binds to nuclear receptors of the steroid superfamily, which includes the vitamin D receptor. It reduces keratinocyte proliferation [36] and also reduces Th17 cells with a concomitant increase in regulatory T cells [37].

The evidence base for the use of acitretin in psoriasis is small and of low quality although more extensive and robust studies had been performed for etretinate. The efficacy of acitretin in psoriasis is dose dependent and NICE guidelines suggest dose escalation with a target dose of 25–50 mg/day, assessing efficacy at 4 months [35]. Low-dose acitretin as monotherapy (10–25 mg daily) is of low efficacy and in one study daily doses of 50 mg or higher were required for significant efficacy [38]. A comparative study between acitretin and etretinate reported a 76% improvement in PASI in 127 patients treated with acitretin 0.54 mg/kg/day for 12 weeks [39]. In a small controlled study of 20 patients, Gisondi *et al.* reported a PASI-75 of 30% in patients treated with acitretin 0.4 mg/kg/day after 24 weeks of therapy [40]. In a comparative study with etanercept, PASI-75 at 12 weeks was achieved in 27% with acitretin 0.4 mg/kg/day [40].

Acitretin is associated with mucocutaneous side effects, which are dose dependent. Retinoids can cause hyperlipidaemia and rarely hepatitis. Acitretin is teratogenic and is contraindicated in pregnancy, and due to its lipophilic nature can persist in adipose tissue for up to 3 years. Current guidelines recommend that women of childbearing age must not become pregnant for 3 years after cessation of acitretin [41], which precludes its use in most women of childbearing age.

There are many reports of acitretin use in combination with other modalities. Retinoids and PUVA appear to act synergistically. The combination reduces the dose of retinoid and the dose of UV radiation needed to achieve remission and is highly effective, with complete remission reported in 94% of patients [**42**]. Acitretin 0.3–0.5 mg/kg combined with NB-UVB or oral 8-MOP PUVA in 60 patients produced PASI-90 at 8 weeks in 57% of patients receiving re-UVB compared with 63% in the re-PUVA group [43]. Similar results have been reported with bath PUVA and acitretin [44].

Acitretin has the advantage of being a non-immunosuppressant. There are a minority of patients in whom immunosuppression is contraindicated. In these patients acitretin monotherapy or in combination with NB-UVB or PUVA can be a highly effective and safe therapy.

Fumaric acid esters (FAE)

FAE were first reported to be effective in psoriasis in 1959 [45]. FAE have been licensed for the treatment of severe psoriasis in Germany since 1995 and for moderate disease since 2009 [41]. The active component, dimethyl fumarate (DMF), was licensed for moderate to severe psoriasis in Europe in 2017 and is also licensed for the treatment of multiple sclerosis [46].

DMF has multiple effects on immune function. It causes a reduction of glutathione with subsequent decreased Th1 cytokine production including IL-12 and IL-23, and a corresponding increase in Th2 cytokines such as IL-4 [47]. FAE also cause altered Langerhans cell function and reduction in NFκB production, with subsequent decreased TNF-α and IL-8 levels [48,49]. A relative reduction in Th17 cells compared with Treg cells has also been proposed [50].

DMF is given according to a gradually increasing dosing schedule to a maximum dose of 240 mg three times daily. DMF treatment for 16 weeks has produced an improvement in PASI of between 50% and 80% [51–53]. Long-term studies have suggested that the efficacy of DMF continues to improve beyond 16 weeks with one large study of 984 patients reporting good responses in up to 80% of patients [54]. The response to DMF is heterogeneous and some patients will achieve long-term control on small doses (<120 mg daily) [55]. DMF has been compared with Fumaderm® and placebo in a randomised placebo-controlled trial. At 16 weeks, 37.5% of patients treated with DMF achieved PASI-75 compared with 15.7% of placebo treated patients and 40% of those receiving Fumaderm.

One study has reported that up to 60% of patients remain on therapy after 4 years [55]. DMF is undergoing trials for the treatment of moderate psoriasis (5–10% BSA).

DMF causes gastrointestinal upset, usually diarrhoea, in about 60% of patients [54]. Tolerance develops in the majority of patients allowing dose escalation. Flushing manifests in 30% of patients and may respond to aspirin. A transient eosinophilia may develop in some patients. A significant issue is that DMF can cause lymphopenia in 53% of patients. Current guidelines suggest dose reduction if the lymphocyte count decreases below 0.8×10^9/L. If the lymphocyte count persists below this level then further dose reductions should be made until the count recovers or consideration should be given to discontinuing treatment. DMF does not cause anaemia or thrombocytopenia. Despite the immunosuppressive nature of FAE there are few reports of serious or opportunistic infections and these appear less than traditional systemics and biologic therapies [56].

Progressive multifocal leukencephalopathy has been described in 19 patients receiving FAE/DMF [57]. The majority of these patients had prolonged lymphopenia (<0.5×10^9/L) for 6 months or more. One case of Kaposi sarcoma has been described in a patient taking FAE. The lesions resolved on stopping the drug and restoration of normal lymphocyte function [58]. DMF should be monitored in a similar fashion to other immunosuppressant drugs. Active infection should be excluded prior to starting the medication and caution should be exercised in using FAE in the setting of systemic malignancy. Prophylactic immunisation with influenza and pneumococcal vaccine should be part of routine management, as should screening for malignancies such as cervical cancer.

DMF may cause proteinuria and this should be screened for routinely. Most cases of proteinuria are stable and do not require dose reduction and/or cessation of the drug. Proximal renal tubule dysfunction may occasionally occur and Fanconi syndrome has been reported rarely [59]. Despite recognised effects on renal function, progression to renal failure is not reported in the literature. Guidelines recommend that renal failure is a contraindication to DMF therapy [41].

NICE recommends DMF after ciclosporin and methotrexate for psoriasis patients in the UK. This contrasts with Germany, Austria and the Netherlands. Its long-term safety and low level of serious infections suggest that it may best be used as a first line therapy as recommended by the European S3 guidelines [60].

Hydroxycarbamide (hydroxyurea)

Hydroxycarbamide is indicated predominantly in lymphoproliferative disorders but has been used occasionally in patients with psoriasis over the past 30 years [61].

There are no randomised controlled trials of hydroxycarbamide in psoriasis. Given this lack of evidence and lack of clinical experience outside a few centres, it is used infrequently. In a retrospective study, Layton et al. reported remission in 52 of 80 patients (61%) with severe psoriasis prescribed 0.5–1.5 g daily [62]. In another small study in which 31 patients with psoriasis received hydroxycarbamide 1–1.5 g daily for 36 weeks, 75% had at least a 35% improvement in PASI, and 50% had a 70% or greater reduction in PASI [63]. There does not appear to be any benefit in increasing the dose beyond 1.5 g/day. Long-term satisfactory control can be achieved in patients with hydroxycarbamide for up to 20 years in some patients.

Hydroxycarbamide is inexpensive and appears well tolerated. It can cause dose-dependent bone marrow toxicity and has a narrow therapeutic window. It is excreted via the kidneys so caution should be used in treating patients with impaired renal function [61]. A raised mean corpuscular volume on full blood count tests is expected and in contrast to when this occurs in patients on methotrexate therapy, it is not a cause for concern. Hydroxycarbamide has been used in the treatment of HIV infection [64] and may be a suitable choice of systemic treatment in psoriasis patients with HIV [65]. Hydroxycarbamide has been reported to be associated with an increased incidence of actinic keratosis and SCC. The majority of these arise in patients with myeloproliferative disorders who are at increased risk of pre-malignant cutaneous lesions [61].

Apremilast

Apremilast is a small molecule inhibitor of phosphodiesterase 4, which modulates pro-inflammatory mediator production. In phase III randomised controlled trials at a dose of 30 mg twice daily, between 33.1% and 28.8% of patients achieved PASI-75 compared with 5% and 5.8% of patients on placebo at week 16 [66,67]. Apremilast may cause diarrhoea and 10% of patients lose >10% of their body weight independent of diarrhoea. One year drug survival was 31% in one large study but no prospective registry data have been reported [68]. The incidence of serious infections appears low, but these have been reported including tuberculosis. Apremilast is also licensed for the treatment of psoriatic arthritis – see later.

Miscellaneous

Tofacitinib

Tofacitinib, an oral inhibitor of Janus kinases JAK1 and JAK3, is currently licensed for the treatment of rheumatoid arthritis and psoriatic arthritis. In a phase II clinical trial in psoriasis, PASI-75 was achieved at 12 weeks in 40.8% of patients receiving 5 mg twice daily and 66.7% of those receiving 15 mg twice daily compared with 2% in the control arm [69]. Tofacitinib is not licensed for the treatment of psoriasis.

Tyrosine kinase 2 inhibitor

A novel oral tyrosine kinase 2 inhibitor, deucravacitinib is licensed for moderate to severe psoriasis. This acts on gene expression of the STAT pathway, leading to a reduction in IL-12 and IL-23 and ultimately Th17 cells. In a phase II study, 75% of patients at a dose of 12 mg daily achieved PASI-75 at week 12 compared with 7% on placebo in patients with moderate to severe psoriasis (PASI >12) [70]. In two phase III studies, deucravacitinib was compared with placebo and apremilast. At week 16, 53.6–58.7% of patients on deucravacitinib 6 mg once daily achieved PASI-75 compared with 35.1–40.2% of patients on apremilast 30 mg twice daily and 9.4–12.7% of patients on placebo [71].

Biologic therapy

The development of biologic therapies or biologics for psoriasis has revolutionised care for patients suffering with this disease. Currently licensed treatments in this category are TNF-α inhibitors (TNFi), the IL-12/IL-23 p40 inhibitor ustekinumab, IL-17 inhibitors and IL-23p19 inhibitors.

The evidence base for their short-term efficacy is robust, based on many well-designed randomised controlled trials. There are direct comparative trials between these agents [1,2,3,4] and indirect comparisons using network meta-analysis [5]. These suggest marked variation in their short-term efficacy. The optimal sequence of biologic treatments is still being developed as longer term efficacy and safety data emerge and guidelines have been published on their use [6]. The evidence derived from clinical trials needs to be interpreted with caution in the clinical setting, due to factors such as the limited duration of the placebo-controlled phase of the trial, and the large number of exclusion criteria when recruiting to trials. Longer term safety data can more reliably be obtained from well-designed treatment registers such as the British Association of Dermatologists Biologics and Immunomodulators Register (BADBIR) [7].

For instance, 30% of patients enrolled in a Spanish severe psoriasis register would have been ineligible for most randomised controlled trials (because of their age, pattern of psoriasis or co-morbidities) and this ineligible group was at increased risk of serious adverse events [8]. A similar report has been published using data from BADBIR. Registers or networks of registers are more powerful for detecting adverse events and were primarily designed to assess the safety of these medications [9,10].

TNF-α inhibitors

TNFi have the advantages, compared with previous conventional treatments, of a different and relatively precise mechanism of action and as a consequence a different safety profile, high response rates (Table 35.6) and efficacy when other approaches have failed.

Table 35.6 Relative short-term efficacy in randomised controlled trials of biologics for psoriasis.

Treatment	Dose	% achieving PASI-75
Adalimumab	40 mg every other week	71–80% at week 16
Etanercept	25 mg twice weekly	34% at week 12
	50 mg twice weekly	49% at week 12
Infliximab	5 mg/kg at weeks 0, 2 and 6	80–88% at week 10
Ustekinumab	45 mg at weeks 0 and 4	67% at week 12
	90 mg at weeks 0 and 4	66–76% at week 12

PASI, Psoriasis Area Severity Index.

Currently, four TNFi are licensed for this indication: adalimumab, certolizumab, etanercept and infliximab. Although they share the same therapeutic target, these agents differ in many respects including their dosing, route of administration, mechanism of action, speed of onset, retention on treatment, immunogenicity and safety. In Europe, the marketing authorisation of each agent for the indication of psoriasis is the same, being limited to moderate/severe disease when other treatments (methotrexate, ciclosporin and phototherapy) have been ineffective, or are contraindicated. Their use is often further restricted because of their greater cost than traditional systemic treatments. The development of biosimilar agents for infliximab, etanercept and adalimumab has led to huge cost reductions in the medications with improved access. In many countries biosimilar availability has led to >70% reduction in the cost of biologics and primary (first-time) use of these agents among biologics.

Infliximab

As has often been the case in the development of new treatments for psoriasis, the potential efficacy of TNFi was first suspected in 2000, when infliximab (a chimeric human–murine monoclonal antibody with affinity for TNF-α) was coincidentally found to improve dramatically the psoriasis of a woman who was receiving the drug for the treatment of Crohn disease [1]. Infliximab binds to soluble TNF-α and TNF-α that is bound to the TNF receptor. Subsequent randomised controlled trials confirmed the rapid onset of action and high efficacy of infliximab in psoriasis compared with placebo [2–4]. Infliximab also has efficacy in psoriatic nail disease and psoriatic arthritis [5]. In contrast to the other TNFi, the drug is given by intravenous infusion and dose is based on body weight (5 mg/kg at weeks 0, 2 and 6 and then every 8 weeks). A response is often seen after the first infusion, and after an induction phase of three infusions 80% of patients achieve PASI-75 at week 10 and 57% achieve PASI-90 compared with 3% and 1% with placebo respectively [3]. This rapid and reliable response makes the drug particularly suitable in urgent circumstances such as erythrodermic psoriasis and generalised pustular psoriasis [6,7]. In the maintenance phase, efficacy is maintained to 50 weeks in randomised controlled trials in the majority of cases [3] although persistence of response is lower with intermittent dosing [8]. In the UK, infliximab is recommended only for use in patients with PASI values >20.

Persistence on infliximab at 4 years was reported in 70% of a registry cohort of 144 Danish psoriasis patients [9]. Antidrug antibodies (ADA) have been reported in a high proportion of individuals treated with infliximab, and correlate with lower serum drug levels, loss of efficacy and the development of infusion reactions [10,11]. Higher serum levels of infliximab and a reduced incidence of ADA have been reported when infliximab is prescribed in combination with methotrexate [10]. Although combination therapy with methotrexate is a licensing recommendation for infliximab in the treatment of rheumatoid and psoriatic arthritis, this has not been prospectively studied in plaque psoriasis.

Infliximab is associated with a higher incidence of serious infections compared with other biologics and systemic therapies [**12**]. These infections tend to be pneumonia and soft-tissue infections although opportunistic infections have also been reported. Infliximab is also associated with an increased risk of activation of latent tuberculosis. Tuberculosis is associated with infliximab, a TNF-α neutralising agent [**13**]. This risk is low although fatalities have been reported and the presentation is often atypical. Tuberculosis reactivation depends on age, cigarette smoking, country of origin and residence among other factors. It is recommended that prior to infliximab therapy, patients are screened for latent tuberculosis using an IGRA test such as Quantiferon and a chest X-ray [14].

Infliximab is also associated with reactivation of hepatitis B infection and fulminant hepatitis has been reported. Patients should be screened for hepatitis B infection and HIV prior to commencing treatment.

Etanercept

Etanercept is a fully human soluble TNF-α receptor fusion protein that binds and neutralises soluble TNF-α. Response is of slower onset than with infliximab, becoming evident after 4–8 weeks of treatment [15,16]. PASI-75 was achieved at 12 weeks in 34% and 47–49% of patients receiving 25 mg twice weekly or 50 mg twice weekly and PASI-90 in 11–12% and 21% of patients at these same doses [17]. The number responding to treatment continues to rise up to 24 months, at which point 59% of patients will have achieved PASI-75 with the higher dose of treatment [15]. Open-label extensions of the phase III trials have revealed the continuing efficacy of etanercept in initial responders for up to 4 years, with some loss of efficacy between 1 and 2 years [18]. A subsequent randomised controlled trial has demonstrated PASI-75 at 12 weeks in 37.5% of patients treated with etanercept 50 mg weekly [18]. The licensed dose of etanercept is 25 mg administered twice weekly or 50 mg administered once weekly. Alternatively, 50 mg given twice weekly may be used for up to 12 weeks followed, if necessary, by a dose of 25 mg twice weekly or 50 mg once weekly, although this dose has not been approved by NICE on pharmacoeconomic grounds. In light of the development of cheaper biosimilar versions of etanercept, the use of etanercept at higher doses should be reconsidered. Etanercept is associated with a lower risk of reactivation of tuberculosis and serious infections than infliximab. It is also effective and licensed for the treatment of psoriatic arthritis.

In head-to-head randomised controlled trials, etanercept at 50 mg twice weekly for 12 weeks and then 50 mg weekly is less effective than ustekinumab, secukinumab, ixekizumab and tildrakizumab [19]. The first line use of etanercept has therefore declined and is not recommended in current guidelines. However, there are many patients who have achieved and continue to achieve excellent safe long-term control of psoriasis on etanercept therapy.

Etanercept has also been found to be an effective treatment in paediatric psoriasis, for which it is licensed in resistant moderate to severe disease. In a randomised controlled trial of 211 patients with psoriasis aged 4–17 years, etanercept 0.8 mg/kg body weight produced PASI-75 at week 12 in 57% of patients compared with 11% of those receiving placebo [20]. Response has been maintained for up to 96 weeks. Etanercept has been combined safely with phototherapy [21], acitretin [22] or methotrexate [23]. In short-term studies of adult patients, in each instance the combination is of greater efficacy than etanercept alone.

Adalimumab

Adalimumab (a fully human monoclonal antibody with affinity for TNF-α) has demonstrated high efficacy in psoriasis and is also licensed for psoriatic arthritis, rheumatoid arthritis, polyarticular juvenile idiopathic arthritis, Crohn disease, ulcerative colitis and hidradenitis suppurativa. The onset of treatment response in psoriasis is rapid, being significant at 2 weeks and maximal between weeks 12 and 16. In phase III trials, PASI-75 and PASI-90 at 16 weeks was seen in 71–80% and 45–51%, respectively, of patients receiving adalimumab 80 mg at week 0 then 40 mg every other week beginning at week 1 [**24**,25], although higher response rates are seen with the unlicensed dose of 80 mg weekly [26]. Open-label extensions of phase III trials have confirmed continuing efficacy of up to 3 years in most initial responders [27]. Adalimumab has shown greater efficacy after 16 weeks of treatment than methotrexate (7.5 mg/week initial dose increasing to a maximum of 25 mg/week as tolerated) [**24**]. Patients on adalimumab therapy may develop ADA, which are associated with reduced serum levels and reduced efficacy. In one small study, serum adalimumab levels at week 4 were predictive of efficacy at 6 months [19]. This has since been replicated in a larger study [28].

Adalimumab is often used in combination with methotrexate in rheumatology patients and azathioprine for IBD in order to improve efficacy and reduce ADA. This is less reported in psoriasis but nonetheless appears an attractive therapeutic proposition.

As with infliximab, adalimumab is associated with an increased risk of tuberculosis reactivation and serious infections but these are low in incidence (about 1.4 per 100 patient years for serious infection). Hepatitis B reactivation has also been described with adalimumab. Opportunistic infections have been reported albeit rarely in psoriasis especially when used as a monotherapy. The concerns regarding adalimumab and cancer development have largely been unfounded.

In short-term head-to-head trials, adalimumab has been shown to be less effective than risankizumab, bimekizumab and guselkumab [29,**30**]. In registry studies, the drug survival of adalimumab for psoriasis is less than ustekinumab, secukinumab and guselkumab [31,32]. Nonetheless, with the availability of cheaper, biosimilar versions of adalimumab, adalimumab will and should continue to be used as a first line biologic for the foreseeable future.

Certolizumab pegol

Certolizumab pegol is a recombinant humanised antibody Fab fragment against TNF-α. In phase III randomised controlled trials, patients with moderate to severe psoriasis were randomised to certolizumab 200 mg every 2 weeks, certolizumab 400 mg every

2 weeks or placebo. The primary outcome measure was PASI-75 at week 16. In CIMPASI-1 66.5% of the 200 mg every 2 weeks group achieved PASI-75 compared with 75.8% on 400 mg every 2 weeks and 6.5% of placebo. Certolizumab was also compared with etanercept and placebo in the CIMPACT study and the 400 mg twice weekly dose achieved higher efficacy than etanercept 50 mg twice weekly at week 12 [33]. As certolizumab is a pegylated monoclonal antibody, it does not have an Fc portion. This may have advantages when treating psoriasis patients during pregnancy [34].

Registries

The development of biologic registries has been a pivotal development in dermatology research and contributed significantly to our knowledge about biologic therapies, systemic therapies and psoriasis. There have been several successful registries in rheumatology and gastroenterology and results from these registries have highlighted several differences between adverse events across diseases and confirmed the importance of individual disease registries.

In the UK and Republic of Ireland the British Association of Dermatologists Biologics and Immunomodulatory Registry (BADBIR) has, to date, recruited >20 000 patients on systemic therapies and biologic therapies.

The primary outcomes of the registry are the incidence of serious infections and cancer in psoriasis patients treated with biologics compared with traditional systemic agents. Valuable information is being reported about long-term efficacy and factors that are associated with clinical outcomes [1,2].

Registries are important sources of real-life data on the treatment of moderate to severe psoriasis. Up to 40% of psoriasis patients are ineligible for clinical trials due to precise inclusion and exclusion criteria required for these trials [3].

The overall incidence of serious infections in psoriasis patients on biologic treatment is approximately between 1.4 and 1.8 per 100 patient years. A serious infection is defined as an infection that results in admission to hospital or death. Several registries have reported higher incidences of serious infections for those patients on infliximab compared with etanercept, adalimumab and ustekinumab and compared with traditional systemic agents [4–6].

The predominant infections reported are respiratory tract and soft tissue. Analysis of infection rates in patients treated with traditional systemic agents compared with adalimumab, etanercept and ustekinumab have shown consistently no significant differences in infection rates between groups. This is surprising and despite the limitations of registry data suggest little if any difference between infection risks. Several factors have been shown to increase infection risk in psoriasis patients treated with biologics. These include age >65, the presence of diabetes and cigarette smoking [4].

The incidence of cancer in psoriasis patients treated with biologics is low [7]. Combined data from several registries has suggested that biologic therapy does not cause cancer [7]. Data from rheumatology registries albeit in small numbers of patients suggest that continuation of TNFis after a cancer diagnosis does not adversely affect prognosis [7]. A decision to continue biologic or systemic therapy after a diagnosis of a solid organ or haematological malignancy should be made on an individual basis and in conjunction with specialist oncological advice.

Biosimilars

Biologic therapies are recombinant proteins that have undergone complex manufacturing processes. Biosimilars are molecules with the same amino acid sequence which are not identical to the originator molecule but have similar efficacy and side effects. Biosimilars are available for infliximab, adalimumab and etanercept. These drugs are significantly less expensive than the originator therapies – up to 90% cheaper in some countries. This has allowed access to biologic therapies in many countries where the cost was too prohibitive previously. Biosimilars have to demonstrate similar efficacy to the originator molecule in one indication usually rheumatoid arthritis for TNFis. There are, however, clinical trials in psoriasis comparing biosimilar adalimumab to originator adalimumab with equivalent efficacy and safety results [8].

IL-12/IL-23 p40 inhibitor

The knowledge that IL-12 expression was increased in psoriasis plaques led to the development of ustekinumab; the first time a monoclonal antibody was designed specifically for the treatment of psoriasis. Ustekinumab is a fully human IgG_1 κ monoclonal antibody against the p40 subunit that is common to both IL-12 and IL-23. Its efficacy in moderate to severe plaque psoriasis was confirmed in two separate randomised controlled trials [1,2]. In the first of these, PASI-75 was achieved at week 12 in 67% and 66% of those receiving ustekinumab 90 mg or 45 mg, respectively, at week 0, 4 and 12, compared with 3% in the placebo arm [1]. In the second pivotal trial, PASI-75 was achieved at week 12 in 76% and 67% of those receiving ustekinumab 90 mg and 45 mg, respectively, as against 4% in those randomised to placebo [2]. In this latter trial, 69% of partial responders (defined as >PASI-50 but <PASI-75) to ustekinumab 90 mg every 12 weeks achieved PASI-75 at week 52 when the injection frequency was increased to every 8 weeks [2]. There is evidence for reduced efficacy in patients with increased body weight, in association with reduced serum drug levels [3] leading to a licensed dose of ustekinumab 45 mg at weeks 0, 4 and then every 12 weeks in those who weigh less than 100 kg, and 90 mg at the same dosing interval in those who weigh more than 100 kg. Ustekinumab has greater efficacy than etanercept 50 mg twice weekly [4]. This trial was the first head-to-head study to compare the efficacy of biologic therapies in inflammatory disease. This has led to the use of head-to-head trials in subsequent psoriasis treatment development.

The drug survival of ustekinumab is superior to adalimumab, etanercept and infliximab in multiple registries [5]. The long-term safety of ustekinumab has been established and early concerns regarding cardiovascular events have proven to be unfounded [6–8]. Safety data from open-label extensions of the original phase III trials reveal no significant cumulative safety signals in up to 5 years of follow-up and this data has been reflected in real-world registry data [6].

There is evidence of an increased response rate to ustekinumab in patients who are HLA-C:06:02 positive [9,10]. There is also preliminary data suggesting that higher serum ustekinumab levels are associated with increased response [11].

Ustekinumab is also effective in psoriatic arthritis especially for dactylitis and enthesitis [12], and Crohn disease [13] albeit at a higher licensed maintenance dose in Crohn disease of 90 mg every 8 weeks.

IL-17 inhibitors

There are six cytokines in the IL-17 cytokine family, IL-17 A–F, and five receptors, IL-17 A–E. mRNA levels of IL-17A, -C and -F are elevated in psoriasis plaques and increased numbers of IL-17A-positive cells are found to be involved in psoriasis skin compared with controls [1]. The cellular source of IL-17 in psoriasis includes lymphocytes but also innate immune cells such as mast cells and innate lymphoid cells. There are currently four IL-17 inhibitors licensed for the treatment of psoriasis (brodalumab, ixekizumab, secukinumab and bimekizumab). Secukinumab and ixekizumab target IL-17A, brodalumab targets a subunit of the IL-17 receptor (IL-17RA), and thereby inhibits IL-17A, IL-17F and IL-E (also known as IL-25), and bimekizumab targets IL-17A and F.

Secukinumab

Secukinumab, a fully human monoclonal antibody to IL-17A, has been evaluated in phase III randomised controlled clinical trials. Given at a dose of 300 mg or 15 mg (administered once weekly for 5 weeks, then every 4 weeks) produced PASI-75 at 12 weeks in 77.1–88.6% and 67–71.6%, respectively. PASI-90 was achieved by 54.2–59.2%, and 39.1–41.9% of patients in the 300 mg and 150 mg groups, respectively. PASI-100 was achieved by 24.1–28.6% of the 300 mg group and 12.8–14.4% of the 150 mg group. Both doses were more effective at 12 weeks than etanercept 50 mg twice weekly in a head-to-head comparison [2]. Secukinumab is also more effective than ustekinumab in head-to-head clinical trials [3]. This has been replicated in real-world patients [4]. Secukinumab is also as effective as adalimumab and licensed for psoriatic arthritis [5] (see Psoriatic arthritis) The majority of clinical trial patients who respond to secukinumab continue to do so for up to 5 years with most maintaining PASI-90 responses in open label extension studies [6].

It appears that secukinumab is less effective as a second-line biologic [7]. In an open-labelled study, where secukinumab was used to treat patients who had failed anti-TNF therapy, the PASI-75 responses were less than reported in clinical trials [8].

In a registry study from Denmark, the 1-year survival of secukinumab was 66.4%, significantly less than ustekinumab or adalimumab. Drug survival was less in patients who had received previous biologic therapy [9]. The drug survival of secukinumab in the BADBIR registry, however, was similar to ustekinumab and better than adalimumab [7].

Ixekizumab

Ixekizumab, a humanised anti-IL-17A monoclonal antibody, is licensed for the treatment of moderate to severe psoriasis and psoriatic arthritis. In phase III randomised controlled trials, ixekizumab 160 mg was given subcutaneously at week 0, followed by 80 mg at week 2 and every 2 weeks for 12 weeks. The PASI-75 response was 89.1% at week 12 [10]. In head-to-head trials ixekizumab is superior to etanercept [10], ustekinumab [11] and guselkumab [12]. In open label extension trials, the majority of patients who respond to ixekizumab maintain long-term efficacy on 80 mg [13]. Preliminary registry data report that the drug survival of ixekizumab is longer than that of secukinumab [9]. Similar to secukinumab, these real-world data suggest that ixekizumab is less effective when used as a second or third line biologic.

Brodalumab

Brodalumab, a fully human IL-17RA monoclonal antibody, is licensed for the treatment of moderate to severe chronic plaque psoriasis. In phase III trials, at week 12, 86% of patients on brodalumab, at the licensed dose of 210 mg every 2 weeks, achieved PASI-75 compared with 8% of patients on placebo. PASI-100 was achieved by 44% of patients compared with 22% on ustekinumab at licensed doses [14]. Brodalumab is effective in phase II trials for psoriatic arthritis but is not licensed for this indication.

In the phase III trial programme there were six suicides in brodalumab treated patients leading to a black box warning in the USA. Long-term follow-up of patients on brodalumab has not shown an increase in suicide rates and the consensus is that these events were not related to brodalumab [15].

Bimekizumab

Bimekizumab is a fully humanised monoclonal antibody to both IL-17A and F. This has been evaluated in phase III trials for the treatment of psoriasis and psoriatic arthritis and has been licensed for the management of psoriasis. At week 16, PASI-90 was achieved in 85% of patients on bimekizumab 320 mg subcutaneously every 4 weeks compared with 4.8% of placebo and 49.7% of ustekinumab patients. This effect was continued to week 52 [16]. Bimekizumab is also more effective than adalimumab and secukinumab in head-to-head trials [17,18]. The incidence of candidal infections is higher with bimekizumab treated patients compared with secukinumab [17]. Monoclonal antibodies to IL-17A, IL-17 receptor and IL-17A/F share common adverse events. From clinical trial data serious infections are similar to those with TNFi. Patients on IL-17 inhibitors are more likely to develop candidal infections than patients on placebo or comparator biologics. These infections tend to be mild and do not necessitate discontinuation of therapy in the majority of patients.

Secukinumab was trialled in Crohn disease in a phase II study. In this study patients on placebo fared better than those on secukinumab. Thus, IL-17 inhibition is contraindicated in active IBD [19]. Long-term safety evaluations in clinical trial patients suggest that the incidence of IBD is comparable to the background population rates which is less than 1% per year. Nevertheless, this is greater than seen with adalimumab and ustekinumab, which are both effective and licensed for the treatment of IBD. Patients starting on IL-17 inhibitors should be asked about a personal or family history of IBD and even if negative on history should be asked about symptoms of IBD while on treatment and investigated accordingly.

It is recommended that patients are screened for tuberculosis prior to treatment with IL-17 inhibitors. Patients with latent tuberculosis should be considered for anti-tuberculosis prophylaxis. To date, however, there are no reported cases of tuberculosis developing while on IL-17 inhibitors and this class may be a safer option for patients with latent tuberculosis [13,20].

IL-23p19 inhibitors

IL-17A is produced predominantly by Th17 cells. IL-23 is essential for the development of Th17 cells and is an attractive target for psoriasis therapy; the IL-23p19 subunit only binds to IL-23. There are three IL-23p19 monoclonal antibody inhibitors licensed for the treatment of moderate to severe chronic plaque psoriasis (guselkumab, risankizumab and tildrakizumab) and one, mirak-izumab, which completed phase III trials but was not licensed for psoriasis.

In phase III trials of guselkumab at a dose of 100 mg subcuta-neously at week 0, 4 and every 8 weeks, 70% of patients achieved a PASI-90 at 16 weeks compared with 2.4% of patients on placebo [1]. Guselkumab has been shown to be superior to adalimumab in head-to-head trials [2] and to be effective in non-responders to ustekinumab [3]. In a head-to-head randomised controlled trial, guselkumab was more effective than secukinumab at 48 weeks in terms of PASI-90 response [4]. In contrast, ixekizumab was more effective than guselkumab in terms of PASI-100 efficacy at 12 weeks in a separate head-to-head study [5]. In this study, at 24 weeks there was no difference in efficacy between ixekizumab and guselkumab. This high level of efficacy has been maintained in open-label exten-sion studies of guselkumab for up to 4 years [6,7]. An interesting feature of guselkumab therapy is a long-lasting effect seen in clinical trial patients even after active treatment withdrawal. Guselkumab is also licensed for psoriatic arthritis. Real world evidence from the BADBIR registry has replicated the excellent persistence of treatment efficacy seen in clinical trials [8].

There is a risk of serious infections with guselkumab which is similar to other biologic agents at approximately 1 per 100 patient years. Il-23 does not appear important in tuberculosis pathogenesis although the summary of product characteristics for guselkumab states that patients should be evaluated for tuberculosis infection prior to initiation of therapy. Rare cases of tuberculosis have been reported with guselkumab therapy [9]. Of interest, guselkumab treatment is not associated with candidal infection or IBD.

With risankizumab, a dose of 150 mg at week 0, 4 and every 12 weeks, 74.8% and 75% of moderate to severe psoriasis patients achieved PASI-90 at week 16 compared with 2–4.9% on placebo [10]. Risankizumab is more effective than ustekinumab [11] and adali-mumab at week 16 [12] in head-to-head trials. In a head-to-head trial when compared with secukinumab, risankizumab was more effective than secukinumab at week 52 [13]. The long-term effi-cacy is maintained in open-label extension studies. Similar to guselkumab, risankizumab treatment leads to significant remission in patients switched to placebo in withdrawal arms of phase II studies [14]. This has led to the concept that perhaps IL-23p19 inhibitors may be disease modifying but further studies are needed to assess this idea.

Tildrakizumab, when used in randomised controlled trials at an earlier end-point of 12 weeks, 62% of patients on 200 mg and 64% of patients on 100 mg at week 0, 4 and every 12 weeks achieved PASI-75 compared with 6% in the placebo group. Tildrakizumab is more effective than etanercept at week 12 [9].

Mirakizumab is a fourth IL-23p19 targeting monoclonal antibody which has undergone phase III trials for psoriasis. In a head-to-head study with secukinumab and placebo, 74.4% of patients on mirak-izumab 250 mg every 4 weeks achieved PASI-90 at 16 weeks com-pared with 6.3% on placebo. This was non-inferior to secukinumab (72.8% PASI-90) at 16 weeks [15].

IL-23p19 inhibitors have very high efficacy levels. In clinical trial patients, there is a slower onset of action compared with IL-17 inhibitors but at 1 year where head-to-head trials have been carried out (guselkumab, risankizumab) there is higher efficacy. At the time of writing long-term data is limited to open-label extension trials and real-world registry data is lacking. Nevertheless, the long-term data from open-label trials suggests a high level of sustained efficacy.

PUSTULAR PSORIASIS

Introduction and general description

Pustular psoriasis is a group of rare diseases characterised by pri-mary, sterile pustules on variably erythematous skin. A clinically diverse range of pustular phenotypes is recognised [1]. It is useful to separate these clinical entities into generalised pustular psoriasis (GPP) and localised pustular psoriasis. GPP is usually acute, often associated with systemic symptoms and may be life threatening. Localised pustular psoriasis is usually chronic, mainly effects acral skin, and comprises palmoplantar pustulosis (PPP) and acroder-matitis of Hallopeau (ACH). European consensus classification criteria and disease definitions have been published [1] (Table 35.7).

Pustular psoriasis is distinct from chronic plaque psoriasis in clin-ical presentation, genetics, immunology and response to treatment. Its place within the family of psoriatic disease is being refined as the molecular genetic basis of these diseases is further resolved [2]. Although pustular psoriasis and plaque psoriasis vulgaris co-exist more frequently than expected by chance, many patients with pustu-lar psoriasis do not have plaque psoriasis. However, there are phases of pustular psoriasis that can be difficult to distinguish clinically from unstable plaque psoriasis. Also, pustules, more readily seen by dermoscopy, may be provoked within plaques of psoriasis vulgaris in the unstable phase of the disease. Although this has sometimes been referred to confusingly as 'localised GPP' [3,4], this is better considered 'plaque psoriasis with pustules' ('psoriasis cum pustu-latione') rather than a form of pustular psoriasis *per se*.

Unlike chronic plaque psoriasis, pustular psoriasis is not asso-ciated with *HLA-C:06:02*. Recent molecular genetic studies have revealed mutations in *IL36RN* in a significant minority of patients with GPP and to a lesser extent in localised pustular psoriasis [5,6,7]. *IL36RN* mutations have not been identified in patients with chronic plaque psoriasis [8].

Generalised pustular psoriasis

Definition

GPP is a rare disease defined by the presence of primary, sterile, macroscopically visible pustules on non-acral skin [1]. It is often relapsing and remitting, with acute flares of cutaneous inflam-mation with systemic symptoms. Less frequent chronic persistent forms occur. There is a relationship between these entities and chronic plaque psoriasis, in that some patients may have phases of plaque psoriasis before or after GPP, but in many GPP occurs as the sole phenotype without plaque psoriasis at any time.

GPP is heterogeneous in its age at onset, genetics, phenotype, pre-cipitants, severity and natural history. Several overlapping clinical subgroups are recognised.

Table 35.7 Consensus definitions for the diagnosis of pustular psoriasis.

	Definition	Sub-classifiers
Generalised pustular psoriasis	Primary, sterile, macroscopically visible pustules on non-acral skin (excludes cases where pustulation is restricted to psoriatic plaques)	Relapsing or persistent ± systemic inflammation ± psoriasis vulgaris
Palmoplantar pustulosis	Primary, persistent, sterile, macroscopically visible pustules on palms and/or soles	± psoriasis vulgaris
Acrodermatitis of Hallopeau	Primary, persistent, sterile, macroscopically visible pustules affecting the nail apparatus	± psoriasis vulgaris

Source: Based on data from [1].

Epidemiology

Incidence and prevalence

GPP is rare. The annual incidence and prevalence in a French population has been estimated as at least 0.64 and 1.76 per million, respectively [9]. The prevalence in Japan has been estimated at 7.46 per million [10]. There is regional variation in the prevalence of GPP, which appears to be more common in North Africa, South East Asia and Japan [11].

Age at onset

There is a wide range in the age at onset, which peaks between 40 and 59 years of age [4]. Infantile and juvenile cases are also reported (Augey 2006). The age at onset is earlier in those with a family history of psoriasis [4], and in those who are homozygous or compound heterozygotes for mutations in *IL36RN* [12].

Sex

In most published series, women outnumber men 2F:M [3,4,9], although this is not consistent in all cohorts [13].

Pathophysiology

Genetic factors

There is often a family history of GPP in those affected and the pattern of inheritance is usually Mendelian suggesting monogenic inheritance, in contrast to the typically polygenic inheritance of chronic plaque psoriasis. In a series of 35 Asian adults with GPP, 29% had a family history of plaque psoriasis and 11% of GPP [5]. Multiplex GPP families with parental consanguinity have been reported, suggesting autosomal recessive inheritance in some families [5,6].

Causal germline mutations in the *IL36RN* gene were identified in 2011 in familial GPP by linkage analysis in Tunisia [5] and in sporadic GPP in the UK by exome sequencing [6]. Subsequently, mutations in *IL36RN* have been identified in a significant minority of all patients with GPP, in the largest series reported to date affecting 23.7% of those affected [12]. Different *IL36RN* mutations have been reported in different ethnic groups with evidence of a founder effect; in Europeans the commonest mutation in *IL36RN* results in the substitution p.Ser113Leu [14–18]. The same mutation is seen in GPP (von Zumbusch), acrodermatitis continua of Hallopeau and to a lesser extent palmoplantar pustulosis. In a North African population p.Leu27Pro was present in the homozygous state in all individuals with GPP, including infantile and juvenile cases, and in patients diagnosed as impetigo herpetiformis [5]. There is some evidence for genotype–phenotype correlation as GPP patients with

IL36RN mutations are more likely to have early-onset disease, and a systemic inflammatory response [19]. In addition, *IL36RN* mutations are present in a higher proportion of GPP patients without concomitant plaque psoriasis; for instance in Japan the commonest mutation (p.Arg10*) was present in the homozygous state or as a compound heterozygote in about 80% of pure GPP but only 10% of GPP with prior plaque psoriasis [17].

Mutations in *AP1S3*, initially identified in ACH [7], are present in about 10% of individuals with GPP [12]. *AP1S3* encodes the σ1C subunit of the adaptor protein complex 1, which is involved in vesicular transport between the transgolgi network and endosomes. Digenic inheritance with mutations in *IL36RN* and *AP1S3* in the same individual has been described [12].

There are occasional reports of mutations in *CARD14* in GPP, particularly in those with coexistent plaque psoriasis [20]. Genetic variants in *MPO*, which encodes myeloperoxidase, have recently been reported in several cases of GPP [21,22] and *SERPINA3*, which encodes serine protease inhibitor A3 [23].

Environmental factors

Environmental factors that may trigger or exacerbate GPP include infection, topical or systemic treatments, psychological stress, pregnancy and hypocalcaemia. Provocation is most obvious in the acute forms. Von Zumbusch's original case in 1909 was provoked by irritating topical therapy [24]. Coal tar and dithranol may provoke pustulation if injudiciously applied when the disease is unstable [25,26]. The most important drug provocation is by corticosteroids. Withdrawal of systemic corticosteroid therapy can precipitate GPP and potent topical corticosteroid under occlusion has also been implicated [25,27]. There are reports of the induction of GPP on starting adalimumab, infliximab and ustekinumab [28–31] and on withdrawal of ciclosporin or ustekinumab [4,32,33]. Other systemic drugs have also occasionally been implicated including terbinafine [34,35] and NSAIDs [4,36]. Some of these instances may now be considered to represent acute generalised exanthematous pustulosis (AGEP), which can be difficult to distinguish from GPP in patients known to have psoriasis [37].

Viral or bacterial infections are common exacerbating factors, reported in 12 of 16 patients with known GPP in one series [5]. Many individuals report deterioration at times of psychological stress [6].

Hypocalcaemia may arise as a consequence of GPP, but triggering of active disease by hypocalcaemia caused by hypoparathyroidism has occasionally been reported [38,39].

GPP may be triggered by pregnancy, which is discussed further below.

Pathogenic mechanisms

GPP appears to result from a primary dysregulation of the innate immune system. While IL-17A, IFN-γ, TNF α, IL-1, IL-36 and interferons are overexpressed in both GPP and chronic plaque psoriasis, lesional skin in GPP expresses relatively more IL-1 and IL-36 and less IL-17A and IFN-γ than in chronic plaque psoriasis [40]. IL-36 comprises three pro-inflammatory cytokines of the IL-1 family (IL-36 α, β and γ) and is expressed by keratinocytes below neutrophilic pustules in GPP. *IL36RN* encodes the IL-36 receptor antagonist (IL36-Ra), which is expressed primarily in the skin and is an antagonist of IL-36 cytokines. In patients with GPP in whom *IL36RN* is mutated, there is an absence of functional IL-36Ra leading to unopposed IL-36 signalling. Mutations in *AP1S3* have also been shown to lead to over-expression of IL-36α via disruption of keratinocyte autophagy [41]. IL-36 acts on keratinocytes to induce neutrophil chemo-attractants CXCL1, CXCL2 and CXCL8 [42]. Neutrophils release neutrophil proteases which further enhance the bioactivity of IL-36 by cleavage, in an auto-inflammatory loop [43]. IL-36 also stimulates the production of interferon α from plasmacytoid dendritic cells which may mediate some of the systemic effects seen in GPP [44].

There is interaction between immune pathways in GPP and plaque psoriasis. In pustular psoriasis, cross talk can occur between IL-36 and the IL-23 axis. IL-36 is upstream of cytokines such as IL-17, TNF-α and IL-22. IL-17A in turn increases the expression of IL-36 in keratinocytes in a positive feedback circuit if the pathway is not checked.

Clinical features

Acute generalised pustular psoriasis (von Zumbusch).

This relapsing and remitting pattern of GPP is named after Leo von Zumbusch, who described a brother and sister who experienced repeated waves of acute erythema and pustulation over many years, sometimes provoked by topical treatment [24]. This is the most acute and severe form of GPP and is clinically and genetically heterogeneous. It may occur as the sole phenotype or arise following chronic plaque psoriasis, acrodermatitis continua of Hallopeau or palmoplantar pustulosis. Japanese diagnostic criteria require each of the following four features for a definitive diagnosis:

1 Systemic symptoms such as fever and fatigue
2 Multiple sterile pustules that sometimes merge to form lakes of pus
3 Kogoj's spongiform pustules on skin biopsy
4 Repeated recurrence [45].

The eruption may be ushered in by a sensation of burning in the skin, which becomes dry and tender. These warning signs – not always present – are followed by an abrupt onset of high fever and severe malaise. Pre-existing lesions become fiery and develop pinpoint pustules (Figures 35.29 and 35.30). Sheets of erythema and pustulation spread to involve previously unaffected skin, the flexures and genital regions being particularly involved. Any configuration or variety of pustular exanthem may occur, for instance isolated pustules, lakes of pus, circinate lesions, plaques of erythema with pustular collarettes or a generalised erythroderma. Waves of pustulation may succeed each other, subsiding into exfoliation of the dried pustules. The nails may become thickened or separated by subungual lakes of pus. The buccal mucosa and tongue may be

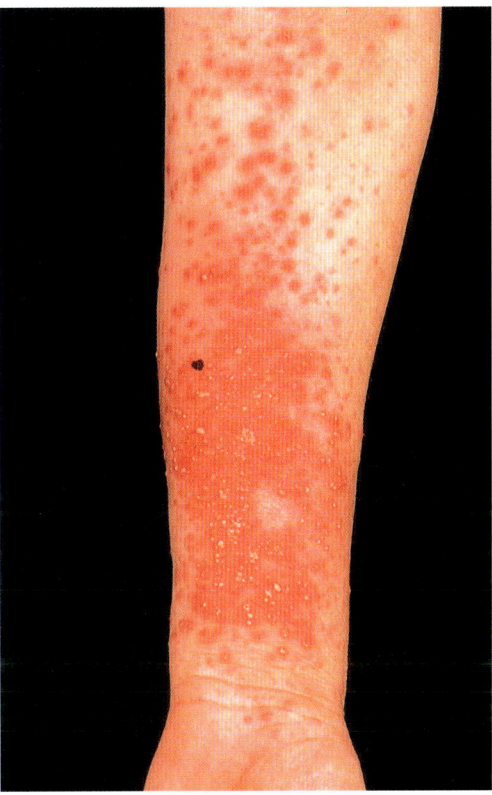

Figure 35.29 Acute generalised pustular psoriasis: pre-existing psoriasis plaques become fiery and develop pinpoint pustules. Courtesy of St John's Institute of Dermatology, London, UK.

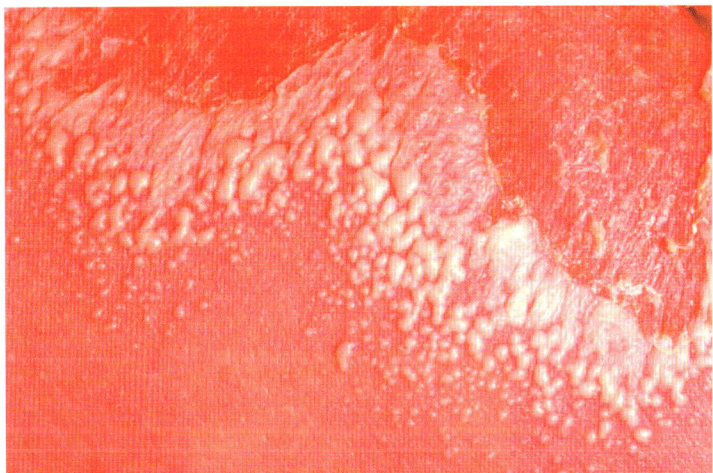

Figure 35.30 Acute generalised pustular psoriasis of von Zumbusch.

involved, the lesions on the latter being clinically and histologically indistinguishable from geographic tongue.

In the acute phase, the affected individual may be systemically unwell. Hypovolaemia and oligaemia can cause acute kidney injury. Hypoalbuminaemia in the acute episode may be profound and associated with hypocalcaemia [46–48]. The absorption of orally administered therapeutic drugs may also be impaired. Abnormalities of liver enzymes are common, occurring in up to a half of patients during the acute episode [13]. Cholestatic jaundice has been reported as a consequence of neutrophilic cholangitis [49,50].

Acute respiratory distress syndrome (psoriasis-associated aseptic pneumonitis) is rare but possibly underreported [51]. It presents with rapidly deteriorating dyspnoea and hypoxia in the absence of infection. If acute GPP lasts more than a few days, telogen effluvium may follow 2–3 months after the height of the illness. Amyloidosis is a rare late complication of repeated flares [52].

GPP may manifest only in pregnancy when it has been referred to as impetigo herpetiformis. This is a very rare entity, first described by Hebra in 1872 [53], 37 years before the report of GPP by von Zumbusch, and the relationship between these diseases has generated controversy subsequently [3,54,55]. Recent molecular genetic studies support the view that impetigo herpetiformis represents GPP triggered by or occurring in pregnancy [5]. Onset is usually in the last trimester of pregnancy, but may be earlier, and has been recorded in the first month of pregnancy and in the first day of the puerperium [56,57]. The disease tends to persist until the child is born, and occasionally long afterwards. The eruption often starts in the inguino-genital region and other flexures, spreading centrifugally, with minute pustules arising on an acutely inflamed area of skin. Constitutional disturbance is characteristically severe, and death may occur due to cardiac or renal failure. The more severe and longstanding the disease, the greater the risks of placental insufficiency leading to stillbirth, or neonatal death. Characteristically, the disease recurs in subsequent pregnancies. Recurrence has been described in up to nine successive pregnancies, and on subsequent use of oral contraceptives [54].

Subacute annular generalised pustular psoriasis. Annular and other patterned lesions may be seen in acute GPP (von Zumbusch) but are more characteristic of the rarer subacute or chronic forms in which lesions are persistent, and without the severe flares of acute GPP [4,58,59]. Lesions begin as discrete areas of erythema, which become raised and oedematous. Pustules appear peripherally on the crest of the advancing edge, become desiccated and leave a trailing fringe of scale as the lesion slowly advances (Figure 35.31). There are generally no systemic symptoms.

Subacute annular GPP is the most common presentation of GPP in infancy and early childhood [60,61]. Although GPP can begin at any age in childhood, in over 25% of cases onset has been in the first year of life [62]. The disease may begin in the first few weeks of life and two cases of congenital GPP have been described [63]. In at least onethird of infantile cases, a history of an eruption diagnosed as seborrhoeic dermatitis, napkin dermatitis or sudden-onset napkin psoriasis is obtained [64,65]. GPP may be localised to flexural areas, for instance the neck, for long periods [66].

Some authors have separated a related pattern, well described by Lapière, as recurrent circinate erythematous psoriasis [67,68]. As with subcorneal pustular dermatosis of Sneddon and Wilkinson, the relation to GPP is not universally accepted, and these conditions are specifically excluded in Japanese diagnostic criteria for GPP [45], while being accepted in European classification criteria [1].

Linear forms of pustular psoriasis are occasionally observed within the context of more generalised pustulosis [69,70].

Histology

The intense inflammation of GPP is characterised by infiltration of masses of neutrophils. Discrete collections of neutrophils in the oedematous stratum spinosum case the characteristic spongiform pustule of Kogoj [71]. There may be acanthosis with elongation of rete ridges. The stratum corneum becomes parakeratotic and subcorneal pustules shed as epidermal turnover is accelerated. Similar features are seen in subacute as in acute patterns but in a less intense form.

Differential diagnosis

There is an extensive differential diagnosis of GPP, comprising eruptions that cause widespread non-follicular pustules. In acute GPP, the presence of fever, leukocytosis and elevated inflammatory markers may lead to a mistaken diagnosis of systemic infection, sometimes leading to a counterproductive discontinuation of necessary immunosuppressive treatment. The differentiation of acute GPP from unstable psoriasis with secondary pustulation (psoriasis cum pustulatione) (Figures 35.32 and 35.33) can be challenging, especially in those with both GPP and plaque psoriasis and requires careful consideration of all available clinical information, including the history, morphology, systemic symptoms, laboratory parameters (peripheral white cell count and acute phase reactants) and genetics. AGEP can also be a difficult differential diagnosis, occurring as an acute, spontaneously healing reaction to drugs, usually antimicrobials [72]. There is an overlap in the immunopathogenesis of GPP and AGEP, but the pustulation usually resolves more rapidly in the latter [73]. A skin biopsy may contribute features that assist in the distinction [74].

Slow centrifugal spread of subacute annular GPP may mimic erythema annulare centrifugum [75,76]. Pemphigus foliaceus and IgA pemphigus can mimic subacute GPP, but histological and immunofluorescence testing will distinguish between them. Occasionally, the bowel bypass syndrome, Sweet syndrome and Behçet syndrome cause difficulties [77,78]. Extensive impetigo, tinea or candidiasis in the immunosuppressed should be remembered.

Classification of severity

The severity of GPP varies greatly between patients and over time. The activity of disease at a given time point has been categorised as mild, moderate or severe based upon the extent of erythema,

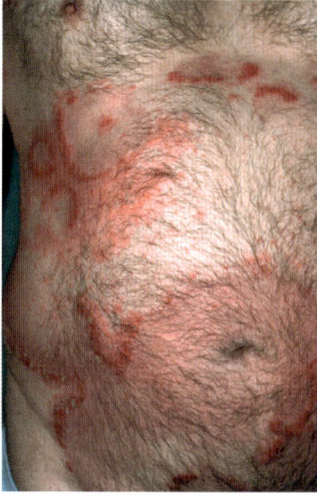

Figure 35.31 Subacute annular generalised pustular psoriasis.

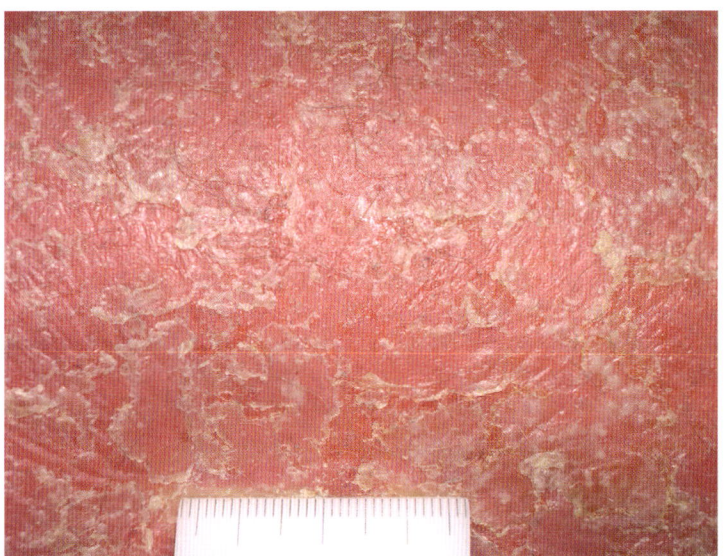

Figure 35.32 Pustulation in unstable psoriasis – 'psoriasis with pustules' – rather than pustular psoriasis.

oedema and pustulation, fever and laboratory abnormalities (leukocytosis, elevated inflammatory markers, and albumin) [45]. Modifications of PGA (GPPGA) and PASI (GPPASI) in which the scaling subscore is replaced by a pustule severity have been validated and used in clinical trials [79,80].

Co-morbidities
GPP frequently co-exists with chronic plaque psoriasis. The mean rate of concurrence of these diseases is reported as 54% in a cohort of 251 GPP patients, with lower concordance in European populations [12]. Inflammatory polyarthritis is common, affecting about onethird of patients [3,4]. Uveitis and keratoconjunctivitis are also reported [4,45]. Components of the metabolic syndrome are common; a large series reported obesity (43%), hypertension (26%), hyperlipidaemia (26%) and diabetes (24%) [4].

Disease course and prognosis
Acute GPP is typically characterised by flares and remissions [1,11]. The frequency and duration of flares varies from patient to patient, and they may be provoked by a known trigger or be spontaneous. Flares tend to last days or weeks without treatment, in one large series ranging from 7 to 60 days with a mean of 16 days [4]. In between flares, there may be more limited areas of GPP, the skin may be clear, or there may be plaque psoriasis. Mortality rates directly attributable to GPP or its associated treatment of 2–16% have been reported [4,9,81]. The prognosis is better when there is a clear trigger, exemplified by acute GPP of pregnancy [54]. GPP developing from acrodermatitis continua of Hallopeau seems to have the worst prognosis [81]. The prognosis is good for subacute annular GPP and, consequently, for GPP in infants and children [62]

Investigations
In the acute phase, the activity of inflammation is reflected in elevated C-reactive protein and erythrocyte sedimentation rate levels [4]. There may be an absolute lymphopenia at the onset of generalised pustular psoriasis followed by a polymorphonuclear

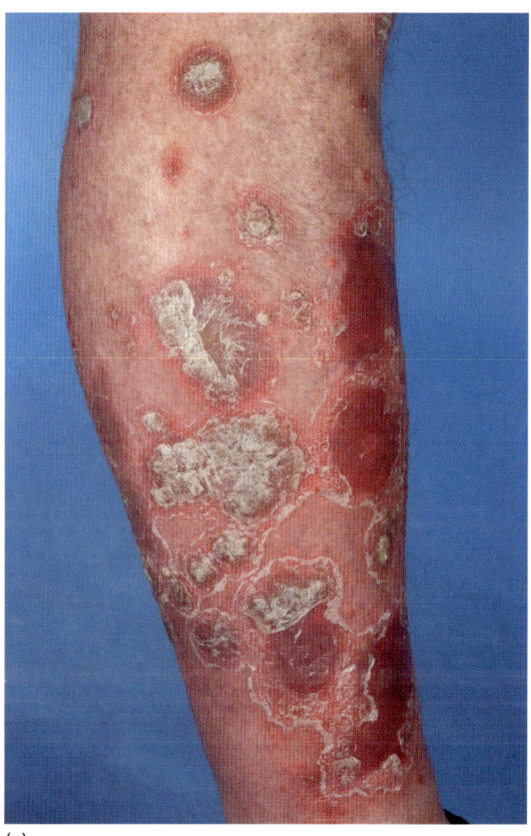

(a)

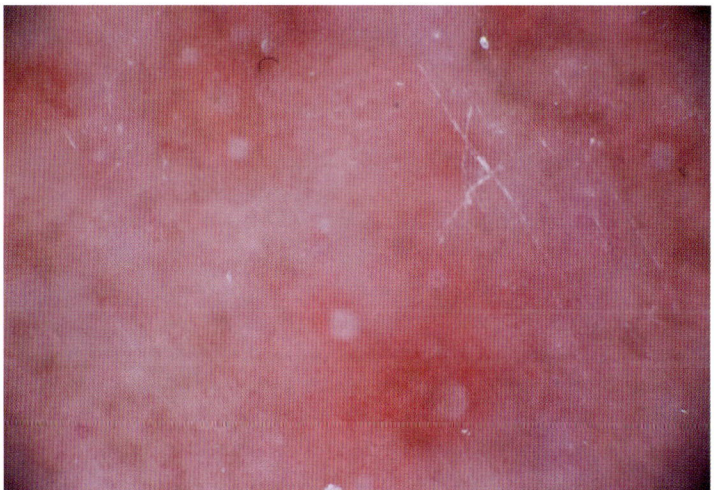

(b)

Figure 35.33 (a) Inflammatory unstable psoriasis; (b) close-up of pustules on dermoscopy.

leukocytosis with a left shift. Liver enzymes, renal function, albumin and calcium levels should be monitored. A skin biopsy may be useful to demonstrate characteristic histological features and exclude other diagnoses.

Management
The treatment of acute GPP often requires in-patient management, and sometimes needs treatment on an intensive care unit. Dermatological management involves topical or systemic drug therapy, general supportive measures and removal of possible provocative

factors. Excessive heat loss must be prevented by maintaining an adequate ambient temperature. Fluid intake should be increased so that the daily urine volume remains adequate. Tar or dithranol can be withdrawn abruptly, but removal of potent topical corticosteroids requires more care. Infection, where present, should be treated with the appropriate antibiotics. When GPP in pregnancy is threatening maternal life, termination or early delivery may be considered.

Topical treatment

Often, bland creams or lotions are best. Weak corticosteroid creams may be helpful in subacute forms. Tar and dithranol are contraindicated.

Systemic therapy

Most cases of GPP require systemic therapy but the quality of the evidence for specific interventions is generally poor, given the rarity of these diseases. Most evidence comes from retrospective surveys and open label cohort studies of drugs licensed for chronic plaque psoriasis. Guidelines for the management of GPP were published in Japan in 2018 and recommend an oral retinoid as treatment of first choice at present, unless contraindicated [45]. In a survey of French dermatology departments in 2005, 89% used acitretin as first line treatment of choice and the authors observed that their widespread introduction as treatment for GPP correlated with a reduction in mortality of the disease [9]. High doses of acitretin (1 mg/kg/day) should be given for rapid control in severe GPP and lower doses of 0.5–0.75 mg/kg/day may be sufficient in milder disease and to maintain remission [45]. Acitretin should not be used for GPP of pregnancy.

Rapid control of GPP can been achieved with high-dose ciclosporin and remission maintained with a lower dose [82,83]. Doses in the range of 2.5–5 mg/kg/day are recommended [45]. Ciclosporin is a suitable first line option for women who are pregnant or in their reproductive years. Methotrexate has a relatively slow onset of action and so is not suitable for treatment flares of the disease. Oral methotrexate needs to be dosed with caution in those with severe disease, particularly if renal or hepatic function is impaired, because of concerns about erratic absorption; parenteral administration should be considered. Methotrexate has been used with success in children with GPP [84]. Oral or parenteral corticosteroids should generally be avoided and used only when urgent control of complications is needed (e.g. acute respiratory distress syndrome). The short-term effects of prednisolone (30–40 mg/day) are good, but serious relapses are liable to occur as the dosage is reduced unless another form of therapy is given simultaneously.

Experience with the use of biologic treatment in GPP is increasing, supported by case reports and small case series. Infliximab was first reported to be effective for GPP in a case report in 2002 [85] and subsequently in several small case series [86]. Subsequently, adalimumab, certolizumab, ustekinumab, secukinumab, ixekizumab, brodalumab, guselkumab and risankizumab have each been assessed in small open-label trials of up to 12 patients with either GPP or erythrodermic psoriasis, with generally favourable results, and on this basis several of these agents have been approved by regulators in Japan, but not in Europe or the USA [87–94].

Based on the central role of IL-36 signalling the pathogenesis of GPP, treatments targeting this pathway are being developed. Spesolimab is a first in class monoclonal antibody against the IL-36 receptor and was shown to be rapidly effective in an open label study of seven patients with GPP, three with an *IL-36RN* mutation and four without [95]. A subsequent randomised placebo-controlled trial in 53 patients with acute GPP demonstrated the clearance of all pustules in 54% of patients at day 8 with a single intravenous infusion of spesolimab (placebo 6%) and clear or almost clear skin on the GPPGA in 43% (placebo 11%) [96,97], leading to licensing for the treatment of GPP flares in Europe, the USA and Japan. Spesolimab has recently completed a trial of subcutaneous maintenance treatment for GPP flare prevention [98].

Palmoplantar pustulosis

Definition and nomenclature

Palmoplantar pustulosis (PPP) is a chronic condition in which multiple sterile pustules occur on the palms and/or soles, often with associated erythema and scaling. The disease is persistent, and very resistant to treatment. The relationship between PPP and plaque psoriasis is controversial [99]. The two diseases occur together more frequently than expected by chance but more usually PPP occurs in isolation. This, and the absence of the genetic associations characteristic of chronic plaque psoriasis, indicate that PPP represents a distinct entity within the family of psoriatic skin diseases.

Synonyms and inclusions

- Chronic palmoplantar pustular psoriasis
- Pustulosis palmaris et plantaris
- Persistent palmoplantar pustulosis

Epidemiology
Incidence and prevalence

PPP is the most common of the entities within the pustular psoriasis family. The prevalence is estimated at 0.005–0.08% in European populations [100] rising to 0.12% in Japan [101].

Age at onset

The onset may be in early adult life, but peaks between the ages of 30 and 50 years, with a mean age at onset of 44 years [**12**,102].

Sex

Approximately 75% of those affected are women [**12**,100,101]. Disease severity may be greater in women than men [103].

Pathophysiology
Genetics

The heritability of PPP is not known precisely but about 8% of cases have a positive family history of PPP [104]. Molecular genetic studies have demonstrated that it is genetically distinct from chronic plaque psoriasis. In particular, PPP is not associated with the major psoriasis susceptibility locus *PSORS1* or *HLA-C:06:02* [105,106]. Mutations in known susceptibility genes for GPP are seen in only about 10% of PPP patients, a lower percentage than in patients with GPP. In the largest study to date, 12 of 234 (5.1%) had mutations in *IL36RN* and 14 of 212 had mutations in *AP1S3* [**12**]. *IL36RN* mutations are more frequently present in the heterozygous state in PPP, rather than the homozygous or compound heterozygotes seen in GPP. *CARD14* mutations have been reported in a few patients with PPP [106–109]. Genetic association with polymorphisms in an autophagy gene (*ATG16L1*) and IL-19 family members have been reported [110,111].

Environmental factors

PPP usually starts without obvious provocation. In 10% of a series of 215 cases seen at the Mayo Clinic it was induced by drugs, especially TNFi [112] although this has also been reported with IL-17 inhibition [113]. PPP is one of the commonest morphologies seen in patients who develop psoriasiform rashes on exposure to TNFi for the treatment of rheumatoid arthritis or Crohn disease [114].

Cigarette smoking is strongly associated with PPP – about 80% of patients are current or previous smokers [**12**], and this group also has more severe disease [103,115,116]. In some instances, the disease improves in those who manage to stop smoking [117].

The pustules in PPP are not infected, although they contain a distinctive microbiome, which may be influenced by smoking [118]. Distant septic foci, particularly in the tonsils or oro-pharynx, have been associated with PPP by some researchers, who have reported an increased production of cutaneous lymphocyte-associated antigen positive T cells in the tonsils of patients with PPP [119,120]. Resolution of PPP following tonsillectomy has been described, with complete resolution of all signs of the disease in 66% of 80 patients 2 years after tonsillectomy in a retrospective analysis at a single institution [121]. The effect was greater in those who stopped smoking after tonsillectomy.

Pathogenic mechanisms

The pathogenesis of PPP is not fully known and is less well understood than chronic plaque psoriasis. Activation of innate immune pathways appears to play an important role. Lesional PPP overexpresses antimicrobial peptides, chemokines including IL-8, and cytokines IL-1β, IL-17A, IL-22, IL-36γ and IL-36RA, some of which derive from the acrosyringium [122–125]. Activation of the IL-17A pathway appears to be important but the pattern of cytokine expression differs from that seen in plaque psoriasis affecting the palms and soles [126]. IL-17A induced IL-36 production of IL-36 cytokines in human keratinocytes has been shown to be enhanced by cigarette smoke extract [115], which may contribute to the strong association with smoking. Lesional gene expression levels of IL-36 cytokines correlate with disease activity measured by palmoplantar pustular psoriasis area severity index (PPPASI) [127].

Clinical features

History

Itching is variable; more often the patient complains of burning discomfort or pain in the lesions. Pain on standing or walking, especially when there is fissuring, and limitation of hand function

have a detrimental effect on patient normal functioning and quality of life.

Presentation

The disease presents as a pustular eruption either diffusely or within well-defined plaques. The disease may be limited to the palms, or to the soles, or both may be affected. On the hands, the thenar eminence is the most common site. Less commonly, the hypothenar eminence or the central palm or the distal palm are involved. On the feet, the instep, the medial or lateral border of the foot at the level of the instep, or the sides or back of the heel are involved. Less frequently, the distal sole or the whole sole is implicated. Digital lesions are less common although associated subungual pustulation is sometimes seen. A striking symmetry of the lesions on the hands or feet is common, but sometimes a solitary lesion persists for months before others appear.

The affected area is dusky red and scaly, and fissures may develop. Removal of scale (e.g. by treatment) leaves a glazed dull red surface. Within this plaque, numerous pustules are present, usually 2–5 mm in diameter. In early disease, dermoscopy can help to identify vesicles, or vesico-pustules within plaques, the lesions arising at the top of dermatoglyphic ridges [122]. Fresh pustules are yellow; older ones are yellow-brown or dark brown as the pustule dries. Normally, pustules in all stages of evolution are seen (Figure 35.34). Eventually, the desiccated pustule is exfoliated. Plaques of psoriasis may be present elsewhere on the body in a minority of patients and may be mild and atypical [128].

Pustular bacterid (of Andrews) (Figure 35.35) was a term first used to describe an acute monomorphic eruption of sterile pustules occurring on the hands and feet [129]. Whether it is a distinct entity or merely an acute variant of PPP is unclear.

Histopathology

There is an infiltrate of inflammatory cells including T lymphocytes, dendritic cells, eosinophils and mast cells in the dermis [130]. Early lesions are vesicles in the absence of spongiosis, that develop into pustules containing mononuclear cells and neutrophils as they become more superficial [131–133]. Early vesicles appear to arise in or near epidermal sweat ducts [122], around which are increased numbers of Langerhans cells [123].

Differential diagnosis

Palmoplantar plaque psoriasis can be difficult to exclude in phases of PPP when pustules are absent, for instance on treatment [128]. Tinea and eczema are common differential diagnoses. Tinea is usually asymmetrical or unilateral and the toe clefts may be involved. Microscopy and culture or PCR will confirm the diagnosis. Secondary infection of eczema may be pustular but is more painful, and Gram stains and culture of pustule contents will establish the diagnosis. Allergic contact dermatitis caused by rubber in footwear should not cause diagnostic difficulties: typically, the insteps are spared. The chronic acropustulosis seen in black infants does not occur in adults.

Classification of severity

The impact of involvement of palmoplantar skin on physical functioning and quality of life is disproportionate to the relatively small

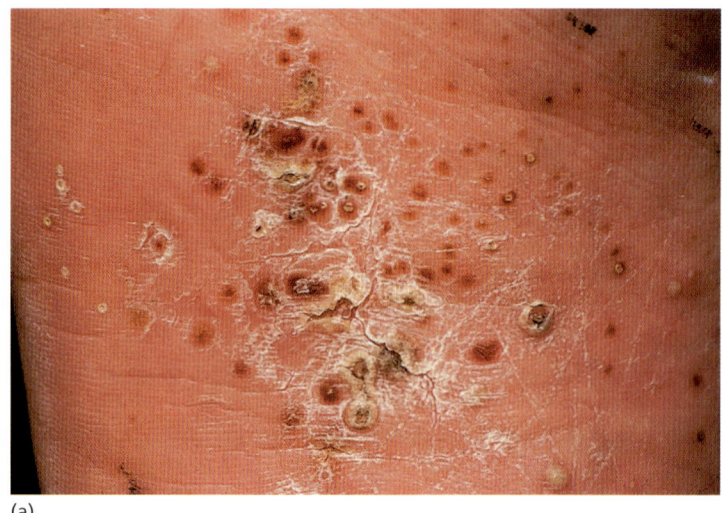
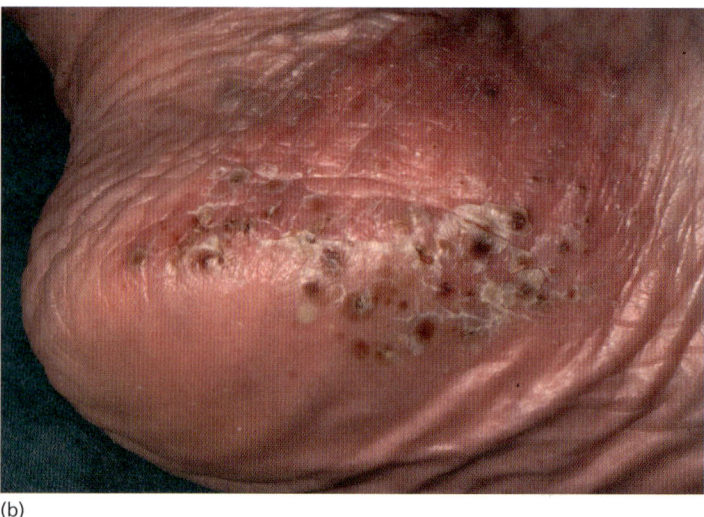

(a)   (b)

Figure 35.34 (a) Palmoplantar pustulosis. Normally, pustules in all stages of evolution are seen. Courtesy of St John's Institute of Dermatology, London, UK. (b) Palmoplantar pustulosis of the heel.

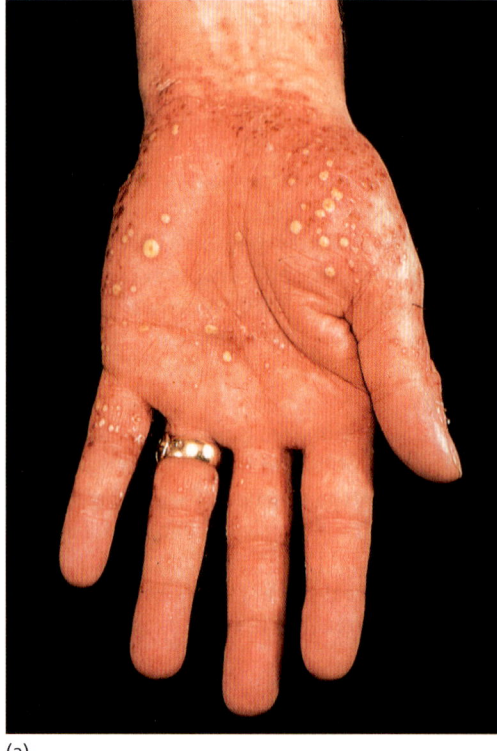
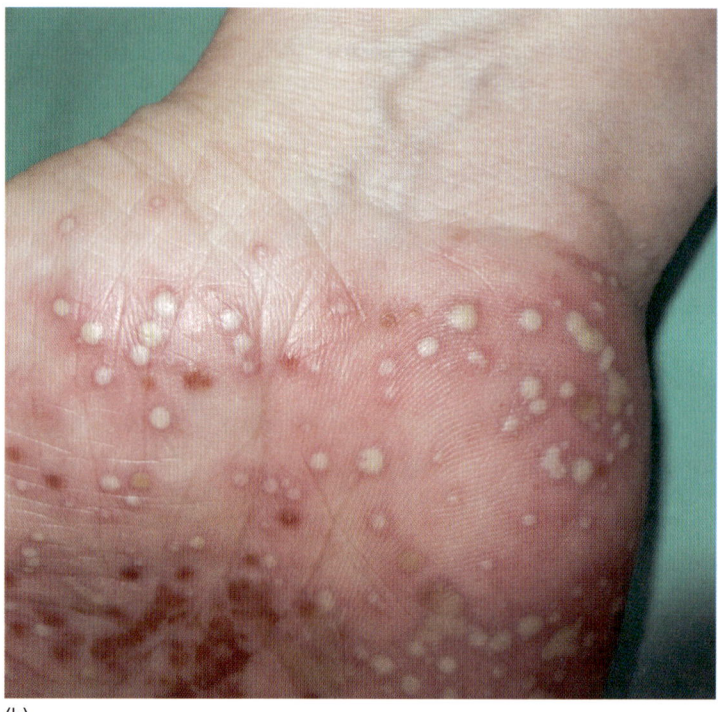

(a)   (b)

Figure 35.35 (a) Acute palmoplantar pustulosis. Courtesy of St John's Institute of Dermatology, London, UK. (b) Acute palmoplantar pustulosis.

area affected [134,135]. In clinical trials, the PPPASI or fresh pustule counts have been used to measure disease severity [136].

Co-morbidities

Between 15% and 35% of patients with PPP develop chronic plaque psoriasis at other sites [12,100] and in those who have both PPP and chronic plaque psoriasis there is a high prevalence of psoriatic arthritis. A distinctive form of arthritis affecting the sternoclavicular joints called pustulotic arthro-osteitis is common in Japanese patients with PPP but appears to be rare in other parts of the world [128]. PPP is a key component of the rare SAPHO syndrome (synovitis, arthritis, pustulosis, hyperostosis, osteitis), in which the articular component also predominantly affects the anterior chest wall [137].

A significant prevalence of autoimmune thyroid disease and the presence of thyroid antibodies have been found in association with PPP [12]. Some patients also have antigliadin antibodies – in one Swedish study of 123 patients, 18% had antigliadin antibodies and some of these experienced an improvement in PPP on a gluten-free diet [138]. Hypertension, hyperlipidaemia and diabetes

PART 4: INFLAMMATORY DERMATOSES

are common associations, although the relative risk has not been determined [139,140].

Disease course and prognosis

The course is usually prolonged. Slow spread or extension may be refractory to all treatment. Sometimes spontaneous remission does occur but is more often temporary than permanent. In one cohort of 59 patients, only nine had a remission for more than a year [102].

Investigations

The diagnosis can usually be made clinically. Skin scrapings for mycological examination may be needed, and occasionally bacterial swabs or patch testing may be indicated.

Management

Effective therapy is elusive and treatment is often as disappointing for the physician as for the patient. There is a pressing need for more effective treatment and for higher quality evidence of efficacy and safety. In view of the finding that PPP is immunogenetically distinct from plaque psoriasis, it is perhaps unsurprising that using conventional psoriasis therapies to treat palmoplantar pustulosis is not ideal. A Cochrane review of treatments for PPP published up to March 2019 has been published [141].

Topical

It is usual to start with topical therapy but this alone is often ineffective. Super-potent topical corticosteroids may be beneficial in the short term. Hydrocolloid gel occlusion can enhance efficacy of moderate potency corticosteroid creams [142,143]. Atrophy, particularly of the skin around the medial longitudinal arch, is a risk. A phase III randomised placebo-controlled trial of the vitamin D analogue maxacalcitol in 188 patients with PPP demonstrated a significant reduction in disease activity, and particularly in the pustule score [144].

Phototherapy

Studies of topical PUVA have failed to demonstrate superiority over placebo. Oral PUVA may be effective in improving PPP and will sometimes clear the disease temporarily; the response is enhanced by combination with an oral retinoid (re-PUVA). There is some evidence for improvement with Grenz ray therapy or excimer laser [141,145,146].

Systemic therapy

Systemic therapies offer the best opportunity for remission, although the evidence base is poor, efficacy is limited, and there are no head-to-head trials [141]. Oral retinoids have established efficacy for remission and maintenance therapy. Most clinical trials were carried out in the 1980s, were small and evaluated etretinate, before the development of acitretin [141]. Response rates with ciclosporin are higher. Many patients will respond in the short term to ciclosporin 2.5 mg/kg/day [147,148] and some patients can be maintained on doses as low as 1 mg/kg/day [149]. The dose should be tapered rather than stopped abruptly in view of rare instances of provoking GPP [150] Low quality evidence of efficacy has been published in small uncontrolled case series with methotrexate, leflunomide, alitretinoin, fumaric acid esters, tofacitinib and apremilast

[151–157]. The longest mean drug survival among conventional systemic treatments in 347 PPP patients treated in five German university departments over a 12-year period was reported for apremilast [158]. In a placebo-controlled clinical trial of apremilast in 90 Japanese patients with PPP, a response (PPASI 50) was seen in 78.3% on apremilast versus 40.9% with placebo ($P = 0.0003$) [159].

Biologic therapy

The effectiveness of TNFi has not been adequately assessed in the treatment of PPP. Only etanercept 50 mg twice weekly has been studied in a small randomised controlled trial in 15 patients, which demonstrated no statistically significant improvement (or deterioration) compared with placebo [160]. A retrospective descriptive study of real life TNFi use in PPP demonstrated improvements with infliximab and adalimumab, but infrequent clearance [161]. Ustekinumab has been reported to be effective in small case series [162,163] but this has not been confirmed in a small placebo-controlled trial [164].

A pilot study of the anti-IL-36 receptor monoclonal antibody spesolimab in 59 patients with PPP demonstrated PPPASI50 at 16 weeks in 31.6% in the active arms compared with 23.8% in the placebo arm (risk difference 0.078; 95% CI –0.190, 0.338) [127]. The primary end point of the trial was not met. In a randomised placebo-controlled study with anakinra (an IL-1 receptor antagonist) for PPP there was no evidence of efficacy compared with placebo.

Secukinumab has been evaluated in a phase IIIb randomised placebo-controlled trial in 237 patients with PPP in Europe [165]. Patients were randomised 1:1:1 to receive secukinumab 300 mg, 150 mg or placebo. At the primary end point at week 16, PPPASI75 was achieved in 26.6% in the secukinumab 300 mg arm compared with 14.1% in the placebo arm ($P = 0.0411$, OR 2.62; 95% CI 1.04–6.60). PPPASI50 was achieved in 52.2% in the secukinumab 300 mg arm compared with 32.9% in the placebo arm ($P = 0.0159$). This response appears to be less than was achieved in trials of chronic plaque psoriasis.

Guselkumab has been evaluated in a phase III randomised placebo-controlled trial in 159 patients with PPP in Japan [133]. Patients were randomised 1:1:1 to receive guselkumab 200 mg, 100 mg or placebo. At the primary end point at week 16, PPPASI75 was achieved in 20.4% in the guselkumab 100 mg arm compared with 3.8% in the placebo arm ($P = 0.01$). PPPASI50 was achieved in 57.4% in the guselkumab 100 mg arm compared with 34% in the placebo arm ($P = 0.02$). On this basis, guselkumab has been licensed for PPP in Japan. No biologic is currently licensed for PPP in Europe or the USA.

Acrodermatitis continua of Hallopeau

Definition and nomenclature

Acrodermatitis continua of Hallopeau (ACH) is a rare chronic sterile pustular eruption initially affecting the nail units of the fingers or toes, from where it slowly extends proximally. It may evolve into GPP [1].

Synonyms and inclusions
- Acropustulosis
- Pustular acrodermatitis
- Acrodermatitis perstans
- Dermatitis repens

Introduction and general description

The relationship between ACH and psoriasis in general and with GPP in particular has been debated since the entity was first recognised by Hallopeau in 1890. Patients with ACH may have additional plaque psoriasis and GPP.

Epidemiology
Incidence and prevalence

This is a rare entity, described in case reports and small case series only. Its incidence and prevalence are unknown.

Age at onset

This may be seen in children. It is rare in young adults and, unlike PPP, not infrequently begins in old age. The mean age at onset in the largest series was 55 years [12].

Sex

ACH is seen more frequently in females [12].

Pathophysiology
Genetics

The frequency of germline *IL36RN* mutations is similar in ACH (18.2%) to GPP, and higher than in PPP [12]. A Lebanese man with ACH has been reported in whom a mutation in *IL36RN* was detected (homozygous p.Ser113Leu). His sister who had acute GPP von Zumbusch without acral involvement had the same *IL36RN* mutation, supporting a view that ACH is a localised variant of GPP [166].

Mutations in *AP1S3* (which were first identified in ACH) [7] were found in about 10% of patients [12]. One patient with a mutation in *MPO* has been reported [21].

Environmental factors

The onset is often attributed by the patient to minor trauma, or infection at the tip of the digit. It may be precipitated or aggravated by oral corticosteroids.

Clinical features
History and presentation

The first lesion starts on a finger or thumb more often than on a toe. It is usually unilateral and remains restricted to one or a limited number of digits [167,168]. The skin over the distal phalanx becomes red and scaly, and pustules develop. The nail folds and nail bed may be involved, leading to nail dystrophy. The proximal edge of the lesion is bordered by a fringe of undermined epidermis, irregular, often sodden and sometimes preceded by a line of vesiculo-pustules. Removal of scale or desiccation of pustules may leave a brighter red, glazed, very sore and painful digit. Slow proximal extension is the rule but this may take several years. Eventually, other digits may be involved. The nail plate may be completely destroyed

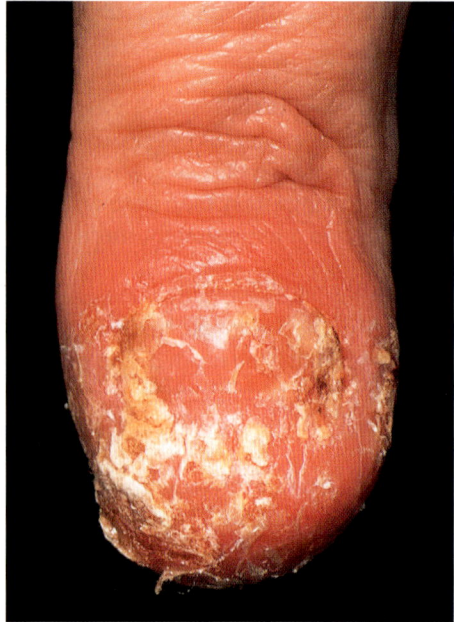
(a)

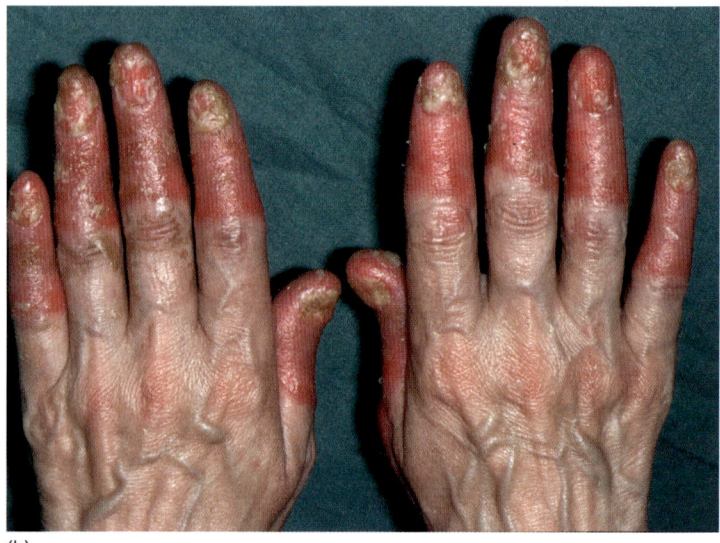
(b)

Figure 35.36 (a) Acrodermatitis continua with destruction of the nail plate. Courtesy of St John's Institute of Dermatology, London, UK. (b) Acrodermatitis continua in the acute phase.

(Figure 35.36). Bone changes can occur with osteolysis of the tuft of the distal phalanx. The free end of the digit may become wasted and tapered, mimicking scleroderma.

Histopathology

The features are similar to those of GPP. In the epidermis, there are numerous subcorneal neutrophilic pustules and spongiform pustules with hypergranulosis and parakeratotic hyperkeratosis. There is a lymphocytic infiltrate in the dermis, which in chronic disease may become atrophic [167].

Differential diagnosis

The distribution of lesions in ACH is distinctive, as is the local destruction of soft tissue, nail apparatus and sometimes the terminal digit. In the earlier stages, staphylococcal infection, pulp infection, herpetic whitlow, tinea or contact dermatitis may be suspected. Candidiasis is only likely to be a problem in the immunocompromised. Parakeratosis pustulosa should be considered in children.

Co-morbidities

In a cohort of 41 patients with ACH, nine had an additional diagnosis of GPP and four of PPP [12]. Chronic plaque psoriasis was present in 46% of cases [12]. Arthritis involving the peripheral joints is present in about 27% of cases [169].

Disease course and prognosis

The usual course is prolonged. Slow spread or extension may be refractory to all treatment. Sometimes spontaneous remission does occur but is more often temporary than permanent.

Investigations

The diagnosis can usually be made clinically. Swabs for bacterial culture should be taken.

Management

ACH is often refractory and the evidence base for treatment is poor, consisting mainly of case reports. Potent topical corticosteroids, tacrolimus or calcipotriol may improve symptoms [167,170–172]. Acitretin or ciclosporin have been reported to be effective in some cases [173]. There are case reports of the efficacy of etanercept, adalimumab, infliximab, ustekinumab, secukinumab, ixekizumab, guselkumab and anakinra [168]. TNFi appear to be more effective in ACH than in PPP [161] although they may need to be given at higher than usual doses or in combination with other systemic treatment [174].

PSORIATIC ARTHRITIS

Definition and nomenclature

Psoriatic arthritis is a seronegative inflammatory arthritis, which occurs in up to 40% of patients with moderate to severe psoriasis. It can be destructive to joints and adds considerably to the impairment of quality of life and symptoms such as fatigue suffered by psoriasis patients [1]. The quality-of-life impairment and disease burden associated with psoriatic arthritis is similar to that seen in rheumatoid arthritis [2]. There is a genetic susceptibility with an increased risk among family members of both psoriasis and psoriatic arthritis [3].

In rheumatology practice, psoriatic arthritis can be differentiated from other forms of arthritis according to CASPAR (Classification Criteria for Psoriatic Arthritis) criteria, with 99% sensitivity and 91% specificity (Table 35.8) [4]. A diagnosis of psoriatic arthritis is made in the presence of an inflammatory articular disease (joint, enthesis or spine) if some or all of the following criteria are met: current psoriasis; personal history of psoriasis; family history of psoriasis in a first- or second-degree relative; nail psoriasis; dactylitis (inflammation of an entire finger or toe) (Figure 35.37); and plain

Table 35.8 Classification of Psoriatic Arthritis (CASPAR) criteria for psoriatic arthritis. To be characterised as having psoriatic arthritis, a patient with inflammatory articular disease (joint, spine or entheseal) must have three or more points from five categories. Each category scores a maximum of 1 point, except category 1, which scores 2 points for current psoriasis.

Psoriasis	Current psoriasis	2
	Personal history of psoriasis	1
	Psoriasis in a first- or second-degree relative	1
Typical psoriatic nail involvement		1
A negative test for rheumatoid factor		1
Dactylitis	Current dactylitis	1
	History of dactylitis	1
Radiological evidence of juxta-articular new bone formation		1

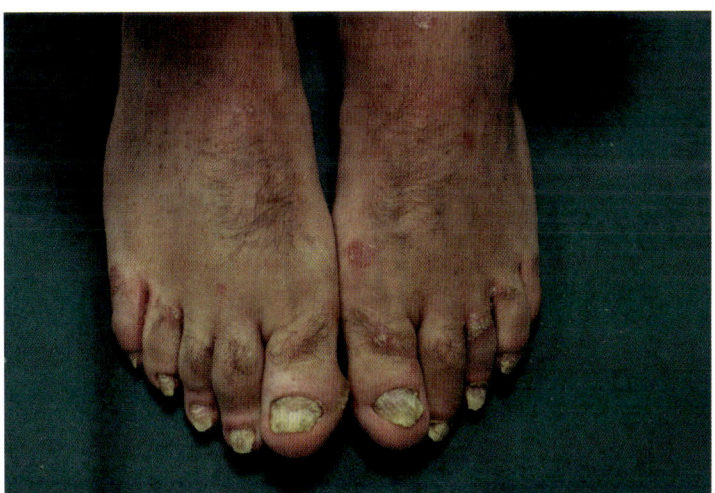

Figure 35.37 Dactylitis.

radiographic evidence of juxta-articular new bone formation on the hands or feet.

Psoriatic arthritis is clinically heterogeneous. It has been traditionally classified according to the criteria of Moll and Wright, although there is considerable overlap between the subtypes [5]. It can occur as peripheral mono- or asymmetrical oligo-arthritis, predominantly affecting the distal interphalangeal joints (Figure 35.38) (a distinguishing feature from rheumatoid arthritis), symmetrical rheumatoid-like pattern, arthritis mutilans (a rare severe deforming arthritis of the hands and feet) (Figure 35.39), axial disease with spondylitis and/or sacro-iliac disease. Although the original classification of Moll and Wright remains valid, several alternative classifications have been proposed [6]. Asymmetric oligo-arthritis is the commonest variety followed by symmetric polyarthritis. A pattern of predominant distal interphalangeal involvement is often found. Spondylitis is reported in 50% of patients and the rare arthritis mutilans is the last classification. This classification is useful, but overlap between the subtypes occurs.

Synonyms and inclusions
- Psoriatic arthropathy

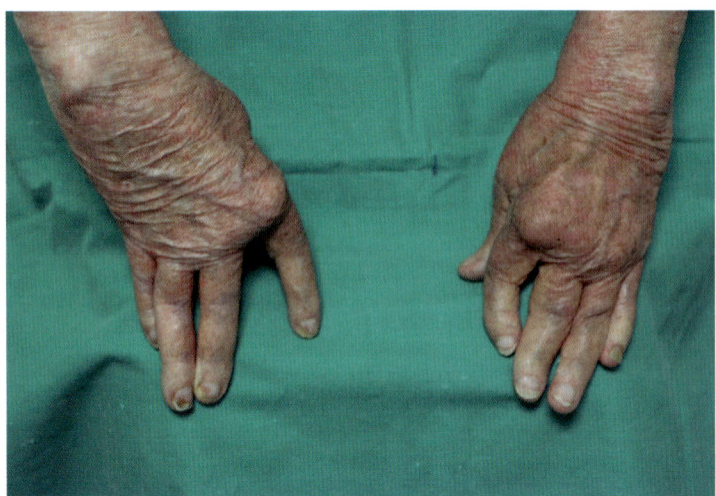

Figure 35.38 Arthritis mutilans.

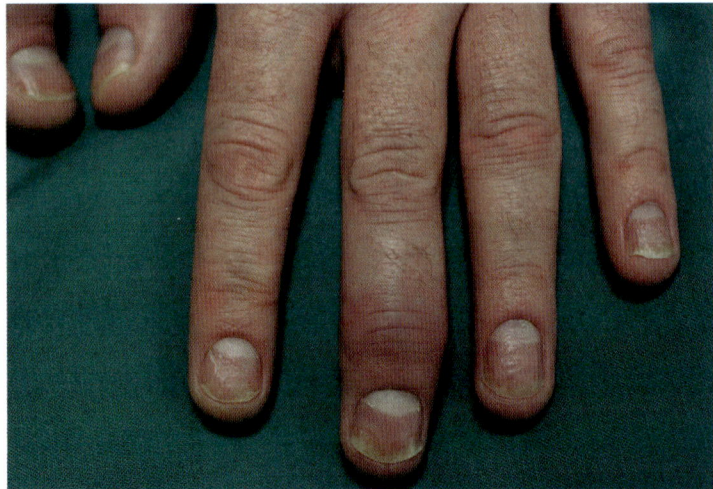

Figure 35.39 Distal interphalangeal involvement.

Epidemiology

Incidence and prevalence

There is a wide variation in the reported annual incidence (<0.01–0.25%) and prevalence (0.5–23.1/100 000) of psoriatic arthritis [7]. This variation probably reflects ethnic variation and methodological differences in the published studies. Arthritis mutilans occurs in between 3 and 5 per million people [7]. It is associated with enthesitis, dactylitis and more severe skin disease and is equally divided between the sexes.

Age at onset

Most patients develop psoriatic arthritis before the age of 40 years. Childhood onset is rare. The incidence appears to be equal between the sexes although men may have more axial disease and less peripheral arthritis. The majority of patients have psoriasis prior to the onset of arthritis. In 70% of patients, the skin features of psoriasis develop prior to joint disease, in 20% of patients, the joint disease presents first and in 10% the skin and joints are affected

concurrently. In a prospective cohort study, the annual incidence of psoriatic arthritis is approximately 2–3% [8].

Associated diseases

There is an association between more severe psoriasis and the development of psoriatic arthritis. For every 1% increase in body surface area involvement with psoriasis, there is a 2% increased risk of psoriatic arthritis [9]. The prevalence of psoriatic arthritis is also increased in patients with nail and scalp psoriasis [3,7].

Ocular diseases occur in up to 30% of patients with psoriatic arthritis. Most of these patients develop conjunctivitis with uveitis. Iridocyclitis, keratoconjunctivitis sicca and cataracts have also been reported [10,11]. Although less well studied than in psoriasis alone, there are associations between psoriatic arthritis and obesity/metabolic syndrome and alcohol misuse [12]. Premature cardiovascular disease is also associated with psoriatic arthritis [9].

Genetics and pathophysiology

Psoriatic arthritis has a strong heritable component. There are no well-powered twin registry studies, but heritability calculated from recurrence risk in first-degree relatives estimates a greater genetic component to psoriatic arthritis than with psoriasis [13]. In common with psoriasis, psoriatic arthritis is associated with MHC alleles, but the nature of the association appears to be different [14]. Although associated with *HLA-C:06:02*, the magnitude of the association is small compared with cutaneous psoriasis. Psoriatic arthritis is also associated with several HLA-B alleles, notably *HLA-B13*, *HLA-B27*, *HLA-B38/39*, *HLA-B57* and *HLA-DRB1*04* [15]. There is evidence that HLA types influence the presentation of psoriatic arthritis. In patients with psoriatic arthritis, HLA-C:06:02 without B27 or B39 is associated with early onset of psoriasis with the subsequent development of psoriatic arthritis 10 years after appearance of the skin disease. In contrast, the presence of HLA-B27 and/or B39 is associated with the simultaneous development of early joint and skin disease. The skin disease also appears to be less severe than in those patients who are HLA-C:06:02 positive [16].

Genome-wide association scans in psoriatic arthritis have replicated many psoriasis susceptibility loci and identified IL-23R as a disease specific locus [17]. Other distinct genetic loci have been reported [18].

Psoriatic arthritis may be triggered by trauma to a joint or tendon – the so-called deep Koebner effect. Cigarette smoking and excess alcohol intake are also associated with the disease. HIV infection is associated with the initiation or worsening of psoriatic arthritis whereas rheumatoid arthritis improves in HIV infection [3]. In contrast to psoriasis, streptococcal infection, medications such as lithium or psychological stress do not appear to be triggers of psoriatic arthritis. Like psoriasis, there is an increased incidence of obesity and the metabolic syndrome in patients with psoriatic arthritis [9].

Pathophysiology

The pathophysiology of psoriatic arthritis is similar to psoriasis with immune activation in the synovium and enthesis of affected joints. There is activation of both innate and adaptive immune cells with overproduction of multiple cytokines including TNF-α, IL-17 and IL-23. Angiogenesis is increased in the synovium and appears to be more prominent than in rheumatoid arthritis. In response to the inflammation, joint fibrosis occurs. There may be erosion of bone with abnormal bone formation occurring simultaneously, resulting in joint deformities and loss of function [3,7]. There is evidence from single RNA sequencing studies that synovial honing CD8+ T cells are important in PsA pathogenesis [19].

There are important differences, however, in the inflammatory process in the joint compared with the skin. IL-17, Th17 cells and IL-23 production appear to be less prominent in psoriatic synovitis compared with the skin [3,7]. These differences in pathophysiology may influence the observed differential therapeutic responses between the skin and joints to systemic and biologic treatments.

Clinical features

The diagnosis of psoriatic arthritis is important and an enquiry regarding joint symptoms should be made at every consultation in patients with psoriasis. Symptoms of inflammatory joint disease (early morning stiffness and joint swelling) should be ascertained. Early morning back stiffness may be the only clinical feature of sacroiliitis or cervical spondylitis. Heel pain (a manifestation of enthesitis of the Achilles tendon) or plantar fasciitis may also be a presenting feature.

Clinical examination may reveal evidence of dactylitis (sausage fingers) or swollen or tender joints. This may affect one joint in an asymmetric pattern or several joints simultaneously. The features may be subtle and diagnosis is often delayed. The nail changes of psoriasis will be present in up to 80% of patients.

Most dermatologists are not proficient at joint examination but a reasonable approach is to examine the joints of the hands and feet for evidence of joint swelling or tenderness and dactylitis. The diagnosis of psoriatic arthritis may be challenging even for an experienced rheumatologist. Several studies have suggested that up to 30% of patients attending specialist psoriasis clinics may have undiagnosed psoriatic arthritis [3,7]. Several screening questionnaires have been developed to assist with the early diagnosis of psoriatic arthritis. These include the Psoriasis Arthritis Screening Evaluation (PASE), the Psoriasis Epidemiology Screening Tool (PEST) and the Toronto Arthritis Screening Questionnaire (ToPAS) tools. Studies assessing these screening tools suggest that they may be beneficial in helping dermatologists to refer patients for appropriate rheumatological assessment [20].

Differential diagnosis

Differential diagnoses include early rheumatoid arthritis, ankylosing spondylitis, gout, osteoarthritis and fibromyalgia. It is important to recognise that patients with psoriatic arthritis often suffer from other musculoskeletal problems.

Classification of severity

Disease severity may be assessed by a variety of measures. These include the American College of Rheumatology (ACR) tender and swollen joint count. The ACR-20 refers to a 20% improvement in swollen and tender joint count and a 20% improvement in patient and physician global assessment, pain, disability and acute phase reactant measurement. ACR-50 and ACR-70 refer to a 50% and 70% improvement, respectively, in these criteria [21]. The Disease Activity Score (DAS) is calculated using swollen and painful joint scores together with the measurement of the erythrocyte sedimentation rate. The Psoriatic Arthritis Response Criteria (PsARC) is defined as a specified improvement in at least two of the following four measures, without worsening of the others: patient global assessment; physician global assessment; tender joint count; and swollen joint count [22]. Axial disease is often assessed using the Bath ankylosing spondylitis disease activity index (BASDAI) [23]. Scores assessing quality of life and dactylitis scores have also been developed [22]. Composite indices that include the severity of cutaneous psoriasis have also been proposed [24,25]. In practice, these composite measures are used predominantly in research settings. Most measures of disease severity for psoriatic arthritis have been adapted from rheumatoid arthritis and controversy exists as to whether they are truly a reflection of severity in psoriatic arthritis. Nonetheless the ACR measures remain those required by licensing agencies for new drug approval for psoriatic arthritis.

Investigations

Investigations include tests for inflammation (including C-reactive protein and erythrocyte sedimentation rate), uric acid, rheumatoid factor (less commonly used) and anticyclic citrillated peptide (CCP) antibodies. Plain X-rays of the hands and feet may be useful in detecting erosive disease but plain X-rays have a low diagnostic sensitivity in early disease. Other imaging modalities such as ultrasound or magnetic resonance imaging (MRI) are useful in assessing enthesitis, and MRI is the modality of choice for assessing axial disease.

Treatment

Psoriatic arthritis should be managed by a rheumatologist and, for complex cases, combined clinics involving a dermatologist and rheumatologist may facilitate management decisions. Early treatment is important as early interventions may prevent irreversible joint damage. Several guidelines have been published which provide treatment algorithms for physicians to assist them in the management of psoriatic arthritis [26–29]. The therapeutic options for psoriatic arthritis are not as broad as those for psoriasis and are influenced by the pattern of the articular disease (Figure 35.40).

The main treatments have been non-steroidal anti-inflammatory drugs (NSAIDs), methotrexate, oral corticosteroids, sulphasalazine, leflunomide, apremilast, TNFi, ustekinumab, IL-17 inhibitors and IL-23p19 inhibitors. A single agent that combines efficacy on both the skin disease and the arthritis is preferred.

NSAIDs are the mainstay of treatment in patients with mild disease. In view of their potential toxicities, the lowest dose should be used for short-term control of symptoms only [26–29]. Oral corticosteroids are used commonly for the control of acute flares of psoriatic arthritis. This may cause instability of concomitant psoriasis and a

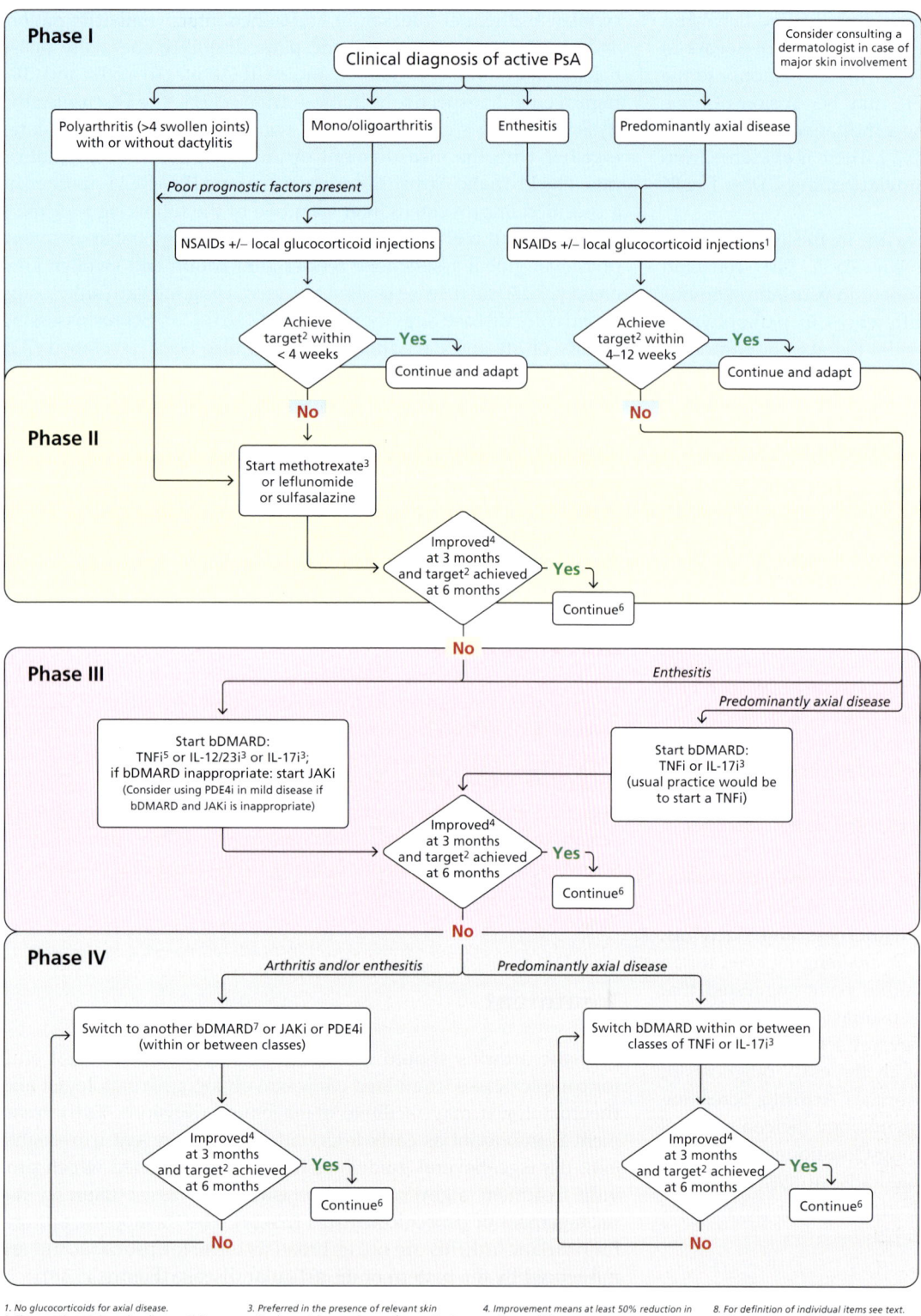

Figure 35.40 EULAR guidelines for management of psoriatic arthritis. Source: Reproduced from Gossec L, Baraliakos X, Kerschbaumer A *et al.* EULAR recommendations for the management of psoriatic arthritis with pharmacological therapies: 2019 update. *Ann Rheum Dis* 2020;79(6):700–12.

slow reduction of the dose is recommended in order to try and avoid deterioration of the skin and/or generalised pustular psoriasis. Joint injections with corticosteroids can provide symptomatic relief but there is little evidence that they prevent bone remodelling and fibrosis. Physiotherapy may also be beneficial.

Systemic therapy

The systemic treatments used for peripheral psoriatic arthritis, enthesitis and dactylitis have limited evidence for their use. Methotrexate has been studied in several trials in psoriatic arthritis. In one randomised controlled trial of methotrexate 15 mg weekly compared with placebo in patients with active psoriatic arthritis, there was no benefit of methotrexate compared with placebo when the ACR-20 criteria and the DAS-28 score were used [30]. The trial did report improvements in patient symptoms. The results of this trial contrast with several smaller studies that have shown positive effects [31,32]. The data have called into question the usefulness of methotrexate monotherapy in managing the acute synovitis of psoriatic arthritis.

Leflunomide has demonstrated efficacy in psoriatic arthritis compared with placebo [33] and in the real-life setting of clinical practice [34]. It does not often, however, have a beneficial effect on psoriasis. Sulphasalazine has been reported as effective in small open trials in psoriatic arthritis but has been disappointing in placebo-controlled trials. Nonetheless it continues to be used in clinical practice. The efficacy of ciclosporin in psoriatic arthritis has not been adequately addressed and its use is not recommended in some guidelines [35]. Axial disease appears to be resistant to treatment with conventional systemic therapy.

Apremilast, a phosphodiesterase 4 inhibitor that has shown efficacy in psoriasis and other inflammatory diseases, is licensed for psoriatic arthritis at a dose of 30 mg twice daily. A phase III trial of 504 patients with psoriatic arthritis compared the effects of apremilast 20 mg twice daily, apremilast 30 mg twice daily and placebo over 16 weeks. The ACR-20 responses were 31%, 40% and 19%, respectively, with significant differences between both doses and placebo [36].

Tofacitinib, a JAK-2 inhibitor, is an oral small molecule therapy that is licensed for rheumatoid arthritis and psoriatic arthritis at a dose of 5 mg twice daily [37]. In a randomised placebo-controlled trial, after 3 months therapy, 50% of patients on tofacitinib 5 mg orally twice daily achieved ACR-20 compared with 61% on tofacitinib 10 mg twice daily and 33% on placebo. In this study, tofacitinib was non-inferior to adalimumab 40 mg subcutaneously every 2 weeks. The majority of patients were on concomitant methotrexate. The long-term safety of tofacitinib in psoriatic arthritis has yet to be established in real-world registries. Tofacitinib is associated with serious infections, herpes zoster reactivation and veno-thromboembolism.

Deucravacitinib, a TYK-2 inhibitor, has undergone phase II trials in psoriatic arthritis. In a double-blind placebo-controlled trial, deucravacitinib at a dose of 6 mg orally once daily or 12 mg once daily had higher ACR-20 responses (52.9% for 6 mg dose and 62.7% for the 12 mg dose at week 16 compared with placebo (31.8%) [38]. Phase III studies are ongoing.

Biologic treatment

Biologic therapies are recommended for patients with active psoriatic arthritis affecting more than three joints who have failed to respond to at least two systemic treatments, or for axial disease that has failed to respond to NSAIDs and/or local corticosteroids [26–29].

Infliximab, at a dose of 5 mg/kg, has been shown to improve psoriatic arthritis compared with placebo. Of patients treated with infliximab, 65% reached the ACR-20 primary end point compared with 10% with placebo. The benefits were maintained to 50 weeks [39]. This study also provided evidence that infliximab improved the quality of life of treated patients and prevented radiological

progression of the disease [40,41]. Concomitant methotrexate has been shown to prolong retention on treatment [42].

Etanercept, at a dose of 25 mg subcutaneously twice weekly, has been shown to improve psoriatic arthritis compared with placebo. In a study of 60 patients over 12 weeks, 87% of patients treated with etanercept met PsARC compared with 23% of placebo-treated patients. ARC-20 was achieved by 73% of patients compared with 13% of placebo patients [43]. In a study comparing etanercept 50 mg twice weekly to 50 mg once weekly in patients with severe psoriasis and psoriatic arthritis, the higher dose of etanercept resulted in better PASI outcomes but the PsARC response at 12 weeks was similar in both groups (77% compared with 76%) [44]. While the combination of methotrexate and etanercept has demonstrated increased efficacy in rheumatoid arthritis, there are no controlled trials assessing this combination in psoriatic arthritis.

Adalimumab, at a dose of 40 mg subcutaneously every 2 weeks, has demonstrated efficacy in psoriatic arthritis compared with placebo. At week 12, 58% of patients treated with adalimumab achieved the primary end point of ACR-20 compared with 14% of placebo patients. Adalimumab improved the joint manifestations, quality of life and skin disease. It also improved radiological progression of the disease [45]. There are no controlled studies on the use of methotrexate with adalimumab in psoriatic arthritis but registry studies suggest that no additional efficacy is achieved by the addition of methotrexate [46].

Golimumab is licensed for psoriatic arthritis but has not been developed for the treatment of cutaneous psoriasis. In a placebo-controlled trial of golimumab in psoriatic arthritis, 48% of patients receiving golimumab 50 mg every 4 weeks and 46% of patients receiving 100 mg every 4 weeks achieved the ACR-20 criteria compared with 9% of placebo patients [47].

Certolizumab, a pegylated humanised TNFi fragment, has shown efficacy in psoriasis, psoriatic arthritis and also in Crohn disease. In a phase III study, 368 patients were randomised to receive certolizumab 200 mg every 2 weeks, certolizumab 400 mg every 4 weeks or placebo for 24 weeks. At week 12, 58% of the certolizumab 200 mg every 2 weeks reached the ACR-20 primary end point compared with 51% of those in the certolizumab 400 mg every 4 weeks group and 24.3% in the placebo group. Certolizumab improved all aspects of the disease including physical function and radiographic progression. The clinical improvements were significant after 1 week of treatment [48].

The IL-17 inhibitors, secukinumab and ixekizumab, are licensed for psoriatic arthritis either as monotherapy or in combination with methotrexate. Brodalumab has been shown to be effective in psoriatic arthritis but due to problems in its phase III programme for psoriasis, it was not developed for psoriatic arthritis. Bimekizumab has completed phase III studies for psoriatic arthritis but at the time of writing has not been licensed for the treatment of psoriatic arthritis.

Secukinumab and ixekizumab have shown positive effects on axial disease and radiographic progression.

In a randomised controlled trial, secukinumab 300 mg was compared with 150 mg, 75 mg and placebo. Secukinumab was given weekly for five doses and thereafter every 4 weeks. The primary end point was 24 weeks. ACR-20 responses were achieved in 54%, 51% and 29% of patients in the 300 mg, 150 mg and 75 mg groups respectively compared with 33% of placebo [49]. On the basis of this trial, secukinumab was licensed at a dose of 150 mg every 4 weeks for psoriatic arthritis compared with 300 mg every 4 weeks for psoriasis.

In a head-to-head trial of 300 mg secukinumab subcutaneously weekly for 5 weeks and then 300 mg every 4 weeks compared with adalimumab at 40 mg every 2 weeks, there was no significant difference in ACR-20 responses at 52 weeks (67% in the secukinumab group and 62% in the adalimumab group) [50].

Ixekizumab

In a randomised placebo-controlled trial ixekizumab given subcutaneously at 80 mg every 2 weeks was compared with ixekizumab 80 mg every 4 weeks and adalimumab in a non-inferior design. The primary outcome was the ACR-20 response at 24 weeks: 62.1% of ixekizumab every 2 weeks treated patients achieved ACR-20 compared with 57.9% of those treated with ixekizumab every 4 weeks compared with 30% of placebo. Non-inferiority to adalimumab was demonstrated [51].

Brodalumab

In a placebo-controlled trial, patients with active psoriatic arthritis were randomised to receive 210 mg (licensed dose for psoriasis) or 140 mg subcutaneously of brodalumab or placebo at weeks 0, 1, 2 and every 2 weeks for 24 weeks. The primary end point was ACR-20 at week 16: 47.9% in the 210 mg group achieved ACR-20 compared with 45.8% in the 140 mg group and 20.9% in the placebo arm [52].

Bimekizumab

Bimekizumab has been evaluated in two phase III trials. In the first randomised controlled trial, patients with psoriatic arthritis who were naïve to biologic therapy were treated with bimekizumab 160 mg every 4 weeks, placebo or adalimumab. At week 16, 44% of patients achieved ACR-50 compared with 10% on placebo and 46% on adalimumab [53]. A second study assessed bimekizumab 160 mg every 4 weeks compared with placebo in patients who did not respond or were intolerant of TNF inhibitors. At week 16, 43% of patient on bimekizumab achieved ACR-50 compared with 7% on placebo [54].

The IL-12/IL-23p40 inhibitor ustekinumab has also been shown to be effective for psoriatic arthritis in a randomised controlled trial: 605 patients were randomised to ustekinumab 45 mg, ustekinumab 90 mg or placebo at week 0, 4, 16 and every 12 weeks thereafter. ACR-20 at week 24 was achieved in 42.4% of the 45 mg group, 49.5% of the 90 mg group and 22.8% of placebo-treated patients. The response was maintained at 52 weeks [55]. Improvements were also seen in dactylitis and enthesitis and in radiological progression of the disease [56]. Ustekinumab is not effective in axial disease.

The IL-23p19 inhibitors guselkumab, risankizumab and tildrakizumab have all shown efficacy for psoriatic arthritis.

Guselkumab is effective and licensed for psoriatic arthritis either alone or in combination with methotrexate. In a placebo-controlled trial, patients with psoriatic arthritis were randomised to receive guselkumab 100 mg at week 0, 4 and every 4 weeks, 100 mg at week 0, 4 and every 8 weeks or placebo. The primary outcome was

ACR-20 at week 24. ACR-20 was achieved in 59% of guselkumab 100 mg every 4 weeks compared with 52% in the guselkumab 100 mg every 8 weeks and 22% of the placebo group. Over 50% of patients were taking concomitant methotrexate [57].

In a similar study that included only biologic-naïve patients, guselkumab 100 mg every 4 weeks and every 8 weeks had similar ACR-20 responses (64%) compared with 31% in the placebo group. In this study, guselkumab was reported as effective in axial disease and prevented radiographic progression [51].

Risankizumab is licensed for the treatment of psoriatic arthritis. It has been evaluated in two phase III trials. The first study compared risankizumab 150 mg at week 0, 4 and week 12 compared with placebo in patients who had an inadequate response to or were intolerant of one or more disease-modifying antirheumatic drugs. At week 24, 57.3% of patients on risankizumab reached ACR-20 compared with 33.5% on placebo [58]. In a second study, which included patients who were resistant to or intolerant of biologic therapies, risankizumab was compared with placebo. At week 24, 51.3% of patients achieved ACR-20 compared with 26.5% on placebo [59].

In a phase IIb placebo-controlled trial 391 patients were randomised to receive tildrakizumab (200 mg every 4 weeks, 200 mg every 12 weeks, 100 mg every 12 weeks, or 20 mg every 12 weeks) or placebo. Preliminary results showed clear efficacy of tildrakizumab in the treatment of psoriatic arthritis as compared with placebo with differences detected in ACR20 and ACR50 at 12 weeks in the groups treated with 200 mg every 4 weeks and every 12 weeks.

Abatacept

Abatacept is a fusion protein that binds to CD80 thereby inhibiting T-cell activation. It is licensed as a monotherapy or in combination with methotrexate for psoriatic arthritis. In a randomised placebo-controlled trial, patients with active psoriatic arthritis were treated with weekly subcutaneous abatacept 125 mg ($n = 213$) or placebo ($n = 211$) for 24 weeks: 39.4% of patients on abatacept achieved ACR-20 compared with 22.3% on placebo (P <0.001). Abatacept is not effective for psoriasis.

The management of psoriatic arthritis has benefited significantly from the development of effective biologic therapies and high-quality data from clinical trials and is outlined in both the GRAPPA and EULAR guidelines. Early diagnosis and appropriate therapy are significant challenges in many health care systems.

There is a need for greater comparative data on biologic efficacy and safety from registries [60]. To date, there seems to be similar drug survival between adalimumab and secukinumab [60].

One of the compelling questions is whether biologic treatment of psoriasis may prevent the development of psoriatic arthritis. There are several studies that suggest that treatment with biologics that are also effective in the treatment of psoriatic arthritis may prevent the development of psoriatic arthritis [61,62]. These studies have multiple limitations but there appears to be a developing picture that biologic treatment of psoriasis, particularly with TNF inhibitors, may reduce the incidence of psoriatic arthritis [63].

There is a need for biomarkers to identify patients at highest risk of the development of psoriatic arthritis so that early effective treatment can be initiated [64]. Several longitudinal studies are assessing this issue.

Key references

The full list of references can be found in the online version at https://www.wiley.com/rooksdermatology10e

Chronic plaque psoriasis (psoriasis vulgaris)

1 Parisi R, Iskandar IYK, Kontopantelis E et al. Global Psoriasis Atlas. National, regional, and worldwide epidemiology of psoriasis: systematic analysis and modelling study. *BMJ* 2020;369:m1590.

2 Lomholt G. Psoriasis. Prevalence, spontaneous course and genetics. A census study on the prevalence of skin disease on the Faroe Islands. Copenhagen: GEC Gad, 1963:31–3.

3 Iskander IYK, Parisis R, Griffiths CEM, Ashcroft DM. Systematic review examining changes over time and variation in the incidence and prevalence of psoriasis by age and gender. *Br J Dermatol* 2021;184:243–58.

17 Duffy DL, Spelman LS, Martin NG. Psoriasis in Australian twins. *J Am Acad Dermatol* 1993;29:428–34.

20 Dand N, Mahil SK, Capon F et al. Psoriasis and genetics. *Acta Derm Venereol* 2020;100:adv00030.

24 Lowes MA, Bowcock AM, Krueger JG. Pathogenesis and therapy of psoriasis. *Nature* 2007;445:866–73.

29 Allen MH, Ameen H, Veal C et al. The major psoriasis susceptibility locus PSORS1 is not a risk factor for late-onset psoriasis. *J Invest Dermatol* 2005;124:103–6.

30 Jordan CT, Cao L, Roberson ED et al. PSORS2 is due to mutations in CARD14. *Am J Hum Genet* 2012;90:784–95.

32 Nair RP, Duffin KC, Helms C et al. Genome wide scan reveals association of psoriasis with IL-23 and NF-kappaB pathways. *Nat Genet* 2009;41:199–204.

34 de Cid R, Riveira-Munoz E, Zeeuwen PLJM et al. Deletion of the late cornified envelope LCE3B and LCE3C genes as a susceptibility factor for psoriasis. *Nat Genet* 2009;41:211–15.

37 Strange A, Capon F, Spencer CC et al. A genome-wide association study identifies new psoriasis susceptibility loci and an interaction between HLA-C and ERAP1. *Nat Genet* 2010;42:985–90.

43 Sigurdardottir SL, Thorleifsdottir RH, Valdimarsson H, Johnston A. The role of the palatine tonsils in the pathogenesis and treatment of psoriasis. *Br J Dermatol* 2013;168:237–42.

44 Diluvio L, Vollmer S, Besgen P et al. Identical TCR beta-chain rearrangements in streptococcal angina and skin lesions of patients with psoriasis vulgaris. *J Immunol* 2006;176:7104–11.

53 Basavaraj KH, Ashok NM, Rashmi R, Praveen TK. The role of drugs in the induction and/or exacerbation of psoriasis. *Int J Dermatol* 2010;49:1351–61.

55 Conrad C, Di Domizio J, Mylonas A et al. TNF blockade induces a dysregulated type I interferon response without autoimmunity in paradoxical psoriasis. *Nat Commun* 2018;9:25.

91 Christophers E, Metzler G, Rocken M. Bimodal immune activation in psoriasis. *Br J Dermatol* 2014;170:59–65.

94 Lande R, Gregorio J, Facchinetti V et al. Plasmacytoid dendritic cells sense self-DNA coupled with antimicrobial peptide. *Nature* 2007;449:564–9.

96 Herster F, Bittner Z, Archer NK et al. Neutrophil extracellular trap-associated RNA and LL37 enable self-amplifying inflammation in psoriasis. *Nat Commun* 2020;11:105.

101 Prinz JC. Human leukocyte antigen-class 1 alleles and the autoreactive T cell response in psoriasis pathogenesis. *Front Immunol* 2018;9:354.

119 Woronoff DI. Die periphere Veranderungen der Haut, um die Effloreszenzen der Psoriasis vulgaris und Syphilis corymbosa. *Derm Wsh* 1926;82:249–53.

121 Nicholas MN, Chan AR, Hessami-Booshehri M. Psoriasis in patients of color: differences in morphology, clinical presentation, and treatment. *Cutis* 2020;106(2S):7–10.

123 Griffiths CEM, Christophers E, Barker JNWN et al. A classification of psoriasis vulgaris according to phenotype. *Br J Dermatol* 2007;156:258–62.

165 Goeckerman WH, O'Leary PA. Erythroderma psoriaticum: a review of 22 cases. *JAMA* 1932;99:2102–5.

186 Clark RA. Skin-resident T cells: the ups and downs of on site immunity. *J Invest Dermatol* 2010;130:362–70.

187 Menon K, Van Voorhees AS, Bebo BF et al. Psoriasis in patients with HIV infection. *J Am Acad Dermatol* 2010;62:291–9.

190 National Institute for Health and Care Excellence (NICE). The Assessment and Management of Psoriasis. Clinical Guideline. Methods, Evidence and Recommendations. NICE, 2012. http://www.nice.org.uk/Cg153.

191 Fredriksson T, Pettersson U. Severe psoriasis – oral therapy with a new retinoid. *Dermatologica* 1978;157:238–44.

196 Finlay AY, Khan GK. Dermatology Life Quality Index (DLQI): a simple practical measure for routine clinical use. *Clin Exp Dermatol* 1994;19:210–16.

204 Finlay AY. Current severe psoriasis and the rule of tens. *Br J Dermatol* 2005;152:861–7.

206 Abuabara K, Azfar RS, Shin D et al. Cause-specific mortality in patients with severe psoriasis: a population-based cohort study in the UK. *Br J Dermatol* 2010;163:586–92.

220 Gudjonsson JE, Thorarinsson AM, Sigurgeirsson N, Valdimarsson H. Streptococcal throat infections and exacerbation of chronic plaque psoriasis: a prospective study. *Br J Dermatol* 2003;149:530–4.

233 Langan SM, Seminara NM, Shin DB et al. Prevalence of metabolic syndrome in patients with psoriasis: a population-based study in the United Kingdom. *J Invest Dermatol* 2012;132:556–62.

234 Armstrong AW, Harskamp CT, Armstrong EJ. Psoriasis and metabolic syndrome: a systematic review and meta-analysis of observational studies. *J Am Acad Dermatol* 2013;68:654–62.

238 Patrick MT, Stuart PE, Zhang H et al. Causal relationship and shared genetic loci between psoriasis and type 2 diabetes through trans-disease meta-analysis. *J Invest Dermatol* 2021;141:1493–502.

246 Jensen P, Zachariae, Christensen et al. Effect of weight loss on the severity of psoriasis. A randomized clinical study. *JAMA Dermatol* 2013;149:795–801.

257 Gelfand JM, Neimann AL, Shin DB et al. Risk of myocardial infarction in patients with psoriasis. *JAMA* 2006;296:1735–41.

266 Fortune DG, Richards HL, Main CJ et al. Pathological worrying, illness perceptions and disease severity in patients with psoriasis. *Br J Health Psychol* 2000;5:71–82.

290 Harder E, Andersen A-MN, Kamper-Jørgensen M, Skov L. No increased risk of fetal death or prolonged time to pregnancy in women with psoriasis. *J Invest Dermatol* 2014;134:1747–9.

Management

1 Iversen L, Eidsmo L, Austad J et al. Secukinumab treatment in new-onset psoriasis: aiming to understand the potential for disease modification - rationale and design of the randomized, multicenter STEPIn study. *J Eur Acad Dermatol Venereol* 2018;32:1930–9.

2 Eyerich K, Weisenseel P, Pinter A et al. IL-23 blockade with guselkumab potentially modifies psoriasis pathogenesis: rationale and study protocol of a phase 3b, randomised, double-blind, multicentre study in participants with moderate-to-severe plaque-type psoriasis (GUIDE). *BMJ Open* 2021;11:e049822.

13 Ashcroft DM, Li Wan Po A, Williams HC, Griffiths CEM. Systematic review of comparative efficacy and tolerability of calcipotriol in treating chronic plaque psoriasis. *BMJ* 2000;320:963–7.

14 Kragballe K, Beck HI, Søgaard H. Improvement of psoriasis by a topical vitamin D3 analogue (MC903) in a double-blind study. *Br J Dermatol* 1988;119:223–30.

35 Ingram JT. The approach to psoriasis. *BMJ* 1953;2:591–4.

38 Rogers S, Marks J, Shuster S et al. Comparison of photochemotherapy and dithranol in the treatment of chronic plaque psoriasis. *Lancet* 1979;i:455–8.

42 Goeckerman WH. The treatment of psoriasis. *Northwest Med* 1925;24:229–30.

Phototherapy

Narrow-Band UVB

4 Almutawa F, Alnomair N, Wang Y et al. Systematic review of UV-based therapy for psoriasis. *Am J Clin Dermatol* 2013;14:87–109.

10 Addison R, Weatherhead SC, Pawitri A et al. Therapeutic wavelengths of ultraviolet B radiation activate apoptotic, circadian rhythm, redox signalling and key canonical pathways in psoriatic epidermis. *Redox Biol* 2021;41:101924.

11 Sigmundsdottir H, Johnston A, Gudjonsson JE, Valdimarsson H. Narrowband-UVB irradiation decreases the production of pro-inflammatory cytokines by stimulated T cells. *Arch Dermatol Res* 2005;297:39–42.

12 Markham T, Rogers S, Collins P. Narrowband UV-B (TL-01) phototherapy vs oral 8-methoxypsoralen psoralen-UV-A for the treatment of chronic plaque psoriasis. *Arch Dermatol* 2003;139:325–8.

PUVA photochemotherapy

5 Wolff KW, Fitzpatrick TB, Parrish JA *et al.* Photochemotherapy for psoriasis with orally administered methoxsalen. *Arch Dermatol* 1976;112:943–50.

8 Rogers S, Marks J, Shuster S *et al.* Comparison of photochemotherapy and dithranol in the treatment of chronic plaque psoriasis. *Lancet* 1979;i:455–8.

9 Griffiths CE, Clark CM, Chalmers RJ *et al.* A systematic review of treatments for severe psoriasis. *Health Technol Assess* 2000;4:1–125.

13 Stern RS, Laird N, Melski J *et al.* Cutaneous squamous-cell carcinoma in patients treated with PUVA. *N Engl J Med* 1984;310:1156–61.

Systemic therapy

3 Warren RB, Mrowietz U, von Kiedrowski R *et al.* An intensified dosing schedule of subcutaneous methotrexate in patients with moderate to severe plaque-type psoriasis (METOP): a 52 week, multicentre, randomised, double-blind, placebo-controlled, phase 3 trial. *Lancet* 2017;389:528–37.

10 Saurat JH, Stingl G, Dubertret L *et al.* Efficacy and safety results from the randomized controlled comparative study of adalimumab vs. methotrexate vs. placebo in patients with psoriasis (CHAMPION). *Br J Dermatol* 2008;158:558–66.

12 Alabas OA, Mason KJ, Yiu ZZN *et al.* Effectiveness and survival of methotrexate versus adalimumab in patients with moderate-to-severe psoriasis: a cohort study from the British Association of Dermatologists Biologics and Immunomodulators Register (BADBIR). *Br J Dermatol* 2023;189:271–8.

14 Otero ME, van den Reek JM, Seyger MM, van de Kerkhof PC, Kievit W, de Jong EM. Determinants for drug survival of methotrexate in patients with psoriasis, split according to different reasons for discontinuation: results of the prospective MTX-CAPTURE. *Br J Dermatol* 2017;177:497–504.

18 Gelfand JM, Wan J, Zhang H *et al.* Risk of liver disease in patients with psoriasis, psoriatic arthritis, and rheumatoid arthritis receiving methotrexate: a population-based study. *J Am Acad Dermatol* 2021;84:1636–43.

27 van der Kraaij G, Busard C, van den Reek J *et al.* Adalimumab with methotrexate vs. adalimumab monotherapy in psoriasis: first-year results of a single-blind randomized controlled trial. *J Invest Dermatol* 2022;142:2375–83.

30 Griffiths CE, Powles AV, Leonard JN *et al.* Clearance of psoriasis with low dose cyclosporin. *BMJ (Clin Res Ed)* 1986;293:731–2.

32 Ellis CN, Fradin MS, Messana JM *et al.* Cyclosporine for plaque-type psoriasis. Results of a multidose, double-blind trial. *N Engl J Med* 1991;324:277–84.

42 Saurat JH, Geiger JM, Amblard P *et al.* Randomized double-blind multicenter study comparing acitretin-PUVA, etretinate-PUVA and placebo-PUVA in the treatment of severe psoriasis. *Dermatologica* 1988;177:218–24.

45 Schweckendiek W. Heilung von. Psoriasis. *Med Monutschr* 1959;13:103–4.

50 Sulaimani J, Cluxton D, Clowry J *et al.* Dimethyl fumarate modulates the Treg-Th17 cell axis in patients with psoriasis. *Br J Dermatol* 2021;184:495–503.

60 Nast A, Smith C, Spuls PI *et al.* EuroGuiDerm Guideline on the systemic treatment of psoriasis vulgaris - Part 1: treatment and monitoring recommendations. *J Eur Acad Dermatol Venereol* 2020;34:2461–98.

71 Armstrong AW, Gooderham M, Warren RB *et al.* Deucravacitinib versus placebo and apremilast in moderate to severe plaque psoriasis: efficacy and safety results from the 52-week, randomized, double-blinded, placebo-controlled phase 3 POETYK PSO-1 trial. *J Am Acad Dermatol* 2023;88:29–39.

Biological therapy

2 Reich K, Armstrong AW, Langley RG *et al.* Guselkumab versus secukinumab for the treatment of moderate-to-severe psoriasis (ECLIPSE): results from a phase 3, randomised controlled trial. *Lancet* 2019;394(10201):831–9.

3 Blauvelt A, Papp K, Gottlieb A *et al.* A head-to-head comparison of ixekizumab vs. guselkumab in patients with moderate-to-severe plaque psoriasis: 12-week efficacy, safety and speed of response from a randomized, double-blinded trial. *Br J Dermatol* 2020;182:1348–58.

9 Mason KJ, Barker JNWN, Smith CH *et al.* Comparison of drug discontinuation, effectiveness, and safety between clinical trial eligible and ineligible patients in BADBIR. *JAMA Dermatol* 2018;154:581–8.

10 Yiu ZZN, Sorbe C, Lunt M *et al.* Development and validation of a multivariable risk prediction model for serious infection in patients with psoriasis receiving systemic therapy. *Br J Dermatol* 2019;180:894–901.

TNF-α inhibitors

1 Oh CJ, Das KM, Gottlieb AB. Treatment with anti-tumor necrosis factor alpha (TNF-alpha) monoclonal antibody dramatically decreases the clinical activity of psoriasis lesions. *J Am Acad Dermatol* 2000;42:829–30.

12 Yiu ZZN, Ashcroft DM, Evans I *et al.* Infliximab is associated with an increased risk of serious infection in patients with psoriasis in the U.K. and Republic of Ireland: results from the British Association of Dermatologists Biologic Interventions Register (BADBIR). *Br J Dermatol* 2019;180:329–37.

13 Keane J, Gershon S, Wise RP *et al.* Tuberculosis associated with infliximab, a tumor necrosis factor alpha-neutralizing agent. *N Engl J Med* 2001;345:1098–104.

24 Saurat JH, Stingl G, Dubertret L *et al.* Efficacy and safety results from the randomized controlled comparative study of adalimumab vs. methotrexate vs. placebo in patients with psoriasis (CHAMPION). *Br J Dermatol* 2008;158:558–66.

30 Warren RB, Blauvelt A, Bagel J *et al.* Bimekizumab versus adalimumab in plaque psoriasis. *N Engl J Med* 2021;385:130–41.

Registries

3 Mason KJ, Barker JNWN, Smith CH *et al.* Comparison of drug discontinuation, effectiveness, and safety between clinical trial eligible and ineligible patients in BADBIR. *JAMA Dermatol* 2018;154:581–8.

Pustular psoriasis

1 Navarini AA, Burden AD, Capon F *et al.* European Consensus Statement on Phenotypes of Pustular Psoriasis. *J Eur Acad Dermatol Venereol* 2017;31:1792–9.

4 Choon SE, Lai NM, Mohammad NA *et al.* Clinical profile, morbidity, and outcome of adult-onset generalized pustular psoriasis: analysis of 102 cases seen in a tertiary hospital in Johor, Malaysia. *Int J Dermatol* 2014;53:676–84.

5 Marrakchi S, Guigue P, Renshaw BR *et al.* Interleukin-36-receptor antagonist deficiency and generalized pustular psoriasis. *N Engl J Med* 2011;365:620–8.

6 Onoufriadis A, Simpson MA, Pink AE *et al.* Mutations in IL36RN/IL1F5 are associated with the severe episodic inflammatory skin disease known as generalized pustular psoriasis. *Am J Hum Genet* 2011;89:432–7.

12 Twelves S, Mostafa A, Dand N *et al.* Clinical and genetic differences between pustular psoriasis subtypes. *JACI* 2019;143:1021–6.

45 Fujita H, Terui T, Hayama K, Akiyama M *et al.* Japanese guidelines for the management and treatment of generalised pustular psoriasis: the new pathogenesis and treatment of GPP. *J Dermatol* 2018;45:1235–70.

CHAPTER 36

Pityriasis Rubra Pilaris

Curdin Conrad

Department of Dermatology, Lausanne University Hospital CHUV, Lausanne, Switzerland

Pityriasis rubra pilaris

Definition and nomenclature

Pityriasis rubra pilaris (PRP) represents a group of rare inflammatory skin disorders of unknown aetiopathology sharing common clinical and histopathological features. The disease is characterised by the appearance of hyperkeratotic follicular papules, which tend to coalesce to diffuse pink or red plaques, and a yellowish palmoplantar keratoderma. It may progress to erythroderma with characteristic distinct areas of uninvolved skin, the so-called 'islands of sparing'. Based on its age of onset, clinical presentation and prognosis, PRP has been classified into distinct subtypes.

Synonyms and inclusions

- Pityriasis pilaris
- Lichen ruber acuminatus

Introduction and general description

Pityriasis rubra pilaris represents a group of papulosquamous skin disorders of unknown aetiopathology. It was first described by Claudius Tarral in 1828 and given its present name by Besnier in 1889 [1]. Literally translated, the name means fine, bran-like scaling (*pityriasis*), redness (*rubra*), and involvement of hair follicles (*pilaris*). In 1980, Griffiths proposed a classification of PRP into five types based on age of onset, clinical presentation and prognosis [2]:

- Type I: classic adult (55% of all cases).
- Type II: atypical adult (5%).
- Type III: classic juvenile (10%).
- Type IV: circumscribed juvenile (25%).
- Type V: atypical juvenile (5%).

In addition, a human immunodeficiency virus (HIV)-associated form of PRP (type VI) has been described [3].

Epidemiology

Incidence and prevalence

Pityriasis rubra pilaris is a rare skin disease. Although no reliable data are available concerning its prevalence, incidences of 1 in 3500–5000 patients presenting in dermatology clinics have been reported in the UK and USA [4].

Age

It has a bimodal age distribution with peaks in the first (juvenile forms) and fifth to sixth decades (adult forms) of life [2]. The rare familial form typically starts in early childhood.

Sex

It occurs equally in men and women.

Ethnicity

Pityriasis rubra pilaris shows no racial predilection.

Associated diseases

Several case reports suggested associations with autoimmune diseases, infections and malignancies. A case series from 2016 showed hypothyroidism in 20% of patients [5]. However, the significance and a causal link for these associations remain unclear. The most convincing association is still HIV (type VI). PRP can represent the first manifestation of infection and might benefit from retroviral therapy, which supports a pathogenic role.

Pathophysiology

The pathogenesis of PRP remains largely unknown. Based on its clinical resemblance to psoriasis, a role of the interleukin 23 (IL-23)–TH17 axis in PRP is suspected. Gene expression analyses of lesional skin samples from PRP patients show a preferential increase of TH17 cytokines [6] and several cases of successful treatment of PRP with biologics typically used for psoriasis have been reported [6,7,8]. These findings suggest that shared pathogenic inflammatory pathways could drive psoriasis and PRP. However, despite the similarities, obvious differences exist between psoriasis and PRP at the clinical, histopathological and molecular levels (Table 36.1). Excellent efficacy of anti-IL-12/IL-23 ustekinumab but a variable response to anti-IL-17A therapy might suggest a role for other IL-17 family members. This notion was further supported by the finding that sustained high levels of IL-17C were associated with anti-IL-17A treatment failure [9]. Interestingly, IL-17C is mainly

Table 36.1 Pityriasis rubra pilaris (PRP) and psoriasis compared.

	PRP	Psoriasis
Scalp scaling	Furfuraceous/bran-like	Adherent
Palmoplantar keratoderma	Characteristic; waxy, yellowish orange	Less common; redness, pustules common
'Islands of sparing'	Characteristic	Uncommon
Cephalocaudal disease progression	Characteristic	Uncommon
Nail pitting and salmon patches	Absent	Common
Munro microabscesses	Absent	Characteristic
Seronegative arthropathy	Rare	Common
Ultraviolet B phototherapy	Poor response	Good response
Topical corticosteroids	Limited response	Good response
Methotrexate	Variable	Good
Tumour necrosis factor α blockade	Variable	Very good to excellent
Interleukin 12 (IL-12)/IL-23 blockade	Probably excellent	Excellent
IL-17 blockade	Variable	Excellent

produced by keratinocytes but not by T cells suggesting that, unlike psoriasis, PRP might not be driven by T cells but rather by keratinocyte-derived type 3 cytokines (equivalent to T-cell-derived TH17 cytokines).

Numerous triggers of PRP have been proposed, including photoaggravation by ultraviolet (UV) exposure, trauma (koebnerisation) and various drugs, as well as bacterial and viral infections.

Pathology

The characteristic histopathological features of fully developed PRP skin lesions are usually modest (Figure 36.1) and include:

- Alternating perpendicular and horizontal ortho- and parakeratosis ('checkerboard' pattern).
- Hyperkeratosis with follicular plugging (keratin-plugged follicles) and parakeratosis adjacent to both sides of the follicular orifice ('shoulder parakeratosis').
- Focal or confluent hypergranulosis.
- Irregular psoriasiform acanthosis.
- Acantholysis may be present.
- Sparse, superficial, dermal, perivascular lymphohistiocytic infiltrate; neutrophils are typically absent.
- Note that in the context of erythrodermic PRP, the epidermis may be thinned with a diminished granular cell layer.

These findings are, although characteristic, not pathognomonic for PRP and not all features are present. However, histopathological examination remains an essential diagnostic criterion to distinguish PRP from psoriasis and other causes of erythroderma.

Genetics

Most PRP cases are sporadic, but familial cases have been reported and associated with gain-of-function mutations in the caspase recruitment domain family member 14 (*CARD14*) gene [10,11]. Variants of the *CARD14* gene, which lead to enhanced and sustained nuclear factor κB (NFκB) activation, have also been described

in psoriasis and account for the psoriasis susceptibility locus 2 (*PSORS2*).

Clinical features
Presentation

The clinical presentation and the course of PRP are largely variable. However, the classic clinical features include hyperkeratotic follicular papules that tend to coalesce into diffuse red to salmon-coloured, dry, scaly plaques, typical islands of sparing (areas of normal skin) and yellowish orange, waxy palmoplantar keratoderma (Figure 36.2).

In adults, PRP typically starts on the face and scalp before spreading in a caudal direction. The disease can be accompanied by pruritus, sparseness of hair, nail involvement and – in the case of prolonged facial involvement – ectropion. Some patients may develop erythroderma.

Among clinical and patient-reported features that influence disease severity in PRP are redness, scaling, palmoplantar involvement, ectropion, itch and pain, as well as lack of sweating.

Clinical variants

Griffiths's classification of PRP into five subtypes, based on the age of onset, the clinical presentation and the prognosis, remains the most commonly used [2]. HIV-associated PRP represents an additional type, later proposed as type VI PRP [3].

Classic adult-onset PRP (type I). Type I PRP represents the classic and most common adult variant that affects *c.*55% of patients, with the highest incidence between 40 and 60 years of age. It typically starts with a pink-red, slightly scaly macule on the face, scalp or neck, which might initially be mistaken for seborrhoeic dermatitis. Within a few weeks or months, more lesions appear, including the classic keratotic follicular papules, which typically progress in a cephalocaudal manner (Figure 36.3). While the follicular lesions are initially discrete, interfollicular redness gradually appears and eventually coalesces into the characteristic orange-red plaques with bran-like scaling and islands of sparing making the diagnosis apparent. The hyperkeratotic follicular papules can be observed both within the sharply demarcated patches and within the adjacent normal skin. Most patients develop a yellowish orange, waxy palmoplantar keratoderma and nail involvement with a thickened nail plate, yellow-brown discoloration and subungual hyperkeratotic debris. Within a few months, the disease can evolve into erythroderma, and with prolonged facial redness ectropion may ensue. Despite its severe disease course and a major impact on the patient's quality of life, type I PRP carries the best prognosis: more than 80% of patients show spontaneous remission within 3 years [4].

Atypical adult-onset PRP (type II). Type II or atypical adult-onset PRP accounts for approximately 5% of all PRP cases [2]. It is characterised by a more chronic disease course, typically more than 20 years (only a minority of patients show clinical resolution within 3 years), but also shows atypical morphological features. Type II PRP does not follow the rapid cephalocaudal progression described for type I. It typically involves the lower extremities and patients often show eczematous lesions with ichthyosiform scaling. The

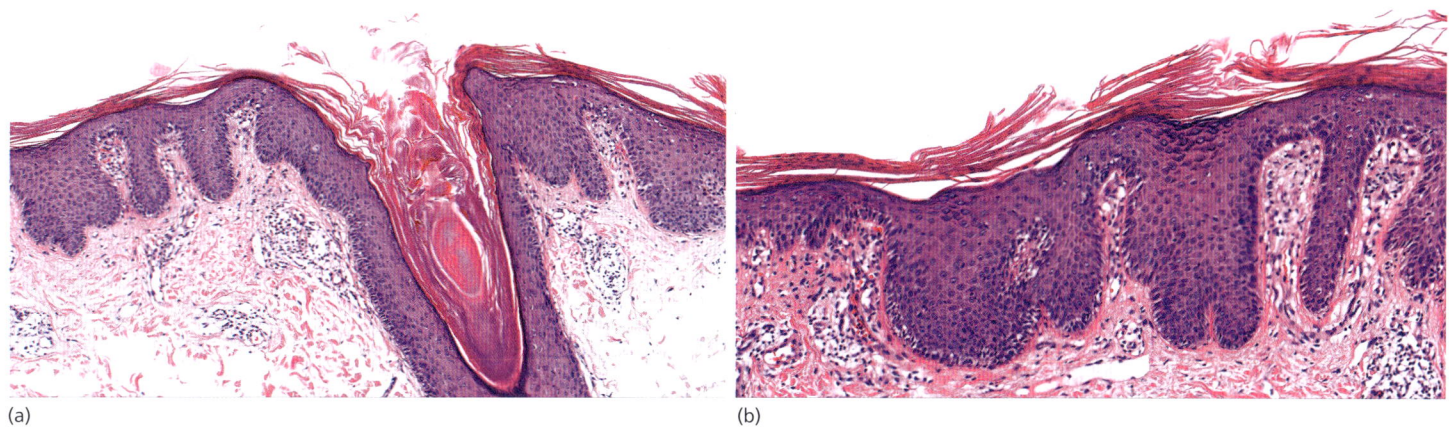

(a)   (b)

Figure 36.1 Microscopic image of pityriasis rubra pilaris. (a) Hyperkeratosis with follicular plugging (keratin-plugged follicles) and parakeratosis adjacent to both sides of the follicular ostium ('shoulder parakeratosis'). There is a scarce, superficial, dermal, perivascular lymphohistiocytic infiltrate and lack of neutrophils. (b) Irregular psoriasiform acanthosis showing alternating ortho- and parakeratosis ('checkerboard' pattern). Courtesy of Emmanuella Guenova.

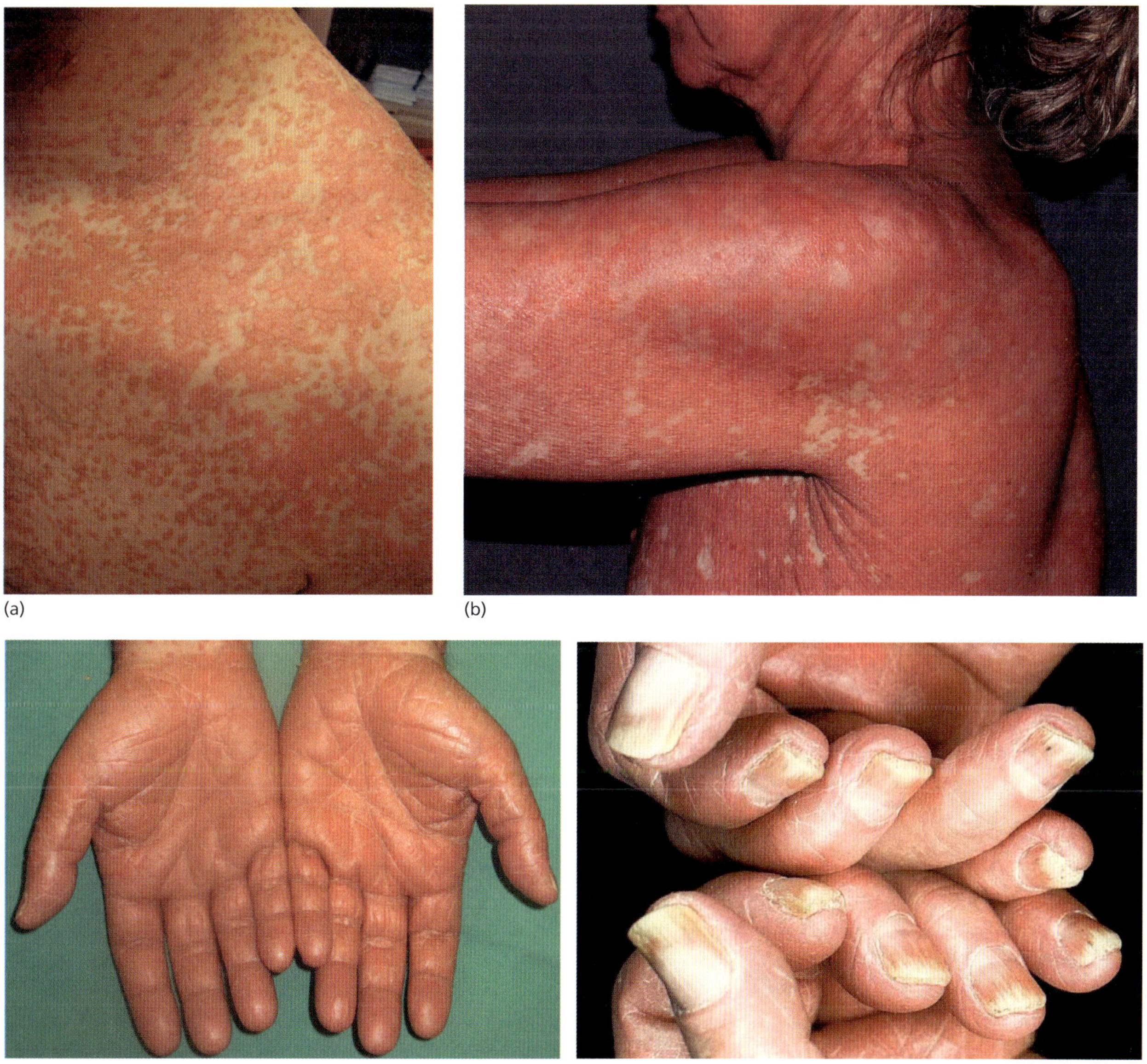

(a)   (b)

(c)   (d)

Figure 36.2 Classic clinical features of pityriasis rubra pilaris include (a) hyperkeratotic follicular papules that tend to coalesce into diffuse red to salmon-coloured, scaly plaques, with (b) typical islands of sparing (areas of normal skin), (c) yellowish orange, waxy palmoplantar keratoderma and (d) thickening of the nails, subungual hyperkeratosis and splinter haemorrhages.

PART 4: INFLAMMATORY DERMATOSES

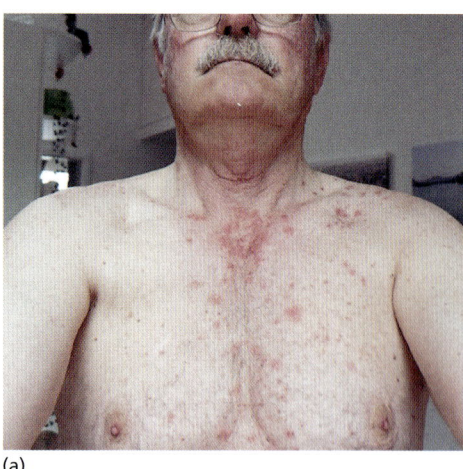 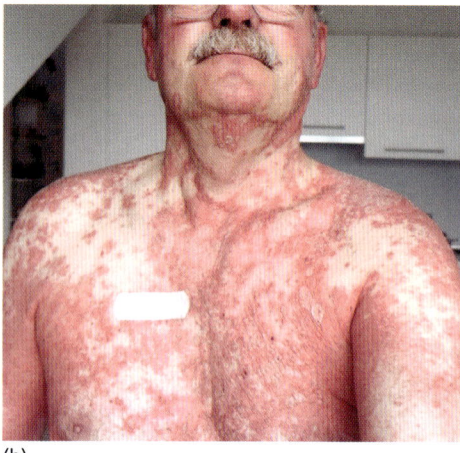 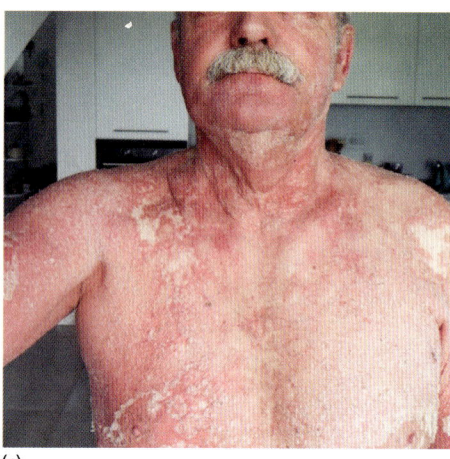

(a) (b) (c)

Figure 36.3 (a–c) Evolution of type I PRP: cephalocaudal progression from limited seborrhoeic dermatitis-like rash on the upper trunk and face to erythroderma with islands of sparing in an elderly man.

palmoplantar keratoderma is coarser than in type I disease, with lamellar scales. Sparseness of body hair is common.

Classic juvenile-onset PRP (type III). Type III or classic juvenile-onset PRP accounts for *c*.10% of all cases (Figure 36.4). It mirrors the clinical features of the adult type I except for a disease onset typically between the ages of 5 to 10 years [12]. The prognosis is favourable; most cases are self-limiting and undergo spontaneous resolution within 1–2 years [4]. However, one study showed that not only type I PRP but also juvenile-onset PRP can persist well beyond the anticipated course of 3 years [5]. Some patients with type III PRP may evolve into type IV PRP and vice versa [12]. Recurrence of type III PRP in later adult life has also been reported [13].

Circumscribed juvenile PRP (type IV). Type IV or circumscribed juvenile PRP accounts for approximately 25% of cases [2] and mainly affects prepubertal children, usually under 12 years of age [12]. It represents the only localised variant and does not show the progression of the classic forms (Figure 36.4). Type IV PRP is characterised by well-demarcated red plaques of grouped hyperkeratotic follicular papules over the elbows and knees and potentially other bony prominences. Palmoplantar keratoderma is often observed but can be absent in some [14]. The prognosis of type IV PRP is uncertain but seems less favourable than the classic adult- and juvenile-onset types. Spontaneous remissions and exacerbations are observed.

Atypical juvenile PRP (type V). Type V PRP or atypical juvenile PRP accounts for *c*.5% of cases and is characterised by its early onset (sometimes present at birth) and a chronic course. Most cases of familial PRP fall under this type [2,10]. Clinical presentation can be similar to type III PRP with follicular hyperkeratosis and ichthyosiform features. Some patients show scleroderma-like changes on the palms and soles.

HIV-related PRP (type VI). Type VI PRP occurs in patients with HIV infection; in some cases, it represents the first clinical manifestation of an infection [3]. Type VI PRP resembles type I but presents distinct clinical features: red follicular papules with conspicuous follicular plugging and spicules are common. Association with acne conglobata and hidradenitis suppurativa, which are linked to follicular occlusion, has been described [3,15,16]. HIV-associated PRP carries a poorer prognosis and tends to be resistant to treatment, but may respond to retroviral treatment [17].

Differential diagnosis

The differential diagnosis largely depends on the subtype of PRP and the stage of disease.

Types I and III PRP can be confused with psoriasis (see Table 36.1). Characteristic features of PRP that help distinguish it from psoriasis include yellowish orange, waxy palmoplantar keratoderma and islands of sparing. The clinical course with progression from head to toe and poor response to phototherapy are further helpful criteria. Histopathological findings eventually help to confirm the diagnosis. In the future, distinct gene expression profiles might guide early diagnostics.

As types II and V PRP present ichthyosiform changes, differential diagnoses include follicular ichthyosis, follicular eczema and erythrokeratoderma.

Type IV PRP shares clinical features with keratosis circumscripta.

For specific signs or symptoms of PRP, the following differential diagnoses should be considered:
- Erythroderma: psoriasis, atopic dermatitis, Sézary syndrome and other cutaneous T-cell lymphomas, drug reactions and other causes of erythroderma.
- Palmoplantar keratoderma: psoriasis, ichthyosis, hereditary palmoplantar keratoderma and erythrokeratoderma.
- Early scalp and facial lesions: seborrhoeic dermatitis or psoriasis.

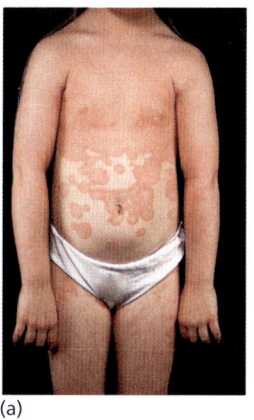 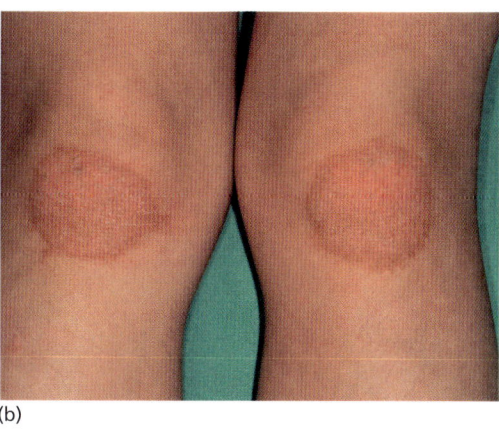 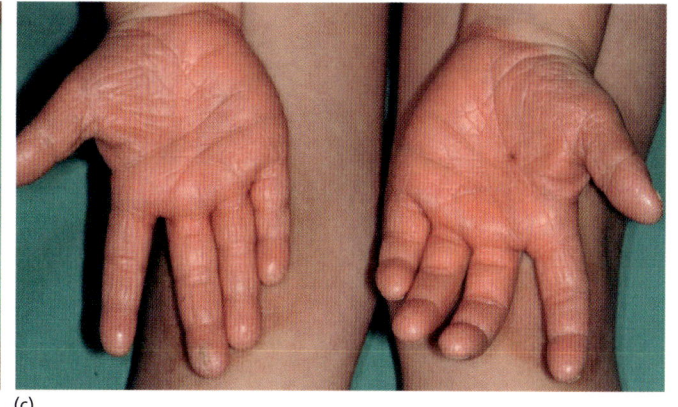

(a) (b) (c)

Figure 36.4 Juvenile pityriasis rubra pilaris (PRP): (a) classic juvenile-onset type III and (b,c) circumscribed juvenile-onset type IV PRP. Note the orange-red skin colouring with cephalocaudal downward extension in type III PRP (a), and the circumscribed areas of red hyperkeratotic plaques over the knees (b) and prominent palmar keratoderma (c) in type IV PRP.

Complications and co-morbidities

In patients with erythroderma, there is a risk for high-output cardiac failure and body temperature dysregulation. Ocular complications in patients with ectropion can range from dry eyes to peripheral ulcerative keratitis [18].

Disease course and prognosis

Disease course and prognosis largely depend on the PRP type. Classic adult type I PRP may progress from limited disease to erythroderma in a matter of weeks and, in rare cases, might persist indefinitely. However, in most affected patients, type I PRP clears spontaneously within 3 years [2]. Type III PRP carries an even better prognosis with remission typically within 1 year, but can persist well beyond this time [5] and recurrence in adult life has been reported [13].

Investigations

Diagnosis is made on clinical features and supported by histology. No other tests are indicated. In the future, analysis of a distinct gene expression might confirm diagnosis.

Management

Due to its rarity, lack of controlled trials and the tendency of PRP to spontaneous resolution, assessing efficacy and the actual value of a therapeutic option remains difficult. Recommendations are largely based on case reports, small case series and retrospective reviews.

In many cases, PRP is self-limiting and, therefore, patients with milder disease might not require treatment. On the other hand, erythrodermic patients may need intense supportive care to prevent electrolyte imbalance, protein loss and temperature dysregulation.

For limited disease and in paediatric patients, topical treatments are promising and include emollients, keratolytic agents (urea, salicylic acid or α-hydroxy acids such as lactic acid), topical retinoids, calcineurin inhibitors and, in particular, topical steroids.

These treatments can improve redness and scaling and might provide symptomatic relief, but it remains unclear whether they can alter the disease course. Phototherapy, with or without oral retinoids, might be an alternative treatment option. However, response to phototherapy is often poor and exacerbation upon UV exposure has been reported [19,20]. Therefore, phototesting should be considered prior to treatment initiation.

Oral retinoids are now considered first line systemic treatment for both adults and children. They provide antiproliferative, antidifferentiative, immunomodulatory and anti-inflammatory effects. In a larger prospective study with isotretinoin, the majority of patients showed marked improvement within 4 weeks [21]. Similar onset of effect was seen for acitretin in a smaller retrospective study [22], but a retrospective analysis suggested lower response rates for acitretin than isotretinoin [23]. Interestingly, alitretinoin, which has the ability to bind to retinoid X receptors in addition to retinoid acid receptors, showed efficacy in patients who previously had failed acitretin treatment [24]. Limitations in the use of oral retinoids include skeletal toxicity in the paediatric population and their teratogenicity.

Methotrexate is a second line systemic therapeutic option, either alone or in combination with retinoids for recalcitrant cases. However, combination therapy increases the risk for hepatic toxicity. Low-dose methotrexate has successfully been used in a case of PRP-induced cicatricial ectropion [25].

In recent years, biologics have increasingly been used in the management of PRP. The choice of biologic agents used for PRP was initially based on its clinical resemblance to psoriasis. Antitumour necrosis factors (anti-TNFs) have been the most widely reported biologics in PRP showing decent efficacy [19,26,27]. However, the response rates were variable and might be slightly overestimated due to a reporting bias. Some small case series have indicated a potential pathogenic relevance for the IL-23–IL-17 axis in PRP [6,7]. Moreover, IL-23 blockers and, in particular, the anti-IL-12/IL-23 ustekinumab have shown great potential with rapid onset of

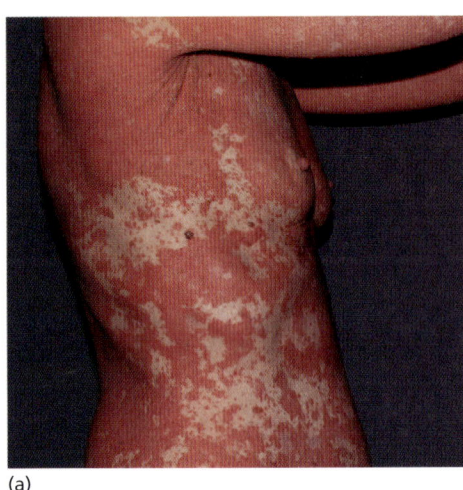
(a)

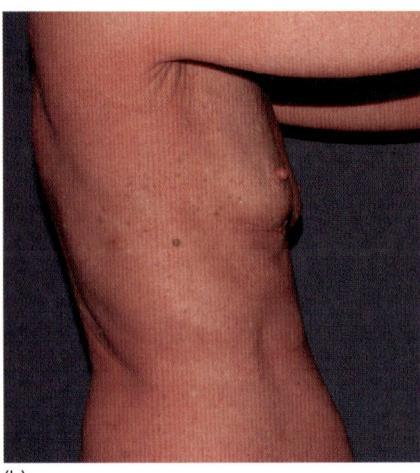
(b)

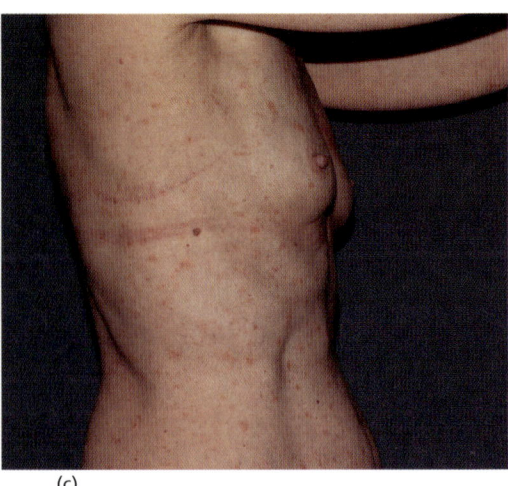
(c)

Figure 36.5 Evolution of type I pityriasis rubra pilaris over 12 months in a 60-year-old woman. (a) An initial progression from extended plaques with 'islands of sparing' to (b) a complete erythroderma and (c) resolution over the ensuing 6 months following ustekinumab therapy.

response, even in patients who had failed previous therapies and in familial PRP associated with *CARD14* mutations [7,**26**,28–30]. Anti-IL-17 treatments, although showing excellent response in a subset of patients, seem to have a more variable response [8,31].

Given their efficacy and superior safety profile, biologics should be considered in patients needing systemic therapy but where retinoids are either contraindicated, lead to side effects or provide insufficient results (Figure 36.5).

- Fumaric acid
- Intravenous immunoglobulins
- Azathioprine

Other treatments
- UVB phototherapy
- Acitretin + UVA1 phototherapy
- Extracorporeal photochemotherapy
- Antiretroviral therapy (for type VI PRP)

Treatment ladder for pityrisasis rubra pilaris

Topical treatments
- Emollients (± urea, salicylic acid, α-hydroxy acids)
- Topical corticosteroids
- Topical retinoids
- Topical vitamin D analogues
- Topical calcineurin inhibitors

Systemic treatments

First line
- Systemic retinoids (isotretinoin, alternatively acitretin, alitretinoin)

Second line
- Methotrexate
- Ustekinumab, potentially anti-IL-23p19

Third line
- Anti-TNF, anti-IL-17, anti-IL-23p19
- Ciclosporine

Key references

The full list of references can be found in the online version at https://www.wiley.com/rooksdermatology10e

2 Griffiths WA. Pityriasis rubra pilaris. *Clin Exp Dermatol* 1980;5:105–12.
6 Feldmeyer L, Mylonas A, Demaria O *et al.* Interleukin 23-helper T cell 17 axis as a treatment target for pityriasis rubra pilaris. *JAMA Dermatol* 2017;153:304–8.
8 Haynes D, Strunck JL, Topham CA *et al.* Evaluation of ixekizumab treatment for patients with pityriasis rubra pilaris: a single-arm trial. *JAMA Dermatol* 2020;156:668–75.
9 Strunck JL, Cutler B, Rajpal B *et al.* Pityriasis rubra pilaris response to IL-17A inhibition is associated with IL-17C and CCL20 protein levels. *J Invest Dermatol* 2022;142:235–9.e1.
11 Fuchs-Telem D, Sarig O, van Steensel MA *et al.* Familial pityriasis rubra pilaris is caused by mutations in CARD14. *Am J Hum Genet* 2012;91:163–70.
19 Engelmann C, Elsner P, Miguel D. Treatment of pityriasis rubra pilaris type I: a systematic review. *Eur J Dermatol* 2019;29:524–37.
26 Napolitano M, Abeni D, Didona B. Biologics for pityriasis rubra pilaris treatment: a review of the literature. *J Am Acad Dermatol* 2018;79:353–9.e11.

CHAPTER 37

Lichen Planus and Lichenoid Disorders

Felix Lauffer[1] and Kilian Eyerich[1,2]

[1] Department of Dermatology and Allergy, Technical University of Munich, Munich, Germany

[2] Department of Dermatology and Venerology, Medical Center, University of Freiburg, Frieburg,Germany; Division of Dermatology and Venereology, Department of Medicine Solna, Karolinska Institutet, Stockholm, Sweden

PART 4: INFLAMMATORY DERMATOSES

Introduction

Historically, lichenoid disorders are viewed as a heterogeneous group of inflammatory skin diseases characterised by a typical clinical phenotype – flat-topped, polygonal papules with fine white surface lines known as Wickham striae – combined with hallmark histopathological changes, namely a dense band of lymphocytes in the upper dermis. More recently, a common pathomechanism of lichenoid disorders has been recognised: type I immune cell killing of basal keratinocytes. A better understanding of pathogenesis leads to novel therapeutic concepts. Lichen planus is the protoype lichenoid disease, but numerous other diseases share this definition, such as graft-versus-host disease (Chapter 38).

Lichen planus

Introduction and general description

Lichen planus (LP), the most typical and best characterised lichenoid dermatosis, is an idiopathic inflammatory skin disease affecting the skin and mucosal membranes, often running a chronic course with relapses and periods of remission. Its prevalence is approximately 0.5% of the population (reviewed in [1]).

Epidemiology

The incidence varies between 0.22% and 1% of the adult population worldwide. LP represented about 1.2% of all new dermatology patients in London and Turin [2], 0.9% in Copenhagen [3] and 0.38% in India [4]. Hypertrophic cases were reportedly to be common in Nigeria [5]. In contrast, oral LP seems to be more frequent with a reported incidence between 1% and 4% of the population [1]. LP is rare in children and commonly affects adults during their fourth to sixth decades. There was an overrepresentation of South Asians in a series of childhood cases in Birmingham, UK [6]. There is no obvious racial predisposition for LP, although a small overrepresentation with patients of Indian subcontinent origin has been suggested, at least in oral disease [7]. Familial cases are unusual but have been reported in association with human leukocyte antigen (HLA)-A3, -A5, -B7, -DR1 and -DRB*0101. The global prevalence of oral LP is 1.01% with increasing prevalence from the age of 40 and a higher prevalence in Europe as compared with Asia [8].

Pathophysiology
Pathology

Lichen planus is thought to be a T-cell-mediated autoimmune disease, possibly targeting the basal keratinocytes, which can be triggered by a variety of situations, including viruses, drugs and contact allergens.

The central pathogenic event in LP is lymphocyte-mediated keratinocyte killing. This cytotoxicity is observed in numerous inflammatory or autoimmune skin diseases, including most lichenoid diseases, cutaneous lupus, graft-versus-host disease and alopecia areata; furthermore, similar cytotoxic events against other cutaneous cells (e.g. melanocytes) cause diseases such as vitiligo. Collectively, lichenoid diseases and further diseases that are caused by lymphocyte-mediated cytotoxicity may be regarded as type I immune response pattern diseases [9]. The physiological and evolutionary significance of cellular cytotoxicity against self is to sacrifice some of the body's cells in order to protect the whole organism. This is particularly relevant in the case of intracellular infections, as well as in premalignant or malignant cancer cells. Type I immunity is mediated by a subset of lymphocytes, the so-called type I immune cells which comprise CD8+ cytotoxic T cells, T helper 1 (Th1) cells, innate lymphoid cells (ILCs) and natural killer (NK) cells or NKT cells [10]. The overarching transcription factor of all these lymphocytes is Tbet; activation of type I cells leads to secretion of cytokines such as interferon γ (IFN-γ) or tumour necrosis factor (TNF). In fact, Tbet and CXCR3-positive type I immune cells dominate the dense cellular infiltrate in the lesional skin in LP [11,12] and chemokines such as CXCL9 released by keratinocytes in response to IFN-γ can be used as a diagnostic biomarker for LP [13].

Rook's Textbook of Dermatology, Tenth Edition. Edited by Christopher Griffiths, Jonathan Barker, Tanya Bleiker, Walayat Hussain and Rosalind Simpson.
© 2024 John Wiley & Sons Ltd. Published 2024 by John Wiley & Sons Ltd.

Type I immune cells orchestrate keratinocyte killing at the basal epidermis via different mechanisms. Usually, these mechanisms occur in parallel; the predominating mechanism most likely depends on the microenvironment. First, type I immune cells induce keratinocyte apoptosis and the inflammatory variant of apoptosis, so-called necroptosis. These mechanisms occur through upregulation of major histocompatibility complex (MHC) class I molecules and adhesion molecules such as intercellular adhesion molecule 1 (ICAM-1) on keratinocytes in response to IFN-γ and/or TNF. This upregulation of cell surface receptors is mediated via JAK (Janus kinase)/STAT (signal transducers and activators of transcription) signalling in keratinocytes. Besides contact-dependent cytotoxicity, type I immune cells may also kill basal keratinocytes via soluble mediators released by granule exocytosis. Granules released by type I immune cells contain membrane-destructing molecules such as perforin and granulysin, and induce cytotoxicity via granzymes that cause cell death via distinct caspase-independent mechanisms within the target cell [14]. Perforin, granulysin and granzymes are all highly overexpressed in LP skin [15]. Finally, type I immune cells release other cytotoxic molecules, among them Fas and TRAIL (tumour necrosis factor-related apoptosis-inducing ligand). Both of these molecules result in keratinocyte death. They have been well studied in the context of contact dermatitis. Taken together, type I immune cells kill basal keratinocytes by apoptosis, necroptosis and the release of cytotoxic granules (Figure 37.1). At least some of these cytotoxic mechanisms require recognition of a cognate antigen by adaptive type I immune cells. The structure of the recognised antigen in most lichenoid diseases of the skin is still not known. A subset of patients seem to react to epidermal structures such as desmogleins or bullous pemphigoid antigen 180 [16]. It is speculated that these antigens are recognised by type I immune cells that had differentiated from naive precursor cells as a response to a virus. These virus-specific T cells now recognise epidermal antigens as potentially harmful because of structural similarities with virus-derived peptides, a process called molecular mimicry [17]. This hypothesis is supported by the observation that hepatitis C virus infections are associated with the development of LP.

Genetics

There is no genetic factor yet identified that strongly predisposes to LP. Nevertheless, there are reports of familial LP and monozygotic twins both affected by this disease [18,19]. Most single nucleotide peptides (SNPs) associated with LP are HLA class I and class II molecules, but none of them has the clinical utility to be mentioned here [19,**20**].

Environmental factors

In the vast majority of LP patients, no causative factor can be identified. However, chronic viral infections, drugs, contact allergens and others have been reported to be associated with LP.

Hepatitis and other viruses. In a meta-analysis, the pooled odds ratio point estimate for the prevalence of hepatitis C in LP patients was 5.4 (95% confidence interval (CI) 3.5–8.3) [21]. Therefore, it is recommended to perform hepatitis screening at first diagnosis of LP. However, there is no clear evidence for a causative relationship and some authors regard the observed association between LP and hepatitis as a regional coincidence in areas with a high prevalence of both [22]. On the other hand, there are case reports describing a new onset of LP after vaccination for hepatitis B [23], indicating that vaccine-mediated type I immune responses might initiate LP development. In line with the cytotoxic immune response pattern mediated by type I immune cells that is the molecular basis of LP, there are associations with several other viruses reported, such as human papillomavirus (HPV), human herpesvirus 7 (HHV-7), varicella-zoster virus (VZV) and Epstein–Barr virus (EBV). LP can also be triggered after vaccination against hepatitis, influenza, or SARS-CoV-2 [19].

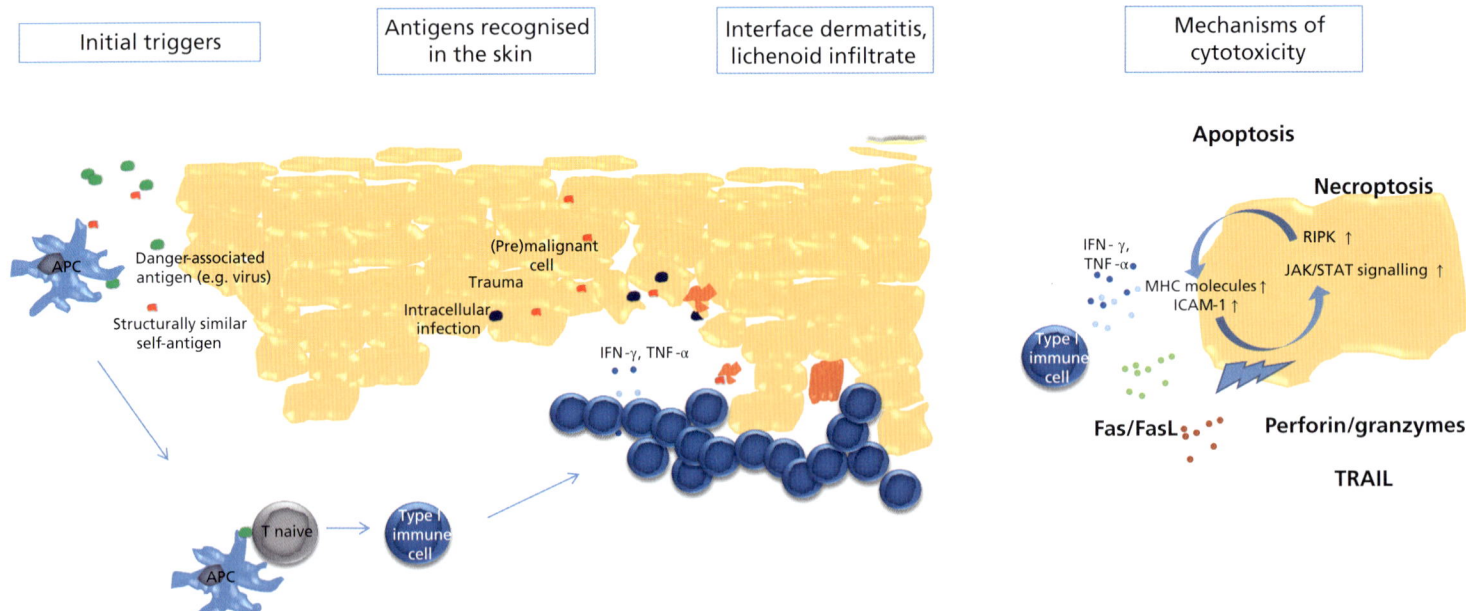

Figure 37.1 Pathogenesis of lichenoid disorders. APC, antigen-presenting cell; RIPK, receptor-interacting serine/threonine kinase 1; for other abbreviations, see text.

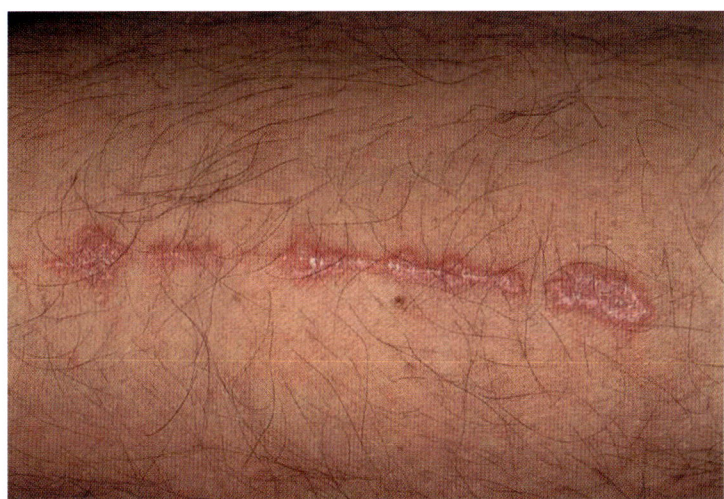

Figure 37.2 Lichen planus induced by mechanical irritation (Koebner phenomenon). Courtesy of University of Munich.

Bacterial or fungal dysbiosis. While the association to viruses is well described, there is less evidence for bacterial and/or fungal colonisation and LP. Microbiome and mycobiome studies suggest possible targets of T-cell activation in oral LP by periodontal pathogens [24].

Mechanical irritation. As for other inflammatory skin diseases, mechanical irritation can induce LP skin lesions (the Koebner phenomenon) (Figure 37.2). Linear LP lesions are suggestive for mechanically induced LP, however they must be distinguished from lichen striatus and inflammatory linear verrucous epidermal naevus (ILVEN), which follow the Blaschko lines.

Drugs. Many drugs have been linked with cutaneous eruptions similar or identical to LP. Often the terms LP-like eruption or lichenoid eruption are used in the context of an adverse drug reaction with features of LP. The list of drugs causing LP and LP-like eruptions has grown steadily and includes several classes, including antimicrobials, antihypertensives, antimalarials, antidepressants, anticonvulsants, diuretics, metals, non-steroidal anti-inflammatory drugs (NSAIDs) and more recently imatinib [25], intravenous immunoglobulin [26], etanercept [26] and adalimumab [27]. These reactions are described in more detail in Chapter 117.

Dental amalgam. Another putative antigen in oral LP is the mercury in dental amalgam [28], however oral contact allergies (allergic contact stomatitis) must be ruled out as it might mimic the clinical picture of mucosal LP. Clear associations between amalgam and oral LP have not been proven [29].

Betel nut. Social use of the betel nut is relatively common in India and South-East Asia. The product that is chewed, betel quid, is a mixture of substances including the areca nut and betel leaf, and is associated with oral LP [30,31].

Lichen planus-like contact dermatitis. While acute contact dermatitis leads to eczematous eruptions, chronic allergen exposure can induce LP-like contact dermatitis. Industry workers exposed

to allergenic chemicals, such as *para*-phenylenediamine, without sufficient protective equipment are at high risk for developing LP-like contact dermatitis. Historically, LP-like eruptions were reported in up to 25% of persons exposed to the chemicals found in colour developer [32]. Furthermore, LP-like lesions have developed on skin exposed to methacrylic acid esters used in the car industry, and more recently from dimethylfumarate, which can be found in sofas [33]. Due to automated equipment these cases are rare nowadays [32].

Clinical features
Presentation

The classic clinical presentation of LP includes primary lesions consisting of firm, shiny, polygonal, 1–3 mm diameter papules with a red to violet colour. More closely, a tracery of thin white lines can be seen on the surface of the lesions, known as Wickham striae (Figure 37.3) [34]. Papules can be isolated or grouped in a linear or annular distribution. Typically, a greyish brown pigmentation can be observed in lesions that have resolved due to deposition of melanin in the superficial dermis. LP can affect any part of the body surface, but is most often seen on the volar aspect of the wrists (Figure 37.4), the lumbar region and around the ankles. The ankles

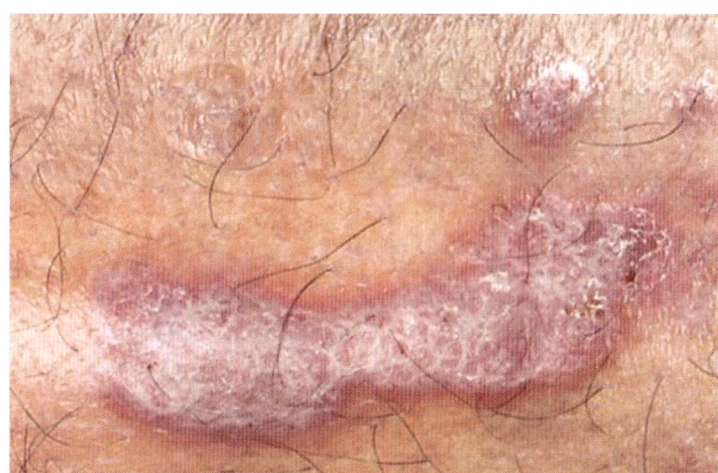

Figure 37.3 Lichen planus. Close up to show Wickham striae. Courtesy of University of Munich.

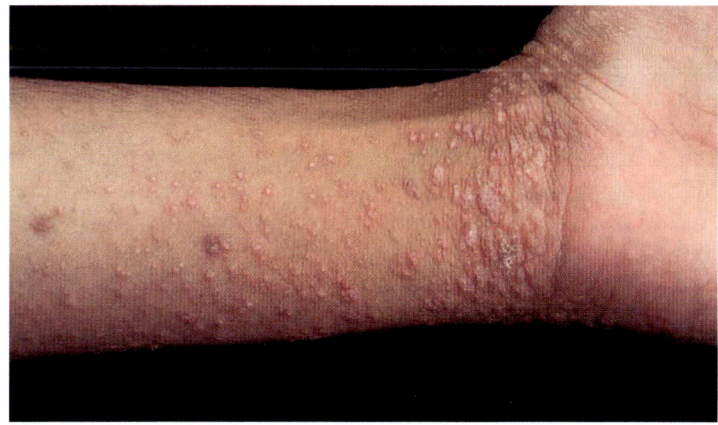

Figure 37.4 Lichen planus. Classic eruption on the volar aspect of the wrist. Courtesy of University of Munich.

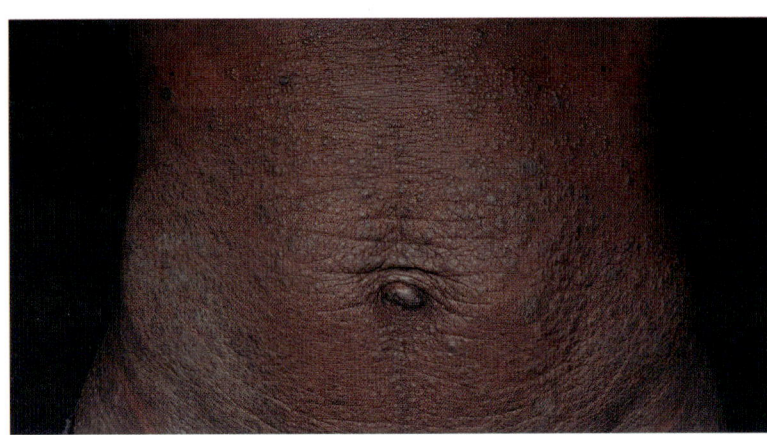

(a)

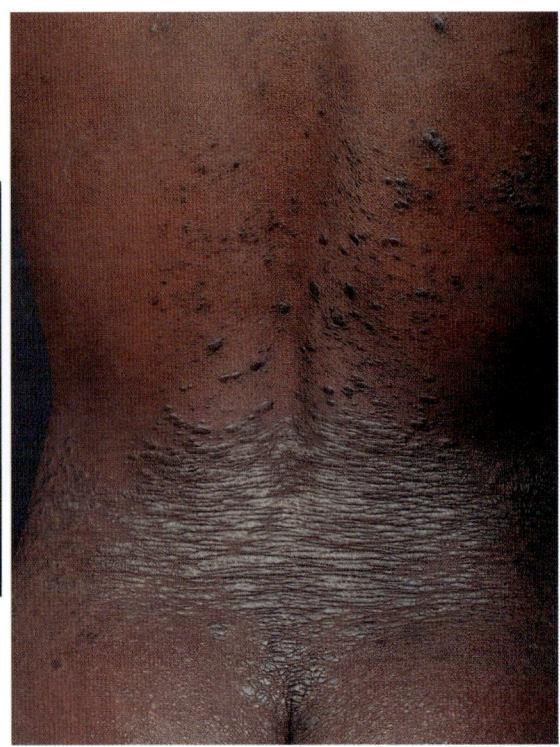

(b)

Figure 37.5 (a, b) Lichen exanthematicus. Courtesy of University of Munich.

and shins are the commonest sites for hypertrophic lesions. Lichen exanthematicus develops rapidly and usually affects the limbs and trunk (Figure 37.5). Annular atrophic LP lesions are especially common on the acral and genital areas (Figure 37.6) and rarely may be the predominant type of lesion present. Lichen planopilaris is a variant in which groups of 'spiny' lesions resembling keratosis pilaris develop around hair follicles of the scalp, leading to a progressive scarring alopecia (Figure 37.7). Lichen planopilaris often occurs solely and sometimes in association with classic LP. When the palms and soles are affected, the lesions tend to be firm and rough with a yellowish hue (Figure 37.8) [35]. Linear LP occurring within the Blaschko lines has also been observed [36]. Rare variants include erosive, flexural LP [37] and isolated lesions of LP on the eyelids [38,39] or lips [40–42].

Mucous membrane lesions are very common, occurring in 30–70% of cases, and may be present without evidence of skin lesions. They are, however, much less common in black people. The buccal mucosa and tongue are most often involved, but lesions may be found around the anus, on the genitalia, in the larynx and, very rarely, on the tympanic membranes or even in the oesophagus. White streaks, often forming a lacework, on the buccal mucosa are highly characteristic (Figure 37.9). They may be seen on the inner surface of the cheeks, on the gum margins or on the lips. On the tongue, the lesions are usually in the form of fixed, white plaques, often slightly depressed below the surrounding normal mucous membrane, especially on the upper surface and edges. Ulcerative lesions in the mouth are uncommon, but may be the site of epitheliomatous transformation (Figure 37.10). There may be striking pigmentation of oral LP in darkly pigmented people [43]. Diabetes is a possible associated disease of oral LP [44,45], and candidiasis may coexist with LP in some patients.

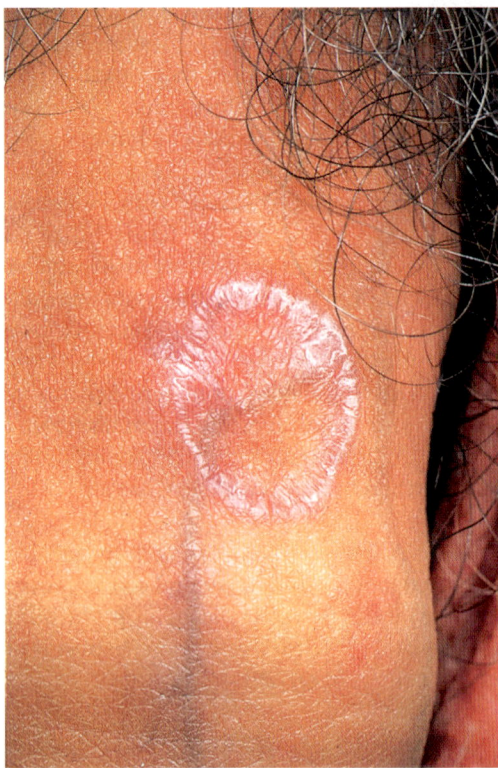

Figure 37.6 Lichen planus showing an annular lesion on the shaft of the penis. Courtesy of St John's Institute of Dermatology, King's College London, UK.

Pruritus is a consistent feature in LP and ranges from occasional mild irritation to more or less continuous, severe itching which interferes with sleep and makes life almost intolerable; very occasionally, pruritus is completely absent. Hypertrophic lesions

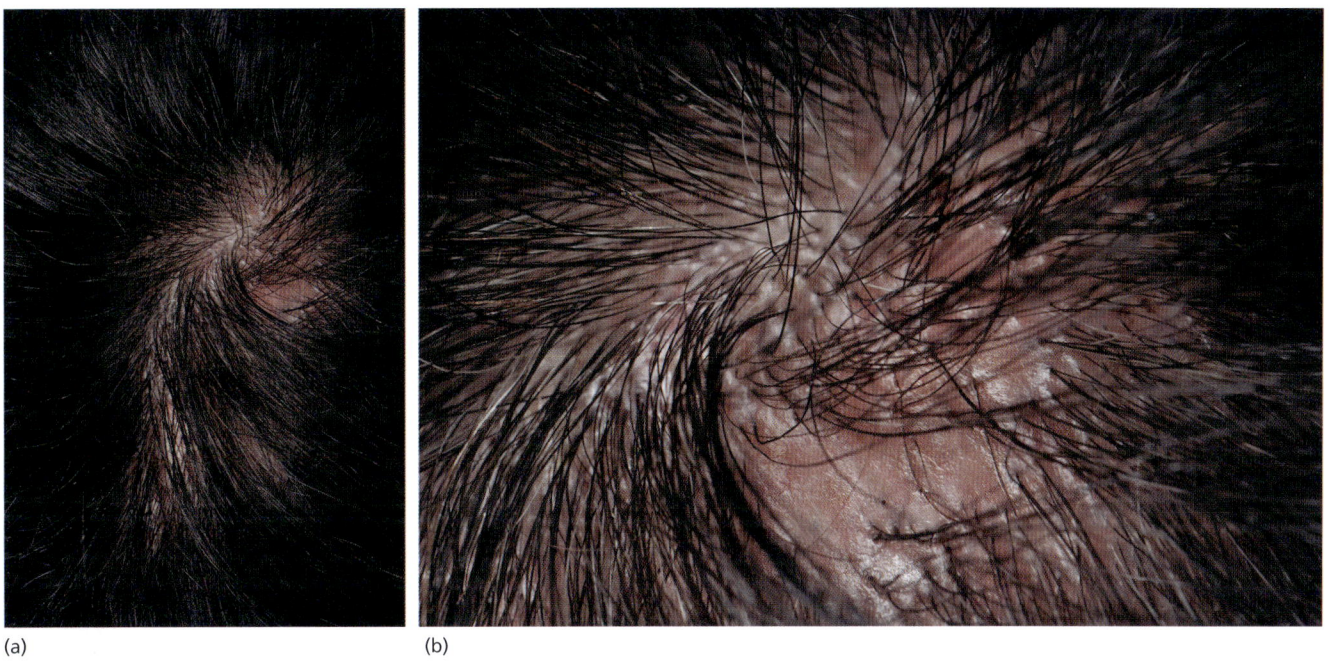

Figure 37.7 (a, b) Lichen planopilaris showing perifollicular redness and hyperkeratosis, tufts of hair within one follicle and scaring alopecia. Courtesy of University of Munich.

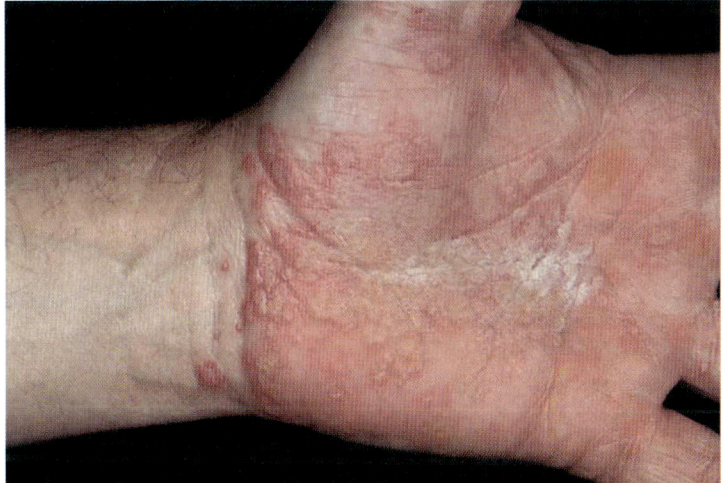

Figure 37.8 Lichen planus of the palm showing hyperkeratosis and a yellow colour. Courtesy of University of Munich.

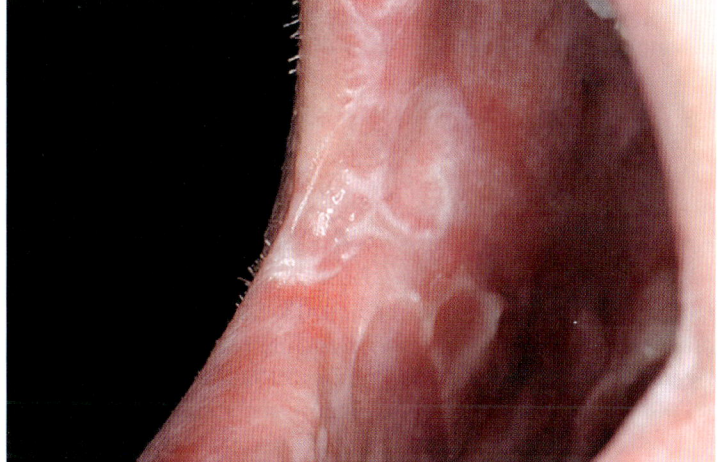

Figure 37.9 Lichen planus on the buccal mucosa showing a lacework of white streaks. Courtesy of the Welsh Institute of Dermatology, University Hospital of Wales, Cardiff, Wales, UK.

usually itch severely. Paradoxically, there is seldom evidence of scratching, as the patient tends to rub to gain relief. Itching at sites without visible skin lesions can occur. Burning and stinging are less frequent. The patient may complain of discomfort, stinging or pain in the mouth; ulcerated lesions are especially painful. Great discomfort may be caused by hot foods and drinks.

Clinical variants

Oral lichen planus. Lesions confined to the mouth, or with minimal accompanying skin involvement, are not uncommon [46–51] and account for about 15% of all cases. Mucosal lichen sclerosis/LP overlap syndrome can also be observed [46]. The prevalence of oral LP ranges between 0.5% and 2.2% in epidemiological studies [47,52].

The lesions do not differ from those found in connection with skin lesions, but, being confined to the mouth, may lead to great difficulty in diagnosis. They are often referred first to a dental surgeon as the most relevant differential diagnosis is epithelial neoplasms of the mucosa. Of note, mucosal LP is regarded as pre-cancerous as the chronic inflammation favours the development of dysplasia and squamous cell carcinoma [53]. Distinct clinical subtypes such as reticular, atrophic, hypertrophic and erosive forms are well recognised, and more than one type may be present [47]. Of these, erosive forms of oral LP severely impact patients' quality of life. On the tongue and buccal mucosa, lesions are most likely to be mistaken for leukoplakia and on the gum margin for gingivitis or chronic candidiasis; the latter conditions may coexist. Other

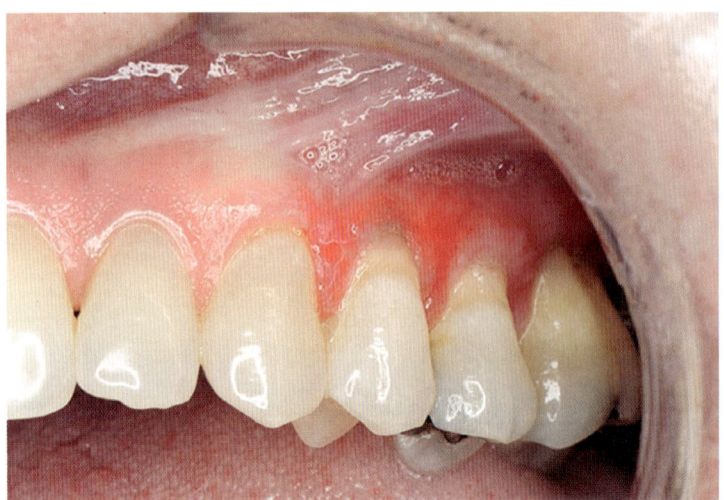

Figure 37.10 Erosive lichen planus of the buccal mucosa. Courtesy of the Welsh Institute of Dermatology, University Hospital of Wales, Cardiff, Wales, UK.

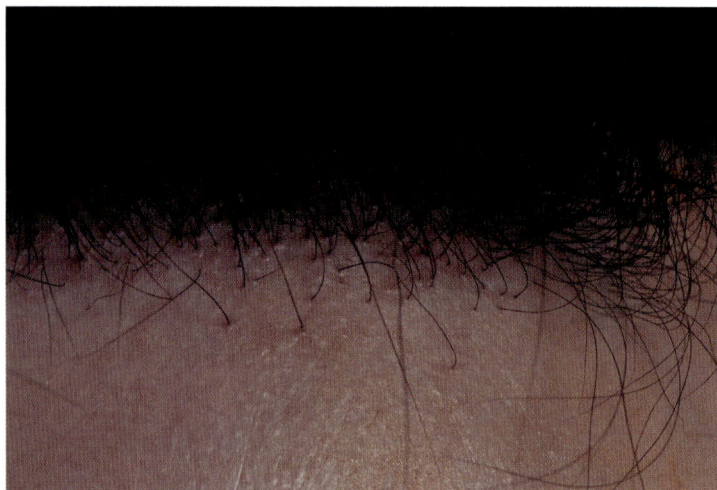

Figure 37.11 Frontal fibrosing alopecia with follicular hyperkeratosis and 'lonely hairs'. Courtesy of University of Munich.

conditions that must be excluded are 'smoker's patches', which characteristically involve the palate, and white-sponge naevi, in which the mucous membrane is thickened, irregularly folded and feels soft to the touch. These occur mainly on the floor of the mouth and histologically many of the prickle cells in the epidermis are vacuolated. It is important to bear in mind the possibility of a lichenoid drug reaction in patients with oral lichenoid changes (Chapter 108). Oral lichenoid reactions may be asymmetrical on the buccal mucosa and occur adjacent to dental amalgam fillings. If patch testing reveals mercury allergy, changing to another type of filling may prove beneficial [54–59]. Very occasionally, LP lesions extend to the larynx or oesophagus [60–64]. Oesophageal LP may result in dysphagia and the formation of benign strictures.

Lichen planus involving genital mucosa. In young men, the lesions of LP are sometimes restricted to the genitalia and/or mouth [65,66]. Genital lesions, which are usually characteristic, may be present on the penile shaft (Figure 37.6), glans penis, prepuce or scrotum. Ulceration is very unlikely, and syphilis can usually be excluded without difficulty. The presence of buccal mucosal lesions will usually confirm the diagnosis. Circumcision may be helpful in resolving LP [65].

Lesions on the female genitalia are common [67–74]; they may occur alone, be combined with lesions in the mouth only, or be part of widespread involvement. The clinical presentation of LP of the vulva spans a spectrum from subtle, fine, reticulate papules to severe erosive disease accompanied by dyspareunia, scarring and loss of the normal vulvar architecture. In these cases, genital LP can be difficult to distinguish from lichen sclerosus. Diagnostic criteria have been proposed [**75**] and include well-demarcated erosions/red areas at the vaginal introitus, the presence of a hyperkeratotic border to lesions and/or Wickham striae in the surrounding skin, symptoms of pain/burning, scarring/loss of normal architecture, the presence of vaginal inflammation and the involvement of other mucosal surfaces. Histologically, a well-defined inflammatory band involving the dermal–epidermal junction and consisting predominantly of lymphocytes and signs of basal layer

degeneration are seen. Coexisting vulval lichen sclerosus and lichenoid oral lesions have been described [76].

Lichen planopilaris.

Synonyms and inclusions
- Follicular lichen planus

Follicular lesions can either appear during the course of typical LP or they predominate, making diagnosis difficult. Follicular lesions occurring in the scalp are accompanied by some scaling and are likely to lead to a scarring alopecia (Figure 37.11). Histologically, a perivascular and perifollicular lymphocytic infiltrate in the reticular dermis, mucinous perifollicular fibroplasia within the upper dermis with an absence of interfollicular mucin, an absence of arrector pili muscles and sebaceous glands, and superficial perifollicular wedge-shaped scarring are characteristic features [77]. Presentation with alopecia of the trunk is recorded [78]. The Graham-Little–Piccardi–Lassueur syndrome comprises the triad of multifocal scalp cicatricial alopecia, non-scarring alopecia of the axillae and/or groin and keratotic lichenoid follicular papules [79–84]. The clinical, histological and immunofluorescence overlap between this syndrome and LP with follicular involvement (lichen planopilaris) suggest that both are variants of LP. Follicular LP must be distinguished by biopsy from keratosis pilaris, Darier disease, follicular mucinosis, lichen scrofulosorum and, in the scalp, from lupus erythematosus.

Frontal fibrosing alopecia is a scalp condition that affects elderly women in particular and frequently involves the eyebrows. Typically it leads to so-called 'lonely hairs', which represent residual hairs within a scarring alopecia of the frontal scalp. It has been regarded by some authors as a clinically distinct variant of lichen planopilaris [85] but is considered by most to be a variant [86], and is certainly associated with mucocutaneous LP [87,88] (Chapter 105).

Hypertrophic lichen planus. This usually develops during a subacute attack, but occasionally only hypertrophic or warty lesions

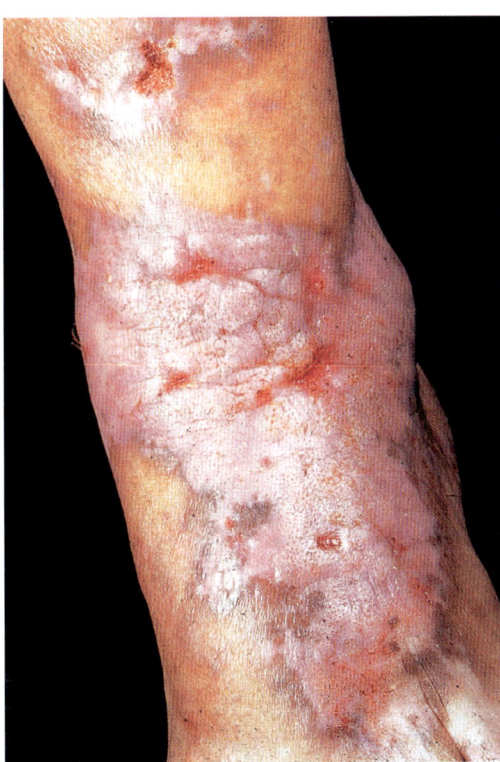

Figure 37.12 Hypertrophic lichen planus of great chronicity occurring on the lower leg and ankle. Courtesy of St John's Institute of Dermatology, King's College London, UK.

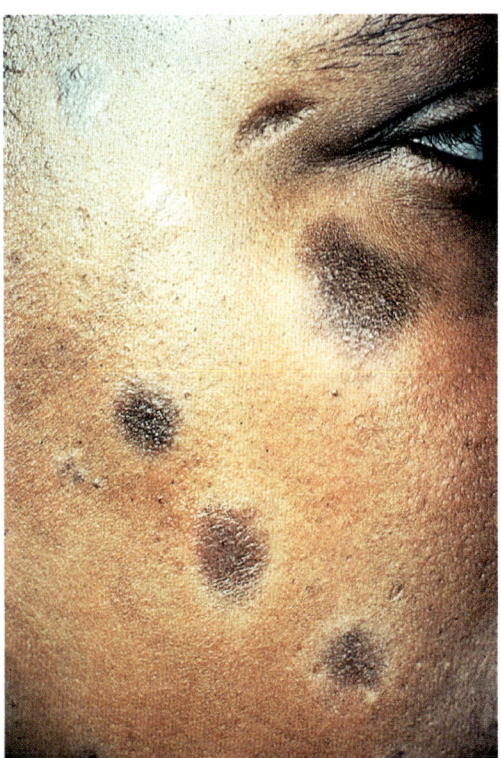

Figure 37.13 Lichen planus actinicus showing well-defined, pigmented, nummular patches on the face. Courtesy of St John's Institute of Dermatology, King's College London, UK.

are found. They most often occur on the lower limbs, especially around the ankles (Figure 37.12); venous stasis has been postulated as an explanation. The development of hypertrophic lesions greatly lengthens the course of the disease as they may persist for many years. When such lesions eventually clear, an area of pigmentation and scarring may remain and there is often some degree of atrophy. They must be distinguished from lichen simplex chronicus and lichen amyloidosus (papular). Multiple cutaneous horns overlying hypertrophic LP are recorded [89], as are keratoacanthoma [90,91] and malignant transformation [92–94] arising in hypertrophic LP, as well as metastatic squamous cell carcinoma [95].

Lichen planus of the palms and soles. Although lesions on the volar aspect of the wrists or at the ankles occur in more than 50% of cases of LP, lesions on the adjacent palms and soles are less common, lack the characteristic shape and colour of lesions elsewhere and are firm to the touch and yellow in hue (see Figure 37.8) [96]. They may be broad sheets or show up as punctate keratoses [97]. Vesicle-like papules are recorded [98]. Itching may be absent. When such changes occur in isolation, diagnosis is very difficult; syphilis, psoriasis, callosities and warts must be excluded.

Actinic lichen planus.

'Actinic' or (sub)tropical LP generally occurs in children or young adults with dark skin living in tropical countries; virtually all cases originate from the Middle East, East Africa or India [99–103]. Lesions occur on exposed skin (usually the face) as well-defined annular or discoid patches, which have a deeply hyperpigmented centre surrounded by a striking hypopigmented zone (Figure 37.13). Erythematous actinic LP has been associated with oral erosive LP and chronic active hepatitis [104]. Sunlight exposure appears to be central to the pathogenesis of actinic LP [105], although evidence for photo-induction of lesions in actinic LP is still lacking [106]. Actinic LP may mimic melasma [107]. There is a histological spectrum comprising a form with features of classic idiopathic LP; an intermediate form (lichenoid melanodermatitis) with foci of spongiosis and parakeratosis; and a more overtly eczematous type [108]. All share striking pigmentary incontinence. Some of these 'hybrids' of actinic LP may not be mere variants of LP.

Lichen planus pigmentosus. This is a pigmentary disorder seen in India or in the Middle East, which may or may not be associated with typical LP papules [109–111]. The macular hyperpigmentation involves chiefly the face, neck and upper limbs, although it can be more widespread, and varies from slate grey to brownish black. It is mostly diffuse, but reticular, blotchy and perifollicular forms are seen [98,111]. The duration at presentation ranged from 2 months to 21 years in one series [111]. Occasionally, there is a striking predominance of lesions at intertriginous sites, especially the axillae [112,113]. The mucous membranes, palms and soles are usually not involved, but involvement of mucous membranes has been observed [114]. LP pigmentosus has been anecdotally reported in association with acrokeratosis of Bazex [115].

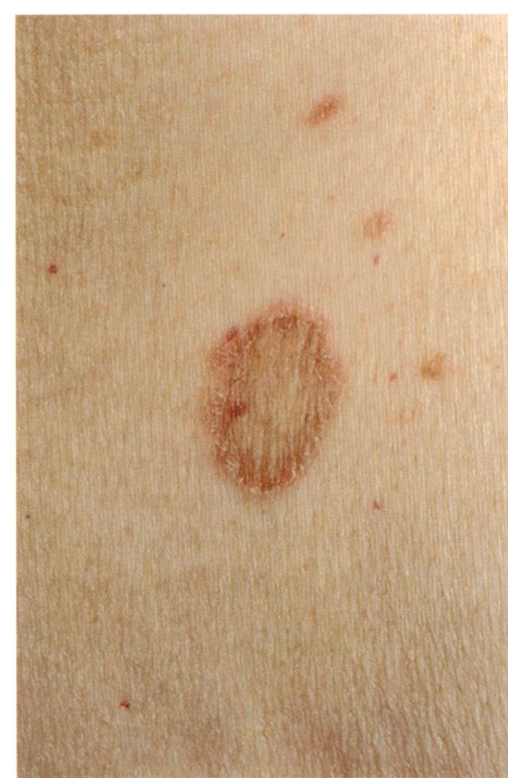

(a)

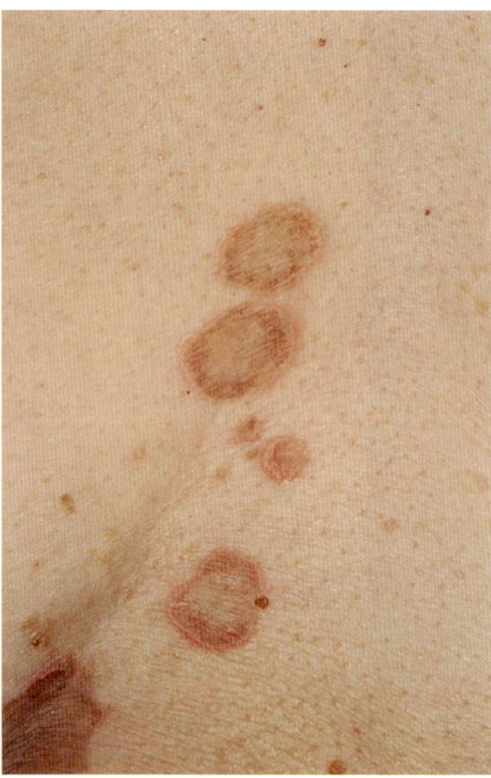

(b)

Figure 37.14 (a, b) Annular lichen planus. Courtesy of the Welsh Institute of Dermatology, University Hospital of Wales, Cardiff, Wales, UK.

Annular lichen planus. Although small annular lesions are common in LP, cases showing a few large annular lesions only are unusual. They may be widely scattered, and usually have a very narrow rim of activity and a depressed, slightly atrophic centre (Figure 37.14) [116]. Much less frequently, the margin is wide and the central area is small. Annular lesions are characteristically found on the penis (see Figure 37.6), sometimes associated with lesions on the buccal mucosa. The differential diagnosis includes granuloma annulare. A distinct entity termed annular lichenoid dermatitis of youth [97,98,117,118] has been described, characterised by persistent, asymptomatic reddish macules and round, annular patches with a red-brownish border and central hypopigmentation, mostly distributed on the groin and flanks, in children and adolescents. Histology reveals an atrophic epidermis and interface dermatitis with necroptosis/apoptosis of the keratinocytes limited to the tips of rete ridges.

Guttate lichen planus. Lesions are widely scattered and remain discrete, they may be all small (1–2 mm across) or larger (up to 1 cm), and individual lesions seldom become chronic (Figure 37.15). Guttate psoriasis and pityriasis rosea must be excluded as a differential. Guttate LP may be regarded as a variant of lichenoid exanthema (see later in this chapter).

Acute and subacute lichen planus with a confluence of lesions. In these forms, small lesions are widely distributed and may simulate eczema. Colour changes may be marked, with individual lesions initially red but progressing rapidly to black as they fade. Successive crops may occur, such that the total time for clearance may be little different from other forms. A small minority clear in under 3 months. The differential diagnosis includes pityriasis rosea

in the earliest phase, and eczema later; once again, drug-induced lichenoid eruptions or lichenoid exanthema may present in this fashion.

'Mixed' lichen planus/discoid lupus erythematosus disease patterns. Discoid lupus erythematosus (DLE) and LP are usually considered as distinct entities with characteristic clinical, histopathological and immunopathological features, with basement membrane deposition of immunoglobulin G (IgG) in DLE [119,120]. However, similarities between LP and DLE have been noted. In addition, there have been several reports of patients showing overlapping features of both disorders [121–126]. Chronic atrophic DLE-like lesions on the head, neck and upper trunk may accompany reticular white lesions in the oral cavity, and combinations of lichenoid or verrucous lesions are seen. Eyelid involvement has been recorded [127]. The association of extensive generalised LP with subacute cutaneous DLE has also been documented [128].

Bullous lichen planus and lichen planus pemphigoides. Lichen ruber pemphigoides was first described by Kaposi in 1892. Bullous LP and LP pemphigoides were in the past differentiated solely on clinical and histological criteria [129] but can now be differentiated using immunofluorescence (IMF) and immunoelectron microscopy. In bullous LP, blisters arise only on or near the lesions of LP, because of maximal interface dermatitis with widespread degeneration of the basal cell layer [130]. Histologically, there is subepidermal bulla formation with typical changes of LP, and direct and indirect IMF is negative [130,131]. The eruption is usually only of short duration [131]. In LP pemphigoides, the LP tends to be acute and generalised and is followed by the sudden appearance of large bullae on both involved and uninvolved skin (Figure 37.16) [132–135].

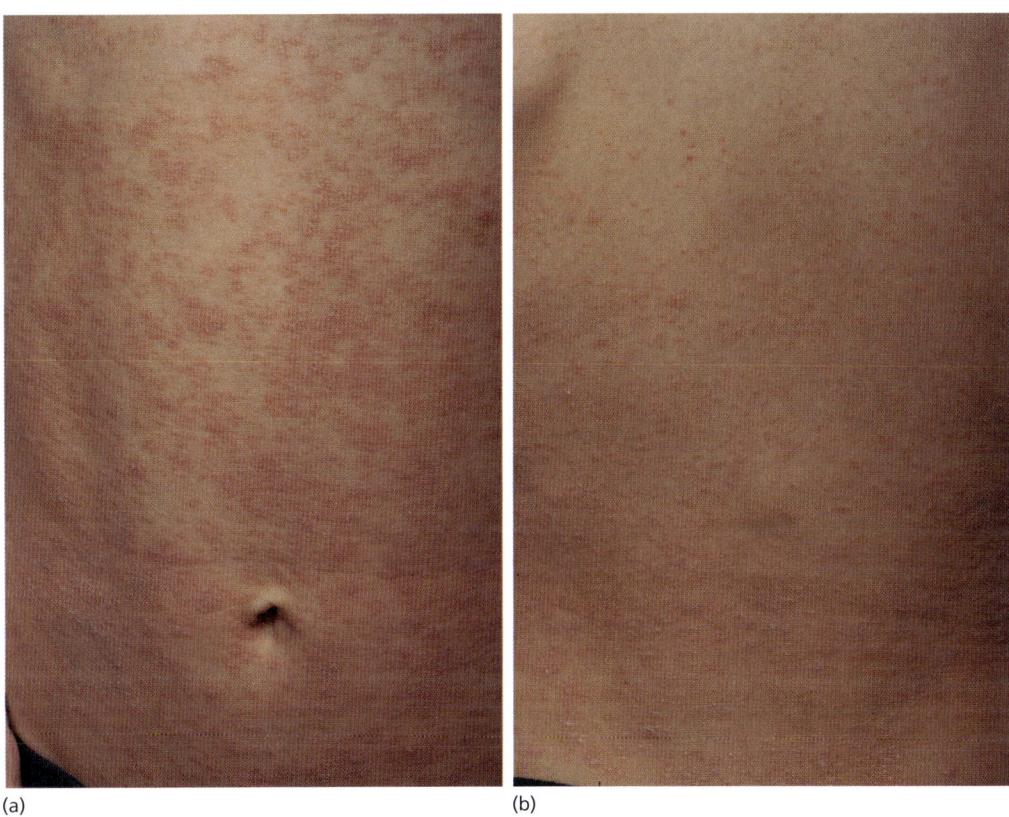

Figure 37.15 (a, b) Guttate lichen planus. Courtesy of University of Munich.

(a)   (b)

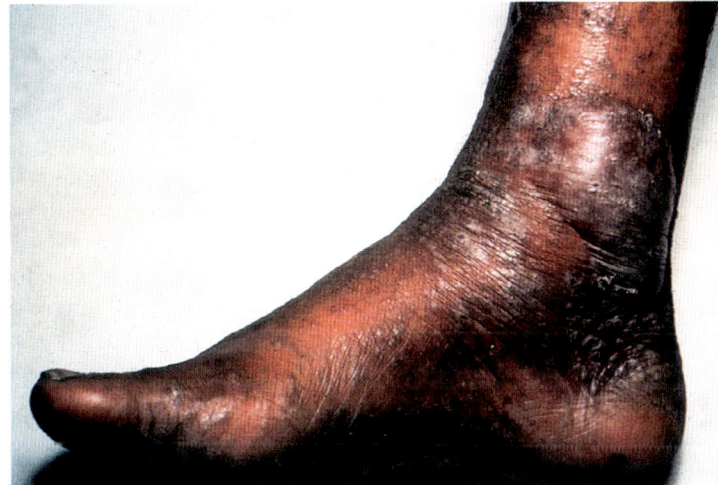

Figure 37.16 Lichen planus pemphigoides showing large bulla arising on and around the vicinity of lichen planus around the ankle. Courtesy of St John's Institute of Dermatology, King's College London, UK.

Occasionally, even in LP pemphigoides, blisters may arise only on the lesions of LP [136]. LP pemphigoides has been precipitated by psoralen and ultraviolet A (PUVA) [137] and has evolved into pemphigoid nodularis [138]. An LP pemphigoides-like eruption has been reported to overlap with paraneoplastic pemphigus [139,140]. In LP pemphigoides, the histology shows a subepidermal bulla with no evidence of associated LP [131]. Direct IMF shows linear basement membrane zone deposition of IgG and C3 in perilesional skin [131,135]. Immunoelectron microscopic studies reveal deposition of IgG and C3 in the base of the bulla and not in the roof as found in bullous pemphigoid [141].

Immunoblotting data have revealed that circulating autoantibodies in LP pemphigoides react with an epitope within the C-terminal NC16A domain of bullous pemphigoid 180 kDa antigen, and with a 200 kDa antigen detected in bullous pemphigoid [142,**143**,144–146]. It seems that epidermal damage from liquefaction degeneration in LP exposes basement membrane antigens, and a consequent stimulation of autoantibody production. The mean age of patients with LP pemphigoides is lower than that of those with classic bullous pemphigoid, and the course of the disease also tends to be less severe.

Lichen nitidus. Lichen nitidus is a rarer condition than classic LP and is characterised clinically by the presence of small papules, which are usually asymptomatic and flesh-coloured, with a flat, shiny surface. The view that lichen nitidus represents a variant of LP tends to be supported by the fact that early, tiny LP papules may be clinically and histopathologically indistinguishable from lichen nitidus. Immunophenotypic studies also reinforce the association between LP and lichen nitidus [147]. However, some authors favour a separation into two dermatoses because of histopathological differences such as parakeratotic papules occurring typically in lichen nitidus [148,149].

Typical lichen nitidus papules are minute, pinpoint to pinhead sized, and have a flat or dome-shaped, shiny surface. They usually remain discrete, although they may be closely grouped (Figure 37.17). They are found on any part of the body but the sites of predilection are the forearms, penis, abdomen (Figure 37.18), chest and buttocks. The eruption is sometimes generalised [150,151]. When the palms or soles are involved, the changes can be those of a confluent hyperkeratosis resembling chronic fissured eczema, or there may be multiple, distinctive, minute papules [152,153].

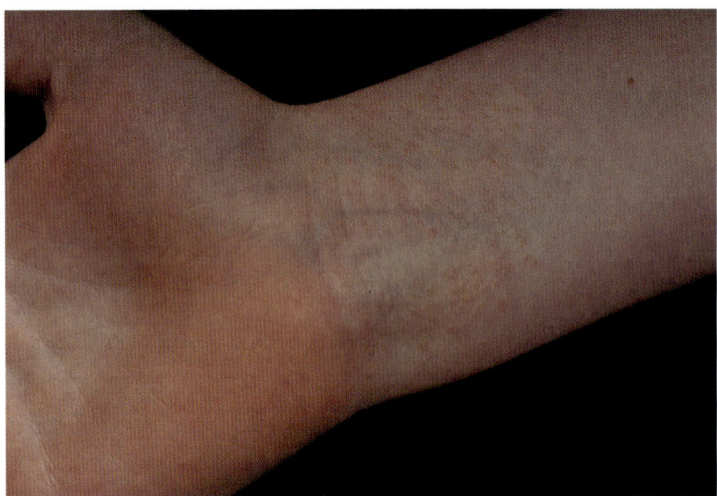

Figure 37.17 Lichen nitidus showing aggregated, pinhead-sized papules. Courtesy of University of Munich.

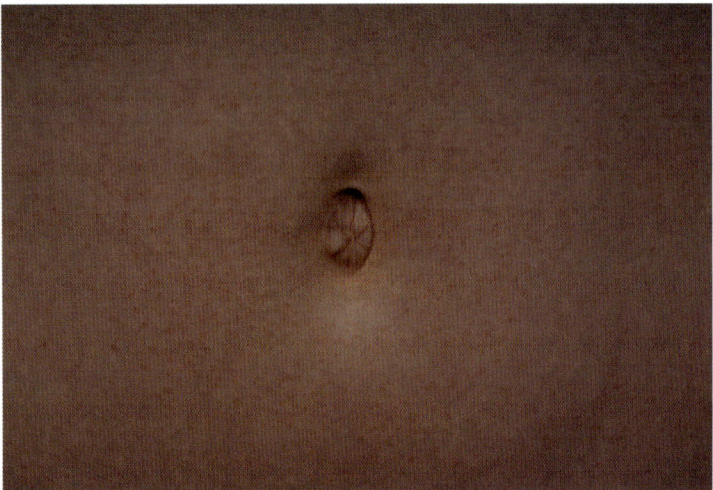

Figure 37.18 Lichen nitidus showing aggregates of pinhead-sized papules on the trunk of a 7-year-old boy Courtesy of University of Munich.

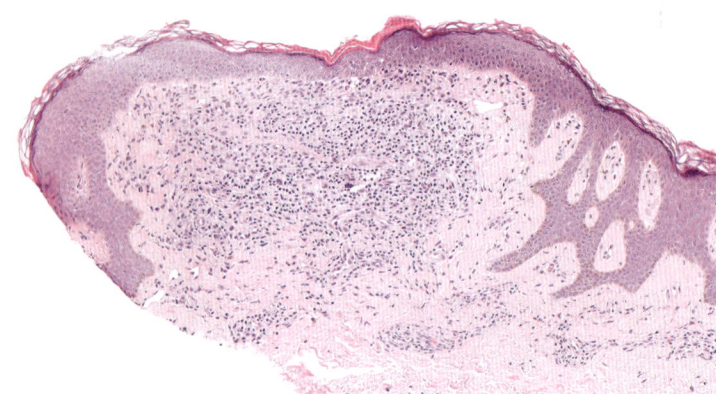

Figure 37.19 Lichen nitidus. Typical histology showing the focally dense infiltrate containing a few giant cells. Magnification 100× (H&E). Courtesy of St John's Institute of Dermatology, King's College London, UK.

On the palms, the minute papules can become purpuric and may occasionally resemble pompholyx. Such cases may lack lesions of lichen nitidus elsewhere, so a biopsy is essential to confirm the diagnosis [152,154].

Linear lichen nitidus has been described but is exceptionally rare [155]. The development of lesions along scratch marks is not uncommon. The lesions are flesh coloured or reddish brown. Although intense pruritus can occur [151], the lesions are generally symptomless. Nail pitting may coexist with lichen nitidus [156], or the affected nails may appear rough due to increased linear striations and longitudinal ridging [152,157]. An actinic variant has been documented [158]. Mucous membrane lesions occur occasionally and are much rarer than in LP. Lichen nitidus must be distinguished from the tuberculid lichen scrofulosorum [159], where there are follicular papules grouped in small patches on the trunk, and from keratosis pilaris, where there are horny follicular papules mainly on the extensor surface of the limbs. In cases of doubt, a biopsy usually clarifies the diagnosis. Lichen nitidus has been described in association with Crohn disease, trisomy 21, congenital megacolon

[160], Niemann–Pick disease type B [161] and therapy with the checkpoint inhibitor nivolumab [162].

The histology of a typical papule is characteristic. The papule is formed by an intense infiltrate situated immediately below the epidermis and is well circumscribed. The infiltrate consists of lymphocytes and histiocytes and there are often a few Langerhans giant cells (Figure 37.19). Plasma cells may be numerous in the infiltrate [163]. The overlying epidermis is flattened and sometimes with liquefaction degeneration of the basal cell layer. The rete ridges at the margin of the infiltrate are elongated and tend to encircle it. Although tuberculoid in appearance, true tubercle formation or caseation never occur. The histology of a palmar lesion may show a deep parakeratotic plug, which distinguishes it from the palmar lesions of LP [154]. Perifollicular granulomas can occur in spinous and follicular lichen nitidus, which may simulate lichen scrofulosorum [159]. Perforating lichen nitidus has also been described [164]. In its characteristic monomorphic form, lichen nitidus is rare, but lesions of lichen nitidus occurring in association with LP are more common. The age incidence tends to be lower than that of LP. Most cases occur in children or young adults. Familial lichen nitidus has rarely been observed [165].

Nékam disease.

Synonyms and inclusions
- Keratosis lichenoides chronica
- Orokeratosis striata lichenoides
- Lichen ruber moniliformis
- Lichen verrucosus et reticularis

The variety of synonyms used implies that there is no complete consensus of agreement about this rare disorder. The great majority of cases are adults between the ages of 20 and 40 years [166], although children are occasionally affected [167]. Nékam disease is characterised by violaceous, papular and nodular lesions typically arranged in a linear and reticulate pattern (Figure 37.20), most marked on the extremities and buttocks, and accompanied by a seborrhoeic dermatitis-like eruption on the face. Nékam's

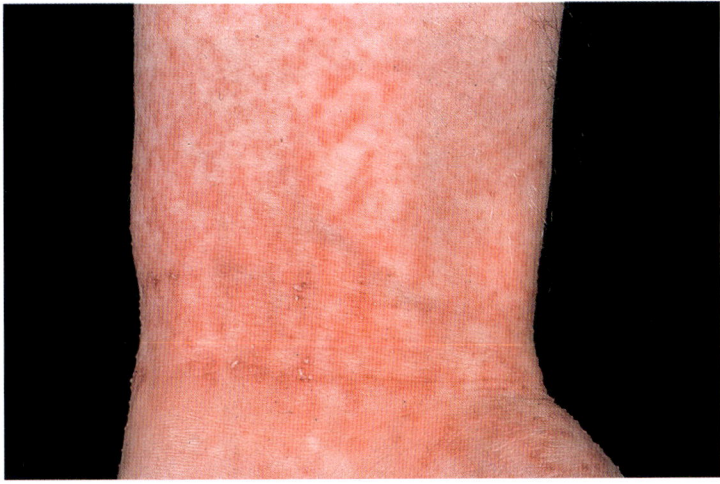

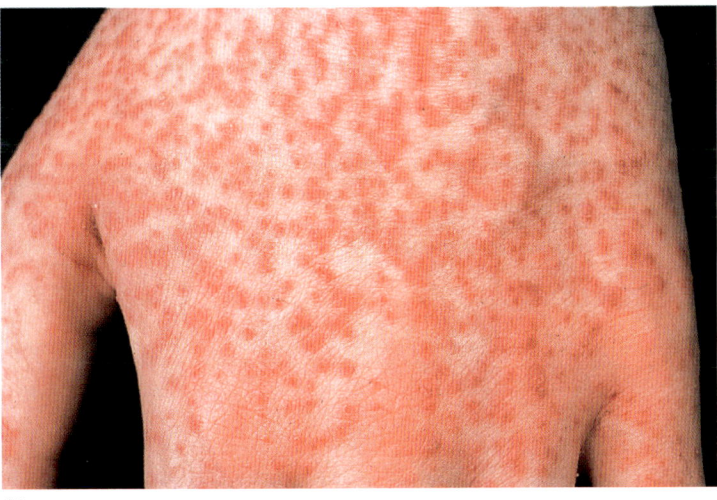

Figure 37.20 Nékam disease. Reticulate keratotic red papules on (a) the volar aspect of the wrist and (b) the dorsum of the hand. Courtesy of St John's Institute of Dermatology, King's College London, UK.

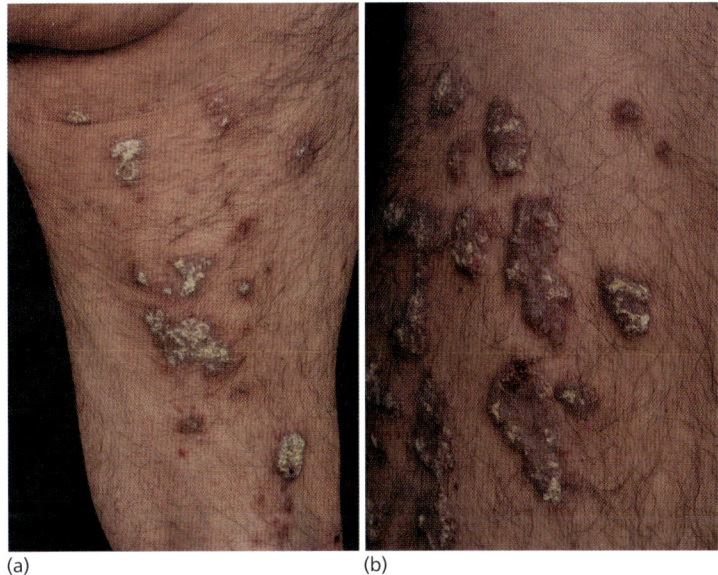

Figure 37.21 (a, b) Nékam disease. Hyperkeratotic plaques on the lower limbs. The patient presented with additional erosive lesions of the oral and genital mucosa. Courtesy of University of Munich.

original case was also associated with palmoplantar keratoderma. The individual lesions are reddish verrucous papules covered by a hyperkeratotic plug that can only be removed with difficulty, revealing irregular indentations and prominent capillary loops [166,168]. In extensive Nékam disease, the lesions tend to be symmetrical bilaterally, mainly involving the antecubital fossae, extensor forearms, lumbo-sacral area and buttocks, posterior thighs, popliteal fossae and less commonly the oral cavity and genitals (Figure 37.21). Oral manifestations occur in 50% of patients – recurrent aphthous ulcers, larger chronic ulcers or erythrokeratotic papules being the commonest oral features [169]. The nails can become thickened, longitudinally ridged and prone to paronychia [170]. Cases have followed trauma [171] and erythroderma [172]. A limited variant of Nékam disease presenting with reddish hyperkeratotic papules and plaques on the face, clearing in the summer months, has been described in two young siblings [173]. Histologically, changes are often non-specific and consistent with a chronic dermatitis, but lichenoid features can be seen [166,168]. Some authors believe that the condition is an unusual variant of LP [166], while others consider it to be a distinct entity [174]. A case of Nékam disease

associated with porokeratotic histology and amyloid deposition may argue against the view that Nékam disease is a subset of LP [175]. A possible association of Nékam disease with glomerulonephritis and lymphoproliferative disorders has been commented on [169].

Complications and co-morbidities

Hair. Alopecia is uncommon in LP, but most often occurs in small areas on the scalp, producing patches of atrophic cicatricial alopecia of fibrosing frontal alopecia, most frequently observed as frontal fibrosing alopecia (see Figure 37.11) [176–180]. It results from follicular destruction by the inflammatory infiltrate, with scarring. Areas of alopecia may continue to appear, or to extend, for months after the skin lesions have faded. The result is one of pseudopelade [177,180]; this is probably best considered as a distinct clinical entity due to a number of independent conditions, of which LP is only one. Lichen planopilaris is more common in women and about half will develop involvement of the glabrous skin, mucous membranes or nails [176]. It may also occur in children [178]. Tumid forms of LP follicularis have been described in which clusters of milium cysts and comedones develop [181]. LP pilaris has been reported in association with dermatitis herpetiformis [182].

Nails. Nail involvement occurs in up to 10% of cases but is usually a minor feature of the disease [183,184]. Most cases present during the fifth or sixth decades. Long-term permanent damage to the nails is rare [185]. Fingernails are more frequently affected than toenails [185], with initial involvement of two or three fingernails before subsequent involvement of the remaining digits. The most common changes are exaggeration of the longitudinal lines and linear depressions due to slight thinning of the nail plate (Figure 37.22). These changes usually occur in the context of severe generalised LP, although skin lesions may not be seen in the vicinity of the affected nail. Elevated ridges may be seen on the nail [184].

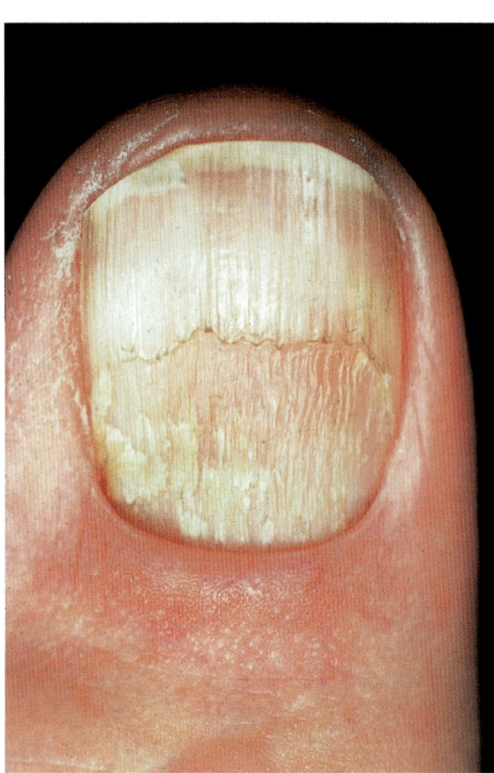

Figure 37.22 Lichen planus of the thumbnail showing thinning of the nail plate and longitudinal lines. Courtesy of St John's Institute of Dermatology, King's College London, UK.

Adhesion between the epidermis of the dorsal nail fold and the nail bed may cause partial destruction of the nail (pterygium unguis) (Figure 37.23a). Rarely, the nail is completely shed; there is usually clinical evidence of LP at the base of the nail before shedding. Nails may partially regrow or be permanently lost (Figure 37.23b) or have longitudinal ridging (Figure 37.23c); the nails of the great toes are the ones most often affected. LP has been shown to cause childhood idiopathic atrophy of the nails [186]. LP of the nails in childhood is rare [187] but may overlap with the condition of twenty-nail dystrophy of childhood (idiopathic trachyonychia); the exact relationship is unclear [188–191,**192**,193]. The rare variant of LP that causes ulceration of the soles is often accompanied by permanent destruction of several toenails. LP of the nail bed may give rise to longitudinal melanonychia [194], hyperpigmentation, subungual hyperkeratosis or onycholysis [184], or changes mimicking the yellow nail syndrome [195,196].

Mucous membranes. Squamous cell carcinoma developing in oral lesions is uncommon but is a potential danger, especially with ulcerated lesions [197–205], although the incidence varies greatly in different series. Lesions may occur on the lip, the buccal mucosa or the gum margin. It has been postulated that the high expression of cyclo-oxygenase 2 reported in oral LP may be of aetiological significance in the development of squamous cell carcinoma [206]. Squamous cell carcinoma arising on cutaneous lesions of LP [207] and ano-genital lesions [208–210] is a rare phenomenon. Cicatricial conjunctivitis [211] and lacrimal canalicular obstruction are recorded [212].

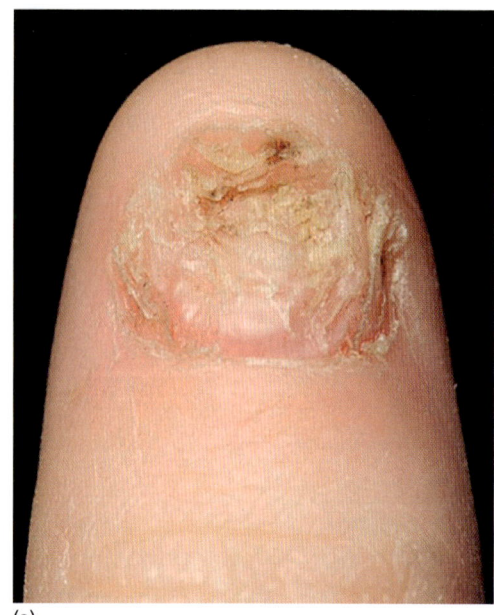

(a)

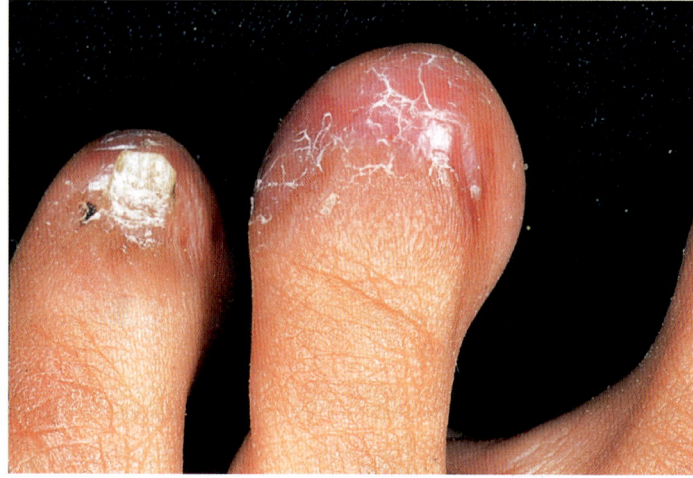

(b)

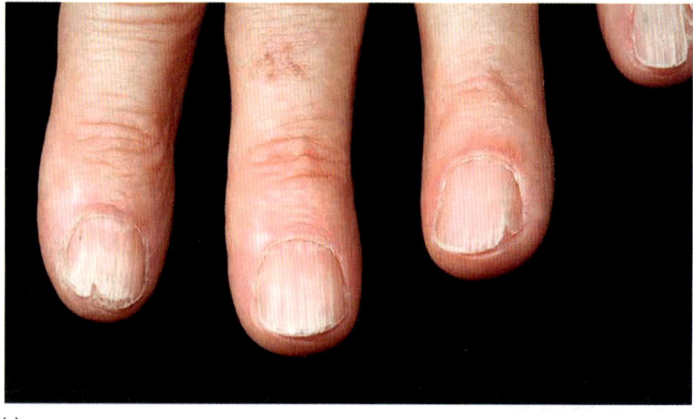

(c)

Figure 37.23 (a) Severe lichen planus of all fingernails showing involvement of the nail fold areas and early pterygium formation. (b) Severe, destructive lichen planus of the toenails. (c) Longitudinal lines. (a) Courtesy of the Welsh Institute of Dermatology, University Hospital of Wales, Cardiff, Wales, UK. (b) Courtesy of St John's Institute of Dermatology, King's College London, UK. (c) Courtesy of University of Munich.

Associated conditions

Lichen planus has been reported in association with diseases of altered or disturbed immunity, including ulcerative colitis [213–215], alopecia areata [215,216], vitiligo [215], dermatomyositis [217], morphoea and lichen sclerosus [218], systemic lupus erythematosus [219,220], pemphigus [219] and paraneoplastic pemphigus [221,222]. In addition, LP has been observed in association with thymoma [216,219,223,224], hypothyroidism [225], myasthenia gravis [214,215,224], hypogammaglobulinaemia [216,217,226], primary biliary cholangitis [227–229], especially in those treated with penicillamine, and primary sclerosing cholangitis [230]. The literature about LP and hepatitis C infection is reviewed in the section on pathogenesis earlier in this chapter. In Italy, possibly because of a higher prevalence of hepatitis B and C infection, patients with LP seem more prone to develop liver disease, including chronic active hepatitis [231,232]. A high prevalence of anticardiolipin antibodies has been documented in patients with hepatitis C-associated oral LP [233]. Elsewhere, the association between LP and chronic active hepatitis or primary biliary cholangitis is unusual and probably coincidental [234–236]. Overall, most patients with LP live to old age, despite an association with autoimmunity disorders [237].

LP has also been associated with diabetes [238]. Anecdotally, LP has occurred in patients with Castleman tumours (giant lymph node hyperplasia) [239] or with generalised lichen amyloidosis [230]. LP has been described in certain tattoo reactions, particularly in those areas where there is coexisting mercury hypersensitivity to the injected dye [241,242].

Disease course and prognosis

Although a few cases evolve rapidly and clear within a few weeks, the onset is usually insidious. In most cases, the papules eventually flatten after a few months, often to be replaced by an area of pigmentation that retains the shape of the papule and persists for months or years. There may be a gradual change in colour from pink to blue to black. The residual pigmentation may be intense, especially in dark-skinned people, or almost imperceptible in fair-skinned individuals. New papules may form while others are clearing. Some papules persist much longer, enlarge and thicken, and develop a roughened surface with a prominent violaceous hue so called hypertrophic LP. Such lesions may resolve with atrophy or scarring. Areas of pigment loss are described in black South Africans.

Investigations

Histology is the most useful investigation to confirm a diagnosis of LP. Dermoscopy is useful in some cases when Wickham striae can be visualised better with the device (Figure 37.24) [243]. Typical features of dermoscopy images of LP include a network of whitish striae with red globules at the periphery [243,244]. Histology is routinely obtained to confirm the diagnosis of LP [**245**,246]. The earliest finding is an increase in epidermal Langerhans cells [**245**], associated with a superficial perivascular infiltrate of lymphocytes and histiocytes, impinging on the dermal–epidermal junction (DEJ). Mild spongiosis is followed by vacuolar alteration and clefting along the DEJ, with accumulation of necrotic keratinocytes (colloid bodies) [247]. The characteristic histological changes are

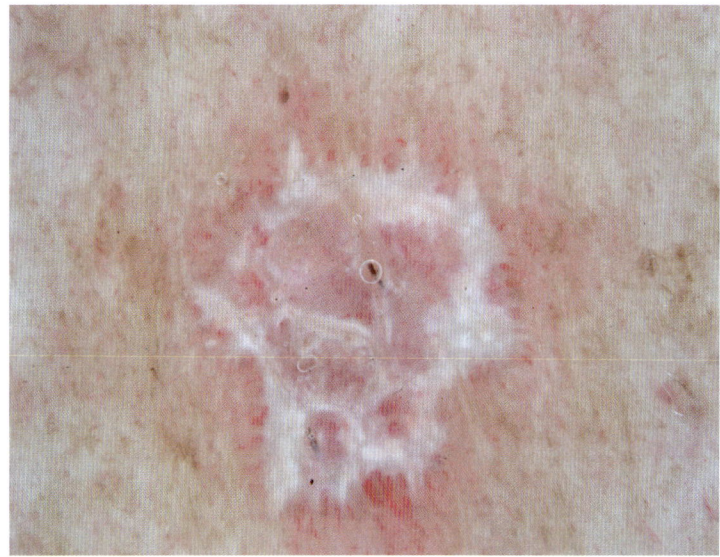

Figure 37.24 Dermoscopy image of lichen planus with typical Wickham striae. Courtesy of Dr Alan Cameron, School of Medicine, University of Queensland, Brisbane, Australia.

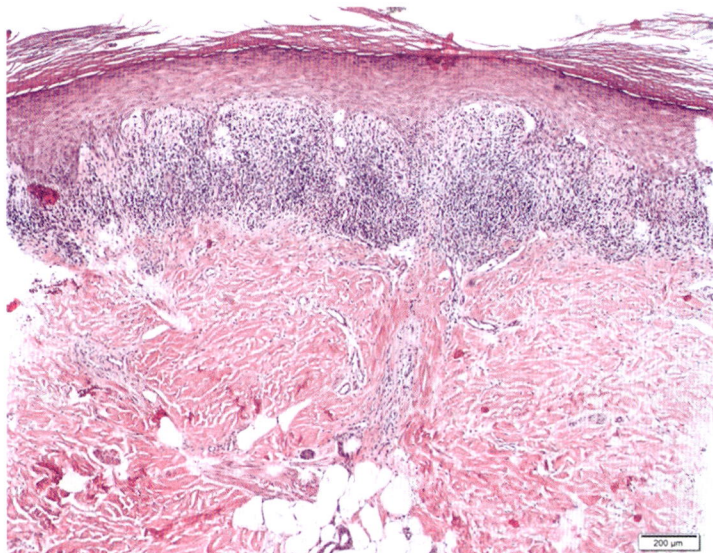

Figure 37.25 Typical histology of lichen planus. Magnification 40× (H&E). Courtesy of University of Munich.

best seen in biopsies of fully developed LP papules (Figure 37.25) [248]. The centre of the papule shows irregular acanthosis of the epidermis, irregular thickening of the granular layer and compact hyperkeratosis. The mid-epidermal cells appear larger, flatter and paler than usual [248]. In oral LP, epithelial proliferation is increased [249]. Parakeratosis is rarely found in idiopathic LP, in contrast to some drug-induced lichenoid tissue reactions. A focal increase in thickness of the granular layer and infiltrate corresponds to the presence of Wickham striae [250]. Degenerating basal epidermal cells are transformed into *colloid bodies* (15–20 μm diameter), which appear singly or in clumps [251–253]. The rete ridges may appear flattened or effaced (*'saw-tooth' appearance*) and focal separation from the dermis may lead to Max Joseph spaces (Figure 37.26). In older or hypertrophic lesions, the number of colloid bodies is considerably reduced. In 'active' LP, a *band-like infiltrate* of lymphocytes and histiocytes, rarely admixed with

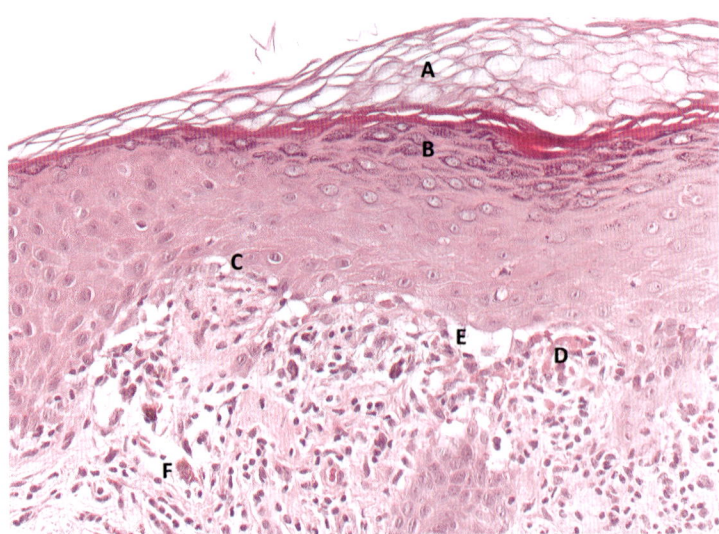

Figure 37.26 Lichen planus: A, orthohyperkeratosis; B, hypergranulosis; C, vacuolated basal keratinocytes; D, cytoid bodies; E, Max Joseph space; F, melanophages. Magnification 200× (H&E). Courtesy of University of Munich.

plasma cells [254,255], obliterates the DEJ. Epidermal melanocytes are absent or considerably decreased in number [248], while *pigmentary incontinence* with dermal melanophages is characteristic. When the disease is becoming inactive, the infiltrate, with melanophages, becomes sparser and is arranged around papillary blood vessels, which may show ectasia and surrounding fibroplasia.

In hypertrophic LP, the epidermis may show a pseudoepitheliomatous appearance with extreme irregular acanthosis. Follicles may be expanded and at times have a cyst-like appearance. The infiltrate may not appear very band-like, but serial sections will usually show foci of basal cell liquefaction and colloid body formation, often around the follicular epithelium. Longstanding cases usually demonstrate coexistent dermal fibrosis adjacent to the inflammatory changes.

In atrophic LP, the epidermis may be greatly thinned almost to the level of the granular layer, although relatively compact hyperkeratosis remains. The rete ridges are usually completely effaced with relatively few colloid bodies. The papillary dermis shows fibrosis and loss of elastic fibres.

In follicular lesions, an infiltrate extends around, and may permeate, the base of the hair follicle epithelium, with follicular keratin plugging (Figure 37.27) [256,257].

In mucosal LP, the epithelium is usually thinned with parakeratosis, although both types of keratinisation may be seen [258,259]. The epithelium may resemble epidermis from the skin, plasma cells may be prominent in the band-like infiltrate and colloid bodies are fewer than in typical cutaneous papular LP. The reddish subtype of oral LP is associated with increased cell proliferation compared with the reticular form [260]. Moderate or severe epithelial dysplasia on oral biopsy should probably be regarded as an increased risk for subsequent cancer development [261].

Bullous LP is rare. Blister formation takes place predominantly between the basal lamina and the cytomembranes of basal keratinocytes (i.e. intrabasal) [251], such that there is a wide separation between the epidermis and infiltrate.

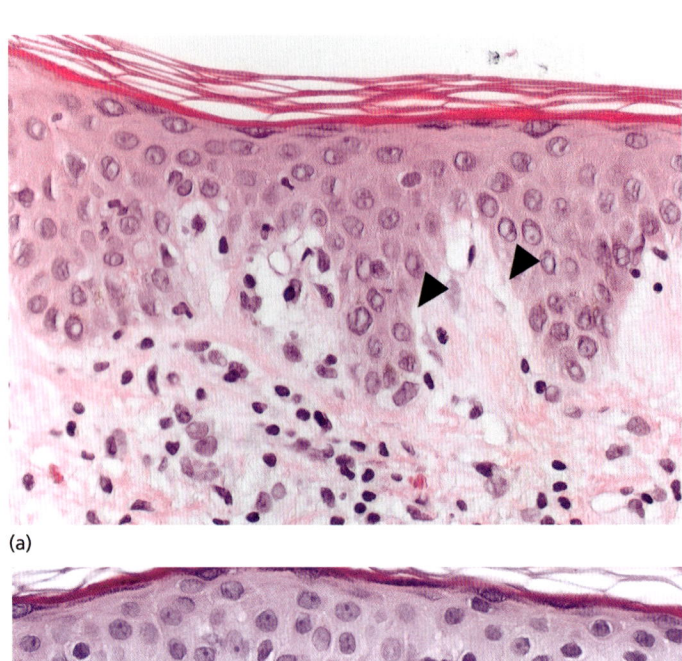

(a)

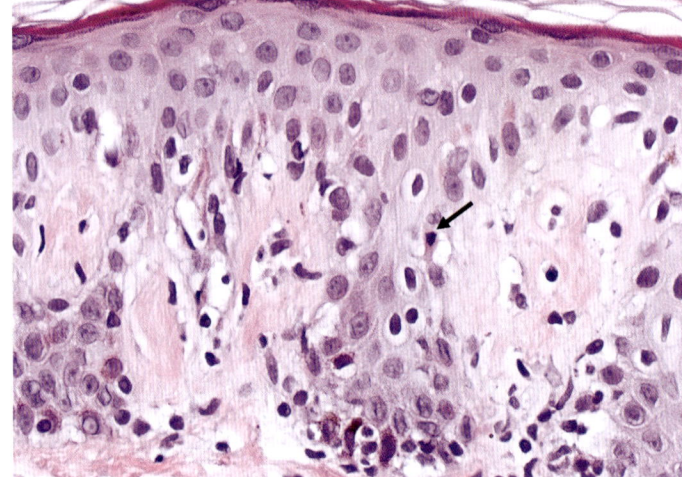

(b)

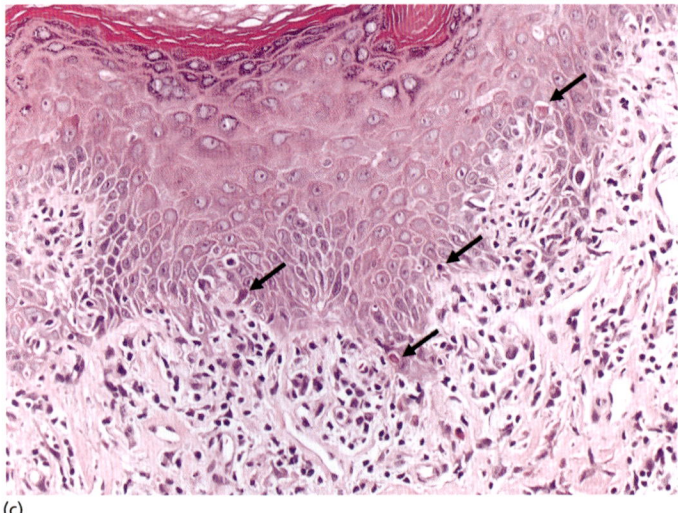

(c)

Figure 37.27 Different types of interface dermatitis. (a) Interface dermatitis *non sensu strictu*: some vacuolated basal keratinocytes (triangles) but no dyskeratotic keratinocytes are detectable. (b) Vacuolar interface dermatitis: prominent vacuolar alterations of the basal layer and single dyskeratotic cells (arrow) are seen. (c) Lichenoid interface dermatitis: a dense subepidermal infiltrate and numerous dyskeratotic keratinocytes (arrows) can be seen. (a, b) Magnification 200× (H&E). (c) Magnification 100× (H&E). Courtesy of University of Munich.

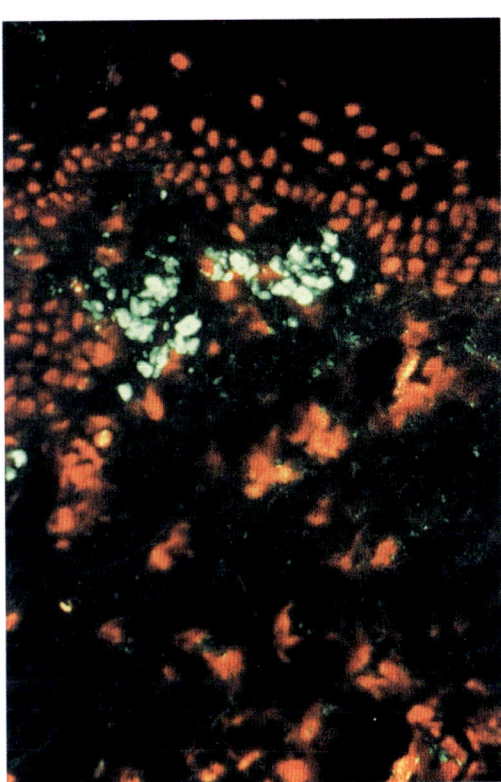

Figure 37.28 Lichen planus: photomicrograph of direct immunofluorescence showing the bright fluorescence of cytoid bodies with anti-IgM. Magnification 100×. Courtesy of St John's Institute of Dermatology, King's College London, UK.

Direct immunofluorescence shows globular deposits of IgG, IgM (Figure 37.28) and occasionally C3 and IgA, representing apoptotic keratinocytes, around the DEJ and lower epidermis, with fibrin deposition at the region of the DEJ [258,262]. Direct IMF studies may be useful in differentiating LP from lupus erythematosus or LP pemphigoides [263,264], and can be carried out on routine histological material [265].

Management

Treatment of LP can represent a challenge and depends on the localisation, clinical form and severity [266]. For cutaneous LP, which can clear spontaneously within 1–2 years, the aim of treatment is to reduce pruritus and time to resolution [267]. Therapeutic abstention is recommended for asymptomatic oral LP. However, painful, erosive LP may need aggressive and long-term treatments [268]. Nail or scalp involvement [269,270], which may induce scars, genital LP [271] and oesophageal and conjunctival involvement, which may induce strictures and fibrosis, require rapid treatment to avoid scarring or avoid a fatal course.

Overall, the level of evidence for treatments used in LP is low [272]. Surprisingly, there is still little evidence for the efficacy of topical or systemic corticosteroids, commonly recommended as first line treatment for LP. Treatment is mainly based on clinical experience. In contrast, for oral LP, there are several randomised controlled trials (RCTs) and one Cochrane review [272–274]. However, most of these trials are small, have used various outcomes and are at high risk of bias. For cutaneous LP, there are only a few small RCTs. No RCT has assessed treatment for genital or nail LP, lichen planopilaris or other lichenoid disorders.

Treatment goals

The goals of therapy of cutaneous LP are to improve itching and induce resolution of the lesions. In mucosal LP, the aims of treatment are to heal erosive lesions to reduce pain and permit normal food intake. Education of the patient should emphasise that oral LP frequently has a chronic course marked by treatment-induced remission followed by relapse [269,272]. Considering the potential higher risk of squamous cell carcinoma in this form of LP, the need for regular clinical surveillance on a long-term basis has also to be explained [275]. Alcohol and tobacco should be avoided as well as spicy or acidic foods and drinks. Good oral hygiene and professional dental care are recommended.

In ano-genital LP, foreskin retraction or removal surgery in uncircumcised men and vaginal dilators in women are used to prevent synechiae formation. Surgery is required after complete resolution of the active lesions if adhesion occurs.

First line

Topical corticosteroids are the first line treatment for limited cutaneous LP. Depending on the sites of the lesions, the use of very potent corticosteroids is required (clobetasol propionate ointment 0.05%) once daily at night until remission. If no evolution is observed after 6 weeks, second line therapy should be considered. After remission, the optimal length of maintenance therapy is unknown and needs to be adapted to each patient. For hypertrophic LP, very potent corticosteroids need to be applied under an occlusive bandage. Oral corticosteroids are the first line treatment for widespread cutaneous LP: prednisolone 0.5–1 mg/kg per day until improvement (usually 4–6 weeks). In a small RCT in which potent corticosteroid cream alone was compared with oral prednisolone (30 mg per day for 10 days) combined with topical corticosteroids, the time to clearing was significantly shorter in the oral prednisolone group (18 weeks versus 29 weeks) than in the topical steroid cream only group. Two patients in the corticosteroid group experienced a severe relapse after treatment withdrawal [276]. After remission, oral corticosteroids should be tapered down slowly.

For other manifestations of LP, treatment recommendations are similar. In mucosal LP, two trials compared tacrolimus ointment 0.1% with clobetasol propionate 0.05%. One found a statistically significant difference favouring tacrolimus [277], while no difference between the two treatment modalities was observed in the other [278]. An RCT comparing pimecrolimus cream 1% to triamcinolone acetonide paste 0.1% found no difference between the two treatments [279]. Thus, calcineurin inhibitors are a safe alternative to topical corticosteroids for mucosal LP. Furthermore, three small RCTs compared topic retinoid (retinoic acid 0.05%, isotretinoin gel and tazarotene) with placebo. Improvement or cure rates were significantly higher in the treated group [280–282]. For widespread mucosal LP, a soluble prednisolone tablet 5 mg dissolved in 15 mL water can be used for a mouthwash 'swish and rinse' three times daily. Oral candidiasis is the most frequent complication of this treatment [283]. If no improvement is observed after 6 weeks, second line therapy has to be considered.

For special locations such as lichen planopilaris or ano-genital LP, corticosteroids may also be given as suppositories, as monthly intralesional injection of triamcinolone acetonide (0.5–10 mg/mL) or as systemic oral corticosteroids (prednisolone 1 mg/kg/day) [271,284,285].

Evidence for therapies used for nail LP is based only on retrospective case series and depends on the number of affected nails. The aims of treatment are to reduce pain and avoid irreversible nail scars. Two-thirds of 142 patients treated with intramuscular injection or oral systemic glucocorticoids and/or intralesional injection or topical glucocorticoids for 6 months were cured or had marked improvement [269,286]. When less than four nails are involved, the recommended treatment is a twice daily application of super-potent corticosteroids (e.g. 0.05% clobetasol propionate ointment) or if lesions are more severe, monthly intralesional injections of triamcinolone acetonide (0.5–10 mg/mL) in the periungual sites. When more than two or three nails are involved, systemic corticosteroids are required. Treatment with oral prednisolone (0.5–1 mg/kg/day) for 4–66 weeks or intramuscular triamcinolone acetonide injection have been reported. Etanercept has been suggested in a case report [287], although LP-like eruptions can be triggered by TNF antagonists [288].

Second line

If corticosteroids are not effective or long-term therapy is needed, numerous therapies have been described. Overall, the level of evidence is low, but phototherapy, retinoids, methotrexate and JAK inhibitors can be regarded second line alternatives [289,290,**291**]. For cutaneous LP, a second line option is photochemotherapy or phototherapy. In a small trial, PUVA used three times weekly on one side of the body was compared with no treatment on the other side. Clearance was observed on the treated side only in 50% of the patients [292]. In a retrospective series, clearance within a mean of 3 months was observed in 70% of patients treated with narrow-band UVB therapy [293]. PUVA phototherapy may also be combined with acitretin but evaluation of this association has not been assessed. Phototherapy can increase the risk of residual hyperpigmentation in dark-skinned patients.

For both cutaneous and mucosal LP, retinoids have been reported to be effective second line treatment options. An RCT showed a rate of regression or remission at 8 weeks significantly higher with acitretin (30 mg per day for 8 weeks) than with placebo [294]. The best level of evidence for methotrexate in cutaneous LP is a prospective series. Complete remission was observed in 14/24 patients at 24 weeks [295].

Finally, insights into the pathogenesis of LP support a role for JAKs in mediating the intracellular signal that leads to upregulation of molecules predisposing keratinocytes to lymphocyte-induced cell death. JAK inhibitors have the potential therefore to become the therapy of choice in the second line treatment of LP. To date, there are only a few case series or case reports that report efficacy of JAK inhibitors [**296**,297], but the level of evidence is not sufficient to give a general recommendation to treat LP. Besides, there is a case series ($n = 5$ patients) reporting benefit of anti-interleukin 17A (anti-IL-17A), anti-IL-12/23 or anti-IL-23 for cutaneous and mucocutaneous LP [298]. The anti-IL-17A antibody secukinumab is currently being investigated for its efficacy in LP in clinical proof-of-concept trials.

Third line

There are four RCTs assessing griseofulvin, hydroxychloroquine or sulfasalazine [299–301]. Because of the risk of bias in these trials, discrepancies of results between studies for griseofulvin and life-threatening adverse reaction for sulfasalazine, these treatments are not generally recommended in cutaneous LP. There is very limited evidence that ciclosporin treatment might have beneficial effects for the treatment of LP [302].

Treatment ladder for lichen planus

First line

- Limited cutaneous LP: very potent corticosteroids (clobetasol propionate ointment 0.05%); potent topical corticosteroids can be used in less severe forms of LP or during maintenance therapy
- Widespread cutaneous LP: prednisolone 0.5–1 mg/kg per day until improvement

Second line

- Methotrexate 15–20 mg SC once a week, evaluation after 12 weeks
- Acitretin 30 mg per day, evaluation after 12 weeks
- PUVA or UVB: two to five times a week, alone or associated with systemic retinoids
- JAK inhibitors (tofacitinib, baricitinb) as labelled for psoriasis, evaluation after 8 weeks

Third line

- Antimalarials (hydroxychloroquine)
- Ciclosporin
- Azathioprine
- Mycophenolate mofetil

Management of clinical variants

Lichen nitidus. As the disease is often asymptomatic and eventually self-limiting, no treatment is required in most cases. However, fluorinated topical corticosteroid preparations may be recommended if treatment is demanded, for example for lesions on the penis, and can be highly successful [303]. Clearance of generalised lichen nitidus has been described with sun exposure [304], PUVA [305], narrow-band UVB phototherapy [306,307] and astemizole [308,309]. Acitretin can lead to a gradual improvement in palmoplantar lichen nitidus [310].

Nékam disease. The course of the dermatosis is chronic and progressive and very resistant to therapeutic approaches but has shown a favourable response to photochemotherapy without [311,312] or with [313] acitretin. Etretinate [314] and photodynamic therapy [315] have been reported to be helpful.

'Mixed' lichen planus/discoid lupus erythematosus disease patterns. Both ciclosporin [316] and acitretin [317] can be of benefit in treating LP/DLE overlap syndrome.

Actinic lichen planus. Actinic LP has been treated with acitretin and topical corticosteroids [318] and with ciclosporin [319].

Bullous lichen planus and lichen planus pemphigoides. Some cases require treatment with systemic steroids or azathioprine and fatalities can occur [318]. A combination of corticosteroids and acitretin has been used [319,320].

Lichen striatus

Definition and nomenclature

Synonyms and inclusions
- Linear lichenoid dermatosis
- Lichen striatus albus

Lichen striatus is a distinctive, usually self-limiting, and asymptomatic inflammatory dermatosis characterised by pink or red papules in a linear distribution that develop in the lines of Blaschko. These usually occur as isolated lesions on the limbs in children aged 5–15 years and generally resolve over 6–12 months. Areas of postinflammatory hypopigmentation may occur and persist for longer. The aetiology is incompletely understood but approximately 40% of cases have a background of atopy. Clustering of cases in families and in winter suggests an infectious agent; potentially, a virus may be involved.

Epidemiology
Incidence and prevalence
The incidence or prevalence is unknown, but, between January 1989 and January 2000, 115 cases were identified at the Paediatric Dermatology Unit, University of Bologna, Bologna, Italy [1].

Age
Over 50% of cases occur in children, usually between the ages of 5 and 15 years, but onset in early infancy and in adults has been reported.

Sex
Females are affected approximately two to three times as frequently as males [1].

Associated diseases
Lichen striatus occurs more often in individuals with atopy; atopy was reported in approximately 43% of cases in a recent series [2].

Pathophysiology
Pathology
As the condition develops in the lines of Blaschko, which represent embryonic migratory patterns of ectoderm (Chapter 8), it has been hypothesised that postzygotic mutation or loss of heterozygosity may lead to cutaneous mosaicism and play a role in its pathophysiology, perhaps predisposing to the effects of an environmental trigger

or an infectious agent. The presence of atopy in approximately 40% of cases is therefore intriguing. On the other hand, the resolution of lichen stratus over a period of months in the majority of cases suggests a temporary phenomenon, leading to the proposal of cutaneous antigenic mosaicism and a localised inflammatory T-cell response, again potentially related to viral infection or injury [3].

Histology
The histological appearances are variable and depend on the stage of disease [3]. Usually, a band-like infiltrate composed of lymphocytes and histiocytes is observed with associated overlying epidermal change including parakeratosis and hyperkeratosis, resembling lichen planus. The earliest change is intercellular oedema, stretching the tonofilament–desmosome complexes and separating the epidermal cells. Like the spongiosis, acanthosis is variable in degree. Dyskeratotic keratinocytes, like the 'corps ronds' of Darier disease, are seen in about 50% of cases. There is often focal liquefactive degeneration of the basal layer. The dermis is oedematous, and the vessels and appendages are surrounded by an infiltrate of lymphocytes and histiocytes, which may be quite dense and extend deeply. Scattered lymphocyte cells often penetrate into the epidermis.

Immunohistochemical studies have revealed a predominance of CD8+ T cells compared with CD4+ T cells [3,4].

Genetics
Familial cases are documented [1,5,6], although whether this relates to clustering related to contact with a common infectious agent remains to be determined.

Environmental factors
Possible triggering factors include infectious agents and trauma. For example, in a retrospective case review of 115 cases from Italy, the majority occurred in the cold season, five had prodromal symptoms of viral infection and two had a preceding history of skin trauma [1]. Other reported triggers include varicella infection [7] and measles, mumps and rubella vaccination [3].

Clinical features
History
The onset is usually sudden. Frequently, there are no symptoms, but pruritus may occasionally occur and is more common in adults. The course is variable. The area affected typically reaches its maximum extent within 2–3 weeks, but gradual extension can continue for several months. Spontaneous resolution can be expected within 6–12 months in most cases, but some lesions may persist for over a year [8]. Resolution may be followed by hypopigmentation or more rarely hyperpigmentation [1,2].

Presentation
The initial presentation is characterised by the sudden appearance of small, discrete, pink, flat-topped, lichenoid papules in a typical linear distribution. In a recent series of 23 patients from Spain, 11 presented with reddish papules [2]. Occasionally, vesicles are observed, but were present in only two out of 24 patients. The lesions extend over the course of a week or more and rapidly

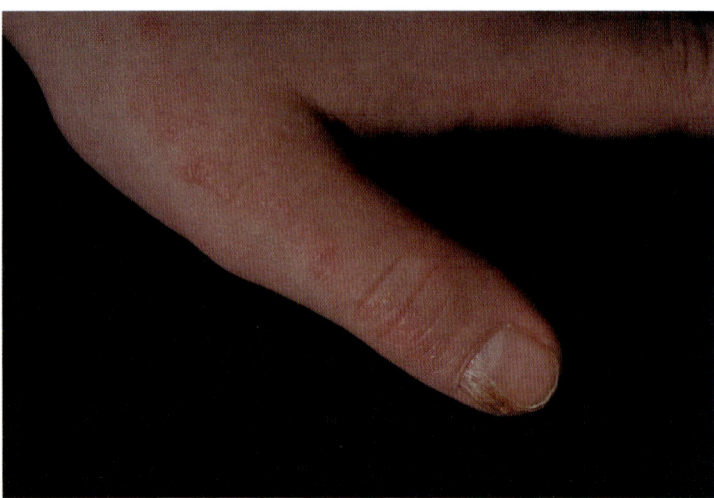

Figure 37.29 Lichen striatus of the hand involving the nail matrix. Note, that only a part of the nail shows the typical longitudinal lines of lichen planus. Courtesy of University of Munich.

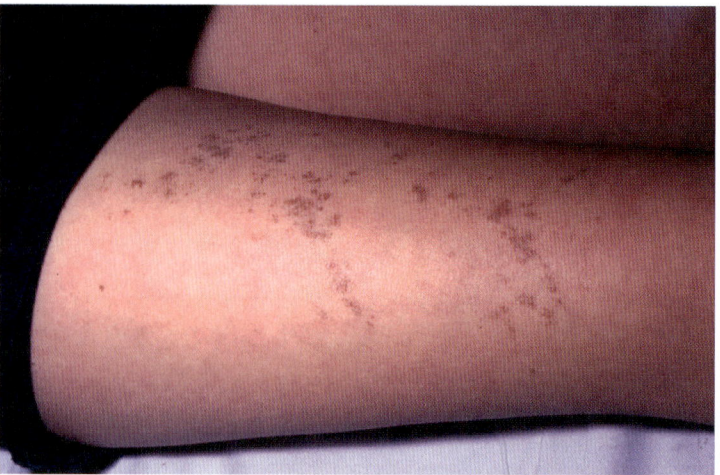

Figure 37.30 Lichen striatus showing parallel linear bands in a zigzag distribution on the thigh of a 15-year-old girl. Histology showed epidermal hyperkeratosis, focal liquefactive degeneration at the dermal–epidermal junction and upper dermal oedema with chronic inflammatory infiltrate in the upper dermis. The eruption resolved spontaneously.

coalesce to form a dull-red to brown, slightly scaly, linear band, usually 2 mm to 2 cm in width, and often irregular. Occasionally, the bands broaden into plaques, especially on the buttocks. The lesion may be only a few centimetres in length or may extend the entire length of the limb or other extremities and may be continuous or interrupted (Figure 37.29).

The initial lichenoid papules are pink rather than violaceous and show no umbilication or Wickham striae. The papules may be hypopigmented in dark-skinned people and hypopigmentation was noted at presentation in one-third of 23 cases reported from Spain [2]. Residual persistent hypopigmentation may occur in some patients. Postinflammatory hyperpigmentation is reported less commonly.

The lesions occur most commonly on one arm or leg, or on the neck, but may develop on the trunk [1]. The abdomen, buttocks and thighs may be involved in single extensive lesions, but multiple lesions are rare, and bilateral involvement is exceptional. Involvement of the nails may result in longitudinal ridging, splitting, onycholysis or nail loss [1,9].

Clinical variants

Parallel linear bands or zosteriform patterns have been recorded (Figure 37.30) and extensive bilateral lesions were reported in two out of 23 patients in the series from Barcelona, Spain [2]. The majority of episodes are solitary, but occasionally repeated episodes can occur in different locations.

Differential diagnosis

Linear inflammatory eruptions that are distributed along Blaschko lines or show a zosteriform distribution, including linear psoriasis, linear Darier disease, linear lichen planus, linear porokeratosis and ILVEN, should be considered in the differential diagnosis. Linear forms of lichen planus and psoriasis can usually be differentiated clinically, even in the absence of typical lesions in other sites, which should always be sought. Linear LP and lichen striatus are considered two ends of one spectrum by some authors,

both clinically and regarding immune mechanism [10,11]. ILVEN (Chapter 73) has many clinical and histological features in common with lichen striatus. However, ILVEN is always pruritic and persists despite periods of relative improvement. The differential diagnosis of hypopigmented lesions includes linear vitiligo or naevoid hypomelanosis [2].

Disease course and prognosis

The disease course is variable. The majority of lesions last for at least 6 months and resolve within 1 year, but lesions may last for just a few weeks or persist for several years, both in children and in adults [1,8]. It may follow a prolonged and/or relapsing course, particularly in adults [1,12]. Postinflammatory hypopigmentation may last for years, particularly in darker skin types. Hypopigmentation may also be the presenting feature in some patients [2]. Lichen striatus presenting in adults tends to be more extensive and symptomatic and may require treatment [12].

Investigations
Skin biopsy may be helpful.

Management
General principles of management
Usually, no treatment is necessary in childhood cases, which are largely asymptomatic and typically spontaneously resolve. In patients with troublesome itch (usually adults), topical corticosteroids are the first line of management. However, in resistant cases or when there are concerns over topical corticosteroid-induced skin atrophy, calcineurin inhibitors may be considered. Because of the rarity of the condition, no trials have been performed, but individual case reports and small case series report positive and prompt symptomatic response and rapid resolution of lesions in response to both tacrolimus and pimecrolimus [4,12,13]. A single case of a response to photodynamic therapy is reported [14]. Nail involvement may respond to potent steroid cream under occlusion.

Treatment ladder for lichen striatus

First line
- Observation and reassurance
- Topical corticosteroids

Second line
- Topical tacrolimus
- Topical pimecrolimus

Lichenoid exanthema

Introduction and general description

In line with our understanding of the lichenoid phenotype to be a consequence of keratinocyte killing by lymphocytes, several triggers have the potential to elicit an acute and most often generalised skin inflammation resembling LP. The border between LP and lichenoid exanthema is not clearly defined as LP can be induced by several drugs and is associated with hepatitis C virus (see earlier in this chapter). The difference is the eliciting antigen. While this is a clearly identified external factor in lichenoid exanthema, LP is most likely an autoimmune disease. This is relevant as it means lichenoid exanthema is self-limited once the trigger is removed while LP tends to be chronic.

Pathogenesis

Several triggers that induce a cytotoxic immune reaction are known to cause lichenoid exanthema. These can be grouped as: (i) infectious triggers; (ii) side effects of drugs; and (iii) a primary mechanism of drugs. Infectious triggers are typically viruses or intracellular bacteria, as clearance of these requires cytotoxic immunity. In the context of the Covid-19 pandemic, numerous patients have been reported to develop lichenoid exanthema. The second group of triggers are unwanted effects of certain drugs. While the exact pathogenesis is unknown, it is obvious that certain drug classes such as gold, β-blockers, angiotensin-converting enzyme blockers or antimalarial drugs preferentially induce lichenoid exanthemas [1]. Also TNF inhibitors and other biologics used to treat psoriasis are associated with lichenoid exanthemas. These reactions are usually classified as 'paradoxical reactions', and a suggested mechanism is the induction of type I interferons in the skin [2]. As for the third group, checkpoint inhibitors targeting either CTLA4 or the PD1 axis are designed to boost the cytotoxic immune response that should ideally be directed against tumour cells. As a consequence of their mode of action, these checkpoint inhibitors cause lichenoid exanthema in up to 25% of all treatments by induction of type I immunity against keratinocyte-derived antigens [1].

Clinical features

The clinical and histological picture of lichenoid exanthemas resembles that of a generalised acute LP. Lesions are mostly small in size and are not confluent in the acute stage (Figure 37.31). Histologically, scattered eosinophils may be present in addition to the classic LP histopathology. More specific diagnostic tools such as

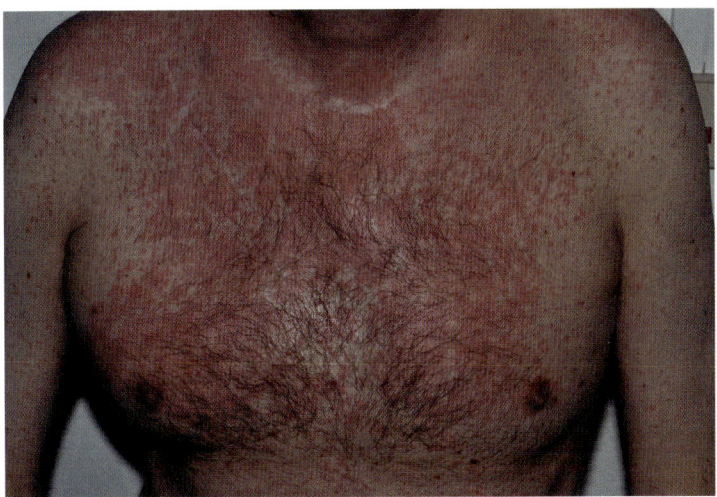

Figure 37.31 Lichenoid exanthema evolving after PD1 checkpoint blockade with nivolumab. Histology showed vacuolated interface dermatitis. Courtesy of University of Munich.

an epicutaneous patch testing or a lymphocyte transformation test are not highly sensitive and specific, but they can be of additional diagnostic value in individual cases.

Management

In contrast to LP, identifying and eliminating the trigger is the highest priority in the management of lichenoid exanthema. Short-term treatments mostly rely on corticosteroids, which may have to be given systemically.

Key references

The full list of references can be found in the online version at https://www.wiley.com/rooksdermatology10e

Lichen planus

8 González-Moles MÁ, Warnakulasuriya S, González-Ruiz I *et al.* Worldwide prevalence of oral lichen planus: a systematic review and meta-analysis. *Oral Dis* 2021;27:813–28.

9 Eyerich K, Eyerich S. Immune response patterns in non-communicable inflammatory skin diseases. *J Eur Acad Dermatol Venereol* 2018;32:692–703.

11 Lauffer F, Jargosch M, Krause L *et al.* Type I immune response induces keratinocyte necroptosis and is associated with interface dermatitis. *J Invest Dermatol* 2018;138:1785–94.

20 Boch K, Langan EA, Kridin K, Zillikens D, Ludwig RJ, Bieber K. Lichen planus. *Front Med* 2021;8:737813.

75 Simpson RC, Thomas KS, Leighton P, Murphy R. Diagnostic criteria for erosive lichen planus affecting the vulva: an international electronic-Delphi consensus exercise. *Br J Dermatol* 2013;169:337–43.

88 Vano-Galvan S, Molina-Ruiz AM, Serrano-Falcon C *et al.* Frontal fibrosing alopecia: a multicenter review of 355 patients. *J Am Acad Dermatol* 2014;70:670–8.

143 Zillikens D, Caux F, Mascaro JM *et al.* Autoantibodies in lichen planus pemphigoides react with a novel epitope within the C-terminal NC16A domain of BP180. *J Invest Dermatol* 1999;113:117–21.

192 Scheinfeld NS. Trachyonychia: a case report and review of manifestations, associations, and treatments. *Cutis* 2003;71:299–302.

207 Sigurgeirsson B, Lindelof B. Lichen planus and malignancy. An epidemiologic study of 2071 patients and a review of the literature. *Arch Dermatol* 1991;127:1684–8.

245 Ragaz A, Ackerman AB. Evolution, maturation, and regression of lesions of lichen planus. New observations and correlations of clinical and histologic findings. *Am J Dermatopathol* 1981;3:5–25.

266 Le Cleach L, Chosidow O. Clinical practice. Lichen planus. *N Engl J Med* 2012;366:723–32.

291 Husein-ElAhmed H, Gieler U, Steinhoff M. Lichen planus: a comprehensive evidence-based analysis of medical treatment. *J Eur Acad Dermatol Venereol* 2019;33:1847–62.

296 Damsky W, Wang A, Olajiju B *et al*. Treatment of severe lichen planus with the JAK inhibitor tofacitinib. *J Allergy Clin Immunol* 2020;145:1708–10.e2.

Lichen striatus

1 Patrizi A, Neri I, Fiorentini C *et al*. Lichen striatus: clinical and laboratory features of 115 children. *Pediatr Dermatol* 2004;21:197–204.

3 Muller CS, Schmaltz R, Vogt T, Pfohler C. Lichen striatus and blaschkitis: reappraisal of the concept of blaschkolinear dermatoses. *Br J Dermatol* 2011;164:257–62.

10 Herd RM, McLaren KM, Aldridge RD. Linear lichen planus and lichen striatus – opposite ends of a spectrum. *Clin Exp Dermatol* 1993;18:335–7.

12 Campanati A, Brandozzi G, Giangiacomi M *et al*. Lichen striatus in adults and pimecrolimus: open, off-label clinical study. *Int J Dermatol* 2008;47:732–6.

14 Park JY, Kim YC. Lichen striatus successfully treated with photodynamic therapy. *Clin Exp Dermatol* 2012;37:570–2.

Lichenoid exanthema

1 Merk HF, Vanstreels L, Megahed M. [Lichenoid drug reactions.] *Hautarzt* 2018;69:116–20.

2 Conrad C, Di Domizio J, Mylonas A *et al*. TNF blockade induces a dysregulated type I interferon response without autoimmunity in paradoxical psoriasis. *Nature Communications* 2018;9:25.

PART 4: INFLAMMATORY DERMATOSES

CHAPTER 38

Graft-versus-host Disease

Tanya N. Basu

Department of Dermatology, King's College Hospital, London, UK

Definition and nomenclature

Graft-versus-host disease (GvHD) is a multiorgan disease process that results from the action of donor-derived immunocompetent T lymphocytes against antigens expressed on the cells of the immunocompromised recipient host. The main organs affected are the skin, liver and gastrointestinal (GI) tract.

GvHD is a major complication of allogeneic haematopoietic stem cell transplantation (HSCT), with an incidence of 25–80% [1,2]. The exact risk depends on factors such as the degree of human leukocyte antigen (HLA) disparity between donor and host, the conditioning regimen intensity and the GvHD prophylaxis used.

There are two major forms of GvHD, acute (aGvHD) and chronic (cGvHD), that were originally defined according to the time of presentation. An overlap variant of these two forms is also described. GvHD can also occur after transfusions of unirradiated blood, such as donor lymphocyte infusion (DLI), solid-organ transplants and maternofetal lymphocyte engraftment.

Synonyms and inclusions
- Acute graft-versus-host disease, acute GvHD (aGvHD)
- Chronic graft-versus-host disease, chronic GvHD (cGvHD)
- GvHD overlap syndrome, sometimes called acute on chronic GvHD

Introduction and general description

Allogeneic HSCT, transplantation of multipotent stem cells, usually derived from bone marrow, peripheral blood or umbilical cord blood, from either a family member or unrelated donor, is used widely for haematological malignancies, but also immunodeficiencies and marrow failure syndromes. The procedure is increasingly

being utilised for other life-threatening conditions such as multiple sclerosis, Crohn disease, systemic lupus erythematosus and systemic sclerosis [3,4].

GvHD is the major cause of morbidity and non-relapse-related mortality following allogeneic HSCT. In most patients, the first and most common site affected by GvHD is the skin.

GvHD has classically been divided into acute and chronic based on time of onset:
- aGvHD – disease presenting within the first 100 days of HSCT.
- cGvHD – disease onset after 100 days of HSCT.

However, clinicians now prefer to define acute and chronic GvHD based on the distinctive clinical features of these diseases rather than a specific time point post-transplant. An overlap syndrome for GvHD is also included in the National Institutes of Health (NIH) consensus diagnostic criteria [5] in which clinical features of both aGvHD and and cGvHD appear together. This is sometimes referred to as 'acute on chronic' GvHD. More recently the term 'progressive GvHD' has been coined where aGvHD leads rapidly to cGvHD [6].

For patients being treated for haematological malignancy, minimising the GvHD without compromising the graft-versus-tumour (also known as graft-versus-leukaemia, GVL) effect remains the focus of active research [7,8].

Epidemiology

Incidence and prevalence
Approximately 10–80% of HSCT recipients will develop aGvHD, depending on the risk factors present [9]. Large retrospective registry studies show recipient HLA mismatching and the use of unrelated donors confers a greater risk of aGvHD, as does gender

mismatch, relative risk (RR 2) of developing grade 2–4 aGvHD [10], total body irradiation (RR 1.4) [11] and older recipient age (age over 40 years; RR 1.4) [11].

The 5-year cumulative incidence of cGvHD in long-term survivors varies from 9 to 80% [1,12]. However, estimates of incidence are somewhat unreliable due to variation in diagnostic criteria. Particular risk factors include gender mismatch between recipient and donor and older recipient and donor age, donor alloimmunisation (e.g. previous pregnancy or transfusions), history of aGvHD and the administration of donor lymphocyte infusions following allograft [13] and Epstein–Barr virus donor seropositivity [14]. GvHD prophylaxis with oral tacrolimus or methotrexate reduces the risk of cGvHD (hazard ratio [HR] 0.35) [9,15], as does the use of reduced intensity conditioning – the reduction in RR depends on the underlying disease and source of stem cells [16].

Pathophysiology

Predisposing factors

Acute graft-versus-host disease
The pathophysiology of aGvHD is well understood and has been elucidated using animal models [17,18], supported by some experimental human studies [19,20]. It is likely that aGvHD arises from a three-stage process:

1 First, toxicity from conditioning chemotherapy or radiotherapy causes tissue damage in the host, resulting in the release of numerous inflammatory cytokines.
2 Second, mature donor lymphocytes from the graft are recruited by these cytokines, leading to their activation and proliferation when contact is made with host and donor antigen-presenting cells (APCs) expressing disparate host antigens such as minor histocompatibility antigens (MiHC).
3 Third, alloreactive T cells expand to form cytotoxic effector T cells that, in turn, induce further tissue injury and release more inflammatory cytokines.

The transplant conditioning regimen used, pre-existing innate immune system defects and GI microbiome all influence aGvHD pathophysiology [21,22,**23**].

Chronic graft-versus-host disease
The pathogenesis of cGvHD has become more clearly understood over the last 5 years, using a combination of mouse model studies and corroborative clinical research [24,25,**26**]. With the wide spectrum of clinical cGvHD phenotypes and the numerous predisposing factors, it is unsurprising that a complex, multistep immune basis is emerging, involving early tissue damage, dysregulated immunity and anomalous tissue repair with fibrosis.

First, early tissue/endothelial cell damage results from conditioning therapies, aGvHD and body irradiation [**26**,27]. Mature naïve donor T lymphocytes (antigen-inexperienced) contribute to tissue damage of the thymus causing thymic disruption. Graft-derived precursor T cells (lymphoid progenitor cells) that migrate to the recipient bone marrow also play a role in immune dysregulation.

The thymic disruption enables autoreactive (against donor antigens) and alloreactive Th17 cell production.

In addition, donor-derived B cells also play a role in cGvHD pathogenesis, triggering further auto- and alloantibody production. The interest in a role for B cells was first sparked by the clinical observations that cGvHD phenotypes can resemble B-cell-mediated autoimmune disease such as scleroderma and Sjögren syndrome [28]. Elevated levels of B-cell activating factor (BAF) cytokines have been detected in cGvHD patient serum [29], and GvHD cannot be induced in B-cell-depleted mice [30]. Furthermore, reduced peripheral regulatory T cells (Tregs) due to thymic damage and exogenous calcineurin inhibitors reduce immune tolerance.

Damage of endothelial cells (that act as a barrier between donor and host cells) allows donor cells to migrate to organs. Macrophage transforming growth factor (TGF)β production (innate immune system activation), stimulated further by the auto- and alloreactive antibodies, in turn activates fibroblast and aberrant collagen production. Hence end-organ fibrosis is found, leading to the clinical manifestations of GvHD [31,32].

Pathology
For aGvHD, skin histopathology shows a lichenoid inflammatory process with a linear arrangement of lymphocytes along the basement membrane zone. The hallmark change, although not pathognomonic, is satellite cell necrosis consisting of apoptotic keratinocytes with tightly associated lymphocytes seen in the epidermis and associated interface vacuolar change. Histology can be indistinguishable from a lichenoid drug eruption (Figure 38.1).

The cutaneous histological changes have been graded for severity (Table 38.1), although cutaneous biopsy is not useful in predicting either clinical severity or outcome [34]. Less severe histological grades may be impossible to differentiate from drug-induced reactions. Scattered eosinophils are found both in drug reactions and in GvHD and only a very high number of eosinophils (16 per 10 high-power fields) excludes GvHD [35].

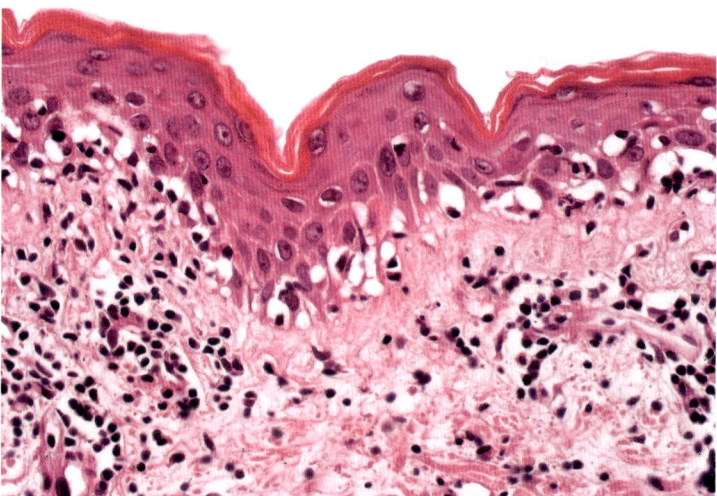

Figure 38.1 Skin histology of acute graft-versus-host disease. Courtesy of Dr Eduardo Calonje, King's College Hospital, London, UK.

Table 38.1 Histological grading of severity of acute graft-versus-host disease.

Histological severity	Description
Grade I	Basal cell vacuolation with or without mononuclear cell infiltration
Grade II	Solitary epidermal cell necrosis, surrounded by mononuclear cells
Grade III	Regional epidermal cell necrosis with bullae
Grade IV	Complete dermal and epidermal separation

Adapted from Pintar 2007 [33]. Reproduced with permission of Thieme.

Now validated panels of immunohistological biomarkers to diagnose GvHD and to predict response to treatment are emerging [36], and this remains an area of active research [37,38]. Prognostic biomarkers include elafin, a keratinocyte-derived protein, which is overexpressed in the skin in cutaneous GvHD [39]. Also, ST2 (suppression of tumorigenicity 2), an interleukin-1 receptor family protein, may predict response to treatment in aGvHD patients [40]. Regenerating islet-derived 3-α (REG3α) levels are raised in patients with gut GvHD [41].

In cGvHD, histological changes depend on the type of skin involvement, which may be lichenoid or resemble scleroderma. Lichenoid cGvHD histology has hyperkeratosis, hypergranulosis, acanthosis, saw-toothed rete ridges, interface dermatitis and dyskeratotic keratinocytes. Periadnexal, particularly peri-eccrine, inflammation may be evident (Figure 38.2).

Of the sclerotic lesions of cGvHD, lichen sclerosus-like lesions show epidermal atrophy, oedema and homogenisation of collagen in the superficial dermis (Figure 38.3). Morphoeaform lesions show thickened dermal collagen fibre bundles with loss of adnexal structures and often no epidermal change. There may be involvement of the fat with thickened septae and lymphocytic infiltrate at the border between dermis and subcutis.

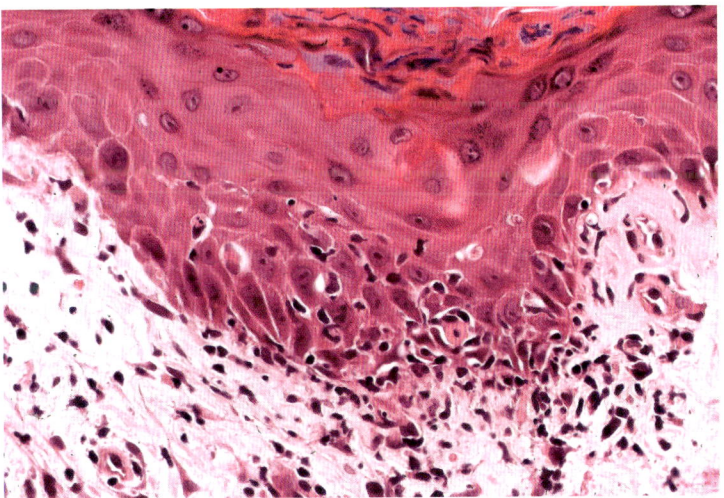

Figure 38.2 Skin histology of chronic lichenoid graft-versus-host disease. Courtesy of Dr Eduardo Calonje, King's College Hospital, London, UK.

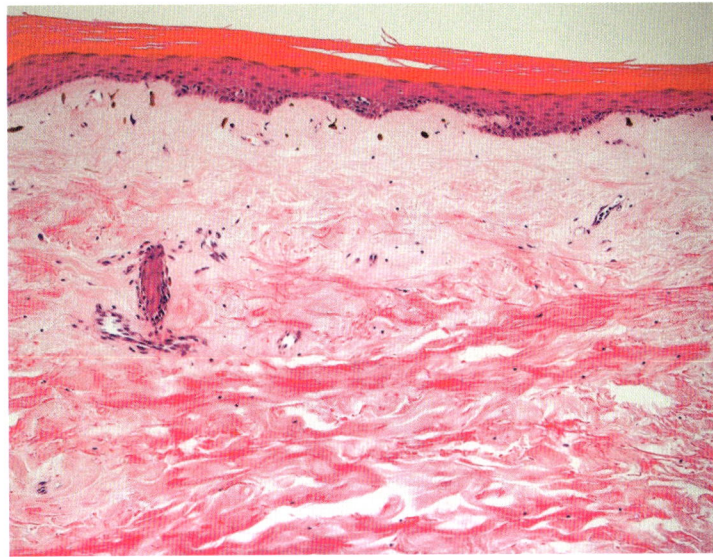

Figure 38.3 Skin histology of chronic sclerodermoid graft-versus-host disease. Courtesy of Dr J.R. Salisbury, King's College Hospital, UK.

Acute graft-versus-host disease

Clinical features

History

aGvHD often occurs 2–4 weeks after HSCT but can present any time after transplantation. Hence aGvHD onset can be classic (onset <100 days post-HSCT), late (>100 days post-HSCT), recurrent or persistent [24]. Pruritus or a burning sensation can precede the skin eruption. Patients may report oral or genital ulceration. Profuse diarrhoea points to GI tract involvement, as do symptoms of nausea, anorexia, vomiting and abdominal pain. Cholestatic symptoms of pale urine, dark stools and right upper quadrant tenderness may also be reported.

Presentation

Typically, red blanching macules develop on the palms, soles (Figure 38.4) or ears. The eruption may appear photoaggravated in distribution affecting the neck (Figure 38.5a,b), upper back and face or it may be folliculocentric.

As aGvHD evolves, lesions become more confluent with a morbilliform appearance. In severe cases, there may be generalised erythroderma (Figure 38.5c), bullae and extensive Nikolsky sign-positive epidermal skin loss with a toxic epidermal necrolysis-like picture.

Orally, xerostoma, redness and ulcers occur but may be difficult to distinguish from chemotherapy-induced mucositis [18].

Differential diagnosis

The differential diagnosis includes adverse drug reaction, viral exanthem and engraftment syndrome.

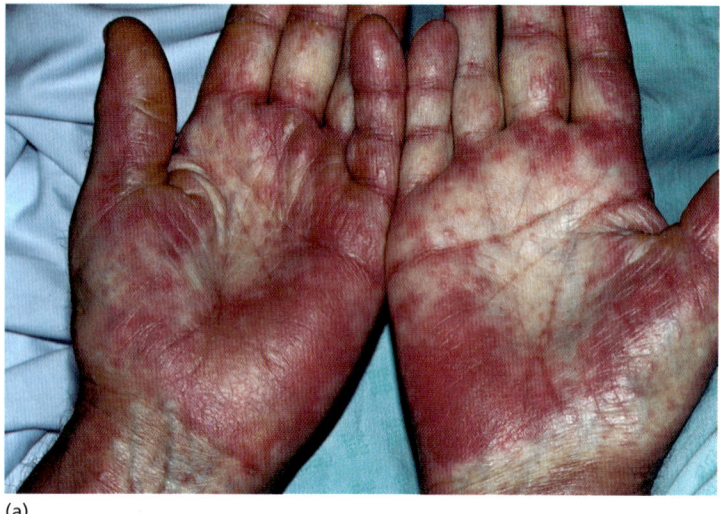

(a)

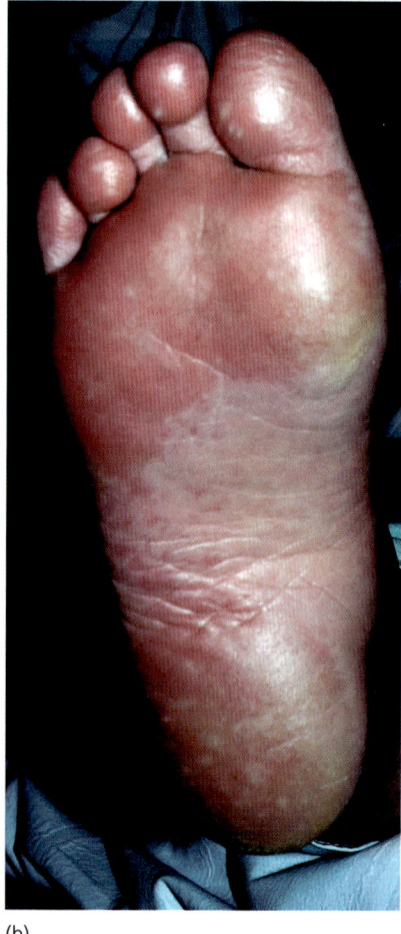

(b)

Figure 38.4 Clinical features of acute graft-versus-host disease: (a) acute palmar erythema; and (b) plantar erythema.

Classification of severity

The validated Glucksberg staging system is the one used most often; the extent of cutaneous involvement, liver and GI involvement are assessed and used to give an overall severity (grade) of aGvHD (Table 38.2 and Box 38.1).

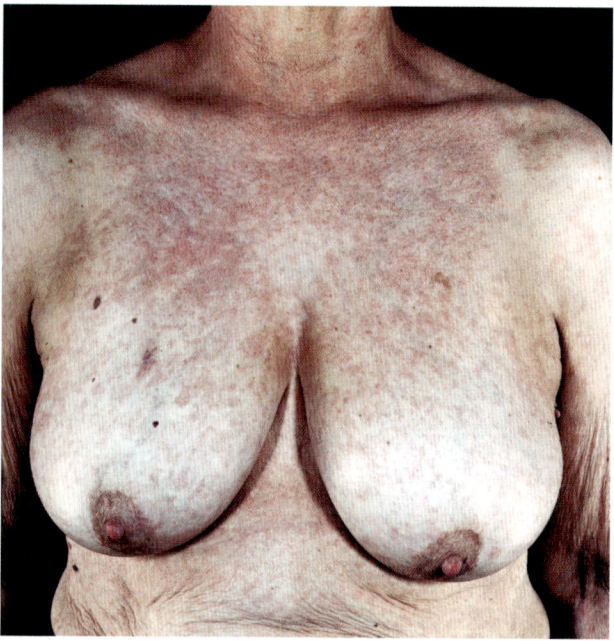

(a)

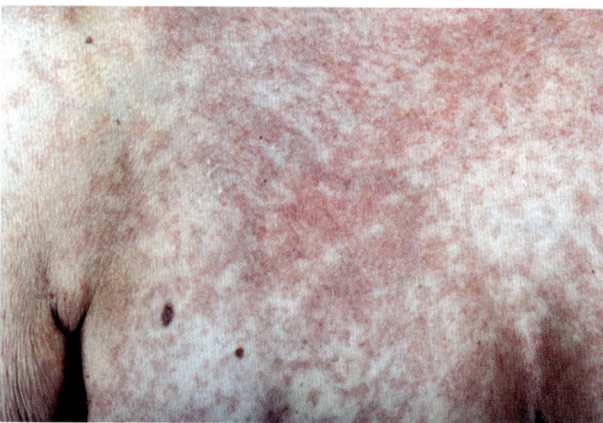

(b)

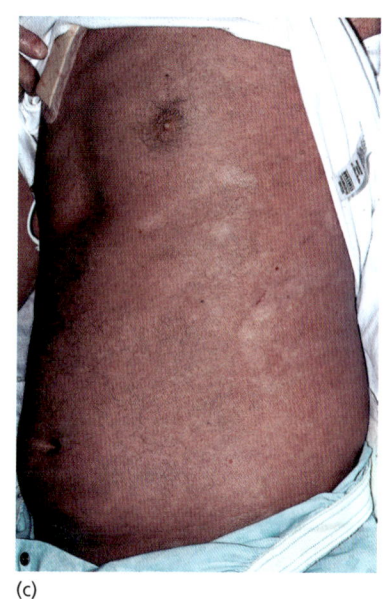

(c)

Figure 38.5 Clinical features of acute graft-versus-host disease: (a) morbilliform exanthem with photoexposed accentuation; (b) morbilliform exanthema with telangiectasia in close-up; and (c) confluent erythroderma.

Table 38.2 Severity grading of acute graft-versus-host disease, Glucksberg score.

Organ	Stage	Description
Skin	1	Maculopapular rash over <25% of body area
	2	Maculopapular rash over 25–50% of body area
	3	Generalised erythroderma
	4	Generalised erythroderma with bullous formation and often with desquamation
Liver	1	Bilirubin 2.0–3.0 mg/dL; SGOT 150–750 IU
	2	Bilirubin 3.1–6.0 mg/dL
	3	Bilirubin 6.1–15.0 mg/dL
	4	Bilirubin >15.0 mg/dL
Gut	1	Diarrhoea >30 mL/kg or >500 mL/day
	2	Diarrhoea >60 mL/kg or >1000 mL/day
	3	Diarrhoea >90 mL/kg or >1500 mL/day
	4	Diarrhoea >90 mL/kg or >2000 mL/day; or severe abdominal pain with or without ileus

Adapted from Glucksberg *et al.* 1974 [42], modified from Thomas *et al.* 1975 [43]. With permission from LWW/Massachusetts Medical Society.
Glucksberg grade:
I – Stage 1 or 2 skin involvement; no liver or gut involvement; ECOG PS 0.
II – Stage 1–3 skin involvement; grade 1 liver or gut involvement; ECOG PS 1.
III – Stage 2 or 3 skin, liver or gut involvement; ECOG PS 2.
IV – Stage 1–4 skin involvement; stage 2–4 liver or gut involvement; ECOG PS 3.
ECOG, Eastern Cooperative Oncology Group; PS, performance status; SGOT, serum glutamic oxaloacetic transaminase.

Complications and co-morbidities

Oral ulceration and diarrhoea can lead to weight loss and dehydration. Skin erosions can lead to secondary infection.

Box 38.1 International Bone Marrow Transplant Registry (IBMTR) severity index for acute graft-versus-host disease

The severity is the highest level that the patient reaches based on separate skin, liver and gastrointestinal staging.

A – Stage 1 skin involvement; no liver or gut involvement
B – Stage 2 skin involvement; stage 1–2 gut or liver involvement
C – Stage 3 skin, liver or gut involvement
D – Stage 4 skin, liver or gut involvement

Disease course and prognosis

The severity grade of GvHD correlates with overall survival. The transplant-related mortality rates for grades 0–IV aGvHD are 28%, 27%, 43%, 68% and 92%, respectively [45].

Investigations

Diagnosis of acute cutaneous GvHD can be challenging and is based on clinical findings. A 4 mm skin biopsy sent for haematoxylin and eosin (H&E) staining can lend support to clinical signs but there are no pathognomonic features. Studies suggest that performing a skin biopsy does not alter whether aGvHD treatment is instigated or not [46]. A peripheral eosinophilia may be present. Serum biomarkers are not routinely measured in clinical practice, but compelling research suggests panels of biomarkers will assist diagnosis and predict treatment response in GvHD [36]. Elafin,

an elastase inhibitor, is validated as a cutaneous GvHD predictive biomarker [39]. The Mount Sinai GvHD International Consortium (MAGIC) has validated an algorithm biomarkers panel combining two GI biomarkers (ST2 and REG3α) that predict GvHD severity and treatment response.

Management

There are few randomised controlled trials of the management of aGvHD and patients should be included in trial protocols wherever possible. Patients with grade 1 disease do not usually require systemic treatment. For grade 1 aGvHD confined to the skin (less than 50% body surface area (BSA) affected), topical corticosteroid and emollient therapy is recommended [2] (Table 38.3) along with optimisation of ongoing prophylactic GvHD immunosuppression (e.g. ensuring therapeutic levels of ciclosporin). Adjunctive antihistamine therapy can help for patients with itch. Topical tacrolimus ointment may be useful in refractory grade 1 aGvHD, but this is not a licensed indication [2].

In addition to the measures for grade 1 aGvHD, patients with grade 2–4 GvHD (>50% BSA skin affected, with or without liver and GI involvement), require systemic glucocorticoid therapy. Although dosing and treatment schedules vary, in the UK 1 mg/kg oral prednisolone is considered first line therapy for grade 2 aGvHD, and 2 mg/kg intravenous methylprednisolone for grade 3–4 disease [2] (Figure 38.6). In responsive patients, this dose may be continued for several weeks and tapered over several months. The minimally absorbable glucocorticoid beclomethasone may be added for patients with GI involvement in whom infection, such as with cytomegalovirus, has been ruled out. Patients with no clinical improvement or worsening of GvHD signs are considered steroid non-responsive after 7 days and second line therapies should be instigated in consultation with a haematologist.

Treatment ladder for Stage 2–4 aGvHD [2]

First line
- Corticosteroids, e.g. prednisolone 1 mg/kg oral or IV
- Oral calcineurin inhibitors (ciclosporin or tacrolimus), dose optimisation

Second line
- Extracorporeal photopheresis (the only commissioned second line treatment in the UK)
- Mycophenolate mofetil
- mTOR inhibitors, e.g. sirolimus

Third line
- Mesenchymal stromal cells
- Alemtuzumab
- Pentostatin

Future treatments/trials
- T-regulatory adoptive immunotherapy strategies
- Itolizumab anti-CD6 [47]
- Bortezomib, a proteosome inhibitor
- Maraviroc CCR5 antagonist

Table 38.3 Topical corticosteroid therapy recommended for grade 1 acute graft-versus-host disease. Generally, a lower steroid usage is recommended in children. Dermatology supervision is advised when using potent steroids on the face. Side effects: prolonged use of topical steroids can thin skin and may cause redness, striae and dyspigmentation. If more than 50 g of very potent steroid is used per week, sufficient steroid may be absorbed through the skin to result in adrenal gland suppression or cushingoid features. Occlusion of steroids will enhance absorption and it is possible that larger amounts of weaker steroids may have the same effect.

Steroid strength	Very potent, e.g. Dermovate	Potent, e.g. Betnovate 0.1%	Moderately potent, e.g. Eumovate	Mildly potent, e.g. 1% hydrocortisone
Face	Should generally be avoided. Use twice daily	Twice daily 4–12 weeks	Twice daily 6–12 months	Twice daily Long-term use acceptable
Body	Twice daily 4–12 weeks	Twice daily Long-term therapy may be appropriate		
Palms and soles	Twice daily May be used under occlusion to enhance efficacy Long-term therapy may be appropriate	Long-term therapy may be appropriate		

Adapted from Dignan *et al.* 2012 [1]. Reproduced with permission of John Wiley & Sons Ltd.

Second line therapies include mycophenolate mofetil (small prospective studies suggest 50–65% efficacy in steroid-resistant aGvHD [48]), and extracorporeal photopheresis (ECP). ECP involves collection, by apheresis, of autologous peripheral lymphocytes that are incubated with 8-methoxypsoralen, ultraviolet A-irradiated and then reinfused. The mechanism of action of ECP is unclear but mouse model studies suggest it may downregulate activated T-cell clones and increase Tregs. There are few studies analysing the efficacy of ECP in aGvHD. One prospective non-randomised study suggests complete response in 82% of patients with cutaneous aGvHD and 62% with GI or liver involvement [49]. Etanercept is a recombinant human tumour necrosis factor (TNF)-α receptor fusion protein. TNF-α is frequently implicated in the evolution of GvHD but no comparative data for efficacy of anti-TNF therapies such as infliximab and etanercept are available [50].

The mTOR inhibitor sirolimus and anti-IL-22 receptor antibodies have also been used. Third line therapies include alemtuzumab (a humanised monoclonal anti-CD52 antibody), pentostatin (a purine analogue) and mesenchymal stromal cells (MSCs). MSCs are bone marrow derived cells that can differentiate into mesenchymal lineage cells and increase numbers of CD4+/CD25+/FOXP3+ regulatory T cells. *Ex vivo* expanded, unmatched MSCs can be used to treat steroid-resistant acute gut GvHD and are particularly used in paediatric patients [51]. Numerous trials are underway to identify targeted aGvHD therapies, such as itolizumab, an anti-CD6 agent showing promising phase 1 results [47].

Chronic graft-versus-host disease

Clinical features

History
Chronic GvHD was historically defined as occurring more than 100 days post-HSCT. However, classical cGvHD can present before 100 days. Chronic GvHD can occur *de novo* (no prior aGvHD), be termed quiescent (occurring after a period of aGvHD inactivity or resolution) or progressive (aGvHD evolving into cGvHD) [6]. The skin is the most common site involved, followed by mucosa, but virtually any organ can be affected. Patients can report the insidious onset of dry, tight or itchy skin. It is important to ask about ocular discomfort and dryness as well as oral discomfort, often noted after eating spicy foods or using toothpaste. Patients may be hesitant to report genital symptoms such as vulvovaginal dryness, itch and discomfort without direct questioning. GI symptoms of nausea, diarrhoea and vomiting, respiratory symptoms of shortness of breath (where infection has been excluded) and musculoskeletal symptoms, including muscle weakness and limited range of movement, are important in this multisystem disease [52].

Presentation
The NIH Consensus project has defined the cutaneous and extracutaneous diagnostic criteria for cGvHD [5]. The skin features considered diagnostic are lichen planus-like lesions on the skin (Figure 38.7) or in the mouth (Figure 38.8a,b), sclerotic skin lesions and poikiloderma. Other distinctive associated clinical signs (not sufficient alone to make the diagnosis) include skin dyspigmentation, nail dystrophy (Figure 38.8c), alopecia, oral ulceration, mucoceles and xerostomia, keratoconjunctiva sicca and myositis.

Skin changes may be sclerotic or non-sclerotic and have traditionally been classified as lichen planus-like (lichenoid) or scleroderma-like (sclerodermoid) (Figures 38.9 and 38.10). In practice, a combination of lichen-planus like violaceous papules (that can be folliculocentric), sclerodermatous and poikilodermatous change is often seen, along with deep fascial involvement that can lead to contractures developing. With dermal involvement, a rippled cellulite appearance on thighs and upper arms can be seen, resembling eosinophilic fasciitis. 'Grooving' of the skin along the path of superficial vessels or between fascial planes can be observed [53]. In addition, lichen sclerosus-like guttate hypopigmented atrophic plaques can be seen (when fibrosis is limited to the papillary dermis) and nummular morphoea-like plaques (when dermal fibrosis has occurred). Morphoea-like plaques exhibit an isomorphic response localising to sites of pressure or trauma such as the waistband, brassiere line or previous Hickman line sites [53]. Non-sclerotic (epidermal) manifestations also occur including eczema-like variants (eczematoid) [54]; papulosquamous, pityriasis rubra pilaris-like, exfoliative and keratosis pilaris-like presentations have been reported [55].

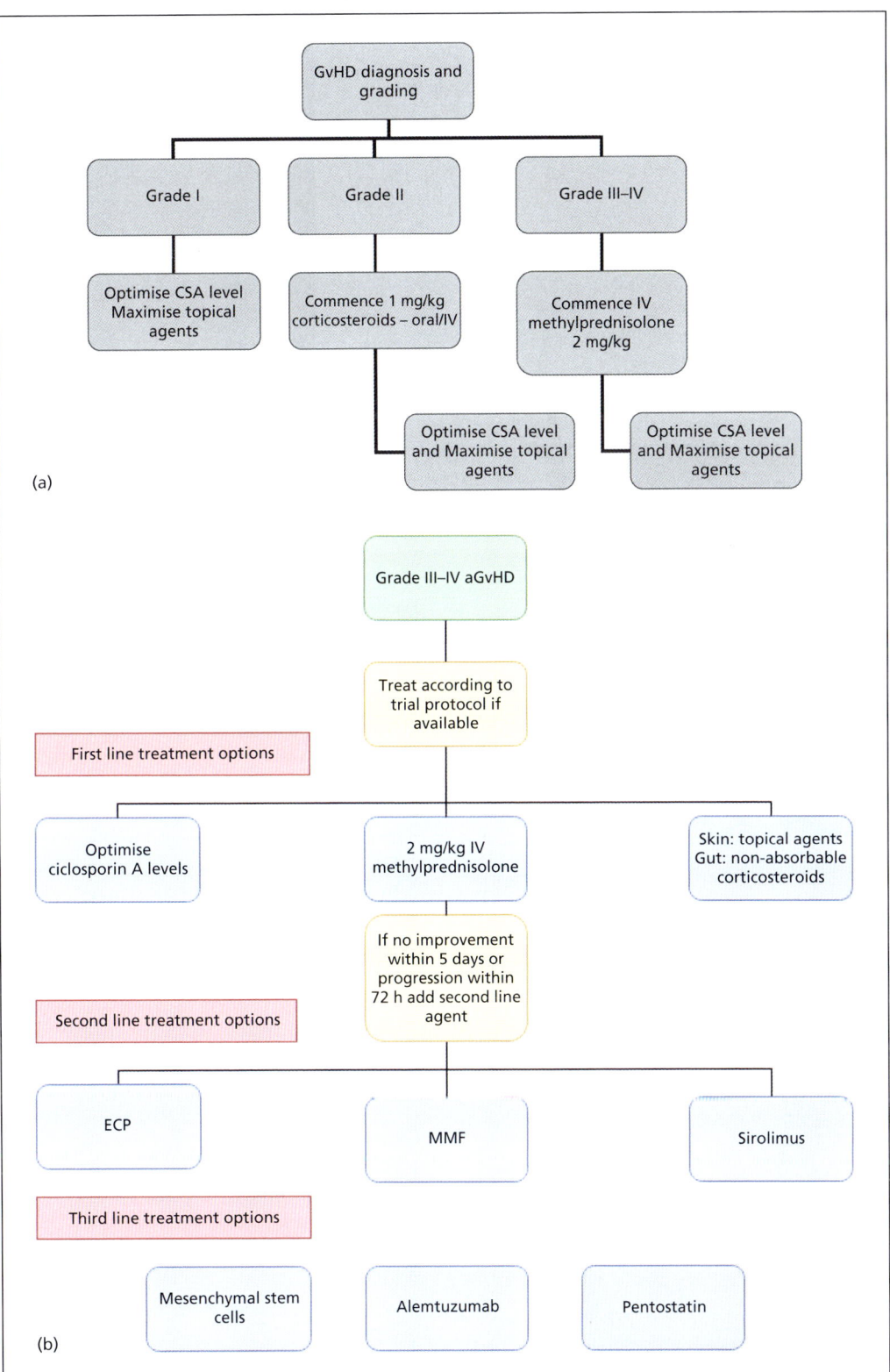

PART 4: INFLAMMATORY DERMATOSES

Figure 38.6 (a) Treatment algorithm summarising initial treatment of acute graft-versus-host disease (GvHD). CSA, ciclosporin. Adapted from Dignan *et al*. 2012 [1]. Reproduced with permission of John Wiley & Sons Ltd. (b) Treatment algorithm for grade III–IV acute graft-versus-host disease (aGvHD) (third-line agents). CSA, ciclosporin; ECP, extracorporeal photopheresis; IL-2, interleukin 2; TNF, tumour necrosis factor; mTOR, mammalian target of rapamycin; MMF, mycophenolate mofetil. Adapted from Dignan *et al*. 2012 [1]. Updated according to Treatments for GvHD following haematopoietic stem cell transplantation Clinical Commissioning policy 2017 (see resources). With thanks to Keya Downward.

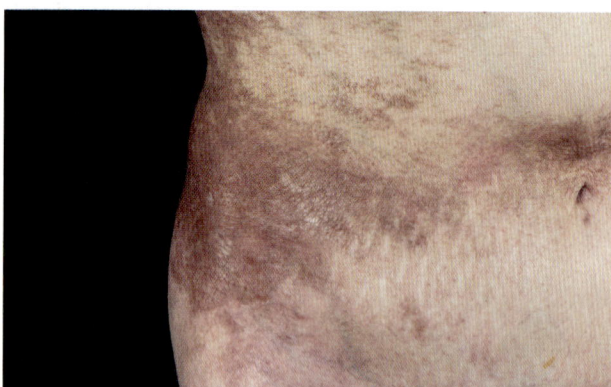

Figure 38.7 Clinical features of lichenoid chronic graft-versus-host disease. Lichenoid skin change accentuated on the flanks, along the waistband site.

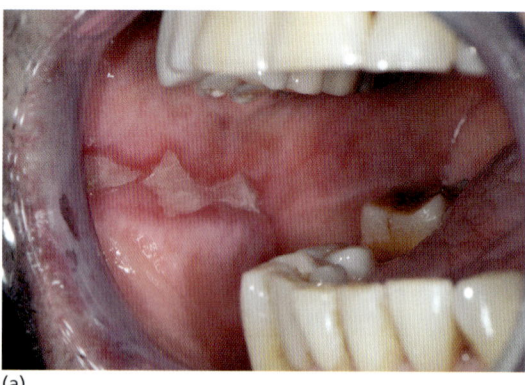

(a)

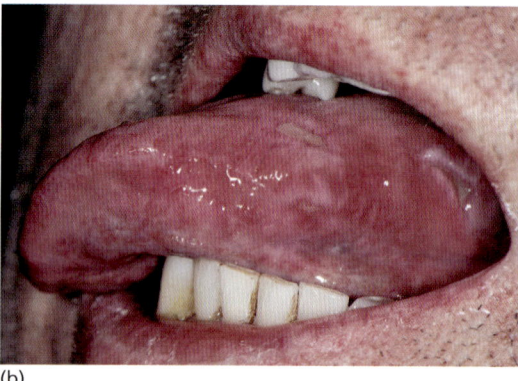

(b)

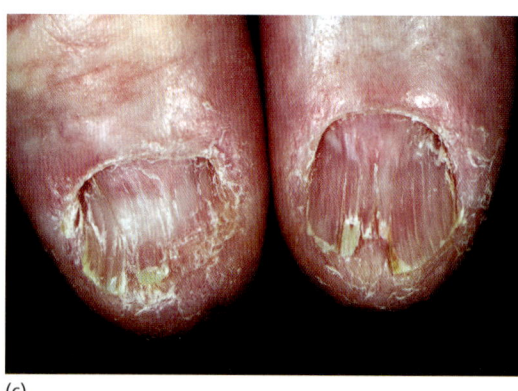

(c)

Figure 38.8 Clinical features of lichenoid chronic graft-versus-host disease (cGvHD). (a) Oral cGvHD with lichenoid buccal change and hyperkeratosis along the bite line. (b) Lichenoid change and ulceration of the tongue. (c) Lichenoid nail changes of cGvHD.

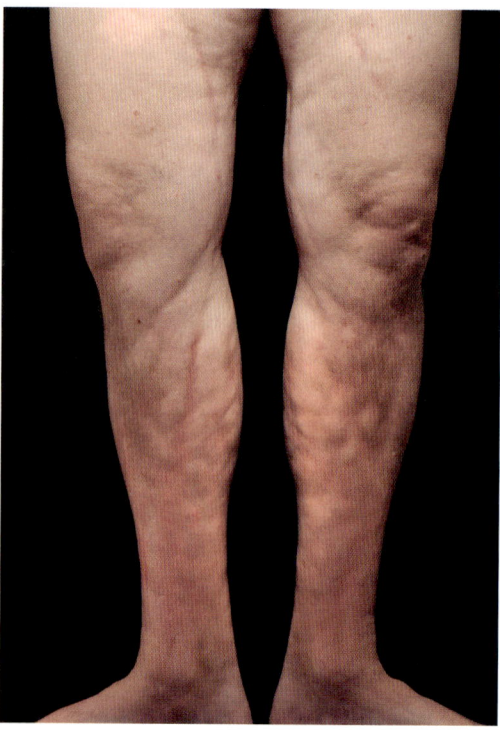

Figure 38.9 Clinical features of chronic sclerodermoid graft-versus-host disease (GvHD). Chronic GvHD showing extensive sclerodermoid changes of the legs with orange peel-like change, woody induration of the skin and venous guttering. Courtesy of Dr F. Child, St John's Institute of Dermatology, London, UK.

Mucosal signs include oral mucoceles and Wickham striae on the lips and buccal mucosa. Minor and major salivary gland damage can result in xerostomia and dental caries [56]. Hence, a systematic oral examination is essential. Genital involvement can lead to vulvovaginal stenosis, labial fusion and resorption and, in men, scarring on the prepuce and glans penis.

In addition, there may be scarring or non-scarring alopecia and nail changes including dystrophy, anonychia and pterygium.

A multidisciplinary team approach is essential to carefully assess for extracutaneous manifestations including GI, hepatic, respiratory and cardiac and musculoskeletal involvement.

Summary of clinical variants of chronic graft-versus-host disease

Cutaneous features:
1 Sclerotic:
   - Sclerodermoid, deep sclerosis/eosinophilic fasciitis-like.
   - Lichen sclerosus-like.
   - Morphoeaform.
2 Lichenoid.
3 Epidermal – eczematoid, papulosquamous, PRP-like (single report).
4 Associated features:
   - Oral lesions – lichenoid, microstomia, mucoceles, sicca symptoms, oral verruciform xanthoma (rare).
   - Hair – scarring or non-scarring alopecia.
   - Nails – dystrophy, anonychia, pterygium.
   - Ocular and genital mucosa – erosions, pain, lichen planus-like or lichen sclerosus-like lesions.

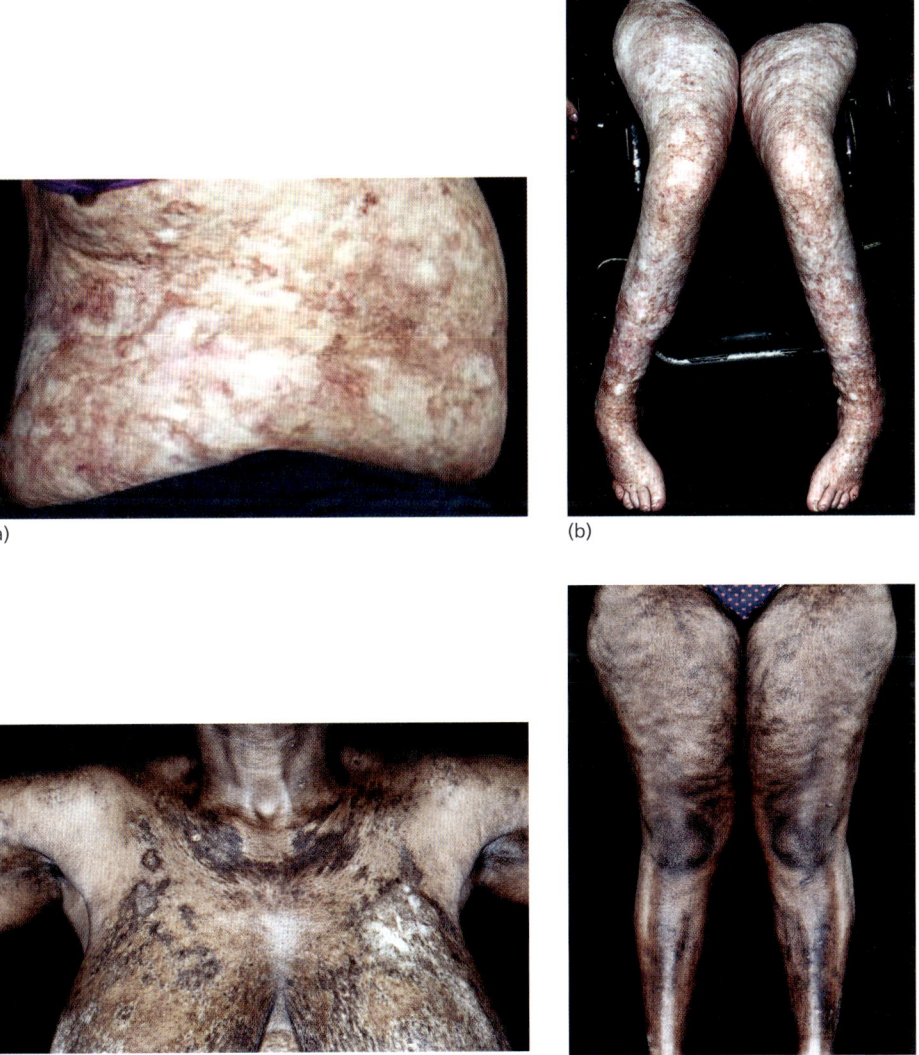

Figure 38.10 Clinical features of chronic sclerodermoid graft-versus-host disease (GvHD). (a, b) Chronic GvHD showing extensive sclerodermoid changes. (c) Chronic GvHD showing extensive sclerodermoid changes with discoid lupus-like change on the chest. (d) Peau d'orange changes on the legs. Courtesy of Tanya Basu.

Extracutaneous features:

Extracutaneous manifestations:

- Liver.
- GI.
- Lung.
- Musculoskeletal (fasciitis, myositis).
- Other, e.g. demyelination.

Differential diagnosis

The differential includes drug-induced lichenoid eruptions, radiation-induced fibrosis and skin sclerosis and morphoea.

Classification of severity

Several systems for grading the severity of cGvHD have been developed. The validated NIH Consensus criteria for cGvHD are the most widely used (Table 38.4). The score includes the number and sites involved and the severity within each affected organ. Using these scores, an overall grade of mild, moderate or severe can be made. It is important to carefully assess the extent of cutaneous and mucous membrane involvement in a systematic way [52], and to allow accurate staging, every 3 months, so response to treatment can be gauged.

Complications and co-morbidities

Sclerotic disease and fascial contractures can cause severe limitation of movement and disability along with other issues such as difficult venous access. Dyspigmentation and poikiloderma can cause profound changes of appearance. The psychological burden of cGvHD and its impact on quality of life can be underestimated in patients who have already had to cope with the impact of malignancy and allogeneic transplant [57].

Disease course and prognosis

Chronic GvHD is the major cause of mortality and morbidity in long-term survivors of HSCT. Severity grading predicts prognosis [58]. Chronic GvHD is associated with a higher treatment-related mortality post-allogeneic transplant (RR 1.8–2.8, 95% CI 1.3–4.1) despite a slightly lower rate of disease relapse (RR 0.5–0.6; 95% CI 0.3–1.0) [59]. Overall survival at 2 years was 97, 86 and 62% for patients with mild, moderate and severe cGvHD, respectively [59].

Table 38.4 Severity grading of chronic graft-versus-host disease, National Institutes of Health (NIH) score.

	Score 0	Score 1	Score 2	Score 3
Performance score (ECOG, KPS or LPS)	Asymptomatic and fully active (ECOG 0, KPS or LPS 100%)	Symptomatic, fully ambulatory, restricted only in physical strenuous activity (ECOG 1, KPS or LPS)	Symptomatic, ambulatory, capable of self-care, >50% of waking hours out of bed (ECOG 2, KPS or LPS 60–70%)	Symptomatic, limited self-care, >50% of waking hours in bed (ECOG 3–4, KPS or LPS <60%)
Skin – clinical features: Maculopapular rash, lichen planus-like, papulosquamous or ichthyotic, hyperpigmentation, hypopigmentation, keratosis pilaris, redness, poikiloderma, erythroderma, sclerotic pruritus, hair involvement, nail involvement	No symptoms	<18% BSA and no sclerotic features	19–50% BSA or superficial sclerotic features (able to pinch)	>50% BSA or deep sclerotic features 'hidebound'/unable to pinch or impaired mobility, ulceration or severe pruritus
Mouth	No symptoms	Mild signs/symptoms not limiting oral intake significantly	Moderate signs/symptoms with partial limitation of intake	Severe signs/symptoms with major limitation of oral intake
Eyes	No symptoms	Mild dry-eye symptoms (using eye drops <×3/day) or asymptomatic but signs of keratoconjunctivitis sicca	Moderate dry-eye symptoms, partially affected ADL (using eye drops ≥×3/day) or punctate plugs, no visual impairment	Severe dry-eye symptoms, significantly affected ADL or unable to work or loss of vision
GI tract	No symptoms	Symptoms (dysphagia, anorexia, nausea, vomiting, abdominal pain, diarrhoea) without significant weight loss (<5%)	Symptoms with 5–15% weight loss	Symptoms with >15% weight loss requiring nutritional supplement for most calorie needs or oesophageal dilatation
Liver	Normal LFT	Elevated BR, AST or ALP <2 × ULN	Elevated BR, AST or ALP 2–5 × ULN	BR or enzymes ≥5 × ULN
Lungs	No symptoms	Mild symptoms (SOB after 1 flight of steps); FEV$_1$ 60–79% or LFS 2	Moderate symptoms (SOB walking on flat ground); FEV$_1$ 40–59% or LFS 6–9	Severe symptoms (SOB at rest or requiring supplemental O$_2$); FEV1 ≤39% or LFS 10–12
Joint/fascia	No symptoms	Mild tightness of limbs, mildly decreased ROM not affecting ADL	Tightness of arms or legs or joint contractures, redness due to fasciitis, moderate reduction in ROM and mild–moderate limitation in ADL	Contractures with significantly decreased ROM and significant limitation of ADL
Genital tract	No symptoms	Symptomatic with mild signs and no effect on coitus/minimal discomfort on examination	Symptomatic with moderate signs and mild dyspareunia or discomfort on examination	Symptomatic with advanced signs (strictures, labial agglutination or sever ulceration) and severe pain on coitus or inability to insert vaginal speculum

Adapted from Filipovitch *et al.* 2005 [5]. Reproduced with permission of Elsevier.

Based upon this information, the overall severity is scored as mild, moderate or severe:

- Mild – involves two or fewer organs/sites with no clinically significant functional impairment.
- Moderate – involves three or more organs/sites with no clinically significant functional impairment or at least one organ/site with clinically significant functional impairment, but no major disability.
- Severe – major disability caused by chronic GvHD.

ADL, activities of daily living; ALP, alkaline phosphatase; AST, aspartate aminotransferase; BR, bilirubin; BSA, body surface area affected; ECOG, Eastern Cooperative Oncology Group; FEV$_1$, forced expiratory volume in 1 second; GI, gastrointestinal; KPS, Karnofsky performance status; LFS, lung function score (includes FEV$_1$ and diffusion capacity of the lung for CO); LFT, liver function tests; LPS, Lansky performance status; ROM, range of motion; SOB, shortness of breath; ULN, upper limit of normal.

Management

Patients should be graded as mild, moderate or severe according to the NIH Consensus criteria and should be assessed for the involvement of other organs [1]. A multidisciplinary approach for patients with cGvHD is essential. Joint care coordinated by a dermatologist or haematologist with input from ophthalmology, gastroenterology, rheumatology and oral medicine, as well as physiotherapy and occupational therapy, is needed [1] (Table 38.3).

Mild or localised cGVHD may not require treatment. Topical corticosteroid therapy is useful in cutaneous cGvHD. If cutaneous disease is extensive or corticosteroid-resistant, there is a role for psoralen with ultraviolet A phototherapy (PUVA) [60].

In moderate or severe disease, 1 mg/kg oral prednisolone is first line treatment, often for 2 weeks then tapering to 0.5 mg/kg after 4–6 weeks, though there are no set guidelines on corticosteroid tapering [1] (Figure 38.11).

Second line treatment is considered if disease progresses despite 1 mg/kg prednisolone for 2 weeks or if corticosteroids cannot be tapered to 0.5 mg/kg after 4–6 weeks. Ciclosporin use must be weighed against the risk of inducing relapse of malignancy

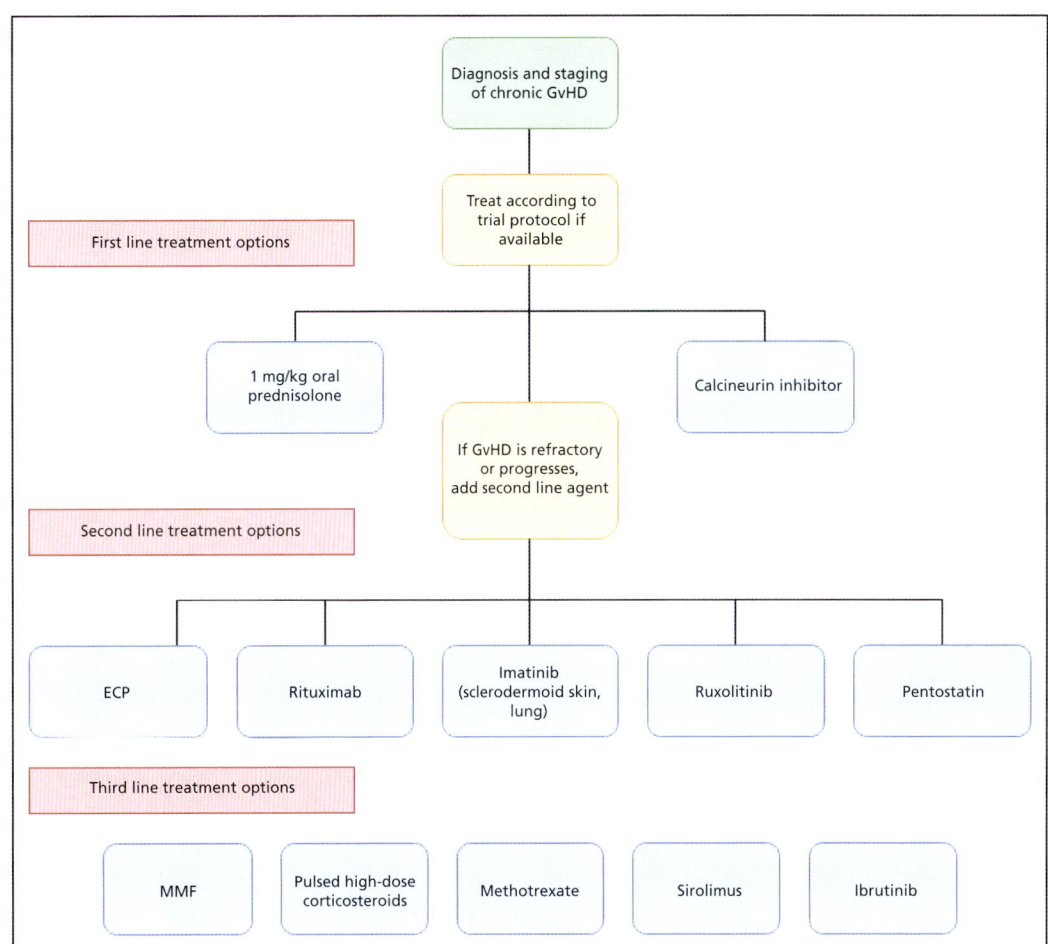

Figure 38.11 An algorithm to show treatment options in chronic graft-versus-host disease (GvHD) to show first, second and third line treatment options. ECP, extracorporeal photopheresis; MMF, mycophenolate mofetil; mTOR, mammalian target of rapamycin. Adapted from Dignan *et al.* 2012 [**1**]. Updated according to Treatments for GvHD following haematopoietic stem cell transplantation Clinical Commissioning policy 2017 (see resources). With thanks to Keya Downward.

PART 4: INFLAMMATORY DERMATOSES

and infectious complications (e.g. driven by Epstein–Barr virus or cytomegalovirus). ECP is not immunosuppressive but evidence for its use in cGvHD remains limited. One prospective randomised controlled trial failed to reach its primary end point but showed a trend for clinical improvement at 12 weeks in patients with sclerodermoid GvHD treated with ECP [**61**]. Retrospective meta-analysis suggests ECP results in overall response rates of 50–65% (approximately 30–35% complete) and approximately 25–35% of patients were able to taper corticosteroid use significantly [**62**]. The REACH3 clinical trial demonstrated efficacy of the Janus kinase (JAK1/JAK2) inhibitor ruxolitinib in glucocorticoid refractory or dependent cGvHD [**63**]. Other treatment options hold promise, including the small molecule tyrosine kinase inhibitor imatinib [**64,65**], and are outlined in the treatment algorithm provided here.

Treatment ladder for moderate or severe cGvHD
[**1**] (Figure 38.11)

First line
- Corticosteroids, e.g. prednisolone 1 mg/kg oral or IV – no standardised tapering regimens

- Oral calcineurin inhibitors – ciclosporin as a steroid sparing agent

Second line
- ECP
- Rituximab
- Imatinib
- Ruxolitinib [**63**]
- Pentostatin

Third line
- Mycophenolate mofetil
- Pulsed high-dose corticosteroids
- Methotrexate
- Sirolimus
- Ibrutinib, Bruton tyrosine kinase inhibitor [**66**]

Others
- Hydroxychloroquine, clofazemine, cyclophosphamide, alemtuzumab, anti-TNF antibodies, thalidomide, alefacept, retinoids, azathioprine, mesenchymal stem cells

Future treatments/trials
- Ixazomib, proteasome inhibitor [**67**]
- Belumosudil, ROCK2 inhibitor [**68**]

Resources

Further information

Acute GvHD management guidelines: http://onlinelibrary.wiley.com/doi/10.1111/j.1365-2141.2012.09129.x/pdf.

Chronic GvHD management guidelines: http://onlinelibrary.wiley.com/doi/10.1111/j.1365-2141.2012.09131.x/pdf.

Clinical Commissioning policy: treatments for GvHD following haematopoietic stem cell transplantation. Reference: NHS England: 16069/P. 2017. https://www.england.nhs.uk/wp-content/uploads/2017/03/gvhd-heamatopoietic-stem-cell.pdf

Patient resources

Leukaemia and Lymphoma Society disease information: http://www.lls.org/diseaseinformation/managingyourcancer/treatmentnextsteps/typesoftreatment/stemcelltransplantation/graftvshostdisease/

Cancer Research UK information site: https://www.cancerresearchuk.org/about-cancer/coping/physically/gvhd

(All sites last accessed April 2022)

Key references

The full list of references can be found in the online version at https://www.wiley.com/rooksdermatology10e

1 Dignan FL, Amrolia P, Clark A *et al*. Diagnosis and management of chronic graft-versus-host disease. *Br J Haematol* 2012;158:46–61.

2 Dignan FL, Clark A, Amrolia P *et al*. Diagnosis and management of acute graft-versus-host disease. *Br J Haematol* 2012;158:30–45.

6 Schoemans HM, Lee SJ, Ferrara JL *et al*. EBMT-NIH-CIBMTR Task Force position statement on standardized terminology & guidance for graft-versus-host disease assessment. *Bone Marrow Transplant* 2018;53:1401–15.

23 Lee MW, Yeon SH, Heo BY *et al*. Impact of pre-transplant use of antibiotics on the graft-versus-host disease in adult patients with hematological malignancies. *Hematology* 2021;26:96–102.

26 MacDonald KP, Hill GR, Blazar BR. Chronic graft-versus-host disease: biological insights from preclinical and clinical studies. *Blood* 2017;129:13–21.

36 Srinagesh HK, Özbek U, Kapoor U *et al*. The MAGIC algorithm probability is a validated response biomarker of treatment of acute graft-versus-host disease. *Blood Adv* 2019;3:4034–42.

49 Greinix HT, Volc-Platzer B, Rabitsch W *et al*. Successful use of extracorporeal photochemotherapy in the treatment of severe acute and chronic graft-versus-host disease. *Blood* 1998;92:3098–104.

52 Carpenter PA. How I conduct a comprehensive chronic graft-versus-host disease assessment. *Blood* 2011;118:2679–87.

61 Flowers ME, Apperley JF, van Besien K *et al*. A multicenter prospective phase 2 randomized study of extracorporeal photopheresis for treatment of chronic graft-versus-host disease. *Blood* 2008;112:2667–74.

63 Zeiser R, Polverelli N, Ram R *et al*. Ruxolitinib for glucocorticoid-refractory chronic graft-versus-host disease. *New Engl J Med* 2021;385:228–38.

CHAPTER 39

Eczematous Disorders

Avad A. Mughal[1] *and John R. Ingram*[2]

[1]Dermatology Department, Neath and Port Talbot Hospital, Swansea Bay University Health Board, Port Talbot, Wales, UK
[2]Department of Dermatology and Wound Healing, Cardiff University, Cardiff, UK

PART 4: INFLAMMATORY DERMATOSES

ASSESSMENT, INVESTIGATION AND MANAGEMENT OF ECZEMATOUS DISORDERS

Eczema

Definition and nomenclature

Eczema, derived from the Greek word 'ε'κζεμα' meaning 'to boil over', is a clinical and histological pattern of inflammation of the skin seen in a variety of dermatoses with widely diverse aetiologies. Clinically, eczematous dermatoses are characterised by variable intensity of itching and soreness, and, in variable degrees, signs including dryness, redness, excoriation, exudation, fissuring, hyperkeratosis, lichenification, papulation, scaling and vesiculation. Histologically, the clinical signs are reflected by a range of epidermal changes including spongiosis (epidermal oedema) with varying degrees of acanthosis and hyperkeratosis, accompanied by a lymphohistiocytic infiltrate in the dermis.

The terms 'dermatitis' and 'eczema' are synonymous, although some authors still use the term 'dermatitis' to include all types of cutaneous inflammation, so that all eczema is dermatitis, but not all dermatitis is eczema [1,2]. Some caution is required when using the term dermatitis, as some patients regard it as implying an occupational cause.

Introduction and general description

Classification based on aetiology has been proposed and is a useful system where the cause is clear, for example patch test-proven allergic contact dermatitis. However, frequently the aetiology is unclear or, as in hand eczema, there are a number of probable contributing aetiologies. Morphology of the condition can be used as a classification like 'nummular' dermatitis (derived from the Latin '*nummus*' meaning 'coin'). However, one morphological pattern of eczema can have a variety of causes. Pompholyx eczema can be due to atopy, irritant or allergic contact dermatitis. In addition, the morphology of an acute presentation, which tends to be oedematous and exudative (Figure 39.1a), may differ from chronic eczema, in which the predominant features are dryness, hyperkeratosis and lichenification (Figure 39.1b).

The *International Statistical Classification of Diseases and Related Health Problems 11th Revision (ICD-11)* is moving towards a composite system based on aetiology, where known, and skin site (Box 39.1). Management of exogenous eczemas is to remove the cause, whereas endogenous eczemas more often require pharmacological intervention. Disorders in which the predominant feature is lichenification are generally regarded as eczematous dermatoses and these are also included in this chapter. Eczema is a common cause of erythroderma and therefore this is also included.

There remain cases of eczema that do not fit any of the described patterns [3]. These are not uncommon and have been termed 'unclassified eczema' [4]. These patients may have a poor prognosis, with a tendency for the disease to become chronic. It is not unusual to see generalised, apparently endogenous, but otherwise unclassified eczema in the elderly [5].

Epidemiology
Incidence and prevalence

In 2010 a worldwide survey of skin disease found there were 230 million cases of eczema with high disease burden [6], while in 2017 dermatitis was found to be the leading skin disease worldwide

Rook's Textbook of Dermatology, Tenth Edition. Edited by Christopher Griffiths, Jonathan Barker, Tanya Bleiker, Walayat Hussain and Rosalind Simpson.
© 2024 John Wiley & Sons Ltd. Published 2024 by John Wiley & Sons Ltd.

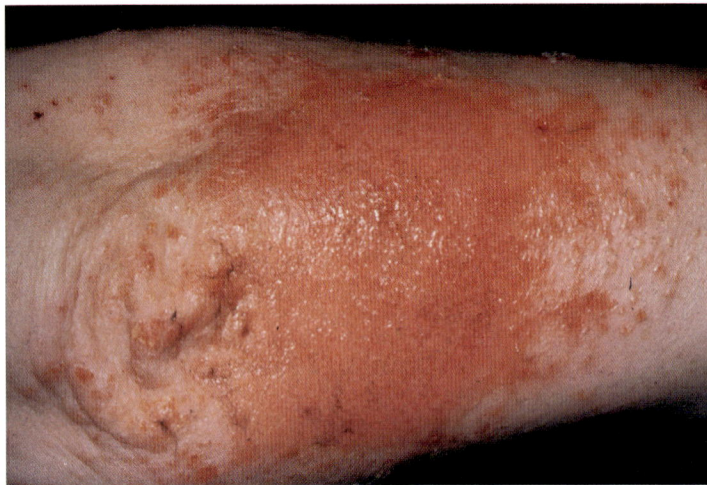

(a)

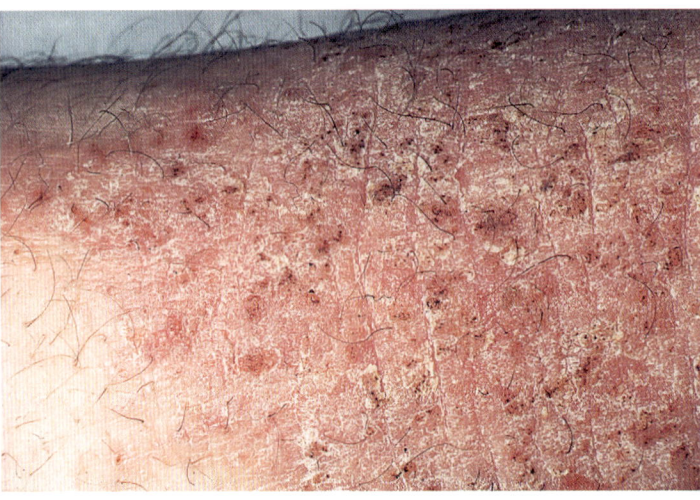

(b)

Figure 39.1 (a) Acute eczema of the arm, with rednessa and marked exudation. (b) Chronic eczema of the arm.

with the highest disability-adjusted life-years score [7]. A review of 66 studies found hand eczema to have a lifetime risk of 14.5% and a 1-year prevalence of 9.1% with a pooled incidence of 7.3 cases/1000 person-years [8]. Head and neck dermatitis exists commonly, with atopic eczema affecting 50% of adults and 79% of children [9]. A meta-analysis of epidemiological studies of contact allergic dermatitis suggests 20% of subjects demonstrate at least one contact allergic reaction, with nickel being the most common allergen at 11% followed by fragrances at 3.5% [10].

Consultations for eczema are a major part of the workload in primary care. Horn [11] recorded the details of 6819 dermatological consultations in a UK general practice of 3000–4000 patients from 1958 to 1985. Eczema patients formed the largest group (19% of the consultations). In a general practice in Belfast, 8% of patients seen during an 8-week period had a dermatological condition. Eczema accounted for 25% of these, of which 63% were considered to be exogenous in origin [12]. Barbarot *et al*. found adult eczema to have a point prevalence of 2.5% in the UK in 2018 [13]. In the UK, two-thirds of eczema cases are diagnosed in primary care, and half in primary care in Canada. In most other countries, dermatologists are mainly responsible for making the diagnosis.

Box 39.1 Classification of the principal forms of eczema

Exogenous eczemas
- Allergic contact eczema (Chapter 127)
- Dermatophytide
- Eczematous polymorphic light eruption (Chapter 126)
- Infective dermatitis
- Irritant eczema (Chapter 128)
- Photoallergic contact eczema (Chapter 126)
- Post-traumatic eczema

Endogenous eczemas
- Asteatotic eczema
- Atopic eczema (Chapter 41)
- Chronic superficial scaly dermatitis
- Eyelid eczema
- Hand eczema
- Juvenile plantar dermatosis
- Metabolic eczema or eczema associated with systemic disease (Chapter 61)
- Nummular dermatitis
- Pityriasis alba
- Seborrhoeic eczema
- Venous eczema

In the UK, eczema consultations account for 10% of the total secondary care dermatology caseload [14].

Age and sex
Most cases of eczema in infants and young children are atopic. In the National Health and Nutrition Examination Survey (NHANES) epidemiological survey in the USA [15], atopic eczema was by far the most common form found up to the age of 11 years; nummular (discoid) and 'dyshidrotic' eczema were recorded, but were much less frequent. Perioral eczema is common in children with atopic eczema (Chapter 41), but it can also occur in non-atopic children. Hand eczema is common in atopic children and uncommon in non-atopic children. Several specific patterns of eczematous change are predominantly found in children; for example, juvenile plantar dermatosis and napkin dermatitis.

Pompholyx and atopic eczema are less common in elderly people, while other forms of eczema assume greater importance. Nummular dermatitis occurs particularly in elderly males in winter, and asteatotic eczema of the trunk and legs is also common. In older factory workers, irritant hand eczema can be very troublesome, although allergic contact dermatitis becomes less common with advancing age. The subject is discussed more fully in Chapter 127.

Ethnicity
Eczematous dermatoses are reported in all ethnic groups with variations in clinical presentation in atopic eczema, but data are limited regarding ethnic differences for non-atopic eczema [16].

Associated dermatoses
Atopic eczema is associated with some forms of non-atopic eczematous dermatoses, in particular hand eczema (Chapter 41).

Pathophysiology

Eczema is a barrier dysfunction of skin. There has been considerable research on the pathogenesis of some types of eczema, particularly allergic contact dermatitis, primary irritant contact dermatitis and atopic eczema. One particular challenge in this research field has been distinguishing non-specific common pathways from specific mechanisms. The interaction of trigger factors, keratinocytes and T lymphocytes seems particularly important in most eczema types.

Allergic contact dermatitis represents a reproducible model of eczema development [17], as discussed in Chapter 127. Eczema may also be provoked in a non-allergic manner, as in irritant contact dermatitis. Three predominant processes occurring in irritant dermatitis are disturbed barrier function, epidermal cell change and release of inflammatory mediators and cytokines.

Certain irritants may provoke a chronic reaction in which an effect on epidermal cell turnover predominates, leading to lichenification, whereas in acute irritant reactions inflammatory mediator and cytokine release is similar to that seen in acute allergic contact dermatitis [18]. More recent studies suggest that even in acute settings differential gene expression for more allergic sensitising molecules is greater than for irritants, reflecting more inflammatory recruitment in allergic dermatitis and more cell turnover (lichenification) in irritancy [19].

After activation of the immune pathway by cytokine release, the accumulation of inflammatory cells progresses, leading to the morphological changes that are apparent histologically and clinically. The histological changes of primary irritant dermatitis are similar to those seen in allergic contact dermatitis, but they appear to proceed more quickly, depending on the concentration of the irritant used. Both intracellular and intercellular oedema are visible throughout the epidermis at 3–6 h, and within 24 h there may be epidermal necrosis, with cellular vacuolation and nuclear pyknosis. In severe forms, the primary epidermal damage may progress to subepidermal blister formation.

Filaggrin is a 37 kDa intracellular protein that binds to and condenses the keratin cytoskeleton, resulting in squame formation [20]. Loss-of-function mutations of the filaggrin gene result in impaired skin barrier function and are linked to atopic eczema and some subtypes of non-atopic eczema (including irritant and allergic contact dermatitis). The Th2 cytokines interleukin 4 (IL-4) and IL-13 have been shown to downregulate filaggrin protein content within the skin and stratum corneum [21].

Predisposing factors

These will be discussed in relation to each subtype of eczema in the relevant sections of this chapter.

Pathology

The histopathological features of eczema, in common with the clinical features, are variable, and depend particularly on whether the disease is acute or chronic [22–25].

In the acute phase (Figure 39.2a), the histological picture is dominated by spongiosis, an intercellular epidermal oedema that leads to stretching and eventual rupture of the intercellular attachments, with the formation of vesicles. The epidermal vesicles commonly occur in discrete foci, but on the thicker skin of palms and soles they tend to become large by coalescence. There is variable

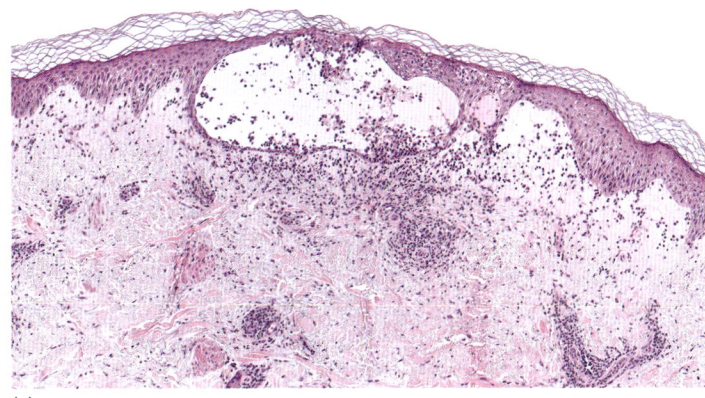
(a)

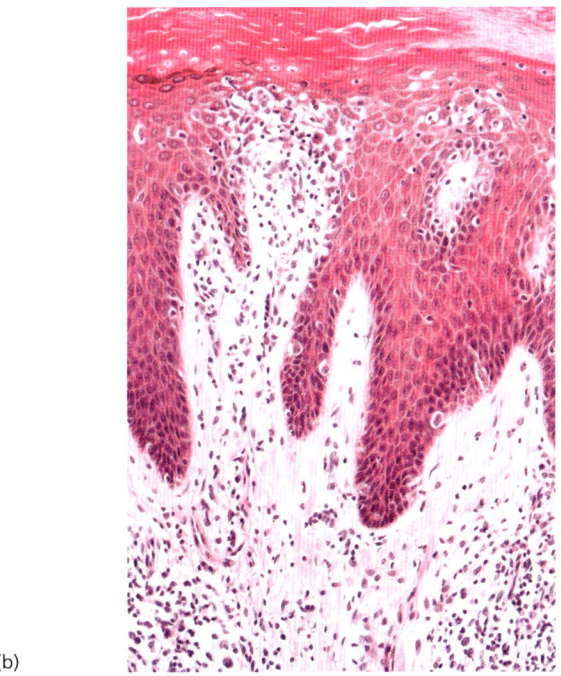
(b)

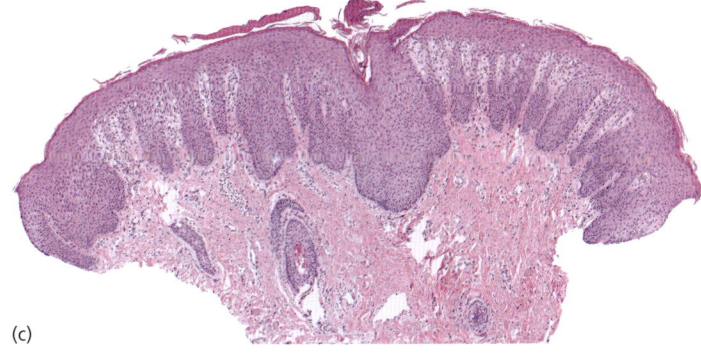
(c)

Figure 39.2 (a) Acute eczema. The epidermis shows distinct vesicle formation. The vesicle contains serum, and a moderate number of inflammatory cells. Magnification 100× (H&E). (b) Subacute eczema. There is irregular acanthosis and patchy spongiosis, with the formation of incipient microvesicles. A few lymphocytes are migrating up from the dermis into the epidermis. Magnification 100× (H&E). (c) Chronic lichenified eczema. There is compact hyperkeratosis, some patchy parakeratosis and irregular acanthosis. Mild spongiosis is seen throughout much of the epidermis, and there is a lymphocytic infiltrate in the upper dermis. Magnification 100× (H&E). Courtesy of Dr E. Calonje.

infiltration of the epidermis by lymphocytes. Increased epidermal mitotic activity leads to acanthosis but, if spongiosis is intense, disintegration of the suprapapillary epidermis may cause clefts to form. The intercellular oedema may be diffuse, but is commonly most intense in the mid-epidermal region. Loosening and disruption of the individual cells occur and some intracellular vacuolation may be found, with displacement of the nucleus from the centre of the cell. Loose, shrunken epidermal cells may resemble histiocytes. Vesicles and the oedematous epidermis may be permeated by mononuclear cells, chiefly monocytes.

In the subacute stage (Figure 39.2b), spongiosis and vesiculation diminish and increasing acanthosis is associated with the formation of a parakeratotic horny layer. This often contains layers of coagulated plasma and pyknotic nuclei of inflammatory cells.

In chronic eczema (Figure 39.2c), hyperkeratosis gradually replaces parakeratosis. Acanthosis is more prominent than spongiosis. Inflammatory cells are less evident in the epidermis, but dermal changes become more prominent. The rete ridges become elongated and broadened, and changes are then those of lichenification.

Vascular dilatation in the dermis is marked in all stages. The papillary vessels are particularly involved, and in lichenification they may become tortuous. The infiltrate is predominantly lymphohistiocytic, although polymorphs and eosinophils may be present in very acute eczema and eosinophils are particularly common in eczematous drug eruptions. In the presence of infection, polymorphs may invade the epidermis. In grossly lichenified eczema, prurigo and exfoliative dermatitis, the infiltrate is mixed and may be so dense that it simulates a granuloma.

The trauma of rubbing or scratching may cause superficial erosions, haemorrhage or subepidermal fibrinoid changes. Although some degree of lichenification is always present during a prolonged attack of eczema, it is particularly prominent in atopic eczema. At times, extreme hyperkeratosis and papillomatosis develop.

With secondary infection, the formation of follicular or subcorneal pustules can simulate the appearance of impetigo, although typical eczematous changes are still visible at the edges of the lesion.

Although spongiosis and a dermal lymphohistiocytic infiltrate are always present at some stage in eczema, the dynamic nature of the changes and their modification by secondary events may make histological diagnosis difficult. All the changes mentioned, with the exception of the spongiotic vesicle, may also be found in burns or simple traumatic lesions of the skin. The distinction between eczema and psoriasis can be especially difficult, particularly on the palms and soles. The presence of more classic disease elsewhere in the body can help to distinguish the two as well as a reduction in granular layer thickness on histology in psoriasis compared with eczema.

Seborrhoeic dermatitis is particularly difficult to distinguish from psoriasis, but the finding of Munro microabscesses is suggestive of the latter. It is generally true that cases which cause diagnostic difficulty clinically often have equivocal histological appearance. The histological features of pityriasis rosea are those of eczema but the clinical features, particularly the distribution, are characteristic.

Other modifications of the histopathological pattern in relation to different clinical subtypes of eczema are described later in this chapter.

Causative organisms

Most eczema subtypes are not thought to be primarily due to infection although they may be complicated by secondary bacterial or viral infection. The exception is infective dermatitis (see later in this chapter). Staphylococcal colonisation of the skin in atopic eczema and possible eczema exacerbation by staphylococcal toxin superantigen production are discussed in Chapter 41.

The variety of skin commensals is reduced in eczematous skin and the predominance of *Staphylococcus aureus* and *Malassezia* species seems to be closely related with increased risk of eczema [26,27].

Genetics

Filaggrin mutations are linked to hand eczema, irritant contact dermatitis and allergic contact dermatitis due to nickel and possibly other allergens [28].

Environmental factors

Irritants and allergens may act as triggers for irritant contact dermatitis and allergic contact dermatitis, respectively. Irritants play a direct role in inducing inflammation through causing or exacerbating barrier dysfuncton. Type IV allergens induce a cell-mediated response either local to the area of contact or systemically. Type I allergens induce a direct mast cell degranulation which initially causes an urticarial or anaphylactoid response. However, sustained exposure may lead to repeated excoriation and subsequent physical barrier dysfunction.

Clinical features

History

The main symptom is pruritus, which may disturb sleep and other elements of quality of life and can affect family members profoundly as well. It is important to note occupation and recreational activities because these may be relevant in terms of irritant and allergen exposures. Restrictions on life may affect compliance which may not always be volunteered [29].

Presentation

Acute eczema presents as an itchy eruption that is typically oedematous, vesicular and may be exudative. The itch may precede any overt change in the skin. In chronic eczema, these features give way to a more stable picture of redness, scaling, excoriation and lichenification. The specific presentation of different subtypes of non-atopic eczema will be discussed in later sections of this chapter.

Secondary dissemination. A characteristic feature of eczematous inflammation is its tendency to spread far from its point of origin and to become generalised [30]. This phenomenon is often termed autosensitisation or, more specifically, autoeczematisation [31]. Generalised spread is especially likely when the primary site of the eczema is on the legs or the feet. There is also a tendency for an eruption beginning on the feet to extend to the hands and vice versa. The eczema may have been present for only a few days, or for many years, before dissemination occurs. The dissemination, which is often preceded by an exacerbation at the primary site, often occurs rapidly. The secondary eruption may at first consist of small oedematous papules, but these soon become obviously eczematous and grouped papulovesicles may become confluent in small plaques. Occasionally, the lesions take the form of red macules or weals. The distribution is usually symmetrical.

The course of the secondary eruption depends largely on the progress of the primary lesion. If the primary lesion remains acutely inflamed, the eruption increases in severity and may become generalised. If the patient is rested and the local lesion is allowed to settle, the secondary eruption will subside, but will often recur very readily if the local lesion relapses. In a small proportion of patients, the generalised secondary eruption evolves into erythroderma, which may become self-perpetuating.

Causes of secondary dissemination have been explored more fully since this was first documented where those such as neurogenic causes were suggested [32]. Reduced microbial resistance and consistent allergic or irritant reaction may go some way to explain this phenomenon, as well as T-cell activation by keratinocyte release of pro-inflammatory cytokines [33].

Conditioned hyperirritability. Here, an area of inflamed skin on one part of the body results in a generalised hyperirritability of the skin at distant sites. There is considerable evidence that eczematous patients are more vulnerable to mild primary irritants than are unaffected people. Conditioned hyperirritability seems to be associated with any focal inflammation of the skin, and it may explain some clinical phenomena such as the tendency for patients suffering from eczema, especially acute eczema, to have a higher proportion of false positive 'irritant' reactions to patch tests. The 'angry back' syndrome, in which a strongly positive patch test response can increase the percentage of false positive reactions on the back at the same time, is an example of this, as is the more common vesicular irritant reaction of atopic individuals to metallic patch test reagents like nickel, cobalt and dichromate.

There may be several mechanisms underlying the dissemination of eczema and conditioned hyperirritability. Circulating activated T lymphocytes are increased in number [34,35]. In addition, peripheral blood mononuclear cells show increased proliferation in the presence of an autologous skin homogenate as compared with control subjects. This suggests that an abnormal cell-mediated immune response against autologous skin antigens could be occurring [36,37].

Differential diagnosis

This will be discussed in relation to each non-atopic eczema subtype covered later in this chapter.

Classification of severity

There are relatively few classifications available for non-atopic eczema. Many disease scores are being developed for body sites, particularly the hands, but none is yet commonly used. However, the dermatology life quality index (DLQI) can be applied to any skin condition [38].

Complications and co-morbidities

A reduction in skin barrier function increases the risk of both bacterial and viral secondary skin infection. However, eczema herpeticum is linked primarily to atopic eczema and filaggrin mutations (Chapter 41).

Disease course and prognosis

Eczema follows a chronic, relapsing, remitting course. Issues specific to each non-atopic eczema subtype will be covered later in this chapter.

Investigations

Most cases of eczema can be diagnosed clinically. The presence of wheeze and other atopic personal and family history help distinguish atopic eczema from other types and predict disease longevity and severity [39]. Secondary infection can be confirmed by taking swabs for culture and sensitivity to identify the causative organism. When dermatophyte infection is suspected, a potassium hydroxide preparation should be examined or scrapings sent to a laboratory for microscopy and culture. Microscopy, or dermoscopic examination of the skin, can also be helpful to confirm a diagnosis of scabies, which is easy to miss in a patient with pre-existing eczema. Biopsy can occasionally be helpful in confirming the eczematous nature of the eruption, and immunofluorescence can help identify less common conditions such as dermatitis herpetiformis or, in older patients, a non-bullous presentation of bullous pemphigoid.

Patch testing in eczema [40–42]

Routine use of patch testing is not indicated for typical presentations of endogenous eczema such as atopic eczema, pityriasis alba and seborrhoeic eczema. This investigation is much more important in atypical, localised or asymmetrical eruptions, and especially in dermatitis affecting the face, hands and feet [42] or when resistant to standard treatment [43]. Contact dermatitis can also mimic other dermatoses like lichen planus.

In apparently endogenous eczema the threshold for patch testing should still be low. Sensitisation commonly develops to topical medicaments, prescribed or self-administered, and this may exacerbate the eruption. Sometimes, topical remedies are concealed or forgotten by the patient, or the reaction they cause is partially suppressed by the concomitant use of topical corticosteroids. At other times, an unexpected positive test points to a 'hidden' or obscure cause, for example fragrances, preservatives, excipients, epoxys or rubber accelerators. Such substances are commonly encountered in the environment and in topical medication. Corticosteroids are particularly troublesome if they are the cause of the allergy as they suppress their own immune reaction and cross-react in a complex manner [44].

Additional battery tests are available as well as the standard. Knowing the allergens on additional batteries is more important than the batteries themselves. In many cases, treatment failure with topicals will warrant testing to topical corticosteroids and medicament excipients and preservatives. Day 7 readings may be necessary if topical corticosteroids are suspected. The observer must be wary of false positive, irritant reactions, especially in the context of conditioned hyperirritability [45]. For this reason it is always wise to allow the acute phase of eczema to subside before patch testing is carried out, or to repeat any positive tests when it has done so. If a contact urticaria is thought to be occurring, the patch tests should be read at 20, 40 and 60 min after application [46].

Even if a positive patch test is judged to be relevant, it does not necessarily follow that exclusion of the substance from the patient's environment will result in a cure. The allergen may be only one of several contributory factors. Chronic inflammatory cycles may continue the symptoms.

Management

It is important to explore previous treatment experiences and gauge how much time and effort the patient will be able to devote to the care of their (or their child's) skin. An additional issue is the attitude of the patient to the risks and potential adverse effects associated with any treatment that may be required. A particularly common problem is an inappropriate level of anxiety about the use of topical corticosteroids, although methods to reduce this are not always successful [47].

Treatments range from conservative and extremely safe approaches such as rest and the application of emollients, to more hazardous treatments such as phototherapy and systemic immunosuppressants (Table 39.1). When an extrinsic cause is identified or suspected this should be removed. In all cases, exposure to irritants should be carefully avoided and the skin should be protected using emollients and appropriate dressings. Psychological support is an important aspect of management at all stages.

Acute eczema

Acute eruptions and exacerbations of eczema cause great alarm and anxiety, and the stress of the situation is usually aggravated by loss of sleep caused by intense pruritus and soreness. Adequate rest is essential, and support from a dermatology day unit is very helpful. An affected leg should be elevated and affected hands should be used as little as possible.

Highly oedematous, vesicular and exudative eruptions such as pompholyx benefit from soaks in an astringent such as a 1 : 10 000

Table 39.1 Indications for therapeutic agents in eczema.

Therapeutic agent	Acute	Subacute	Chronic
Rest, sedation	++	+	±
Wet dressings and soaks	++	±	−
Wet wrap bandaging	++	+	±
Paste bandages	±	+	++
Sedative antihistamines	++	++	+
Emollients	++	++	++
Corticosteroids, local	+	++	+
Pimecrolimus (topical)	+	++	++
Tacrolimus (topical)	+	++	++
Tar, ichthammol, etc.	±	+	++
Polythene occlusion	±	+	+
Intralesional steroids	−	±	+
Habit reversal therapy	−	±	+
X-ray therapy	−	−	±
UVB phototherapy	−	+	+
PUVA phototherapy	−	+	+
UVA1 phototherapy	−	+	+
Systemic corticosteroids	±	±	−
Ciclosporin	+	+	±
Azathioprine	−	+	+
Methotrexate	−	+	+
Alitretinoin (hand eczema)	−	+	+
Mycophenolate mofetil	−	+	+
Dupilumab	−	+	+

PUVA, psoralen and UVA; UV, ultraviolet.

solution of potassium manganate (VII), or alternatively Burow solution BP, which contains the astringent aluminium acetate. These are difficult to use outside of specialist units in the secondary care setting. Liberal applications of bland emollients, such as white soft paraffin, are soothing. Moderate or potent topical corticosteroids are generally used, at least for a few days, to speed resolution of an acute episode at least until it clears and for a few days beyond to prevent relapse. Severity should be the guide as to potency of the steroid as well as body site [48]. More severe disease requires higher potency of steroids. Topical calcineurin inhibitors such as tacrolimus and pimecrolimus may also have a role. Tacrolimus ointment 0.1% is probably similar in potency to potent topical corticosteroids [49], while pimecrolimus has a lower potency [50]. When practical, tubular bandaging can be used to help keep topical medications in place. The wet wrapping technique, in which a layer of wet tubular bandage (e.g. Tubifast®) is covered with a dry layer, can be particularly soothing. Paste bandages achieve a similar effect to the wet bandage (e.g. Viscopaste® or Ichthopaste®). Hazards include a risk of hypothermia, although, in moderation, the cooling effect is highly beneficial. All paraffin-based products are a fire risk and smoking should be strictly prohibited. Emollients and other medications can be applied under the bandaging as required. Paste bandages are infused with their own emollient but more can be applied on top. The penetration of topical corticosteroids can be significantly increased by this form of occlusion, enhancing both beneficial and adverse effects. Mild or moderate corticosteroids should be used for the face and genital areas. Potent or very potent corticosteroids are required, at least initially, for acute pompholyx on the hands or feet.

When secondary infection is present, or staphylococcal contamination of the skin is thought to be an aggravating factor, oral antibiotics may be required. Topical preparations containing antibiotics or antiseptics in combination with steroids can also be helpful. These compound formulations should only be used when there is an indication for each constituent in order to avoid unnecessary exposure to the risks of sensitisation and the emergence of bacterial resistance [51]. Emollients applied before bed have been found to be the most useful therapy to aid sleep [52].

Subacute eczema

If an acute eczema has failed to clear almost completely in 3–4 weeks with adequate topical therapies, perpetuating factors such as exposure to a sensitising agent and concordance with treatment should be considered. Dermatology day unit review or admission to hospital can often be helpful in these circumstances. Paste bandages are of particular value in occluding areas that are frequently excoriated, as in many lower leg eczemas. These must be applied carefully to ensure that they are firm, but not so tight as to cause discomfort or to restrict blood flow. Corticosteroids under polythene occlusion for a few days may be helpful at this stage to reduce pruritus. Topical immunomodulators such as tacrolimus and pimecrolimus are alternatives.

Chronic eczema

First line therapy for chronic eczema is the frequent application of emollients and avoidance of irritants such as soap and relevant allergens if identified. Daily application of topical corticosteroids is required to treat flares, the choice of potency being determined by eczema severity, skin site and, in children, patient age. Once a flare has been treated successfully, the frequency of application of topical corticosteroids should be reduced gradually to prevent rebound flares. A subsequent period of twice-weekly application may be needed to maintain remission in flare-prone individuals [53]. Topical calcineurin inhibitors are applied in a similar way [53] and may be needed to avoid skin atrophy for individuals who have had prolonged exposure to corticosteroids in areas such as the face. Alternatively, topical corticosteroids could be used to induce remission and topical calcineurin inhibitors can be used for maintenance.

Various modalities of phototherapy have been successfully in chronic eczema resistant to topical therapy, especially for atopic eczema. These include narrow-band ultraviolet B (UVB) [54], psoralen and UVA (PUVA) [54] and UVA1 [55].

In the most severe cases, oral immunosuppressive therapy may be required. Systemic corticosteroids act rapidly, improving symptoms within a day or two, but there is the risk of eczema relapse when treatment is discontinued [56], although this is reduced when the cause is an external agent [57]. Longer-term treatment is provided by ciclosporin [56], azathioprine [58] and methotrexate [59]. Mycophenolate mofetil has also been used, but evidence is limited to pilot studies [60]. All of these systemic modalities require careful monitoring. Alitretinoin, an oral retinoid, has been licensed for chronic hand eczema for a period of 6 months following a large randomised controlled trial (RCT) [61]. However, the evidence for the use of phototherapy and systemic immunosuppressants for non-atopic eczema is largely extrapolated from trials for atopic eczema (Chapter 41).

Dupilumab is the first biologic therapy licensed for use in atopic eczema and targets the IL-4 receptor and can be used where standard systemic therapies fail [62]. Other biologic therapies since include tralokinumab and lebrikizumab which target IL-13 and nemolizumab which targets IL-31 [63].

Small molecule inhibitors of Janus kinase (JAK) cytokine receptors on the cytosolic side of the cell membrane block signal transduction and are collectively known as JAK inhibitors. Baricitinib targets JAK1 and JAK2, while abrocitinib and upadacitinib are selective JAK1 inhibitors [64].

Treatment ladder for eczema

First line
- Avoidance of irritants and allergens
- Liberal use of emollients and soap substitutes

Second line
- Topical corticosteroids and topical calcineurin inhibitors

Third line
- Phototherapy, oral immunosuppressants, alitretinoin (hand eczema) and biologics

---

Nummular dermatitis

Definition and nomenclature

Nummular dermatitis is characterised by circular or oval plaques of eczema with a clearly demarcated edge. It should be distinguished from an irregular, patchy form of eczema in which the lesions are not clearly demarcated. The condition is poorly defined, however, because many eczema patients have one or two circular or oval lesions and few patients with nummular dermatitis have circular lesions alone [1,2].

Synonyms and inclusions
- Discoid eczema
- Nummular eczema

Introduction and general description

Nummular dermatitis is often referred to as discoid eczema. It tends to be a chronic problem, undergoing relapses and remissions. The evidence base for treatment is largely based on studies of atopic eczema, due to a paucity of studies specifically investigating this subtype of non-atopic eczema.

Epidemiology

Incidence and prevalence

A study of over 20 000 people, from 1 to 74 years of age, in the USA, who were examined for skin disease by trained observers, found the prevalence of nummular dermatitis to be 2 per 1000 [3]. An American study found this prevalence to be fairly consistent over the 15 years they reviewed [4]. There was also a greater proportion in the non-white and non-African American cohorts.

Age

Nummular dermatitis tends to affect women in early adulthood, whereas in men onset is commonest in the older age groups. Prevalence steadily increases with age in men.

Associated diseases

Some authors have found a high incidence of atopy in patients with nummular dermatitis [5], but others have found the inverse [6], and levels of immunoglobulin E (IgE) are often within the normal range [7]. However, lesions of similar morphology may undoubtedly occur as part of atopic eczema as there are no definitive criteria for diagnosis.

Pathophysiology

The pathophysiology of nummular dermatitis is unknown but *Staphylococcus aureus* infection has been associated. It is unclear if this has a direct role in pathogenesis or is secondary to it.

Pathology

Histology shows a subacute dermatitis indistinguishable from other forms of eczema, with spongiotic vesicles and a predominantly lymphohistiocytic infiltrate [8,9]. Eosinophils may also be present in the upper dermis.

Electron microscopic studies have shown that the intense intercellular oedema leads to a reduction in the number of desmosomes between the cells of the basal layer, whereas those in the stratum spinosum are mostly preserved.

Causative organisms

Some authors have stressed the role of infection [10,11]. As in other forms of eczema, heavy colonisation of the lesions by staphylococci may increase their severity, even in the absence of clinical evidence of infection [10,11]. However, allergic sensitivity to staphylococci or micrococci may be responsible, at least for secondary dissemination [12].

Nummular dermatitis has been shown to demonstrate the Koebner phenomenon in scar sites [13].

Genetics

There may be an indirect link via atopy.

Environmental factors

There may be a clinically relevant underlying allergic contact dermatitis to allergens like formaldehyde in about one-third of patients [14]. Dry skin due to low environmental humidity is sometimes associated with nummular dermatitis [15], particularly in the elderly [16]. An association between excessive alcohol intake and nummular dermatitis has been reported [17].

Nummular dermatitis has occurred rarely as a result of sensitivity to aloe [18], depilating creams [19] and mercury [20], and in patients taking methyldopa [21]. In addition, oral gold therapy in the form of sodium aurothiomalate and auranofin has been associated with nummular dermatitis in a dose-dependent manner, with resolution on discontinuing the drug and recurrence after rechallenge [22].

Clinical features
Presentation

Nummular dermatitis presents as coin-shaped plaques of closely set, thin-walled vesicles on a red base. This arises, quite rapidly, from the confluence of tiny papules and papulovesicles. These may occur, in the phase of very acute dissemination, as individual lesions on the trunk or limbs at the same time as localised plaques are being formed. In the acute phase the lesions are dull red, very exudative or crusted and highly pruritic (Figure 39.3). They progress towards a less vesicular and more scaly stage, often with central clearing and peripheral extension, causing ring-shaped or annular lesions. As they fade, they leave dry, scaly patches.

After a period of between 10 days and several months, secondary lesions occur, often in a mirror-image configuration on the opposite side of the body. It is very characteristic of this disease that plaques which have apparently become dormant may reactivate, particularly if treatment is discontinued prematurely.

Clinical variants

There are a number of variants:
- Nummular dermatitis: exudative type.
- Nummular dermatitis: dry type.
- Nummular dermatitis of the hands.
- Exudative discoid and lichenoid chronic dermatosis.

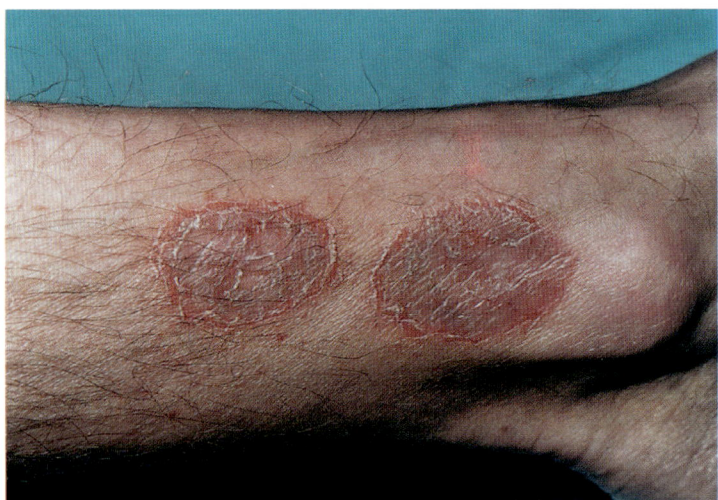

Figure 39.3 Nummular dermatitis of the lower leg. Courtesy of Dr W. A. D. Griffiths, Epsom Hospital, Surrey, UK.

In 'exudative' nummular dermatitis the skin lesions resemble the acute phase of the more typical form of the condition, with leakage of serous fluid and crust formation. This variant usually represents the more severe end of the disease spectrum and may require oral antibiotic treatment.

'Dry' nummular dermatitis is an uncommon variant, consisting of multiple, dry, scaly, round or oval discs on the arms or legs, but also with scattered microvesicles on a red base on the palms and soles [23]. Itching is minimal, in contrast with other forms of nummular dermatitis, and the condition persists for several years, with fluctuation or remission. It is notably resistant to treatment.

Nummular dermatitis of the hands affects the dorsa of the hands or the backs or sides of individual fingers. It often develops as a single plaque, which may occur at the site of a burn or a local chemical or irritant reaction. Secondary lesions may occur on the hands, fingers or forearms, but generalised spread is uncommon. It is a not uncommon form of irritant occupational dermatitis, but may also occur without occupational exposure. An atopic history appears to be more frequent in young women with hand nummular dermatitis than in other forms of the disease.

Exudative discoid and lichenoid chronic dermatosis [24] has no rigid criteria, but it is a widespread, extremely pruritic eruption, characterised by discoid lesions with 'lichenoid' and exudative phases, which either coexist or alternate rapidly with each other (Figure 39.4). After a chronic course of months or years the condition ends in spontaneous cure. It occurs predominantly in adult males of Jewish ancestry, usually between the ages of 40 and 60 years. More than 100 cases have been reported [25], but some authors deny its existence as a distinct entity and consider it to be a variant of nummular dermatitis [26]. The scarcity of reports of this entity over the last three decades lends support to this contention.

Differential diagnosis

When lesions of nummular dermatitis clear in the centre they may simulate tinea infection. Therefore, skin scrapings could be examined for the presence of mycelia. In psoriasis, the lesions are dry, the scaling is more prominent and irritation is milder. Pityriasis

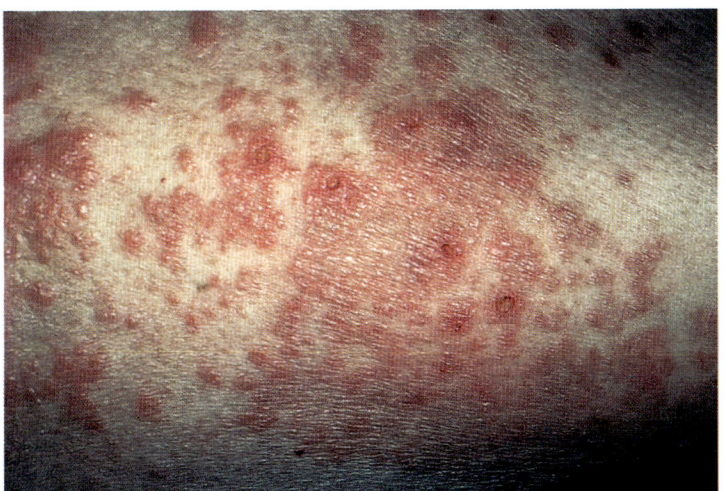

Figure 39.4 Exudative discoid and lichenoid chronic dermatitis. Courtesy of Dr A. Warin, Royal Devon and Exeter Hospital, Exeter, UK.

rosea may transiently resemble nummular dermatitis, but usually presents with the history of a herald patch and characteristic oval patches with long axes parallel to the ribs. Contact dermatitis to ellipsoid objects such as the back of watches or pendants can be distinguished by its localisation and shape.

Table 39.2 gives the diagnostic features of a number of types of discoid lesions that should be considered in the differential diagnosis.

Disease course and prognosis

All forms of nummular dermatitis are chronic, with partial remission during which plaques tend to clear in their centres. Relapse may occur at variable intervals and most are worse during the colder months of the year. A review of 325 cases showed that most either cleared within a year or persisted for many years [27]. More recent studies confirm a relapsing/remitting course over months to years [28].

Investigations

Exogenous contact dermatitis should be suspected if the condition is unusually severe and persistent or if patches are few, asymmetrical or of unusual configuration. Irritants and, occasionally, sensitisers may provoke this discoid type of response. When the history suggests this, patch tests should be performed.

In a study from the North American Contact Dermatitis Group (2012), 1.9% of their patch test patients had nummular eczema with 23.9% testing positive from that group, making nummular dermatitis less likely to have coexisting allergic contact dermatitis than other dermatoses [29]. Interestingly, the most common contact allergen worldwide, nickel (II) sulphate, was slightly underrepresented in terms of relevance in those with nummular dermatitis in this study. Preservatives such as formaldehyde (and its releasers), methylisothiazolinone and propylene glycol and fragrance mix I are slightly more prevalent and relevant as allergens. This is in contrast to other studies which found the metals nickel (II) sulphate, potassium dichromate (VI) and cobalt (II) chloride as well as the hair dye paraphenylene diamine to be the most common [29].

Management

General considerations such as the avoidance of irritants apply, as with other forms of eczema. Bed rest and removal from a stressful environment can be helpful. Ambient conditions of low humidity should be corrected.

Emollients and topical corticosteroids are useful. In the early stages, a potent or very potent topical corticosteroid may be needed and combination with a topical antiseptic or antibiotic can be considered. Treatment failure can occur if the corticosteroid potency is too low. A course of a broad spectrum oral antibiotic, such as oxytetracycline or clarithromycin, is often helpful in severe exudative cases.

Treatment ladder for nummular dermatitis

First line
- Emollients
- Topical corticosteroid ± topical or oral antibiotic

Second line
- Topical calcineurin inhibitor

Third line
- Phototherapy (narrow-band UVB/PUVA), oral immunosuppressants including methotrexate [30] or oral steroids
- Biologic therapy (dupilumab) [31]

Resources

Patient resources

British Association of Dermatologists, patient information leaflets: https://www.bad.org.uk/for-the-public/patient-information-leaflets

DermNet NZ, discoid eczema: https://dermnetnz.org/topics/discoid-eczema/

Medscape, nummular dermatitis: https://emedicine.medscape.com/article/1123605-overview

NHS Choices, discoid eczema: https://www.nhs.uk/conditions/discoid-eczema/ (All last accessed September 2023.)

Asteatotic eczema

Definition and nomenclature

This is eczema developing in very dry skin, usually in the elderly. Asteatotic refers to decreased or non-existent sebum production on the skin.

Synonyms and inclusions
- Eczéma craquelé
- Eczema craquelatum
- Winter eczema
- Xerotic eczema

Table 39.2 Diagnosis of some discoid skin lesions.

Disease	Distribution	Features	Histology	Course and evolution
Tinea corporis	Limbs or trunk	Oval or round, itchy Scraping produces scale for mycology	PAS stain shows fungus	Progresses and spreads steadily until treated
Nummular dermatitis	Limbs more than trunk	Oval or round, very itchy	Eczema, often intense changes	Variable, fluctuant or intermittent
Pityriasis alba	Face, proximal limbs	Depigmentation	Very mild eczema	Spontaneous remission after 1 or more years
Pityriasis rosea	Trunk	Oval herald patch followed by wider eruption	Non-specific chronic dermatitis	Spontaneous resolution
Chronic superficial dermatitis	Limbs more than trunk	Oval or round, no infiltration	Epidermal eczematous	Very chronic, benign, no fluctuations
Prelymphomatous eruption	Flank, trunk, proximal limbs	Angular, bizarre, infiltrated, interdigitated, itchy	Dermal infiltrate	Persistent, may change to lymphoma
Mycosis fungoides	Flank, trunk and limbs, may be asymmetrical with unusually shaped lesions	Polymorphic oval, round in patch stage	Monoclonal lymphocytic infiltrate with Pautrier microabscesses	Persistent, can progress to plaque and tumour stages
Bowen disease (squamous cell carcinoma *in situ*)	Any body site	Singular, non-itchy, oval but can be asymmetrical	Non-invasive neoplastic spindle cells	Continues to grow, 5% can become invasive
Porokeratosis	Trunk and limbs	Single or multiple ring-like lesions with raised edge	Cornified protrusion at edge (cornoid lamella)	Persistent, potential for malignant transformation

PAS, periodic acid–Schiff.

Introduction and general description

Asteatotic eczema usually affects the legs, arms and hands of elderly people in the context of dry skin. A characteristic 'crazy-paving' pattern is observed on the legs in particular, resulting in the synonym of eczéma craquelé. It may flare during winter due to a reduction in humidity associated with central heating. Management centres on the restoration of skin hydration.

Epidemiology
Incidence and prevalence

In a Finnish study of 552 patients aged 70–93 years, 80% were found to have skin disease of which nearly 21% was asteatotic eczema, which was the most common eczema [1]. However, multiple skin diseases coexisted in 39% of cases.

Age

Elderly people are predominantly affected and prevalence increases with increasing age.

Sex

The Finnish study suggested asteatotic eczema was more common in women than men over 70 years of age [1].

Ethnicity

All ethnicities can be affected. Individual study cohorts have had too little ethnic diversity to date in order to draw significant comparisons.

Associated diseases

Asteatotic eczema may be a presenting sign of myxoedema [2]. It can also be due to zinc deficiency [3]. Any condition that leads to dry skin such as nephrotic syndrome and diuretic therapy can exacerbate asteatotic eczema [4].

Skin with decreased sensation from surgery or other desensitisation has also demonstrated signs of asteatotic eczema, possibly due to decreased neuronal activity reducing glandular secretions [5].

Pathophysiology
Predisposing factors

At present, the relevant factors in the production of asteatotic eczema can be considered to be (i) a naturally 'dry' skin and a lifelong tendency to chapping; (ii) a further reduction in lipid with age, illness, malnutrition or hormonal decline; (iii) increased transpiration relative to the environmental water content; (iv) loss of integrity of the water reservoir of the horny layer; (v) chapping and degreasing (and perhaps cell damage) by industrial or domestic cleansers or solvents; (vi) low environmental humidity and dry, cold winds increasing convection loss; and (vii) repeated minor trauma leading to inflammation and further disorganisation of the surface aqueous/lipid balance. Percutaneous absorption through the degreased and damaged epidermis is increased, and contact irritants and sensitisers may further damage and irritate the skin.

Hospital admission can result in more frequent assisted washing in those previously unable to self-care, which will further exacerbate loss of skin lipid [6].

Pathology

The condition is thought to be due to a decrease in skin surface lipid. The amino acid content of the skin is lower in more severe cases [7]. A decrease in the keratohyaline-derived natural moisturising factor may also be important [8]. Older patients have a decrease in sebaceous and sweat gland activity necessary to keep the water content high in the epidermis and maintain structural integrity [9]. This leads to barrier dysfunction and an eczematous response.

Hyposteatosis occurs in many conditions of maldevelopment, malnutrition and atrophy of the skin, but does not necessarily lead to eczema. The part played by the loss of fluid from the skin has been underappreciated in the past. The relationship between the transpiration rate and the lipid layer has been the subject of many studies [10]. Using excised skin it was shown that removal of these lipids increased water loss by 75-fold, and that this returned to normal when they were restored. The implications for treatment are obvious.

The histopathological features are those of a mild, subacute eczema, with a varying amount of dermal infiltrate. When vesicular or nummular dermatitis supervenes, the changes are more marked, and are as seen in the latter disease.

Genetics
No specific genetic mutations have been documented in the literature to date.

Environmental factors
A patient will often ascribe the onset to an event or change in life that is quite trivial, for example the installation of central heating or a particularly cold, dry winter [11]. In industry, years of contact with degreasing agents may be tolerated until, usually in the 50–60-year age group, some small additional hazard precipitates a disabling dermatitis.

Diuretics sometimes appear to be an important contributory factor in elderly people [12].

Clinical features
History
Irritation in this form of eczema is often intense, and worse with changes of temperature, particularly on undressing at night.

Presentation
The condition occurs particularly on the legs, arms and hands. The asteatotic skin is dry and slightly scaly. The surface of the backs of the hands is marked in a criss-cross fashion. The finger pulps are dry and cracked, producing distorted prints and retaining a prolonged depression after pressure ('parchment pulps'). On the legs the pattern of superficial markings is more marked and deeper ('crazy-paving' pattern or eczéma craquelé) (Figure 39.5). In some patients the fissures may become haemorrhagic. The borders of this irregular reticulation become red and slightly raised, and

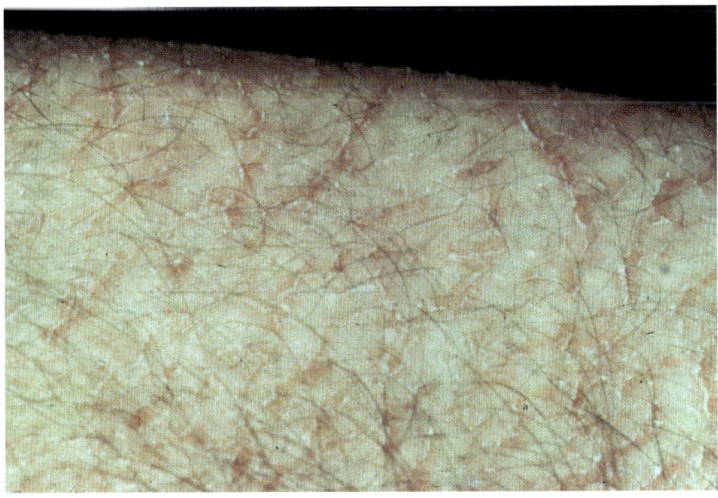

Figure 39.5 Asteatotic eczema demonstrating an eczéma craquelé appearance.

frank eczematous changes finally develop. Similarly, on the hands, localised areas become chapped or itchy, and eventually form eczematous patches.

Clinical variants
Extensive or generalised forms involving the trunk as well as the legs are rare but should raise the suspicion of malignancy. Cases have been reported in association with malignant lymphoma [13], angioimmunoblastic lymphadenopathy [14], anaplastic gastric adenocarcinoma [15] and spheroidal cell carcinoma of the breast [16].

Differential diagnosis
Asteatotic eczema has a characteristic appearance thus the differential diagnosis is limited to other forms of eczema.

Classification of severity
There are no specific severity classification systems.

Complications and co-morbidities
Secondary infection is possible due to a reduction in skin barrier function. Nummular dermatitis can also occur on a background of asteatotic eczema, although the relationship between the two conditions is uncertain.

Disease course and prognosis
Without treatment, the condition is usually chronic, relapsing each winter and clearing in the summer, but eventually becoming permanent. Scratching, rubbing or contact irritants and sensitisers cause further eczematous changes or spread, or a more diffuse vesiculosquamous eruption occurs.

Investigations
There are no specific investigations unless generalised asteatotic eczema is present. Patch testing may be useful as with any recalcitrant or localised dermatitis.

Management
Central heating should be humidified where possible, and abrupt temperature changes avoided. Wool is usually poorly tolerated and possibly damaging due to irritation. Baths are best restricted and should not be hot. Soap substitutes should be used for bathing to prevent further skin lipid loss and irritation. Emollients should be used after bathing and during the day.

Weak topical corticosteroids are often prescribed. Among the older remedies, ichthammol is of value.

Treatment ladder for asteatotic eczema

First line
- Humidify environment and avoid sudden temperature changes

Second line
- Emollients and soap substitute

Third line
- Mild topical corticosteroids; pimecrolimus 1% [17]

Resources

Patient resources

DermNet NZ, eczéma craquelé: https://www.dermnetnz.org/topics/asteatotic-eczema/ (last accessed September 2023)

Dermatitis and eczema of the hands

Definition and nomenclature

The term hand eczema implies that the dermatitis is largely confined to the hands, with only minor involvement of other areas. If the eczema is widespread and the hands appear to be involved only coincidentally, it is preferable to refer to hand involvement as part of the widespread eczema. In defining the entity of hand eczema, both patients and clinicians have described similar characteristics of it being thickened, red, itchy and frustrating to treat [1].

Synonyms and inclusions

- Hyperkeratotic palmar eczema is also known as 'tylotic eczema'
- Pompholyx hand eczema is also known as 'vesicular eczema of palms and soles'. When pompholyx occurs on the palms, it may be called 'cheiropompholyx', and when on the soles, 'podopompholyx'
- The term 'dyshidrotic eczema' as an alternative to pompholyx hand eczema has been dropped because no causal relationship with the sweat glands or sweating has been demonstrated

---

Introduction and general description

Hand eczema is a common and distressing condition, and has a particular impact on quality of life due to its effects on dexterity, appearance and social and occupational functioning [2,3]. Up to 30% of occupational medical practice relates to hand eczema, with important issues regarding medical litigation, worker's compensation and disability. Hand eczema is often the reason for referral to specialised contact dermatitis clinics; 28% of UK patch test patients were found to present with affected hands [4].

In a comprehensive review of published data, the mean annual cost per patient of hand eczema was found to be between €1712 and €9712, with the majority (70%) being due to absence from work [5].

No single classification of hand eczema is completely satisfactory. As with eczematous dermatoses in general, classification is based partly on aetiology (Box 39.2) and partly on morphology (Box 39.3). Several different morphological forms are seen clinically as fairly consistent entities, but some of these entities can have several different causes. Conversely, a single cause can sometimes produce several different morphological patterns.

Hand eczema can also be subdivided into acute and chronic forms with 3 months being the cut-off (some authors saying 6 months [6]).

Most cases of hand eczema have a multifactorial aetiology. This not only makes treatment difficult, but it can cause considerable problems in medicolegal cases, for example occupational dermatitis in which negligence is alleged against an employer.

Box 39.2 Hand eczema: aetiological possibilities to be considered

Exogenous
- Contact irritants:
  - Chemical (e.g. soap, detergents, solvents, foods)
  - Physical (e.g. friction, minor trauma, cold dry air)
- Contact allergens:
  - Delayed hypersensitivity (type IV) (e.g. chromium, nickel, rubber accelerators, acrylates)
  - Immediate hypersensitivity (type I) (e.g. seafood, dust)
  - Protein contact dermatitis/contact urticaria
- Ingested allergens (e.g. drugs, possibly nickel, chromium)
- Infection (e.g. following bacterial infection of hand wounds)
- Secondary dissemination (e.g. dermatophytide reaction to tinea pedis)

Endogenous
- Idiopathic (e.g. discoid, hyperkeratotic palmar eczema)
- Immunological or metabolic defect (e.g. atopic)
- Psychosomatic: stress aggravates, but may not be causative
- Dyshidrosis: increased sweating aggravates, but may not be causative

---

Box 39.3 Morphological patterns of hand eczema

- Apron eczema
- Chronic acral dermatitis
- Nummular dermatitis (discoid eczema)
- Fingertip eczema
- 'Gut' eczema
- Hyperkeratotic palmar eczema
- Pompholyx
- Recurrent focal palmar peeling
- Ring eczema
- 'Wear and tear' dermatitis (dry palmar eczema)
- Other patterns (e.g. patchy vesiculosquamous)

Epidemiology

Incidence and prevalence

Minor degrees of hand eczema are very common, and virtually everyone suffers from mild dryness and chapping at some time or another. Studies on incidence and prevalence rely heavily on self-reporting which may underestimate true prevalence.

In a pooled study of data covering over 150 000 individuals, the lifetime prevalence of hand eczema was found to be 14.5% with a 1-year prevalence of 9.1% and a point prevalence of 4.0% [7]. The annual incidence was 7.3/1000 person-years. The majority of these data were from Nordic countries with some from other European states [7]. A UK study looking at computerised data from primary care (as read codes) recorded a 1-year prevalence of 0.4% [8]. This study also estimated that most do not seek help for their hand eczema, leading to underestimation of the true prevalence.

Age

The prevalence of hand eczema is higher in adults than children. Quaade et al. showed a lifetime prevalence of 8.9% in children and adolescents compared with 15.6% in adults; however confidence intervals were wide for both [7]. The 1-year prevalence for children and adolescents was 7.0% and for adults 9.7% with narrower, non-overlapping confidence intervals [7]. There were no data for differences in incidence.

The UK study showed increased prevalence with age, children aged 0–18 years having a 1-year population period prelevance of 0.203% and adults over 19 years of 0.397%. The annual incidence for those under 18 years of age was 1.956/1000 person-years and over 19 was 2.877/1000 person-years [8]. This study showed a peak for women aged between 20 and 39 years and men aged 60–69 years.

Sex

Hand eczema has a higher incidence in women than men. In one study the incidence was 8.7/1000 person-years in women and 4.7/1000 person-years in men [7]. The UK study also found the incidence in women to be higher than men at all ages.

Ethnicity

Hand eczema is a common problem in all ethnic groups. No studies have specifically reviewed differences. It should be noted that diagnosis can be more difficult in darker pigmented skin as the redness is not as clear, but dry, scaling skin and hyperkeratosis contrast more.

Associated diseases

About 50% of hand eczema patients have atopy [6]. The most common site of atopic eczema in the adult is the hands, and in some patients the hands alone may be involved. The atopic state may first become apparent with the development of hand eczema in an adolescent or young adult when they are exposed to school, hobby or occupational irritants. There is no specific topographical pattern, although the feet may also be involved [9,10]. The atopic diathesis may also predispose to a discoid pattern of hand eczema in young adults.

While rare, acrokeratosis neoplastica (Bazex syndrome) can mimic palmar and plantar eczema and may be indicative of internal malignancy [11]. This should be considered in the elderly and red flag symptoms should be asked about.

Pathophysiology

Predisposing factors

Having one or more positive patch test reactions, atopic eczema and employment with wet work are all predisposing factors. A proportion of atopic individuals are known to carry filaggrin gene mutations, as discussed in the genetics section.

The role of stress in aggravating hand eczema is difficult to evaluate, and the disease itself is stressful [12]. Many patients give a convincing account of exacerbations at times of acute anxiety, frustration or grief. The role of hormonal factors is also difficult to assess. Occasionally, there is a history of premenstrual exacerbation or deterioration during pregnancy.

Inflammatory pathways

The cellular inflammatory pathways of irritant contact dermatitis and allergic contact dermatitis follow a more innate lymphoid cell 1 (ILC1) cytokine profile with IL-1, IL-2, tumour necrosis factor α (TNF-α) and T helper 1/17 (Th1/17) cells predominating [13]. In contrast, atopic hand eczema follows an ILC2 pathway with IL-4, IL-13 and Th2/22 cells predominating early, although late and chronic inflammation can have more of an ILC1 pathway. These pathways are thought to inhibit each other, producing no net increase in the prevalence of contact dermatitis among atopic individuals despite increased barrier dysfunction.

Pathology

In general, the differences between the various forms of hand eczema are clinical rather than histological, but the considerably thickened horny layer and the presence of numerous sweat glands modify the histological features of eczema on the hands.

Causative organisms

This is not applicable, except for secondary bacterial infection.

Genetics

Twin studies suggest hereditary factors play a role in the development of hand eczema [14], with atopic diathesis the commonest endogenous cause [15]. Loss-of-function mutations of the filaggrin gene underpin the link with atopy and are associated with early onset and persistence of hand eczema in atopic subjects [16]. Carriers of filaggrin gene mutations are more likely to develop digital fissures (chapping) than those who do not carry the mutation [17]. In a 3-year prospective observational cohort study of 459 patients with occupational irritant contact dermatitis on the hands, those with atopy and filaggrin mutations had more sick leave and a threefold higher rate of job loss compared with controls [18,19]. Filaggrin gene mutations have also been linked with an increased susceptibility to chronic irritant contact dermatitis in case–control studies [20] and chronic hand eczema characterised by combined allergic and irritant contact dermatitis [21].

Environmental factors

Contact irritants are the most common exogenous cause of hand eczema [22], but contact allergens including chromate, epoxy glues and rubber are also important (Chapter 127). For external causes 70% are irritant contact dermatitis with 25% being allergic. Protein contact dermatitis accounts for about 5% [3]. All patterns of hand eczema are possible in contact allergy. Most dermatitis usually affects the dorsa of the hands (Figure 39.6), as can contact irritant and atopic eczema [23]. Certain occupations are particularly likely to provoke hand eczema. The problem of occupational eczema in hairdressers, beauticians, fish industry workers, farmers, construction workers, dental and medical personnel, metal workers and caterers has provoked many studies to determine its prevalence and to develop programmes for the prevention of hand dermatitis.

Health care workers have had an increase in both facial and hand irritant dermatitis due to the wearing of personal protective equipment and frequent hand sanitisation in the Covid-19 era. A survey of 114 health care workers in a surgical centre in April 2020 found acute hand dermatitis in 90.4% while hand eczema was reported in only 14.9% [24].

Type I allergic reactions to certain proteins may also give rise to hand eczema as well as to contact urticaria. In mild cases they

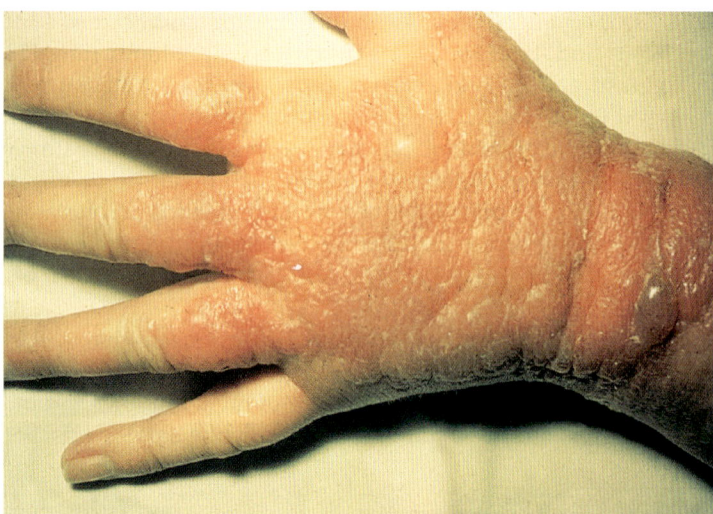

Figure 39.6 Bullous eczema due to contact allergy to rubber gloves.

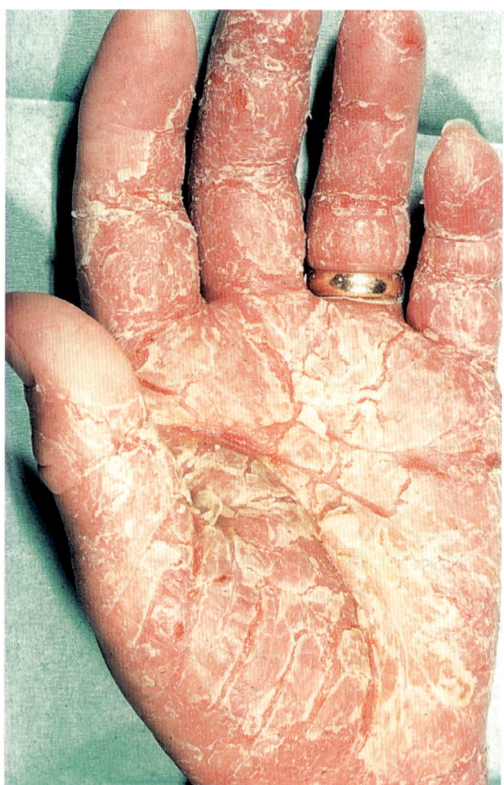

Figure 39.7 Hyperkeratotic palmar eczema.

provoke a vesicular eczema of the fingers, particularly among those who prepare seafood. In a Scandinavian study, one-third of restaurant food handlers with hand dermatitis had seafood contact urticaria [25]. Among health care workers, reactions to natural rubber latex protein found in latex gloves are a particular problem. The reactions range from contact urticaria to rhinitis, asthma and anaphylaxis [26].

Oral ingestion of allergens such as nickel, chromium or myroxylon pereirae (balsam of Peru) has been reported to provoke or aggravate hand eczema in sensitised subjects, although the importance of this phenomenon is controversial [27]. Contact proteins from foods may be ingested from airborne particles in kitchens when preparing foods [28]. Cold and dry air may play some part [29] and smoking is also an independent risk factor for all types of hand eczema [30].

Clinical features
History
Particular attention should be given to the patient's occupational and recreational activities because these may indicate potential contact allergies. Occupational involvement is suggested by improvement associated with leave from work or suspension of other activities. Health care workers are particularly vulnerable due to hand hygiene protocols in the Covid-19 era [31]. Current hand-protection strategies should also be elicited.

Hand eczema often has a severe impact on quality of life due to pruritus, painful fissuring, loss of dexterity and impairment of social functioning. Median dermatology life quality index (DLQI) scores [32] in patients attending patch test clinics were found to be 7 and 8 in males and females, respectively [33].

Presentation
This will be discussed in relation to each clinical variant next.

Clinical variants
Hyperkeratotic palmar eczema. This condition is a distinct form of hand eczema characterised by highly irritable, scaly, fissured, sharply demarcated hyperkeratotic patches on the palms and palmar surfaces of the fingers (Figure 39.7) [22]. It is common, and 2–5% of all applications for permanent disability pensions in some western European countries are due to hyperkeratotic hand eczema. It occurs more commonly in men and at an older age of onset compared with atopic eczema, is more likely to be associated with foot symptoms and is more common in smokers.

Pompholyx. Pompholyx (acute recurrent vesicular hand eczema) is a form of eczema of the palms and soles in which oedema fluid accumulates to form visible vesicles or bullae (Figure 39.8). As a result of the thick epidermis in these sites, the blisters tend to become relatively large before they burst. Pompholyx probably accounts for about 5–20% of all cases of hand eczema [22]. There is some debate whether the term pompholyx should be reserved for typical cases in which the attacks resolve and recur. Chronic, recurrent vesiculation without periods of remission may be termed chronic vesicular dermatitis. It is not related to allergic or irritant contact but is linked to atopy.

Apron eczema. This condition is a type of hand eczema that involves the proximal palmar aspect of two or more adjacent fingers and the contiguous palmar skin over the metacarpophalangeal joints, thus resembling an apron (Figure 39.9) [34]. This pattern of hand eczema may be irritant, allergic or endogenous.

Chronic acral dermatitis. This is a distinctive syndrome affecting patients in middle age. A chronic, intensely pruritic, hyperkeratotic, papulovesicular eczema of the hands and feet is associated with grossly elevated IgE levels in subjects with no personal or family

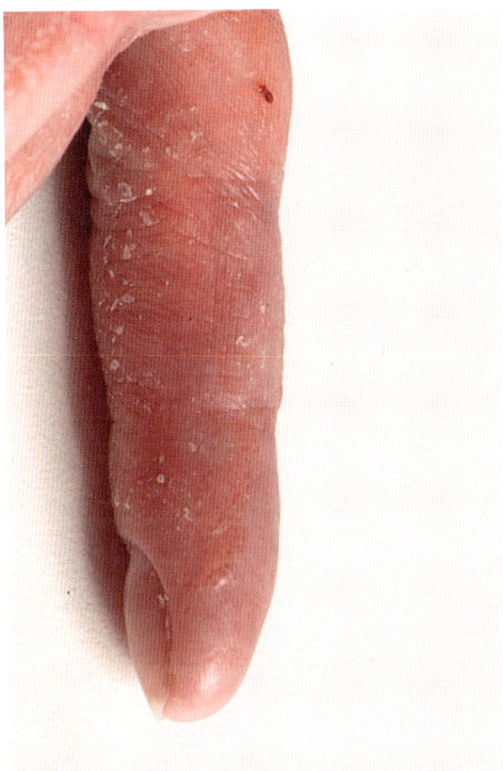

(a)

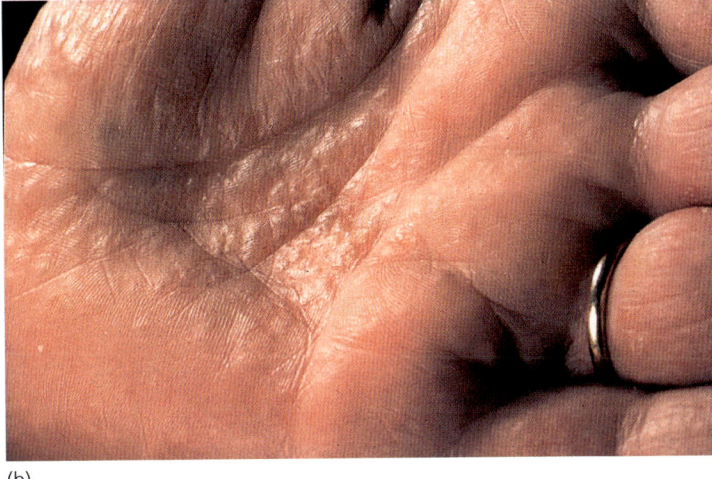

(b)

Figure 39.8 Pompholyx eczema. (a) Small vesicles coalescing into blisters on the lateral aspect of a finger. (b) Confluent vesicles of the palm.

history of atopy. The condition responds to oral corticosteroids, but the response to topical therapy is poor [22].

Nummular dermatitis. This is also known as discoid eczema (see section on nummular dermatitis earlier in this chapter).

Fingertip eczema. This condition presents a characteristic pattern, involving the palmar surface of the tips of some or all of the fingers. The skin is dry, cracked and sometimes breaks down into painful fissures (Figure 39.10). Usually remaining localised, it may occasionally extend along the palmar surfaces of the fingers to merge with palmar eczema. Two patterns may be distinguished.

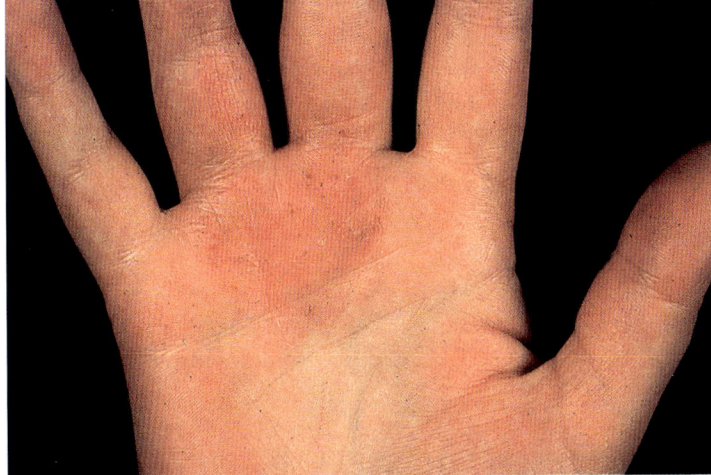

Figure 39.9 Apron eczema, showing the characteristic distribution.

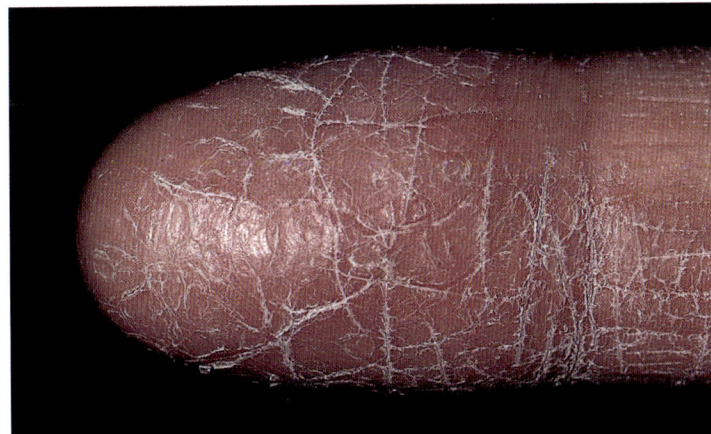

Figure 39.10 Fingertip eczema in a patient with wear and tear eczema. Courtesy of Dr D. A. Burns, Leicester Royal Infirmary, Leicester, UK.

The first and most common involves most or all of the fingers, mainly those of the dominant hand, and particularly the thumb and forefinger. The condition is usually worse in the winter and generally improves on holiday. Fingertip eczema is usually a cumulative irritant dermatitis in which degreasing agents combine with trauma as causative factors; patch tests are typically negative or not relevant. The second pattern preferentially involves the thumb, forefinger and third finger of one hand. This is usually occupational and may be either irritant (e.g. in newspaper delivery employees) or allergic (e.g. to colophony in polish). Methacrylate allergy among nail technicians has been increasing and due to the precision nature of the work can present as fingertip eczema [35]. The condition usually involves the dominant hand, but there may be allergy to onions, garlic [36] and other kitchen products held in the non-dominant hand when being cut. In these cases, patch testing (and 20 min contact tests) may be rewarding.

'Gut'/slaughterhouse eczema. Workers who eviscerate and clean pig carcasses are at risk of developing vesicular eczema which starts in the finger webs and spreads to the sides of the fingers. This is a mild, self-limiting condition, which clears in a week or two, even if the patient remains at work, but it can recur at intervals. Workers in Danish bacon factories call this 'fat eczema', although there is little evidence that it is due to fat, and prick tests to pig fat extracts are negative [37]. The pathogenesis is unknown, but some slaughter workers have developed contact urticaria from exposure to animal blood [38].

Patchy vesiculosquamous eczema. In a large group of cases, a mixture of irregular, patchy, vesiculosquamous lesions occurs on both hands, usually asymmetrically. In contrast to the lesions of hand nummular dermatitis, the degree of activity and distribution of the lesions vary. Nail changes are common if the nail folds are affected.

Recurrent focal palmar peeling. The condition is sometimes a mild form of pompholyx; it is also known as desquamation en aires, keratolysis exfoliativa or ringed keratolysis of the palms. During the summer months, small areas of superficial, white desquamation develop on the sides of the fingers and on the palms or on the feet (Figure 39.11). These areas appear abruptly and expand before peeling. There is little or no irritation, and vesicles as such are not seen. The condition is probably not rare, but because it is relatively asymptomatic it is not seen very often by dermatologists. Some patients subsequently develop true pompholyx.

Ring eczema. This characteristic pattern particularly affects young women and rarely men. The condition usually starts soon after marriage or childbirth. An irritable patch of eczema begins under a ring – usually a broad wedding ring – and typically spreads to involve the adjacent side of the middle finger and the adjacent area of the palm. It may remain confined to these sites but is occasionally followed by the appearance of discoid patches elsewhere; or a more diffuse vesicular eczema may develop. Despite the clearly defined demarcation of the initial eruption, these patients are not sensitive to gold or copper, although nickel, cobalt and even chromium sensitivity is more commonly found on patch testing than might be expected; only rarely can 'white gold' alloys be implicated. Ring dermatitis has been described as the clinical presentation of fragrance sensitisation [39]. Transference of the ring to the other hand is often rapidly followed by the appearance of eczema at the new site and, once affected, patients may find that wearing of the ring for only a few minutes, even without washing, causes irritation. This type of hand eczema is probably due primarily to concentrations of soap and detergent beneath rings (which may tighten on fingers immersed in hot water), but microtrauma, especially friction, may also play a role. Very rarely, radioactive gold in a ring may cause radiation dermatitis that mimics this type of wedding ring eczema [40].

Differential diagnosis

The diagnosis of hand eczema is usually self-evident, but the distinction from psoriasis can be very difficult and may only become apparent over time with the development of psoriasis at other sites. In some cases, even biopsy does not allow a clear distinction to be made. In most cases of psoriasis on the hands, however, the silvery nature of the scale, involvement of the knuckles, sharply demarcated 'scalloped' edges to the redness along the borders of the hands and fingers, and the relative absence of pruritus are helpful pointers to the diagnosis. A family history of psoriasis and the presence of nail pits in the absence of nail fold lesions are also suggestive.

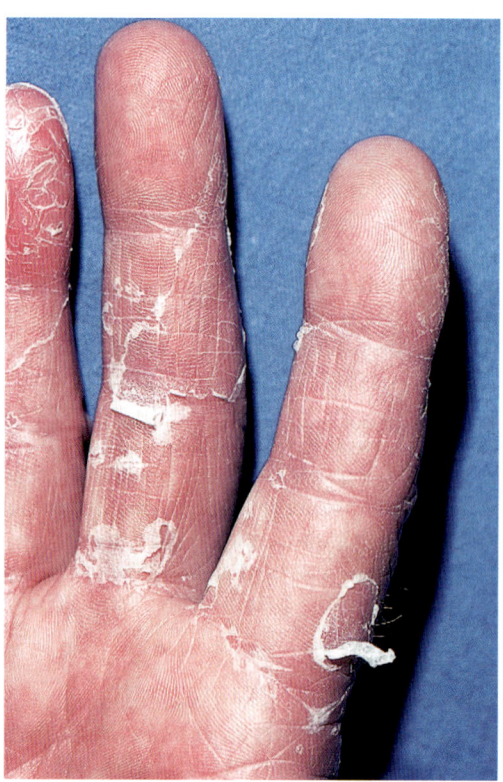

(a)

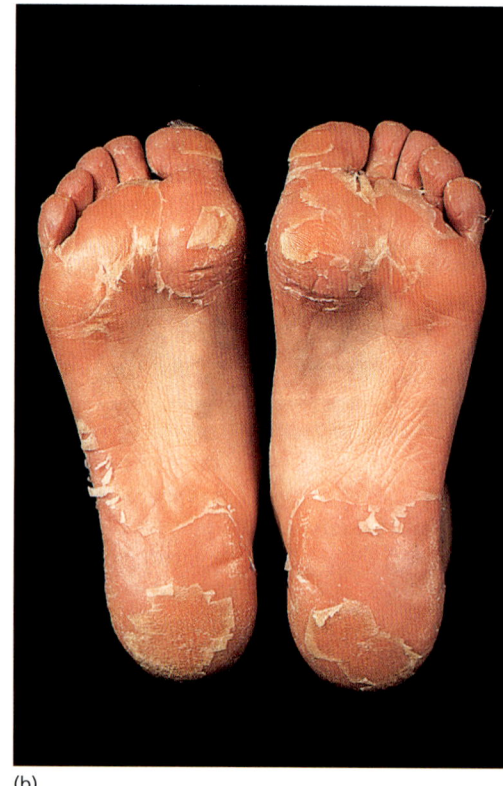

(b)

Figure 39.11 Recurrent focal palmar peeling. (a) Well-established lesions on the hands. (b) Lesions on the feet. (a) Courtesy of Dr A. Marsden, St George's Hospital, London, UK.

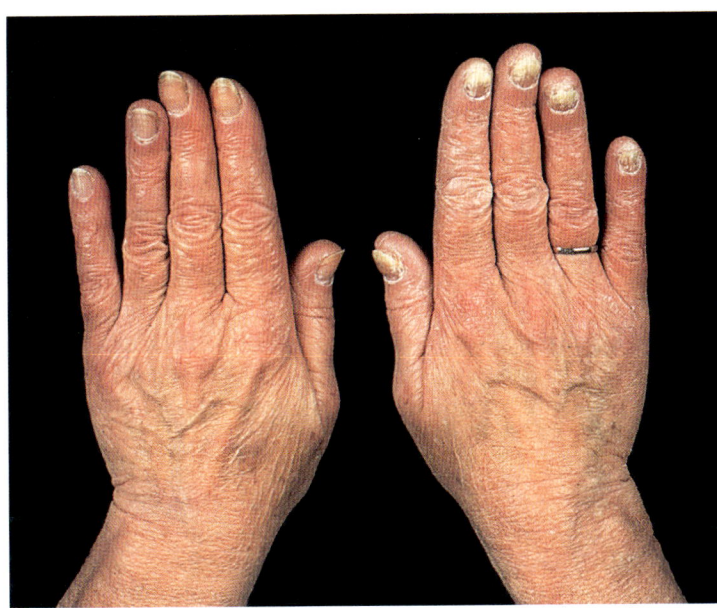

Figure 39.12 *Trichophyton* infection of the hands that failed to respond to topical corticosteroids. Note the nail involvement.

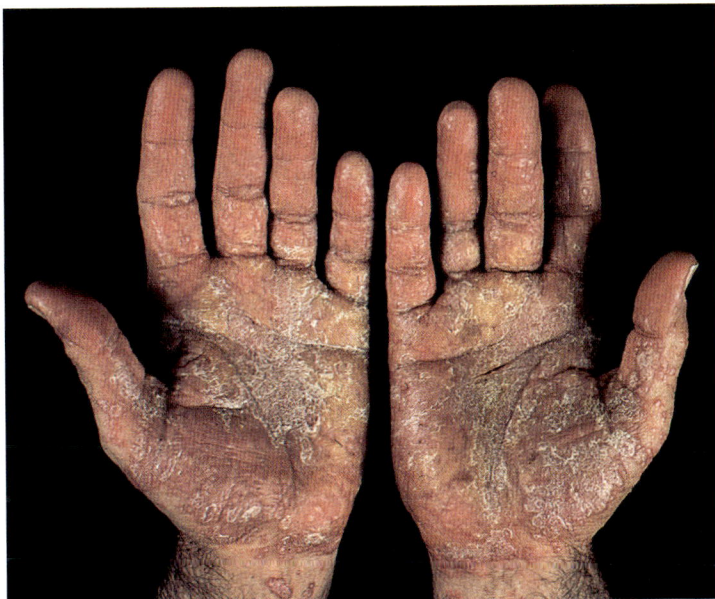

Figure 39.13 Lichen planus mimicking hyperkeratotic hand eczema, but the margins are well demarcated and the lesions on the left wrist are characteristic of lichen planus.

Tinea manuum can be missed, particularly when it is extensive (Figure 39.12) or secondarily infected. Unilateral scaling of the palm should always suggest a possible *Trichophyton* infection, and a discoid plaque due to *T. verrucosum* is sometimes seen in farmers. Partial treatment with topical corticosteroids can mask the typical appearance if misdiagnosed (tinea incognito).

Lichen planus (Figure 39.13) and pityriasis rubra pilaris may resemble eczema on the hands, but usually present with typical lesions at other sites.

Pompholyx eczema can resemble palmoplantar pustulosis. Clinically, the two conditions are distinguished by the presence of vesicles in the former and sterile pustules that resolve with characteristic brown marks in the latter. A pustular bacteride secondary to bacterial infection elsewhere in the body is a less common differential. Repeated attacks of pompholyx may produce hyperkeratotic lesions that mimic psoriasis vulgaris. Pemphigoid, linear IgA disease and pemphigoid gestationis occasionally present with blisters on the palms that mimic pompholyx.

Scabies (particularly crusted scabies) may present on the hands but is likely to exist elsewhere on the body and in close contacts with the same symptoms. Crusted scabies may be confused with hyperkeratotic hand eczema.

Hand, foot and mouth disease (coxsackie A16 viral infection) presents with typical oval lesions in all three sites and is self-limiting. It can be confused with pompholyx. Management with topical corticosteroids and moisturisers may appear to 'cure' it but it usually resolves spontaneously.

Secondary syphilis also presents with palmar hand lesions (Chapter 29).

A total skin examination should be performed in any case of hand eczema where the diagnosis is in doubt. There may, for example, be evidence of nickel allergy or tinea pedis, or small patches of psoriasis of which the patient is unaware.

Classification of severity

A photographic guide for assessing the severity of chronic hand dermatitis has been developed and validated, mainly for use in clinical trial settings [41]. In daily practice, measurement of quality of life using a dermatology-specific index can be done by clinicians to quantify disease severity. UK National Institute for Health and Care Excellence (NICE) guidelines for alitretinoin for chronic hand eczema require a DLQI score [33] to be measured [42,43]. Some more recent studies have used the hand eczema severity index (HECSI) which is an objective measure of examination features complementing the subjective scoring of the DLQI [44].

Complications and co-morbidities

Secondary bacterial infection of hand eczema may occur, usually associated with a sudden deterioration, pain and/or exudate from the affected areas. In pompholyx eczema, infection may also be indicated by the new onset of pustules rather than vesicles, usually in association with pain.

Disease course and prognosis

Unless a responsible allergen can be identified and removed, the prognosis of hand eczema for an individual is uncertain. Even if a relevant allergen is identified, it may be difficult to avoid all contact with the hands for allergens such as nickel and fragrance. Atopy, sensitisation to one or more contact allergens and extent of disease are all risk factors for a worse prognosis [3]. Smoking is also associated with a worse prognosis.

Following an acute attack of pompholyx, about one-third of patients experience no further episodes, one-third suffer from recurrent episodes and in the remainder the condition develops into a chronic, possibly hyperkeratotic phase. Those forms of hand eczema that are due in part or wholly to the effects of irritants carry a particularly poor prognosis unless these irritants can be completely removed. Patients who have suffered from severe hand eczema will often remain vulnerable to mild irritants for several months after the eczema has apparently cleared. Interdigital dermatitis has been shown to be a potential precursor to more severe hand dermatitis in hairdressers. Recognition of this sign by the patient may allow early intervention to prevent progression of the disease [45].

A questionnaire follow-up answered by 868 of 1115 persons with hand eczema, identified 15 years previously in a population-based study, found that 44% had experienced hand eczema in the previous year [46]. For about 5%, the hand eczema had resulted in a major life change such as long sick leave periods, early retirement or a change of occupation.

Investigations

A circumscribed and asymmetrical area of scaling and vesiculation of the palm or sole should suggest the possibility of dermatophytosis, and scrapings should be examined for fungus. If the redness is limited to one or two interdigital clefts, or is asymmetrical, or involves the dorsal skin to any extent, the possibility of contact dermatitis must be considered and investigated by patch testing. If there are immediate symptoms on wearing latex gloves, then type I latex hypersensitivity should be excluded with latex prick testing and specific IgE to latex (in the context of a total IgE).

Management

Chronic hand eczema

Management of chronic hand eczema, defined as persisting for at least 3 or 6 months, is similar to eczema affecting other skin sites and involves the avoidance of irritants, frequent application of emollients and use of topical corticosteroids when indicated.

Avoidance of irritants is particularly difficult for patients with hand eczema because they are so ubiquitous and the very function of the hand is contact. Patient education is of paramount importance and this can be reinforced by printed or online advice sheets. Gloves usually provide the best protection against irritants and allergens; the optimal choice of glove should be considered in terms of the material, size and weight depending on the individual's particular needs. Natural rubber latex (NRL) gloves generally give good protection for housework. In patients with a latex allergy, nitrile or polyvinyl chloride household gloves should be worn instead. It should be noted that some allergens, such as acrylates and epoxy resins, can penetrate vinyl or rubber gloves [47]. Gloves that develop holes should be discarded immediately and, if sweating makes the condition worse, it may be helpful to wear cotton gloves beneath the protective ones.

In an occupational setting, gloves are often worn for a significant amount of time to protect against exogenous agents such as hair dyes and preservatives. Allergens like hair dyes penetrate NRL gloves after 90 min and vinyl ones after 40 min [48]. In general, nitrile gloves offer the most resistance to penetration but no gloves prevent absorption completely. Changing gloves frequently helps prevent this but there may be an added factor of being allergic to contents in the glove itself. Latex allergy is on the decline, but rubber accelerators designed to speed up the hardening of glove materials can be found in both NRL and nitrile glove types. The most common accelerators are thiuram mix, mercapto mix and mercaptithiobenzole and carba mix.

Barrier creams are used to prevent hand eczema of occupational origin, however in practice they may not be applied effectively [49], and the debate continues about their actual benefit [50]. A Cochrane review of interventions such as emollients and barrier creams for preventing occupational irritant hand dermatitis found generally positive results but no statistical significance was reached [51].

Emollients should be applied frequently, and containers should be left at convenient locations at home and at work so that they are readily available. In general, choice of emollient is directed by the patient to ensure maximal compliance. Soap substitutes should be used in place of soap for all hand washing. Patients should be warned that some topical preparations sold over the counter by pharmacists as antipruritics or emollients can contain irritants such as alcohol or propylene glycol.

Topical corticosteroids are required for all but the mildest cases of hand eczema. For severe hand eczema, potent or very potent topical corticosteroids may be needed. Applying topical corticosteroids at night (in bed) can increase contact time as the hands are used less. Painful fissures of the fingertips are a particular therapeutic problem and these can be treated with corticosteroid-impregnated adhesive tape, which provides both physical protection and local delivery of topical corticosteroid.

In difficult, unresponsive cases the use of a topical corticosteroid under occlusion may be considered. The corticosteroid is applied at bedtime, and polythene gloves, sealed at the wrist with sticky tape, are worn overnight. This can be an effective treatment, but it greatly increases the risk of atrophy and secondary bacterial infection and should be discontinued as soon as the eczema shows satisfactory improvement. After improvement with daily corticosteroid use, it is safe to use a potent corticosteroid cream intermittently to prevent relapse [52].

If hand eczema does not respond to topical corticosteroid therapy, the diagnosis should be reviewed, particularly with regard to the possibility of tinea. The patient should be asked again about exposure to irritants or allergens, and the possibility of contact sensitisation to medicament bases, preservatives or the corticosteroid itself should be considered, with patch testing if necessary.

Topical calcineurin inhibitors provide a further option for treating hand eczema. In a left/right comparative trial with 16 subjects, topical tacrolimus 0.1% proved similar in efficacy to mometasone furoate [53]. Calcipotriol has also been used to good effect in hand eczema, although traditionally it was used for psoriasis.

Intradermal injection of triamcinolone (10 mg/mL) into recalcitrant, localized patches of hand eczema may also be beneficial [54]. For pompholyx eczema, iontophoresis has been used successfully [55]. Tar and Grenz rays have gone out of favour considering newer therapies and risk of malignancy [56].

At present, the retinoid alitretinoin (9-*cis* retinoic acid) is the only licensed systemic therapy for chronic hand eczema. It interacts with both retinoid X and retinoic acid receptors and has been shown to improve chronic hand eczema [57]. In the UK, NICE has approved alitretinoin for patients who have severe chronic hand eczema, defined by the physician's global assessment and a DLQI of 15 or more, and in whom potent topical corticosteroid therapy has failed [43].

A small RCT involving 29 patients with hyperkeratotic hand eczema suggested some benefit from acitretin [58], however this is unsuitable for women of child-bearing age due to its long half-life and teratogenicity. An RCT of 41 patients compared ciclosporin (licensed for atopic eczema) 3 mg/kg daily with a potent topical corticosteroid, betamethasone diproprionate, and found no significant difference between the two groups [59]. Ciclosporin can be used for up to 6 months according to European guidelines [60]. A brief report of an RCT comparing azathioprine 50 mg daily and a very potent topical corticosteroid with the very potent topical corticosteroid alone suggested possible additive benefit from low-dose azathioprine [61], but effectiveness was limited.

Oral PUVA therapy and UVB therapy have been used to treat chronic hand eczema; there is no evidence to suggest that UVB is better than PUVA or that oral PUVA is any better than topical PUVA [56]. Topical hand PUVA soaks are frequently used in clinical practice although there is only limited published evidence for hand eczema. Methotrexate is now well established as a treatment for both eczema and psoriasis, but there is limited evidence for effectiveness in hand eczema.

Dupilumab is an IL-4 receptor α-inhibitor, blocking the Th2 cytokines of atopy. Relatively low-powered retrospective and prospective studies have demonstrated improvement in hand eczema but, in many cases, atopic eczema was also present or it was unclear if it was present.

Emerging therapies in eczema include the JAK and tyrosine kinase (TYK) inhibitors. Topical delgocitinib, a JAK1, JAK2, JAK3 and TYK2 inhibitor in early development, has shown some positive results in a phase II trial [62]. A 2022 case report has demonstrated the successful use of baricitinib in hand eczema [63].

Acute hand eczema

For hand eczema that presents acutely, it is important to eliminate any precipitant, for example a contact allergen. Emollients should be applied copiously and, if the eruption involves exudate or pompholyx vesicles, then dilute potassium manganite (VII) soaks are helpful. Large bullae may be aspirated using a sterile syringe. Systemic antibiotics will be required if secondary bacterial infection develops and empirical therapy with flucloxacillin to provide cover for staphylococci is generally effective, pending culture and sensitivity results from swabs.

Treatment ladder for dermatitis and eczema of the hands

First line
- Hand care advice
- Irritant and allergen avoidance
- Emollients
- Soap substitute

Second line
- Potent or very potent topical corticosteroids, steroid-impregnated tape

Third line
- Alitretinoin/PUVA/azathioprine/ciclosporin/methotrexate

Resources

Patient resources

British Association of Dermatologists, patient information leaflets: https://www.bad .org.uk/for-the-public/patient-information-leaflets
DermNet NZ, hand dermatitis: https://dermnetnz.org/topics/hand-dermatitis/ (Both last accessed September 2023.)

Dermatitis and eczema of the lower legs

Definition and nomenclature

Dermatitis and eczema of the lower legs are subclassified by *ICD-11* as venous eczema, stasis dermatitis and allergic contact dermatitis. Lower limb venous eczema encompasses the skin changes that result from venous hypertension. Stasis dermatitis relates to the skin changes that result from reduced lower leg venous flow.

Synonyms and inclusions
- Venous eczema is also known as varicose eczema
- Eczema and dermatitis are used interchangeably

Introduction and general description

Venous eczema and stasis dermatitis both result from dysfunctional venous and lymphatic drainage of the lower legs. There is a great deal of overlap between the two skin conditions, which share the same clinical features, and they are distinguished by the presence or absence of venous hypertension. Allergic contact dermatitis of the lower legs is a common complication of both skin conditions.

Epidemiology

Incidence and prevalence

The combined prevalence of venous eczema and venous stasis is estimated to be between 3% and 11% of the population [1,2].

Age

Venous eczema patients are usually middle-aged or elderly. The incidence in the over-seventies is 70% [20].

Sex

There is an increased incidence in females, which may be due to hormonal effects and the tendency for deep-vein thrombosis (DVT) to occur during pregnancy.

Ethnicity

Venous eczema affects all ethnicities.

Associated diseases

There is an association between venous eczema and allergic contact dermatitis.

Pathophysiology

Predisposing factors

Venous eczema is more likely after a previous DVT and in the presence of venous stasis, which is itself linked to obesity, immobility and previous cellulitis [2]. In a study of 170 people with varicose veins, 27% went on to develop eczematous changes [3].

Pathology [4–7]

In venous eczema, the oxygen content in the femoral venous blood of the leg affected by venous hypertension is increased, and the venous blood in such limbs has a faster circulation time than normal [8,9]. These observations could be explained by the development of arteriovenous shunts in the affected areas, but the use of radioactively labelled macroaggregates or microspheres has failed to provide any evidence for such shunts.

An alternative explanation for these findings has been provided by Browse and Burnand [5], who suggested that the high ambulatory venous pressure within the calf muscle pump is transmitted to the capillary circulation in the skin and subcutaneous tissues of the calf. This distends the local capillary bed and widens the endothelial pores, thus allowing fibrinogen molecules to escape into the interstitial fluid, where they form a fibrin sheath around the capillaries. This layer of fibrin presumably forms a pericapillary barrier to the diffusion of oxygen and other nutrients that are essential for the normal vitality of the skin. The hypothesis that pericapillary fibrin impedes oxygen diffusion has been supported by a study using positron emission tomography [10].

It has also been suggested that cutaneous inflammation in venous hypertension may result from increased sequestration of leukocytes in the venules, with a consequent release of proteolytic enzymes and free radicals which produce tissue damage [6]. In normal subjects, leukocytes are sequestered in the limb when venous pressure is elevated; in patients with venous insufficiency the effect is enhanced, with increased endothelial contact and adhesion of white cells [11]. This effect may be related to an increase in the expression of adhesion molecules intercellular adhesion molecule 1 (ICAM-1) and vascular cell adhesion molecule 1 (VCAM-1) on the vascular endothelium in affected skin [12].

Causative organisms

This is not applicable except in cases of secondary infection where standard organisms such as *Staphylococcus* and *Streptococcus* are implicated.

Genetics

No strong genetic links have been identified to date.

Clinical features

History

Venous eczema may develop suddenly or insidiously. It may occur as a late result of DVT, cellulitis or recent surgery.

Presentation

Venous eczema and stasis dermatitis are both red, scaly and often exudative eruptions usually seen around the ankle and lower leg (Figure 39.14). Occasionally, similar changes occur at other sites of venous hypertension such as the pendulous skin over an obese

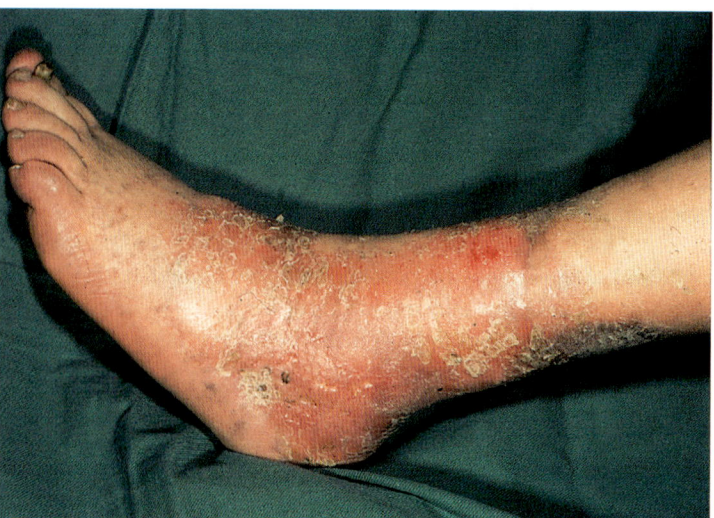

Figure 39.14 Venous (gravitational) eczema.

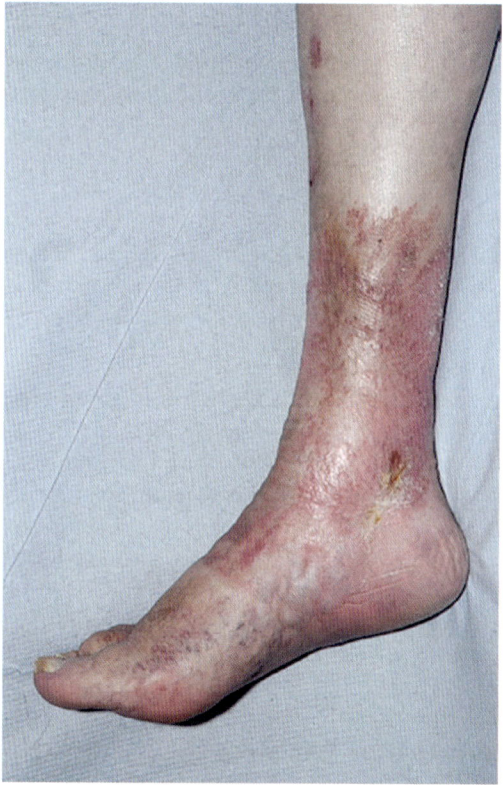

Figure 39.15 Venous eczema of the ankle with ulceration at the medial malleolus.

abdomen or in association with an ateriovenous fistula in the upper limb [13]. The eczema is often accompanied by other manifestations of venous hypertension, including dilatation or varicosity of the superficial veins, oedema, purpura, haemosiderosis and ulceration (Figure 39.15), or small patches of white, atrophic, telangiectatic scarring ('atrophie blanche'). These changes, which occur in various combinations, are discussed in more detail in Chapter 102. Leashes of dilated venules around the dorsum of the foot or ankle are particularly common. There may be a subepidermal vascular proliferation producing purple papules around the ankle, which may resemble Kaposi sarcoma [14].

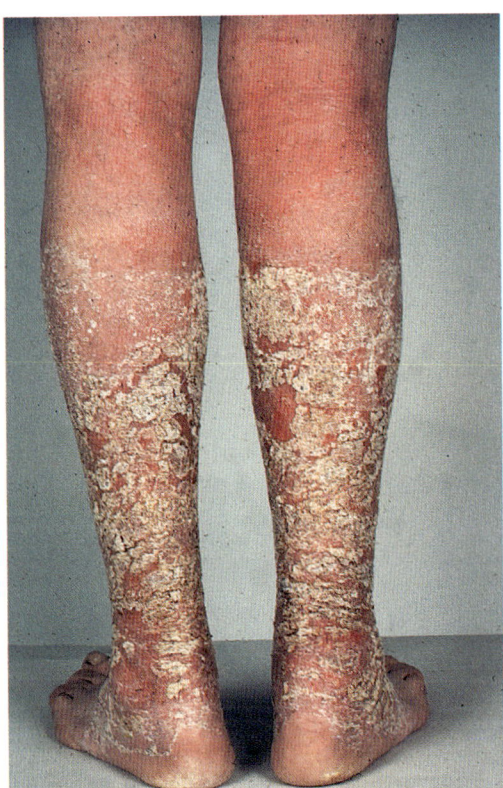

Figure 39.16 Contact eczema of the lower legs due to allergy to paste bandages.

Clinical variants

Secondary patches of eczema may develop on the other leg, even when it is not affected by obvious venous insufficiency. Generalised secondary dissemination may occur, and occasionally this can progress to erythroderma.

Differential diagnosis

In children or young adults, atopic eczema may manifest as licheni-fied patches around the ankle or behind the knees. Allergic contact dermatitis of the lower legs is usually due to topical medicaments and components of dressings (Figure 39.16). Patch testing is often indicated. An infected ulcer may be complicated by infective eczema spreading from the edge of the ulcer, which should respond to appropriate antibiotic therapy. Nummular dermatitis is common on the lower leg, usually on the anterior or anterolateral aspect. Asteatotic eczema commonly affects the legs of elderly patients.

Psoriasis may present as a single, irritating plaque on the leg, but is usually scalier and clearly marginated. Hypertrophic lichen planus of the lower leg may occasionally be mistaken for eczema if there are no characteristic lesions elsewhere. Dermatophyte infection may present as diffuse redness and scaling and may be difficult to recognise, particularly if it has been treated with topical steroids. Profuse actinic keratoses may cause red, irritable patches on the lower legs in sunny climates. In the late stage of borreliosis, the leg can feel heavy, with thick cyanotic itchy skin that may mimic the changes of venous hypertension [15].

Classification of severity

The Clinical Etiological Anatomical Pathological (CEAP) classification is a linear system that divides venous eczema by the presence or absence of signs [16]. However, some signs do not necessarily follow in order and this classification is not routinely used (Chapter 102).

Complications and co-morbidities

Allergic contact dermatitis. Clinically this may present as an eczematous eruption with a sharp, linear cut-off matching the application of a topical therapy, wound dressing or compression hosiery. Allergic contact dermatitis is a common complication of venous eczema, possibly because of the large number of antigen-presenting cells in the inflamed skin [17] and the resultant barrier dysfunction, and also because of prolonged contact with topical therapies and compression hosiery. The most common allergen is myroxylon pereirae (balsam of Peru) followed by fragrances, topical antibiotics and components of dressings [18]. Like venous eczema, this too is more common in women and polysensitisation is also more common due to multiple exposures [19]. Allergic contact dermatitis of the lower leg is covered in more detail in Chapter 127.

Secondary infection. This usually presents as a sudden worsening of eczema. If cellulitis ensues, the patient may experience pain and increased skin temperature and swelling of the affected area, as well as malaise and rigors if infection becomes systemic. The mode of antibiotic administration depends on the severity of the infection, ranging from topical antibiotics for mild infection, oral for moderate and intravenous for severe.

Lipodermatosclerosis. Chronic venous insufficiency may result in lipodermatosclerosis, described in more detail in Chapter 101.

Venous ulceration. There is an association between venous eczema and venous ulceration because these are both the result of venous hypertension. Ulcer healing is inhibited by both venous eczema and stasis dermatitis, in part due to chronic lower leg swelling. Itch is a common symptom often overlooked [20].

Disease course and prognosis

Venous eczema is a chronic condition that undergoes relapse and remission. Long-term improvement may be provided by effective lower limb compression, if tolerated, or in some cases by varicose vein surgery.

Investigations

Ankle brachial pressure index (ABPI) measurement is required prior to consideration of compression therapy. An ABPI of more than 0.8 in the absence of vessel calcification due to diabetes or atherosclerosis, which can give a falsely high reading, indicates suitability for graduated compression bandages (Chapter 102).

Management

Any underlying venous hypertension and/or pedal oedema should be controlled. Obese patients should be encouraged to lose weight. Well-fitted support stockings or firm bandages can be helpful if worn regularly and care is taken to avoid the formation of a band at the top of the leg. The legs should be elevated as effectively as possible. Exercise also encourages flow away from peripheral circulation [21]. As a preventative measure, compression postvenous thrombosis can reduce the risk of developing venous eczema as well as reduce the risk of further thrombi [22].

Mild topical corticosteroids may be used to relieve irritation, but the use of potent corticosteroids should be limited to short periods of a few days as they may cause cutaneous atrophy and increase the risk of ulceration. Topical tacrolimus has been reported to be effective [23]. However, when necessary, the inflammation should be reduced. Bacterial infection must be treated where appropriate, but the risk of sensitisation to topical antibiotics and antiseptics should be borne in mind; systemic antibiotics may be preferable. Bacteria cultured from a swab do not necessarily have a pathogenic role. If trauma is thought to be playing a part, and the patient cannot resist scratching, a paste bandage may be helpful.

> ### Treatment ladder for dermatitis and eczema of the lower legs
>
> #### First line
> - Skin care, including leg elevation and exercise
> - Emollients
> - Topical corticosteroids
>
> #### Second line
> - Compression hosiery
>
> #### Third line
> - Referral to a vascular surgeon to consider surgical intervention

Resources

Patient resources

British Association of Dermatologists, patient information leaflets: https://www.bad .org.uk/for-the-public/patient-information-leaflets

DermNet NZ, Leg dermatitis: https://dermnetnz.org/cme/dermatitis/leg-dermatitis/

National Institute for Health and Care Excellence, Clinical Knowledge Summaries, Venous eczema and lipodermatosclerosis: https://cks.nice.org.uk/topics/venous-eczema-lipodermatosclerosis/ (All last accessed September 2023.)

Dermatitis and eczema of the eyelids

Definition

This is eczema affecting predominantly the eyelids and is covered in more detail in Chapter 107.

Introduction and general description

This is a common and distressing clinical presentation [1,2]. The skin is an organ of communication as well as other established functions. When people communicate 'with their eyes' it is not the eyeball itself offering that information but the configuration of the eyelids, brows and periorbital skin that does so.

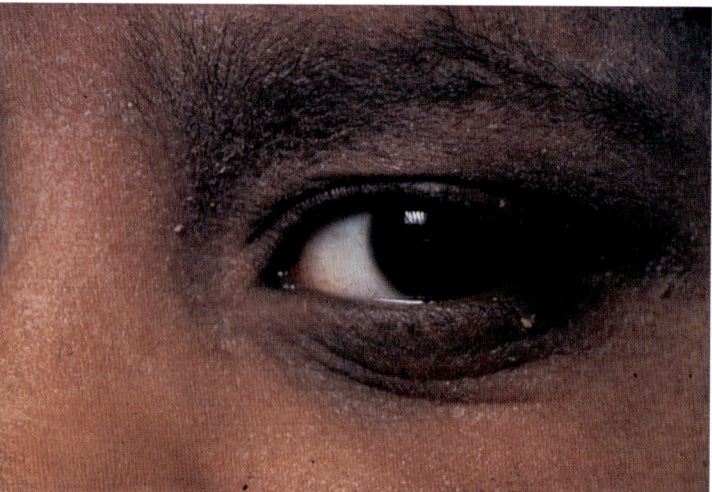

(a)

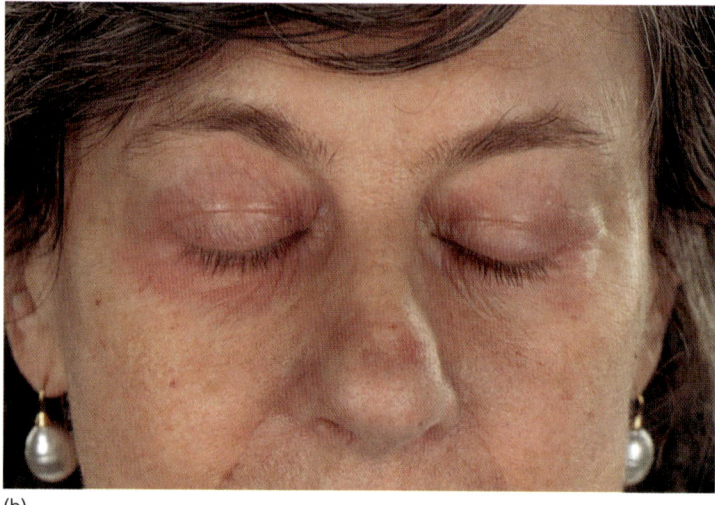

(b)

Figure 39.17 (a) Eyelid atopic eczema (note the infraorbital Dennie–Morgan fold). (b) Allergic contact dermatitis of the eyelid due to the airborne fragrance linalool.

The delicate skin of the eyelid is only 0.55 mm thick and contains a complex layer of musculature, vasculature and secretory organs [3]. Unlike other areas of the body, there is no subcutaneous fat and the skin is firmly attached to the underlying tarsal plate [4]; the remaining skin is loosely attached to underlying structures. The skin thickness changes from the eyelid to the periorbital and facial skin. The most common cause of eyelid dermatitis and periorbital dermatitis is contact dermatitis, followed by atopic dermatitis (Figure 39.17). It is likely that many cases represent mild atopic eczema without other manifestations [5]. Several studies have reported a female preponderance [6].

Other dermatoses like seborrhoeic dermatitis, rosacea or lupus may also underlie the presentation or indeed be a differential. Dermatomyositis should also be considered. Contact allergy to various components of eye make-up, nail varnish, fragrance, rubber [7] or ophthalmic medicaments [8] is responsible for some cases. Allergy to nickel in spectacle frame screws may cause eczema near the temples and periorbital areas. In some cases the cause remains obscure.

Eyelid eczema can also be complicated by the presence of concomitant eye diseases associated with eczema such as allergic conjunctivitis, keratoconus and cataract [9].

The skin of the rest of the face varies subtly from the eyelids and periorbital skin with changes in apocrine glands and vasculature.

Pathophysiology
The thin nature of the eyelid predisposes to diffusion of potential allergenic substances across the epidermis, more so than with other body sites. Concomitant dermatoses of the eyelid can also worsen this, with inflammation reducing barrier function and increasing diffusion capacity. Rubbing the eyelids due to itch exacerbates this further.

Allergic contact dermatitis of the eyelids can be from direct application of allergenic substances such as make-up, transfer of substances on the hands or even from volatile airborne allergens. Despite a larger area of facial skin being exposed, the eyelids may be the only areas manifesting dermatitis due to the different nature of the skin and possible concentration of previously sensitised cutaneous memory T cells in that area. However, allergens can migrate and manifest in adjacent skin [6].

The most common allergens reported are metals such as nickel or gold sodium thiosulphate [10], although relevance may not be significant. This is followed by fragrances such as *Myroxylon pereirae* that are often contained in make-up products. Topical medications can also cause problems with either the medications themselves or the preservatives contained in them [11,12].

Investigation
Patch testing should be considered when reviewing a patient with eyelid dermatitis as allergic contact dermatitis is the most common cause. Due to the different nature of eyelid skin, prepreparing the back to increase diffusion capacity may be necessary with tape stripping. However, if ruled out or the allergen is not relevant, clinical diagnosis of the differentials may be all that is required.

Management
When the condition is not amenable to removal of the cause, treatment with hydrocortisone cream is often effective. Topical calcineurin inhibitors (tacrolimus, pimecrolimus) can be particularly useful in this setting, and avoid the risks of inducing atrophy, rosacea or raised intraocular pressure associated with prolonged use of topical corticosteroids.

Crisaborole is a topical boron based phosphodiesterase 4 inhibitor which has as yet weak evidence for reducing inflammation in eczema. Because it is not a corticosteroid, skin atrophy and telangiectasia are less of a problem, making it more acceptable in sensitive sites such as the eyelids [13].

Treatment ladder for dermatitis and eczema of the eyelids

First line
- Patch test
- Avoid allergens/irritants (if relevant)
- Emollient

Second line
- Hydrocortisone 21-acetate 1% cream

Third line
- Tacrolimus 0.03% or 0.1% ointment or pimecrolimus 1% cream

Juvenile plantar dermatosis

Definition and nomenclature
This condition is characterised by shiny, dry, fissured dermatitis of the plantar surface of the forefoot.

Synonyms and inclusions
- Forefoot eczema
- Peridigital dermatosis
- Dermatitis plantaris sicca
- Atopic winter feet

Introduction and general description
The first record of this condition appeared in 1968, and since then it has been described under a variety of names depending on the authors' beliefs concerning pathogenesis and the possible association with atopy. The name 'juvenile plantar dermatosis' has the merit of making no presumptions about cause.

Epidemiology
Incidence and prevalence
There is little up-to-date information on incidence and prevalence, possibly due to differences in coding and classification. A review of 389 children aged 0–16 years referred to a paediatric dermatology clinic over 19 years found juvenile plantar dermatosis in 8 of them (15.4%) [1]. However, this study is skewed by the referral indication being suspected contact dermatitis.

Age
It occurs mainly in children aged 3–14 years. Only occasional cases are seen in adults or infants.

Sex
There is a slight preponderance of male children.

Associated diseases
An association with atopy has been proposed but the evidence for this is not convincing. In a controlled study, a personal or family history of eczema or other atopic illness was no more common in cases than in controls [2].

Pathophysiology [3,4]
Some authors consider juvenile plantar dermatosis to be an irritant contact dermatitis caused by excessive humidity and maceration of the skin leading to a barrier compromise [5]. Histology shows a mild, non-specific eczema. An inflammation of eccrine sweat ducts can be identified in many cases [6].

Genetics

It has been reported in identical twins [7].

Environmental factors [2,3,5,8–10]

It seems likely that changes in fashion, and the resulting changes in the composition of children's socks and shoes, may have been responsible for the emergence of this disease. Waxing and waning fashions for the use of synthetic materials such as nylon and plastics, compared with more porous natural materials such as cotton, wool and leather, may have been the cause. However, the exact pathogenesis of the disease remains uncertain [8]. Occasional cases have occurred in children wearing open leather sandals and cotton socks. Many of the affected children are keen on dancing or sports, and this suggests that friction and enhanced sweating may be playing some part.

Clinical features

The presenting features of juvenile plantar dermatosis are redness and soreness on the plantar surface of the forefoot, which assumes a shiny, 'glazed' and cracked appearance (Figure 39.18). The condition is most severe on the ball of the foot and toe pads and tends to spare the non-weight-bearing instep. The toe clefts are normal and this helps to distinguish the condition from tinea pedis. The symmetry of the lesions is a striking feature. Occasionally, the disease can affect the hands, resulting in sore, shiny, fissured palms or fingertips. This is more likely in atopic subjects [11].

Most cases will clear spontaneously during childhood or adolescence, but the condition may persist into adulthood [12].

Investigations

The diagnosis is clinical, although skin scrapes to exclude fungus and patch tests to exclude footwear allergy may be helpful if there is any doubt. Consultation with the manufacturer of the shoes may help to identify potential allergens. Fungal infections and erythrasma typically affect the interdigital spaces whereas allergic contact dermatitis typically does not.

Management

Patients are usually advised to change from non-porous footwear to 100% cotton socks and leather shoes or sandals, although this strategy may not resolve the problem [2,5,12,13]. A variety of topical preparations may help, including urea preparations, Lassar paste, white soft paraffin, tar or tacrolimus ointment, but no single preparation is always effective [3,14–16].

Treatment ladder for juvenile plantar dermatitis

First line
- Change to leather footwear and cotton socks/open sandals

Second line
- Emollients, including urea-containing preparations

Third line
- Lassar paste/tar/tacrolimus ointment (Protopic™)

MISCELLANEOUS SPECIFIED ECZEMATOUS DERMATOSES

Infective dermatitis

Definition and nomenclature

Infective eczema is caused by microorganisms or their products, and that by definition clears when the organisms are eradicated (Figure 39.19). This should be distinguished from infected eczema in which eczema due to some other cause is complicated by secondary bacterial or viral invasion of the skin (Figure 39.20). In practice, however, the two conditions can coexist, and the distinction may be difficult.

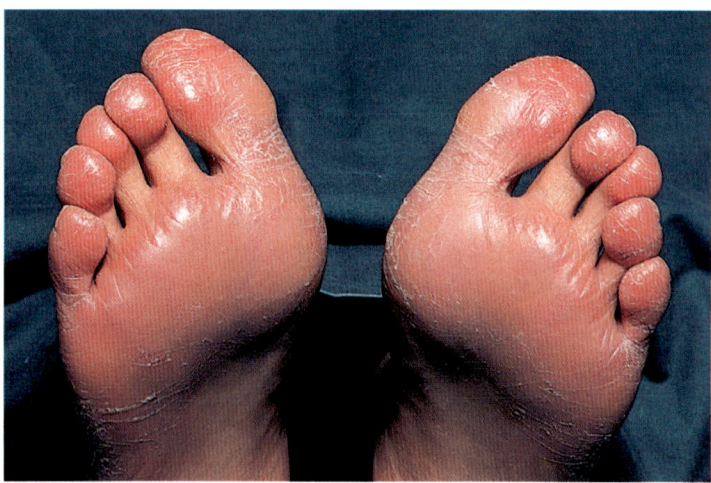

Figure 39.18 Juvenile plantar dermatosis, showing the characteristic glazed appearance of the forefoot skin.

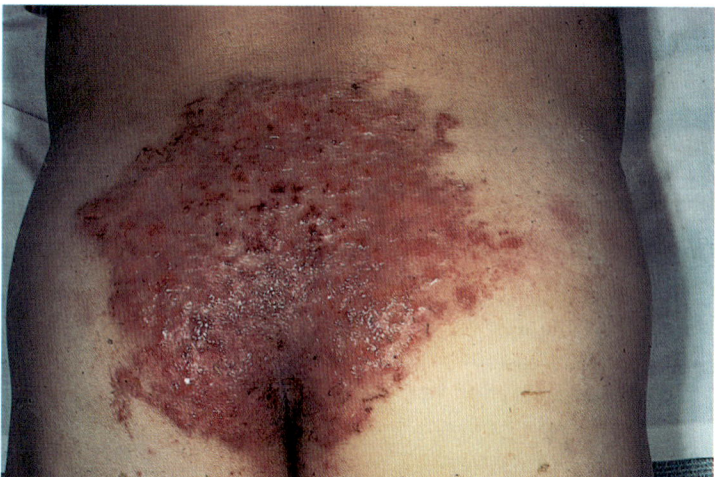

Figure 39.19 Infective eczema in a non-atopic man. Histology of this localised rash showed eczema, and *Staphylococcus aureus* was repeatedly isolated. There was no response to topical corticosteroid therapy but the condition cleared rapidly with oral flucloxacillin.

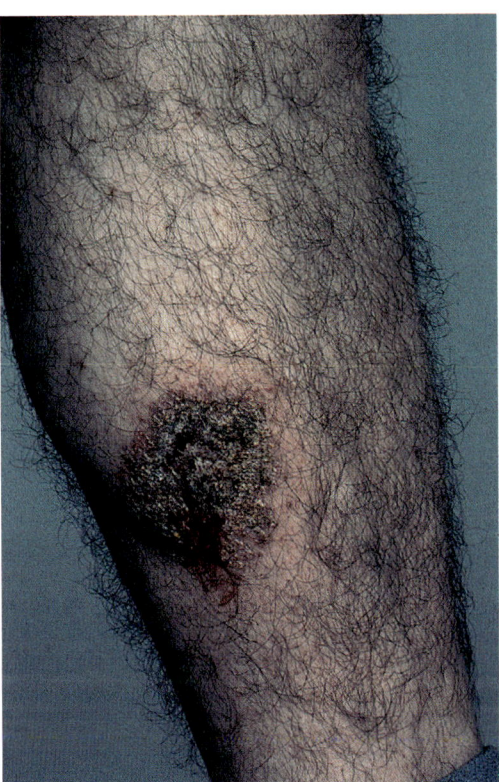

Figure 39.20 Infected dermatitis. This man had a patch of nummular dermatitis that became secondarily infected with *Staphylococcus aureus*.

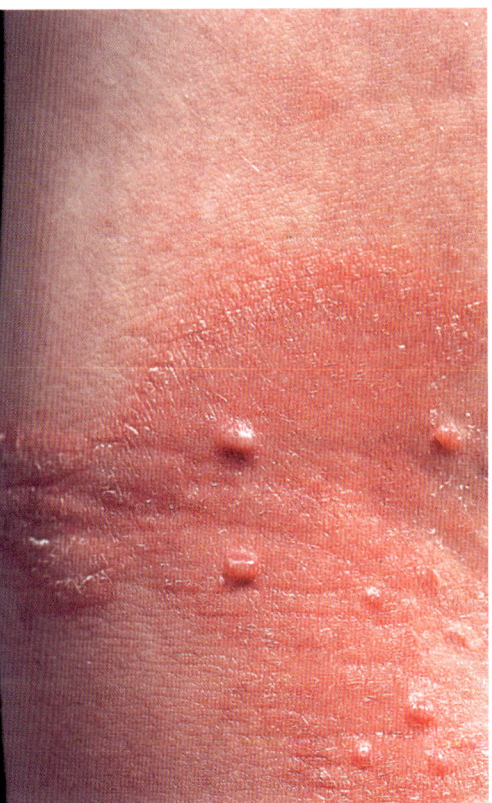

Figure 39.21 An area of eczematisation developing around lesions of molluscum contagiosum. The skin had previously appeared normal, and it returned to normal when the molluscum infection cleared. Courtesy of Dr D. A. Burns, Leicester Royal Infirmary, Leicester, UK.

Synonyms and inclusions
- Microbial eczema

Introduction and general description

Infective dermatitis is a controversial entity and some dermatologists never make the diagnosis. This is because the bacterial flora of an eczematous lesion differs quantitatively from that of normal skin [1] and the demonstration that organisms are present does not establish that they are modifying the lesion. The distinction between colonisation and infection can be very difficult, but the presence of an increased venous C-reactive protein level may offer a useful clue [2]. The skin is a distinct ecosystem with interactions between microbial flora, secretions and keratinocytes [3]. In a way, the stratum corneum could be viewed as the product of a holocrine secretion.

Nevertheless, cases are seen occasionally in which bacterial or viral invasion of the skin seems to occur as the primary event and is followed by secondary eczematisation which can spread for several centimetres beyond the area of obvious infection. The patches of eczema that occasionally develop around lesions of molluscum contagiosum are a good example (Figure 39.21). The pearly papules of molluscum are the initiating event and eczema can develop in the surrounding skin some days later, even when the lesions have not been scratched or traumatised. The eczema generally clears when the molluscum lesions subside. Similarly, eczematous skin is occasionally seen around infected wounds; this clears with antibiotic treatment alone.

Pathophysiology

The mechanism by which microorganisms cause eczema is not understood. Bacterial antigens can promote a cytotoxic reaction in the skin, but this is perhaps more likely to aggravate or perpetuate than initiate the eczematous process [4–7]. Bacterial superantigens such as staphylococcal protein A and enterotoxin B [7] may be profound immune stimulants and may aggravate atopic eczema (Chapter 41). They induce a T-cell response without being presented on the usual major histocompatibility complex (MHC) molecule and recognised by the T-cell receptor (TCR). Instead, they bind to non-active site aspects of both molecules in a non-immune recognition manner [8]. Bacterial antigens may play this role in a variety of syndromes, including nummular dermatitis, and not merely in infective dermatitis. Cultured staphylococci applied topically to human skin can also provoke an eczematous delayed hypersensitivity reaction [9,10].

It is accepted that eczematous reactions can occur as an allergic reaction to a fungal infection elsewhere in the skin (dermatophytide).

Pathology

The histological picture of infective eczema is generally of subacute or chronic eczema in which spongiosis is combined with acanthosis, hyperkeratosis and patchy parakeratosis. The dermis shows inflammatory changes, with polymorphonuclear and lymphocytic infiltration invading the epidermis to a variable extent. In some stages, subcorneal pustulation may be conspicuous.

Clinical features

The distinction between infective and infected eczema can be difficult.

Infected eczema. This shows redness, exudation and crusting. Exudation may be profuse, generating crusting, or slight, with the accumulation of layers of somewhat greasy, moist scale, beneath which the surface is raw and red. The margin is characteristically sharply defined, and the horny layer is often split to form an encircling collaret. There may be small pustules in the advancing edge and in flexures, often a deep and persistent fissure. This may spread to distal sites of existing eczematous skin with possible systemic symptoms.

Infective eczema. This usually presents as an area of advancing redness, sometimes with microvesicles. It is seen predominantly around discharging wounds or ulcers, or moist skin lesions of other types. It is relatively common in patients with venous leg ulcers, but care must be taken to distinguish it from contact dermatitis due to the application of topical medicaments.

Tinea pedis may also become eczematous due to the overgrowth of Gram-negative organisms [11]. Infective dermatitis may also complicate chronic threadworm infestation, pediculosis or scabies. It is not always clear how much of the eczematous change is due to repeated scratching, secondary impetigo or a direct response to the infestation.

Clinical variants

Infective dermatitis of the forefeet is a distinctive pattern of eczema that mainly affects the interdigital spaces on the dorsum of the medial toes. Staphylococci or streptococci can be cultured, and the lesions respond to antiseptic or antibiotic therapy [12]. This condition seems to occur particularly in patients with poor standards of hygiene, and is predisposed by hyperhidrosis and heavy footwear. In children, the condition must be distinguished from juvenile plantar dermatosis.

Management

Factors predisposing to infection should be sought and eliminated when possible. Although topical antibacterial agents are effective in mild forms of infective eczema due to bacteria, systemic antibiotics may be needed. In acute exudative lesions, potassium manganate (VII) ($KMnO_4$) soaks are helpful for the first 2 or 3 days, in combination with a systemic antibiotic.

Treatment ladder for infective dermatitis

First line
- Treat primary cause (e.g. ulcer) or modify footwear if relevant

Second line
- Topical antibiotics (for mild presentations)

Third line
- Systemic antibiotics (also potassium manganate (VII) soaks for forefeet variant)

Pityriasis alba

Definition

This is a pattern of dermatitis in which hypopigmentation is the most conspicuous feature. Redness and scaling usually precede the development of hypopigmentation but these are often relatively mild.

Epidemiology

Incidence and prevalence

The incidence of pityriasis alba has been estimated to be between 1.9% and 5.2% in children [1].

Age

Pityriasis alba occurs predominantly in children between the ages of 3 and 16 years.

Sex

The sexes are equally susceptible.

Ethnicity

Pityriasis alba presents more commonly in those with darker skin type [2].

Associated diseases

It is often a manifestation of atopic eczema, but is not confined to atopic individuals.

Pathophysiology

Sun-exposed sites are at higher risk. Pityriasis alba can be associated with excessive washing, long bathing and exfoliation reducing skin defensive mechanisms.

The histological changes are unimpressive – acanthosis and mild spongiosis, with moderate hyperkeratosis and patchy parakeratosis. There may be follicular plugging, spongiosis and sebaceous gland atrophy [3–6]. On electron microscopy there are reduced numbers of active melanocytes and a decrease in the number and size of melanosomes in affected skin [5]. Although pigment is reduced, melanocyte numbers are not and may even be increased relative to healthy skin [7].

Clinical features [4,7–9]

The individual lesion is a rounded, oval or irregular hypopigmented patch that is usually poorly demarcated. Lesions are often slightly red with a raised edge and have fine scaling. Initially, the redness may be conspicuous and there may even be minimal serous crusting. Later, the redness subsides completely and, at the stage at which the lesions are commonly seen by a physician, they show only persistent fine scaling and hypopigmentation. It is this that usually induces the patient to seek advice. The hypopigmentation is most conspicuous in pigmented skin, and in lighter skins may become more evident after sun tanning (Figure 39.22).

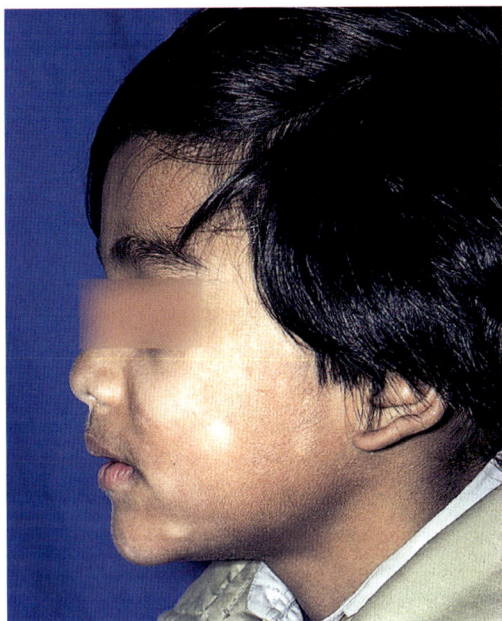

Figure 39.22 In pityriasis alba the failure of the affected patches to tan may first bring them to the patient's notice. Courtesy of Dr A. Marsden, St George's Hospital, London, UK.

In classic pityriasis alba there are usually several patches ranging from 0.5 to 2 cm in diameter, but they may be larger, especially on the trunk. In children the lesions are often confined to the face but can affect the neck, shoulders, trunk and limbs. A pigmenting pityriasis alba is found in the Middle East and darker skin types in South Africa. These lesions are blue from deep melanin with a halo of depigmentation and can coexist with classic pityriasis alba [1]. Extensive pityriasis alba affects teenagers and young adults, more often females. Lesions of extensive pityriasis alba are typically larger than other variants at 2 cm and are not limited to the face.

Differential diagnosis

The age incidence, fine scaling and distribution of the lesions usually suggest the diagnosis. Conspicuous hypopigmentation may lead to a misdiagnosis of vitiligo. Naevus depigmentosus most commonly presents at birth or before 3 years of age and most often causes single, well-marginated lesions on the trunk [10]. Naevus anaemicus is also detected most commonly at birth. However, this condition may be difficult to distinguish from pityriasis alba when it occurs on the face and in cases of later onset. Nummular dermatitis in an atopic child is intensely pruritic, and the lesions are larger and more oedematous. In older children and adults, early trunk lesions may be mistaken for psoriasis, but the distribution and the relatively mild scaling should exclude this diagnosis. Mycosis fungoides, although relatively rare, may present with lesions clinically resembling pityriasis alba [11]. This condition may also be difficult to distinguish histologically and so follow-up and repeated biopsies are sometimes required.

Disease course and prognosis

The course is extremely variable. Most cases persist for some months, and some may still show hypopigmentation for a year or more after all scaling subsides. Recurrent crops of new lesions may develop at intervals. The average duration of the common facial form in childhood is a year or more.

Management

Response to treatment is often disappointing, mainly because the pigmentation takes a long time to recover. However, complete repigmentation is the normal outcome. The scaling may be reduced by a bland emollient cream. Reduction in excessive skin care and washing may remove precipitating factors. Mild topical corticosteroids are helpful if inflammation persists. Topical tacrolimus and pimecrolimus are effective in facial atopic eczema and seem likely to prove helpful, if required, in pityriasis alba [12]. Sunblock will help reduce the contrast with surrounding skin.

Treatment ladder for pityriasis alba

First line
- Emollient
- Sun protection
- Reduction of excessive skin care

Second line
- Mild topical corticosteroids

Third line
- Topical tacrolimus or pimecrolimus

Chronic superficial scaly dermatitis

This is a chronic condition with round or oval, red, slightly scaly patches on the limbs and trunk, histologically showing mild eczematous changes with little or no dermal infiltrate (Figure 39.23). It is characterised as small plaque parapsoriasis (EA95 in *ICD-11*) and is covered extensively in Chapter 134.

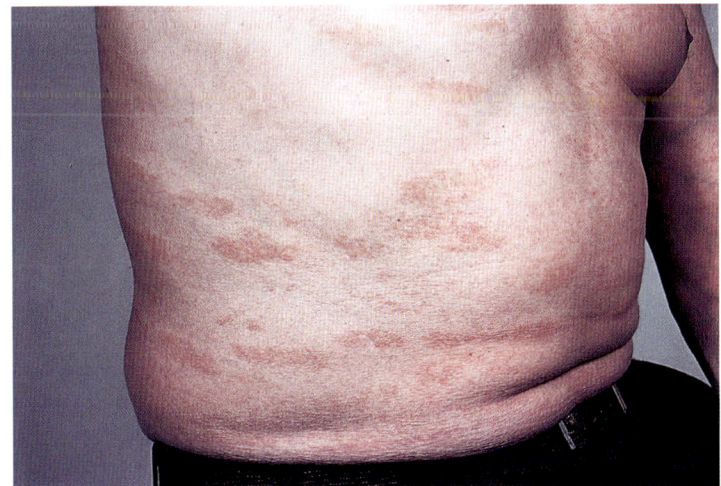

Figure 39.23 Chronic superficial scaly dermatitis.

PART 4: INFLAMMATORY DERMATOSES

PART 4: INFLAMMATORY DERMATOSES

Dermatophytide

This is a reaction, at a remote site, to a dermatophyte infection [1–3], covered extensively in Chapter 32.

Halo dermatitis

Definition and nomenclature

Halo dermatitis is the occurrence of an eczematous ring surrounding a melanocytic naevus.

> **Synonyms and inclusions**
> • Meyerson naevus
> • Meyerson phenomenon

Introduction and general description

Meyerson [1] described two patients with multiple, pruritic, papulosquamous lesions surrounding melanocytic naevi (Figure 39.24). More than 20 similar cases have since been described [2–4], mainly in young adults. Histology shows a benign naevus surrounded by a dermal lymphocytic and eosinophilic infiltrate, with overlying acanthosis, spongiosis and parakeratosis. One case developed during treatment with interferon α-2b in a patient with dysplastic naevus syndrome and Behçet disease [5]. The condition usually resolves spontaneously within a few months, without involution of the naevus. It differs from Sutton halo depigmentation, although the two conditions have been reported to coexist in the same patient and in one case progression to Sutton naevus occurred [6]. Similar changes are not infrequently seen around seborrhoeic keratoses [7] and other elevated skin lesions [8] and are termed the Meyerson phenomenon.

Murray Williams warts

Multiple seborrhoeic keratoses occurring in areas of resolved eczema have only occasionally been reported since the phenomenon was described by Williams in 1956 [1,2]. Multiple seborrhoeic keratoses arise in the few months following resolution of the eczema and tend to gradually resolve by 5–6 months. It has been reported following allergic contact dermatitis [3].

OTHER RELATED DERMATOSES

Lichen simplex and lichenification

Definition and nomenclature

Lichen simplex is an eczematous dermatosis characterised by a small number of heavily thickened (lichenified) plaques or, very often, a single lesion. Lichen simplex chronicus of genital regions is covered in more detail in Chapters 110 and 111.

> **Synonyms and inclusions**
> • Circumscribed neurodermatitis

Introduction and general description

Lichenification is a change in appearance and texture of the skin associated particularly with pruritic dermatoses. Mild or early lichenification presents as a rather subtle coarsening of the skin surface markings on a background of dry and usually red skin. As the condition progresses, the skin becomes markedly thickened and hyperkeratotic (Figure 39.25). Lichenification may occur spontaneously, when it is known as lichen simplex, or may occur as a secondary consequence of eczema and other inflammatory dermatoses.

Epidemiology
Age
The peak incidence is between 30 and 50 years of age, but it is seen at any age from adolescence onwards. Secondary lichenification of atopic eczema can occur in any age group and broadly mirrors the prevalence of atopic eczema in the particular age group.

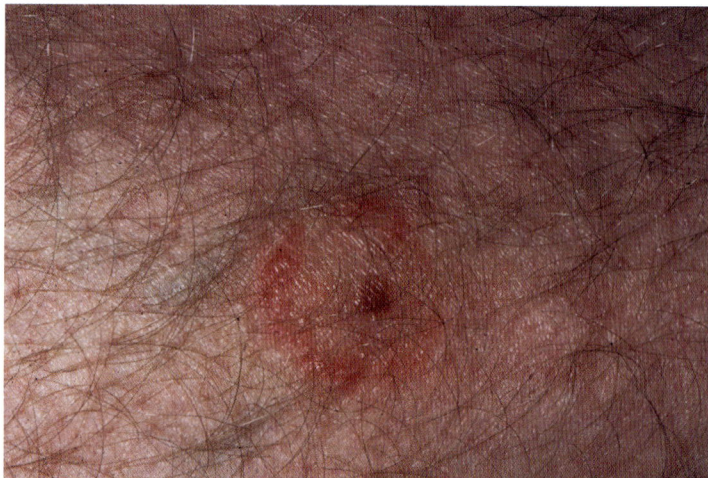

Figure 39.24 Halo dermatitis showing eczema around a mole.

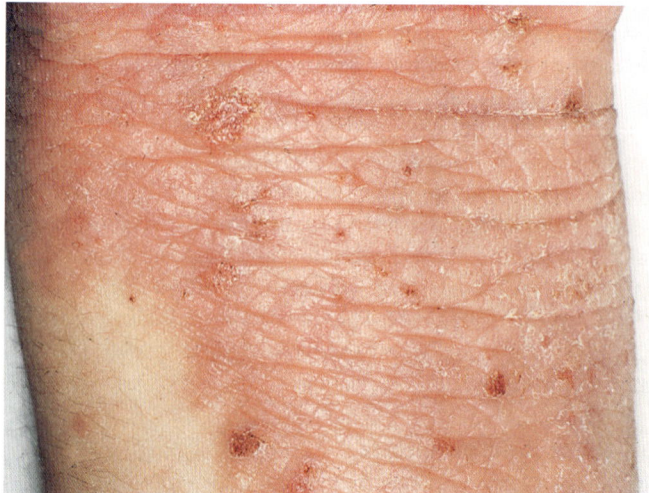

Figure 39.25 Lichenification of the arm in a patient with atopic eczema.

Sex
Women are affected by lichen simplex more often than men.

Ethnicity
There is no conclusive evidence of a link with particular ethnicities.

Associated diseases
A dermatomal pattern of lichen simplex chronicus has been described as the initial presentation of an intramedullary neoplasm with syringomyelia [1].

Pathophysiology
Predisposing factors
Patients with lichen simplex are more readily conditioned to scratch following an itch stimulus than are control subjects [2]. Lichenification frequently occurs as a manifestation of atopic eczema [3] but is not universally present and lichen simplex occurs in many individuals who show no stigmata of atopy. In the predisposed subject, emotional tensions play an important role in favouring the development of lichen simplex and ensuring its perpetuation [4].

Pathology [5,6]
The histological changes of lichen simplex vary with site and duration. Acanthosis and variable degrees of hyperkeratosis are usually observed. The rete ridges are lengthened. Spongiosis is sometimes present, and small areas of parakeratosis are occasionally seen. There is hyperplasia of all components of the epidermis [7]. The labelling index has been shown autoradiographically to be over 25%, but the transit time is longer than in psoriasis [8].

The dermis contains a chronic inflammatory infiltrate, and in very chronic lesions there may be some fibrosis. Silver impregnation techniques show proliferation of the Schwann cells, which may make up an appreciable proportion of the cellular infiltrate.

In very chronic lesions, especially in giant lichenification, the acanthosis and hyperkeratosis are gross, and the rete ridges are irregularly but strikingly elongated and widened.

Genetics
There are no specific genetic links reported for lichen simplex.

Environmental factors
Lichenification can arise as a result of allergic contact dermatitis. Lichen simplex has been linked in a case series to allergic contact dermatitis to hair dye [9].

Clinical features
History
In all forms of lichenification, pruritus is a prominent symptom, and is often out of proportion to the extent of the objective changes. It may develop in paroxysms of great intensity. Scratching tends to give initial satisfaction, but is then continued until the skin is sore. There then follows a refractory period before another intense bout of pruritus; however, habit can perpetuate excoriation [10].

Presentation
In lichen simplex, single and multiple sites are involved with about equal frequency. Almost any area may be affected, but the

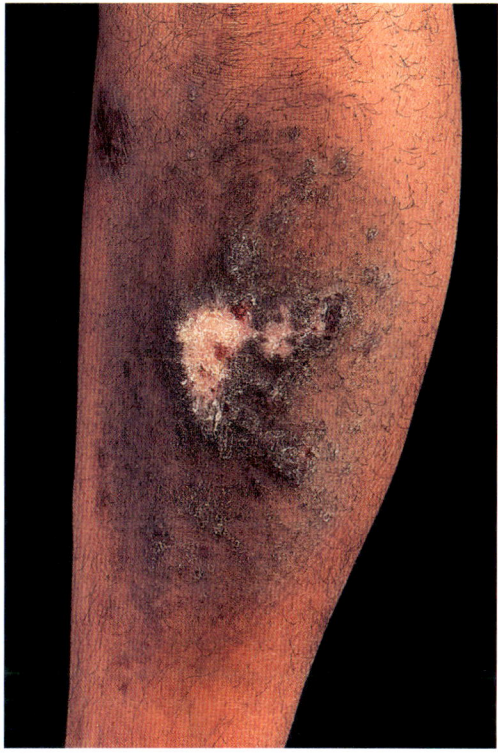
(a)

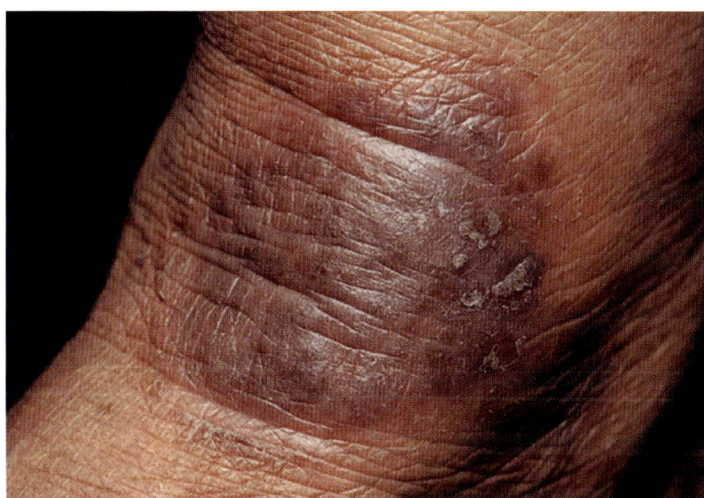
(b)

Figure 39.26 Lichen simplex. (a) On the lower leg. (b) On the ankles. (a) Courtesy of Dr D. A. Burns, Leicester Royal Infirmary, Leicester, UK.

commonest sites are those that are conveniently reached. The usual sites are the nape of the neck, lower legs (Figure 39.26a) and ankles (Figure 39.26b), sides of the neck, scalp, upper thighs, vulva, pubis or scrotum and extensor forearms. In lichenified eczema and secondary lichenification, the sites are those affected by the primary dermatosis, for example limb flexural sites in atopic eczema.

During the early stages of lichen simplex, the skin is red and slightly oedematous, and normal skin markings are exaggerated. The redness and oedema subside and the central area becomes scaly and thickened and sometimes pigmented. Surrounding this central plaque is a zone of lichenoid papules and beyond this an

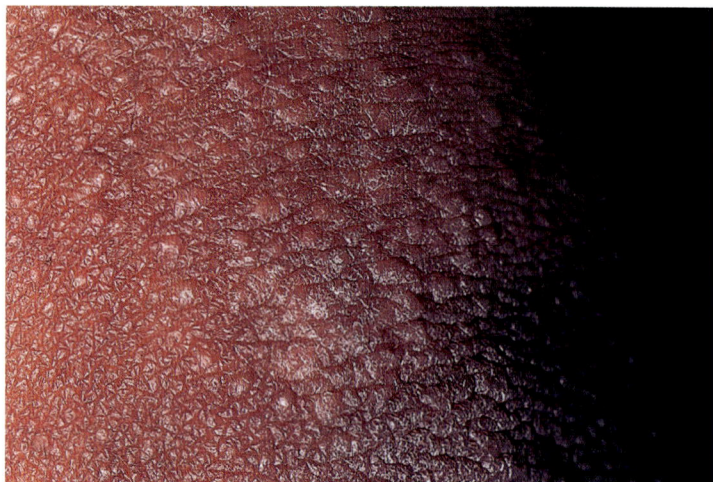

Figure 39.27 Follicular papules of lichenification adjacent to the elbow.

indefinite zone of slight thickening and pigmentation merging with normal skin. These features may be greatly modified by the site and duration of the lesion. In mild cases, follicular eczematous papules may be seen, particularly on the forearms and elbow regions of children (Figure 39.27).

Clinical variants
Lichen simplex of the nape of the neck (lichen nuchae) is usually confined to women. The plaque may be limited to a small area around the midline of the nape or may extend some distance into the scalp and over the neck. Scaling is often profuse and psoriasiform, and episodes of secondary infection are frequent. The fold behind the ear may also be involved. Scaling, crusting and fissuring are more evident than the usual changes of lichenification. Other regions of the scalp are less often affected. The presenting manifestation is an area of scaling, with twisted, broken hairs. The epidermal thickening may be great enough to form a nodule.

If lichenification occurs at sites where the subcutaneous tissues are lax and excoriation continues for many years, solid tumour-like plaques may be formed, with a warty, cribriform surface. This variant is known as giant lichenification of Pautrier [11] and occurs mainly in the genito-crural region.

The descriptive term pebbly lichenification has been applied to a distinctive clinical variant, consisting of discrete, smooth nodules, seen occasionally in atopic and seborrhoeic subjects, and in photo-dermatitis. Clinically it may simulate lichen planus.

Differential diagnosis
The morphological diagnosis of lichenification is usually characteristic. However, lichen planus, lichen amyloidosis and psoriasis are differential diagnoses that may be elicited by checking other anatomical sites. Sometimes, however, no conclusive diagnosis is possible on either clinical or histological grounds. A patient with psoriasis may develop lichen simplex that combines the histological features of both conditions.

Once the diagnosis of lichenification has been established its causation must be carefully investigated. Secondary lichenification complicates persistent skin lesions of many types. It occurs on the lower leg in the presence of venous insufficiency, in atopic eczema, in asteatotic eczema, in low-grade chronic contact dermatitis and in some chronic infections with *Trichophyton rubrum*. Symmetrical lesions may suggest secondary lichenification from a contact dermatitis.

Complications and co-morbidities
An association has been reported between lichen simplex and depression and dissociative experiences [12].

Disease course and prognosis
Lichen simplex tends to follow a chronic course unless the itch–scratch cycle can be broken.

Investigations
Skin scrapings for mycological investigation may be indicated. Suspicion of allergic contact dermatitis should be investigated by patch testing.

Management
A careful psychological history should be taken to elucidate any underlying problems. The nature of lichen simplex and the need to break the scratching habit should be explained. Sedative antihistamines may be helpful and antibiotics may be necessary if secondary infection is present.

Neurological itch stimulus and inflammation may both need to be addressed [13]. A potent or very potent topical corticosteroid can be very helpful in some cases but seems to have no effect in others.

On an arm or leg it is useful to apply an occlusive zinc paste bandage, if tolerated, which prevents scratching and improves skin hydration. Self-adhesive, steroid-impregnated tape (e.g. fludroxycortide tape) can often be effective for localised lesions. Alternatively, a potent steroid ointment under polythene occlusion, for short periods, may also be considered. Modest improvement has also been shown with 5% doxepin cream [14].

For solitary, circumscribed, chronic lesions, dermal infiltration with triamcinolone (10 mg/mL) can be effective. Improvement has been reported with cislosporin and methotrexate [15].

Response has also been reported to capsaicin cream [16]. Gabapentin, pregabalin and opioid receptor antagonists have been used in nodular prurigo and may have a role in lichen simplex. More recently, the biologics nemolizumab and dupilumab have also been used in nodular prurigo as well as opioid receptor modulators such as naloxone and naltrexone [17].

Treatment ladder

First line
- Patient education

Second line
- Topical corticosteroids, including impregnated adhesive tape

Third line
- Zinc paste bandages for limbs or intralesional triamcinolone for solitary lesions

Resources

Patient resources

DermNet NZ, lichen simplex: https://dermnetnz.org/topics/lichen-simplex/ (last accessed September 2023).

Erythroderma

Definition and nomenclature

Erythroderma is the term applied to any inflammatory skin disease that affects more than 90% of the body surface.

Synonyms and inclusions

- Exfoliative dermatitis (although the degree of exfoliation is sometimes quite mild)

Introduction and general description

Erythroderma is included in this chapter because eczema is one of the commonest underlying causes. Erythroderma may be the initial presentation of eczema in an individual or, more commonly, arises in the context of longstanding eczema.

Epidemiology

Incidence and prevalence

The most recent study estimated the European annual incidence at 1 to 2 per 100 000 population [1]. An Indian study found incidence to be 20 per 19 000 person-years, while in Tunisia the rate was 30–44 per 100 000 [2].

Age and sex

It is more common in middle age between 41 and 61 years with a male to female ratio of 2–4 : 1 [3].

Ethnicity

There have been no specific ethnic variations reported.

Associated diseases

This will vary depending on the underlying cause of the erythroderma.

Pathophysiology

Predisposing factors [4–8]

The main causes of erythroderma in adults are listed in Table 39.3 and are discussed here. The figures vary somewhat with the age of the population, and are based on several published studies. In younger people, for example military personnel, there will be a larger proportion due to drug allergies [8]. Drugs commonly causing erythroderma are listed in Chapter 118. In some communities, the incidence of erythroderma may be higher because of self-medication and use of herbal remedies such as St John's wort [9]. The causes of erythroderma in the newborn are considered in Chapter 114.

Other rare causes of erythroderma include sarcoidosis [10], Hailey–Hailey disease [11], pemphigoid [12], toxic shock syndrome

Table 39.3 Causes of erythroderma and relative prevalence in adults [3–7,54]. These data are an approximation of different studies worldwide.

Condition causing erythroderma	Relative prevalence (%)
Eczema of various subtypes	20.0
Psoriasis	27.0
Lymphoma and leukaemias	11.0
Drugs (including phenylbutazone, phenytoin, carbamazepine, gold salts, lithium, cimetidine)	12.0
Unknown	14.0
Hereditary disorders (ichthyosiform erythroderma, pityriasis rubra pilaris)	2.0
Pemphigus foliaceus	3.0
Other skin diseases (lichen planus, dermatophytosis, crusted scabies, dermatomyositis)	11.0

[13], lupus erythematosus [14], angioimmunoblastic lymphadenopathy [15] and dermatomyositis [16]. Graft-versus-host disease may progress to erythroderma in some cases. A related disorder was reported in Japan, where cases of fatal erythroderma occurred following major surgery. It was suggested that these cases were examples of post-transfusion graft-versus-host disease [17].

Erythroderma has occasionally been reported with seroconversion following human immunodeficiency virus (HIV) infection [18]. In established acquired immune deficiency syndrome (AIDS), erythroderma may arise from a variety of causes including seborrhoeic dermatitis, lymphoma or an unknown cause [19]. However, it should be noted that CD4+ T lymphocytopenia has been associated with erythroderma in the absence of HIV infection [20].

Pathology

Histopathology can help identify the cause of erythroderma in up to 50% of cases, particularly if multiple skin biopsies are examined [21]. The histological appearances vary depending upon the severity and duration of the inflammatory process. In the acute stage, spongiosis and parakeratosis are prominent, and a non-specific inflammatory infiltrate permeates a grossly oedematous dermis to a variable depth. In the chronic stage, acanthosis and elongation of the rete ridges become more prominent.

In erythroderma due to lymphoma the infiltrate may become increasingly pleomorphic and eventually acquire specific diagnostic features such as a band-like lymphoid infiltrate at the dermal–epidermal junction, with atypical cerebriform mononuclear cells and Pautrier microabscesses [22]. In other cases, however, it remains non-specific throughout its course, and the distinction can be difficult. Patients with Sézary syndrome often show some features of chronic dermatitis, and benign erythroderma may occasionally show some features suggestive of lymphoma. Immunophenotyping of the lymphoid infiltrate may not solve the problem as it generally shows features of mature T cells in both benign and malignant erythroderma [23].

In psoriasis, papillomatosis and clubbing of the papillary zones may be seen, and in pemphigus foliaceus, superficial acantholysis will be present. In ichthyosiform erythroderma and pityriasis rubra pilaris, repeated biopsies from carefully selected sites may reveal their characteristic features.

The causes of congenital erythroderma depend on the nature of the disorders of the stratum corneum such as dysregulated lipid metabolism and transport as well as keratin structure. Acquired erythroderma, despite its many different causes, tends to have certain common elements such as raised serum IgE and a predominance of ILC2 cytokines like IL-4 and IL-13. This favours a Th2 cell type. There is also increased expression of adhesion molecules like VCAM-1, ICAM-1, E-selectin and P-selectin on the endothelial cells near erythrodermic skin, facilitating the extravasation of inflammatory cells to the tissues [1].

Genetics
This will depend on the underlying condition.

Clinical features
History and presentation
Acquired erythroderma developing in primary eczema or associated with a lymphoma is often of sudden onset. Patchy red skin, which rapidly generalises, may be accompanied by fever, shivering and malaise. Hypothermia may develop.

The redness extends rapidly, and may be universal in 12–48 h. Scaling appears after 2–6 days, often first in the flexures, but it varies greatly in degree and character from case to case. The scales may be large or fine and bran-like. At this stage the skin is bright red, hot and dry and palpably thickened. The intensity of the redness may fluctuate over periods of a few days or even a few hours. Irritation is sometimes severe, but a sensation of tightness is more characteristic. Many patients complain of feeling cold, especially when the redness is increasing. The redness can be less visible in darker pigmented skin; however this can contrast more greatly the dry and flaky skin giving an appearance of being covered in ash.

When the erythroderma has been present for some weeks, the scalp and body hair may be shed and the nails become ridged and thickened and they may also be shed. The periorbital skin is inflamed and oedematous, resulting in ectropion, with consequent epiphora. In very chronic cases there may be pigmentary disturbances, especially in darker skin, where patchy or widespread loss of pigment is often seen.

The degree of enlargement of the lymph nodes in the absence of an underlying malignant lymphoma is variable. They are usually slightly or moderately enlarged and of rubbery consistency, but in some cases the enlargement may be gross. It is important that this dermatopathic lymphadenopathy is not mistaken for lymphoma. In difficult cases, lymph node biopsy may be advisable, but the pathologist must be told that the patient is erythrodermic for a reliable histological interpretation to be made.

The general picture is modified according to the nature of any underlying disease and the patient's age and general physical condition.

Clinical variants
Clinical variants are considered in terms of the underlying cause of the erythroderma. Papuloerythroderma of Ofuji is also discussed as a distinct clinical variant.

Eczematous dermatoses. Generalisation of an eczema occurs most frequently in the sixth and seventh decades when venous eczema is

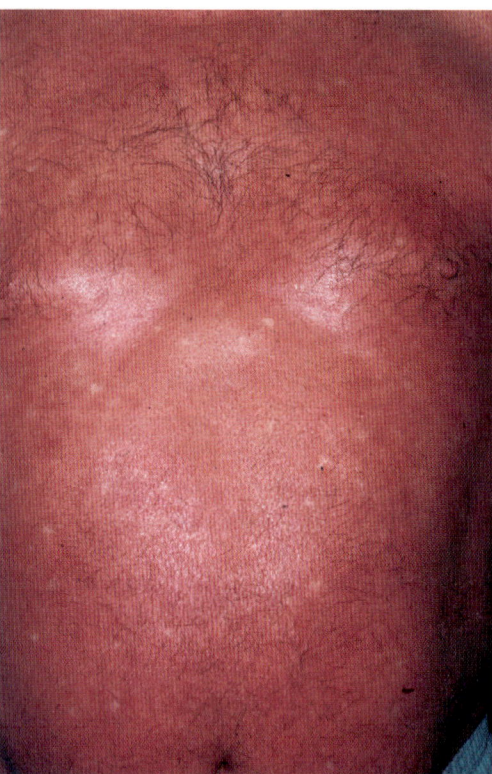

Figure 39.28 Erythrodermic psoriasis.

a common precedent. However, atopic erythroderma may occur at any age, although it is uncommon in neonates [55]. Exacerbation of existing lesions usually precedes the generalisation, which follows the usual pattern. Pruritus is often intense.

Psoriasis. In erythrodermic psoriasis (Figure 39.28) the clinical picture may be highly desquamative, but when the erythroderma is fully developed the specific features of psoriasis are often lost. In some cases, crops of sterile miliary pustules may develop at intervals, and transition to generalised pustular psoriasis may occur, especially in cases treated with potent topical corticosteroids or systemic steroids that are abruptly stopped [24]. Emotional stress, intercurrent illness and phototherapy overdosage may also precipitate erythroderma.

Lymphoma, leukaemia and other malignancy. Cutaneous T-cell lymphoma is the commonest malignancy to cause erythroderma (Figure 39.29), followed by Hodgkin disease. Non-Hodgkin lymphoma, leukaemias and myelodysplasia have also been reported as causes. Association with other internal malignancies has been observed less often [7].

Pruritus is often very severe. The erythroderma is universal, and infiltration of the skin may be so severe that the patient's facial features are deformed. Rubbing and scratching may produce secondary lichenification. Enlargement of lymph nodes may be considerable, even if histologically they are not infiltrated by lymphoma.

A biopsy of involved skin may show only non-specific features initially, and may need to be repeated several times before infiltration with atypical lymphocytes becomes evident. A skin biopsy

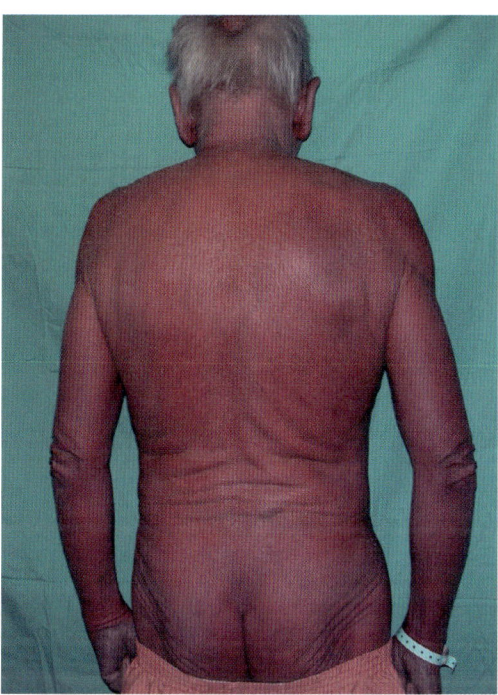

Figure 39.29 Erythroderma in Sézary syndrome. Courtesy of Dr B. Dharma, University Hospitals Coventry and Warwickshire, UK.

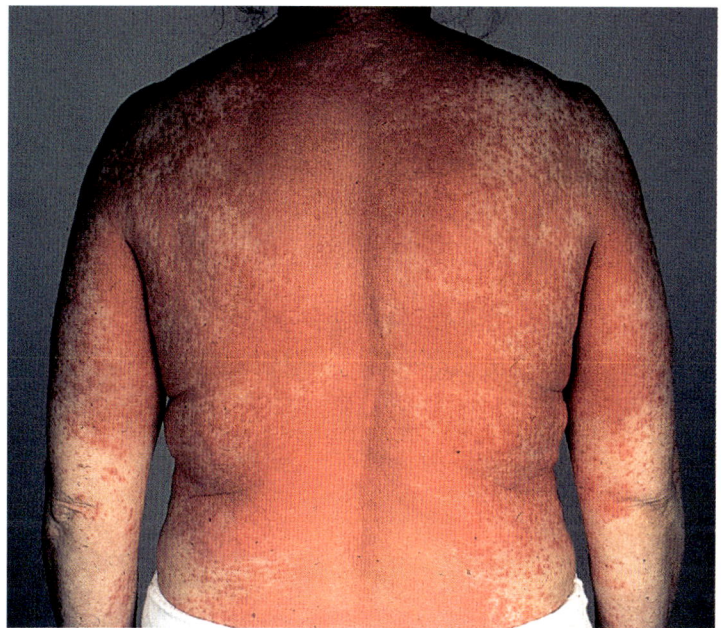

Figure 39.30 Widespread drug rash. This will progress rapidly to erythroderma if the drug is continued.

for analysis of T-cell receptor gene rearrangement, to determine whether clonality is present in the infiltrate, may be helpful [25,26]. Lymph node biopsy may be diagnostic of lymphoma but often shows only the features of dermatopathic lymphadenopathy. There may be hepatosplenomegaly. A differential white blood cell count should be performed and the blood examined for abnormal cells. Eosinophilia may suggest Hodgkin disease. Atypical lymphocytes with cerebriform nuclei (Sézary cells) are often observed in erythroderma regardless of cause. When they constitute more than 20% of the circulating peripheral blood mononuclear cells they become diagnostic of the leukaemic variant of cutaneous T-cell lymphoma known as Sézary syndrome. Large Sézary cells (15–20 μm in diameter) are diagnostic even in small numbers [27]. The demonstration of a clonal T-cell population in the peripheral blood by analysis of T-cell receptor genes, using polymerase chain reaction, appears to offer high diagnostic specificity for Sézary syndrome. The sensitivity also appears high, but on occasion the test may need to be repeated if initial results are negative and this diagnosis is still suspected [27].

Drugs. Among the more commonly implicated drugs are phenylbutazone, phenytoin, carbamazepine, cimetidine, gold salts and lithium [28]. The eruption may start as a generalised eczema, or scarlatiniform or morbilliform redness, often accompanied by some irritation, which increases steadily in severity. Skin redness may first appear in the flexures or over the whole skin (Figure 39.30). This group has the best prognosis of all the causes of erythroderma [4,29], often resolving in 2–6 weeks [30]. However, it is important to remember that the cutaneous manifestations of drug hypersensitivity may be accompanied by the involvement of other organs, for example haematological abnormalities, hepatitis, nephritis or pneumonitis. An example is the DRESS syndrome (drug reaction with eosinophilia and systemic symptoms; Chapter 118) which is a type IVb hypersensitivity reaction [31].

Erythroderma of unknown origin. This is rarely below 10% of cases despite thorough investigation [1,5,6,30]. The cutaneous changes may precede any other evidence of a lymphoma by many months or years. If these cases are excluded, the remaining patients with chronic erythrodermas of unknown origin consist mainly of elderly men, in whom the condition runs a very long course with partial and temporary remissions, sometimes also known as the 'red man syndrome'. It is characterised by marked palmoplantar keratoderma, dermatopathic lymphadenopathy and a raised serum IgE [32,33]. This condition is not established erythrodermic cutaneous T-cell lymphoma, which is occasionally referred to as 'l'homme rouge'.

The three commonest causes of idiopathic protracted erythroderma are probably atopic eczema of the elderly, intake of drugs overlooked by the patient and pre-lymphomatous eruptions [5].

Ichthyosiform erythroderma. This congenital erythroderma is usually present from birth or early infancy. Non-bullous ichthyosiform erythroderma is an autosomal recessive condition with multiple gene defects. Children are born with a thick collodion membrane in 90% of cases which sheds over the proceeding weeks [34]. The erythroderma then presents. They may have eclabium and ectropion; it is important to check the external auditory canal for obstruction with skin debris [35].

Pityriasis rubra pilaris. The erythrodermic forms may begin in childhood or adult life. The presence of follicular, horny plugs on the knees and elbows, and on the backs of the fingers and toes, is distinctive. In many cases, scattered islands of normal skin persist in the erythrodermic regions, and horny plugs may be evident around their margins. These normal pale 'islands' of sparing are highly suggestive of the diagnosis; the skin on the palms and soles often has an orange discoloration. See Chapter 36.

Pemphigus foliaceus. Moist, crusted lesions on the face and upper trunk often precede the development of the erythroderma. Scaling is conspicuous, moist and adherent. Crops of thin-walled bullae may erupt, especially on the limbs. Taking a biopsy for immunofluorescence will be difficult as perilesional skin needs to be taken. See Chapter 50.

Lichen planus. Erythrodermic lichen planus is very rare but lichenoid reactions to gold, quinine and other drugs have resulted in erythroderma. As the initial redness and oedema subside, individual violaceous papules may be revealed. The buccal mucous membrane may show typical lacy, bluish white streaks. It is very rare but possible to present in children [36]. See Chapter 37.

Dermatophytosis. Generalised erythroderma has very rarely resulted from chronic infection with organisms such as *Trichophyton violaceum*.

Norwegian scabies. The heavily crusted hands and feet, with thickened nails, characteristic of Norwegian scabies may occasionally be accompanied by generalised redness and scaling. The condition is often mistaken for erythrodermic psoriasis. The occurrence of scabies in others in the same environment, or in the medical or nursing staff caring for the patient, may reveal the diagnosis.

Papuloerythroderma of Ofuji [37–41]. This differs from ordinary erythroderma in that papulation is prominent, it tends to spare the face and flexures, and is often intensely pruritic. It is not yet clear whether this represents a distinct disease or a reaction pattern. Although most cases are idiopathic, several have been reported in association with other diseases including atopy, malignancies, infections and drugs [42]. It is more common in later life, with ages at diagnosis ranging from 57 to 100 years. Many cases occur in the eighth or ninth decades. Males are predominantly affected, with the male to female ratio estimated at 4.7 : 1 [38].

Histological features are usually non-specific. In the epidermis there are generally mild degrees of acanthosis, spongiosis, hyperkeratosis and focal parakeratosis with marked lymphohistiocytic infiltration of the dermis, predominantly perivascular in distribution, and eosinophils are often conspicuous. A mild degree of epidermotropism has been observed and, rarely, plasma cells and multinucleate giant cells may be present. Immunofluorescence is negative.

The erythroderma typically begins with an eruption of brownish red, flat-topped papules that become confluent (Figure 39.31a). The limbs and trunk are affected and the face and flexures tend to be spared. A characteristic and distinctive pattern of sparing of the abdominal flexures has been termed the 'deck-chair sign' [39], indicating a similarity to the distribution of sunburn in one who has been sitting out in a deckchair for too long (Figure 39.31b). The lesions sometimes develop along scratch marks. Pruritus is a consistent feature and ranges from moderate to very severe. Additional features often observed include hyperkeratosis and fissuring of the palms and soles, and benign lymphadenopathy. There is usually

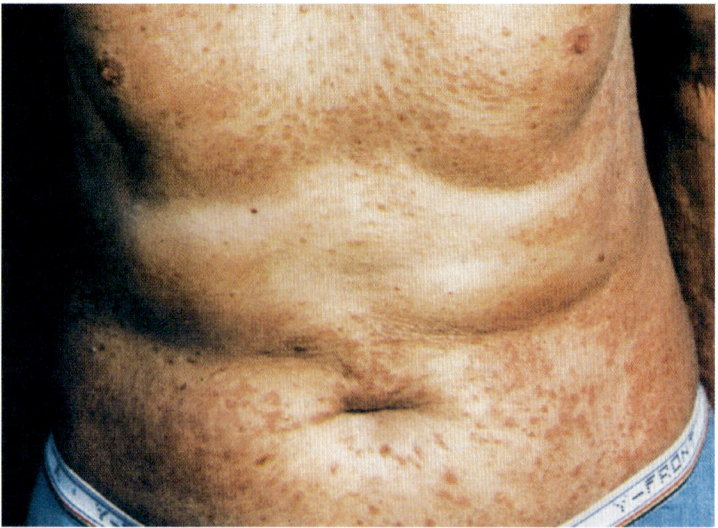

(a)

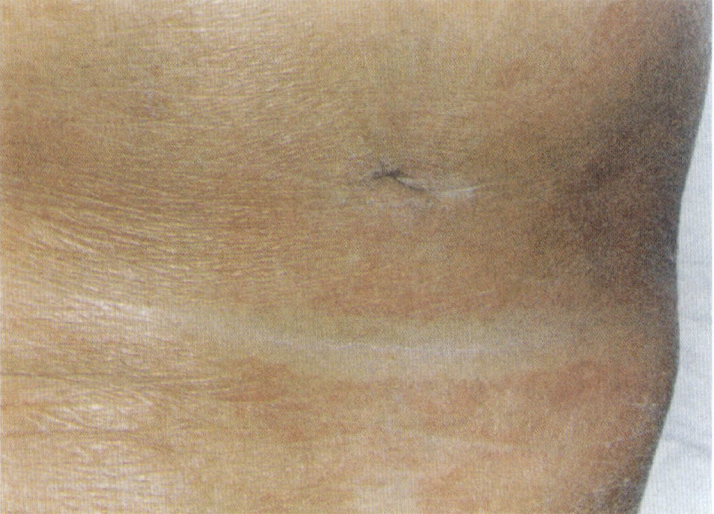

(b)

Figure 39.31 Papuloerythroderma of Ofuji. (a) The papules. (b) The 'deck-chair sign' (sparing of the body folds). Courtesy of Dr M. J. Tidman, Edinburgh Royal Infirmary, Edinburgh, UK.

circulating eosinophilia and a raised IgE, as well as a mild degree of absolute or relative lymphocytopenia. In terms of prognosis, papuloerythroderma typically persists for many years, although some cases have remitted.

Reports of papuloerythroderma occurring in association with malignancies, which have included T-cell [40,41] and B-cell [41] lymphomas and gastric [41], lung [41], colon [43], prostate [38] and hepatocellular [44] carcinomas, would suggest that this eruption may sometimes occur as a paraneoplastic phenomenon. There are also several reports that papuloerythroderma may progress into mycosis fungoides [38,45,46], in one case 11 years after the onset of symptoms [47]. In some cases, papuloerythroderma therefore seems to be a presentation of cutaneous T-cell lymphoma. One case developed into psoriasis [38]. Papuloerythroderma has also been reported in association with HIV infection [48,49] and, in one case, biliary sepsis [50].

In terms of management, emollients, topical corticosteroids and antihistamines have produced a response, although slow, in some cases. The condition can respond well to oral prednisolone, although high doses are sometimes required. PUVA, including bath PUVA, has proved effective in several reports. Azathioprine [51], ciclosporin [52] and etretinate [53] may be effective. Retinoids or phototherapy may be preferable to immunosuppressants because of the possible progression to cutaneous T-cell lymphoma and association with malignancy. However, papuloerythroderma is sometimes very refractory to treatment. In paraneoplastic cases, treatment of the malignancy can resolve the eruption [42].

Allergic contact dermatitis [3,54]. Widespread exposure to contact allergens presenting as erythroderma is not common and can be the result of a systemic contact dermatitis.

Differential diagnosis
See Table 39.3 for possible underlying causes.

Classification of severity
By definition, erythroderma involves more than 90% of the body surface. No subclassifications are used.

Complications and co-morbidities
The main complications of erythroderma are haemodynamic and metabolic disturbances. Blood flow through the skin is markedly increased and this can result in high-output cardiac failure, especially in elderly patients [55,56]. The increased skin perfusion may lead to hypothermia [57]. Fluid loss by transpiration is much increased and is roughly proportional to the basal metabolic rate. Hypoalbuminaemia is in part due to increased protein loss from exfoliated scale, which may reach 9 g/m^2 of body surface or more each day [58]. This in turn results in peripheral oedema. Immune responses may become altered, reflected by an increase in γ-globulins or CD4+ T lymphocytopenia in the absence of HIV infection [20]. Pain may also be a feature not often considered.

Disease course and prognosis
Erythroderma is a potentially fatal condition. Current mortality rates are probably lower than historically reported, varying from 18% to 64% [4,6,8], but erythroderma remains particularly dangerous in elderly people. Cutaneous, subcutaneous and respiratory infections are common and pneumonia remains the commonest cause of death [24]. Complications resulting from systemic treatment of the erythroderma also contribute to mortality rates.

The more frequent forms of erythroderma, including eczematous, psoriasis or of unknown origin, may continue for months or years and often follow a relapsing–remitting course [24].

Investigations
The greatest diagnostic yield to determine an underlying cause is obtained from multiple skin biopsies; however, characteristic histological features are often lacking despite this [59]. A detection of T-cell clonality in the skin or peripheral blood should be sought if lymphoma is suspected, as described earlier.

Management
Treatment in hospital is frequently necessary, especially in acute and fulminant cases, because some patients may develop profound loss of homeostasis. In these cases the protein and electrolyte balance, circulatory status and body temperature require close monitoring. Appropriate fluid intake should be maintained and cardiac failure must be treated if it develops. Hypothermia can be corrected with emollients and warm blankets. All non-essential drugs should be withdrawn if they might be responsible for the erythroderma. Patients should be monitored for infection to ensure timely instigation of antibiotics if needed. Analgesia may be needed but opioids can worsen pruritus.

The cutaneous inflammation should be treated in the first instance with greasy emollients in order to restore skin barrier function. These need to be applied very frequently initially as excessive xerosis leads to rapid absorption. Other topical treatments should be used with caution because systemic absorption is greatly increased. The majority of patients will improve over a week or two with this regimen, during which time the diagnosis of the underlying condition will probably be established. Systemic therapy is usually necessary and will depend on the underlying cause identified. Systemic corticosteroids should be avoided for erythroderma due to psoriasis to avoid pustular transformation [24]. In erythroderma due to psoriasis, second line treatments may be necessary such as methotrexate, acitretin or biologics [3]. Ciclosporin will achieve a rapid improvement but caution should be taken over the renal function, especially with the potential of haemodynamic compromise.

Erythroderma is a skin emergency. Many of the underlying causes can be addressed once a level of resolution with basic measures has been achieved.

> **Treatment ladder for erythroderma**
>
> **First line**
> - Consider hospital or day unit admission
> - Withdraw or switch medications that may be implicated as a cause
> - Monitor and correct loss of homeostasis including temperature and fluid balance
> - Treat any secondary infection
> - Frequent application of greasy emollients
> - Analgesia if needed
>
> **Second line**
> - Systemic therapy dependent on underlying cause

Key references

The full list of references can be found in the online version at https://www.wiley.com/rooksdermatology10e

Assessment, investigation and management of eczematous disorders
Eczema

14 Schofield J, Grindlay D, Williams H. *Skin Conditions in the UK: A Health Care Needs Assessment*. Nottingham: Centre of Evidence Based Dermatology, University of Nottingham, 2009.
16 Langan SM, Irvine AD, Weidinger S. Atopic dermatitis. *Lancet* 2020;396:345–60.

Dermatitis and eczema of the hands

2 Moberg C, Alderling M, Meding B. Hand eczema and quality of life: a population-based study. *Br J Dermatol* 2009;161:397–403.

3 Agner T, Elsner P. Hand eczema: epidemiology, prognosis and prevention. *J Eur Acad Dermatol Venereol* 2020;34(Suppl. 1):4–12.

20 De Jongh CM, Khrenova L, Verberk MM *et al*. Loss-of-function polymorphisms in the filaggrin gene are associated with an increased susceptibility to chronic irritant contact dermatitis: a case–control study. *Br J Dermatol* 2008;159:621–7.

51 Bauer A, Schmitt J, Bennett C *et al*. Interventions for preventing occupational irritant hand dermatitis. *Cochrane Database Syst Rev* 2010;Issue 6:CD004414.

57 Ruzicka T, Lynde CW, Jemec GB *et al*. Efficacy and safety of oral alitretinoin (9-cis retinoic acid) in patients with severe chronic hand eczema (CHE) refractory to topical corticosteroids: results of a randomized, double-blind, placebo-controlled, multicentre trial. *Br J Dermatol* 2008;158:808–17.

Dermatitis and eczema of the eyelids

11 Mughal AA, Kalavala M. Contact dermatitis to ophthalmic solutions. *Clin Exp Dermatol* 2012;37:593–7, quiz 597–8.

Juvenile plantar dermatosis

12 Jones SK, English JSC, Forsyth A *et al*. Juvenile plantar dermatosis – an 8-year follow-up of 102 patients. *Clin Exp Dermatol* 1987;12:5–7.

Other related dermatoses
Erythroderma

1 Tso S, Satchwell F, Moiz H *et al*. Erythroderma (exfoliative dermatitis). Part 1: underlying causes, clinical presentation and pathogenesis. *Clin Exp Dermatol* 2021;46:1001–10.

CHAPTER 40

Seborrhoeic Dermatitis

Sarah Wakelin and Anastasia Therianou

Imperial College Healthcare Trust, London, UK

PART 4: INFLAMMATORY DERMATOSES

Synonyms and inclusions

- Seborrhoeic eczema
- Sebo-psoriasis
- Pityrosporal dermatitis
- Dandruff
- Pityriasis capitis

Introduction and general description

Seborrhoeic dermatitis (SD) is a common, chronic skin disease characterised by red or pink patches with superficial scaling. It affects areas with a high density of sebaceous glands – namely the scalp, face, central chest and anogenital region. Dandruff is generally regarded as the mildest form of SD localised to the scalp and lacking visible inflammation [1]. The diagnosis is based on clinical findings. SD has a predilection for the skin folds including large flexures and submammary areas, and the distribution is usually symmetrical. A variant of SD may affect young infants; the disease otherwise occurs at any time from puberty throughout adult life. The cause remains unclear, but the skin surface microbiome, in particular lipophilic *Malassezia* yeasts, sebum secretion and individual susceptibility, appear relevant [2]. Sebo-psoriasis is a psoriasis-like variant of SD with coarser, well-defined scaling and inflammation in an SD distribution. It may represent koebnerisation of psoriasis into areas of SD.

Epidemiology

SD is a common dermatosis globally, but estimates of its true prevalence in different populations are still limited by a lack of validated diagnostic criteria. A retrospective case note study of 50 237 first attendances at the dermatology out-patients in a Greek teaching hospital reported an overall prevalence of 4% [3] and a recent large study by dermatologists of 161 269 German employees identified SD in 3.2% (men 4.6%, women 1.4%) [4]. The authors found age-related increases in the prevalence of SD. These are likely to explain the higher prevalence of 14.3% in the Rotterdam study of 5498 participants whose median age was 67.9 years [5]. SD is approximately twice as common in men than women [4,5]. It is unclear whether this relates to sebum excretion, differences in skin care or other factors. An increased rate of SD has been reported in fair skin [5] with lower rates in skin of colour [6]. This may be due to an under recognition of inflammation in darker skin, or related to racial variation in stratum corneum ultrastructure and barrier function. Dandruff (pityriasis capitis) has been estimated to affect up to half of the world's population post puberty and is associated with stratum corneum dysfunction [7].

An infantile variant of SD and pityriasis capitis ('cradle cap') is well recognised. An Australian study of preschool children found a peak prevalence of approximately 72% in the first 3 months of life with most cases clearing by 1 year of age [8]. Similarly, a high prevalence of 56% was also found in a study of infants in Northern India [9]. SD occurs frequently and early in the course of HIV infection with rates of 35% in early disease, increasing to 85% in patients with AIDS [10] in whom it may be widespread [11]. A twofold increase in the rate of SD has also been reported in HTLV-1 seropositive Brazilian patients [12]. Higher rates of SD have been found in organ transplant recipients [13,14] increasing with duration of immunosuppression [13]. The prevalence of SD is also increased in patients with chronic neurological disease, including Parkinson disease (PD) [15], spinal cord injury [16] and a 31% prevalence of SD was reported in a study of 71 children with Down syndrome [17].

Rook's Textbook of Dermatology, Tenth Edition. Edited by Christopher Griffiths, Jonathan Barker, Tanya Bleiker, Walayat Hussain and Rosalind Simpson.
© 2024 John Wiley & Sons Ltd. Published 2024 by John Wiley & Sons Ltd.

This may be due to lack of facial movement and reduced clearance of sebum in patients with the aforementioned conditions.

Pathophysiology

The pathogenesis of SD is not clearly understood. While much attention has focused on the role of *Malassezia* yeasts, these are the main fungal component of the normal skin microbiome so they are not conventional pathogens. The situation is complicated by the existence of multiple species and strains of *Malassezia*. *M. globosa* and *M. restricta* are the commonest species on the head and neck and have been most frequently associated with SD. Sebum plays a key role in SD as a nutrient for *Malassezia* and source of inflammatory mediators. Release of lipases from these lipid-dependent organisms leads to formation of oleic acid (OA) which has irritant effects on the epidermis and can lead to SD-like changes in the absence of the yeast. Alterations in the bacterial microbiome have also recently been identified in SD [18,19]. Variations in individual susceptibility are important, especially skin barrier function, which can be affected by environmental factors such as climate and skin care. The importance of the host's immune response to the yeast is highlighted by the high prevalence of SD in those with HIV infection and other forms of immunosuppression. Genetic studies have so far failed to show any clear genetic predisposition, but SD shares an association with the LEC3 gene cluster similar to atopic eczema and psoriasis. *Malassezia* may have complex interactions with the skin's innate immune system and potentially relevant mechanisms include release of immunoregulatory indole metabolites, oxidative stress and activation of Th17 immunity, which plays a key role in defence against fungi and inflammation.

Causative organisms

A connection between fungi and SD was first proposed by Louis-Charles Malassez in 1874 [20] whose name is given to the genus of lipophilic yeasts that are present in lesional skin in SD and dandruff. A pathogenic role in SD was supported by studies showing that their clearance with antifungal agents leads to the remission of SD [21] and relapse of SD and dandruff is associated with reappearance of *Malassezia* [22]. In addition, antifungal activity is a common mechanism of many treatments for SD. However, *Malassezia* are part of the normal skin microbiome and how the yeast–host interaction changes from a commensal to pathogenic relationship remains a conundrum [23]. Intrinsic host factors such as altered sebum, impaired skin barrier and an aberrant host response may be more relevant than the yeast itself [24]. Genetic engineering of *Malassezia* is now possible and should help elucidate the mechanisms that may lead to pathogenicity [25].

Malassezia have undergone confusing nomenclature changes since their identification, including renaming as *Pityrosporum* (*-ovale, orbiculare and pachydermatis*) in the 1950s. Contemporary molecular phylogenetic and genomic studies have revealed the complexity of this genus which it is now agreed comprises 18 species and numerous functionally distinct strains. At least 10 species have been identified on human skin. Different species have been associated with SD, atopic eczema, pityriasis versicolor, dandruff, psoriasis and folliculitis [26].

Understanding of the skin mycobiome (fungal community) is being revolutionised by advances in molecular techniques which overcome the limitations of culture-based methods. These have identified *Malassezia* as the predominant organism at all body sites except the feet [27]. Skin colonisation starts within hours of birth, increasing with time and acquiring an adult diversity type similar to the mother's within the neonatal period. [28]. In childhood, fungal diversity is broader, with profound alteration during puberty, presumably due to increased sebaceous gland activity and altered sebum composition [29]. The proportion of *Malassezia* species varies according to body site and geographic variations have also been reported, but these may be affected by methodology. Culture in particular favours rapid-growing species such as *M. sympodalis* over *M. restricta*. *M. globosa* and *M. restricta* are the predominant species on the head and facial sites and have been most commonly associated with SD and dandruff. *M. sympodialis, M. furfur, M. sloofiae, M. obtuse* and most recently *M. arunalkei* have also been isolated from SD patients [22,30,**31**]. Detailed genotypic analysis of *M. globosa* and *M. restricta* suggests that specific strains are associated with SD compared with healthy controls [32,33]. There is conflicting evidence on whether the quantity of yeast correlates with disease severity in SD [**31**]. Alterations in the bacterial microbiota have also been identified in areas of SD, with predominance of *Staphylococcus* and *Acinetobacter, Streptococcus* or *Pseudomonas*, so other microbes may also be relevant in the dysbiosis of this disease [18,19].

Malassezia have several pro-inflammatory effects that may be relevant in SD pathogenesis [**34**]. Having evolved for a nutrient-poor environment, the yeast possesses many hydrolytic enzymes including extracellular lipases, phospholipases, acid sphingomyelinases and proteases that allow it to utilise skin lipids and proteins [35,36]. Increased secretion of lipases and phospholipases has been found *in vivo* in patients with SD [37] and liberated but unconsumed free fatty acids such as OA have direct irritant effects on the skin and arachidonic acid, a precursor of pro-inflammatory mediators. OA causes increased desquamation of keratinocytes and impaired barrier function, and can trigger dandruff in susceptible individuals [38]. It also promotes yeast growth and development of hyphae *ex vivo* [39]. The activity of *Malassezia* lipases varies according to skin pH and *M. restricta* lipase 5 has been speculated to play a role in severe disease as its activity increases at the higher skin surface pH associated with diseased skin [40]. Changes in the proteolytic balance may also influence the effects of fatty acids, as increased kallikrein 5 (KLK5) has been identified in the stratum corneum in dandruff [41], whereas absence of its neutralising peptidase was associated with high susceptibility to OA-induced 'dandruff' in a mouse model [42].

In vitro studies have shown that *Malassezia* elicit secretion of a range of cytokines (IL-1b, IL-6, IL-8, IL-10, TNF-α and TGF-β) from isolated keratinocytes and peripheral blood mononuclear cells [**26**,43]. However, the results vary according to the clinical and experimental context. The thick cell wall of *Malassezia* is characterised by a lipid-rich outer layer and its components are recognised by various membrane-bound receptors on immune cells. It remains unclear how these influence commensalism, inflammation and adaptive immunity [**26**]. Figure 40.1 summarises alterations in the skin microbiome and inflammatory response (described in more detail later) that occur in SD compared with normal skin.

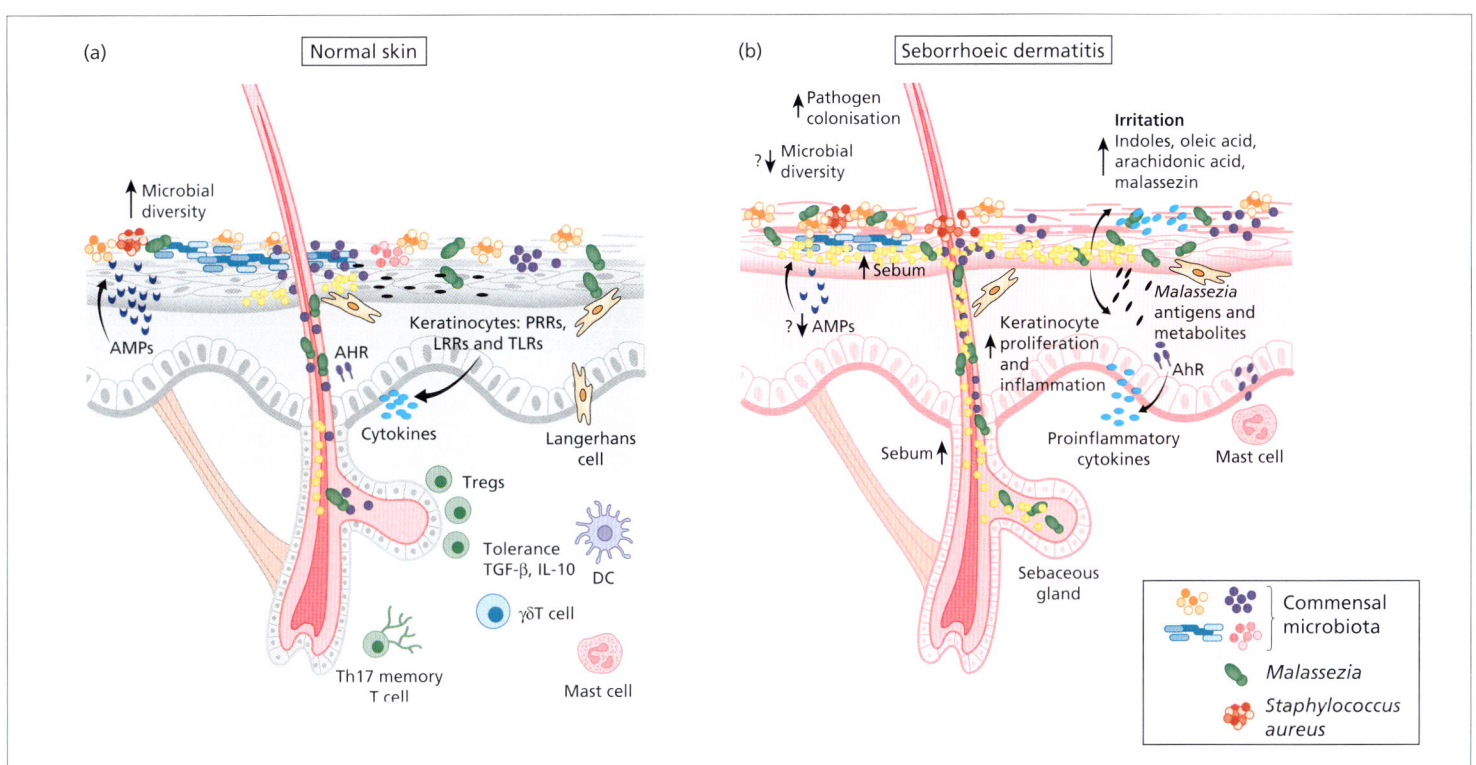

Figure 40.1 The skin microbiome and inflammatory response in normal skin and seborrhoeic dermatitis (SD). In the healthy state (a) the skin maintains high microbial diversity when compared with SD (b). Keratinocytes sense microbial populations through recognition of microbial pathogen-associated molecular patterns (PAMPs) motifs via their pattern recognition receptors (PRR), leucine-rich repeats (LRR) and Toll-like receptors (TLR), as shown in (a). The binding of PAMPs to PRRs, LRRs and TLRs triggers innate immune responses, resulting in the secretion of antimicrobial peptides that can rapidly inactivate a diverse range of pathogens including fungi and bacteria. Langerhans cells interact with microbial antigens in the epidermis to detect barrier breach and maintain homeostasis. The skin tolerance is dependent on regulatory T cells (Tregs), a subset of lymphocytes that control the immune response to antigens via release of inhibitory cytokines including TGF-ß and IL-10. In SD, alteration in sebum content favours expansion of *Malassezia* as the dominant species that may cause the disease (b). Increased *Malassezia* colonisation and secretion of lipases convert sebum and stratum corneum fatty acids into by-products such as oleic acid and arachidonic acid which irritate and cause inflammation in the skin. Indole metabolites such as malassezin, a potent ligand of the aryl hydrocarbon receptor, may alter gene expression, leading to keratinocyte proliferation and inflammation. Accumulation of histamine in SD lesions suggests mast cell degranulation. Reproduced from Vijay Chandra, Srinivas, Dawson and Common 2021 [**26**].

The host response to *Malassezia* may also be influenced by a range of immunoregulatory metabolites secreted by the yeast. *M. furfur* strains isolated from the skin of patients with SD have been found to produce increased levels of bioactive indolic substances from tryptophan metabolism [44] including formylindolocarbazole, indolocarbazole, malassezin and pityriacitrin. These are potent ligands for the aryl hydrocarbon receptor, a nuclear receptor and transcription regulator with pleiotropic effects including modulation of Toll-like receptor function [45,46] and regulation of oxidative stress. Increased oxidative stress may play a pathogenic role in SD [47] leading to high levels of squalene peroxides as found in dandruff-affected scalps [48]. Normal function of the NADPH (nicotinamide adenine dinucleotide phosphate) oxidative system is important in the oxidative burst for phagocyte microbe killing. A defect in the neutrophil cytosolic factor 1 (NCF1) component of this pathway was speculated to play a role in the severe, early-onset SD observed in two sisters with autosomal recessive chronic granulomatous disease [49].

TH-17 immunity could be relevant as it protects host barriers against fungal infection as well as having pro-inflammatory effects. Indeed, application of *Malassezia* in a mouse model of SD was found to trigger rapid induction of IL-17 expression by innate immune cells

followed by fungal elimination within about 2 weeks [50]. Increased IL-17 expression has also been observed in a Mpzl3 knockout mouse model of SD [51]. However, although IL-17 pathway defects underlie chronic mucocutaneous candidiasis, SD is not a notable feature of this disease. Most recently, *Malassezia* has been shown to increased production of IL-18, an IL-1 type pro-inflammatory cytokine, in an *ex vivo* human skin model of SD [39].

Sebum is a key pathogenic factor in SD although the sebum excretion rate is not increased in affected individuals compared with healthy controls. Abnormalities in epidermal surface lipids have been considered to be secondary to *Malassezia* rather than a primary abnormality because they are absent in non-lesional skin [22]. However, an increased sebum excretion rate, combined with facial immobility, has been thought to account for the high prevalence of SD in patients with PD [31] in whom high yeast densities have been demonstrated [52]. Polymorphisms in lipid-regulating genes have been found to confer an increased risk of PD and this may in part explain the association with SD. These include *LRRK2* and *PINK1* which increase lipid droplet size and a variant of the *SNCA* gene that increases lipase susceptibility of lipid droplet coatings [53].

Depletion and disorganisation of stratum corneum lipids have been found in ultrastructural studies of dandruff, and this subclinical barrier defect may predispose to further inflammation [2]. Raised levels of cathepsin S and histamine have been identified in scalp samples from patients with SD/dandruff [54] and may play a role in the pruritus that usually accompanies the disease [55]. In addition, changes in epidermal morphology with increased thickness, convolution and increased expression of Ki-67 [56] indicate that dandruff is a hyperproliferative state, despite its lack of overt inflammation.

Genetics

Unlike in atopic eczema and psoriasis, there is no clear understanding of the inheritance or genetic basis of SD. An association between SD and HLA alleles A*32, DQB1*05 and DRB1*01 has been reported [57]. However, a more recent search of candidate genes and genome-wide association study (GWAS) of 4500 participants of whom 15% had SD did not show any specific locus for SD, but suggested some overlap with psoriasis and atopic eczema, particularly in the *LCE3* gene cluster. The GWAS identified two significant single nucleotide polymorphisms in the *MAT4* gene that is expressed in hair follicle keratinocytes and close to the *PRIT* gene that modulates TRPV1 and TRPV8, which are involved in itch and epidermal homeostasis respectively [58].

There are a handful of reports of rare gene mutations or protein deficiencies associated with SD in humans and in animal models [59]. These include mutations in *ACT1* (involved in IL-17 signalling), complement component C5 in Leiner disease, nuclear factor (NF)-κB essential modulator (NEMO), which regulates NF-κB signalling, and SKT4, which is important for lymphocyte maintenance. A mutation within a zinc finger transcription factor ZNF750 – a master regulator of late epidermal differentiation – has been reported in a family with an autosomal dominant, early-onset, severe SD-like rash [60], suggesting that primary skin barrier defects may be relevant in SD. Studies of the knockout mouse Mpzl3 which lacks the promotor required for ZNF750 binding and develops an early-onset rash resembling SD [61] should aid further study of this topic.

Environmental and lifestyle factors

SD has been reported to occur more commonly in winter, when skin barrier function is impaired due to low temperature and humidity, and although a disease of sebum-rich areas, it is often accompanied by generalised skin dryness [5]. It is not clear if ultraviolet (UV)-induced immunosuppression plays any role in the improvement of SD in summer [5,62] because this was proposed to be the reason for a high rate of facial SD observed in alpine mountain guides in one study [63].

Skin care and grooming practices may affect SD because cosmetic products contain various components that can influence the skin microbiome. Proteins, lipids and carbohydrates can promote microbial growth while biocides have an inhibitory effect. Use of cosmetics was speculated to account for the lower level of *Malassezia* observed in healthy young Japanese women [64]. Hair styling practices may also be important and a study of African American girls up to the age of 15 found a significant association between SD and use of hair extensions and infrequent hair oil application [65]. The choice of oil may be important because a study of *Malassezia* cultures in the presence of a wide range of cosmetic ingredients found that natural oils, especially olive and avocado oils, waxes, primary alcohols and certain fatty acid esters, promoted growth whereas other ingredients including lanolin, paraffin and silicone-based substances, polymers and fatty alcohol ethers had no effect [66]. However, coconut oil has been reported to help dandruff [67], so the effects may be different when cosmetics are applied to the skin. This complex topic deserves further exploration.

The Rotterdam study included evaluation of dietary patterns in 4397 participants. The authors found that a high fruit intake was associated with a lower prevalence of SD whereas a western dietary pattern in females was associated with more SD [68]. An association between SD and vitamin D deficiency has also been reported [69]. No association between SD prevalence and alcohol or smoking was found in the Rotterdam study, whereas a case-crossover study reported an association between flares and higher alcohol consumption as well as psychological stress [70].

Clinical features

History

SD usually starts in adolescence or early adult life with localised inflammation and superficial flaking of the skin. Affected areas may be asymptomatic or intensely itchy and symptoms may be disproportionate to the clinical signs, especially on the scalp. The condition usually runs a chronic, relapsing course.

Presentation

Facial SD typically affects the cutaneous folds – nasolabial, ear creases, eyelids and glabellar area – and medial eyebrows (Figures 40.2 and 40.3). Fine scaling of the skin with localised red or pink patches is often present around the alar creases and nasal side walls and posterior ear folds. The ear canals often have light scaling and inflammation – otitis externa may occur with secondary bacterial or *Candida* infection. Scalp involvement ranges from mild small grey–white scales without underlying red or pink patches (i.e. dandruff) to a more inflammatory eruption with thicker, yellow, greasy scales and crusts. Similar changes can occur in the beard (Figure 40.4). Inflammation of the anterior eyelid margin (anterior blepharitis) may occur in SD, presenting with flaky debris around the base of eyelashes which can fall into the eye, leading to conjunctival irritation and red eye [71]. Consequent meibomian gland loss may lead to dry eye disease [72].

On the torso, several forms of SD may occur. In men, involvement of the presternal area is typical with petaloid (petal-shaped) lesions that may be localised (Figure 40.5). More widespread involvement may extend to the upper back, umbilicus, axillae, groins and submammary area. In the large flexures, the affected areas may appear glazed and pink (Figure 40.6). 'Pityriasiform' SD is a more inflammatory and widespread variant, involving the torso and sometimes the limbs. Anogenital involvement may occur in both genders. Endogenous vulvar dermatitis is not always classified further, but in one study 40% of women also had extragenital features of SD [73].

Hypopigmentation may be a prominent feature of SD in darker-skinned individuals with little obvious inflammation. In adults, arcuate and petaloid lesions may affect the hairline and

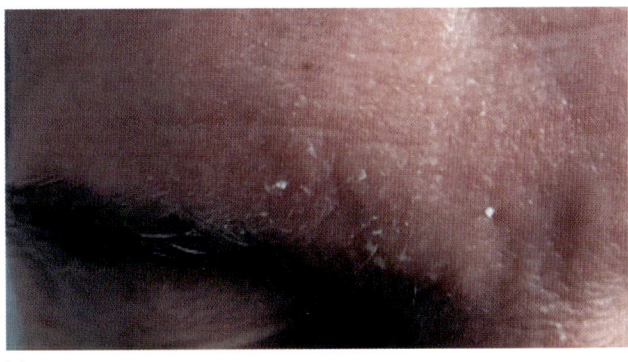
(a)

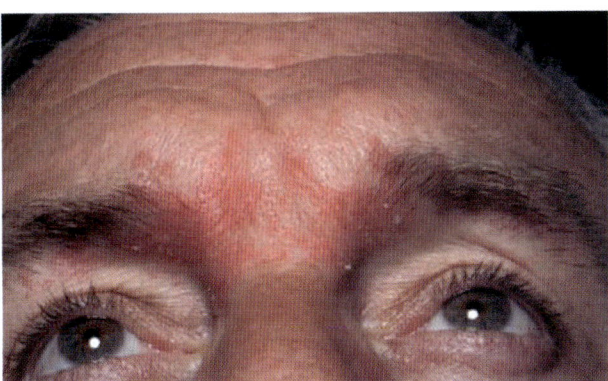
(b)

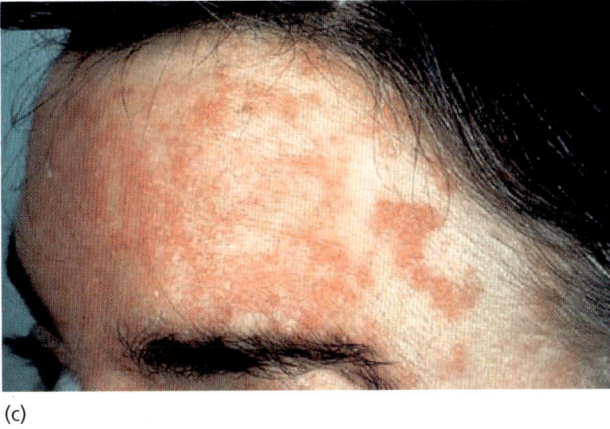
(c)

Figure 40.2 Facial seborrhoeic dermatitis. (a) Early changes of scaling and mild erythema in the medial eyebrow. (b) Pronounced inflammation of medial brows and glabellar folds. (c) Diffuse involvement of the forehead, eyebrows and scalp margin.

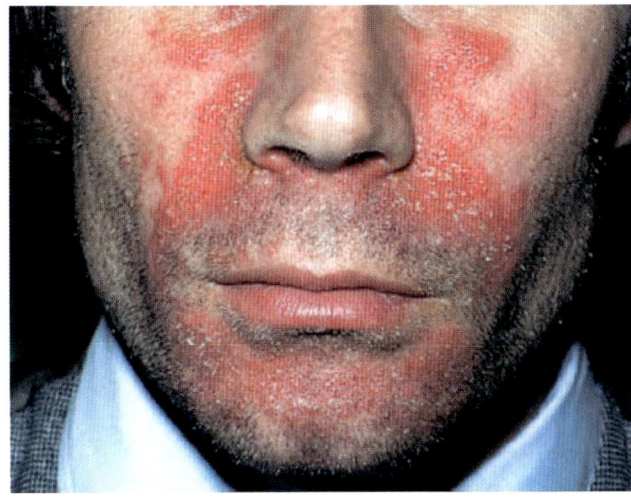

Figure 40.3 Severe facial seborrhoeic dermatitis with prominent involvement of the naso-labial grooves.

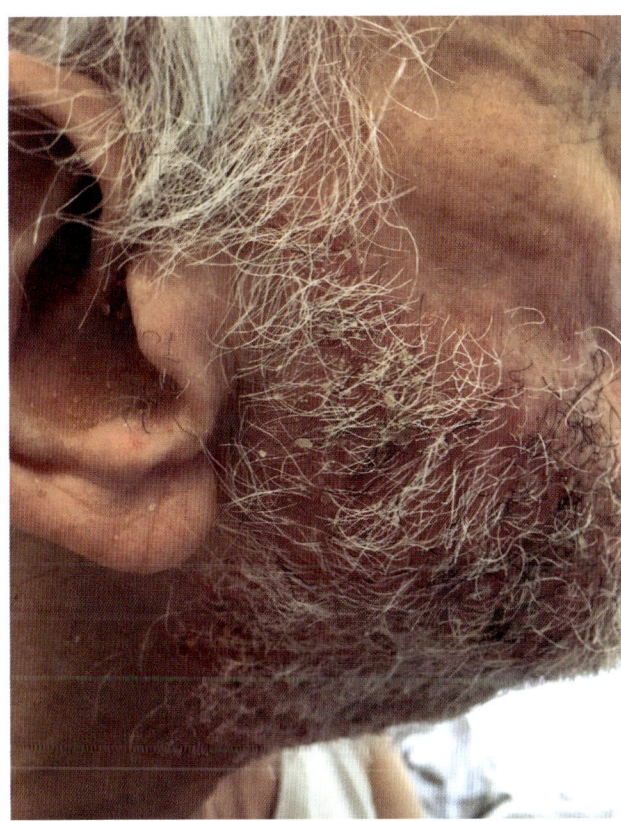

Figure 40.4 Seborrhoeic dermatitis of the beard area.

face with multiple pale or pink polycyclic coalescing lesions with little scale [74]. A hyperpigmented variant termed 'seborrhoeic melanosis', in which typical SD areas show hyperpigmentation with epidermal acanthosis and hyperpigmentation on dermoscopy, has been reported in Indian patients [75] (Figure 40.7).

Clinical variants

Infantile SD presents with cradle cap and/or napkin dermatitis. It usually appears by the age of 3 months, disappearing spontaneously by 1 year of age. Additional involvement of the eyebrows, paranasal areas and large flexures is often present and this distribution has been considered helpful in distinguishing infantile SD from atopic eczema [76]. Darker-skinned children usually present with

mild erythema, flaking and hypopigmentation rather than a typical cradle cap and often have overlapping features of atopic eczema [74]. The distinction between infantile SD and atopic eczema is not always clear-cut. A retrospective study of infants with SD found that a higher-than-expected number developed atopic eczema within a short period of time [77]. The features of infantile SD also overlap with so-called psoriasiform napkin dermatitis (see Chapter 35).

In adults, SD may occur in association with other common dermatoses with a predilection for the sebaceous areas including

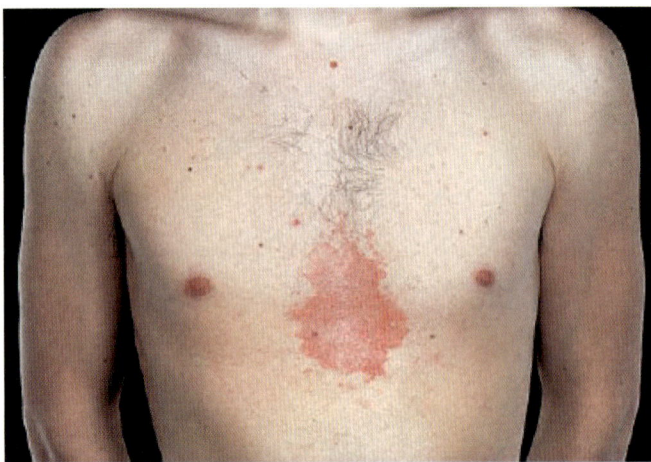

Figure 40.5 Seborrhoeic dermatitis of the presternal area. Courtesy of Dr D. A. Burns, Leicester Royal Infirmary, UK.

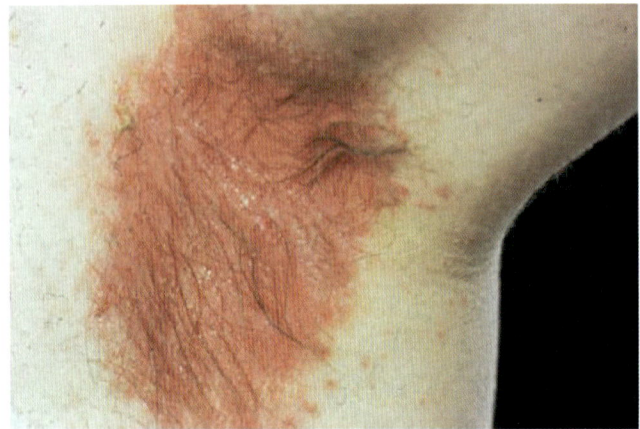

Figure 40.6 Seborrhoeic dermatitis of the axilla. The large flexures may become secondarily infected.

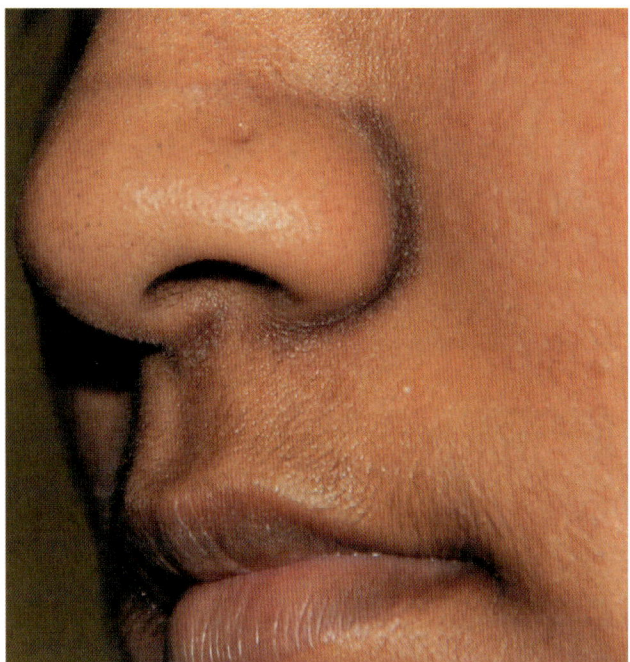

Figure 40.7 Post-inflammatory hyperpigmentation in seborrhoeic dermatitis of the nasal crease ('seborrhoeic melanosis'). Courtesy of Dr S. B. Varma.

acne, rosacea, pityriasis versicolor and pityrosporum folliculitis [76], as well as onychomycosis and tinea pedis [4]. Widespread SD may rarely evolve into an exfoliative dermatitis with erythroderma (Chapter 35).

Differential diagnosis

The diagnosis of SD is usually straightforward, but in atypical cases the differential diagnosis is wide. Scalp scaling is a common feature of psoriasis, but psoriatic scaling is usually well-circumscribed, thicker and silvery. General examination of the skin should be carried out to look for nail changes and typical plaques of psoriasis. The term 'sebopsoriasis' has been used to describe patients with psoriasiform scaling in an SD distribution, but this entity is not clearly defined. Scaling is more pronounced than in SD and individuals may have plaque psoriasis elsewhere. It may represent koebnerisation of psoriasis into areas of SD (Chapter 35). It has been reported to arise in HIV-positive men established on antiretroviral therapy with an undetectable viral load [78]. Allergic contact dermatitis may mimic or complicate SD at various sites including the face. Patch testing should be considered in atypical

cases and in patients with eyelid dermatitis. Mild cases of Darier disease and Hailey–Hailey disease may be misdiagnosed as SD due to their predilection for sebaceous areas and large flexures, respectively. In Darier disease, lesions are typically more dome-shaped and papular. If either disease is suspected, a skin biopsy is indicated. Perioral dermatitis also typically affects the naso-labial folds with superficial scaling. Presence of inflammatory papules in a diamond-shaped distribution in the periocular area and periocular papules are helpful diagnostic features. Pemphigus foliaceus and pemphigus erythematosus may affect seborrhoeic areas on the face and torso, mimicking SD. If suspected, skin biopsy and immunofluorescence studies are indicated.

Pityriasis rosea may mimic the pityriasiform variant of SD in which there is no herald patch, and involvement beyond the torso is typical. Early cutaneous T-cell lymphoma may present with SD-like lesions. Erythrasma may mimic SD of the large flexures.

The differential diagnoses in infants include psoriasis, histiocytosis, zinc deficiency, acrodermatitis enteropathica and Leiner disease (erythroderma desquamativum) in which SD is typically severe and widespread and occurs in association with recurrent infections, failure to thrive and deficiencies of various complement components. SD-like changes may also be a feature of biotinidase deficiency [79], a rare, inherited neurocutaneous disorder that leads to reduced levels of biotin (vitamin B7).

Prepubertal children with scalp scaling should be carefully examined for hair loss and broken hairs to exclude tinea capitis. Pediculosis is also a common infestation in this age group so those with itchy scalps should be inspected for lice and their eggs.

Drug-induced/exacerbated seborrhoeic dermatitis

A range of drugs may produce SD-like eruptions, including those containing sulphydryl groups (captopril, D-penicillamine, sodium aurothiomalate) [80] and other gold salts, lithium, buspirone, methyldopa, chlorpromazine and cimetidine. A longitudinal study of patients with hepatitis C virus infection treated with interferon-α and ribavirin found that SD was one of the most frequent mucocutaneous complications [81]. SD-like rashes [82,83] and reactivation of SD [84] have been reported in patients receiving recombinant IL-2. SD-like eruptions may also feature among the range of adverse skin reactions to targeted chemotherapeutic drugs including the epidermal growth factor inhibitor erlotinib [85,86], the multikinase inhibitors sorafenib [87] and sunitinib [88], dasitinib [89] and the *BRAF* inhibitor vemurafenib [90], which has also been reported to cause pityriasis amiantacea [91]. Topical 5-fluorouracil has been reported to trigger or exacerbate SD at distant sites and flares may also be induced by systemic therapy [92].

New-onset SD and sebopsoriasis have been reported in patients with severe atopic eczema treated with dupilumab [93] and a retrospective study of 1000 patients treated with this anti-IL-4/IL-13 biologic reported that 4.2% developed new or worsening non-specific head and neck dermatitis [94].

Classification of severity

The severity of SD and dandruff is highly variable. Unlike atopic eczema and psoriasis there is no validated scoring system, so many studies have simply used descriptive categories. Some studies have used a clinical score termed the SD area severity index (SDASI) that was proposed by a Turkish group in 2007 and based on the psoriasis area severity index (PASI) [95].

Complications and co-morbidities

SD is one of the most common HIV-associated dermatoses and occurs early in the course of HIV disease [96]. It may therefore be an initial clinical marker of HIV infection. SD is one of several 'indicator diseases' that should prompt testing for HIV in order to decrease the probability of late HIV diagnosis [97,98]. Late HIV diagnosis is associated with a poorer response to antiretroviral treatment and increased rates of HIV transmission. SD may also develop as part of an immune reconstitution inflammatory syndrome in HIV-infected patients starting highly active antiretroviral therapy [99]. The German employees study reported that when controlling for age and sex, adults with SD had an increased prevalence of folliculitis, contact dermatitis, intertriginous dermatitis, rosacea, acne, pyoderma, tinea corporis, pityriasis versicolor and psoriasis [4]. This supports the concept that SD is associated with a broader susceptibility to dysbiosis and inflammation.

Patients commonly report that an outbreak of SD is preceded by a stressful event [100–102] and this has been supported by findings of a case–control and case-crossover study [70]. One study of 150 patients with psychiatric disorders reported that the higher rate of SD was entirely ascribable to patients with depression [103]. Other studies have specifically reported higher anxiety scores among adults with SD [101,104].

A case–control study of 50 dermatology outpatients with SD found high rates of somatisation, depression, anxiety and neuroticism [105]. However, this may reflect increased health care-seeking behaviour among people with these personality traits, because the Rotterdam study found no significant association between

SD and depression [5]. SD has also been associated with anorexia nervosa [106].

It is difficult to separate out the role of disease, lifestyle, nutrition and psychological problems in these situations. In patients over the age of 65, SD was found to be independently associated with age and loss of self-sufficiency, suggesting a role of senescence [107]. Although there have been reports of an association between SD and features of the metabolic syndrome, namely hypertension [108] and higher body fat content [109], this was not confirmed in the recent Rotterdam study [5].

Quality of life

As with other inflammatory dermatoses, SD has been reported to be associated with an impaired quality of life (QoL). High disease severity and facial involvement have been found to have greater impact [110]. A multicentre Spanish study of 2159 adults showed a mean Skindex-29 global score of 20.5 [101], which is in the range of mild impairment [111]. A smaller study of 312 outpatients with SD in China found a higher mean Skindex-29 score of 33.97 with severe emotional problems in nearly half of all patients [112].

Disease course and prognosis

Longitudinal studies are lacking, but SD is usually a chronic condition, punctuated with flares, which requires long-term/maintenance treatment.

Investigations

The diagnosis of SD is usually made on clinical grounds without the need for diagnostic tests. HIV testing should be considered if the history indicates.

Dermoscopy/trichoscopy may help distinguish scalp SD from psoriasis, with SD showing a characteristic vascular pattern of arborising vessels, atypical vessels and the absence of red dots and globules (which are features of psoriasis) [113] (Figure 40.8). White scales and red and yellowish areas can also be seen [114].

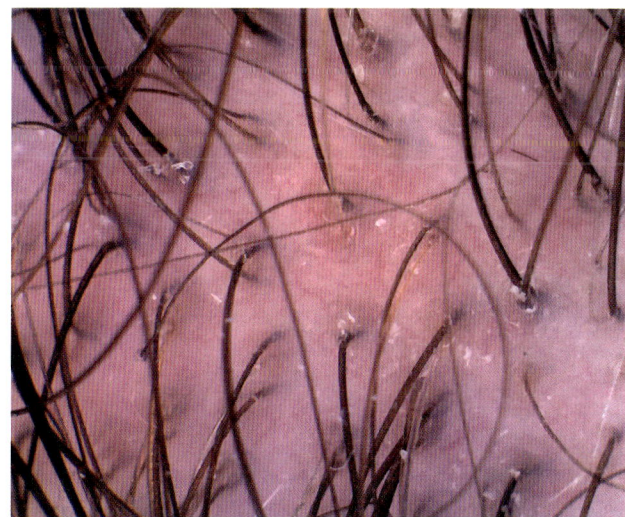

Figure 40.8 Trichoscopy of seborrhoeic dermatitis showing dilated vessels, redness and scaling.

Histology is not diagnostic and usually shows overlapping features of psoriasis and chronic dermatitis. Spongiosis is a helpful distinguishing feature, but less evident in older lesions where psoriasiform features of follicular plugs of orthokeratosis and parakeratotic cells and uneven rete ridges predominate [115]. Shoulder parakeratosis and a more prominent lymphocytic infiltrate favour SD [116]. The perifollicular infiltrate includes increased numbers of dendritic cells [117]. The primary histological lesion of SD first identified by Civatte [118], then later by Pinkus and Mehregan [119], is the 'squirting papilla' which involves capillary dilatation in the papillae, followed by migration of granulocytes into the epidermis where they incite spongiosis.

Immunohistochemistry including Ki-67, keratin 10, caspase-5 and GLUT-1 was not helpful in differentiating psoriasis from SD [116]. Presence of nucleated cells in dandruff permits DNA extraction and forensic identification of an individual from a single skin squame [120].

Management

There is no definitive cure for SD. Long-term maintenance treatment may be required but some patients only use treatment intermittently for acute, symptomatic flares. Although successful treatment improves symptoms and can improve quality of life, it is important to explain that some symptoms may remain or recur because this helps set a realistic expectation and can free the patient from a life overly limited by their condition [121]. A range of topical agents may be used and systemic therapy is rarely indicated. The treatment approach depends on patient age, disease severity and distribution. Three broad categories of topical therapy are antifungals, keratolytics and anti-inflammatory/immunomodulatory agents. Many plant-derived treatments have also been proposed.

Topical antifungals

Topical antifungals are the first line therapy of therapy for SD due to their safety in all ages. The 2015 Cochrane systematic review of topical antifungals for SD in adolescents and adults concluded that ketoconazole 2% and the broad spectrum antifungal ciclopirox olamine 1% had similar remission failure rates but were superior to placebo [122]. The long-established azoles, miconazole and clotrimazole, were found to have comparable efficacy with topical steroids in short-term studies but there was an overall lack of evidence comparing one antifungal to another or for symptom clearance beyond 4 weeks. Small studies have reported benefit with 2% sertaconazole [123,124] whereas 1% bifonazole was found to lack efficacy in a high-quality randomised controlled trial (RCT) [125,126]. Despite lacking activity against *Malassezia* species, topical use of the allylamines terbinafine [127] and naftitine [128] has been reported to be effective in SD, suggesting that other mechanisms may be involved.

The availability of different formulations improves patient choice and may aid adherence. For example, 2% ketoconazole foam [129] was found to be popular and effective as a long-term treatment of SD for up to 52 weeks. When treating scalps, it is important to consider hair texture and grooming practices. White patients may prefer antifungal foams, gels and sprays, whereas black patients prefer ointment or oil preparations [130]. African American women may be cautious about use of ketoconazole shampoo due to concerns about hair fragility [74]. Although most *Malassezia* species are sensitive to azole drugs, long-term use of antimicrobials may drive resistance. Indeed, a recent study identified ketoconazole-resistant *M. restricta* strains from patients with severe dandruff. Possible mechanisms include multiplication of genes involved in ergosterol synthesis and oxidative stress responses and overexpression of drug efflux proteins [131].

Other antifungal active agents present in antidandruff shampoos include zinc pyrithione, piroctone olamine and coal tar. Selenium sulfide has both antifungal and keratolytic effects and is available in several formulations such as shampoo, lotion, cream foam and suspension [71,132]. Topical antifungals often have low efficacy in dandruff due to poor bioavailability and short duration at the site of application. Newer formulations such as liposomes and nanoparticles should aid drug delivery and improve efficacy [133].

Keratolytics

Topical keratolytics break down corneocyte bonds and are helpful in removing adherent scale with improved penetration of topical agents. They include salicylic acid, sulphur, coal tar (which also has antiproliferative and cytostatic effects), urea, lactic acid and propylene glycol. Some keratolytic agents also inhibit growth of fungi and have been found to reduce signs of scalp SD but may cause stinging [134]. Although these agents have been used for many years there is little robust evidence of their efficacy, particularly in infantile SD and cradle cap [135]; topical salicylic acid is contraindicated in infancy due to toxicity.

Topical anti-inflammatory agents

Topical corticosteroids may be used as monotherapy or in combination with antifungals where the results are superior to antifungal monotherapy [136]. Short-term use of a mild topical corticosteroid is recommended by the National Institute for Health and Care Excellence (NICE) for SD in adults when topical antifungal therapy has failed [137] (Table 40.1). Concerns about atrophy limit the long-term use of corticosteroids, especially in delicate sites such as the eyelids, and topical calcineurin inhibitors have emerged as an effective alternative for treatment and maintenance. High-quality RCT evidence supports the use of pimecrolimus and tacrolimus in facial SD [126] although neither is licensed for this indication. Improvement is apparent within 2 weeks of starting topical calcineurin inhibitors and a reduction in severity of subsequent SD relapses has been noted [138]. One RCT found that maintenance treatment with twice weekly 0.1% tacrolimus was effective (and superior to once a week treatment) compared with vehicle [139] and a long-term 24-week study reported longer remissions than with ciclopirox olamine 1% cream twice a week in adults with facial SD [140]. Application site adverse effects are common with topical calcineurin inhibitors and include flushing, burning and irritation. Patients should be forewarned and reassured that this does not indicate an allergic reaction.

There is high-quality evidence for the efficacy of topical lithium in reducing the severity of clinical symptoms and signs of SD [126] and one study of patients with facial SD reported that 8% lithium

Table 40.1 Summary of NICE recommendations for the treatment of seborrhoeic dermatitis.

Type of seborrhoeic dermatitis	First line therapy	Second line therapy	Additional therapy
Scalp and beard	2% ketoconazole shampoo or selenium sulphide shampoo twice a week for a month, then once or twice a week for symptom control	Medicated shampoos with zinc pyrithione, coal tar or salicylic acid	Topical keratolytic or mineral/olive oil for the removal of scale and crust Potent topical corticosteroid scalp application for 4 weeks if there is severe scalp itch
Face and body in adults	Ketoconazole 2% cream OD/BD, clotrimazole 1% cream BD/TDS, econazole 1% cream BD, miconazole 2% cream BD Use as above for at least 4 weeks, then less frequently	Mild topical corticosteroids for 1–2 weeks	Antifungal shampoo, e.g. 2% ketoconazole, as a body wash Hygiene measures for eyelid involvement using cotton buds moistened with baby shampoo
Severe	Review diagnosis, consider specialist referral, HIV testing		
In infants	Removal of scalp crusts with baby shampoo and gentle brushing. Overnight soak of petroleum jelly or warmed vegetable oil if needed. Daily bathing with soap substitute	Topical imidazole cream: clotrimazole 1% cream BD/TDS, econazole 1% cream BD, miconazole 2% cream BD	Topical corticosteroids not routinely advised but may be used for certain infants with nappy rash

Adapted from National Institute for Health and Care Excellence [**137**].

gluconate was more effective than 2% ketoconazole in inducing complete remission [141]. Anti-inflammatory effects include inhibition of pathways such as glycogen synthase kinase 3 beta (GSK3β), nuclear factor (NF)-κB and signal transducers and activation of transcription (STAT) [142]. Lithium salts also precipitate free fatty acids thereby limiting their availability for growth of lipid-dependent yeasts [143].

Other treatments reported to be of benefit in facial SD include 4% nicotinamide cream [144] and metronidazole 0.75% gel [145], which may be particularly useful in patients with coexistent acne/rosacea. A small open study has reported efficacy of 2% crisaborole, a phosphodiesterase (PDE) 4 inhibitor approved for atopic eczema [146], and another highly potent PDE4 inhibitor, roflumilast, is in a phase 3 clinical trial for use in SD. Photodynamic therapy with indole-3-acetic acid, which has sebum-reducing, anti-inflammatory and antimicrobial activity, has been proposed as an option for both SD and acne [147,148]. Promiseb™ also marketed in Europe as Sebclair® – a non-prescription, non-steroidal emollient with reported antifungal and anti-inflammatory properties – showed similar efficacy in facial SD to desonide, a mild-potency steroid, in a 28-day trial [149].

Many herbal treatments have been reported to be of benefit in dandruff/SD [133] but for most the level of evidence is very low. High-quality evidence exists for 30% aloe vera extract [150], 5% tea tree oil (*Melaleuca alternifolia* extract) [151] and 4% *Quasia amara* extract [152] in the treatment of facial SD [**126**]. In infantile SD, short-term treatment with a moisturiser containing the liquorice derivative licochalcone was reported to be equally effective to 1% hydrocortisone in a split-site, double-blind study [153]. Phytocannabinoids have been found to have anti-inflammatory and sebosuppressive actions which suggest therapeutic potential in SD [154]. A 2-week open study reported improvement in scalp SD and psoriasis with a shampoo containing 0.075% cannabidiol [155]. However, phytocannabinoids have complex actions on the human hair follicle and may inhibit growth [156], so further study is needed.

Systemic treatment

Oral antifungal therapy is occasionally advocated for recalcitrant or widespread SD, although high-quality studies are lacking [**157**]. Itraconazole has been the most frequently reported oral treatment for SD and a pulse regimen has generally been associated with good clinical and mycological responses. An RCT of oral itraconazole 200 mg daily for 1 week followed by 200 mg daily for the first 2 days of the month was more effective than placebo, though an improved quality of life was observed in both groups [158]. A small open study reported improvement with narrow-band UVB therapy in all 18 SD patients treated [159], but the median time for relapse was 3 weeks, thus benefit appears short lived. Low-dose oral isotretinoin may be an (unlicensed) option in those with severe seborrhea and an RCT showed improvement in SD [160]. Despite clinical similarities between infantile SD and inborn errors of biotin synthesis, oral biotin supplements were not found to be effective in normal infants [**135**].

Looking to the future, antimicrobial peptides may provide another treatment option for SD [132,161]. *In vitro* studies of a modified synthetic antimicrobial peptide, P5, found this to be three or four times more potent against *M. furfur* than ketoconazole or itraconazole, with additional anti-inflammatory properties, inhibiting keratinocyte expression of IL-8 and TLR2 [162]. Other possibilities include lipase inhibitors [163] and selective inhibitors of *Malassezia* carbonic anhydrase include natural polyphenols [164].

Key references

The full list of references can be found in the online version at https://www.wiley.com/rooksdermatology10e

2 Borda LJ, Wikramanayake TC. Seborrhoeic dermatitis and dandruff: a comprehensive review. *J Clin Investig Dermatol* 2015;3;10.13188/2373–1044.1000019.
4 Zander N, Sommer R, Schafer I et al. Epidemiology and dermatological comorbidity of seborrhoeic dermatitis: population-based study in 161 269 employees. *Br J Dermatol* 2019;181:743–8.

5 Sanders MGH, Pardo LM, Franco OH, Ginger RS, Nijsten T. Prevalence and determinants of seborrhoeic dermatitis in a middle-aged and elderly population: the Rotterdam Study. *Br J Dermatol* 2018:178:148–53.

23 LeibundGut-Landmann S, Dawson TL Jr. *Malassezia*: a skin commensal yeast impacting both health and disease. *Front Cell Infect Microbiol* 2021;11:659219.

24 Wikramanayake TC, Borda LJ, Miteva M, Paus R. Seborrheic dermatitis – looking beyond *Malassezia*. *Exp Dermatol* 2019;28:991–1001.

26 Vijay Chandara SH, Srinivas R, Dawson TL, Common JE. Cutaneous *Malassezia*: commensal, pathogen or protector? *Front Cell Infect Microbiol* 2021:10:Article 614446.

31 Adalsteinsson JA, Kaushik S, Muzumdar S, Guttman-Yassky E, Ungar J. An update on the microbiology, immunology and genetics of seborrhoeic dermatitis. *Experimental Dermatology* 2020;29:481–9.

34 Gaitanis G, Velegraki A, Mayser P, Bassukas ID. Skin diseases associated with *Malassezia* yeast: facts and controversies. *Clin Dermatol* 2013;31:455–63.

126 Gupta AK, Versteg SG. Topical treatment of facial seborrheic dermatitis: a systematic review. *Am J Clin Dermatol* 2017;18:193–213.

135 Victoire A, Magin P, Coughlan J, van Driel ML. Interventions for infantile seborrhoeic dermatitis (including cradle cap). *Cochrane Database Syst Rev* 2019; Issue 3: CD011380.

137 National Institute for Health and Care Excellence (NICE). Clinical knowledge summary. Seborrhoeic dermatitis. https://cks.nice.org.uk/topics/seborrhoeic-dermatitis/ (last accessed February 2022).

157 Gupta AK, Richardson M, Paquet M. Systematic review of oral treatments for seborrheic dermatitis. *J Eur Acad Dermatol Venerol* 2014;28:16–26.

CHAPTER 41

Atopic Eczema

Michael R. Ardern-Jones[1], Carsten Flohr[2] and Nick J. Reynolds[3]

[1] University Hospitals Southampton NHS Foundation Trust and University of Southampton, UK
[2] King's College London and St John's Institute of Dermatology, UK
[3] Newcastle Hospitals NHS Foundation Trust and Newcastle University, UK

PART 4: INFLAMMATORY DERMATOSES

Definition, nomenclature and classification

Concise definition and diagnostic criteria

Atopic eczema, which is synonymous with atopic dermatitis, is a difficult condition to define robustly because it lacks a diagnostic test, except skin biopsy, and shows variable clinical features across patients of different ages and ethnicities. The following definition is in accord with most consensus groups: atopic eczema is an itchy, chronically relapsing, inflammatory skin condition that often starts in early childhood (usually before 2 years of age) [1,2] (Box 41.1). The rash is characterised by inflammation (redness in light skin and often increased pigmentation in dark skin) and skin surface change (fine scaling, excoriations and lichenification from recurrent scratching, oedema/papulation, oozing/crusting in case of skin infections and vesicle formation). It typically has a flexural distribution (Box 41.1 and Box 41.2) but non-flexural involvement is common in infants and those with skin of colour. The eruption is frequently associated with other atopic conditions in the individual or other family members [1–3]. In patients harbouring a filaggrin mutation, the main genetic predisposing factor, clinical features may additionally include ichthosis vulgaris, keratosis pilaris and hyperlinear palms (Table 41.1).

Box 41.1 Clinical features of atopic eczema

- Itching
- Macular erythema
- Papules or papulovesicles
- Eczematous areas with crusting
- Lichenification and excoriation
- Hyper- or hypopigmentation
- Dryness of the skin
- Secondary infection

Rook's Textbook of Dermatology, Tenth Edition. Edited by Christopher Griffiths, Jonathan Barker, Tanya Bleiker, Walayat Hussain and Rosalind Simpson.
© 2024 John Wiley & Sons Ltd. Published 2024 by John Wiley & Sons Ltd.

Box 41.2 Diagnostic criteria of atopic dermatitis (eczema)

In order to qualify as a case of atopic eczema with the UK diagnostic criteria, the child:

Must have:
- An itchy skin condition in the last 12 months

Plus three or more of:
- Onset below age 2[a]
- History of flexural involvement
- History of a generally dry skin
- Personal history of other atopic disease[b]
- Visible flexural dermatitis as per photographic protocol

[a] Not used in children under 4 years
[b] In children aged under 4 years, history of atopic disease in a first degree relative may be included

Table 41.2 Different names that have been used for atopic eczema.

Prurigo diathésique	Besnier (1892)
Névrodermite diffuse	Brocq (1902)
Prurigo Besnier	Rasch (1903)
Eczéma constitutionel	Brocq (1927)
Early and late exudative eczematoid	Rost (1928)
Eczema infantum	
Eczema flexurarum	
Neurodermatitis disseminate and pruriginosa	
Hay fever eczema–asthmatic eczema	
Neurodermitits	Rost and Marchionini (1932)
Atopic dermatitis	Wise and Sulzberger (1935)
Endogenous eczema	Korting (1954)
Neurodermitis constitutionalis sive atopica	Schnyder and Borelli (1967)
Neurodermitis atopica sive constitutionalis	Wuthrich (1983)
Pure-mixed atopic eczema	Wuthrich (1989)
Atopiforme dermatitis	Bos (1998) (2002)
Extrinsic-intrinsic atopic eczema	Wuthrich (1989)
IgE-mediated–non-IgE-mediated atopic eczema	
Allergic–non-allergic atopic eczema dermatitis syndrome	Johansson et al. (2001) [5]

Adapted from Novak et al. (2003) [6].

Synonyms and inclusions

Debate has added to the already wide variety of historical names for the condition (Table 41.2). Gradually, as the understanding of the association with atopy and allergic immune responses grew, 'atopic dermatitis' became the accepted name. More recently, 'atopic eczema' has become widely used. It is likely that molecular biomarkers such as filaggrin status will become more central to the disease description.

Classification links: ICD-10: L20; ICD-11: 215767047; MIM: 603165.

Introduction and general description

Atopic and non-atopic eczema

One of the difficulties in defining atopic eczema arises from the impreciseness of its association with atopy and the nature of atopy itself. Atopic eczema and disorders that cause anaphylaxis, for example those resulting from insect stings and food allergies, may be associated with IgE antibodies and are therefore grouped with the atopic diseases. Such grouping is not ideal, as individuals with atopic eczema can have a normal total IgE level (see later) [7], and atopic eczema is rarely attributable to a specific allergic reaction. It is still a matter of debate whether the group with dermatitis and normal IgE levels, termed intrinsic atopic eczema or non-atopic dermatitis, can be distinguished clinically and prognostically from extrinsic atopic dermatitis. Thus, positive skin tests for allergen-specific IgE responses or raised levels of allergen-specific IgE titres in serum are found in 40–90% of patients (extrinsic atopic dermatitis) [8,9]. However, not all cases of atopic eczema have high levels of IgE and some studies suggest that 'non-atopic' atopic eczema (known as intrinsic atopic dermatitis) may represent >50% of cases [9–11], but with time atopic features become more prevalent and the intrinsic form may be found in only 5.4% of adult patients [12]. Furthermore, the predisposition to extrinsic atopic eczema is associated with genetic abnormalities in the gene encoding filaggrin [13].

Because current understanding supports a principal role of the epidermis in disease pathogenesis (Figure 41.1), some experts have questioned the word 'atopic' in the title. The European Academy of Allergy and Clinical Immunology proposed a definition of: 'Atopy is a personal or familial tendency to produce IgE antibodies in response to low doses of allergens, usually proteins, and to develop typical symptoms of asthma, rhinoconjunctivitis or

Table 41.1 Clinical features associated with Filaggrin gene status [4].

Skin phenotype or clinical feature	FLG null homozygotes[a] (n = 9), n (%)	FLG null heterozygotes (n = 98), n (%)	FLG wild-type homozygotes (n = 671), n (%)
Flexural eczema	5 (55.6)	16 (16.3)	95 (14.2)
Ichthyosis vulgaris	9 (100)	3 (3.1)	0 (0)
Milder ichthyosis	2 (22.2)	23 (23.5)	30 (4.5)
Xerosis	0 (0)	32 (32.7)	163 (24.3)
Keratosis pilaris	9 (100)	59 (60.2)	201 (30.0)
Hyperlinear palms	9 (100)	73 (74.5)	84 (12.5)
Clinically normal skin	0 (0)	10 (10.2)	281 (41.9)

Genotyping results for all six of the screened mutations (R501X, 2282del4, R2447X, S3247X, 3702delG, 3673delC) were available for these 778 children out of the 792 children included in this cohort study. Analysis is performed using a combined null genotype, in which the different FLG null mutations are considered to be equivalent, on the basis of their equivalent effects demonstrated in previous biochemical and immunohistochemical studies. [a]The group of FLG null homozygotes includes one R501X homozygote and eight compound heterozygotes.

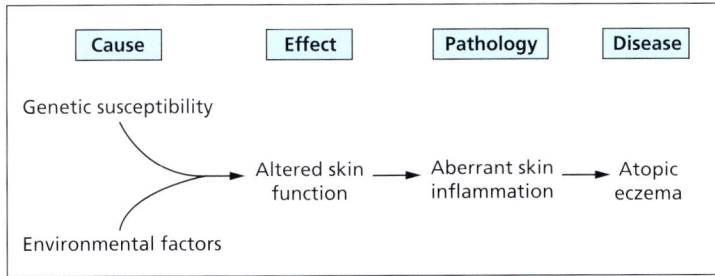

Figure 41.1 Schematic of the pathophysiology of atopic eczema.

eczema/dermatitis' [14]. Based on this, the World Allergy Organization suggested that 'eczema' should be used as an umbrella term and subdivided it into atopic eczema and non-atopic eczema [15]. However, this definition did not achieve international consensus. Here, we use the term 'atopic eczema' in keeping with the latest ICD-11 nomenclature.

Diagnostic criteria

Hanifin and Rajka [16] proposed major and minor diagnostic criteria based on their clinical experience. These criteria allow a uniformity of diagnosis for hospital-based and experimental studies but were considered not helpful for population-based studies [17]. Consequently, Williams coordinated a UK working party to refine the criteria of Hanifin and Rajka into a repeatable and validated set of diagnostic criteria for atopic eczema which were shown to have an 80% positive predictive value and 97% negative predictive value in UK populations [18,19] (Box 41.2). These diagnostic guidelines appear to be valid for adults, children and non-white ethnic groups suffering from atopic eczema [20], and have been validated in various population settings, including in skin of colour. They were primarily developed for epidemiological studies and, of necessity, exclude some signs that could be useful for diagnosis in individuals but are not common enough for use when assessing large populations. More recently, other modifications of the diagnostic criteria have been proposed, but these have been less rigorously validated [21,22].

Epidemiology

Prevalence across the life course

Some of the most valuable atopic eczema prevalence and trend data have come from the International Study of Asthma and Allergies in Childhood (ISAAC) [23–26]. With close to two million children from 106 countries, ISAAC is the biggest and only allergy study that has taken a truly global approach. These data showed that prevalence varied greatly between geographical settings; for instance, from fewer than 2% in Iran to over 16% in Japan for those aged 6–7 years. In addition, a systematic review of 69 cross-sectional and cohort studies has confirmed that atopic eczema is now a worldwide phenomenon with life-time atopic eczema prevalence of well over 20% in many affluent country settings [27]. There is also good evidence for an increase in prevalence in low-income countries, in particular in Africa and East Asia [27]. The Global Burden of Disease (GBD) project showed similar prevalence

patterns recently, not just for children but also in adult populations. Apart from the well-established overall high prevalence of atopic eczema in children and young adults, the GBD project also found a gradual increase in the prevalence of atopic eczema in middle aged and older adults (Figure 41.2) [28]. This may be due to a gradual decline in the hydrophilic properties of the skin barrier in older age. These observations are also consistent with reports from large population-based studies in the UK and the USA, suggesting that adult atopic eczema may be more common than previously believed, and likely includes both persisting or recurring disease from childhood and new-onset adult disease [29–31]. Further research is required to better characterise adult atopic eczema.

Disease severity

In public health terms, the severity distribution of atopic eczema is more significant than its total prevalence (which may include many mild asymptomatic cases), as severity is likely to determine those who use, or need to use, available health services. Few studies have rigorously examined the severity distribution of atopic eczema in the community, but indications are that severe cases are unusual, affecting fewer than 5% of total cases [29,32,33]. Even for those with moderate-to-severe disease who receive treatment with systemic immunosuppressants, a strong negative effect of atopic eczema on quality of life remains [34,35].

Age and sex

In the majority of cases, atopic eczema starts during infancy (usually younger than 2 years of age) [18], although age of onset might be later, even into adulthood [35,36]. Minor sex differences, with a slightly higher prevalence among females, have been noted previously, but this is not a consistent finding [29,37].

Morbidity and cost

According to GBD data, atopic eczema is the skin disease with the highest burden in terms of disability adjusted life years (DALY) among all skin diseases, ranking 25th among all diseases [38]. Cases of atopic eczema often achieve the highest morbidity scores on generic disability measures when compared with other skin diseases, and the health state utilities of severe atopic eczema are comparable to rheumatoid arthritis and multiple sclerosis [38]. Furthermore, impairment of quality of life appears to be directly related to the severity of atopic eczema [39]. The psychological morbidity associated with a lifetime of scratching, sleep loss and the stigma of a visible skin disease can also affect families to a considerable degree, and there are significant associations with attention-deficit-hyperactivity disorder, anxiety and depression [40–42]. These associations are more pronounced with more severe disease, also including suicidality [43].

Assessing the economic burden of atopic eczema is complex as it consists of costs for medical care and non-medical care and indirect costs (e.g. loss of education and workdays). The degree to which medical costs are an individual (out-of-pocket) burden or a collective one depends largely on the health care system. This diversity is reflected in the studies on this subject. Firstly, two studies from the USA reported direct and indirect costs totalling about USD 3300 per person per year (PPPY) for children and adults in 2013 [44,45]. Three European studies reported out-of-pocket costs for medical care as

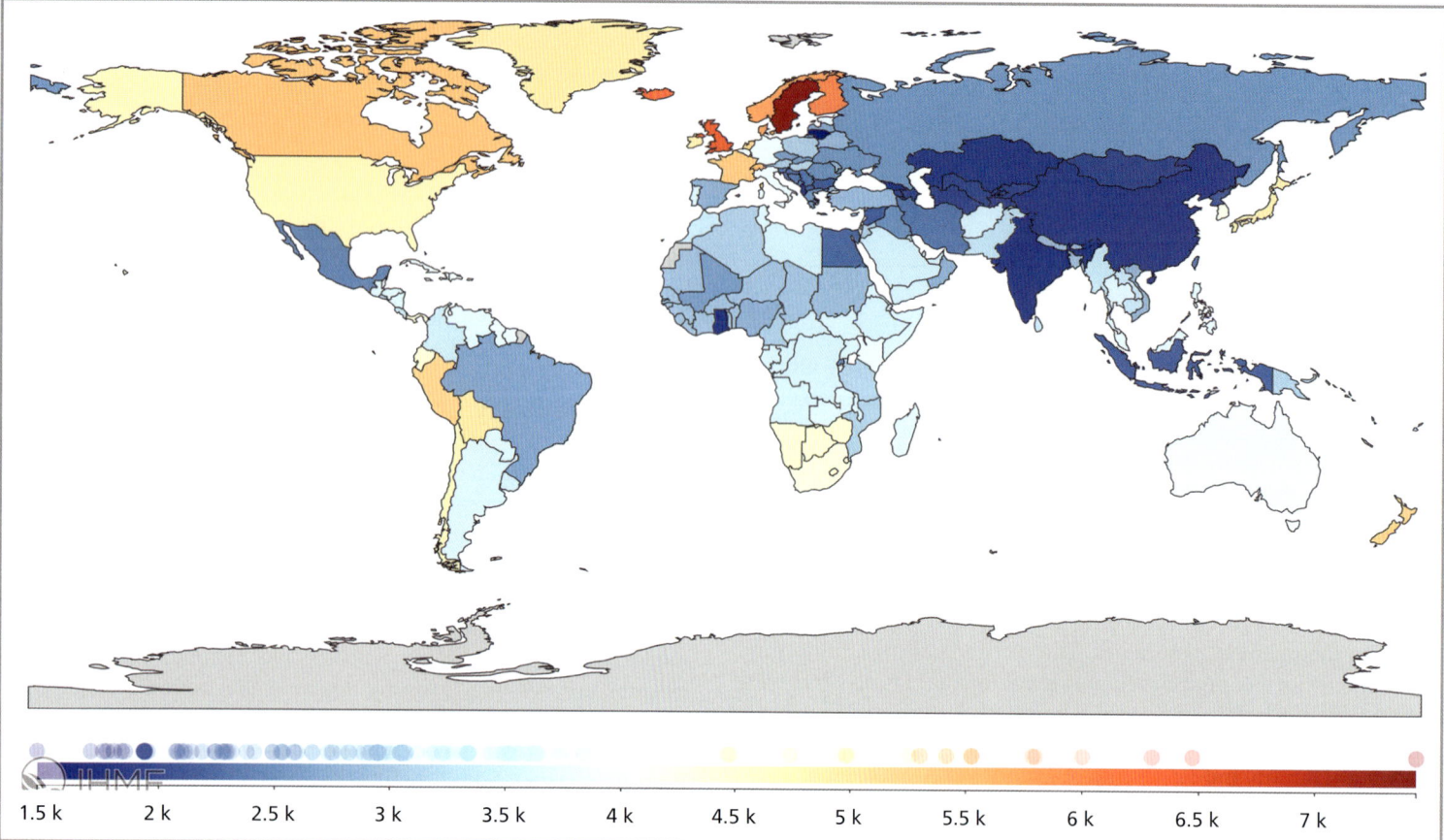

Figure 41.2 The global age-standardised prevalence of atopic dermatitis in all individuals per 100 000 persons. Blue areas indicate low prevalence and red areas indicate high prevalence. Source: Global Burden of Disease project 2017 data, Institute for Health Metrics and Evaluation, University of Washington, Seattle, WA, USA. Reproduced from Laughter *et al.* (2021) [28].

USD 1500 PPPY for Italian children (2016), €351 for French adults (2018) and €927 for adults with moderate-to-severe atopic eczema in nine European countries (2018) [46–48]. In the latter study, German patients' costs were higher for atopic eczema than for psoriasis and rheumatoid arthritis (€941, €224 and €628, respectively). Similar cost estimates have been published for Singapore, the Asia Pacific region, Thailand, South Korea and Vietnam [49,50]. Understandably, cost increases with disease severity.

What can we learn from prevalence surveys?

Population-based surveys show significant atopic eczema prevalence differences not only between but also within countries, suggesting environmental rather than genetic factors as the main drivers of changes in disease burden [51] (Figure 41.2). Significant changes in the burden of disease over short periods of time, such as observed before-and-after German reunification, offer opportunities to detect environmental risk factors. While the incidence of atopic eczema was stable among pre-schoolchildren in West Germany after the country's reunification, East Germany saw a more than doubling in the number of newly diagnosed atopic eczema cases in children up to the age of 6 years from 9.6% in 1991 to 23.4% in 1997 [52]. Similar observations can be made in association with urbanisation in developing countries and by studying migrant populations, who move from regions of low to high disease prevalence, typically adopting the atopic eczema risk of their new environment.

Such changes in disease risk identified by standardised methodology and diagnostic criteria have been attributed to the adoption of a 'western' lifestyle [51]. However, the precise lifestyle and other environmental ingredients that are responsible remain to be determined.

Pathophysiology

Atopic eczema is a complex disorder, reflecting interplay between genetics, epigenetic factors and the environment, including the skin microbiome. These disease drivers coalesce to result in aberrant epithelial barrier formation and dysregulated immunity in the skin giving rise to cutaneous inflammation. In turn, atopic inflammatory processes can alter epidermal function, indicating that epidermal barrier function and the cutaneous immune system regulate each other. By better understanding the mechanistic pathways in individual patients, we will be better placed to stratify therapies to disease endotypes [53]. Key pathways are summarised in Figure 41.3.

Genetic influence

The importance of genetic factors in determining the expression of the atopic phenotype is reflected in data from twin studies. Thus, monozygotic twins have a concordance rate of 0.72, whereas dizygotic twins have a concordance rate of only 0.23 [54–56]. These

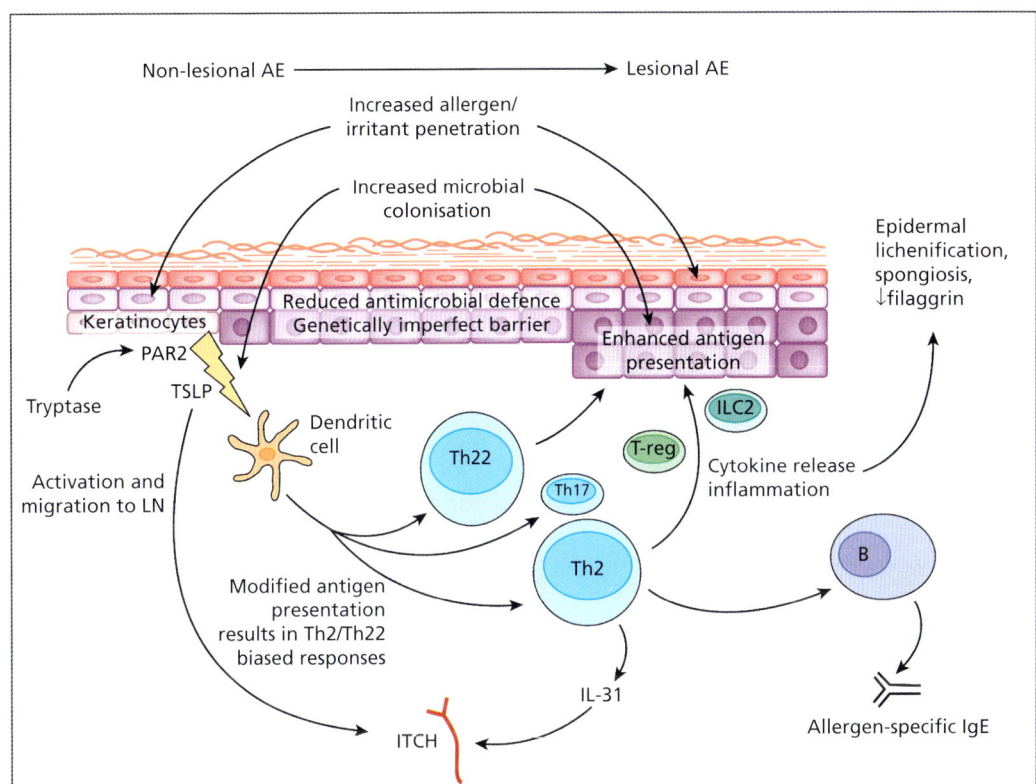

Figure 41.3 Pathophysiology of atopic eczema (AE). LN, lymph node; TSLP, thymic stromal lymphopoietin.

findings have been further validated by a more recent systematic review of 35 155 twin pairs and suggest overall heritability to be approximately 75% [57]. Therefore, although an undoubted central genetic effect is clear, it is important to consider that one quarter of cases have strong environmental factors significant in causality.

Genome-wide association studies (GWAS) compare cohorts of individuals with disease to control populations. These studies utilise DNA chip analysis to compare up to 2.4 million single nucleotide polymorphisms (SNP) and associate SNP allele frequencies with disease status. To date GWAS have identified 25 loci of relevance, but cumulatively these only account for 20% of the heritability of atopic eczema [58], suggesting that there is much left to discover. Of these loci, most have not been fully characterised to define the functional genetic effect. However, the regions contain genes implicated in immunity and skin barrier formation. The immune-related genes regulate T-cell activation and type 2 differentiation, perhaps suggesting that there is genetic regulation of the 'predisposition' to type 2 cytokines, rather than excessive 'normal' immune activation along the type 2 cytokine pathway.

To address the gap in heritability and discovery by GWAS, recent approaches have begun to utilise whole genome and whole exome sequencing to identify rare genetic variants. To date the cohorts studied have been small and have replicated the gene encoding filaggrin (FLG) as well as identifying new genes [59,60], but as cost reduces, it is expected that this approach will provide increasingly important data.

Filaggrin genetics and the epidermal barrier in atopic eczema

In individuals without atopic eczema who have no skin barrier defect, there is full integrity of the epidermis, marked by minimal transepidermal water loss (TEWL) and adequate protection against microbes and environmental allergens. Data demonstrating skin barrier function is defective in lesional > non-lesional atopic eczema > controls [61,62] and that impaired barrier function parallels disease severity [63] support the view that the skin barrier is critical in pathogenesis of the disease. A landmark paper in 2006 identified the association of loss-of-function variants of FLG in approximately 50% of severe atopic eczema, thus underlining the critical role of the epidermal barrier in pathogenesis [64]. Filaggrin is encoded within the epidermal differentiation complex (EDC) on 1q21, which comprises a large number of diverse proteins critical for skin barrier formation including loricrin, involucrin and S100 proteins. Profilaggrin, made up of 10–12 repeats of filaggrin monomers, is expressed in keratinocytes where it makes up the dominant component of keratohyalin granules in the stratum granulosum. All atopic eczema associated FLG mutations reported to date are nonsense mutations which insert a premature stop codon or frameshift resulting in absent or reduced profilaggrin and subsequently filaggrin expression. The keratinocyte undergoes terminal differentiation to form the stratum corneum, during which dephosphorylation of profilaggrin is followed by cleavage with matriptase and other proteases [65]. This process requires inhibition of LEKTI, a serine protease inhibitor expressed at epithelial and mucosal surfaces and frees filaggrin monomers which bind and aggregate keratin bundles and intermediate filaments to form the cellular scaffold in corneocytes and squames. Mutations in SPINK5, which encodes LEKTI, determine Netherton syndrome, and variants in the gene have also been associated with atopic eczema [66–68]. Metabolism of filaggrin monomers, higher in the stratum corneum, releases component amino acids that have been reported to contribute to epidermal water retention through their hygroscopic properties ('natural moisturising factor'). Further reduction of the histidine-rich protein to trans-urocanic acid and pyrrolidone-5-carboxylic acid (PCA) is important in maintaining the epidermal pH gradient [69]. At least 20 *FLG* variants have been identified in European populations, but two (R501X and 2282del4) account for 80% of all *FLG* alleles and are present in 7–10% of the population [69]. In Asian populations a different repertoire of *FLG* variants exists. The clinical phenotype of *FLG* loss-of-function variants is described in Table 41.1.

The risk of *FLG* mutation status on atopic eczema can be gleaned from the estimated 30% of ichthyosis vulgaris individuals who suffer concomitant atopic eczema. Genetic studies have shown that this equates to an odds ratio (OR) for homozygous mutations or compound heterozygote cases of 85.9 (20.1–367.6) [70]. Indeed, more than 30 studies have replicated the association between *FLG* mutations and atopic eczema. The majority of these have been case–control studies where cases have been recruited from dermatology outpatients and therefore generally more severe disease. Meta-analyses estimate an overall allelic risk (increased risk of atopic eczema for those carrying one *FLG* mutation and one wild-type gene) of 3.39–4.78 [71,72]. However, family studies and population-based studies that are more likely to indicate the background risk of atopic eczema from a *FLG* null allele show an odds ratio of 1.99–2.19 [71,72]. A meta-analysis, pooling data from high risk and low risk cohorts, has suggested that 20% of individuals with atopic eczema carry *FLG* mutations [71] and in those with heterozygote filaggrin mutations, atopic eczema only develops in approximately 42% of cases [73]. Therefore, although the strong association with atopic eczema and *FLG* variants is unprecedented for complex diseases, there remains a significant genetic component of atopic eczema associated with other genes, which is likely to reflect complex interactions between multiple common variants.

FLG variants also confer a risk of asthma and peanut allergy but only in the context of atopic eczema [74–76] and sensitisation to food allergens in infancy in association with *FLG* mutations has been shown to predict childhood asthma [77]. In addition to atopic eczema, *FLG* deficiency has been reported to confer a risk of eczema herpeticum [78].

Proteomic approaches to identify the protein signature of atopic eczema skin have been limited but have shown evidence of reduced expression of epidermal barrier proteins including S100/A11 [79], reduced tight junction proteins including Claudin 1 and 23 [80], and increased inflammatory proteins related to dendritic cell markers and T-cell activation [81]. Knockdown and proteomic studies in an epidermal equivalent model indicated that filaggrin deficiency in the absence of inflammation was sufficient to alter the expression level of proteins relevant to atopic eczema pathogenesis, including kallikrein 7 and cyclophilin A [82]. Recent studies have suggested that tape strip approaches to sample the skin non-invasively offer a useful approach for future proteomic studies in atopic eczema [83].

Lipids

It has been recognised for many years that reduced extracellular lipids and impaired ceramide production are characteristic of atopic eczema epidermal barrier defects. Increased activity of serine proteases in the epidermis is analogous to what is seen in Netherton syndrome [84]. Recent work comparing body sites in atopic eczema

and controls has shown that body sites regulate skin lipid profile, and that there are differences in individuals with atopic eczema including higher levels of ceramide species [85]. Early findings have suggested that these differences may be exacerbated by *FLG* mutations.

Environmental risk and protective factors
Climate

One potential explanation for prevalence differences between populations is climate – an area that has received little attention with regard to atopic eczema. Based on the ISAAC Phase One data set, an ecological analysis was conducted using information on long-term climatic conditions in the different study areas from the World Weather Guide [86]. Variables that were examined included latitude, altitude, average outdoor temperature and relative outdoor humidity. The results, which were adjusted for countries' gross national per capita income (GNP), suggest that symptoms of atopic eczema correlate positively with latitude and negatively with annual outdoor temperature but none of the other factors. These findings have been supported by cross-sectional studies in Spain [87] and Taiwan [88] and could be due to direct climatic influences, especially UV radiation exposure, as also suggested by a recent ecological analysis in a US cohort [89,90]. UV radiation has a well-established immuno-suppressive effect [91], partly because it facilitates the conversion of the skin barrier filaggrin (*FLG*) breakdown product trans-urocanic acid into the immuno-suppressive cis-urocanic acid isoform [92] and is an effective therapy for atopic eczema.

Research that has looked at flare factors in established atopic eczema supports this notion, as lower outdoor temperatures, especially in combination with skin irritants, can contribute to disease worsening, whereas indoor conditions seem less important [93,94]. However, the relationship between outdoor climate and disease flares is complex with some children reporting worsening in summer and others in winter, as shown in a small longitudinal study among German children [95]. The effects of outdoor temperature, UV radiation and humidity as well as seasonal changes in pollen counts are likely to interact, and further studies, which also take skin barrier function, *FLG* status and hydration status as well as bacterial skin colonisation into account, are required. Shifts in atopic eczema prevalence through climate change, in particular the interaction between UV radiation, air pollution, outdoor temperature, humidity and pollen count, are expected and will be an important area for future research [96].

Urban vs rural living

Another important place for epidemiological investigations are areas where people of a similar ethnic makeup and genetic background show significant prevalence differences within close geographical proximity [97]. A systematic review of 26 studies showed good evidence of higher disease burdens in cities compared with the countryside, and this was particularly the case in less affluent settings [98]. Where an attempt has been made to identify responsible environmental risk factors linked to urbanisation, differences in hygiene-related exposures (parasitic, bacterial and viral infections, vaccination, antibiotics and farm environment), environmental pollution, including smoking, allergen exposure and sensitisation, diet, and infant feeding practices have received particular attention.

Diet

Given how uncommon atopic eczema and other allergies still are in most developing nations, an important question is whether consumption of a 'western' affluent diet (i.e. high intake of refined grains, cured and red meats, as well as saturated and unsaturated fatty acids) leads to an increase in atopic eczema risk. This was explored in ISAAC Phase Three and a consistent protective effect was found between frequent consumption of fresh fruits (1–2×/week) and atopic eczema risk (adjusted OR = 0.81, 0.67–0.97), whereas the opposite was true for fast food consumption (≥3×/week, adjusted OR = 1.70, 1.48–1.95) [99]. An ecological analysis based on the ISAAC data set came to similar conclusions, showing a consistent inverse association between atopic eczema prevalence and per capita consumption of vegetables, protein from cereal and nuts, as well as all fresh and frozen fish, even after adjustment for GNP [100].

The latter finding is supported by a number of longitudinal studies that suggested a high fish intake during pregnancy lowers atopic eczema risk in the offspring up to 5 years of age by 25–43% [101,102]. Similar risk reductions have been described in children with a high fish intake during late infancy [103,104]. These results have been attributed to fish being rich in anti-inflammatory n-3 polyunsaturated fatty acids (n-3 PUFA). Western diets have become low in n-3 PUFAs over past decades with a corresponding increase in pro-inflammatory n-6 PUFA, such as linoleic acid [105,106].

A Cochrane systematic review of the benefit of maternal dietary interventions during pregnancy or lactation concluded that during pregnancy there was a low likelihood of any dietary intervention reducing the risk of the child's development of atopic diseases but that there was evidence that this was associated with adverse outcomes on maternal or fetal nutrition or both. Similarly, during breastfeeding, no strong evidence supports the role of dietary modification to lower the risk of atopic eczema or allergic sensitisation [107]. Similarly, no role for dietary supplements for established atopic eczema has been shown [51].

Breastfeeding and delayed weaning

Breastfeeding has been advocated as a way of preventing allergies, including atopic eczema. For instance, the World Health Organization (WHO) recommends that babies are exclusively breastfed for 6 months, and most European ministries of health advocate at least 4 months of exclusive breastfeeding to aid allergy prevention [108]. It is therefore conceivable that differences in the length of breastfeeding and the age infants are weaned onto solids could explain part of the atopic eczema prevalence differences between study populations. However, data from cross-sectional studies in developed and developing countries, including 51 119 schoolchildren in ISAAC Phase Two, offer little support for this notion [25]. Furthermore, a meta-analysis of 27 prospective cohort study populations failed to show a statistically significant benefit with exclusive breastfeeding (pooled OR = 0.89, 0.76–1.04) [109]. However, the promotion of breastfeeding, as opposed to exclusive breastfeeding, does appear to have a protective effect into adolescence [110,111].

Obesity and physical exercise

Increasing numbers of children in affluent settings are overweight. Three studies, including a UK cohort study and a substantial worldwide series of cross-sectional surveys based on the ISAAC Phase Three data set, found an association with obesity for all atopic eczema (OR = 1.42, 1.23–1.64) and severe atopic eczema (OR= 1.94, 1.52–2.46) at 13–14 years, while no association was detected in a number of other cross-sectional studies [112–116]. The ISAAC analysis also examined the effect of TV viewing (≥5 h), which showed a positive relationship with atopic eczema risk (OR = 1.16, 1.06–1.28), and this was stronger in obese vs overweight vs normal/underweight children in a dose-response fashion [117]. It remains unclear whether the positive associations seen are causal, for instance due to inflammation mediated by adipokines such as leptin, or related to dietary factors, which could facilitate atopic eczema through oxidative stress pathways, as diets excluding antioxidant food, such as fruits and vegetables, are related to increased obesity and atopic eczema.

Pollution and tobacco smoke

A population-based cross-sectional survey among more than 300 000 Taiwanese schoolchildren with sophisticated, objective measurement of traffic-related air pollutants, including nitrogen oxides (NO_2) and carbon monoxide (CO), suggested that air pollution may contribute to atopic eczema risk, but this association, albeit statistically significant, was weak (OR = 1.12, 1.04–1.22) [88]. Similarly, a cohort study among 3000 schoolchildren in West Germany with repeat objective pollutant measurements reported that NO_2 exposure was positively associated with physician-diagnosed atopic eczema at age 6 years (OR = 1.18, 1.00–1.39) [118]. Furthermore, a French cross-sectional survey among more than 5000 schoolchildren in six cities showed a stronger positive relationship with fine particle pollution (OR = 2.51, 2.06–3.06) [119]. Other work has shown similar positive associations with measures of outdoor pollution [118,120]. There is less evidence that atopic eczema risk in the offspring increases in association with maternal smoking during pregnancy or environmental tobacco exposure postnatally [121–125].

The Hygiene Hypothesis

The notion that microbial exposure might influence the development of atopic eczema originally stemmed from the observation that disease risk is inversely related to sibship size, an effect that has been observed in many different settings, since the original description in a large UK birth cohort in the late 1980s [126,127,**128**,129,130]. There have been two systematic reviews on microbial exposure and atopic eczema risk [131,132]. Individual risk factors, including pets and farm animals because of their potential link with endotoxin exposure, are briefly discussed below.

Basic hygiene

One large birth cohort study (n >10 000), the Avon Longitudinal Study of Parents and Children (ALSPAC), has examined the question whether general hygiene measures at age 15 months, such as frequency of washing and use of household cleaners and wet wipes, are weakly associated with atopic eczema between 2.5–3.5 years of age, and a proportional increase in disease risk was found per increase in hygiene score (adjusted OR = 1.04, 95% CI 1.01–1.07) [133]. However, a Japanese cohort with 865 mother–infant pairs found an inverse relationship between a daily bath or shower vs washing less frequently (adjusted OR = 0.26, 0.10–0.77) [134]. None of these studies took potential gene–environment interactions between hygiene practices, skin barrier gene mutation inheritance and skin barrier (dys)function into account, and microbial exposures were not measured objectively.

Day care

There is consistent evidence that day care attendance is associated with increased microbial exposure, in particular respiratory tract infections, and there are some cohort studies that have reported a reduction in atopic eczema risk in children attending day care facilities during the first year of life [135–137]. However, others have found the opposite effect [138–140], and day care attendance in the first 2 years of life has been identified as the main risk factor to explain the atopic eczema prevalence gradient between East and West Germany [140].

Farm environment and animals

The influence of farm environments and animals have also been extensively studied but no convincing protective effect of living on a farm has been found *per se* [141–146]. Interestingly, consumption of unpasteurised farm milk during the first 2 years of life is an independent protective factor against atopic eczema development [144,145], even in non-farming families [147]. This inverse relationship is independent of a family history of allergic disease. Once the raw cow's milk is boiled, the protective effect is lost. The mechanism for these properties of unpasteurised farm milk remains uncertain and could either be related to microbial contamination or other constituents of unprocessed cow's milk [147–149]. In addition, direct contact with farm animals reduces atopic eczema risk in early life in some settings [150], especially where mothers have regular *direct* contact with farm animals during pregnancy, and this protective effect appears even stronger in those who are exposed both pre- and postnatally [150,151], suggesting that perinatal priming of the immune system may be of particular importance.

Pets

Like farm animals, pets have been implicated as potentially protective against atopic eczema. A meta-analysis of studies revealed an almost uniform protective effect of dog exposure (pooled OR = 0.61, 0.50–0.74), especially where this occurred in early life [152]. The picture is less clear for cats. Although the same meta-analysis showed a protective effect (pooled OR = 0.83, 0.74–0.95), study heterogeneity was significant. It is interesting to note that where *FLG* skin barrier mutation inheritance was taken into account, there was a significantly higher risk of atopic eczema in those with *FLG* mutations compared with wild-type children, suggesting that cat sensitisation can be facilitated by an impaired skin barrier and then contribute to atopic eczema risk [153–155].

Endotoxin exposure

Some have argued that the risk reduction seen with farm animal and pet exposure, in particular during pregnancy, is due to endotoxins, a group of lipopolysaccharides found on the cell surface of Gram-negative bacteria, not least because endotoxins are known to be inducers of interleukin (IL)-10 and interferon (INF)-gamma [156]. Birth cohort studies have suggested an up to 50% reduction in atopic eczema risk associated with endotoxin exposure [132]. However, this effect tended to be confined to high endotoxin exposure levels [25].

Helminth parasites

Helminth parasites, such as hookworm and *Ascaris lumbricoides*, are potential candidates to explain prevalence gradients between rural and urban areas of tropical developing countries, where such infections remain endemic in the countryside but become rare, once the life cycle of the parasite is interrupted due to improved hygiene. There is some support for this from cross-sectional studies, but the relationship between helminth parasites and the effect on the immune system of their human hosts is rather complex and depends on the type and burden of the parasite (host invasive helminths and a higher parasite burden have a stronger immuno-modulatory effect) as well as the timing of infection, especially if this occurs in early life or during pregnancy [157]. The strongest evidence for a protective effect of helminth infections on the risk of atopic eczema comes from a double-blind randomised controlled trial with deworming therapy conducted among >2500 pregnant mothers during the last trimester of pregnancy in a helminth-endemic area in Uganda, which found an approximately two-times increased atopic eczema risk up to 1 year of age in the intervention groups [158]. Interestingly, loss of helminth exposure does not appear to affect atopic eczema risk later in life [159,160], further supporting the notion that perinatal priming of the immune system can provide protection against atopic eczema [157].

Childhood infections and vaccinations

The protective effect of parasitic infections does not apply to childhood vaccinations, including the BCG vaccine, or common viral and bacterial infections, which are the common infection-related exposures in affluent settings [106]. As for antenatal infections, a British historical cohort study, using a general practitioner research database, examined the effect of infections during pregnancy on atopic eczema in the offspring and found a small increase in risk associated with two or more antenatal infections (adjusted HR = 1.16, 95% CI 1.07–1.26) [161]. However, a more recent analysis based on historical data on acute viral respiratory infection notifications in former Eastern Germany suggested the opposite: a reduction in atopic eczema risk associated with exposure to prenatal viral respiratory infections. This effect was particularly strong for exposures during the last trimester (adjusted HR = 0.70, 0.52–0.95) and extended into the postnatal period up to 7 months of age [162], but this finding has not been replicated in a number of more recent cohorts from New Zealand, the Netherlands and Germany, which found either positive or no association between infections in early life and subsequent development of atopic eczema [132].

Where specific viral and bacterial childhood infections, such as chickenpox, mumps, whooping cough and measles, have been examined, the majority of studies have shown either positive or no associations, although a US case–control study suggested a 50% risk reduction with parent-reported chickenpox infection that occurred between 0 and 8 years of age (adjusted OR = 0.57, 0.34–0.96);

this effect was particularly strong for children with moderate to severe atopic eczema and was associated with a reduced risk of allergic sensitisation [25]. However, these studies typically rely on parent-reported exposures, rarely take vaccination history into account and also tend to ignore concomitant antibiotic prescribing as an important confounding factor.

Antibiotics

Schmitt *et al.* examined the complex relationship between respiratory, gastrointestinal and ear infections, as well as antibiotic prescribing and atopic eczema risk and found that it was the antibiotics that seemed causally linked to an increased risk of developing atopic eczema rather than the infections themselves [163]. A recent systematic search identified 17 studies on the association between postnatal antibiotic exposure and the development of atopic eczema in the offspring and found an overall risk increase of 41% in those who received at least one course of antibiotics in early life (pooled OR = 1.41, 1.30–1.53) [164]. This association remained significant when only longitudinal studies (*n* = 10) were taken into account (pooled OR = 1.40, 1.19–1.64). There was also a significant dose-response association, suggesting a 7% risk increase in atopic eczema risk with each additional antibiotic course (pooled OR = 1.07, 1.02–1.11), an effect that was particularly strong for broad spectrum antibiotics vs penicillins. It is possible that the risk increase associated with antibiotics is due to changes in the host microbiota, leading to an altered development of the infant's immune system or enhanced immune responses to environmental allergens.

The microbiome of the gut and skin

There is some evidence using conventional culture-based techniques that the early gut microflora of children who later develop atopic eczema has more *Staphylococcus aureus* and coliforms and fewer lactobacilli and bifidobacteria [165]. However, culture-based methods miss around 80% of human bacteria compared with culture-independent approaches (e.g. next generation pyrosequencing) that study bacterial DNA directly and these new technologies promise a deeper understanding of the interactions between the host microbiome of the gut, the skin, the respiratory tract and the immune system.

Having been sterile *in utero*, the infant's skin, gut and respiratory tract quickly become colonised with a broad range of bacterial species postnatally. It is not surprising that environmental factors, such as mode of delivery and feeding practices (breastfeeding vs formula milk and time of weaning), influence the host microbiota in the immediate postnatal period [166]. In addition, exposure to antibiotics alters the natural balance of the host bacterial communities and encourages the emergence of 'nosocomial' species, such as certain types of staphylococci. It is well established that *S. aureus* is a major cause of skin infection, disease exacerbation and chronicity in atopic eczema [167,168]. There is also evidence from animal models to support the role of the skin microbiota in the (dys)regulation of the cutaneous immune system [169]. Next generation sequencing has confirmed the cross-sectional association between atopic eczema and *S. aureus* colonisation. Disease flares are associated with a significant fall in skin microbiota diversity and an increase in the relative abundance of *S. aureus*. Interestingly, *S. aureus* elimination does not appear to be the main reason why atopic eczema improves after

a flare, and antimicrobial and anti-inflammatory therapy enhances bacterial diversity. Early-life colonisation with commensal staphylococci is associated with a lower risk of developing atopic eczema [170]. At the gut interface, there is an association between low diversity of the infant gut microbiota in early life and an increase in atopic eczema risk during infancy, especially in high-risk children [171]. The main environmental risk factor impacting the gut microbiota in early life is mode of delivery, with caesarean section being associated with a reduced abundance of bacterial flora as well as a higher risk of developing atopic eczema. Increased relative abundance of *Clostridium sensu stricto* at 3 months was associated with the presence of atopic eczema on examination at ages 3 and 12 months in a UK study [172].

Immune dysregulation

A variety of primary immune deficiencies including Wiskott–Aldrich syndrome, hyper IgE (Job) syndrome and Omenn syndrome give rise to eczematous lesions, which suggests that immunological dysfunction alone can result in cutaneous inflammation typical of atopic eczema. However, individuals with atopic eczema are not systemically immunocompromised and show balanced profiles of immunological subsets in blood as compared with controls [**173**–175]. Furthermore, atopic eczema patients can make appropriate responses to systemic infection and vaccination [176] and do not suffer increased mortality. Thus, it seems most likely that any immunological dysfunction is confined to the skin and this deduction is borne out by detailed investigations as described below.

Biopsy of developing lesions of atopic eczema reveals that T cells infiltrate the skin early in the disease process [177,178]. The cellular infiltrate in early lesional atopic eczema is comprised predominantly of T lymphocytes (CD4+:CD8+ ratio = 7 : 1) but eosinophils are also present, albeit at lower frequencies [179,180]. The immunological bias towards type 2 cytokine responses (IL-4, -5 and -13) in atopic eczema is well established in early lesional atopic eczema skin as compared with non-lesional or control skin [181,182]. The cytokine profiles in atopic eczema at least partly explain the pathology of the disease: IL-4 and IL-13 downregulate filaggrin expression in keratinocytes thereby inducing further epidermal barrier disruption [183]. Furthermore, IL-4 is known to downregulate expression of cutaneous defensins [184] and increase expression of bacterial adhesion molecules, both of which facilitate *S. aureus* colonisation [185,186].

Exposure of antigen through 'healthy' skin induces Th2 responses in atopic eczema but not in controls. Furthermore, Th2 polarisation is not dependent upon *FLG* mutations [**173**]. Thus, it seems that altered immune regulation in atopic eczema epidermis plays a key role in mediating Th2 responses critical to pathogenesis and that this is distinct from the role of filaggrin deficiency. It seems reasonable to surmise that a combination of both epidermal barrier disruption and altered epidermal immune function are required for the manifestation of the disease.

In chronic as opposed to acute atopic eczema lesions IL-5, granulocyte macrophage colony stimulating factor (GM-CSF), IL-12 and IFN-γ predominate. IL-5 and GM-CSF production are important in promoting the growth and survival of eosinophils and macrophages whereas IL-12 is important for the polarisation of IFN-γ producing

Th1 cells which induce keratinocyte apoptosis associated with epidermal spongiosis [187]. A Th17 signature is also present in chronic atopic eczema and is reduced in line with improvements in disease severity following treatment with ciclosporin [**188**]. IL-22 (from Th22 cells) is increasingly recognised as a key cytokine in atopic eczema pathology as it is detected at high levels in lesions of chronic disease and is known to enhance keratinocyte proliferation and reduce expression of antimicrobial proteins [189–192] as well as downregulate filaggrin expression [193]. Single cell transcriptomic studies showed enrichment of cytotoxic T cells expressing IL-13, IL-22 and IFN-γ (Tc IL13/IL22) in lesional atopic eczema skin and increased clonality of Tc IL13/IL22 cells [**194**]. Additionally, a shared macrophage programme (Mac-2) between fetal skin and atopic eczema was identified although similar changes were also found in psoriasis. Increased numbers of Mac-2+ cells in atopic eczema lesional skin were reduced 12 weeks into therapy with methotrexate in line with clinical response [**194**]. In view of the highly regulated mechanisms for activation of T cells through interaction between the T-cell receptor and its cognate MHC:peptide ligand, the precise pathway to T-cell activation in atopic eczema remains poorly understood. While antigen specificity to environmental allergens can be demonstrated and these interactions account for associated allergen specific IgE synthesis, T cells in the skin are polyclonal [**195**], and aero- or food allergen avoidance has been disappointing as a therapeutic option, suggesting that T-cell activation is not constrained to one or even a few antigens [196–198]. Additionally, there is no evidence of a primary abnormality in dendritic cell function, which would result in type 2 skewing of T-cell responses. Dendritic cells (DCs) in atopic eczema have a highly upregulated expression of the high affinity IgE receptor (FcεR1) [199,200] but this most likely reflects higher circulating levels of total IgE [199].

The long-standing consensus of the role of type 2 cytokines in atopic eczema has been recently validated by the development of anti-IL4Ra therapy (dupilumab), which is highly effective in approximately two-thirds of cases. Therefore, understanding the drivers of type 2 cytokine production offers the next therapeutic horizon. There is strong evidence that the keratinocyte derived IL-7-like cytokine thymic stromal lymphopoietin (TSLP) can directly induce neuronal triggering of itch [201] and also epidermal programming of cutaneous DCs, via increased expression of OX40, to induce the generation of inflammatory Th2 cells characterised by the co-production of TNF-α in addition to the classical Th2 cytokines [202]. Indeed, mice that have TSLP overexpressed in the epidermis spontaneously develop an inflammatory skin condition that resembles atopic eczema. Therefore, it seems that the epidermis is critical to regulation of Th2 responses. However, TSLP expression in non-lesional atopic eczema skin has been found to be normal, thus constitutive overactivity of this pathway is an unlikely primary dysfunction in the condition. Other important immune-related neurosignalling molecules critical to itch in eczema include IL-31, and inhibition of this with monoclonal antibody therapy has proven the importance of this pathway [203]. Histamine H1 and H4 receptors and TRPV1 (vanilloid receptor 1) channels also regulate itch in atopic eczema and although improvement in skin inflammation is minimal with H1 antihistamines, studies are underway to examine the potential to block H4.

Microbial responses

Patients with atopic eczema are particularly susceptible to certain cutaneous infections [204], the most common being *S. aureus*. However, human papillomavirus-induced warts, fungal infections, viruses (such as HSV1 and 2, vaccinia, coxsackie A and the pox virus of molluscum contagiosum) are also frequent pathogens causing, in some cases, severe complications.

Innate immunity is compromised in atopic eczema, as demonstrated by reductions in keratinocyte-derived antimicrobial peptides (cathelicidin LL-37, β-defensin 2 and β-defensin 3) [**205**,206–207], neutrophil chemoattractant IL-8 [206], and inducible nitric oxide synthetase (iNOS) [206], which mediates pathogen death through release of NO [208]. Further antimicrobial compromise occurs as a result of defective dermcidin-derived antimicrobial peptides, produced by eccrine glands [209]. Production of IgA, a key epithelial antimicrobial immunoglobulin, is also reduced in the sweat and tears of atopic eczema patients [210,211], which may help to explain the concordance between staphylococcal growth on both mucosal and skin surfaces in these patients.

Most individuals with atopic eczema have *S. aureus* identifiable on skin swabs, often at very high density, and more often present on lesional than non-lesional skin [212,213]. Furthermore, *S. aureus* present on the skin of atopics is significantly more likely to express superantigen than in non-atopics, and indeed the levels of superantigen expression correlate with disease severity [214–216]. In support of the role of superantigen, eczematous responses were found to be elicited by concomitant exposure of skin to staphylococcal superantigen and house dust mite allergen in humans in a patch test model. In contrast, either superantigen or allergen alone failed to induce positive reactions, suggesting a synergistic enhancement of allergen-specific responses by superantigen [217]. Further work has demonstrated that keratinocytes show enhanced allergen presentation to T cells following exposure to staphylococcal enterotoxin B (SEB)-stimulated peripheral blood mononuclear cells (PBMC) *in vitro* through upregulation of HLA class II and ICAM-1 expression [**218**], providing evidence of a potent adjuvant effect of staphylococcal products for human allergen-specific Th2 responses. Furthermore, staphylococcal superantigen has been documented to reduce regulatory T-cell activity in humans [219] and to confer T-cell steroid resistance [220], both of which may contribute to the association with more severe atopic eczema.

Herpes simplex virus poses an increased risk for individuals with atopic eczema and superficial dissemination on the skin known as 'Kaposi varicelliform eruption' or eczema herpeticum, which, although rare, has long been recognised as a complication more prevalent in people with atopic eczema. Interest in the genetic basis for eczema herpeticum has identified multiple risk genes including filaggrin (combined null mutation vs controls, OR = 10.1, 4.7–22.1; vs individuals with atopic eczema without eczema herpeticum OR = 2.2, 1.3–3.8) [78], TSLP [221], INF regulatory factor (IRF) 2 (OR 0.46–0.66) [222], INF-α receptor 1 [223] and INF-γ receptor 1 [223]. Further work, characterising gene expression (RNA sequencing) in immune cells in atopic eczema has shown a defect in type I and III IFNs mediated by IRF 3 and 7 inhibition [224].

Innate immune cells

The role of natural killer (NK), gamma delta (γδ) T cells and other innate immune cells has been of interest in atopic eczema research because of their potent ability to secrete cytokines including those classically associated with a type 2 cytokine profile. Previous work has suggested that type 1 cytokine secreting NK and γδ T cells in atopic eczema patients undergo selective apoptosis leading to a predisposition to type 2 cytokine skewing [225]. A subset of innate immune cells (nuocytes; innate lymphoid cells (ILCs)) have been shown to secrete type 2 cytokines (ILC2s) in atopic eczema and in human skin after allergen challenge in an IL-33 dependent manner, but that E-cadherin, which is expressed on keratinocytes and Langerhans cells, can bind receptors on the surface of the ILC2s resulting in downregulated cytokine secretion. These data suggest that downregulated E-cadherin expression as seen in atopic eczema and in models of filaggrin gene knock-down may be an important mechanism which licenses ILC2 type 2 cytokine production in the skin in the context of a defective epithelial barrier [226]. Observed reductions in ILC2 activity in allergic contact dermatitis may suggest that rather than purely activators of atopic inflammation, these cells may play a regulatory role in the skin [227].

IgE, allergy and the 'atopic march'

The term 'atopic march' describes the progression within an individual from atopic eczema to other atopic diseases including allergic rhinitis, food allergy and asthma. The association between atopic eczema and subsequent development of these conditions has been shown in multiple longitudinal studies [228–234]. Inter-relationships between atopic conditions have also been shown [235–238]. Whether this progression from atopic eczema to other atopic conditions is causal or reflects co-manifestation is the subject of significant debate. Indeed, some groups have challenged the impact of the atopic march, for instance finding in a longitudinal study of 9801 children that progression through atopic diseases only occurred in approximately 7% of cases [239]. Other reports have suggested that adjustment for early life wheeze and sensitisation abrogates the association between atopic eczema and asthma [240,241] while others found this nullified only asthma in girls [241] yet none of these studies controlled for filaggrin status [35]. Whether sensitisation should truly be considered a confounding factor is uncertain. However, it seems clear that in individuals with atopic eczema and sensitisation, there is an increased risk of asthma in childhood.

This observation has raised the intriguing possibility that sensitisation through the skin is critical for asthma pathogenesis and that the impaired skin barrier in atopic eczema is to blame. As a consequence, a number of studies have examined the potential to prevent atopic eczema by early use of emollients, but so far, these studies have shown no evidence that this approach reduces the risk of atopic eczema or allergic disorders [242,243].

Previous studies have associated total IgE, specific IgE and number of IgE mediated allergic reactivities with atopic eczema severity. Although not all cases of atopic eczema have high levels of IgE (intrinsic atopic dermatitis), identification of specific-IgE to environmental allergens beyond those from aeroallergens and foods may be extended by testing to microbes which colonise the skin and cutaneous autoantigens [244–246]. Both intrinsic and extrinsic atopic eczema demonstrate raised levels of circulating eosinophils [9]. This gives rise to the question: is there any meaningful difference between individuals with the same clinical phenotype (atopic eczema) who have raised levels of IgE as compared with those who do not? The answer to this question is currently unclear.

One possible explanation for the high levels of IgE is that production may be induced by *S. aureus* antigens [247]. Staphylococci colonise the skin of atopic eczema patients, and exotoxins with superantigen properties have been isolated from them and contribute to IgE production [**205**,248,249]. Some staphylococcal exotoxins are superantigens [250], which activate a greater number of lymphocytes than those stimulated by specific antigen, resulting in a 'superstimulation'.

Direct examination of the role of IgE in atopic eczema is illustrated through studies of omalizumab, anti-IgE, therapy that has been shown to be ineffective in its treatment [251]. This emphasises the consensus that IgE does not play a major role in atopic eczema pathogenesis. Therefore, allergic sensitisation is likely to be a secondary phenomenon in atopic eczema, which acts as an important trigger for disease flares and possibly disease chronicity but is not the primary defect. Hence, diagnostic tests to identify key allergens of relevance to disease flares are of limited clinical utility.

Food allergy

The prevalence of food allergy in atopic eczema varies with age and severity of the condition [252]. In a study of 4453 1-year-old children, 20% with atopic eczema were food allergic compared with 4% of those without (P <0.001) [253]. However, data for older children and adults are far fewer and less convincing. The prevalence of food allergy associated with atopic eczema has been estimated to be approximately 30–40% in unselected infants with the disease [254], but even in those confirmed as allergic by challenge testing, the benefit to atopic eczema of dietary avoidance is much lower [255]. Confusion often surrounds the nature of the reaction. Immediate urticarial reactions secondary to food, arising in an individual with atopic eczema, inevitably lead to a deterioration following increased scratching. Therefore, food allergen avoidance can be beneficial to atopic eczema in allergic individuals even if not 'curative'. Allergic responses to milk, egg, wheat, soy, peanut and fish account for 85% of reactions in this group [256,257]. Data from double-blind placebo-controlled food challenges have shown that more than 90% of food allergic reactions arise within 2 hours and are urticarial in nature, frequently involving concomitant gastrointestinal and respiratory reactions [256–258], while it seems that screening with skin prick tests has a reasonable negative predictive value for benefit from food avoidance. Indeed, screening for IgE to foods has been shown to have little utility in predicting onset of food allergy in atopic eczema [259].

It therefore seems possible that the eczematous inflammation in early onset eczema facilitates transcutaneous sensitisation through environmental exposure to food protein in house dust and through direct contact with food protein contaminated hands, for instance through moisturiser application [260,261]. This is currently an area of intensive research, as the prevention of atopic eczema and changes in skin care practices may well prevent the development of food allergy.

While it is important to take a good history looking for immediate and delayed type reactions to foods in infants and younger children and to perform allergy testing accordingly to identify potential foods that are contributing to disease flares and chronicity, routine implementation of exclusion diets is not advocated [197,198,262].

Allergic contact dermatitis

Allergic contact dermatitis (ACD) describes immune responses principally targeting chemicals applied directly to the skin. Although ACD is an important consideration (see later), and demonstrates clinical and histological similarities to atopic eczema, the immunophenotypes are distinct and there is no suggestion that in general atopic eczema reflects unidentified ACD.

Autoimmunity

Autoimmunity in atopic eczema is a relatively underexplored area of research in disease pathogenesis [263]. A variety of autoantigens have been characterised in atopic eczema as well as the presence of autoreactive T cells and IgE against autoallergens, which correlate with disease activity [245,264,265]. It has been suggested that scratching may release membranous and intracellular antigens from keratinocytes which result in Th2 responses and IgE targeting self-proteins. Whether autoreactivity is a primary disease mechanism or develops secondary to the chronic exposure to skin-derived antigens remains to be established. However, it is thought that once present, autoreactivity may contribute to the chronicity and severity of the dermatitis. A recent systematic review of this area estimated that autoreactivity, as defined by demonstration of the presence of IgE specific for self-proteins, is evident in 25% of atopic eczema and is associated with more severe disease [245].

Pruritus

The sensation of itch is central to atopic eczema. Non-histaminergic signalling is thought to be more relevant for chronic itch conditions. Protease activated receptor-2 (PAR2) has been shown to be overexpressed in atopic eczema skin [266] and this receptor, along with PAR4, have been implicated in itch triggered by mast cell tryptase, trypsin and thrombin [267] as well as TSLP release from keratinocytes [201]. Undoubtedly, pruritus is closely linked to the inflammatory component of atopic eczema as suggested by rapid resolution of itch with anti-inflammatory treatments such as ciclosporin and the novel biologics and selective janus kinase (JAK)

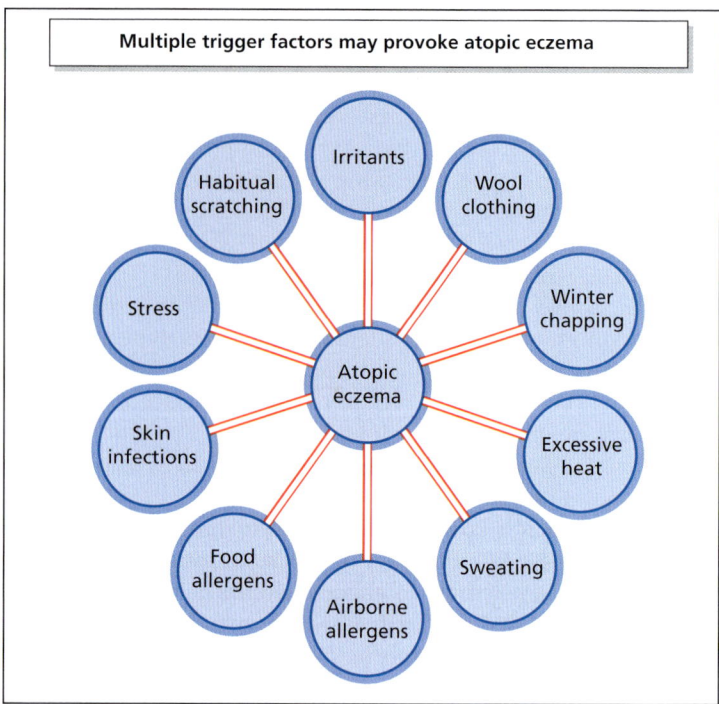

Figure 41.4 Trigger factors for atopic eczema.

inhibitors. Cytokines, such as TSLP and IL-31 are thought to be critical to the pathogenesis of itch in atopic eczema [201].

Overexpression of IL-31 in mice led to progressively worsening itch, excoriation and dermatitis [268–270], and in humans, levels of IL-31 correlate with disease severity [271]. The receptor for IL-31 is expressed by keratinocytes and infiltrating macrophages [272] and IL-31 expression is strongly induced by staphylococcal superantigen [273], thereby linking changes in the cutaneous microbiome with atopic eczema itch.

Clinical features

Important aspects to the history (Table 41.3)

The majority of patients with atopic eczema will present with symptoms in childhood, usually younger than 2 years of age and typically between 2 and 6 months, but it may start at any age, even within the first few weeks of life and during adulthood. The

Table 41.3 History at the initial assessment.

Atopic eczema history	Impact on quality of life (consider visual analogue scales)	Personal and family history of atopic disease	Trigger factors (Figure 41.4)
Age of onset	Patient's/carer's assessment of severity	Asthma	Exposure to irritants, e.g. bubble bath, etc.
Areas of skin affected	Sleep	Hay fever	Skin infections
Severity	Itch	Food allergies	Dry skin
Dietary history	Effects on family dynamic	–	Food allergens
Seasonal variation	–	–	Contact allergens
Response to previous treatment	–	–	Exposure to pets or animals
Current treatment	–	–	Air-borne allergens
Frequency of flares	–	–	
Frequency of skin infections	–	–	

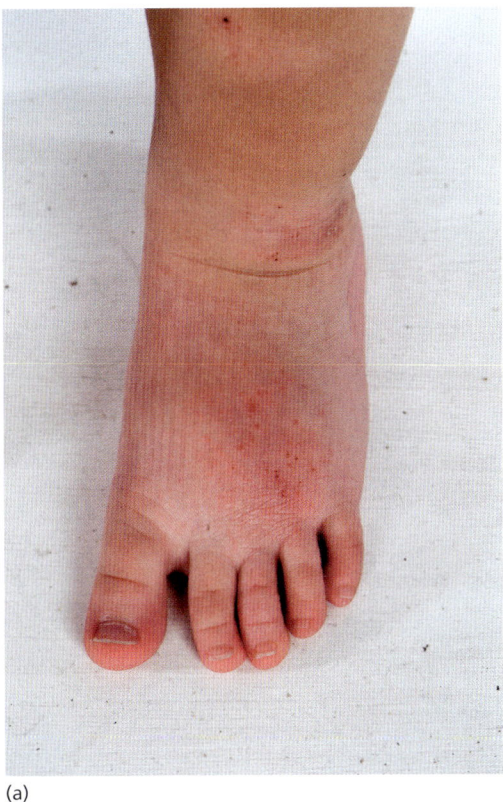

(a)

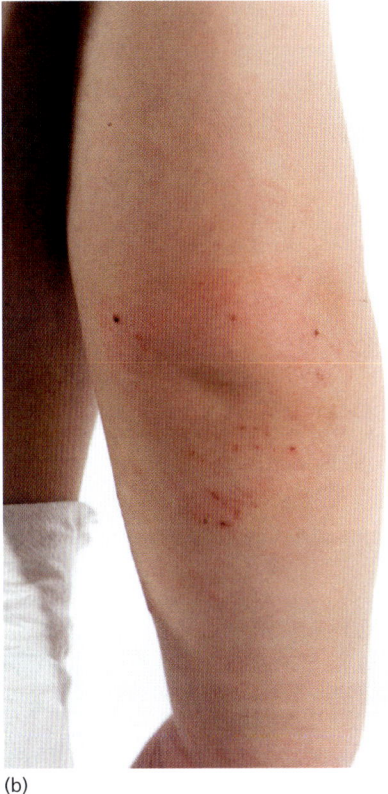

(b)

Figure 41.5 Active eczema and papulovesicules (a) adjacent to hypopigmentation and (b) Affecting extensor dermatitis in an infant.

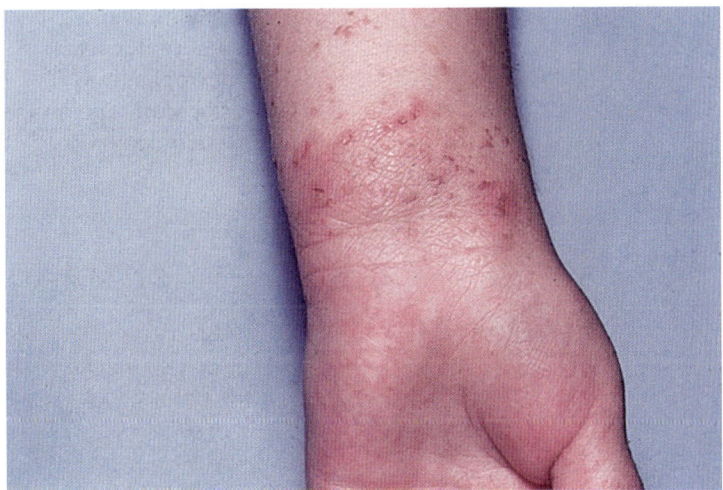

Figure 41.6 Flexural atopic eczema of the wrist in a child, with papulovesicles and an ill-defined border.

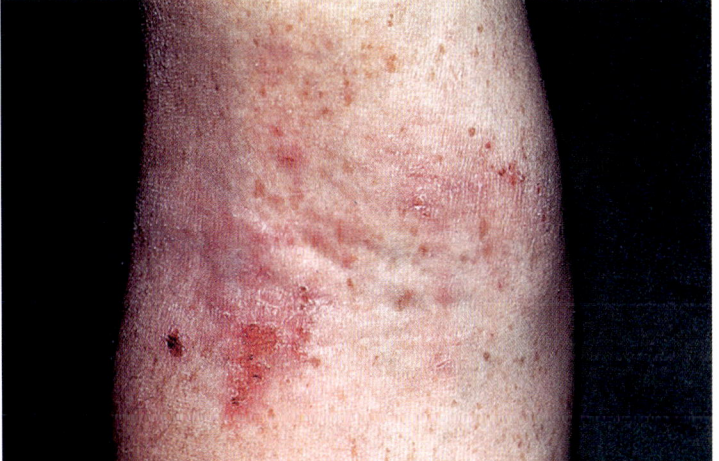

Figure 41.7 Adult flexural dermatitis.

cardinal symptom is itch associated with a chronic fluctuating rash with a range of features. Itch often causes significant sleep disturbance, irritability and distress and can be aggravated by warmth, sweating, bathing, exercise, emotional upset and woollen clothes worn against the skin. The skin is inflamed and may be painful.

Clinical features present at all ages

Although the clinical phenotype and distribution of atopic eczema changes with age and varies according to ethnic background, atopic eczema is characterised by a typical constellation of clinical signs. Acute atopic eczema is symmetrical with ill-defined, slightly raised inflamed areas that may be weepy. Papulation and oedema are mostly seen in acute eczematous inflammation (Figures 41.5 and 41.6). Flexural changes are distinctive, particularly over the limbs (Figure 41.7). In the chronic phase, thickening of the skin typically occurs which may progress to lichenification, with accentuation of skin markings and hyperpigmentation, especially in those with darker skin types (Figure 41.8). Secondary changes may be observed as a result of scathing or rubbing. Yellow crusting and oozing indicate secondary infection (Figure 41.9).

PART 4: INFLAMMATORY DERMATOSES

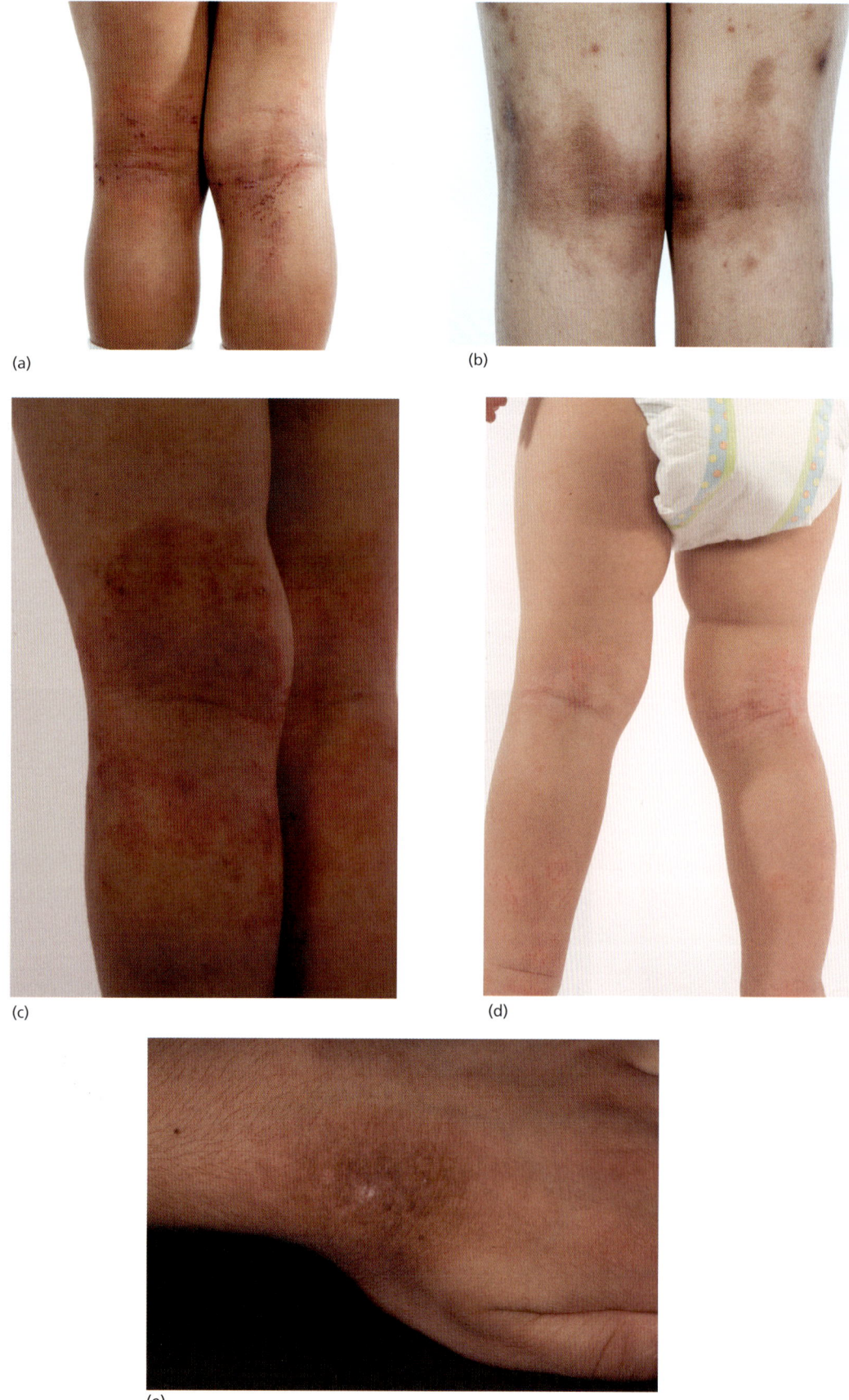

(a)

(b)

(c)

(d)

(e)

Figure 41.8 (a) Lichenification, crusting and excoriation in the popliteal fossae. (b) Post-inflammatory hyperpigmentation. (c) Flexural dermatitis causing hyperpigmentation. (d) Flexural dermatitis. (e) Lichenification.

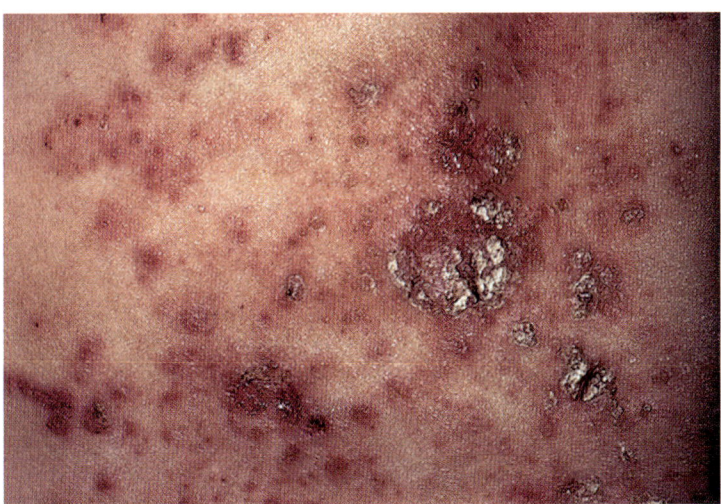

Figure 41.9 Atopic eczema: erythema, papules, excoriations, crusting and secondary infection.

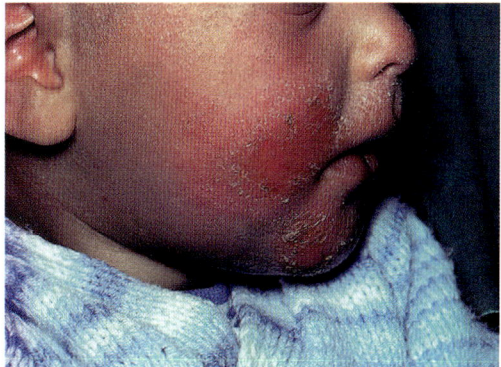

Figure 41.10 Atopic eczema: infantile phase.

Dry skin

This is a common feature of atopic eczema and features prominently in its management. It is likely that it occurs because of increased water loss through an abnormal stratum corneum, which may also correlate with disease activity. The dry skin is a consequence of abnormal ceramide and sphingosine synthesis and has an important role in the development of the skin inflammation. Ichthyosis vulgaris and keratosis pilaris may also be seen in association with the condition, with loss-of-function variants of the skin barrier protein filaggrin being the link between these conditions and atopic eczema (Table 41.1).

Endotypes

In line with many immune-mediated inflammatory diseases, there is an increasing emphasis on delineation of specific subgroups within the atopic eczema disease spectrum, called 'endotypes'.

'Endotype' refers to a subgroup of patients with atopic eczema who show distinct genetic or molecular profiles and can be broadly subdivided into 'disease endotypes' and 'drug endotypes'. 'Disease endotypes' are separated by their clinical features (e.g. flexural versus discoid versus follicular), while 'drug endotypes' are associated with underlying pharmacology, mechanism of action, efficacy and adverse effects. As there is intense interest in focusing drug development on molecular mechanisms of disease, the connectivity and overlap between disease and drug endotypes will increase.

The association between ichthyosis vulgaris and atopic eczema has been known for many years (hyperlinear palms were, for instance, noted back in 1981) [274]. Interestingly, the association between hyperlinear palms and ichthyosis vulgaris combined with atopic eczema was first reported in 1981 [275] and subsequently linked to underlying *FLG* mutations in 85–100% of individuals [4]. Further studies delineated that the constellation of palmar hyperlinearity, keratosis pilaris, flexural eczema and ichthyosis/xerosis were strongly associated with *FLG* mutations [276,277], essentially defining a filaggrin-related endotype of atopic eczema. Additionally, irritant hand dermatitis, involvement of exposed skin sites and susceptibility to water hardness has also been associated with filaggrin-related endotype of atopic eczema [277–279].

Importantly, filaggrin-associated atopic eczema is linked to a number of clinically relevant outcomes. Thus, for example, patients with filaggrin loss of function mutation tend to have early onset disease that is more chronic and severe. This endotype is also associated with atopic asthma, allergic rhinitis and peanut allergy [280–282] with subjects carrying filaggrin mutations showing district longitudinal disease clustering and time courses of atopic eczema persistence [35]. In addition, patients with atopic eczema carrying the *FLG* R501X mutation have a greater risk of eczema herpeticum [78]. Interestingly, *FLG* mutations also influence the cutaneous microbiome and the skin microbiome in healthy subjects carrying a *FLG* mutation is shifted towards that seen in patients with atopic eczema [283].

More recently, distinct clinical phenotypic differences in patients from different ethnic backgrounds have been associated with particular molecular endotypes [284]. For example, innate immune activation and Th1 and Th17 pathway activation was attenuated in African American patients compared with European American participants [285].

Infantile phase

During infancy, atopic eczema is commonly present on the face (Figure 41.10) but also commonly occurs elsewhere in a flexural and non-flexural/extensor distribution (Figure 41.5).

Childhood phase

Beyond infancy, the sites most characteristically involved are the elbow and knee flexures (Figure 41.8a–d), the sides of the neck, wrists and ankles (Figure 41.8e and Figure 41.6). The extensor distribution is commoner in black and Asian patients (Figures 41.11 and 41.12), but these patient groups also frequently show flexural involvement. In addition, discoid patches can occur (Figure 41.13). Involvement of the hands, sometimes with vesiculation (pompholyx) can also be present (Figures 41.14 and 41.15). Acute generalised or localised vesiculation should always suggest the possibility of secondary bacterial or viral infection (eczema herpeticum).

Adult phase

The picture is essentially similar to that in later childhood, with lichenification, especially of the flexures and hands. Frequently, facial and hand involvement is more problematic in adulthood and many adults find the flexural inflammation less troublesome.

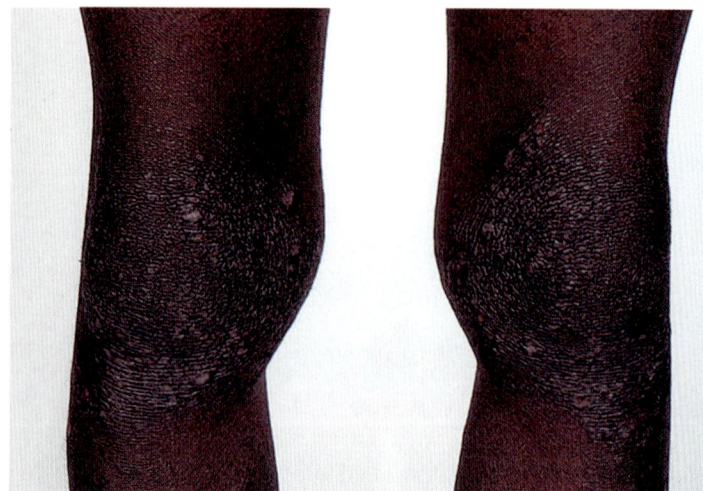

Figure 41.11 Marked lichenification on the knees in an African child. The popliteal fossae were spared.

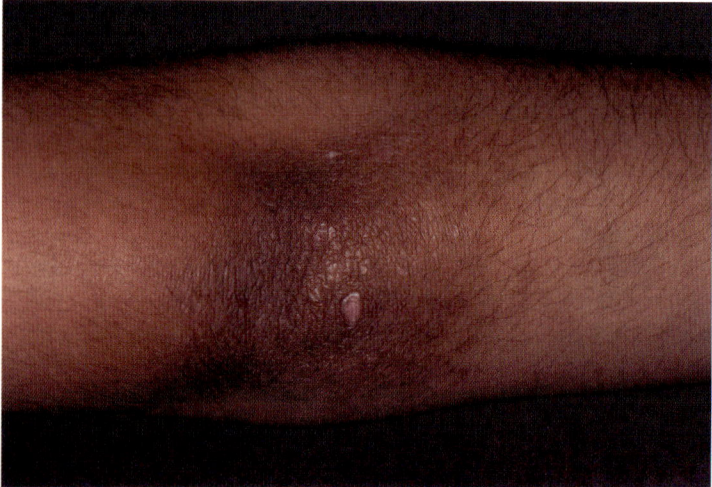

Figure 41.12 Persistent lichenification in an extensor distribution.

Skin of colour

The presentation of atopic eczema in skin of colour is as equally variable as in light coloured skin. A key difference from fair skin is the reduced redness evident in inflamed dark skin (Figure 41.11). Therefore, clinicians may have to rely on the symptoms of itch to grade inflammatory activity. As with other conditions affecting skin of colour, there is an increased risk of pigmentary changes after therapy and/or disease resolution. Although potent topical corticosteroids can modify (reduce) pigmentation in prolonged treatment, mostly post-inflammatory hypopigmentation is due to the inflammation rather than the treatment as suggested by the fact that most areas where topical corticosteroids are applied do not suffer any pigmentary abnormality, and that at sites where topical calcineurin inhibitors are used, pigmentary abnormalities have been identified after completed treatment.

Coloured skin shows some specific variants of atopic eczema including follicular and discoid patterns. Post-inflammatory changes of lichenified eczema often show hyperpigmentation (Figure 41.12).

Measuring disease severity

The classic concept of disease treatment determined by the preference of the attending physician is becoming largely redundant and health care systems are increasingly requiring measures of disease severity to justify specific treatments and reimbursement. Interestingly, in the USA, driven in large part by the Food and Drug Administration, the 'Investigator Global Assessment' (IGA) remains the gold standard measure of severity and encompasses five points: clear, almost clear, mild, moderate and severe. In Europe, greater emphasis is placed on 'objective' scores, which take into account clinical signs (e.g. redness, papulation/oedema, lichenification and scratch marks) as well as body surface area involvement.

The Harmonising Outcome Measures for Eczema (HOME) initiative has led the global consensus on measurements for atopic eczema severity measures used in clinical trials (http://www.homeforeczema.org) and has provided guidance on which tools to use. The cross-disciplinary group, which includes patients, has selected specific key outcomes, which include both objective (doctor/nurse scored) and subjective measures (patient reported) of disease severity (Table 41.4).

It is widely accepted that the measures of quality of life are critical in understanding how the condition affects individuals with atopic eczema. It is important that clinicians undergo training in scoring atopic eczema to reduce interobserver variability.

Clinical variants

The clinical phenotype of atopic eczema changes with age and ethnic background and may include, for example, non-flexural patterns, such as discoid and follicular eczema, as already outlined above. Similarly, nodular prurigo lesions can occur in atopic eczema, more commonly in those with skin of colour (Chapter 81).

Infra-auricular dermatitis is quite frequently seen in atopic eczema patients and infra-auricular fissures appear to be quite specific to the condition. The sides of the neck may show a striking reticulate pigmentation, sometimes referred to as 'atopic dirty neck' (Figure 41.16).

Localised patches of atopic eczema can occur on the nipples, especially in adolescent and young women, often associated with skin infection. Involvement of the vermilion of the lips and the adjacent skin is commonly an additional manifestation. Follicular lichenified papules (Figure 41.17a) are a frequent feature in black and Asian patients. A distribution on the face and neck may correlate with areas of maximal thermal sweating or *Malassezia furfur* colonisation and sometimes sensitivity.

Photo-aggravation or sensitivity may occur. Management of such cases requires a combination of approaches used for ordinary atopic eczema and for photosensitivity. Pityriasis alba and juvenile plantar dermatosis are more commonly seen in people with atopic eczema.

Hand involvement

Hand involvement is common and its prevalence increases with age. A patchy, somewhat vesicular and lichenified eczema is a common manifestation of atopic eczema in childhood. The nails are often involved, resulting in coarse pitting and ridging. A more diffuse, chronic lichenified eczema of the hands is frequently found in cases of extensive atopic eczema which persists into adult life (Figure 41.17b). Involvement of the feet is also common.

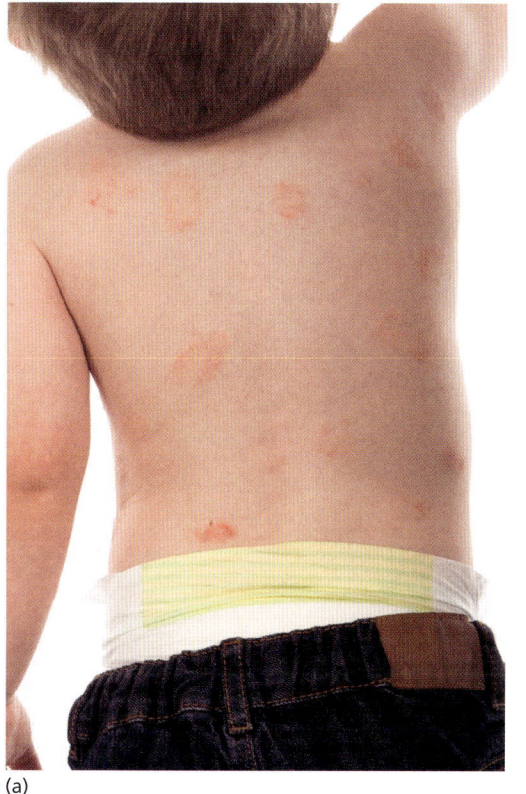

(a)

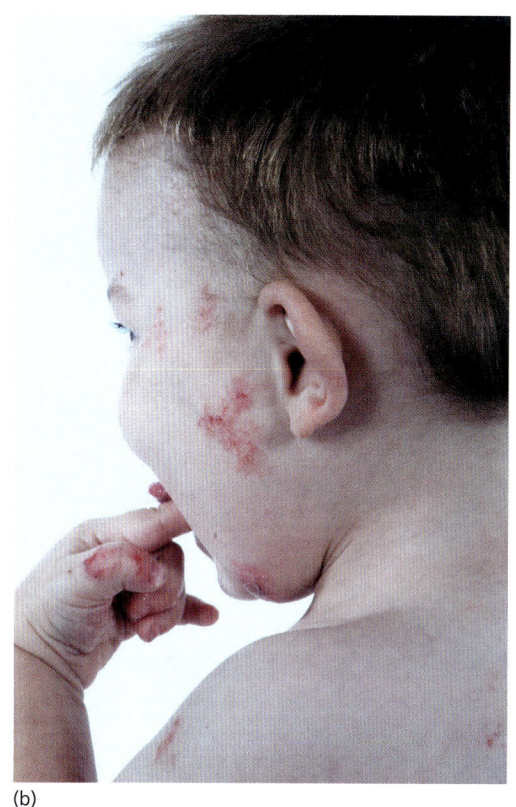

(b)

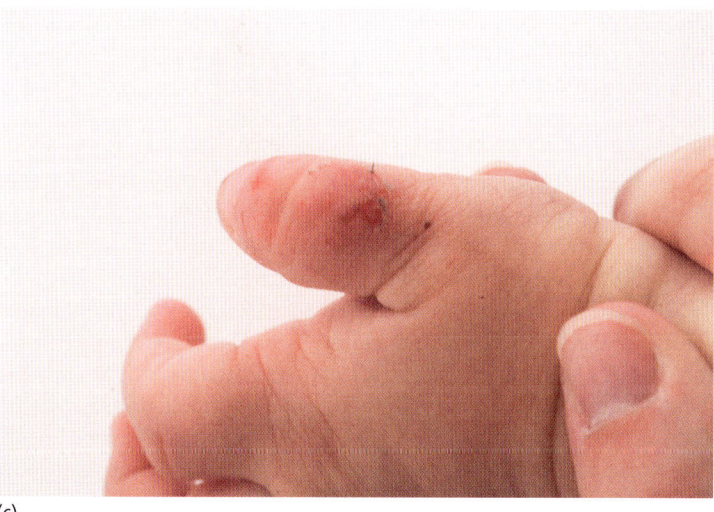

(c)

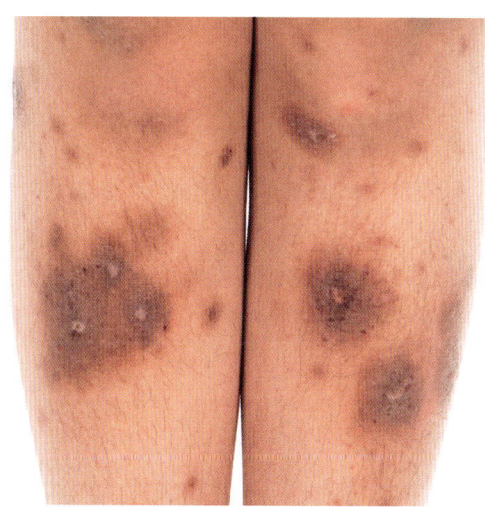

(d)

Figure 41.13 (a) Discoid eczema lesions. (b) Discoid lesions on the face. Saliva is a common irritant in young children. (c) Discoid lesion aggravated by thumb sucking. (d) Postinflammatory hyperpigmentation and lichenification in a discoid pattern.

A previous history of atopic eczema, and more particularly hand involvement, is a highly significant risk factor for the development of occupational dermatitis particularly if associated with loss-of-function filaggrin mutations. Atopics may be at risk of occupational food-related hand dermatoses.

Pityriasis alba

Pityriasis alba describes poorly defined patches of post-inflammatory hypopigmentation usually identified on the cheeks of children with atopic eczema. The skin scale is usually minimal. At the time of presentation, it is unusual to demonstrate active inflammation although the child will usually give a history of preceding itch at the site. The differential diagnosis of vitiligo is often questioned but the anatomical preference and incomplete loss of pigment in the context of an individual with atopic eczema is usually clear. Treatment is to prevent inflammation by strategies to treat before eczema arises, for example with twice weekly mild potency topical corticosteroids or calcineurin inhibitors. Pityriasis alba is self-limiting.

White dermographism

This phenomenon is poorly understood but reflects vasospasm in superficial cutaneous vessels in response to scratching. While this is

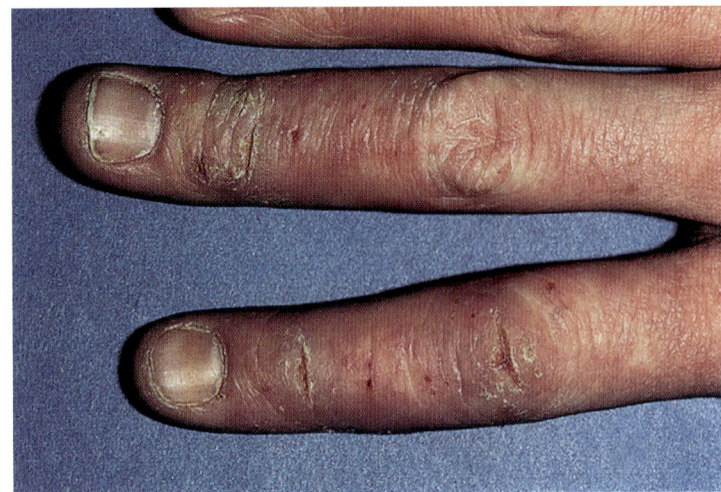

Figure 41.14 Atopic eczema of the fingers of a child.

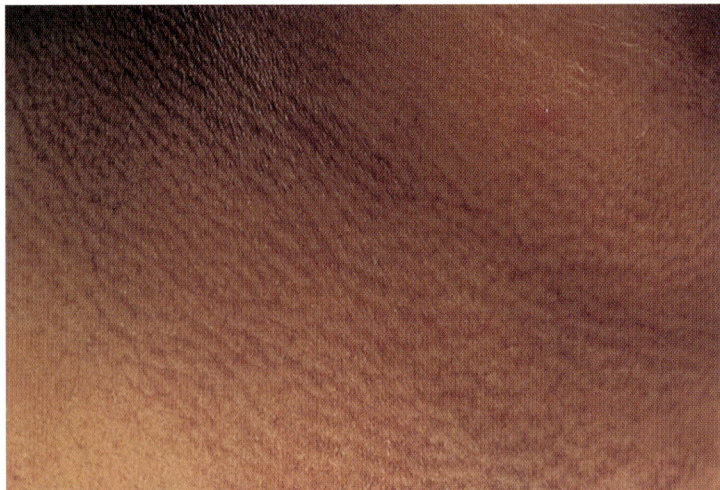

Figure 41.16 Atopic 'dirty neck'; reticulate pigmentation on the neck of a patient with longstanding atopic eczema.

an unusual complaint, patients can identify 'white lines' where they scratch.

Sweating

Many patients are aware that sweating induces itching and aggravates their condition. This may reflect altered sensations associated with the neuropeptides released in the neurogenic control of sweat glands. Altered inflammatory responses to acetylcholine are described above, and increased numbers of nerve fibres have been described around the sweat glands in atopic non-lesional skin compared with lesional and healthy control skin [286]. Sweating responses to neurogenic stimuli are altered in atopic eczema sufferers, although there is lack of agreement between findings, and diverse methods have been used to quantify sweat production. Sweating in response to cholinergic stimulation was found to be reduced in volume by one group [287,288] but normal in volume, although of more prolonged duration by another group [289].

A possible explanation for the differences comes from the study of Eishi *et al.* [290], who measured both direct cholinergic effects on sweat glands and distant effects mediated via the axon reflex. They found that directly induced sweat production hardly differed from that in healthy controls, whereas axon reflex induced sweating was of lower volume with a longer latency. In a study of the response to adrenergic stimulation, sweating was similar between atopic eczema patients and non-atopic controls at low concentrations of adrenaline, but at higher concentrations sweating in non-atopic individuals was increased compared with a decrease in atopic eczema patients [291]. Sweating in response to the thermal stress of sitting in a heated room was found to be reduced in atopic eczema patients [292]. However, there was no difference in sweating responses induced by hard cycling on a bicycle ergometer between atopic eczema sufferers and healthy controls [293].

Another way in which sweating may induce itching and aggravate eczema is related to the observation that there may be IgE-mediated allergic reactivity to components of sweat [294]. Thus, skin challenges with autologous sweat induced positive responses in 56 of 66 (84%) patients compared with three of 27 (11%) healthy controls. Also, basophils were induced to release histamine

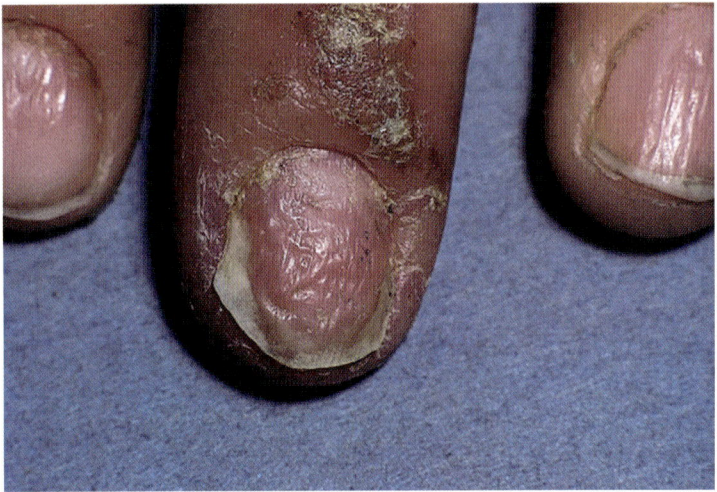

Figure 41.15 Nail involvement in atopic eczema in childhood.

Table 41.4 Preferred measures of disease severity, impact on quality of life and disease control for use in clinical trials.

Disease measure		Validated preferred assessment tool
Clinician measured disease severity		Eczema Area and Severity Index (EASI)
Patient-reported symptoms	Short-term control	Patient-Oriented Eczema Measure (POEM)
		Numerical Rating Scale (NRS-11), for peak itch over past 24 hours
	Long-term control	Recap of Atopic Eczema (RECAP) or Atopic Dermatitis Control Test (ADCT)
Quality of life		Dermatology Life Quality Index (DLQI), Childrens DLQI (CDLQI), Infants Disease Quality of Life (IDQoL)

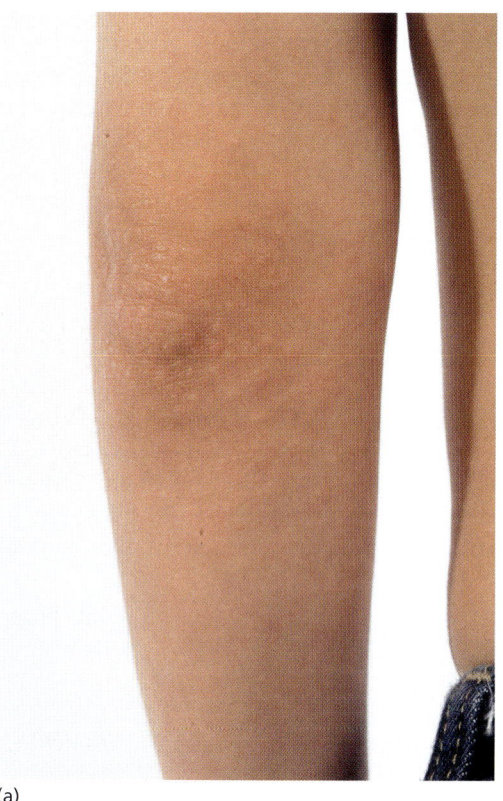

(a)

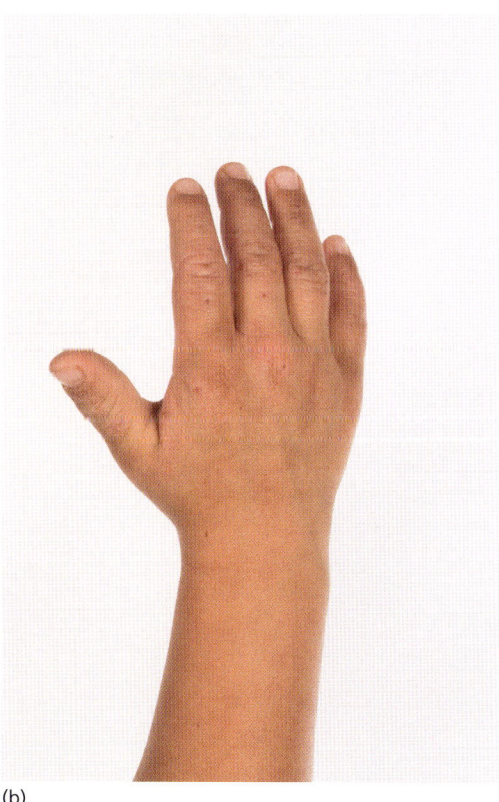

(b)

Figure 41.17 (a) Follicular lichenification on the surface. (b) Atopic hand eczema.

in an IgE-dependent process [294]. The nature of the sweat reactivity has been suggested to be IgE mediated although this does not seem compatible with the lack of response to antihistamines [295,296].

Endocrine and psychological factors

Patients with atopic eczema commonly complain that their condition is exacerbated by episodes of psychological stress, a situation that is also found in many inflammatory dermatological conditions. Buske-Kirschbaum *et al.* [297] showed that formal stressing of people who experience recurrent herpes simplex lesions could significantly increase the recurrence rate of cold sores, and that there was also a rise in plasma levels of TNF-α. The role and mechanisms of psychosocial stress on the clinical course of atopic eczema still remain to be elucidated. When volunteers are subjected to formal stress tests in the form of public speaking and performance of mental arithmetic, a wide range of endocrinological changes occur. These include increased production of adrenaline, ACTH, corticotrophin releasing factor (CRF) and cortisol, and reduced production of growth hormone, prolactin and progesterone [298]. The stress-induced rise in free cortisol is reportedly lower in patients with atopic eczema [299].

Another humoral influence that appears to modulate atopic eczema is mediated by sex steroids. One third of 133 patients questioned claimed there was a significant premenstrual flare of atopic eczema [300]. Pregnancy exacerbated eczema in 52% of women, whereas it ameliorated eczema in 24% [301]. It has been proposed that a possible mechanism by which sex steroids alter susceptibility to inflammatory skin diseases is by modification of sensitivity to anti-inflammatory effects of glucocorticoids (GC). In a comparison of differences in susceptibility between men and women, Rohleder *et al.* [301] psychologically stressed volunteers; women were tested in the luteal phase of the menstrual cycle. Sensitivity to GC was assessed *in vitro* by measurement of dexamethasone inhibition of lipopolysaccharide-stimulated production of IL-6 and TNF-α. Salivary cortisol levels increased equally between the sexes. However, in men, GC sensitivity was markedly increased one hour after stress, whereas GC sensitivity decreased significantly in women. Similarly, lipopolysaccharide-induced cytokine production decreased in response to stress in men but increased in women. It is not clear whether this is the result of the increased cortisol production suppressing cytokine production in men or a change in responsiveness to lipopolysaccharide itself. Hence, the premenstrual flares of atopic eczema could reflect the reduced sensitivity to the anti-inflammatory effects of endogenous cortisol.

Psychosocial aspects

Atopic eczema has a profound effect, equal to or greater than that of asthma and diabetes, on many aspects of patients' lives and the lives of their families [302]. The psychological disturbance caused by atopic eczema is increasingly recognised and may be amenable to specific interventions. In children, the most troublesome symptoms are itching, distress at bath time and difficulty going to sleep. Itching, scratching and sleep disturbance in moderate to severe atopic eczema results in impairment in quality of life to an equivalent degree as rheumatoid arthritis or multiple sclerosis. Severe atopic eczema promotes family dysfunction, causing exhaustion, sleep deprivation and emotional distress and may predispose to later

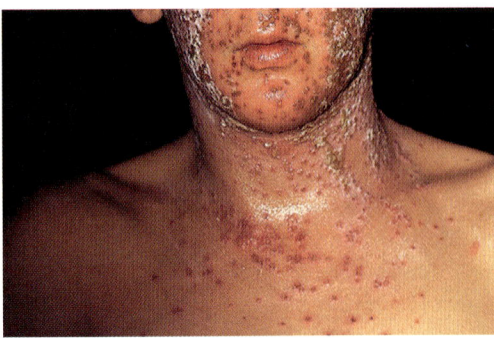

Figure 41.18 Eczema herpeticum.

problems with mental health. Indeed, partial sleep disturbance is increasingly recognised to result in neurocognitive impairment. Teasing because of abnormal skin appearance can lead to concerns over contagion and social exclusion. This in turn can lead to negative effects on self-image and self-esteem, particularly during adolescence. Higher trait anxiety and stress vulnerability are also recognised in atopic eczema patients [303]. Attention deficit hyperactivity disorder (ADHD) is commoner in children with atopic eczema. Depression, anxiety, conduct disorder and autism are similarly increased in frequency in atopic eczema. Topical steroid phobia is common and leads to reduced adherence to treatment [304].

Complications and other associated diseases
Bacterial infections
Secondary bacterial infection with staphylococci or streptococci is common [305]. It contributes to disease exacerbations, even without grossly visible purulent exudate. Widespread impetigo may sometimes closely mimic Kaposi varicelliform eruption and any acute vesicular eruption in an atopic person should suggest the diagnosis of secondary bacterial or viral infection.

Viral infections
Patients with atopic eczema, both active and quiescent, are liable to develop acute generalised infections with herpes simplex virus (eczema herpeticum) (Figure 41.18) [306]. Such episodes may present as a severe systemic illness with high fever and a widespread eruption. However, there may be no systemic disturbance, and at times the eruption may be localised, often to areas of pre-existing atopic eczema. The individual lesions start as the characteristic viral papulovesicles, but not necessarily with herpetiform grouping. There may then be rapid evolution to a state in which extensive purulent exudate masks the initial papulovesicles, or superficial scattered erosions may be the only clue to the cause of a rapid deterioration of the AE. The differential diagnosis includes bacterial impetigo and chickenpox. Herpes zoster and chickenpox behave as in those without atopic eczema.

The population level frequency of molluscum contagiosum in atopic eczema patients is not clear. However, the clinical impression is that widespread molluscum contagiosum is more common in children with atopic eczema. Additionally, there is good evidence that common HPV-associated warts are more common in children with atopic eczema.

Food allergy
Both immediate and delayed atopic eczema flares due to food sensitisation occur, in the case of immediate reactions usually associated with other symptoms (urticarial wheals, gastrointestinal upset, wheezing or rhinitis and conjunctivitis). Gastrointestinal reflux is a common feature of detailed type hypersensitivity to foods associated with atopic eczema in infancy. For further details on the association between food allergy and atopic eczema see above.

Asthma
Atopic eczema, in particular in those with early onset, more severe and persistent disease, allergic sensitisation and a family history of atopy, is an important risk factor for the development of allergic airways disease, including asthma. This is most likely due to a combination of shared genetic loci, shared environmental risk factors (e.g. environmental pollutants and irritants) and percutaneous sensitisation to aeroallergens through an abnormal and inflamed cutaneous barrier [307].

Allergic rhino-conjunctivitis
Allergic rhino-conjunctivitis is a common co-morbidity in those with atopic eczema, affecting well over 50% of those with moderate-to-severe disease [308]. The main sources of sensitisation are tree and grass pollen as well as house dust mite, leading to either seasonal or more perennial symptoms. The severe itching of the eyes and/or nose commonly exacerbates periorbital eczema, with disease flares typically seen during the pollen season in an airborne pattern (face, head and neck) in patients where aeroallergen sensitisation plays an important role. Better symptom control of rhino-conjunctivitis can lead to improved atopic eczema and close working with allergists as part of a multidisciplinary team approach is advocated in those who are significantly affected.

Ocular surface disorders (Chapter 107)
A number of ocular changes can occur in atopic eczema [308]. The Dennie–Morgan fold (Figure 41.19) is often present as a fold of skin under the lower eyelids. However, this change is not specific to eczema, and is commonly seen in non-atopic black children.

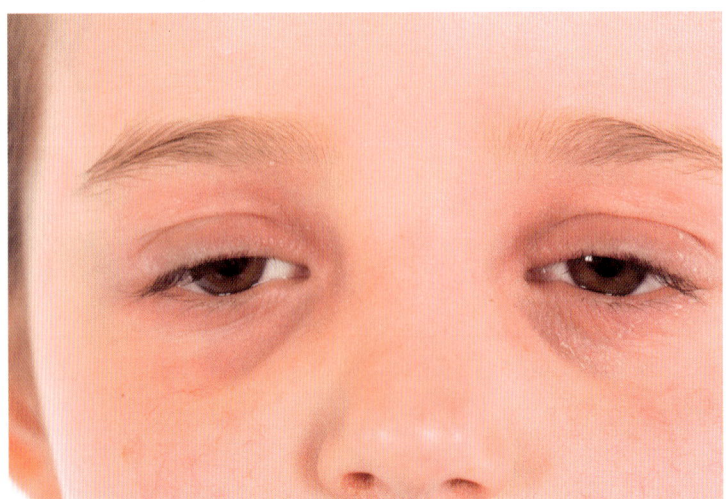

Figure 41.19 Periorbital dermatitis with Dennie–Morgan fold.

Eye lid eczema, conjunctival irritation, atopic keratoconjunctivitis and superficial punctate keratopathy are common in patients with atopic eczema [308] and until recently (with the advent of dupilumab) were probably under-reported. Herpes simplex infection should be considered within the differential diagnosis, as this may lead to severe complications if unrecognised and not managed appropriately.

Ocular surface disease induced by dupilumab appears more common in real-life studies (~25%) [309–311] compared with reports from randomised controlled trials (RCTs) [312] and appears more frequent in patients with a past history of atopic keratoconjunctivitis [313]. A spectrum of clinical presentations have been observed from a mild conjunctivitis with dry eyes and a superficial punctate keratitis to a more severe conjunctivitis associated with blepharitis, limbitis and ectropion in some cases [310,311,314].

Histopathological examination has shown distinct features compared with allergic conjunctivitis with reduced intra-epithelial goblet cells, which may account for mucin deficiency and stability of the tear film. Symptoms may be troublesome and include stinging, burning, tearing, photophobia and eyelid swelling [309]. Pre-treatment with artificial tears containing hyaluronate, topical antihistamine/ketotifen drops and early intervention with topical steroid drops/ointment (in conjunction with ophthalmologists) may reduce incidence and severity [309,310,315], but adds considerable burden to the patient. The management of severe ocular surface disease requires referral and ideally a close working relationship with ophthalmology.

Keratoconus [29], or conical cornea, is a rare but important condition, most frequently diagnosed in adolescence. It may occur in the absence of any other disease or in association with atopic eczema. It is due to a degenerative change and thinning of the cornea, which is forced outwards by the intraocular pressure, giving rise to marked visual disturbances. Onset is in childhood, and after some years progress of the disease becomes arrested. Eye rubbing is significantly associated with keratoconus, suggesting a potential link to eyelid involvement and the need for appropriate treatment [316]. Contact lenses may be helpful to improve visual acuity but many cases require surgical treatment. During early stages, corneal cross-linking may arrest disease progression. However, in severe cases with corneal scarring, corneal keratoplasty may be required [317]. Cataract associated with atopic eczema (Figure 41.20) is thought to arise due to a combination of rubbing and the use of topical corticosteroids. There is some association with disease severity, IgE levels and also with a polymorphism in the IFNγR1 gene [318]. Although both posterior and anterior subcapsular cataracts are more common, and in line with population prevalence, posterior cataract is most common in atopic eczema. The prevalence of anterior cataract is significantly more common in atopic eczema than in the population as a whole [319]. It occurs in up to 10% of the more severe adolescent and adult cases. It may start in early childhood or up to the age of 30 years, but the peak incidence is between 15 and 25 years. It is almost always bilateral. The appearances on slit lamp examination are characteristic but not diagnostic. In the early stages, translucent globules and small opacities appear at the pole in front of the posterior capsule and also in the anterior subcapsular zone. The final appearance may resemble a mature cortical senile cataract. Ophthalmological management of the cataract is not specific for

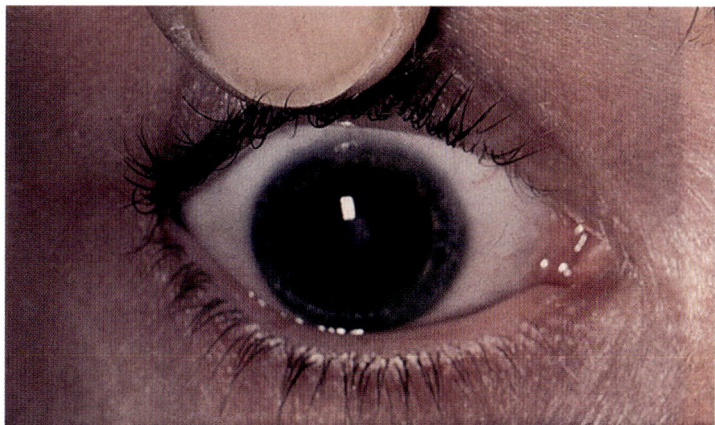

Figure 41.20 Atopic cataract.

atopic eczema, although subsequent control of periocular atopic eczema is important.

Retinal detachment has been reported, particularly in Japanese patients with atopic eczema, and appears to be identical to the retinal detachment seen following trauma [33]. Although one of the most severe eye complications, the incidence in atopic eczema may be decreasing [320].

Developmental

Growth delay may be associated with atopic eczema, but it is usually only seen in severely affected children. It used to be seen in severe cases before the advent of corticosteroid therapy and can therefore be mainly attributed to the disease, rather than the treatment. While inappropriate use of topical corticosteroids can induce inhibition of the pituitary axis (Cushing syndrome) in both children and adults, there is no evidence that the appropriate use of topical corticosteroids affects growth adversely [321].

Cardiovascular

A systematic review of the literature including 19 studies concluded that there was an independent, albeit small association in terms of absolute risks, with increased risk of cardiovascular disease [322,323]. The effects of atopic eczema reported in cross-sectional studies were particularly heterogeneous, with no evidence for pooled associations with angina, myocardial infarction, heart failure or stroke.

Malignancies

It has been suggested that atopic eczema is associated with a reduced overall cancer risk, potentially due to more active immune surveillance in those with Th2 inflammation. However, the literature is heterogeneous, and the results depend on study type (generally population-based studies vs case–control and other cross-sectional analyses) and the cancer type examined [324]. At the same time, chronic inflammation has also been associated with an increase in malignancy risk. Atopic eczema has been reported to be associated with lymphoma in cohort studies, including cutaneous T-cell lymphoma [325]. This may at least in part be due to the potential misdiagnosis of cutaneous T-cell lymphoma as atopic eczema. However, these findings are not consistent across all studies, similar to reports on the association between atopic eczema and other skin cancers, such as malignant melanoma.

Urticaria

Urticaria is more common in those with an atopic background, including atopic eczema. Chronic urticaria, when significant, can be an important contributor to atopic eczema flares, especially in those with dermographism, as the additional histamine release leads to more itching and scratching.

Autoimmune diseases

Several studies have shown an increased susceptibility to autoimmune disease in people with atopic eczema including alopecia areata, rheumatoid arthritis and inflammatory bowel disease, but have often been restricted to adult atopic eczema patients in hospital settings [326–328].

Differential diagnosis

A number of other common conditions need to be considered and are listed in Box 41.3. Scabies should always be excluded and can cause confusion when superimposed on pre-existing atopic eczema. In the first few months of life, the differentiation of infantile seborrhoeic dermatitis from atopic eczema can be difficult, although with time the distinction becomes apparent. Immunodeficiency states should also be considered in infants in whom the disease is unusually severe, when there are recurrent systemic and cutaneous infections, and if there is failure to thrive, malabsorption or petechiae (Box 41.4). An eruption resembling atopic eczema, with or without other atopic disorders, and sometimes with raised IgE levels may be found in several rare disorders (Box 41.4).

In adults, flexural eczema may be a consequence of secondary dissemination of other types of eczema, for example in nickel allergy and occupational contact dermatitis; occasionally contact dermatitis can mimic atopic eczema in children.

Box 41.3 Common disorders that may mimic atopic eczema

- Scabies
- Infantile seborrhoeic dermatitis
- Contact dermatitis
- Skin lymphoma
- Rare primary immunodeficiencies

Box 41.4 Rare disorders that may have an atopic eczema-like rash

- Hyper-IgE syndrome
- Hypereosinophilic syndrome
- Agammaglobulinaemia
- Anhidrotic ectodermal dysplasia
- Ataxia telangiectasia
- Netherton syndrome (ichthyosis, bamboo hairs)
- Phenylketonuria
- Wiskott–Aldrich syndrome (infections and thrombocytopenia)

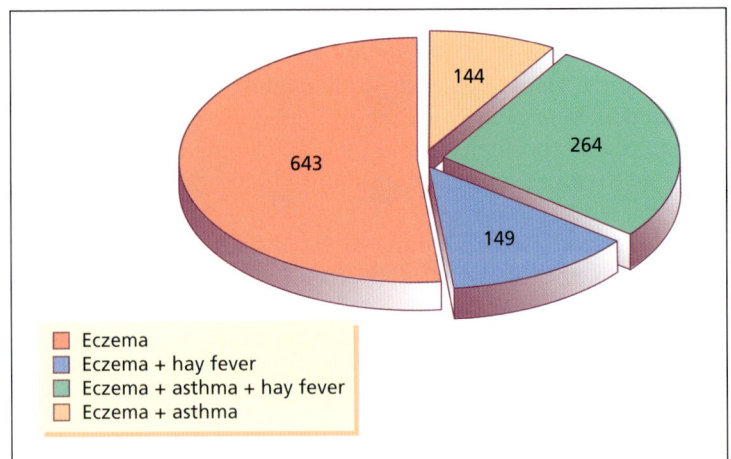

Figure 41.21 (a) Lip-lick cheilitis. (b) Lip-lick dermatitis with mild impetiginisation. (c) Lip-lick dermatitis with hyperpigmentation.

Other patterns of eczema
Infantile seborrhoeic dermatitis

This condition is discussed in Chapter 40. It normally starts earlier than atopic eczema and it may be possible to distinguish between the two conditions clinically. However, there are a number of children who present with what appears to be seborrhoeic dermatitis and then progress to typical atopic eczema.

Allergic contact dermatitis (see earlier)

It is clear that atopic eczema patients are at greater risk of developing irritant contact dermatitis than non-atopic individuals and this risk may be increased in patients with filaggrin mutations. However, there is a dispute about whether they are at greater risk of developing allergic contact dermatitis. Nonetheless, patients can develop sensitivity to a variety of contact allergens such as topical medicaments, including topical corticosteroids, fragrances and metals. There is also a risk of protein contact sensitivity, such as that associated with latex in rubber gloves (Chapter 128).

Lip-lick cheilitis

Synonyms and inclusions

- Perioral eczema
- 'Lick eczema'

Moist or fissured eczema around the mouth is common in children with atopic eczema. It can also occur as a result of food allergy and in children with no known atopy. Frequently spreading some distance around the mouth, it may become secondarily infected and crusted, and cause hyperpigmentation in darker skin (Figure 41.21). Its persistence, and perhaps its origin, is attributable to habits of lip licking, thumb sucking, dribbling or chapping. It is easily transformed into true perioral dermatitis by the application of potent corticosteroids. The regular application of 1% hydrocortisone ointment is usually most helpful. Contact sensitivity, for example to toothpaste ingredients, can occasionally be demonstrated.

Primary disease prevention advice

Ways to reduce the incidence or severity of atopic eczema have been explored as early as the perinatal period [329]. For many years, these attempts centred around allergen avoidance. However, partly driven by disappointing results but also an improved understanding of the role of allergic sensitisation in the development of atopic eczema, we are increasingly moving away from strict allergen avoidance towards methods of tolerance induction.

Infant feeding and dietary allergen avoidance

The role of breastfeeding promotion and its protective effect has already been discussed earlier, and there is no evidence that routine dietary allergen avoidance either during pregnancy or postnatally prevents atopic eczema, even in high-risk infants. Along the lines of food allergen avoidance, partially and extensively hydrolysed (hypoallergenic) formulas have also been studied, and it has been suggested that prolonged feeding with a hydrolysed formula, compared with a cow's milk formula, may result in an around 30% reduction in infantile atopic eczema. However, there is no evidence to support feeding with a hydrolysed formula for the prevention of atopic eczema *per se* compared with breast-feeding.

However, there is some evidence that maternal and infant pre- and probiotic (especially lactobacilli and bifidobacteria) supplementation during pregnancy and breastfeeding reduces the risk of atopic eczema in the offspring, an effect that may be mediated by the gut microflora by up to 50%. However, these studies are hampered by methodological diversity, and it is therefore difficult to recommend a specific probiotic preparation to pregnant mothers.

House dust mite avoidance

The association between house dust mite (HDM) and atopic eczema is strong: 50–80% of atopic eczema patients show sensitisation to HDM; experimental cutaneous HDM exposure can induce atopic eczema flares in the atopy patch test; and inhalation of HDM allergen can provoke eczematous skin lesions in pre-disposed patients. However, even the most rigid methods to reduce HDM exposure have shown mixed results on disease activity, even in sensitised individuals. Somewhat paradoxically, a longitudinal study showed that children with allergic mothers who were randomised to receive mite allergen-impermeable mattress covers actually had a higher occurrence of atopic eczema and a recent systematic review found no evidence for prevention by HDM avoidance [330]. Interestingly, and consistent with the latter trial and similar to work on endotoxin and parasite exposure, there is evidence that high environmental HDM levels in early life reduce atopic eczema risk.

Water hardness

Given the association between exposure to hard domestic water and development of atopic eczema in infancy in those with *FLG* mutation inheritance, it is possible that installation of a water softener in early life can prevent the development of atopic eczema. This is currently assessed in the SOFtened watER eczema prevention trial in the UK [331] (SOFTER: https://www.isrctn.com/ISRCTN71423189).

Preventing skin barrier breakdown

Skin barrier dysfunction plays a major role in atopic eczema development and dry, cracked skin is often the precursor of eczematous skin inflammation. Children carrying the *FLG* skin barrier gene show an increase in TEWL, even before atopic eczema develops. Intensive emollient use in early life in addition to soap and detergent avoidance may therefore be a powerful and cheap method of primary prevention, especially in children who carry skin barrier gene mutations and show early signs of skin barrier impairment, such as dry skin and an increase in TEWL.

Several pilot studies using daily emollients from early life showed a promising reduction in the development of atopic eczema. However, two large randomised controlled trials with an emollient intervention have shown no benefit, even in children with a family history of atopic eczema [242,243]. Others are working on new barrier enhancing topical and systemic preparations, which are able to upregulate *FLG* expression in the epidermis and improve skin barrier function as a potential means of disease prevention but also causative treatment.

Occupational advice

A number of occupational aspects are relevant to atopic eczema patients because they run a significant risk of developing occupational contact dermatitis. Atopy amplifies the effects of irritant and allergen exposure in several professions such as hairdressers, nurses, metalworkers, mechanics and cleaners, where hand eczema is a very common disease [332]. The risk for hand eczema in atopic eczema patients is increased about fourfold [333]. Physicians should inform atopic eczema patients about this increased risk and provide good guidance about prophylactic skin protection and irritant/contact allergen avoidance. All dermatologists treating adolescent patients with atopic eczema should advise them early about the occupational aspects of their skin disease and suitable career choices.

Investigations

The initial diagnosis of atopic eczema is rarely aided by investigations. The role of diagnostic testing for allergenic triggers of atopic eczema has best been examined in the context of food allergy. A prospective study of 107 children with atopic eczema who had never ingested egg compared the outcome of an oral challenge with egg against skin prick test or detection of serum specific IgE. While the detection of specific IgE or positive skin prick test >3 mm or serum specific IgE 0.35 kU/L are sensitive and specific for diagnosing type 1 allergic reactions to egg, it is important to recognise that positive oral challenge reactions to egg yolk arose with negative skin prick tests or specific IgE measurements in 20% and 30% of cases respectively [334]. Furthermore, negative oral challenge reactions were observed in 6% of cases with positive skin or serum tests. These findings have been replicated in multiple subsequent studies and it is recognised that there is no evidence that either wheal size or specific IgE level predict likelihood of relevance in atopic eczema and that many individuals with a positive test for IgE lack clinical reactivity [335]. Therefore, even in the context of immediate hypersensitivity, e.g. anaphylaxis, where avoidance is mandatory,

PART 4: INFLAMMATORY DERMATOSES

correlation between diagnostic tests and clinical benefit of allergen avoidance in atopic eczema is poor. Thus, diagnosis of food-induced atopic eczema is best diagnosed by the gold standard challenge exposure. Certain important differences from challenge testing for immediate hypersensitivity is required, including the need to wait 48 hours to assess deterioration of eczema, before introduction of an alternative allergen, and the importance of stabilising topical therapy before and during the test.

To explore allergens implicated in atopic eczema further, and to replicate the skin exposure better, development of the 'atopy patch test' (APT) initially ignited great interest as a tool to detect clinically relevant allergic sensitisations [336]. However, its use remains controversial, in particular due to the risk of skin irritation and the lack of standardisation [337]. Thus, for food allergy, where challenge testing is feasible, the APT adds minimal benefit to the work-up.

Suspicion of allergic contact dermatitis should be considered in all cases failing to respond to standard therapy and investigated by patch testing. Topical drugs along with emollients are frequent sensitisers and should be included in the patch test series. In addition, positive responses can be elicited in atopic eczema sufferers to *Malassezia* yeasts [338–341]. The clinical relevance of allergy to *Malassezia* yeast is indicated by studies showing that treatment with itraconazole to eradicate the yeast resulted in improvement of the atopic eczema comparable to that obtained with betamethasone valerate [340,342]. Patch testing is increasingly recognised as important in children with atopic eczema [343]. Recent evidence suggests that allergic contact dermatitis in atopic eczema is identified at least as frequently as in controls [344]. Apart from nickel allergy [345] there is a lack of association between *FLG* mutations and individuals with atopic eczema who develop allergic contact dermatitis [346]. This is in line with experimental data which suggest that immunological sensitisation in atopic eczema may be underestimated by patch testing due to impaired cutaneous responsiveness to haptens in atopic eczema [347] (Chapter 127).

If there is failure to thrive or one suspects immunodeficiency with atopic eczema, the appropriate investigations should be performed, for example Ig levels and subclasses, IgE levels, white cell count, platelets, complement levels and function, and T-, B- and phagocyte cell numbers and functions. If clinically appropriate, one may also consider testing for HIV or HTLV-1.

Bacteriology and virology swabs may be helpful in identifying causes for deterioration of atopic eczema. Although atopic eczema skin is often colonised by *S. aureus*, bacterial culture can identify antibiotic resistance and detect β-haemolytic streptococci. Patients with severe furuncles or deeper skin infections should have swabs to identify *S. aureus* producing Panton–Valentine leukocidin toxin because of the risk of systemic infections. Herpes simplex is usually readily confirmed by polymerase chain reaction, but it can also be identified by culture, a Tzanck smear, an immunofluorescence slide test or electron microscopy. Treatment should not be delayed.

Management

Treatment should be tailored to an individual's needs, bearing in mind age, gender, social conditions, sites of involvement and severity. A treatment strategy based on consistent advice and cooperation between health carers, including experienced nurses, and the patient should be developed. However, recent years have seen the emergence of several new treatment approaches that hold promise for the near future. Management is summarised in Figure 41.22.

First Assessment

In all settings the initial assessment is very important. Although over 80% of suffers have mild disease it is important to take a comprehensive history of the patient's disease, family history, recognised trigger factors and the home environment (Table 41.3).

Examination should include an assessment of the whole skin to assess severity, complications and comorbidities. Additionally, measurement of the impact on the patient's quality of life should be considered (Table 41.4).

First line treatment (Table 41.5)

In most patients (for simplicity, the term patient will be used to include interactions with individuals, parents and carers), even with severe atopic eczema, initial management comprises advice and education, advice on the reduction of trigger factors, use of bathing/showering with emollients, regular emollient application, and suppression of inflammation with a topical corticosteroid to induce remission. An explanation about the role of barrier dysfunction in the pathogenesis of atopic eczema helps to reinforce the critical role of emollients. In all cases, emollients should be maintained during remission and in more severe cases maintenance of topical anti-inflammatory therapy is valuable to reduce the frequency of flares (see later). Almost always this can be initiated as a written home treatment plan.

Often there is significant reluctance to use topical corticosteroid therapy, so called steroid phobia [348]. Frequently patients arrive at the consultation requesting, often inappropriate, identification and management of allergy (usually dietary) and need to be persuaded to leave with the appropriate use of topical corticosteroid therapy.

General advice and education

In order to develop a treatment strategy, the patient's specific requirements should be discussed, and achievable aims agreed. These may include improvement in a range of factors, such as reducing itch, improving sleep, reducing absenteeism from school/work or improving family interactions.

It is the clinician's responsibility to determine a balance between effective control of the condition and improved quality of life, and safe long-term therapy.

Clear and consistent advice from doctors, nurses, pharmacists, self-help groups and national support groups is also very helpful in achieving these aims. Information about current knowledge of the disease, the types of trigger factors, the treatment options and their likely benefits and risks and demonstration of the use of topically applied medications, bandages or wet wraps may improve compliance and disease control. However, there is still debate about the value of formal education programmes in improving patient outcomes [349,350].

Reduction of trigger factors

Atopic eczema can be aggravated by a variety of trigger factors acting in concert (Figure 41.4). These will vary at different ages

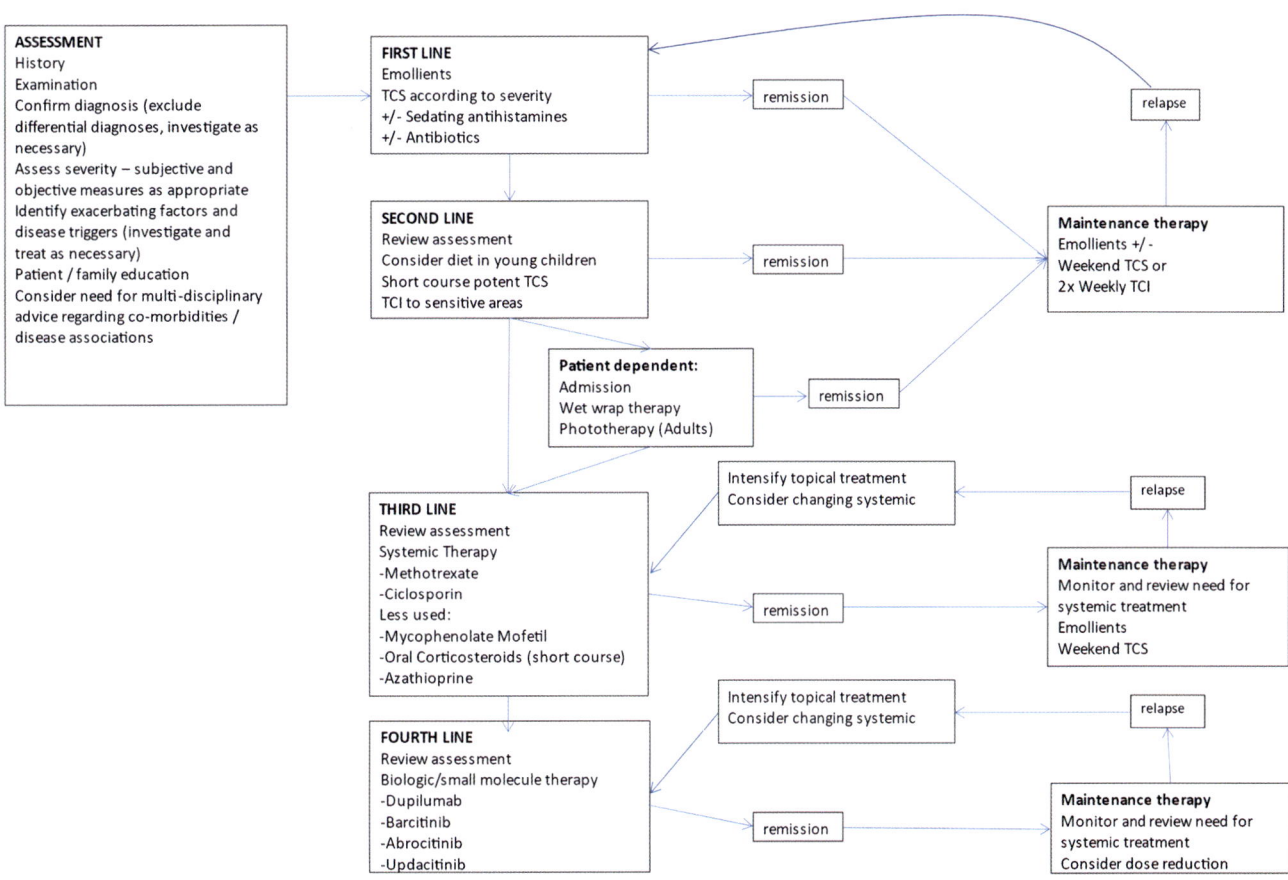

Figure 41.22 Atopic eczema treatment algorithm. TCS, topical corticosteroids; TCI, topical calcineurin inhibitors.

Table 41.5 First line therapy in atopic eczema.

Severity	Clear	Mild	Moderate	Severe
Treatment for body	Emollients	Emollients	Emollients	Emollients
		Mild potency topical corticosteroids	Moderate potency topical corticosteroids (use for axillae and groin flares for 7–14 days only) Night-time sedating antihistamines (if sleep disturbed) Oral antibiotics (if clinically infected)	Potent topical corticosteroids (use for axillae and groin flares for 7–14 days only) Night-time sedating antihistamines (if sleep disturbed) Oral antibiotics (if clinically infected)
Treatment for face and neck	Emollients	Emollients alone or mild potency topical corticosteroids	Emollients Mild potency topical corticosteroids Night-time sedating antihistamines (if sleep disturbed) Oral antibiotics (if clinically infected)	Emollients For severe flares, use moderate potency topical corticosteroids for 3–5 days only Night-time sedating antihistamines (if sleep disturbed) Oral antibiotics (if clinically infected)

(Figure 41.23), between patients, and may differ at various times in an individual patient.

All patients have dry skin; soaps and detergents can further damage the barrier and exacerbate the eczema. Avoidance of irritants, soap substitutes and emollients are particularly important for these patients. Many patients will suffer seasonal exacerbations and will recognise summer or winter deterioration. In those with summer worsening, photosensitivity should be considered. Simple measures

such as turning down the central heating, not heating the bedroom, avoiding contact of wool with the skin and wearing cotton clothing may also make life more comfortable.

Formal dietary manipulation is rarely necessary but should be discussed. Many patients have already started a restricted diet before seeing a doctor, so dietary assessment is important to confirm adequate nutrition. If the patient clearly identifies aggravating foods then avoidance should be tested. Airborne allergens are also

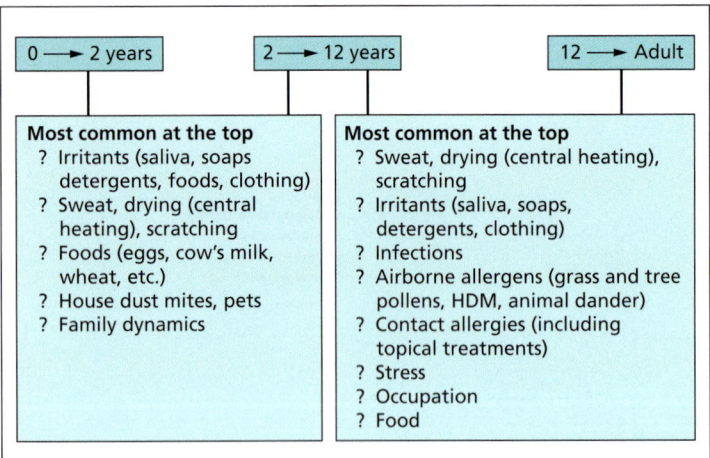

Figure 41.23 The spectrum of trigger factors at different ages. Adapted from Katayama *et al.* 2011 [13]. Reproduced with permission from the Japanese Society of Allergology.

often aggravating factors (see earlier), but again formal manipulation of the environment is not required for most patients. A further consideration with the concept of allergen avoidance is that of tolerance. There is a complex relationship between levels of exposure and tolerance, and it seems that high levels of exposure may be important for induction of tolerance. Thus, allergen avoidance regimens may in fact increase allergic responses on accidental allergen exposure due to loss of tolerance.

Most patients with atopic eczema are sensitised to HDM, but allergen avoidance is challenging and a systematic review of interventions such as mattress covers, vacuuming and acaricidal sprays showed only modest treatment responses in sensitised individuals [196].

Not only can stress aggravate atopic eczema, but the severely affected child is also a source of stress to the whole family. The doctor's role in giving simple reassurance and listening to family problems should not be underestimated. Stress can respond to treatment and the atopic eczema can be improved by using a variety of cognitive behavioural techniques and group therapy [351].

Parents should be advised about the risk of herpes simplex infection in a child with atopic eczema and told to avoid contact of active cold sores with the child's skin.

Topical therapy
Bathing and showering
Bathing is soothing for the majority of patients and is helpful as long as the skin is moisturised immediately afterwards. The frequency of bathing or showering is an individual choice and clear evidence as to the benefit or otherwise of frequent or infrequent regimes is lacking [352]. Foaming detergents (bubble bath and shower gels) and soaps should be avoided [353,354] and a soap substitute emollient used for cleansing. Dispersible bath oils can be helpful for some patients but do not maintain skin hydration and their use was not shown to benefit standard management of atopic eczema in a randomised clinical trial [355]. One previous study has convincingly shown that dilute bleach baths reduced the *S. aureus* bioburden and improved the overall disease severity score [356] but four other studies did not show convincing results to support this intervention [357].

Emollients
Emollients have been the mainstay of treatment regimens for atopic eczema for the last century. They undoubtedly have a low adverse event profile and therefore their liberal application is recommended. However, as with many older treatments, evidence for their benefit is limited. A recent systematic review demonstrated the heterogeneity in reported studies, but did find evidence to support the role of emollients in improving atopic eczema disease severity when combined with anti-inflammatory treatment, extending time between flares, and reducing the requirement for topical corticosteroids [358]. As discussed earlier, two large studies have independently confirmed no evidence that emollient application can act as a means for primary prevention of atopic eczema [242,243].

Important gaps in clinical trial evidence remain including which emollients are most effective and how to personalise their use. In general, in chronic lesions of atopic eczema, ointments are preferred, particularly when lichenification is prominent. In certain individuals, ointments can cause irritation and less oily preparations may be required. If lesions are exudative then creams or lotions may be required for a short time until ointments become more appropriate. One must be careful of preparations that contain irritants or surfactants such as sodium lauryl sulphate [359]. In order to identify the emollient that best suits an individual it may be useful to provide small quantities of several agents, so that they may choose which they prefer. A generous quantity (150–250 g per week for children through to 500 g per week for adults) should then be prescribed to encourage their frequent use throughout the day. There is no evidence that the order of application of emollient and topical corticosteroid affects response rates.

Since the recognition of the importance of barrier function in atopic eczema there are numerous 'designer emollients' being researched containing ingredients such as ceramide. There are suggestions that these can be effective in barrier repair and suppression of inflammation. However, there are limited studies and few comparisons with standard paraffin-based emollients.

Topical suppression of eczematous inflammation
Topical corticosteroids are the predominant treatment for the inflammation of atopic eczema and if applied correctly are very safe. Anxiety among both the general public and family doctors about potential adverse effects of topical corticosteroids has led to undertreatment of the skin in many sufferers. The strength and mode of application of the topical corticosteroids depends on the severity of the dermatitis, the sites to be treated and the age of the patient.

Once daily treatment in the evening, with morning application of emollients, may be as effective as twice daily corticosteroid treatment. There appear to be no differences in efficacy or side effects between pulsed potent corticosteroid creams and the continuous use of mild topical corticosteroids in patients with mild to moderate disease [360]. Corticosteroid-resistant or infected or crusted dermatitis may respond better to corticosteroid/antibiotic or corticosteroid/antiseptic combinations. However, in young children there is some concern about the potential systemic toxicity of some antiseptics, such as clioquinol, and the risk of bacterial resistance development, especially if large surface areas are to be treated [361].

Monitoring corticosteroid use

Complications related to systemic absorption of topical corticosteroids are very rare but prolonged application of potent or very potent preparations can induce adrenal suppression [362]. It is advisable to educate patients about the quantities to apply, for example the fingertip unit [363]. A strip of ointment measured from the distal phalangeal crease to the tip of the finger will treat two palm-sized areas of skin. It is also helpful to ask how long a standard 30 g tube of ointment has lasted. Even with limited dermatitis in a child, 10 g per week would not be excessive. Local side effects, such as permanent telangiectasia on the cheeks in babies and striae of the breasts, abdomen and thighs in adolescents, may be minimised if appropriate corticosteroid strengths are used. Particular care is required around the eyes, as glaucoma and cataracts have been associated with periocular topical steroids, but evidence for this effect is weak [364]. When there are concerns about side effects the topical calcineurin inhibitors, pimecrolimus and tacrolimus may prove to be helpful (see later).

Itch and antihistamines

Itch is the most important symptom of atopic eczema for patients and is associated with significant loss of quality of life. The use of emollients and reduction of trigger factors remains the initial approach. Emollients will usually provide short-term relief (2–4 hours) that can be beneficial before sleep, but for longer benefit, treatment with anti-inflammatory preparations is required. In atopic eczema, itch is initiated by inflammatory mediators and cytokines in the skin and this underlines why the priority in treating itch is controlling the inflammation.

Sometimes first generation oral antihistamines can be used for their sedative properties where sleep loss is significant, but it is important to acknowledge that antihistamine action is not beneficial in atopic eczema, as histamine is not the main mediator of pruritus in the disease [365,366].

Infection and antibiotics

Although 90% of patients with atopic eczema are colonised with *S. aureus*, exudation and pustule formation often implies staphylococcal and sometimes streptococcal infection of the skin. Topical or oral antibiotics may be beneficial for short periods (when there is clinical evidence of infection) but a randomised clinical trial showed no benefit from this approach [367] and therefore oral antibiotics are best reserved for those with signs of severe infection.

Topical calcineurin inhibitors

Topical calcineurin inhibitors (TCI) do not cause the cutaneous side effects of skin atrophy, striae, telangiectasia and bruising that may been seen with prolonged or inappropriate corticosteroid use. Therefore, they are particularly useful for eczema at sensitive sites such as the face, or as steroid-sparing agents where large quantities of topical corticosteroids are required [368,369].

Tacrolimus ointment use is licensed for patients aged 16 years and above at 0.1% strength and for children between 2 and 15 years of age at 0.03% strength. However, in practice the higher strength is commonly used in younger age groups where a potent anti-inflammatory effect is needed. Pimecrolimus 1% cream may be considered for use in corticosteroid-resistant facial dermatitis in children between 2 and 16 years. Generally, all TCIs are perceived as second line agents, but conditions of use vary. Many studies have demonstrated their efficacy. Tacrolimus 0.03% is considered to be more effective than mild potency topical corticosteroids but has less than moderate potency, whereas tacrolimus 0.1% is as effective as moderate potency topical corticosteroids [370]. Pimecrolimus 1% cream is less effective than moderate potency corticosteroids [370].

Both preparations can cause stinging and burning on initial application. This sensation often settles with continued use and can often be avoided through the initial use of topical corticosteroids.

The US Food and Drug Administration placed a black box warning on TCI because of widespread off-label use in under 2-year-olds and the theoretical risk of skin malignancy based on evidence from transplant patients and animal studies at 25–50 times the maximum recommended human dose. Since initial concerns over the risk of lymphoma and skin cancer, 10-year data do not show an increased risk [371,372]. Indeed, in recent studies of vitiligo tacrolimus and phototherapy were combined [373]. Although these concerns appear to be disproven, they should be discussed with patients.

New topical treatments

Crisaborole is a topical phosphodiesterase 4 (PDE_4) inhibitor that was shown to be effective for the treatment of mild–moderate atopic eczema compared with vehicle [374]. Active comparator trials are currently lacking. Use of crisaborole was approved for the treatment of atopic eczema in adults and children by the US Food and Drug Administration in 2016 and the European Medicines Agency (EMA) in 2020 although the EMA subsequently withdrew marketing authorisation. Further topical (PDE_4) inhibitors are under development.

Topical JAK inhibitors

JAK inhibitors (JAKi) target proteins in the Janus kinase-signal transducer and activator of transcription (JAK–STAT) pathway and inhibit downstream inflammatory cytokine production. They can be used orally or topically and are discussed under the section on novel small molecules below.

Maintenance therapy

The majority of patients will respond to initial treatment regimens. At follow-up, the importance of continuing to reduce exposure to trigger factors, as far as is practical, should be discussed. Particularly in children, one needs to strike a balance between social and physical development and avoidance of trigger factors.

The continuous use of emollients should be emphasised, as often in mild disease prolonged control can be obtained with the addition of very intermittent use of topical corticosteroids. In more severe disease, the addition of twice-weekly application of potent topical corticosteroids to the healed areas (the 'weekender approach') can safely and significantly reduce relapses [375]. If relapse occurs then topical corticosteroids should be used daily again for a week and then stepped down to the 'weekender approach' once more.

TCI have also been used to maintain control by twice weekly applications [375]. Adding mid-week use of tacrolimus ointment to the topical corticosteroid 'weekender approach' has been used to improve control of severe atopic eczema [376].

Unresponsive disease

Patients who fail to respond should be reviewed to check adherence, as this is the commonest cause for treatment failure in the management of atopic eczema even in severe disease and especially in children. Adherence can be improved by taking a structured approach to the consultation to address trust between doctor and patient/family, giving clear instructions with written action plans and, in resistant cases, employing psychological techniques such as shortening gaps between follow ups, and using rewards [377]. Anxieties about the treatment such as steroid phobia may be preventing appropriate therapy and can occur in all demographics [378–380]. It is also important to check that significant trigger factors have not been missed, to exclude recurrent or antibiotic-resistant infection and to consider more intensive treatment.

Intensive topical treatment

The potency of topical corticosteroid treatment can be increased for a short period. In-patient treatment is rarely used but can be particularly helpful in children with severe disease to both improve disease control but also explore the parental engagement with treatment protocols. During admission, the skin frequently improves using the same treatment that was unsuccessful as an out-patient.

Wet-wrap technique

This can be a useful technique for the control of severe atopic eczema in younger children. Classically, two layers of absorbent tubular bandage are applied to the skin. The inner layer is pre-soaked in warm water and the outer layer is dry. A generous quantity of a low potency topical corticosteroid is applied to the skin before the dressings. The dressings can be used overnight or changed every 12–24 h. More recently, the widespread availability of elasticated garments has prompted most centres to switch the regimen to application of topical therapy under a warm damp inner and an outer dry garment. This regimen can be used in hospital or for short-term out-patient treatment. Caution should be employed when applying moderate to high potency topical corticosteroids under the wet-wrap because suppression of the hypothalamopituitary axis can occur [381]. Regimens using emollient only under the wet dressings have become popular but are somewhat less effective.

Localised areas of severe lichenification can be treated with occlusive colloid dressings or paste banding that is left on for several days [382].

Phototherapy

Numerous types of phototherapy have undergone trials for the treatment of moderate to severe atopic eczema and show efficacy, albeit to a lesser degree than psoriasis. These include broad-band ultraviolet B (UVB), narrow-band UVB, medium- and high-dose UVA1 and PUVA [383]. Currently, narrow-band phototherapy seems to be the preferred option for chronic disease [384]. Its use in adults is supported by a strong evidence base and narrow-band UVB also appears effective in children. On average, disease activity is reduced by approximately 30–50% at the end of a typical 24-treatment course. Moreover, improvement may be maintained for several months. Patients should continue with routine topical corticosteroids and emollients. Acute flares of atopic eczema should be treated with intense topical treatment prior to narrow-band

UVB phototherapy and secondary infection should also be treated beforehand. A careful history prior to phototherapy should exclude photosensitive eczema. Assessment of the patient's minimal erythema dose (MED) may help to reduce burning episodes and optimise dosimetry.

The availability of medium- and high-dose UVA1 is generally restricted to specialist units but UVA1 may also improve acute atopic eczema [385]. A practical consideration is the relative timing of the use of phototherapy and topical/systemic immunosuppressant therapy because of the concerns about skin cancer development in later life. Home phototherapy under consultant guidance may be considered for patients who are unable to travel for phototherapy. In general, phototherapy courses should be limited to one per annum.

Third line therapy for atopic eczema

A number of interrelated clinical and holistic factors contribute to the decision process leading to the initiation of systemic therapy [386]. These include disease severity, patient and carer education over optimal use of topical treatments, adherence, sites affected, failure of first line and second line treatments to control the atopic eczema adequately (including the occurrence of repeated flares), avoidance of trigger factors, side effects from first line and second line treatments, patient choice, age of patient and co-morbidities. In addition, it is important to consider potential modifying factors that may account for lack or loss of therapeutic response such as secondary infection, allergic contact dermatitis and also re-evaluation of clinical differential diagnoses. If phototherapy is impractical, ineffective or there is rapid relapse then this may again lead to the consideration of systemic treatment. Finally, the development of unacceptable side effects from a primary therapy such as marked skin atrophy from overuse of topical corticosteroids or intolerability of TCI may again feed into the decision-making process.

Patients should receive adequate information about the proposed systemic treatments including their side-effect profile and proposed duration. This is particularly relevant if systemic therapy is being considered to gain rapid control of a severe acute flare. Systemic agents, such as ciclosporin, used in this situation may not be so suitable for longer term maintenance therapy.

The choice of systemic therapy is complicated by a relative lack of licensed medication for moderate-to-severe atopic eczema and a lack of comparative trial data particularly with respect to longer term maintenance therapy.

Of therapies available in clinical practice, randomised controlled trials provide evidence of efficacy for ciclosporin, azathioprine, methotrexate and mycophenolate mofetil, biologics (dupilumab, lebrikizumab, tralokinumab) and the selective JAK-kinase inhibitors abrocitinib, baracitinib and upadacitinib.

The introduction of biologics and small molecule inhibitors significantly changed the therapeutic landscape. In the UK, these drugs have been approved by NICE in circumstances when 'the disease has not responded to at least one systemic immunosuppressant, such as ciclosporin, methotrexate, azathioprine and mycophenolate mofetil, or these are not suitable' [387]. However, in some European countries, such as Germany, and the USA (dupilumab), the prescribing of these drugs does not depend on prior systemic therapy and therefore they are often used as first line systemics, depending on local funding arrangements. In the UK, care pathways have also changed with fewer patients cycling through several conventional systemics before commencing a novel systemic agent.

Conventional systemic agents
Ciclosporin
Ciclosporin is an effective treatment in both adults and children. An initial dose of 2.5–3.5 mg/kg/day is recommended with a maximal daily dose of 5 mg/kg/day [388] but there is a narrow therapeutic index. Virtually all patients respond rapidly with a reduction in disease severity by approximately 55% at 6–8 weeks [389–391]. However, symptoms recur rapidly when the drug is discontinued [390]. In the UK, ciclosporin is licensed for an 8-week course from age 16. Longer term use of ciclosporin is associated with an increased side-effect profile, in particular renal function impairment. However, if the dose can be reduced down to or below 2.5 mg/kg and regular monitoring of renal function and blood pressure are satisfactory, ciclosporin may be continued, typically for up to 1 year. Longer term use for inflammatory skin disease is not recommended [392].

Low-dose ciclosporin may be used 'off label' in severe and refractory disease in children [393,394] and is the commonest first line conventional systemic agent prescribed in Europe and the USA [395].

Azathioprine
The short-term use of azathioprine for the control of moderate-to-severe atopic eczema is supported by a good evidence base [396,397]. Its onset of action is slower than ciclosporin. An improvement in disease activity of approximately one third can be expected over the first 3 months of therapy, matched by improvements in patient orientated symptoms (including itch and quality of life) [398,399]. Clinical improvement may be maintained for several months after discontinuation of azathioprine therapy [397,399]. However, with the introduction of newer therapies, the use of azathioprine is declining, in part because of concerns over longer term potential side effects, such as risk of malignancy [400].

The dosage of azathioprine should be adjusted according to the patient's ability to metabolise the drug as determined by the activity of the enzyme thiopurine methyltransferase (TPMT) measured in red blood cells [388,396]. Patients with absent TPMT activity should not receive azathioprine; those with normal or high TPMT activity should receive azathioprine at a dose of 1–3 mg/kg/day, and those with low TPMT activity should receive azathioprine as a dose of 0.5–1 mg/kg/day [396]. TPMT-based dosimetry for patients with low TPMT activity appears to maintain efficacy, minimise side effects and has potential safety benefits [396]. Regular blood monitoring is still required for patients receiving azathioprine as TPMT polymorphisms account for only 65% of azathioprine induced neutropenia [396]. It is also important to bear in mind the potential for drug interactions with commonly prescribed drugs such as allopurinol [396]. 6-mercaptopurine may be considered in patients who are intolerant of azathioprine as imidazole moiety has been implicated in azathioprine-induced gastrointestinal side effects [396].

Formal trial data are lacking in children but azathioprine is prescribed as a first line systemic treatment in approximately one fifth of cases of severe eczema in children across Europe but less commonly in the USA [395,401]. Nevertheless, longer term continuation of azathioprine should be used with caution in children in view of

potential concerns regarding the potential risk of malignancy and photosensitivity [402].

Methotrexate
The use of systemic methotrexate for atopic eczema is supported by a moderate evidence base [403], typically at a dose of 15 mg per week in adults and a therapeutic dose of 0.4 mg/kg/week in paediatric patients. Methotrexate appears equally efficacious as azathioprine [397]. Also, and similar to azathioprine, methotrexate has a relatively slow onset of action but may result in persistent improvement after discontinuation. Clinical experience suggests that it may be better tolerated than azathioprine and has also shown to have clinical utility and efficacy in children [404]. While non-specific symptoms such as nausea, headache and a feeling of tiredness, are most common, serious side effects such as bone marrow suppression, liver and pulmonary fibrosis should be monitored for carefully [405].

Mycophenolate mofetil
For patients who have failed to respond or are intolerant of azathioprine and/or methotrexate, mycophenolate, may be considered as a fourth line agent, with dosage up to 2 g/day [388]. Importantly, enteric-coated mycophenolate mofetil (1.4 g daily) appeared as efficacious as ciclosporin (3 mg/kg/day) as maintenance treatment for 30 weeks [364]. Side-effects include gastrointestinal disturbance, leukopenia, lymphopenia and anaemia, which should be monitored appropriately. In the UK, prescribing of mycophenolate to treat atopic eczema has declined significantly because of its lesser efficacy as compared with methotrexate and availability of newer highly effective therapies.

Alitretinoin (9-cis retinoic acid)
Alitretinoin has been established as an efficacious systemic treatment for chronic hand eczema patients. An open study has also suggested benefit in more general atopic eczema [406].

Biologics for atopic eczema
There is no evidence to support the efficacy of anti-TNF therapy in atopic eczema. Omalizumab, a monoclonal antibody against IgE, has shown some benefit for asthma but variable outcomes in studies of atopic eczema. A small open study of six patients reported a benefit of rituximab following two infusions of 1000 mg, 2 weeks apart, but confirmatory reports are lacking.

IL-4/IL-13 inhibitors
Dupilumab is a fully human monoclonal antibody to the alpha subunit of the IL-4 receptor that inhibits IL-4 and IL-13 signalling. It was the first biologic to receive a licence for atopic eczema. Dupilumab is highly effective based on short-term RCTs (risk ratio (RR) compared with placebo for achieving 75% improvement in Eczema Area and Severity Index (EASI75) 3.04, 95% confidence interval (CI) 2.51–3.69; improvement in mean difference compared with placebo Patient Orientated Eczema Measurement (POEM) 7.30, 95% CI 6.61–8.00 (≤16 weeks). While comparative RCTs against abrocitinib and upadacitinib suggest that the JAK1 inhibitors may be more effective, the studies were not designed to explore superiority. However, dupilumab also appears safer than other agents over the short term [407]. Common adverse events included conjunctivitis,

nasopharyngitis and injection-site reactions. A systematic review and metanalysis of observational studies covering 3303 atopic eczema patients supported the short-term efficacy of dupilumab in the real-world [408]. However, side effects appeared more frequent than reported in RCTs. For example, conjunctivitis was reported in 26.1% of subjects. Patients with a previous history of ocular surface disease may be more at risk of developing ocular adverse events. Close liaison with ophthalmic colleagues is indicated and prophylactic topical eye therapy may be helpful (see earlier). On the other hand, the evidence from longer term studies for sustained efficacy is of low certainty [407]. There are currently no concerns over longer term adverse events apart from those noted earlier. However, clinical trials are not powered to detect rare but important adverse events. Further data will emerge from post-market surveillance studies and national/international registries that have been established. There is currently a lack of data about biomarkers that may help to predict clinical response and adverse events from dupilumab. Dupilumab has been explored as a therapy for nodular prurigo and to date the data looks promising [409].

New biologics in late phase trials

A number of new biologic therapies targeting key cytokines implicated in atopic eczema pathogenesis are in late phase clinical trials (Tables 41.6 and 41.7) and some of these are now licensed and in clinical practice (e.g. tralokinumab). Anti-IL-13 agents (e.g. lebrikizumab and tralokinumab) look promising [410–412]. Although comparison between placebo-controlled trials is difficult and depends on selection criteria, wash-out periods and in particular the concomitant topical therapies used, these drugs may not be as effective as dupilumab (Table 41.6) [407] although the evidence suggests that lebrikizumab may be more effective than tralokinumab. Side-effect profiles are similar to dupilumab. IL-31 plays an important role in itch and rapid improvement in itch was reported in trials of anti-IL-31 therapy (nemolizumab) [413]. Improvement in disease activity appears a little slower with overall improvement of 31–56%. TLSP is an important keratinocyte-derived cytokine that triggers itch and immune cell activation [201] (Figure 41.24). Consequently, it was a logical target for therapeutic development. An RCT of anti-TSLP (tezepelumab) though showed that just 24% of subjects achieved EASI75 and the primary end point was not achieved [414]. IL-22 is a cytokine produced by Th17, Th22 cells and innate lymphocytes that regulates keratinocyte proliferation and cell survival and has been implicated in the epithelial thickening response of atopic eczema [415]. Although the RCT of anti-IL-22 (fezakinumab) did not meet its primary endpoint, subset *post hoc* analysis identified a responsive sub-group with severe eczema [416]. Interestingly, the most severe patients with high baseline IL-22 expression showed the most pronounced transcriptomic improvements to fezakinumab [417].

New small molecules
JAK inhibitors

Increased understanding about the inflammatory cascade in atopic eczema led to the application and development of systemic and topical agents that target the JAK/STAT pathway. In particular, engagement of Th2 and other key cytokines involved in the pathogenesis of atopic eczema including IL-4, IL-5, IL-13, IL-22,

IL-31 and TSLP with their receptors leads to activation of specific JAK/STAT molecules [418]. This signal transduction pathway regulates important cellular processes relevant to atopic eczema including immune cell activation, eosinophil apoptosis, mast cell homeostasis, keratinocyte proliferation and differentiation, and itch. Hence JAKi would be expected to exert broader immunological effects than biologics targeting single molecules. The first generation of JAKi (e.g. tofacitinib) bound to and inhibited all three JAKs. The development of relatively selective drugs targeting specific components of this pathway represents a potentially important advance, given that the use of non-selective JAKi in other fields resulted in significant systemic adverse events (including stroke, myocardial infarction, venous embolic events and death). JAKi currently in clinical practice include abrocitinib, baricitinib and upadacitinib. However, studies comparing the clinical outcomes of JAKi to other systemic agents and biologics in atopic eczema are currently limited. This lack of evidence hinders clinical decision making. However, until long-term safety studies are available, concerns over cardiovascular and venous embolic events may mitigate against the use of these agents in 'at risk populations'.

Baricitinib is an oral selective JAK1-2 inhibitor that was approved for atopic eczema by the EMA and authorities in Japan in 2020. Metanalysis of three RCTs with topical steroids showed baracitinib was superior to placebo for EASI75 with a risk difference (RD) of 0.16, (95% CI 0.10–0.23) at 16 weeks [419]. An RD of 0.16 means that the 'risk' of achieving EASI75 is 16% more likely with baricitinib compared with placebo. Side effects appear more common than targeted therapies and include acne, nasopharyngitis, upper respiratory tract inflammation, elevated blood creatine phosphokinase levels and headache. Baricitinib was approved for rheumatoid arthritis in 2017; treatment-emergent infections including herpes zoster and deep venous thrombosis has been reported as a rare event in this context [420,421]. Pooled analysis across eight RCTs, involving 2531 subjects, identified two major adverse cardiovascular and two venous thrombosis events and one death [422]. Notably, the NICE appraisal committee commented in 2021 that 'baricitinib was not a "step change" in the same way as dupilumab', although the sequence of use of the two systemic agents is currently left to physician choice [423].

Upadacitinib and abrocitinib are oral selective inhibitors of JAK1. One RCT of upadacitinib showed significant superior efficacy to placebo for the primary end point percentage improvement in EASI score from baseline to week 16 [424] but was rated by the Cochrane risk-of-bias tool (RoB) for randomised trials as having 'some concerns' [407]. In a comparative study against dupilumab, a greater proportion of subjects in the upadacitinib group achieved the primary endpoint of EASI75 at week 16 ($n = 692$) [425]. The side effect profile appeared similar to baricitinib. Abrocitinib appeared as effective as dupilumab in a phase 3 study ($n = 838$) [**426**]. Side effects appeared similar to other JAKi (Table 41.6). Upadacitinib is also currently licensed for rheumatoid arthritis and reports from this field should be monitored.

Histamine 4 (H4) receptor is a recently discovered receptor subtype that contributes to histamine-induced inflammation and pruritus. A RCT showed that the H4 receptor inhibitor ZPL389 did not achieve the primary end point of significant change in NRS

Table 41.6 Conventional systemic agents, biologics and novel small molecules in clinical practice or in late phase clinical trials.

Drug	Therapeutic target	Approved for atopic dermatitis?	Estimated efficacy (mean % reduction in eczema severity scores)	Dose range	Common or serious side effects	Recommended monitoring	Relative effect (Cochrane review) [407]
Conventional systemic agents							
Azathioprine	TPMT	No	2–39% [304]	Adult: 1–3 mg/kg/day Paediatric: 1–4 mg/kg/day (based on TPMT activity)	Bone marrow suppression, haematological and LFT abnormalities, skin and other malignancies; drug interactions	TPMT prior to initiation; FBC, U&Es, LFTs every 3 months	
Ciclosporin	Calcineurin	No in USA, yes in Europe	53–95% [304]	Adult and paediatric: 2.5–5 mg/kg in split doses	Renal impairment; hypertension; drug interactions	FBC, U&Es, LFTs every 3 months	
Methotrexate	Folic acid antagonist	No	42% [304]	Adult: 7.5–25 mg weekly orally or by subcutaneous injection Paediatric: 0.2–0.7 mg/kg weekly orally or by subcutaneous injection	Hepatoxicity, haematological abnormalities, teratogen, gastrointestinal intolerance, nausea and fatigue; drug interactions	FBC, U&Es, LFTs every 3 months	
Mycophenolate	Purine biosynthesis	No		1.0–1.5 g orally twice daily Paediatric: 30 50 mg/kg daily	Gastrointestinal, teratogen	FBC, U&Es, LFTs every 3 months	
Biologics							
Dupilumab	Alpha subunit of IL-4 receptor	Yes	98% at week 16 [419]	Adult: 600 mg loading followed by 300 m/alternate weeks	Injection site reactions and ocular surface disease	FBC, U&Es, LFTs every 12 months	RR 3.04 (2.51–3.69) (8 RCTs; 1978 participants)
Tralokinumab	IL-13	Yes	56% EASI75 week 16 [431]		Viral upper respiratory tract infection, conjunctivitis, headache and injection-site reaction		RR 2.54 (1.21–5.34) (1 RCT; 153 participants)
New small molecules							
Baricitinib	JAK1 and JAK2	Yes	Metanalysis of three RCTs with topical steroids allowed showed baricitinib superior to placebo for EASI75 RD of 0.16 (95% CI 0.10–0.23) and EASI90 RD 0.14 (95% CI 0.09–0.20) at 16 weeks [419]	2–4 mg OD	Acne, nasopharyngitis, upper respiratory tract inflammation, elevated blood creatine phosphokinase levels and headache; treatment-emergent infections including herpes zoster and DVT in rheumatoid arthritis [420,421]		
Upadacitinib	JAK1	Yes	Phase 3 study EASI75 responses at week 24: 71% 30 mg OD upadacitinib compared with 61.1% dupilumab [425]	1 mg OD or 30 mg OD	Upper respiratory tract infection, worsening of atopic dermatitis and acne		
Abrocitinib	JAK1	Yes	Phase 3 study EASI75 response at week 12: 70.3% (200 mg abrocitinib), 58.7% (100 mg abrocitinib), 58.1% (dupilumab) and 27.1% (placebo) groups [426]	100 mg OD or 200 mg OD	Upper respiratory tract infections, nausea, acne, herpes simplex, herpes zoster, thrombocytopenia		

CI, confidence interval; DVT, deep vein thrombosis; EASI, Eczema Area and Severity Index; FBC, Full blood count; JAK, Janus kinase; LFT, liver function test; OD, once daily; RCT, randomised controlled trial; RD, risk difference; RR, risk ratio; TPMT, thiopurine methyltransferase; U&E, urea and electrolytes

PART 4: INFLAMMATORY DERMATOSES

Table 41.7 New drugs for atopic dermatitis in late phase trials.

Drug	Therapeutic target	Estimated efficacy (mean % reduction in eczema severity scores)	Dose range	Common or serious side effects	Relative effect EASI75 short-term follow-up (Cochrane review) [407]
Biologics					
Fezakinumab	IL-22	14% (NS); 22% in severe subset post hoc at 12 weeks [416]	Loading dose of 600 mg followed by 300 mg every 2 weeks IV	Facial cellulitis, viral upper respiratory tract infections	
Lebrikizumab	IL-13	Phase II studies; 55% achieved EASI75 but high placebo response in TREBLE (TCS allowed) [411] 41% at week 16 (monotherapy, no TCS) [410]	125 mg every 4 weeks (250 mg LD), 250 mg every 4 weeks (500 mg LD), or 250 mg every 2 weeks (500 mg LD at baseline and week 2)	Injection-site reactions, herpesvirus infections and conjunctivitis	RR 1.40 (0.83 to 2.36) 1 RCT; 46 participants)
Nemolizumab	IL-31	31–56% (systematic review) [413]	0.1–2 mg/kg q4w; 10–90 mg q4w	No difference compared with placebo	
Tezepelumab	TLSP	65% achieved EASI50 and 24% EASI75 at week 12 but large placebo response and not statistically significant [414]	80 mg every 2 weeks, plus TCS	Injection-site erythema	
New small molecules in late phase trials					
ZPL389	Histamine 4 receptor	50% reduction in EASI score compared with 27% for placebo at week 8 [430]	30 mg once daily	Similar to placebo	
New topical agents					
Delgocitinib	Pan JAKi	52% improvement in modified EASI50 and 28% improvement in modified EASI75 at week 52 [431]	0.5% ointment	Nasopharyngitis, eczema herpiticum	
Tofacitinib	JAK3 (+JAK1/2)	82% at week 4 [432]	2% ointment		

EASI, Eczema Area and Severity Index; IV, intravenous; JAK, Janus kinase; JAKi, JAK inhibitor; LD, loading dose; NS, not significant; q4w, every 4 weeks; RCT, randomised controlled trial; RR, risk ratio; TCS, topical corticosteroid; TLSP, thymic stromal lymphopoietin.

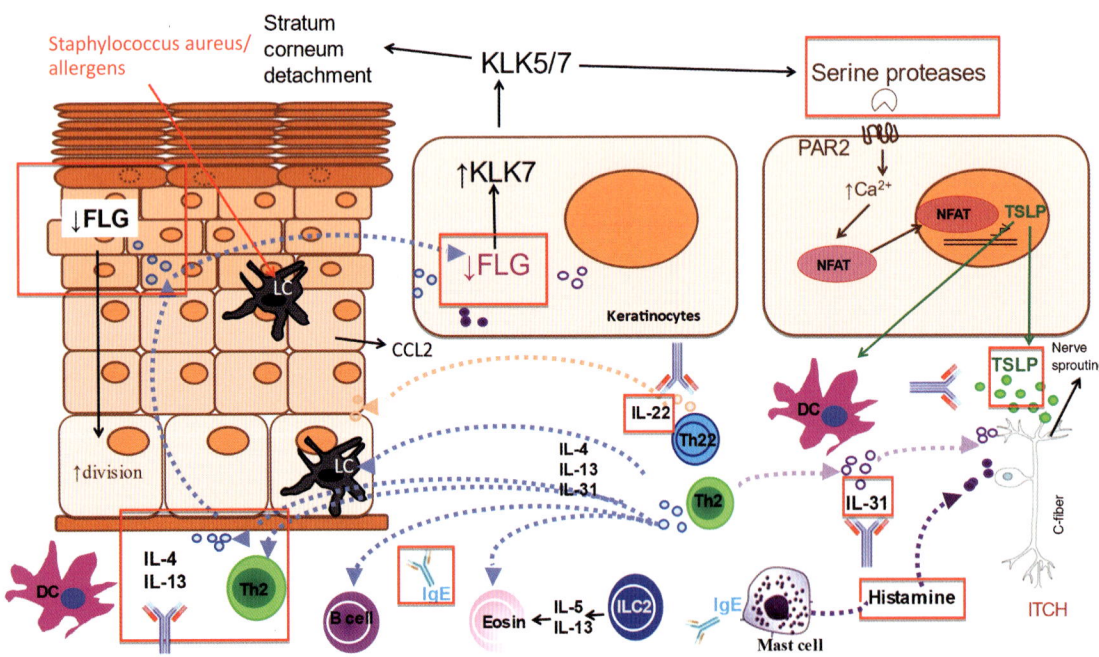

Figure 41.24 Targeting of key pathophysiological pathways (red boxes) by biologic and novel therapies in atopic eczema.

score for pruritus or secondary end point of reduction in EASI score compared with placebo from baseline to week 8. ZPL389 induced 50% reduction in EASI score compared with 27% for placebo. Further larger studies are required.

A variety of topical JAKi have been developed. RCTs have shown that topical cerdulatinib, delgocitinib, elgocitinib, ifidancitinib, ruxolitinib and tofacitinib are effective in treating atopic eczema in adults [427]. However, most studies are of limited duration (1–4 weeks) and active compactor trials are limited. Longer studies (≥12 weeks) are to date confined to delgocitinib, ruxolitinib and tofacitinib. Active compactor trials are to date confined to delgocitinib and ruxolitinib. Their side-effect profile within RCTs appears good and largely confined to local adverse reactions. Compared with oral JAKi, systemic side effects are limited although nasopharyngitis has been reported (delgocitinib).

Delgocitinib is a topical pan-JAKi, not yet approved in the USA or Europe for atopic dermatitis, but is approved in Japan. Clinical response is dose dependent and >50% of subjects achieved EASI75 response at higher doses (3%) with rapid improvement in symptoms including itch [427]. A recent phase 3 study reports promising results for the use of delgocitinib in moderate to severe hand eczema [428].

Key references

The full list of references can be found in the online version at https://www.wiley.com/rooksdermatology10e

28 Laughter MR, Maymone MBC, Mashayekhi S *et al*. The global burden of atopic dermatitis: lessons from the Global Burden of Disease Study 1990–2017. *Br J Dermatol* 2021;184:304–9.

64 Palmer CN, Irvine AD, Terron-Kwiatkowski A *et al*. Common loss-of-function variants of the epidermal barrier protein filaggrin are a major predisposing factor for atopic dermatitis. *Nat Genet* 2006;38:441–6.

128 Apfelbacher CJ, Diepgen TL, Schmitt J. Determinants of eczema: population-based cross-sectional study in Germany. *Allergy* 2011;66:206–13.

173 Newell L, Polak ME, Perera J *et al*. Sensitization via healthy skin programs Th2 responses in individuals with atopic dermatitis. *J Invest Dermatol* 2013;133:2372–80.

188 Clayton K, Vallejo A, Sirvent S *et al*. Machine learning applied to atopic dermatitis transcriptome reveals distinct therapy-dependent modification of the keratinocyte immunophenotype. *Br J Dermatol* 2021;184:913–22.

194 Reynolds G, Vegh P, Fletcher J *et al*. Developmental cell programs are co-opted in inflammatory skin disease. *Science* 2021;371(6527).

195 Brunner P, Emerson R, Tipton C *et al*. Nonlesional atopic dermatitis skin shares similar T-cell clones with lesional tissues. *Allergy* 2017;72:2017–25.

203 Ruzicka T, Hanifin JM, Furue M *et al*. Anti-interleukin-31 receptor A antibody for atopic dermatitis. *N Engl J Med* 2017;376:826–35.

205 Ong PY, Ohtake T, Brandt C *et al*. Endogenous antimicrobial peptides and skin infections in atopic dermatitis. *N Engl J Med* 2002;347:1151–60.

218 Ardern-Jones MR, Black AP, Bateman EA, Ogg GS. Bacterial superantigen facilitates epithelial presentation of allergen to T helper 2 cells. *Proc Natl Acad Sci U S A* 2007;104:5557–62.

426 Bieber T, Simpson EL, Silverberg JI *et al*. Abrocitinib versus placebo or dupilumab for atopic dermatitis. *N Engl J Med* 2021;384:1101–12.

PART 4: INFLAMMATORY DERMATOSES

CHAPTER 42

Urticaria

Clive E. H. Grattan[1] and Alison V. Sears[1,2]

[1]St John's Institute of Dermatology, Guy's and St Thomas' NHS Foundation Trust, London, UK
[2]Kingston Hospital, Kingston-upon-Thames, London, UK

Urticaria, 42.1	Key references, 42.19

Urticaria

Definition and nomenclature

The term urticaria defines an illness that may present with short-lived itchy weals, angioedema or both [1]. It also describes an eruption of weals. It may be spontaneous or inducible. There may be overlap between patterns of urticaria. Similarly, angioedema is used as a disease term and as a physical sign.

Synonyms and inclusions
- Weals (hives or nettlerash)
- Angioedema (angioneurotic oedema, Quincke's oedema)
- Spontaneous (idiopathic) urticaria
- Inducible (physical, cholinergic and contact) urticarias

Terminology

A *weal* is a descriptive term for transient, well-demarcated, superficial red, skin-coloured or pale swellings of the dermis due to reversible exudation of plasma in the skin that fade, usually within hours, without leaving a mark (Figure 42.1). Weals are usually very itchy and often associated with a surrounding red flare when they arise.

Angioedema swellings are deeper than weals affecting, primarily, subcutaneous or submucosal tissues (Figure 42.2) but merging with weals may be seen. They are usually painful, rather than itchy, poorly defined and normal in colour. They can occur anywhere on the skin, mouth or genitalia and usually last longer than weals. Angioedema presenting without weals may be mast cell mediated (e.g. spontaneous urticaria) or, much less commonly, bradykinin mediated (e.g. hereditary angioedema, angiotensin-converting enzyme-induced angioedema), when involvement of the larynx and bowel may occur.

Anaphylaxis is a sudden, severe, life-threatening reaction due to systemic mast cell activation, usually involving the skin with flushing, weals or angioedema.

Classification

Urticaria may be acute (the disease resolving in less than 6 weeks) or chronic (continuous disease lasting for 6 weeks or more). Recurrent intermittent or episodic presentations of urticaria also occur [2]. They are often included within the definition of chronic urticaria [1,3] but the terms can be used to describe disease behaviour (e.g. acute intermittent or chronic intermittent) for the purpose of clinical care. The acute and chronic terminology is usually applied to spontaneous urticaria but inducible urticarias may also be acute or chronic, depending on their duration. The main types of urticaria and differential diagnoses of urticarial rashes are shown in Box 42.1.

Box 42.1 Main subtypes of urticaria and differential diagnoses of urticarial rash

Subtypes
- Spontaneous urticarias:
  - Acute
  - Intermittent (episodic)
  - Chronic (syn. 'idiopathic')
- Inducible urticarias (including physical, cholinergic and contact urticarias)

Differential diagnoses
- Urticarial vasculitis
- Autoinflammatory syndromes with urticarial rash
- Hereditary and acquired angioedema without weals (bradykininergic)

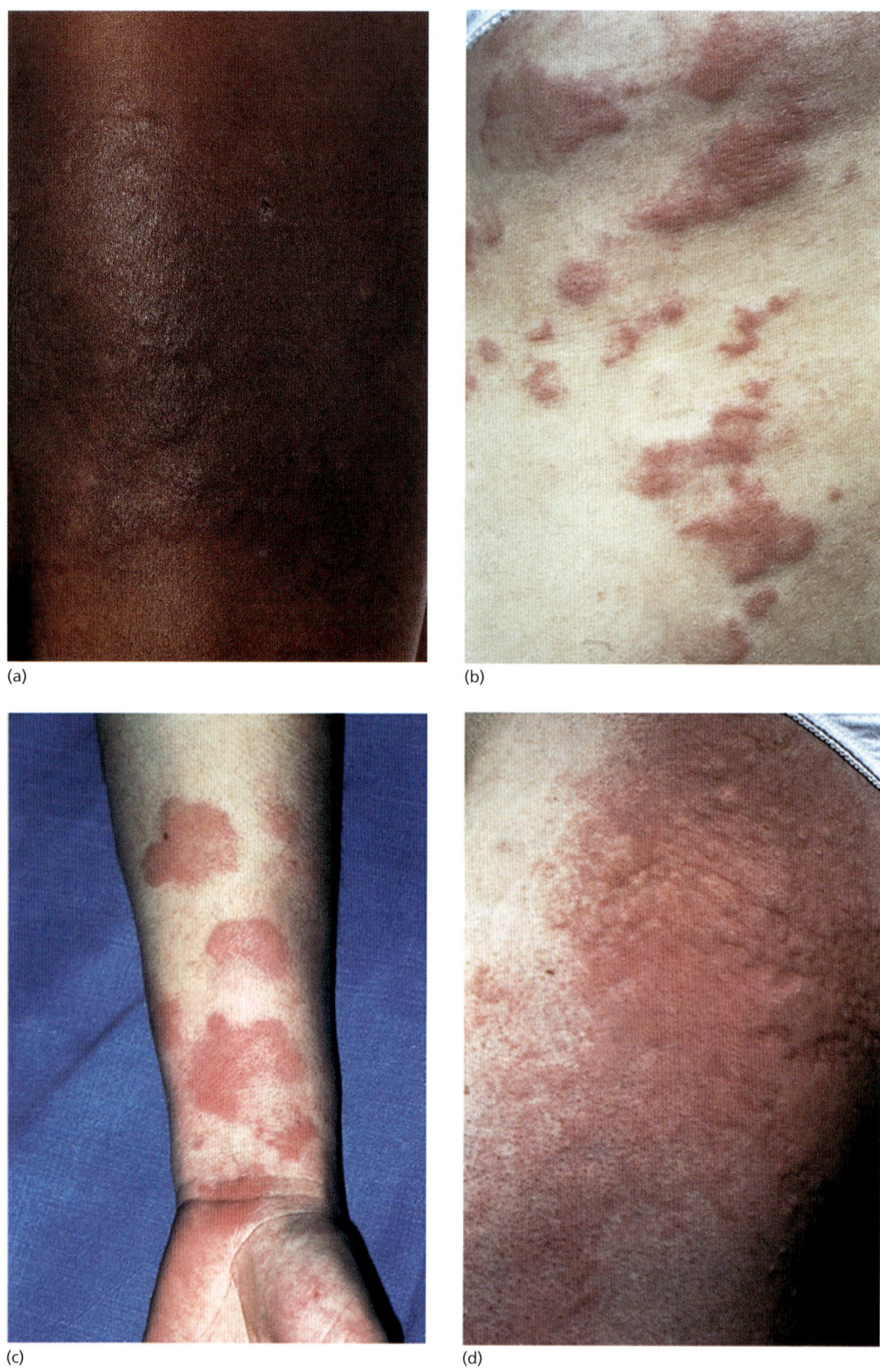

(a)

(b)

(c)

(d)

Figure 42.1 (a–d) Different morphology of urticarial weals. Courtesy of St John's Institute of Dermatology, London, UK.

Introduction and general description

Urticaria has been recognised since the days of Hippocrates. The term dates back to the 18th century, when the stinging and burning was likened to the sting of a nettle (*Urtica dioica*) by Cullen and Bateman [4].

Epidemiology
Incidence and prevalence

Early studies suggested that one in five of the general population may develop some form of urticaria over their lifetime, although this figure may be an overestimate [5]. A point prevalence between

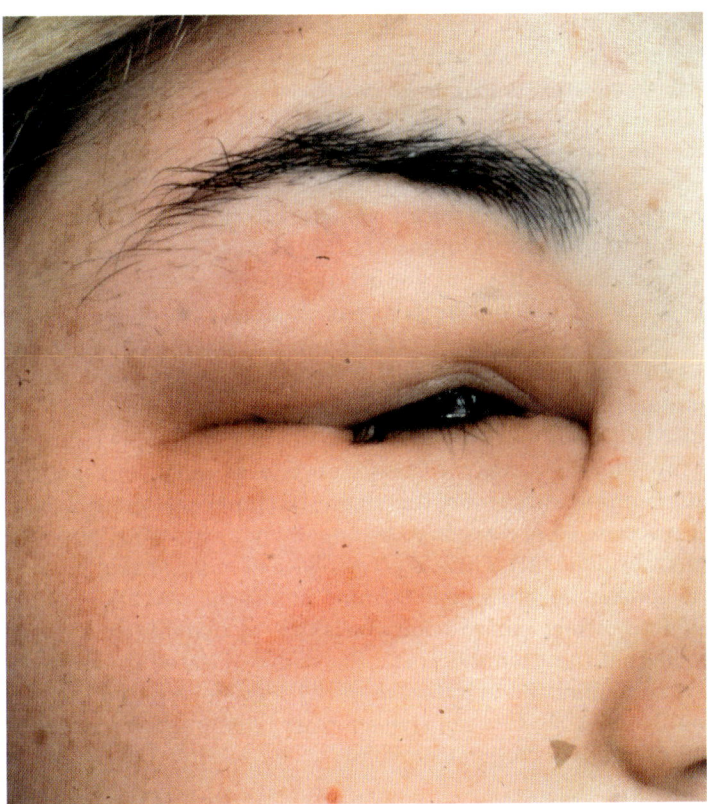

Figure 42.2 Angioedema of the eyelid. Courtesy of St John's Institute of Dermatology, London, UK.

0.5% and 1.0% for chronic spontaneous urticaria has been proposed [5]. Lifetime prevalence estimates range from 0.6% [6] to 1.8% [7]. A 1-year prevalence estimate in European children was 0.75% [8]. Regional differences in point prevalence of chronic urticaria were identified in a recent meta-analysis (Asia 1.4%, Europe 0.5%, North America 0.1%) [9].

Age
Urticaria may occur at any age. Acute spontaneous urticaria often presents in childhood but the peak incidence of chronic spontaneous urticaria is in the fourth to fifth decades [5].

Sex
Women outnumber men by 2 : 1 with chronic spontaneous urticaria but there is no consistent sex difference in acute spontaneous urticaria or the inducible urticarias.

Ethnicity
No difference in prevalence has been reported for race or ethnic groups although data on this are scarce.

Associated diseases
Autoimmune disease. An association between chronic spontaneous urticaria and autoimmune thyroid disease was first reported by Leznoff and Sussman [10] and confirmed subsequently by many others. The association is particularly strong at 30% for patients with a positive basophil histamine release test as a marker of functional autoantibodies [11]. There also appears to be a higher frequency of autoimmune disease in patients with autoimmune urticaria [12]. The most frequent organ-specific autoimmune co-morbidities after thyroid disease (Hashimoto disease being more common than Graves disease) are pernicious anaemia and vitiligo followed by coeliac disease, rheumatoid arthritis and insulin-dependent diabetes [13]. Little evidence is available on the co-morbidity of systemic lupus erythematosus with chronic spontaneous urticaria, with estimates ranging from 0% to 21.9% in a systematic review [14].

Infection. The association of chronic urticaria with infection is less clear. The older literature suggests that chronic 'idiopathic' urticaria may be associated with chronic infections, especially dental, and *Candida* infections of the bowel, but in the authors' experience this occurs rarely, if at all. A meta-analysis of therapeutic trials for patients with active *Helicobacter pylori* infection and chronic urticaria showed that those who responded to eradication treatment were more likely to go into remission of urticaria than those who did not respond [15]. Bowel parasitic infection as a cause of chronic urticaria is rare in developed countries but should always be considered in countries where it is endemic. The evidence linking chronic urticaria and infections has been reviewed [16]. These authors described a link between *H. pylori* and a positive autologous serum skin test (ASST). They drew attention to the relatively high frequency of upper respiratory tract viral infections (47%) with acute urticaria and concluded that the evidence base to link viral, bacterial, parasitic and fungal infection with chronic urticaria is lacking. Chronic spontaneous urticaria patients were more often diagnosed with protozoa and had a significantly higher risk of toxocariasis seropositivity and *Anisakis simplex* sensitisation when compared with healthy controls [17].

Malignancy. Although there have been anecdotal reports of urticaria occurring with systemic malignancies, no overall association was found in a large epidemiological study [18]. An increased risk of cancer (standardised incidence ratio 2.2), including haematological malignancies (standardised incidence ratio 4.1), especially non-Hodgkin lymphoma, was observed in a retrospective population-based cohort study using data from a national health insurance research database in Taiwan [19]. Anecodotal series of patients with chronic urticaria that cleared after treatment of cancer provide indirect evidence for a possible link [20].

Pathophysiology
Urticaria is primarily a mast cell-driven disease, although the importance of cross-talk between the cutaneous mast cell and the inflammatory infiltrate and the relevance of T helper 2 (Th2) cell inflammation is increasingly being recognised in chronic spontaneous urticaria. A range of immunological and non-immunological stimuli can degranulate cutaneous mast cells *in vivo* and *in vitro* (Figure 42.3), releasing histamine, tryptase and preformed cytokines and generating eicoanoids. Cross-linking of mast cell-bound specific immunoglobulin E (IgE) by exogenous allergens may be relevant to acute spontaneous urticaria, but type I allergy is probably never the cause of continuous chronic spontaneous disease. Binding of pathogen-associated molecular patterns (PAMPs) on microbes to Toll-like receptors on mast cells may be relevant to the pathogenesis

NON-IMMUNOLOGICAL   IMMUNOLOGICAL

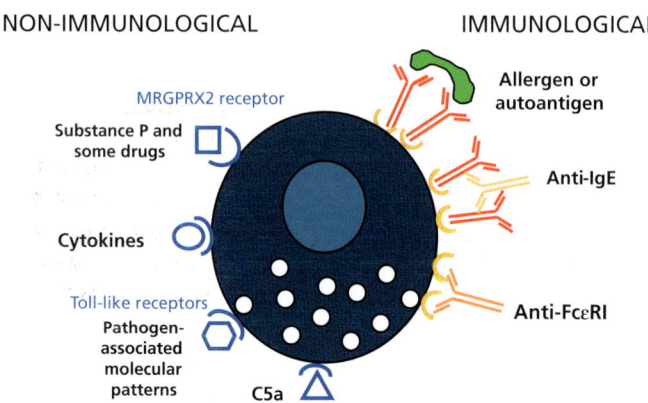

Figure 42.3 Immunological and some non-immunological mast cell degranulation stimuli. The mast cell responds with degranulation to non-immunological as well as immunological stimuli *in vitro*. It is often difficult, if not impossible, to know the exact cause of degranulation *in vivo*.

of acute urticaria, which is more often linked to acute viral or bacterial infections than any other aetiology, but experimental proof for this is lacking.

There is convincing evidence of functional IgG autoantibodies against IgE or the high-affinity IgE receptor in 25–30% of patients with chronic spontaneous urticaria. They cause degranulation of healthy donor basophils and cutaneous mast cells *in vitro* and *ex vivo* [21,**22**,23,24]. C5a complement is a cofactor for mast cell degranulation *in vitro* [25]. The subclass of IgG appears to determine functionality: IgG1 and IgG3 are closely linked with histamine release from basophils, but IgG2 and IgG4 are not [26]. The autoimmune hypothesis of chronic spontaneous urticaria proposes that functional autoantibodies are of direct pathogenic importance. Circumstantial and indirect evidence is available to support this hypothesis [27]. A proportion of patients with chronic spontaneous urticaria show upregulation of activation markers on circulating basophils [28] with reduced responsiveness to anti-IgE stimulation that appears to recover with spontaneous disease remission [29]. While type I allergy is exceptional as a cause of chronic spontaneous urticaria, IgE antibodies have been described against self-antigens including thyroid peroxidase (TPO) [30], interleukin 24 (IL-24) [31] and eosinophil peroxidase [32], giving rise to the concept of autoallergic urticaria [**33**].

Weals and angioedema result from transient vasopermeability and vasodilatation of the dermal and subcutaneous vasculature following the release of preformed and newly synthesised mast cell mediators. Histamine is the major preformed mediator in most patients. Newly formed mediators include prostaglandin D2 and platelet-activating factor. Preformed tumour necrosis factor α (TNF-α) upregulates adhesion molecules with recruitment of acute inflammatory cells, including neutrophils and eosinophils, into the weal. Basophils are likely to contribute to prolongation of the weal response by releasing histamine after migrating into the weals. Other cyokines are almost certainly involved. Increased peripheral blood levels of IL-8 and IL-10 [34] have been found in acute urticaria. IL-6 and IL-8 were found to be increased within induced cold urticaria weals by sampling dermal fluids using microdialysis [35]. The role of infiltrating T cells in relation to other inflammatory cells has been reviewed [36]. Increased expression of Th2-initiating

cytokines has been shown in lesional skin biopsies [37]. IL-17 in plasma and lesional skin biopsies supports a pathogenic role of Th17 lymphocytes [38]. Increased vascular markers are expressed in lesional skin [39].

Activation of H_1 receptors on nerve endings induces itch, with redness, oedema and flare from binding receptors on the smooth muscle cells of small blood vessels. However, activation of H_2 receptors in skin, including smooth muscle cells, contributes to redness and wealing but not itch or flare. H_3 receptors, identified on inhibitory neurons in the brain, act as inhibitory autoreceptors by reducing biosynthesis and release of histamine; they have not been identified in human skin. Although H_4 receptor activation on granulocytes, including mast cells, leads to scratching behaviour in mice [40], there is currently no evidence of its relevance to urticaria symptoms. Compared with normal controls, cutaneous mast cells from chronic urticaria release more histamine spontaneously and in response to non-specific degranulating agents such as codeine and morphine [41]. There is no evidence of reduced skin histamine metabolism by *N*-methylhistamine in chronic urticaria, although reduced metabolism of dietary histamine by diamine oxidase in the bowel has been reported [42]. Tryptase is released in conjunction with histamine. It can induce mast cell degranulation and cleave C3 to C3a and C3b. C3a can activate mast cells, and C3b can activate the alternative complement pathway.

Predisposing factors
No predisposing genetic or environmental factors for developing spontaneous or inducible urticarias have emerged to date. However, several polymorphisms have been linked to aspirin-sensitive urticaria and a very strong association between patients with functional autoantibodies and human leukocyte antigen (HLA) DR4 in patients with chronic spontaneous urticaria has been described (see 'Genetics' later in this chapter).

Aetiology
Although some cases of acute urticaria can be ascribed to type I hypersensitivity, infection, food or drug intolerance, the cause in at least 60% of patients remains unknown and may be multifactorial. The cause of acute urticaria in more than 50% of patients presenting to a city 'walk-in' dermatology centre remained unexplained after investigation [43]. In the others, the most common preceding event was an upper respiratory tract infection, followed by drug ingestion, but food allergy or intolerance was rare.

Approximately 50% of patients with chronic spontaneous urticaria will react with a red weal response to intradermal injection of their own serum known as the ASST response [44] as evidence of autoreactivity. Around half of these will have functional autoantibodies on the basophil histamine release assay [45]. A much smaller number will show evidence of dietary pseudoallergens, including food additives, histamine and salicylates [46], or chronic infection as aggravating factors that may be augmenting their illness. A cause will not be identified, even after looking for functional autoantibodies (where this option is available to clinicians) in at least 50% of patients with chronic spontaneous urticaria. Some of these may have autoallergic urticaria defined by specific IgE against autoantigens, although no commercial test is currently available for this. The term 'idiopathic' is still favoured by some specialists for patients with chronic spontaneous urticaria to reflect increasing understanding of the complex events resulting in clinical disease activity beyond the presence or absence of detectable serum histamine release autoantibodies *in vitro*. Although the trigger for inducible urticarias is defined by challenge testing, the underlying cause of the mast cell releasability remains unknown, except in allergic contact urticaria where skin or mucosal contact with the relevant allergen elicits local mast cell degranulation with mediator release. The response of some patients with inducible urticarias to omalizumab (anti-IgE) suggests that IgE directed against neoantigens generated by the inducing stimulus could be a factor. However, other mechanisms are needed to explain the rapid onset and offset of wealing that characterise this group of patients, with the exception of delayed pressure urticaria.

Acute spontaneous urticaria

Allergic. Any drug, food, foreign substance from blood transfusion, injection, implant, contactant and inhalant should be considered as a potential allergen (Box 42.2). Acute urticarial reactions from drugs are common, usually occurring within hours of drug administration in presensitised patients, although it should be noted that *urticarial* drug reactions (i.e. reactions with an urticarial component) are not synonymous with acute urticaria due to a drug. It is often difficult to know whether acute urticaria following infection treated with antibiotics is due to the infection or the drug and it may merit investigation later to confirm or exclude antibiotic allergy.

Box 42.2 Potential causes of acute urticaria

- Idiopathic
- Infections:
  - Viral, e.g. upper respiratory tract infections, hepatitis B and C, SARS-CoV-2 (Covid-19)
  - Bacterial, e.g. *Streptococcus pyogenes*
  - Parasitic, e.g. *Anisakis simplex*
- Foods, e.g. cow's milk, hen's egg, nuts, seeds, lipid transfer proteins, alpha gal
- Drugs, e.g. β-lactam antibiotics
- Stings, e.g. bee, wasp venoms
- Blood products, e.g. transfusions
- Vaccines
- Contactants, e.g. latex

Acute urticarial reactions to food are believed to be common and many go unreported [47]. Urticarial reactions may not be to the main food itself but to other ingredients, such as seeds or spices. Rarely, allergic reactions to food occur only if intake is followed by exercise, with neither food nor exercise alone inducing weals (food-dependent exercise-induced anaphylaxis) [48]. Substances reported to cause this include wheat and shellfish. Wheat-dependent exercise-induced anaphylaxis is associated with IgE against omega-5-gliadin (a gluten component). Delayed reactions have also been described to galactose alpha-1,3-galactose (alpha gal) in red meat after IgE sensitisation from exposure to cetuximab or tick bites [49].

Non-allergic. These include the following.

1 *Histamine liberators.* Mast cell histamine release is non-immunological and may occur after first exposure. Examples include morphine, codeine, neuromuscular blocking agents, such as atracurium, and antibiotics, such as polymyxin and vancomycin. Iodinated radiocontrast dyes may cause non-allergic anaphylaxis. Exactly how radiocontrast media, low- and high-molecular dextran plasma expanders cause these reactions is not known. Complement activation is thought to play a role in serious dextran reactions.

2 *Pseudoallergic reactions.* Intolerance reactions are not substance-specific and may occur in response to unrelated compounds in the same individual. The severity of reaction is usually dose related. Drug causes include aspirin and other non-steroidal anti-inflammatory agents. By inhibiting the cyclo-oxygenase (COX-1) pathway of arachidonic acid metabolism, pro-inflammatory lipoxygenase pathway products leukotriene C_4, D_4 and E_4 are generated with inhibition of prostaglandin E_2, which is inhibitory for immunological mast cell degranulation [50].

Alcohol-induced urticaria is rare; the mechanism of causation is unknown, but appears not to be allergic [51]. Alcoholic beverages can aggravate urticaria non-specifically. White wines are often treated with sulphites, which have rarely been reported to cause urticaria and anaphylaxis [52,53]. Some red wines contain measurable concentrations of vasoactive amines including histamine, which could aggravate urticaria, but cutaneous symptoms relate poorly to histamine content [54].

Food may also contain vasoactive amines including histamine (such as in cheese, fish, processed meat, tomatoes, pineapple and avocados) or histamine-releasing substances (such as in strawberries). Histamine generated in scombroid fish (underprocessed tuna, mackerel or swordfish) by histidine decarboxylase from bacteria can cause acute flushing, urticaria, vomiting and diarrhoea. High levels of histamine can usually be found in affected fish [55].

Infections. Urticaria may follow non-specific viral infections, Epstein–Barr [56] or acute hepatitis B viral infections, Covid-19 [57], anisakiasis (infection by a fish parasite in presensitised individuals) [58], streptococcal throat infections in children and, rarely, *Campylobacter jejuni* infections [59].

Chronic spontaneous urticaria

Idiopathic. Nearly all patients were considered to have 'idiopathic' urticaria before autoimmunity was recognised as a cause in some patients. Clinical experience suggests that chronic urticaria is often a multifactorial disease and that its day-to-day activity is determined by aggravating factors (see 'Clinical features' later in this chapter) over and above its primary aetiology.

Allergic. IgE-mediated allergy is probably never the cause of chronic spontaneous urticaria in adults, except in the rare event that unrecognised food allergy might present with recurrent weals over a period of 6 weeks or more until the cause is suspected and withdrawn.

Autoallergic. The response of many patients with chronic spontaneous urticaria to anti-IgE (omalizumab) and the finding of autoantigen-specific IgE in the blood of some patients with urticaria suggests that autoallergy is a potential mechanism for spontaneous urticaria. Demonstrating a weal and flare response by passive transfer of IgE anti-TPO from a patient with chronic spontaneous urticaria to healthy controls followed by skin testing with recombinant TPO supports the concept of potential functionality for these autoantibodies [60]. An animal model is not available and the proportion of patients with chronic spontaneous urticaria driven by autoallergy is currently unknown.

Autoimmune. The concept of autoimmune urticaria is based on indirect and strong circumstantial evidence [27] for functional IgG against the high-affinitiy IgE receptor on mast cells and basophils or cell-bound IgE, but an animal model has not been developed. No routine tests are available to clinicians although the basophil histamine release assay or basophil activation tests using sera of patients incubated with healthy donor basophils are commercially available in some countries. Low total IgE and raised IgG anti-TPO appear to be useful surrogate markers of functional autoantibodies and are widely available [61].

Pseudoallergic. Food additives, natural salicylates, amines, spices, green teas and alcohol may aggravate existing chronic spontaneous urticaria in up to 30% of patients [37,62] but are very rarely the cause. A 3-week trial of a low pseudoallergen diet (Table 42.1) may be considered as a diagnostic investigation [1] in well-motivated patients.

Infection and infestation-related. The incidence of bacterial infections, such as dental sepsis, sinusitis, urinary tract and gallbladder infections, in chronic urticaria varies in different series. If present, treatment of the infection usually does not cure urticaria. *Helicobacter pylori* infection of the stomach, which has variable prevalence worldwide, has been associated with chronic spontaneous urticaria [13]. Linear urticated lesions may follow migration of *Ancylostoma* and *Strongyloides* worms but are not urticaria. *Toxocara canis* antibodies have been associated with chronic urticaria, but a causal relationship is unproven [63].

Pathology

The histology of weals is usually non-specific, with vascular and lymphatic dilatation, oedema and a variable perivascular cellular dermal infiltrate consisting of lymphocytes, neutrophils and eosinophils (Figure 42.4). The number of mast cells in chronic spontaneous urticaria biopsies is probably increased but the evidence from studies is inconsistent. In one study, dermal mast cells in weals of chronic urticaria were increased by 10 times [64] compared with non-urticated skin, using conventional histochemical stains, but this increase was not confirmed in a study using tryptase and chymase as markers [65]. Tryptase-positive mast cells were increased in chronic spontaneous urticaria biopsies compared with controls but there was no difference between lesional and non-lesional skin [39]. In the majority of weals, there is a sparse perivascular infiltrate,

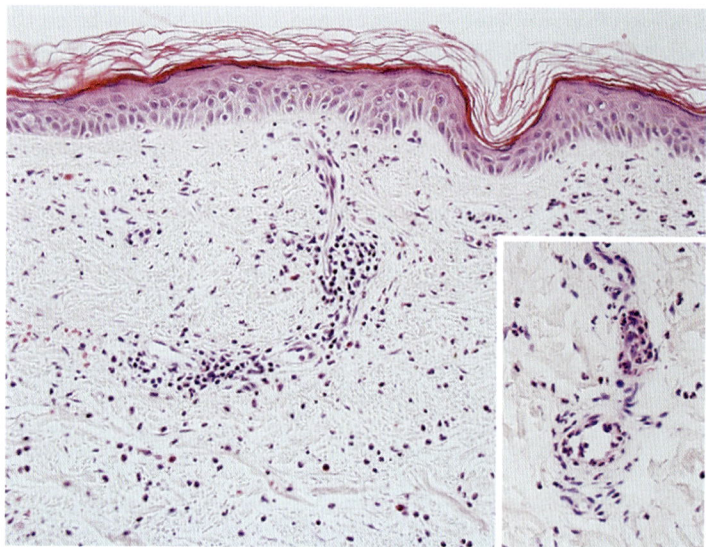

Figure 42.4 Histology of a spontaneous weal from a patient with chronic spontaneous urticaria showing dermal oedema with a moderate perivascular and interstitial mixed inflammatory infiltrate, including intravascular neutrophils (inset), lymphocytes and a few eosinophils but no vasculitis. Courtesy of Dr Alistair Robson, St John's Institute of Dermatology, London, UK.

Table 42.1 Low pseudoallergen diet.

Food type	Allowed	Not allowed
Carbohydrate	Organic (preservative-free) bread, potatoes, rice, flour (not self-raising), pasta *without* egg, plain cereals (e.g. porridge, muesli without fruit, Cornflakes)	All others, e.g. pasta *with* egg, noodles, popcorn, fruit muesli, potato chips and crisps, biscuits, cakes
Fat and oils	Butter, cold-pressed plant oils (e.g. olive, sunflower)	All others, e.g. margarine, mayonnaise, butter substitute
Dairy	Fresh milk, cream, white cheese (e.g. Brie), fromage frais, Gouda (small amounts)	All others, e.g. yoghurt, Cheddar, Stilton, Gorgonzola, Parmesan
Meat, fish, eggs	Fresh meat without seasoning, organic eggs	All others, e.g. non-organic eggs, fish, seafood, processed and smoked meats (e.g. sausages, meat pies, smoked salmon)
Vegetables	All vegetables and salads, except those listed as not allowed	Tomatoes and tomato products, peas, spinach, sweet peppers, olives, mushrooms, artichokes, rhubarb
Fruits	None	All fresh, dried and sugared fruits (e.g. glace cherries), fruit juices
Herbs, spices and nuts	Salt, sugar, onions, chives, all nuts (unless allergy has been shown, and avoid walnuts)	All others, e.g. curries, chillies, garlic, coriander
Desserts, spreads and sweets	None except honey	All others, e.g. jams, Nutella, toppings, sweets, chewing gum
Drinks	Milk, water, coffee, black tea (Indian and Ceylon)	All others, e.g. beer, wine, spirits, herbal and green teas (Japanese or China), fruit squashes and cordials

Adapted from Zuberbier *et al.* 1995 [83].

predominantly of helper T lymphocytes [66,67] with a TH$_0$ cytokine profile expressing mRNA for IL-4, IL-5 and interferon γ (IFN-γ) [68]. Th2 initiating cytokines IL-33, IL-25 and thymic stromal lymphopoetin were identified in lesional but not non-lesional skin [37]. In a minority of weals, neutrophils are a conspicuous feature within the vessel walls or scattered in the dermis [69]. Eosinophils may play a more important role than their sparse numbers seen on light microscopy would suggest, as extracellular eosinophil major basic protein is frequently deposited in spontaneous weals [70] and they stain for activation markers [71]. The spectrum of cellular changes may depend on the age of weals and their underlying cause. Biopsies are generally performed if individual weals are persistent, and they may show features of delayed pressure urticaria or urticarial vasculitis. In delayed pressure urticaria, the infiltrate is denser, with neutrophils often present in early weals and eosinophils extending deep into the fat in early and late weals. These cellular changes correlated with moderate upregulation of the vascular endothelial adhesion molecules E-selectin, intercellular adhesion molecule 1 (ICAM-1) and vascular cell adhesion molecule 1 (VCAM-1) on perivascular cells [72]. Urticaria with histological evidence of small-vessel vasculitis (venulitis) is defined as urticarial vasculitis (Chapter 44).

Genetics

There is a highly significant linkage of HLA DRB1*04 (DR4) and its associated allele DQB1*0302 (DR8) with histamine-releasing autoantibody-positive chronic spontaneous urticaria [73]. Polymorphisms of the FcεRIα promoter [74] and leukotriene C$_4$ synthetase genes [75] have been associated with aspirin-sensitive urticaria. Families with cholinergic urticaria have been reported. Mutations in *ADGRE2* have been reported in hereditary vibratory angioedema [76].

Environmental factors

Urticaria is a worldwide illness. Prevalence of infection as a co-morbidity will vary between countries and communities: for example, bowel parasites (tropical countries), hepatitis C (South-East Asia), anisakiasis (Mediterranean) or *Helicobacter pylori* (eastern Europe). Environmental triggers of inducible urticarias (e.g. heat, cold, sun, water) that provoke the rash should be mimimised where possible.

Clinical features
History

Taking a thorough history is essential in the assessment of a patient with urticaria to make a diagnosis (often in the absence of lesions at the time of examination) and to understand possible causes, co-morbidities, aggravating factors and the impact of disease on quality of life. As a rule, itchy weals erupt anywhere, anytime, spontaneously and fade without a mark over 24 h or less, although giant or coalescing weals may last longer. Completing health-related quality of life scores such as the dermatology life quality index (DLQI) [77] or disease-specific tools such as the chronic urticaria quality of life questionnaire (CU-Q2oL) [78] is very helpful and should be considered an essential step in the initial assessement of a patient with urticaria (see also section on classification of severity later in this chapter).

Presentation of spontaneous urticaria

The itchy red macules develop into weals consisting of well-defined red or skin-coloured, raised areas of superficial skin oedema often with initial pale centres and a surrounding red flare. They may occur anywhere on the body, including the scalp, palms and soles, in variable numbers and sizes, ranging from a few millimetres to lesions covering large areas, and of varying shapes including rounded, annular, serpiginous and bizarre patterns due to the confluence of adjacent lesions (see Figure 42.1). Very rarely, bullae may form when oedema is intense. Patients tend to rub rather than scratch, so excoriation marks are unusual, but occasionally bruising may result which may be seen particularly on the thighs. Weals may be more pronounced in the evenings or premenstrually.

Around 50% of patients with chronic spontaneous urticaria describe angioedema associated with wealing at some time in their illness and less than 10% describe angioedema without weals. These deep swellings, which may be the same colour as normal skin, occur most frequently on the face, affecting the eyelids and lips, but any other area of the body may be affected, such as the ears, neck, hands, feet and genitalia. Mucosal swellings may also occur inside the oral cavity on the buccal mucosa, tongue and pharynx, but laryngeal involvement is fortunately rare and not life-threatening in chronic spontaneous urticaria. Angioedema may be preceded by an itching or tingling sensation, but it is not always itchy and may be painful. It may last from hours to days and the swellings resolve without skin dryness, unlike acute contact dermatitis, which may resemble angioedema on the face but typically resolves over days rather than hours with scaling and may last up to a week.

Aggravating factors (Box 42.3). Even though a specific cause of urticaria may not be identified in individual patients, it may be possible to identify non-specific aggravating factors in chronic urticaria, such as heat and clothing pressure or dietary pseudoallergens in spontaneous urticaria, avoidance of which can help to minimise exacerbations through lifestyle changes.

Box 42.3 Aggravating factors for spontaneous urticaria

- Physical:
  - Pressure
  - Overheating (passive or active)
- Infections, e.g. upper respiratory tract infections
- Drugs:
  - Non-steroidal anti-inflammatory drugs (common)
  - Opiates (rarely)
- Dietary pseudoallergens:
  - Natural salicylates
  - Histamine
  - Food additives
  - Spices
  - Alcohol
- Menses (especially premenstrual)
- Stress

Drugs. Aspirin and other related non-steroidal anti-inflammatory drugs (NSAIDs), such as ibuprofen, naproxen or diclofenac, can aggravate urticaria and asthma by non-allergic mechanisms. Patients usually react with either urticaria or asthma, but not both [79]. The percentage of patients whose urticaria is exacerbated by aspirin (acetylsalicylic acid) varied from 20% to 30% in different studies [40,80].

Dietary pseudoallergens. There are many reports that food additives aggravate chronic urticaria, but the high incidence of 33% from self-reporting [81] has not been confirmed in double-blind studies [82]. Only 19% of in-patients responding to a low pseudoallergen diet reacted to double-blind placebo-controlled challenge with food additives [83]. The most frequently implicated food additives are tartrazine (E102) and other azo dyes, including sunset yellow (E110). Reactions to benzoate preservatives (E210–219) and antioxidants, such as butylated hydroxytoluene (E321) and butylated hydroxyanisole (E320), are reported less often. Sulphites (E223–228), monosodium glutamate (E621) and sorbic acid are very rare causes of urticaria, which is usually of the acute type. The sensitivity to additives gradually lessens as the urticaria resolves and may disappear. There is also a literature on histamine, histamine liberators and salicylate-rich foods aggravating chronic urticaria but strict avoidance is difficult and benefit is uncertain. Diets are becoming less popular with the introduction of effective pharmacological and biologic treatments.

Infections. Chronic spontaneous urticaria is often temporarily exacerbated by upper respiratory tract viral infections. This may be a non-specific effect of circulating pro-inflammatory cytokines or chemokines.

Menstrual cycle and pregnancy. Urticaria may worsen premenstrually, but if urticaria occurs predominantly or only premenstrually, it may be due to progesterone sensitivity [84] or more rarely oestrogen sensitivity [85], usually on an autoimmune basis. Skin prick and intradermal testing may confirm progesterone sensitivity [86]. A non-immune mechanism has been suggested for 'autoimmune' progesterone urticaria [87]. Chronic spontaneous urticaria may remit or worsen during pregnancy but often recurs after delivery. Half the chronic urticaria patients surveyed rated their chronic urticaria as improved, 30% worse and 20% unchanged [88]. Exacerbations were most common in the first or third trimesters.

Stress. Psychological factors appear to play a contributory role in a proportion of patients, and flare-ups of urticaria do occur at times of psychological stress [89]. Psychological factors are often wrongly thought to contribute to angioedema because of the historical term 'angioneurotic oedema', which implied something very different when it was first introduced. The importance of psychological factors is challenging to evaluate scientifically. Depression and anxiety are found more frequently in chronic urticaria as co-morbidities [90]. A meta-analysis showed that almost one in three chronic urticaria patients have an underlying psychiatric disorder but there was little evidence that treatment improved urticaria activity [91]. Depression may reduce the threshold for pruritus [92], and the effect of chronic urticaria on quality of life should not be underestimated [93].

Presentation of inducible urticarias

The inducible urticarias are a distinct subgroup of urticarias in which a specific stimulus induces reproducible wealing. This feature is the basis of diagnosis and classification (Box 42.4). Cholinergic urticaria occurs in response to sweating caused by an active or passive increase in core temperature, so it is frequently included in the inducible urticaria group, but it may also be triggered by emotional and gustatory sweating. The currently accepted challenge procedures for the diagnosis of inducible urticarias are summarised in Box 42.5 [94].

Box 42.4 Classification of inducible urticarias by eliciting stimulus

Mechanical
- Skin stroking:
  - Immediate:
    - Symptomatic dermographism (always itchy)
    - Simple dermographism (physiological, no itch)
    - Cholinergic dermographism
    - Red dermographism (punctate weals after skin rubbing)
  - Delayed
- Vibration:
  - Acquired vibratory angioedema
  - Familial vibratory angioedema

Thermal
- Cold contact:
  - Immediate:
    - Primary cold contact urticaria (idiopathic)
    - Secondary cold contact urticaria (to cryoproteins)
  - Delayed (rare)
  - Localised
- Heat contact (rare)
- Generalised chilling:
  - Reflex cold urticaria (drop in body core temperature)
  - Cold-dependent cholinergic urticaria (after exercise in the cold)
- Generalised overheating:
  - Exercise-induced anaphylaxis (active overheating only)
  - Food- and exercise-induced anaphylaxis (e.g. after omega-5-gliaden in gluten or shrimp in IgE presensitised individuals)

Cholinergic urticaria (sweating induced)
- Overheating (passive (e.g. showering, bathing/hot rooms) or active (exercise)
- Stress
- Spicy foods (gustatory)

Others
- Solar
- Aquagenic
- Contact urticarial:
  - Allergic (immunological)
  - Non-allergic (non-immunological)

Box 42.5 Challenge procedures for inducible urticarias

- *Symptomatic dermographism*: skin stroking stimulus, read after 5–10 min:
  - Frictest® (Moxie GmbH, Berlin) on volar forearm
  - Calibrated dermographometer on upper back at ≤36 g/mm^3
- *Delayed pressure urticaria*: read after 2–6 h and the following day:
  - Calibrated dermographometer (HTZ, East Grinstead, UK) over the scapula at 100 g/mm^2 for 70 s
  - Weighted rod (1.5 cm diameter, 2.5 kg anterior thigh, 20 min)
- *Cold urticaria*: localised cold stimulus, usually volar forearm, read after 10 min:
  - Melting ice cube in a thin polythene glove or bag, 5 min standard (up to 20 min for non-reactors)
  - TempTest® (Moxie GmbH, Berlin) for 5 min, read at 10 min
- *Heat urticaria*: localised heat stimulus, usually volar forearm, read after 10 min:
  - TempTest for 5 min, read at 10 min
  - Warm water in a glass or copper beaker, 38–44°C for 5 min
- *Cholinergic urticaria*: aim to bring out a sweat, read after 5–10 min:
  - Passive heating in a bath or shower (maximum temperature 42°C)
  - Exercise to the point of sweating in a warm environment
- *Solar urticaria*: exposure to sunlight or solar simulator, read after 10 min:
  - Ultraviolet A (UVA) (2.4–4.2 J/cm^2)
  - Broad-band UVB (0.024–0.042 J/cm^2)
  - Monochromator light testing (specific wavelengths of UVB (290–320 nm) and UVA (320–400 nm))
- *Aquagenic urticaria*: room temperature water contact on normally affected skin:
  - Wet towel or cloth applied for 5 min, read at 5–10 min
  - Water immersion at any temperature for 5 min, read at 5–10 min
- *Vibratory angioedema*: inspect for angioedema 10 min after vibratory challenge:
  - Laboratory vortex mixer
  - Other vibratory stimulus relevant to the story, e.g. jogging on the spot

The frequency of inducible urticarias in the general population is unknown, but they accounted for 19% of urticaria cases in a dermatology clinic [95], with dermographism making up 9% and cholinergic urticaria 4%. However, mixtures of various types of inducible urticaria or of an inducible urticaria with spontaneous urticaria are common – for example, dermographism or delayed pressure urticaria in patients with spontaneous chronic urticaria.

Wealing caused by inducible stimuli usually occurs within minutes at the site of exposure and persists for less than 30–60 min (e.g. symptomatic dermographism and cold contact urticaria). However, sometimes a generalised stimulus affecting the whole body is necessary (reflex type, e.g. cooling the body core temperature to induce reflex cold urticaria and a rise in core temperature to induce cholinergic urticaria). In a few forms of physical urticaria, a delay of several hours from the physical stimulus occurs before weals appear – for example, delayed dermographism, delayed pressure urticaria and the rare delayed cold urticaria.

If the stimulus is sufficiently great or the patient is very sensitive, angioedema and systemic reactions may occur from mediator release in many forms of inducible urticaria but this is not seen in symptomatic dermographism.

Urticaria due to mechanical forces

Dermographism. This includes the following.

- *Symptomatic dermographism* (syn. factitious urticaria). The triple response of local redness due to capillary vasodilatation, followed by oedema and a surrounding flare due to axon reflex-induced dilatation of arterioles after stroking the skin, first described by Lewis [96], is commonly elicited in chronic urticaria patients and may be seen in healthy individuals. This is known as simple (or physiological) dermographism. However, in less than 5%, it is accompanied by severe itching and a low threshold for wealing (symptomatic dermographism). Dermographism has been successfully transferred when IgE [97] (and occasionally IgM [98]) in patients' sera has been injected into normal recipients. It has been proposed that mast cells sensitised with immunoglobulins (especially IgE) react to a neoantigen induced by mechanical stimulation of the skin and release their mediators. Neuropeptides may contribute to the reaction through binding the MRGPRX2 receptor on skin mast cells.

Symptomatic dermographism can occur at any age, but the greatest incidence is in young adults. Patients complain of wealing and itching at sites of trauma, friction with clothing or scratching the skin. The itching is disproportionately severe without antihistamines compared with wealing and is often worst at night. The eliciting stimulus determines the shape of the weals (Figure 42.5). They are often linear from scratching or stroking but large patches at the sites of repeated scratching are also seen. There is no association with systemic disease or food allergy [99]. Dermographism is usually idiopathic, but may sometimes follow a drug reaction (e.g. penicillin [100]) or an infestation, including scabies. Dermographism may last for months or years, or be present intermittently.

Symptomatic dermographism is most easily diagnosed by using a calibrated instrument, the dermographometer, which has a spring-loaded stylus, the pressure of which can be adjusted to a predetermined setting. Stroking the skin at a tip pressure of

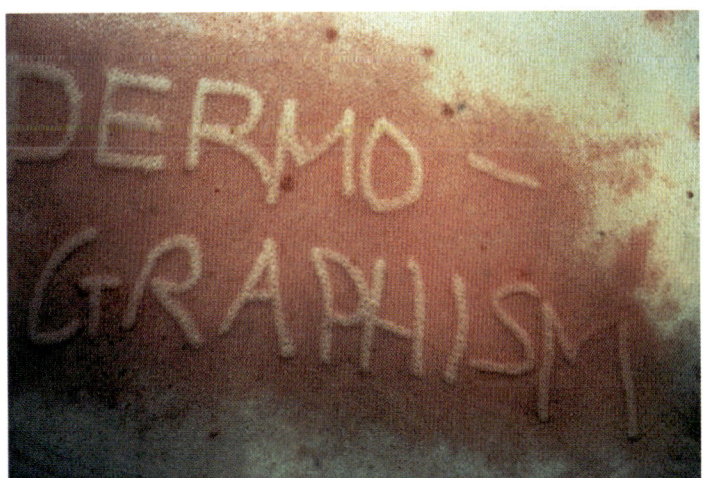

Figure 42.5 Dermographism, meaning 'skin writing'. Courtesy of St John's Institute of Dermatology, London, UK.

less than 36 g/ mm^2 [94] induces a linear itching weal within 10 min. Treatment of symptomatic immediate dermographism with low-sedating H$_1$ antihistamines is often effective, but some patients do not respond.

- *Other forms of dermographism.* Much less common forms of dermographism exist, including red dermographism, where repeated rubbing is necessary to induce small punctate weals [101]. *Cholinergic dermographism* is seen in some patients with cholinergic urticaria, whose dermographic response consists of a red line studded with punctate weals characteristic of cholinergic weals [102]. *Delayed dermographism* is rare. After normal fading of an immediate dermographic response, a weal returns in the same site, but is usually tender and persists for up to 48 h. The mechanism is unknown, but it is closely related to pressure urticaria in which a delayed dermographic response is not unusual [103].

Not all dermographism is urticaria. *White dermographism* (due to capillary vasoconstriction following light stroking of the skin) occurs normally but is particularly pronounced in atopic eczema.

Delayed pressure urticaria. Delayed pressure urticaria [104–106] in its predominant form is uncommon (about 2% of urticarias) but pressure exacerbation occurs to some degree in about a third of patients with chronic spontaneous urticaria, although they may be unaware of this unless directly questioned. Patients with predominantly delayed pressure urticaria nearly always have a component of chronic spontaneous urticaria. Wealing occurs at sites of sustained pressure applied to the skin after a delay of 30 min to 9 h, but usually 4–8 h, and lasts 12–72 h.

Weals occur frequently under tight clothing, on the hands after manual work, on the buttocks and lower back after sitting (Figure 42.6) and on the feet after walking. Lesions may be itchy, but are often tender or painful, particularly on the soles and scalp. The severity is variable, but it may be accompanied by systemic symptoms of malaise, flu-like symptoms, arthralgia, myalgia and leukocytosis. The condition may be mistaken for urticarial vasculitis or angioedema.

The diagnosis can usually be made by careful questioning and can be confirmed by testing. Objective testing is performed by using a dermographometer set at 100 g/mm^2 pressed perpendicularly on the upper back for 70 s, or rods with a convex end diameter of 1.5 cm weighted with 2.5 kg for 20 min or 4.5 kg for 15 min on the back or thighs [94]. A positive response is when indurated lesions are present at test sites at 6 h. Areas of delayed pressure urticaria may be refractory to further pressure-induced lesions for up to 48 h.

The prognosis is variable. The symptoms fluctuate in severity; they may show spontaneous improvement, or last for many years.

Vibratory angioedema. Vibratory urticaria is a very rare form of urticaria, which was first described in its familial form [107]. It is associated with a missense mutation in the *ADGRE2* gene [76]. Any vibratory stimulus such as jogging, vigorous towelling or using lawnmowers induces a localised red itchy swelling within minutes, lasting less than a few hours. If the stimulus is severe, generalised redness and headache may occur. Vibratory angioedema may occur in an acquired form [108].

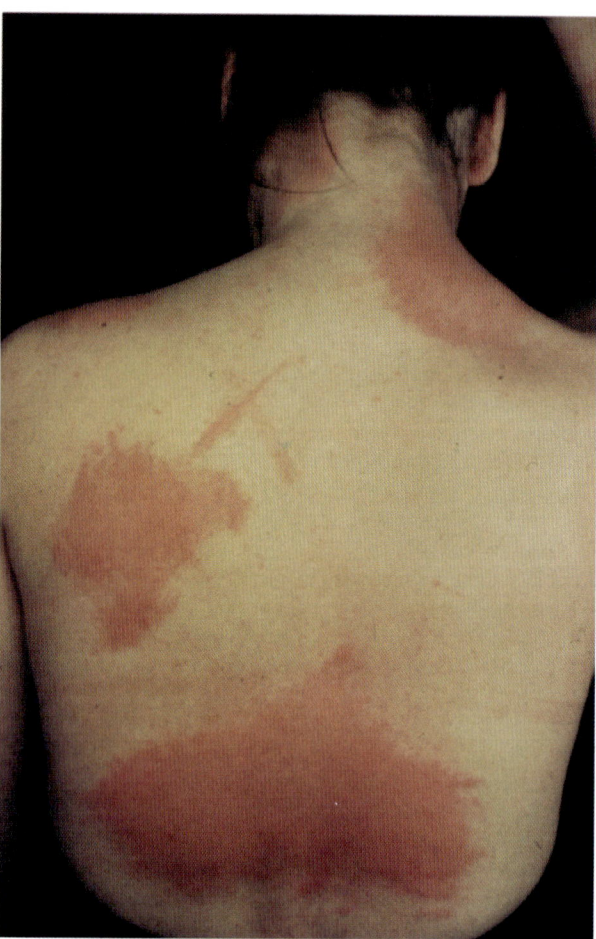

Figure 42.6 Extensive delayed pressure urticaria over the back after sitting against a hard surface. Induced delayed dermographism is also seen on the upper back. Courtesy of St John's Institute of Dermatology, London, UK.

Temperature-dependent urticaria

Heat contact urticaria. Heat contact urticar (syn. heat urticaria) is one of the rarest forms of inducible urticaria [109–111]. Localised warming of skin at temperatures from 38 to 44°C for 2–5 min induces wealing at the test site lasting 1 h.

Cold contact urticaria. Cold contect urticaria (syn. cold urticaria) encompasses a variety of syndromes in which cold induces urticaria [112,113]. Idiopathic cold contact urticaria is the most common, comprising 96% of a series of cold urticaria patients [114], while others are rare. What is known and what is unknown at the present time have been reviewed recently [115]. In some patients with idiopathic cold contact urticaria, the serum can passively transfer the cold urticarial response to normal recipients. This autoantibody is usually IgE [116], but IgM has been reported. It is important to warn against cold water bathing due to the risk of anaphylaxis and drowning. Treatment with low-sedation antihistamine is helpful. Induction of tolerance by repeated graduated exposures to cold has been used [117], but is time consuming and not always effective.

A genetic defect in factor XII has been reported in familial cold urticaria that appears to be bradykinin rather than mast cell dependent and unrelated to mutations in the *NLRP3* gene seen in familial cold autoinflammatory syndrome [118]. Cold urticaria is also a regular feature of PLCγ₂-associated antibody deficiency and immune dysregulation (PLAID) [119]. This is a rare, complex, mast cell driven, dominantly inherited disorder with a high frequency of positive antinuclear antibodies, granulomatous rash and negative ice cube test.

- *Primary cold contact urticaria.* This includes immediate and delayed types. *Immediate primary cold contact urticaria* is by far the commonest form, occurring at any age but most frequently in young adults. It may be preceded by non-specific upper respiratory tract viral infections, infectious mononucleosis or insect stings. Itching and wealing of the skin occur on cold exposure within minutes and last up to 1 h. Cold winds and cold rain are particularly effective stimuli. Sometimes, the mouth and pharynx may swell after drinking cold liquids. Systemic symptoms include flushing, palpitations, headache, wheezing and loss of consciousness, and drowning is a risk of cold water bathing. Diagnosis is made by the application of a melting ice cube in thin plastic (or Clingfilm®) onto the skin for 5–20 min; wealing occurs within 10 min, usually during rewarming (Figure 42.7a). Sometimes a more extensive local challenge, such as immersion of a forearm in iced cold water, is necessary to induce a response. A Peltier-based temperature-testing device (TempTest®, Moxie GmbH, Berlin) allows temperature thresholds to be established for individual patients (Figure 42.7b) as well as cold stimulation time as a measure of severity [120].

  Delayed primary cold contact urticaria, where wealing occurs after a delay of hours after cold contact, is very rare [121]. A familial form has been reported [122].

- *Secondary cold contact urticaria.* Cold urticaria secondary to cryoproteins is rare. It is usually associated with other manifestations such as Raynaud phenomenon, purpura or skin necrosis. Cryogobulinaemia may be idiopathic or occur in autoimmune collagen vascular disease, chronic lymphocytic leukaemia, myeloma and in infectious disease, including viral hepatitis and Epstein–Barr virus infections. Cold urticaria is said to occur in only 3% of people with cryoglobulinaemia [123]. Blood samples for cryoprotein estimation must be kept warm until laboratory testing. Treatment is directed against the underlying condition. Cryofibrinogen occurred in the blood of 3.4% of a large hospital population [124] and in 3% of patients in cold urticaria [125]. Its significance in relationship to cold urticaria remains to be determined. Cold agglutinins are not usually associated with cold urticaria [126]. Cold haemolysins have not been detected.

- *Systemic cold urticaria.* In generalised reflex cold urticaria, widespread wealing occurs in response to cooling of the core body temperature, but a local ice cube test is negative [127]. Testing is performed by placing the patient, in lightweight clothes, in a cold room at 4°C for 30 min. In cold-induced cholinergic urticaria, additional exercise is necessary in the cold room to induce weals.

- *Familial cold autoinflammatory syndrome.* This rare form is inherited as an autosomal dominant trait and is now known to be caused by the same gene mutation as Muckle–Wells syndrome (Chapter 45). The ice cube test is negative.

Cholinergic urticaria. Cholinergic urticaria is a very distinctive type in which characteristic small weals appear in association with sweating. It accounts for about 5% of chronic urticaria, and often presents in adolescents. Wealing occurs on stimulation of sweating, whether induced by a rise in core temperature, emotion or gustatory stimuli.

The pathogenesis is still not clear. It is thought to be related to stimulation of the cholinergic postganglionic sympathetic nerve supply to the sweat glands. Increased histamine levels have been detected in the blood of patients with cholinergic urticaria. It was originally proposed that acetylcholine can release histamine, perhaps in an indirect way, but such a mechanism is conjectural. Passive transfer tests with sera of affected individuals are sometimes positive, probably due to an immunoglobulin [128]. Such an antibody may prime the mast cell for activation. An allergy to

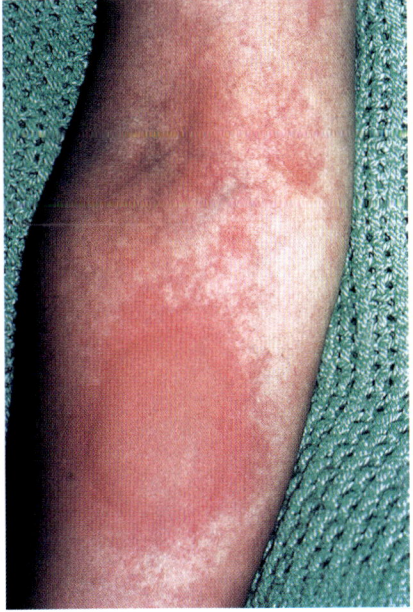

Figure 42.7 (a) Wealing following application of a melting ice cube for 20 min. (b) The critical temperature threshold of 16°C using TempTest®. (a) Courtesy of St John's Institute of Dermatology, London, UK.

(a) (b)

sweat itself has been proposed [129]. It has also been proposed that cholinergic urticaria should be classified into two subtypes based on intradermal skin test reactions to autologous sweat and serum [130]. Decreased levels of the protease inhibitor antichymotrypsin have been detected in the serum of some patients [131].

The disease typically occurs in adolescents of either sex and may be worse in the winter months [132], for instance after exercising in the cold. It has been reported to occur in families [133] and often occurs in atopics. The patient complains of itching weals that appear within minutes of exertion, when overheated or after emotional disturbances or even after eating spicy food. The weals characteristically are small, 1–3 mm across, and may coalesce (Figure 42.8). Sometimes the red component is more pronounced, especially in the 'blush areas', and is confluent and studded with weals. Oblique lighting is helpful for observing the weals, especially in darker skin types. The lesions persist for an hour or so. Spontaneous urticaria may be associated with cholinergic urticaria. Although micropapular weals resembling those of cholinergic urticaria can occur in spontaneous urticaria, these usually last for hours. Cholinergic angioedema has been reported [134]. Cholinergic pruritus without weals has been described [135] but is rare. In cholinergic erythema, multiple small red macules are distributed symmetrically on the trunk and limbs, increasing in number after exercise. Individual macules are short-lived, but appear at different sites over a prolonged period, giving the overall impression of a persisting rash [136].

The diagnosis of cholinergic urticaria is best confirmed by provocation, with the appearance of typical itchy weals on a red background after warming – for example in a hot bath at 42°C for 15 min, to raise the core temperature by 0.7–1°C – or exercise in a hot environment [94]. A few patients find that if they can bring on a severe attack by mild exertion they can achieve freedom for up to 24 h afterwards, analogous to temporary desensitisation. In some patients with cholinergic urticaria, systemic symptoms of flushing, faintness or asthma may occur [137–139]. Rarely, a generalised eruption resembling cholinergic urticaria may be provoked by systemic chilling [140].

Exercise-induced anaphylaxis. Exercise-induced anaphylaxis does not appear to be associated with cholinergic urticaria and cannot be reproduced by hot bathing. It occurs in patients sporadically and unpredictably. It appears to be a distinct entity [141]. It is possible that some are examples of unrecognised food-dependent exercise-induced anaphylaxis.

Other types of inducible urticaria

Solar urticaria. Weals develop at the site of exposure within minutes of exposure to visible, long- or short-wave ultraviolet radiation (Figure 42.9) [142–144] and usually fade within 2 h, in contrast to polymorphic light eruption, in which urticated lesions appear hours later and last for days. A rare, delayed form has been described [145]. The cause of solar urticaria is usually unknown (idiopathic) but can be secondary to porphyrias [146].

Aquagenic urticaria. Contact with water at any temperature induces an eruption resembling cholinergic urticaria, although the weals are few in number and are surrounded by a wide flare (Figure 42.10) [147]. Other urticarias that can also be induced by water, such as cold urticaria, cholinergic urticaria and dermographism, must be excluded. This is a different entity from aquagenic pruritus, in which there is water-induced itching but no wealing [148].

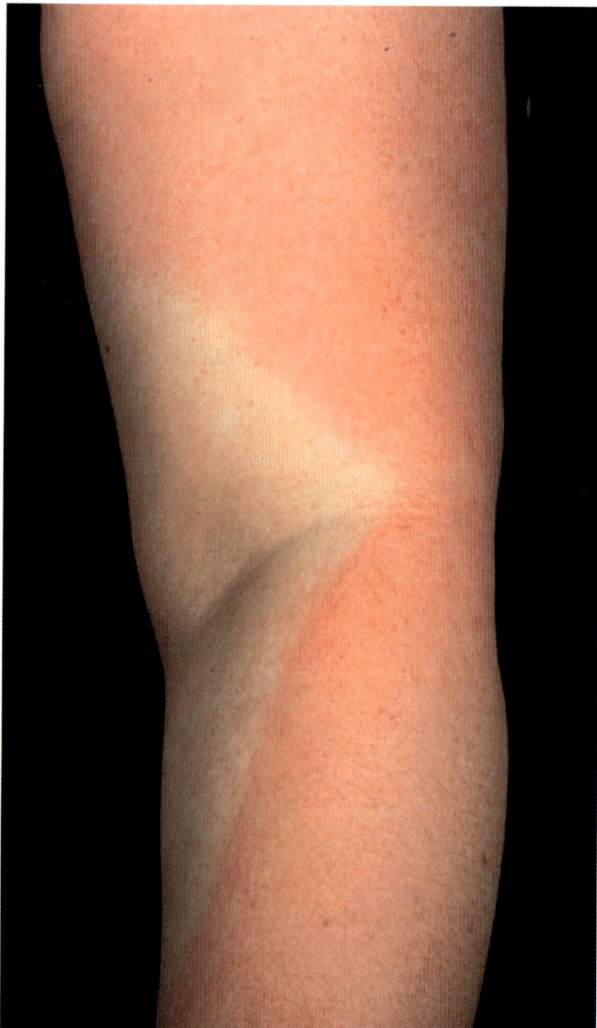

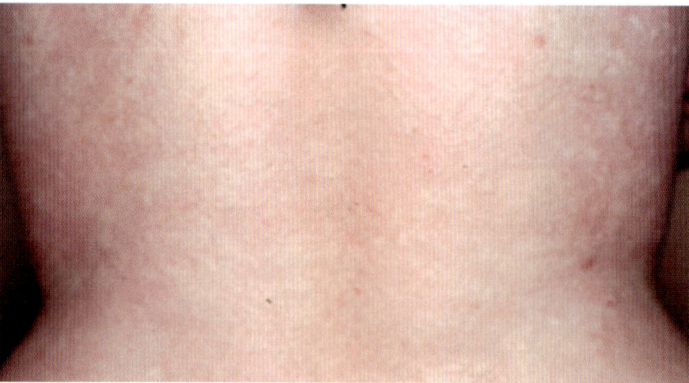

Figure 42.8 Close-up of small monomorphic lesions of cholinergic urticaria on the back. Courtesy of Norfolk and Norwich University Hospital, UK.

Figure 42.9 Solar urticaria.

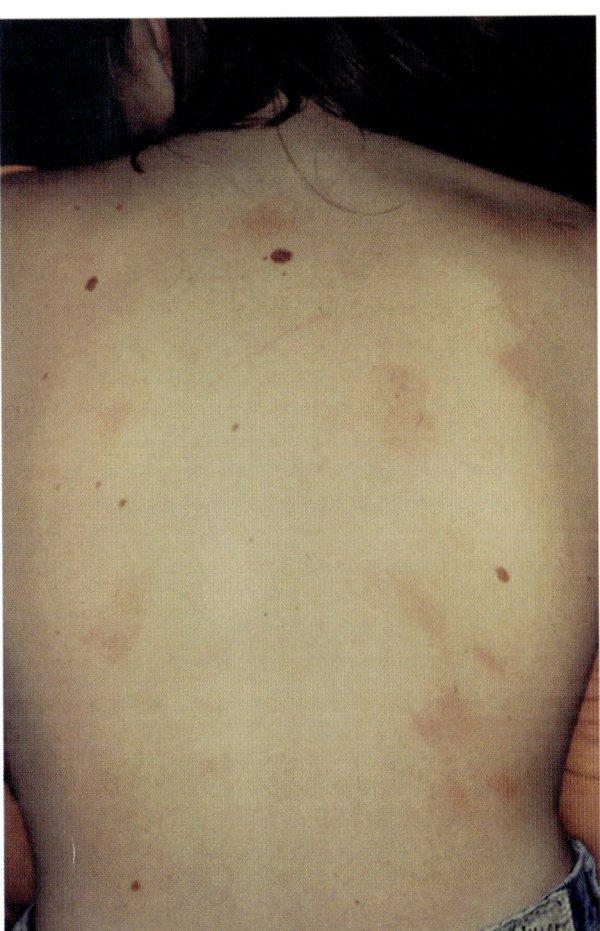

Figure 42.10 Aquagenic urticaria on the back after swimming, showing a few small papular weals surrounded by wide flares. Courtesy of Norfolk and Norwich University Hospital, UK.

Contact urticaria. This is now included with the inducible urticarias [1]. Contact urticaria is quite common, but is not usually a cause of hospital referral unless there is an occupational problem, for instance latex allergy due to glove use. The term simply means urticaria resulting from skin or mucosal contact with the provoking substance. It may be allergic or non-allergic (also called immunological and non-immunological). The range of chemical, plant, animal and food exposures causing contact urticaria is very wide (Box 42.6) [149].

- *Allergic.* Percutaneous or mucosal penetration of an allergen to which the individual has already developed specific IgE will provoke a type I hypersensitivity response involving mast cell degranulation with histamine release. This results in an immediate, localised weal and flare resolving within 2 h, generalised urticaria or even anaphylaxis if the individual is extremely hypersensitive. It is easily missed when it is responsible for exacerbations of a pre-existing eczema, for example in atopic children. Weals occur at sites of contact with the allergen, usually on the hands and face. The commonest causes are foods (e.g. nuts, fish, fruits) or latex. Diagnosis can be confirmed *in vitro* by detecting specific IgE against whole allergens or components (e.g. ImmunoCAP® fluoroimmunoassay) if there is a history of anaphylaxis, or by skin prick testing. Management is largely directed at avoidance of the allergen.

Box 42.6 Some causes of contact urticaria

Allergic (immunological)
- Foods:
  - Cow's milk
  - Cod
  - Kiwi fruit
  - Peanuts
  - Spices
  - Celery
- Animals:
  - Saliva
  - Moths/caterpillars
  - Urine
- Human:
  - Semen
- Other:
  - Fragrance
  - Latex

Non-immunological
- Histamine liberators:
  - Cobalt
  - Dimethyl sulphoxide
- Vasoactive:
  - Nettle stings
  - Jellyfish stings

Undetermined action
- Bleaching agent:
  - Ammonium persulphate
- Fragrance:
  - Balsam of Peru
- Flavouring agents:
  - Cinnamic acid
  - Cinnamic aldehyde
- Preservatives:
  - Benzoic acid
  - Sorbic acid

Oral allergy syndrome is a form of allergic contact urticaria involving the mouth, characterised by immediate itching, swelling and burning after eating a wide range of fresh fruits, including apples, pears, cherries, plums, celery, spices and hazelnuts [150]. Eating cooked, dried, peeled or bottled fruit does not often cause symptoms. The symptoms are due to cross-reactions between profilins (ubiquitous pan-allergens in plants, including grass and mugwort in north Europe) and pathogenesis-related protein 10 (PR10) (e.g. Bet v 1, the major allergen in silver birch pollen) and homologous proteins in plants, especially fruits. Oral allergy syndrome therefore occurs in patients with respiratory allergies to common pollens (pollinosis). Diagnosis is by skin prick testing with the fresh fruit. ImmunoCAP and skin prick testing with commercial standardised solutions may be negative. Fortunately, the condition rarely progresses to angioedema, and treatment with antihistamines is not usually necessary.

- *Non-allergic.* This form of contact urticaria may be caused by direct injection of vasoactive chemicals by plants (e.g. nettles) or animals (e.g. caterpillars, jellyfish). A more common form though is from exposure to cosmetics (e.g. cinnamic aldehyde, balsam of Peru) or food additives (e.g. sorbic acid, benzoic acid) in foods such as tomato ketchup. Occupational exposures include ammonium persulphate in hairdressing. The reaction may take up to 45 min to develop and is thought to be due to prostaglandin D_2 formation rather than histamine release, since it can be blocked by NSAIDs. The relevant investigation is either a prick test or patch test, read at 20 min rather than 48 h.

Presentation of chronic urticaria

A comprehensive history is essential for the diagnosis and elucidation of any causative factors as weals are often not present at the time of consultation. Performing an extensive panel of investigations in addition to a standardised questionnaire was found to add little to making a final diagnosis [151]. Information should be obtained regarding the onset, duration and course of the disease. The duration of individual weals and presence of purpura are important. Weals lasting more than 24–48 h, particularly if painful or tender, suggest urticarial vasculitis or delayed pressure urticaria, but can occur in spontaneous urticaria. Purpura, although rare, suggests urticarial vasculitis, but can occur rarely in spontaneous urticaria, especially on the legs. Dermoscopy of weals may demonstrate the presence of linear vessels in urticaria compared with red-purple dots or globules seen in urticarial vasculitis [152]. Drawing a line around the outline of a weal with daily phone photographs can be useful to determine its duration. The location, numbers and shapes of weals vary and are usually not helpful in differentiating most urticarias, except for the typical small, monomorphic, short-lasting weals of cholinergic urticaria and the linear weals of dermographism. The occurrence of angioedema should be noted, particularly if it has affected the oro-pharynx with difficulty in swallowing or breathing. Enquiry should be made for systemic symptoms sometimes associated with severe chronic spontaneous urticaria, including malaise, headache, abdominal pain, arthralgia, wheezing and syncope [153]. Possible precipitating or aggravating factors – including physical factors such as heat, cold, localised pressure on the skin, friction and sunlight – should be sought directly. It is important to ask about any association with recent acute infection, drugs, non-prescription medicines and foods, although the latter are rarely a cause for chronic urticaria. A family history of atopy, autoimmunity or angioedema may be relevant. Enquiry should be made about drug intake including NSAIDs.

Differential diagnosis

The diagnosis of urticaria is rarely a problem. Weals are distinguished by their evanescent nature and normal overlying epidermis without scaling. Papular urticaria, erythema multiforme and pre-bullous eruptions must be distinguished. Acute contact dermatitis, lymphoedema and collagen vascular disease (such as dermatomyositis) may mimic angioedema, but these conditions last longer than 24–48 h.

Classification of severity

The severity of chronic spontaneous urticaria is assessed by a composite 42-point urticaria activity score (UAS-7) of itch intensity and weal numbers over a week [154]. The angioedema activity score (AAS) [155] is applicable to both histaminergic and bradykininergic angioedema. Relevant quality of life scores include the generic dermatology quality of life score (DLQI) [78], the disease-specific health-related quality of life score (CUQ2oL) [79], validated in several European languages, and the angioedema quality of life score (AE-QoL) [156]. The urticaria control test (UCT) [157] and quality of life scores can be used in the assessment of both spontaneous and inducible urticarias.

Complications and co-morbidities

There are no long-term complications of urticaria. The illness resolves without damage in everyone but can last for decades. There is some limited evidence from the literature of potential extra-cutaneous organ disease in chronic urticaria (respiratory, musculoskeletal, central nervous system, cardiac, gastrointestinal) [158]. Whether this represents chance or causal association is not yet clear. The main concern of angioedema affecting the oro-pharynx is acute respiratory compromise with suffocation, but this is not a known risk of chronic spontaneous urticaria.

Metabolic syndrome (increased body mass index, cardiovascular disease, hyperlipidaemia and type 2 diabetes) has been proposed as a co-morbidity in patients with chronic urticaria [159] as well as autoimmune disease, malignancy and infections (see 'Associated diseases' earlier in the chapter) and mental health disorders (see 'Stress' earlier in the chapter). Atopic disorders are more frequent in chronic spontaneous as well as acute urticaria, raising the possibility of a predisposition to developing a Th2 phenotype. Korean patients with chronic spontaneous urticaria had a 4.7-fold higher likelihood of developing allergic rhinitis, drug or other allergies, or asthma than expected [160]. Adolescents with chronic spontaneous urticaria had significantly more food allergy, allergic rhinitis, atopic dermatitis and asthma [161]. Children with a history of early-onset atopic dermatitis are at increased risk of chronic spontaneous urticaria later [162].

Burden of chronic urticaria on the patient and to society

A recent review identified the limitations imposed by chronic urticaria on daily life, work and sports activities, interfering with life within the family and in society, including performance at school and work (6% absenteeism and 25% presenteeism), and a high consumption of medical resources and indirect costs (including loss of earnings) [**163**].

Disease course and prognosis

Acute attacks may last a few hours or days and be of great severity. There is no way to predict the duration of an initial attack at its onset. Chronic cases where no diagnosis is established may last for weeks, months or even years, or be intermittent with repeated episodes occurring over decades. The severity is often greatest at the onset, with subsequent waning. New lesions appear daily or at irregular intervals, and there may be periodic exacerbations, sometimes associated with intercurrent infections or NSAID intake. In general, natural improvement occurs even in the absence of diagnosis or treatment. Of patients with weals alone attending a specialist clinic 50% can be expected to clear within 6 months of onset, but 50% of those with associated angioedema can still be expected to have their condition 10 years later (Figure 42.11) [164]. Another survey

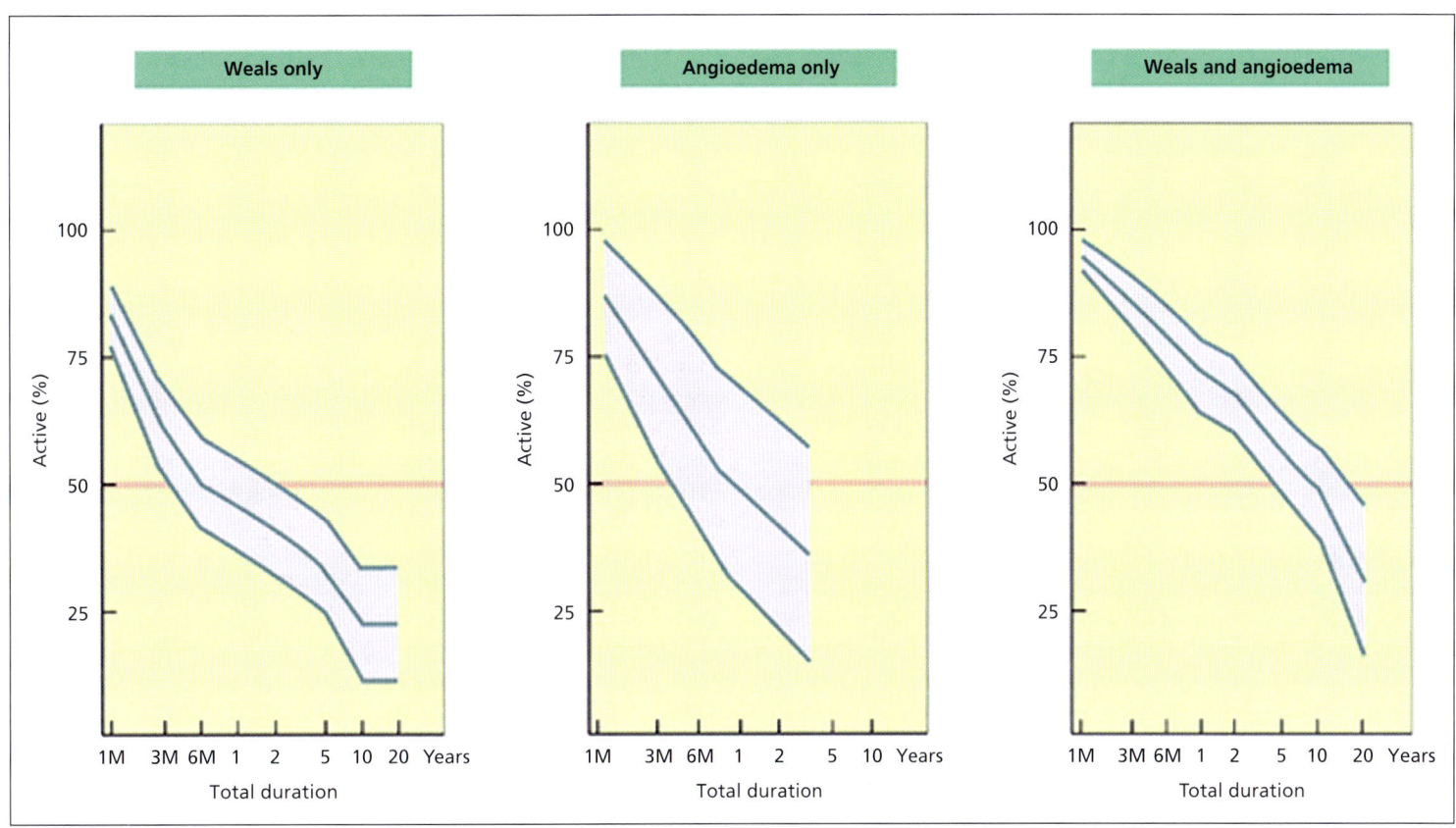

Figure 42.11 The natural history of urticaria in 554 hospital patients. The expected percentage of patients with active urticaria, with 95% confidence limits, by the total duration of disease (log scale). Reproduced from Champion *et al.* 1969 [164].

of the prognosis of patients attending a tertiary referral clinic in the Netherlands confirmed the poor outlook for many patients with chronic urticaria, especially those with cold urticaria [165]. The prognosis for patients in primary care is likely to be better than for those patients whose disease is bad enough to be referred to secondary or tertiary clinics. Studies of chronic urticaria in children suggest that it may run a more protracted course, with more than 30% of patients still requiring treatment after 5 years [166].

Investigations (Box 42.7)

Box 42.7 Investigation of spontaneous urticaria

Acute urticaria
- Infection:
  - Throat swab if pharyngeal symptoms
  - Other appropriate samples for suspected viral or bacterial infection
- Drugs:
  - Withdraw suspected drugs
- Foods:
  - Investigate for IgE sensitisation (skin prick tests or ImmunoCAP® where appropriate from the history)

Chronic urticaria

H_1 antihistamine responsive
- Full blood count, ESR or CRP
- Others, as indicated by the presentation

H_1 antihistamine unresponsive
- Thyroid autoantibodies (all patients)
- Thyroid function tests (all patients)
- Additional tests dependent on clinical presentation:
  - C4 complement (angioedema without weals)
  - Non-organ-specific autoantibodies (if associated autoimmune disease possible)
  - Total IgE
  - Basophil histamine release assay or basophil activation tests (if functional autoantibodies suspected)
  - *Helicobacter pylori* (stool antigen or urea breath test)
  - Stool for ova, cysts and parasites (foreign travel)
  - Chest X-ray ± other imaging (if lymphoma considered)
- Optional tests for extensive work-up when other tests non revealing:
  - 25-hydroxycholecalciferol (vitamin D)
  - D-dimer
  - 3-week trial of a low pseudoallergen diet

CRP, C-reactive protein; ESR, erythrocyte sedimentation rate; IgE, immunoglobulin E.

Acute urticaria

In patients with potentially life-threatening reactions to an allergen, confirmation is by ImmunoCAP fluoroimmunoassay, which measures serum allergen-specific IgE to the allergen or skin prick testing, for example for peanut sensitisation. In most cases of acute urticaria in which no cause is suggested in the history, investigation rarely provides an answer. Prick testing is possibly risky if there is a history of anaphylaxis. The clinical relevance of the results of skin prick and ImmunoCAP tests needs careful assessment.

Chronic spontaneous urticaria

A thorough history of the rash and any associated systemic symptoms is essential. It is useful to identify any associated inducible urticaria, especially delayed pressure urticaria, by appropriate testing. If weals persist and are painful, with systemic symptoms of fever or arthralgia, urticarial vasculitis should be considered and a skin biopsy performed of a spontaneous lesion, preferably one that is 12–15 h old. Direct immunofluorescence may provide additional information if complement and immunoreactants are found within blood vessel walls of early lesions. Patients frequently suspect allergy to foods, but this is rarely if ever found in adults with chronic spontaneous urticaria. Routine allergy testing in continuous chronic urticaria is therefore of no value. A food diary may be helpful, especially in episodic urticaria, but it should be remembered that the time interval may vary from minutes with allergy and up to 24 h with dietary pseudoallergens, and the substance may have been consumed regularly for years. If the patient suspects food additives, or if they have improved substantially on elimination of the substance or on a diet free of food additives, challenge testing can be carried out on a single-blind placebo-controlled basis. This is performed when the patient is in relative remission. A low pseudoallergen diet may be helpful for some patients [84], especially if antihistamines have failed or are not accepted.

A full blood count and erythrocyte sedimentation rate (ESR) should be performed routinely. An elevated ESR suggests the possibility of an underlying systemic disease (lupus erythematosus, urticarial vasculitis, macroglobulinaemia, autoinflammatory syndromes), and an eosinophilia should prompt a search for parasitic disease. C-reactive protein (CRP) and D-dimers may be increased in severe chronic spontaneous urticaria but a CRP >30 mg/L would suggest an autoinflammatory disease. Thyroid function tests and thyroid autoantibodies are worthwhile as around 14% of patients with chronic spontaneous urticaria may have thyroid autoimmunity [10]. Clinical experience indicates that the proportion of severe chronic urticaria patients with thyroid autoimmunity is higher than this and it may be a useful surrogate marker for autoimmune urticaria [167], particularly in the presence of a low total IgE [168].

Further tests depend on the history. Routine biochemistry, complement levels, serum proteins and electrophoresis, serum immunoglobulins, non-organ-specific and organ-specific autoantibodies, specific IgE and fastidious searching for evidence of infection are not indicated [169]. There is currently no simple clinical test for serum histamine-releasing autoantibodies. The ASST appears to be a reasonably sensitive and specific marker for a positive serum basophil histamine release assay [170], but is no longer much used since it is not specific for functional autoantibodies and there are regulatory concerns about skin testing with blood products. The basophil histamine release assay and basophil activation tests are useful to demonstrate functional autoantibodies indirectly but are not routinely available and are not specific for chronic urticaria. C4 complement should be measured as a screening test for hereditary or acquired C1 esterase inhibitor deficiency

if angioedema presents without weals. It is reduced and rarely, if ever, reaches normal values even between attacks of C1 esterase deficiency angioedema. Functional C1 esterase inhibitor is reduced in hereditary and acquired disease. A lesional skin biopsy should be considered if weals persist for more than 48 h and do not respond to antihistamines. Urticarial vasculitis or delayed pressure urticaria is then suspected.

Management (Figure 42.12)

Advances in the pharmacological treatment of chronic urticaria have transformed management for patients with severe disease; however, treating the cause (where one can be identified), avoidance of aggravating factors and triggers and managing co-morbidities are important. Explanation and non-specific measures, including the wearing of loose-fitting clothing and application of soothing creams containing menthol, may be helpful. Patients should minimise identifiable aggravating factors including overheating, stress and alcohol. Aspirin, aspirin-containing compounds and other NSAIDs should be avoided if possible. Paracetamol is usually a satisfactory alternative. Selective COX-2 inhibitors may be tolerated by aspirin-sensitive patients if an anti-inflammatory drug is essential. If food additives, colourings or preservatives are suspected to be a problem, diets excluding these substances may be of value for a limited number of patients. Pharmacological therapies can be first, second or third line, the choice of treatment depending upon the response to previous measures and the degree of impairment in quality of life for the patient. The strongest quality of evidence is for non-sedating H_1 antihistamines and omalizumab (anti-IgE) and these dominate current evidence-based guidelines [171,172]. However, there remain a place for low-evidenced treatments that can be targeted at specific indications and a need for better, safer, cost-effective treatments for the different presentations of acute and chronic urticaria in the future. Even though many treatments suppress the symptoms of urticaria, there are currently no cures.

First line

Non-sedating second-generation H_1 antihistamines are the first line treatment of all types of urticaria. They are rapidly absorbed, reaching peak serum concentrations in 1–3 h, and are often effective for mild disease as monotherapy. However, some are metabolised in the liver, and some active metabolites have a longer half-life than the parent compound (e.g. desloratadine, the active metabolite of loratadine). The main pharmacokinetic and clinical properties of second-generation antihistamines currently licensed in the UK are summarised in Table 42.2.

The second generation of potent, specific, low-sedation H_1 antihistamines are now the treatment of choice. Their main advantage is low sedation at doses recommended by the manufacturer and with minimal anticholinergic side effects, although an occasional individual may develop sedation with any of them. They are at least as effective as hydroxyzine and generally as effective as each other. There is no evidence that tolerance develops. Very rarely, antihistamines appear to make urticaria worse. This has been reported anecdotally with cetirizine but clinical experience suggests that most if not all antihistamines may be implicated in those who are affected.

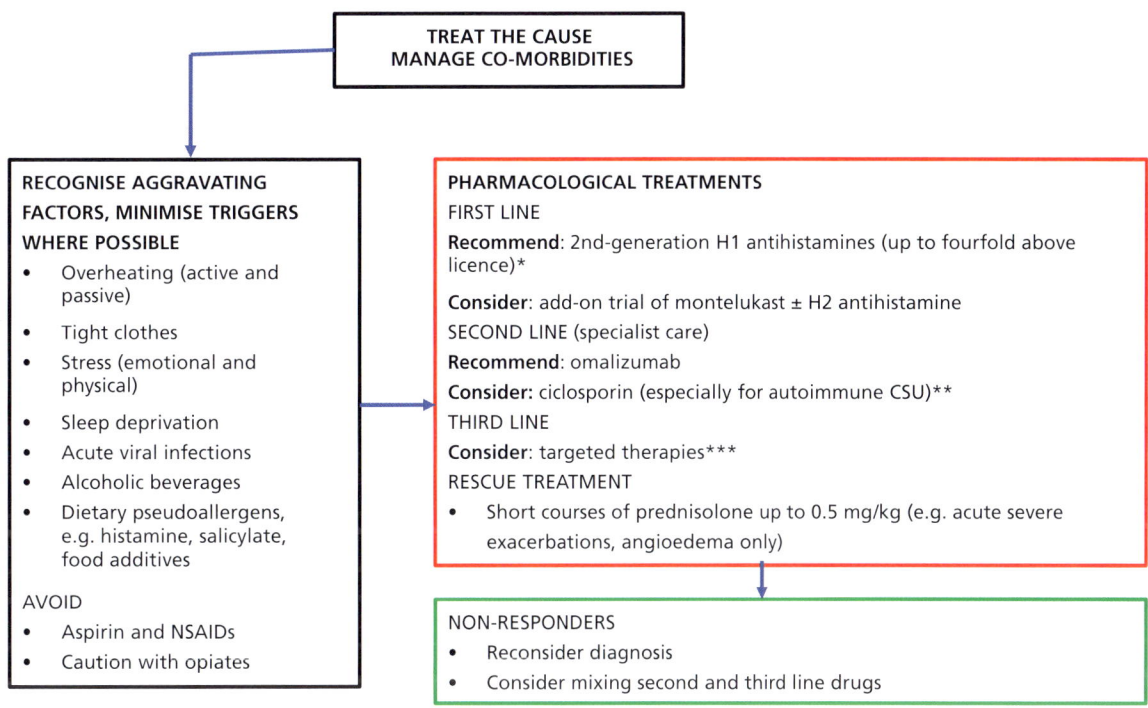

```
                    ┌─────────────────────────┐
                    │   TREAT THE CAUSE        │
                    │   MANAGE CO-MORBIDITIES  │
                    └─────────────────────────┘
```

RECOGNISE AGGRAVATING FACTORS, MINIMISE TRIGGERS WHERE POSSIBLE

- Overheating (active and passive)
- Tight clothes
- Stress (emotional and physical)
- Sleep deprivation
- Acute viral infections
- Alcoholic beverages
- Dietary pseudoallergens, e.g. histamine, salicylate, food additives

AVOID
- Aspirin and NSAIDs
- Caution with opiates

PHARMACOLOGICAL TREATMENTS

FIRST LINE

Recommend: 2nd-generation H1 antihistamines (up to fourfold above licence)*

Consider: add-on trial of montelukast ± H2 antihistamine

SECOND LINE (specialist care)

Recommend: omalizumab

Consider: ciclosporin (especially for autoimmune CSU)**

THIRD LINE

Consider: targeted therapies***

RESCUE TREATMENT

- Short courses of prednisolone up to 0.5 mg/kg (e.g. acute severe exacerbations, angioedema only)

NON-RESPONDERS

- Reconsider diagnosis
- Consider mixing second and third line drugs

* See caution about up-dosing above licence (text)
** Increased anti-TPO and low IgE as potential surrogate markers for positive basophil histamine release or activation assays
*** Low-evidence drugs used off-label for targeted phenotypes (see Box 42.8)

Figure 42.12 Management of chronic spontaneous urticaria. CSU, chronic spontaneous urticaria; IgE, immunoglobulin E; NSAIDs, non-steroidal anti-inflammatory drugs; TPO, thyroid peroxidase.

Acrivastine (adult dose 8 mg three times a day) has a rapid onset and duration of action and is excreted predominantly in the urine.

Cetirizine (adult dose 10 mg/day) is poorly metabolised in the liver and is excreted, predominantly in the urine, unchanged. It is also rapidly absorbed. It is more sedative than placebo in some studies and is best taken at night. There are no studies to show that its active enantiomer, levocetirizine, has an advantage in the treatment of chronic urticaria.

Fexofenadine (adult dose 180 mg/day) is the active metabolite of terfenadine (now withdrawn) but appears to be devoid of cardiotoxicity at clinically relevant doses and has the widest therapeutic window of the second-generation antihistamines in terms of being least likely to cause sedation.

Loratadine (adult dose 10 mg daily) is a derivative of azatadine. Although loratadine is metabolised in the liver by cytochrome P450, so far not clinically proven, relevant drug interactions have been reported. It is not clear whether its metabolite, desloratadine (adult dose 5 mg daily), offers a clinical advantage in urticaria.

Rupatadine (adult dose 10 mg daily) is a low-sedation antihistamine that is also effective in chronic urticaria. It should not be administered with other drugs that inhibit CYP3A4 such as erythromycin or ciclosporin.

Low-sedation antihistamines are used to control the symptoms of urticaria but do not influence the disease course. Individual response is variable, but adequate dose and timing in relationship to maximal urticarial activity are important. If one antihistamine does not work it is worth trying another. Increasing the dose of second-generation H_1 antihistamines up to fourfold above licence in adults when lower doses do not provide adequate symptom control has become common practice. This is a strong recommendation in the latest international consensus paper on urticaria [171] and in the guidelines of the British Association of Dermatologists [172]. Although it used to be common practice to recommend additional sedating antihistamines at night when sleep was disturbed, there is evidence that this is no more effective than increasing the dose of a second-generation antihistamine and it may cause unwanted sedation the following day [173].

The use of classic antihistamines is limited by their side effects, including sedation, anticholinergic properties and paradoxical excitation in children. There may be carry-over effects of sedation in the morning and patients should be warned of this. Hydroxyzine is the most potent of the classic antihistamines. Twenty-five milligrams of hydroxyzine is equivalent to 10 mg of cetirizine. A few classic antihistamines are available for parenteral administration (e.g. chlorphenamine, promethazine).

Adverse effects of antihistamines. Sedation is the major risk of classic antihistamines and may be seen in some patients with second-generation antihistamines, particularly at above licensed doses. Concerns about the potential cardiotoxicity of antihistamines have receded since terfenadine and astemizole were withdrawn from the market. Elucidation of the *HERG1* gene encoding the major K^+ cardiac repolarisation channels offers a molecular understanding of the cardiotoxic properties of terfenadine and astemizole, which block the channels at clinically relevant concentrations [174]. Mizolastine, which also undergoes limited conversion by hepatic

Table 42.2 Properties of currently licensed non-sedating H$_1$ antihistamines in the UK.

(a) Pharmacokinetic properties

Name	T_{max} (h)	$T\frac{1}{2}$ (h) Adults	$T\frac{1}{2}$ (h) Children	$5 \times T\frac{1}{2}$ (days)	Principal elimination
Acrivastine	1.5	1.5		<1	Renal
Bilastine					
Cetirizine	0.5–1	10		2	Renal
Levocetirizine	0.9	8	6	2	Renal
Loratadine	1 (2 h after food)	(8.4)		(2)	Hepatic (CYP3A4)
Desloratadine	3	27		6	Hepatic
Fexofenadine	1–3	11–15		3	Biliary
Mizolastine	1.5	13		3	Hepatic
Rupatadine	0.75	5.9		1.25	Hepatic

(b) Clinical properties

Drug	Dose (mg)	Age (years)[a]	Sedation	Metabolism	Interaction Drug	Interaction Food
Acrivastine	24	>12	–	–	–	–
Bilastine						
Cetirizine	5–10	≥2	+/–	–	–	–
Levocetirizine	5	≥2	+/–	–	–	–
Fexofenadine	180	≥12	–	–	–	+
Loratadine	5–10	≥2	–	+	+	–
Desloratadine	1.25–5	≥1	–	+	–	–
Mizolastine	10	≥12	–	+	+	–
Rupatadine	10	≥12	–	+	+	+

[a] Current UK licence.

CYP3A4, is able to block HERG1 channels to some degree. Its use with drugs that prolong the Q-T interval – such as amiodarone, quinidine, neuroleptic drugs and tricyclic antidepressants – and with electrolyte disturbance should be avoided. The classic antihistamines hydroxyzine and diphenhydramine may induce Q-T prolongation, emphasising that higher than licensed doses of these antihistamines should be used only with caution.

Antihistamines in pregnancy. Antihistamines cross the placenta. There is no reliable evidence that they are teratogenic, but they should be avoided in pregnancy and particularly in the first trimester if possible. Current guidelines on urticaria support the use of cetirizine and loratadine beyond the first trimester of pregnancy if the benefits of an antihistamine are considered to outweigh any risks of administration for an individual patient [171,172]. Chlorphenamine has been used based on its long availability and excellent safety record. However, cardiotocography demonstrates reduced fetal heart rate consistent with sedation during treatment of pregnant women with first-generation antihistamines, although it is not clear whether this has long-term effects.

Antihistamines in childhood. The principles of prescribing of antihistamines in childhood are the same as for adults, with second-generation non-sedating antihistamines being preferred. Doses should follow the relevant manufacturer's recommendations.

Second line
Omalizumab. Large phase III studies of omalizumab (anti-IgE) showed very good results in H$_1$ antihistamine-unresponsive chronic spontaneous urticaria [175,176]. The patient population in the pivotal GLACIAL study took H$_1$ antihistamines at above approved doses with or without H$_2$ antihistamines and montelukast, comparing 300 mg omalizumab every 4 weeks versus placebo. The data were used by the National Institute for Health and Care Excellence (NICE) as the basis for subsequent approval in the UK of omalizumab for severe chronic spontaneous urticaria not responding to full-dose H$_1$ antihistamines with montelukast at 300 mg every 4 weeks. Subsequent studies showed that omalizumab is effective and safe in patients with chronic spontaneous urticaria treated for 48 weeks and that most patients retreated with omalizumab after relapse following withdrawal regained symptomatic control. Omalizumab reduced angioedema-burdened days per week by threefold when compared with placebo in patients with chronic spontaneous urticaria and angioedema, with first recurrence of angioedema after 57–63 days with omalizumab and <5 days with placebo [177]. Shortening dose intervals or increasing the dose can benefit patients with inadequate response to standard-dosed omalizumab. Patients with partial response to omalizumab treatment experienced substantial or complete response when switched to 450 mg/month or 600 mg/month where funding allows [178]. A systematic review of more than 40 studies including several investigator-initiated randomised controlled trials showed that omalizumab treatment in patients with chronic inducible urticaria results in substantial or complete response in most patients [179]. The evidence for the efficacy of omalizumab in patients with chronic inducible urticaria when used off-label is strongest for symptomatic dermographism, cold urticaria, solar urticaria and cholinergic urticaria.

Ciclosporin. Ciclosporin at 2.5–3.5 mg/kg/day for 1–3 months improved or temporarily cleared severe urticaria in the majority of patients [180,181] and its efficacy has been confirmed in a randomised placebo-controlled study at 4 mg/kg/day for 4 weeks [182]. Fewer therapeutic failures occurred with a reducing dose of ciclosporin over 4 months than over 8 weeks [183], although the optimal dose and duration of treatment have yet to be defined.

Rescue medication
Corticosteroids. Oral corticosteroids are effective in severe urticaria at high doses (e.g. prednisolone 0.5 mg/kg/day) and may be used as rescue treatment over 1–3 days for angioedema in chronic urticaria. Prolonged use should be avoided because of the risk of side effects. Oral corticosteroids have been used for disease control in severe delayed pressure urticaria and urticarial vasculitis, but every attempt should be made to minimise their dose and duration.

Epinephrine. Epinephrine (syn. adrenaline) (300–500 µg by intramuscular injection) may be needed very rarely for anaphylaxis complicating chronic urticaria (e.g. cold urticaria or food- and exercise-induced anaphylaxis) or histaminergic non-hereditary angioedema causing respiratory compromise in acute urticaria. It acts rapidly by vasoconstriction and by stabilising mast cells through β-adrenoceptor stimulation.

Third line (targeted therapies)

Beyond antihistamines, it is often possible to use additional treatments off-label that have been shown by clinical experience or limited trial evidence to benefit specific presentations of urticaria or specific populations (Box 42.8).

Box 42.8 Targeted therapies

Pharmacological
- Antidepressants:
  - Doxepin
- H$_2$ antidepressants:
  - Famotidine
  - Nizatadine
  - Cimetidine
- Anticoagulants:
  - Warfarin
  - Heparin
- Immunosuppressives:
  - Methotrexate
  - Mycophenolate
  - Azathioprine
- Immunomodulators:
  - Hydroxychloroquine
  - Plasmapheresis
  - Intravenous immunoglobulins
- Leukotriene receptor anatagonist:
  - Montelukast
- Sulphones
  - Dapsone
  - Sulphasalazine

Non-pharmacological
- Phototherapy/PUVA
- Diet
- Psychological

PUVA, psoralen and ultraviolet A.

Pharmacological treatments

H$_2$ antihistamines. Combining an H$_2$ antihistamine with a non-sedating H$_1$ antihistamine may be more effective for redness and wealing (but not itch) although there is little published evidence from clinical trials. Famotidine or nizatidine as alternatives to ranitidine (currently unavailable) are preferable to cimetidine, which has antiandrogenic side effects and potential drug interactions.

Leukotriene receptor antagonists. These have been shown to benefit aspirin-sensitive urticaria and may be of value in delayed pressure urticaria and autoimmune urticaria when added to antihistamines [184].

Doxepin. Doxepin, a tricyclic antidepressant with H$_1$ and H$_2$ antihistaminic activity, may be used at night in a starting dose of 10–30 mg, but it also reacts with α-adrenergic receptors and should not be taken with monoamine oxidase inhibitors. It may help with sleep disturbance and anxiety but is unlikely to be effective as an antidepressant at the lower doses used for urticaria.

Anabolic steroids. Danazol may be beneficial for patients with refractory cholinergic urticaria [185], but it is more likely to be tolerated by men than women because it potentially has unwanted virilising effects.

Thyroxine. Thyroxine has been reported to reduce urticarial activity in some clinically euthyroid patients with thyroid autoimmunity but clinical experience has been disappointing [186].

Sulphonamides. Sulphasalazine [187] and dapsone [188] may be useful for delayed pressure urticaria, especially when oral corticosteroids are otherwise required for disease control, although the literature on these useful agents is small.

Tranexamic acid. Tranexamic acid may suppress non-histaminergic idiopathic angioedema [189].

Immunomodulatory and immunosuppressive treatments. Plasmapheresis improved six out of eight patients with autoimmune urticaria for 3–8 weeks only [190], highlighting the likely relevance of functional autoantibodies to disease activity. Intravenous immunoglobulin infusions, at 0.4 g/kg/day for 5 days (total 2 g), improved 9 out of 10 patients, 2 of whom remained clear for 2 years [191], but controlled studies are unavailable. Open studies of tacrolimus [192] and mycophenolate mofetil [193] suggest that they may have similar efficacy in severe chronic spontaneous urticaria. There is an anecdotal literature on methotrexate [194] and cyclophosphamide [195]. Azathioprine was found to be non-inferior to ciclosporin [196].

Non-pharmacological treatments. Narrow-band ultraviolet B phototherapy may help some patients with chronic urticaria [197], especially those with symptomatic dermographism [198], although controlled studies are needed. Cold desensitisation may be effective for well-motivated patients with cold contact urticaria [199]. There is an anecdotal literature on 'curative' antibiotic therapy for the same group [200]. A whole person treatment approach to explore unique meanings and emotional states resulted in a significant clinical benefit for symptoms in a small series of patients with chronic urticaria [201]. Autologous blood or serum injection was no better than placebo for chronic spontaneous urticaria in a recent meta-analysis [202].

Key references

The full list of references can be found in the online version at https://www.wiley.com/rooksdermatology10e

Urticaria

22 Hide M, Francis DM, Grattan CE, Hakimi J, Kochan JP, Greaves MW. Autoantibodies against the high-affinity IgE receptor as a cause of histamine release in chronic urticaria. *N Engl J Med* 1993;328:1599–604.

27 Konstantinou GN, Asero R, Ferrer M *et al*. EAACI taskforce position paper: evidence for autoimmune urticaria and proposal for defining diagnostic criteria. *Allergy* 2013;68:27–36.

33 Kolkhir P, Church MK, Weller K, Metz M, Schmetzer O, Maurer M. Autoimmune chronic spontaneous urticaria: what we know and what we do not know. *J Allergy Clin Immunol* 2017;139:1772–81.

PART 4: INFLAMMATORY DERMATOSES

36 Giménez-Arnau AM, DeMontojoye L, Asero R *et al*. The pathogenesis of chronic spontaneous urticaria: the role of infiltrating cells. *J Allergy Clin Immunol Pract* 2021;9:2195–208.

60 Sánchez J, Sánchez A, Cardona R. Causal relationship between anti-TPO IgE and chronic urticaria by *in vitro* and *in vivo* tests. *Allergy Asthma Immunol Res* 2019;11:29–42.

94 Magerl M, Altrichter S, Borzova E *et al*. The definition, diagnostic testing, and management of chronic inducible urticarias – the EAACI/GA(2) LEN/EDF/UNEV consensus recommendations 2016 update and revision. *Allergy* 2016;71:780–802.

163 Gonçalo M, Gimenéz-Arnau A, Al-Ahmad M *et al*. The global burden of chronic urticaria for the patient and society. *Br J Dermatol* 2021;184:226–36.

171 Zuberbier T, Abdul Latiff AH, Abuzakouk M *et al*. The international EAACI/GA^{2}LEN/EuroGuiDerm/APAAACI guideline for the definition, classification, diagnosis, and management of urticaria. *Allergy* 2022;77:734–66.

172 Sabroe RA, Lawlor F, Grattan CEH *et al*. British Association of Dermatologists' Clinical Standards Unit. British Association of Dermatologists guidelines for the management of people with chronic urticaria 2021. *Br J Dermatol* 2022;186:398–413.

CHAPTER 43

Recurrent Angio-oedema without Weals

Clive E. H. Grattan[1] *and Marcus Maurer*[2]

[1]St John's Institute of Dermatology, Guy's and St Thomas' NHS Foundation Trust, London, UK
[2]Institute of Allergology, Charité – Universitätsmedizin Berlin, corporate member of Freie Universität Berlin and Humboldt-Universität zu Berlin and Fraunhofer Institute for Translational Medicine and Pharmacology ITMP, Allergology and Immunology, Berlin, Germany

Recurrent angio-oedema without weals

Synonyms and inclusions

- Angio-oedema was known historically as Quincke's oedema or angioneurotic oedema
- Angio-oedema due to acquired C1-INH deficiency was formerly known as AAE but this term is now recommended for all types of non-HAE [1]

Definition and nomenclature

Angio-oedema is a deep, localised and self-limiting swelling of the skin and submucosal tissues due to a temporary increase in vascular permeability resulting from vasoactive mediators.

Angio-oedema *without* weals should be considered separately from angio-oedema *with* weals. The former may be a presentation of the uncommon but very important bradykinin-induced angio-oedemas, including hereditary angio-oedema (HAE), or the much more common mast cell mediator-induced angio-oedema, sometimes also called histaminergic angio-oedema. The latter falls within the spectrum of spontaneous or inducible urticarias (Chapter 42) resulting from mast cell degranulation. Bradykinin-induced angio-oedema may cause fatal laryngeal obstruction or painful bowel obstruction, sometimes presenting as an acute abdomen. Mast cell mediator-induced angio-oedema, by comparison, is a common presentation of spontaneous urticaria and may occur without weals. It affects the skin and/or oropharynx, but life-threatening laryngeal involvement in chronic urticaria does not occur even though patients may describe throat symptoms and the bowel is never affected.

The spectrum of disease includes HAE and acquired angio-oedema (AAE). The former is always bradykinin mediated and is usually linked to C1-esterase inhibitor (C1-INH) deficiency or impaired function. The latter is either mast cell mediator mediated in patients with urticaria, or bradykinin mediated in patients with angio-oedema due to acquired C1-INH deficiency or angiotensin-converting enzyme inhibitor (ACE inhibitor)-induced angio-oedema (Table 43.1). It is nearly always possible to distinguish between these subtypes of angio-oedema, or at least suspect the correct diagnosis, by careful history taking and appropriate blood tests.

Introduction and general description

Angio-oedema without weals affects the subcutaneous and submucosal tissues rather than the dermis. Almost any part of the body may be involved, but the most common sites are the lips (Figure 43.1), eyelids and genitalia due, in part, to the laxity of the dermal and subcutaneous tissues at these sites. The tongue and pharynx may also be affected, but this is much less common in mast cell mediator-induced angio-oedema than bradykinin-induced angio-oedema. Individual lesions may be either single or multiple, unilateral or symmetrical, and may appear suddenly. Itching is often absent. The lesions last from a few hours to several days. They resolve without scaling or dryness.

Mast cell mediator-induced angio-oedema

Mast cell mediator-induced angio-oedema without weals is mainly spontaneous (syn. histaminergic, idiopathic). Around 5% of patients with chronic spontaneous urticaria develop angio-oedema without weals. Delayed pressure urticaria weals are usually deep and may resemble angio-oedema. A rare presentation of inducible urticaria, vibratory angio-oedema, appears to be caused by IgE-independent vibration-induced mast cell degranulation.

Hereditary angio-oedema

This is a rare disorder, accounting for fewer than 2% of all cases of angio-oedema without weals. A family history is usually, but not always, present because up to 25% of cases appear to result from *de novo* mutations of C1-INH. However, it must be remembered

PART 4: INFLAMMATORY DERMATOSES

Table 43.1 The different types of angio-oedema presenting without weals.[a]

Mast cell mediator induced	Bradykinin induced
Chronic spontaneous urticaria without weals	Hereditary angio-oedema (HAE)
• *Known causes* Type 1 and Type IIb autoimmunity	• Type I (C1-INH *concentration* low)
	• Type II (C1-INH *activity* low)
• *Unknown cause* (idiopathic)	• HAE with normal C1-INH
Chronic inducible urticarias (only rarely present with pure angio-oedema), e.g.	Acquired angio-oedema
	• Acquired C1-INH deficiency
• Vibratory angio-oedema	• Drug induced (e.g. ACE inhibitor)
• Cholinergic urticaria spectrum	

[a] In some patients, acquired angio-oedema is idiopathic and not linked to mast cell mediators or bradykinin. The prevalence of this entity is unknown and it is poorly defined as there are no diagnostic tests.

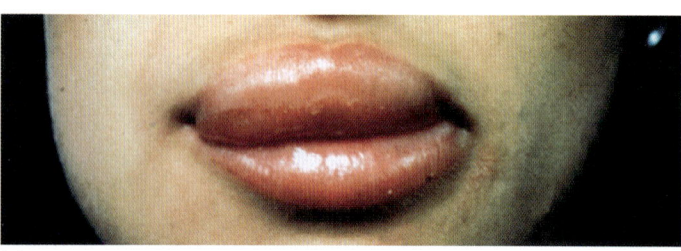

(a)

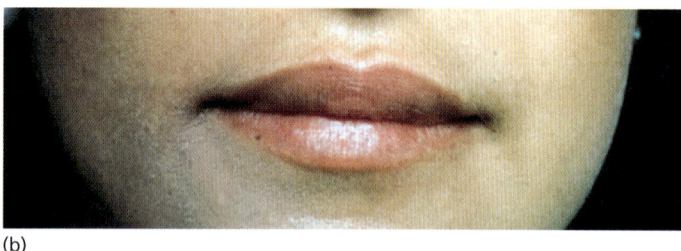

(b)

Figure 43.1 Spontaneous mast cell mediator-induced angio-oedema of the lips, (a) during and (b) 3 days after an attack. Courtesy of St John's Institute of Dermatology.

that a family history of urticaria is not infrequent because the estimated lifetime prevalence of all types of urticaria (acute and chronic) is in the region of 20%. Spontaneous urticaria can also occur in an HAE patient as an exceptional event. HAE due to C1-INH deficiency (CI-INH-HAE) is the most common form of HAE. It results from a quantitative (Type 1, approximately 85% of patients) or functional (Type 2, approximately 15%) deficiency of C1-INH. C1-INH, which is synthesised in the liver, is the main plasma serine-protease inhibitor in the contact system, the activation of which through Factor XII (FXII) results in the generation of bradykinin. Types 1 and 2 C1-INH-HAE are caused by mutations in the C1-INH gene, *SERPING 1*, and show autosomal dominant inheritance [2].

Several types of HAE with normal C1-INH (nC1-INH-HAE) have been reported [3]. The clinical appearance of nC1-INH-HAE is similar to that of C1-INH-HAE but most patients are female and their C1-INH and complement levels are normal. As of now, six types of nC1-INH-HAE have been linked to distinct mutations. The genes

affected include *F12* (Factor XII) [4], *PLG* (plasminogen) [5], *ANGPTI* (angiopoietin-1) [6], *KNG1* (kininogen-1) [7], *MYOF* (myoferlin) [8] and *HS3ST6* (heparan sulfate 3-O-sulfotransferase 6) [9]. FXII-HAE, PLG-HAE and KNG1-HAE are considered to be bradykinin-mediated forms of recurrent angio-oedema with excess formation of bradykinin, whereas ANGPT1-HAE and MYOF-HAE are held to be due to vascular endothelial growth factor (VEGF) receptor modulation and VEGF signal transduction.

Angiotensin-converting enzyme inhibitor-induced angio-oedema

ACE inhibitors (ACEi) may cause angio-oedema by inhibiting ACE (kininase II) resulting in reduced bradykinin metabolism (Figure 43.2). Most cases develop within 3 weeks of commencing treatment, but can occur at any time, even more than 10 years after starting. It is a class effect seen with all ACEi and only occasionally with angiotensin receptor blockers. Angio-oedema affects predominantly the face and oropharynx. Symptoms may be severe and laryngeal involvement may be life threatening. Gliptins and mTor inhibitors augment the risk of angio-oedema with ACEi [10,11]. Sacubitril-valsartan is an angiotensin receptor-neprilysin inhibitor combination drug (ARNI) used in the management of heart failure with reduced ejection fraction. ARNIs should not be given to patients with previous angio-oedema to an ACEi, because they cause angioedema at rates similar to ACEi.

Epidemiology
Incidence and prevalence
Mast cell mediator-induced angio-oedema is the commonest presentation of angio-oedema without weals, representing 5–10% of patients with chronic spontaneous urticaria. The prevalence of HAE types 1 and 2 is around 1:50 000 (i.e. a lifetime prevalence of 0.002%) without evidence of any sex, ethnic or racial differences [2]. More than 400 and 100 patients with FXII-HAE and PLG-HAE have been reported, respectively. Only a few families with ANGPT1-HAE, KNG1-HAE, MYOF-HAE and 3-OST-6-HAE have been described as of now. ACE inhibitor-induced angio-oedema affects up to 1% of patients on treatment with a 3.5–4.0–fold higher incidence in those with an Afro-Caribbean ethnicity [1]. Angio-oedema due to acquired C1-INH deficiency is extremely rare; its prevalence is unknown.

Age
Mast cell mediator-induced angio-oedema can present at any age but more often in the fourth or fifth decades of life in line with chronic spontaneous urticaria. Over 75% of patients with HAE will have had their first attack by the age of 15 years although onset may be delayed until adult life [12]. ACE inhibitor-induced angio-oedema is predominantly a problem of older people requiring antihypertensive treatment.

Sex
Mast cell mediator-induced angio-oedema and ACE inhibitor-induced angio-oedema [1] are more common in women. There is no sex bias for HAE types I or II, but HAE with normal C1-INH presents mainly in women.

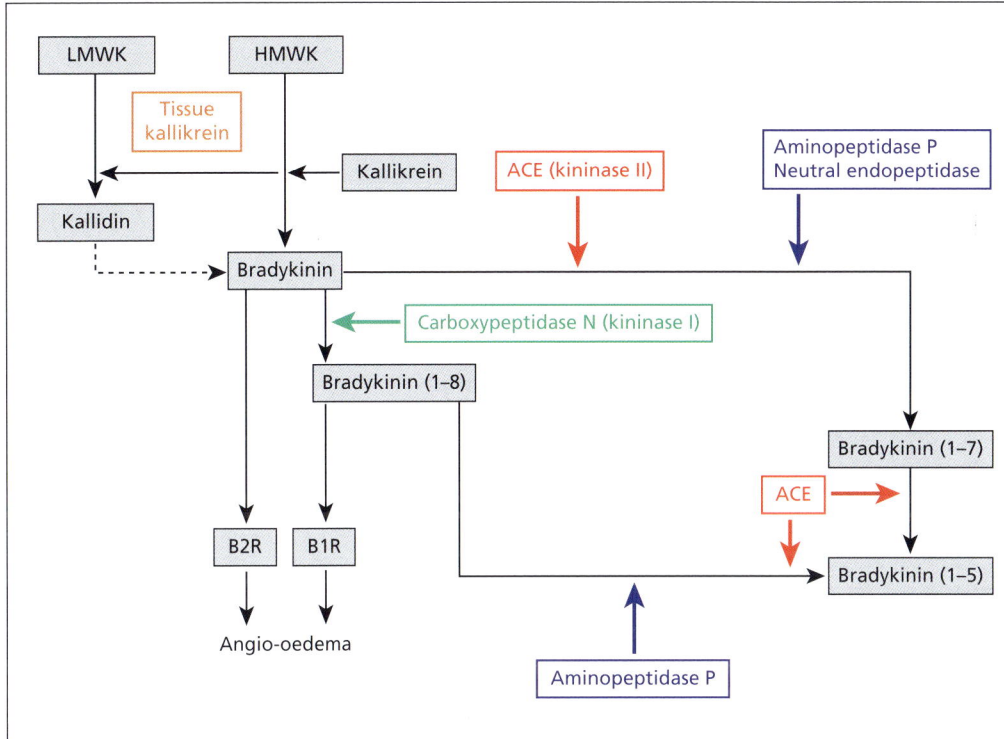

Figure 43.2 Bradykinin formation and breakdown. Bradykinin is formed predominantly from high-molecular-weight kininogen (HMWK) by plasma kallikrein. Binding of bradykinin to the B2 receptor (B2R) on the endothelium of small blood vessels causes vasodilatation and vasopermeability. Bradykinin is broken down by a multistage process primarily involving angiotensin-converting enzyme (ACE), also known as kininase II. LMWK, low-molecular-weight kininogen.

Ethnicity
There is no known racial or ethnic predilection for any type of angio-oedema without weals except for ACE inhibitor-induced angio-oedema where the incidence can be as high as 4% in patients of Afro-Caribbean ancestry taking an ACE inhibitor.

Associated diseases
Mast cell mediator-induced angio-oedema is associated with thyroid autoimmunity in common with spontaneous urticaria [13]. Although a weak association between HAE with autoimmune diseases, including Sjögren syndrome and systemic lupus erythematosus, has been proposed [14], a large case–control study found no increase in the prevalence of autoimmune disease in HAE [15]. However, the severity and effectiveness of long-term treatment of HAE were influenced by the autoimmune disorder in affected patients.

Pathophysiology
Mast cell mediator-induced angio-oedema without weals
Most cases are due to mast cell degranulation as evidenced by their response to H$_1$ anti-mast cell mediator drugs and omalizumab, a monoclonal antibody that specifically binds to free human immunoglobulin E. The cause of degranulation is held to be auto-allergic and autoimmune mechanisms with functional IgE and IgG autoantibodies in common with spontaneous urticaria (Chapter 42). Stress, infections and non-steroidal anti-inflammatory drugs are held to trigger mast cell mediator-induced angio-oedema in some patients. A few patients with angio-oedema resembling C1-INH deficiency with normal investigations, no family history and no response to H$_1$ antihistamines are thought to have idiopathic

non-histaminergic angio-oedema but little is known about this entity because it is difficult to diagnose (see footnote to Table 43.1).

ACE inhibitor-induced angio-oedema
ACE cleaves bradykinin and ACE inhibitors prevent this resulting in an increase in bradykinin levels. However, several enzymatic pathways are involved in bradykinin degradation and the pathophysiology is more complicated than is often assumed (Figure 43.2).

Acquired idiopathic angio-oedema
In some patients, acquired angio-oedema is idiopathic and not linked to mast cell mediators or bradykinin. The prevalence of this entity is unknown and it is poorly defined as there are no diagnostic tests.

Hereditary angio-oedema
Patients with HAE types I and II are deficient in a natural inhibitor of C1-INH, which is made under genetic control in the liver. It has an autosomal dominant pattern of inheritance. It seems to require the activity of both alleles of *SERPING1* to maintain normal levels. The inhibitor is present either in reduced amounts (Type I) or, in 15% of affected families, in an inactive form, although it can be detected in normal amounts immunologically (Type 2). NC1-INH-HAE, which was initially referred to as HAE type III or oestrogen-dependent angioedema [16] because the original cases were exclusively in women, results from mutations that do not affect C1-INH. The diagnosis of HAE with normal C1-INH is defined by a family history of recurrent angio-oedema without weals in more than one generation with normal C1-INH and confirmed by genetic testing.

C1-INH is a natural inhibitor of the activated first component of complement, kallikrein and the fibrinolytic and intrinsic coagulation systems. Attacks are triggered by stimuli that activate FXII (Hageman factor) and hence consume the deficient inhibitor. This C1-INH deficiency may be detected antigenically, but functional assays are necessary to confirm type II HAE. Most components of complement are normal, but C_4 is nearly always low during, after and usually between attacks. The diagnostic work-up in patients suspected of having HAE should therefore include measurements of C_4 as well as C1-INH levels and function. There is no clear correlation between the clinical severity and laboratory abnormalities.

Angio-oedema due to acquired C1-INH deficiency

Two types are recognised. Type 1 is due to continuous activation of complement by lymphoproliferative disease, including paraproteinaemia due to increased catabolism of C1-INH. Type 2 is due to autoantibodies that recognise C1-INH and inactivate it without triggering its target proteases. Both forms will have reduced antigenic and functional C1-INH levels.

Infections

There is some evidence that HAE may be destabilised by *Helicobacter pylori* infection of the stomach [17].

Genetics

Types I and II HAE are inherited as an autosomal dominant trait on chromosome 11q 12.1. Over 500 different mutations of the gene controlling C1-INH (*SERPING1*) have been identified. Gain-of-function mutations of *F12* that have been described in about 20% of patients with nC1-INH-HAE relate to north European ancestry [18]. NC1-INH-HAE has autosomal dominant inheritance. Other types of C1-INH-HAE are linked to mutations in *PLG*, *ANGPT1*, *KNG1*, *MYOF* and *HS3ST6*. A missense variant in *ADGRE2* has been described in patients with autosomal dominant vibratory angio-oedema [19] presenting with or without weals.

Environmental factors

All types of HAE are aggravated by oestrogen in contraceptive and hormone replacement therapies [20] but not non-steroidal anti-inflammatory drugs (NSAIDs).

Clinical features

Mast cell mediator-induced angio-oedema

The presentation of mast cell mediator-induced angio-oedema without weals is the same as angio-oedema that presents in patients with spontaneous urticaria who also exhibit weals (Chapter 42). Oro-pharyngeal involvement is unusual and life-threatening laryngeal oedema does not occur. Abdominal angio-oedema does not occur.

ACE inhibitor-induced angio-oedema

Swellings are confined to the face and oropharynx. Larnygeal angio-oedema may occur and may be fatal without prompt recognition and treatment. Rare abdominal symptoms due to small bowel oedema have been reported [21].

Hereditary angio-oedema

The clinical picture of HAE usually facilitates strong suspicion of the diagnosis before laboratory confirmation. There are recurrent swellings of the skin and mucous membranes throughout life, often associated with nausea, vomiting, colic and urinary symptoms. These attacks may occur regularly every few days or weeks or may be less frequent. Abdominal symptoms may occur in the absence of skin changes and cause great diagnostic difficulty. In one series [22], 34% of patients had undergone abdominal surgery. Pharyngeal, laryngeal and even bronchial involvement are especially significant and dominate the prognosis. The skin and mucosal lesions are often solitary and may be painful. They seldom itch and they may occur spontaneously or after trauma; dental trauma and intubation are especially hazardous. Weals do not occur, but many patients exhibit a rather distinctive reticulate erythema, perhaps with minimal oedema, which occurs prodromally [23] (Figure 43.3). A few patients have a relatively minor disability and most patients are severely debilitated. In other families, before the advent of modern therapy, over 20% of patients used to die of respiratory obstruction before early middle age, and fatalities still occur and remain a risk [24].

Clinical variants

Systemic capillary leak syndrome (syn. Clarkson syndrome). This is a rare syndrome in which there are dramatic recurrent episodes of exudation of fluid into various organs including the skin. Angio-oedema has been reported. A severe shock-like state may ensue and the eventual mortality is high. There is an IgG paraproteinaemia [25].

Episodic angio-oedema with eosinophilia (syn. Gleich syndrome) [26]. Recurrent episodes of angio-oedema associated with pyrexia, blood eosinophilia and infiltration of the dermis with eosinophils have been described. There is no evidence of systemic involvement

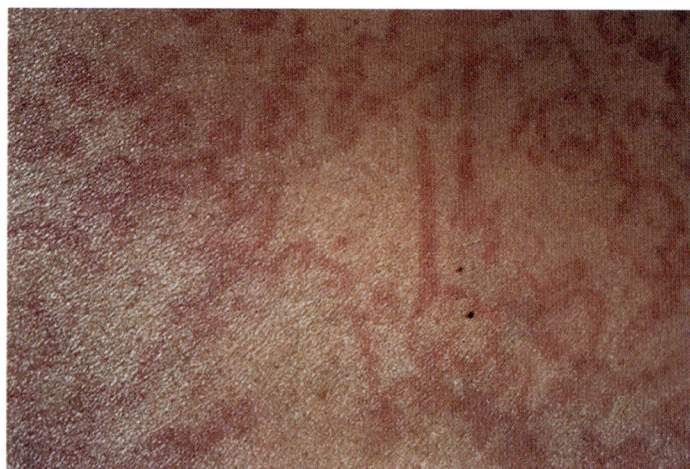

Figure 43.3 Reticulate prodromal erythema seen in some families with hereditary angio-oedema (HAE). 'Chicken-wire' reticulate erythema/urticaria, non-pruritic, on the trunk of a woman aged 38 years who had had numerous episodes over many years, each one lasting many hours or even days. Many attacks, but not all, were followed within 24 h by classical attacks of HAE, confirmed by history and laboratory confirmation of C1-esterase deficiency. Courtesy of Dr A. P. Warin.

or progression to a cardiomyopathy, in contrast to hypereosinophilic syndrome where this is a recognised complication. Each episode resolves with prednisolone treatment. During an attack, elevated serum levels of interleukin 5 (IL-5) have been demonstrated in some cases [27] and IL-6 in others [28].

Other differential diagnosis. Other differential diagnosis of angio-oedema without weals includes oro-facial granulomatosis, acute dermatitis (especially of the eyelids), cellulitis, connective tissue diseases and idiopathic scrotal oedema.

Assessment of disease activity and impact on patients
Scoring systems for patients for patients with recurrent angio-oedema without weals have been published and are used and useful in routine clinical practice. They include the angio-oedema activity score (AAS, for disease activity) [29], the angio-oedema quality of life questionnaire (AE-QoL for disease impact) [30] and the angio-oedema control test (AECT for disease control) [31]. They are also suitable for use in patients with recurrent angio-oedema and weals.

Disease course and prognosis
Chronic mast cell mediator-induced angio-oedema usually lasts for several months to years. Spontaneous resolution is the rule. HAE is lifelong with variations in activity corresponding to environmental factors, lifestyle, drugs (especially exogenous oestrogens and ACE inhibitors) and endogenous factors (e.g. puberty and pregnancy). The main risk of HAE is suffocation and death [24]. Treatment of the underlying B-cell lymphoproliferative disorder may lead to resolution of type 1 acquired C1-INH deficiency. ACE inhibitor-induced angio-oedema remits after discontinuation of the drug but may take up to 6 months to subside after stopping. The reason for this is unknown.

Investigations
In patients with mast cell mediator-induced angio-oedema, spontaneous and inducible forms should be considered. They can occur in the same patient. Severe inflammatory disorders should be ruled out by checking C-reactive protein (CRP) and a white blood cell differential. Patients with frequent attacks and/or longstanding disease should be checked for underlying causes.

C_4 complement is a good screening blood test for HAE types I and II, especially during attacks. It should be less than 30% of mean normal in affected patients [12]. Measurement of functional C1-INH is necessary to diagnose type II HAE. Both C_4 and C1-INH will be normal in nC1-INH HAE. C_4 and functional C1-INH are low in acquired C1-INH deficiency and C1q is also reduced. The laboratory profile of the different types of angio-oedema without weals is shown in Figure 43.4.

Management
The management of mast cell mediator-induced histaminergic angio-oedema is essentially the same as for chronic spontaneous urticaria patients with weals, except that oro-pharyngeal lesions may occur and cause great distress. Non-sedating, second-generation H_1 antihistamines are the first line treatment. They should be used on a daily basis until spontaneous remission. Higher than standard doses (up to fourfold) may be required to achieve sufficient protection [32] (Chapter 42). Omalizumab (anti-IgE) is licensed in Europe and the USA for the use of anti-histamine refractory cases of chronic spontaneous urticaria and should be considered as third line therapy. Emergency treatment with epinephrine is discussed along with anaphylaxis in Chapter 42.

The treatment of recurrent angio-oedema due to C1-INH deficiency is completely different and is discussed here. H_1 antihistamines, steroids and epinephrine are ineffective for HAE

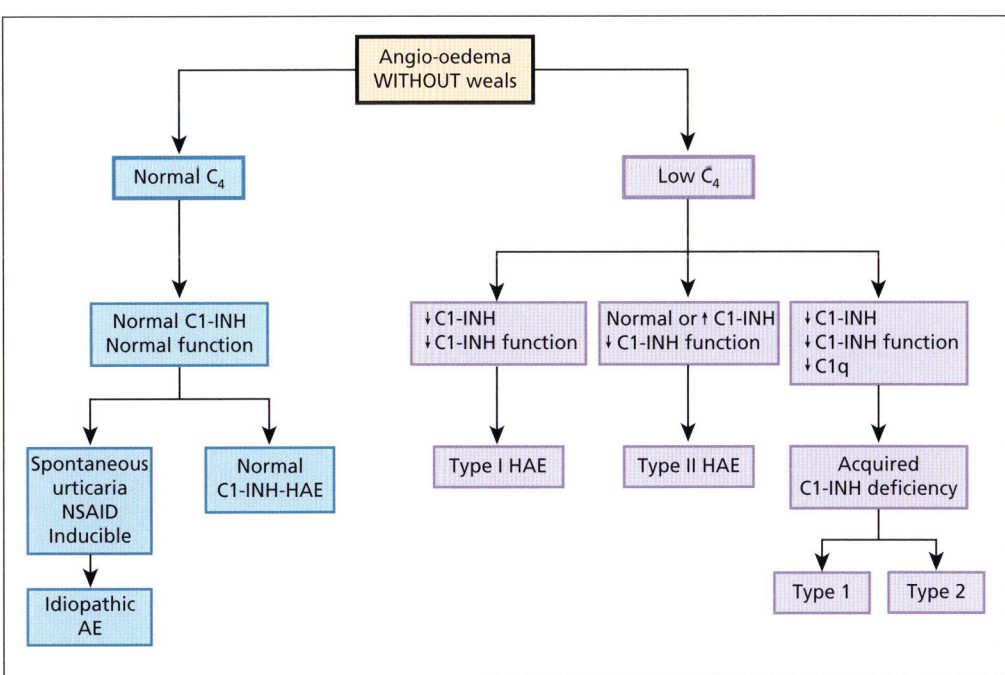

Figure 43.4 Laboratory profiles of different types of angio-oedema without weals. HAE, hereditary angio-oedema; NSAID, non-steroidal anti-inflammatory drugs.

or angio-oedema due to acquired C1-INH deficiency. Oestrogen therapies, such as the oral contraceptive pill, and ACE inhibitor may induce or exacerbate HAE and should be avoided. Management should be considered under emergency treatment of an established attack, short-term and long-term prophylaxis (Box 43.1).

Box 43.1 Treatment summary for angio-oedema without weals

Mast cell mediator-induced angio-oedema
- As for chronic spontaneous urticaria (Chapter 42)

Bradykinin-induced angio-oedema
- Hereditary types 1, 2, HAE with normal C1-INH[a]
  - Emergency
    - Icatibant (bradykinin receptor 2 antagonist) (SC)
    - Plasma-derived C1-INH (IV)
    - Recombinant C1-INH (IV)
    - Ecallantide (kallikrein inhibitor) (SC)
  - Short-term prophylaxis
    - Plasma-derived C1-INH (IV)
  - Long-term prophylaxis
    - Plasma-derived C1-INH (IV or SC)
    - Lanadelumab (SC)
    - Berotralstat (PO)
    - Tranexamic acid (PO)
    - Anabolic steroids (danazol) (PO)
- Acquired C1-INH deficiency
  - Emergency
    - Plasma-derived C1-INH
    - Icatibant (bradykinin receptor 2 antagonist)[a]
  - Prophylaxis
    - Plasma-derived C1-INH
    - Tranexamic acid
    - Anabolic steroids
    - ? Rituximab[a]
- ACE inhibitor-induced angio-oedema
  - Stop and avoid all ACE inhibitors
  - ? Icatibant[a]

[a] Unlicensed use.

Emergency treatment of hereditary angio-oedema

Purified plasma-derived C1-INH (pdC1-INH) given by bolus intravenous infusion based on body weight or the bradykinin 2 receptor antagonist, icatibant, given by subcutaneous injection [33] are the primary emergency treatments for oro-facial or laryngeal oedema and abdominal attacks. Twenty units/kg body weight of pdC1-INH is recommended. Self-administration by patients at the first sign of an attack is now encouraged since it leads to more rapid resolution of symptoms and less risk of progression of swellings. Symptom relief should be seen within 30–90 min of administration but it may take 6–8 h for complete resolution. C1-INH is also available as a recombinant product prepared from the milk of transgenic rabbits [34]. A 60-amino-acid kallikrein inhibitor produced by recombinant DNA technology, ecallantide [35], given by subcutaneous injection is available only in the USA and a few

other countries. Solvent detergent-treated plasma, or, when not available, fresh frozen plasma containing C1-INH, can be given in an emergency if other products are unavailable.

Short-term prophylaxis of hereditary angio-oedema

Plasma-derived C1-INH concentrate should be given shortly before medical procedures involving trauma, especially dental work or intubation during general anaesthetic [3]. For relatively minor dental procedures, such as dental cleaning, ensuring availability of pdC1-INH or icatibant should be sufficient. Where C1-INH is not available, anabolic steroids and plasmin inhibitors, including tranexamic acid, may also be used for short-term prophylaxis, for example 48 h before and 2–5 days after dental surgery, at the higher dose ranges [12].

Long-term prophylaxis of hereditary angio-oedema

Plasma-derived C1-INH replacement therapy and the plasma kallikrein inhibitors lanadelumab (SC) and berotralstat (PO) are the preferred prophylactic treatment for HAE patients where they are available. For pdC1-INH patients, twice-weekly subcutaneous or intravenous infusions are sufficient in most patients to greatly reduce or completely prevent the occurrence of attacks. With lanadelumab, a fully human, monoclonal antibody (IgG1/κ-light chain) against kallikrein, given every 2 weeks or 4 weeks subcutaneously, most patients experience complete response. Once-daily berotralstat, a small molecule oral kallikrein inhibitor, also protects from attacks. Both are approved for HAE patients aged 12 years or older.

Attenuated androgens/anabolic drugs such as danazol and stanozolol are second-line prophylactic options and should only be used when pdC1-INH, lanadelumab or berotralstat is not available. They are still used in adults but may not work or be tolerated, especially by women in whom androgenic side effects including menstrual irregularities, acne and hirsutism may be unacceptable. They stimulate production of the deficient inhibitor by the liver under the control of the remaining functioning C1-INH allele in heterozygotes. The usual starting dose of danazol is 100–200 mg daily but lower doses may be effective in some patients [12]. Tranexamic acid, an antifibrinolytic that inhibits activation of plasminogen to plasmin at 2.0–4.5 g daily, has been found to help some patients, but is contraindicated by a past history of thrombosis or inherited thrombophilia. Epsilon aminocaproic acid (not available in the UK), 12–18 g daily is also used. Antifibrinolytics are less effective than anabolic steroids but may be useful where C1-INH, lanadelumab and berotralstat are unavailable and androgens are contraindicated, especially for short-term prophylaxis and in children.

Treatment of angio-oedema due to acquired C1-inhibitor deficiency

Icatibant and C1-INH are the treatment of choice. Lanadelumab and berotralstat may be of benefit but there are no reports to support this. Danazol is helpful in some cases, but not the autoantibody type, which also fails to respond to replacement therapy but may be helped by tranexamic acid and corticosteroids. Rituximab has been reported to give longlasting improvement [36].

Resources

Patient resource

https://haei.org (last accessed October 2022).

Key references

The full list of references can be found in the online version at https://www.wiley.com/rooksdermatology10e

1 Cicardi M, Aberer W, Banerji A *et al*. Classification, diagnosis and approach to treatment for angioedema: consensus report from the Hereditary Angioedema International Working Group. *Allergy* 2014;69:602–16.

2 Maurer M, Magerl M, Ansotegui I *et al*. The international WAO/EAACI guideline for the management of hereditary angioedema – the 2017 revision and update. *Allergy* 2018;73:1575–96.

3 Maurer M, Magerl M. Differences and similarities in the mechanisms and clinical expression of bradykinin-mediated vs. mast cell-mediated angioedema. *Clin Rev Allergy Immunol* 2021;61:40–9.

12 Gompels MM, Lock RJ, Abinun M *et al*. C1-INHibitor deficiency: consensus document. *Clin Exp Immunol* 2005;139:379–94.

18 Bork K. Hereditary angioedema with normal C1-INHibitor activity including hereditary angioedema with coagulation factor XII gene mutations. *Immunol Allergy Clin North Am* 2006;26:709–24.

22 Agostoni A, Cicardi M. Hereditary and acquired C_1-inhibitor deficiency: biological and clinical characteristics in 235 patients. *Medicine* 1992;71:206–15.

24 Bork K, Hardt J, Witzke G. Fatal laryngeal attacks and mortality in hereditary angioedema due to C1-INH deficiency. *J Allergy Clin Immunol* 2012;130:692–7.

31 Weller K, Donoso T, Magerl M *et al*. Validation of the Angioedema Control Test (AECT) – a patient-reported outcome instrument for assessing angioedema control. *J Allergy Clin Immunol Pract* 2020;8:2050–7.

PART 4: INFLAMMATORY DERMATOSES

CHAPTER 44

Urticarial Vasculitis

Karoline Krause[1] and Clive E. H. Grattan[2]

[1] Institute of Allergology, Charité – Universitätsmedizin Berlin, corporate member of Freie Universität Berlin, Humboldt-Universität zu Berlin, and Berlin Institute of Health, Germany
[2] St John's Institute of Dermatology, Guy's and St Thomas' NHS Foundation Trust, London, UK

PART 4: INFLAMMATORY DERMATOSES

Definition and nomenclature

Urticarial vasculitis is a rare disease characterised clinically by urticarial lesions with histological evidence of leukocytoclastic vasculitis. Clinicopathological correlation is essential for diagnosis.

Synonyms and inclusions
- Urticarial vasculitis
- Urticarial venulitis
- McDuffie syndrome

Introduction and general description

Urticarial vasculitis is a rare immune-mediated disease characterised by continued wealing associated with histopathological evidence of leukocytoclastic vasculitis [1]. If associated with systemic involvement, urticarial vasculitis can lead to substantial morbidity [2]. Distinguishing between hypocomplementaemic (HUV) and normocomplementaemic urticarial vasculitis (NUV) is important since the former may have multisystem involvement, including nephritis and lung disease, whereas the latter usually runs a benign and, ultimately, self-limiting course. Urticarial vasculitis is a complex dynamic process with incompletely understood pathophysiology [3]. The diagnosis relies on both clinical features and a lesional skin biopsy and can be challenging in clinical practice for both clinicians and histopathologists because there is considerable overlap with its main differential diagnosis of chronic spontaneous urticaria [4,5]. Additionally, thorough laboratory work-up is essential in patients with urticarial vasculitis in view of potential multisystem involvement and the possibility of identifying associated diseases relevant to its pathogenesis [6]. Successful management of urticarial vasculitis can be difficult and includes antihistamines, oral corticosteroids, immunomodulating and immunosuppressive agents [7]. Also, biological agents have been used in the treatment of urticarial vasculitis [8,9].

Epidemiology

Incidence and prevalence
The lifetime prevalence of urticarial vasculitis has not been studied but may be in the region of 0.025% (estimated as 5% of the estimated prevalence of chronic urticaria). It is a rare disease that occurs in about 1–20% of patients presenting with a chronic urticarial illness [2,10,11]. The use of different diagnostic criteria has resulted in considerable variation in the reported frequencies of urticarial vasculitis in patients with chronic urticarial disease [10]. A US based population study reported an incidence of 0.5 per 100 000 person-years [12].

Age
Urticarial vasculitis may occur at any age but shows a peak incidence in the fourth decade of life [4,13]. The incidence of hypocomplementaemic variants including urticarial vasculitis syndrome (HUVS) peaks in the fifth decade [14]. All forms are rare in children [15].

Sex

Women are more often affected than men. Studies with a sizeable number of patients reported 57–80% of participants to be females [16,17,18].

Ethnicity

Ethnic predisposition to urticarial vasculitis is unknown; it has been reported primarily in European, American and Asian populations [4,7,16].

Associated diseases

Several diseases are associated with urticarial vasculitis [1] although it is unknown whether these represent causality or coincidence.

Common associations with urticarial vasculitis are attributed to connective tissue diseases including systemic lupus erythematosus [19] and Sjögren disease [20]. Chronic hepatitis B and C are frequent associations [13,21] although other infections such as infectious mononucleosis [22] and Lyme borreliosis [23] have been also linked. Serum sickness represents an acute form of urticarial vasculitis [6]. Recently, a number of case reports described urticarial vasculitis during or after Covid-19 infection [24–26].

Urticarial vasculitis has been reported in association with haematological disorders (essential cryoglobulinaemia and idiopathic thrombocytopenia) and malignancies (non-Hodgkin lymphoma, acute non-lymphocytic leukaemia, acute myelogenous leukaemia, B-cell chronic lymphocytic leukaemia [27] and immunoglobulin A (IgA) myeloma) [7,28,29]. An association between urticarial vasculitis and adenocarcinoma of the colon has also been described in a single case report [30]. Although urticarial vasculitis has been reported in Schnitzler syndrome [31] it is now accepted that the histopathological changes seen in Schnitzler syndrome [32] and other urticarial autoinflammatory syndromes should be regarded as a neutrophilic urticarial dermatosis (NUD) rather than vasculitis (Chapter 45).

Pathophysiology

Urticarial vasculitis is a type III hypersensitivity reaction, in which intravascular antigen–antibody complexes result in complement activation. Its pathophysiology is incompletely understood mainly due to great interpatient variability and the scarcity of sequential histological studies of disease development and progression. Several factors are thought to be of pathogenic importance in this disease, including circulating immune complexes, complement activation via the classical pathway, mast cell activation, production of pro-inflammatory cytokines, endothelial cell activation and damage as well as inflammatory cell infiltration, neutrophil karyorrhexis and fibrin deposition [2,3,33,34].

Urticarial vasculitis predominantly affects postcapillary venules in the superficial dermis. The vascular endothelial damage is thought to be mediated by circulating immune complexes [34]. Deposition of IgG and IgM and C3 within and around the vessel wall and at the dermoepidermal junction is a common feature [13,17].

Hypocomplementaemia in urticarial vasculitis is consistent with complement activation via the classical complement pathway caused, presumably, by circulating immune complexes [1,34].

Patients with HUVS usually have IgG autoantibodies directed against the collagen-like region of C1q (anti-C1q) and low levels of C1q [2].

A spectrum of autoantibodies has been observed in urticarial vasculitis including antinuclear antibodies, extractable nuclear antigens [35], antiphospholipid [19] and antiendothelial antibodies [36]. Skin autoreactivity to patient's serum has been reported occasionally in urticarial vasculitis [37] although there has been no systematic study to ascertain how commonly this occurs. The pathogenic importance of these observations is unclear and further research may elucidate their clinical relevance.

Mast cell activation is thought to occur early in the formation of vasculitic lesions [33]. This is associated with the release of the pro-inflammatory cytokine tumour necrosis factor-α [33]. Interleukin (IL)-6 and IL-1 receptor antagonist are also increased in the serum of patients with urticarial vasculitis [8].

The mechanisms of activation and damage of endothelial cells in urticarial vasculitis are poorly understood. Microscopically, endothelial cell involvement is characterised by swelling and necrosis [10,38]. Endothelial cell activation is reflected by upregulation of cell adhesion molecules [3,33]. In vasculitis, endothelial cell activation is known to result in the loss of anticoagulant and fibrinolytic properties, thereby leading to fibrin deposition and fibrinoid degeneration of the affected vessels. Also, activation of endothelial cells contributes to the recruitment of inflammatory cells into the perivascular infiltrate [39]. Unresolved questions remain as to whether this activation is caused by antiendothelial antibodies, complement activation or transmigration of inflammatory cells.

The dynamic nature of the inflammatory infiltrate has been reported [33,40]. In serial biopsies from a patient with exercise-induced urticarial vasculitis, eosinophils were the first cells recruited at 3 h, followed by neutrophil predominance at 24 h [33]. Histological studies have shown extracellular deposition of eosinophil peroxidase and neutrophil elastase. Neutrophil-rich infiltration with leukocytoclasis is a common feature [18]. As described in other autoimmune diseases of the skin such as lupus erythematosus, neutrophil extracellular trap formation, that is web-like structures of decondensed chromatin, histones, and antimicrobial peptides released by neutrophils, were shown in lesional skin of urticarial vasculitis too [41].

Lymphocytes are thought to be the predominant cells in the perivascular infiltrate in the lesions older than 48 h [2,40]. Other authors have reported lymphocyte-dominated infiltrates in younger lesions as well [42]. The true relevance of lymphocytic infiltration to the vasculitic process needs to be clarified further [43].

Predisposing factors

Urticarial vasculitis is considered to be of unknown cause in the majority of patients [4] with only few hard data on predisposing factors (see Genetics and Environmental factors later).

Pathology

Classical histopathological features of fully developed urticarial vasculitis are: (i) endothelial cell damage and swelling and loss of integrity of the vessel wall; (ii) fibrin deposits in the affected postcapillary venules; (iii) neutrophil- or lymphocyte-predominant perivascular infiltrate with leukocytoclasis; and (iv) erythrocyte extravasation [10,**44**]. However, not all of these features may be present at the same time, thereby causing diagnostic uncertainty. Furthermore, the well-recognised continuum of histological changes between urticaria and urticarial vasculitis [5,45] may contribute to uncertainty over diagnosis. In addition, differences in weal duration and body sites may further complicate the histological classification of skin biopsies.

Immunoglobulin G, IgM and/or C3 within or around the vessels of lesions is seen more often in patients with hypocomplementaemic than NUV [**13**]. Immunoglobulin deposits can also be found at the dermal–epidermal junction [17]. However, the detection of immunoglobulins or complement within vessel walls largely depends on the duration of weals and timing of biopsy. Thus, negative immunofluorescence does not rule out a diagnosis of urticarial vasculitis [**46**]. There may be eosinophil predominance in NUV, whereas patients with HUV have more neutrophil-rich perivascular infiltrates [47].

Lymphocytic predominance in perivascular infiltration is often seen in skin biopsy specimens from lesions older than 48 h [2]. Lymphocytic vasculitis is not a common feature in urticarial vasculitis [43] and the histological diagnosis in these cases should be based on the histological evidence of vessel damage with fibrinoid degeneration [10].

Genetics

The genetic basis of urticarial vasculitis is largely unknown. It is not known to be familial but the concordance of HUVS was described in identical twins [48]. Homozygous mutations in *DNASE1L3* encoding an endonuclease have been identified in two families with autosomal recessive HUVS [49]. Mutations in *DNASE1L3* were also linked to familial forms of systemic lupus erythematosus [50].

Environmental factors

Potential causes or triggers include drugs, infections and physical factors. Drugs implicated in the development of urticarial vasculitis include cimetidine, diltiazem, procarbazine, potassium iodine, fluoxetine, procainamide and etanercept [**1**,7,10]. Infections include hepatitis B and C, infectious mononucleosis, Lyme disease and lately Covid-19. Rarely, the disease is induced by physical factors such as exercise and exposure to sun or cold [**1**].

Clinical features

History

In some cases, infection or drug intake may precede the onset of urticarial vasculitis. Patients complain of recurrent weals which are typically painful rather than itchy, lasting longer than 24 h and often leaving residual hyperpigmentation (Figure 44.1) [2]. Patients often complain about fatigue, malaise, musculoskeletal symptoms or fever associated with weals [**16**].

Presentation

Although the duration of the weals is typically longer than 24 h, in some patients, the weals in urticarial vasculitis are indistinguishable from those in chronic urticaria. Evidence suggests that urticarial vasculitis may be an underlying process in 20% of patients with clinical

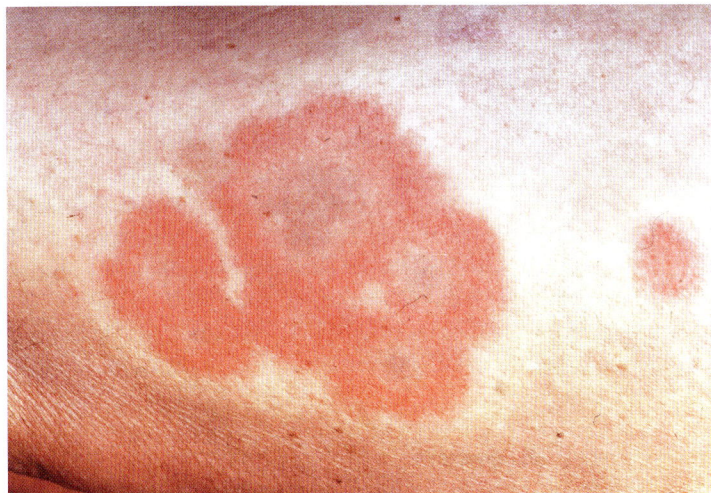

Figure 44.1 Urticarial vasculitis lesions resembling weals of chronic spontaneous urticaria. These sometimes fade to leave bruising.

presentations of chronic urticaria resistant to treatment with antihistamines [**11**]. Of note, two recent studies reported longer weal duration as well as occasional bruising in a subgroup of patients with chronic spontaneous urticaria showing no signs of vasculitis upon skin histopathology [5,**18**]. In addition to weals, other cutaneous signs in urticarial vasculitis may include livedo reticularis, Raynaud phenomenon and very occasionally bullous lesions [10,**14**]. Angioedema occurs in the majority of patients (51–70%) [**14**,**18**].

Joint involvement is common; usually arthralgia and joint stiffness and, rarely, arthritis or synovitis [**16**,51]. Patients with HUV may present with gastrointestinal features including nausea, vomiting, abdominal pain, intestinal bleeding or diarrhoea [**16**]. Also, gastrointestinal complaints are frequent in children [15]. Some patients develop transient or persistent microscopic haematuria and proteinuria [**13**]. Pulmonary symptoms may include cough, dyspnoea or haemoptysis and occasionally the development of chronic obstructive pulmonary disease [52]. Leukocytoclastic vasculitis has been detected on lung biopsy in these patients [**1**]. The pulmonary involvement tends to be more severe in smokers [**1**]. Other clinical presentations may include lymphadenopathy, splenomegaly or hepatomegaly as well as ocular involvement with uveitis, conjunctivitis and scleritis [**14**]. Rare neurological (pseudotumour cerebri, optic nerve atrophy) manifestations and rhinitis or chondritis may occur [**1**,**14**]. Of interest, a few case reports suggested a distinct association of cardiac valvulopathy, Jaccoud arthropathy with HUV [53].

Clinical variants

Urticarial vasculitis can be divided into the following subtypes: NUV, HUV and HUVS. The normocomplementaemic variant represents the most common and mildest form (about 80% of patients) and usually comes without organ involvement [7].

Hypocomplementaemic disease tends to be more severe [54]. Some authors suggest that HUV and HUVS could be part of a disease continuum ranging from isolated vasculitic lesions with low complement levels to a more systemic disease with organ involvement and anti-C1q antibodies [**14**]. Hypocomplementaemia is often associated with long duration, systemic symptoms and underlying disease such as lupus erythematosus. Inflammation of the skin is characterised by diffuse neutrophil-rich infiltrates [7]. Anti-C1q antibodies are not specific to HUVS. For instance, they may be a useful marker of overall disease activity in systemic lupus erythematosus and particularly of renal involvement [55]. They are not always accompanied by complement consumption, especially at low titres.

HUVS is the most severe subtype identified in about 5% of patients with urticarial vasculitis of more than 6 months' duration [2] with the following diagnostic criteria: (i) biopsy-proven vasculitis; (ii) arthralgia or arthritis; (iii) uveitis or episcleritis; (iv) recurrent abdominal pain; (v) glomerulonephritis; and (vi) decreased C1q or presence of anti-C1q autoantibodies [54]. Also, neurologic manifestations may occur. Not all systemic features are required to make a diagnosis.

Differential diagnosis

In clinical practice, chronic spontaneous urticaria is the most important differential diagnosis of urticarial vasculitis. The continuum of histological changes between urticaria and urticarial vasculitis has been well recognised and confirmed by a series of patients with intermediate histological features [5,56]. This suggests that there may not be a clear-cut histological distinction between these two conditions. Therefore, the concept of minimal diagnostic histological criteria for urticarial vasculitis has been introduced. Some authors suggest that leukocytoclasis and/or fibrin deposition with or without erythrocyte extravasation may be sufficient for diagnosis in difficult cases [10]. A recent study developed a quantitative histological tool, the urticarial vasculitis score, to differentiate urticarial vasculitis from urticaria by combining the three criteria leukocytoclasia, fibrin deposits and extravasated erythrocytes [18]. Clinically, the additional use of dermoscopy may discriminate urticarial lesions in urticarial vasculitis (showing purpuric patches) from those in chronic spontaneous urticaria (no purpuric patches) [57,58]. Besides urticaria, other differential diagnoses of urticarial vasculitis are urticarial autoinflammatory diseases such as Schnitzler syndrome and cryopyrin-associated periodic syndrome [59]. Schnitzler syndrome is an acquired disease of unknown cause that starts around the age of 50 years. It is characterised by recurrent urticarial rash combined with a variety of systemic symptoms including fever, fatigue, arthralgia and bone pain. Laboratory work-up reveals monoclonal gammopathy (IgM, rarely IgG) as a defining feature [60]. Cryopyrin-associated periodic syndrome is caused by a mutation in NLRP3 and usually starts in early childhood. In addition to the recurrent urticarial rash, fever and musculoskeletal complaints it presents with eye inflammation and sensoneurinal hearing loss [61]. As opposed to urticarial vasculitis, urticarial autoinflammatory diseases do not show leukocytoclastic vasculitis but neutrophil-rich infiltrates only upon skin histology [62].

Classification of severity

Severity of urticarial vasculitis varies from mild to life-threatening; there is no established consensus on the severity grading. A patient-reported urticarial vasculitis activity score (UVAS) has been developed for research applications [8]. Patients with cutaneous involvement only are considered to have milder disease. Patients with severe urticarial vasculitis present with hypocomplementaemia, systemic involvement or treatment-refractory disease. HUVS is at the very severe end of the spectrum [2].

Complications and co-morbidities

Patients with urticarial vasculitis may present with renal involvement (most often microscopic haematuria or proteinuria) at disease onset or later in the disease course but it rarely progresses to renal failure. Renal biopsy may reveal glomerulonephritis [63]. Patients with urticarial vasculitis, who have deposits of immunoglobulins or complement at the dermal–epidermal junction on direct immunofluorescence, are more likely to develop glomerulonephritis [64].

Chronic obstructive pulmonary disease is considered as a life-threatening late complication of urticarial vasculitis [2]. Further complications include uveitis and scleritis due to ocular involvement. Also, biopsy-proven gastrointestinal vasculitis has been reported in a patient with HUVS [65].

Connective tissue diseases and haematological malignancies are potential co-morbidities in urticarial vasculitis [7]. More than 50% of patients with HUVS develop systemic lupus erythematosus [16,66]. In some patients, urticarial vasculitis can be the first presentation of these diseases while in others urticarial vasculitis can present in the context of these diseases. Lately, thyroid autoimmune disease has also been linked to urticarial vasculitis [67].

Disease course and prognosis

In most patients, urticarial vasculitis is a self-limiting disease but in some it may last for several years [10]. Patients with NUV limited to the skin tend to have a benign disease with a good prognosis. Conversely, HUV is associated with a more severe course and more frequent systemic involvement [2]. The most severe course is described for HUVS with a high risk for the development of systemic lupus erythematosus [66]. In HUVS, chronic obstructive pulmonary disease (COPD) or laryngeal angio-oedema can be a life-threatening complication [2].

Prognosis in urticarial vasculitis depends on the presence of systemic involvement. Systemic involvement may occur early on although late-onset complications have been described. A recent study from Sweden reported a 10-year survival rate of 83% in patients with HUV. Reasons for disease-associated deaths were COPD and renal failure [68].

Investigations (Table 44.1)

Lesional skin biopsy of lesions over 12 hours old is the cornerstone of the diagnosis of urticarial vasculitis (Figure 44.2). Several skin biopsies may be required for the confirmation of the diagnosis of urticarial vasculitis [10]. Routine use of direct immunofluorescence on frozen lesional tissue is not recommended unless HUV/HUVS is suspected, in which case, an early lesion (<3 h) should be selected.

All patients with urticarial vasculitis should undergo a laboratory work-up consisting of full blood count, blood biochemistry and C-reactive protein or erythrocyte sedimentation rate. Urinalysis and liver function tests are essential in the laboratory work-up for systemic involvement [4]. Transient or permanent microscopic haematuria or proteinuria can be observed. In the case of abnormal urinalysis, 24-h urine protein and creatinine clearance should be checked. Complement profile (C3, C4, C1q and anti-C1q antibodies)

Table 44.1 Diagnostic work-up in urticarial vasculitis.

Initial work-up	Extended work-up (dependent on clinical presentation)
Lesional skin biopsy (diagnostic)	Direct immunofluorescence studies of skin biopsy
Full blood count	C1q anti-C1q antibodies
C-reactive protein, erythrocyte sedimentation rate	Cryoglobulins
Biochemical profile	Hepatitis B and C serology
C3, C4 complement components (serial testing)	Thyroid function and autoantibodies
Antinuclear antibodies	24-h urine protein and creatinine clearance
Anti-extractable nuclear antigens	Serum protein electrophoresis
Circulating immune complexes	Chest X-ray, lung function tests
Urinalysis	Assessment of visual acuity and slit lamp examination

Table 44.2 Therapeutic algorithm in urticarial vasculitis.

First line treatments	Second line treatments	Third line treatments
Non-sedating H1 antihistamines	Dapsone	Azathioprine
Short trial of corticosteroids	Colchicine	Ciclosporin
	Hydroxychloroquine	Mycophenolate mofetil
		Methotrexate
		Intravenous immunoglobulins
		Cyclophosphamide
		Omalizumab
		Interleukin antagonists
		Rituximab
		TNF antagonists

Adapted from Black 1999 [10], Berg *et al.* 1988 [69], Kolkhir *et al.* 2019 [7].

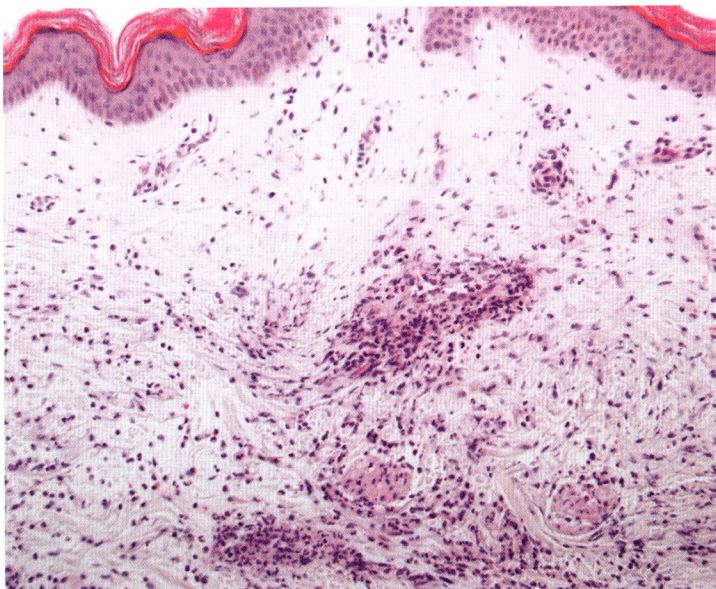

Figure 44.2 Urticarial vasculitis – histopathology of lesional skin typically shows a heavy mixed infiltrate within and around blood vessels with predominant neutrophils, leukocytoclasia and evidence of structural vasculitis of postcapillary venules associated with fibrin deposition (H&E, high power).

is important for differentiating between normocomplementaemic and hypocomplementaemic disease. Antibody screen in patients with urticarial vasculitis should include antinuclear antibodies, antibodies against extractable nuclear antigens, rheumatoid factor and circulating immune complexes. Testing for hepatitis B and C is important [1].

The extent of the laboratory work-up should be guided by the patient's history and presentation. For example, suspicion of pulmonary involvement should trigger a work-up including chest X-ray and lung function testing. If eye involvement is suspected, ophthalmic examination should be performed.

Management

Management of urticarial vasculitis is mostly based on case reports, small patient series and a few open-label, non-controlled studies.

There is no general agreement on a stepwise approach to the treatment of urticarial vasculitis; however, some guidance can be derived from published experts' opinions and experience [7,10,14].

First line therapy for urticarial vasculitis largely depends on disease severity and organ involvement. In normocomplementaemic mild disease, the use of standard-dosed or up-dosed H1 antihistamines is well-established [4,69] (Table 44.2). However, a recent meta-analysis demonstrated efficacy in only 24% of cases [7]. Still, antihistamines may be beneficial in reducing pruritus and burning sensations and their use is often combined with other anti-inflammatory/immunosuppressive therapies. High efficacy on cutaneous and extracutaneous symptoms was shown for oral corticosteroids (prednisolone at doses of 0.5–1 mg/kg/day) in all subtypes of urticarial vasculitis [14,15,69]. Nevertheless, their prolonged use should be avoided in view of their toxicity. For non-responders, immunomodulators such as dapsone 75–100 mg/day, colchicine 1.0–1.5 mg/day and/or hydroxychloroquine 200–400 mg/day can be used as second line treatments [7,69] and to taper the doses of oral corticosteroids. For severe refractory cases and patients with HUV or HUVS, immunosuppressive agents (e.g. methotrexate, ciclosporin, mycophenolate mofetil, cyclophosphamide, azathioprin), may be beneficial [1,14,69].

Other approaches such as intravenous immunoglobulins, pentoxifylline and plasmapheresis have also been used [4].

Recently, several biological therapies have shown promise for urticarial vasculitis in anecdotal reports or small series. So far, the best evidence exists for anti-IgE (omalizumab) treatment. A number of cases and non-controlled studies showed favourable clinical responses in the majority of patients with NUV [9,70,71]. As in chronic spontaneous urticaria, non-response was linked to lower total IgE levels [9]. Mixed responses were reported for anti-IgE treatment in HUV and/or systemic involvement [72]. Also, anti-IL-1 with anakinra (IL-1 receptor antagonist) or canakinumab (humanised anti-IL-1β) was beneficial in several reported cases [73,74] and an open-label study [8]. A patient with urticarial vasculitis associated with cutaneous lupus erythematosus was treated with anti-IL-6 (tocilizumab) with favourable outcome [75]. Furthermore, B cell-targeted treatment with rituximab (anti-CD20) was shown to be effective in therapy-refractory (hypocomplementaemic) urticarial vasculitis with organ involvement [76]. Likewise, anti-TNF blockers may be used, if first and second line therapies fail [7].

Integration of biological agents into the management protocol for urticarial vasculitis in the future may help overcome the issue of toxicity associated with the use of conventional treatments for urticarial vasculitis, especially long-term oral corticosteroids.

The choice of treatment should take co-morbidities and disease associations into account. Stratification of patients in terms of systemic involvement and prognosis may facilitate more targeted and individualised treatment approaches in the future.

At present, there is a strong need for double-blind placebo-controlled studies to evaluate the efficacy of conventional and novel therapeutic approaches to urticarial vasculitis. This may be achievable by collaborative multicentre and multidisciplinary efforts given the rarity and complexity of this disease. From a clinical perspective, a consensus on the management of urticarial vasculitis is much needed and would harmonise the treatment approaches to this rare condition.

Resources

Patient resources

http://www.vasculitisfoundation.org/education/forms/urticarial-vasculitis/ (last accessed February 2022). http://www.vasculitis.org (last accessed February 2022).

Key references

The full list of references can be found in the online version at https://www.wiley.com/rooksdermatology10e

1 Venzor J, Lee WL, Huston DP. Urticarial vasculitis. *Clin Rev Allergy Immunol* 2002;23:201–16.

7 Kolkhir P, Grakhova M, Bonnekoh H, Krause K, Maurer M. Treatment of urticarial vasculitis: a systematic review. *J Allergy Clin Immunol* 2019;143:458–66.

11 Tosoni C, Lodi-Rizzini F, Cinquini M *et al*. A reassessment of diagnostic criteria and treatment of idiopathic urticarial vasculitis: a retrospective study of 47 patients. *Clin Exp Dermatol* 2009;34:166–70.

13 Mehregan DR, Hall MJ, Gibson LE. Urticarial vasculitis: a histopathologic and clinical review of 72 cases. *J Am Acad Dermatol* 1992;26:441–8.

14 Jachiet M, Flageul B, Deroux A *et al*. The clinical spectrum and therapeutic management of hypocomplementemic urticarial vasculitis: data from a French nationwide study of fifty-seven patients. *Arthritis Rheumatol* 2015;67:527–34.

16 Dincy CV, George R, Jacob M, Mathai E, Pulimood S, Eapen EP. Clinicopathologic profile of normocomplementemic and hypocomplementemic urticarial vasculitis: a study from South India. *J Eur Acad Dermatol Venereol* 2008;22:789–94.

18 Puhl V, Bonnekoh H, Scheffel J *et al*. A novel histopathological scoring system to distinguish urticarial vasculitis from chronic spontaneous urticaria. *Clin Transl Allergy* 2021;11:e12031.

44 Carlson JA. The histological assessment of cutaneous vasculitis. *Histopathology* 2010;56:3–23.

46 Frumholtz L, Laurent-Roussel S, Lipsker D, Terrier B. Cutaneous vasculitis: review on diagnosis and clinicopathologic correlations. *Clin Rev Allergy Immunol* 2021;61:181–93.

58 Garcia-Garcia B, Auban-Pariente J, Munguia-Calzada P, Vivanco B, Argenziano G, Vazquez-Lopez F. Development of a clinical-dermoscopic model for the diagnosis of urticarial vasculitis. *Sci Rep* 2020;10:6092.

CHAPTER 45

Autoinflammatory Diseases Presenting in the Skin

Dan Lipsker[1], Clive E. H. Grattan[2] and Christopher R. Lovell[3]

[1]Faculté de Medicine, Université de Strasbourg, Strasbourg, France
[2]Norfolk and Norwich University Hospital, Norwich; St John's Institute of Dermatology, Guy's and St Thomas' NHS Foundation Trust, London, UK
[3]Department of Dermatology, Royal United Hospital and Royal National Hospital for Rheumatic Diseases, Bath, UK

Introduction

Autoinflammatory diseases are characterised aetiologically by abnormal activation of the innate immune system and clinically by recurrent inflammation and, in many cases, fever and rash. Cutaneous clinical features may include urticarial reactions, oedema, erysipelas-like lesions, pustulosis, pyoderma gangrenosum, chilblain and livedo. The majority of these conditions are rare, hereditary, monogenic syndromes. There is also an increasing number of complex, polygenic, inflammatory disorders in which abnormalities of the innate immune system play an important pathogenic role. These conditions typically present later in life and include, among others, Schnitzler syndrome and adult-onset Still disease. The neutrophilic dermatoses (Chapter 49) can also be considered as autoinflammatory syndromes. Some adult-onset autoinflammatory disorders result from acquired somatic mutation in haematopoietic cells, such a *UBA1* mutation in the VEXAS (Vacuoles, E1 enzyme, X-linked, Autoinflammatory, Somatic) syndrome, the hallmarks of which are fever, relapsing polychondritis and Sweet syndrome in adult men [1].

Neutrophilic urticarial dermatosis is the most typical dermatological presentation of those autoinflammatory syndromes that present with an urticarial or maculopapular rash [2,3].

The dermatological signs of monogenic autoinflammatory syndromes and related complex disorders are illustrated in Table 45.1.

For all the genetic autoinflammatory syndromes and related complex disorders, diagnosis is suspected on clinical or clinico-pathological grounds and confirmed by more specific analyses. Skin biopsy is helpful and demonstrates the nature of the inflammatory infiltrate, which can provide some guidance to treatment strategies. In patients with recurrent fever and rash for example, the finding of a neutrophilic infiltrate strongly points to cryopyrinopathies or Schnitzler syndrome [4].

Acute phase reactants, neutrophils and C-reactive protein (CRP) levels are usually increased. Serum amyloid A levels are also increased and this is predictive of an increased risk of amyloidosis, the major complication of many autoinflammatory syndromes.

Genetic diagnosis is often the next step and will be guided by the clinical context. Other investigations will depend on the specific disorder, as for example hearing tests in the cryopyrinopathies.

HEREDITARY MONOGENIC AUTOINFLAMMATORY SYNDROMES

Definition

Monogenic autoinflammatory syndromes encompass a group of rare hereditary disorders, the commonest of which is familial Mediterranean fever (FMF) (Tables 45.2 and 45.3). They typically present in early childhood and are characterised by seemingly unprovoked bouts of recurrent inflammation. Inflammatory flares can occur in many organs, especially the skin, joints, eyes and serous membranes. An underlying genetic abnormality predisposes the affected individual to activation of the innate immune system and an exaggerated inflammatory response to exogenous or endogenous triggers. Markers of autoimmunity are classically absent.

Introduction and general description

The spectrum of individual monogenic, autoinflammatory syndromes has dramatically expanded in the last 15 years. They include the periodic (hereditary) fever syndromes, a range of syndromes of which pustular eruptions form a component, disorders with Behçet disease-like or inflammatory bowel disease (IBD)-like presentations, type I interferonopathies, granulomatous disorders and disorders of keratinisation. It is continuously expanding as new entities are being described and/or characterised genetically, sometimes in only a few individuals or families. Some autoinflammatory syndromes will also include a part of autoimmunity and/or immune deficiency or even allergy [5]. The term autoinflammation has been immensely helpful to nosologically delineate, within the broad group of inflammatory diseases, those that do not need intervention of the adaptive immune system. However, diseases that are exclusively autoinflammatory are rare. Autoinflammation should therefore rather be conceptualised as a mechanism explaining part or all the clinical manifestations in each patient, than explaining the disease *per se*. It then remains a helpful concept guiding therapeutic choices. The most relevant of these entities are summarised in Tables 45.1, 45.2 and 45.3. They are usually classified either by clinical criteria, especially mode of inheritance, major signs and type of rash, pattern of recurrence and duration of the inflammatory flare, or according to the genetic abnormality. Another meaningful way to classify them is according to the main inflammatory pathway that is involved and their response to treatment; it is particularly useful to separate those entities that are responsive to interleukin (IL)-1 blockade, tumour necrosis factor (TNF)-blockade or JAK-inhibition.

The detailed phenotypical analysis and the pathogenic deciphering of monogenic autoinflammatory syndromes have led to a new classification of inflammatory diseases in general [5,6]. The same mechanisms which contribute to inflammation in these rare diseases are shared by many more common late-onset sporadic or polygenic disorders. Their relevance reaches far beyond an understanding of their role just in this group of diseases. Skin lesions can be the presenting sign or one of the main clinical findings in many of these disorders, thus it is important that dermatologists are familiar with them [7].

Epidemiology

Some entities such as chronic infantile neurological and articular (CINCA) syndrome (syn. neonatal onset multisystem inflammatory disease (NOMID)) start in the newborn while others can present for the first time from early childhood to late adulthood, e.g. FMF or TNF receptor-associated periodic syndrome (TRAPS). Epidemiological and clinical features of the major monogenic autoinflammatory syndromes are summarised in Table 45.3.

FMF and TRAPS are the two most common monogenic autoinflammatory syndromes. Prevalence of FMF, the commonest, depends on genetic background. The highest prevalence rates are found in the Sephardic Jewish, Turkish, Armenian and Arab populations: prevalence rates of 1 : 248 to 1 : 1000 and carrier rates of 1 : 3 to 1 : 7 are reported [8]. The incidence of TRAPS in German children has been estimated as 0.56 per million person-years [9]. The same German investigators found an incidence rate of meval-onate kinase deficiency (MKD) manifesting as hyper–IgD syndrome (HIDS) of 0.39 per million person-years [10]. The other monogenic autoinflammatory syndromes are even rarer and some have so far been described only in a few families.

Pathophysiology

Those disorders result from exaggerated activation of the innate immune system, which can occur on multiple levels [5]:
- Activation of inflammasome and associated inflammatory pathways (e.g. FMF, cryopyrinopathies).
- Dysregulation of NFκB pathway (e.g. Blau syndrome, HA20).

Table 45.1 Key dermatological signs and entities occurring in hereditary monogenic autoinflammatory syndromes and related acquired/complex disorders.[a]

Predominant skin and/or mucosal manifestation	Hereditary autoinflammatory syndrome (transmission)/treatment of choice[b]	Related acquired sporadic or complex disorder
Maculopapular rashes, red plaques, erysipela-like lesions, migratory eruption, periorbital oedema, various types of non-urticarial rashes Histopathology variable; lymphocytic (MVKD), neutrophilic (FMF), monocytic (TRAPS)[c], atypical (CANDLE) or mixed infiltrates	*FMF* (AR>AD)/colchicine, IL-1 inhibitor *TRAPS* (AD)/NSAID, steroids on demand, etanercept, IL-1 inhibitor *MVKD* (AR)/NSAID, steroids on demand, IL-1 inhibitors, etanercept, tocilizumab *Other:* CANDLE ORAS	Delayed pressure urticaria Gout Some drug reactions Yao syndrome
Urticarial rashes Histopathology variable; some eruptions characterised by a neutrophilic infiltrate	Neutrophilic urticarial dermatosis *CAPS*[4] (AD)/IL-1 inhibitor *NLRP12-AID*[d] (AD)/IL-1 inhibitor *NOCARH syndrome*[e] (AD)/IL-1 inhibitor/IFNγ-inhibitor Non-neutrophilic urticaria *NLRC4-AID*[d] (AD)/NSAID, steroids, IL-1 inhibitor, IL-18 inhibitor, anti-IFNγ *PLAID*[d] (AD)/avoidance of cold temperatures, oral glycopyrrolate/IgIV *Vibratory urticaria* (AD)/antihistamines Rarely presenting as urticaria TRAPS MVKD	Schnitzler syndrome Adult-onset Still's disease Systemic-onset juvenile idiopathic arthritis Cystic fibrosis-associated episodic arthritis
Pustules (aseptic) Histopathology generally not helpful	**Bone involvement with multifocal osteomyelitis** *DIRA* (AR)/IL-1 inhibitor *Majeed syndrome* (AR)/IL-1 inhibitor **Pyoderma gangrenosum usually present** *PAPA* (AD) spectrum disorders/IL-1 inhibitor, glucocorticoids, TNFα-inhibitor *PAAND* (AD)/IL-1 inhibitor, TNFα-inhibitor, IL-6 inhibition **Behçet disease-like or inflammatory bowel disease phenotype, mucosal ulcerations usually present** *ADAM17-deficiency* (AR)/?/IL-1 inhibitor *IL-10 signalling defects* (AR)/?/HSCT HA20 **Monogenic forms of pustular psoriasis** *DITRA* (AR)/acitretin, TNFα-inhibitor, IL-36 inhibitor *CAMPS* (AD)/classic treatments of psoriasis or of pityriasis rubra pilaris, especially ustekinumab and acitretin *AP1S3* (AD)/IL-36 inhibitor **Other** *ORAS* *SAVI* *AGS*	Generalised pustular psoriasis Impetigo herpetiformis SAPHO syndrome Acne fulminans
Ulceration (nosology = pyoderma gangrenosum in most cases) Histopathology: neutrophilic infiltrate	**Authentic pyoderma-gangrenosum** PAPA PAAND CAIN **Pyoderma gangrenosum-like necrotising fasciitis** NFκB1 associated necrotising neutrophilic dermatosis (FANF) (AD)/steroids, IL-1 inhibitors, TNF inhibitors **Other** PFIT	Pyoderma gangrenosum 'idiopathic' or occurring in the setting of a nosologically characterised inflammatory disease Necrotising fasciitis
Oedematous plaque (nosology = Sweet syndrome) Histopathology: neutrophilic infiltrate	Majeed syndrome MVKD	Sweet syndrome either 'idiopathic' or occurring in the setting of a nosologically characterised inflammatory disease or in patients with myelodysplasic syndromes with acquired mosaic *MEFV* or *UBA1* (VEXAS syndrome) mutations
Deep dermal and subcutaneous nodules and plaques as manifestations of panniculitis; lipodystrophy Histopathology variable; septal and/or lobular lymphohistiocytic, neutrophilic, atypical or mixed infiltrates	*PRAAS (AR)/CANDLE*[f] (AR > AD)/JAK inhibitors, glucocorticoids *SIFD* (AR)/TNF inhibitors, IgIV *ORAS*[f] (AR)/TNF inhibitors *SAMD9L-SAAD*[f,g] (AD)/JAK inhibitors, glucocorticoids/HSCT *NEMO-NDAS*[h] (XL)/?/TNF inhibitors?/HSCT Other DADA2	Dermatomyositis, Barraquer–Simons syndrome, lupus panniculitis Recurrent lipoatrophic panniculitis of children

(continued)

PART 4: INFLAMMATORY DERMATOSES

Table 45.1 (continued)

Predominant skin and/or mucosal manifestation	Hereditary autoinflammatory syndrome (transmission)/treatment of choice[b]	Related acquired sporadic or complex disorder
Aphthous stomatitis and mucosal ulceration Biopsy usually not performed	*HA20* (AD)/colchicine, TNFα-inhibitor, IL-1-inhibitor, IL-6 inhibitor, glucocorticoids *RELA haploinsufficiency* (AD)/colchicine, TNFα-inhibitor, IL-1-inhibitor, IL-6 inhibitor, glucocorticoids NFκB1-*associated Behçet disease* (AD)/colchicine, TNFα-inhibitor, IL-1-inhibitor, IL-6 inhibitor, glucocorticoids *CAIN* (AR)/dapsone/colchicine/IL-1 inhibitors *HOIL-1 deficiency* (AR)/TNF inhibitors, steroids, HSCT *CRIA*/IL-6 inhibitors *PFIT*/IgIV, colchicine, antibiotics/HSCT Other IL-10 signalling defects SIFD MVKD TRAPS DADA2 SAVI PRAAS	Behçet disease Inflammatory bowel disease PFAPA
Violaceous areas of skin with telangiectasia and surface alterations (atrophy, scales, ulceration, crusts, necrosis, scarring) on fingers, toes, nose, cheeks, ears (nosology = vasculopathy or chilblain-like) Histopathology: dermal lymphocytic infiltrate with characteristic perisudoral topography (inflammatory chilblain pattern) and/or enlarged vessels and/or vasculitis and/or thrombosis of superficial dermal vessels ('small vessel') Raynaud phenomenon	*SAVI* (AD and AR)/JAK inhibitors *AGS* (AR or rarely AD)/JAK inhibitors, reverse transcriptase inhibitors *PRAAS*	Lupus erythematosus Dermatomyositis Antiphospholipid syndrome Levamisole-induced vasculopathy Symmetric peripheral gangrene ANCA+ vasculitis
Livedo, nodules, digital necrosis (nosology = vasculopathy) Histopathology: vasculitis and/or thrombosis of deep dermal vessels (medium-sized vessel)	*DADA2* (AR)/TNFα-inhibitor, HSCT	Vasculitis Sneddon syndrome
Granulomatous disorder (clinical manifestations protean: papules, plaques, nodules, ulceration, ichthyosis-like, …) Histopathology: sarcoidal (Blau, PLAID) or interstitial granulomatous dermal infiltrate (APLAID)	*Blau syndrome* (AD)/ glucocorticoids/TNFα-inhibitor *APLAID* (AD)/?/ TNFα-inhibitor/IL-1 inhibitor/IgIV *PLAID*	Sarcoidosis Crohn's disease Combined variable immunodeficiency Granuloma annulare Interstitial granulomatous dermatitis Other granulomatous disorders
Disorders of keratinisation Histopathology variable, sometimes highly characteristic (e.g. cornoid lamella in porokeratosis)	*Familial porokeratosis*/?/topical retinoids/imiquimod/laser *Familial keratosis lichenoides chronica*/?/acitretin/dapsone/ methotrexate/phototherapy *Multiple self-healing palmoplantar carcinoma*/?/acitretin *NAIAD* (AD or AR)/?/acitretin/IL-1 inhibitor *CARD-14 associated papulosquamous eruption*/ustekinumab	Porokeratosis, all types Keratosis lichenoides chronica/lichen planus/ lupus erythematosus /keratoacanthoma/squamous cell carcinoma Pityriasis rubra pilaris

AD, autosomal dominant; AGS, Aicardi-Goutières syndrome; APLAID, autoinflammation and PLCγ 2–associated antibody deficiency and immune dysregulation; AR, autosomal recessive; CAIN, CCAAT enhancer binding protein ε (C/EBPε)-associated autoinflammation and immune impairment of neutrophils; CAMPS, card14 mediated psoriasis; CANDLE, chronic atypical neutrophilic dermatosis with lipodystrophy and elevated temperature; CAPS, cryopyrin-associated periodic syndrome; CRIA, cleavage resistant RIPK1-induced autoinflammatory; DADA2, deficiency of adenosine deaminase 2; DIRA, deficiency of interleukin 1 receptor antagonist; DITRA, deficiency of interleukin 36 receptor antagonist; FANF, familial autoinflammatory necrotising fasciitis; FMF, familial Mediterranean fever; HA20, Haploinsufficiency of *A20*; IFN, interferon; IL, interleukin; NAIAD, NLRP1-associated autoinflammation with arthritis and dyskeratosis; NEMO-NDAS, NFκB essential modulator-Δ-exon 5-autoinflammatory syndrome; NFκB1, nuclear factor κ light-chain enhancer of activated B-cells 1; NLRC4-AID, NLR family, caspase recruitment domain-containing 4-auto inflammatory disease; NLRP12-AID, NLR family, pyrin domain-containing 12-auto inflammatory disease; NOCARH, neonatal onset of pancytopenia, autoinflammation, rash and episodes of haemophagocytic lymphohistiosis; NSAID, non-steroidal anti-inflammatory drugs; ORAS, otulin-related autoinflammatory syndrome; PAAND, pyrin-associated autoinflammation with neutrophilic dermatosis; PAPA, pyogenic arthritis-pyoderma gangrenosum-acne; PFAPA, periodic fever, aphthous stomatitis, pharyngitis and cervical adenitis; PFIT, periodic fever, immunodeficiency and thrombocytopenia; PLAID, PLCγ 2-associated antibody deficiency and immune dysregulation; PRAAS, proteasome associated autoinflammatory syndromes; SAMD9L-SAAD, sterile alpha motif domain-containing protein domain 9 like associated autoinflammatory disease; SAPHO, synovitis, acne, pustulosis, hyperostosis and osteitis; SAVI, STING-associated vasculopathy with onset in infancy; SIFD, sideroblastic anaemia with B-cell immunodeficiency, periodic fevers and developmental delay; TNF, tumour necrosis factor; TRAPS, TNF receptor-associated periodic syndrome; UBA1, ubiquitin-like modifier-activating enzyme 1; XL, X-linked.

[a] Other autoinflammatory disorders, such as those characterised by pigmentary changes (e.g. X-linked pigmentary reticulate disorder, AGS/dyschromatosis symetrica hereditary, H-syndrome), or by ectodermal dysplasia (NEMO-AID) were not included in the table.

[b] In case of multiple occurrences in the table, transmission and treatment are only specified in the main category.

[c] Extensive soft tissue masses histologically consistent with mononuclear myofasciitis have also been reported in one patient with SIFD.

[d] Cold-induced urticaria.

[e] The few published photographs suggest that the rash might be a neutrophilic urticarial dermatosis.

[f] Can evolve to lipodystrophy.

[g] SAMD9L-SAAD is a newly recognised type 1 interferonopathy with a dermatological presentation similar to CANDLE, but with a more severe interstitial lung disease. Patients develop B and NK-cell cytopenia.

[h] NEMO-NDAS: those patients have a phenotype of ectodermal dysplasia with lymphohistiocytic panniculitis, progressive B-cell lymphopenia and hypogammaglobulinaemia.

Table 45.2 Selected autoinflammatory syndromes: terminology and international classification.

Disease/gene	ICD-11	MIM	Orphanet	Synonyms and inclusions
Familial Mediterranean fever (FMF)/*MEFV*	4A60.0	134610/249100	ORPHA342	Periodic disease Benign paroxysmal peritonitis Benign recurrent polyserositis Familial paroxysmal polyserositis
Tumour necrosis factor receptor 1 associated periodic syndrome (TRAPS)/*TNFRSF1A*	4A60.2	142680	ORPHA32960	Familial hibernian fever Autosomal dominant periodic fever Familial periodic fever
Familial cold autoinflammatory syndrome (FCAS)/*NLRP3*	4A60.1	120100	ORPHA47045	Familial cold urticaria
Muckle–Wells syndrome/*NLRP3*	4A60.1	191900	ORPHA575	Urticaria-deafness-amyloidosis
Chronic infantile neurological cutaneous and articular syndrome (CINCA)/ neonatal onset multisystem inflammatory disease (NOMID)/*NLRP3*	4A60.1	607115	ORPHA1451	Prieur–Griscelli syndrome Infantile-onset multisystem inflammatory disease (IOMID)
Pyogenic arthritis-pyoderma gangrenosum-acne (PAPA) syndrome/*PSTPIP1*	4A60.Y	604416	ORPHA69126	Familial recurrent arthritis
Deficiency of interleukin 1 receptor antagonist (DIRA) syndrome/*IL-1RN*	4A60.Y	612852	ORPHA210115	Sterile multifocal osteomyelitis with periostitis and pustulosis Autoinflammatory disease due to IL-1 receptor antagonist deficiency
Mevalonate kinase deficiency/ hyperimmunoglobulinaemia D with recurrent fever/*MVK*	4A60.Y	251170/260920	ORPHA343	Hyper-IgD syndrome (HIDS) Partial MKD Hyperimmunoglobulinaemia D with periodic fever
Chronic atypical neutrophilic dermatosis with lipodystrophy and elevated temperature (CANDLE)/*PSMB8*	4A60.Y	256040	ORPHA325004/ 2615	Nakajo–Nishimura syndrome Asian autoinflammatory syndrome Joint contractures-muscular atrophy-microcytic anaemia-panniculitis-induced lipodystrophy syndrome . Proteasome-associated autoinflammatory syndrome 1 (PRAAS1)
Aicardi-Goutières syndrome (AGS)/multiple genes, AR: *TREX1, SAMHD1, RNASEH2A, RNASEH2B, RNASEH2C, ADAR1* or AD: *IFIH1*	4A60.Y	225750/610181/ 610329/610333/ 612952/615010/ 615846	ORPHA51	Familial infantile encephalopathy with intracranial calcifications Pseudotoxoplasmosis syndrome Cree encephalitis
STING-associated vasculopathy with onset in infancy (SAVI)/*STING1*	4A60.Y	615934	ORPHA425120	
Blau syndrome/*NOD2*	4A60.Y	186580/609464	ORPHA90340	Early-onset sarcoidosis Autoinflammatory granulomatosis of childhood NOD2-related systemic autoinflammatory granulomatosis Granulomatous arthritis of childhood Juvenile systemic granulomatosis Caspase recruitment domain containing protein 15 deficiency *CARD15* deficiency Familial juvenile sarcoidosis Jabs syndrome
PLCγ 2-Associated Antibody Deficiency and Immune Dysregulation (PLAID)/*PLCγ 2*	4A60.Y	614468	ORPHA300359	Familial atypical cold urticaria Familial cold urticaria with common variable immunodeficiency Familial cold autoinflammatory syndrome 3
Autoinflammation and PLCγ 2–associated antibody deficiency and immune dysregulation (APLAID)/*PLCγ 2*	4A60.Y	614878	ORPHA324530	
Haploinsufficiency of A20 (HA20)/*TNFAIP3*	4A60.Y	616744	ORPHA476102	Behçet-like disease due to HA20 Behçet disease due to haploinsufficiency of A20 Autoinflammatory syndrome, familial, Behçet-like (AISBL)
NLRC4-Associated autoinflammatory disease (NLRC4-AID)/*NLRC4*	4A60.Y	616115/616050	ORPHA576349/ 436166	NLRC4-related cold autoinflammatory syndrome NLRC4-MAS (macrophage activating syndrome) Syndrome of colitis and autoinflammation associated with mutations of NLRC4 (SCAN4) Periodic fever-infantile enterocolitis-autoinflammatory syndrome Familial cold autoinflammatory syndrome 4 Autoinflammation with infantile enterocolitis (AIFEC)
Deficiency of adenosine deaminase 2 (DADA2)/*ADA2*	4A60.Y	615688	ORPHA404553	Vasculitis, autoinflammation, immunodeficiency, and haematological defects syndrome (VAIHS) Childhood onset polyarteritis nodosa

Table 45.3 Epidemiology, clinical features and treatment of selected autoinflammatory syndromes.

Disease	Mode of inheritance	Predominant ethnic group	Age at onset	Typical duration of flare	Typical frequency of flares	Typical/distinctive clinical features	Treatment
FMF	AR (rare AD variant)	Eastern Mediterranean	Childhood to early adulthood	1–3 days	Variable	Colchicine responsiveness; Pseudo-appendicular pain; Erysipelas-like redness	Colchicine; Anti-IL-1 (e.g. Anakinra)
TRAPS	AD	Northern European; numerous other ethnic groups	Childhood/early adulthood; rarely late onset	>7 days; may be prolonged over many weeks	Variable	Longer duration of attack; migratory myalgia with overlying redness periorbital oedema	Steroids on demand; Anakinra; Etanercept
MVK deficiency/HIDS	AR	Northern European	Infancy	3–7 days	1–2 monthly	Palpable lymph nodes; diarrhoea; triggered by vaccinations	Steroids on demand; Anti-TNF; Anti-IL-1; Anti-IL-6
FCAS	AD	Northern European	Childhood	24 h	Depend on exposure to cold	Triggered by exposure to cold; Neutrophilic urticarial dermatosis; Conjunctivitis; Thirst and transpiration; Excellent response to anakinra	Cold avoidance; Anti-IL-1
MWS	AD	Northern European	Neonatal/infancy	Continuous; worse in the evening	Often daily	Neutrophilic urticarial dermatosis; Hearing loss; Spectacular response to anakinra	Anti-IL-1
CINCA	Sporadic	Northern European	Neonatal/infancy	Continuous	Continuous	Neutrophilic urticarial dermatosis; Dysmorphia; Aseptic meningitis; Deforming arthropathy; Spectacular response to anakinra	Anti-IL-1
PAPA	AD	European	Childhood	Intermittent	Variable	Pathergy; Notion of familial pyoderma gangrenosum; Migratory arthritis in early childhood	Anti-TNF; Anti-IL-1
DIRA	AR	Puerto Rico; Brazil; Lebanon; Newfoundland; Europe; Turkey	Neonatal/infancy Rarely late childhood/early adolescence	Continuous	Continuous	Pustules; Osteolytic bone lesions/osteomyelitis; Spectacular response to anakinra	Anakinra; Anti-TNF
CANDLE	AR	Japan; Israel (Ashkenazi Jews), Spain, North America, Bangladesh	Infancy	Continuous	Continuous	Exacerbated in winter; Plaques with atypical myeloid infiltrate; Pernio-like lesions; Lipoatrophy; Basal ganglia calcification	JAK inhibitors
AGS	AR (rare AD variant)	Numerous ethnic groups	Neonatal/infancy	Continuous	Continuous	Pernio-like lesions; Pseudo-TORCH syndrome; Psychomotor regression; Glaucoma; Basal ganglia calcification	JAK inhibitors; Reverse transcriptase inhibitors
SAVI	AD and AR	Numerous ethnic groups	Infancy	Continuous	Continuous	Cold-exposed skin areas: violaceous lesions, chilblain, telangiectases, blisters, ulcerations, necrosis; Interstitial lung disease; Recurrent fever; Growth retardation; Myositis	JAK inhibitors

	Inheritance	Ethnic groups	Age of onset	Course	Course	Clinical features	Treatment
Blau syndrome	AD	Numerous ethnic groups	Childhood	Continuous	Continuous	Granulomatous dermatitis Uveitis Arthritis	Steroids Anti-TNF
PLAID	AD	European	Neonatal/infancy	Continuous	Continuous	Early-onset cold-induced evaporative urticaria Ulcerative self-resolving neonatal lesions in cold sensitive regions Later, plaques and nodules (histology = sarcoid type or diffuse granulomatous inflammation of the dermis) Immune deficiency Autoimmunity Atopy	Avoiding cold temperatures Glycopyrrolate IgIV
APLAID	AD	European, Mexican	Neonatal/infancy	Continuous	Continuous	Early-onset blistering skin lesions with vesicles, pustules, boggy pustular masses, papules and plaques Histology = interstitial granuloma annulare with transepidermal elimination of basophilic material Eye inflammation Inflammatory bowel disease Interstitial pneumontis	Steroids Anakinra IgIV
HA20	AD	European, Turkish, numerous other ethnic groups	Childhood, adolescence	Continuous	Continuous	Orogenital ulcers Ocular inflammation Polyarthritis Recurrent fever Early-onset inflammatory bowel disease	Colchicine Thalidomide Steroids Methotrexate TNFα-inhibitor IL-6 inhibitors
NLRC4-AID	AD	European, Japanese, other ethnic groups	Neonatal, infancy (AIFEC phenotype) Childhood (FACS4 phenotype)	Continuous	Continuous or intermittent in the AIFEC variant Depend on exposure to cold in the FACS4 variant	AIFEC variant: Inflammatory bowel disease Signs similar to CINCA Macrophage activating syndrome Increase in markers of inflammation with high ferritin levels FACS4 variant: Cold-induced urticaria (histopathology different from CAPS, lymphohistiocytic infiltrate) Eye inflammation Recurrent fever Extremely high IL-18 levels in both phenotypes	NSAID Steroids Anakinra IgIV Cyclosporine Severe disease: Recombinant IL-18 binding protein IFNγ-inhibitor
DADA2	AR	Georgian Jewish, Turkish and numerous other ethnic groups	Childhood to adulthood	Continuous	Continuous	Fever Livedo Nodules (polyarteritis nodosa) Stroke Immune deficiency Haematological manifestations	TNFα-inhibitor HSCT

AD, autosomal dominant; AGS, Aicardi-Goutières syndrome; APLAID, autoinflammation and PLCγ 2–associated antibody deficiency and immune dysregulation; AR, autosomal recessive; CANDLE, chronic atypical neutrophilic dermatosis with lipodystrophy and elevated temperature; CAPS, cryopyrin-associated periodic syndromes; CINCA, chronic infantile neurological cutaneous and articular syndrome; DADA2, deficiency of adenosine deaminase 2; DIRA, deficiency of interleukin 1 receptor antagonist; FCAS, familial cold autoinflammatory syndrome; FMF, familial Mediterranean fever; HSCT, haematological stem cell transplantation; IgIV, intravenous immunoglobulins; IL, interleukin; MVK, mevalonate kinase; NLRC4-AID, NLR family, recruitment domain-containing 4 autoinflammatory disease; NSAID, non-steroidal anti-inflammatory drugs; PAPA, pyogenic arthritis-pyoderma gangrenosum-acne; PLAID, PLCγ 2-associated antibody deficiency and immune dysregulation; SAVI, STING-associated vasculopathy with onset in infancy; TNF, tumour necrosis factor; TRAPS, TNF receptor-associated periodic syndrome.

7

- Dysregulated type 1 interferon signalling (e.g. Aicardi-Goutières syndrome, CANDLE, SAVI).
- Protein misfolding and endoplasmic reticulum stress (e.g. TRAPS; see Tables 45.2 and 45.3).

Activation can involve gain of function mutations of receptors or signal transduction elements or loss of function mutations of regulatory elements. Multiple mechanisms are involved since defective DNA, RNA or protein processing, transport or metabolism induce accumulation of increased or abnormal (e.g. misfolded) substrates that will activate the innate immue system. Many diseases with abnormal intracellular protein metabolism (e.g. those involving ubiquination) result in autoinflammatory syndromes.

Many environmental factors can induce flares of the different monogenic autoinflammatory syndromes, including trauma, cold temperature and common infections.

The pathological hallmark of many monogenic autoinflammatory syndromes with cutaneous manifestations, those that are most frequently encountered by dermatologists, is a neutrophilic (aseptic) dermatosis. Neutrophilic urticarial dermatosis (NUD) is a term coined to describe the combination of an urticarial eruption with infiltration by neutrophils: it is strongly suggestive of a monogenic autoinflammatory syndrome, or of complex disorders with an underlying autoinflammatory mechanism [2,3]. Patients with NUD often have fever and joint pain, as well as biological markers of inflammation with leukocytosis and elevated CRP. Nuclear dust (leukocytoclasia) and marginating of neutrophils along collagen bundles resembling urticarial vasculitis is typical. Foci of interstitial collagen degeneration, reminiscent of interstitial granulomatous dermatitis, can be present. In addition to the aforementioned features dilated dermal vessels filled with neutrophils are a hallmark of cryopyrin-associated periodic syndrome.

Other important pathological findings of monogenic autoinflammatory syndromes include:
- Vasculopathy, either thrombotic or inflammatory, especially in the type 1 interferonopathies and DADA2.
- Granulomas, in Blau syndrome or phospholipase Cγ 2-associated disorders.
- Disorders of keratinisation: keratinocytic autoinflammatory disorders is a relatively new concept and includes entities such as linear porokeratosis or NLRP1-associated autoinflammation with arthritis and dyskeratosis.

Hereditary periodic fevers

Cryopyrin-associated periodic syndrome

Introduction and general description
Cryopyrin-associated periodic syndrome (CAPS) is a paradigm of IL-1 mediated autoinflammation [11]. The syndrome includes three partially overlapping entities related to mutations in the NLRP3/CIAS1 gene: familial cold autoinflammatory syndrome (FCAS), MWS and CINCA/NOMID. Within the CAPS spectrum, FCAS is the least severe entity while CINCA is the most severe. A closely related syndrome to the milder FCAS/MWS variants has been described in patients with a NLRP12 mutation [12].

Pathophysiology
These autosomal dominant disorders are associated with predominantly missense mutations in the NLRP3/CIAS1 gene encoding a death domain protein known variously as NLRP3, NALP3 or cryopyrin. This protein is expressed in epithelial cells of the skin and mucosa, granulocytes, dendritic cells and in T and B lymphocytes. A variety of danger signals, including 'pathogen-associated molecular patterns' (often referred to as PAMPs) induce association of NLRP3 with other members of the death domain superfamily to form a cytosolic protein complex which has been named the 'inflammasome' [13]. This results in activation of caspase 1, which cleaves biologically inactive pro-IL-1β into biologically active IL-1β. It also upregulates NFκB expression and thereby increases IL-1 gene expression and overproduction of IL-1β protein. IL-1β is a major pro-inflammatory cytokine and the key mediator of the manifestations of CAPS. This assumption is supported by the observation that IL-1 blockade (e.g. anakinra; see Table 45.3) induces rapid and complete response in patients with CAPS.

All patients with CAPS have a persistent neutrophilia, chronic anaemia and raised acute phase proteins.

Histopathology
In CAPS, an urticarial rash with a neutrophilic intravascular, perivascular, peri-eccrine and interstitial infiltrate on histopathological evaluation is typical. In the authors' experience, leukocytoclasia is frequent in patients with NUD in the context of Schnitzler syndrome but much less so in children with CAPS; intravascular accumulation of neutrophils in enlarged dermal vessels is characteristic of CAPS [2,4].

Clinical features
The three disorders usually start in the newborn or during early infancy with fever, fatigue, a 'flu-like syndrome' and rash [11]. Late-onset has been described in patients with somatic mosaicism (detected in blood) [14]. The flares are triggered by exposure to cold in FCAS and partially in MWS, while they are continuous in CINCA. Typically, a non-itchy symmetrical urticarial rash without angio-oedema arises on the trunk and limbs during the day as fever and malaise develop (Figure 45.1).

FCAS is characterised by rash, fever, conjunctival redness, joint pain, intense fatigue, thirst and transpiration occurring 1–2 h after exposure to cold. The flare lasts up to 24 h. Patients may experience profuse sweating, thirst, dizziness and nausea.

In MWS, cold dependency of flares is less marked, but patients develop sensorineural hearing loss and polyarthritis and are at risk of AA amyloidosis.

CINCA (NOMID) is the most severe CAPS syndrome and is characterised by continuous flares with neutrophilic aseptic meningitis, dysmorphism, mental retardation, sensorineural deafness and deforming arthropathy. Children present in the first few weeks of life with urticated erythematous papules and plaques, often in a figurate pattern. Lesions feel tight and warm and are generally not pruritic. The facies is characteristic, with frontal bossing, midfacial hypoplasia and saddle nose. Arthralgia can progress to a large joint polyarthritis with joint enlargement and loss of function. Radiologically, there is abnormal endochondral ossification, leading to

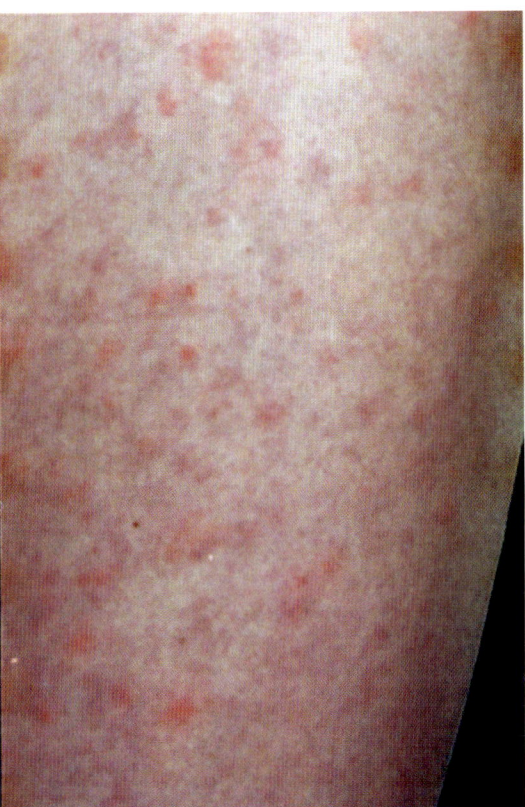

Figure 45.1 Cryopyrin-associated periodic syndrome (CAPS): non-itchy symmetrical urticarial weals lasting hours on the thigh after cold exposure in a patient with familial cold autoinflammatory syndrome (FCAS).

calcified masses in the joints [15]. The risk of renal impairment from amyloidosis is greatest in these patients.

Investigations

Diagnosis is based on typical clinical and biological findings and it is helpful if these are supported by the Eurofever/printo classification criteria [16]; evidence of an autosomal dominant mutation in the *NLRP3/CIAS1* gene is helpful, but the mutation will not be present in all patients. Cold stimulation tests (ice cube, immersion) can be negative, as exposure to cold air is the usual trigger. Regular high frequency audiograms and eye examinations are necessary, especially in patients with the Muckle–Wells phenotype [17].

Differential diagnosis

In newborns with a severe systemic disorder and uticarial rash, NLRC4-AID (presence of IBD and MAS) and NOCARH (neonatal onset of pancytopenia, autoinflammation, rash and episodes of haemophagocytic lymphohistiosis) syndrome (presence of cytopenia) should also be considered. In children with cold-induced urticaria: NLRP12-AID [12], NLRC4-AID [18] and PLAID (PLCγ 2-associated antibody deficiency and immune dysregulation) [19] are the main other diagnostic considerations. Cold-induced urticaria is however 'idiopathic' in most cases.

Management

See Table 45.3.

Tumour necrosis factor associated periodic syndrome

Introduction and general description

Tumour necrosis factor associated periodic syndrome (TRAPS), an autosomal dominant disorder, is one of the more common monogenic autoinflammatory syndromes and can be caused by mutations which affect the ability of the tumour necrosis factor (TNF) receptor to bind circulating TNF. AA amyloidosis is a feared complication of TRAPS.

Pathophysiology

TRAPS is associated with mutations in the gene for TNF receptor superfamily 1A (*TNFRSF1A*), encoding a p55 TNF receptor (TNFR1). It is thought that intracellular accumulation of misfolded mutant protein leads to endoplasmic reticulum stress and enhanced inflammatory responses through constitutive activation of various immune pathways [20]. This observation explains why IL-1 blockade is often more effective than TNF blockade (see Table 45.3).

Histopathology

A deep perivascular monocytic infiltrate is characteristic. Lesional skin biopsy usually reveals a perivascular and interstitial mononuclear cell infiltrate with CD68+ histiocytes and CD3+ lymphocytes in TRAPS [21].

Clinical features

TRAPS usually first manifests in childhood or adolescence and is characterised by episodes of pyrexia lasting 1–3 weeks (mean, 13 days) [21,22] associated with abdominal or chest pain, myalgia, arthralgia, conjunctivitis and periorbital oedema [23]. Late-onset cases can be the consequence of somatic mosaicism [24].

A migratory redness is present in 60–80% of patients [22]. Red macules and patches, most commonly on the extremities, coalesce and expand centrifugally into extensive oedematous dermal plaques, which typically overlie an area of local muscle tenderness, representing contiguous inflammation extending from muscle to skin. Usually only one anatomical area is affected in any single episode.

A variety of other skin manifestations unassociated with muscle pain have been described. They may resemble urticaria, hereditary angio-oedema or erysipelas. Residual ecchymoses may be noticed after resolution of the inflammatory component [21]. Arthralgia may also occur, but this rarely progresses to a destructive arthritis.

Investigations

Diagnosis relies on the typical clinical context and the Eurofever/printo classification criteria are helpful [16]. It is supported by detecting autosomal dominant mutations in the *TNFRSF1A* gene.

Management

See Table 45.3.

Familial Mediterranean fever

Introduction and general description

Familial Mediterranean fever (FMF) is an autoinflammatory disease associated with mutations in the *MEFV* gene, which encodes for pyrin. This results in enhanced IL-1β production.

Pathophysiology

The pathophysiology of FMF is less clear than that of CAPS. FMF is usually an autosomal recessive disorder related to gain of function mutations in the *MEFV* gene, although rare dominant mutations exist [25]. *MEFV* encodes pyrin, which probably plays an important role in the modulation of caspase 1, and thus the production of IL-1β and IL-18.

Histopathology

A sparse neutrophilic infiltrate in the upper dermis is the hallmark of the erysipelas-like erythema (ELE) of FMF [26,27]. Leukocytoclasia can be present but without significant vasculitis. Histiocytes and eosinophils can also be present.

Clinical features

FMF usually presents in childhood or early adulthood and generally before the age of 30, with recurrent flares of fever, abdominal pain, sometimes mimicking an acute abdomen, pleurisy and large joint arthritis lasting between 1 and 3 days. The major risk is the development of inflammatory AA amyloidosis but this risk can be largely prevented by continuous treatment with colchicine. Diagnosis is based on the Livneh or Tel Hashomer criteria (Box 45.1) [28,29] and is supported by the Eurofever/printo classification criteria [16].

Box 45.1 Tel Hashomer criteria set for the diagnosis of familial Mediterranean fever (FMF)[a]

Major criteria

Typical attacks
1 Peritonitis (generalised)
2 Pleuritis (unilateral) or pericarditis
3 Monoarthritis (hip, knee, ankle)
4 Fever alone

Minor criteria

1–3 Incomplete attacks involving one or more of the following sites:
1 Abdomen
2 Chest
3 Joint
4 Exertional leg pain
5 Favourable response to colchicines

Supportive criteria
1 Family history of FMF
2 Appropriate ethnic origin
3 Age <20 years at disease onset
4–7 Features of attacks:
4 Severe, requiring bed rest
5 Spontaneous remission
6 Symptom-free interval
7 Transient inflammatory response, with one or more test result(s) for white blood cell count, erythrocyte sedimentation rate, serum amyloid A and/or fibrinogen
8 Episodic proteinuria/haematuria
9 Unproductive laparotomy or removal of white appendix
10 Consanguinity of parents

From Livneh *et al.* 1997 [22] © American College of Rheumatology/JohnWiley & Sons.
[a] The requirements for diagnosis of FMF are ≥1 major criteria, or ≥2 minor criteria, or ≥1 minor criterion plus ≥5 supportive criteria, or ≥1 minor criterion plus ≥4 of the 5 supportive criteria. Typical attacks are defined as recurrent (≥3 of the same type), febrile (rectal temperature of 38°C or higher) and short (lasting between 12 h and 3 days). Incomplete attacks are defined as painful and recurrent attacks that differ from typical attacks in one or two features, as follows: (1) the temperature is normal or <38°C; (2) the attacks are longer or shorter than specified (but not shorter than 6 h or longer than a week); (3) no signs of peritonitis are recorded during the abdominal attacks; (4) the abdominal attacks are localised; and/or (5) the arthritis is in joints other than those specified. Attacks are not counted if they do not fit the definition of either typical or incomplete attacks.

Skin involvement is absent in more than 50% of patients but occurs more frequently in those with an early age of onset of symptoms. The most typical cutaneous finding is the so-called 'ELE' [26,27,30,31] (Figure 45.2). It consists of a warm swollen redness more often than a circumscribed plaque. The redness is usually localised to the distal lower limbs, typically in the perimalleolar area or the dorsum of the foot. It may be either unilateral or bilateral and symmetrical. Physical effort seems to be a triggering factor for some patients. Fever can be present and thus initial differential diagnosis from cellulitis or erythema nodosum is difficult, if the context of FMF is not known.

ELE usually regresses spontaneously within 3 days, especially with bed rest. If ELE is the first manifestation of FMF, a very rare situation, patients seem to have a somewhat less severe phenotype [30], although patients with ELE usually have a more severe disease [32]. Other cutaneous manifestations of FMF include acute scrotal inflammation, localised redness of the face or of the palmoplantar regions with secondary desquamation, scattered non-vasculitic purpura on the face, trunk and extremities or vasculitic purpura related to IgA vasculitis (Henoch–Schönlein) or polyarteritis nodosa: these

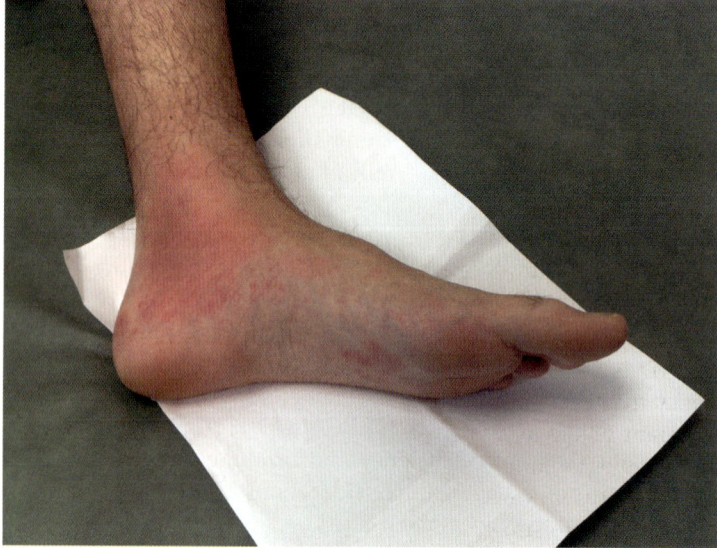

Figure 45.2 Familial Mediterranean fever (FMF): oedematous warm, swollen erythema on the ankle. Courtesy of Dr Barzilai, Tel Hashomer, Israel.

occur much more often in children than in adults [33,34]. It is noteworthy that patients with FMF are at increased risk of vasculitis [33] and thus a diagnosis of IgA vasculitis in a child should not rule out the possibility of associated FMF [34].

Investigations

Diagnosis is supported by detection of a pathogenic autosomal recessive *MEFV* gene mutation; a rare dominant variant also exists.

Management

See Table 45.3.

Pyrin-associated autoinflammation with neutrophilic dermatosis

Synonyms and inclusions

- This entity is recorded under the heading: neutrophilic dermatosis, acute febrile (#608068) in OMIM
- Familial autoinflammation with neutrophilic dermatosis

Pyrin-associated autoinflammation with neutrophilic dermatosis (PAAND) is a dominant disorder caused by mutations in the same *MEFV* gene that is mutated in FMF, leading to activation of the pyrin inflammasome. It has childhood onset with fever that can last several weeks, joint and muscle pain, skin lesions and increase in acute phase reactants [**35**].

Skin manifestations include numerous types of aseptic neutrophilic dermatoses: pyoderma gangrenosum, pustules, aseptic skin abscesses, acne, hidradenitis suppurativa, neutrophilic panniculitis; it is thus a differential diagnosis of pyogenic arthritis-pyoderma gangrenosum-acne (PAPA) spectrum disorders.

Just as in FMF, inflammatory (AA) amyloidosis can be a serious complication [36], and the aim of treatment should be control of inflammation.

Treatment relies on anakinra and in case of poor response, TNF inhibitors or IL-6 inhibitors [36].

Mevalonate kinase deficiency with recurrent fever and hyper-IgD syndrome

Pathophysiology

Mutations in the mevalonate kinase (*MVK*) gene may result in a partial or complete inability to metabolise mevalonic acid. *MVK* plays a key role in the biosynthesis of cholesterol and non-sterol isoprenoids. How deficiency results in inflammation is not fully understood but it seems that shortage of isoprenoids is associated with a predisposition to inflammatory attacks.

MKD is inherited in an autosomal recessive pattern. The deficiency may be partial or complete. Partial MKD is associated with recurrent fevers and usually but not always with overproduction of immunoglobulin D (HIDS). Complete deficiency (MVK activity <1%) induces mevalonic aciduria, a severe form of MKD associated with dysmorphism, growth retardation, neurological impairment, recurrent febrile flares and early death if untreated; treatment relies on bone marrow transplantation. These entities overlap and there is a continuous spectrum between HIDS and mevalonic aciduria [37].

Clinical features

The disease usually first presents in infancy and almost always before 3 years of age. It manifests with recurrent flares of 3–7 days duration with fever, chills, headache, polyarthralgia, abdominal pain with diarrhoea and bilateral cervical tender lymphadenopathy. Enlargement of the axillary or inguinal lymph nodes and spleen occurs less frequently. Immunisation, surgery, trauma and stress are classic triggering factors. Importantly, it does not respond to colchicine. The frequency of flares diminishes in adulthood. An increase of acute phase reactants is observed during the inflammatory flares and increased IgA and IgD levels are characteristic although not specific: IgD levels can be normal.

Dermatological findings occur in about two thirds of patients [38]. Aphthous stomatitis is the most common mucocutaneous manifestation, occurring in 60% of patients [39]. Different types of cutaneous involvement have been reported: red macules, maculopapular rashes (sometimes referred to as 'morbilliform'), urticaria, purpura and erythema nodosum. Macules, papules and plaques are intermittent and sometimes painful. Lesions are usually referred to as being fixed and not migrating. Pigmentary sequelae can persist after redness has cleared. The trunk, extremities, buttocks and face can be involved. Telangiectasia has been reported in two patients, but neither type nor anatomical site was specified [40].

Amyloidosis is a very rare complication, but patients are at increased risk of severe infection (especially pneumococcal) and of macrophage-activating syndrome. There is probably an increased risk of renal angiomyolipoma [40].

Investigations

Diagnosis is supported by the Eurofever/printo classification criteria [**16**] and the presence of mevalonate aciduria with increased excretion of mevalonic acid during attacks.

Management

See Table 45.3.

Autoinflammatory diseases with granuloma

Autoinflammatory granulomatosis of childhood (Blau syndrome)

Introduction and general description

This rare autosomal dominant multisystem disorder is a monogenic autoinflammatory disorder due to mutations in the pattern recognition receptor gene *NOD2* (*CARD15*). The first reports of a familial granulomatous disorder characterised by early-onset chronic granulomatous arthritis, uveitis and rash appeared simultaneously by Blau [41] and Jabs [42]. Sporadic cases were originally reported under the name of early-onset sarcoidosis but subsequently shown to be genetically indistinguishable from the familial form: transmission from affected mother to child has been documented. Diagnosis is based on typical clinicopathological findings and confirmed by detecting mutations in the *NOD2* (*CARD15*) gene.

Pathophysiology

NOD2 is a member of a family of pattern recognition receptors involved in innate immune defence against invading pathogens. It is hypothesised that the mutations responsible for this disorder confer gain of function, promoting inflammation and ultimately increasing activation of NFκB and release of a range of inflammatory cytokines including IL-1β, IL-6 and IFNγ, the latter being possibly the key mediator of the disease [43].

Clinical features

Presentation is characterised by early onset, usually before 4 years of age, of chronic granulomatous polyarthritis and a rash. Arthritis affects principally the peripheral joints (wrists, knees, ankles and proximal interphalangeal joints) and may be accompanied by tenosynovitis. Cystic swelling on the dorsal side of the wrists or the ankle is highly characteristic. Uveitis develops in 80% of cases at a median age of about 4 years [44]. If untreated, joint destruction and blindness can occur.

The rash presents during the first 10 years of life, sometimes as early as the neonatal period, as a widespread papular eruption. The primary lesion is a discrete skin-coloured or slightly yellowish to red-brown coloured papule measuring 1–5 mm in diameter. Individual papules are grouped, sometimes in linear arrays, and can be confluent: they usually first involve the face and extremities, and later spread to the trunk. They may fade spontaneously then recur and can leave pitted scars as a result of follicular atropho-derma. Histopathologically, there is a non-caseating granulomatous inflammatory infiltrate located in the adventitial dermis. Ichthyosiform skin changes, erythema nodosum and leukocytoclastic vasculitis have all been reported in patients with Blau syndrome.

Management

See Table 45.3.

Autoinflammation and PLCγ 2-associated antibody deficiency and immune dysregulation (APLAID)

APLAID is a dominant disorder caused by mutations in the *PLCγ 2* gene resulting in hyperactivation of the PLCγ2 pathway [45]. PLCγ 2 plays a key role in the regulation of immune responses. Patients have early-onset blistering skin lesions, eye inflammation (conjunctivitis, episcleritis, uveitis), IBD, interstitial pneumonitis, joint pain and recurrent upper airway infection related to humoral immunodeficiency with almost absent switched memory B cells.

Dermatological findings include [45–48]: early-onset papules that evolve to pustular or vesiculobullous blistering lesions with crusts that can mimic epidermolysis bullosa, as well as boggy pustular masses, especially on the back of the hands, that ulcerate and evolve with time to plaques, sometimes with cribriform scarring. At some stage, a co-existence of pustules, papules and plaques is present. Cutis laxa-like lesions have been reported. Histopathological evaluation of the infiltrated lesions can show an interstitial granuloma annulare rich in neutrophils, with leukocytoclasia and sometimes transepidermal elimination of basophilic material through follicular channels. Mucin is present in the areas of degenerated collagen.

Management

See Table 45.3.

PLCγ 2-associated antibody deficiency and immune dysregulation (PLAID)

PLAID is also a dominant disorder due to mutation of *PLCγ 2* [49]. Skin involvement is characterised by early-onset pruritus, red macules and urticaria after generalised exposure to cold air or evaporative cooling, but with a negative cold stimulation time test [50,51]. Vesiculobullous eruptions in the first days of life on the colder areas of the body such as the tip of the nose, the ears and the fingers, sometimes evolving into crusted ulcerations, can occur; the lesions usually resolve spontaneously but in a few patients the rash worsens with time and leads to destruction of ear and nose cartilage [49]. Plaques and nodules sparing the warmer regions of the body appear; the latter can also involve the mucosa. Histopathology of urticarial lesions shows a slight increase in dermal mast cells. Biopsy of the plaques reveals sarcoid type granulomas or diffuse granulomatous inflammation of the dermis. Additional immunologic abnormalities are often present: antibody deficiency, recurrent infections, autoimmune disease (vitiligo, Hashimoto's thyroiditis) and symptomatic allergic disease (rhinitis, asthma).

Management

See Table 45.3.

Autoinflammatory syndromes with pustulosis

Deficiency of interleukin 1 receptor antagonist

Introduction and general description

Deficiency of interleukin 1 receptor antagonist (DIRA) is an autosomal recessive disorder related to a deficiency of the naturally occurring antagonist of the IL-1 receptor (IL-1Rn) [52,53]. The result is an excess of IL-1-mediated inflammation.

Clinical features

DIRA presents in neonates with aseptic pustular dermatitis, multifocal osteomyelitis and periostitis. Fever is usually absent, but acute phase reactants are elevated during flares. Grouped pustules appear on a red base in the newborn or within the first 3 weeks; these may then develop yellowish crusts [52,53]. The lesions can be localised or widespread, including face and scalp involvement. Bullae with hypopyon can be present. The skin may become diffusely red and ichthyotic with diffuse desquamating scales. Oral mucosa and nails can be affected, with pitting and onychomadesis. One child also developed pyoderma gangrenosum [52]. Late-onset forms (adolescence) have been reported [54].

Investigations

Diagnosis relies on clinical and radiological findings (widened ribs and clavicles, osteolytic lesions of the long bones) and is supported by detecting a homozygous or compound heterozygous loss of function mutation in the *IL-1RN* gene [52,53].

Management
See Table 45.3.

Deficiency of interleukin 36 receptor antagonist (DITRA)

> **Synonyms and inclusions**
> • Deficiency of IL-36 receptor antagonist (DITRA)
> • Infantile pustular psoriasis

Severe early-onset pustular psoriasis has been associated with homozygous or compound heterozygous mutations in the gene encoding IL-36 receptor antagonist, *IL36RN*. This is discussed fully in Chapter 35.

Pyogenic sterile arthritis, pyoderma gangrenosum and acne syndrome

Introduction and general description
Pyogenic sterile arthritis, pyoderma gangrenosum and acne (PAPA) syndrome is a rare autosomal dominant pustular autoinflammatory disorder affecting principally the skin and joints [55]. It is due to mutations in the *PSTPIP1* gene which encodes a protein which is involved in the inflammatory pathway associated with other autoinflammatory disorders such as FMF [56]. Indeed, the *PSTPIP1* gene encoded protein binds to pyrin and exerts a dominant negative effect on its activity [56].

Many related pyoderma gangrenosum (PG)/acne syndromes have been reported under different acronyms [57]: PASH (Pyoderma gangrenosum, Acne, Hidradenitis Suppurativa), PAPASH (PASH with pyogenic arthritis), PsAPASH (PASH with psoriatic arthritis), PASS (PG, acne, seronegative spondyloarthritis, with or without hidradenitis suppurativa), PAC (PG, acne, ulcerative colitis) and PAMI (*PSTPIP1*-associated myeloid-related proteinaemia inflammatory syndrome). They should nosologically be considered as PAPA spectrum disorders.

Clinical features
It presents in early childhood with a recurrent painful sterile pauciarticular non-axial arthritis, often apparently precipitated by trauma and occasionally resulting in significant joint destruction. By puberty, joint symptoms tend to subside while skin manifestations predominate. Pyoderma gangrenosum is variable; pathergy may occur. PAPA should be considered in every patient with a familial history of pathergy and/or pyoderma gangrenosum. Severe nodular acne develops in most from puberty onwards [58]. Hidradenitis suppurativa may also be associated [59]. PAAND can mimick PAPA syndrome [60].

Investigations
Typical presentation and genetic testing for mutations in the *PSTPIP* gene.

Management
See Table 45.3.

Type 1 interferonopathies

They include the different genetic variants of the Aicardi-Goutières syndrome (AGS), proteasome associated autoinflammatory syndromes (PRAAS) such as CANDLE, and SAVI. Those disorders are IFN-mediated and are referred to as 'type 1 interferonopathies'. Typical manifestations are calcifications of basal ganglia (AGS), interstitial lung disease (SAVI), muscle involvement, glaucoma, glomerular nephropathy, lymphopenia; CRP levels are usually normal or only mildly elevated. Autoantibodies can be present. Irreversible end-organ damage is common. Typical skin manifestations pointing to type 1 interferonopathies are cold-sensitivity with inflammatory (e.g. chilblains) or vasculopathic (e.g. telangiectasia, violaceous skin areas evolving into ulceration and necrosis) changes in cold-exposed areas (fingers, toes, tip of the nose, ears) that can progress to tissue loss and scarring. Neutrophilic panniculitis is another skin finding present in some in patients with a high interferon type 1 gene score [61]. Interferonopathies involve mainly small vessels, while medium-sized vessels are involved in DADA2. Classic immunosuppressors and most biologicals (anti-IL-1, TNF and IL-6) are not helpful. JAK-inbitors are the treatment of choice.

Aicardi-Goutières syndrome

Introduction and general description
Aicardi-Goutières syndrome (AGS) comprise a group of six recessively inherited (*TREX1, SAMHD1, RNASEH2A, RNASEH2B, RNASEH2C, ADAR1*) and one dominantly inherited (*IFIH1*) monogenic disorders characterised by inflammation affecting particularly the brain and the skin [62,63]. Mutations in some genes that are responsible for recessive AGS (e.g. *TREX1, SAMHD1*) can give rise to dominant familial chilblain lupus erythematosus [64,65] and possibly minor forms of AGS (*TREX1, ADAR1* [66]).

Clinical features
The most severe forms of AGS mimic TORCH (Toxoplasmosis, Other agents, Rubella, Cytomegalovirus, Herpes) syndrome. Signs include neonatal encephalopathy with severe developmental delay, axial hypotonia, peripheral hypertonia with spasticity, microcephaly, progressive cerebral atrophy and basal ganglia calcifications; and loss of previously acquired skills in case of postnatal onset [62,63]. Fever and hepatosplenomegaly, as well as abnormal liver tests, can be present. Lymphocytosis with elevated IFNα level in an aseptic cerebrospinal fluid are typical. Signs of autoimmunity such as arthritis, presence of antinuclear antibodies, lymphopenia and thrombocytopenia can appear.

In this context, the following skin findings are highly suggestive: acral redness, red papules and plaques typical of chilblains on hands, feet, ears; more rarely are necrotic acral lesions, Raynaud phenomenon and livedo reticularis.

Histopathological analysis of acral papuloerythematous lesions is consistent with chilblains [67].

AGS6 is caused by homozygous or compound heterozygous mutations in *ADAR1*, the gene involved in dyschromatosis symmetrica hereditary, explaining overlap between those two entities [68]. AGS7 is caused by mutations in *IFIH1* and can display

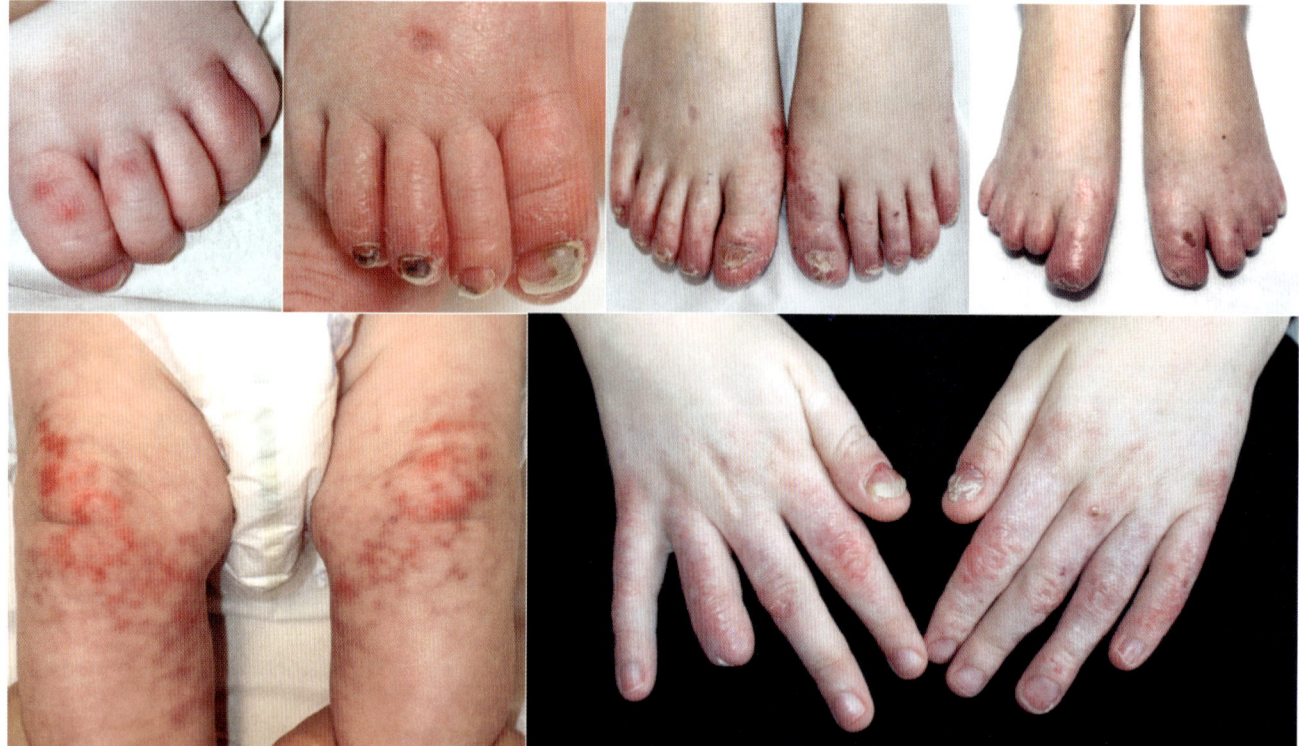

Figure 45.3 Acral erythematous and atrophic lesions that can evolve to amputation of distal phalanges in patients with STING-associated vasculopathy with onset in infancy (SAVI); one patient with livedo. Courtesy of Professor Didier Bessis, Montpellier, France.

overlapping features with Singleton–Merten syndromes and at least in one family multiple lentigines were part of the clinical spectrum [69].

Investigations
Diagnosis relies on clinical findings. It is supported by high interferon levels in cerebrospinal fluid and confirmed by genotyping.

Management
See Table 45.3.

STING-associated vasculopathy with onset in infancy

Introduction and general description
STING-associated vasculopathy with onset in infancy (SAVI) is a dominant disorder caused by gain of function mutations in stimulator of interferon cGAMP interactor 1 or *STING1* (formerly *TMEM173*) encoding STING, a sensor of cytosolic DNA that activates IRF3 and induces transcription of IFN-1 related genes [70]. A recessive form of SAVI has also been reported [71].

Clinical features
SAVI is characterised by neonatal-onset of recurrent fever with rash, failure to thrive and interstitial lung disease that can progress to end-stage respiratory failure, contributing to the high mortality rate [72]. Arthralgia and arthritis are common. During flares, acute phase reactants are elevated. Patients have autoantibodies, such as ANA, ANCA and antiphospholipid antibodies. Rare cases of adult-onset SAVI have been reported manifesting as

ANCA-associated vasculitis in one family [73]. *STING1* mutations also account for isolated lung fibrosis and isolated familial chilblain lupus [74]. Some patients have recurrent infections and present as common variable immunodeficiency.

Skin signs are usually the first manifestations. The most typical lesions are violaceous, scaly and atrophic skin areas, that can ulcerate and/or progress to necrosis of the extremities, the cheeks, the ears and the nose [70]. Telangiectatic erythema, acral cyanosis or livedoid erythema in cold-sensitive areas are other typical manifestations. Livedo reticularis, Raynaud phenomenon, periungual erythema are also often present. Digital gangrene and nasal perforation can occur. Vesicles or blisters can appear on cold-exposed sites. Localised, or more often generalised, pustules have been reported, as well as oral ulcers. Nails can become dystrophic or be completely destroyed and alopecia areata may occur [73]. The skin lesions can evolve to definitive damage of the fingers and the toes with amputation, as well as tissue loss and scarring of the ears and the nose (Figure 45.3). On the face, redness is situated in the cold-sensitive areas on the tip of the nose and on the middle part of the cheeks, below the malar area, thus it is relatively different from the malar rash observed in systemic lupus erythematosus. Histopathological evaluation reveals a mixed pattern, consisting of a prominent dermal inflammatory infiltrate with features of leukocytoclastic vasculitis and microthrombotic angiopathy of small dermal vessels.

Investigations
Diagnosis relies on clinical, biological and imaging findings and is supported by genotyping.

Management

See Table 45.3.

Chronic atypical neutrophilic dermatosis with lipodystrophy and elevated temperature

Introduction and general description

Chronic atypical neutrophilic dermatosis with lipodystrophy and elevated temperature (CANDLE) is an autosomal recessive syndrome, first reported in Japan as Nakajo–Nishimura syndrome, and is characterised by abnormal signalling in the interferon pathways. It is related to a mutation in the *PMSB8* gene, which encodes the ß5i subunit of the immunoproteasome: the latter is highly expressed in haematopoietic cells and is involved in protein degradation [75]. Diagnostic criteria have been published by authors in Japan [76]. *PMSB8* mutation is also found in the JMP syndrome (joint contractures, muscle atrophy, microcytic anaemia and panniculitis-induced childhood-onset lipodystrophy), which shares clinical features with CANDLE [77]. *PMSB4, PSMB9, PSMA3* and *POMP* are other proteasome genes identified as causing PRAAS/CANDLE. *POMP* mutations cause an autosomal dominant disorder [78]. SAMD9L-SAAD is a newly recognised type 1 interferonopathy with a dermatological presentation similar to CANDLE, but with a more severe interstitial lung disease, B and NK-cell cytopenia [61].

Histopathology

There is a dense dermal infiltrate of mononuclear cells intermingled with mature and immature neutrophils, with karyorrhexis [79]. Mononuclear cells were found to be 'atypical' because of a large vesicular elongated or kidney-shaped nucleus, scant eosinophilic cytoplasm and frequent mitotic figures. There are foci of interstitial collagen degeneration. Immunohistochemistry reveals the mononuclear cell component is either myeloperoxidase positive, Leder staining positive (naphthol AS-D chloroacetate esterase or specific esterase, which specifically identifies cells of the granulocyte lineage from the early promyelocyte stage to mature neutrophils) or CD68+ and CD163+ and was thus interpreted as being composed of immature neutrophils/myeloid precursors and activated macrophages. This infiltrate is admixed with eosinophils.

Clinical features

Children usually present in early life with recurrent fever, rash and arthralgia or arthritis. These may first develop within 2 or 3 weeks of birth but then continue episodically during the first year of life with violaceous or red, often annular and oedematous plaques on the face and trunk and over the interphalangeal joints. Each episode lasts from a few days to several weeks and resolves with purpura or pigmentation [77,79].

Later these children develop persistent violaceous periorbital oedema and swelling of the fingers and toes reminiscent of perniosis; later still, recurrent episodes of panniculitis evolve to lipoatrophy. Other signs include thickened lips, hypertrichosis, mouth ulcers and muscle atrophy. Enlarged lymph nodes, spleen and/or liver with abnormal liver function tests are frequently found. Chondritis and episcleritis, aseptic meningitis, parotiditis, as well as inflammation in other organs are further possible

complications. Basal ganglia calcification can occur. Acute phase reactants are raised and liver and often muscle enzymes are elevated.

Without treatment, up to 50% of patients die before adulthood. The remainder risk development of muscle atrophy, cardiac arrhythmias and dilated cardiomyopathy.

Investigations

These are genetic testing for mutations in the *PMSB8* and other proteasome genes and imaging of the basal ganglia for calcification.

Management

See Table 45.3. First-line treatment should include JAK inhibitors [80].

Behçet disease-like or inflammatory bowel disease-like autoinflammatory syndromes

There is a growing number of monogenic autoinflammatory disorders with features suggestive of early-onset Behçet disease or IBD. Some of these diseases also display immune deficiency and/or autoimmunity. Mucocutaneous manifestations include aphthous stomatis and numerous aseptic neutrophilic infiltrates: pustules, Sweet syndrome, pyoderma gangrenosum, as well as early-onset periorificial redness with fissuring.

Haploinsufficiency of A20

Haploinsufficiency of A20 (HA20) is a dominant disorder caused by mutations in the *TNFAIP3* gene encoding protein A20, a crucial negative regulator of inflammation, leading to increased NFκB signalling [81]. The clinical triad of orogenital ulcers, ocular inflammation and non-deforming polyarthritis is characteristic. Other manifestations include recurrent fever, hepatosplenomegaly, gastrointestinal ulcers, serositis, pharyngitis, retinal vasculitis and central nervous system vasculitis. It is a cause of early-onset IBD with perianal lesions [82]. Acute phase reactants are elevated during flares. Age of onset is usually before 10 [83]. Several organ-specific autoimmune diseases can occur: cytopenia, type 1 diabetes, Hashimoto thyroiditis, glomerulonephritis, interstitial lung disease. Some systemic autoimmune diseases, such as systemic lupus erythematosus, can also occur. Autoantibodies can be present. HA20 is a heterogeneous disorder as some patients will only have autoimmune manifestations [84] or immune deficiency [85].

Dermatological manifestations are very common: oral and genital ulcerations, as well as gastrointestinal ulcerations. Numerous neutrophilic aseptic dermatoses can occur: pustules, abscesses, erythema-nodosum-like lesions. Pathergy can be present. Histopathology of skin lesions is a neutrophilic dermatosis and mucin deposition has been reported.

Management

See Table 45.3.

PART 4: INFLAMMATORY DERMATOSES

RELA haploinsufficiency

Synonyms and inclusions
- Mucocutaneous ulceration, chronic (CMCU)

It is a dominant disorder caused by mutations of *RELA* which encodes RelA, a subunit of NFκB [86]. The subunit RelA/NFκB1 constitutes the predominant form of NFκB, critical for cell survival. Patients have a Behçet disease-like presentation reminiscent of A20 (*TNFAIP3*) haploinsufficiency, with mucosal ulceration, IBD, fever and elevated acute phase reactants. Oral and genital ulcers are the most common dermatological manifestations. Some patients with RELA haploinsufficiency will not have autoinflammatory manifestations, but rather autoimmunity [87].

Treatment with steroids and TNF inhibitors is efficient for the autoinflammatory variant.

NLRC4-associated autoinflammatory disease

This group of autosomal dominant disorders is related to gain of function mutations in *NLRC4* leading to constitutive activation of the NLRC4 inflammasome and increased secretion of active IL-1β and IL-18. It is characterised by extremely high IL-18 levels. It includes NLRC4-associated macrophage activating syndrome (NLRC4-MAS) [88,89] and familial cold autoinflammatory syndrome 4 (FCAS4) [90]. NLRC4-MAS is a multisystemic disease starting early in life with chronic IBD (AIFEC: autoinflammation and infantile enterocolitis), that usually subsides over time. Patients can have severe inflammation with signs similar to CINCA/NOMID and they are prone to develop MAS. FCAS4 is very reminiscent of FCAS with urticaria, arthralgia, ocular inflammation and fever after exposure to cold stimuli. Painful nodules can occur on lower extremities, especially in adult patients. Histopathological evaluation of urticarial lesions reveals a lymphohistiocytic infiltrate, different from the neutrophilic infiltrate seen in CAPS [91]. Biopsy of a nodular lesion reveals a deep dermal and subcutaneous septal and lobular lymphohistiocytic infiltrate.

Management
See Table 45.3.

Nuclear factor κ light-chain enhancer of activated B-cells 1 (NFκB1)-autoinflammatory disease

Synonyms and inclusions
- Familial autoinflammatory necrotising fasciitis
- Immunodeficiency, common variable, 12

This comprises different dominant disorders due to *NFκB1* mutations, encoding p105, resulting in increased expression of IL-1 and sometimes TNF and IFNγ. Those patients have common variable immune deficiency with autoimmunity, and some of them have an associated autoinflammatory phenotype, which can either be a Behçet-like disease, or a necrotising neutrophilic dermatosis phenotype, reminiscent of postoperative pyoderma gangrenosum (familial autoinflammatory necrotising fasciitis, FANF) [92,93].

Manifestations of immune deficiency and autoimmunity start in infancy and include recurrent respiratory tract infections with bronchiectasis, diarrhoea, lymphadenopathy, splenomegaly, thyroiditis, and autoimmune cytopenias. They have hypogammaglobulinaemia, deficient production of specific antibodies, and decreased classed-switched memory B cells [94]. Those with Behçet disease-like have immune deficiency and mucocutaneous ulcerations, sometimes gastrointestinal inflammation, arthritis, and uveitis. They often have leukocytosis.

Dermatological manifestations of patients with the Behçet-like variant are aphthae of the oral and genital mucosa, as well as ulcerations of the oesophagus. Pathergy can be present. Aseptic necrotising-fasciitis-like lesions characterise the patients with FANF.

Interestingly, mutations in *NFκB2* were also reported in patients with common variable immune deficiency and autoimmunity (vitiligo, alopecia areata) and recently in a patient with a neutrophilic panniculitis [95].

If immune deficiency is present, treatment includes antibiotics and intravenous immunoglobulins. Behçet-like manifestations are treated like classic Behçet disease, with potential utility of IL-1 and TNF-inhibitors.

ADAM17 deficiency

Synonyms and inclusions
- Inflammatory skin and bowel diseases, neonatal, 1

An extremely rare recessive disease related to *ADAM17* mutations encoding TNF-α converting enzyme which is necessary for the cleavage and secretion of different molecules including TNF-α, epidermal growth factor, transforming growth factor-β and some desmogleins. Affected patients have neonatal onset of IBD, mild cardiomyopathy and rashes [96].

Skin findings include pustules, peri-orificial redness with fissuring and evolution to exfoliative dermatitis. Hair was reported as fragile, nails are thickened and paronychia common. Skin infections were reported as frequent and overall prognosis as good. Histopathology reveals a perifollicular and epithelial T-cell infiltrate.

IL-10 signalling disorders (IL-10/IL-10R colitis)

Synonyms and inclusions
- Inflammatory bowel disease 28, early onset, autosomal recessive
- Inflammatory bowel disease 25, early onset, autosomal recessive

Different disorders with aberrant IL-10 signalling, as for example autosomal recessive mutations of the gene encoding the IL-10 receptor α (IL-10RA) or β (IL-10RB), are causes of early-onset IBD [97]. Those patients often have folliculitis, perianal abscesses and enterocutaneous fistula. Treatment of choice is haematopoietic stem cell transplantation.

Miscellaneous monogenic autoinflammatory syndromes

This group includes a growing number of autoinflammatory diseases that will probably be more accurately classified in the coming years.

CCAAT enhancer binding protein ε (C/EBPε)-associated autoinflammation and immune impairment of neutrophils (CAIN)

CAIN is a recessive disorder caused by gain of function mutations in *CEBPE* encoding C/EBPε, a transcription factor expressed in myeloid and lymphoid lineage, that regulates cellular differentiation and function of late myeloid lineage as well as the inflammasome. The disease is characterised by neutrophil dysfunction, hyposegmented neutrophils, recurrent abscesses, mild bleeding (epistaxis, haematomas after needle sticks) and recurrent fever [98]. It starts after adolescence with recurrent attacks of abdominal pain, fever and an increase in acute phase reactants lasting 4–5 days. Flares recur every 2–4 weeks. Recurrent purulent skin, and mucosal and upper respiratory tract infection were reported, but it was not documented whether those were authentic infections or recurrent aseptic abscesses. Other findings include episcleritis, myalgia, joint pain, pleurisy and aphthous colitis.

Dermatological findings include crater-like buccal ulcerations, pyoderma gangrenosum, purulent paronychia with lymphangitis and recurrent skin abscesses.

Treatment modalities are not defined but if neutrophil modulators such as dapsone or colchicine are not effective, IL-1 inhibitors could potentially be helpful.

Cleavage resistant RIPK1-induced autoinflammatory syndrome

> **Synonyms and inclusions**
> * Autoinflammation with episodic fever and lymphadenopathy (AIEFL)

Cleavage resistant RIPK1-induced autoinflammatory (CRIA) syndrome is a dominant disorder related to *RIPK1* mutations resulting in early-onset fever occurring every 2–4 weeks, of 1–7 days duration, continuing through adulthood, with enlarged lymph nodes, and hepatosplenomegaly in some individuals [99,100]. Fever can reach temperatures as high as 41°C with coincident chills, headaches and hallucinations. Joint pain and gastrointestinal symptoms (abdominal pain, nausea, diarrhoea, constipation, loss of appetite, weight loss) are common. Oral ulcerations have been reported. Tocilizumab is the treatment of choice.

Deficiency of adenosine deaminase 2

Introduction and general description
Deficiency of adenosine deaminase 2 (DADA2) is a recessive disorder related to biallelic hypomorphic mutations in *ADA2* (formerly *CECR1*) encoding ADA2, a growth factor in the myeloid lineage promoting differentiation into anti-inflammatory macrophages

[101,102]. The deficit promotes differentiation towards the pro-inflammatory M1 subset. ADA2 also plays a role in the homeostasis of endothelial cells and its deficiency promotes vascular damage.

Clinical features
Affected patients can have persistent and/or recurrent fever, livedo and/or nodules, and ischaemic and/or haemorrhagic stroke [101,102,**103**]. Vasculitis and inflammation can affect multiple organs, which explains intestinal, cardiac, hepatological, neurological and renal manifestations. Acute phase reactants are increased in about 50% of patients.

Other presentations include:
* Haematological manifestations: hypogammaglobulinaemia, marrow aplasia, pure red cell aplasia, immune thrombocytopenia and neutropenia.
* Immunodeficiency, and some patients will present as common variable immunodeficiency.
* Lymphoproliferation with generalised lymphadenopathy and splenomegaly.

The disease usually starts early in life (about 80% before age 10), although a few cases with adult-onset have been reported. The male to female ratio is close to 1. In some patients, the disease is indistinguishable from polyarteritis nodosa and DADA2 can be considered as a monogenic variant of polyarteritis nodosa.

Skin manifestations are the most common feature of DADA2, present in approximately 75% of patients. Livedo reticularis or more often livedo racemosa is a typical manifestation (Figure 45.4). Biopsy

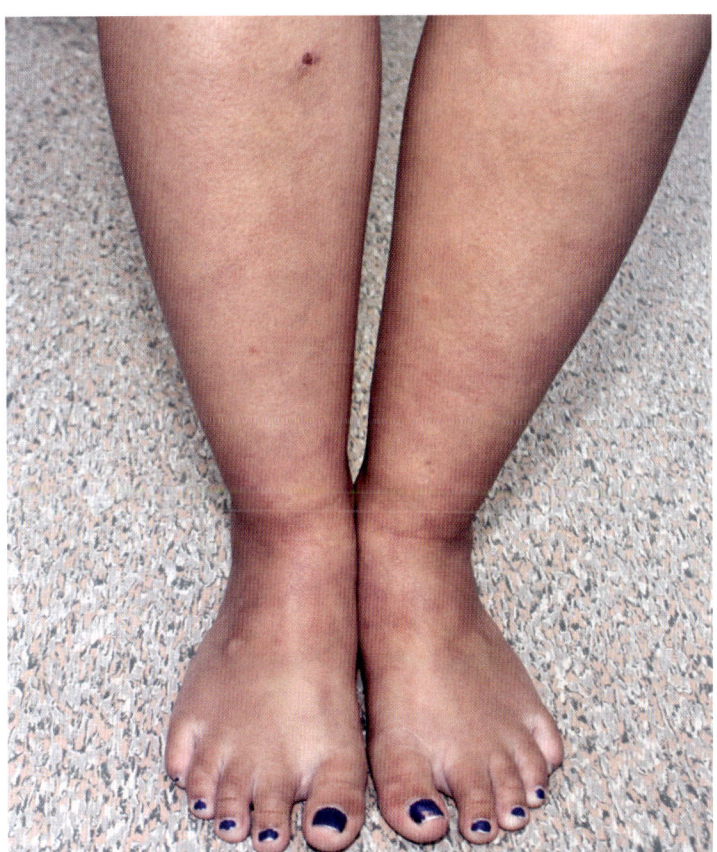

Figure 45.4 Racemosa type livedo in a patient with deficiency of adenosine deaminase 2 (DADA2). Courtesy of Professor Didier Bessis, Montpellier, France.

reveals an interstitial infiltrate of neutrophils and macrophages, with perivascular T cells without vasculitis. Nodules are another typical manifestation, displaying histopathological features of non-granulomatous vasculitis of small and medium-sized vessels in the skin. Other findings include digital necrosis and skin ulcers, Raynaud phenomenon, aphthous ulcers and poorly described rashes.

Management
See Table 45.3.

HOIL-1 deficiency

It is a recessive disorder caused by *HOIL-1* mutations, encoding Hoil-1, a component of linear ubiquitin chain assembly complex (LUBAC) [104,105]. Mutations destabilise expression of the entire LUBAC complex, the consequences of which are defective activation of the immune signalling with failure of B cells to upregulate on one hand, and increased IL-1 susceptibility of peripheral blood monocytes on the other hand. Thus, patients combine an immune deficiency syndrome with recurrent bacterial infections and an autoinflammatory syndrome with recurrent fever, failure to thrive, gastrointestinal symptoms (diarrhoea with blood and mucus), lung involvement and lymphadenopathy. Patients also develop amylopectinosis (intracellular glycogen inclusions) by a mechanism so far not understood. Cutaneous manifestations are erythroderma and exfoliative dermatitis as well as 'eczema' and oral ulcerations.

Majeed syndrome

Synonyms and inclusions
- Chronic recurrent multifocal osteomyelitis, congenital
- Dyserythropoietic anaemia, and neutrophilc dermatosis

This is a rare autosomal recessive monogenic autoinflammatory disorder related to germline *LPIN2* mutations, in which chronic recurrent multifocal osteomyelitis (CRMO) is associated with dyserythropoietic anaemia and a neutrophilic dermatosis resembling Sweet syndrome [106,107]. It is mainly reported in the Arab and Turkish literature, more rarely in Indian and Chinese patients and IL-1 inhibition is treatment of choice [108].

NLRP1-associated autoinflammation with arthritis and dyskeratosis

Synonyms and inclusions
- Autoinflammation with arthritis and dyskeratosis

Introduction and general description
NLRP1-associated autoinflammation with arthritis and dyskeratosis (NAIAD) can be caused by homozygous or heterozygous mutations of the *NLRP1* gene, encoding NLRP1, a key inflammasome in the skin. It is a paradigm of autoinflammatory keratinisation diseases.

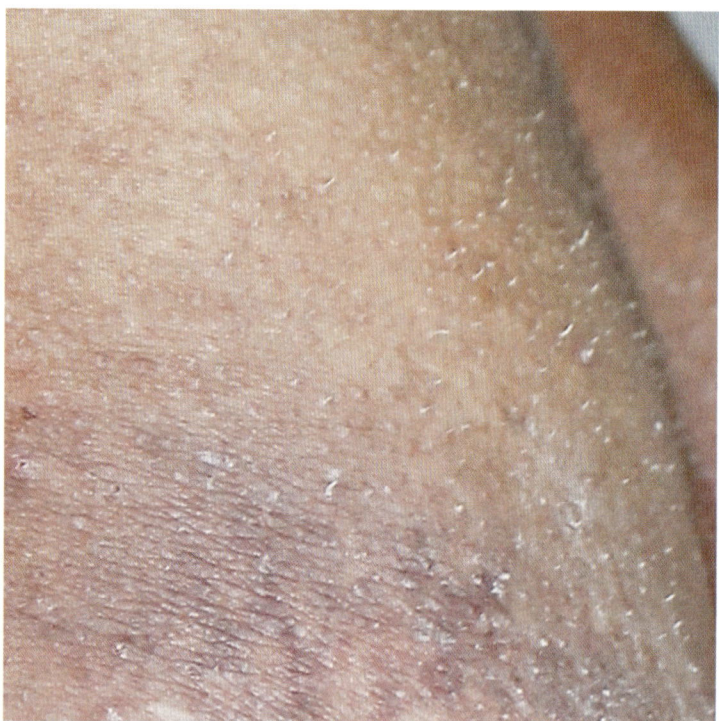

Figure 45.5 Multiple minute digitate keratosis in a patient with NLRP1-associated autoinflammation with arthritis and dyskeratosis (NAIAD). Courtesy of Professor Didier Bessis, Montpellier, France.

Clinical features
The disease starts during childhood with a recurrent fever lasting 3–4 days, polyarthritis, repeated infections, eye involvement (xerophthalmia with punctate keratitis, photophobia with corneal dyskeratosis, or uveitis) and keratotic skin lesions [109]. In some families, failure to thrive and hepatosplenomegaly were reported. CRP is elevated during flares, low titre antinuclear antibodies, elevated titres of IgA, IgG or IgE, neutrophilia, and a high transitional B-cell level are present. Vitamin A deficiency is common. Organ autoimmunity was reported in a few individuals (immune haemolytic anaemia, thyroiditis).

Dermatological findings include diffuse xerosis with multiple minute digitate keratosis (Figure 45.5) covering extensive areas of limbs, shoulders and flanks, with brownish purple pigmented macules with indistinct edges present in the area of keratotic lesions. Other reported skin lesions are: symmetric tender warty keratotic lesions on soles and in the larynx; comedo-like papules and vermiculated atrophic scars on the cheeks; perifollicular cylindrical keratotic sheaths (hair casts) on hair of the vertex and occipital region. Histopathological hallmarks are acanthosis with scattered to confluent dyskeratotic keratinocytes of the supra-basal layers. In some areas, the granular cell layer is completely replaced by dyskeratotic keratinocytes. Some patients with NAIAD go on to develop hidradenitis suppurativa (Professor D. Bessis, personal communication).

Investigations
Diagnosis relies on clinical features and genotyping.

Management
Treatment relies on acitretin and anakinra.

Neonatal onset of pancytopenia, autoinflammation, rash and episodes of haemophagocytic lymphohistiosis (NOCARH) syndrome

NOCARH syndrome is related to a heterozygous mutation in the cell division cycle 42 (*CDC42*) gene. The syndrome associates neonatal onset of persistent fever, rash, hepatosplenomegaly, pancytopenia, transaminitis and persistently elevated markers of inflammation [110]. Patients go on to develop often fatal haemophagocytic lymphohistiocytosis; high ferritin and IL-18 levels are found, features shared with NLRC4-AID and X-linked inhibitor of apotosis (XIAP) deficiency. Most patients have mild dysmorphism (frontal bossing, hypertelorism, nasal bridge depression). The eruption is urticarial with petaloid and/or polycyclic confluence of lesions. Histopathology reveals perivascular lymphocytic and neutrophilic infiltration [111]. The disease is severe with no established treatment; IL-1 inhibition was very efficient in a few patients [111] and IFNγ inhibitors could be helpful [110].

Otulin-related autoinflammatory syndrome

Synonyms and inclusions
- Autoinflammation, panniculitis and dermatosis syndrome (AIPDS)
- Otulopenia

Otulin-related autoinflammatory syndrome (ORAS) is a rare recessive autoinflammatory disease related to mutations in the *OTULIN/FAM105B* gene encoding otulin, a deubiquitinase acting as negative regulator of the NFκB pathway by counter regulating LUBAC [112]. Affected individuals have early-onset fever, failure to thrive, joint and abdominal pain, diarrhoea, lymphadenopathy and elevated acute phase reactants. Cutaneous manifestations include red plaques and nodules, pustules and lipoatrophy. Histopathological evaluation of skin findings is poorly documented and was reported as 'panniculitis' and 'neutrophilic dermatosis'. Authentic vasculitis has been documented in some patients [105,113]. Untreated, ORAS can be fatal. TNF inhibitors are a very efficient treatment.

Periodic fever, immunodeficiency and thrombocytopenia syndrome

Synonyms and inclusions
- Lazy leukocyte syndrome

Periodic fever, immunodeficiency and thrombocytopenia (PFIT) syndrome is a recessive disorder caused by *WDR1* gene mutations, encoding WDR1 which regulates actin assembly [114]. It is characterised by recurrent fever, oral ulcers, intermittent thrombocytopenia and immune deficiency. Flares of fever last 3–7 days, and they recur with a periodicity of 6–12 weeks. Raised acute phase reactants, leukocytosis, hyperferritinaemia and thrombocytopenia are present during the flares. Other findings in WDR1-deficient patients include intellectual impairment, recurrent infections, abnormal herniation of nuclear lobes in the neutrophils on blood smear and aberrant T-cell activation and B-cell development.

Oral ulcers are the most typical dermatological manifestation; they can be very severe and induce microstomia because of scarring. Poorly described skin ulceration resembling pyoderma gangrenosum have been reported. As WDR1 is an actin skeleton regulator similar to the Wiscott–Aldrich protein, WDR1 deficiency might possibly also be associated with an enhanced risk of malignancy, especially myelodysplasia and acute leukaemia, although this has so far not been demonstrated.

Treatment has yet to be defined; colchicine, steroids and anakinra were not efficient. IgIV and antibiotics are administered for recurrent infections. Haematopoietic stem cell transplantation could be the treatment of choice for some patients.

Sideroblastic anaemia with B-cell immunodeficiency, periodic fevers and developmental delay (SIFD)

SIFD is a recessive disorder caused by mutations of *TRNT1*, encoding the nucleotidyl transferase enzyme. Mutations are responsible for a spectrum of diseases ranging from neonatal onset to adult presentation, but the severe form is often a lethal disorder [115]. Manifestations include recurrent fever, failure to thrive, developmental delay, diarrhoea, vomiting and sideroblastic anaemia, cataract and sensorineural deafness. Hypogammaglobulinaemia is usually present. Dermatological manifestations include oral ulcers, red nodules and plaques on the trunk and limbs. Biopsy revealed neutrophilic infiltrates of the deep dermis and the hypodermis, with enlarged septa. Numerous atypical myeloid cells can be present raising the question of leukaemia cutis [116]. Partial response was reported with TNF inhibitors.

VEXAS (vacuoles, E1 enzyme, X-linked, autoinflammatory, somatic) syndrome

Introduction and general description
VEXAS syndrome is a paradigm of an acquired autoinflammatory syndrome arising from myeloid lineage restricted somatic mutation in *UBA1*, an X-chromosome gene encoding ubiquitin-like modifier-activating enzyme 1 (*UBA1*), first identified in 2020 [1].

Clinical features
VEXAS syndrome is the cause of a late-onset systemic inflammatory disease in men. Patients develop fever, elevated concentrations of C-reactive protein and haematological abnormalities, which can be subtle, such as isolated macrocytosis or thrombopenia. Vacuoles are present in the bone marrow. Most patients go on to develop an overt myelodysplastic syndrome. Some have polyarteritis nodosa or giant cell arteritis. Thromboembolic complications are common. The cutaneous expression of VEXAS are relapsing polychondritis, Sweet syndrome and interstitial granuloma annulare (D. Lipsker, personal observation).

VEXAS syndrome should be considered in every adult man with otherwise unexplained systemic inflammation and minor haematological abnormalities such as macrocytosis and/or thrombopenia. The diagnosis can be confirmed by demonstrating a pathogenic mutation in the *UBA1* gene.

Management

VEXAS patients are extremely resistant to treatment and the disease is often exacerbated by IL-1 inhibitors. Corticosteroids, anti-IL-6 and azacytidine are the treatments of choice.

Vibratory urticaria

Autosomal dominant vibratory urticaria related to *ADGRE2* mutations is just briefly mentioned here (Chapter 42), as it is also an autoinflammatory disorder [117]. One of the most serious complications is recurrent angioedema of the hypopharynx related to snoring.

COMPLEX AND POLYGENIC AUTOINFLAMMATORY DISEASES PRESENTING WITH URTICARIAL OR MACULOPAPULAR RASH

Schnitzler syndrome

Introduction and general description

This syndrome, first reported by Liliane Schnitzler in 1972, is now considered as a paradigm of a sporadic acquired autoinflammatory disorder manifesting usually in an adult patient, typically aged 50 years or older [118,119]. It comprises a chronic urticarial eruption with a persistently raised monoclonal IgM, plus at least two of the following features: recurrent fever above 40°C, bone or joint pain (especially over the ilium or tibia), lymphadenopathy, hepatomegaly or splenomegaly, neutrophilia, elevated acute phase reactants or abnormal bone imaging (e.g. osteocondensation, particularly around the knee joint) (Table 45.4). Although arthralgia is common, arthritis is rare.

Pathophysiology

For the following reasons, Schnitzler syndrome is regarded as a late-onset acquired autoinflammatory syndrome:

Table 45.4 Clinical and biological findings in patients with Schnitzler syndrome.

	%
Urticarial rash	100
Elevated ESR (≥30 mm/h)	95
Fever	93
Monoclonal IgM gammopathy	89
Kappa light chain	89
Arthralgia/arthritis	77
Leukocytosis (≥10 000 × 10⁹/L)	76
Bone pain	68
Abnormal bone morphology[a]	62
Palpable lymph nodes	47
Pruritus	45
Liver and/or spleen enlargement	34

[a] As usually assessed by conventional X-rays. ESR, erythrocyte sedimentation rate. From Simon *et al.* [122]/John Wiley & Sons.

- Strong clinicopathological similarities with CAPS.
- High spontaneous and lipopolysaccharide-induced IL-1 release from peripheral blood mononuclear cells of affected patients [120].
- Dramatic and immediate responsiveness to IL-1 inhibitors.

Histopathology

This shows a mainly interstitial neutrophilic skin infiltrate.

Clinical features

A recurrent urticarial rash is usually the first sign (Figure 45.6), although some patients will first complain of bone and/or joint pain [**121**]. Skin lesions include non-pruritic macules, papules or plaques, particularly on the trunk. Most patients will also develop fever. Therefore, Schnitzler syndrome should be suspected in any patient with a recurrent urticarial rash and/or fever and/or fatigue and/or general malaise and/or increase in acute phase reactants and/or joint and/or bone pain and/or enlarged lymph nodes, liver or spleen and/or a neutrophilic infiltrate on biopsy [4,122]. Immunoelectrophoresis is then mandatory.

An IgG variant of Schnitzler syndrome has been reported but whether it is true Schnitzler syndrome is a matter of debate [123].

The rash is typically NUD. Validated diagnostic criteria (the 'Strasbourg criteria'), summarised in Box 45.2, underline the diagnostic importance of the neutrophilic skin infiltrate [122,124].

Box 45.2 Schnitzler syndrome: Strasbourg diagnostic criteria

Obligate criteria
- Chronic urticarial rash
- Monoclonal IgM or IgG

Minor criteria
- Recurrent fever[a]
- Objective findings of abnormal bone remodelling with or without bone pain[b]
- A neutrophilic dermal infiltrate on skin biopsy[c]
- Leukocytosis and/or elevated CRP[d]
  Definite diagnosis if:
- Two obligate criteria *and* at least two minor criteria if IgM, and three minor criteria if IgG
  Probable diagnosis if:
- Two obligate criteria *and* at least one minor criterion if IgM, and two minor criteria if IgG

[a] A valid criterion if objectively measured. Must be >38°C, and otherwise unexplained. Occurs usually – but not obligatory – together with the skin rash.
[b] As assessed by bone scintigraphy, MRI or elevation of bone alkaline phosphatase.
[c] Corresponds usually to the entity described as 'neutrophilic urticarial dermatosis' [2]; absence of fibrinoid necrosis and significant dermal oedema.
[d] Peripheral blood neutrophils >10 000/mm³ and/or C-reactive protein >30 mg/L. From Simon *et al.* [122]/John Wiley & Sons.

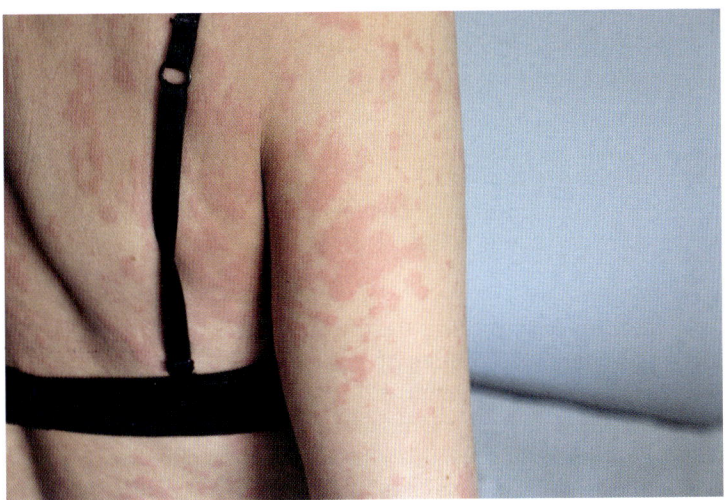

Figure 45.6 Schnitzler syndrome: the non-itchy symmetrical urticarial eruption resembles the weals of chronic spontaneous urticaria.

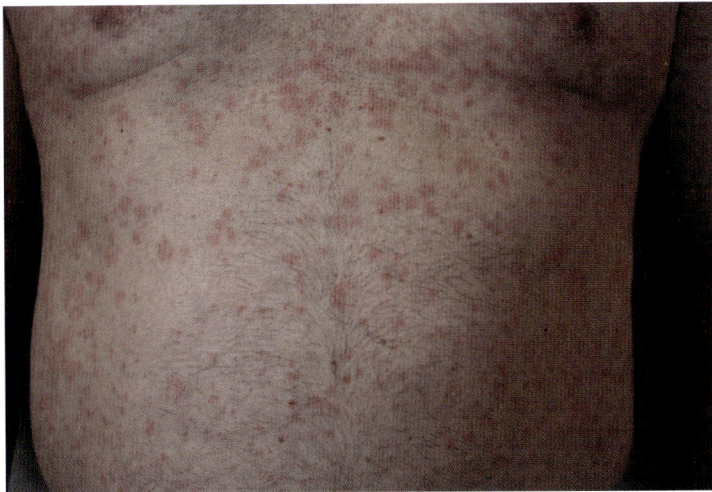

Figure 45.7 Adult-onset Still disease: the rash is a subtle salmon-coloured maculopapular exanthem.

Differential diagnosis

The main differential diagnosis is systemic adult-onset Still disease, but patients with the latter entity usually have a very high ferritin concentration (of which only a low proportion is glycosylated) and lack a monoclonal gammopathy [121]. Hypocomplementaemic urticarial vasculitis, cryoglobulinaemia and systemic lupus erythematosus are usually easily ruled out. Mosaic CAPS syndrome should be ruled out in younger patients or patients with eye or ear involvement [14].

Disease course and prognosis

Frequency and intensity of the clinical manifestations, mainly pain, rash and fever, as well as persistent elevation of acute phase reactants, determine the severity of the disease. Profound alteration in quality of life, refractory inflammatory anaemia and AA amyloidosis are severe complications of Schnitzler syndrome [118,121,125].

Between 15% and 20% of patients will develop a B-cell lymphoproliferative disorder, a percentage close to patients with monoclonal IgM gammopathies in general. Rarely reported and possibly coincidental co-morbidities include: autoimmune peripheral neuropathy; C4 deficiencies; nodular regenerative hyperplasia of the liver; pancreatitis; pseudoxanthoma elasticum; impairment of renal function; antiphospholipid antibodies; and hearing loss [121,125].

Disease course is protracted and only two patients with spontaneous remission have appeared in the published literature [118,126]. Prognosis depends on the development of AA amyloidosis or haemoproliferative disorder.

Management

Patients with altered quality of life or persistent inflammation (CRP >30 mg/L) should be treated with anti-IL1 agents, e.g. anakinra.

Adult-onset Still disease

Synonyms and inclusions
- AOSD
- Wissler–Fanconi syndrome

Adult-onset Still disease (AOSD) is rare. It occurs in young to middle-aged adults with 75% of cases presenting before the age of 50 years [127]. The cause is unknown. Patients are as likely to present to rheumatologists as dermatologists with intermittent episodes of high fever (>39°C) for at least a week, severe pharyngitis, lymphadenopathy, arthralgias and a salmon-coloured maculopapular exanthem (Figure 45.7), which typically appears with the onset of fever in the evenings and decreases in the morning.

Arthritis is generally less prominent in AOSD than in systemic-onset juvenile idiopathic arthritis (SoJIA). There appear, however, to be two phenotypes in adults. In addition to the classical systemic febrile form, a more indolent variant has been described in which arthritis predominates [127]. A variant in which more persistent pruritic papules and plaques develop on the trunk, neck, face or extensor limbs has also been described [128–130]. Such persistent lesions, qualified or 'atypical', have been associated with a worse prognosis [131]. Persistent eyelid oedema sometimes mimicking dermatomyositis and flagellate lesions are other rare manifestations [132]. Histopathological changes of evanescent lesions are characterised by an interstitial and perivascular neutrophil-dominant mixed infiltrate or a mild lymphocytic infiltrate, possibly depending on timing of biopsy. In the case of persistent lesions, epidermal involvement is frequent (acanthosis, spongiosis and superficial necrotic keratinocytes).

A neutrophil leukocytosis is present during the attacks. Very high serum ferritin levels (approximately 1000 µg/L) help to distinguish this rare entity from other complex autoinflammatory syndromes, urticarial vasculitis and infectious disease. With catastrophic antiphospholipid syndrome, septic schock, macrophage activating syndrome and severe Covid-19, AOSD belongs to the hyperferritinaemic syndromes [133].

Treatment relies on corticosteroids, methotrexate and IL-1 and IL-6 antagonists.

Systemic-onset juvenile idiopathic arthritis

Synonyms and inclusions
- SoJIA
- Still disease

Introduction and general description

Systemic-onset juvenile idiopathic arthritis (SoJIA) occurs in children. The presentation is similar to AOSD with spiking fevers and a maculopapular rash, but the occurrence of arthritis is a mandatory diagnostic criterion. The lack of autoantibodies or HLA associations suggests that SoJIA is a polygenic autoinflammatory disease rather than an autoimmune disorder [134,135]. A monogenic autosomic recessive form of SoJIA with an underlying mutation in *LACC1* has been described; its protein product regulates metabolism within macrophages [136].

Histopathology

Skin biopsy reveals a perivascular and interstitial dermal infiltrate of neutrophils and monocytes [129,130].

Clinical features

Classical features include high spiking fever once or twice daily associated with equally evanescent salmon pink macules on the trunk and lower legs. There may be a history of sore throat, arthralgia or serositis.

Laboratory investigations typically reveal neutrophilia, raised ferritin and abnormal liver function tests. Oligo- or polyarthritis may antedate other symptoms; it is slowly progressive. Macrophage activating syndrome and severe lung involvement with alveolar proteinosis and/or endogenous lipoid proteinaemia are serious complications [137].

In a subset of children, more persistent pruritic papules and plaques develop on the trunk, neck, face or extensor limbs. These may be urticated or violaceous [128,130]. Histologically, a distinctive distribution of dyskeratotic keratinocytes is seen in the stratum corneum [128,130]. Similar findings have been reported in adults.

Management

Methotrexate has been the mainstay of management of juvenile idiopathic arthritis, although blockade of IL-1 and IL-6 with drugs such as anakinra or tocilizumab is especially valuable in this systemic variant [138]. Macrophage activation syndrome is a potentially fatal complication of Still disease. Expansion of haemophagocytic macrophages and lymphocyte activation leads to a cytokine storm, which requires steroids, cyclosporine and specific anticytokine therapy such as IL-1 or IL-18 blockade and/or JAK inhibitors [139].

Synovitis, acne, pustulosis, hyperostosis and osteitis syndrome

Synonyms and inclusions
- Synovitis, acne, pustulosis, hyperostosis and osteitis (SAPHO) syndrome
- Pustulopsoriatic hyperostotic spondylarthritis

Introduction and general description

The association of synovitis, acne, pustulosis, hyperostosis and osteitis was first described in 1987 [140]. Together with CRMO, it resembles monogenic syndromes such as Majeed syndrome (see earlier) but no genetic basis has been determined as yet. Synovitis, acne, pustulosis, hyperostosis and osteitis (SAPHO) syndrome is rare, with a prevalence of fewer than four per 10 000. Female children and young adults are predominantly affected.

Clinical features

Skin manifestations are commoner in adults than in children. A neutrophilic palmoplantar pustulosis is the commonest dermatosis. Acne conglobata, acne fulminans and hidradenitis suppurativa occur predominantly in men [141]. Pyoderma gangrenosum and Sweet syndrome are rare.

There may be associated IBD and systemic features such as fever in around 10% of patients [142]. Musculoskeletal changes can occur without skin lesions [140]. Bone pain can be severe and recurrent, often worse at night. The sternoclavicular joint is most affected, although it can involve other sites such as the thoracic spine and mandible [143]. Long bone involvement is commoner in children [142], whereas adults may develop synovitis at remote sites [144–146]. There may be associated soft-tissue swelling and redness, raising the possibility of a suppurative osteomyelitis. Radiological features may support this misdiagnosis; the affected bones show osteosclerosis with cortical thinning and a narrowed medullary canal with blurring and irregularity of the external surface. Bone histology reveals a sterile inflammatory infiltrate [145,146]. *Cutibacterium acnes* and other organisms have been isolated in bone lesions, although their significance remains uncertain [147].

Management

Treatment of the musculoskeletal symptoms includes non-steroidal anti-inflammatory drugs, corticosteroids and bisphosphonates, notably intravenous pamidronate [148,149]. Several biological agents have been used to good effect, including anti-TNF and anti-IL-1 drugs and more recently ustekinumab (anti-IL-12/IL-23), anti-IL-17 and JAK inhibitors [149–153].

Yao syndrome

Synonyms and inclusions
- NOD2-associated autoinflammatory disease

Yao syndrome is a sporadic disease occurring in patients in their forties characterised by recurrent fever, fatigue, rash, polyarthritis (hip, ankle, shoulder, wrist), sicca syndrome (without anti-SSA/SSB antibodies), serositis and abdominal pain or diarrhoea. The skin findings are pruritic or non-pruritic macules, patches, papules or plaques on the face, trunk and extremities, and oedema of lower extremities [154]. Biopsy reveals a spongiotic dermatitis with a moderate perivascular lymphohistiocytic dermal infiltrate. Treatment relies on topical or low dose oral corticosteroids. Some variants in the *NOD2* gene seem to confer susceptibility.

Resources

Further information
Eurofever Project https://www.printo.it/eurofever/index (last accessed May 2023).

Patient resources
Autoinflammation Network (ANEV) http://autoinflammation.net/en/home_en/ (last accessed May 2023).

National Organization for Rare Disorders (NORD) https://www.rarediseases.org/rare-disease-information/rare-diseases (last accessed May 2023).

Key references

The full list of references can be found in the online version at https://www.wiley.com/rooksdermatology10e

1 Beck DB, Ferrada MA, Sikora KA *et al.* Somatic mutations in *UBA1* and severe adult-onset autoinflammatory disease. *N Engl J Med* 2020;383:2628–38.

2 Kieffer C, Cribier B, Lipsker D. Neutrophilic urticarial dermatosis: a variant of neutrophilic urticaria strongly associated with systemic disease. Report of 9 new cases and review of the literature. *Medicine (Baltimore)* 2009;88:23–31.

5 Savic S, Caseley EA, McDermott MF. Moving towards a systems-based classification of innate immune-mediated diseases. *Nat Rev Rheumatol* 2020;16:222–37.

16 Gattorno M, Hofer M, Federici S *et al.* Classification criteria for autoinflammatory recurrent fevers. *Ann Rheum Dis* 2019;78:1025–32.

35 Masters SL, Lagou V, Jéru I *et al.* Familial autoinflammation with neutrophilic dermatosis reveals a regulatory mechanism of pyrin activation. *Sci Transl Med* 2016;8(332):332ra45.

61 de Jesus AA, Hou Y, Brooks S *et al.* Distinct interferon signatures and cytokine patterns define additional systemic autoinflammatory diseases. *J Clin Invest* 2020;130:1669–82.

70 Liu Y, Jesus AA, Marrero B, Yang D *et al.* Activated STING in a vascular and pulmonary syndrome. *N Engl J Med* 2014;371:507–18.

103 Meyts I, Aksentijevich I. Deficiency of adenosine deaminase 2 (DADA2): updates on the phenotype, genetics, pathogenesis, and treatment. *J Clin Immunol* 2018;38:569–78.

109 Grandemange S, Sanchez E, Louis-Plence P *et al.* A new autoinflammatory and autoimmune syndrome associated with NLRP1 mutations: NAIAD (*NLRP1*-associated autoinflammation with arthritis and dyskeratosis). *Ann Rheum Dis* 2017;76:1191–8.

121 Lipsker D, Veran Y, Grunenberger F *et al.* The Schnitzler syndrome. Four new cases and review of the literature. *Medicine (Baltimore)* 2001;80:37–44.

CHAPTER 46

Mastocytosis

Clive E. H. Grattan[1] *and Deepti H. Radia*[1,2]

[1] St John's Institute of Dermatology, Guy's and St Thomas' NHS Foundation Trust, London, UK
[2] Department of Haematology, Guy's and St Thomas' NHS Foundation Trust, London, UK

Mastocytosis

Definition and nomenclature

Mastocytosis is a rare condition characterised by too many neoplastic mast cells in the skin and other tissues. A bone marrow biopsy usually reveals an aberrant mast cell immunophenotype, with clonal mast cells expressing mutations in *KIT* encoding the receptor for stem cell factor (KIT).

The term maculopapular cutaneous mastocytosis (MPCM) used in the World Health Organization (WHO) classification of mastocytosis embraces urticaria pigmentosa and telangiectasia macularis eruptiva perstans (TMEP). This is logical because some patients with extensive urticaria pigmentosa have a marked red, patchy component (Figure 46.1) and the original descriptions of TMEP included classic lesions of urticaria pigmentosa (see Clinical features later in this chapter).

Classification

The 2016 WHO classification of mastocytosis [1] is shown in Box 46.1.

Most cases presenting to dermatology clinics with skin lesions will be cutaneous in children or indolent systemic in adults. However, the distinction between cutaneous and systemic disease is becoming blurred by finding clonal *KIT* mutations in the peripheral blood of most adults and some children with cutaneous signs of mastocytosis who have not had a bone marrow biopsy. Aggressive systemic mastocytosis (ASM) and mast cell leukaemia (MCL) are rare. Patients with systemic mastocytosis with an associated haematological (non-mast cell lineage) neoplasm (SM-AHN), ASM or MCL are said to have advanced SM. Within the advanced systemic mastocytosis category up to 70% of the patients may have an AHN, most commonly myeloid. It should be noted that the WHO classification carries no implication that one pattern will naturally evolve to another more serious form although this may occur.

Introduction and general description

The first description of mastocytosis was made by Nettleship and Tay in 1869 [2]. The term urticaria pigmentosa was used by Sangster

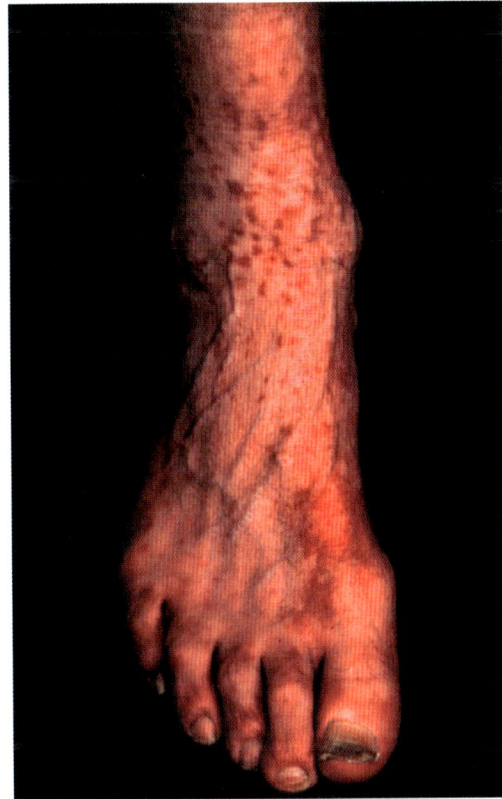

Figure 46.1 Patient with maculopapular cutaneous mastocytosis showing urticaria pigmentosa and telangiectasia macularis eruptiva perstans.

to describe the skin lesions in 1878 [3], but it was not until 1936 that the term 'mastocytosis' was proposed by Sézary to describe skin and systemic involvement together [4].

Distinguishing between cutaneous and systemic mastocytosis in patients presenting with skin lesions depends on further investigation, including bone marrow biopsy and blood tryptase measurements. Most adult cases will have systemic disease when investigated by bone marrow biopsy but other tissues, including the gut and liver, may be involved (see criteria for the diagnosis of systemic mastocytosis later in this chapter). Those with confirmed

---

Box 46.1 Classification of mastocytosis (World Health Organization 2016 revision)

Cutaneous mastocytosis (CM)
- Maculopapular cutaneous mastocytosis (MPCM)[a]:
  - Monomorphic (usually adults)
  - Polymorphic (usually children)
- Mastocytoma
- Diffuse cutaneous mastocytosis (DCM)

Systemic mastocytosis (SM)
- Indolent systemic mastocytosis (ISM)
- Smouldering indolent systemic mastocytosis
- Systemic mastocytosis with an associated haematological (non-mast cell lineage) neoplasm (SM-AHN)
- Aggressive systemic mastocytosis (ASM)
- Mast cell leukaemia (MCL)

Mast cell sarcoma

[a] Urticaria pigmentosa and telangiectasia macularis eruptiva perstans (TMEP) are not included in the WHO classification. They should be considered as useful descriptive terms within MPCM.

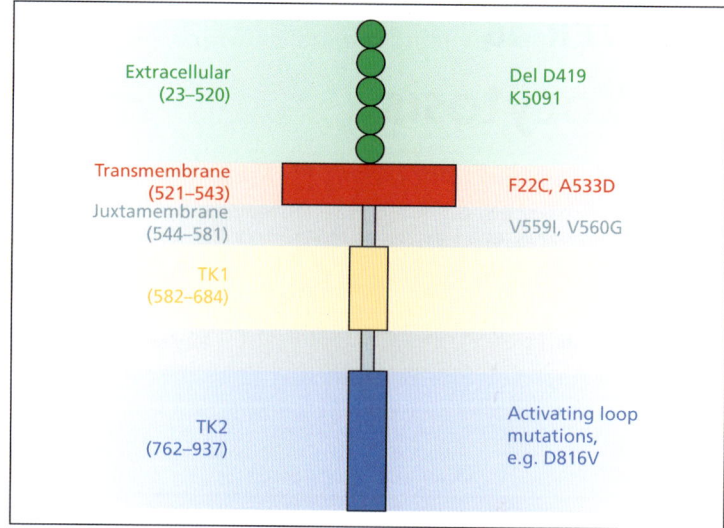

Figure 46.2 Schematic diagram of KIT, the receptor for stem cell factor on mast cells.

skin involvement who have not been investigated with bone marrow for systemic disease are said to have 'mastocytosis in the skin' [5]. About 10% of patients with systemic mastocytosis do not have skin lesions (known as bone marrow mastocytosis (BMM) in patients with indolent systemic disease). Some will present with anaphylaxis, especially after hymenoptera stings.

Aetiopathogenesis

The symptoms of mastocytosis are primarily due to mast cell mediator release. There is increasing evidence that mast cells accumulate in tissues as a direct consequence of acquiring a gain-of-function mutation of *KIT*, which encodes the transmembrane receptor for stem cell factor (KIT). Activation of KIT enhances the survival and migration of tissue mast cells. Several amino acid substitutions have been described in KIT, the commonest being D816V in the intracellular TK2 domain (Figure 46.2). About 90% of adults with systemic mastocytosis have this mutation. Extracellular, transmembrane and juxtamembrane mutations have also been reported, especially in childhood mastocytosis where the common activating D816V mutation is less frequently present [6]. Three of six children were found to have a novel dominant inactivating mutation in codon 839 [7]. Another study, using archived skin biopsies, reported a mutation of codon 816 (exon 17) in 42% of children with cutaneous mastocytosis and mutations outside exon 17 in 44%. There was no clear phenotype–genotype correlation or relationship between familial versus spontaneous disease [8]. KIT is also expressed on haemopoietic stem cells and melanocytes, which might be relevant to the development of myeloproliferative and myelodysplastic disorders in mastocytosis. The reason for hyperpigmentation in lesions of urticaria pigmentosa is unclear.

Epidemiology

Incidence and prevalence

Mastocytosis is uncommon. Population estimates suggest a lifetime prevalence in the region of 1 in 10 000 to 1 in 30 000 including children and adults although reliable data are not available. The incidence of new cases of mastocytosis is bimodal with about one third of cases presenting in childhood.

Age

The majority of childhood mastocytosis cases present in the first 2 years of life. Adults generally present between their third to sixth decades [9].

Sex

There is no gender difference.

Ethnicity

Most of the reported cases of mastocytosis have been in white people but whether this represents a greater susceptibility of white-skinned individuals to develop the disease or a reporting bias is unknown.

Associated diseases

Despite a higher incidence of anaphylaxis in systemic than cutaneous mastocytosis [10], there is no increase in atopy [11] or specific sensitisation to inhalant, food or sting allergens. Hereditary alpha tryptasaemia (HAT) is more prevalent in mastocytosis than in the general population [12] and may be an augmenting factor for anaphylaxis. About 20% of adults with indolent systemic mastocytosis (ISM) have osteoporosis [13] and a higher proportion have osteopenia. Osteosclerosis, osteolysis and bone cysts may occur. Vertebral fractures are seen in about 20% of patients with osteoporosis, especially in men. The lifetime risk of adults developing an associated non-mast cell haematological disorder should become clearer as cumulative data from the European Competence Network Registry become available but it has been estimated at around 20% of adults with ISM [14].

Pathophysiology
Pathology
Skin. Dermal mast cell numbers are increased in cutaneous mastocytosis [15]. The epidermis is normal apart from an increase in melanin. The mast cells are usually oval or spindle shaped (Figure 46.3a) with granules that stain metachromatically with toluidine blue but may be large and clustered in mastocytoma (Figure 46.3b). They are also well demonstrated by Giemsa, tryptase, CD117 or chloroacetate esterase (Figure 46.3a, inset) stains

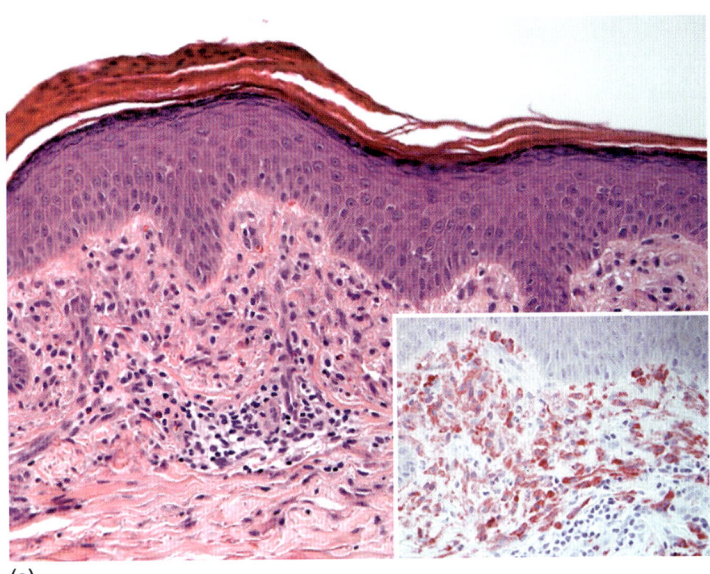

(a)

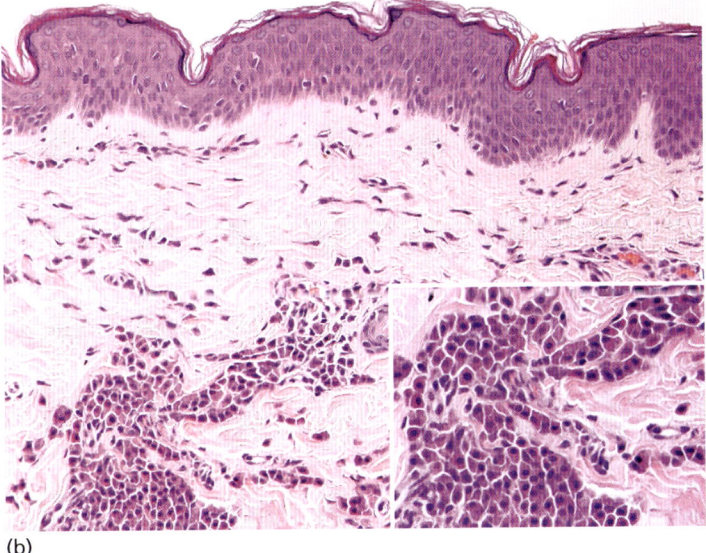

(b)

Figure 46.3 Histopathology of skin lesions. (a) Urticaria pigmentosa in an adult showing mast cell infiltrates predominantly around blood vessels and skin appendages in the papillary dermis. Magnification 100× (H&E); inset stained with chloroacetate esterase, magnification 400×. (b) Skin biopsy of a child with mastocytomas showing large numbers of well-defined dermal mast cells in clusters. Magnification 100× (H&E); inset with detail, magnification 200× (H&E). Courtesy of Alistair Robson.

in formalin-fixed biopsies. Mast cell infiltrates are predominantly found around blood vessels and skin appendages in the papillary dermis. In urticaria pigmentosa, they are increased up to 15-fold above normal [16], estimated to be around 40 mast cells/mm² [17]. A careful technique when taking the skin biopsy, to minimise traumatic degranulation, is important. Injecting local anaesthetic around the lesion to be biopsied may yield a higher number of mast cells identified by granule stains. Full-thickness infiltration of the skin or a band-like involvement of the upper dermis are seen in mastocytomas and diffuse cutaneous mastocytosis. By contrast, mast cells are confined to superficial capillaries and dilated venules in TMEP and may be only slightly increased over the numbers seen in normal skin.

Bone marrow. Bone marrow involvement typically presents with focal aggregates of mast cells seen on biopsy (Figure 46.4). The infiltration may be diffuse and spindle shaped. Mast cell infiltration of the marrow is often accompanied by increased numbers of immature neutrophils, phagocytosing macrophages, eosinophils and lymphocytes and sometimes by fibrosis [1,18]. Clonal mast cells typically co-express the aberrant markers CD25 and/or CD2 with tryptase, CD117 or both. The prognostic role of CD30 positivity is currently uncertain.

Genetics
Most mastocytosis is sporadic but familial mastocytosis has been reported [19]. Most of these families had urticaria pigmentosa, but four cases of TMEP occurred in three generations of one family, with an autosomal dominant pattern of inheritance. Heritability associated with germline mutations is extremely rare [17]. Eight germline *KIT* mutations have been reported, mainly in exons 8, 9, 10, 13 and 17 in contrast to somatic mutations that are mainly in exon 17. In families with autosomal dominant mastocytosis, patients usually have increased tryptase levels, systemic features and a chronic course [17]. Germline mutations in *KIT* have been reported in a few cases of familial mastocytosis with gastrointestinal stromal tumours [20].

Clinical features
Cutaneous mastocytosis
Maculopapular cutaneous mastocytosis
Urticaria pigmentosa
This is the commonest pattern of cutaneous mastocytosis in adults and children. Urticaria pigmentosa developed in the first year of life in 84% of 67 children [21]; the most common age of onset for adult disease is 20–40 years. Numerous reddish brown or pale monomorphic maculopapules, plaques or nodules appear in a symmetrical distribution anywhere on the body, with the highest concentration usually being on the lower trunk (Figure 46.5) and thighs (Figure 46.6). Lesions may be seen in the hairline of children and on the neck of adults but it is unusual for the face to be affected. They characteristically urticate within minutes of gentle rubbing (Darier sign) in children and some adults causing localised pruritus, redness and wealing (Figure 46.7), which subside within an hour. Gentle skin stroking does not produce wealing between lesions of urticaria pigmentosa (Figure 46.8). Stroking lesional and perilesional skin with a calibrated dermographometer at 20–36 g/mm² provides a useful

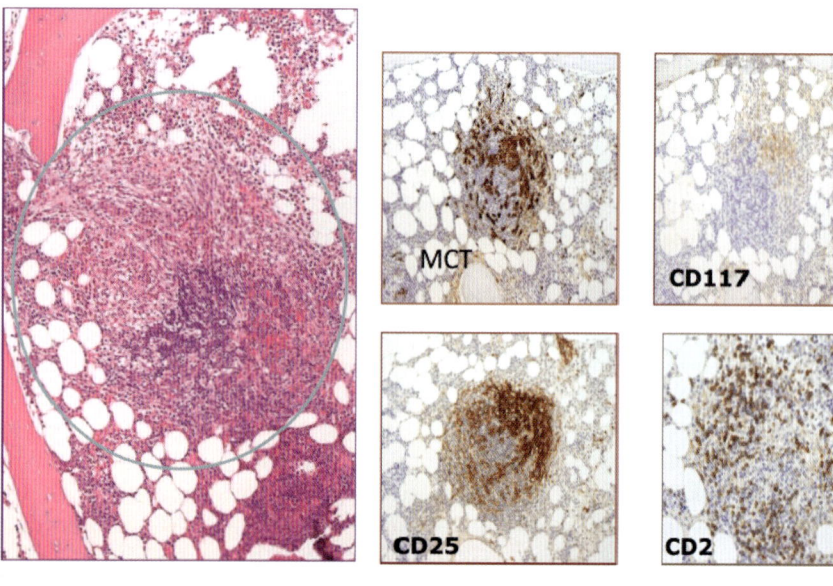

Figure 46.4 Systemic mastocytosis involving the bone marrow (H&E). Malignant whorls of rounded and spindle-shaped mast cells are seen infiltrating the bone marrow in a paratrabecular distribution (circle). Expression of CD2, CD25 and mast cell tryptase (MCT) is seen. Courtesy of Dr Deepti Radia.

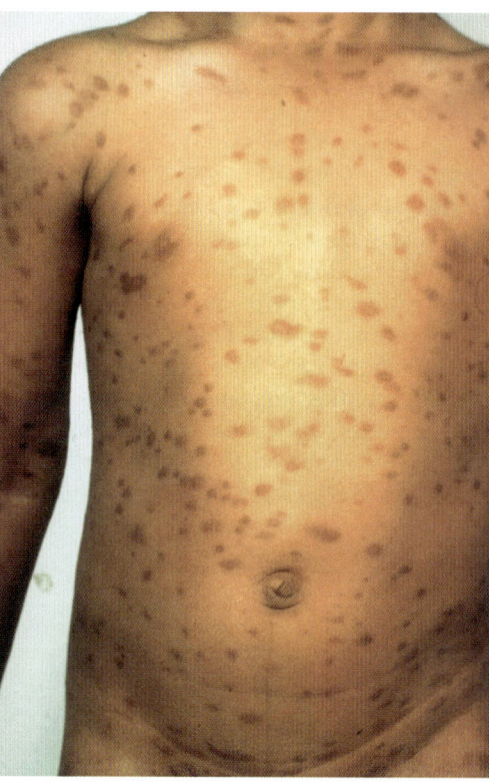

Figure 46.5 Urticaria pigmentosa lesions on the trunk of a child. Courtesy of St John's Institute of Dermatology.

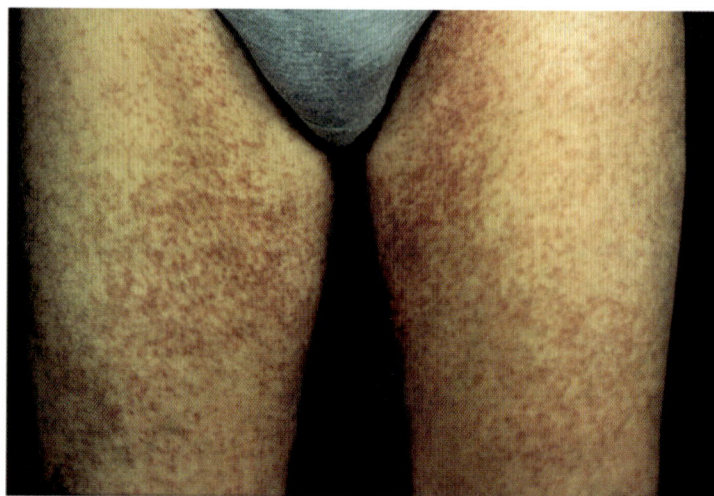

Figure 46.6 Monomorphic urticaria pigmentosa on the thighs of an adult. Courtesy of St John's Institute of Dermatology.

demonstration of selective wealing within lesions. A positive result can substitute for skin biopsy in very young children. However, the Darier sign is not always demonstrable, especially in the adult form of urticaria pigmentosa with a long history of the disorder or a child with resolving lesions; nor is it 100% specific for mastocytosis, since it has been described very rarely in juvenile xanthogranuloma [22] and acute lymphoblastic leukaemia of neonates [23]. Lesions may blister in infancy, and this may be the presenting feature, but heal without scarring. Bullous mastocytosis is not a specific clinical pattern. It is most often seen in infants with mastocytomas

and diffuse cutaneous mastocytosis due to intense subepidermal oedema resulting from mast cell degranulation. A recent consensus statement recommended that urticaria pigmentosa should be subdivided into two variants: a monomorphic variant with small maculopapular lesions, which is typically seen in adult patients, and a polymorphic variant with larger lesions of variable size and shape, which is typically seen in paediatric patients (Box 46.1). Clinical observation suggests that the monomorphic variant, if present in children, often persists into adulthood, whereas the polymorphic variant may resolve around puberty [24].

Flushing occurs in about 50% of patients, alcohol intolerance and pruritus in slightly less [25]. Other symptoms may include heat or cold intolerance, recurrent diarrhoea, acid dyspepsia and urinary frequency. Depression and headache are common. Wheezing is often quoted but is, in reality, extremely rare as a presentation of mastocytosis. Syncope due to hypotension is usually a presenting feature of anaphylaxis. Early studies indicated that about 60% of adult patients have bone marrow involvement [26,27] but it is now thought that the proportion of adults with skin lesions

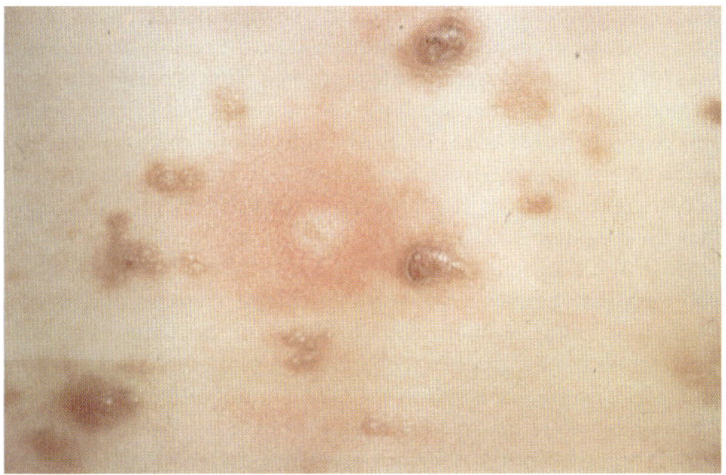

Figure 46.7 Positive Darier sign in a nodule of urticaria pigmentosa in a young child. Courtesy of Norfolk and Norwich University Hospital.

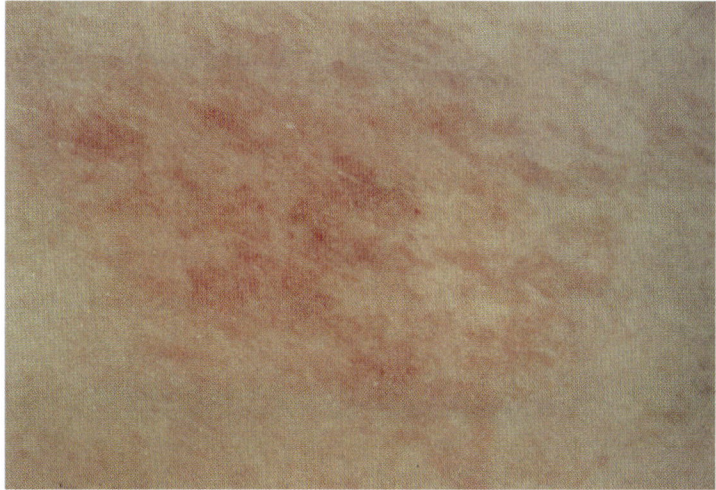

Figure 46.9 Telangiectasia macularis eruptiva perstans. Courtesy of St John's Institute of Dermatology.

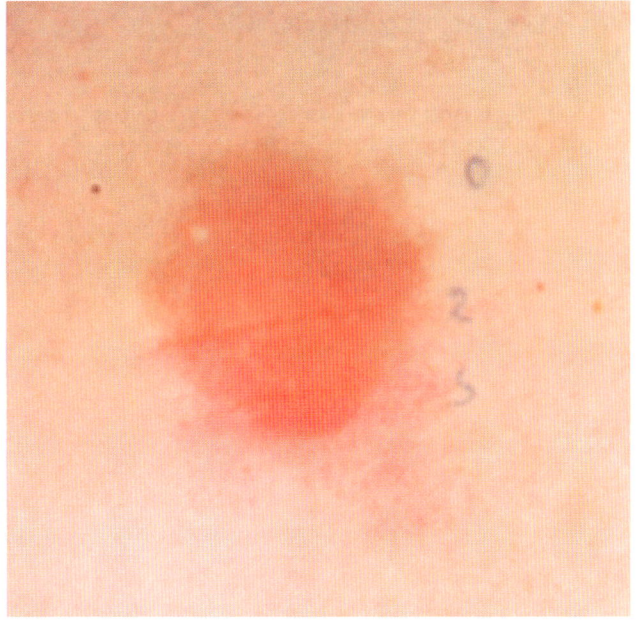

Figure 46.8 Wealing is confined to the lesion of urticaria pigmentosa, not the adjacent skin at three different settings of a calibrated dermographometer (0, 2, 5).

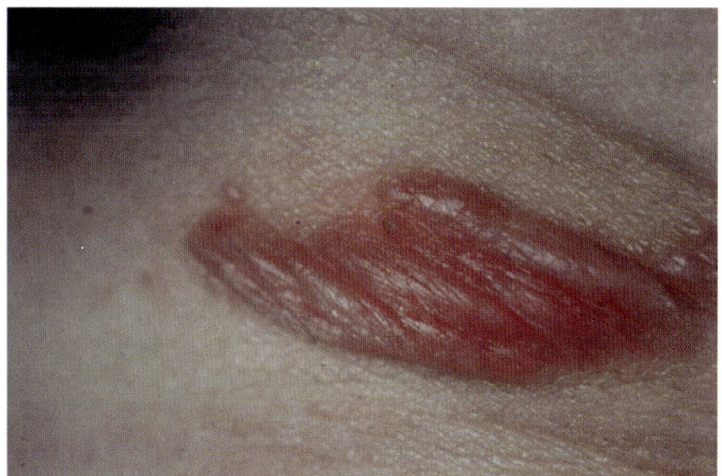

Figure 46.10 Pink mastocytoma in an infant. Courtesy of St John's Institute of Dermatology.

who have ISM is as high as 90–95% [9]. There is no obvious relationship between finding ISM on biopsy and symptomatology or prognosis [26]. Using sensitive molecular genetic techniques (e.g. digitial droplet polymerase chain reaction, ddPCR) on bone marrow aspirate, blood or skin, up to 95% of adults with MPCM have evidence of a clonal mast cell disease [28]. Clearance or fading of urticaria pigmentosa was observed in 12 of 106 adult patients with confirmed bone marrow involvement who were followed for 12–20 years, with a parallel overall improvement in the patients' well-being [29].

Telangiectasia macularis eruptiva perstans. Fixed red patches may rarely be the predominant clinical feature of cutaneous mastocytosis. Patients are usually adults presenting with persistent red patches that usually do not show obvious telangiectasia, especially on the trunk, which flush but usually do not urticate on rubbing (Figure 46.9). Finding excess mast cells on skin biopsy will confirm the clinical suspicion, although they are usually not numerous. It has been discussed whether the term TMEP should include patients with urticaria pigmentosa or should be restricted to those without it [30]. Whether the very rare 'pure' TMEP without urticaria pigmentosa carries a better overall prognosis when it is restricted to the skin is unclear. It tends to be persistent and unresponsive to treatment.

Mastocytoma. Cutaneous mastocytosis may present with red, pink or yellowish nodules or plaques in infancy or early childhood, measuring up to 3–4 cm in diameter (Figure 46.10). They are usually solitary. About 15% of young children will present with mastocytomas [31]. If multiple, the lesions can be difficult to distinguish from nodular urticaria pigmentosa. They tend to blister if rubbed, especially in the napkin area of infants and flushing can be induced by rubbing a solitary mastocytoma [32]. Nearly all mastocytomas involute over the first few years of childhood.

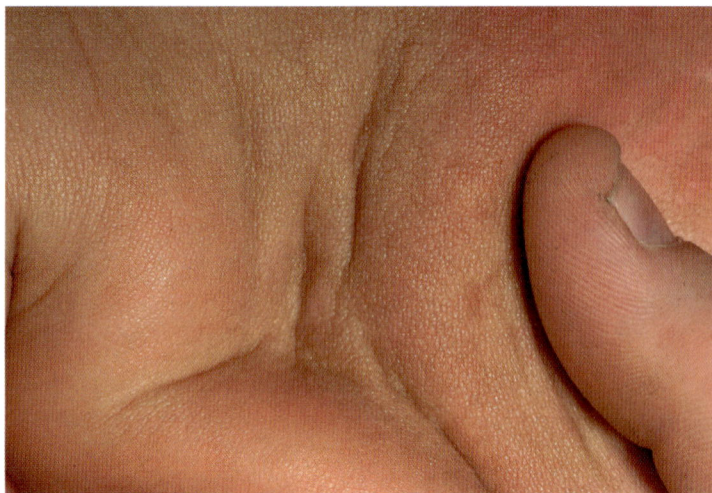

Figure 46.11 Diffuse cutaneous mastocytosis on the back.

Diffuse cutaneous mastocytosis. This is a very rare form of mastocytosis in which mast cells infiltrate the entire skin diffusely. It usually presents in the neonatal period. The skin tends to be thickened and doughy in consistency (Figure 46.11) but may be smooth. Skin colour may be normal or almost red. Pigmentation is usually absent. Blistering after minor trauma or scratching is common and pruritus for the child may be intense. The epidermis may be lost temporarily due to the intense dermal oedema over a large area and can resemble impetigo. Patients with this type of mastocytosis are at risk of systemic disease and severe complications including anaphylaxis and diarrhoea [33], but it usually improves naturally over childhood and may resolve.

Systemic mastocytosis

Patients must meet at least one major and one minor, or three minor, criteria from the WHO criteria (Box 46.2) to be diagnosed with systemic disease [1].

Box 46.2 World Health Organization criteria for systemic mastocytosis

Systemic mastocytosis is defined by finding 1 major + 1 minor *or* 3 minor criteria on bone marrow biopsy

1 **Major:** multifocal aggregates of at least 15 mast cells in bone marrow or other organ (not skin)
2 **Minor:**
   a. More than 25% of mast cells in infiltrates are spindle shaped or atypical in bone marrow biopsy or other tissue, *or* >25% of mast cells in bone marrow aspirate smears are immature or atypical
   b. Activating mutations in *KIT* (e.g. codon 816) in bone marrow, blood or other tissue (not skin)
   c. Coexpression of CD117 with CD2 and/or CD25 in bone marrow mast cells, blood or other tissue (not skin)
   d. Serum tryptase >20 µg/L (unless associated with clonal myeloid disorder)

Not all patients with proven bone marrow involvement will be symptomatic, but in those who are nausea, cramping, hyperacidity, diarrhoea, palpitations, hypotension, syncope, headache, dyspnoea (and occasionally wheeze in children), itch, fatigue and 'brain fogginess' may feature as significant symptoms. This is partly due to the release of cutaneous mast cell mediators which have distant effects and partly to direct local effects of infiltration in other tissues, such as the gastrointestinal tract. Bone pain, bone cysts, premature osteoporosis, osteosclerosis or spontaneous fractures should prompt further investigation.

Most adult patients investigated for urticaria pigmentosa with bone marrow biopsy will have ISM. Blood tryptase and urinary methylhistamine or methylimidazole acetic acid may be useful markers for bone marrow involvement. A persistent blood tryptase of 20 µg/L or greater is one of the WHO minor criteria for the diagnosis of systemic mastocytosis [1]. However, a persistently raised blood tryptase is not diagnostic of systemic mastocytosis since it can occur in other conditions, including myeloproliferative neoplasms, hereditary α-tryptasaemia, chronic kidney disease and rarely in chronic spontaneous urticaria (Box 46.3) [34,35]. A diagnosis of systemic mastocytosis may be made in patients with a tryptase of less than 20 µg/L if other criteria are met.

Box 46.3 Reasons for a persistently raised blood tryptase in a patient without skin lesions

Haematological
- Systemic mastocytosis
- Chronic myeloid leukaemia
- Myelodysplastic syndrome
- Myeloproliferative neoplasm
- Others, e.g. eosinophilic and basophilic leukaemias

Increased copy number of the *TPSAB1* gene
- Hereditary α-tryptasaemia

Others
- Renal failure
- Chronic spontaneous urticaria

An algorithm for the assessment of patients with an elevated blood tryptase without skin lesions of mastocytosis is shown in Figure 46.12 [35].

Although there is a risk of progression of ISM to SM-AHN or aggressive systemic mastocytosis, the literature indicates that this is unusual and there are no reliable markers to identify subgroups of patients at greater risk of this. Mast cell leukaemia is much more likely to present to a haematologist *de novo* than to a dermatologist, with changes in the peripheral blood picture against a background of being unwell with lymphadenopathy or organomegaly.

Monoclonal mast cell activation syndrome

Patients with evidence of episodic mast cell activation who show evidence of clonality on bone marrow biopsy (CD25 expression on mast cells and/or *KIT* D816V mutation) but do not meet the criteria for systemic mastocytosis are said to have monoclonal mast cell activation syndrome. There is an implication that these patients are at risk of developing systemic mastocytosis and, as a consequence, should be under review.

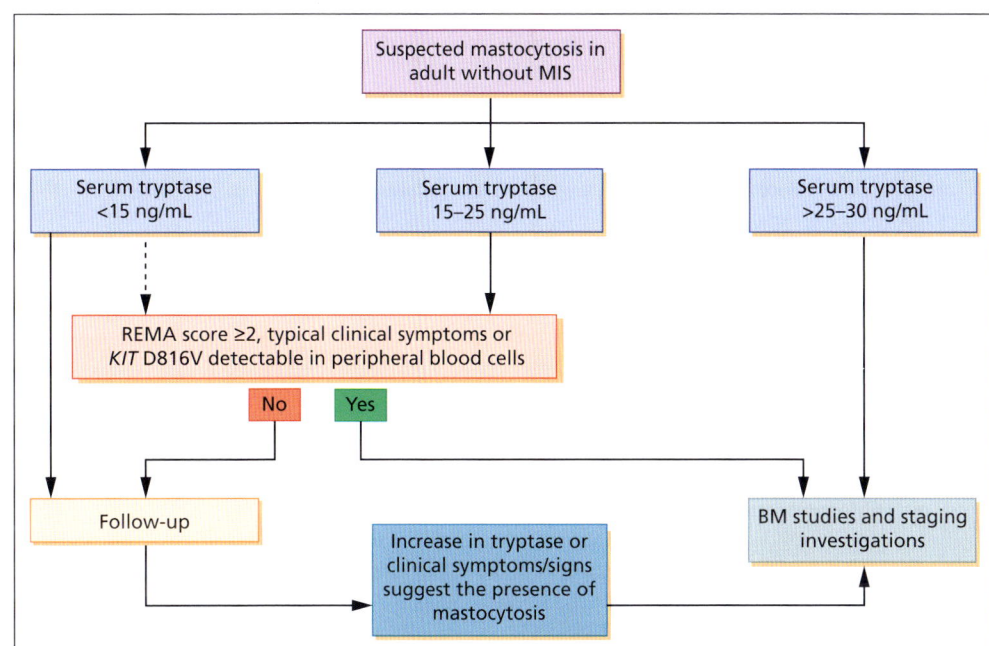

Figure 46.12 Algorithm for the assessment of patients with a raised tryptase but no evidence of mastocytosis in the skin (MIS). BM, bone marrow; REMA, Red Española de Mastocitosis.

Mast cell activation syndrome

Patients may present with episodic symptoms of systemic mast cell mediator release. The term 'mast cell activation syndrome' has been applied to patients with primary clonal mast cell disease (mastocytosis or monoclonal mast cell activation syndrome), mast cell activation secondary to known causes (e.g. immunoglobulin E (IgE) mediated or non-IgE mediated anaphylaxis), or idiopathic anaphylaxis [36]. Mast cell activation syndrome may be considered when patients present with mast cell mediator symptoms in at least two body systems (e.g. skin/respiratory/gastrointestinal/ cardiovascular), respond to antimast cell mediator therapies and can be shown to have evidence of mast cell mediator release during an episode (rise and fall in blood tryptase or increase in urinary histamine breakdown products including N-methyl histamine, leukotriene C_4 or prostaglandin 11βPGF2-α (a metabolite of prostaglandin D_2)).

Co-morbidities

In a population-controlled study of the national Danish registry for systemic mastocytosis, there was an increased risk of solid cancers, including melanoma and non-melanoma skin cancers, and venous thromboembolism in addition to known increased risks of anaphylaxis and osteoporosis [37]. Anaphylaxis after bee and wasp stings and drugs (including some anaesthetic agents) is increased in adults, especially with systemic mastocytosis, but may be multifactorial and unpredictable.

Disease course and prognosis

Most mastocytomas resolve in the first decade. Over 50% of children with urticaria pigmentosa clear by adolescence. In a review of 67 paediatric cases, five resolved over 2 years of follow-up and 20 improved but did not clear over a mean period of 6 years [38]. Complete regression of skin lesions is mostly seen in mastocytomas and paediatric MPCM [17]. Spontaneous resolution of cutaneous

mastocytosis was observed in about 10% of adults [39]. The main problems likely to be experienced by patients relate to the risks of anaphylaxis and osteoporosis. Patients with ISM/smouldering systemic mastocytosis have a better overall survival than those with advanced systemic mastocytosis. Prognostic scores for systemic mastocytosis have been developed to predict and improve outcomes and now include the mutational landscape in these patients in addition to the *KIT* D816V mutation; additional mutations including the presence of *SRSF2*, *ASXL1* and *RUNX1* confer a poorer prognosis. The prognosis of advanced mastocytosis with an associated blood disorder will relate to the associated haematological disorder, and management will be directed primarily towards this.

Investigations

A skin biopsy should be done to confirm a clinical diagnosis of mastocytosis in the skin in adults although observation alone is often appropriate in very young children unless there is diagnostic doubt, especially those with a solitary mastocytoma, in whom systemic disease is very unlikely and those with a convincing positive Darier sign. As a general rule, children with mastocytomas and urticaria pigmentosa do not require extensive investigation if they are well. Taking a history, examination for hepatosplenomegaly, full blood count and differential, liver function, ImmununoCAP® for IgE sensitisation to bee and wasp venoms, and tryptase with skin biopsy (unless there are clinical reasons for not doing so) is sufficient.

A full blood count, biochemical profile, total IgE with specific IgE to bee and wasp venoms, vitamin D and tryptase should be performed at presentation in adults (Box 46.4). A dual-energy X-ray absorptiometry (DEXA) scan should be done at baseline and every 3–5 years in adults but not children. A blood count, liver profile and tryptase should be done annually at least when systemic disease is either suspected or proven (Figure 46.13). Other investigations should be guided by the clinical presentation.

Box 46.4 Protocol for the diagnostic work-up of adults with suspected mastocytosis

Initial assessment
- *History*, to include specific enquiry about:
  - Allergic reactions, including *Hymenoptera* stings and bites
  - Bowel symptoms, including dyspepsia, diarrhoea and abdominal pain
  - Bone pain
- *Examination*, to *include*:
  - Head to toe skin assessment (including melanoma)
  - Abdominal and lymph node examination
  - Blood pressure and weight
  - Clinical photography
- *Standard investigations*, to include:
  - Skin biopsy:
    - Atraumatic sample of lesional skin using a 4 mm punch biopsy (with an option of accompanying normal skin biopsy for comparative mast cell number counts) if the clinical diagnosis is uncertain
    - Local anaesthesia (preferably ring block)
    - Formalin preservative for routine histopathology and mast cell stains
  - Blood tests:
    - Full blood count
    - Clinical chemistry profile
    - Tryptase
    - Vitamin D
    - Total IgE with ImmunoCAP® for specific IgE to bee and wasp venoms (and other relevant allergens, as suggested by the history)
    - DEXA (not in children)
  - Urine assays, none routinely

Further investigations (to be guided by the initial assessment)
- If full blood count is abnormal (e.g. unexplained eosinophilia, persistent leukocytosis or cytopenias), refer for further assessment by the haematology department
- If random tryptase is above 20 ng/mL on at least two occasions or there is a high clinical suspicion of systemic disease, refer for staging work-up to include:
  - Bone marrow biopsy and *KIT* D816V mutational analysis (adults, and children only if clinically necessary)
  - X-rays of thoraco-lumbar spine if fracture or collapse is suspected in adults with indolent systemic mastocytosis, especially men
  - If hepatosplenomegaly, perform an abdominal ultrasound scan proceeding to CT scan when appropriate
- If allergic disease is suspected on the history, especially in the context of anaphylaxis, refer for a full allergy assessment
- If peptic ulceration is suspected, refer for gastroscopy
- If there is bone pain, refer for X-ray examination (and ongoing referral to metabolic bone disease specialist)
- Repeat blood tryptase annually for monitoring if the initial level is greater than the laboratory normal range

CT, computed tomography; DEXA, dual-energy X-ray absorptiometry; IgE, immunoglobulin E.

Bone marrow examination is not obligatory in the absence of other features, such as anaemia, persistent leukocytosis, unexplained eosinophilia, hepatosplenomegaly or lymphadenopathy. Blood tryptase is a useful surrogate marker for bone marrow involvement but not diagnostic of systemic disease without other features being present [1]. A basal tryptase of 20 μg/L on at least two occasions in patients with skin lesions is a useful threshold for bone marrow biopsy in adult patients, although the significance of a raised tryptase in very young children with extensive skin involvement is less certain [40]. Adults may have ISM with a blood tryptase less than 20 μg/L. An abdominal ultrasound scan may be informative for suspected hepatosplenomegaly but should not form part of the routine investigation. Thoraco-lumbar spine X-rays should be performed in adult patients with systemic mastocytosis if the patient is symptomatic with vertebral bone pain. Current evaluation of highly sensitive mutation analysis enabling the detection of *KIT* D816V in peripheral blood leukocytes is increasingly being used and may, in future, provide a useful non-invasive test in children or adults with borderline tryptase levels [41,42].

Management (Box 46.5)

Most patients presenting to dermatology clinics with cutaneous mastocytosis or ISM will have an excellent prognosis, particularly children, thus it is important to provide reassurance about the nature and prognosis of the condition. A retrospective study from the Mayo Clinic of 159 adult patients showed no difference in lifetime survival between those with and those without ISM [43]. Management hinges on the avoidance of trigger factors for mast cell degranulation, symptomatic relief with antimast cell mediator drugs, provision of epinephrine, immunotherapy when appropriate (e.g. venom allergy) and early detection of systemic disease causing significant blood or bone complications. No cure is currently available but there is increasing evidence of the benefit of cytoreductive therapies in patients with organ dysfunction (B findings) or damage/failure (C findings) including tyrosine kinase inhibitors.

The flushing and itching experienced by many patients with cutaneous mastocytosis are due to the release of mast cell mediators. This can be exaggerated by physical stimuli, such as extremes of temperature, towelling, massage or alcohol. Potential triggers of mast cell degranulation include known allergens, non-steroidal anti-inflammatories, opiates, *Hymenoptera* venoms (even in the absence of IgE sensitisation), iodinated contrast media (especially ionic), dextrans and some muscle relaxants (Box 46.6). The impact of skin lesions on quality of life should not be underestimated.

Up to 50% of adults and 20% of children experience one or more episodes of anaphylaxis [17] so epinephrine autoinjectors should be prescribed for all adults with mastocytosis, especially those with proven or suspected systemic disease, children with widespread cutaneous mastocytosis and those with relevant IgE sensitisations, such as to bee or wasp venoms. Oral antihistamines are helpful for milder attacks of flushing or pruritic weals without respiratory difficulty or hypotension. Venom immunotherapy for patients with *Hymenoptera* sting anaphylaxis should be for life [44]. Fatal cardiovascular collapse during general anaesthesia has been reported [45]. Prophylactic corticosteroids and antihistamines before general anaesthesia are usually given [46] but will not prevent mast cell degranulation.

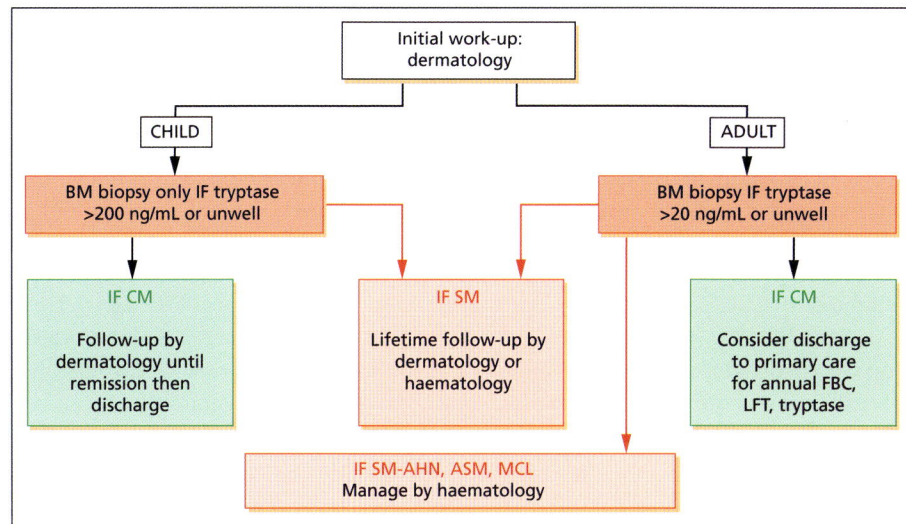

Figure 46.13 Algorithm for reviewing adults and children with mastocytosis. ASM, aggressive systemic mastocytosis; BM, bone marrow; CM, cutaneous mastocytosis; FBC, full blood count; LFT, liver function test; MCL, mast cell leukaemia; SM, systemic mastocytosis; SM-AHN, systemic mastocytosis with an associated haematological (non-mast cell lineage) neoplasm.

Box 46.5 Summary of management options for mastocytosis

- Avoid triggers of mast cell degranulation (Box 46.6)
- Treat systemic and skin symptoms due to mast cell mediator release:
  - Non-sedating (second generation) H_1 antihistamines (up-dosing allowed in line with chronic urticaria)
  - H_2 antihistamines (hyperacidity or dyspepsia)
  - Proton pump inhibitors
  - Sodium cromoglycate (orally for bowel symptoms)
- Consider skin-directed treatments for symptoms and for improving the appearance of lesion:
  - Topical corticosteroids (e.g. 0.05% clobetasol propionate cream twice daily for up to 6 weeks for urticaria pigmentosa on the body in adults but avoiding the face)
  - Topical 4% sodium cromoglycate cream for children, especially for bullous mastocytosis (if available)
  - Narrow-band ultraviolet B phototherapy or photochemotherapy (PUVA)
- Cytoreductive treatments for systemic mastocytosis with organ dysfunction or failure:
  - Oral corticosteroids (short term)
  - Interferon-α
  - Cladribine
  - KIT tyrosine kinase inhibitors
    - Imatinib (not effective for D816V-positive systemic mastocytosis)
    - Midostaurin
    - Avapritinib
    - Investigational drugs (e.g. masitinib)
- Manage complications:
  - Osteopenia and osteoporosis:
    - Vitamin D and calcium supplements
    - Bisphosphonates
- Haematological (chemotherapy protocols for AHN)
- Anaphylaxis (epinephrine autoinjectors should be offered to all adults with mastocytosis and children with extensive cutaneous mastocytosis)

AHN, associated haematological neoplasm; PUVA, psoralen and ultraviolet A.

Box 46.6 Potential mast cell degranulating stimuli

- Physical triggers (especially rubbing, heat or exertion)
- Non-steroidal anti-inflammatory drugs (e.g. aspirin, ibuprofen, diclofenac)
- Some general anaesthetic drugs:
  - Some non-depolarising muscle relaxants (e.g. atracurium, mivacurium)
  - Opiates (e.g. morphine, codeine)
  - Plasma volume expanders (e.g. dextrans)
  - Anticholinergics (e.g. hyoscine)
- Radiocontrast media (especially iodine-based ionic agents)
- Insect and snake venoms (allergic and non-allergic effects)
- Other allergens (e.g. latex)
- Alcohol

First line

Antihistamines. Non-sedating H1 antihistamines are the mainstay of therapy for mast cell mediator symptoms and may be given at higher than licensed doses. Itching and flushing can be controlled by antihistamines in many patients but can be refractory to treatment. Ketotifen has theoretical mast cell stabilising properties and is preferred by some patients but is often sedating. H_2 antihistamines and proton pump inhibitors are used for gastrointestinal symptoms, including indigestion.

Second line

Mast cell stabilising and anti-inflammatory drugs. Abdominal pain, nausea and diarrhoea also respond to sodium cromoglycate; however, this has little if any value for other systemic symptoms because it is not absorbed from the gut in any significant amount [47]. Aspirin and other non-steroidal anti-inflammatory drugs have been reported to ameliorate prostaglandin-mediated flushing in some patients, but must be introduced with caution, under cover of antihistamines and with initial observation, if there is any history of intolerance.

Photochemotherapy and phototherapy. Although oral psoralen and ultraviolet A (PUVA) may help pruritus and wealing and improve the appearance of urticaria pigmentosa [48], the benefits are only temporary so the risks of long-term treatment need to be considered carefully. The mechanism for improvement is not certain, but probably involves a reduction of mast cell numbers in the papillary dermis and of total histamine content in lesional skin [49], with some cosmetic improvement due to tanning. Narrow-band UVB therapy may be effective for pruritus when PUVA is not tolerated.

Topical corticosteroids and calcineurin inhibitors. Potent or very potent topical corticosteroids applied under polythene occlusion for 2 weeks or used without occlusion twice daily for 6 weeks in adults, or intralesional injection of corticosteroids into mastocytomas, can lead to clearance of mast cells and a reduction of pigmentation for at least a year [50]. Steroid atrophy is an important risk of continued treatment, especially in body flexures. Restriction to limited areas, such as the forearms and legs, will minimise significant adrenocortical suppression. Improvement was observed with 1% pimecrolimus cream in a small series of young children with cutaneous mastocytosis studied retrospectively [51], but efficacy of topical calcineurin inhibitors has not been confirmed in controlled studies.

Omalizumab. Omalizumab may be effective for recurrent anaphylaxis in systemic mastocytosis and improving mast cell mediator-related symptoms, especially in the skin, when insufficiently controlled by conventional therapy [52].

Third line

Cytoreductive treatment. Oral corticosteroids at high doses can offer temporary symptomatic improvement for patients with ASM. Patients with ISM who are symptomatic despite maximal antimast cell mediator treatments and those with advanced mastocytosis should be considered for cytoreductive or targeted treatments. Interferon α, usually given in combination with oral corticosteroids [53,54], and cladribine have been found to result in partial remissions in some patients but the latter can cause severe myelosuppression with risk of infections [55].

Tyrosine kinase inhibitors (TKIs) demonstrate efficacy in patients with advanced systemic mastocytosis, while imatinib shows efficacy in *KIT* D816V negative patients or those with unknown mutational status and in patients with a well-differentiated systemic mastocytosis variant with F522C transmembrane mutation/wild type *KIT*. Midostaurin – an oral multikinase inhibitor of wild type and D816V-mutated *KIT* as well as *FLT*3 and *PGRFR*α/β – has been approved for patients with advanced systemic mastocytosis demonstrating decreases in overall mast cell burden, a reduction in spleen size, and decreases in bone marrow mast cell burden with improved symptom scores [56]. The US Food and Drug Administration recently approved avapritinib (June 2021), an oral directed *KIT* D816V inhibitor for patients with advanced systemic mastocytosis. Significant reductions were seen in mast cell burden, with improved clearance of mast cell aggregates and a reduction in *KIT* allele burden becoming undetectable in some patients.

Finally, allogeneic bone marrow transplantation is an option for those patients with a suitable donor and more so with the promising results shown in the clearance of mast cells with the new TKIs. Treatment of an associated haematological disorder should be undertaken as appropriate for that disorder and the overall prognosis is usually that of the latter.

Resources

Patient resources

UK Masto: http://www.ukmasto.org/ (last accessed October 2022).

Key references

The full list of references can be found in the online version at https://www.wiley.com/rooksdermatology10e

1 Valent P, Akin C, Metcalfe DD. Mastocytosis: 2016 updated WHO classification and novel emerging treatment concepts. *Blood* 2017;129:1420–7.

5 Valent P, Akin C, Escribano M *et al*. Standards and standarization in mastocytosis: consensus statements on diagnostics. Treatment recommendations and response criteria. *Eur J Clin Investig* 2007;37:435–53.

9 Brockow K. Epidemiology, prognosis, and risk factors in mastocytosis. *Immunol Allergy Clin North Am* 2014;34:283–95.

10 Brockow K, Jofer C, Behrendt H, Ring J. Anaphylaxis in patients with mastocytosis: a study on history, clinical features and risk factors in 120 patients. *Allergy* 2008;63:226–32.

14 Akin C, Valent P. Diagnostic criteria and classification of mastocytosis in 2014. *Immunol Allergy Clin North Am* 2014;34:207–18.

17 Lange M, Hartmann K, Carter MC *et al*. Molecular background, clinical features and management of pediatric mastocytosis: status 2021. *Int J Mol Sci* 2021;22:2586.

18 Pardanani A, Tefferi A. Systemic mastocytosis in adults: a review on prognosis and treatment based on 342 Mayo Clinic patients and current literature. *Curr Opin Hematol* 2010;17:125–32.

35 Valent P, Escribano L, Broesby-Olsen S *et al*. Proposed diagnostic algorithm for patients with suspected mastocytosis: a proposal of the European Competence Network on Mastocytosis. *Allergy* 2014;69:1267–74.

36 Akin C. Mast cell activation syndromes. *J Allergy Clin Immunol* 2017;140:349–55.

43 Lim KH, Tefferi A, Lasho TL *et al*. Systemic mastocytosis in 342 consecutive adults: survival studies and prognostic factors. *Blood* 2009;113:5727–36.

46 Royal College of Anaesthetists (RCoA). *Mastocytosis and Anaesthesia, Advice for Patients*. London: RCoA, 2014 (reviewed 2017). http://www.rcoa.ac.uk/media/6656 (last accessed October 2022).

56 DeAngelo DJ, George TI, Linder A *et al*. Efficacy and safety of midostaurin in patients with advanced systemic mastocytosis: 10-year median follow-up of a phase II trial. *Leukemia* 2018;32:470–8.

CHAPTER 47

Reactive Inflammatory Erythemas

Ruth Murphy

Sheffield University, Sheffield; Sheffield Teaching Hospitals NHS Foundation Trust, Sheffield, UK

PART 4: INFLAMMATORY DERMATOSES

Introduction

Cutaneous annular erythemas may be classified as either (i) those due to a specific skin disorder such as psoriasis and tinea corporis; or (ii) a cutaneous inflammatory reaction to a trigger such as a drug, infection or malignancy or in some cases an unknown cause. Cases where no trigger is identified are described as idiopathic annular erythemas. This chapter describes the known patterns of reactive inflammatory erythemas, namely erythema multiforme (EM), annular erythema of infancy, necrolytic migratory erythema (NME), erythema annulare centrifugum, erythema chronicum migrans, erythema gyratum repens and erythema marginatum. When assessing a patient with a likely reactive erythema, knowledge of local disease prevalence and local use of therapeutics will be useful. For example, the advancement of immunotherapy for the treatment of metastatic melanoma with checkpoint inhibitors and the evolution of new infections such as SARS-CoV-2 are two recently identified triggers for these reactive erythemas. By inference, therefore, disease associations will be influenced by local population health and socioeconomic factors and will vary with geography and over time.

In contrast, the decline in streptococcal infections in certain parts of the world has made erythema marginatum relatively less common. When assessing a patient presenting with annular lesions, first decide whether this is specific to a known dermatological diagnosis such as psoriasis or whether it is a reactive erythema. It is also important to elicit a very comprehensive medical history including current and recent medication, symptoms of infection and occult malignancy, as the rash may herald the opportunity for early detection and treatment of an underlying cause. If a reactive erythema is considered likely, then identifying the subtype might be helpful, although there may be overlap between these. In the sections that follow the types of reactive erythemas are described and some of their associated triggers, with cross-referencing to other relevant chapters.

Erythema multiforme

Introduction and general description

Erythema multiforme is an immune-mediated disease characterised by target lesions that can occur anywhere on the skin and mucous membranes. They occur most commonly on the extremities on the hands and feet. Causality, for instance associations with infections, autoimmune disease and drugs, might be found but not always.

EM, Stevens–Johnson syndrome (SJS) and toxic epidermal necrolysis (TEN or Lyell syndrome) were considered to form a spectrum from mild to severe cases. There has been a re-evaluation of this concept and a tendency to consider EM minor and EM major as part of one spectrum, commonly following infections (especially with herpesvirus) where it is often recurrent in nature. Sometimes EM is due to drug reactions and in many cases no underlying cause is found.

SJS and TEN are discussed in detail in Chapter 118 and are more closely linked to drug sensitivities, although cases of TEN in children secondary to mycoplasma and herpesvirus infections have been reported. SJS and TEN may be regarded as severe variants of a single disease [1,2–5]. In this chapter, we will describe EM and its associated drug and infection triggers.

EM is best regarded as a self-limiting cytotoxic dermatitis resulting from cell-mediated hypersensitivity most commonly to drugs or infection. It presents clinically with a spectrum of macular, papular or urticarial lesions, as well as the classic acral iris or 'target lesions' (Figure 47.1). Lesions may involve the palms or trunk, as well as the oral and genital mucosal membranes, which are associated with erosions. On the other hand, SJS, first described in 1922, comprises extensive EM of the trunk and mucous membranes (Figure 47.2), accompanied by fever, malaise, myalgia and arthralgia [6,7]. Lyell first reported TEN in 1956 [8], which was characterised by extensive, sheet-like skin erosions with widespread purpuric

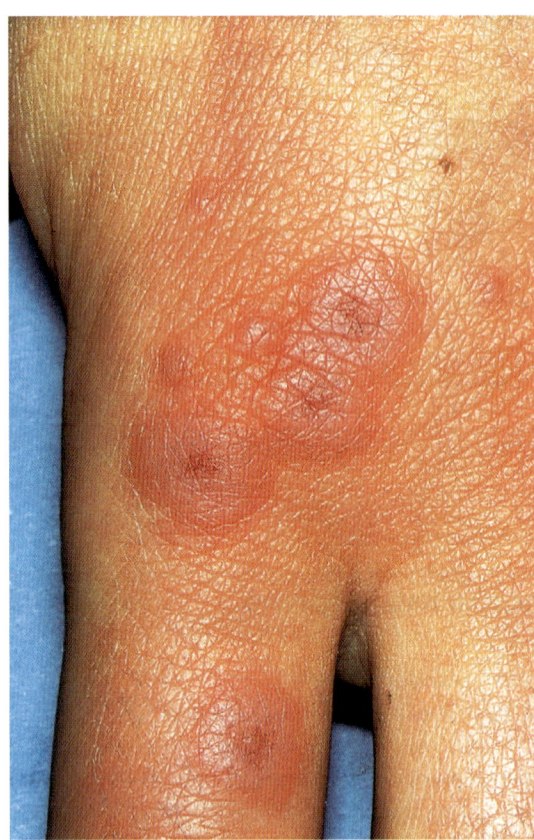

Figure 47.1 Classic target lesion in erythema multiforme.

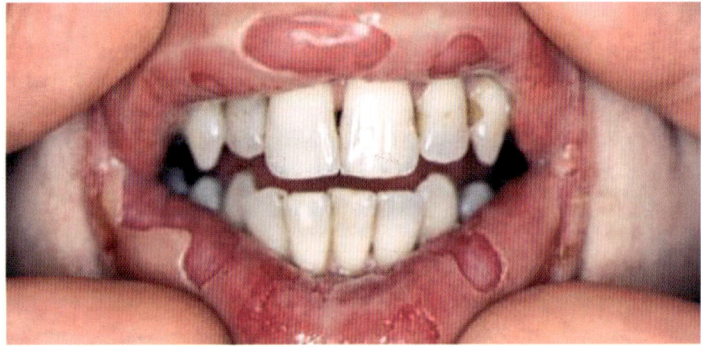

Figure 47.2 Mucosal lesions in erythema multiforme.

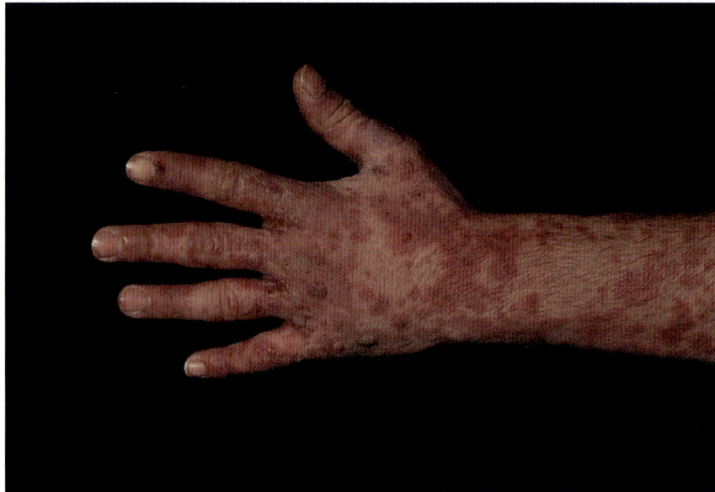

(a)

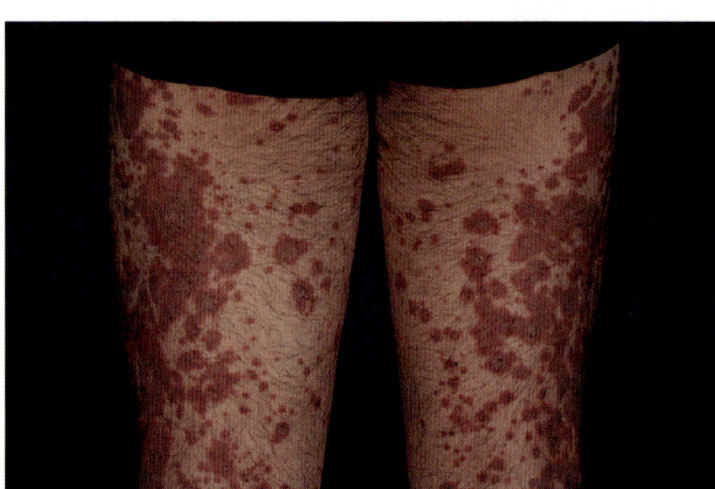

(b)

Figure 47.3 (a) Widespread acutely inflamed target lesions, including blisters, in erythema multiforme on the hands and arm in a 33-year-old Asian man. (b) Classic target lesions in erythema multiforme on the thighs in an adult white man.

macules or flat, atypical target lesions (Figure 47.3), accompanied by severe involvement of the conjunctival, corneal (Figure 47.4), irideal, buccal, labial and genital mucous membranes [9,10].

EM major occurs in younger males, frequently recurs, has less fever and milder mucosal lesions, and lacks an association with collagen vascular diseases, human immunodeficiency virus (HIV) infection or cancer. Herpes simplex is associated with SJS in up to 10% of cases and may be recurrent [10]. SJS, with occasional skin blisters and erosions covering less than 10% of the body's surface area, is differentiated from TEN, in which, typically, sheet-like erosions involve more than 30% of the body surface. However, there are several cases (10–20% in adults, and a higher percentage in children) that even experienced clinicians and histopathologists are unable to classify as they seem to have features of both groups. As such each case requires careful and ongoing evaluation for

disease progression, especially if more than 10% of body surface area is affected and/or there are signs of systemic disease, especially in the first few days of presentation, and escalation in disease management if indicated (Chapter 118).

Pathophysiology

Immunology

The clinical reaction pattern of EM is associated with many different triggering factors in genetically predisposed individuals. The immune profile of lesional skin from both infection-associated and drug-triggered EM gives clues to the pathogenesis. Human leukocyte antigen (HLA) studies have shown an association with HLA-B62 (B15), HLA-B35 and HLA-DR53 in recurrent cases of EM [1–3]. Immune complexes, both in the skin and circulation [4,5], autoantibodies against epithelial cells [6] and autoantibodies against desmosomal plaque proteins desmoplakin I and II, with suprabasal acantholysis, have also been demonstrated [7,8]. CD4+ T cells have been found in the dermis and CD8+ T cells in the epidermis of lesional skin.

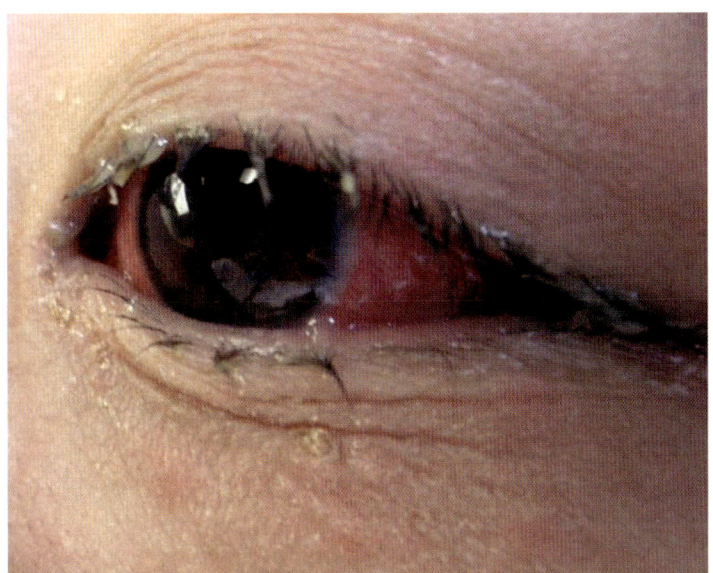

Figure 47.4 Eye involvement in erythema multiforme.

Herpesvirus-infected peripheral blood mononuclear cells (PBMCs) induce upregulation of CD54+ and major histocompatibility complex class I molecules in adjacent, non-infected, human dermal microvascular endothelial cells *in vitro*, and a consequent increased endothelial binding of PBMCs [9]. Herpes simplex virus (HSV) DNA has been identified in lesions of herpes-induced EM [10,11]. It has been proposed that PBMC antigen-presenting cells (macrophages, dermal dendritic cells or Langerhans cells) phagocytose HSV DNA and transport fragments to distant skin sites. This leads to recruitment of HSV-specific CD4+ T helper 1 (Th1) cells, thereby enhancing interferon α (IFN-α) production [12–14]. Thereafter an inflammatory cascade is initiated that includes the expression of IFN-α-induced genes, increased sequestration of circulating leukocytes, monocytes and natural killer (NK) cells, and the recruitment of autoreactive T cells. By extrapolation, drug hapten-specific T cells could be involved in the pathogenesis of drug-induced EM. PBMCs obtained from a patient with carbamazepine-induced EM at the time of disease showed increased binding to intercellular adhesion molecule 1 (ICAM-1) positive heterologous keratinocytes, and to autologous keratinocytes *in vitro*, which could be inhibited completely by antibodies to lymphocyte function-associated antigen 1 (LFA-1), the ligand for ICAM-1 [15]. Perforin-positive cells may mediate apoptotic cell death in EM and SJS [16]. Monocyte chemotactic protein 1 (MCP-1), RANTES (regulated upon activation, normal T-cell expressed and secreted), macrophage IFN-α-inducible gene (Mig) and IFN-α-inducible protein 10 (IP-10) were expressed by basal keratinocytes above, and mononuclear cells within, inflammatory foci. These cytokines contribute to the cell-specific and spatially restricted recruitment of mononuclear cells in the acute inflammation of EM [17]. Recently, EM major has been reported after the sequential use of two immune checkpoint inhibitors, nivolumab and ipilimumab, for the treatment of advanced melanoma. These drugs work by reversing the imbalance of antitumour self-tolerance and enhance T-cell response, which in this report blocked both the PD-1 (programmed cell death protein 1) and CTLA-4 (cytotoxic T-lymphocyte-associated protein 4) pathways.

Triggering factors

Potential triggering factors are listed in Box 47.1 [1–4,5,6–24,25,26]. The most common association is with a preceding herpes simplex infection (facial or genital) [1–3] or with a *Mycoplasma* infection [4,5], especially when conjunctival and corneal involvement occurs. Other viral or bacterial infections and vaccination have also been incriminated. More recently SARS-CoV-2 has been associated with EM-type lesions in adults and children, often in association with peripheral chilblain-like lesions [25,26]. Other cases are caused by drugs but in up to 50% no associated trigger may be identified.

Box 47.1 Some triggers of erythema multiforme

Viral infections [1]
- Herpes simplex virus [2,3]
- *Mycoplasma* infections [4,**5**]
- Acquired immune deficiency syndrome
- Adenovirus [6]
- Cytomegalovirus [7,8]
- Hepatitis B [9]
- Infectious mononucleosis [10,11]
- Lymphogranuloma inguinale
- Milker nodules
- Mumps
- Orf [12]
- Poliomyelitis
- Psittacosis
- SARS-CoV-2 [**25,26**]
- Vaccinia
- Varicella [13]
- Variola

Bacterial infections
A wide range has been recorded including rickettsiae [14]

Fungal infections [15,16]
- Histoplasmosis [17,18]

Drug reactions
- Including vaccinations

Contact reactions
Miscellaneous
- Carcinoma, lymphoma, leukaemia
- Granulomatosis with polyangiitis
- Lupus erythematosus (Rowell syndrome)
- Polyarteritis nodosa
- Polymorphic light eruption [19]
- Pregnancy, premenstrual, 'autoimmune progesterone dermatitis' [20]
- Sarcoidosis [21]
- X-ray therapy [22–24]

Drug reactions

Erythema multiforme was regarded as a well-recognised pattern of adverse cutaneous drug reaction [1–7]. As new drugs develop, EM-type lesions are reported in association with them. However, in a prospective study of cases of EM, only 10% were drug related [2]. In another study, antecedent medication use, especially cephalosporins, was recorded in 59% of EM patients and 68% of

SJS patients [4]. Perhaps all too frequently, and controversially, drugs are implicated on inadequate evidence; description of some reactions as 'EM like' does not help in this regard. Confirmation of drug sensitivity really necessitates re-exposure to the drug, which may carry an unacceptable risk and is not usually performed, which makes diagnosis uncertain.

Some of the drugs with notoriety for triggering EM are shown in Box 47.2. These range from historical and infrequently used therapies to the newer agents and include antibiotics, anticonvulsants, non-steroidal anti-inflammatory drugs, statins, immunotherapy and vaccinations [8–55,**56**–**58**].

Box 47.2 Drugs reported as causing erythema multiforme

Antibiotics
- Cephalosporins:
  - Ceftazidime
- Erythromycin
- Penicillins and ampicillin
- Quinolones
- Rifampicin
- Sulphonamides:
  - Co-trimoxazole
  - Sulfadoxine–pyrimethamine
- Sulphones
- Tetracyclines
- Thiacetazone
- Vancomycin

Antifungal preparations
- Griseofulvin
- Nystatin
- Terbinafine

Antiretroviral drugs
- Abacavir
- Nevirapine

Non-steroidal anti-inflammatory drugs
- Fenbufen
- Ibuprofen
- Paracetamol (acetaminophen)
- Pyrazolone derivatives:
  - Antipyrine
  - Phenylbutazone
  - Phenazone
- Salicylates
- Sulindac

Immunotherapy
- Ipilimumab
- Nivolumab
- Pembrolizumab

Metals and other elements
- Arsenic
- Bromides
- Gold
- Iodides
- Mercury

Anticonvulsants
- Barbiturates
- Carbamazepine
- Hydantoin derivatives
- Lamotrigine
- Trimethadione

Antihypertensives
- Furosemide
- Hydralazine
- Minoxidil
- Thiazide diuretics

Statins
- Pravastatin
- Simvastatin

Drugs acting on the central nervous system
- Lithium
- Mianserin
- Phenothiazines
- Trazodone

Miscellaneous
- Allopurinol
- Chlorpropamide
- Codeine
- Cyclophosphamide
- Danazol
- Methaqualone
- Nitrogen mustard
- Pentazocine
- Phenolphthalein
- Progesterone
- Topical agents (see text)
- Vaccination

Topical agents triggering erythema multiforme-like reactions

Allergic contact dermatitis may present with EM-like reactions [1]. The substances involved are usually potent sensitisers such as *Primula obconica* [2,3], poison ivy [4], a variety of weeds [5], laurel oil [6], *Alpinia galanga* (spicy edible Thai ginger) [7], diphenyl-cyclopropenone and bromofluorene [8–10]. A large number of topical medications can induce EM-like eruptions, including balsam of Peru, chloramphenicol, econazole, ethylenediamine, furazolidone, mafenide acetate cream used to treat burns, the muscle relaxant mephenesin, neomycin, nifuroxime, promethazine, scopolamine, sulphonamides, ophthalmic anticholinergic preparations (scopolamine hydrobromide and tropicamide drops), vitamin E, the antimycotic agent pyrrolnitrin, as well as proflavine, topical steroids [11,12], topical nitrogen mustard [13], sesquiterpene lactones in herbal medicine [14], bufexamac [15] and phenylbutazone [16], nitroglycerin patch [17], tea tree oil [18] and *para*-phenylenediamine, including in a henna tattoo [19–21]. A topical ketoprofen-containing tape provoked a photocontact dermatitis and subsequent EM [22].

EM has been reported with use of rubber gloves [23] and with blister beetle dermatitis [24]. In addition, contact with several environmental substances may induce EM-like reactions [25], including nickel, formaldehyde, trichloroethylene, phenyl sulphone derivative, the insecticide methyl parathion, a glyphosate pesticide [26], epoxy compounds, trinitrotoluene, cutting oil [27] and bisphenol A [28].

Pathology [1–5]

Although some authors refer to 'epidermal' and 'dermal' subtypes of EM, this is just a function of the timing of the biopsy in relation to the development of the lesion. The most important changes are necrotic keratinocytes in the epidermis which can be zonal and in the upper dermis – that is, a spectrum belonging to the lichenoid, band-like or cytotoxic CD8+ T-cell reaction patterns. The pathology of EM is variable and may overlap with fixed drug eruption and SJS, and is most florid in TEN, requiring good clinicopathological correlation to guide diagnosis. The timing of the biopsy in the evolution of the reactive erythema is important and is described later in this chapter.

Initially in EM there is a dermal, angiocentric, mixed infiltrate with progressive alignment and tagging of cytotoxic lymphocytes along the dermal–epidermal junction. This results in degenerative alterations in the basal keratinocytes and, with chronicity, progressive squamatisation and dyskeratosis. Some cases have prominent dermal inflammatory changes, with an interstitial and perivascular lymphohistiocytic infiltrate, sometimes with eosinophils if drug related, papillary oedema and vasodilatation. Rarely, red blood cell extravasation can occur without vasculitis. There is vacuolar liquefaction degeneration of the basal layer, epidermotropism of CD8+ lymphocytes, subepidermal blister formation and often, if chronic, individually necrotic apoptotic cells (Figure 47.5) and pigmentary incontinence with papillary melanophages. Such changes occur especially in classic EM with target lesions. In more severe bullous cases, there are subepidermal bullae (Figure 47.6) and necrosis of the whole epidermis, as in TEN. The histology of oral lesions is similar to that in the skin, and there may be a spectrum of similar pathological changes with very marked degenerative changes in the epithelium [6].

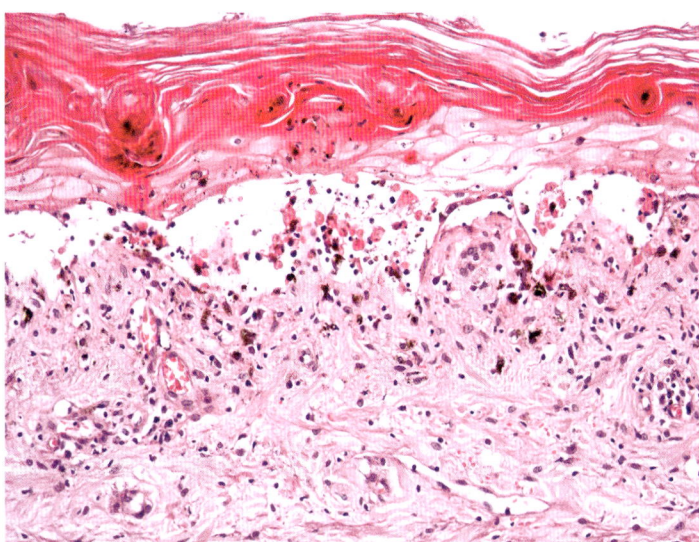

Figure 47.6 Subepidermal blister in erythema multiforme. Courtesy of Dr E. Calonje.

Clinical features [1–4]

Erythema multiforme can occur at any age, including in neonates [5,6] or young children [7]. In general, the course is that of an eruption developing over a few days and resolving in 2–3 weeks usually without scarring. Repeated attacks associated with recurrent herpes simplex are frequent and are optimally managed with adjunctive antiviral medication to suppress future outbreaks.

Lesions of EM classically evolve as macular, papular or urticarial lesions, developing into the classic iris or target lesions (see Figure 47.1), with a preferential distribution on the distal extremities. Lesions may involve the palms or trunk, as well as the oral (Figure 47.7) and genital mucous membranes. The lesions are dull red, flat or slightly raised maculopapules, which may either remain small or increase in size to reach a diameter of 1–3 cm in 48 h. Target lesions are usually less than 3 cm in diameter, rounded and have three zones: a central area of dusky redness or purpura, a middle paler zone of oedema and an outer ring of redness with

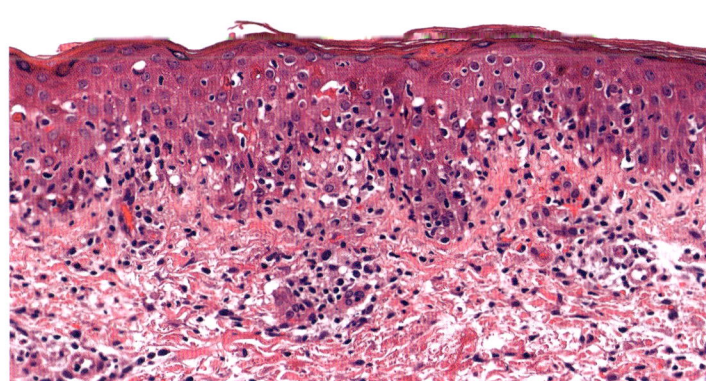

Figure 47.5 Necrosis of individual keratinocytes, exocytosis of lymphocytes and hydropic degeneration of basal cells in erythema multiforme (H&E). Courtesy of Dr E. Calonje.

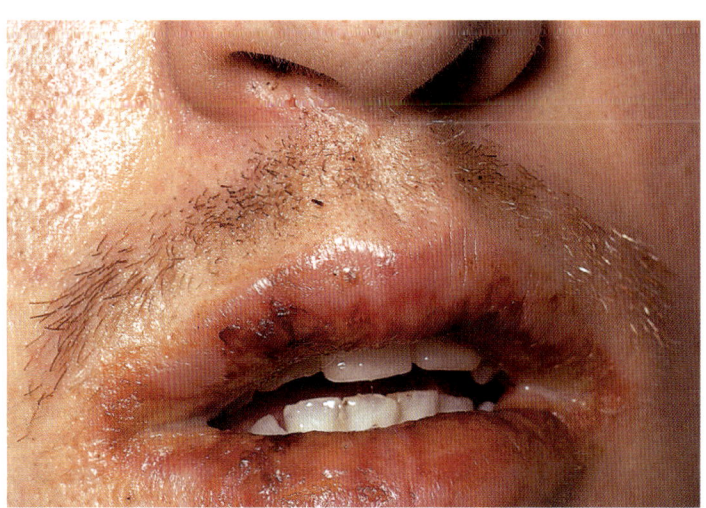

Figure 47.7 Erythema multiforme minor. Mucosal lesions.

a well-defined edge. Atypical target lesions have only two zones. The lesions appear in successive crops for a few days and fade in 1–2 weeks, sometimes leaving dusky discoloration. Lesions may be either few or profuse.

Characteristically, the dorsa of the hands, palms, wrists, feet and extensor aspects of the elbows and knees are affected, less commonly the face. Sometimes the outbreak is localised to just the lips or hands. There may be occasional red or pink lesions, erosions or bullae limited to the mucous membranes while the patient is otherwise well. Photoaggravation of EM is well recognised in association with HSV and statins [8,9].

Because the diagnosis of EM depends on the clinical and pathological appearance, criteria for the diagnosis of atypical cases are difficult to apply. However, there are cases where the clinical picture is atypical, but the histology nevertheless shows the characteristic changes. EM-like lesions have been reported in the setting of acute generalised exanthematous pustulosis [10]. Lesions, many centimetres in diameter, may remain stationary or enlarge slowly over several weeks or months (persistent EM) [11,12]. On rare occasions, cases with otherwise typical morphology and histology may develop lesions almost continuously rather than episodically [11]. EM along the Blaschko lines has been reported [13], as has disseminated granuloma annulare following EM minor [14].

Rowell syndrome comprises lupus erythematosus associated with EM-like skin lesions, and immunological findings of speckled antinuclear antibodies, anti-La or anti-Ro antibodies, and a positive test for rheumatoid factor [15–20]. However, the wide acceptance of this syndrome as a distinct entity is not universal [20].

Differential diagnosis

The differential diagnosis is wide and is that for most bullous disorders, particularly when there is predominantly mucosal involvement and obvious blistering clinically. Drug eruptions, such as vancomyin-induced linear immunoglobulin A (IgA) disease [21] and lupus erythematosus, must be excluded, along with pemphigoid and other autoimmune bullous conditions, and toxic erythemas of unknown cause [22,23]. Stem cell transplantation reactions may be difficult to differentiate from EM [24]. The distinction between atypical EM and urticarial vasculitis can be difficult but histology should be helpful. Kawasaki disease (Chapter 26) may resemble EM, but the characteristic red lips, strawberry tongue, red and swollen palms and soles and lymphadenopathy should permit a clinical diagnosis. The differential diagnosis of mouth lesions is considered elsewhere (Chapter 108).

Management [1,2]

Management is dependent on the extent of the disease. Localised bullous forms may be self-limiting or require topical corticosteroids for limited disease and/or oral corticosteroids if more widespread and symptomatic relief is required [3–5]. Ocular involvement requires early referral to an ophthalmologist. In the more severe cases, good nursing is of paramount importance and such cases may require the sort of attention used for TEN, in a dermatological high-dependency unit or intensive therapy or burns unit. The value of systemic corticosteroids is still debated [1,2,6,7], but relief of systemic symptoms such as fever is achieved. For more severe cases, prednisolone at an initial dosage

of 30–60 mg/day, decreasing over a period of 1–4 weeks, may be used [4,5].

Antiviral therapy with agents such as aciclovir for EM triggered by overt herpes simplex infections tends to be disappointing once the eruption has appeared; this is also true for recurrent cases, even when prescribed at the first sign of recurrent herpes. However, long-term prophylactic use may be quite helpful [8–10]. A dosage of 200 mg three times daily may be appropriate, but smaller or larger doses may be needed. Relapses tend to occur when the drug is omitted. It is of interest that some patients who suffer from recurrent EM without overt herpes infection can be helped by prophylactic aciclovir, implying that recurrent herpes infection may nevertheless be responsible [11]. Aciclovir has also been reported to prevent recurrent polyarthritis associated with EM [12]. Burnett *et al.* found the HSV DNA polymerase and VP5 protein was expressed in 75% of those with HSV-associated EM [13].

Thalidomide has been used in a few cases to prevent relapses of recurrent EM [14–16]. Other drugs used mainly in idiopathic or postherpetic EM have included dapsone [17,18], azathioprine [17], mycophenolate mofetil [19] and ciclosporin [20].

Erythema annulare centrifugum

Definition and nomenclature

Erythema annulare centrifugum (EAC) is a figurate dermatitis that is typically characterised by annular, polycyclic, red or pink plaques with scaling behind the advancing edge (Figure 47.8). Lesions first appear as red indurated papules that slowly enlarge to form a ring as the central area flattens and fades. The lesions may be static, have a varied rate of expansion (typically 2–3 mm/day) and the extension may be irregular, producing arciform segments [1–6]. EAC can have a variable maximum size (6–8 cm), different degrees of induration (from flat to cord like) and the lesions may either have an overlying scale, be vesicular or have no surface change. Lesions may be solitary or, more often, multiple and last from a few days to months or years. Itching is variable, but seldom intense. The commonest sites are the buttocks, thighs and upper arms, but any areas may be involved. Purpura and pigmentation may occur within the lesions.

Synonyms and inclusions

- Erythema perstans
- Erythema gyratum perstans
- Annular erythema of infancy
- Erythema figuratum perstans
- Erythema simplex gyratum

Introduction and general description

There has been great controversy as to the classification of the gyrate erythemas [7] and since its initial description, the term EAC has grown to include several histological and clinical variants. Several authors have suggested a classification of two types of gyrate erythema, a superficial (pruritic, scaling) and a

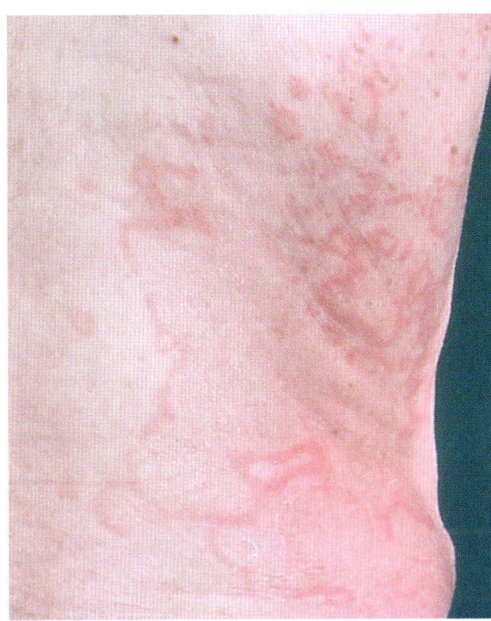

(a)

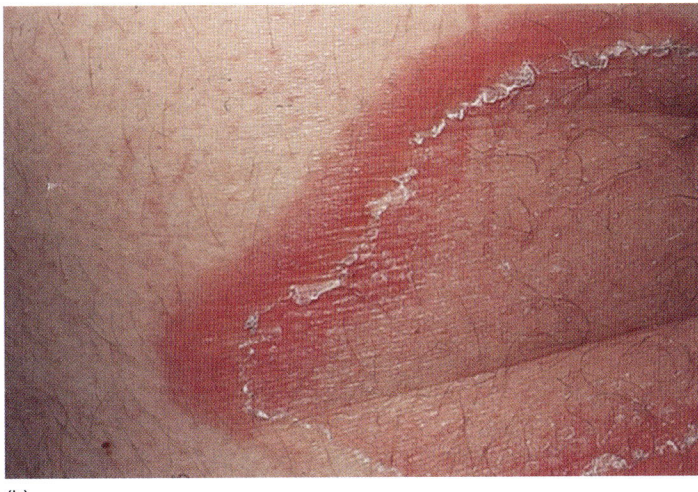

(b)

Figure 47.8 Erythema annulare centrifugum. (a) Multiple polyclic annular lesions, some of which have an urticated edge. (b) Close-up view of a lesion.

deep (non-pruritic, non-scaling) type, but in this chapter EAC is considered to include all the gyrate erythemas, except for erythema marginatum, erythema chronicum migrans and erythema gyratum repens.

Epidemiology
Incidence and prevalence
There is approximately one case per 100 000 population per year [5].

Age
It can occur at any age.

Sex
There is no difference between sexes.

Ethnicity
There is no obvious predilection.

Associated diseases
Erythema annulare centrifugum is a reactive process most probably associated with a concurrent infection. It can also be associated with drugs or malignancy [3–6]. Many of the described associated causes may be coincidental but the infective causes may be viral (Epstein–Barr virus), including more recently SARS-CoV-2 [8], bacterial (streptococcal infections, *Escherichia coli*), mycobacterial, fungal (dermatophytes) or parasitic. Several systemic diseases (thyroid and liver) have also been associated with EAC but in the majority of cases no underlying cause is identified.

Pathophysiology
Predisposing factors
Many disease states have been associated with EAC and it is possible that the association is coincidental, since there is a lack of good evidence for true disease association. In some cases the eruption is likely to be an unusual presentation of diseases mimicking EAC. The most common underlying association is concurrent infection, and usually this is within the skin, with dermatophytosis being implicated in up to 48% of cases. The causes described in the literature are summarised in Table 47.1 [1–6,8–32].

Pathology
A spectrum of non-specific histological findings is seen in EAC and clinicopathological correlation is critical [33]. The characteristic

Table 47.1 Reported causes and associations of erythema annulare centrifugum.

Cause	Associations
Idiopathic [1–6]	
Familial	Dominant inheritance [9], twins [10]
Infantile onset	Annular erythema of infancy [11]
Bacterial infections [1–6]	Mycobacteria, streptococci, *Escherichia coli*, syphilis, *Pseudomonas* septicaemia [12]
Viral infections [1–6]	Epstein–Barr virus, HIV, herpes simplex, herpes zoster [13], molluscum contagiosum [14], viral hepatitis, SARS-CoV-2 [8]
Fungal infections [1–3]	*Candida* [15], dermatophytosis
Parasitic infections	*Ascaris lumbricoides* [16], *Phthirus pubis* [17]
Drugs [1–6]	Acetazolomide, amitriptyline [18], ampicillin, chloroquine, cimetidine, co-trimoxazole, finasteride, gold [19], hydrochlorothiazide, hydroxychloquine [20], non-steroidal anti-inflammatory drugs [21], penicillins, salicylates, spironolactone
Endocrine	Autoimmune progesterone dermatitis [22], hyperthyroidism, pregnancy
Neoplasia:	
Keratinocyte	Squamous cell carcinoma
Haematological [3]	Acute myelogenous leukaemia, chronic lymphocytic leukaemia [23], hypereosinophilic syndrome [24], lymphomas [25,26], myeloma
Internal [3,5,27]	Breast, bronchial, naso-pharyngeal, ovarian, prostatic and gastric carcinomas
Autoimmune [1,5]	Autoimmune hepatitis, lupus erythematosus, polyglandular autoimmune disease type 1 [28], relapsing polychondritis [29], Sjögren syndrome [30]
Miscellaneous	Appendicitis [31], blue cheese, cholestatic liver disease, inflammatory bowel disease, sarcoidosis [32]

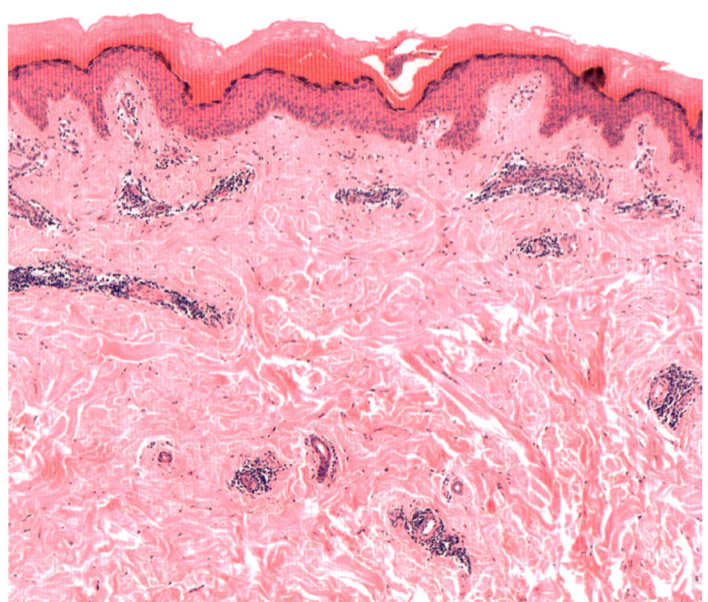

Figure 47.9 Histology of erythema annulare centrifugum showing a perivascular 'sleeve-like' lymphohistiocytic infiltrate. Courtesy of Dr Florence Deroide, The Royal Free Hospital, London, UK.

histological feature in EAC is a perivascular 'sleeve-like' lymphohistiocytic infiltrate which may be mainly superficial, mainly deep or mixed (Figure 47.9). The pathological changes may be entirely within the dermis, whereas in other cases there is a much more obvious epidermal change (spongiosis and parakeratosis). There is dispute about whether these represent two separate diseases or a continuous range. A study of 82 biopsies from 73 patients suggested that EAC with a superficially situated infiltrate is different to that with a deeper dermal infiltrate [6]. The superficial pattern was associated clinically with a collarette of scale that was not seen in the deeper pattern. Histologically, the superficial pattern was more likely to have spongiosis, parakeratosis, epidermal hyperplasia and papillary dermal oedema, while the deeper pattern more commonly had a sleeve-like infiltrate, melanophages and individual necrotic keratinocytes. However, neither pattern appeared to have any consistent association to systemic disease nor to the timing of the biopsy in relation to the evolution of the lesions. Thus, the clinical utility of this histological distinction is unclear.

Eosinophils may occasionally be seen around superficial vessels. Significant peripheral eosinophilia raises the possibility of parasitic infection as the underlying cause. A very rare eruption that has clinical features of EAC but with a frank eosinophilic infiltrate has been described under the name 'eosinophilic annular erythema' [34,35]. It has been suggested that this may be a variant of Wells syndrome (eosinophilic cellulitis). Other cases described as EAC have shown a pseudolymphomatous reaction pattern with positive staining to spirochaetes and this would extend the spectrum of EAC [36].

Genetics
No genetic cause is known.

Clinical features
Presentation
The presentation is with expanding polycyclic, annular, red plaques that may expand by up to 2–3 mm per day with central clearing (Figure 47.8).

Differential diagnosis
There are multiple annular dermatoses that could enter the differential diagnosis; these include tinea corporis, subacute cutaneous lupus erythematosus, annular sarcoidosis, necrolytic migratory erythema, granuloma annulare, cutaneous T-cell lymphoma, granuloma faciale, drug eruptions, erythema multiforme, erythema gyratum repens, erythema marginatum and Wells syndrome (eosinophilic cellulitis).

Disease course and prognosis
It may be of variable duration, lasting from days to decades, with a mean of 2.8 years.

Investigations
These are aimed at excluding alternative diagnoses and identifying an underlying cause. As fungal infections are the commonest cause, a culture of affected skin and nails should be undertaken if a dermatophyte infection is suspected. Biopsy of lesional skin and direct immunofluorescence will help to confirm the diagnosis and to exclude differential diagnoses. Additional investigations would include a full blood count, liver and thyroid function tests, abdominal ultrasound and chest X-ray. An antinuclear antibody profile, serum angiotensin-converting enzyme (ACE) and HIV serology should also be checked. If a malignancy is suspected, positron emission tomography/computed tomography (PET/CT) scanning should be undertaken.

Management

> **Treatment ladder for erythema annulare centrifugum**
>
> **First line**
> The first goal is to identify and treat any underlying condition, but if this is not possible treatment with moderately potent or potent topical corticosteroids or topical calcipotriol [37] is appropriate
>
> **Second line**
> - Topical tacrolimus [38]
> - Phototherapy
>
> **Third line**
> - Chloroquine or hydroxychloroquine
> - Systemic steroids

Annular erythema of infancy

Definition

There is some doubt as to whether annular erythema of infancy (AEI) represents a separate entity or whether it is merely EAC occurring in a younger individual. AEI occurs in young children where the primary lesion adopts an annular, arcuate or polycyclic form, with a circinate or polycyclic pattern. The condition usually resolves spontaneously over a few weeks without any scarring or pigmentary changes. Several mechanisms have been postulated to explain the annular pattern of the lesion. The clinical morphology is the same as EAC and although one has to consider the spectrum of diseases associated with EAC, underlying malignancy is rare and annular erythemas in general are more common in children than adults.

Introduction and general description

Annular erythema of infancy was first described as a distinct dermatosis in 1981 [1] and further cases have been reported [2–4,5,6]. The lesions are identical to those of EAC with asymptomatic, red, maculopapular lesions enlarging and evolving into variably sized, single or grouped annular plaques, predominantly localised to the face, trunk and proximal limbs with a scaly edge (Figure 47.10). Individual lesions last from days to weeks and there may be a cyclical pattern of new lesions appearing every 5–6 weeks. The eruption may start in infancy or in teenage years, is self-limiting and has no associated systemic symptoms. An autosomal dominant inherited form has been described [7].

Epidemiology
Pathology

The appearances are typically the same as in cases of EAC with a dermal perivascular and interstitial lymphocytic infiltrate (Figure 47.11). There have been reports of a prominent eosinophilic infiltrate [3,4] and an associated peripheral blood eosinophilia [8]. A neutrophilic variant has also been reported [6,9,10].

Causative organisms

Heavy intestinal colonisation with *Candida albicans* [11], concurrent Epstein–Barr virus [12] and *Malassezia* infections [13] have been documented.

Clinical features
Presentation

Polycyclic, annular, red plaques that may expand by up to 2–3 mm per day with central clearing and a scaly edge.

Differential diagnosis

This includes familial annular erythema, urticaria, erythema gyratum atrophicans, neonatal lupus erythematosus [14], erythema chronicum migrans, tinea corporis, mycosis fungoides [15] and annular lichenoid dermatitis of youth [16].

Disease course and prognosis

Annular erythema of infancy is self-limiting.

Investigations

Investigations include microscopy and culture of skin scrapings, antinuclear antibodies including antibodies to dsDNA and extractable nuclear antigen (Ro, La, Sm and RNP), electrocardiogram and skin biopsy and serology for Lyme disease.

Management

Treatment ladder for annular erythema of infancy

First line
- Any associated infection should be treated

Second line
- Potent topical steroids

Third line
- Topical tacrolimus

Erythema chronicum migrans

This is considered one of the most common annular erythemas in paediatric patients where Lyme disease is endemic. This disorder is caused by a bite from a tick of the genus *Ixodes* and infection by the *Borrelia burgdorferi* spirochete. It is reported to occur in up to 90% of children infected by Lyme disease [1,2]. Lyme disease is described in detail in Chapter 26. It is an important diagnosis to make and treat with antibiotics to prevent systemic disease. Children should be treated with antibiotics such as doxycycline, ampicillin or azithromycin depending on their age, weight and antibiotic sensitivity [3].

Erythema marginatum

Definition

Erythema marginatum is an annular and sometimes polycyclic, serpiginous, red eruption. Together with carditis, migratory polyarthritis, chorea and subcutaneous nodules it is one of the Duckett Jones major criteria for the diagnosis of rheumatic fever [1]. Erythema marginatum occurs in about 10% of patients with rheumatic fever [2,3,4,5].

Epidemiology
Incidence and prevalence

Erythema marginatum as a manifestation of rheumatic fever is now predominantly a disease of developing countries and the incidence declines as socioeconomic conditions improve.

Age

It is most common in children between the ages of 5 and 15 years.

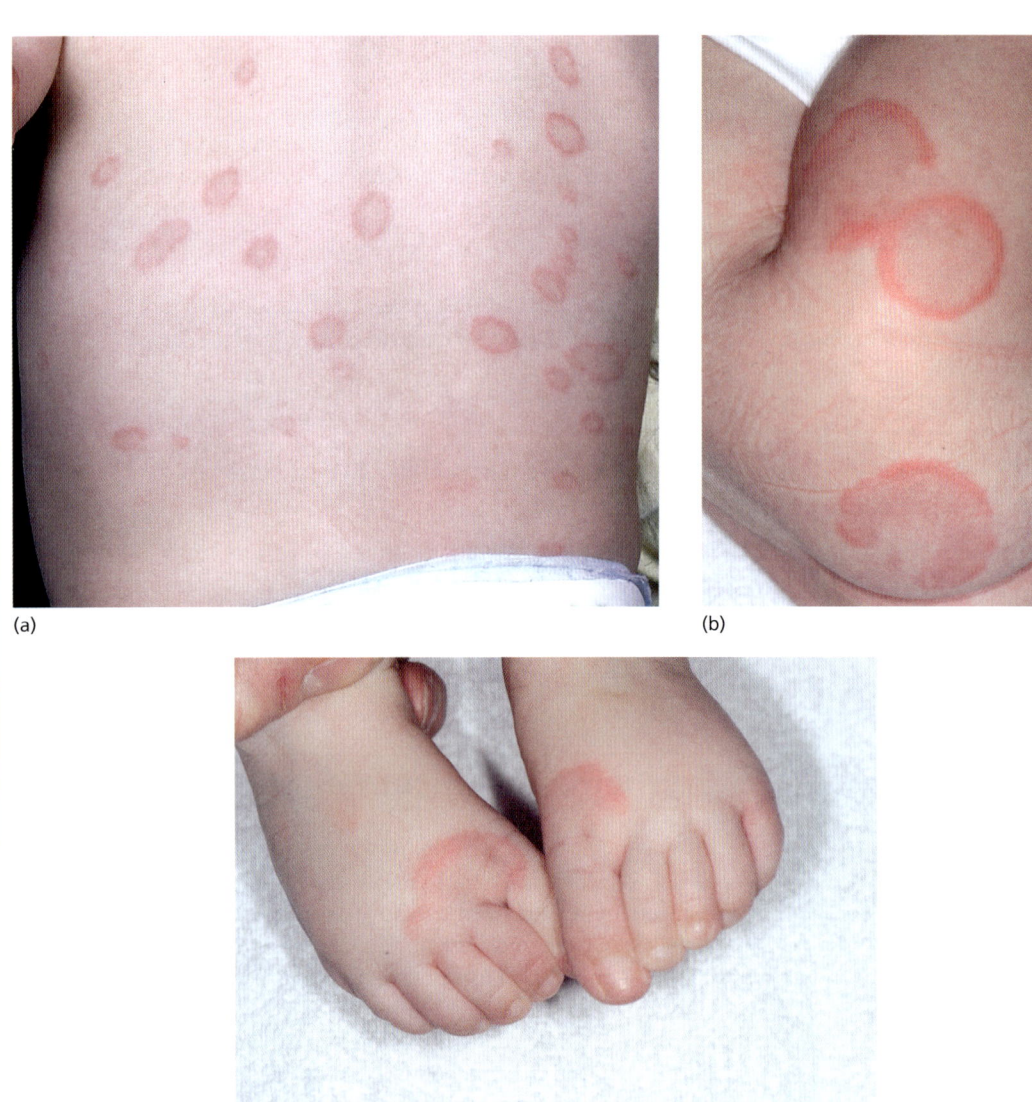

(a)

(b)

(c)

Figure 47.10 Scattered lesions of annular erythema of infancy on (a) the back, (b) the upper leg and (c) the feet. (b, c) Courtesy of Dr Jane Ravenscroft, Consultant Dermatologist, Queen's Medical Centre, Nottingham, UK.

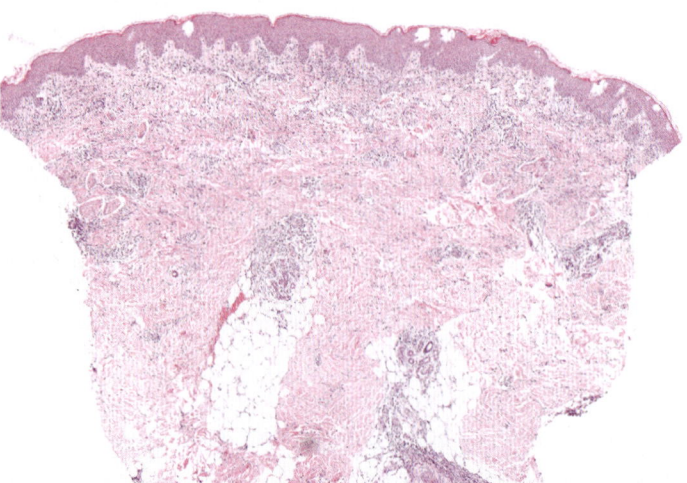

Figure 47.11 Histopathology of lesional skin showing upper dermal and perivascular lymphohistiocytic infiltrate. Courtesy of Dr Jane Ravenscroft, Consultant Dermatologist, Queen's Medical Centre, Nottingham, UK.

Sex
There is no difference between the sexes.

Associated diseases
These include rheumatic fever, psittacosis [6] and angioedema (C1 inhibitor deficiency acquired or hereditary) [7,8]. A firm diagnosis of rheumatic fever requires that two major or one major and two minor criteria are satisfied (Box 47.3), in addition to evidence of recent streptococcal infection.

Pathophysiology
Pathology
The histological features are non-specific and include a perivascular polymorphous infiltrate of neutrophils and mononuclear cells in the papillary dermis and upper portion of the reticular dermis [9]. Nuclear debris suggestive of leukocytoclasia is often present but vasculitis is not seen. There are reports of cases devoid of neutrophils where the infiltrate consisted of a sparse, superficial, perivascular, mononuclear infiltrate composed entirely of lymphocytes and histiocytes.

Box 47.3 Duckett Jones criteria for the diagnosis of rheumatic fever

Major criteria
- Carditis: all layers of cardiac tissue are affected (pericardium, epicardium, myocardium, endocardium). The patient may have a new or changing murmur, with mitral regurgitation being the most common, followed by aortic insufficiency
- Polyarthritis: migrating arthritis that typically affects the knees, ankles, elbows and wrists. The joints are severely painful and symptoms are dramatically responsive to anti-inflammatory medicines
- Chorea: also known as Sydenham chorea or St Vitus dance. There are abrupt, purposeless movements. This may be the only manifestation of acute rheumatic fever and its presence is diagnostic. May also include emotional disturbances and inappropriate behaviour
- Erythema marginatum: a non-pruritic rash that commonly affects the trunk and proximal extremities, but spares the face. The rash typically migrates from central areas to the periphery and has well-defined borders
- Subcutaneous nodules: usually located over bones or tendons, these nodules are painless and firm

Minor criteria
- Fever
- Arthralgia
- Previous rheumatic fever or rheumatic heart disease
- Raised acute phase reactants, e.g. leukocytosis, elevated erythrocyte sedimentation rate and C-reactive protein
- Prolonged P-R interval on electrocardiogram

Causative organisms
It is predominantly associated with a β-haemolytic streptococcal infection but has also been described in association with psittacosis.

Clinical features
Presentation
The lesions of erythema marginatum can be distinguished from other annular erythemas due to their transient clinical presentation. These typically begin as red macules or papules (which may be urticated) that spread peripherally and may merge to produce the typical serpiginous, polycyclic annular eruption. As the lesions advance, sometimes with a rapid spread of 2–10 mm in 12 h, the pattern may change sometimes within an hour, completely resolving and then reappearing. The edges become raised and red, and the centre clears. These lesions are neither pruritic nor painful and sometimes go unnoticed by the patient; they may fade and reappear within hours or may persist intermittently for weeks to months. The rash blanches on pressure, is transient and tends to migrate from one part of the body to another. It is associated with rheumatic fever but this only occurs in 1–18% of patients.

Differential diagnosis
This includes annular erythema, urticaria, toxic erythema and erythema multiforme.

Complications and co-morbidities
Rheumatic fever is an autoimmune inflammatory process that develops as a sequela of a streptococcal infection, most often pharyngeal infection with rheumatogenic group A streptococci in a susceptible individual. The disease manifests as polyarthritis, carditis, chorea, erythema marginatum and/or subcutaneous nodules. Carditis, the most serious complication, occurs in 30–45% of rheumatic fever patients and leads to chronic rheumatic heart disease which is characterised by progressive and permanent valvular lesions.

Investigations
Erythema marginatum is part of a clinical syndrome for which no specific tests exist. However, to aid the diagnosis the following would be appropriate: full blood count, urea and electrolytes, liver function tests, erythrocyte sedimentation rate, C-reactive protein and ferritin, throat swab, antistreptolysin O titre, psittacosis serology, blood cultures, electrocardiogram and echocardiography and skin biopsy.

Management

Treatment ladder for erythema marginatum

First line
- Aspirin or non-steroidal anti-inflammatory drugs
- Penicillin or erythromycin

Erythema gyratum repens

Definition
Erythema gyratum repens is a rare, distinctive, figurate eruption consisting of mobile, concentric, often palpable, red, wave-like bands, which give a 'wood-grain' appearance to the skin [1]. A peripheral scale or collarette may be present. Lesions often commence on the limbs and the whole torso may be affected. There is often associated severe pruritus, and sometimes ichthyosis and bullae may develop within the red area. The lesions migrate from day to day, usually changing position by about 1 cm per day. See also Chapter 148.

Introduction and general description
Erythema gyratum repens has long been considered to be a paraneoplastic cutaneous eruption, but a similar or possibly identical eruption has been described in the absence of malignancy. Unfortunately, histological appearances are not diagnostic. The clinical features are distinctive, and patients should be investigated to exclude underlying neoplasia.

Originally, 80% of cases were described as having an associated underlying internal malignancy [2,3,4,5]. Six per cent of patients have a tumour of unknown primary origin but, if identified, resection of the tumour often results in resolution of the eruption.

More recently, an erythema gyratum repens-like eruption has been reported in the absence of an underlying malignancy and may be associated with pityriasis rubra pilaris, psoriasis, ichthyosis, connective tissue diseases and, on occasion, is drug induced [6,7].

Epidemiology
Age
It usually presents after the age of 40 years, characteristically in the seventh decade with a mean age of 63 years. However, it has been reported to occur from age 16 to 75 years.

Sex
The male to female ratio is 2 : 1.

Ethnicity
It has been reported to occur predominantly in white people.

Associated diseases
Although erythema gyratum repens is strongly associated with underlying malignancy, it has also been described in association with infections, drugs and autoimmune disease [8]. The most frequent underlying malignancies in descending order are carcinoma of the lung (47%) followed by oesophagus, breast, stomach, kidney, cervix, pharynx, urinary bladder, uterus and/or cervix, pancreas, prostate and haematological neoplasia. Treatment of the cancer may result in clearance of the eruption, and tumour recurrence or metastases can precipitate a recurrence. Erythema gyratum repens has also been described in the absence of an underlying malignancy associated with pityriasis rubra pilaris [9], psoriasis, ichthyosis, mycobacterial infections, connective tissue diseases (lupus erythematosus, Sjögren syndrome, rheumatoid arthritis and scleroderma) and the hypereosinophilic syndrome. An erythema gyratum repens-like eruption may be a manifestation of another cutaneous disease, diagnosis being made on histology (lupus erythematosus, immunobullous disorder [10], mycosis fungoides, erythrokeratoderma variabilis, urticarial vasculitis and neutrophilic dermatosis). Close clinicopathological correlation is required, but the caveat of a patient presenting with erythema gyratum repens is that there is an underlying malignancy present even if this cannot be diagnosed at presentation, so ongoing surveillance is warranted.

Pathophysiology
Pathology
The histological features are not diagnostic. There is a superficial and occasionally deep perivascular lymphohistiocytic infiltrate in the papillary dermis associated with hyperkeratosis, parakeratosis, acanthosis and spongiosis. Granular deposits of IgG and C3 have been found at the basement membrane zone of both involved and uninvolved skin, supporting the concept that this dermatosis has an immunological pathogenesis [11].

Clinical features
Presentation
Regular waves of redness spread over the body to produce a series of concentric, figurate bands in a pattern resembling wood grain. The characteristic feature is the way the rings, swirls or waves appear within existing lesions to form a concentric pattern of sequential eruptions, with day to day migration of the leading edge by about 1 cm. Scaling, typically at the trailing edge, and itch are usually prominent. This contrasts with the more common 'annular erythemas' of the EAC pattern, in which each lesion is usually a distinct ring or arc with variable but mostly without prominent scaling, and not in a concentric arrangement. Hyperkeratosis of the palms occurs in about 10% and has been reported in both paraneoplastic and idiopathic cases.

Differential diagnosis
The diagnosis can be challenging and relies on the clinical history and examination since the histology is not pathognomic. Differential diagnoses include EAC, erythema multiforme, necrolytic migratory erythema, subacute cutaneous lupus erythematosus, lupus erythematosus gyratum repens, erythema chronicum migrans, tinea corporis, erythrokeratoderma variabilis, subacute annular (Lapière) variant of psoriasis and pityriasis rubra pilaris, all of which may morphologically present with erythema gyratum repens-like lesions. Diagnosis is therefore often one of exclusion.

Disease course and prognosis
This is dependent on the underlying disease. If associated with malignancy it may recur if the neoplasia relapses.

Investigations
Useful investigations include a full blood count, biochemistry, antinuclear antibody profile, chest X-ray, mammogram, cervical smear, prostate-specific antigen, CT scan of the thorax, abdomen and pelvis and, if indicated, endoscopy or colonoscopy and PET scan.

Management

Treatment ladder for erythema gyratum repens

First line
- Identify the underlying disease with extensive investigation to exclude neoplasia

Second line
- Treat the underlying disease

Necrolytic migratory erythema

Definition and nomenclature
Necrolytic migratory erythema (NME) is, in most cases, considered to be a paraneoplastic cutaneous eruption associated with a pancreatic neuroendocrine tumour (NET) – an α-cell pancreatic islet cell tumour (with an anatomical predilection towards the tail of the pancreas). These tumours are described as 'glucagonoma' secreting glucagon. The eruption can precede the diagnosis of glucagonoma by several years and may be misdiagnosed as an atypical eczematous/psoriasiform eruption before the characteristic histopathological features are identified [1,2–5]. The triad of unusual

dermatosis, recent-onset diabetes and weight loss should trigger consideration of NME. It may occur in the setting of glucagonoma associated with multiple endocrine neoplasia or glucagon-secreting tumours (bronchial or naso-pharyngeal carcinomas) or in the absence of a glucagon-secreting tumour (pseudoglucagonoma syndrome) with pancreatic insufficiency, coeliac disease and intestinal malabsorption syndromes, inflammatory bowel disease, cirrhosis, non-pancreatic malignancies and myelodysplastic syndrome [6].

Synonyms and inclusions
- Glucagonoma syndrome
- Pancreatic islet cell tumour
- Pseudoglucagonoma syndrome
- Pancreatic neuroendocrine tumours

Introduction and general description

Pancreatic neuroendocrine tumours are rare, representing 3–5% of all pancreatic malignancies. Hormonally active NETs are classified by the hormonal products they produce (e.g. insulinomas, gastrinomas, glucagonomas) and are associated with a myriad of clinical syndromes including hypoglycaemia, diarrhoea and peptic ulceration. NME is the hallmark cutaneous manifestation of a glucagonoma but may, in its absence, also occur in association with other diseases [7]. The key features of the 'glucagonoma syndrome' are NME and diabetes.

Epidemiology

Incidence and prevalence

More than 400 cases of glucagonoma have been reported in the literature to date. The estimated incidence has been reported to be 2.4/100 million population per year [8], but other authors have reported an incidence of 1 in 20 million [9].

Age

The median age at diagnosis has been reported at 53.5 years with a range of 19–84 years; the median time from onset of symptoms to diagnosis was 39 months [6].

Sex

Males and females appear to be equally affected.

Pathophysiology

The pathogenetic mechanism of NME is not certain, but the condition could possibly be due to amino acid deficiency (particularly histidine and tryptophan) caused by high glucagon levels [3] or by intestinal protein loss or malabsorption. There may be contributory roles for essential fatty acid and zinc deficiencies, but abnormal zinc levels or response to zinc supplementation are not consistent, and treatment with amino acid infusions may lead to a resolution of the skin eruption [6]. It is characteristic that all skin changes disappear after complete surgical removal of the tumour where this is the cause [10], and correction of malabsorption secondary to coeliac disease is usually effective [2].

Pathology

A skin biopsy should be taken from the edge of early lesions and, in view of the evolving nature of the eruption, serial biopsies

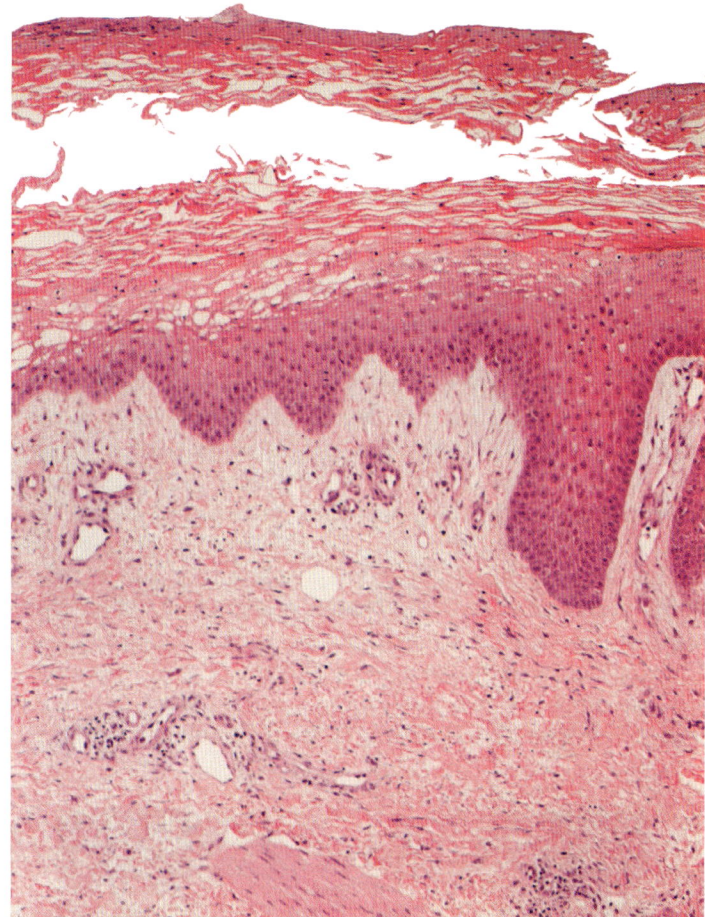

Figure 47.12 Necrolytic migratory erythema showing necrosis and separation of the upper layers of the epidermis. Courtesy of Dr Ed Rytina, Addenbrooke's Hospital, Cambridge, UK.

may be required. Histology shows parakeratosis with loss of the granular cell layer, necrosis and separation of the papillary epidermis with vacuolar degeneration of the keratinocytes, dyskeratotic keratinocytes and the presence of neutrophils (Figure 47.12). Many cases may just have local or diffuse parakeratosis, creating a vast differential diagnosis. Early lesions may present as a 'dyskeratotic dermatitis' with superficial perivascular inflammation in the dermis, and minor spongiosis and dyskeratotic or vacuolated epidermal cells [11,12]. In the dermis, a mild perivascular lymphocytic and histiocytic infiltrate occurs. Older lesions show various degrees of dyskeratosis, acanthosis and a lymphocytic infiltrate in the dermis. Direct immunofluorescence reveals staining of apoptotic keratinocytes with immunoglobulins, fibrinogen and C3. The histological changes are similar to those observed in acute zinc deficiency, in which cell degeneration and the formation of clefts and vesicles are predominant at the level of the basal layer of the epidermis.

Clinical features

History

Most cases of NME have an underlying glucagonoma and patients present with weight loss (67%), anaemia (33%), glucose intolerance (56%), diarrhoea (20%), venous thrombosis (10%), malaise and oral symptoms including angular cheilitis and glossitis [9]. In those patients with NME in the absence of a glucagon-secreting tumour (pseudoglucagonoma syndrome) underlying diseases include chronic pancreatitis, alcoholic liver disease, gastrointestinal malabsorption, hepatic cirrhosis and aberrant glucagon-secreting tumours such as bronchial or naso-pharyngeal carcinomas.

Presentation

Necrolytic migratory erythema may present initially with a non-specific itchy or tender macular patch of red skin with a predilection for the groin, genitalia or buttocks (Figure 47.13). It then evolves to form a centrifugally extending, annular, red eruption with a crusted edge that may be itchy, burning, painful, blistered or eroded. It often displays a fluctuating or cyclical pattern and predominantly affects the flexural sites on the lower abdomen, groins, buttocks and thighs. Eczematous or psoriasiform features may be seen. Central areas may heal over 7–14 days, leaving postinflammatory hyperpigmentation. Perianal and genital lesions are common and one-third of patients have angular cheilitis and painful, beefy-coloured glossitis [8]. Twenty per cent of patients with glucagonomas will also exhibit neurological and/or psychiatric disturbances such as dementia, psychosis, agitation, paranoid delusions, ataxia and hyperreflexia [13]. Patients may also present with thromboembolic complications such as pulmonary embolus or deep vein thromboses and rarely dilated cardiomyopathy.

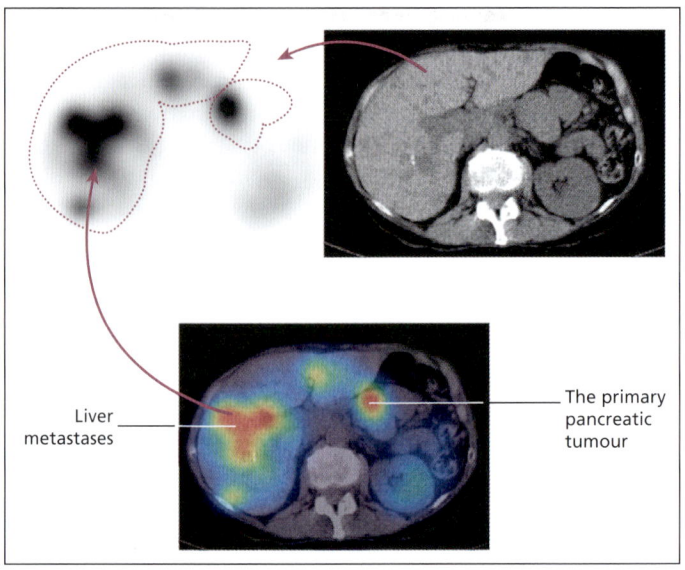

Figure 47.14 Single-photon emission computed tomography (SPECT), CT and fused SPECT/CT images showing the primary pancreatic tumour and liver metastases. Courtesy of Dr S. Navalkissoor, The Royal Free Hospital, London, UK.

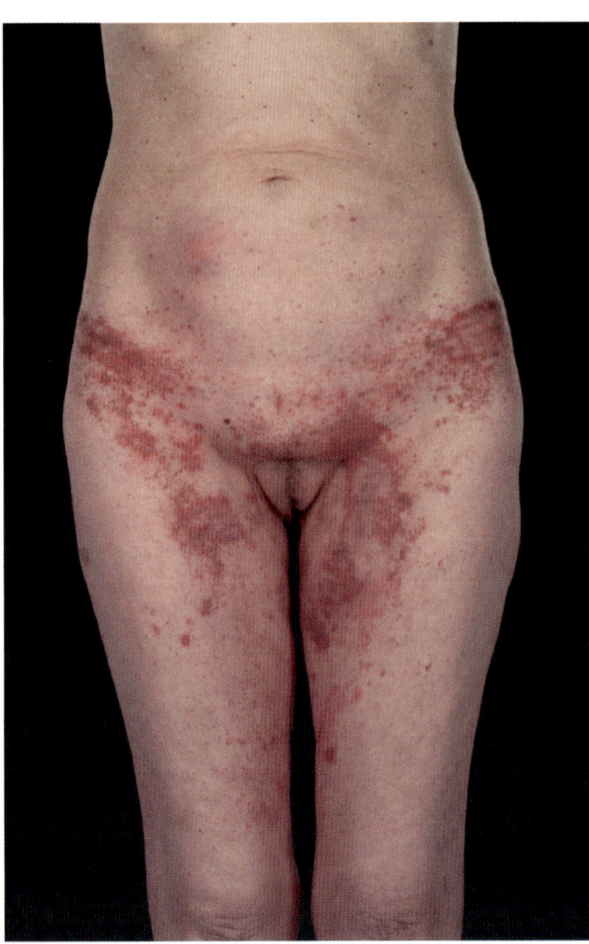

Figure 47.13 Necrolytic migratory erythema in the groin area.

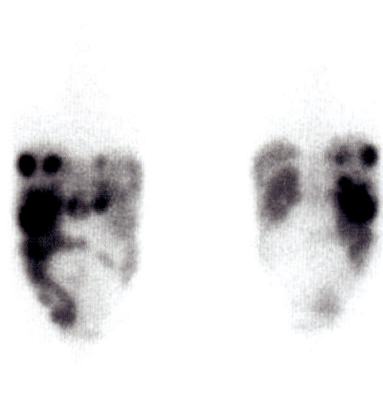

(a)   (b)

Figure 47.15 ^{111}In-DTPA octreotide scan showing abnormal uptake in the liver and upper abdomen in a patient presenting with necrolytic migratory erythema secondary to a glucagonoma. (a) Anterior image; (b) posterior image. Courtesy of Dr S. Navalkissoor, The Royal Free Hospital, London, UK.

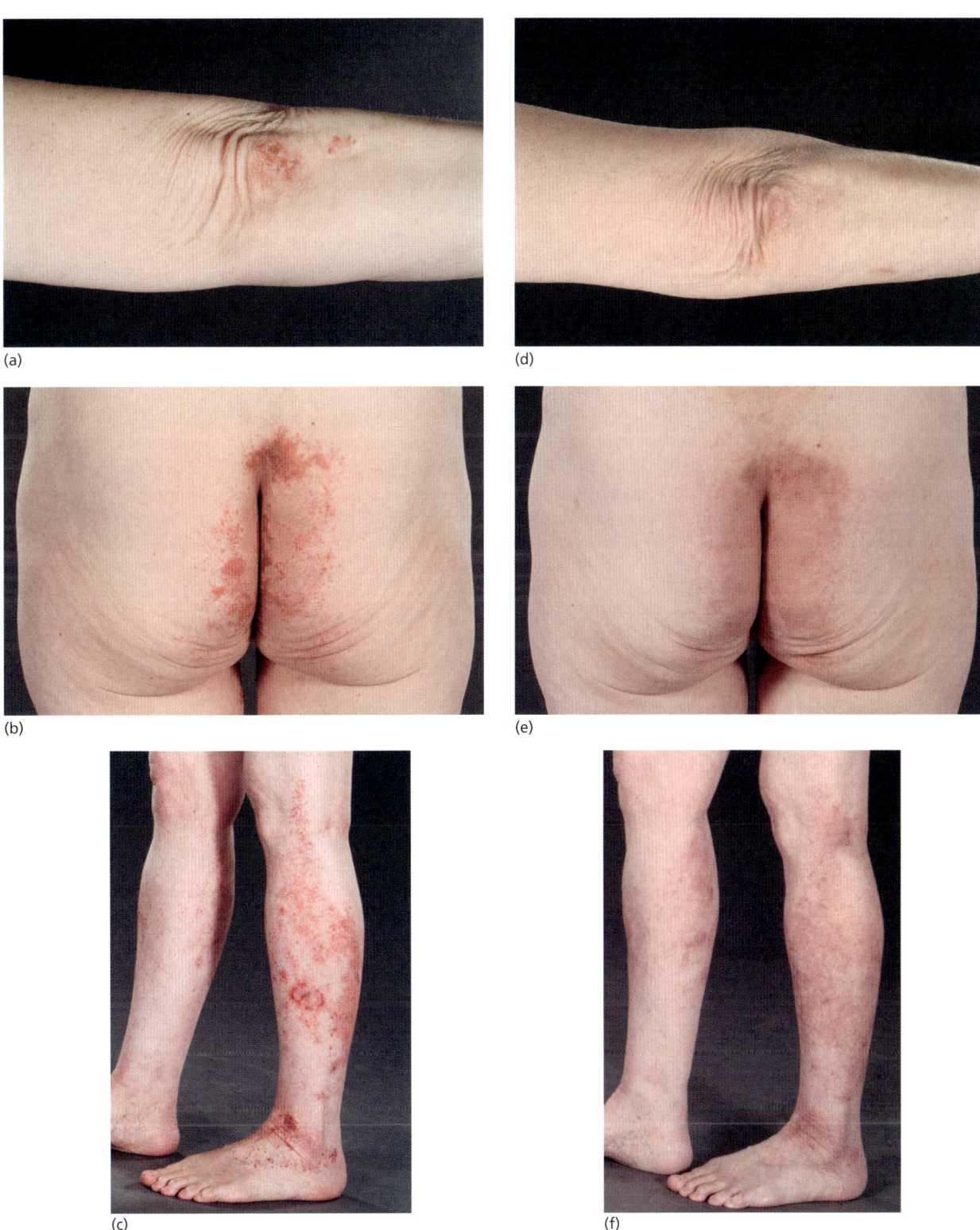

(a)

(d)

(b)

(e)

(c)

(f)

Figure 47.16 Necrolytic migratory erythema pre-treatment (a–c) and (d–f) post-treatment with octreotide.

Clinical variants

Necrolytic acral erythema presents with well-demarcated, acral (mainly hands and feet but can affect forearms, knees and lower legs), dusky discoloration with peripheral blister formation progressing to form keratotic erythrokeratoderma-like chronic inflammation. Histology is that of a necrolytic process, but the distribution and laboratory tests (positive hepatitis C serology and normal glucagon) confirm the diagnosis [14].

Differential diagnosis

The differential diagnosis can include eczema, impetiginised eczema, psoriasis, pemphigus foliaceous, annular lesions of pustular psoriasis and subcorneal pustular dermatosis.

Classification of severity

A TNM staging classification for pancreatic NETs derived from the staging algorithm for exocrine pancreatic adenocarcinomas has been proposed, but this has not yet been validated [15].

Disease course and prognosis

Fifty per cent of patients with NME secondary to glucagonoma will have metastatic disease (to liver, regional or cervical lymph nodes, bone and lung) at the time of diagnosis, in part because of the invariable delay in reaching a diagnosis. Because of the rarity of glucagonoma, the 5-year survival rate has not yet been determined. However, one study reported an overall median survival of 66 months in a group of 12 patients [16], and in another study half of those with metastatic disease survived 10 years and up to 21 years in one published case [17]. The skin changes resolve after complete surgical removal of the tumour and following treatment with the somatostatin analogue octreotide [5].

Investigations

Useful investigations include a full blood count, biochemistry and glucose, serum glucagon level, skin biopsy, abdominal ultrasound, CT scan of the chest, abdomen and pelvis, PET/CT scan, coeliac axis angiography and single photon emission CT (SPECT) (Figure 47.14). Somatostatin receptor imaging using ^{111}In-octreotide (octreotide is a somatostatin analogue and is taken up by NETs as they overexpress somatostatin receptors) can also be useful (Figure 47.15).

Management

> #### Treatment ladder for necrolytic acral erythema
>
> #### First line
> - Surgery is the cornerstone of management for pancreatic endocrine tumours, but curative surgery is rarely obtained in most cases because of metastatic disease at time of presentation
>
> #### Second line
> - Somatostatin is a polypeptide produced by gastrointestinal paracrine cells and inhibits the release of hormones such as glucagon. Long-acting somatostatin analogues (e.g. lanreotide or octreotide) provide good control of symptoms (Figure 47.16) but do not influence tumour growth
>
> #### Third line
> - Chemotherapy with 5-fluorouracil, dacarbazine, streptozocin or doxorubacin
> - Embolisation of hepatic metastases
> - Peptide receptor radioligand therapy
> - Everolimus (an oral inhibitor of mammalian target of rapamycin) [18]
> - Sunitinib (multitargeted tyrosine kinase inhibitor) [19]

Wells syndrome

Synonyms and inclusions
- Eosinophilic cellulitis
- Bullous cellulitis with eosinophilia

Introduction and general description

Wells syndrome is a rare disorder of uncertain aetiology first described in 1971 by Wells [1]. Multiple triggers and diseases have now been reported in association with the disorder, such as infection (mycoplasma), insect bites, haematological disorders (chronic lymphocytic leukaemia), medications such as non-steroidal anti-inflammatory drugs, Covid-19 vaccination and targeted immunotherapies including ustekinumab, infliximab and adalimumab [3–5]. The exact pathogenesis remains unclear, although recent case series reporting successful treatment with baracitinib suggest upregulation of JAK2/STAT5 signalling pathways [6]. In addition, interleukin-5 blockade with mepolizumab in resistant cases suggests a role for interleukin-5 in disease severity and upregulation of the TH2 pathway in disease pathogenesis [7].

Pathophysiology
Pathology

The classical histology shows an eosinophil-rich diffuse inflammatory infiltrate with characteristic 'flame figures' (Figure 47.17). This is associated with marked dermal oedema and in some cases there may be evidence of intradermal and subepidermal blisters with negative immunofluorescence.

Clinical features
Presentation

Affected individuals present at any age with annular red/pink plaques, blisters and nodules which feel warm and are described by the patient as both itchy and burning. Lesions characteristically remit after 4–8 weeks but typically may continue to relapse over months to years [2] (Figure 47.18).

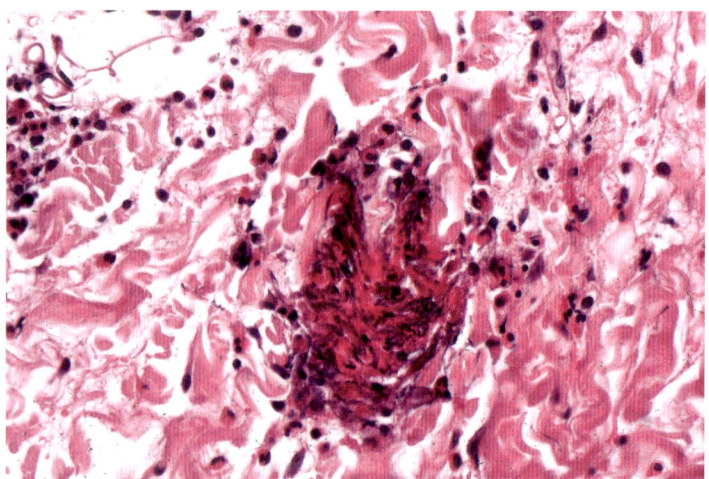

Figure 47.17 Wells syndrome. Note formation of flame figures in which numerous eosinophilic granules cover collagen bundles. Courtesy of Eduardo Calonje.

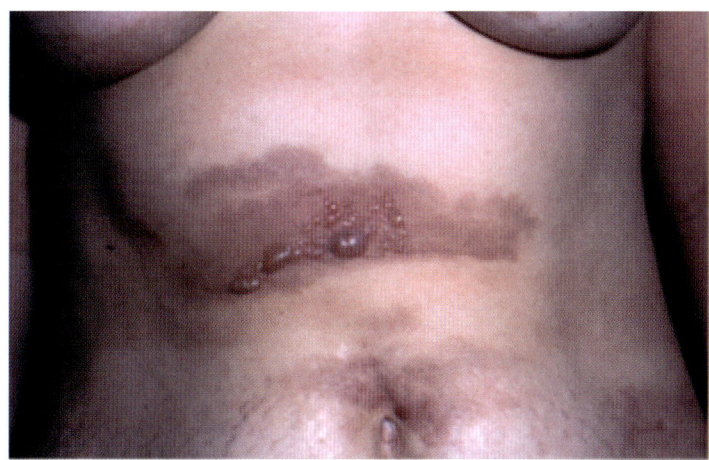

Figure 47.18 Wells syndrome. Lesions may be bullous and often resolve to leave a green discoloration of the skin.

Differential diagnosis

The varied morphology of the lesions can pose a diagnostic challenge as they can resemble annular erythema of infancy and eosinophilic annular erythema. The characteristic histology of Wells syndrome histology from an affected area showing the eosinophilic dermal infiltration and 'flame figures' can aid diagnosis. However, clinicopathological overlap with other annular erythemas may be observed.

Treatment

The rarity and heterogeneity of Wells syndrome means there is limited and inconsistent evidence about the best approaches to treatment. Most of the evidence is at the level of case series or case reports. Systemic corticosteroids have historically been the mainstay of therapy, often with limited success. Dapsone and hydroxychloroquine are often cited as steroid-sparing agents. More recent case series, however, are beginning to report treatment success with JAK pathway inhibition with baricitinib [6]. There are additional case reports of success with dupilumab [8] and with mepolizumab for resistant cases [7]. Omalizumab has been reported to induce long-term remission [9].

Key references

The full list of references can be found in the online version at https://www.wiley.com/rooksdermatology10e

Erythema multiforme
Introduction and general description
2 Roujeau JC. The spectrum of Stevens–Johnson syndrome and toxic epidermal necrolysis: a clinical classification. *J Invest Dermatol* 1994;102:S28–30.
3 Assier H, Bastuji-Garin S, Revuz J, Roujeau JC. Erythema multiforme with mucous membrane involvement and Stevens–Johnson syndrome are clinically different disorders with distinct causes. *Arch Dermatol* 1995;131:539–43.
4 Roujeau JC. Stevens–Johnson syndrome and toxic epidermal necrolysis are severity variants of the same disease which differs from erythema multiforme. *J Dermatol* 1997;24:726–9.
5 Auquier-Dunant A, Mockenhaupt M, Naldi L *et al*. Correlations between clinical patterns and causes of erythema multiforme majus, Stevens–Johnson syndrome, and toxic epidermal necrolysis: results of an international prospective study. *Arch Dermatol* 2002;138:1019–24.
10 Wolkenstein P, Revuz J. Toxic epidermal necrolysis. *Dermatol Clin* 2000;18: 485–95, ix.

Pathophysiology
Triggering factors
5 Grosber M, Alexandre M, Poszepczynska-Guigné E *et al*. Recurrent erythema multiforme in association with recurrent Mycoplasma pneumoniae infections. *J Am Acad Dermatol* 2007;56(Suppl. 5):S118–19.
25 Torrelo A, Andina D, Santonja C *et al*. Erythema multiforme-like lesions in children and COVID-19. *Ped Dermatol* 2020;37:442–6.
26 Demibraş A, Elmas OF, Atasoy M, Türsen Ü, Lotti T. A case of erythema multiforme major in a patient with COVID 19: the role of corticosteroid therapy. *Dermatol Ther* 2020;33:e13899.

Drug reactions
56 Utsunmiya A, Oyama N, Hasegawa M. A case of erythema multiforme major developed after sequential use of two immune checkpoint inhibitors, nivolumab and ipilimumab for advanced melanoma: possible implication of synergistic and/or complementary immunomodulatory effects. *Case Report Dermatol* 2018;10:1–8.
57 Khicher S, Weinberger J. Vancomycin-associated erythema multiforme. *Am J Therapeutics* 2020;27:e674–5.
58 Rodriguez-Pazos L, Sanchez-Aguilar D, Rodriguez-Granados MT *et al*. Erythema multiforme photoinduced by statins. *Photodermatol Photoimmunol Photomed* 2010; 26:216–18.

Annular erythema of infancy
1 Peterson AO, Jarratt MD. Annular erythema of infancy. *Arch Dermatol* 1981;117:145–8.
5 Toonstra J, de Witt RFE. 'Persistent' annular erythema of infancy. *Arch Dermatol* 1984;120:1069–72.

Erythema chronicum migrans
1 Gerber MA, Shapiro ED. Diagnosis of Lyme disease in children. *J Pediatr* 1992; 121:157–62.
3 National Institute for Health and Clinical Excellence (NICE). *Lyme Disease. NG95*. London: NICE, 2018. https://www.nice.org.uk/guidance/ng95 (last accessed September 2023).

Erythema marginatum
1 Dajani AS, Ayoub E, Bierman FZ *et al*. Guidelines for the diagnosis of rheumatic fever: Jones criteria updated 1992. *Circulation* 1993;87:302–7.
2 Abt AF. Erythema annulare rheumaticum. *Am J Med Sci* 1935;190:824–33.
3 Keil H. The rheumatic erythemas; a critical survey. *Ann Intern Med* 1937–38;11:2223–72.

Erythema gyratum repens
1 Gammel JA. Erythema gyratum repens. *Arch Dermatol Syphilol* 1953;66:494–505.
3 Thomas I, Schwartz RA. Cutaneous paraneoplastic syndromes: uncommon presentations. *Clin Dermatol* 2005;23:593–600.
5 Eubanks LE, McBurney E, Reed R. Erythema gyratum repens. *Am J Med Sci* 2001;321:302–5.

Necrolytic migratory erythema
1 Guillausseau PJ, Villet R, Kalloustian E *et al*. [Glucagonomas. Clinical, biological, anatomopathological and therapeutic aspects (general review of 130 cases).] *Gastroenterol Clin Biol* 1982;6:1029–41.
7 Virani S, Prajapati V, Devani A *et al*. Octreotide-responsive necrolytic migratory erythema in a patient with pseudoglucagonoma syndrome. *J Am Acad Dermatol* 2013;68:e44–6.
15 Strosberg JR, Cheema A, Weber J *et al*. Prognostic validity of a novel American Joint Committee on Cancer Staging Classification for Pancreatic Neuroendocrine Tumors. *J Clin Oncol* 2011;29:3044–9.
18 Yao JC, Shah MH, Ito T *et al*. Everolimus for advanced pancreatic neuroendocrine tumors. *N Engl J Med* 2011;364:514–23.
19 Raymond E, Dahan L, Raoul J-L *et al*. Sunitinib malate for the treatment of pancreatic neuroendocrine tumors. *N Engl J Med* 2011;364:501–13.

CHAPTER 48

Adamantiades–Behçet Disease

Christos C. Zouboulis

Departments of Dermatology, Venereology, Allergology and Immunology, Staedtisches Klinikum Dessau, Brandenburg Medical School Theodor Fontane and Faculty of Health Sciences Brandenburg, Dessau, Germany

Adamantiades–Behçet disease

Definition and nomenclature

Adamantiades–Behçet disease (ABD), otherwise known as Behçet disease, is a multisystem inflammatory disease of unknown aetiology, classified as a systemic vasculitis and as a neutrophilic dermatosis involving all types and sizes of blood vessels. It is characterised clinically by recurrent courses of oral aphthous ulcers, genital ulcers, skin lesions (papulopustules, erythema nodosum) and iridocyclitis/posterior uveitis. It is occasionally accompanied by arthritis and vascular, neurological, gastrointestinal or other manifestations [1,2].

Synonyms and inclusions

- Behçet disease
- Behçet syndrome
- Malignant aphthosis

Epidemiology
Incidence and prevalence

Adamantiades–Behçet disease has a worldwide occurrence with varying prevalence, being endemic in eastern and central Asian and eastern Mediterranean countries (along the so-called Silk Road) and rare in northern European countries, central and southern Africa, the Americas and Australia [3]. A prevalence of 660 patients per 100 000 inhabitants has been reported in northern Jordan [4], 80–420 patients per 100 000 inhabitants in Turkey (Anatolia and Istanbul 420/100 000) [3,5], 7–30/100 000 in the rest of the Asian continent (Japan 14–31/100 000, Korea 32.8–35.7/100 000 [6], northern China 14/100 000, Saudi Arabia 20/100 000 and Iran 17/100 000), 3.6/100 000 in Egypt [7] and 1.5–7.5/100 000 in southern Europe [3]. In northern European populations (0.27–1.18/100 000), the USA (0.75/100 000) [3,8] and South America (Colombia 1.10/100 000) [9], the disease is rare. An unexpectedly high estimated prevalence has recently been reported from the UK (14.6/100 000) [10] and southwest USA (8.9–10.6/100 000) [11]. A meta-analysis of publications between 1974 and 2015 assessed an estimated prevalence of 10.3/100 000 inhabitants for all studies, 119.8/100 000 for Turkey, 31.8/100 000 for the Middle East, 4.5/100 000 for Asia and 3.3/100 000 for Europe [12]. The increasing estimated prevalence of the disease is due to its chronic character [6]. On the other hand, the annual incidence is low with 0.05 new cases/100 000 inhabitants in Poland (2014) [13], 0.75–1.0/100 000 in Japan (1990) and Germany (2005) [14], 2.4/100 000 in Taiwan [15] and 4.0/100 000 from 2006 to 2015 in Korea [16] and is steadily declining (from 8.15/100 000 in 2004 to 1.51/100 000 in 2017 in Korea [17] and from 8.9/100 000 in 1984 to 7.5/100 000 in 1990 in Japan [18]) together with a decreasing disease severity.

Age

Adamantiades–Behçet disease most often affects patients in their twenties and thirties; however, early and late onsets (first year of life to 72 years of age) have been reported. Juvenile disease rates are 2–5% in different ethnic groups [19]; its prevalence was estimated to be 0.17/100 000 in France and 0.42/100 000 in the UK [20], and the annual incidence 0.05/100 000 in the UK. Pediatric ABD also differs from adult ABD in the frequency and distribution of clinical findings, as well as through lower disease severity score and better outcome [19]. While gastrointestinal system involvement, neurological findings, arthralgia and positive family history are more common in children, genital and vascular lesions are more common in adult patients.

Sex

In contrast to old Japanese and Turkish reports of male predominance, the male to female ratio has decreased drastically in the last 30 years. In the years 1983–2012 significant proportional declines occurred with respect to male sex, complete type of the disease and the major presenting features (genital ulcers, ocular involvement and skin lesions) in 3674 hospital-based patients of the Korean registry, whereas the mean patient age rose progressively, as did the frequencies of joint, gastrointestinal and central nervous system manifestations [21]. Currently, both sexes are equally affected; a male predominance is still observed in Arab populations, whereas female predominance is evident in Korea, China, some northern European countries and the USA.

Ethnicity

Some ethnic populations, such as those of Turkmen and Mongol descent, are more often affected.

Associated diseases

Recurrent aphthous stomatitis (benign aphthosis) is an associated disease.

Pathophysiology

The aetiology of the disease remains unknown, although genetic factors, infectious agents, environmental pollution, immunological mechanisms and endothelial and clotting factors have been implicated and studied intensively [22,23–25]. The endemic occurrence along the historical Silk Road, the major involvement of certain ethnic groups (mostly of Turkmen and Mongol descent) and associated immunogenetic data support the hypothesis that the disease followed the migration of these old nomadic tribes. On the other hand, the wide variation of disease prevalence in the same ethnic group living in different geographic areas indicates an additional environmental triggering factor. Therefore, transfer of genetic material and/or an unknown exogenous agent may have been responsible for the expansion of the disease.

Pathology

Characteristic histopathological features of ABD are vasculitis and thrombosis (Figure 48.1). Biopsies from early mucocutaneous lesions show a neutrophilic vascular reaction with endothelial swelling, extravasation of erythrocytes and leukocytoclasia or a

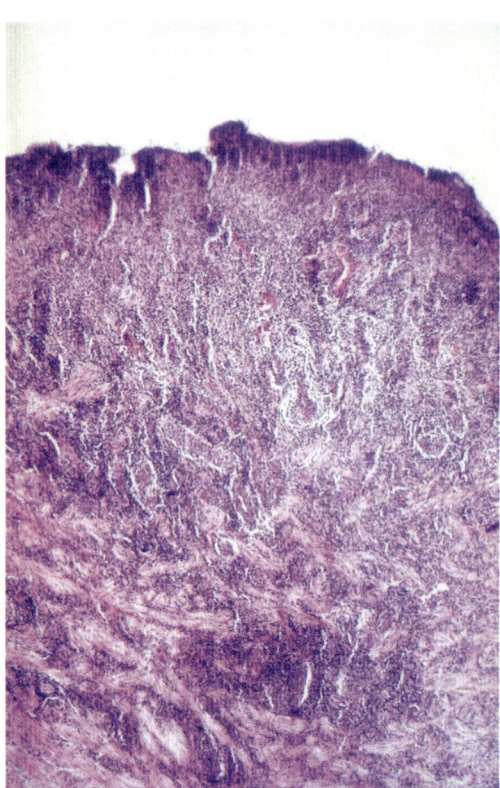

Figure 48.1 Abundant mixed inflammatory infiltrate dominated by neutrophils in an oral ulcer of Adamantiades–Behçet disease.

fully developed leukocytoclastic vasculitis with fibrinoid necrosis of the blood vessel walls [1,14]. There are reports of lesions, especially ocular ones, that consist primarily of a lymphocytic perivasculitis due to lymphangiogenesis [26]. The neutrophilic vascular reaction should be considered the predominant histopathological finding [27]. Aneurysms can also develop in large arteries as a result of vasculitis of the vasa vasorum with penetration of the lamina elastica.

Causative organisms

Adamantiades–Behçet disease is not considered contagious as no horizontal transmission has ever been reported. However, viral and bacterial infections have been implicated in initiating immunopathological pathways, leading to the onset of the disease [22,23,24,28].

Viral agents. Early theories of the pathogenesis of ABD proposed a viral or other infectious aetiology [3]. Partial transcription of herpes simplex virus type 1 (HSV-1) DNA in patients' peripheral blood lymphocytes has been reported [22,24]. HSV-1 DNA was detected in patients' saliva and oral and genital ulcers, and HSV-1 antibodies were found in patients' sera.

Bacterial agents. Disease activity has been known to correlate with bacterial infection, particularly with streptococci [22,24]. *Streptococcus sanguinis* dominates the flora of the oral mucosa in patients with the disease and appears to be the most relevant *Streptococcus* strain as a provoking factor for initiation of the disease [28]. *Streptococcus* antigens and antistreptococcal antibodies are frequently found in the oral mucosa and serum of patients. The involvement of immunoglobulin A protease-producing *S. sanguinis* is proposed as an explanation for a chronic infection leading to initiation of ABD. High titres of the immunogenic *S. sanguinis* antigen KTH-1 have been detected in patients. In addition, exposure of the patients to *Streptococcus* antigens may be a major provoking factor for disease activity [29]. The lipoprotein of *Mycoplasma fermentas* MALP-404 was found in the sera of patients with ABD but not in healthy controls [30]. Interestingly, MALP-404 contains a peptide motif, which can be presented by human leukocyte antigen B51 (HLA-B51). A possible role for bacterial stimulation of monocytes via Toll-like receptor 2 (TLR-2) producing neutrophil-stimulating pro-inflammatory factors in ABD was detected. Moreover, markedly higher expression at the mRNA and protein level of TLR-2, TLR-3, TLR-4 and TLR-8 was observed in patients with active ABD as compared with controls [31].

Genetics

There is no specific mode of Mendelian transmission in ABD [22,23,24]. Familial occurrence with regional differences has been reported, being more frequent in Korea (15%) than in Japan or China (2–3%), and in Arab countries, Israel and Turkey (2–18%) than in Europe (0–5%). An earlier disease onset in children compared with their parents and a higher frequency of familial cases in juveniles than in adults has been observed. ABD heritability has been estimated to be at least 16% [32]. In a Korean study, a familial incidence of 3.57/104 person-years was calculated; familial risks were higher within generation (sibling–sibling) versus between generations (parent–offspring) [33]. Formal twin studies have not been reported.

A significant association exists between the disease and HLA-B51 in Japan, the Middle East and the Mediterranean countries; however, this relationship is not as strong in western countries [34]. The allele also seems to be associated with a more severe prognosis [35]. Its exact role in the disease mechanism is still unknown, although it may be involved in disease development through specific antigen presentation, molecular mimicry with microbial antigens or participation in linkage disequilibrium with a presently unknown susceptibility gene [36,37]. Various KIR alleles (natural ligands of HLA-B51) and their functional polymorphisms influence the risk of presenting with various subtypes of ABD [38]. Among the 24 described alleles, HLA-B5101 and -B5108 have most frequently been associated with ABD [39]. Shared amino acid residues (defining the Bw4 epitope) are crucial for antigen binding and natural killer cell interactions [40], and Bw4 was also reported to contribute to the severity of the disease [41]. Genes possibly associated with the disease have been localised on chromosome 6 in the region between the tumour necrosis factor (TNF) gene and HLA-B or -C genes, including the major histocompatibility complex class I chain A gene (A6 allele) and genes for heat shock proteins (HSPs) [23,34,39,42]. In addition, a novel susceptibility locus mapped to 6p22-23 was detected [39]. Associations on chromosomes 1p31.3 (interleukin 23R (IL-23R)/IL-12RB2) and 1q32.1 (IL-10) were found by genome-wide association studies [40,43]. A haplotype association of IL-8 gene with ABD was also detected [44]. Polymorphisms in genes encoding for host effector molecules may contribute to the disease susceptibility and/or severity of the disease, such as in IL-23R reported in a Chinese Han population [45]. New gene associations with *ERAP-1*, *CCR1–CCR3*, *KLRC4* and *STAT4* genes have been reported [46].

Another genome-wide association study has shown that *ERAP-1* is associated with ABD, and that *ERAP-1* is epistatic with HLA-B*51 allele [47]. Therefore, the activation of immune response could depend on the antigen presentation to T cells in the context of the HLA-B*51. The latter is able also to activate an innate immune response interacting with natural killer and γδT cells. Moreover, polymorphisms of *ERAP-1* could lead to an unfolded protein response, thus favouring an autoinflammatory process [48].

A next-generation sequencing study in 60 Egyptian ABD patients and 160 controls revealed the following gene associations for ABD: HLA-B*51:08 (odds ratio (OR) 19.75), HLA-B*15:03 (OR 12.15), HLA-C*16:02 (OR 6.53), HLA-A*68:02 (OR 3.14) [24,49]. By contrast, HLA-A*03:01 (OR 0.13) and HLA-DPB1*17:01 (OR 0.27) were found to be protective. A strong linkage disequilibrium between HLA-B*51:08, -C*16:02 and -A*02:01 was found. In another genetic association study in ABD with 9444 multinational patients and controls, two novel genetic susceptibility loci, a risk locus in IFNGR1 (OR 1.25) and another within the intergenic region LNCAROD/DKK1 (OR 0.78), were detected and six previously identified susceptibility loci were confirmed (IL-10, IL-23R, IL-12A-AS1, CCR3, ADO and LACC1) [50]. Last, HLA-26 has been shown to be associated with ocular lesions [51].

Immunogenetic factors
Immunological mechanisms are considered to play a major role in the pathogenesis of ABD [**22**,23,39,42]. The disease has currently been classified among the autoinflammatory disorders [48]. An inverse correlation between the degree of DNA methylation and FKBP5 mRNA expression in ABD was shown [52]. FKBP5 is the gene that plays an important role in the TNF-α nuclear factor κB (NFκB) signalling pathway.

Autoimmune mechanisms. The major microscopic finding at most sites of active disease is an immune-mediated occlusive vasculitis [25]. The pathergy reaction (see 'Clinical features' later in this chapter) is induced by the rapid accumulation of neutrophils (hyperchemotaxis) and later by T lymphocytes and monocytes/macrophages at the needle-prick sites. A Th17 polarisation was confirmed with five highly connected clusters enriched in T- and B-cell activation pathways and two clusters enriched in type I interferon (IFN), JAK/STAT and TLR signalling pathways [53]. The identified gene classes (vascular damage, blood coagulation and inflammation) are involved in the pathogenesis of the typical features of ABD. Patients' lymphocytes also express CD29 molecules and bind to endothelial cells in active disease. In addition to defective T-cell immunity, B-cell activation is impaired. Circulating immune complexes, together with enhanced neutrophil migration, may be involved; the diversity of T cells indicates that specific T-cell responses to several antigens may lead to the variety of symptoms [54]. Tropomyosins and the 160 kDa polypeptide kinectin have been detected as autoantigens in ABD [55,56]. In a transcriptome analysis of CD8+ T-cell subsets in patients with ABD, COL5A1 expression was significantly associated with CD8+CD27–CD28– T cells and TRPV3 and ARHGEF10 with CD8+CD27+CD28+ T cells [57]. A genome-wide association study identified CCR1 and IL-10 loci as contributing to M1 macrophage-predominant inflammation in ABD [58]. Current single-cell analyses highlighted the pro-inflammatory contribution of C1q-high monocytes to the disease [59].

Heat shock proteins. Increased levels of HSP-specific antibodies in the serum have been found in ABD [24,60,61]. T cells respond to 60 kDa HSP, and four different peptide determinants within 60 kDa HSP identified by T-cell epitope mapping have been suggested to be involved in the pathogenesis of the disease.

Cytokine mediators. Various pro-inflammatory cytokines, such as IL-1, -6, -8, -12, -18, -22, -23, -33, -38 and TNF-α, are elevated in the sera of patients with active ABD [62–73]. In particular, IL-8 seems to play an important role, can also be released by endothelial cells, has a potent effect on the inflammatory response and is a sensitive marker of disease activity [62–64,68,70]. Cytokine release may be dependent on the involved organ [60,61,64,67].

Endothelial cells. The endothelium seems to be the primary target, or it may only be involved as an innocent bystander of pathological changes of the immune system [74]. An immunoglobulin M type, 47 kDa, cell surface HSP against endothelial α-enolase has been identified in the serum of patients with ABD [29,75]. Plasma endothelin 1 concentrations were found to be significantly increased, perhaps indicating vasoconstriction and being the direct result of elevated synthesis by injured vascular endothelial cells. Thrombomodulin, a cell surface glycoprotein of vascular endothelium, which is also increased in the plasma of patients with active disease, potentially damages the endothelial cells.

Oxidative stress-mediated circulating haematopoietic progenitor cell dysfunction in ABD may counteract the cells' vascular repair function, thereby contributing to the pathogenesis and the progression of vascular disease in ABD [76].

Covid-19. In contrast with other immunological diseases, ABD patients presented a lower prevalence of Covid-19 compared with the general population [77] and when infected they exhibited a low Covid-19 severity without flares of ABD [78].

Clinical features
History
Hippocrates of Kos (460–377 BC) used the designation στοματα αφθωδεα, ελκωδεα (oral aphthous ulcers) in a probable first description of a patient with the disease (Epidemion book III, case 7). The disease is named after Benediktos Adamantiades, a Greek ophthalmologist, and Hulûsi Behçet, a Turkish dermatologist, who, in 1931 and 1937, respectively, described patients with the characteristic clinical complex and argued for this to be a single clinical entity [79]. The first international multidisciplinary conference was organised by two dermatologists, M. Monacelli and P. Nazarro, in 1964 in Rome, Italy.

Presentation
Adamantiades–Behçet disease is a chronic, recurrent, multisystem and, occasionally, life-threatening disorder [1,3]. Recurrent oral aphthous ulcers, recurrent genital ulcers, skin manifestations, ocular lesions and arthritis/arthropathy are the most frequent clinical features. Vascular, neurological, gastrointestinal, psychiatric, pulmonary, renal and cardiac manifestations, epididymitis and other findings can also occur. The clinical picture usually develops within a few months after the presenting sign. Both an acute multisystem presentation and long-term development of the disease over years are possible.

Diagnosis of ABD is based on clinical signs as neither a pathognomonic laboratory test nor histological characteristics are available. There are several sets of diagnostic criteria, the most popular among the older ones being the criteria of the International Study Group [80] and those of the Behçet's Disease Research Committee of Japan [81]. However, there have been several problems with these criteria, including their performance in selectivity and specificity, so that both of them have been revised. The currently published Revised International Criteria for Behçet's Disease provides the most accurate diagnosis (Table 48.1) [82,83].

Clinical variants/phenotypes
It has been proposed that different populations with ABD should be stratified using cluster analysis and association studies. The main clinical phenotypes described are the 'mucocutaneous and articular', 'vascular', 'neurological and ocular' and 'gastrointestinal' ones [84,85].

Mucocutaneous and articular phenotype. Recurrent oral aphthous and genital ulcers are the most frequently observed mucosal manifestations. Oral aphthous ulcers are the presenting sign in more

Table 48.1 Revised international criteria for Adamantiades–Behçet disease.

Clinical feature	Points[a]
Ocular lesions (recurrent)	2
Oral aphthosis (recurrent)	2
Genital aphthosis (recurrent)	2
Skin lesions (recurrent)	1
Central nervous system lesions	1
Vascular manifestations	1
Positive pathergy test[b]	1

Adapted from ITR-ICBD 2013 [**82**].
[a] Scoring: a score ≥4 indicates Adamantiades–Behçet disease.
[b] Although the main scoring system does not include a pathergy test, where pathergy testing is conducted, a positive result may be included for one extra point.

than 80% of patients (Figure 48.1) [1,14,42]. Although recurrent aphthous stomatitis is a common disorder, only a few patients progress to ABD, and it is not possible to determine in whom or when the transition may occur [86]. Typically, lesions are multiple, painful, 1–3 cm in diameter and sharply margined with a fibrin-coated base and surrounding erythema (Figure 48.2). Oral aphthous ulcers usually heal without scarring (92%). Genital ulcers may not recur as often and usually heal with a characteristic scar (64–88%) (Figure 48.3). Spontaneous healing of aphthae occurs within 4 days to 1 month; genital ulcers may persist longer. Large oral ulcerations can also be associated with problems such as pharyngeal involvement, dysphagia and dyspnoea or fistulae involving the pharynx, larynx, trachea or oesophagus. Genital ulcers can occur on the penis, scrotum, vagina, labia and urethra, and also in the anal, perineal and inguinal regions.

Skin lesions that should be accepted as diagnostically relevant in ABD should be confined to pustular vasculitic lesions (including pathergy lesions), erythema nodosum-like lesions, Sweet disease-like lesions, pyoderma gangrenosum-like lesions and palpable purpuric lesions of necrotising venulitis. All lesions are characterised in their early stages by a neutrophilic vascular reaction. Acneform lesions or follicle-based pustules should not be considered relevant [27].

Systemic lesions. Ocular involvement is the major cause of morbidity in patients with ABD. The most diagnostically relevant lesion is posterior uveitis (also called retinal vasculitis), which can lead to blindness (Figure 48.4). Just over 4% of Japanese ABD patients present with posterior uveitis, making it the one of the six diseases in Japan most likely to exhibit uveitis [87]; compared with previous surveys between 1994 and 2003, the rate of ABD has decreased [88]. Other ocular lesions include anterior uveitis, hypopyon (pus in the anterior chamber of the eye, which is now – due to early treatment – uncommon) and secondary complications such as cataract, glaucoma and neovascular lesions [89]. Retinal inflammation can lead to vascular occlusion and, ultimately, tractional retinal detachment. Severe vitreous involvement, chronic cystoid macular oedema and possible – presumably also vasculitic – involvement of the optic nerve can result in loss of vision. Recurrent vasculitic changes can ultimately lead to ischaemic optic nerve atrophy.

The characteristic arthritis is a non-erosive, asymmetrical, sterile, seronegative oligoarthritis; however, symmetrical polyarticular

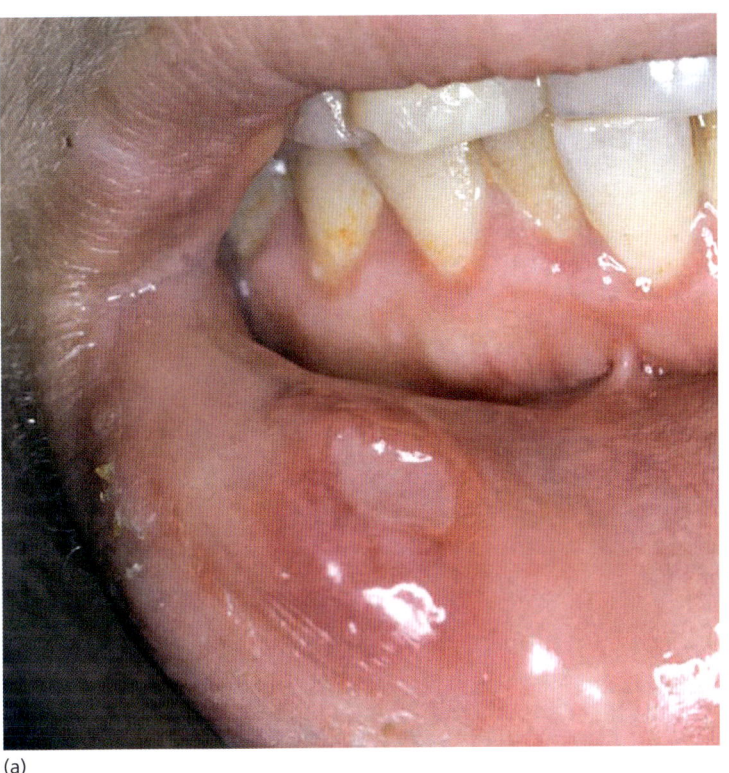
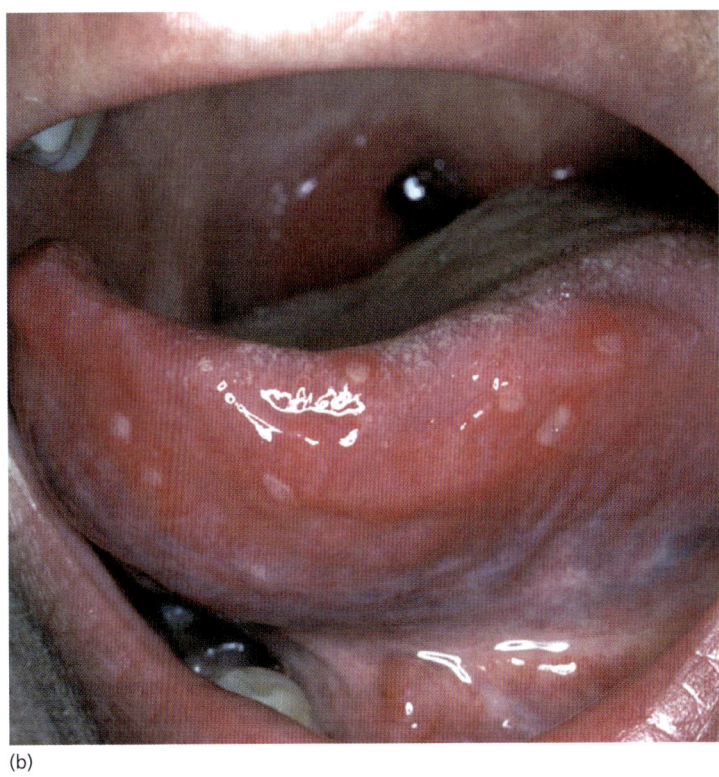

(a)   (b)

Figure 48.2 Single (a) and multiple (b) oral aphthous ulcers. (a) Reproduced from Altenburg *et al.* 2006 [14] with permission of John Wiley & Sons.

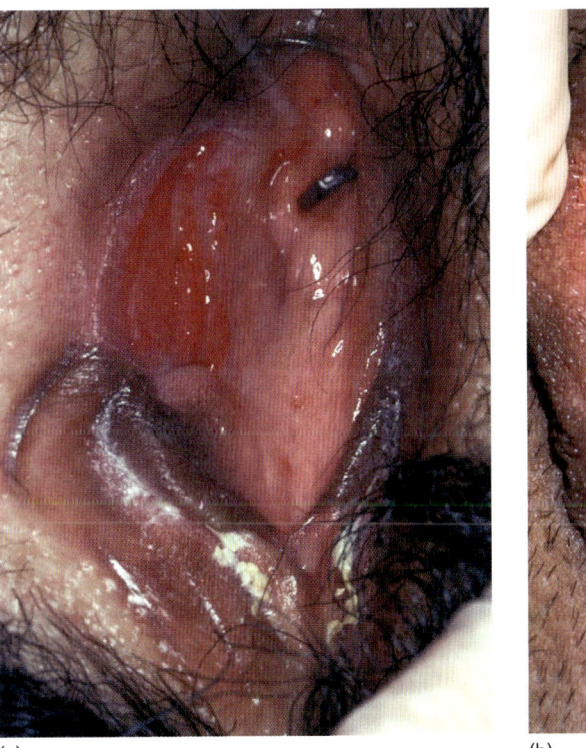
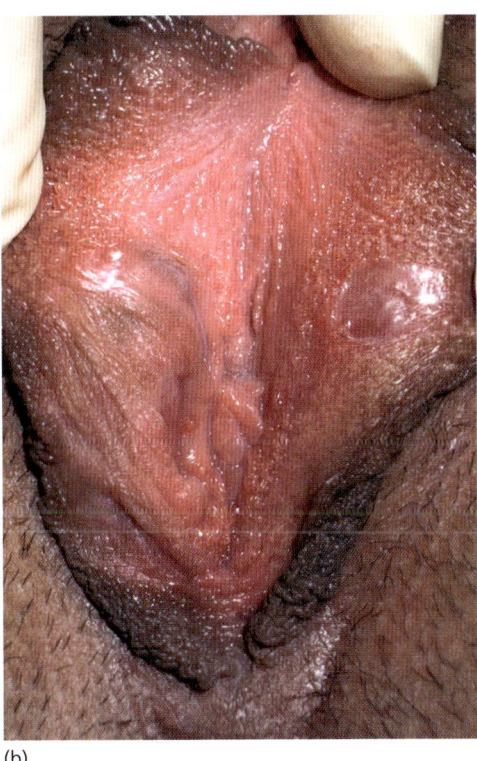

Figure 48.3 Genital ulcer (a) healing with a demarcated flat scar (b).

(a)   (b)

involvement is common. Joint manifestations frequently occur first in one knee or ankle and then the other as a migratory monoarthritis, then in both joints simultaneously, and finally affecting nearly all joints. An HLA-B27-positive erosive sacroiliitis has to be excluded.

Systemic vascular involvement can be significant and includes venous occlusions and varices, arterial occlusions and aneurysms, often being migratory. Cases of large-vein thrombosis (inferior vena cava, cranial venous sinuses) or large-artery aneurysms are

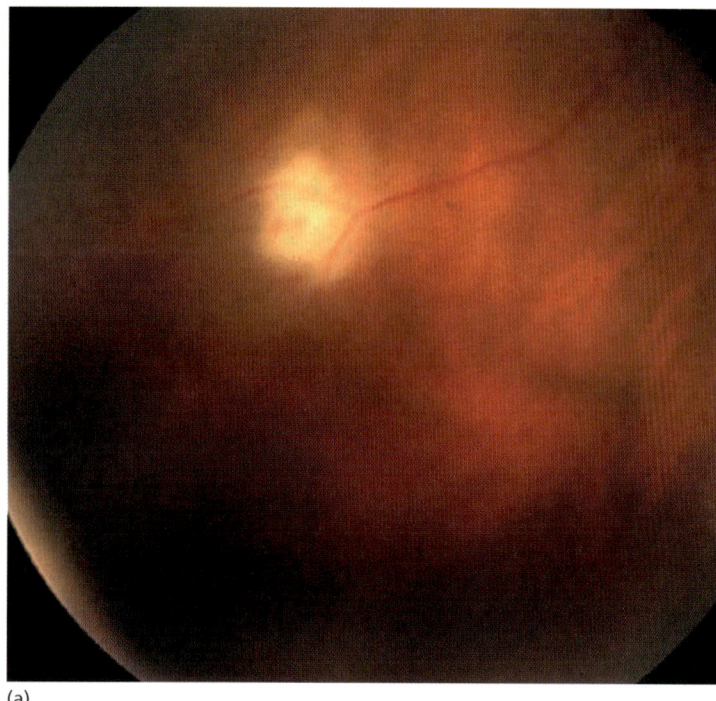

(a)

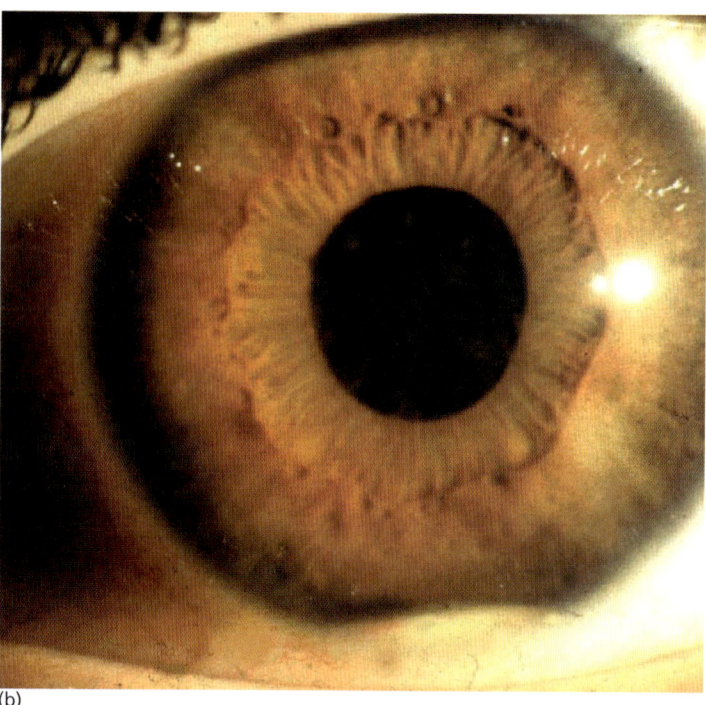

(b)

Figure 48.4 (a) Posterior uveitis with remarkable reduction of intact arterioles due to thrombosis and/or interstitial bleeding. (b) Hypopyoniritis as a result of recurrent iritis. Reproduced from Altenburg *et al*. 2006 [**14**] with permission of John Wiley & Sons.

potentially fatal [**1**,**14**]. Arterial involvement is rather rare and usually presents in the form of thromboses and, less often, of aneurysms, resulting from multicentric arteritis. Pulmonary artery aneurysms are the principal feature of pulmonary involvement in ABD, occasionally resulting in coughing and haemoptysis. Cardiac involvement can include myocarditis, coronary arteritis, endocarditis and valvular disease. A wide spectrum of renal manifestations can occur, varying from minimal change disease to proliferative glomerulonephritis and rapidly progressive crescentic glomerulonephritis. Immune complex deposition is thought to be responsible for the underlying pathogenesis in some cases of glomerulonephritis. Gastrointestinal complaints can be a symptom for aphthae throughout the gastrointestinal tract and can rarely result in perforation and peritonitis (0.5%). The distribution of intestinal ulcers (ileo-caecal and colorectum), erythrocyte sedimentation rate >24 mm/h, persistence of inflammation despite treatment and poor compliance are independent risk factors for poor outcomes in non-surgical intestinal ABD patients [90]. Inflammatory bowel disease has to be excluded. Sterile prostatitis and epididymitis can be present in male patients without genital ulcers.

Significant neurological manifestations occur in approximately 10% of patients and may be delayed in onset. Meningoencephalitis, cerebral venous sinus thrombosis, benign intracranial hypertension, cranial nerve palsies, brainstem lesions and pyramidal or extrapyramidal lesions have been described. Poor prognosis is associated with a progressive course, relapses after treatment, repeated attacks and cerebellar symptoms or parenchymal disease. Neurological manifestations usually present with severe headache. Further symptoms include gait disturbance, dysarthria, vertigo and diplopia, as well as hyperreflexia, epileptic seizures, hemiplegia, ataxia or a positive Babinski reflex. Psychiatric symptoms, such as depression, insomnia or memory impairment, are also signs of neurological involvement.

Differential diagnosis [14,91]
There are many possible differential diagnoses (Box 48.1).

Classification of severity
A severe course, including blindness, meningoencephalitis, haemoptysis, intestinal perforation and severe arthritis, occurs in approximately 10% of patients. Lethal outcome has been seen in 0–6% of affected patients in different ethnic groups. Central nervous system and pulmonary and large-vessel involvement, as well as bowel perforation, are the major life-threatening complications; death may also result as a complication of immunosuppressive therapy.

Complications and co-morbidities
Ophthalmic and neurological sequelae are leading causes of morbidity, followed by severe vascular and gastrointestinal manifestations. Their effects on morbidity may be cumulative.

Disease course and prognosis
The clinical course of ABD is variable. There can be a delay of up to several years before the diagnosis is made, and this may influence the prognosis [92]. Mucocutaneous and joint manifestations usually occur first. Recurrent erythema nodosum and HLA-B51 positivity are risk factors for the development of superficial thrombophlebitis and vision loss; superficial thrombophlebitis, ocular lesions and male sex are risk factors for the development of systemic vessel involvement [35,93,94]. Blindness can often be prevented with early aggressive therapy of posterior uveitis, such as TNF-α

Box 48.1 Differential diagnoses for Adamantiades–Behçet disease

- Oculocutaneous/mucocutaneous syndromes
- Erythema multiforme exudativum and variants, including Stevens–Johnson syndrome
- Vogt–Koyanagi–Harada syndrome
- Reactive arthritis
- Bullous autoimmune diseases: pemphigus vulgaris, cicatricial mucous membrane pemphigoid, epidermolysis bullosa acquisita
- Viral infections (herpes, coxsackie, echo)
- Syphilis
- Articulomucocutaneous syndromes
- Systemic lupus erythematosus
- MAGIC syndrome (mouth and genital ulcers with inflamed cartilage)
- Yersiniosis
- Arthropathic psoriasis
- Gastrointestinal/mucocutaneous syndromes
- Ulcerative colitis, Crohn disease
- Tuberculosis
- Bowel-associated dermatitis–arthritis syndrome
- Aphthae
- Recurrent aphthous stomatitis
- Cyclic neutropenia
- Herpes oralis/labialis/genitalis recidivans
- Genital ulcers
- Ulcus vulvae acutum (Lipschütz ulcer)
- Sexually transmitted infections
- Uveitis
- Other forms of uveitis
- Arthritis
- Ankylosing spondylitis
- Juvenile rheumatoid arthritis
- Central nervous system manifestation
- Multiple sclerosis
- Neuro-Sweet disease
- Lung manifestation
- Sarcoidosis

inhibitors, high-dose ciclosporin A and high-dose intravenous and intraocular corticosteroids. Spontaneous remissions of certain or all manifestations of the disease have been observed. In a study with 245 ABD patients with a mean follow-up of 35 years starting at the age of 16, 63.2% of the patients no longer fulfilled the diagnostic criteria of ABD, 51.8% of them were in sustained remission, and 36.2% of them were asymptomatic [90]. Predictors of sustained remission were remission induction in the first 2 years of treatment, adherence to therapy and treatment for more than 6 years. Poor outcome was observed in 31.8% of patients. HLA-B51 positivity, male sex, obesity, early development of systemic signs and having active severe disease are the risk factors of poor outcome [35,92]. Onset in childhood does not necessarily predict a poor prognosis. In a 3-year follow-up comparison of Turkish patients with ocular involvement during the years 1990–94 and 2000–04 [95], disease was milder at referral – as has been reported for Korean patients [5]. Posterior segment involvement was less common and visual acuity was better. The follow-up revealed no significant difference in number of uveitis attacks in the first 3 years, but fewer eyes lost useful vision, no patient became legally blind and fewer severe ocular complications occurred in the 2000s [95].

Disease duration (≤60 months), neutrophil : lymphocyte ratio (≥2), C-reactive protein (≥10 mg/L), erythrocyte sedimentation rate (≥20 mm/h) and albumin : globulin ratio (<1.5) are independent risk factors of disease activity in ABD patients [96].

Investigations

Pathergy test

A positive pathergy test (hyperreactivity reaction) manifests within 48 h as a red papule (>2 mm) or pustule at the site of a skin needle prick or after intracutaneous injection of 0.1 mL isotonic salt solution using a 20-gauge needle without prior disinfection of the injection site. The skin prick is generally placed at an angle of 45 degrees 3–5 mm intracutaneously on the volar forearm. Redness without infiltration is considered a negative finding. Provoked oral aphthae and genital ulcers after injection or injury (such as chorioretinitis in the corneal region of the eye after photocoagulation of the ocular fundus region) can be considered as positive pathergy phenomena. Broader pathergy phenomena also include the occurrence of aneurysms around vascular anastomoses as well as a local recurrence of ulcers after resection of affected bowel segments. Although a positive pathergy reaction is a sign of ABD, it is not pathognomonic, as it can also occur in patients with pyoderma gangrenosum, rheumatoid arthritis, Crohn disease and genital herpes infection.

Radiological findings

Scintigraphic evidence of arthritis is found in 50% of the patients [14]. Cranial magnetic resonance imaging allows documentation of hypodense or atrophic changes in the brain. Electroencephalographic detection of diffuse α-waves is considered a positive finding. Vascular lesions can be detected by angiography.

Diagnostic tests

An ophthalmological examination with fundus evaluation after mydriasis should be performed regularly in ABD patients, even without ocular symptoms, since initial retinal vessel changes can develop asymptomatically. The diagnostic tests of other organs reported here have to take place following respective symptoms.

Management

A multidisciplinary approach in the management of ABD patients is mandatory. The choice of treatment for patients with ABD depends on the site and severity of the clinical manifestations of the disease [97]. Recurrent aphthae are most often treated with palliative agents such as mild diet, avoidance of irritating agents and potent topical glucocorticoids and local anaesthetics [98,99,100–104]. Lately, topical hyaluronic acid 0.2% gel applied twice a day over 30 days has been found to be effective (Box 48.2) [101]. For the topical treatment of genital ulcers and skin lesions, corticosteroid and antiseptic creams can be applied for up to 7 days. Painful genital ulcerations can be managed by topical anaesthetics in cream. Corticosteroid injections (triamcinolone acetonide 0.1–0.5 mL/lesion) can be helpful in recalcitrant ulcerations. They can also be beneficial

PART 4: INFLAMMATORY DERMATOSES

Table 48.2 Systemic treatment of Adamantiades–Behçet disease with grade A evidence of effectiveness (randomised, double-blind, placebo-controlled trial against placebo unless otherwise mentioned).

Drug and reference	Dose	Indications
Methylprednisolone [108]	40 mg/every 3 weeks IM	Erythema nodosum (in females), but not oro-genital ulcers
Rebamipide [109]	300 mg/day PO (caveat: pregnancy, lactation)	Oral ulcers
Colchicine [110]	1 mg/day PO (caveat: pregnancy, lactation – induces oligozoospermia)	Oral aphthous ulcers, genital ulcers, folliculitis, erythema nodosum
Colchicine [111]	1.5 mg/day PO	Erythema nodosum and arthralgia
Colchicine [112,113]	1–2 mg/day PO	Genital ulcers, erythema nodosum, arthritis (females), arthritis (males) Ineffective: does not reduce the use of immunosuppressives
Colchicine versus colchicine + benzathine penicillin [114]	1–2 mg/day PO; 1.2 mega units × 3/week IM	Combined treatment more effective in reducing frequency of arthritic episodes, duration and frequency of oral ulcers and erythema nodosum, and frequency of genital ulcers
Colchicine versus colchicine + benzathine penicillin [115]	1 mg/day PO;1.2 mega units/month IM	Combined treatment more effective than colchicine or penicillin alone
Zinc sulphate [116]	300 mg/day PO	Mucocutaneous lesions
Dapsone [117]	100 mg/day PO (caveat: pregnancy, lactation; methaemoglobin increase: ascorbic acid 500 mg/day)	Oral ulcers, genital ulcers, skin lesions, pathergy test, arthritis, epididymitis
Azathioprine [118]	2.5 mg/kg/day PO (caveat: pregnancy, lactation, severe liver disease, bone marrow depression, severe infection, children)	Oral ulcers, genital ulcers, arthritis, recent-onset ocular disease Prevents the development of new eye lesions
Interferon-α2a [119]	6 × 10⁶ IU × 3/week SC (caveat: pregnancy, lactation – induces psychotic signs, psoriasis, myopathy)	Oral ulcers, genital ulcers, papulopustular lesions, erythema nodosum, articular symptoms
Interferon-α [120]	1000 and 2000 IU/day PO	Ineffective
Thalidomide [121]	100 mg/day or 300 mg/day PO (caveat: pregnancy, lactation – induces polyneuropathy; minimised at 25 mg/day)	Oral ulcers, genital ulcers, papulopustular lesions
Ciclosporin A versus colchicine [122]	10 mg/kg/day PO; 1 mg/day PO (caveat: lactation, renal insufficiency – induces pathological central nervous system findings)	Ocular manifestations, oral ulcers, skin lesions, genital ulcers (stronger and sustained effectiveness of ciclosporin A versus colchicine)
Ciclosporin A versus conventional treatments (prednisolone, chlorambucil) [123]	10 mg/kg/day PO	Ocular attacks (conventional therapy superior in controlling oral ulcers, genital ulcers and arthritis)
Ciclosporin A versus conventional treatments (prednisolone, chlorambucil) [124]	10 mg/kg/day PO	Hearing loss (25%) (significant improvement under ciclosporin A versus any other conventional treatment)
Ciclosporin A versus conventional treatments (prednisolone, azathioprine) [125]	5 mg/kg/day PO	Oral ulcers, genital ulcers, cutaneous lesions, thrombophlebitis, articular and neurological symptoms (significant improvement under ciclosporin A versus any other conventional treatment)
Ciclosporin A versus cyclophosphamide pulses [126]	5 mg/kg/day PO	Visual acuity (significant improvement under ciclosporin A but not under cyclophosphamide)
Cyclophosphamide + corticosteroids versus corticosteroids [127]	1 g/month IV; 2 g/month IV	Combined more effective in eye disease
Etanercept [128]	25 mg × 2/week PO (caveat: pregnancy, lactation)	Oral ulcers, nodular skin lesions, papulopustular lesions (not pathergy test)
Rituximab versus cytotoxic combination therapy [129]	Two 1000 mg PO courses (15-day interval)	Significant improvement in total adjusted disease activity index (under rituximab but not under cytotoxic combination treatment)
Aciclovir [130]	800 mg × 5/day for 1 week + 400 mg × 2/day PO for 11 weeks	Ineffective
Azapropazone [131]	900 mg/day over 3 weeks PO	Arthritis
Daclizumab (anti-CD25) [132]	1 mg/kg/fortnight IV	Ineffective (eye disease)
Apremilast [**133**]	30 mg × 2/day PO (caveat: diarrhoea, nausea, headache)	Oral aphthous ulcers (reduction of number)

Table 48.3 Systemic treatment of Adamantiades–Behçet disease (ABD) with grade B evidence (well-conducted open clinical trial) or grade C evidence (small open clinical trial) of effectiveness.

Drug and reference	Dose	Indication
Corticosteroids [**2**,42,**97**]	5–60 mg/day prednisolone equivalent PO 100–1000 mg/day over 1–3 days IV (alone or in combinations) (caveat: diabetes – induces psychosis)	Active disease Acute exacerbation (particularly uveitis, neurological manifestations)
Indomethacin [**2**,43]	100 mg/day PO	Mucocutaneous lesions, arthritis
Pentoxifylline [**97**]	300–400 mg × 1–3/day PO	Oral ulcers (particularly in children)
Irsogladine [134]	2–4 mg/day PO	Recurrent aphthous ulcers
Ciclosporin [**97**,135]	3–6 mg/kg/day PO (serum levels: 100–150 ng/mL) (caveat: lactation, renal insufficiency – induces pathological central nervous system findings)	Uveitis, mucocutaneous signs, thrombophlebitis, acute hearing loss
Sulfasalazine [**97**]	1.5–3 g/day PO	Gastrointestinal ulcers
Thalidomide [**97**,136]	2 mg/kg/day PO; increased to 3 mg/kg/day if necessary or decreased to 1–0.5 mg/kg/day PO according to response (caveat: neurotoxicity)	Intestinal involvement (in children)
Tacrolimus [**97**]	0.05–0.2 mg/kg/day PO (serum levels: 15–25 ng/mL)	Refractory uveitis
Interferon-α [137–139]	9×10^6 IU × 3/week or $3–9 \times 10^6$ IU × 5/week SC (3×10^6 IU × 3/week SC maintenance dose) (caveat: pregnancy, lactation – induces psychotic signs, psoriasis, myopathy)	Ocular lesions, long-term visual prognosis, arthritis, vascular lesions
	$1.5–3 \times 10^6$ IU × 3/week SC according to body weight	Cortico-dependent uveitis in children
Cyclophosphamide [**2**,42,**97**]	1 g/month IV bolus (caveat: haemorrhagic cystitis give mesna 200 mg)	Uveitis, neurological manifestations
Cyclophosphamide + azathioprine + prednisolone [140]	Cyclophosphamide 1 g/month IV (for 6 months); azathioprine 2–3 mg/kg/day IV (for 2–3 months); prednisolone 0.5 mg/kg/day IV (for 2–3 months)	Improvement of visual acuity (44%), active posterior uveitis (73%) and retinal vasculitis (70%) of eyes. Improvement of total adjusted disease activity index in 72% of patients
Chlorambucil [**97**]	0.1 mg/day PO (2 mg/day maintenance dose) (caveat: cumulative toxicity)	Neurological manifestations, uveitis, thrombosis, mucocutaneous lesions
Methotrexate [**2**,42] Methotraxate + prednisolone [141]	7.5–20 mg × 1/week PO (caveat: pregnancy, lactation, severe bone marrow depression, liver dysfunction, acute infections, gastrointestinal ulcers, kidney insufficiency) 7.5–15 mg × 1/week PO; 0.5 mg/kg/day PO	Severe mucocutaneous lesions, arthritis, progressive psychosis or dementia Improvement of visual acuity (46.5%), active posterior uveitis (75.4%) and retinal vasculitis (53.7%) of eyes. Improvement of total inflammatory activity index in 74% and total adjusted disease activity index in 69.4% of patients
Infliximab [142–148]	5 mg/kg IV on days 1, 7, 14 and 28 and every 2 weeks/ 4 weeks/6 weeks subsequently (caveat: pregnancy, lactation)	Acute uveitis, refractory posterior uveitis, neurological manifestations, intestinal involvement
Infliximab (long-term) [149,150]	3–5 mg/kg IV at 0, 2, 6 and then every 4–8 weeks over 2–3 years	Remission of uveitis refractory to conventional immunosuppressant agents (73.2%)
Adalimumab [151–153]	160 mg on day 1 SC, 80 mg on day 14 and 40 mg every 2 weeks	Refractory ocular lesions, arthritis, mucocutaneous lesions; effectiveness in intestinal manifestations (84.6%) – recurrence after discontinuation
Gevokizumab (anti-IL-1β) [154]	0.3 mg/kg IV	Severe uveitis
Apremilast [155]	30 mg × 2/day PO	Articular disease refractory to colchicine and DMARDs
Apremilast [156]	30 mg × 2/day PO over 3 months (caveat: diarrhoea, nausea)	Refractory oral ulcers and ABD current activity form
Tofacitinib [157]	5 mg × 2/day PO	Refractory vascular and articular involvement
Tocilizumab [158]	8 mg/kg/4 weeks IV	Refractory ocular, neurological and vascular disease as well as secondary amyloidosis
IL-2 [159]	0.5 million IU/day SC for 5 consecutive days	Partial reduction of disease activity
Ustekinumab [160]	90 mg SC on days 1, 28 and every 12 weeks	Aphthous oral ulcers

DMARDs, disease-modifying antirheumatic drugs.

PART 4: INFLAMMATORY DERMATOSES

on panuveitis and cystoid macular oedema as a single intravitreal injection (triamcinolone acetonide 4 mg) [102,103].

Box 48.2 Treatments of oral aphthous ulcers

General
- Mild diet
- Avoidance of hard, spicy or salty nutrients and irritating chemicals, such as toasted bread, nuts, oranges, lemons, tomatoes, spices (pepper, paprika, curry), alcohol- or CO_2-containing drinks, mouthwashes and toothpastes containing sodium lauryl sulfate[a]
- An association of active smoking with a decrease of recurrence of oral aphthous ulcers and of the incidence of the disease has been described [162]

Topical
- Caustic solutions (silver nitrate 1–2%; tinctura myrrha 5–10% weight/volume; H_2O_2 0.5%; methyl violet 0.5%) once or twice a day
- Antiseptic and anti-inflammatory preparations (amlexanox 5% in oral paste once a day[a]; triclosan 0.1% mouthwash solution and in toothpastes[a]; amyloglucosidase- and glucose oxidase-containing toothpastes[a]; hexetidine 1%, chlorhexidine 1–2% mouthwash solutions; benzydamine; camomile extracts), 3% diclofenac in 2.5% hyaluronic acid[a]; hyaluronic acid 0.2% gel; tetracycline mouthwash (as glycerine solution 250 mg/5 mL glycerine) for 2 min 4–6 times a day[a] (caveat: pregnancy); minocycline 0.2% mouthwash; doxymycine in isobutyl cyanoacrylate[a]
- Corticosteroids (triamcinolone mucosal cream, ointment or paste 0.1%; dexamethasone mucosal paste or solution 0.5 mg/5 mL; betamethasone pastilles) once a day or during the night (ointment/paste); intrafocal infiltrations with triamcinolone suspension (5–10 mg/mL) 0.1–0.5 mL per lesion
- Anaesthetics (lidocaine 2–5%; mepivacaine 1.5%; tetracaine 0.5–1% gel or mucosal ointment) BD or TDS (caveat: allergy)
- 5-Aminosalicylic acid (5% cream) TDS reduces the duration of lesions and pain intensity
- Ciclosporin 500 mg solution as a mouthwash TDS is effective as a topical immunosuppressive drug
- Sucralfate suspension 1 g/5 mL once a day[a] for oral aphthous and genital ulcers

[a] Small, randomised, double-blind, placebo-controlled trial against placebo.

Patients with mucocutaneous lesions resistant to topical treatment, those with systemic involvement and patients with markers of poor prognosis are candidates for systemic treatment [97,104,105,**106,107**]. Several compounds have been found to be effective in randomised, double-blind, placebo-controlled trials (Table 48.2) [**99,107**,108–132,**133**]. Additional treatments have been successful in studies with a lower grade of evidence (Table 48.3) [**2**,42,**97**,134–160]. Oral and intravenous prednisolone can be combined with other immunosuppressants, colchicine, dapsone, sulfasalazine or IFN-α. A synergistic effect with ciclosporin A has been described in patients with ocular involvement. Prednisolone is one of the few medications that can be used during pregnancy. Colchicine can be combined with immunosuppressants and IFN-α. A rapid relapse often occurs after discontinuing

dapsone, ciclosporin A, IFN-α or infliximab [117,135,137,142]. Among biologics, large clinical studies have shown that TNF-α inhibitors and IFN-α are effective and safe treatment options for refractory and major organ involvement, such as ocular, neurological, vascular and gastrointestinal [161]. Anakinra and ustekinumab seem to be promising agents for refractory mucocutaneous disease. IL-1 inhibitors and tocilizumab may be alternatives for the treatment of patients with refractory eye involvement. However, data for the treatment of major organ involvement are still insufficient.

Treatment ladder for Adamantiades–Behçet disease

Mucocutaneous lesions [163]

First line
- *Topical*: antimicrobial agents, sucralfate, corticosteroids
- *Systemic*: corticosteroids, colchicine, colchicine + benzathine penicillin, apremilast (aphthous ulcers)

Second line
- *Topical*: anti-inflammatory agents, amlexanox
- *Systemic*: dapsone, azathioprine, thalidomide, anti-tumour necrosis α (TNF-α) agents

Third line
- *Topical*: anaesthetics, silver nitrate
- *Systemic*: zinc sulphate, rebamipide, pentoxifylline, methotrexate, ciclosporin A, interferon α (IFN-α), other biologics

Since the effectiveness of topical treatment is generally limited to the application area, it should almost always be combined with systemic therapy.

Ocular disease [164,165]

First line
- *Topical*: corticosteroids + mydriatics ± cycloplegic agents
- *Systemic*: corticosteroids, ciclosporin A, azathioprine, adalimumab

Second line
- Infliximab, IFN-α, other biologics

Third line
- Cyclophosphamide, methotrexate

Topical treatment as a sole agent should be restricted to patients with mild uveitis (anterior uveitis).

Articular involvement

First line
- Colchicine, colchicine + benzathine penicillin or anti-inflammatory analgesics

Second line
- Azathioprine, corticosteroids

Third line

- Methotrexate, salazopyrine, IFN-α, anti-TNF-α agents, other biologics

Vascular involvement

First line

- Corticosteroids

Second line

- Azathioprine, methotrexate, cyclophosphamide, anticoagulation, surgical intervention

Third line

- Anti-TNF-α agents, other biologics

Central nervous system involvement

First line

- Corticosteroids

Second line

- Azathioprine, cyclophosphamide, anti-TNF-α agents

Third line

- Methotrexate, anticoagulation, other biologics

Gastrointestinal involvement [166]

First line

- Sulfasalazine, corticosteroids, anti-TNF-α agents

Second line

- Azathioprine

Third line

- Other biologics

Prevention

Patients with severe or progressive recurrent aphthous stomatitis should be followed up for years as potential candidates for ABD, particularly those patients with familial occurrence of the disease.

Patients with suspected ABD should be referred early for specialist advice. Male patients with systemic involvement as a presenting sign and/or an early age of onset should be treated systemically because of the poor prognosis.

Key references

The full list of references can be found in the online version at https://www.wiley.com/rooksdermatology10e

1 McCarty MA, Garton RA, Jorizzo JL. Complex aphthosis and Behçet's disease. *Dermatol Clin* 2003;21:418.

2 Suzuki Kurokawa M, Suzuki N. Behçet's disease. *Clin Exp Med* 2004;4:10–20.

3 Zouboulis CC. Epidemiology of Adamantiades–Behçet's disease. In: Zierhut M, Ohno S, eds. *Immunology of Behçet's Disease*. Lisse: Swets and Zeitlinger, 2003:1–16.

12 Maldini C, Druce K, Basu N, LaValley MP, Mahr A. Exploring the variability in Behçet's disease prevalence: a meta-analytical approach. *Rheumatology (Oxford)* 2018;57:185–95.

14 Altenburg A, Papoutsis N, Orawa H *et al*. Epidemiology and clinical manifestations of Adamantiades–Behçet disease in Germany – current pathogenetic concepts and therapeutic possibilities. *J Dtsch Dermatol Ges* 2006;4:49–66.

19 Vaiopoulos AG, Kanakis MA, Kapsimali V, Vaiopoulos G, Kaklamanis PG, Zouboulis CC. Juvenile Adamantiades–Behçet's disease. *Dermatology* 2016; 232:129–36.

22 Zouboulis CC, May T. Pathogenesis of Adamantiades–Behçet's disease. *Med Microbiol Immunol* 2003;192:149–55.

82 International Team for the Revision of the International Criteria for Behçet's Disease (ITR-ICBD). The International Criteria for Behçet's Disease (ICBD): a collaborative study of 27 countries on the sensitivity and specificity of the new criteria. *J Eur Acad Dermatol Venereol* 2013;28:338–47.

84 Seyahi E. Phenotypes in Behçet's syndrome. *Intern Emerg Med* 2019;14:677–89.

85 Bettiol A, Hatemi G, Vannozzi L, Barilaro A, Prisco D, Emmi G. Treating the different phenotypes of Behçet's syndrome. *Front Immunol* 2019;10:2830.

97 Bonitsis NG, Altenburg A, Krause L *et al*. Current concepts in the treatment of Adamantiades–Behçet's disease. *Drugs Fut* 2009;34:749–63.

99 Alpsoy E. New evidence-based treatment approach in Behçet's disease. *Pathol Res Intern* 2012;2012:871019.

106 Hatemi G, Silman A, Bang D *et al*. Management of Behçet disease: a systematic literature review for the European League Against Rheumatism evidence-based recommendations for the management of Behçet disease. *Ann Rheum Dis* 2009;68:1528–34.

107 Comarmond C, Wechsler B, Cacoub P *et al*. Traitement de la maladie de Behçet. *Rev Méd Interne* 2014;35126–38.

133 Hatemi G, Mahr A, Ishigatsubo Y *et al*. Trial of apremilast for oral ulcers in Behçet's syndrome. *N Engl J Med* 2019;381:1918–28.

163 Nakamura K, Iwata Y, Asai J *et al*. Guidelines for the treatment of skin and mucosal lesions in Behçet's disease: a secondary publication. *J Dermatol* 2020;47:223–35.

CHAPTER 49

Neutrophilic Dermatoses

Philip J. Hampton and Stephanie Ball

Newcastle Hospitals NHS Trust, Newcastle upon Tyne, UK

PART 4: INFLAMMATORY DERMATOSES

Pyoderma gangrenosum

Definition and nomenclature

Pyoderma gangrenosum (PG) is a rare non-infectious, auto-inflammatory neutrophilic dermatosis commonly associated with underlying systemic disease. Diagnosis is based on typical clinical features and the exclusion of other cutaneous ulcerating diseases. The classic ulcerative type presents as a rapidly expanding painful ulcer with a purple undermined edge (Figure 49.1).

Synonyms and inclusions

PG can be usefully classified either by aetiology or by clinical phenotype

Aetiology
- Classic – associated with underlying inflammatory conditions
- Malignancy associated
- Drug induced
- Idiopathic

Clinical phenotype classification
- Classic ulcerative
- Peristomal
- Pustular
- Bullous
- Vegetative (granulomatous superficial)
- Extracutaneous
- Atypical

   Historically some other conditions have been included within the PG classification but this may change with more understanding of the underlying aetiology:
- Neutrophilic dermatosis of the dorsal hand
- Pyodermatitis–pyostomatitis vegetans

Introduction and general description

PG is a reactive non-infectious dermatosis that shares many common features with other neutrophilic dermatoses. It is now regarded as an autoinflammatory condition whereby the triggering of the inflammatory process begins with abnormal activation of the innate immune system, distinct from an autoimmune process involving T cells or antibody production. Once the inflammation has been triggered a wide selection of other inflammatory mechanisms can be recruited [1,2] (for paper test). A number of syndromic variants of PG have also been identified such as PASH (Pyoderma, Acne, Suppurative Hidradentis), which have been linked to mutations in genes controlling elements of the innate immune system (see later).

Although classic PG is the most common presentation, several clinical variants have been described. Diagnostic criteria were originally published for the classic form in 2004 [3]. These criteria have been updated more recently by Maverakis *et al.* [4]. A Delphi consensus exercise led to the generation of one major and eight minor criteria. The presence of the major and at least four minor criteria maximised discrimination, yielding sensitivity and specificity of 86% and 90%, respectively (Table 49.1).

Another scoring system, the Paracelsus score, has also been published [5] and uses a similar list of criteria to the Maverakis diagnostic criteria, with each being given points based on predictive power. The score has been shown to be effective and sensitive for PG diagnosis.

Epidemiology
Incidence and prevalence
The best population-based estimate of incidence comes from a study of the UK general practice research database which suggests that the incidence is 0.63 (95% confidence interval (CI) 0.57–0.71) per 100 000 person-years [6].

Age
The incidence of PG increases with age, with a median age of 59 (interquartile range 41–72) years [6].

Sex
PG is more common in females: 59–76% of cases [7].

Rook's Textbook of Dermatology, Tenth Edition. Edited by Christopher Griffiths, Jonathan Barker, Tanya Bleiker, Walayat Hussain and Rosalind Simpson.
© 2024 John Wiley & Sons Ltd. Published 2024 by John Wiley & Sons Ltd.

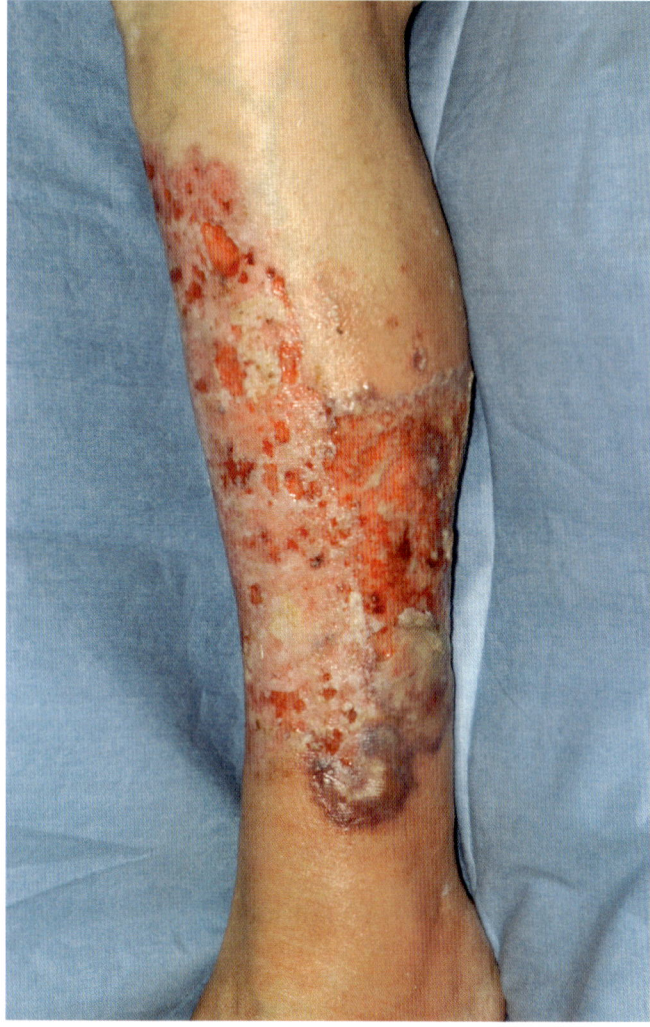

Figure 49.1 Ulcerative pyoderma gangrenosum large plaque on lower leg.

Table 49.1 Maverakis diagnostic criteria for classic ulcerative pyoderma gangrenosum.

Major	Biopsy of ulcer edge showing neutrophilic infiltrate
Minor	Exclusion of infection
	Pathergy
	History of papule, pustule, or vesicle ulcerating within 4 days of appearing
	Personal history of inflammatory bowel disease or inflammatory arthritis
	Peripheral redness, undermining border, tenderness
	Multiple ulcerations (at least one on lower leg)
	Cribriform or wrinkled paper like scars at healed sites
	Decrease in ulcer size within 1 month of initiating immunosuppression

Table 49.2 Syndromes associated with pyoderma gangrenosum (PG).

Syndrome		Gene
PAPA	Pyogenic arthritis, PG, acne	PSTPIP1
PASH	PG, acne, severe suppurative hidradenitis	PSTPIP1, NCSTN
PASS	PG, acne, suppurative hidradenitis, seropositive spondyloarthritis	Unknown
PAPASH	Pyogenic arthritis, PG, acne, suppurative hidradenitis	PSTPIP1

NCSTN, nicastrin; PSTPIP, proline-serine-threonine phosphatase-interacting protein 1.

Ethnicity

There is no association of PG with ethnicity.

Associated diseases

As with other neutrophilic dermatoses, there are classic accepted diseases that occur in association with PG in 33–75% of cases [8–10], suggesting an aetiopathological link. There is some evidence that the pustular form of PG may be associated mainly with inflammatory bowel disease (IBD) and the bullous form with haematological malignancies; the vegetative form is usually not associated with underlying disease [11].

Estimates vary but the most frequent disease associations [6,7,12,13] include IBD, with a similar incidence of Crohn disease and ulcerative colitis, present in up to 65% of cases [10]. Rheumatoid arthritis and seronegative arthritides, which may themselves be IBD related, occur in about 10–20% of cases; haematological malignancy or monoclonal gammopathy in up to 19% and other visceral malignancies in 5% [7].

Other co-morbidities of PG that may either predispose to the condition or result from the disease itself or its treatment include diabetes, depression, peripheral vascular disease and possibly obesity [7].

Furthermore, there are numerous case reports of disease associations, which due to rarity and overlapping disease entities remain of uncertain significance. These include thyroid disease, spondylitis, osteoarthritis, psoriatic arthritis, chronic active hepatitis, hepatitis C viral infection, primary biliary cirrhosis, systemic lupus erythematosus, complement deficiency, hypogammaglobulinaemia, hyperimmunoglobulin E syndrome, AIDS, sarcoidosis, Takayasu arteritis, hidradenitis suppurativa, acne conglobata and chronic obstructive pulmonary disease [7,12].

A number of syndromes are now recognised as having an association with PG, cystic acne and either hidradenitis or inflammatory arthritis (Table 49.2) [14,**15,16**,17–19].

Mutations in the gene proline-serine-threonine phosphatase-interacting protein 1 (PSTPIP1) have been identified. This protein interacts with the pyrin inflammasome and mutations lead to a reduced threshold for innate immune activation. It seems likely that a combination of a reduced threshold for inflammation, other genetic predispositions and environmental factors could together explain these syndromes. There is likely to be great heterogeneity in the aetiology which remains incompletely defined [20]. PSTPIP1-associated autoinflammatory diseases (PAIDs) are now a recognised entity [21].

Pathophysiology

Predisposing factors

Pathergy is the phenomenon whereby skin trauma provokes lesions or the first onset of the disease at the site of injury. This most frequently follows surgical wounds or penetrating injury. Pathergy is likely to play a role in peristomal PG. In patients with ulcerative colitis, the incidence of extraintestinal manifestations, including PG, is independently promoted by smoking and by appendicectomy [22].

The development of peristomal PG is predisposed to by female sex, high body mass index (BMI) and the presence of autoimmune disorders [23].

Pathology

Skin biopsies should be taken (for histology and culture) to exclude other causes of ulceration, but histology is not diagnostic. The value of a skin biopsy is the exclusion of other diseases that mimic PG (see Differential diagnosis) [24]; there is no typical histopathology of PG. Early lesions display neutrophilic pustules but in general the features are non-specific. Typical findings include central necrosis and ulceration of the epidermis and dermis surrounded by an intense inflammatory cell infiltrate, with a more peripheral mixed to chronic inflammatory cell infiltrate [24,25]. Each clinical variant has additional, more specific, histopathological findings: in the ulcerative variant of PG, there is a massive dermal–epidermal neutrophilic infiltrate with suppuration/abscess formation; in pustular PG, a perifollicular neutrophilic infiltrate with subcorneal pustule formation; the bullous variant shows a neutrophilic infiltrate with intraepidermal vesicle formation; and in vegetative PG, there is a granulomatous reaction with peripheral palisading histiocytes and giant cells [12]. The presence of vasculitis in PG is an area of debate. Many investigators have reported findings consistent with a neutrophilic vascular reaction or leukocytoclastic vasculitis, fibrinoid necrosis, segmental necrotising vasculitis, granulomatous vasculitis and lymphocytic vasculitis [24,25]; this may be secondary to ulceration. If vasculitis is evident, true vasculitides and infective causes should be excluded, including culture and staining of biopsy tissue for fungi, mycobacteria and other organisms.

Pathomechanism of pyoderma gangrenosum

The pathomechanism of PG is complex and multifactorial [2,10,26]. Many phenomena, including its association with IBD, its aggressive local destruction of tissues and the pathergy phenomenon, suggest a cascade of inflammatory events, including activation of innate immunity, autoinflammatory pathways, neutrophil dysfunction, recruitment of the adaptive immune response and tissue destruction. Overactivation of numerous cytokines is reported including interleukin (IL)-1β, tumour necrosis factor (TNF), IL-8, IL-17, IL-23, VEGF, CCR5, CXCR3, matrix metalloproteinases (MMPs) and chemokines with neutrophil trafficking and activation. PG is not usually associated with vasculitis, but patients with positive tests for either C-antineutrophilic cytoplasmic antibody (C-ANCA) or P-ANCA are occasionally reported in drug-induced PG, typically with thiouracils [27]

There are five components to the pathogenesis of PG.

Genetic predisposition. Most of the genetic factors predisposing to PG remain unclear [10]. Genetic variations promoting the development of IBD and inflammatory arthritis are likely to influence the inflammation of PG [28]. Mutations in JAK/STAT pathways that predispose to haematological malignancies may also be associated with PG [29]. Gene mutations in *PSTPIP1* have been shown to be influential in some PG acne syndromes [20]. It seems likely that further gene variations in elements of the innate immune system may influence the threshold for triggering PG [30].

Activation of the innate immune system. Activation of innate immunity is suggested by the finding of overexpression of IL-1β and its receptor [31] and by the occurrence of PG in genetic autoinflammatory syndromes such as PAPA and PASH [32]. The successful

treatment of PG by canakinumab also supports the involvement of IL-1β [33].

Neutrophil activation. Neutrophils play a key role in the development of PG and other neutrophilic dermatoses. Clonality in neutrophils infiltrating skin lesions has also been demonstrated in 81% of 15 patients with Sweet syndrome and PG [34]. Neutrophil chemotaxis was impaired in five patients with PG [35]; IL-6 can induce accumulation of neutrophils and is elevated in PG lesions [36]. The neutrophil chemokine IL-8 has been identified in lesions of PG and can produce similar lesions in an animal model [37]. It appears to be produced by fibroblasts from the PG ulcer [38]. Overexpression of IL-8, chemokine (C-X-C motif) ligand (CXCL) 1/2/3, CXCL 16 and regulated upon activation normal T cell expressed and secreted (RANTES) have been shown to be overexpressed in PG lesions [31].

Recruitment of other inflammatory pathways. Clonal expansion of T cells has been shown in peripheral blood in five patients with PG [39]. Clonal expansion of γ and β T-cell receptors have been found in PG associated with haematological disease with splenomegaly [40]. The antigen to which T cells are responding is unknown and could be an autoantigen, microbial antigen or a shared epitope. A putative autoantigen, M(r) 40 K epithelial autoantigen, was identified in the skin, colonic mucosa and biliary epithelium, and has been considered speculatively as a relevant autoantigen linking extraintestinal manifestations of IBD [41]. Cell-mediated defects include cutaneous anergy to *Candida*, streptokinase and purified protein derivative, as well as altered production of macrophage inhibition factor (MIF) by lymphocytes [42].

The expression of inflammatory cytokines in tissue affected by PG has been investigated, with increases in IL-17, TNF-α, IL-8, IL-36a and IL-23 reported [43,44]

Data regarding the involvement of antibody-mediated inflammation and immunofluorescence findings in PG are conflicting. Several studies have shown positive direct immunofluorescence of lesional skin [13,25,45]. The most frequently observed pattern is perivascular or intravascular deposition of C3 or IgM, but deposition of C3 at the dermal–epidermal junction also occurs [45]. However, other studies have shown negative immunofluorescence [46,47] and the positive findings may be non-specific reactive changes following ulceration of the skin. The positive response of PG to intravenous immunoglobulin (IVIG) has suggested antibody involvement, although IVIG has multiple anti-inflammatory mechanisms in addition to antibody depletion [48].

Tissue destruction. Although the primary pathology appears to be a neutrophilic pustule, tissue destruction can be rapid and extensive. Once the skin becomes ulcerated, the appearance of acute and chronic perivascular inflammatory cell infiltrates may be secondary to the ulceration rather than a primary event. However, a series of 58 skin biopsies revealed a mild to moderate perivascular lymphocytic infiltrate associated with endothelial swelling in early lesions [13]. Necrosis was a feature of more developed lesions with a dense lymphocytic infiltration surrounding as well as involving the blood vessels. Bister *et al.* [49] examined 24 skin biopsies and found a pattern of abundant MMP expression, particularly MMP 9 and 10 and TNF-α, which could lead to tissue destruction and degradation of the stromal matrix needed for migration and healing. They also found similar expression of MMPs to that found in ulcerative lesions of IBD. Thus, TNF-α was proposed, and proved to be an important target for therapy.

Causative organisms

Although no pathogen has ever been attributed to causing PG, bullous PG-like skin lesions were reproduced by injection of heat-killed *Escherichia coli* in a patient with IBD and previous PG [50]. This suggests that gut flora antigens presenting in the skin of a susceptible individual might have importance while not fulfilling Koch postulates for primary causation.

Genetics

The genetic basis of PG has not been elucidated but is likely to be complex and heterogeneous. Mutations in genes regulating inflammation may play a direct role and mutations in genes predisposing to PG-associated diseases will also be relevant. Defilippis *et al.* [10] have summarised publications relating to gene mutations and PG. One specific example of clues to the pathogenesis of PG comes from the association of PG with the PAPA syndrome in which a mutation was found in the *PSTPIP1/CD2BP1* gene on chromosome 15 [51], which encodes for a proline/serine/threonine-interacting protein 1. This autoinflammatory syndrome (Chapter 45) links to other cryopyrine syndromes as CD2BP1, now known as PSTPIP1, which binds pyrin [52,53]. Thus, a defect in negative regulators of inflammation links the pathology of PAPA with familial Mediterranean fever [54]. Genetic factors are suggested by the occurrence of PG in siblings [55] and familial clustering of cases [56].

Environmental factors

Skin trauma (pathergy) can induce lesions of PG in 25% of cases.

Drug-induced PG is a relatively new concept and remains poorly understood. Most reported cases relate to colony-stimulating factors (Sweet syndrome) and small-molecule tyrosine kinase inhibitors [57]. Possible mechanisms include effects on neutrophil migration and function, inflammation and keratinocyte apoptosis.

Clinical features
History

Brocq first described PG in 1916 [58]. It was later described in 1930 by Brunsting *et al.* [59]. The prevalence of PG in IBD was discussed by Greenstein *et al.* in 1976 [60].

Presentation

PG can have a variety of clinical presentations. Diagnostic criteria have been proposed for the cutaneous lesions of classic ulcerative PG, as discussed earlier.

Clinical variants

Classic ulcerative PG [8,13,61,62]. This is the commonest and best recognised variant of PG, presenting with small, tender, red-blue papules (Figure 49.2), plaques or pustules that evolve into painful ulcers with characteristic violaceous undermined edges (Figure 49.3). There may be granulation tissue, necrosis or purulent

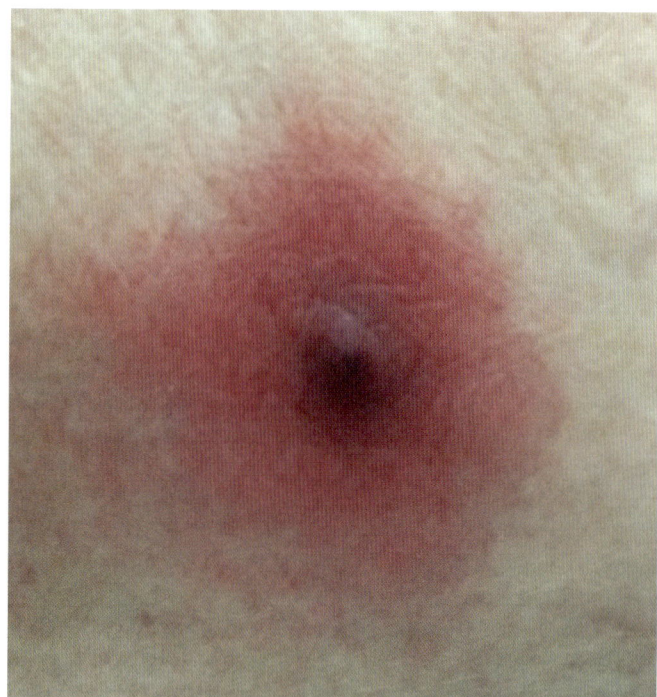

Figure 49.2 Early lesion of pyoderma gangrenosum.

exudate at the ulcer base. Lesions may be solitary or multiple and occur most commonly on the legs (in 70%), but may affect any body site including the genitals and mucosae. Healing usually occurs with an atrophic cribriform (sieve-like) scar (Figure 49.4). Associated symptoms include fever, malaise, myalgia and arthralgia.

Parastomal PG. Parastomal or peristomal PG may arise as a pathergic response to the trauma of stoma formation surgery, stoma appliances and faecal irritation. It is most common with ileostomy for active IBD [23] and the risk is greater with high BMI, female sex and autoimmune disorders [23] (Figure 49.5). General surgeons must be aware of the phenomenon to avoid inappropriate resiting of stomas following ulceration complications.

Pustular PG. Pustular PG is a variant that often occurs during acute exacerbations of IBD [63–65]. Discrete painful pustules, with a surrounding halo of redness, develop on normal skin [66]. These pustules commonly arise with a scattered distribution on the extensor aspects of the limbs. Other painful pustular eruptions in this spectrum [67] of IBD need to be distinguished, including bowel-associated dermatitis–arthritis syndrome (BADAS, Chapter 45), subcorneal pustular dermatosis and pyostomatitis vegetans where the pustules are predominantly mucosal.

Bullous PG. This atypical presentation presents with rapidly arising, superficial, haemorrhagic bullae, often located on the arms. It shares clinical and histopathological findings with Sweet syndrome, but typically ulcerates and heals with scarring. Bullous PG is especially associated with myeloproliferative disorders [68]. Bullous PG, associated with an older age group, upper limb distribution and haematological malignancy with quicker remission, was termed atypical PG in the series of Bennett *et al.* [8]. Other reports describe areas of

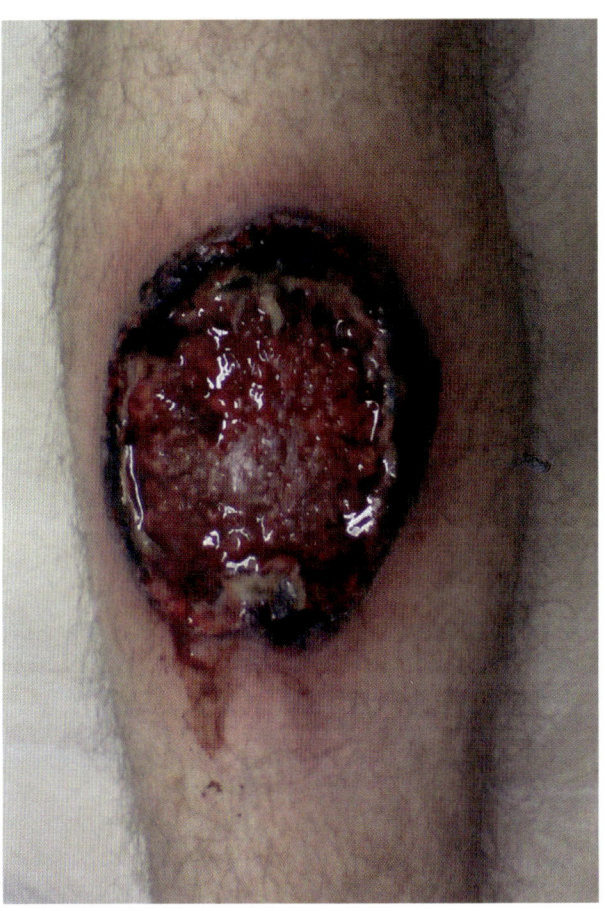

Figure 49.3 Classical pyoderma gangrenosum.

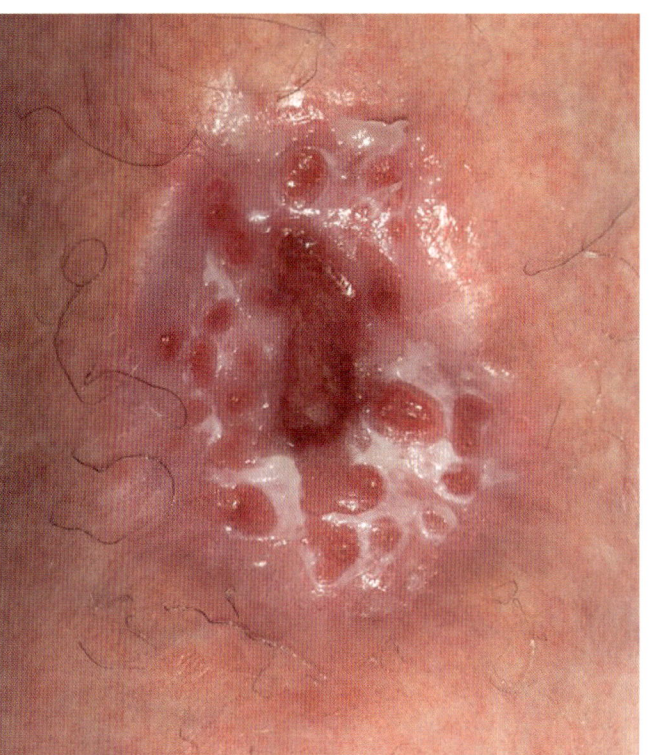

Figure 49.4 Healing ulcer of pyoderma gangrenosum with the beginning of cribriform (sieve-like) scarring.

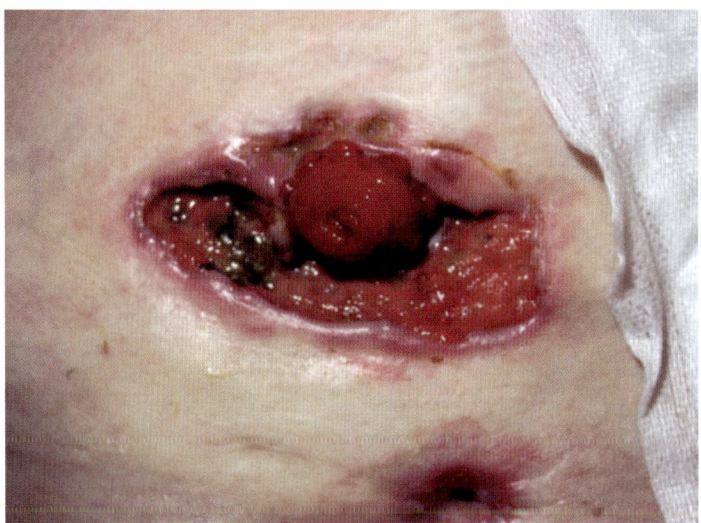

Figure 49.5 Peristomal pyoderma gangrenosum.

concentric bullae that rapidly become confluent and ulcerate [69,70]. PG can precede the onset or detection of the myeloproliferative disorder, and patients with bullous PG should be investigated with a high index of suspicion for a haematological malignancy [71,72].

Vegetative or granulomatous superficial PG. This is a variant of PG with superficial lesions with a granulomatous histology [73,74]. Most cases begin as a single superficial ulcer with granulations and an elevated edge (Figure 49.6). A review of all reported cases in 2005 [74,75] found the lesions were most often located on the trunk (52%) and had a lower incidence of associated conditions. This variant also tended to be more responsive to therapy. Although 39% required systemic corticosteroids, many healed with topical or intralesional corticosteroids, minocycline or dapsone. Very few cases required other forms of systemic immunosuppression.

Neutrophilic dermatosis of the dorsal hand. See later in this chapter.

Extracutaneous PG. PG is not exclusive to the skin and, although rare, PG and other neutrophilic dermatoses can involve other organs, often with aseptic abscesses, most commonly in the lungs [76–78]. Also, PG may affect the bones [79,80], liver [81], heart, brain, gastrointestinal tract [82] and muscle [83]. See also Aseptic abscess syndrome later.

Differential diagnosis

PG is a diagnosis of exclusion with a wide range of alternative pathologies that can appear similar. Ninety-five patients with lesions masquerading as PG were reviewed by Weenig *et al.* (2002) [84]. In non-classic PG, biopsy and culture are important and there should be targeted enquiry, examination and investigation for differential diagnoses. These include vascular occlusive or venous disease, vasculitis, cancer, primary infection, drug-induced or exogenous tissue injury, and other inflammatory disorders, fungi, atypical mycobacteria and opportunistic infections [84], sporotrichosis [85], fusariosis, mycosis fungoides

PART 4: INFLAMMATORY DERMATOSES

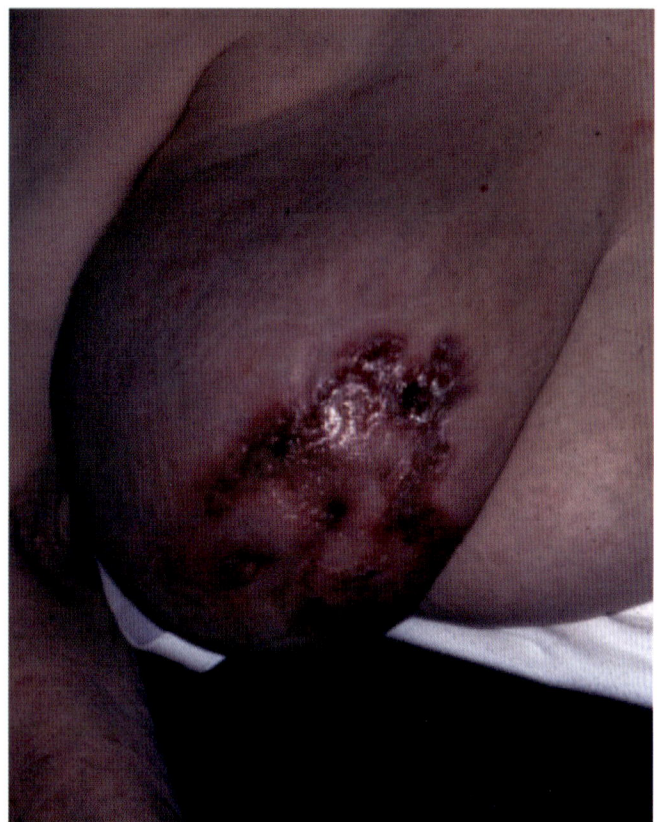

Figure 49.6 Superficial granulomatous or vegetative pyoderma gangrenosum.

[86], mucormycosis [87], histoplamosis [88], blastomycosis [89] and drug-induced, including nicorandil [90].

Classification of severity

A simple measure of the size of skin ulceration or measuring the longest axis of the wound and perpendicular maximum width can be used to monitor therapy and with the formula length × width × 0.785 [91] can be used to approximate to an ellipse, which has been used as a measure in clinical trials and is an important predictor of healing and a confounder in clinical studies. An inflammation scale has been developed for quantifying the degree of inflammation in PG [92]; this was modified in recent trials to include the degree of exudate [91]. Patient-reported outcome measures (PROMS) are also important in documenting disease severity, and measures such as dermatology life quality index and pain visual analogue scale can be useful in the management of PG.

Complications and co-morbidities

PG has a significant all-cause mortality – 16% over 8 years [7]. In an epidemiological study of a large UK database, including 313 cases of PG over 16 years, the relative risks of mortality were compared with those of normal subjects and those with either IBD without PG or rheumatoid arthritis without PG. The risk of death for those with PG was three times higher than that for general controls, 72% higher than that for IBD controls, with a borderline increase compared with RA controls [6]. This suggests an independent risk of PG, but it is not possible to determine whether this is due to complications of PG such as infection, management of PG with potent immunosuppressive agents or a combination of these factors.

Associated diseases are discussed earlier; patients also have co-morbid diseases that may predispose to leg ulceration or that are found in association with other chronic inflammatory conditions. These include anaemia, renal impairment, thyroid disease, obesity, diabetes [93], depression and peripheral vascular disease [7].

Disease course and prognosis

PG is a chronic condition often taking many months or years to completely resolve [93,94]. Once healed, PG may be recurrent in 16–61% of cases [9,78,95] and consideration should be given to long-term systemic preventative therapy.

Investigations

Investigations should be guided by a thorough clinical evaluation. Skin biopsy is not diagnostic in PG but is required to exclude other conditions that may mimic PG. As many of these conditions are infective, it is advisable to send tissue for culture for bacterial, atypical mycobacterial, viral and fungal pathogens to rule out other causes.

Due to the possibility of association with an underlying malignancy, it is important for the clinician to make a firm diagnosis of the triggering mechanism of the PG. If no inflammatory condition, malignancy or drug trigger can be identified, appropriate investigations to exclude an underlying malignancy or undiagnosed inflammatory condition are needed. Investigations will be guided by the individual clinical circumstances. A thorough work-up should include examination for lymphadenopathy, blood count, biochemical profile, blood culture, ulcer tissue culture, chest X-ray, other X-rays as indicated, endoscopy, bone marrow aspirate and CT scan [66].

Management

Management of PG is often complex and will depend on co-morbidities, associated diseases and the site and extent of the lesions (Table 49.3). The basic principles consist of:
- 1a: Induction of remission
- 1b: Analgesia
- 2a: Maintenance of remission
- 2b: Wound healing

The importance of analgesia and wound healing must be emphasised, as often much attention is given to the choice of immunosuppression. Optimising the conditions for wound healing is important from the start. Frequent review is needed to ensure adequate analgesia and also to judge when the inflammation has been controlled and the healing phase has begun. At this stage the immunosuppression can often be slowly reduced and more attention paid to optimisation of wound healing.

The evidence base for treating PG is almost entirely anecdotal and subject to publication bias. There have only been two randomised clinical trials (RCTs) for PG treatment. In 2006 infliximab was shown to be superior to placebo [**96**] and in 2015 ciclosporin (4 mg/kg/day) was shown to be equivalent to prednisolone (0.75 mg/kg/day) [**97**].

The number of suggested therapies is indicative of the difficulty in achieving a successful outcome for these patients. The potential of new biologic drugs is probably not being harnessed as it should be due to a lack of clinical trials, although analysis of real-life data and use of registries could be employed to inform treatment decisions.

Table 49.3 Treatment of pyoderma gangrenosum.

Oral – conventional	Biologic/small-molecule inhibitor	Target cytokine
Prednisolone 0.5–1 mg/kg	Infliximab	TNF-α
Ciclosporin 5 mg/kg	Adalimumab	TNF-α
Combined prednisolone and ciclosporin	Etanercept	TNF-α
Pulsed prednisolone 1 g/day for 5 days	Ustekinumab	IL-12, IL-23
Methotrexate	Guselkumab	IL-23
Mycophenolate mofetil	Ixekizumab	IL-17
Dapsone	Brodalumab	IL-17R
Tetracyclines	Secukinumab	IL-17
Thalidomide	Anakinra	IL-1
Tacrolimus	Canakinumab	IL-1β
Cyclophosphamide	Gevokizumab	IL-1β
Chlorambucil	Tocilizumab	IL-6
Azathioprine	Tofactinib	JAK 1 and 3
Colchicine	Ruxolitinib	JAK-2
	IVIG	

IL, interleukin; IVIG, intravenous immunoglobulin; JAK, Janus kinase; TNF, tumour necrosis factor.

Where PG is associated with specific diseases (e.g. Crohn), controlling activity of the underlying condition is thought to be important and may influence therapeutic decision making. Biologics targeting IL-17, IL-23 and IL-1β are not being investigated due to the difficulty and low profitability in conducting clinical trials in rare diseases. The lack of a licence then makes it very hard to get approval for treatment in most health care systems. There are numerous reviews and case series examining outcomes of therapy [2,9,94,95,98–101].

The available treatments can be divided into three groups.

First line

As PG occurs most frequently on the legs and can be associated with vascular disease and obesity, consideration should be given to providing the most favourable conditions for wound healing, including compression in some instances. Supportive therapy will include attention to dressings, pain relief and topical agents for cleansing, debriding and keeping the wound moist. For smaller lesions, potent topical corticosteroids [102], intralesional corticosteroids [102] and topical tacrolimus [103,104] can be used.

Second line

For more severe disease or for PG not responding to simple measures, systemic therapies are often required, with corticosteroids being the most frequently used and the mainstay of therapy. Systemic prednisolone and ciclosporin either alone or in combination are preferred treatments [98,99]. A large multicentre RCT compared ciclosporin 4 mg/kg/day and prednisolone 0.75 mg/kg/day in 121 subjects and found no difference between these monotherapies, with only 50% achieving complete healing on either therapy over 6 months of follow-up [97]. Many other anti-inflammatory or immunosuppressive drugs are used as alternative therapies, combination or maintenance therapies (Table 49.3). Second line immunosuppressive drugs are frequently used as steroid-sparing agents. PG often requires prolonged treatment courses and all efforts must be made to minimise steroid side effects.

Third line
Biologics
Anti-TNF-α. The lack of licensed indications for biologics for PG and cost mean that most patients will first receive a non-biologic systemic therapy. However, growing evidence suggests that anti-TNF biologic therapy should be considered more often as first line therapy (particularly for those with associated IBD) with 92% healing rates in a systematic review, although this may have been subject to reporting bias [105]. A growing body of evidence supports superiority of anti-TNF therapy to oral prednisolone. A retrospective observational study of 67 IBD patients with associated PG found that oral corticosteroids were used in 76% and that 29 of 31 (93.5%) subjects treated at some point with anti-TNF therapy infliximab or adalimumab healed in 4–8 weeks, while for prednisolone 38% definitively healed over a 1–3-month period. Infliximab or adalimumab was used in 75% of cases in this series since 2000. Biologics were first line treatments in 14% [106]. An RCT which randomised only the first dose of infliximab provided strong evidence for the efficacy of infliximab [96]. Overall, there are more series and reports of successful therapy with infliximab than for any other biologics [107–111], although adalimumab has been beneficial in case reports [112–116] and in a series of three patients [117]. Etanercept has also been successful in case reports and small case series [118–121]. However, paradoxical onset of PG has also occurred with etanercept [122] and with adalimumab [123].

Other biologics. Ustekinumab has been reported as effective [124] and guselkumab has been reported as effective in a case of severe ulcerating lower leg PG [125–128,**129**]. The use of IL-17 blocking biologics has been reported, although clinicians must remember the potential adverse effect of IL-17 blockade in IBD [130]. In PAPA syndrome associated with PG, treatment with IL-1RA agents has been successful including anakinra [17] and canakinumab [131]. In PASH syndrome, anakinra was found to be helpful [**15**] (see Table 45.3, Chapter 45). Gevokizumab, anti-IL-1β, has shown benefit in a small pilot study of six patients [**2**].

JAK/STAT inhibitors. Both tofactinib and ruxolitinib have been reported to play a significant role in healing recalcitrant PG. Tofacitinib has been used in patients with Crohn disease-associated PG [132] and ruxolitinib in a patient with polycythaemia vera [133]. The impact on the underlying associated conditions may, however, have played a key role in the successful treatment.

IVIG. Seven out of 10 patients responded to IVIG in one case series [134]. A systemic review of IVIG for PG reported complete or partial response in 43 of 49 cases [48]. Concurrent diagnoses included malignancy (22 cases), IBD (12 cases), post-traumatic (11 cases) and autoimmune (8 cases). Despite the lack of evidence for antibody-mediated inflammation in PG the success of IVIG, which decreases antibody half-life, raises the possibility of antibody-mediated inflammation. IVIG also reduces complement-mediated tissue destruction.

Alternative therapies. Although surgery should be avoided in the inflammatory stage and can frequently induce PG, skin grafting can be very successful if the inflammation has already resolved following systemic therapy such as with corticosteroids [135,136]. Previous editions of this book have discussed case reports of therapies such as topical nicotone, topical sodium cromoglycate and hyperbaric oxygen, but these should now be regarded as historical rather than recommended options.

Sweet syndrome

Definition and nomenclature
Sweet syndrome is an inflammatory neutrophilic dermatosis characterised by tender, tumid, red, dermal nodules and plaques with a predilection for the arms, upper body and face. The syndrome is often associated with peripheral neutrophilia and fever and may occur primarily or as a cutaneous manifestation of systemic disease. Histological features classically display a striking band of dermal oedema overlying a dense neutrophilic infiltrate.

Synonyms and inclusions
- Acute febrile neutrophilic dermatosis
- Gomm–Button disease

Introduction and general description
In 1964, R.D. Sweet used the term acute febrile neutrophilic dermatosis in describing a case series of eight women with progressive red plaques, fever and non-specific infection, all of whom had similar skin histology changes of neutrophilic infiltrates with oedema [1]. Over the following decades, understanding of the presentation and spectrum of this constellation of symptoms – subsequently named Sweet syndrome – has expanded, though the exact aetiology is not fully understood and oral corticosteroids still remain the mainstay of treatment. The pathogenesis is likely to rely on a number of factors dependent on the underlying cause, including various inciting factors, genetic or acquired, impacting on cell signalling pathways to lead to an increase in neutrophil production and migration and accumulation into tissues [2]. Three subtypes are recognised as follows:

- *Classic.* Classic Sweet syndrome (CSS) is the most common subtype with a female predominance, no racial predilection, and is often idiopathic, though it can be associated with underlying infection, autoimmune and/or inflammatory conditions, and pregnancy [2,3]. CSS usually presents with fever and tender red plaques and nodules affecting the face, neck and upper extremities, and atypical bullous lesions can occur.
- *Malignancy-associated.* This subtype was first described by Cohen and Kurzrock in 1993, although case reports detailing what we now know as malignancy-associated Sweet syndrome (MASS) date back to 1955, before Sweet himself published the defining characteristics of the syndrome [4,5]. MASS can follow, fall concurrently with or even precede a diagnosis of cancer; it accounts for around 21% of all Sweet syndrome diagnoses and can occur secondary to both haematological or solid organ malignancies, but most commonly acute myelogenous leukaemia [3,5]. Lesions are more often vesicular, bullous or ulcerative [6]. Patients

are also more likely to have abnormalities in their full blood count – usually anaemia or deranged platelet count.
- *Drug-induced.* The least common of the subtypes, drug-induced Sweet syndrome (DISS) was first reported in 1986 [7]. While a number of culprit medications have been reported, the most common are granulocyte-colony-stimulating factor (G-CSF), azathioprine and all-*trans* retinoic acid (ATRA) [2,8,9].

Epidemiology
Incidence and prevalence
Sweet syndrome occurs worldwide. Cohen and Kurzrock attempted to estimate the proportion of cases associated with malignancy, and in reviewing 15 studies found 96/448 (21%) had either solid organ or haematological malignancy [4]. A recent UK study by Gopee *et al.* [10] retrospectively reviewed 64 cases, finding a female to male ratio of 2.8:1 for CSS, associated underlying infection in 17 (27%) of CSS, inflammatory conditions in 8 (12.5%) and no identifiable trigger in 24 cases (37.5%). MASS accounted for 20% of the cohort, with a far higher proportion of patients with a haematological rather than solid organ malignancy (85% compared with 15%). Three per cent of the cohort had DISS [10].

Age
Sweet syndrome occurs at any age but most commonly affects people between 30 and 60 years of age [11]. The mean age of onset in the previously mentioned study was 54 years [10].

Sex
The disease is more common in females with a ratio of 4:1 female to male.

Ethnicity
There is no confirmed racial predilection although a high number of publications exist in the Japanese literature. However, this may represent reporting bias.

Associated diseases
Associated diseases are numerous and somewhat dependent on the different subtypes of Sweet syndrome (Table 49.4) [8,12,13]. The original paper by Sweet proffered an association with a non-specific gastrointestinal or respiratory infection. Streptococcal respiratory tract infections, gastrointestinal infections caused by *Salmonella* and *Yersinia* and mycobacterial infections are all confirmed triggers for Sweet syndrome. Other reported associations of CSS include IBD [14–16], sarcoidosis [17–19], rheumatoid arthritis [20], Behçet disease [21] and erythema nodosum [22]. A non-bullous Sweet-like neutrophilic dermatosis in patients with lupus erythematosus has also been described [23–25].

Cohen *et al.* have calculated that 10–20% of cases of Sweet syndrome have an associated malignancy, the vast majority of these being haematological [6,8]. The syndrome can occur either as a paraneoplastic phenomenon or a sentinel of evolving malignancy that is otherwise undetectable, the latter particularly proving an issue in cases associated with solid organ cancer. This can prove to be challenging in deciding who and how to investigate. Acute myelocytic leukaemia and promyelocytic leukaemia are the most common

Table 49.4 The wide variety of diseases that have been associated with Sweet syndrome.

Category	Examples	Comment
Infections	Streptococcal and upper respiratory tract Gastrointestinal (especially *Salmonella, Yersinia*) Mycobacterial infections (including vaccinations) Many others	Upper respiratory tract infections: *Salmonella* and *Yersinia* are well-documented causes of 'classic' Sweet syndrome See also text for discussion of human granulocytic anaplasmosis
Inflammatory bowel disease	Ulcerative colitis Crohn disease	Well-documented causes of 'classic' Sweet syndrome
Endocrine	Pregnancy Autoimmune thyroid disease	Pregnancy and thyroid disease are relatively well documented
Immunological disorders	Collagen vascular disorders: lupus erythematosus, Sjögren syndrome, others Others: autoimmune thrombocytopenic purpura, pemphigus	
Haematological malignancy and related conditions, immunodeficiencies	Acute myelogenous leukaemias Myelodysplastic conditions, polycythaemia Aplastic anaemia Fanconi anaemia Monoclonal gammopathy Lymphomas (various, less common) Chronic granulomatous disease Congenital deficiencies: neutropenia, T-cell immunodeficiency, complement deficiency	Strong evidence linking leukaemias and myelodysplastic disorders Some series suggest a significant association with paraproteinaemias; chronic granulomatous disease, see text
Other malignancies	Genito-urinary Breast Gastrointestinal Prostate Larynx Many others	No specific site association apparent other than the haematological group
Other medical conditions	Sarcoidosis Rheumatoid arthritis Still disease SAPHO	Many reports of sarcoidosis
Medications	Numerous; the most consistently associated agents are: • Colony-stimulating factors (including recent pegylated types) • Neutrophil-maturation drugs (all-*trans* retinoic acid) • Other haematological treatments (imatinib mesylate, bortezomib) • Contraceptives • Propylthiouracil Physical treatments for haematological malignancy have also been implicated, in a patient having splenic irradiation	Although most colony-stimulating factor-related Sweet syndrome has been reported in patients with haematological malignancy, there are also several reports of the same phenomenon in other contexts (e.g. congenital immunodeficiencies) As with vasculitis, there may be positive ANCA with thiouracils
Other neutrophilic dermatoses and related conditions	Pyoderma gangrenosum Neutrophilic dermatosis of the dorsal hands Erythema elevatum diutinum Relapsing polychondritis Neutrophilic eccrine hidradenitis Subcorneal pustular dermatosis Erythema nodosum Behçet disease Vasculitis (various)	In some cases, several are associated either concurrently or sequentially
Mucosal manifestations of Sweet syndrome	Oral or genital mucosa ulceration Ocular inflammation especially conjunctivitis, also nodular episcleritis	Oral lesions especially in cases with haematological malignancy; conjunctivitis mainly in classic Sweet syndrome
Systemic manifestations of neutrophilic dermatoses, and deeper variants	Bone, muscle, tendons, neuro-Sweet, heart, lung, liver, intestine, spleen, kidney, subcutaneous (Sweet panniculitis)	
Unusual consequences of Sweet syndrome	Acquired cutis laxa, mid-dermal elastolysis, elastophagocytosis	Several cases of acquired cutis laxa

ANCA, antineutrophilic cytoplasmic antibody; SAPHO, synovitis, acne, pustulosis, hyperostosis, osteomyelitis.

malignancies reported although chronic myeloid leukaemia [26], multiple myeloma [27,28] and myelodysplastic syndrome have also been described as triggers. Principally, solid organ tumours implicated in Sweet syndrome include adenocarcinomas of the breast, gastrointestinal tract and urinary tract [3,6,29,30].

Pathophysiology
Predisposing factors
Acquired predisposing factors tend to be the various associated conditions which are generally diseases of excessive inflammation or, in the case of malignancy-associated disease, one of a baseline pro-inflammatory state and conditions in which malignant transformation of neutrophils or dysfunction of their progenitors may increase susceptibility to developing Sweet syndrome. Under these conditions, alterations in pro-inflammatory cell signalling pathways and cytokine production may produce a lower threshold for neutrophil proliferation [2].

Pathology
Proliferation of neutrophils in the bone marrow is not enough to cause Sweet syndrome alone, and tissue neutrophil levels are controlled by the following variables, with disruption leading to development of Sweet syndrome:
- Bacterial or fungal triggers for neutrophil migration
- Bone marrow granulopoiesis
- Bone marrow neutrophil storage
- Bone marrow release (and movement from the marginated granulocyte pool of the liver and spleen)
- Transendothelial migration
- Rate of neutrophil destruction

While the exact triggering factor of Sweet syndrome is yet to be determined, haematological malignancy and use of G-CSF, ATRA and fms-like tyrosine kinase 3 (FLT3 inhibitor) demonstrate one proposed mechanism [2].

Significantly increased serum G-CSF levels have been found in patients with Sweet syndrome, particularly those with active disease [31]. Furthermore, many different malignancies can produce G-CSF, which may partly explain the existence of MASS [32,33,34–37]. Exogenous administration of G-CSF is a main cause of DISS. It is thought that G-CSF therapy for haematological malignancies may encourage differentiation and maturation of leukaemic neutrophils which then migrate to the skin [2,38,39]. ATRA therapy leads to promyelocyte differentiation in acute promyelocytic leukaemia and may, in a similar fashion to G-CSF, lead to increased numbers of mature dermal neutrophils in the dermis [40].

Neutrophilic clonality in Sweet syndrome may be secondary to malignant transformation of dermal neutrophils (in the case of haematological malignancy) or non-malignant aggregations of neutrophils in the skin which are derived from a dysfunctional progenitor [2,41]. *FLT-3* gene mutations have been found in 39% of patients with acute myeloid leukaemia and Sweet syndrome, both in leukaemic cells and in dermal neutrophils. This gene encodes tyrosine kinase 3 receptors within the bone marrow and regulates progeny, survival and differentiation of myeloid progenitor cells, and thus mutation results in persistent activation and proliferation [2,42–44].

One further possibility in CSS could be that an individual may fail to respond to an infection either promptly or effectively, leading to a greater stimulus for granulocyte migration and increased neutrophil production with the sequela of developing Sweet syndrome [31]. An immune reaction to a drug, pathogen, tumour or even UV exposure or trauma may lead to a cytokine cascade in which Sweet syndrome is the end point. The presence of pathergy in this condition, and the enduring efficacy of corticosteroids in the management of Sweet syndrome, would support this proposed mechanism [2]. A number of cytokines have been shown to be increased in Sweet syndrome including (but not limited to) IL-1(α and β), IL-2, IL3, IL-6, IL8 and interferon-gamma [8,31,45]. Many of these cytokines are produced by Th1 cells that may play a significant role in activation and aggregation of neutrophils in the dermis. Th17 cells have also been identified as having a role in Sweet syndrome in recruitment and aggregating of neutrophils via production of pro-inflammatory cytokines such as IL-17 [46].

The classic and diagnostic histopathological features are a dense infiltrate of neutrophils in the dermis and prominent dermal papillary oedema (Figure 49.7). Subepidermal vesicles may be seen. The infiltrate, while predominantly neutrophilic, can also include lymphocytes, histiocytes and eosinophils. While the inflammatory infiltrate is usually in a diffuse dermal band, perivascular patterns can occur. Genuine vasculitis is not seen, although leukocytoclasis is a common finding and endothelial swelling but without fibrinoid necrosis is also seen. Although the overlying epidermis is usually normal, the neutrophilic infiltrate may spread into it or occasionally to adipose tissue [47,48].

Causative organisms
Most patients presenting with classic Sweet syndrome have a fever and a history of infection. Upper respiratory tract infections commonly precede the appearance of the skin lesions by 1–3 weeks [8]. Intestinal infection by *Yersinia* has also been reported [49]. There are a few reports of triggering infectious associations such as tuberculosis [50], *Campylobacter* [51] and sporotrichosis [52].

Genetics
The Sweet syndrome variant 'neutrophilic dermatosis of the dorsal hands' has been reported in HLA-B54 positive Japanese patients [53]. Elsewhere, heterozygous mutations of *MEFV* (the defective gene in familial mediterranean fever (FMF)) has been identified in some patients with Sweet syndrome, and the two conditions concurrently [54,55]. *MEFV* codes for expression of pyrin, an amino acid protein produced in leukocytes which activates an inflammasome complex in response to pathogens. When an *MEFV* mutation exists, reduction in the amount or function of pyrin means the inflammatory response is poorly controlled and an autoinflammatory state ensues (Chapter 45). Further genetic mutations in isocitrate dehydrogenase-1 have been implicated in MASS, and mutations in genes coding for protein tyrosine phosphatase non-receptor type 6 (PTPN6) have also been identified in mouse models and humans with Sweet syndrome [56–58].

Environmental factors
Drug-induced Sweet syndrome is an established phenomenon that can be divided into two main types: (i) G-CSF associated; and

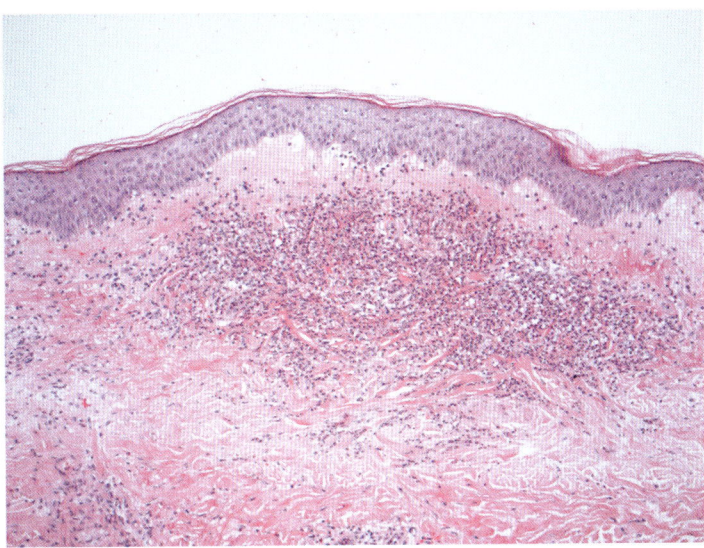

(a)

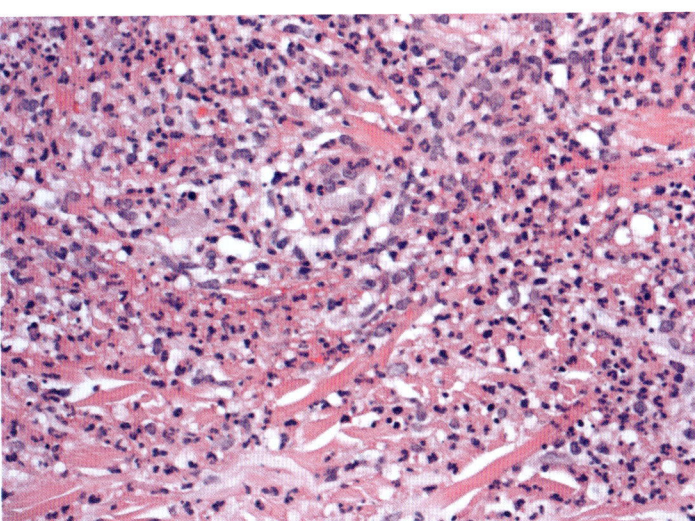

(b)

Figure 49.7 (a,b) Histology of classic Sweet syndrome revealing a normal epidermis overlying confluent papillary dermal oedema and a band-like inflammatory cell infiltrate throughout the reticular dermis. On higher-power (b) it is apparent the infiltrate is predominantly composed of neutrophils, and neutrophilic debris is also seen as well as histiocytes and occasional eosinophils. (a) H&E ×10. (b) H&E ×40.

(ii) other drugs. G-CSF-triggered Sweet syndrome is more commonly described [38,59,60]. For other drugs a true association can only be confirmed if recurrence occurs on rechallenge. For obvious reasons, this is often not done, which leaves uncertainty about many proposed drug associations. The duration between drug exposure and disease was examined by Walker and Cohen who suggested that there should be a close relationship between drug ingestion and clinical symptoms [9].

Cohen has produced a detailed summary of DISS reports [8]. Medicines with possible associations to Sweet syndrome include antibiotics, anticonvulsants, highly active antiretroviral therapy (HAART), antihypertensives, chemotherapeutic agents, colony-stimulating factors, contraceptives, diuretics, non-steroidal anti-inflammatory drugs (NSAIDs) and retinoids.

Clinical features
History
The clinical history may establish the specific subtype of Sweet syndrome and identifying the trigger is important in directing further investigations [10]. Specific questioning must elucidate whether the following are present:
- Any prior history of fever or infective symptoms
- Pregnancy
- Inflammatory conditions
- Current or previous malignant disease
- New medication administration

Presentation
The classic appearance is of tender red papules, nodules and subsequent plaque formation predominantly distributed over the head and neck, upper trunk and upper limbs. MASS may have a more widespread distribution. The plaques are classically tumid and oedematous, and as the inflammatory process progresses may become studded with pseudovesicles (Figure 49.8) or pseudopustules. Definite vesicles and pustules, developing into ulceration, may occur. Patients will often have a fever and feel unwell, although this is not always the case. Figures 49.9 and 49.10 show the typical red plaques that characterise Sweet syndrome.

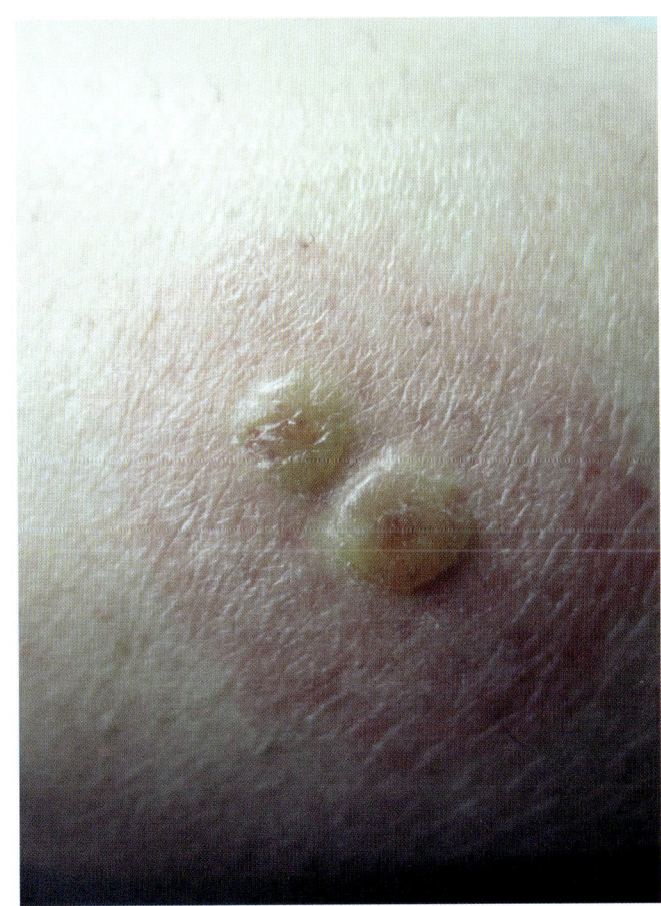

Figure 49.8 Sweet syndrome. Pseudovesicles may occur within the inflammatory plaques.

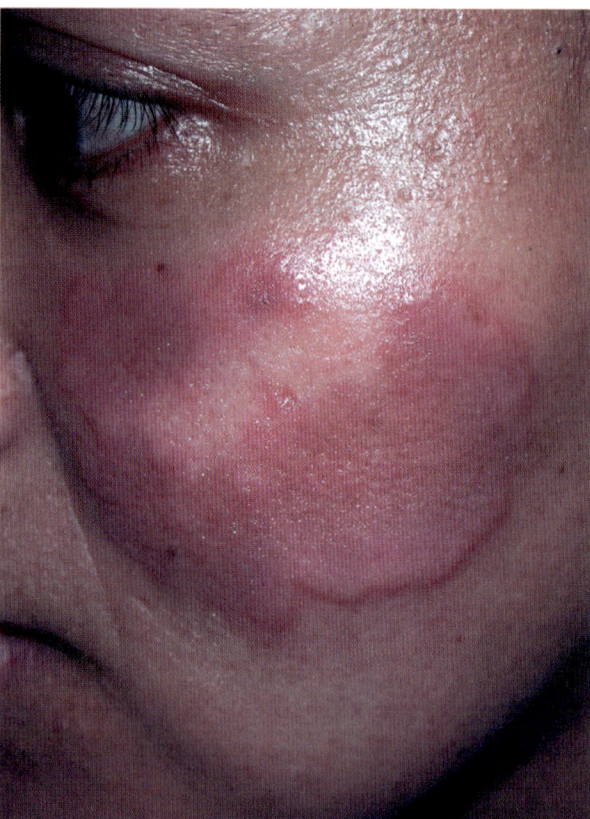

Figure 49.9 Sweet syndrome. The face is often affected.

An associated arthralgia is described in approximately one-third of patients. Ocular involvement is also relatively common with conjunctivitis, panuveitis and episcleritis occurring [61,62].

Most organs have been reported to be affected by Sweet syndrome [8]. The specific involvement of other organs is known as extracutaneous Sweet syndrome. Central nervous system involvement or 'neuro-sweets' may involve, although not be limited to, benign encephalitis; aseptic meningitis; brainstem lesions; and psychiatric symptoms [63,64]. Respiratory involvement may include neutrophilic inflammation of the bronchi or aseptic pulmonary effusion with abundant neutrophils [65].

Spontaneous resolution may occur, often within 3 months, or a pattern of fluctuating exacerbations may be seen in untreated cases.

Clinical variants

Neutrophilic dermatosis of the dorsal hands. This entity is generally accepted as a variant of Sweet syndrome with identical clinical lesions, histology, HLA type [53], demographic features and disease associations [66]. It is characterised by bluish or haemorrhagic papules, bullae and nodules on the dorsal hands (Figures 49.11 and 49.12). In 50% of cases, typical Sweet syndrome lesions are seen at other sites and the condition responds promptly to prednisolone or dapsone. Clinical distinction from PG – especially the bullous variant – and pustular vasculitis may be difficult [53,66–69]. Cases have been associated with myeloproliferative disorders, occult malignancy, IBD and rheumatoid arthritis. It has been suggested that this variant may have a greater association with malignancy [70].

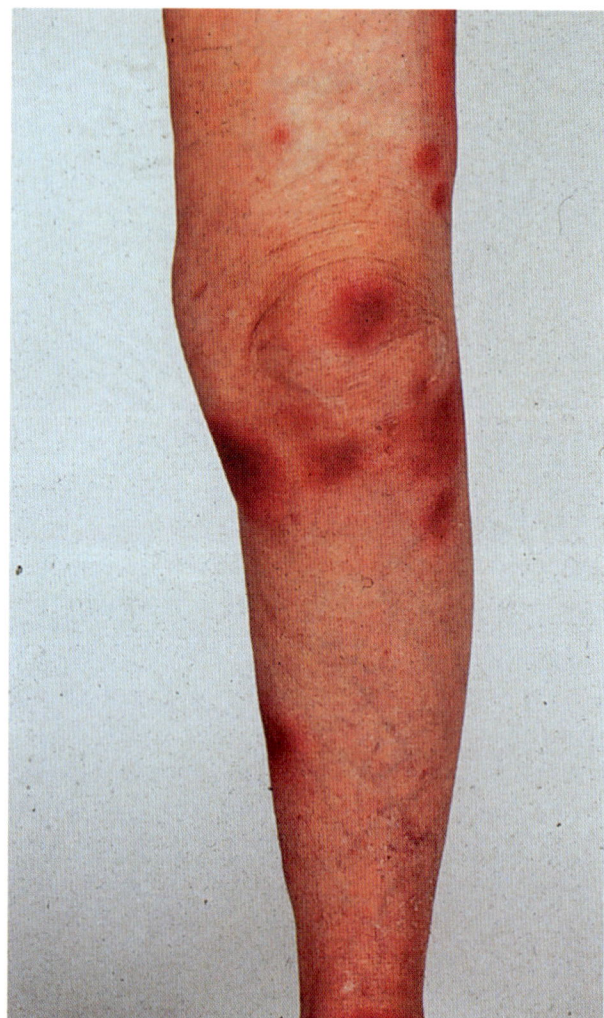

Figure 49.10 Sweet syndrome. Multiple large lesions on the leg.

Subcutaneous Sweet syndrome. This entity presents with erythema nodosum-like tender, subepidermal nodules on the extremities, usually the legs. There are a number of reports of atypical lesions with Sweet syndrome histology presenting in patients with haematological malignancy [8,71]. These are best defined within the entity of subcutaneous Sweet syndrome.

Histiocytoid Sweet syndrome. This variant is characterised by an infiltrate composed of large histiocytoid mononuclear cells (i.e. they look like histiocytes; Figure 49.13). Immunohistochemical staining for myeloperoxidase is positive, suggesting they are immature myeloid cells and neutrophil precursors [72]. Haematological malignancy-associated, idiopathic and drug-induced cases have been reported. Clinically, they may resemble classic Sweet syndrome or may present with subcutaneous erythema nodosum-type lesions.

Diagnostic criteria for Sweet syndrome have been suggested, initially by Su and Liu in 1986, and later modified by von den Driesch in 1994 [7,73] (Box 49.1). Both major criteria and two minor criteria are required for diagnosis. Walker and Cohen developed separate criteria for DISS [9,74].

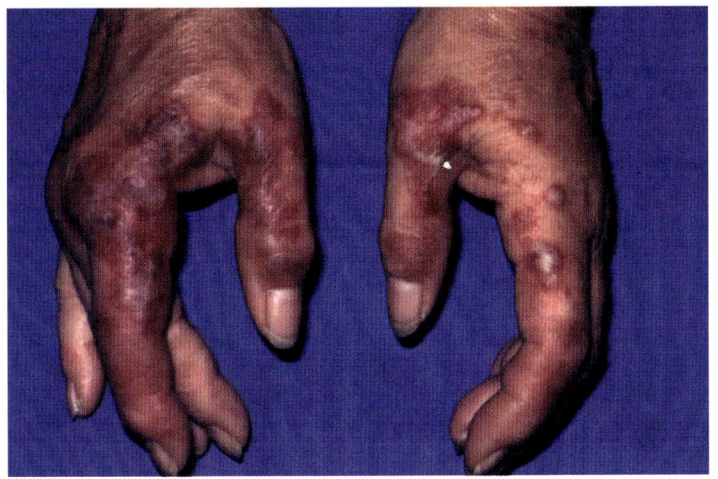

Figure 49.11 Neutrophilic dermatosis of the dorsal hands.

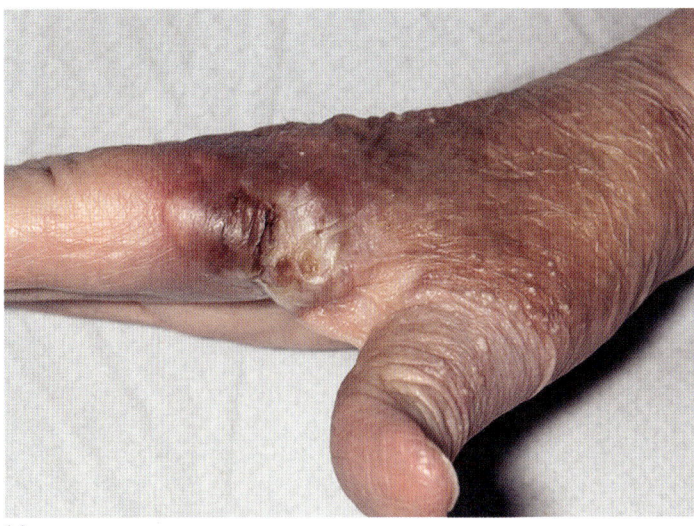

(a)

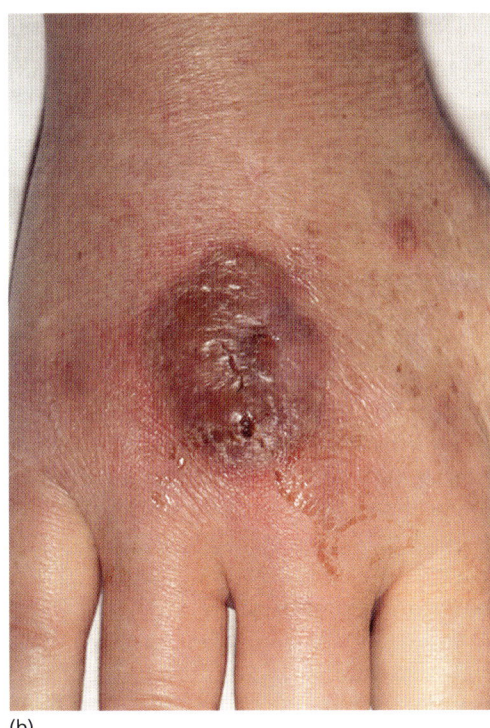

(b)

Figure 49.12 (a,b) Bullous variants of neutrophilic dermatosis of the dorsal hands.

Box 49.1 Diagnostic criteria for Sweet syndrome

Major criteria
1 Abrupt onset of tender or painful red plaques, or nodules, occasionally with vesicles, pustules or blisters
2 Predominantly neutrophilic dermal infiltrate in the absence of leukocytoclastic vasculitis

Minor criteria
1 Preceded by a non-specific respiratory or gastrointestinal tract infection or vaccination or associated with:
   • Inflammatory diseases such as chronic autoimmune disorders, infections
   • Haemoproliferative disorders or solid malignant tumours
   • Pregnancy
2 Fever >38°C
3 Abnormal laboratory values at presentation (three of four required: ESR >20 mm, leukocytes >8000, neutrophils >70%, elevated C-reactive protein)
4 Excellent response to treatment with systemic corticosteroids or potassium iodide

Diagnostic criteria for drug-induced Sweet syndrome
Criteria 1 and 2 are the same as the major criteria for Sweet syndrome diagnosis. However, the remainder must also be satisfied to meet criteria for a diagnosis of drug-induced Sweet syndrome.
3 Fever > 38°C
4 Temporal relationship between drug ingestion and clinical presentation OR temporally related recurrence post oral challenge
5 Temporally related resolution of lesions following drug withdrawal or treatment with systemic corticosteroids

---

Differential diagnosis

There is a long list of clinical and histological differential diagnoses for Sweet syndrome described in detail by Cohen [8]. The following conditions should always be considered:
1 Clinical.
   • Infectious disorders: erysipelas, cellulitis, herpes simplex.
   • Inflammatory: panniculitides, pyoderma gangrenosum, syphilis, tuberculosis.
   • Neoplastic: metastases.
   • Reactive erythemas: erythema nodosum, erythema multiforme, urticarial.
   • Systemic disease: Behçet disease, cutaneous lupus, bowel bypass syndrome.
   • Vasculitis: erythema elevatum diutinum, polyarteritis nodosa, granuloma faciale.
2 Histological.
   • Leukaemia cutis (particularly in the histiocytoid variant).
   • Leukocytoclastic vasculitis.
   • Neutrophilic eccrine hidradenitis.

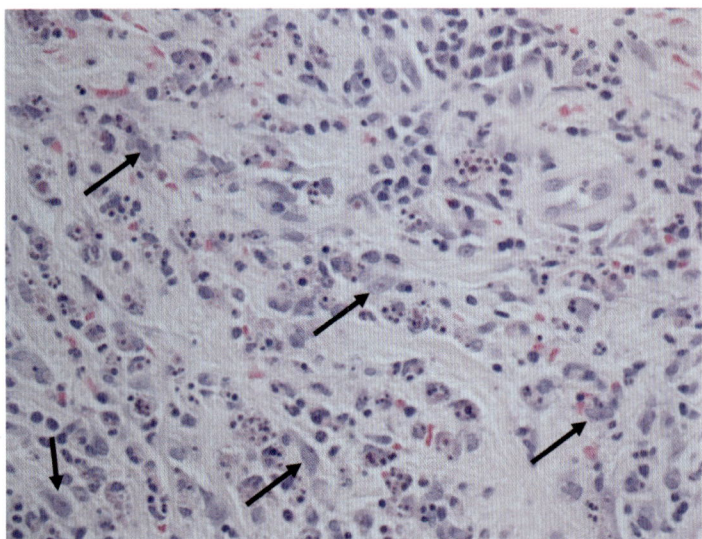

Figure 49.13 High-power image of the dermal infiltrate in lesional skin of a patient with histiocytoid Sweet disease. The arrows point to large, immature histiocyte-like 'histiocytoid' cells of myeloid lineage. H&E ×40.

Classification of severity

There is no formal grading system for Sweet syndrome. Details to be recorded include the type of lesions and their distribution, the presence of extracutaneous signs such as ocular disease and any history of symptoms related to Sweet syndrome such as fever, shortness of breath, arthralgia, myalgia or arthritis.

Complications and co-morbidities

In the vast majority of cases, Sweet syndrome resolves with no sequelae. Severe skin lesions with ulceration or with delayed treatment can lead to scarring. Extracutaneous involvement can rarely lead to complications such as systemic inflammatory response syndrome with pleural effusion [75].

Disease course and prognosis

Without treatment, the disease will often resolve within 3 months. Approximately one-third of cases will recur. The response to corticosteroids is usually rapid.

Gopee *et al.* [10] recommend discharging patients who are classifiable into subtypes of CSS, DISS or MASS once they have been managed, referred to other clinical services as appropriate, and their lesions have resolved. However, due to the risk that Sweet syndrome may be the sentinel of a yet undetectable malignancy or another underlying condition, they recommend repeating full blood count on a 6-monthly basis and following up patients who are unclassifiable and without a clear trigger for 24 months [10].

Investigations

Historically, there has been a lack of guidelines centred around classification, investigation and management of patients with Sweet syndrome, which has led to patients being either over- or under-investigated with potential delays in diagnosis of relevant underlying conditions. Gopee *et al.* [10] have suggested an investigation algorithm that is guided by disease subtype and potential triggers.

Baseline investigations include the following:
- Lesional skin biopsy.
- Serology including full blood count, ESR, C-reactive protein, renal and liver function, thyroid profile, rheumatoid factor, antinuclear antibodies and extractable nuclear antigens, anti-DS DNA, ASO titre, blood film, serum electrophoresis.
- Chest X-ray.
- Urinalysis and microscopy.
- Pregnancy test (if appropriate).

Additional tests should be guided by clinical subtypes and extracutaneous symptoms. Targeted investigations including imaging with CT or positron tomography–CT may be required if possible underlying malignancy is suspected after assessment of 'red flag' symptoms, lifestyle factors such as smoking and results of national cancer screening [10]. However, literature to date discourages aggressive investigation without a reasonable clinical suspicion in the absence of other potential triggers for Sweet syndrome [3,10]. Cohen *et al.* in 1993 [6], Cohen in 2007 [8] and Jung *et al.* in 2022 [76] made specific recommendations regarding exclusion of malignancy, including a full clinical history and medical examination including examination of the lymph nodes and mouth, and furthermore considering assessments of the breasts and pelvis in women and the prostate and testicles in men [6,8].

Management

First line

For mild cases of localised disease, topical treatments may be tried. In the majority of cases, systemic agents are needed and prednisolone is the most common first choice, typically 0.5–2 mg/kg daily within a period of 4–6 weeks [77]. Appropriate guidelines for the prevention of osteoporosis must be adhered to, as well as consideration of gastric protection. If remission has not been induced after 3 months, a second line anti-inflammatory agent should be added.

Second line

There is no evidence base to determine which of the three second line drugs (dapsone, potassium iodide and colchicine) should be tried first. Dapsone requires pre-treatment assessment of glucose-6-phosphate dehydrogenase (G6PD) activity, and close monitoring of haemoglobin levels and reticulocyte count to detect haemolysis. A cautious approach is often beneficial with lower doses such as 50 mg taking time to be effective, but not triggering haemolysis. Haematological side effects are more frequent with doses of 100 mg or more.

Colchicine may be poorly tolerated due to gastrointestinal side effects such as nausea, vomiting and diarrhoea. The side effects are generally dose related.

Third line

NSAIDs such as indomethacin may be effective. In 1997 one study treated 18 patients with indomethacin, with clearance of lesions in 17 of 18 subjects within 7–14 days [78]. Other, older agents mentioned in the literature include chlorambucin, cyclophosphamide, thalidomide, clofazamine and interferon-α. However, these all relate to case reports and small studies only [8].

The advent of monoclonal antibodies has heralded novel therapeutic approaches in the management of Sweet syndrome. It is worth highlighting the caveat that these agents should be used with caution when possible infection is underlying the inflammatory process, and unfortunately patients have died due to disseminated infective processes after initiation of biologic agents [70,79]. Furthermore, in cases of malignancy-associated Sweet syndrome, biologic therapies would usually be an inappropriate choice of treatment due to the significant and enduring immunosuppressive effects.

Anti-TNF-α agents are effective for patients with Sweet syndrome, particularly in those with coexistent inflammatory bowel disease. Infliximab is the most used biologic agent in the management of recalcitrant Sweet syndrome, either as monotherapy or in combination with oral corticosteroids [15,78,80]. Adalimumab and etanercept have also been reported as effective in managing patients with Sweet syndrome, the former also being used with success in patients who fail to respond adequately to infliximab [81–85].

To date, ustekinumab is ineffective and no anti-IL-17 biologic agents have as yet been reported in the use of Sweet syndrome [86]. Anti-IL-1 (anakinra) has been used successfully alongside prednisolone in the treatment of refractory Sweet syndrome (including failure to respond to anti-TNF agents) [87–89].

While biologic treatments are felt to be efficacious, reports of paradoxical Sweet syndrome in patients receiving anti-TNF treatment for IBD or inflammatory arthritis exist [90,91].

Treatment ladder

First line
- Systemic corticosteroids (0.5–2 mg/kg prednisolone for 4–6 weeks)
- Potent topical or intralesional corticosteroids may be tried for mild localised disease [92]

Second line
- Dapsone (50–100 mg/day) [93]
- Potassium iodide (300 mg three times each day) [94]
- Colchicine (0.5 mg three times each day) [95,96]

Third line
- Anti-TNF agents +/− oral corticosteroids (including infliximab, adalimumab or etanercept) [79]
- Anakinra +/− oral corticosteroids [79]
- Indomethacin, ciclosporin, clofazamine, IVIG [78,97–99]

Bowel-associated dermatitis–arthritis syndrome

Definition and nomenclature
Bowel-associated dermatitis–arthritis syndrome (BADAS) is defined by the presence of pustular vasculitic lesions associated with blind loops of bowel or other causes of stasis of bowel content.

Synonyms and inclusions
- Bowel-associated dermatosis–arthritis syndrome

Introduction and general description
BADAS was first described in 1971 as pustular vasculitis, cutaneous lesions and serum sickness-like reactions in patients who had undergone jejuno-ileal bypass surgery for morbid obesity [1–3]. The term has been extended to include the same syndrome in patients with inflammatory bowel disease (IBD), those who have had creation of a blind loop following surgery for peptic ulcer disease [4] or with other causes of stasis of bowel content, such as in achalasia or related to a defunctioning colostomy, or in complex IBD [5]. Recently PASH syndrome (pyoderma gangrenosum acne and hidradenitis suppurativa) has been described following bowel bypass bariatric surgery [6].

Epidemiology

Pathophysiology
Vascular damage secondary to bowel flora antigen-associated circulating immune complexes is thought to be the pathogenesis of the cutaneous lesions. In these patients, peptidoglycans from gastrointestinal flora may be the antigenic trigger for immune complex-mediated vessel damage [1]. Therapeutic response to antimicrobials in some cases supports this concept and immune complexes have been demonstrated [4,7].

Predisposing factors
BADAS may be related to jejuno-ileal bypass [1–3,8], gastric resection [4], blind loops (Bilroth II or Roux-en-Y) [4,9], defunctioning ileo-anal pouch procedures [10] and bilio-pancreatic diversion [11]. It has also been related to other bowel disease: ulcerative colitis [4]; Crohn disease [4]; diverticulitis of the colon [12]; jejunal diverticula [13]; appendicitis [14]; and achalasia of the cardia [15].

In some cases, there are combined causes (e.g. surgery for IBD). In most instances related to surgery, the loop of bypassed bowel, or a blind loop, is contiguous with the intestine, but may be separated as a defunctioning segment of bowel [10].

Pathology
The changes noted in the dermal blood vessels from early lesions of pustular vasculitis in patients with BADAS are similar to those in biopsies from patients with Sweet syndrome [4,7,8,9] and Behçet disease. Several cases have clinical and pathological overlap with other neutrophilic dermatoses.

Clinical features
Presentation
The cutaneous manifestations of BADAS usually begin as small macular lesions that progress to papules and then pustules on a purpuric base, most often on the arms and the upper body (Figure 49.14). The pustules measure 0.5–1.5 cm in diameter (Figure 49.15) and typically occur in crops, with each crop lasting up to 2 weeks, and recurring at intervals of several months [1,4,8]. Other clinical presentations include erythema nodosum-like

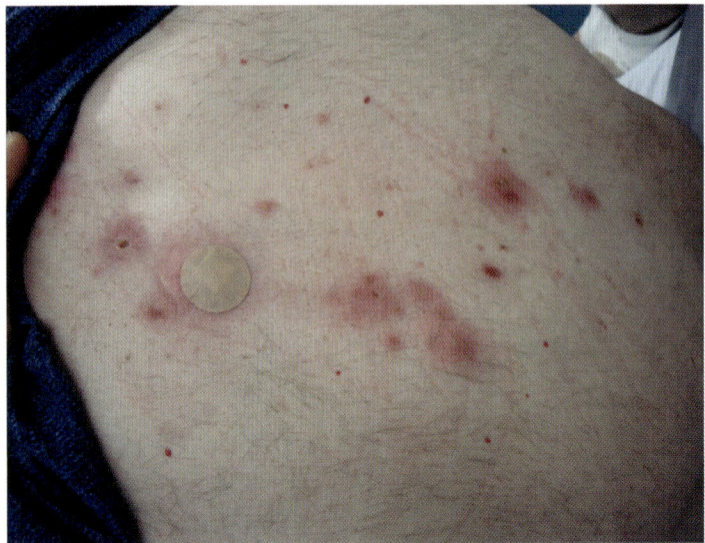

Figure 49.14 BADAS showing crops of large pustules on an erythematous purpuric base on the trunk.

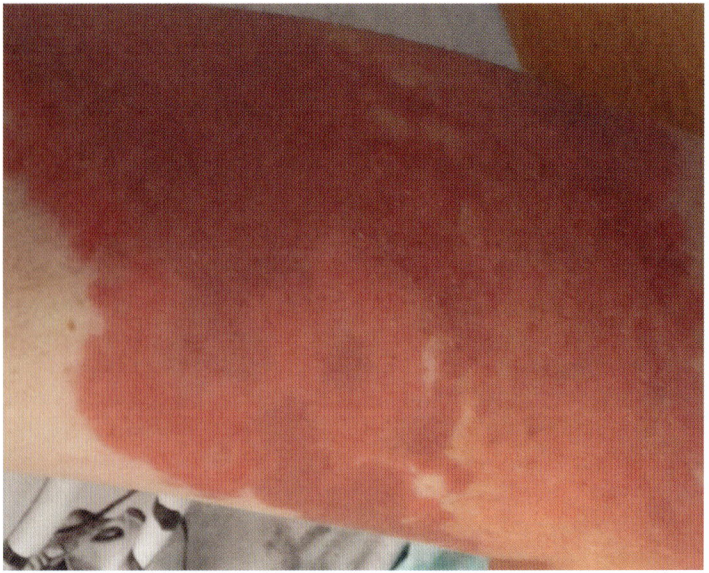

Figure 49.16 Urticarial plaques in BADAS associated with inflammatory bowel disease.

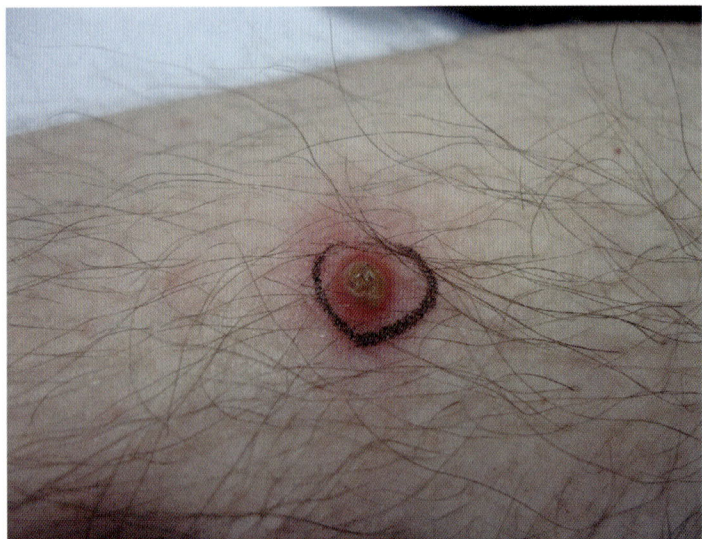

Figure 49.15 A typical initial lesion in BADAS showing a large deep pustule on an erythematous base.

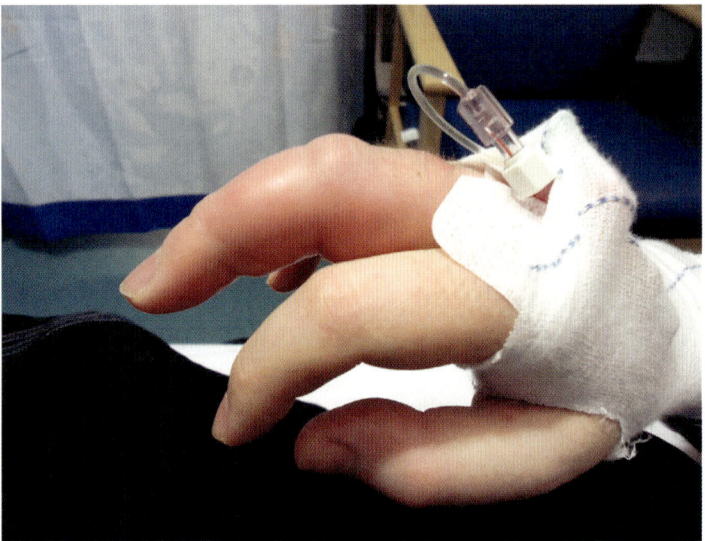

Figure 49.17 Acute inflammatory distal arthritis with tenderness and swelling in BADAS.

lesions, urticarial plaques (Figure 49.16) and also larger pyoderma gangrenosum-like pustular lesions. Pathergy occurs in BADAS as it does in other neutrophilic dermatoses. The cutaneous lesions may be preceded by fever, flu-like symptoms, myalgia or gastrointestinal upset. Arthralgia or non-erosive polyarthritis affecting the hands, wrists and other peripheral joints is common (Figure 49.17); ocular involvement such as episcleritis [16] (Figure 49.18) and haematuria or proteinuria [8,14] may also occur. Rarely, severe skin lesions and marked systemic manifestations may occur [17].

Differential diagnosis

It is important to distinguish between BADAS and Behçet disease (Chapter 48), as both may include oral aphthae and lesions of pustular vasculitis.

Investigations

Clinicopathological evaluation of skin lesions is required but does not exclude lesions of Behçet disease or early lesions of either; some patients appear to exhibit a spectrum of neutrophilic dermatoses. Pustules should be swabbed for microbiological assessment. It is advisable to perform urinalysis in patients with BADAS as, unlike classic Sweet syndrome, there may be haematuria or proteinuria, possibly representing an immune complex-mediated glomerulonephritis [8].

Management

For patients with BADAS following bowel bypass surgery, surgical correction of bowel anatomy often eliminates the signs and symptoms. In other cases, such as patients with blind loops, surgical correction may be difficult and resolution of symptoms is therefore less likely.

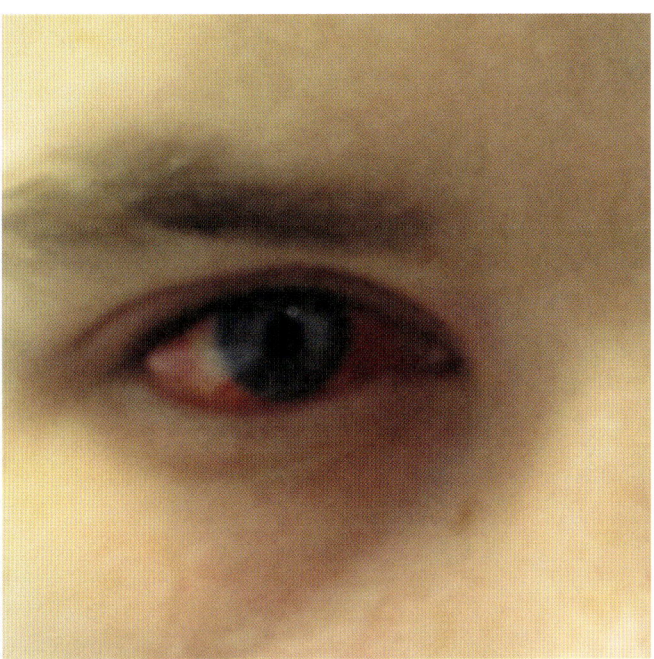

Figure 49.18 BADAS-associated episcleritis.

First line

Manifestations of BADAS may often be controlled by systemic tetracycline, metronidazole, ciprofloxacin or erythromycin [1,7,11]; this further suggests the important role of bowel bacterial colonisation in triggering the systemic response in BADAS.

Second line

Systemic corticosteroids are usually unnecessary for the treatment of BADAS but may be justified depending on the degree of skin, joint or systemic symptoms, or to concurrently treat IBD. Other treatments including oral colchicine [18], dapsone [16] and mycophenolate [10] have been used; systemic immunosuppressants may need to be combined with an appropriate antibiotic. In cases associated with IBD, control of the underlying condition is important. Treatment with biologic drugs has been reported including ustekinumab [19,20].

Subcorneal pustular dermatosis

Definition and nomenclature

This is a rare neutrophilic dermatosis, with sterile subcorneal pustules typically affecting the flexural areas of the trunk and proximal extremities.

Synonyms and inclusions
- Sneddon–Wilkinson disease

Epidemiology
Incidence and prevalence

A rare condition with about 200 cases described. It occurs most frequently in adults aged 40–60 years.

Sex

The disease is more common in females with a ratio of 4 : 1 female to male.

Associated diseases

Subcorneal pustular dermatosis is associated with benign monoclonal gammopathy, more commonly immunoglobulin A (IgA) [1] (occasionally IgG), IBD [2], multiple myeloma, lymphomas, PG [3], rheumatoid arthritis [4] and connective tissue disease, including systemic lupus erythematosus.

Pathophysiology

The pathogenesis is obscure. The condition is characterised by subcorneal accumulation of neutrophils. It has also occurred at injection sites of GM-CSF in a patient with IgA myeloma [5]. Excessive production of TNF-α has also been linked with the lesions, as has neutrophil activation [6]. Thus, subcorneal pustular dermatosis has much in common with other neutrophilic dermatoses. However, it has also been considered to overlap with pemphigus, although in most cases immunofluorescence is negative. In a subgroup, IgA is deposited in the upper dermis and is directed against the extracellular domains of desmocollin 1 [7,8,9]. The relationship between intercellular IgA pemphigus and classic subcorneal pustular dermatosis is unclear [10,11].

Pathology

Biopsies from early lesions show a perivascular inflammatory infiltrate with occasional eosinophils. The pustules sit on the surface of the epidermis rather than within it, spongiosis and spongiotic pustules are absent and acantholysis is only seen in old lesions [12,13]. Immunofluorescence in the classic form is negative [14] but may be positive to IgA in a subgroup [15–17] (Figure 49.19).

Causative organisms

Culture of the pustules is sterile.

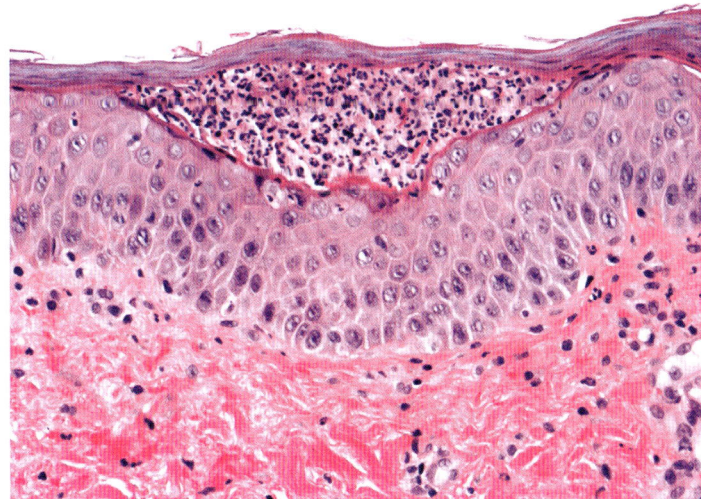

Figure 49.19 Subcorneal pustular dermatosis. Histology showing subcorneal neutrophils. Pustules sit on the surface of the epidermis without spongiosis or acantholysis. Courtesy of Dr Ehab Hussain, Aberdeen Royal Infirmary, Aberdeen, UK. H&E ×10.

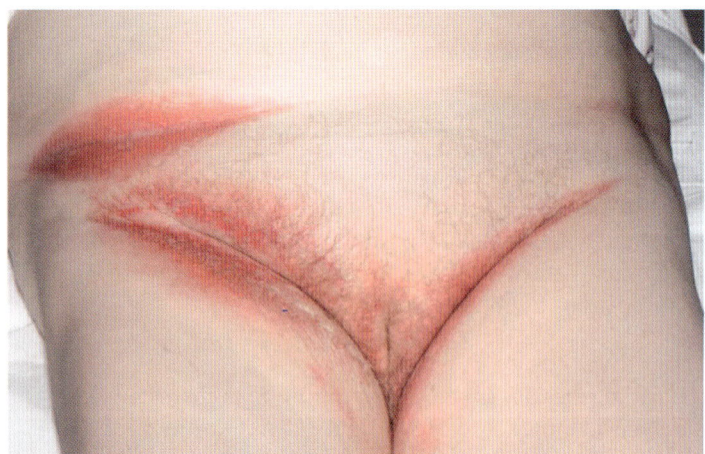

Figure 49.20 Subcorneal pustular dermatosis, showing flexural distribution notably in the groins.

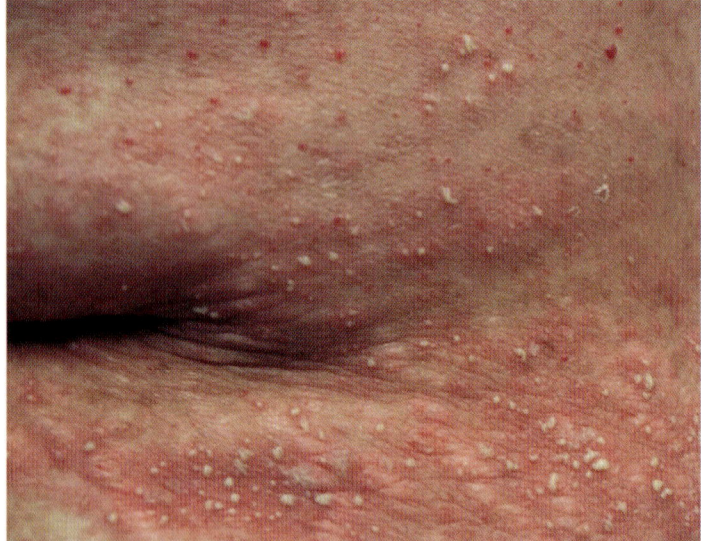

Figure 49.21 Typical appearance of pustules in subcorneal pustular dermatosis.

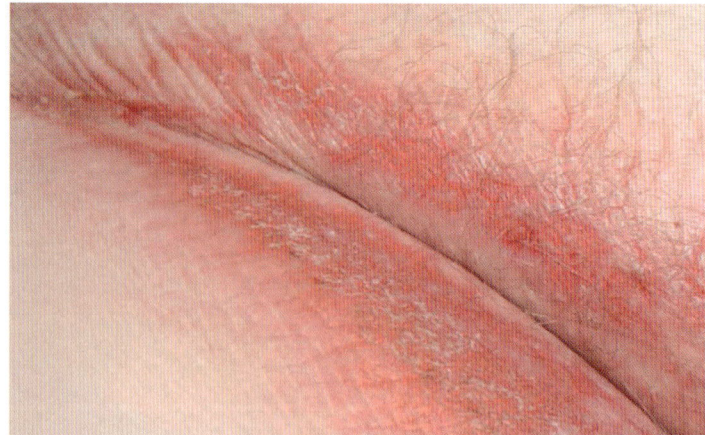

Figure 49.22 Subcorneal pustular dermatosis. Pustules may rupture and be inconspicuous in the skin folds.

IgA pemphigus and acute generalised exanthematous pustulosis (AGEP).

In pustular psoriasis, the presence of spongiform pustules on histology is characteristic. These are not found in subcorneal pustular dermatosis [18], although cases are described where histopathology was indistinguishable from pustular psoriasis [19,20]. These features are also helpful in distinguishing AGEP, which occurs in a febrile subject with a history of recent drug exposure. Immunofluorescence will identify pemphigus. In one report, 10 of 23 patients originally diagnosed with subcorneal pustular dermatosis developed classic lesions of pustular psoriasis or chronic plaque psoriasis 3–40 years after onset [21].

Disease course and prognosis
The condition is benign but chronic with an average duration of 5.8 years [12], although serious associated disease may have a worse prognosis.

Investigations
Investigations should include skin biopsy. It is important to biopsy early pustules and to avoid sampling later lesions, where pustules may have burst, and also to perform immunofluorescence. Bacterial culture of skin swabs should be taken to exclude impetigo and laboratory investigation for underlying associated pathologies should be guided by clinical signs. Investigations to exclude myeloma and other associated conditions are also recommended [22].

Management
As with other neutrophilic dermatoses, therapy for the condition needs to be considered along with therapy directed at any associated disease. Mostly, the basis for recommending therapy is based on anecdote and the distinction between the classic form and IgA subcorneal pemphigus is not always clear in case reports. Response to therapy in these different types might be expected to differ as one of them involves humoral autoimmunity.

First line
Dapsone 50–150 mg daily is the treatment of choice leading to either a partial or a complete response [23].

Clinical features
History
Subcorneal pustular dermatosis was first described in 1956 [12,13].

Presentation
The eruption occurs with acute flares lasting for several days or weeks. The distribution is mainly in the flexures of the trunk and proximal limbs, including axillae, groins, submammary area, neck and inframammary and apron area, sparing the face and mucous membranes (Figure 49.20). Lesions are oval, pea-sized flaccid pustules on a normal or red base (Figure 49.21). A characteristic fluid level with pus in the lower half and clear fluid in the upper half may be seen. Pustules may be isolated or grouped and coalescent to form annular or serpiginous patterns. Successive waves may pass over the same area [13]. In the flexures, these pustules may rupture, thereby becoming indistinct (Figure 49.22).

Differential diagnosis
The differential diagnosis includes impetigo, pustular psoriasis, pemphigus foliaceus, dermatitis herpetiformis, intercellular

Second line

Some cases respond to potent topical or oral corticosteroids but overall these are not particularly effective. Acitretin [24] and tacalcitol have been used effectively [25].

Narrow-band UVB phototherapy [26] has been very effective as have psoralen and UVA (PUVA) [27,28] and retinoids plus PUVA (RePUVA) [29]. Ciclosporin in combination with prednisolone was helpful in one severe case [30].

Third line

Ketoconazole has been reported to be of benefit [31]. Sulfapyridine has been used successfully [32]. There are also reports of effective use of anti-TNF therapy alone [33] or in combination, including etanercept [34,35]. Adalimumab has been used successfully [33]. Infliximab can produce a rapid response [36] and has also been used in combination with standard immunosuppression [37].

Other neutrophilic dermatoses and variants

Pyodermatitis–pyostomatitis vegetans

> **Synonyms and inclusions**
> - Mycosis-like pyoderma
> - Pyoderma vegetans

Definition

Pyodermatitis–pyostomatitis vegetans (PD-PSV) is a disorder distinct from PG in which there is oral mucosal thickening with multiple pustules and 'snail track' superficial ulceration on a red base (at any site, especially the gingivae, the tongue is less affected), and also pustular skin lesions.

Pathophysiology

Little is known about the pathogenesis of this disorder. Although there are similarities with other neutrophilic dermatoses, the differences are clinical and histological, particularly the unexplained eosinophilia which may hold clues to the aetiology.

Predisposing factors

The strongest association, particularly for oral lesions, is with IBD, particularly ulcerative colitis [1]. Leukaemias, lymphoma, diabetes, acne conglobata, hidradenitis suppurativa and dissecting cellulitis, immunosuppression and malnourishment are also associated.

Pathology

Histology shows intraepithelial and/or subepithelial abscesses containing large numbers of eosinophils [2]. Although deeper tissues have a mixed inflammatory infiltrate including neutrophils, eosinophils are prominent and there is often an associated peripheral blood eosinophilia. Skin lesions show pseudoepitheliomatous hyperplasia and neutrophilic microabscesses with negative immunofluorescence [3,4].

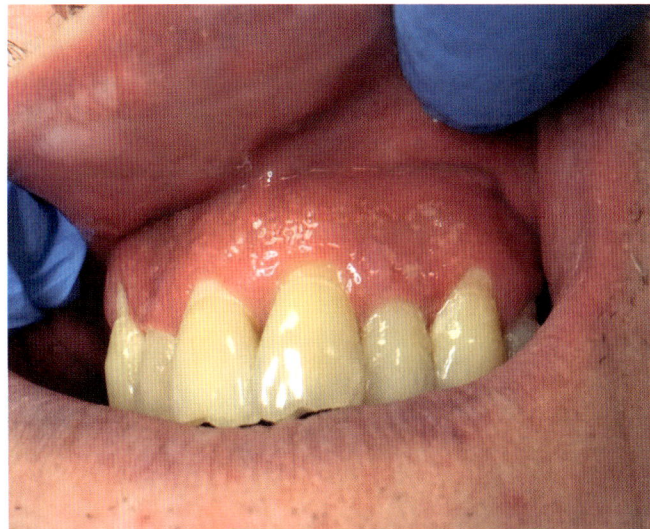

Figure 49.23 Pyostomatitis vegetans.

The pathogenesis is as yet unknown, although immunological and microbial factors have been suggested as possible aetiological factors. Various bacteria have been reported as causative and the disorder may represent an abnormal response to infection. In one case, antibodies to BP230 antigen were found [5].

Clinical features

Typical presentation includes extensive oral mucosa involvement (Figure 49.23) [6] characterised by multiple friable, yellow-cream pustules, on a thickened red base, which ulcerate and form a classic 'snail track' appearance. The skin lesions, if present, are often flexural and clinically suggestive of pemphigus vegetans with verrucous plaques studded with pustules [7,8]. There may be associated dorsal hand lesions that are morphologically very similar to neutrophilic dermatosis, and a rash resembling Sweet syndrome. Lesions may display pathergy.

Investigations

Laboratory findings include raised inflammatory markers and peripheral eosinophilia in two-thirds of patients [3]. Bacterial, viral and fungal cultures, including tuberculosis and atypical mycobacterium, are typically negative [1,3,9]. Direct and indirect immunofluorescence are often negative or weakly positive in PD-PSV [1,9]. Histology characteristically reveals intraepithelial and subepithelial splitting with numerous eosinophils and neutrophils forming microabscesses, leading to ulceration. Possible diagnostic clues include raised IgE in some cases, and eosinophilia which is present in 50–90% of cases.

Management

First line

Systemic prednisolone is usually effective [10,11]. Dapsone and sulfapyridine can be helpful [3] and can be used as steroid-sparing agents. The oral disease may respond to topical corticosteroids [12] or tacrolimus [13,14]. Antiseptic, anaesthetic and steroid mouth washes can assist in providing symptomatic relief.

Second line

Prednisolone and ciclosporin have been used successfully in cases where dapsone was ineffective [15]. Azathioprine in combination with oral steroids and monotherapy with adalimumab have been effective [16]. Crohn disease-associated cases have been treated successfully with a combination of methotrexate and infliximab [17,18].

Amicrobial pustulosis of the skin folds

> **Synonyms and inclusions**
> - Amicrobial pustulosis associated with autoimmune diseases
> - Amicrobial pustulosis
> - Follicular impetigo or pyodermatitis vegetans associated with lupus erythematosus or other autoimmune diseases

Introduction and general description

Most cases occur in patients with systemic lupus erythematosus [19,20], but can occur with coeliac disease and other autoimmune conditions including autoimmune thyroid disease [21,22] and autoimmune hepatic disease [19]. Cases have also been reported in association with Crohn disease [23], Sjögren disease and IgA nephropathy [24,25].

Pathophysiology

Extensive gene expression in lesions was reported in a single case [26].

Clinical features

This is a condition of rapidly evolving small semi-confluent pustules that predominantly affect the flexures with one major or minor skin fold usually affected, that is the face or scalp (causing alopecia) [27] (Figures 49.24, 49.25 and 49.26).

Investigations

Neutrophilic epidermal and ostial exocytosis occurs with spongiform pustules and a neutrophilic dermal infiltrate. Positive direct

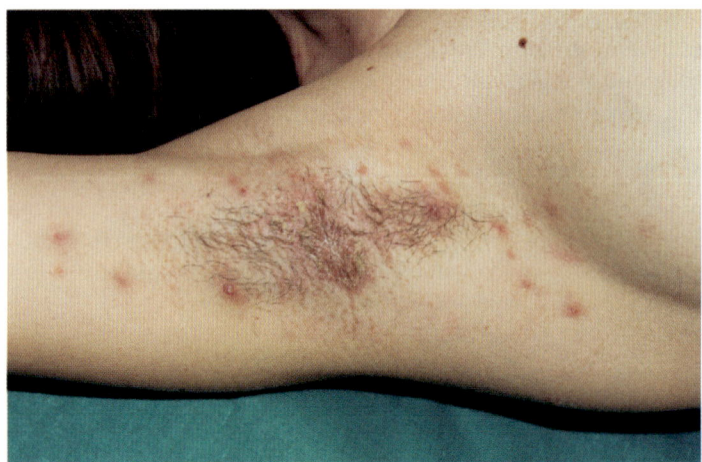

Figure 49.24 Sterile pustules, erosions and crusts on the axillary fold of a patient with amicrobial pustulosis of the skin folds. Courtesy of Professor A.V. Marzano, Fondazione IRCCS Ca' Granda Ospedale Maggiore Policlinico, Università degli Studi di Milano, Milan, Italy.

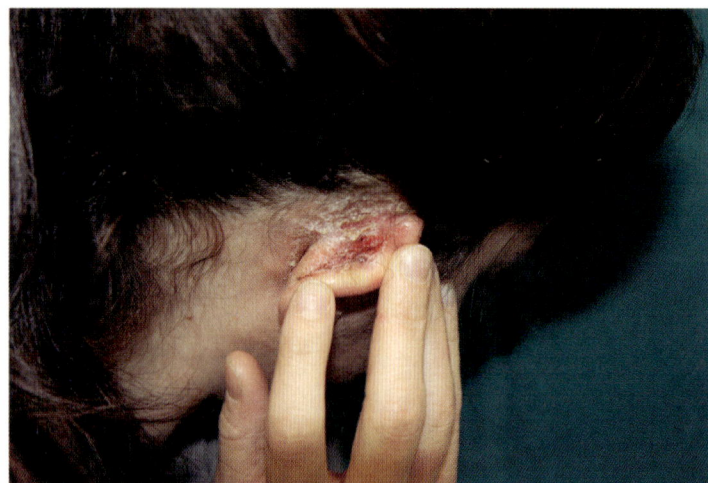

Figure 49.25 Amicrobial pustulosis of the skin folds. Erosions and crusts extensively involving the retro-auricular region. Courtesy of Professor A.V. Marzano, Fondazione IRCCS Ca' Granda Ospedale Maggiore Policlinico, Università degli Studi di Milano, Milan, Italy.

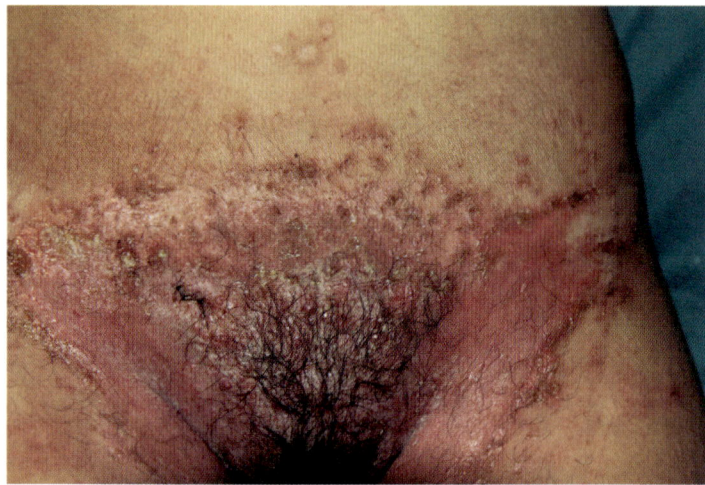

Figure 49.26 Amicrobial pustulosis of the inguinal folds. Erosive and exudating lesions, partially covered by crusts, symmetrically involving the inguinal folds and extending to the genital region. Courtesy of Professor A.V. Marzano, Fondazione IRCCS Ca' Granda Ospedale Maggiore Policlinico, Università degli Studi di Milano, Milan, Italy.

immunofluorescence for IgM, C3 and less often IgG is variable and may be in the endothelium or a lupus band.

Diagnostic criteria

The following criteria have been proposed. Essential criteria include pustulosis involving one or more major skin fold, one or more minor folds in the ano-genital area, a histological pattern of intraepidermal spongiform pustules and a mainly neutrophilic dermal infiltrate, and negative culture from an unopened pustule. Minor criteria include an association with one or more autoimmune disorders, positive antinuclear antibodies 1:160 or higher and the presence of autoantibodies (anti-extractable nuclear antigens (ENA), anti-dsDNA, anti-smooth muscle, anti-mitochondrial or anti-endomesial [20]).

Differential diagnosis

This includes subcorneal pustular dermatosis, pustular forms of psoriasis and erosive pustular dermatosis of the scalp [28].

Management
First line
Oral corticosteroids are effective in most cases.

Second line
Dapsone or ciclosporin is sometimes used; oral zinc was effective in two cases. Topical corticosteroids and colchicine have also been reported as useful in some cases. Cimetidine and ascorbic acid have been advocated as safe treatments in some patients [20]. Complete remission after anakinra has been reported in one case where IL-1α was demonstrated to be involved [26].

Aseptic abscess syndrome

Introduction and general description

As with many of the neutrophilic dermatoses, systemic aseptic abscesses may occur and may precede the onset of the cutaneous manifestations. The term neutrophilic abscess syndrome is now more frequently applied to describe this phenomenon that often occurs in association with IBD [29,30,31]. Joints, pulmonary and intra-abdominal neutrophilic infiltrates or abscesses may occur, and bone, muscle, lymph nodes, ocular and brain involvement are possible [32,33]. Patients are often misdiagnosed with bacterial infections, leading to inappropriate antibiotic therapy [34].

Pathophysiology

In a series of 38 patients with aseptic abscess syndrome, 57% were associated with Crohn disease and 20% with neutrophilic dermatoses, this condition being linked in some cases to mutations in the promoter of the *PSTPIP1* gene similar to those found in the PAPA syndrome [33].

Management

Systemic corticosteroids are usually an effective therapy and they have been used in combination with infliximab followed by etanercept [35].

Key references

The full list of references can be found in the online version at https://www.wiley.com/rooksdermatology10e

Pyoderma gangrenosum

2 Alavi A, French LE, Davis MD, Brassard A, Kirsner RS. Pyoderma gangrenosum: an update on pathophysiology, diagnosis and treatment. *Am J Clin Dermatol* 2017;18:355–72.

4 Maverakis E, Ma C, Shinkai K *et al*. Diagnostic criteria of ulcerative pyoderma gangrenosum: a Delphi consensus of international experts. *JAMA Dermatol* 2018;154:461–6.

5 Jockenhöfer F, Wollina U, Salva KA, Benson S, Dissemond J. The PARACEL-SUS score: a novel diagnostic tool for pyoderma gangrenosum. *Br J Dermatol* 2019;180:615–20.

15 Braun-Falco M, Kovnerystyy O, Lohse P, Ruzicka T. Pyoderma gangrenosum, acne, and suppurative hidradenitis (PASH) – a new autoinflammatory syndrome distinct from PAPA syndrome. *J Am Acad Dermatol* 2012;66:409–15.

16 Calderón-Castrat X, Bancalari-Díaz D, Román-Curto C *et al*. PSTPIP1 gene mutation in a pyoderma gangrenosum, acne and suppurative hidradenitis (PASH) syndrome. *Br J Dermatol* 2016;175:194–8.

23 Wu XR, Mukewar S, Kiran RP, Remzi FH, Hammel J, Shen B. Risk factors for peristomal pyoderma gangrenosum complicating inflammatory bowel disease. *J Crohns Colitis* 2013;7:e171–7.

30 Marzano AV, Borghi A, Meroni PL, Cugno M. Pyoderma gangrenosum and its syndromic forms: evidence for a link with autoinflammation. *Br J Dermatol* 2016;175:882–91.

31 Marzano AV, Fanoni D, Antiga E *et al*. Expression of cytokines, chemokines and other effector molecules in two prototypic autoinflammatory skin diseases, pyoderma gangrenosum and Sweet's syndrome. *Clin Exp Immunol* 2014;178:48–56.

96 Brooklyn TN, Dunnill MG, Shetty A *et al*. Infliximab for the treatment of pyoderma gangrenosum: a randomised, double blind, placebo-controlled trial. *Gut* 2006;55:505–9.

97 Ormerod AD, Thomas KS, Craig FE *et al*. Comparison of the two most commonly used treatments for pyoderma gangrenosum: results of the STOP GAP randomised controlled trial. *BMJ* 2015;350:h2958.

105 Agarwal A, Andrews JM. Systematic review: IBD-associated pyoderma gangrenosum in the biologic era, the response to therapy. *Aliment Pharmacol Ther* 2013;38:563–72.

129 Nunes G, Patita M, Fernandes V. Refractory pyoderma gangrenosum in a patient with Crohn's disease: complete response to ustekinumab. *J Crohns Colitis* 2019;13:812–13.

Sweet syndrome

1 Sweet RD. An acute febrile neutrophilic dermatosis. *Br J Dermatol* 1964;76:349–56.

2 Heath MS, Ortega-Loayza AG. Insights into the pathogenesis of Sweet's syndrome. *Front Immunol* 2019;10:413.

3 Villarreal-Villarreal CD, Ocampo-Candiani J, Villarreal-Martínez A. Sweet syndrome: a review and update. *Actas Dermosifiliogr* 2016;107:369–78.

8 Cohen PR. Sweet's syndrome – a comprehensive review of an acute febrile neutrophilic dermatosis. *Orphanet J Rare Dis* 2007;2:34.

9 Walker DC, Cohen PR. Trimethoprim-sulfamethoxazole-associated acute febrile neutrophilic dermatosis: case report and review of drug-induced Sweet's syndrome. *J Am Acad Dermatol* 1996;34:918–23.

10 Gopee NH, Charlton FG, Hampton PJ. Sweet syndrome: a retrospective study of 64 cases and proposal of an algorithmic approach to improve investigation and management. *Skin Health Dis* 2021;1:e23.

33 Chan MP, Duncan LM, Nazarian RM. Subcutaneous Sweet syndrome in the setting of myeloid disorders: a case series and review of the literature. *J Am Acad Dermatol* 2013;68:1006–15.

47 Ratzinger G, Burgdorf W, Zelger BG, Zelger B. Acute febrile neutrophilic dermatosis: a histopathologic study of 31 cases with review of literature. *Am J Dermatopathol* 2007;29:125–33.

74 Nofal A, Abdelmaksoud A, Amer H *et al*. Sweet's syndrome: diagnostic criteria revisited. *J Dtsch Dermatol Ges* 2017;156:1081–8.

77 Molinelli E, Brisigotti V, Paolinelli M, Offidani A. Novel therapeutic approaches and targets for the treatment of neutrophilic dermatoses: management of patients with neutrophilic dermatoses and future directions in the era of biologic treatment. *Curr Pharm Biotechnol* 2021;22:46–58.

Bowel-associated dermatitis–arthritis syndrome

1 Ely PH. The bowel bypass syndrome: a response to bacterial peptidoglycans. *J Am Acad Dermatol* 1980;2:473–87.

2 Shagrin JW, Frame B, Duncan H. Polyarthritis in obese patients with intestinal bypass. *Ann Intern Med* 1971;75:377–80.

3 Drenick EJ, Ament ME, Finegold SM, Passaro E, Jr. Bypass enteropathy: an inflammatory process in the excluded segment with systemic complications. *Am J Clin Nutr* 1977;30:76–89.

4 Jorizzo JL, Apisarnthanarax P Subrt P et al. Bowel-bypass syndrome without bowel bypass. Bowel-associated dermatosis-arthritis syndrome. *Arch Intern Med* 1983;143:457–61.

7 Jorizzo JL, Schmalstieg FC, Dinehart SM *et al*. Bowel-associated dermatosis-arthritis syndrome. Immune complex-mediated vessel damage and increased neutrophil migration. *Arch Intern Med* 1984;144:738–40.

9 Dicken CH. Bowel-associated dermatosis-arthritis syndrome: bowel bypass syndrome without bowel bypass. *Mayo Clin Proc* 1984;59:43–6.

10 Cox NH, Palmer JG. Bowel-associated dermatitis-arthritis syndrome associated with ileo-anal pouch anastomosis, and treatment with mycophenolate mofetil. *Br J Dermatol* 2003;149:1296–7.

12 Brouard MC, Chavaz P, Borradori L. Acute pustulosis of the legs in diverticulitis with sigmoid stenosis: an overlap between bowel-associated dermatosis-arthritis syndrome and pustular pyoderma gangrenosum. *J Eur Acad Dermatol Venereol* 2004;18:89–92.

14 Prpic-Massari L, Kastelan M, Brajac I, Cabrijan L, Zamolo G, Massari D. Bowel-associated dermatosis-arthritis syndrome in a patient with appendicitis. *Med Sci Monit* 2007;13:CS97–100.

15 Tucker SC, Chalmers RJ, Andrew SM, Odom NJ. Pustular vasculitis secondary to achalasia of the cardia. *Br J Dermatol* 2000;142:373–4.

18 Tu J, Chan JJ, Yu LL. Bowel bypass syndrome/bowel-associated dermatosis arthritis syndrome post laparoscopic gastric bypass surgery. *Australas J Dermatol* 2011;52:e5–7.

Subcorneal pustular dermatosis

8 Lutz ME, Daoud MS, McEvoy MT, Gibson LE. Subcorneal pustular dermatosis: a clinical study of ten patients. *Cutis* 1998;61:203–8.

12 Sneddon IB, Wilkinson DS. Subcorneal pustular dermatosis. *Br J Dermatol* 1956;68:385–94.

13 Sneddon IB, Wilkinson DS. Subcorneal pustular dermatosis. *Br J Dermatol* 1979;100:61–8.

18 Wolff K. Subcorneal pustular dermatosis is not pustular psoriasis. *Am J Dermatopathol* 1981;3:381–2.

20 Sanchez NP, Perry HO, Muller SA. On the relationship between subcorneal pustular dermatosis and pustular psoriasis. *Am J Dermatopathol* 1981;3:385–6.

23 Cheng S, Edmonds E, Ben-Gashir M, Yu RC. Subcorneal pustular dermatosis: 50 years on. *Clin Exp Dermatol* 2008;33:229–33.

26 Orton DI, George SA. Subcorneal pustular dermatosis responsive to narrowband (TL-01) UVB phototherapy. *Br J Dermatol* 1997;137:149–50.

27 Bauwens M, De CA, Roseeuw D. Subcorneal pustular dermatosis treated with PUVA therapy. A case report and review of the literature. *Dermatology* 1999;198:203–5.

37 Voigtlander C, Luftl M, Schuler G, Hertl M. Infliximab (anti-tumor necrosis factor alpha antibody): a novel, highly effective treatment of recalcitrant subcorneal pustular dermatosis (Sneddon-Wilkinson disease). *Arch Dermatol* 2001;137:1571–4.

Other neutrophilic dermatoses and variants

1 Femiano F, Lanza A, Buonaiuto C, Perillo L, Dell'Ermo A, Cirillo N. Pyostomatitis vegetans: a review of the literature. *Med Oral Patol Oral Cir Bucal* 2009;14:E114–17.

2 Hegarty AM, Barrett AW, Scully C. Pyostomatitis vegetans. *Clin Exp Dermatol* 2004;29:1–7.

15 Brinkmeier T, Frosch PJ. Pyodermatitis–pyostomatitis vegetans: a clinical course of two decades with response to cyclosporine and low-dose prednisolone. *Acta Derm Venereol* 2001;81:134–6.

19 Mendez-Flores S, Charli-Joseph Y, Saeb-Lima M, Orozco-Topete R, Fernandez SM. Amicrobial pustulosis of the folds associated with autoimmune disorders: systemic lupus erythematosus case series and first report on the association with autoimmune hepatitis. *Dermatology* 2013;226:1–4.

20 Marzano AV, Ramoni S, Caputo R. Amicrobial pustulosis of the folds. Report of 6 cases and a literature review. *Dermatology* 2008;216:305–11.

26 Amazan E, Ezzedine K, Mossalayi MD, Taieb A, Boniface K, Seneschal J. Expression of interleukin-1 alpha in amicrobial pustulosis of the skin folds with complete response to anakinra. *J Am Acad Dermatol* 2014;71:e53–6.

27 Lagrange S, Chosidow O, Piette JC, Wechsler B, Godeau P, Frances C. A peculiar form of amicrobial pustulosis of the folds associated with systemic lupus erythematosus and other auto-immune diseases. *Lupus* 1997;6:514–20.

29 Marzano AV, Menicanti C, Crosti C, Trevisan V. Neutrophilic dermatoses and inflammatory bowel diseases. *G Ital Dermatol Venereol* 2013;148:185–96.

31 Wallach D, Vignon-Pennamen MD. From acute febrile neutrophilic dermatosis to neutrophilic disease: forty years of clinical research. *J Am Acad Dermatol* 2006;55:1066–71.

33 Andre MF, Aumaitre O, Grateau G et al. Longest form of CCTG microsatellite repeat in the promoter of the CD2BP1/PSTPIP1 gene is associated with aseptic abscesses and with Crohn disease in French patients. *Dig Dis Sci* 2010;55:1681–8.

CHAPTER 50

Immunobullous Diseases

Enno Schmidt[1] *and Richard Groves*[2]

[1]Department of Dermatology and Lübeck Institute of Experimental Dermatology, University of Lübeck, Lübeck, Germany
[2]Clinical Immunodermatology, St John's Institute of Dermatology, Guy's and St Thomas' NHS Foundation Trust, London, UK

PART 4: INFLAMMATORY DERMATOSES

Introduction

The immunobullous disorders represent a group of conditions characterised by antibody-mediated autoimmune responses against structural elements of the skin resulting in blistering of the skin and/or mucosae. Antibody targets include proteins in the hemidesmosomes basement membrane zone and superficial dermis (pemphigoid group), desmosomes (pemphigus group) and epidermal and tissue-type transglutaminase (dermatitis herpetiformis). If left untreated, immunobullous disorders are associated with significant morbidity and mortality and thus prompt, accurate diagnosis and treatment are mandatory. Therapeutic options include corticosteroids, steroid-sparing immunosuppressants such as azathioprine, mycophenolate mofetil and anti-inflammatory agents such as dapsone and tetracyclines. In severe and/or refractory patients, intravenous immunoglobulin, immunoadsorption and anti-B-cell agents such as rituximab may be of benefit. Indeed, recently international and European guidelines have recommended the use of rituximab as first line treatment in moderate and severe pemphigus vulgaris and foliaceous.

Pemphigus

Definition, nomenclature and classification

Pemphigus is a group of chronic autoimmune blistering diseases characterised by the presence of antibodies against desmosomal adhesion proteins.

Classification links (as appropriate)

- ICD-10: L10.0 – L10.5
- Snomed CT: 49420001
- OMIM: 169610
- Orphanet: ORPHA704

Introduction and general description

The term 'pemphigus' derives from the Greek *pemphix* meaning blister or bubble. Several distinct subgroups of pemphigus have emerged and their relevant autoantigens have been characterised. The primary pathogenic antibodies are directed against desmogleins 1 and/or 3, members of the cadherin family of calcium-dependent cell–cell adhesion molecules that contribute to the structure of the desmosome. The two main clinical variants are pemphigus vulgaris (PV) and pemphigus foliaceus (PF) [1]. Characteristic immunopathological features of the various pemphigus disorders are summarised in Table 50.1.

Epidemiology
Incidence and prevalence
The incidence of pemphigus is low but variable worldwide, ranging from 0.5 to 16/million/year (reviewed in [2]). PV is generally the commoner form, although there is some geographical variation in the incidence of the different subtypes; thus, PV is more common in Europe, the USA and India whereas PF is more common in Brazil and Africa. Recent data from the UK suggests that the incidence of PV may be increasing [3], although the reasons behind this are uncertain.

Rook's Textbook of Dermatology, Tenth Edition. Edited by Christopher Griffiths, Jonathan Barker, Tanya Bleiker, Walayat Hussain and Rosalind Simpson.
© 2024 John Wiley & Sons Ltd. Published 2024 by John Wiley & Sons Ltd.

Table 50.1 The intraepidermal immunobullous diseases: immunopathology.

Disease	Direct IMF findings	Indirect IMF substrate	Target antigens	Antigen location
Pemphigus vulgaris and pemphigus vegetans	Intercellular IgG and C3	Mucosa (e.g. primate oesophagus)	Desmoglein 3, desmoglein 1, rarely desmocollins	Desmosome
Pemphigus foliaceus	Intercellular IgG and C3	Normal human skin	Desmoglein 1	Desmosome
IgA pemphigus	Intercellular IgA and C3	Normal human skin	Desmoglein 1, desmoglein 3, sometimes desmocollins	Desmosome
Paraneoplastic pemphigus	Intercellular and subepidermal IgG, C3	Mucosa, normal human skin, transitional epithelia (e.g. rat bladder)	Multiple (desmoglein 1, desmoglein 3, envoplakin, desmoplakin I/II, periplakin, epiplakin, a2 macroglobulin-like 1, BP230)	Desmosome, BMZ; stratified, simple and transitional epithelia

BMZ, basement membrane zone.

Age

Pemphigus can occur at any age but is usually seen between the fourth and sixth decades of life [4], although there is some variability in different countries. In Iran, North India and Pakistan patients with PV have a relatively low age of onset of disease (mean c.40 years of age) [5–7]. In endemic PF in Tunisia, young women tend to be affected [8]. Although pemphigus is rare in childhood it has been reported in children as young as 3 years of age [9]. Children usually develop PV rather than PF [10,11] and the disease may be severe [4].

Sex

Men and women are equally affected, alalthough some studies have suggested a slight female preponderance [7,8,12].

Ethnicity

PV has been reported in all ethnic groups, but is more common in Ashkenazi Jews, Mediterranean, Iranian and Indian populations [13]. Genetic variations are likely to play a major role.

Associated diseases

PV has been associated with many other autoimmune diseases, particularly thyroid disease and rheumatoid arthritis [14,15]. A novel disease cluster of PV, thyroid disease, rheumatoid arthritis and type 1 diabetes has recently been described [16] and there is increasing recognition of a link between pemphigus and neuro-psychiatric disease [17–19]. Paraneoplastic pemphigus occurs in association with haematological malignancy and is described in more detail below.

Pathophysiology

Pemphigus target antigens and the desmoglein compensation hypothesis. The principal target antigens in pemphigus are desmogleins 1 and 3, which are expressed in skin and in mucosal tissue (reviewed in [20]). However, the distribution of the two proteins varies in different epithelia, such that in skin there is high-level expression of desmoglein 1 throughout the epidermis whereas desmoglein 3 is found only in the basal and immediate suprabasal layers. In oral epithelium, desmoglein 3 is expressed throughout all layers whereas desmoglein 1 is only present at a low level. The two desmogleins act cooperatively and consequently antibodies against desmoglein 1 are unable to destabilise oral mucosa whereas they have a marked effect in skin where there is little desmoglein 3 to compensate [21]. In contrast, antibodies against desmoglein 3 lead to severe oral mucosal blistering as there is little desmoglein 1. Consequently, patients with PF, who have anti-desmoglein-1 antibodies alone, exhibit skin blistering without mucosal involvement. In PV, where anti-desmoglein-3 antibodies predominate there is generally marked mucosal blistering.

T cells in pemphigus. While pemphigus is conventionally considered to be a prototypic antibody-mediated disorder, and thus heavily B-lymphocyte dependent, there is increasing evidence that antibody-specific T cells also play a role in pathogenesis [22]. Antibody production generally requires T-cell help and the significant MHC class-II associations of pemphigus imply a T-cell role in the development of pathogenic antibodies. Antigen-specific Th1 and Th2 cells are present in patients with pemphigus and interestingly seem to be modulated by therapy [23]. Very recently, genetically modified T cells have been shown to have utility in highly specific B-cell depletion in patients with pemphigus [24].

Pemphigus antibodies. The predominant class of tissue-bound pemphigus antibody in pemphigus is IgG, which can be demonstrated on direct and indirect immunofluorescence (IF) testing (Figure 50.1). Less commonly IgM, IgA and IgE antibodies are present. There is now considerable evidence confirming the pathogenicity of the IgG fraction of pemphigus sera. Consistent with this, early observations suggested that there was a correlation between intercellular antibody titre and severity of disease [25]. Subsequently, passive transfer experiments with purified IgG autoantibodies derived from pemphigus sera were shown to induce blister development with histological and immunological features typical of pemphigus [26]. *In vitro*, IgG purified from pemphigus patient sera demonstrates a direct effect on dissociation of keratinocyte monolayer cultures [27].

Although there is a large body of evidence that supports the role of desmoglein 1 and 3 as targets for pathogenic antibodies in pemphigus, other antigenic targets have been implicated. Thus, some patients have active pemphigus with intercellular antibodies detectable on direct or indirect IF but have negative desmoglein antibodies as assessed by specific ELISA assays. One explanation for this is that in some patients there may be significant non-desmoglein targets and antibodies against desmocollins, plakoglobin, E-cadherin, collagen XV11/BP180 and acetylcholine receptors have been reported [28]. Indeed, acetylcholine receptor antibodies have been found in up to 85% of pemphigus patients [29]. These antibodies may weaken desmosomal junctions by inducing phosphorylation of adhesion molecules and prevent desmosomal reassembly.

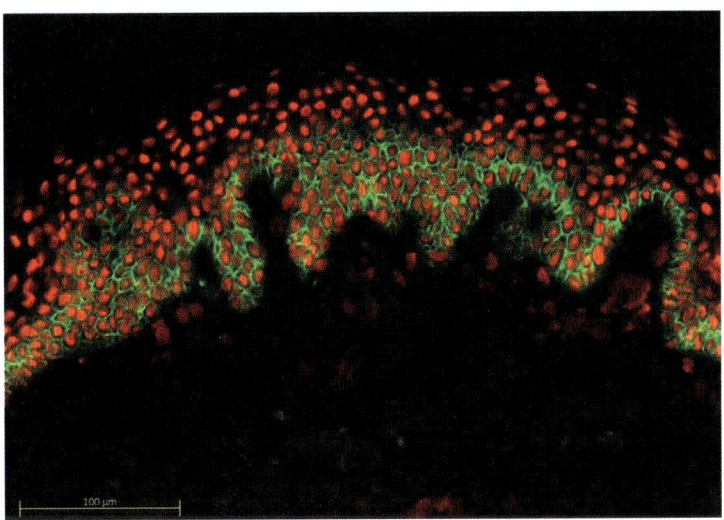

Figure 50.1 Direct immunofluorescence of pemphigus vulgaris. Antibody is deposited around the cell membrane of epidermal keratinocytes.

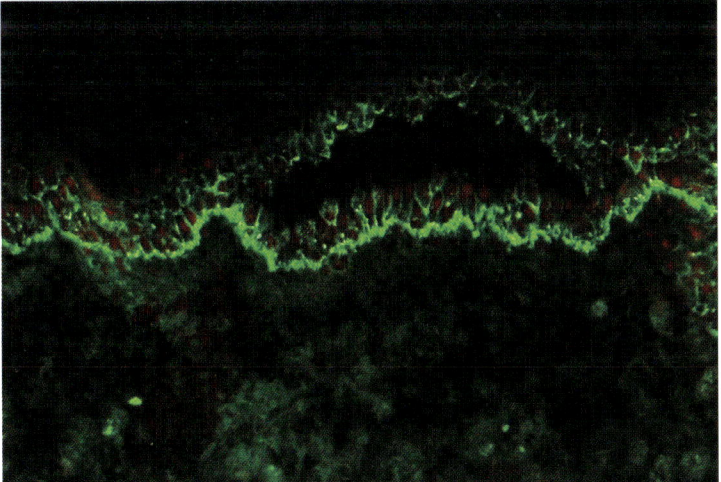

Figure 50.2 Direct immunofluorescence of paraneoplastic pemphigus. Intercellular antibody deposition is seen as in pemphigus vulgaris but in addition there is labelling of the basement membrane zone as a result of the broad-spectrum antibody response.

In paraneoplastic pemphigus (reviewed in [30,31]) there is particularly good evidence that antibodies develop against multiple epidermal antigens in addition to desmogleins 1 and 3. Not only are these antibodies directed against desmosomal proteins such as desmoplakins 1 and 2, envoplakin and periplakin but also constituents of the hemidesmosome including the 230-kD bullous pemphigoid antigen-1. Consequently, direct IF of tissue from paraneoplastic pemphigus patients has features of pemphigus as well as basement membrane labelling (Figure 50.2).

Acantholysis. The key pathological process in PV and PF is separation of keratinocytes from one another, a change known as acantholysis. While acantholysis is not pathognomonic of pemphigus, all subtypes of the disease demonstrate this feature to some degree. A number of mechanisms have been suggested to be involved including steric hindrance by anti-desmoglein antibodies [32], protease activation [33], disruption of intracellular signalling pathways [34,35], and redistribution of desmoglein expression [36]. Some features of apoptosis may also play a role and can be detected in pemphigus skin lesions [37] and is induced by PV-IgG in cultured keratinocytes [38]. Pemphigus antibodies can trigger secretion of factors from keratinocytes which are involved in apoptosis such as Fas ligand. However, evidence of apoptosis is seen late in development of the pemphigus lesions and after acantholysis. More recently a new term 'apoptolysis' has been proposed to explain acantholysis and keratinocyte damage in pemphigus [39]. It is suggested that there are a series of events that follow binding of autoantibodies to pemphigus antigens resulting in epidermal growth factor receptor activation with initiation of cell death cascades, basal cell shrinkage, degradation of structural proteins and apoptosis of acantholytic cells.

The true mechanism for acantholysis is most likely a combination of multiple molecular and structural events and further work is needed to clarify this.

Genetics

The genetic basis of pemphigus is complex [40,41]. Familial cases have been reported but are few [42,43]. The presence of low titres of anti-desmoglein antibodies in healthy relatives of patients with PV has been shown to be as high as 70% in some studies [44,45] suggesting genetic control of the relevant immune response.

The primary genetic association in pemphigus in a number of populations appears to be with class II HLA alleles. Many population studies have shown strong associations between PV and HLA DRB1*04 and *14 alleles and with DQB1*0503 and *0302 [13]. Some class I HLA genes have been implicated in PV including HLA-A10 and HLA-B38 [46,47].

Interestingly, desmoglein 3 polymorphisms have been observed in association with HLA class II pemphigus susceptibility alleles, which may contribute to development of PV [48]. Other non-HLA genes which have been implicated include the immunoglobulin heavy chain [49] and pemphigus-relevant cytokine genes such as interleukin (IL)-10 [50].

Although the MHC clearly has a role in pemphigus susceptibility, this alone cannot explain disease development as: (a) not all pemphigus patients have the disease associated alleles; and (b) healthy relatives of patients may have the relevant HLA allele(s) but do not develop disease. This supports the notion that pemphigus is most likely a multifactorial disease with a polygenic genetic component.

Environmental factors

A role for environmental factors in the pathogenesis of pemphigus is underscored by the recognition of an endemic form of the disease (fogo selvagem, reviewed in [51–54]) in several parts of the world, most notably rural Brazil and Tunisia. The disease is clinically and immunological similar to PF, although it tends to affect children and young adults rather than the older population affected by sporadic PF. The majority of patients live near rivers and black flies (*Simulium* spp.) have been thought to be involved in disease pathogenesis [55]. In endemic areas as many as 50% of normal individuals have anti-desmoglein-1 antibodies.

A number of reports have suggested that smoking may have a protective or beneficial role in pemphigus [56,57]. Human keratinocytes have both nicotinic and muscarinic receptors for acetylcholine [58] and these receptors may play a role in regulating keratinocyte cell–cell adhesion.

Pesticides have also been postulated as possible triggers in disease development and an increased risk of pemphigus has been shown in exposed individuals [59]. Organophosphate pesticides block the acetylcholine breakdown pathway and so may lead to acetylcholine accumulation with resulting loss of cell–cell adhesion in the epidermis [60]. Pesticides implicated in contact pemphigus include glyphosate [61] and dihydrodiphenyltrichlorethane [62].

A link between diet and disease development in pemphigus has been suggested but difficult to substantiate. Although garlic has been proposed as a trigger for disease development [63] – and has been shown to induce acantholysis *in vitro* [64] – this area remains controversial.

Drug-induced pemphigus

Drug-induced pemphigus is rare [65]. Most cases have been in association with drugs containing a thiol group such as penicillamine although non-thiol drugs including angiotensin converting enzyme inhibitors and glibenclamide have also been implicated [66]. An additional group of drugs that may be responsible for induction of pemphigus are those with a phenol group such as cephalosporins, rifampicin, pyritinol, phenobarbital and aspirin; both PV and PF can occur. While immune check point inhibitor therapy has generally been associated with the development of subepidermal immunobullous disease, pemphigus has also been reported [67,68].

Historically, penicillamine has been the most common culprit in drug-induced pemphigus which may occur in 3–10% of patients on the drug, typically after around 1 year of exposure [69]. Penicillamine-induced pemphigus tends to occur in individuals with other autoimmune disorders such as rheumatoid arthritis suggesting that immune dysregulation may be an underlying factor [70], although of course penicillamine tends to be used in patients with underlying immunologically mediated inflammatory disease. Genetic factors may also play a role as an increase in frequency of HLA-B15 has been reported in penicillamine-induced pemphigus [71]. In some patients, simple withdrawal of the drug is insufficient to induce remission, although in others treatment with corticosteroids and immunosuppressive medication may be required.

Clinical features

Pemphigus vulgaris

Nearly all patients have mucosal lesions and PV presents with oral lesions in 50–70% of patients. These may precede cutaneous lesions by months or be the only manifestation of the disease. Intact bullae are rare in the mouth and more commonly patients have ill-defined, irregularly shaped buccal or palatal erosions that are slow to heal (Figure 50.3). The erosions extend peripherally with shedding of the epithelium. Other mucosal surfaces may be involved, including the conjunctiva, nasopharynx, larynx, oesophagus [72], urethra, vulva and cervix [73].

Most patients develop cutaneous lesions. Involvement occasionally remains localised to one site but more commonly becomes widespread. The disease has a predilection for the scalp, face, neck, upper chest and back (Figures 50.4 and 50.5). Flaccid blisters filled with clear fluid either arise on normal skin or a reddish base. The

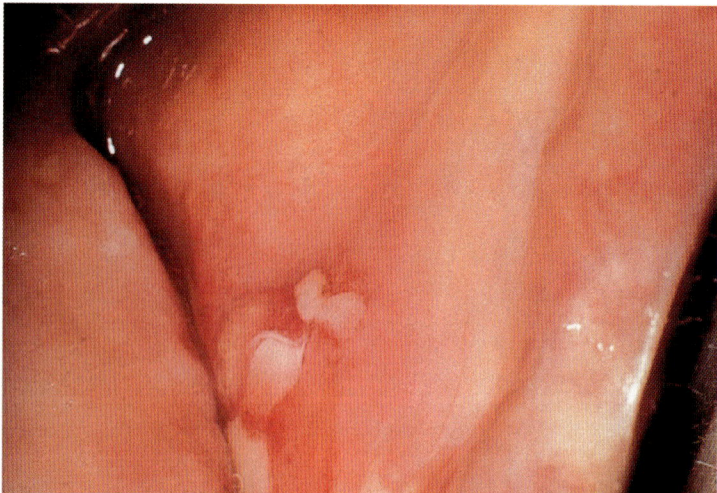

Figure 50.3 Pemphigus vulgaris. Mucosal erosions are an early sign in pemphigus vulgaris, often preceding the cutaneous changes. Courtesy of Dr R.J. Pye, Addenbrooke's Hospital, Cambridge, UK.

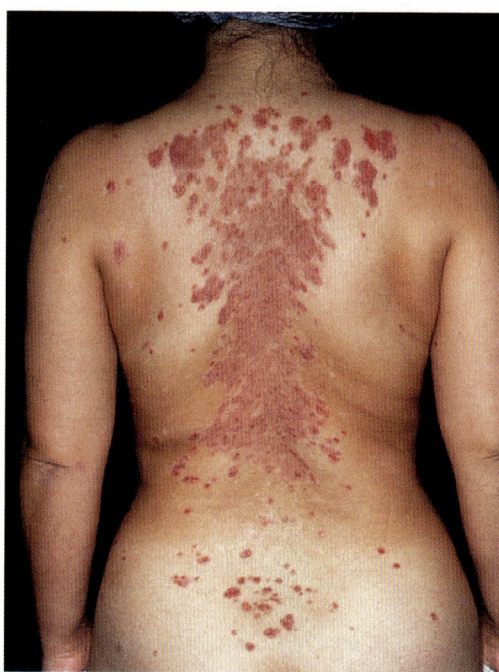

Figure 50.4 Pemphigus vulgaris. Cutaneous lesions typically affect the chest and back in addition to the scalp. Courtesy of Dr R.J. Pye, Addenbrooke's Hospital, Cambridge, UK.

contents may become turbid or the blisters rupture, producing painful erosions that extend at the edges as more epidermis is lost. At this stage, firm sliding pressure with a finger will separate normal-looking epidermis from dermis, producing an erosion – the Nikolsky sign – although this is not specific for pemphigus. Healing occurs without scarring, but pigmentary change may occur in resolving lesions.

Lesions in skin folds may form vegetating granulations (Figure 50.6) and flexural PV merges with its variant pemphigus vegetans. Nail dystrophies, acute paronychia and subungual haematomas have been observed in pemphigus [74,75]. Occasional patients are described with typical PV type lesions confined to the skin

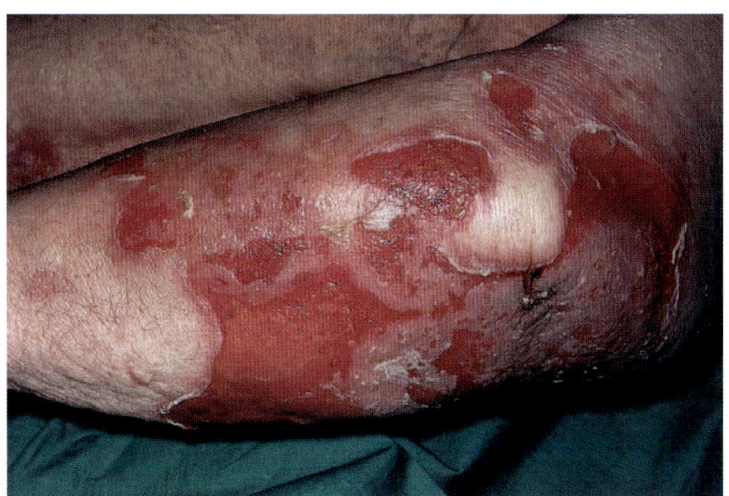

Figure 50.5 Pemphigus vulgaris. Because bullae occur within the epidermis they are fragile and frequently break down to leave widespread erosions. Courtesy of Dr R.J. Pye, Addenbrooke's Hospital, Cambridge, UK.

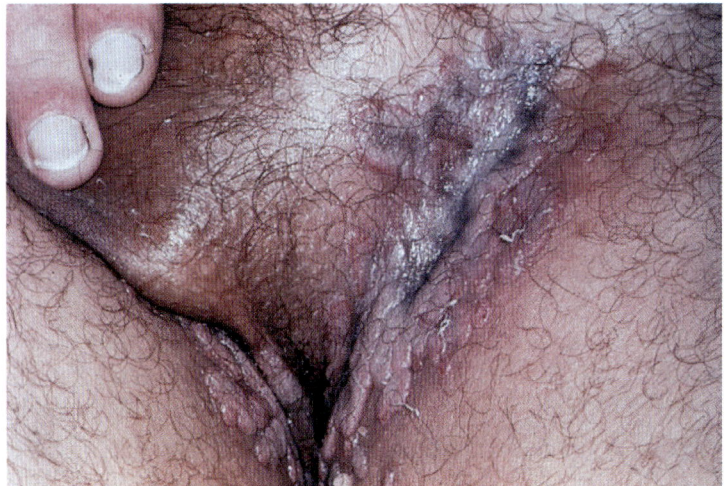

Figure 50.6 Pemphigus vegetans. Vegetating lesions typically occur in the flexures, often without evident blistering. Courtesy of Dr R.J. Pye, Addenbrooke's Hospital, Cambridge, UK.

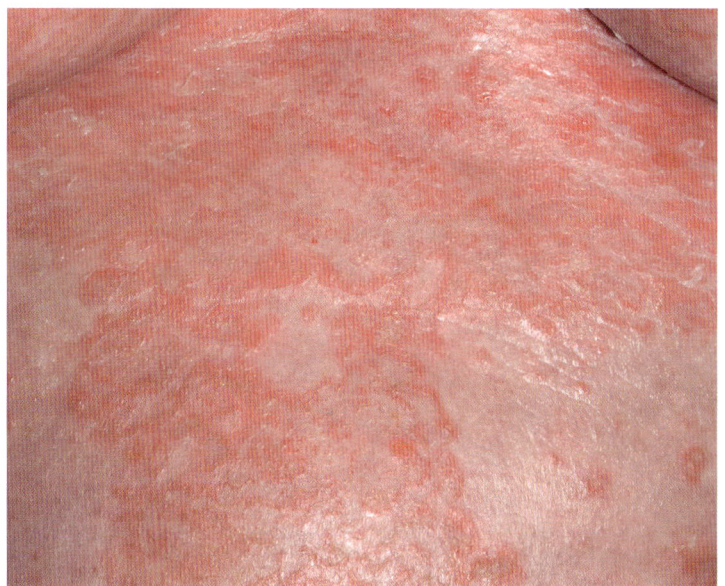

Figure 50.7 Pemphigus foliaceus. There are superficial erosions, frequently without obvious bullae.

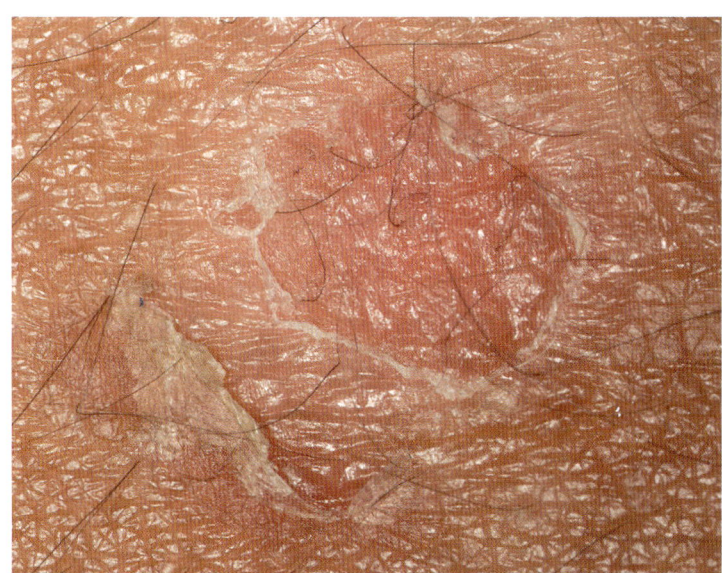

Figure 50.8 Pemphigus foliaceus. Lesions frequently have a fine superficial scale, sometimes as a collarette.

and sparing the mucosae despite the presence of antibodies to desmoglein-3 [76,77]. Additionally, some patients will undergo phenotypic and immunological conversion from PV to PF or vice versa over the course of their disease [78–80].

Pemphigus may deteriorate in pregnancy and the puerperium, and close observation is required at this time. In some patients, initial presentation is in pregnancy. Severe pemphigus in pregnancy may be associated with fetal prematurity and death, but it is difficult to separate the effects of treatment from those of the disease [81,82]. Generally, the baby is healthy although neonatal pemphigus may occur (as IgG crosses the placenta) with mucosal or mucocutaneous lesions which are generally short-lived [81].

Pemphigus foliaceus

PF is often regarded as less severe than PV, although it can be as challenging to manage. The onset is usually insidious with scattered, scaly lesions involving the 'seborrhoeic' areas of the scalp, face, chest and upper back (Figure 50.7). Individual lesions typically have a fine collarette of scale (Figure 50.8). Localised disease slowly extends. Blistering may not be obvious because the cleavage is superficial and the small flaccid blisters rupture easily. Scales separate leaving well-demarcated, crusted erosions surrounded by erythema, sometimes with small vesicles along the borders. In severe cases the patient may become erythrodermic with crusted, oozing red skin (Figure 50.9).

Although the antibodies in PF can cross the placenta, the neonate is not usually affected. In two cases in which the neonate did develop PF, both mother and neonate had very high antibody titres.

Clinical variants

Pemphigus vegetans. Pemphigus vegetans is a rare variant of PV characterised by vegetating erosions, primarily in flexures [83].

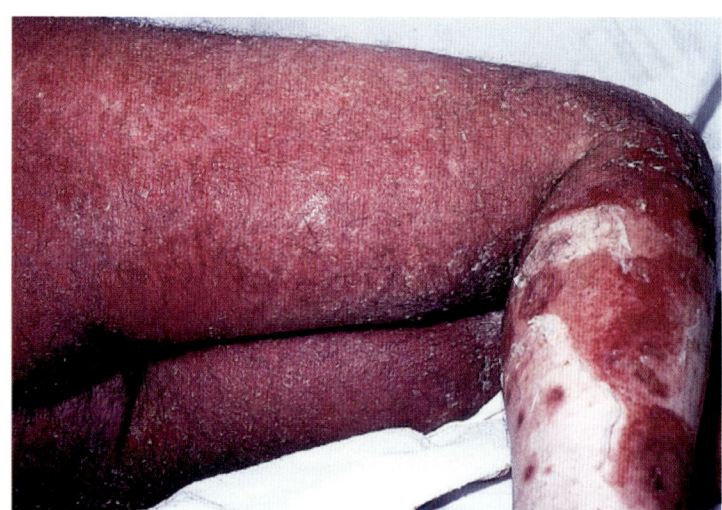

Figure 50.9 Pemphigus foliaceus. Occasionally pemphigus foliaceus becomes widespread and can result in erythroderma.

Two subtypes are recognised that represent a clinical spectrum from the severe Neumann type to the milder Hallopeau type [84]. Patients have circulating IgG antibodies against desmoglein-3, as in PV. In some cases antibodies in patients with pemphigus vegetans react with desmocollin molecules [85,86]. The mechanism by which antibody deposition leads to the vegetating change remains unclear.

The vegetating lesions are hyperkeratotic, papillomatous and acanthotic. Some suprabasal clefts may contain eosinophils but few acantholytic cells are present. Intraepidermal eosinophilic abscesses may be present in older lesions. Early lesions in the Neumann type show suprabasal acantholysis and intraepidermal vesicles without eosinophils. Eosinophilic spongiosis or eosinophilic microabscesses are common in the early pustular lesions of the Hallopeau type. The dermis contains a heavy infiltrate of lymphocytes and eosinophils with few neutrophils.

The disease chiefly affects middle-aged adults. Involvement of the oral mucosa is almost invariable, often with cerebriform changes on the tongue. Elsewhere, lesions are primarily flexural, although vegetations may occur at any site. In the Neumann type, vesicles and bullae rupture to form hypertrophic granulating erosions, which bleed easily. The lesions evolve into vegetating masses exuding serum and pus. The edges are studded with small pustules. Erosions at the edge of the lesions induce new vegetations, which eventually become dry, hyperkeratotic and fissured. In the Hallopeau type, pustules rather than vesicles characterise early lesions but these soon progress to vegetating plaques.

Pemphigus herpetiformis. This is a rare and atypical variant of pemphigus that clinically resembles dermatitis herpetiformis [87,88]. Widespread clusters of pruritic papules and vesicles develop on a reddish background. Biopsies show subcorneal pustules, eosinophilic spongiosis or features of dermatitis herpetiformis often without acantholysis but IF studies reveal intercellular staining. Patients possess circulating IgG autoantibodies which recognise either desmoglein-1 or desmoglein-3 and some patients sera recognise desmocollins 1 or 3 [89,90]. The condition may evolve into classical PF but has also been described preceding PV [91]. In general, the clinical course is benign.

Pemphigus erythematosus. Pemphigus erythematosus is a localised variant of PF, originally described by Senear and Usher [92]. Patients have immunological features of both lupus erythematosus and pemphigus, with granular IgG and C3 at the basement membrane zone, intercellular IgG and C3 in the epidermis and circulating antinuclear antibodies. The antibodies recognise desmogleins together with Ro, La and double-stranded DNA antigens [93]. Progression to systemic lupus erythematosus is rare. Pemphigus erythematosus may be associated with myasthenia gravis or thymoma [94].

Reddish, scaly lesions over the nose and cheeks in a butterfly distribution simulate cutaneous lupus erythematosus or seborrhoeic dermatitis. Sunlight may exacerbate the disease. Lesions on the trunk, either localised or generalised, are similar to those in PF.

Paraneoplastic pemphigus/paraneoplastic autoimmune multi-organ syndrome (PAMS). Paraneoplastic pemphigus has been reported in association with a variety of neoplasms, almost exclusively of haematological origin [30]. The commonest association is with non-Hodgkin lymphoma but chronic lymphocytic leukaemia, Castleman disease, thymoma and Waldenström macroglobulinaemia have all been associated. Immunofluorescence changes are characteristic, with features of both pemphigus and pemphigoid reflecting the broad spectrum of circulating anti-epithelial antibodies [95], characteristically including antiplakin antibodies detected in serum using transitional epithelium as a substrate [96]. The early histopathology is frequently lichenoid [97].

Paraneoplastic pemphigus is characterised clinically by severe stomatitis, conjunctivitis, which may be scarring and oesophageal, genital mucosal and flexural involvement together with bullous and erosive lesions elsewhere [98]. The respiratory tract may be severely affected in some patients. Because of this multiorgan involvement, the term paraneoplastic autoimmune multiorgan syndrome has been proposed [31,99]. Cutaneous lesions may be variable with erosions or blistering as in PV, although tense pemphigoid-like blisters may occur as well as erythema multiforme or lichenoid changes.

IgA pemphigus. Two histological forms of IgA pemphigus have been described; an intraepidermal neutrophilic type and a subcorneal pustular dermatosis type, both of which may be clinically indistinguishable from subcorneal pustular dermatosis (Sneddon-Wilkinson disease) [100]. Both are characterised by the deposition of IgA (in some also with IgG) within the epidermis and, in some patients, by detectable circulating antiepidermal IgA antibodies. In the subcorneal pustular dermatosis type, antibodies appear to be directed against desmocollin-1 [101], although the target in the intraepidermal neutrophilic type is uncertain. Some patients seem to have IgA anti-desmoglein 1 or 3 antibodies also [102,103].

The disease chiefly affects adults [104], although childhood cases have been reported [105]. Patients with both histopathological types have flaccid vesicles or pustules arising on either red or normal skin. The lesions may be intensely pruritic and show a circinate or annular configuration with central clearing, evolving to crusted or scaly red macules. The sites of predilection are the axillae and groin although the trunk, face, scalp and proximal limbs may be affected. While some patients are indistinguishable from Sneddon–Wilkinson disease, others may resemble PF or pemphigus herpetiformis. Flexural, oozing, verrucous plaques mimicking pemphigus vegetans have been described in a child [106]. Mucosal involvement is unusual. Most run a chronic, indolent course.

The most frequently reported association is with monoclonal IgA gammopathy in the subcorneal type, a feature it has in common with classical subcorneal pustular dermatosis. Other cases have been linked with HIV infection [107], inflammatory bowel disease [108], rheumatoid arthritis and thiol drugs [109].

Differential diagnosis

PV. Patients with mucosal lesions are likely to present to dental surgeons, oral surgeons or gynaecologists. Erosions may simulate acute herpetic stomatitis, erythema multiforme, aphthous ulcers, lichen planus or mucous membrane pemphigoid. Bullae are transient in the mouth and biopsies of erosions may not be diagnostic. The diagnosis is less difficult when the patients have cutaneous blisters or erosions, although pemphigoid and its variants, linear IgA disease and erythema multiforme, may need to be ruled out. Blisters in pemphigoid are typically more tense than in pemphigus and may be haemorrhagic. Vegetating, pustular lesions in flexures must be differentiated from chronic infections or Hailey–Hailey disease (benign familial pemphigus). Vegetating plaques mimicking pemphigus vegetans may occur in IgA pemphigus and paraneoplastic pemphigus and the hyperkeratotic lesions of chronic pemphigus vegetans may simulate cutaneous tumours. The histological differential diagnosis of PV includes Darier disease, Hailey–Hailey disease (benign familial pemphigus) and transient acantholytic dermatosis (Grover disease). These conditions have distinctive clinical features in addition to negative IF studies. Eosinophilic spongiosis may be an early histological manifestation of either pemphigus or bullous pemphigoid. Immunofluorescence studies are required to confirm the diagnosis.

PF. This may resemble seborrhoeic dermatitis or impetigo, but the histological and immunopathological features are diagnostic. Pemphigus erythematosus needs to be distinguished from both seborrhoeic dermatitis and chronic cutaneous lupus erythematosus. PF may occasionally simulate dermatitis herpetiformis both clinically and histologically, but immunopathological studies differentiate the two. Histological features may not be diagnostic in the early stages. Eosinophilic spongiosis may be an early manifestation. Immunofluorescence studies should always be performed if pemphigus is suspected.

Paraneoplastic pemphigus: in most patients the diagnosis (and treatment) of the underlying malignancy precedes the development of pemphigus, but this is not universally the case. The clinical differential diagnosis will include PV, erythema multiforme, graft versus host disease, lichen planus and viral infections including herpes simplex.

Classification of severity

A number of severity indices (reviewed in [110]) including the pemphigus disease area index (PDAI [111]) and the autoimmune bullous skin disorder intensity score (ABSIS [112]) have been proposed in order to standardise assessment of patients with autoimmune blistering disorders, the most frequently used being PDAI [113,114]. At the time of writing, an investigator global assessment (IGA) score is being developed for PV and PF to fulfil the FDA requirements in clinical trials.

Disease course and prognosis

Pemphigus in its various forms typically has a chronic course with an average disease duration of 10 years [115]. However, there is great variability in disease length in patients. Various factors have been suggested to influence this including the site and severity of initial disease, with oral involvement an adverse prognostic factor [116–118]. Immunologically, the presence of both anti-desmoglein 1 and 3 antibodies tends to associate with more active disease [119]. Recent data suggest that early age of onset and Asian ancestry associate with more prolonged disease activity [120]. While pemphigus was associated with a high mortality in the era before systemic steroids this has improved hugely, although there is still an excess mortality in treated patients related to the effects of immunosuppression and associated disorders (reviewed in [2]).

Investigations
Histopathology

The earliest histological changes consist of intercellular oedema with loss of intercellular attachments in the basal layer. Suprabasal epidermal cells separate from the basal cells to form clefts and blisters. Basal cells remain attached to the basement membrane but separate from one another and stand like a 'row of tombstones' on the floor of the blister. Blister cavities contain rounded-up acantholytic cells, which can be found in smears taken from the base of a blister or an oral erosion (Tzank preparation). Clefting may extend into the walls of adnexae. Blistering is preceded by eosinophilic spongiosis in some cases. The superficial dermis has a mild, superficial, mixed inflammatory infiltrate that may include eosinophils.

Direct immunofluorescence microscopy

Direct IF is the most accurate way to diagnose mucosal pemphigus [121,122]. Specimens may be transported to a suitable laboratory in Michel's medium if facilities for snap-freezing and storage of the tissues are not available locally [123].

The diagnosis of pemphigus is confirmed by direct IF which shows IgG and often C3 deposited on the surface of keratinocytes throughout the epidermis in perilesional skin (Figure 50.2). IgG1 and IgG4 are the most common subclasses; IgM and IgA are present less frequently than IgG.

Serological assays

Circulating pemphigus autoantibodies are detected by indirect IF in over 80% of patients. The use of more than one substrate improves sensitivity, oesophageal mucosal substrates being preferable for the detection of antibodies to desmoglein-3 [124] whereas normal human skin shows higher sensitivity for the detection of antibodies against desmoglein-1. Rat bladder, which is a transitional epithelium devoid of desmoglein proteins, has proven a useful indirect IF substrate in the diagnosis of paraneoplastic pemphigus [125].

Recombinant desmogleins (Dsg1 and Dsg3) have been used to develop sensitive and specific ELISA assays for the serological diagnosis of pemphigus [126]. Using ELISA over 95% of PV patients have detectable desmoglein-3 antibodies and around 50% have desmoglein-1 antibodies. In appropriate dilutions, anti-desmoglein ELISA assays can be used to monitor disease activity [127,128]. Pemphigus-like circulating intercellular antibodies have been reported in conditions such as thermal burns [129], toxic epidermal necrolysis [130] and in first-degree relatives of pemphigus patients [131,132].

Management

General principles of management

Because of the rarity of the pemphigus group of diseases, progress with informative randomised, controlled trials has been slow. However, systemic corticosteroid therapy remains the mainstay of therapy, generally in combination with a steroid-sparing immunosuppressant. Treatment has been the subject of a number of reviews [1,133–135].

Topical therapy

Patients who present with oral disease and mild cutaneous involvement may remain in this localised phase for months. Potent topical or intralesional steroids may reduce the requirement for oral steroids. Good oral hygiene, including treatment of periodontal disease, is important.

In patients with widespread blistering, intensive nursing care is mandatory. Opportunist infection is the major cause of death in patients with widespread blistering who are also immunosuppressed, and potassium permanganate and topical antiseptics may help reduce the risk of cutaneous infection. Liberal use of emollients will reduce frictional stress on affected skin.

Corticosteroids

Prednisolone, together with a steroid-sparing adjuvant, is the initial treatment for most patients with PV. Prednisolone 0.5–1 mg/kg/day in combination with adjuvant immunosuppression and appropriate topical therapy is sufficient to initiate disease control in many patients [136]. There seems to be little benefit in using higher doses [137]. Once control is established the steroid dose should be titrated according to clinical response.

Patients with generalised disease may require aggressive immunosuppression to suppress blistering and a major difficulty in managing these patients is achieving a balance between the risks associated with high-dose steroid therapy and those of poorly controlled disease. In this situation intravenous (IV) pulses of either 1 g methylprednisolone or 100 mg dexamethasone are safer alternatives, often together with intravenous immunoglobulin (IVIG), immunoadsorption or plasmapheresis. While steroid pulses have been shown to be useful in some studies [138], in others they did not show benefit [139,140].

Azathioprine

Azathioprine has been widely used in the management of pemphigus at a dose of 2–3 mg/kg/day and multiple case series support its use. The combination of prednisolone and azathioprine is more effective than prednisolone alone both in terms of mortality and remission [141]. One randomised, controlled trial of pemphigus treatment found azathioprine to be the most effective steroid-sparing agent, followed by cyclophosphamide (pulse

therapy) and mycophenolate mofetil [136]. Another trial found azathioprine and mycophenolate mofetil to be equally effective [142]. Potential adverse effects of azathioprine include bone marrow suppression, nausea and liver dysfunction and careful blood monitoring is therefore mandatory, particularly in the early stages of treatment. Azathioprine toxicity is more frequent in patients with low levels of activity of the enzyme thiopurine methyl transferase (TPMT) and activity of the enzyme should be checked prior to treatment wherever possible [143]. In patients with low levels of TPMT, azathioprine dose should be adjusted accordingly and avoided in patients who have absent TPMT.

Mycophenolate mofetil

Mycophenolate mofetil (1–3 g/day) has been found helpful as a steroid-sparing agent [142,144,145] in pemphigus. Mycophenolate mofetil is a pro-drug of mycophenolic acid and has a relatively selective effect on T and B lymphocytes through its effect on inhibition of inosine monophosphate dehydrogenase. A double-blind randomised controlled study comparing azathioprine and mycophenolate showed no significant difference in efficacy between the two drugs although there was a trend towards fewer adverse effects and more rapid remission in the mycophenolate group [142]. Adverse effects of mycophenolate include bone marrow suppression and gastrointestinal symptoms and, as with azathioprine, patients require close monitoring in the early stages of treatment. Gastrointestinal symptoms may respond to the use of enteric-coated delayed release mycophenolic acid in place of mycophenolate mofetil.

Cyclophosphamide

Cyclophosphamide is a potent anti-B-cell agent with significant activity in pemphigus and other antibody-mediated autoimmune diseases [146,147]. Its use is limited by its significant adverse effects, including gonadal failure, haemorrhagic cystitis, bone marrow suppression and an increased risk of bladder cancer. It is consequently generally reserved for the rare patients who have failed to respond to rituximab and conventional immunosuppression with azathioprine or mycophenolate mofetil. Monthly IV pulses of cyclophosphamide with dexamethasone combined with low-dose oral cyclophosphamide have been used, as has daily oral treatment [148].

IVIG

IVIG is a potentially attractive treatment option because of its relative lack of immunosuppressive effects in comparison with most other pemphigus treatments. It is generally used at a dose of 2 g/kg split over 3–5 days and treatment may need to be continued monthly for prolonged periods [149]. Its mechanisms of action have not been fully elucidated yet. One of its main effects is the blockage of the neonatal Fc receptor (FcR) preventing the recycling of IgG from the endothelium to the circulation. In addition, IVIG may have anti-idiotypic effects [150]. A multicentre double-blind controlled study in Japan has confirmed its effectiveness [151]. While IVIG is generally well tolerated it can cause headaches, 'flu-like' symptoms and hypotension. Anaphylaxis may occur in patients with complete IgA deficiency, which should be excluded prior to treatment.

Rituximab

Depletion of B lymphocytes using the anti-CD20 monoclonal antibody rituximab has been shown to be effective in the management of pemphigus in several case series. Initial regimens used $375\,mg/m^2$ weekly for 4 weeks but two infusions of $1\,g$, 2 weeks apart have now become established [152–154]. The mechanism of action of rituximab is likely through B-cell regulatory pathways as plasma cells, which are responsible for antibody production, do not express the CD20 molecule. Interestingly, T-cell responses to desmogleins are suppressed following rituximab therapy suggesting a broader mechanism of action than simply on the B-cell pathway [23]. Onset of action of rituximab is typically 8–16 weeks following the first infusion, although it may take longer and improvement may persist for 12–18 months. Rituximab may be combined with conventional steroid therapy and adjuvant immunosuppression, although care needs to be taken to avoid excessive immunosuppression and increased infection risk. In some centres immunoadsorption has been combined with rituximab [155].

The place of rituximab in the hierarchy of pemphigus treatment is evolving and its first line use has been explored. In one recent study, first line use of rituximab was compared against standard corticosteroid therapy. Complete remission off treatment was seen in 89% of patients in the rituximab group, compared with 34% in the corticosteroid group. In addition, in the rituximab arm, the cumulative prednisone dose and the number of severe adverse events were significantly lower compared with the prednisone alone arm [156]. In another study comparing the effect of rituximab and mycophenolate, sustained complete remission was observed in significantly more patients in the rituximab arm compared with the mycophenolate mofetil arm [157]. Based on the available data a large international panel of experts and the S2 guidelines of the European Academy of Venereology and Dermatology (EADV) have recommended the use of rituximab as first line treatment in moderate and severe PV and PF [158,159].

In general, rituximab is well tolerated. Infusion reactions may occur but seem less frequent than when the drug is used in the treatment of B-cell malignancies. Infection has been reported [160], and particular care needs to be taken to avoid reactivation of viral hepatitis – patients should be rigorously screened prior to treatment [161]. Late onset neutropenia is recognised but uncommon [162].

Immunoadsorption and plasmapheresis

Removal of circulating antibodies by plasmapheresis was first used in 1978 [163] and is theoretically an attractive way of managing pemphigus in the acute stage, although other studies have not shown benefit [164]. More recently, selective immunoadsorption of IgG using columns containing protein A or other immunoglobulin binders [165–167] has been effective at inducing remission in pemphigus patients, but concomitant immunosuppression with steroids, steroid sparing adjuvants or anti-B-cell therapy is required to prevent rebound increase in the synthesis of antibody [168,169].

Other therapies

Although initial case reports were suggestive of the benefit of ciclosporin in pemphigus [170,171], more recent studies cast doubt on this [172]. Topical ciclosporin mouthwash may be helpful in severe oral pemphigus [173].

Gold may have a modest effect in pemphigus [174,175], although toxic effects limit its utility. Dapsone has been advocated as an adjunct in some patients with mild disease [176] and a recent prospective, placebo-controlled study showed a modest steroid-sparing effect [177]. Dapsone may be of particular utility in pemphigus herpetiformis and in IgA pemphigus [104]. Acetretin has been used in conjunction with prednisolone in pemphigus vegetans [178].

Methotrexate is now seldom used, although there is some suggestion that it may have a steroid-sparing effect and moderate doses of methotrexate may permit withdrawal of prednisolone in steroid-dependent patients [179,180].

Other therapies that have been used in resistant cases of pemphigus include extracorporeal photopheresis [181,182] and the tumour necrosis factor (TNF) inhibitors infliximab [183] and adalimumab [184] have also been reported as beneficial, although autoimmune bullous disease has been reported as a consequence of TNF blockade [185]. Tetracycline antibiotics with or without nicotinamide may be helpful as steroid-sparing agents in some patients [186,187].

Many novel therapies are currently under investigation, including repurposing existing drugs such as veltuzumab and ofatumumab with higher binding affinities to CD20, novel anti-B cell agents [188] and cell-based therapies designed to eliminate pathogenic B-cell clones [189].

SUBEPIDERMAL IMMUNOBULLOUS DISEASES

Introduction

These bullous disorders include pemphigoid diseases and dermatitis herpetiformis. Pemphigoid diseases are characterised by autoantibodies against structural proteins of the dermal–epidermal junction (DEJ), while in dermatitis herpetiformis, the autoantigen is epidermal transglutaminase (TG, TG3) with most sera also reacting against TG2 (tissue-type TG) [1,2–5]. Via proteins of the DEJ, the cytoskeleton of the basal keratinocytes is linked to the extracellular matrix of the dermis (Chapter 2). Binding of pemphigoid autoantibodies to their target antigens leads to the separation of epidermis and dermis. In bullous pemphigoid (BP), mucous membrane pemphigoid, and the inflammatory variant of epidermolysis bullosa acquisita (EBA), considerable progress has been made to understand this complex process.

Subepidermal bullous diseases share some clinical characteristics, such as tense blisters and erosions and, in contrast to pemphigus, a negative Nikolsky sign, i.e. friction of non-lesional skin does not lead to intraepidermal disruption and visible erosion. These disorders are, however, heterogeneous with regard to the clinical presentation, target antigen(s), autoantibody isotype, and immunopathology. Importantly, prognosis and treatment may vary considerably, and therefore require exact diagnosis.

The target antigen(s) have been identified on the molecular level in most of the distinct entities, among them BP, by far the most common pemphigoid disorder, mucous membrane pemphigoid, linear IgA disease, pemphigoid gestationis, anti-p200 pemphigoid, EBA, bullous systemic lupus erythematosus, lichen

PART 4: INFLAMMATORY DERMATOSES

Table 50.2 Pemphigoid diseases. Autoantibody specificities and diagnostically relevant clinical signs.

Disease	Autoantibody	Clinical signs of diagnostic relevance
Bullous pemphigoid (BP)	*BP180*[a] *NC16A*, *BP230*	Tense blisters, erosions[b], urticarial plaques, intense pruritus, old age (>75 years); no predominant mucosal involvement
Mucous membrane pemphigoid	*BP180*[a], *laminin 332*, *BP230*, α6β4 integrin[c]	Predominant mucosal involvement; oral and ocular mucosae are most frequently affected
Linear IgA disease (LAD)	*LAD-1*[d], BP230 (IgA reactivity)	Tense blisters, erosions; no predominant mucosal involvement
Pemphigoid gestationis	*BP180*[a] *NC16A*, *BP230*	Red macules, papules, rarely vesicles, intense pruritus; pregnancy or post-partum period
Anti-p200 pemphigoid	*Laminin β4* *Laminin γ1*	Tense blisters, erosions; <75 years of age; no predominant mucosal involvement
Epidermolysis bullosa acquisita	*Type VII collagen*	Mechanobullous (like epidermolysis bullosa) and inflammatory variant (like BP or LAD)
Bullous systemic lupus erythematosus (SLE)	Type I: *type VII collagen*[b] Type II: BP180[a], BP230, *laminin 332*	SLE present; tense blisters, erosions; no predominant mucosal involvement; excellent response to dapsone
Lichen planus pemphigoides	*BP180*[a] *NC16A*, *BP230*	Tense blisters independent of lichen planus lesions
Cicatricial pemphigoid	BP180[a], *BP230*, *laminin 332*	Blisters and erosions that heal with scarring and/or milia formation. No predominant mucosal involvement

Main target antigens are indicated in bold. For target antigens in italics, commercial detection systems are available. Modified from [1].
[a] Also termed type XVII collagen.
[b] In about 20% of patients, blisters and erosions are absent and eczematous lesions, red macules and urticarial plaques are seen.
[c] Reactivity against α6β4 integrin needs further confirmation.
[d] The soluble ectodomain of BP180.

planus pemphigoides and cicatricial pemphigoid (Table 50.2). Pemphigoid gestationis is detailed in Chapter 113. In addition, small numbers of patients with a pemphigoid disease characterised by renal insufficiency and autoantibodies against the α5 chain of type IV collagen or with autoantibodies against different not fully characterised antigens, among them 105 kDa, 168 kDa and 285 kDa proteins, have been reported [6–10]. New target antigens are still being described and it seems likely that many more yet only poorly characterised or undiscovered molecules within the DEJ may function as autoantigens in subepidermal blistering diseases.

Bullous pemphigoid

Definition, nomenclature and classification
BP is not only the most common disorder within the group of subepidermal immunobullous disorders but also represents the most frequent autoimmune blistering disease in general. BP mainly affects elderly people although younger patients may also be affected, and often starts with pruritus and urticated and reddish lesions. Later, tense blisters are characteristic both on reddish and on normal skin. Mucosal involvement only develops in a minority of patients and is not predominant. Histopathology of a lesional biopsy reveals subepidermal splitting. Autoantibodies, chiefly IgG, recognise two proteins of the DEJ, BP180 (type XVII collagen) in almost all patients and, in about half of them, BP230. The typical clinical features and immunopathology of BP are summarised in Table 50.2.

Classification links
• ICD-10: L12.0

Introduction and general description
BP was first differentiated from pemphigus in 1953 by Walter Lever who described intraepidermal split formation and loss of cell adherence between keratinocytes (acantholysis) as the histopathological hallmark of pemphigus, whereas he coined the term 'pemphigoid' for conditions in which a subepidermal split formation was present [11]. A decade later, Jordon *et al.* demonstrated that in BP, tissue-bound and serum autoantibodies against proteins of the DEJ were present [12]. Further milestones in the understanding of BP included the immunochemical characterisation of the hemidesmosomal target proteins BP180 (type XVII collagen, also termed BPAG2) and BP230 (BPAG1-e), the cloning of their genes, and the demonstration that autoantibodies against BP180 are pathogenic [13–17].

Epidemiology
Incidence and prevalence
The reported incidence of BP ranges between 2.5 and 76 new cases/million/year depending on the studied population. The lowest incidences have been reported from Romania (2.5/million/year) [18], Kuwait (2.6/million/year) [19], Poland (4.5/million/year) [20] and Singapore (7.6/million/year) [21]. In Scotland, Italy and Switzerland, the incidences range from 10.0 to 14.0/million/year [22,23], whereas higher incidences of 20 to 24 new cases/million/year have been recently estimated in Germany, France, Guadeloupe and the USA (Olmsted County, Minnesota) [24–27]. An even higher incidence of 66 and 76/million/year was reported in the UK and of 71/million/year in Sweden based on data registries [28,29,30]. Interestingly, in Germany, France, the USA (Olmsted County, Minnesota) and the UK, the incidence of BP appears to have increased considerably within the last 20 years (between 0.2-fold and 4.8-fold) [24,26–28,29,31–33]. This may be due to: (i) the increasing age of the general population, (ii) the increased prevalence of debilitating neurological disorders (shown to be major risk factors for BP [34]), (iii) the increasing use of diuretics, psycholeptics and dipeptidyl peptidase 4 inhibitors (DPP4-inhibitors) that were associated with BP [35], (iv) improved diagnostic assays, and (v) increased awareness of prodromal and non-bullous forms of BP.

The prevalence of BP has been calculated to be 26/100 000 in 2014 and 48/100 000 people in 2017 in Germany and England, respectively [29,36].

Age

BP is predominantly a disease of the elderly with a mean age at disease onset between 69 and 83 years [24,37–41]. A somehow lower mean age of 64 years at disease onset was reported from China [42]. The incidence significantly rises with age to 190–312/million/year in individuals older than 80 years of age [22,23,28,31]. With the changing age structure of many populations worldwide even more people are expected to suffer from BP in the coming decades. In individuals younger than 50 years, BP rarely occurs (incidence of <0.5/million/year) [23,28,31,43]. Only about 80 cases of BP in children and adolescents have been described and the prevalence of BP in minors was estimated to be 5/million persons below the age of 18 years [44–47]. In contrast, a retrospective study from Israel has indicated that BP in the first year of life occurs with an estimated incidence rate of 23.6/million infants under the age of 1 year/year [48].

Sex

A slight female predominance (52–60% of BP patients) was observed [24,28,39,40]. After age adjustment the incidence was, however, higher in men [24,43] due to the generally higher life expectancy of women and the increasing incidence of BP with age.

Ethnicity

The incidence varies considerably between different countries (see earlier). In England, the incidence was highest in patients of Asian ethnicity [29]. Most likely, both genetic and environmental factors may contribute to the wide range of incidence. In addition, different diagnostic standards and health care systems may influence reported incidence. In New York, USA, the only difference seen between white patients and those with skin of colour was the significantly lower age in the latter [49].

Associated diseases

Neurological and psychiatric disorders including cognitive impairment, Parkinson disease, stroke, epilepsy, multiple sclerosis, and uni- and bipolar disorders have been associated with BP [34,37,38,41,50–54]. In fact, between a third and half of all BP patients suffer from neurological diseases (odds ratios 2.4–10.6) [37,41,50,53,51] considerably increasing disease burden in this elderly patient population. These findings are intriguing since both target antigens, BP180 and BP230, are expressed in the central nervous system [55,56] and mice with mutations in the dystonin gene encoding for various isoforms of BPAG1 including the epithelial isoform BP230 develop severe dystonia and sensory nerve degeneration [57]. Three studies based on patient registries in Germany, England and Taiwan, including more than 11 000 BP patients, identified a clear association with haematological malignancies including various lymphomas and leukaemias [58,59,60]. Furthermore, significant associations with cardiovascular disease (mainly hypertension), other autoimmune diseases (in particular dermatitis herpetiformis and coeliac disease), ulcerative colitis, diabetes mellitus, allergic asthma and psoriasis have been reported in different populations [60–66].

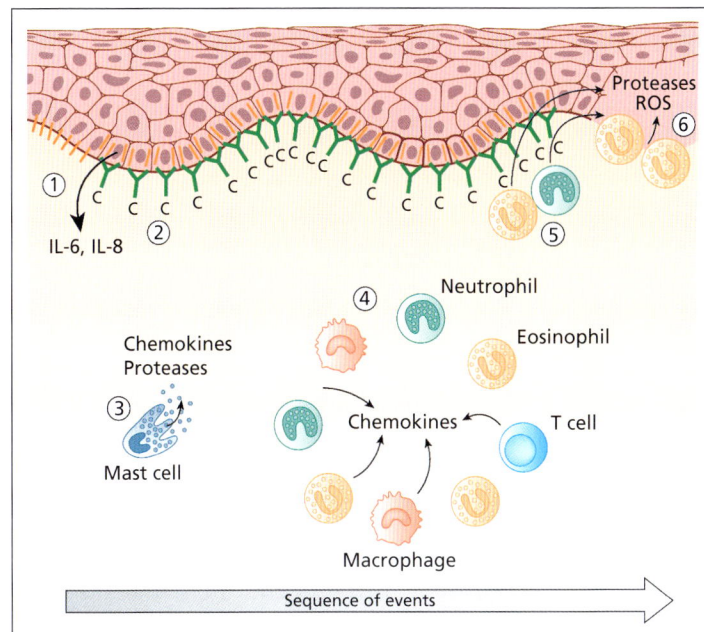

Figure 50.10 Sequence of events leading to blister formation in bullous pemphigoid. Binding of autoantibodies (green) against BP180 (orange) initiates Fc-independent events resulting in the secretion of IL-6 and IL-8 from basal keratinocytes as well as in internalisation and decreased expression of BP180 (1). Complement is activated at the dermal–epidermal junction (DEJ) (2) and mast cells degranulate (3). Complement activation and chemokine gradients trigger the infiltration of inflammatory cells into the upper dermis (4). Their secretion of additional inflammatory mediators further increases the inflammatory reaction. Finally, granulocytes at the DEJ release reactive-oxygen species and proteases (5) that ultimately induce dermal–epidermal separation (6). Adapted from Schmidt and Zillikens 2013 [1] © Elsevier.

Pathophysiology

Summary

The pathogenic importance of humoral and cellular autoimmunity against BP180 has clearly been demonstrated. Both Fc receptor-independent and, importantly, Fc-receptor-mediated effects were shown to be essential for blister formation in BP using *in vitro*, *ex vivo* and various animal models. More specifically, complement activation at the DEJ and the activation of mast cells appeared to be crucial to attract neutrophils and macrophages at the DEJ. Subsequent release of reactive oxygen species and various proteases then induced dermal–epidermal splitting (Figure 50.10). Targeting mast cells, neutrophils, complement activation and the cytokine network may open novel therapeutic avenues for this disease [67].

Autoantibodies. In nearly all BP patients, autoantibodies bind to BP180 (also termed type XVII collagen and BPAG2) (see Chapter 2) [68]. The extracellular portion of the 16th non-collagenous domain (NC16A) located directly adjacent to the cellular membrane is the immunodominant region in BP and is recognised by autoantibodies in 75–90% of BP patients [69–75]. The importance of anti-BP180 NC16A reactivity is further highlighted by the observation that serum levels of BP180 NC16A-specific IgG antibodies correlate with the disease activity in BP patients [68,72,75–78]. IgG4 and IgG1 are the major IgG subclasses of anti-BP180 NC16A antibodies [79]. The majority of patients also raises IgG antibodies against epitopes outside the NC16A domain [68,80,81] while initial reactivity appeared to target the NC16A [82]. IgG reactivity with C-terminal epitopes appeared to be associated with mucosal involvement and more severe skin disease, whereas the intracellular domain was preferentially targeted at an early clinical stage [81,83].

The majority of BP patients also develop, beside IgG, IgA and IgE anti-BP180 reactivity [79,84–88]. Serum anti-BP180 NC16A IgE occurs in about half of BP patients and correlates with disease activity within the same patient [88,89]. IgE anti-BP180 NC16A was also associated with a longer duration for remission and requirement for more intensive therapies [84].

BP230 (also known as BPAG1-e, and BPAG1) is recognised by 50–70% of BP sera [90–96] (Chapter 2). As for BP180, B-cell epitopes are not equally distributed on the molecule but preferentially localise to the globular C-terminal domain of BP230 [68,94,97]. In addition to IgG reactivity, IgE antibodies against BP230 were detected in the majority of BP sera [88,98].

Cellular immune response. In contrast to the humoral immune response, the cellular immune response has been less widely studied in human BP [99]. T- and B-cell reactivity against the NH_2-terminal portion of the BP180 ectodomain is associated with severe BP, while the central portion is more frequently recognised in patients with limited disease. In contrast, combined T- and B-cell response against the COOH- and NH_2-terminal globular domains of BP230 were found in less than 50% [100]. The response to the BP180 ectodomain is restricted to the DQβ1*0301 allele [101,102]. Autoreactive T cells in BP patients produced a Th1/Th2 mixed cytokine profile [100,101]. Reports of circulating and skin T regulatory cells in BP patients are conflicting with increased and decreased numbers being reported [103–106]. The number of peripheral follicular helper T cells, a T-cell subset known to be pivotal for B-cell activation, was higher in patients with active disease compared with those in healthy volunteers and BP patients in remission and correlated with serum levels of anti-BP180 antibodies [107]. More recently, the potential role of Th17 cells in BP was highlighted [104]. Increased numbers of IL-17A+ cells were found in BP skin lesions; the main source has been identified as granulocytes and T cells, respectively [108,109].

Cytokines and chemokines. Elevated levels of IL-1β, IL-2, IL-4, IL-5, IL-6, IL-8, IL-10, IL-15, IL-16, IL-17, IL-21, eotaxin, MCP-4, TNF-α, CCL-2, CCL 10 and CCL-18 have been found in the sera and/or blister fluids of BP patients (reviewed in [110–112]). Serum levels of TNF-α, IL-6, IL-8, IL-15, IL-17, IL-21, IL-23, CCL-2, CCL 10, CCL17, CCL18 and eotaxin correlated with the extent of BP skin lesions [107,110–114] pointing to a pathological relevance of these mediators [115]. The assumption that Th2-type cytokines are important in human BP is supported by the increased frequency of cutaneous lymphocyte-associated antigen-positive IL-4- and IL-13-producing cells in the peripheral blood [116].

Functionally relevant pathogenic mechanisms. Data about the functionally relevant pathogenic mechanisms in BP have been generated by *in vitro* studies using cultured human keratinocytes, *ex vivo* studies using cryosections of human skin, and, importantly, various animal models.

When cultured normal human keratinocytes were treated with anti-BP180 IgG a signal-transducing event leading to a dose- and time-dependent release of IL-6 and IL-8 was observed [117]. In the same model, internalisation and creased expression of BP180 and weakening of keratinocyte attachment in response to anti-BP180 IgG were seen [118,119]. Recently, release of IL-6 and IL-8 and reduction of the number of hemidesmosomes was also seen after incubation with anti-BP180 IgE [120] (Figure 50.10).

Using cryosections of normal human skin, BP180 NC16A-specific IgG induced a dermal–epidermal separation when co-incubated with leukocytes from healthy volunteers [121]. This effect was mediated by the Fc portion of autoantibodies and the Fcγ receptors IIA and IIIA on human neutrophils resulting in the release of matrix metalloproteinase-9 and neutrophil elastase [121–123]. Both enzymes were found in blister fluid and lesional biopsies from BP patients and were capable to degrade BP180 [124–126].

Passive transfer of rabbit IgG raised against the murine homologue of the human BP180 NC16A domain into neonatal wild-type mice produced clinical, histopathological and immunopathological alterations similar to those seen in BP patients [16]. In this model, blister formation was dependent on the activation of complement [127,128], degranulation of mast cells [129], recruitment of macrophages [129] and neutrophils [130], and the release of various proteases including the plasminogen/plasmin system [131], mast cell proteinase-4 [132], matrix metalloproteinase-9 [133], α1-proteinase inhibitor [134] and neutrophil elastase [65–68,135,136]. More specifically, in the early stages of blistering, matrix metalloproteinase-9 is mainly activated by plasmin, which is formed by activation of plasminogen by tissue plasminogen activator and/or urokinase plasminogen activator. Plasmin and the mast cell-specific serine protease-4 can activate matrix metalloproteinase-9 which then inactivates α1-proteinase inhibitor, the physiological inhibitor of neutrophil elastase. The unrestrained activity of neutrophil elastase is then responsible for the degradation of structural proteins of the DEJ including BP180 (Figure 50.10). A recent passive transfer model in adult mice highlighted the importance of FcγR IIB, FcγR III and FcγR IV [137].

Subsequently, further mouse models were developed that allowed exploration of additional pathogenic mechanisms. Among these models, three distinct lines of transgenic mice that expressed human BP180 in murine skin elegantly replicated essential features of human BP [17,138,139]. In one of these models, the complement dependency of experimental BP was questioned when the passive transfer of F(ab')$_2$ fragments of human BP led to skin fragility in Col17-humanised mice [140]. Subsequently, two 'active' mouse models were developed that do not depend on the transfer of anti-BP180 antibodies: wild-type mice were immunised with recombinant murine NC15A and in the second model, Rag-2$^{-/-}$/COL17$^{m-/-,h+}$ mice (immunocompromised mice expressing human BP180) received splenocytes from wild-type mice that had been immunised by grafting of COL17$^{m-/-,h+}$ mouse skin and subsequently developed anti-BP180 antibodies and a blistering phenotype [141,142]. In the latter model, the importance of NC16A-reactive CD4+ T cells has corroborated previous *in vitro* studies with human cells that showed a restriction of NC16A-reactive CD4+ T cells to the HLA-DQB1*301 allele [101,143].

In several mouse models of BP, complement-independent formation of skin lesions has been observed [140,144,145] reshaping the previous picture of complement being a prerequisite of blister formation in BP.

The functional importance of IL-17A was indicated when IL-17A-deficient mice were largely protected from the otherwise pathogenic effect of anti-BP180 IgG and prophylactic administration of an IL-17A-blocking antibody led to significantly fewer skin lesions in wild-type mice [108]. Further anti-inflammatory agents have shown anti-inflammatory activity in the mouse models of BP-like inflammatory EBA (see later) and may prove valuable future treatment options also for BP.

Experimental evidence for the pathogenic role of IgE anti-BP180 autoantibodies was provided in three mouse models [146–148] supporting the data observed in BP patients shown above. In one model, eosinophils were identified as drivers of anti-BP180 IgE-mediated pathology [148]. Later findings were supported by the observation that eosinophils can induce dermal–epidermal separation after incubation of cryosections of human skin treaded with anti-BP IgG [149].

Compared with BP180, the pathogenic relevance of autoantibodies against BP230 is less well defined. Studies on the correlation of serum anti-BP230 autoantibodies with disease have been contradictory, most of them finding no correlation between serum anti-BP230 levels and disease activity [68,82,92]. However, the injection of a monoclonal anti-BP230 IgG antibody in mice resulted in subepidermal splitting [150]. The latter finding was corroborated by the induction of subepidermal blistering in immunodeficient Rag2$^{-/-}$ mice after transfer of splenocytes from BPAG1e (BP230)$^{-/-}$ mice that had been immunised with the recombinant C-terminus of BPAG1e (BP230) [151].

Predisposing factors

Several triggers have been implicated in BP onset including trauma [152,153], burns [154], skin grafting [155,156], radiotherapy [157,158], and UV radiation including sunlight [159], UVA1 [160], PUVA [161] and photodynamic therapy [162]. Furthermore, about 20 case reports have described the association of vaccination with the onset of BP, most frequently against influenza [153,163]. Nevertheless, an epidemiological study over 9 years in Spain did not find a higher incidence of admissions for BP in the 10-week influenza vaccination period compared with the rest of the year [164].

Numerous case reports and several case–control studies have described the triggering of BP by drugs. A recent meta-analysis reported significant associations with aldosterone antagonists, DPP-4 inhibitors (gliptins; most frequently vildagliptin), anticholinergics and dopaminergic medication [35]. It is recommended to omit these drugs in BP patients [165]. Not unsurprisingly, BP has been reported following anti-PD-1/PD-L1 therapy [166]. Immune checkpoint inhibitor-induced BP was reported to occur after a median of 6–9 months and to have a longer pruritic phase without skin lesions, to be less likely to present with tense blisters and more likely to present with peripheral eosinophilia [167,168].

Mice with dysfunctional BP180 spontaneously developed elevated serum IgE, anti-basal membrane zone reactivity, an eosinophil-rich skin inflammation, and microscopic subepidermal blistering [169,170]. How far degradation of BP180 in an elderly

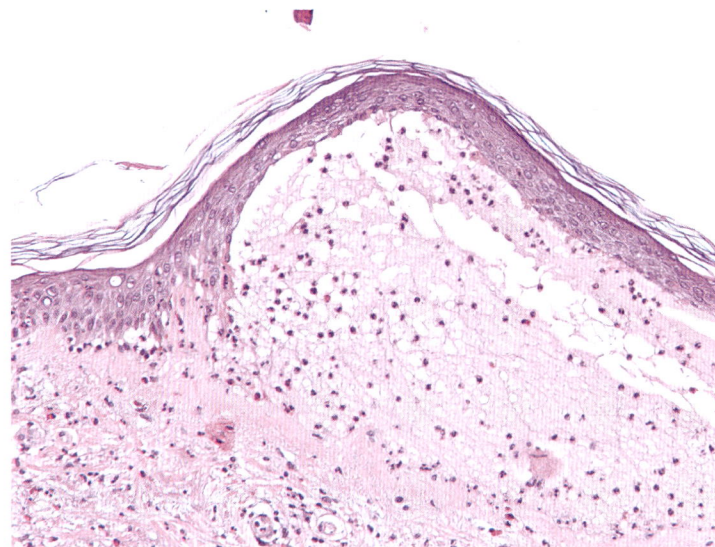

Figure 50.11 Histopathology of bullous pemphigoid. Lesional skin biopsy with subepidermal splitting and a dense inflammatory infiltrate of eosinophils and neutrophils in the upper dermis.

individual may contribute to the induction of anti-BP180/BP230 reactivity and BP remains to be determined.

Pathology

Histopathology. Light microscopy of *lesional* skin typically shows a subepidermal blister with a dense eosinophil-rich infiltrate within the papillary dermis and along the DEJ that usually also includes neutrophils, macrophages and T lymphocytes (Figure 50.11). The histopathological picture may vary considerably with the clinical picture and the age of the lesion. Patients with a predominant lymphocytic infiltration had a higher BPDAI score and those with predominantly neutrophil infiltration revealed lower serum levels of anti-BP180 NC16A IgG levels [171].

Electron microscopy. By electron microscopy the split was shown to occur within the lamina lucida.

Tissue-bound autoantibodies. Tissue-bound autoantibodies can be visualised by direct IF microscopy of a perilesional biopsy in almost all patients. Linear deposits of IgG (IgG4 and IgG1 are the predominant subclasses) and/or C3, and to a lesser extent of IgA and IgE, are seen along the DEJ (Figure 50.12) [172]. This binding pattern is observed in all pemphigoid disease. For further differentiation of the anti-DEJ staining, the n- versus u-pattern analysis can be performed [173] (Figure 50.12b, insert). At higher magnification and in thin sections (4 μm), IgG deposition appears serrated with arches closed at the top referred to as an 'n-serrated' pattern. In all pemphigoid disease except EBA, an n-serrated pattern is seen. Alternatively, the perilesional biopsy is treated with 1 M NaCl solution to induce an artificial split in the DEJ at the lamina lucida level [174]. Autoantibody specificities can then be detected, similarly to indirect IF microscopy, on 1 M NaCl-split skin (see later; Figure 50.13). Further, although not routinely available, computer-aided fluorescence overlay antigen mapping (FOAM) [175] and double IF labelling of tissue-bound and defined antigens

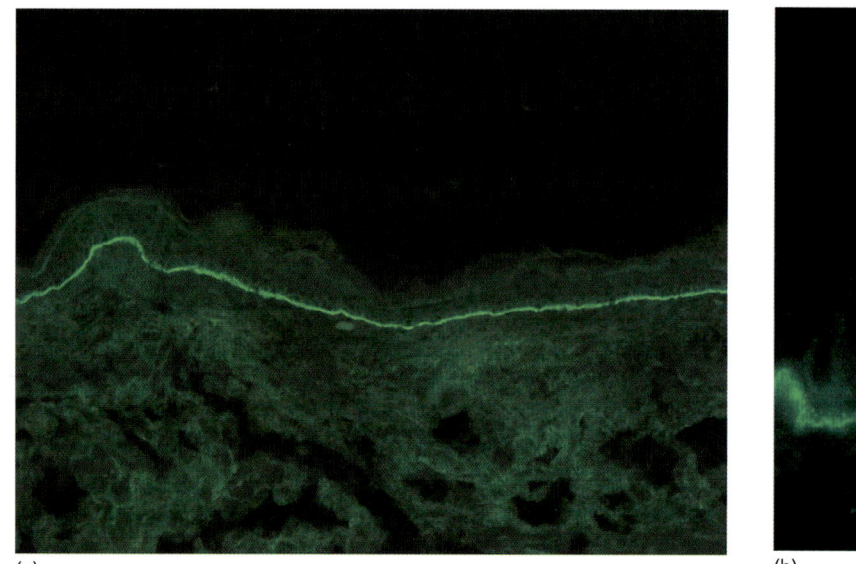
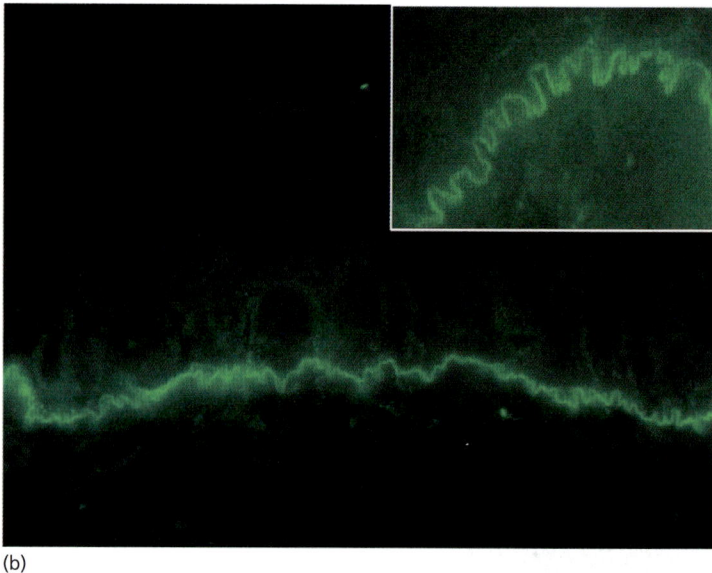

(a)   (b)

Figure 50.12 Direct immunofluorescence microscopy of bullous pemphigoid. In a perilesional biopsy, linear binding of IgG at the dermal–epidermal junction is seen (a). At higher magnification and in thin sections (4 μm), IgG deposition is no longer linear but appears curved with arches closed at the top referred to as 'n-serrated' pattern (b; insert).

Bullous pemphigoid

Mucous membrane pemphigoid

Pemphigoid gestationis

Linear IgA disease

BP180   α6β4 integrin
BP230

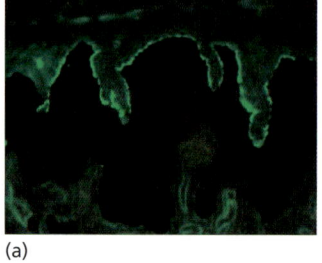
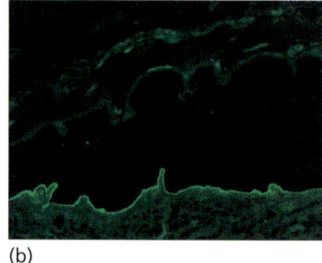

Mucous membrane pemphigoid

Laminin 332

Anti-p200 pemphigoid

Laminin β4, laminin γ1

Epidermolysis bullosa acquisita

Type VII collagen

(a)   (b)

Figure 50.13 Serological screening for autoantibodies in pemphigoid diseases: indirect immunofluorescence microscopy on 1 M NaCl-split human skin. Autoantibodies against BP180, BP230, and α6β4 integrin show a linear binding at the roof of the artificial split (a). Antibodies to laminin 332, laminin γ1/ p200 antigen and type VII collagen label the floor (b). The specific disorders and the corresponding target antigens are indicated to the left of (a) and to the right of (b).

of the DEJ analysed by laser scanning confocal microscopy [176] can be used to differentiate BP from anti-laminin 332 pemphigoid, anti-p200 pemphigoid, for example, and EBA.

The detection rate of IgG in paraffin sections of BP is poor and in a recent meta-analysis only reached 75% and 86% for C4d and C3d, respectively [177]. As such, paraffin sections cannot be recommended in the routine diagnosis of tissue-bound immunoreactants and may be reserved for selected cases when a biopsy specimen for direct IF is not available

Serum autoantibodies. Major characteristics of serum autoantibodies have been described above (see Pathophysiology). Circulating autoantibodies can be detected by: (i) indirect IF microscopy on monkey oesophagus, 1 M NaCl-split human skin and a commercial IF BIOCHIP™ mosaic (described later); (ii) immunoelectron microscopy [178] (not routinely available); (iii) commercial ELISA systems; and (iv) various in house ELISA, immunoblotting and immunoprecipitation analyses using cell-derived or recombinant forms of BP180 and BP230 [172].

Indirect IF microscopy has traditionally been performed on monkey oesophagus with a sensitivity of 60–70% [12,95,179]. Higher

sensitivities between 70% and 95% were obtained with normal human skin in which splitting of the DEJ had been induced by incubation in 1 M NaCl solution [96,179–182]. Moreover, in this technique, BP autoantibodies bind to the roof of the artificial split and can therefore be differentiated from autoantibodies in anti-laminin 332 pemphigoid, anti-p200 pemphigoid and EBA (Figure 50.13). While IF binding signals by direct IF appear to be mainly due to anti-BP180 antibodies, signals by indirect IF on oesophagus and salt-split skin correlate with anti-BP230 antibodies [183,184]. More recently, a BIOCHIP™ mosaic has become available (Euroimmun, Luebeck, Germany). This indirect IF microscopy test allows the simultaneous analysis of several substrates including monkey oesophagus, salt-split skin, BP180 NC16A, a C-terminal stretch of BP230, desmoglein 3 and desmoglein 1 in a single incubation field (Figure 50.14). This BIOCHIP™ mosaic has been shown to provide a similar diagnostic accuracy compared with the routine multistep procedure and can be extended by cells recombinantly expressing laminin 332 and type VII collagen, respectively [185,186].

BP180 NC16A- and BP230-specific ELISA systems are available by two companies (Euroimmun; MBL, Nagoya, Japan) [74,75,94,187]. Both BP230 ELISA systems are based on recombinant C-terminal

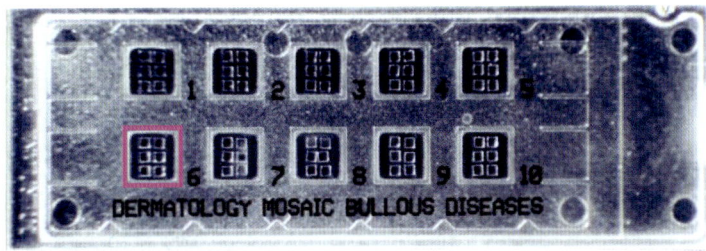

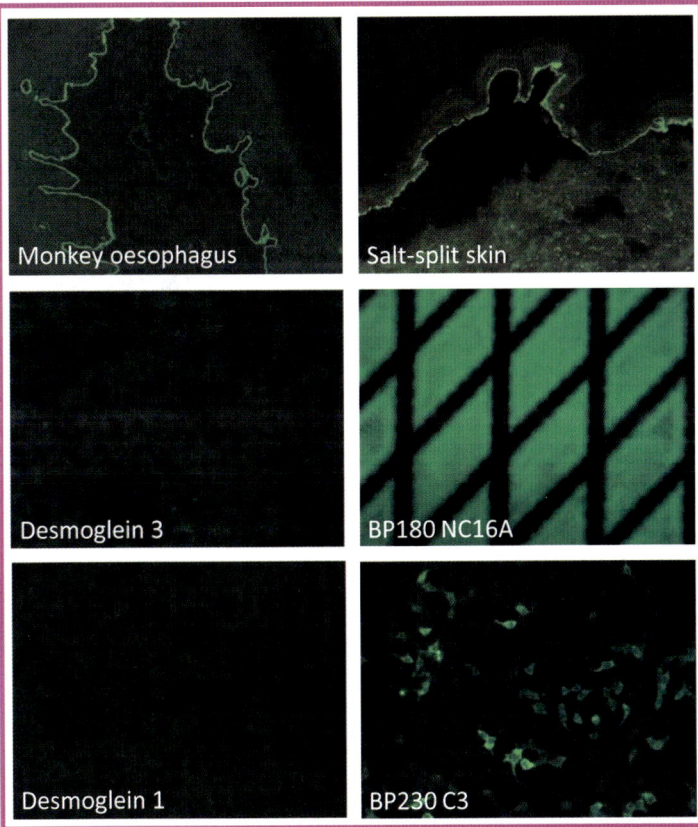

Figure 50.14 Serological screening for autoantibodies in pemphigoid diseases: indirect immunofluorescence microscopy using a BIOCHIP Mosaic™. Ten incubation fields each with six different BIOCHIPs are placed on a standard-sized slide (upper panel). This technology allows the simultaneous testing for serum autoantibodies against various substrates including monkey oesophagus, salt-split human skin, recombinant BP180 NC16A and mammalian cells expressing the ectodomains of desmoglein 1 and 3, and the C-terminus of BP230 (lower panels) in patients with suspected autoimmune blistering diseases. Here, serum from a patient with bullous pemphigoid binds to monkey oesophagus, the roof of salt-split human skin, BP180 and BP230, but as expected not to desmoglein 1 or 3. This commercially available assay has a high agreement compared with the conventional multistep approach and similar specificities and sensitivities as the corresponding ELISA assays [185]. Adapted from [185] with kind permission from BioMed Central.

fragments that in one ELISA is combined with an N-terminal fragment. By the combined use of the BP180 and BP230 ELISA, the diagnostic sensitivity can be increased by 4–8% to 87–91% compared with application of the BP180 ELISA alone [94–96]. Low serum levels of anti-BP180 or -BP230 antibodies may also be found in about 4% of dermatological patients not suffering from BP, in particular in the elderly and patients with chronic pruritus [188–191]. In all patients with low serum levels of anti-DEJ antibodies and in all patients with chronic pruritus of unknown aetiology older than 70 years of age, direct IF microscopy is mandatory to exclude BP [192].

Interestingly, 6–18% of patients with Alzheimer disease or multiple sclerosis have antibodies against epitopes mainly outside the NC16A domain of BP180 [193,194]. Non-NC16A anti-BP180 reactivity has also been associated with a non-inflammatory variant of BP [195,196]. Combining different detection systems, autoantibodies against BP180 can be found in virtually all BP sera [68,197]. Currently, no standardised widely available assay for the detection of anti-BP180 antibodies outside the NC16A domain is available and the pathogenic relevance of these antibodies has not been demonstrated yet.

Genetics
Data about a genetic background in BP are sparse and partly inconsistent. In 21 white patients a significant association with DQB1*0301 was detected [198], an observation that was partly confirmed by the demonstration that the primary response of CD4-positive T cells to BP180 *in vitro* is restricted to DQB1*0301 [101]. DQB1*0301 has also been reported as the susceptibility allele for BP in Chinese Hans, Iranian and Brazilian people, and male white people, as well as Japanese patients with DDP-4 inhibitor-associated BP [199–204]. In contrast, in 25 patients from northern China, DRB1*08 and DRB1*08/DQB1*06 were detected with a lower frequency compared with controls [205] and in 23 Japanese BP patients, HLA-DRB1*04/DQA1*0301/DQB1*0302, DRB1*1101/DQA1*0505/DQB1*0302, DRB1*1101 and DQB1*0302 were associated with BP [206]. The first genome-wide association study in BP including 446 BP patients and 433 age-and sex-matched controls with Germany ancestry revealed a strong association with DQB1*0301 and DQA1*05:05 after deep sequencing of the HLA locus and confirmation with other cohorts [207].

Environmental factors
No environmental factors have been discovered so far. Trigger factors are described in Predisposing factors, earlier.

Clinical features
History
A prodromal non-bullous phase usually precedes the development of tense generalised blisters. This prodromal phase may last for several weeks or even months. In this stage, clinical diagnosis is difficult. Pruritus, from mild to intractable, is typical and may even occur without skin lesions. In the prodromal phase, excoriated papules, eczematous or urticarial lesions, haemorrhagic crusts and excoriations prevail.

Presentation
The bullous stage is characterised by intense pruritus accompanied with widespread tense blisters and vesicles on apparently normal or reddish skin (Figure 50.15). Frequently, partly haemorrhagic crusts and urticated and infiltrated erythematosus plaques with an occasionally annular or figurate pattern are present (Figure 50.16) [208]. The blisters may reach a diameter of many centimetres and contain a clear sometimes haemorrhagic exudate; the Nikolsky sign is negative. Pruritus, which may be incapacitating, is almost constantly present [179]. Blisters are typically symmetrically distributed and may persist for several days. After mechanical irritation, erosions and yellowish or haemorrhagic crusts develop.

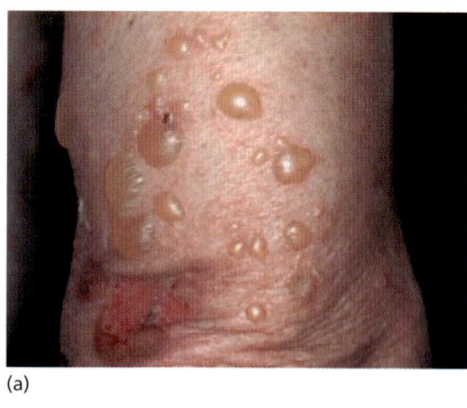

(a)

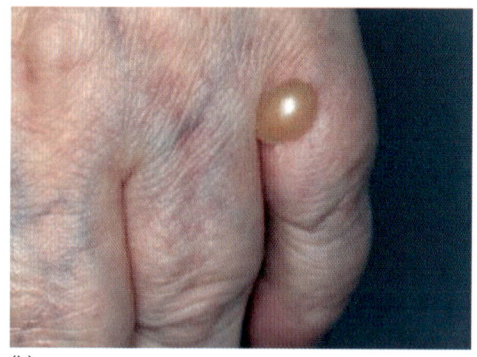

(b)

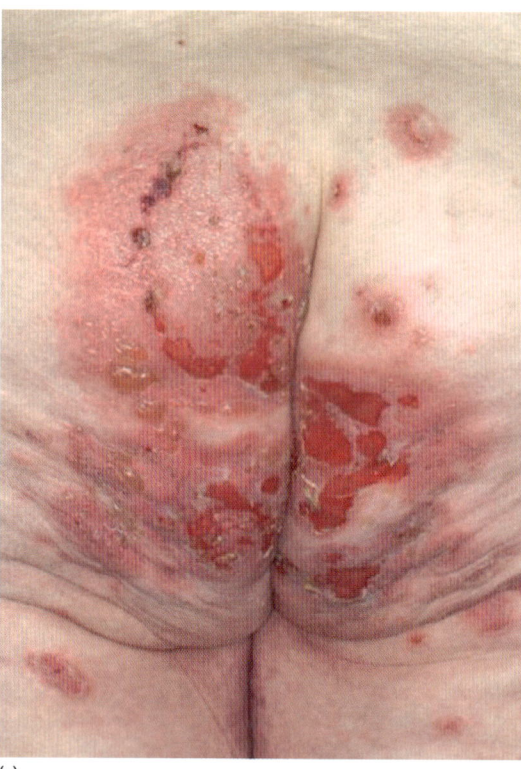

(c)

Figure 50.15 Classical bullous pemphigoid. Tense blisters and erosions on the arm (a), hand (b), and gluteal region (c). Blisters may arise on erythematous (a, c) or otherwise normal skin (b).

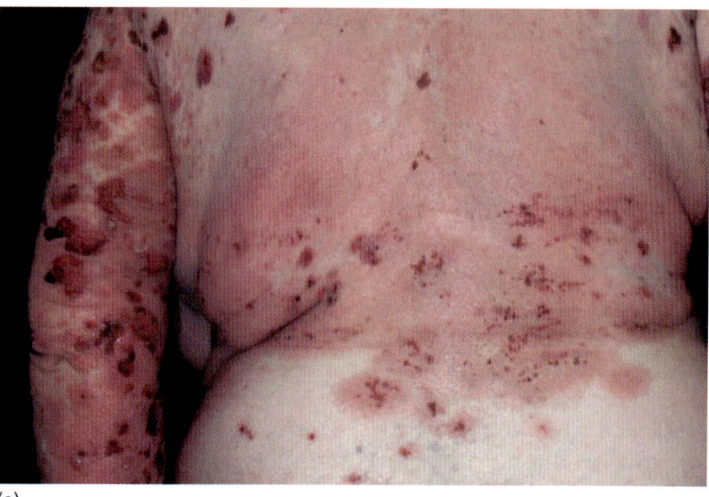

(a)

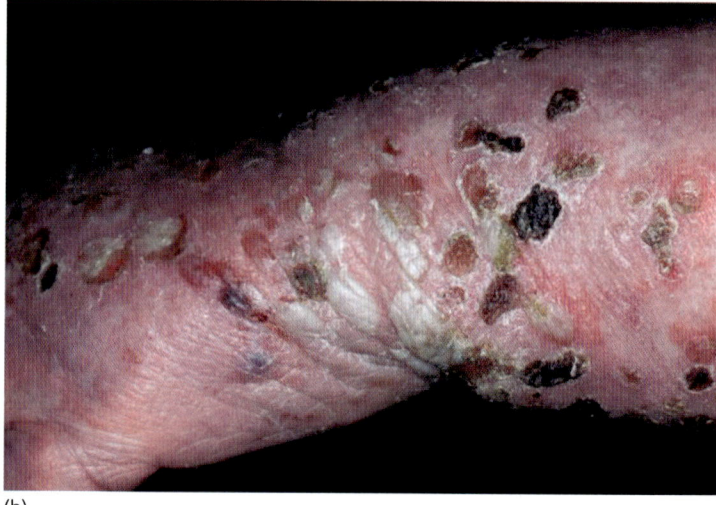

(b)

Figure 50.16 Classic bullous pemphigoid. Tense blisters, erosions, and partly haemorrhagic crusts on back and left arm (a) and left hand (b).

Predilection sites involve the flexural aspects of the limbs and abdomen [209]. In the intertriginous regions, vegetating plaques may occur. Mucosal lesions develop in 10–20% of cases, mostly in the oral cavity [210–212], and were associated with lack of anti-BP230 serum reactivity and lower levels of peripheral eosinophils compared with BP patients without mucosal lesions [212,213]. The mucosae of eyes, nose, pharynx, oesophagus and ano-genital areas are rarely affected (reviewed in [214,215]). Without severe superinfection all lesions heal without scarring. Red macules may persist at the sites of previous blisters for many weeks or months. Milia formation only rarely occurs.

Clinical variants

Cutaneous manifestations of BP can be highly polymorphic. This notion has led to the description of several clinical variants (reviewed in [215]). In all of them, direct IF microscopy of a perilesional biopsy reveals linear deposits of IgG and/or C3 at the DEJ. At present, the fine specificities of serum autoantibodies were not shown to differ from the classical form.

Several clinical variants of BP have been described with a variety of different denominations, such as dyshidrotic [216], prurigo nodularis-like [217,218], prurigo-like [219], erythrodermic, ecthyma gangrenosum-like [220], intertrigo-like, papular, eczematous,

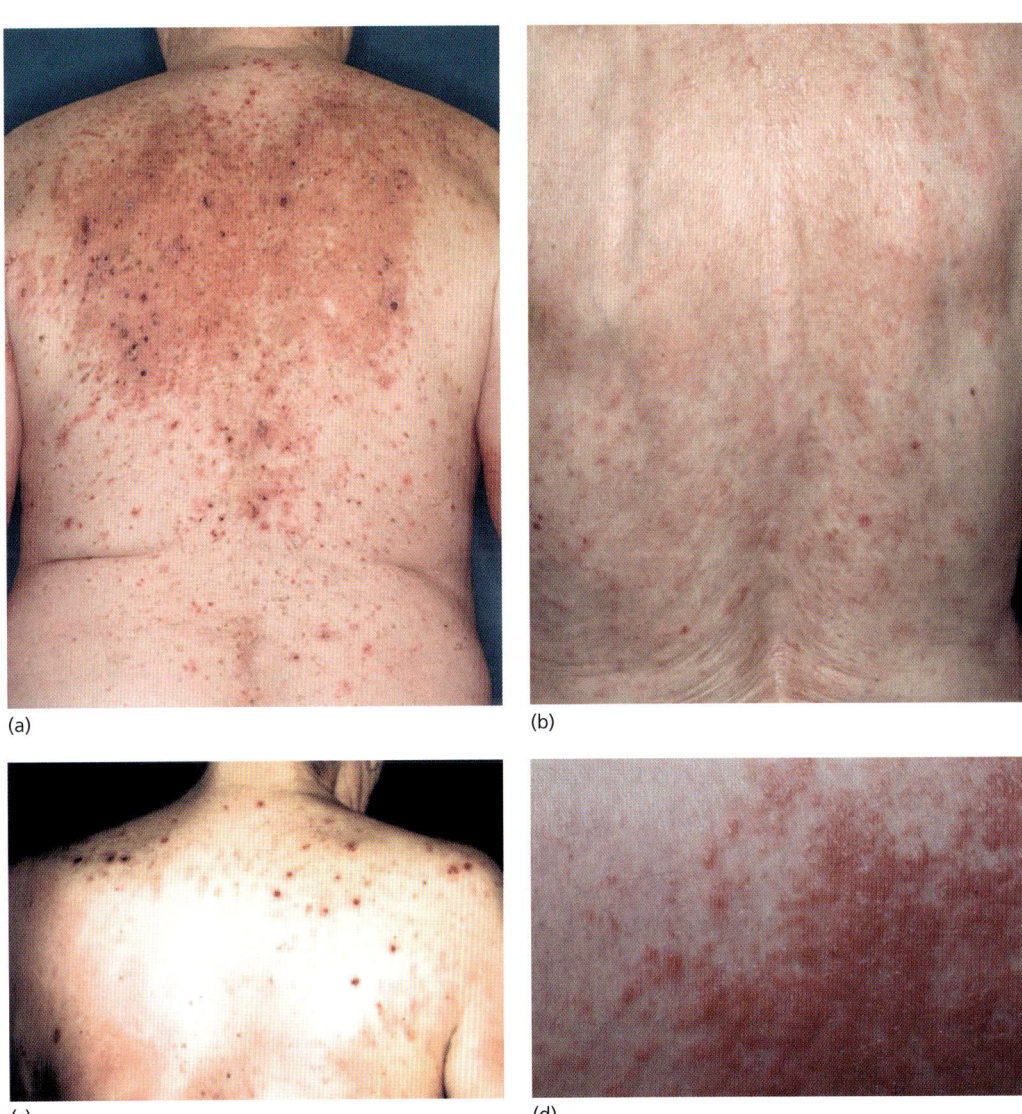

Figure 50.17 Clinical variants of bullous pemphigoid. Eczematous lesions with some erosions and crusts (a, b), prurigo-like variant with multiple excoriated papules (c), and papular variant (d).

lymphomatoid papulosis-like, vegetating [221–223], vesicular [224] and toxic epidermolysis-like pemphigoid [225,226] (Figures 50.17 and 50.18). Some forms, such as prurigo-like, papular, eczematous, vesicular and erythrodermic pemphigoid may later develop tense blisters and transform into the classical type. In a prospective study, 20% of patients presented with a non-classical BP variant at the time of diagnosis [210]. In a systematic review, reddish urticarial plaques and papules/nodule were with 52% and 21%, respectively, the most common clinical manifestations of non-bullous BP. About 10% of these patients developed blisters during the later course of the disease [227].

Localised bullous pemphigoid. In some patients, the disease is limited to certain body parts, most frequently the lower extremities notably the pretibial area [228–230]. Also, other regions such as the flexures, palms, soles, the genital area and the umbilicus have been described [231,232] as well as around stomata and haemodialysis fistulae (Figure 50.19) (see Predisposing factors, earlier). Localised lesions may remain as such or develop into classical BP.

Childhood bullous pemphigoid. Two peaks of incidences of BP in childhood were reported: in the first year of life (infantile BP) and around the age of 8 years [48]. Multiple cases with a close association with preceding vaccinations were reported, most of them in infants. Due to the high rate of vaccinations in this age group, a causative relation is difficult to confirm. In infants, the distribution of the lesions is often acral, in particular palmar and plantar [48]. In older children, involvement of the genital region occurs in almost half of the cases [48] (Figure 50.20). No immunopathological differences between BP in childhood and adults have been reported. Autoantibodies mainly target the NC16A domain of BP180 [233]. Generally, infants and children with BP have a good prognosis with remissions within weeks to a few months under therapy. For treatment, systemic corticosteroids are usually combined with dapsone or sulphapyridine [47,234].

Differential diagnosis

BP must be differentiated from other blistering autoimmune dermatoses (see Investigations, later; Figure 50.21). Diagnostic hallmarks are summarised in Table 50.2. In brief, diseases of the

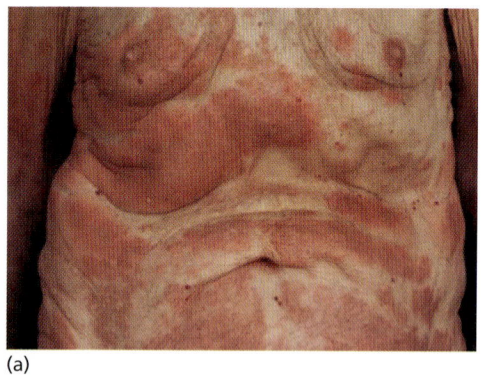

(a)

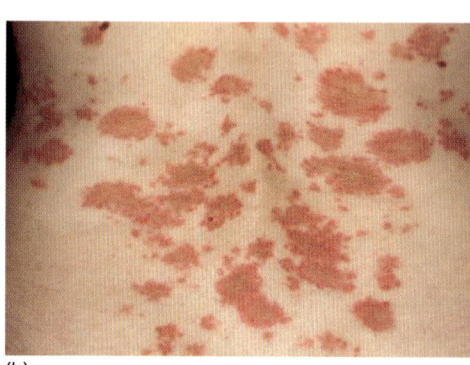

(b)

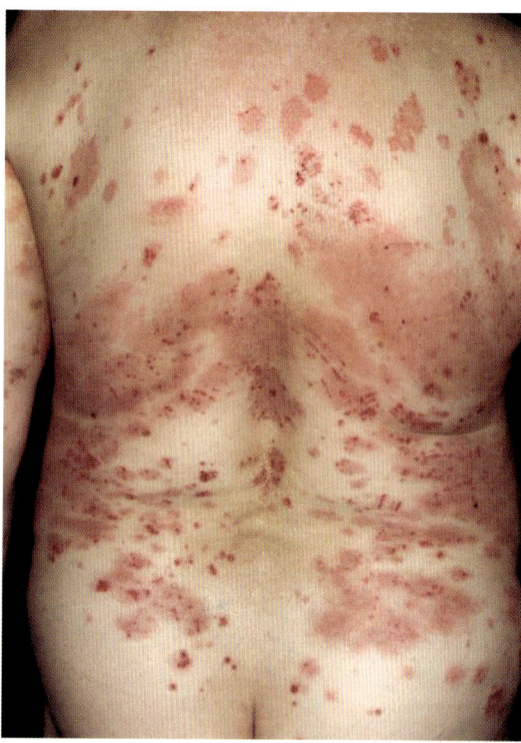

(c)

Figure 50.18 Clinical variants of bullous pemphigoid. Urticarial and erythematous plaques (a–c) accompanied by erosions and excoriations (c).

pemphigus group can be easily differentiated on the basis of distinctive clinical (positive Nikolsky sign) and immunopathological features. Mucous membrane pemphigoid is differentiated from BP by its predominant involvement of mucosal surfaces [235]. In contrast, the distinction of BP from linear IgA disease, EBA and anti-p200/laminin γ1 pemphigoid based simply on clinical and histopathological features is usually impossible and requires direct IF microscopy (for linear IgA disease) and serological analyses (for the latter two entities). In dermatitis herpetiformis, direct IF microscopy findings, and particularly the serological profile (presence of anti-transglutaminase 1 and 2 as well as anti-gliadin IgA antibodies), are often required for diagnosis [208].

Furthermore, in the non-bullous prodromal stage or in atypical presentations, BP can closely resemble a variety of dermatoses including localised or generalised drug reactions, contact and allergic dermatitis, prurigo, urticaria, urticarial vasculitis, arthropod reactions, scabies, ecthyma or even pityriasis lichenoides. A detailed patient history, clinical evaluation, histopathological features and, above all, direct IF microscopy and serology, are essential to distinguish these disorders from BP [208].

Classification of severity
An international panel of experts has recently proposed outcome measures for clinical studies and a clinical scoring system, the *BP Disease Area Index* [**236**]. The index records severity of: (i) skin lesions separately for classical lesions, i.e. erosions and blisters, and atypicial lesions such as red macules, urticaria and others in 12 body regions; (ii) mucosal lesions; and (iii) pruritus. In an international prospective study, cut-offs defining mild, moderate and severe disease based on the 25th and 75th percentiles has proposed BPDAI activity scores of 20 and 57 [237]. The guideline of the German Society of Dermatology proposed involvement of <10%, 10–30%, and >30% of the body surface as classification for mild, moderate and severe BP [**165**].

Currently, an investigator global assessment (IGA) score is being validated to fulfil the FDA requirements in clinical trials.

Complications and co-morbidities
Patients with BP have a significantly higher risk for septicaemia, pulmonary and urinary tract infections, embolism, osteoporosis, and pathological fractures compared with controls [238–241]. Co-morbidities at the time of diagnosis are detailed in Associated diseases, earlier.

Disease course and prognosis
Untreated BP runs a chronic, self-limiting course over a number of months and, more frequently, years. Relapses are frequent and appear in about half of the patients [208] and were associated with extensive disease, dementia and high serum levels of anti-BP180 NC16A antibodies at the time when treatment was omitted [242,243]. The disease duration is usually 3–6 years, with most patients achieving complete remission off treatment.

The first-year mortality rates range from 10% to 40%, which is about two- to sixfold higher compared with age- and sex-matched controls [24,28,37,42,210,244]. Mortality varies considerably between different populations (outpatients versus inpatients, different countries, secondary or tertiary referral centres), and treatments, e.g. a 1-year mortality as high as 41% was observed in patients with extensive disease treated with prednisolone 1 mg/kg/day [**245**], while it was only 8% when class IV topical corticosteroids were combined with methylprednisolone 0.5 mg/kg/day and dapsone [246].

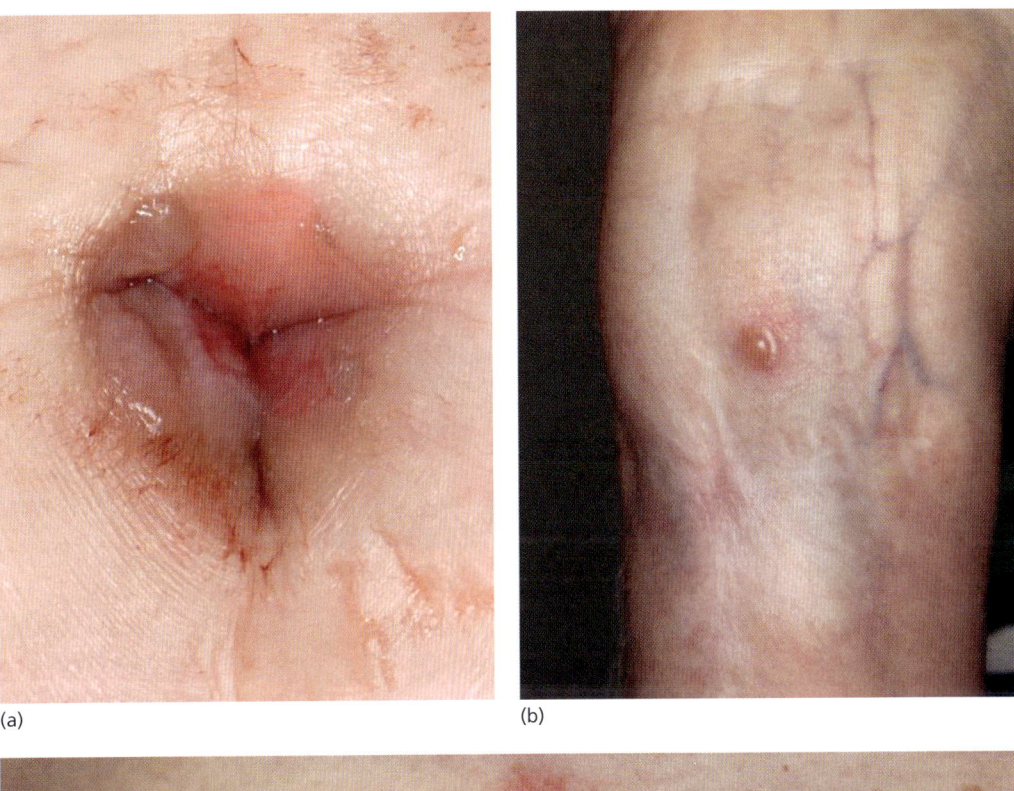

(a)   (b)

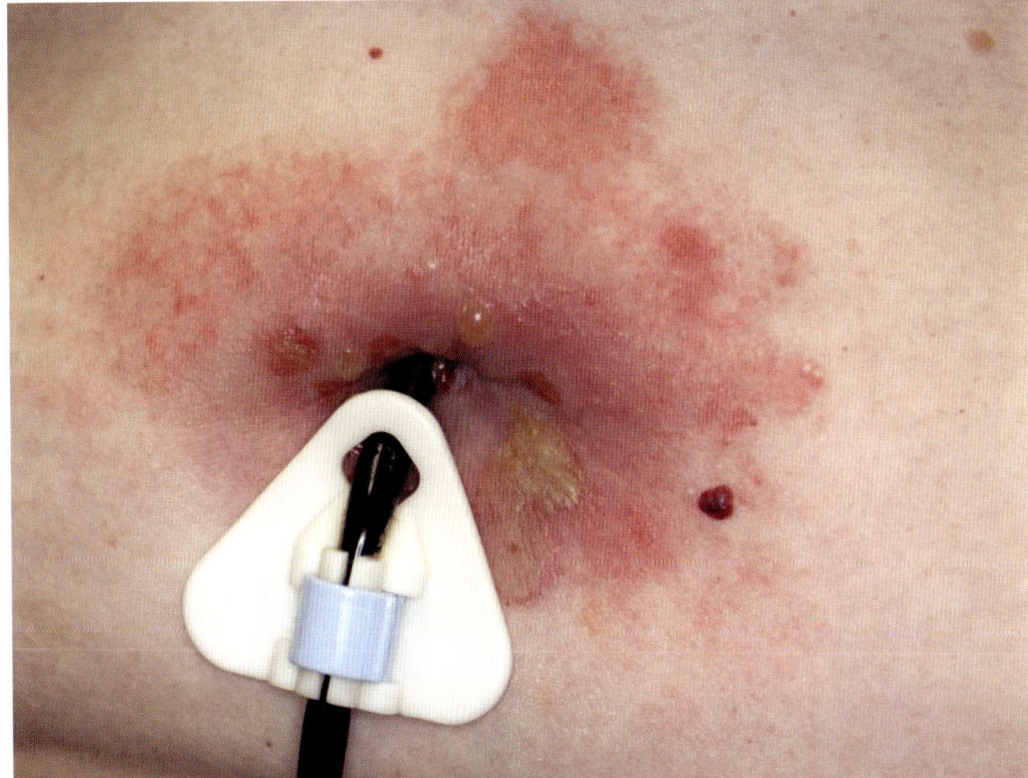

Figure 50.19 Localised bullous pemphigoid. Tense blisters and erosions limited to the umbilical area (a). Single tense blister at the site of major surgery (b). Eczema, erosions and tense blisters restricted to the site of percutaneous endoscopic gastrostomy (c).

(c)

In a meta-analysis, the pooled 1-year mortality was 23.5%, with higher rates in Europe compared with the USA and Asia [247]. Another meta-analysis calculated the 1-year standardised mortality ratio to 2.93 with no significant differences between the tree continents [248].

Risk factors for lethal outcome are old age (greater than 80 years), extensive disease, high doses of prednisolone (>35 mg/day), serum albumin levels of less than 3.6 g/dL, a Karnofsky score of 40 or less, and the presence of heart disease, diabetes, or neurological diseases, dementia, and elevated anti-BP180 antibodies [37,39,40,249–252].

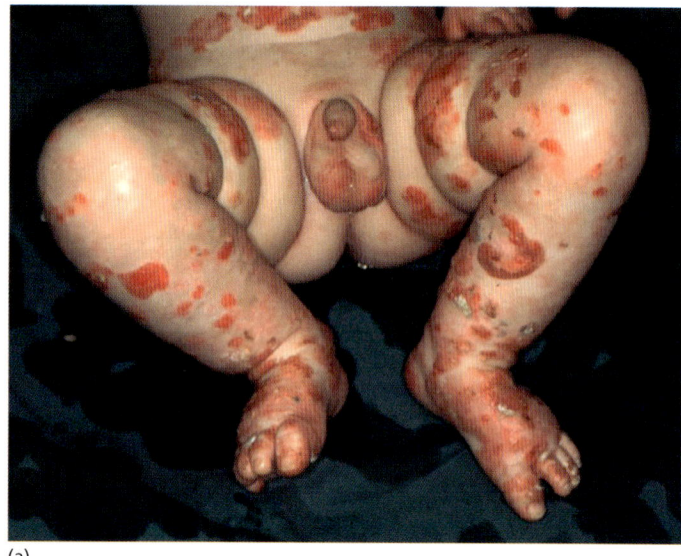

(a)

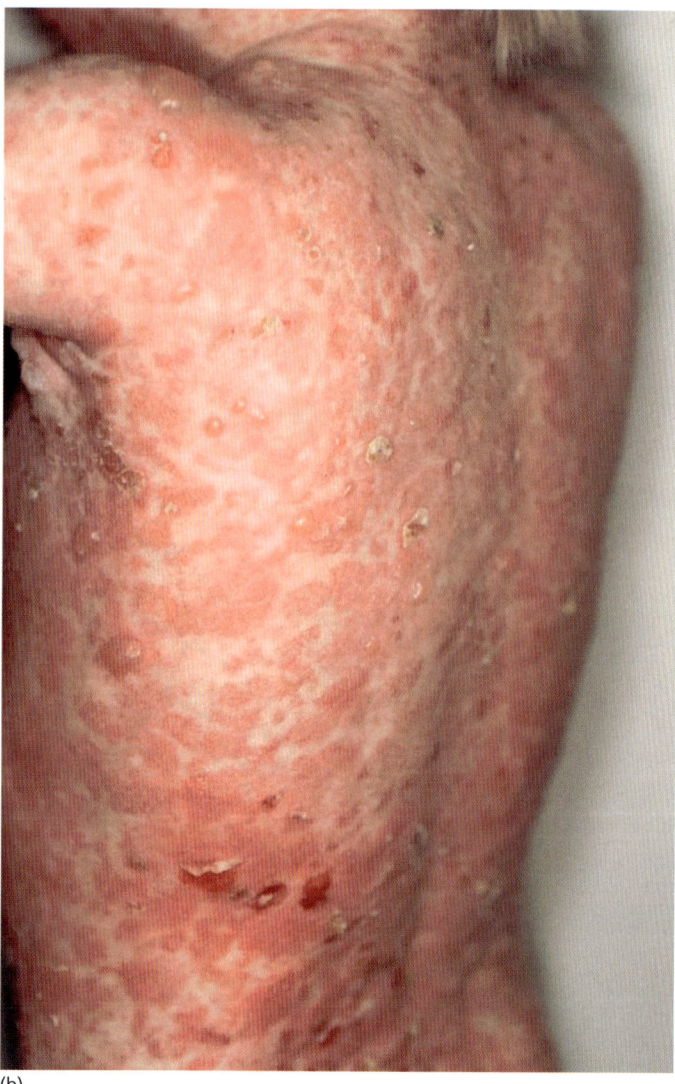

(b)

Figure 50.20 Childhood bullous pemphigoid. Disseminated tense blisters, erosions and crusts on the lower abdomen, genitalia and lower extremities in an infant (a). Generalised erythema, numerous tense vesicles and some erosions on the back of a 3-year-old boy (b).

Investigations and diagnosis

The diagnosis is based on the combination of the clinical picture, direct IF microscopy and serology (Figure 50.21) [1,172,208,253]. Direct IF microscopy and the serological assays are described above in more detail (see Pathology, earlier). About 90% of patients can be diagnosed based on the clinical picture and commercially available BP180- and B230-specific serological tests such as ELISA and indirect IF microscopy [94–96,172,185,186].

Histopathology cannot differentiate BP from other pemphigoid diseases such as anti-laminin 332 mucous membrane pemphigoid and anti-p200/ laminin γ1 pemphigoid in all cases [254,255]. The knowledge of the histopathological spectrum of BP, however, allows the histopathologist to arrange for direct IF microscopy and appropriate serological analyses to obtain a definite diagnosis.

Table 50.3 summarises the recommendations of the S2k guideline of the German Society of Dermatology for diagnosis of BP [256].

Management

The aim of treatment is to suppress disease activity with the minimum dose of drugs necessary. BP patients are elderly, with usually several co-morbidities, are commonly on many drugs and susceptible to adverse reactions.

Topical and systemic steroids are the mainstay of treatment. Very potent topical corticosteroids (0.05% clobetasol propionate ointment) should be considered in all patients. For localised BP, the lesional application of very potent topical corticosteroids is often sufficient.

Controlled randomised trials. Only 13 controlled prospective studies on treatment of BP have been published including oral corticosteroids (in several studies), the long-term whole-body use of very potent topical corticosteroids (in two), azathioprine (in three), plasmapheresis (in two) as well as mycophenolate mofetil, doxycycline, nicotinamide plus tetracycline dapsone, IVIG and mepolizumab (Table 50.4) [257,**258**,259–261].

Joly *et al.* showed in patients with moderate BP that clobetasol propionate 0.05% ointment (40 g/day applied over the whole body, tapering over 12 months) was as effective and safe as oral prednisolone 0.5 mg/day [245]. In a subsequent study, lower doses of this high-potent topical corticosteroid (10–30 g daily, tapering over 4 months) did not differ in the time to achieve disease control compared with the more intensive topical regimen and was associated with less severe adverse events but more relapses in patients with moderate disease [262]. In patients with extensive disease, treatment with oral prednisolone at an initial dose of 1.0 mg/kg/day resulted in significantly more severe adverse events compared with application of long-term very potent topical corticosteroids [**245**].

In a pragmatic study design, Williams *et al.* showed that the treatment with doxycycline 200 mg/day was within a preselected 37% acceptable margin not inferior compared with prednisolone 0.5 mg/kg/day (in both groups ≤30 g/week class 3 topical corticosteroids was allowed within the first 3 weeks) with respect to treatment success after 6 weeks (defined as ≤3 fresh blisters/erosions) and was associated with significantly less severe adverse events after 52 weeks [**258**]. Since after 6 weeks 74% of patients achieved disease control, clinical efficacy of doxycycline has been shown indirectly.

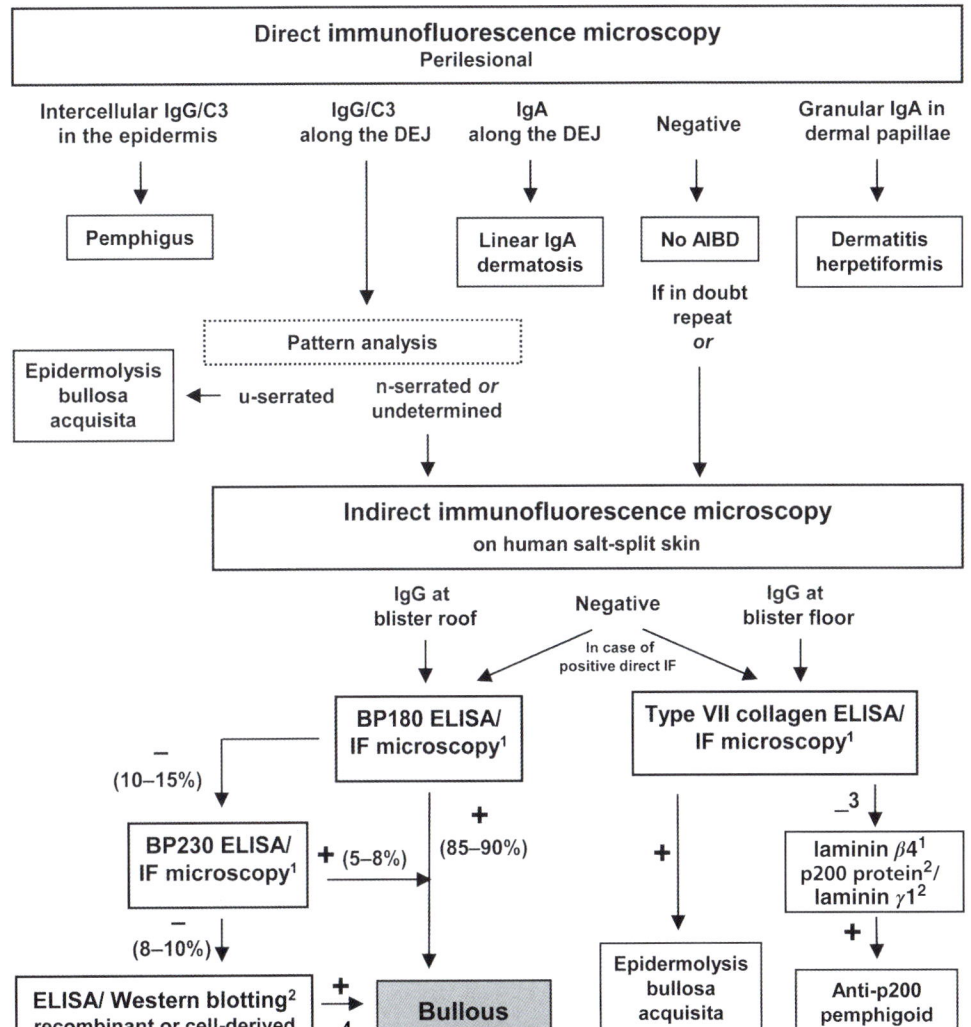

Figure 50.21 Diagnostic pathway for bullous pemphigoid. The diagnostic gold standard is still direct immunofluorescence (IF) microscopy of a perilesional biopsy. About 90% of patients can be diagnosed based on the clinical picture and serological tests. 1, Commercially available assay; 2, only available in specialised diagnostic centres; 3, reactivity with laminin 332 has only been described in individual patients without predominant mucosal manifestations; 4, with positive direct IF microscopy and epidermal binding of IgG by indirect IF microscopy on salt-split skin or n-serrated/undetermined IgG binding by direct IF microscopy and no reactivity against p200 antigen, laminin γ1 and type VII collagen.

Controlled randomised trials with dupilumab (anti-IL-4αR), benralizumab (anti-IL-5R), bertilimumab (anti-eotaxin 1), nomacopan (anti-C5a/LTB4), avdoralimab (anti-C5aR1) and efgartigimod (anti-FcRn inhibitor) are performed or scheduled.

Other clinical studies. Larger uncontrolled studies were performed with chlorambucil (prospective) as well as with dapsone, methotrexate and low-dose oral cyclophosphamide (all retrospective) [246,270–273]. In addition, in small patient cohorts and individual cases, the successful use of erythromycin [274], ciclosporin [275], leflunomide [276], rituximab [277–279], immunoadsorption [280–282], omalizumab [279,283], dupilumab [284] and nomacopan (anti-C5a/LTB4) has been reported [285].

Treatment guidelines. Guidelines from different national and international organisations have been established including the

Brazilian, British, French, German, Italian and Japanese dermatological societies as well as the EADV [165,286,**287**,288–290,**291**].

British colleagues proposed the lesional application of topical clobetasol propionate 0.05% ointment with or without prednisolone 0.3 mg/kg/day or the combination of the topical corticosteroid with anti-inflammatory antibiotics, e.g. doxycycline, tetracycline, minocycline and erythromycin as initial treatment for mild disease [287]. For moderate and severe disease, they recommend: (i) topical clobetasol propionate 0.05% (5–15 g twice daily to the whole skin surface); (ii) prednisolone 0.5–1.0 mg/kg/day plus lesional topical corticosteroid; or (iii) the combination of the topical corticosteroid with anti-inflammatory antibiotics.

German colleagues recommend topical clobetasol propionate 0.05% for mild BP, and for moderate BP the same regimen alone or, if required, combined with systemic treatment. For severe BP, the combination of topical clobetasol propionate 0.05% and

Table 50.3 Diagnosis of bullous pemphigoid (BP) according to the recommendations of the S2k guideline of the German Society of Dermatology [256].

BP can be diagnosed in case of the following constellations:
- Compatible clinical picture and positive direct IF microscopy and reactivity with BP180[a] and/or BP230[a]
- Compatible clinical picture and positive direct IF microscopy and epidermal binding of IgG by indirect IF microscopy on salt-split skin
- Clinical picture with tense blisters and epidermal binding of IgG by indirect IF microscopy on split skin or monkey oesophagus and reactivity with BP180[a] and/or BP230[a]
- Clinical picture with tense blisters and corresponding histopathology and epidermal binding of IgG in indirect IF microscopy on salt-split skin
- Compatible clinical picture and corresponding histopathology (with subepidermal cleavage) and reactivity with BP180[a]
- Clinical picture with tense blisters and pronounced reactivity with BP180[a] (e.g. > 3 times the lower detection threshold)

---

[a] In commercial assays (ELISA or indirect IF microscopy). IF, immunofluorescence.

systemic treatment is recommended. As systemic treatment, prednisolone at an initial dose of 0.5 mg/kg/day is recommended with or without azathioprine, dapsone, doxycycline, methotrexate or mycophenolate. Dapsone, doxycycline or methotrexate can also be used without the systemic corticosteroid. In refractory patients, immunoadsorption/plasmapheresis, rituximab or IVIG is recommended [165]. The EADV guideline was updated in 2022 [291].

Management algorithm

Most clinicians would treat localised and mild BP with lesional, very potent topical corticosteroids alone (see Treatment ladder, below). For moderate BP, very potent topical corticosteroids can be combined with oral prednisolone ≤0.5 mg/kg/day, dapsone or doxycycline (see Treatment ladder, below). For severe BP, the combination of very potent topical corticosteroids with prednisolone 0.5 mg/kg/day and dapsone, doxycycline, methotrexate, azathioprine or mycophenolate is proposed. The corticosteroid-sparing agent may be chosen depending on personal experience; the highest evidence has been provided for doxycycline and dapsone. In refractory patients, immunoadsorption/plasmapheresis, rituximab or IVIG may be added (see Treatment ladder, below).

Treatment ladder for bullous pemphigoid[a]

Localised and mild disease[b]
- Lesional very potent topical corticosteroids 2×/day

Moderate disease[b]
First line
- Very potent topical corticosteroids on the whole body surface 2×/day[c]

Second line
- Very potent topical corticosteroids on the whole body surface 2×/day[c]

plus
- Doxycycline 200 mg/day *or*
- Dapsone 1.0–1.5 mg/kg/day (with normal glucose-6-phosphate dehydrogenase levels)

or
- Prednisolone 0.5 mg/kg/day tapering
- *with or without* doxycycline or dapsone

Third line
- Very potent topical corticosteroids on the whole body surface 2×/day[c] *or*
- Prednisolone 0.5 mg/kg/day tapering

plus
- Azathioprine 2.5 mg/kg/day (with normal TPMT activity) *or*
- Methotrexate 10–20 mg/week *or*
- Mycophenoles (mofetil 2 g/day, gastroresistant mycophenolic acid 1.44 g/day)

Severe disease[b]
First line
- Very potent topical corticosteroids on lesions ×2/day

plus
- Prednisolone 0.5 mg/kg/day tapering

with
- Doxycycline *or* dapsone *or* second line azathioprine, methotrexate *or* mycophenoles
  In case of insufficient response increase prednisolone to 0.75 mg/kg/day, and if still insufficient to 1.0 mg/kg/day
  In refractory patients, add immunoadsorption, rituximab or IVIG

[a]Guidelines differ considerably [299]; here, the preferred approach of the authors is presented.
[b]Localised and mild disease has been defined as involvement of <10% of body surface of BPDAI <20, moderate disease as involvement of 10–30% of body surface or BPDAI between 20 and 57, and severe disease as >10 new lesions per day, involvement of >30% of body surface or BPDAI >57 [165,237,245].
[c]If not possible, prednisolone 0.5 mg/kg/day tapering can be used. IVIG, intravenous immunoglobulin; TPMT, thiopurine methyl transferase.

Mucous membrane pemphigoid

Definition, nomenclature and classification

An international consensus conference defined mucous membrane pemphigoid (MMP) as an immunobullous disease with autoantibodies against components of the DEJ and predominant mucosal involvement [1] (Table 50.2). Previously, the term cicatricial pemphigoid was used synonymously for MMP. Currently, cicatricial pemphigoid only refers to the rare clinical variant in which mucous membranes are not predominantly affected and skin lesions heal with scarring (see Rare pemphigoid variants) [1]. Due to this definition, there is some overlap with linear IgA disease (in patients with predominant IgA anti-DEJ antibodies) and EBA in patients with autoantibodies against type VII collagen) [2] (Figure 50.22). Later patients are now classified as MMP irrespective of the predominant autoantibody isotype or specificity [3,4]. The previously used synonym benign MMP has been abandoned. Patients with single site

Table 50.4 Randomised controlled trials in bullous pemphigoid.

Year	Intervention	Number of patients	Outcome	Comment
2020 [261]	Mepolizumab (anti-IL-5 antibody) 750 mg every 4 weeks over 12 weeks versus placebo; both with standard oral corticosteroids	30	No difference between number of relapses at weeks 16 and 36 and the median time until relapse	No evidence to support mepolizumab
2017 [259]	Azathioprine 1.5–2.5 mg/kg/day versus dapsone 1.5 mg/kg/day; both with methylprednisolone 0.5 mg/kg/day	54	The primary endpoint, i.e. time until complete tapering of methylprednisolone was not significantly different between the two arms; the cumulative methylprednisolone dose was lower in the dapsone arm ($P = 0.06$)	Underpowered study which indicated the corticosteroid-sparing potential of dapsone
2017 [**258**]	Mild to severe disease: doxycycline 200 mg/day versus prednisolone 0.5 mg/kg/day; both combined with topical mometasone furoate ≤30/week for the first 3 weeks	253	Treatment success at week 6 in 92% of the prednisolone group compared with 74% in the doxycycline arm; difference was not significantly inferior to the predefined 25% margin; at week 52 significantly less severe adverse events in patients started with doxycycline	Both primary endpoints were met; doxycycline was non-inferior to prednisolone after 6 weeks and resulted in less severe adverse effects after 52 weeks. Unusual study design that evaluated the treatment approach rather than the efficacy of the drugs
2017 [260]	Patients refractory to prednisolone 0.4 mg/kg/day: single cycle of IVIG 2 g/kg versus placebo	56	Disease activity score at day 15 was significantly lower in the IVIG group	IVIG has clinical efficacy in BP
2009 [262]	Moderate disease: topical clobetasol propionate 0.05% 40 g/day for 1 year (high dose) versus topical clobetasol propionate 0.05% 30 g/day for 4 months (low dose) Extensive disease: low-dose versus high-dose regimen	312	Moderate disease: twofold lower risk for death and severe adverse events in the low-dose group. More relapses in the low-dose group (51% versus 32%) Extensive disease: no difference in efficacy and adverse events	1-year mortality: 28–45%
2006 [292]	Azathioprine 2 mg/kg/day versus mycophenolate mofetil 2 g/day; both with methylprednisolone 0.5 mg/kg/day	73	No difference in time to healing of all lesions and cumulative corticosteroid dose (primary endpoints). More patients with elevated liver enzymes in the azathioprine arm	
2002 [**245**]	Moderate disease: topical clobetasol propionate 0.05% 40 g/day for 1 year versus prednisolone 0.5 mg/kg/day Extensive disease: topical clobetasol propionate 0.05% 40 g/day for 1 year versus prednisolone 1.0 mg/kg/day	341	Moderate disease: no difference in efficacy and adverse events Extensive disease: lower 1-year mortality (primary endpoint) and less severe adverse events with topical steroids	Landmark study that showed the efficacy of topical corticosteroids and the high risk of long-term higher dose (1 mg/day) prednisolone
1994 [293]	Nicotinamide 3 × 500 mg/day plus oxytetracycline 4 × 500 mg/day versus prednisolone 40–80 mg/day	20	Less adverse events in the tetracycline arm. No difference in efficacy	Low number of patients
1993 [294]	Prednisolone 1 mg/kg/day versus prednisolone 1 mg/kg/day plus azathioprine 100–150 mg/day versus prednisolone 1 mg/kg/day plus plasmapheresis (x4 one- to fivefold plasma volume within 2 weeks)	100	No difference in efficacy (disease control after 4 weeks and 6 months). More severe adverse events in the azathioprine arm	Termination of the study following interim analysis after 6 months due to severe adverse events in 30% of patients, in 14% fatal
1993 [295]	Prednisolone versus methylprednisolone, 1.0–1.5 mg/kg/day prednisolone equivalent	57	No difference in efficacy after 5 days. After 10 days less pruritus in the methylprednisolone group. Four severe adverse events within the first 10 days	Double blinded; only 10 days follow-up
1984 [296]	Prednisolone 0.75 mg/kg/day versus prednisolone 1.25 mg/kg/day for 3 weeks, then tapering	46	No difference in efficacy after 21 and 51 days (complete healing of lesions) and number of adverse events	
1984 [297]	Prednisolone 0.3 mg/kg/day versus prednisolone 0.3 mg/kg/day plus plasmapheresis (x8 1.5-fold plasma volume within 2 weeks). When no response after 1 week, prednisolone 1 mg/kg/day	41	Higher efficacy in the plasmapheresis group (more patients could be treated with the initial prednisolone dose, lower cumulative steroid dose)	Only mild adverse reactions of plasmapheresis
1978 [298]	Prednisolone 30–80 mg/day versus prednisolone 30–80 mg/day plus azathioprine 2.5 mg/kg/day	25	Lower cumulative steroid dose with azathioprine after follow-up of 3 years	Long follow-up time

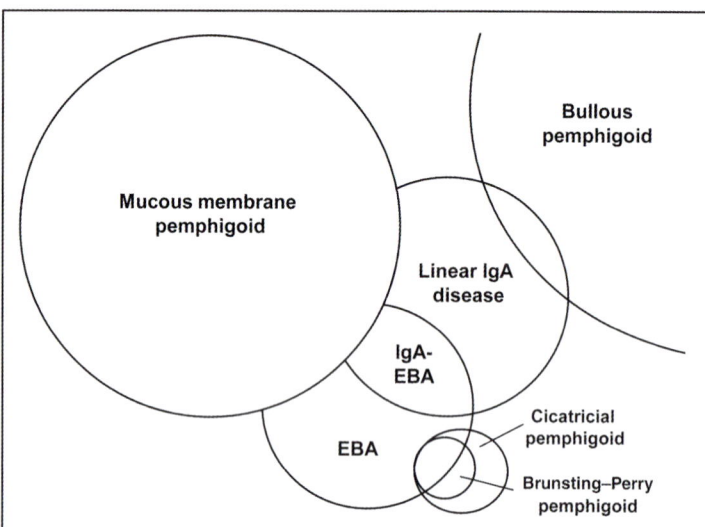

Figure 50.22 Diagnostic overlap between mucous membrane pemphigoid (MMP), linear IgA disease, epidermolysis bullosa acquisita (EBA), cicatricial pemphigoid and bullous pemphigoid. MMP is diagnosed in any patient with predominant mucosal lesions and antibodies against proteins of the basal membrane zone of surface-close epithelia irrespective of the autoantibody isotype and specificity [3]. Brunsting–Perry pemphigoid can be regarded as variant of cicatricial pemphigoid or EBA. The size of the circles approximates the incidence of the diseases.

involvement are termed ocular MMP, oral MMP, laryngeal MMP, etc., for example.

Classification links
- ICD-10: L12.1

Introduction and general description

MMP is the second most frequent autoimmune blistering disease in Central Europe. By definition, it predominantly affects the mucous membranes, most frequently the oral cavity followed by conjunctivae, nasopharynx, skin, the anogenital region, larynx and oesophagus [1,3,5,6]. Severe complications may arise with laryngeal and oesophageal involvement; conjunctival lesions result in scarring with a high risk of vision impairment and, ultimately, blindness.

The disease was first differentiated from pemphigus and BP in 1953 by Walter Lever as benign MMP or pemphigus conjunctivae [7]. Earlier reports of the disease are available by Wichmann (1798), Cooper (1858), Morris and Roberts (1889), and Thost (1911) [8–10].

As defined in the 1st International Consensus on MMP in 2002 [1] and elaborated in the S3 guideline of the EADV in 2021 [3,4], diagnosis is based on the clinical presentation of predominant mucosal manifestations and the detection of linear deposits of IgG and/or IgA and/or C3 at the DEJ by direct IF microscopy of a perilesional biopsy. Serum autoantibodies are only present in low titres compared with BP and detectable in 50–60% of patients. In about half of the patients, indirect IF microscopy on salt-split human skin, the standard screening test for serum autoantibodies in pemphigoid diseases, is negative [11,12]. In MMP, four target antigens have been well characterised on the molecular level: BP180 (type XVII collagen), BP230, laminin 332 and type VII collagen [2,4]. Additional data are required to confirm studies that described α6β4 integrin as

target antigen in MMP [4]. Reactivity with laminin 332 was shown to be associated with a malignancy in 25–30% of patients [4,13–18]. The clinical features and immunopathology are summarised in Table 50.2.

Epidemiology
Incidence and prevalence
In the early 1990s, the incidence was determined to be 0.9 and 1.3/million/year in Germany and France, respectively. Ten years later, the incidence appeared to have increased to 2.0/million/year in Germany [19–21]. In a prospective study, the incidence in the state of Schleswig-Holstein, Germany, was 2.1/million/year in 2016 [22]. The incidence of ocular MMP was calculated to be 0.7 and 0.8/million/year in the Australia/ New Zealand and UK, respectively [23,24]. In 2014, the prevalence of MMP has been calculated to be 24.6/million inhabitants in Germany [25].

Age
MMP is a disease of late middle to old age with a mean age of onset between 60 and 70 years [6,25–29]. It very rarely affects children and teenagers with only a few cases reported [30,31,32].

Sex
In a compilation of a large case series, a female predominance of 1.5- and 2.3-fold was reported [26,29].

Ethnicity
No geographical or racial predilection was observed.

Associated diseases
In several patient cohorts, 25–30% of patients with anti-laminin 332 antibodies presented with a solid cancer [13,14–17]. Recently, in a bicentric study with more than 150 MMP patients, a 6.8-fold higher risk of malignancy was calculated in anti-laminin 332 MMP patients compared with the general population [18]. In this study also, ocular lesions were associated with an increased risk of internal malignancies [18]. The S3 EADV guideline recommends a tumour search in every MMP patient with laminin 332-specific serum IgG [4]. No association with a malignancy was found in MMP patients overall irrespective of the target antigen as well as in patients with anti-α6β4 reactivity [33–35]. In some patients, an association with other autoimmune disorders such as thyroid diseases, rheumatoid arthritis, systemic lupus erythematosus and polyarthritis nodosa was observed [1,36].

Pathophysiology
Four different target antigens in patients with MMP have been recognised at the molecular level: BP180 (in about 75% of patients) [11,37], laminin 332 [38] (formerly termed laminin 5 and epiligrin; in 10–20%) [11,39–41], BP230 (in 25%; nearly exclusively in conjunction with anti-BP180 reactivity) [42] and type VII collagen (in <5% of patients) (Table 50.2) [4]. Reactivity against multiple antigens has repeatedly been reported [37,43–45]. In contrast to BP, C-terminal epitopes on BP180 are predominantly recognised in MMP rather than the NC16A domain, which is targeted by about 50% of BP180-reactive sera [11,37,43,46,47–50]. In about a

third of BP180-reactive sera, additional reactivity against epitopes on the intracellular portion of the molecule were described [11]. Antibodies against laminin 332 mainly react with the α3 chain with frequent reactivities against more than one chain [4]. Autoantibodies against an additional structural protein of the DEJ, α6β4 integrin, have been reported. IgG against α6 integrin was associated with oral lesions and reactivity against β4 integrin with ocular involvement [51–53]. Reactivity against α6β4 integrin, however, awaits confirmation by independent laboratories [4].

Autoantibodies in MMP may be IgG, IgA or of both isotypes [11,12,54–56]. A dual IgG and IgA autoantibody reactivity and antibodies against laminin 332 were associated with a more severe clinical phenotype [39,57]. Reactivity with BP180NC16A was more frequent in monosite mucosal lesions [18]. Higher disease activity was also linked to reactivity with multiple BP180 epitopes, and the HLA class II alleles DQB1*301, DRB1*04 and DRB1*11 [12,37].

The pathogenic relevance of autoantibodies in MMP has been demonstrated both *in vitro* and *in vivo*. Incubation with anti-BP180 NC16A IgG resulted in more prominent BP180 depletion in cultured skin compared with oral keratinocytes, whereas IgG against the BP180 C-terminus, which alone was not pathogenic in this *in vitro* system, led to BP180 depletion from both skin and oral keratinocytes when co-incubated with anti-BP180 NC16A IgG [58]. This observation was explained by the higher BP180 expression in oral compared with skin keratinocytes as well as the impaired interaction of the BP180 C-terminus with collagen type IV in oral keratinocytes upon treatment with IgG against the BP180 C-terminus [58,59]. The pathogenic relevance of antibodies against the BP180 C-terminus has not yet been shown *in vivo*.

Passive transfer of anti-laminin 332 IgG to neonatal or adult mice induced subepidermal blisters of skin and mucous membranes reproducing clinical, histological and immunopathological features of human MMP [60]. Of note and in contrast to BP, injection of Fab fragments against laminin 332 resulted in lesion formation and lesions could also be induced in mice lacking complement, mast cells or T cells, suggesting that such anti-laminin 332 antibodies elicit epidermal detachment in an Fc-independent manner [60,61]. In contrast, injection of IgG against the murine α6β43 chain in adult mice resulted in predominant oral and conjunctival as well as skin lesions. Lesion formation was completely dependent on Fcγ receptors and drastically reduced in C5a receptor-deficient mice [62]. In the latter model, dapsone significantly mitigated the development of both oral and skin lesions [63].

Antibodies to the α6 and β4 subunits of α6β4 integrin were shown to induce separation along the DEJ in organ cultures of oral and conjunctival mucosa [52,64–66] and injection of rabbit IgG against intracellular fragments of β4 integrin in neonatal mice induced subepidermal skin blisters [67].

Limited data about the role of T cells are available in MMP. In a subgroup of patients, peripheral T cells released IFNγ after stimulation with NC16A peptides [68].

Since scarring is the major pathogenic process in conjunctival disease, fibrosis has been intensively studied in biopsies and cultured conjunctival fibroblasts. Various profibrotic factors were identified, including heat shock protein 47, connective tissue growth factor, TGF-β, IL-4, IL-5, IL-13 and TNF-α [69–71].

Predisposing factors

No predisposing factors are known. It may be speculated that in the subgroup of anti-laminin 332 MMP associated with solid cancers, pathological expression of laminin 332 in the tumour tissue may have triggered the autoimmune disease.

Pathology

Histopathology. Histological examination of a blister is helpful only if the blister is intact and recent. Biopsy of an erosion is not adequate. Blisters in the mouth and on the skin show subepithelial or subepidermal blister formation, but often lack distinctive and diagnostic features. There are usually fewer eosinophils present in the cutaneous lymphohistiocytic infiltrate than in BP. However, MMP cannot be differentiated from other pemphigoid diseases based on histopathology [9,72]. At a later stage, fibrosis, the distinctive feature of MMP, may develop. The conjunctiva shows epithelial metaplasia, reduced numbers of goblet cells, and an lymphocytic infiltrate with plasma cells and an increased number of mast cells in the substantia propria, fibrosis of the lamina propria accompanied by inflammatory cells and an appearance of granulation tissue in the submucosa [73].

Tissue-bound autoantibodies. Tissue-bound autoantibodies can be visualised by direct IF microscopy of a perilesional biopsy. Linear deposits of IgG, C3 and/or IgA at the DEJ are diagnostic together with a compatible clinical phenotype (Figure 50.12) [1]. For further differentiation of the anti-DEJ staining, the n- versus u-pattern analysis can be performed [15] (Figure 50.12, insert). In all pemphigoid disease except EBA, an n-serrated pattern is seen. Alternatively, the biopsy is treated with 1 M NaCl solution to induce an artificial split in the DEJ at the lamina lucida level [74]. Autoantibody specificities can then be detected in a similar way to indirect IF microscopy on 1 M NaCl-split skin (see later; Figure 50.13). A further, not routinely available method is the double IF labelling of tissue-bound and defined antigens of the DEJ analysed by laser scanning confocal microscopy [75] that differentiates anti-laminin 332 MMP from BP, anti-p200 pemphigoid and reactivity with type VII collagen. The sensitivity of detection of linear C3d or C4d at the DEJ in paraffin-embedded issue biopsies was about 50% significantly lower compared with the same approach in BP [76].

Serum autoantibodies. Major characteristics of serum autoantibodies have been described above (see Pathophysiology, earlier).

For routine analysis of circulating autoantibodies, indirect IF microscopy on 1 M NaCl-split human skin is most appropriate (Figure 50.13). Its sensitivity of 50–70% is considerably lower as in BP [11,77–79]. Reactivity depends on the target antigen(s) and can be epidermal (most cases), dermal, or both (Figure 50.13). Monkey oesophagus, a BIOCHIP™ mosaic (Figure 50.14) and ELISA systems for anti-BP180 NC16A and anti-BP230 antibodies and a BIOCHIP™ mosaic with recombinant laminin 333 are commercially available [4,80,81,82].

Using skin from patients with epidermolysis bullosa that lack laminin 332 or type VII collagen expression by indirect IF in comparison with normal skin is an elegant method to detect antibodies against the two antigens [83]. Furthermore, indirect immuno-electron microscopy (rarely available) [84] and various in-house

ELISA, immunoblotting and immunoprecipitation analyses using cell-derived or recombinant forms of BP180, BP230, laminin 332, α6β4 integrin and type VII collagen are used in specialised laboratories.

Genetics

Associations with HLA-DQB1*03(01) [85–90], DRB1*04 [89] and DRB1*11(01) [88,89] have been reported. In contrast, a decreased frequency of the HLA-DRB1*02 allele was noted [88]. In MMP with ocular involvement, associations with HLA-DQB1*03(01) [85,87,91–93], DRB1*04 [87] and HLA-B12 [94] were found. In a genome-wide association study with British and German patients, the β-galactocerebrosidase (GALC) gene was associated with susceptibility to MMP [95].

Environmental factors

No environmental factors have been discovered so far.

Clinical features
Presentation

MMP most frequently affects the oral cavity (in 85% of patients) followed by conjunctivae (65%), skin (25–30%), nasal cavity (40–20%), anogenital area (20%), pharynx (20%), larynx (5–10%) and oesophagus (5–15%) [1,3,5,6,27]. Involvement of the trachea, urethra and anal canal has been reported in individual patients [96–98]. At all affected body sites except the oral cavity, lesions tend to heal with scarring. The various clinical manifestations of MMP have been extensively reviewed in the EADV S3 guideline [3].

The extent of oral lesions may vary considerably from mild almost asymptomatic erosions and chronic gingivitis to extensive extremely painful ulcers (Figure 50.23). Nasal lesions may present as haemorrhagic crusts and epistaxis, and can finally lead to disfiguring fibrosis and septum perforation. Pharyngeal lesions manifest with odynophagia, with initial involvement of the larynx as hoarseness. Oesophageal disease becomes symptomatic with dysphagia, odynophagia and heartburn. Genital lesions usually present with erosions (Figure 50.24). Scarring may lead to labial fusion and introital shrinkage with end-stage scarring that may be indistinguishable from lichen sclerosus [99]. Skin lesions may either resemble BP or heal with scarring and milia formation (Figure 50.25).

Ocular lesions usually start unilaterally with subtle symptoms such as burning, dryness and foreign body sensation, and may proceed to scar formation causing shortening of the inferior fornix, symblepharon, trichiasis, neovascularisation and, finally, blindness (Figure 50.26) (reviewed in [3,69]). Within 2 years, the disease is usually bilateral [5]. All patients with MMP should be seen by an ophthalmologist to recognise subtle changes by slit-lamp examination and measurement of the fornix depth (Figure 50.27). The latter is an objective clinical parameter for disease activity. In patients without initial ocular involvement, the annual risk for developing eye lesions was 5% over the first 5 years [6]. Of interest, ocular lesions have recently been associated with internal malignancies [18].

So far, reactivity with a specific target antigen has not been linked with a specific clinical presentation. Some data about a more frequent oral and pharyngo-laryngeal involvement in patients with anti-laminin 332 reactivity have been presented [100]. Of note,

because 25–30% of patients with anti-laminin 332 MMP have a solid cancer is present, a thorough tumour search is required in patients with this subtype of MMP [3].

Clinical variants

Oral pemphigoid. The term oral pemphigoid is used when the disease is restricted to the oral cavity. The predominant symptoms upon presentation include discomfort, burning, gingival bleeding, mucosal peeling and difficulty in eating. Desquamative gingivitis is the most frequent manifestation. Extragingival lesions present as reddish patches, erosion and blisters [3,101].

Ocular pemphigoid. When MMP is confined to the conjunctivae, which is found in about 20% of patients, the term ocular pemphigoid is applied [1,6]. Many patients initially complain of redness, tearing, burning, decreased vision and foreign body sensation. By the time of diagnosis, most patients have moderate to severe conjunctival inflammation with advanced cicatrising disease and symblepharon formation [3].

Vulvar pemphigoid. This rarely reported entity is characterised by recurrent blistering confined to the vulva of young girls, which does not result in scarring [102,103]. This form usually responds well to topical corticosteroids.

Differential diagnosis

The oral lesions, which may appear first, must be differentiated from PV, paraneoplastic pemphigus, oral lichen planus, Behçet disease, Stevens–Johnson syndrome and bacterial gingivitis [6]. Pemphigus can be excluded by direct IF microscopy or serologically. Lichen planus and Stevens–Johnson syndrome may be diagnosed histopathologically or, more easily, when skin or nail involvement is present.

For ocular disease, in particular when the conjunctivae are the only site of manifestation (ocular pemphigoid) and direct IF microscopy is negative (in about 20% of ocular pemphigoid), diagnosis can be challenging. Ocular rosacea, chronic anti-glaucoma therapy, conjunctival lichen planus, Stevens–Johnson syndrome, toxic epidermal necrolysis, Sjögren syndrome, graft-versus-host disease, chronic allergic conjunctivitis, severe atopic dermatitis, trauma, and viral and bacterial infections need to be excluded [4,6,23,69,104].

Classification of severity

Several classifications for ocular involvement of MMP have been proposed (reviewed in [3]). The classification of Foster is relatively simple and may also be applied by dermatologists [105]. The Mondino and Tauber systems require the measurement of fornix depth and better allow the documentation of disease progression (Table 50.5) [106–109]. An international panel of experts has recently proposed definitions for outcome measures and a clinical scoring system, the MMP Disease Area Index. The index records severity of skin lesions at 12 anatomical sites, scalp, mucosal lesions at 10 sites and both eyes [110]. The Oral Diseases Severity Score has also been validated for oral lesions in MMP [111].

The S3 guideline has defined mild and moderate MMP as diseases limited to the oral mucosa with or without skin involvement

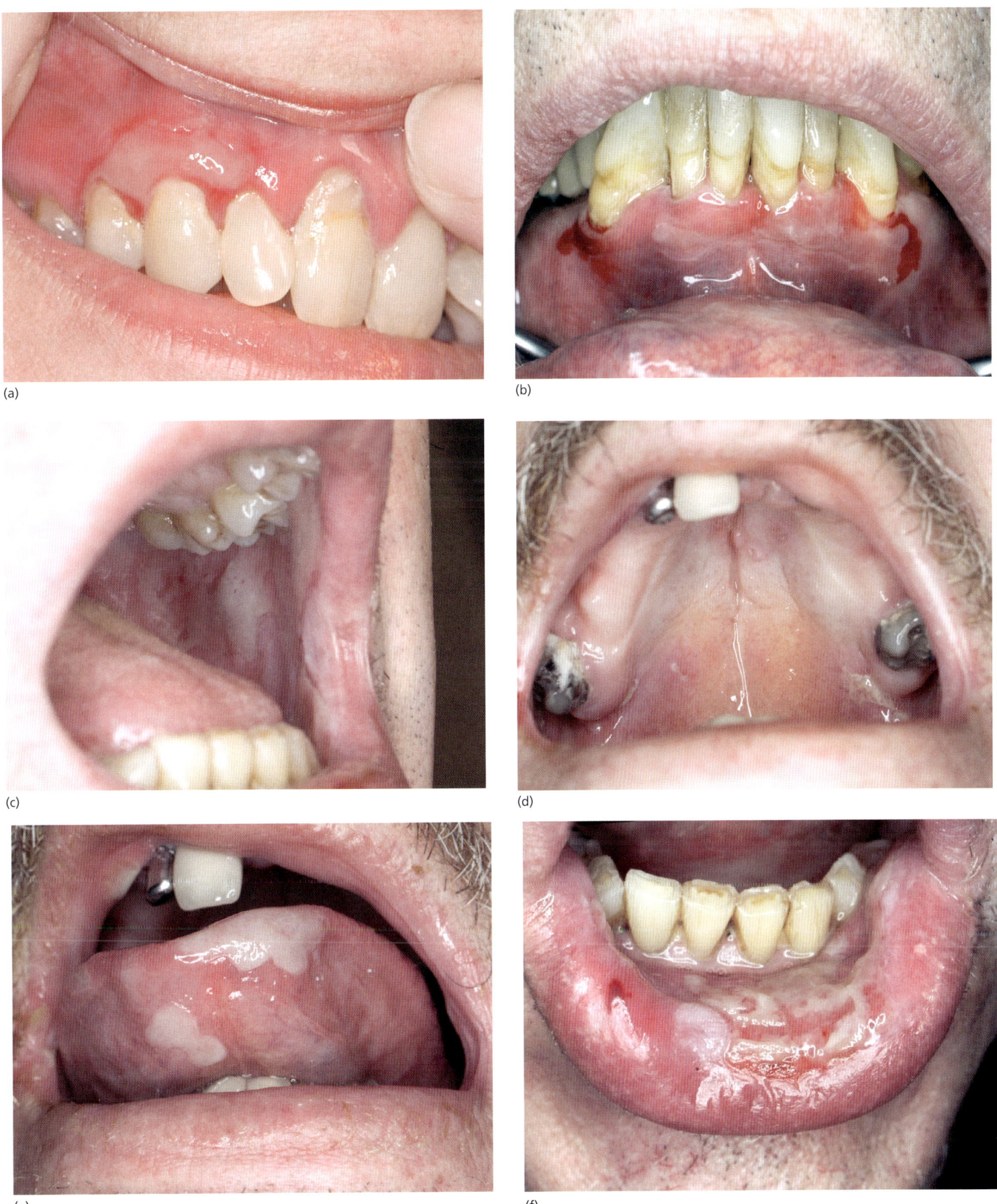

(a)

(b)

(c)

(d)

(e)

(f)

Figure 50.23 Oral lesions in mucous membrane pemphigoid.

PART 4: INFLAMMATORY DERMATOSES

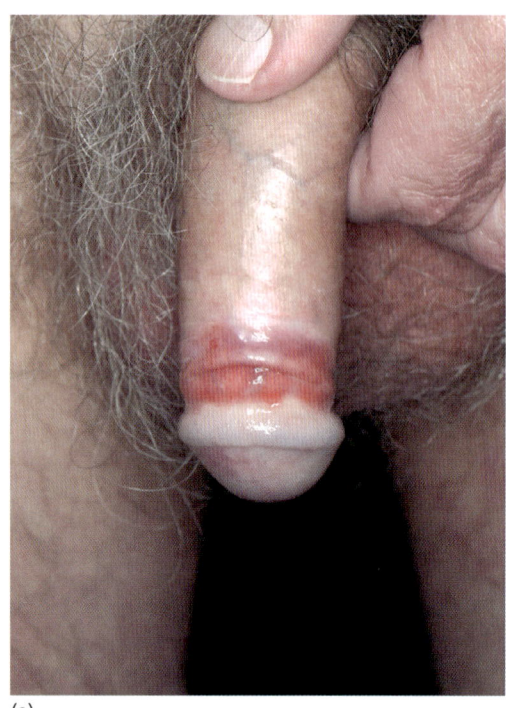

(a)

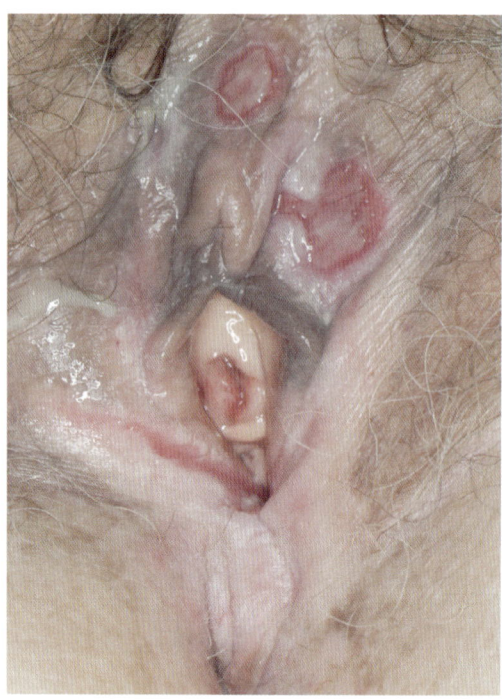

(b)

Figure 50.24 Genital involvement in mucous membrane pemphigoid.

Table 50.5 Classification of ocular disease in mucous membrane pemphigoid.

Stage	Foster [105]	Mondino [106–108]	Tauber [109]
I	Subconjunctival scarring/fibrosis	Loss of inferior fornix 0–25%	Subconjunctival scarring/ fibrosis
II	Shortening of fornix	25–50%	Shortening of fornix a–d describes loss of inferior fornix depth **a.** 0–25% **b.** 25–50% **c.** 50–75% **d.** 75–100%
III	Symblepharon	50–75%	Symblepharon a–d describes horizontal involvement by symblephara **a.** 0–25% **b.** 25–50% **c.** 50–75% **d.** 75–100%
IV	Ankyloblepharon	75–100%	Ankyloblepharon

replacing the term 'low-risk' MMP of the 2002 consensus. Severe MMP is now defined as MMP affecting an extraoral/cutaneous site replacing the term 'high-risk' MMP [1,3,4].

Complications and co-morbidities

Ocular inflammation and fibrosis can lead to the destruction of the tear ducts, corneal ulceration, corneal pannus and, ultimately, blindness. If laryngeal involvement is severe, life-threatening stenosis can occur requiring tracheotomy [112]. Deafness from involvement of the middle ear has been reported [27] as well as carcinoma arising from chronic oral and oesophageal lesions [113].

In 25–30% of patients with anti-laminin 332 MMP, a solid cancer develops [3].

Disease course and prognosis

MMP is typically a chronic and progressive disease. The disease often extends over many years with periods of activity and extension followed by quiescent phases. Unlike BP and linear IgA disease, MMP rarely goes into spontaneous remission except in localised oral disease [9,114,115]. Patients with dual IgG and IgA anti-DEJ autoantibodies were shown to have a more severe and persistent disease [12].

Investigations and diagnosis

Diagnosis is based on the combination of the clinical picture, direct IF microscopy, and serology. In contrast to BP, diagnosis is complicated by the generally lower amounts of autoantibodies both tissue-bound and circulating. In ocular involvement, close collaboration with an ophthalmologist experienced with the disease is mandatory for diagnosis, treatment decisions and follow-up.

Direct IF microscopy is the major diagnostic test for MMP with a sensitivity between 70% and 88% [4,116,117]. Indistinguishable from BP, deposition of IgG and/or C3 and, to a lesser degree, of IgA along the DEJ is detected. Serration pattern analysis (Figure 50.12, Figure 50.33) is not helpful in mucosal biopsies to differentiate deposition of anti-type VII collagen antibodies from other antibody specificities [118]. In ocular MMP, detection of autoantibodies by direct IF microscopy may fail in up to 20% [6,119]. The site for biopsy often presents a challenge. Direct IF of a biopsy from skin was more sensitive than from conjunctiva in MMP with ocular involvement, biopsies from normal buccal mucosa revealed a

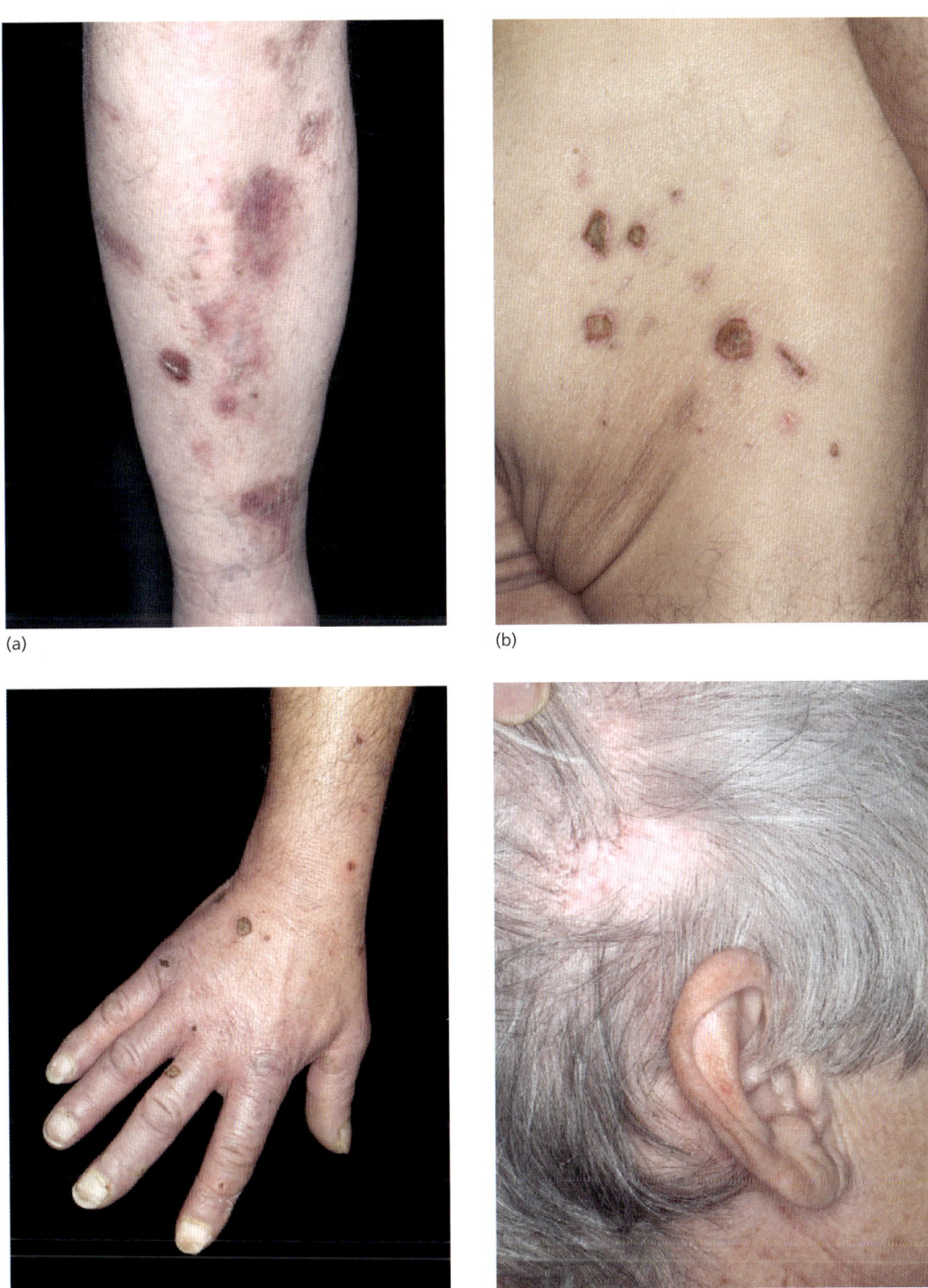

(a)

(b)

(c)

(d)

Figure 50.25 Skin lesions in mucous membrane pemphigoid. Brownish erythema, erosions and some crusts on the right thigh (a). Erosions, ulcerations and some atrophic scars on the right buttock (b). Multiple crusted erosions on the right hand (c). Atrophic alopecic scar on the right occiput (d). Of note, all patients had concurrently predominant mucous membrane lesions (not shown).

similar sensitivity compared with perilesional oral mucosa, and importantly, repeated biopsies for direct IF increased the sensitivity from 70% to 95% [117,120,121]. According to the S3 guideline [4], we recommend a perilesional skin biopsy in patients with skin involvement, and in patients without skin involvement the intact buccal mucosa as the biopsy site. This also applies for patients without oral lesions. If negative, a repeated biopsy preferentially from another mucosal site is recommended. If a conjunctival biopsy is required on suspicion of ocular pemphigoid, to avoid the risk of

disease exacerbation, infiltration anaesthesia should be avoided, biopsy size limited to 2 × 3 mm, the upper fornix or limbus chosen as the biopsy site, and surgery may follow topical treatment with corticosteroids and antibiotic for 1 week.

By indirect IF microscopy on salt-split skin, epidermal and/or dermal staining of the artificial split is seen depending on the target antigen (Figure 50.13). In contrast to BP, MMP sera contain anti-DEJ reactivity at low titres (1:10–1:40) and in a lower percentage (50–80%) [4,5,11,12,43]. In about 60% of MMP sera, IgA autoantibodies can be

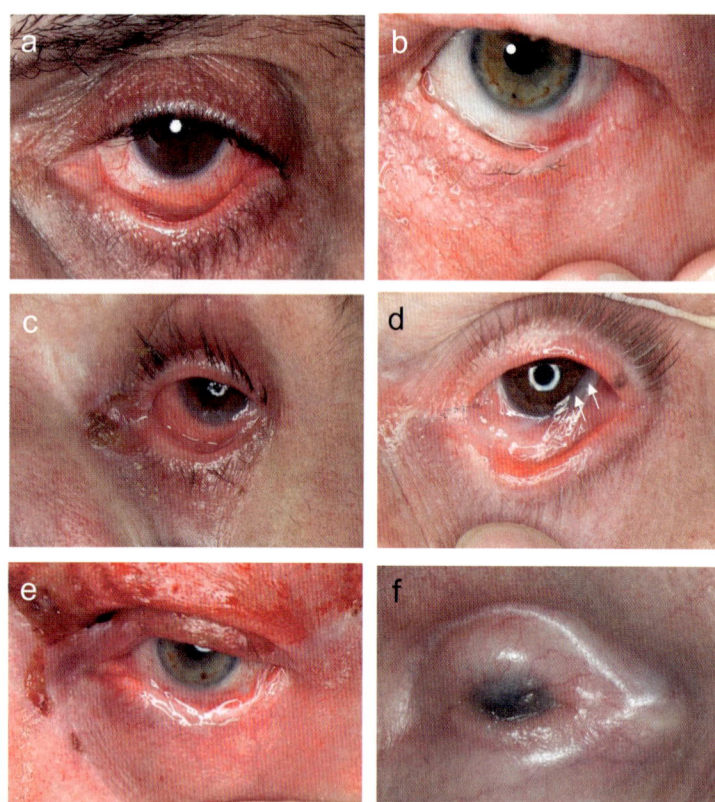

Figure 50.26 (a) Ocular disease in mucous membrane pemphigoid. Conjunctival hyperaemia, inferior fornix shortening and loss of the plica in early disease (Foster II, Mondino II, Tauber IIb). (b) Loss of the temporal fornix and symblepharon with loss of lashes (Foster III, Mondino III, Tauber IId). (c) Intensive conjunctival injection with discrete shortening of the inferior fornix and periocular erosions and crusts. (d) Shortening of the inferior fornix and limbal scarring (white arrows. (e) Complete loss of inferior fornix with some symblephara and loss of lashes (Foster III, Mondino IV, Tauber IId, IIIb). (f) End stage disease showing a 'frozen globe' and keratin covering the dry surface (Foster IV, Mondino IV, Tauber IV) (f).

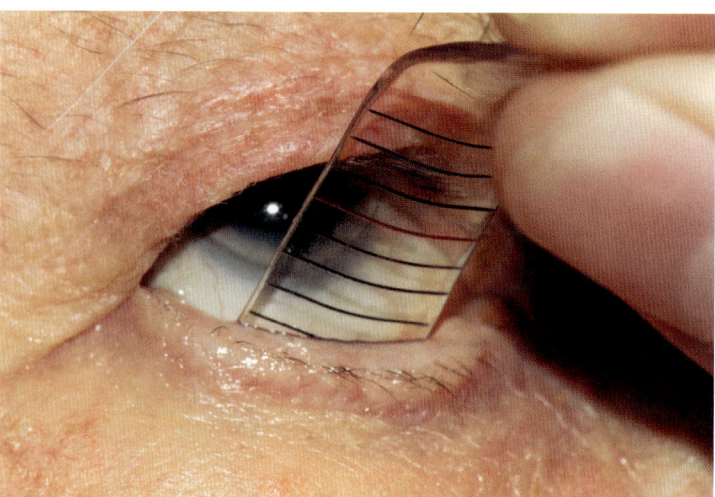

Figure 50.27 Fornix meter. Measurement of the fornix depth by an experienced ophthalmologist is important for objective assessment of ocular disease activity. Courtesy of Dr Gerd Geerling, Department of Ophthalmology, University of Düsseldorf, Germany.

detected [11,12,37,43,122,123] and in 10–30% of sera, autoantibody reactivity is restricted to the IgA isotype [11,116,123]. Due to the relatively low indirect IF microscopy reactivity it is also recommended to use antigen-specific highly standardised test systems to detect serum autoantibodies in indirect IF-negative patients. Commercial test systems for serum IgG against BP180 NC16A, BP230, type VII collagen and, more recently, against laminin 332 are available [4]. Latter indirect IF assay is based on the BIOCHIP™ technology and uses a human cell line recombinantly expressing laminin 332 on the cell surface. In a large multicentre study, this method revealed a sensitivity of 84% and a specificity of 100% (Figure 50.28) [81]. Due to the associated malignancy in 25–30% of patients, detection of anti-laminin 332 serum IgG is recommended in every patient with negative indirect IF on salt-split skin or dermal binding [4]. IgA and IgE antibodies against laminin 332 have also been reported in individual MMP patients [124,125]. Elegantly, indirect IF microscopy on laminin 332-deficient skin can be applied in salt-split skin-reactive sera [83].

So far, no widely available assay for antibodies against the BP180 C-terminus has been established. For detection of these antibodies, various assays based on recombinant fragments or cell-derived forms of BP180, including the soluble ectodomain of BP180 (LAD-1) in conditioned concentrated medium of cultured keratinocytes, as well as, for example, extract of human oral mucosa, amniotic membrane and cultured oral keratinocytes are employed in specialised laboratories [11,37,41,43,46–50,123,126–128]. Immunoblotting with bovine gingiva lysate, hemidesmosomal-rich extract, and recombinant fragments have been used to determine serum α6β4integrin-specific antibodies in three specialised laboratories [51–53,129]; currently, this service is limited to anti-β4 integrin IgG in one of them.

Lesional histopathology facilitates differentiation of MMP from PV and is helpful to evaluate differential diagnoses if direct IF and serology are negative [4].

The diagnostic work-up in MMP is summarised in Figure 50.29.

Management
General principles of management
The treatment of MMP is challenging for several reasons: (i) only three controlled therapeutic trials have been conducted; (ii) clinical response to immunosuppression in patients with severe disease, in particular with ocular lesions, is poor; and (iii) conjunctival fibrosis is irreversible and, in contrast to other pemphigoid diseases, causes permanent damage when treatment is delayed or ineffective [1,73]. In fact, conjunctival, laryngeal and oesophageal scarring may even continue for some time after inflammation has been successfully treated. The primary treatment aim is to stop the inflammation without delay. Management of MMP warrants a multidisciplinary approach involving specialists from dermatology, ophthalmology, otorhinolaryngology, gastroenterology and gynaecology/urology [4].

Controlled randomised trials. In all three trials, only ocular involvement was studied. One trial with 24 patients showed a superior effect of oral cyclophosphamide 2 mg/day plus prednisolone 1.0 mg/kg/day versus prednisolone 1.0 mg/kg/day alone. The other trial included 40 patients and compared dapsone 2 mg/kg/day and cyclophosphamide 2 mg/day with response in 14 and 20 patients, respectively [73,130]. In a more recent study with 30 MMP patients from Egypt, the IV administration of the anti-TNF-α drug pentoxifylline in combination with corticosteroid and

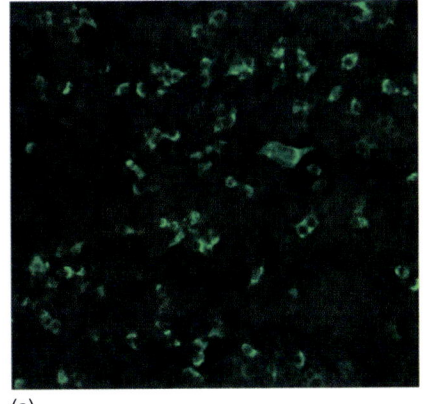
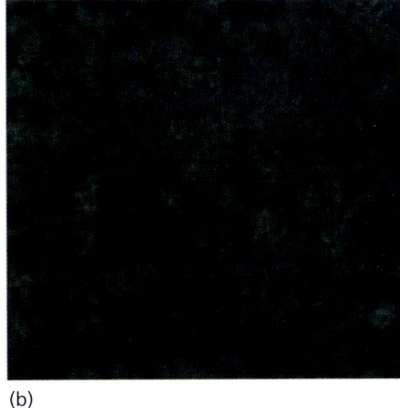

(a) (b)

Figure 50.28 Biochip™ mosaic for detection of serum anti-laminin 332 IgG. HEK293 cells recombinantly express the laminin 332 heterotrimer on their cell surface. IgG reactivity is seen with an MMP serum (a) but not a normal human serum (b). Of note, transfection of cells is suboptimal to also provide laminin 332-negative cells as an internal negative control.

cyclophosphamide pulses was more effective than corticosteroid and cyclophosphamide pulses alone [131].

Other clinical studies. Larger uncontrolled studies showed efficacy of the sulpha drugs dapsone, sulphapyridine and sulphamethoxy-pyridazine (in oral, ocular and generalised MMP) [130,132], cyclophosphamide (ocular, oral and generalised MMP) [130,133], minocycline (oral MMP) [130], topical mitomycin (ocular MMP) [134,135], methotrexate (ocular MMP) [136,137], mycophenolate mofetil (ocular MMP) [138,139] and IVIG (ocular and oral MMP) [140–142].

A retrospective study with 115 patients with ocular lesions (223 eyes) reported the highest efficacy for cyclophosphamide followed by mycophenolate, azathioprine and dapsone, with the lowest number of adverse reactions for mycophenolate and the highest for azathioprine [139]. In a similarly designed study with 15 MMP patients, colchicine was identified as the most effective drug in combination with prednisolone 40 mg/day compared with azathioprine, cyclophosphamide, tetracycline and dapsone [143].

Since the first use of rituximab in severe treatment refractory MMP that led to healing of all oral lesions but could not prevent progression of ocular disease [144], data from more than 100 patients, mostly with generalised MMP, are available [145]. The two largest studies included 24 and 25 cases [146,147]. All 24 rituximab-treated patients reached disease control (as defined in [110]) compared with 40% of 25 MMP patients treated with conventional immunosuppression [147]. A systematic review, including the latter two studies, concluded that in about 70% of the 112 included rituximab-treated MMP patients, all lesions had healed, which is about 10–20% fewer compared with pemphigus [148–150]. Of note, relapses occurred in about a third of rituximab-treated MMP patients [145,147,151,152]. To this end, five rituximab-unresponsive patients rapidly achieved complete remission on IVIG [153]. In the above-mentioned systematic review, complete remission was reported in 62% of 154 MMP patients treated with IVIG and 71% of seven patients following use of TNF-α inhibitors [145].

In addition, individual patients were successfully treated with the proteasome-inhibitor bortezomib and the JAK1/2 inhibitor baricitinib, respectively [154,155].

Comprehensive overviews about all published clinical studies were provided by the Cochrane Collaboration (until 2005) and, more recently, the S3 guideline [4,156].

Treatment guidelines. National guidelines for the management of MMP have been proposed by French, Japanese and Brazilian societies of dermatology [157–159]. The recommendations of the EADV S3 guideline are presented later [4].

In mild and moderate MMP, i.e. in patients with lesions limited to the mouth with or without skin involvement, high-potency topical corticosteroids as adhesive paste, mouthwash or spray are proposed as first line therapy either alone or in combination with dapsone, methotrexate or doxycycline [4]. In refractory oral MMP, intralesional triamcinolone has been applied successfully [160]. High-potency topical corticosteroids are also recommended as first line approach for genital MMP, in particular in vulvar MMP in minors. Secondary infection of oral and genital mucosae with candida is common and should be treated with antifungal therapy. Oral hygiene, including patient instructions and professional periodontal therapy, is recommended since periodontal plaques and bleeding in oral MMP are significantly reduced if recommendations are followed [161]. In all other forms of severe MMP, defined as MMP with extraoral manifestations excluding the skin, systemic medication in addition to topical treatment is recommended [4].

Management algorithm

The treatment ladder is modified from the EADV S3 guideline [4].

In ocular involvement, close cooperation with an ophthalmologist experienced in MMP is required to monitor ocular disease activity, adjust topical treatment including corticosteroids, tetracyclines, cyclosporine and lubricants, as well as surgical therapy for control of trichiasis [4]. Treatment of ocular MMP, i.e. in patients with lesions limited to the eyes, is detailed elsewhere [4,162–164].

Treatment ladder for mucous membrane pemphigoid

Oral pemphigoid (mild and moderate MMP)[a]

Mild

First line
- Oral hygiene *and*
- Topical high-potency topical corticosteroids

Second line
- As in moderate oral MMP

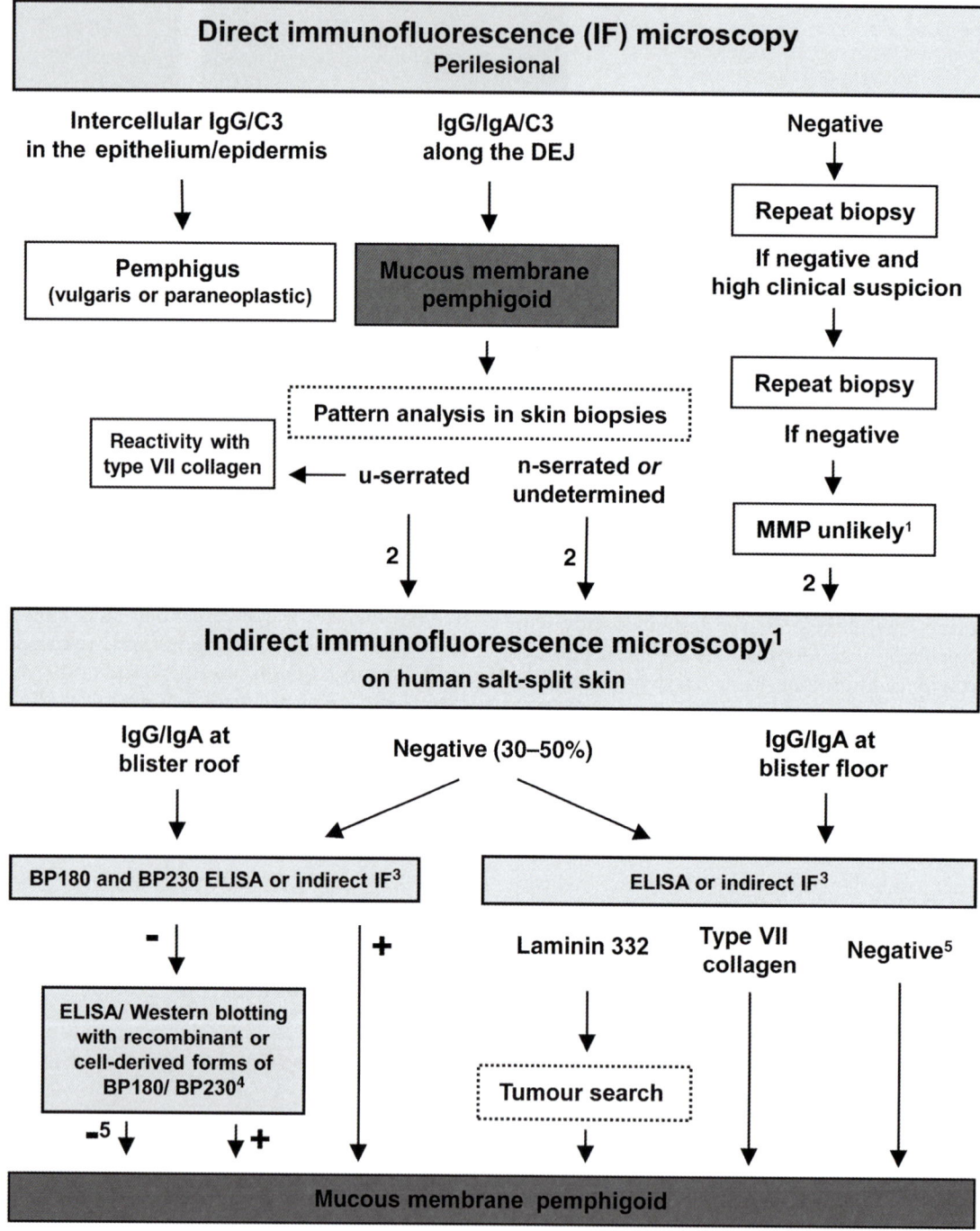

Figure 50.29 Diagnostic pathway for mucous membrane pemphigoid (MMP) (adapted from the EADV S3 guideline). 1, Unlike in ocular MMP; in ocular MMP, the combination of direct immunofluorescence (IF) and serology is negative in up to 20–50% of patients; 2, serum autoantibodies are recommended to be determined irrespective of the direct IF result; 3, commercially available (for IgG antibodies); 4, only available in specialised diagnostic centres; 5, with positive direct and/or indirect IF microscopy.

Moderate

First line
- As in mild oral MMP *plus*
- Dapsone 1.0–1.5 mg/kg/day[b] *or*
- Tetracyclines, e.g. doxycycline 200 mg/day or minocycline 50 mg/day

Second line
- As in severe oral MMP

Severe
- As in moderate oral MMP *plus*
- Prednisolone 0.5 mg/kg/day tapering *plus*
- Mycophenoles (mofetil 2 g/day, gastroresistant mycophenoloic acid 1.440 g/day)

Severe MMP[a]

First line
- Dapsone 1.0–1.5 mg/kg/day[2] *plus* prednisolone 0.5–1.0 mg/kg/day tapering[c]
- in case of rapid progression in conjunctivae, larynx or oesophagus *plus*
- Cyclophosphamide (50 mg/day p.o. *or* 500–50 mg/ 3–4 weeks IV)[d]

Second line
- Prednisolone 0.5–1.0 mg/kg/day tapering[c] *plus*
- Dapsone 1.0–1.5 mg/kg/day[b] *or* mycophenoles (see above) *plus*
- Rituximab 2× 1 g

Third line
- *plus* IVIG

[a] As defined by [3,4].
[b] With normal glucose-6-phosphate-dehydrogenase level.
[c] Alternatively, IV dexamethasone pulses (100 mg on 3 consecutive days every 3–4 weeks) can be applied.
[d] After disease control has been achieved, mycophenolates (mofetil 2 g/day, gastroresistant mycophenoloic acid 1.440 g/day) can be given.

Linear IgA disease

Definition, nomenclature and classification

This pemphigoid disease is defined by its main immunopathological feature, the exclusive or predominant binding of IgA along the DEJ (Table 50.2). Linear IgA disease (LAD) is the most frequent autoimmune blistering disease in infants and children. For this age group, several terms have been designed (see Synonyms and inclusions). It later became clear that, immunopathologically, diseases in children and adults are identical, although some clinical features may slightly differ. The use of the term LAD for both age groups is therefore recommended. Some overlap is seen with BP (in patients with dual IgG and IgA deposition along the DEJ) and EBA (in patients with IgA autoantibodies against type VII collagen) [1,2]. The recent EADV S3 guideline for mucous membrane pemphigoid has classified patients with predominant mucosal lesions irrespective of the autoantibodies isotype as MMP [3,4] (Figure 50.22).

Synonyms and inclusions
- Linear IgA bullous dermatosis

Adults:
- Linear IgA disease of adults
- IgA bullous pemphigoid

Children:
- Chronic bullous disease/dermatosis of childhood
- Linear IgA disease of childhood
- Benign chronic bullous dermatosis of childhood

Classification links (as appropriate)
- ICD-10: L12.2 (chronic bullous dermatosis of childhood), L12.8 (other pemphigoid disorders)

Introduction and general description

Tense blisters, vesicles and annular erythema are the clinical hallmarks. Frequently, blisters are arranged annularly, a formation referred to as 'crown of jewels' or 'string of pearls' and mucous membrane lesions are present. Skin lesions have the same morphology in children and adults. However, they arise more abruptly in children and predilection sites are different [5,6].

LAD was first differentiated from dermatitis herpetiformis in 1975 by Chorzelski and Jablonska by the finding of linear deposits of IgA antibodies at the DEJ by direct IF microscopy [7–9]. The linear deposits of predominant or exclusive IgA antibodies at the DEJ are still the diagnostic hallmark of LAD [1]. As for the other pemphigoid diseases, indirect IF microscopy on human salt-split skin is an appropriate screening test for serum IgA antibodies in suspected LAD [10,11]. Immunodominant epitopes were later localised on the ectodomain of BP180 [12,13]. Reactivity with type VII collagen, BP230, laminin 332 and various not molecularly characterised antigens have also been described [14,15–21].

The clinical features and immunopathology are summarised in Table 50.2.

Epidemiology

Incidence and prevalence

An incidence of 0.25–1.0 patients with LAD/million/year was reported in Central Europe, Singapore and Kuwait [22–25]. In a prospective study, the incidence in the state of Schleswig-Holstein, Germany, was 1.0/ million/year in 2016 [26]. LAD is the most frequent autoimmune blistering diseases in children, while the majority of LAD patients are adults. In 2014, the prevalence of LAD has been calculated to be 10.3/million inhabitants in Germany [27]. In minors, the prevalence was 24.5/million in the age group below 18 years of age [28]. The incidence appeared to be higher in developing countries such as Malaysia, India, Thailand, Tunisia, Mali, South Africa and Uganda [29–35]. It may be speculated that this is related to the different age distribution of the populations with up to half of the population being minors in these countries [29].

Age

LAD is the most frequent immunobullous disorder in children [36]. As such, two peaks of onset are recognised, below the age of 5 and between the age of 60 and 65 years [5,27].

Sex

A slight female predominance was observed [5]. However, larger studies are lacking.

Ethnicity

No geographical or racial predilection was observed.

Associated diseases

A slightly higher frequency of lymphoproliferative disorders and non-lymphoid malignancies as well as ulcerative colitis compared with the general population has been found [37–39]. A recent literature review showed that in 94% of LAD patients with concomitant ulcerative colitis, the colitis preceded the autoimmune blistering diseases indicating that the bowel disease most likely triggers the immunobullous disorder [40]. Of interest, BP180, the only target antigen identified in these LAD patients, is also expressed in the basement membrane zone of colon. Furthermore, numerous case reports with a variety of concomitant diseases in LAD have been published [6].

Pathophysiology

The major *target antigen* is the ectodomain of BP180. Initially, two target molecules in LAD were described. Zone *et al.* reported a 97 kDa protein in the extract of human epidermis and dermis termed the linear IgA bullous dermatosis antigen (LABD) 97 and Marinkovich *et al.* a 120 kDa protein in the conditioned culture supernatant of human keratinocytes, referred to as linear IgA antigen-1 (LAD-1) [12,13]. Later, it became clear that both antigens represent C-terminal portions of BP180 [41,42] (Figure 50.30). The N-termini of both antigens were localised within the NC16A domain of BP180 [43]. LAD-1 has different N-termini since the shedding of this fragment from the cell surface is mediated by at least three different sheddases (ADAM 9, 10, and 17) [44] producing BP180 fragments with different cleavage sites between Asp514 and Ala531 [42,43,45] (Figure 50.30). Some of them may function as neoepitopes [45,46]. LABD97 appears to be generated from BP180 by plasmin [47].

In contrast to BP and MMP, the BP180 NC16A domain is targeted in only 20% of LAD patients [48]. Exclusive IgA reactivity against the NC16A domain has only been described in individual patients [48,49]. Most patients react with multiple epitopes on the BP180 ectodomain [48,50]. In line with this, NC16A-specific T cells have been identified in LAD patients [51].

IgA antibodies in LAD were reported to be exclusively of the IgA1 subclass [52]. In fact, the majority of LAD sera, in addition to IgA anti-BP180 antibodies, also contain IgG antibodies against BP180 [50,53]. Interestingly, in most BP sera, IgA anti-BP180 antibodies can also be detected [53]. The two diseases may thus be regarded as different ends of a continuous spectrum with some overlap [53] (Figure 50.22). This notion is supported by the finding that the isotype of anti-DEJ reactivity was associated with the age of the patients: in younger patients, IgA autoantibodies predominated,

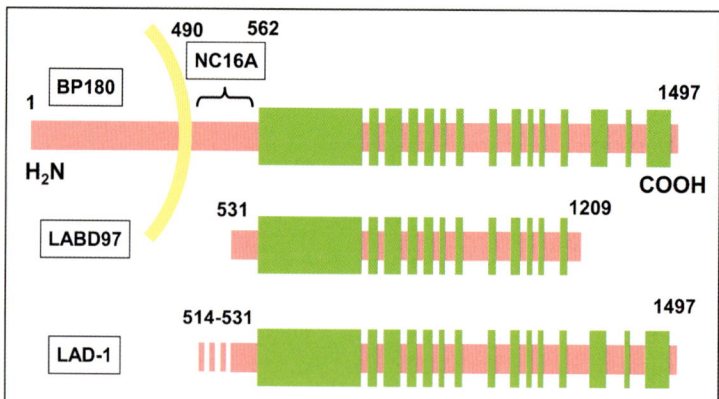

Figure 50.30 Schematic diagram of BP180 (type VII collagen) and its cell-derived fragments recognised by linear IgA disease (LAD) sera. Most LAD sera contain IgA reactivity against two fragments of the BP180 ectodomain, the 97 kDa linear IgA bullous dermatosis antigen (LABD97) and the 120 kDa linear IgA disease antigen 1 (LAD-1). While LABD97 is present in extract of human epidermis and dermis, LAD-1 is shed by ADAM 9, 10, and 17 from membrane-bound full-length BP180 of cultured human keratinocytes and, depending on the particular ADAM, has different N-termini. In only about 20% of LAD sera, IgA antibodies against the extracellular portion of the 16th non-collagenous domain (NC16A), the immunodominant region in bullous pemphigoid and pemphigoid gestationis, are found. Green boxes, collagenous domains; yellow, cell membrane. Amino acid numbers are depicted above the molecules.

whereas in older patients preferentially anti-DEJ antibodies of the IgG isotype were found [29]. For patients with equal IgG and IgA reactivity against the DEJ, the diagnosis 'mixed immunobullous dermatosis' or 'linear IgA/IgG bullous dermatosis' was proposed [54,55] (see Clinical variants, later).

The mechanism of blister formation in LAD is not fully understood but is likely to involve IgA- and complement-mediated neutrophil chemotaxis. The pathogenic role of autoantibodies was first suggested by the adherence of stimulated human neutrophils along the DEJ after preincubation with LAD serum [56]. In line with this, in cultured human skin samples, the incubation with LAD sera resulted in dermal–epidermal separation [57]. In both approaches, the direct effect of serum proteases or IgG antibodies could not be excluded. The injection of monoclonal IgA anti-LAD-1 antibodies in human skin grafted onto SCID mice leading to microscopic subepidermal splitting in some of the mice, was the first direct proof of the pathogenic potential of IgA antibodies in LAD [58]. In line, monoclonal IgA against type VII collagen induced dermal–epidermal separation in normal human skin after incubation with normal human leukocytes [59].

In conjunction with anti-BP180 antibodies, IgA reactivity against BP230 can be found in some LAD sera [18,60]. Predominant or exclusive IgA antibodies against type VII collagen have been reported in a number of patients [15,19,61,62]. These patients can be attributed to the sublamina densa variant of LAD [63] and may also be diagnosed as IgA EBA (see below) (Figure 50.22). In individual patients, IgA antibodies against laminin 332 and the p200 antigen were reported [16,17,64].

Predisposing factors

LAD can be triggered by various drugs, most frequently vancomycin (in 50–60% of reported cases), followed by penicillins, non-steroidal anti-inflammatory drugs and phenytoin (all in about

5% of reported cases) [5,37,65–70]. In line, in a retrospective study with 69 drug-associated LAD patients retrieved from the French Pharmacovigilance network, 57% patients used vancomycin [**71**]. Of note, in some cases of vancomycin-induced LAD, IgA reactivity only reacted by indirect IF microscopy on human skin as well as with recombinant type VII collagen by immunoblotting and ELISA when sera were co-incubated with vancomycin [72]. A large number of other drugs were also associated with the onset of LAD [6,70,**71**,73]. Furthermore, infections, trauma, vaccination, UV-radiation exposure and building work in the home were also reported as precipitating factors [5,37,69,74–76].

Pathology

Histopathology of a lesional biopsy typically shows subepidermal splitting and in the majority of patients, an infiltrate with neutrophils in the papillary dermis sometimes forming microabscesses as typically seen in dermatitis herpetiformis. In about a quarter of patients, eosinophils predominate and in about 50% of patients, lymphocytes are present [5,62,77,78] (Figure 50.31). Similar alterations may be seen in other pemphigoid diseases including BP, MMP and anti-p200 pemphigoid. Accumulation of IL-8 was observed in the epidermis and perivascularly and of IL-5 at the site of blistering [78].

Tissue-bound autoantibodies can be visualised by direct IF microscopy of a perilesional biopsy. Linear deposits of IgA, frequently accompanied by weaker staining of IgG and/or C3, at the

DEJ are diagnostic (Figure 50.32). By serration pattern analysis, a u-serrated pattern is seen with anti-type VII collagen autoantibodies (Figure 50.33). In all other autoantibody specificities, an n-serrated pattern is observed [61,79–81] (Figure 50.12, insert).

By direct immunoelectron microscopy three binding patterns of IgA autoantibodies have been described; at the lamina lucida, at or below the lamina densa, and, reported by Prost *et al.*, above and below the lamina lucida in a so-called mirror image [82–85]. These observations have led to the concept of classifying LAD in a lamina lucida type and a sublamina densa type. The latter type is most likely characterised by autoantibodies against type VII collagen [**63**] and may also be classified as IgA EBA.

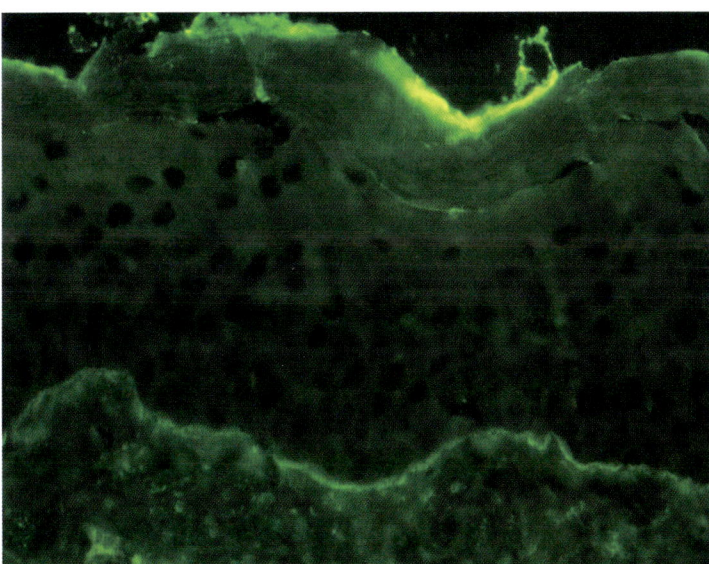

Figure 50.32 Direct immunofluorescence microscopy of a perilesional biopsy in linear IgA disease. Linear deposition of IgA at the dermal–epidermal junction.

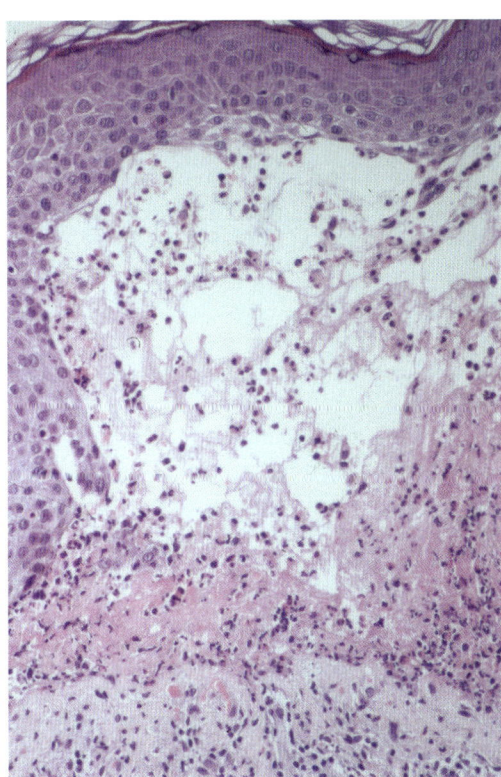

Figure 50.31 Lesional histopathology of linear IgA disease. H&E staining shows subepidermal splitting with a dense inflammatory infiltrate in the blister cavity and the underlying upper dermis composed of neutrophils, eosinophils and some lymphocytes. A similar histopathological pattern may also be seen in bullous pemphigoid, mucous membrane pemphigoid and anti-p200 pemphigoid.

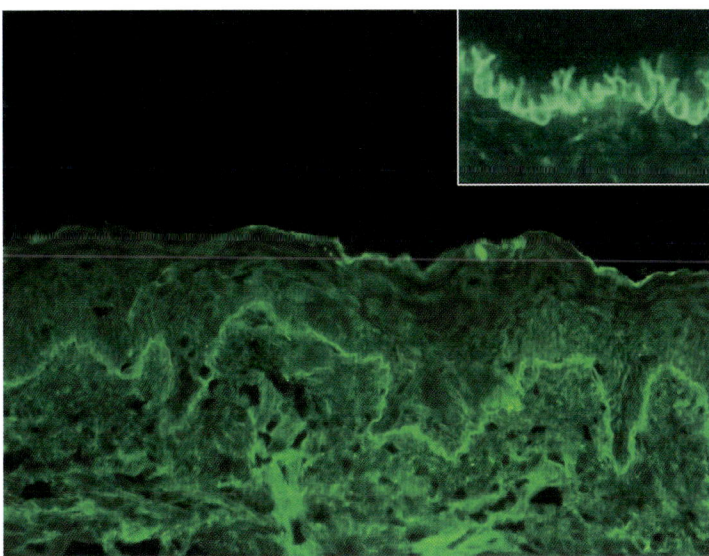

Figure 50.33 Direct immunofluorescence microscopy of a perilesional biopsy of a patient with epidermolysis bullosa acquisita. Linear deposition of IgG at the dermal–epidermal junction. A u-serrated pattern is seen (inset) with IgA reactivity in IgA epidermolysis bullosa acquisita (not shown).

Genetics

The only study on the genetic susceptibility of LAD identified an association with HLA-B8, HLA-Cw7, DR3, DR2 and the TNF2 allele as well as in children, with B8, DR3, DQ2, and also TNF2 [86]. In addition, five of 20 South African children with LAD (all black Africans) had the B8 allele, which is uncommon in this population [31].

Environmental factors

No environmental factors have been discovered so far. Trigger factors were described in Predisposing factors, earlier.

Clinical features
Presentation

In both children and adults, the individual lesions are similar, including tense blisters and vesicles, urticated plaques, erosions and red macules (Figures 50.34 and 50.35) [5]. Blisters and vesicles frequently arise in an annular pattern with blistering along the edge of lesions forming the so-called 'string of pearls', 'crown of jewels', or 'cluster of jewels' sign (Figure 50.36a) [6]. Of note, this sign is not pathognomonic for LAD and may also be seen in BP (Figure 50.36b). Pruritus is variable from absent to severe. In children, lesions arise more abruptly compared with adults and tend to involve the perioral area and perineum in addition to the other predilection sites, trunk and limbs. The latter localisations are mainly involved in adult patients [5,87]. Mucosal involvement is common (in about 60–70% of patients) with mostly oral erosions and ulcers; nasal crusting and genital lesions may also occur [5,62]. When mucous membrane lesions are predominant, MMP is diagnosed [3,4] (Figure 50.22). As in BP, lesions tend to heal without scarring unless extensive superinfection occurs. Milia formation is uncommon.

Clinical variants
Mixed immunobullous disease and linear IgA/IgG bullous dermatosis. For patients with equal IgA and IgG deposits at the DEJ,

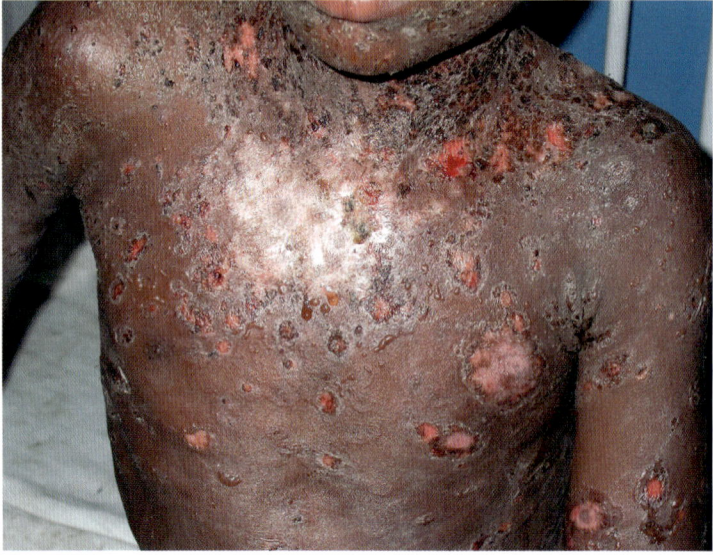

Figure 50.34 Linear IgA disease. Erosions and tense blisters on the trunk in a Ugandan child. Lesions were also present on the face.

as defined by direct or indirect IF microscopy, these two terms have been proposed [54,55,88]. No specific clinical phenotype was identified in these entities. Since in most LAD patients, IgG autoantibodies against proteins of the DEJ can also be found [50,53,54,88,89] and most BP sera also contain IgA autoantibodies, these cases may represent the centre of an LAD-BP spectrum.

Sub-lamina densa variant and IgA EBA. The sub-lamina densa variant as defined by the direct immunoelectron microscopical appearance, dermal binding of IgA along the floor of the artificial blister by indirect IF microscopy of human salt-split skin, or IgA reactivity against type VII collagen, is a rare subtype comprising 2–9% of LAD patients [90,91]. Classification of this variant as LAD or EBA is currently debated [2]. In a study with four patients with this variant, they appeared to differ from patients with the lamina lucida subtype with respect to higher co-morbidities and refractory treatment responses [91].

Differential diagnosis

In young children, bullous impetigo may resemble initial lesions. Hereditary epidermolysis bullosa is often present at birth and the family history is helpful. The adult disease may be confused with atypical erythema multiforme, neurotic excoriations and prurigo.

In both age groups, dermatitis herpetiformis (antibodies against epidermal and/or tissue transglutaminase with granular deposits of IgA in the dermal papillae by direct IF microscopy), BP (autoantibodies against the DEJ preferentially of the IgG isotype and reactivity against BP180 and/or BP230), MMP (predominant mucosal involvement) and EBA (reactivity against type VII collagen) need to be distinguished. Key clinical and immunopathological features of these diseases are detailed in the corresponding chapters and summarised in Table 50.2.

Classification of severity

No scoring system for the quantification of disease activity has been validated in LAD. The BPDAI score, developed for BP, or the ABSIS score may be applied [92,93].

Complications and co-morbidities

No specific complications and co-morbidities related to the pemphigoid disease have been described.

Disease course and prognosis

Patients with LAD almost always respond well to treatment. Preliminary data suggest a more refractory course in patients with the sub-lamina densa variant [91]. Relapses may occur over the next 2–4 years but are usually less severe than the initial disease episode. During pregnancy, the disease appears to improve with relapses within a few months post-partum [94]. Most children go into complete remission within 2 years of disease onset and only very rarely does the disease persist after puberty [5,95,96]. Drug-induced LAD usually heals within 4–8 weeks after discontinuation of the drug. Some cases, however, have persisted for months [97].

Investigations and diagnosis

Diagnosis is based on the combination of the clinical picture and direct IF microscopy. Linear deposits of predominant or exclusive

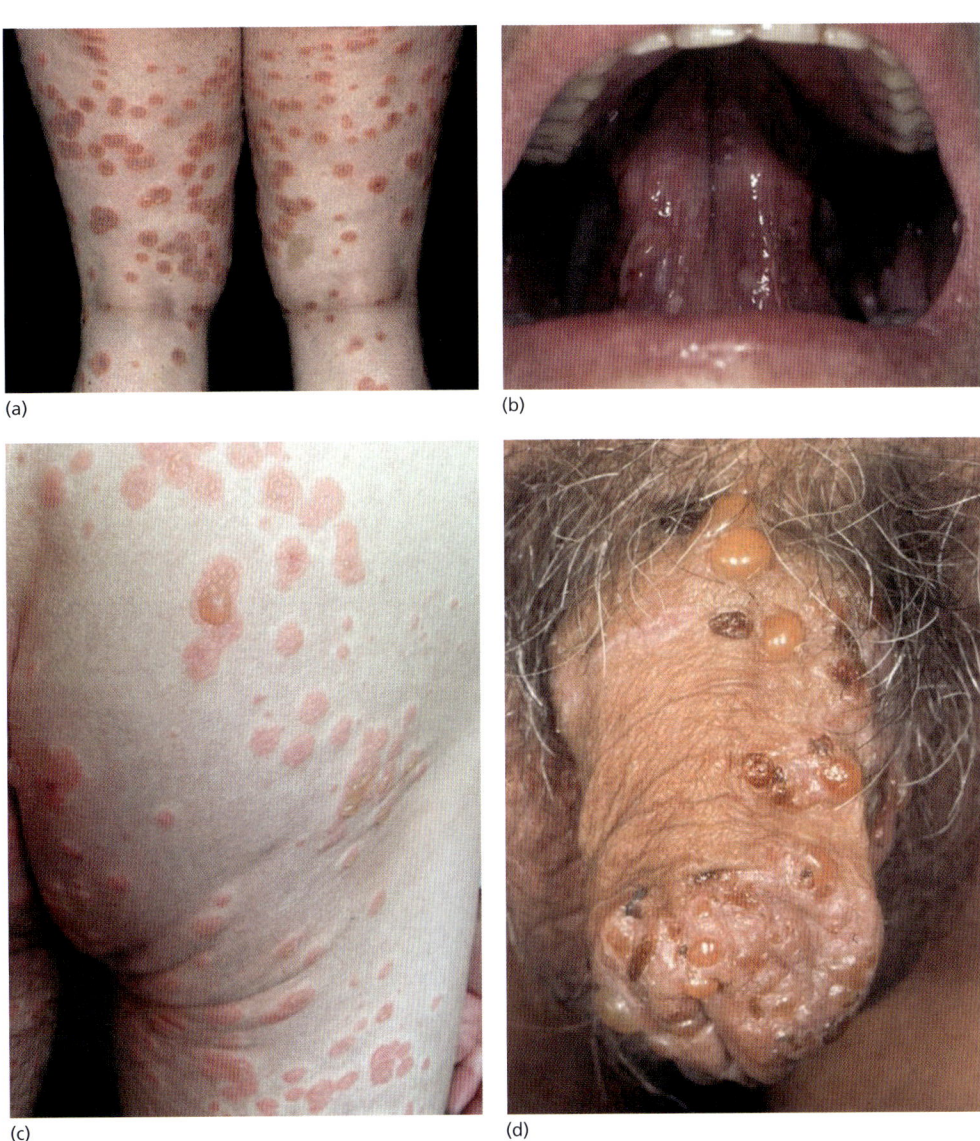

Figure 50.35 Linear IgA disease. Tense blisters in an annular pattern on the thighs (a), erosions on the tongue (b), erythema and blisters on the right gluteal region (c), and tense blisters and crusted erosions on the penis (e) in adult patients.

PART 4: INFLAMMATORY DERMATOSES

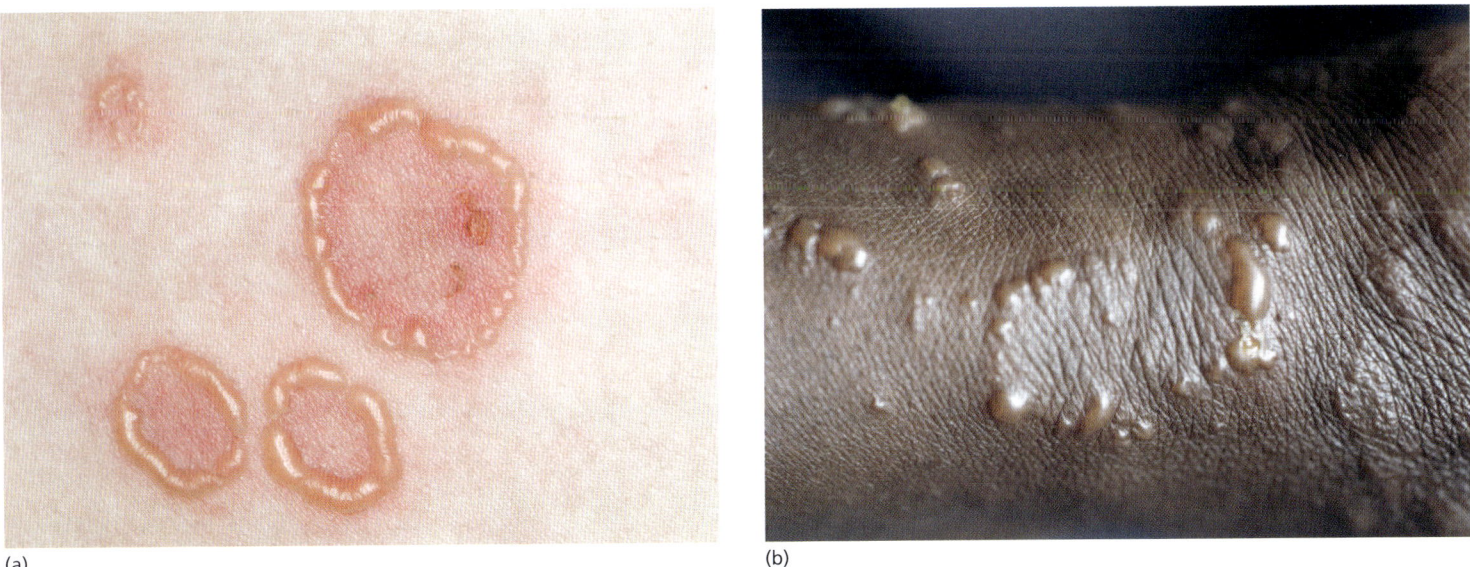

Figure 50.36 'Cluster of jewels' or 'string of pearls' sign. The peculiar appearance of vesicles in an annular pattern or along the edge of a lesion is frequently seen in linear IgA disease (a). However, it is not pathognomonic and may also be observed in bullous pemphigoid (b).

IgA deposits at the DEJ are diagnostic for LAD. Patients meeting these criteria and predominant mucosal involvement are diagnosed as MMP [3,4]. Whether patients with predominant IgA reactivity against type VII collagen are classified as sub-lamina densa type of LAD or as IgA EBA will be clarified in the EADV S2k guideline of LAD.

For screening of serum autoantibodies, indirect IF microscopy on monkey oesophagus or, even more sensitive and informative, on 1 M NaCl-split human skin, can be used. The latter assay usually reveals IgA binding at low titres (1:10–1:40) with a sensitivity of 60–70% [10,11,21,48,90] and can differentiate anti-BP180/BP230 reactivity (epidermal binding) from anti-type VII collagen reactivity (dermal binding) (Figure 50.13). Blister fluid can be applied as an alternative to serum and may be easier to obtain in a child [98].

To pinpoint the fine specificities of serum autoantibodies, various assays, all of them not commercially available, can be performed. Antibodies against the ectodomain of BP180 can be detected by immunoblotting with extracts of epidermal, dermal and amniotic membrane (LADB-97) [13,62], conditioned medium of cultured keratinocytes and extract of amniotic membrane (LAD-1) [12,62,90,99,100] and various recombinant fragments [50,99,101], as well as by ELISA [102]. Assays for serum antibodies against type VII collagen are described in the Epidermolysis bullosa acquisita section, later.

Management
General principles of management
No prospective controlled clinical trial or larger case series have been reported. Patients usually respond well to treatment. When drug-induced LAD is suspected, in particular in patients using vancomycin, penicillins, non-steroidal anti-inflammatory drugs or phenytoin, the drug needs to be suspended before treatment is initiated. In localised or limited disease potent topical corticosteroids may suffice. Otherwise, dapsone 1.0–1.5 mg/kg/day in combination with potent topical corticosteroids is regarded as first line treatment [1,87,103,104]. Glucose-6-phosphate dehydrogenase deficiency should be excluded before dapsone is prescribed. The most frequent adverse events are anaemia (a reduction of haemoglobin of 1–2 g/dL can be expected), methaemoglobulinaemia and increased liver enzymes. Agranulocytosis is rare but can be fatal and at least monthly blood counts are required. In cases of fever, agranulocytosis needs to be excluded [105]. Sulphapyridine and, often better tolerated, sulphamethoxypyridazine are an alternative to dapsone. Some patients may require concomitant low-dose prednisone (0.25–0.5 mg/kg/day) to suppress blister formation [1,103]. In refractory patients, erythromycin, colchicine, flucloxacillin, methotrexate, cyclosporine, tetracycline and nicotinamide, IVIG, azathioprine, mycophenolates and immunoadsorption have been employed successfully [106].

Guidelines of both the French and Brazilian Societies of Dermatology recommend dapsone as first line treatment followed by sulphones. While the French guideline reserves topical corticosteroids for severe and refractory cases, the Brazilian colleagues recommend them as the first line approach in mild LAD [104,107].

Treatment ladder for linear IgA disease[a]

First line
- Dapsone 1.0–1.5 mg/kg/day[b] *plus*
- Potent topical corticosteroids

Second line
- Other sulpha drugs (sulphapyridine, sulphamethoxypyridazine) *plus*
- Potent topical corticosteroids

Third line
- *plus* prednisolone 0.25–0.5 mg/kg/day

Fourth line
- Mycophenoles (mofetil 2 g/day, gastroresistant mycophenolic acid 1.440 g/day) *plus*
- Prednisolone 0.25–0.5 mg/kg/day

In refractory cases
- *plus* IVIG 2 g/kg/month *or plus*
- Immunoadsorption

[a]In the sub-lamina densa type/reactivity with type VII collagen, the treatment ladder for epidermolysis bullosa acquisita (see later) is recommended.
[b]With normal glucose-6-phosphate-dehydrogenase level.

Anti-p200 pemphigoid

Definition, nomenclature and classification
Anti-p200 pemphigoid is a distinct subepidermal bullous skin disease characterised by autoantibodies against a 200 kDa protein (p200) of the DEJ detected by Western blotting with extract of human dermis or epidermis. Clinically, patients resemble bullous pemphigoid, but tend to be younger and show more hand and foot involvement [1,2]. Laminin γ1 is recognised by 70–90% of anti-p200 pemphigoid sera while, recently, laminin β4 was identified as a major autoantigen of this disease [2–4].

Synonyms and inclusions
- Anti-laminin β4 pemphigoid
- Anti-laminin γ1 pemphigoid

Classification links (as appropriate)
- Anti-p200 pemphigoid has no specific ICD and can be encoded as ICD-10 L12.8 (pemphigoid diseases not otherwise classified)

Introduction and general description
Anti-p200 pemphigoid was first described in 1996 by Zillikens and Hashimoto [5,6]. Subsequently, the p200 protein was shown to be

an acidic non-collagenous N-linked glycoprotein that was localised within the lower lamina lucida outside of hemidesmosomes by electron microscopy [5,6–9]. The p200 protein is different from all major target antigens of the DEJ including BP180, BP230, α6β4 integrin, laminin 332, laminin 331, type VII collagen and nidogen [1,3,10]. It is synthesised by both keratinocytes and dermal fibroblasts [10]. In 2009, Dainichi *et al*. reported that 90% of anti-p200 pemphigoid sera contained antibodies against the C-terminal 245 amino acids of laminin γ1 and coined the term anti-laminin γ1 pemphigoid [3]. Subsequently, 70–90% of anti-p200 patients were reported to recognise laminin γ1, while the pathogenic role of anti-laminin γ1 antibodies remained enigmatic [2,11,12]. Recently, laminin β4 was described as autoantigen of this disease targeted by nearly all patients [4,13].

Traditionally diagnosis is made by the detection of autoantibodies against the p200 protein by Western blotting against an extract of the upper portion of human dermis [1,5]. Alternatively, epidermal extract or recombinant laminin γ1 can be applied by Western blotting or [3,11,14]. Recently, an indirect IF assay based on the BIOCHIP™ technology using recombinant laminin β4 became widely available [13]. The detection of the target antigen(s) is of importance, since serum autoantibodies in anti-p200 pemphigoid label the dermal side of the artificial blister by indirect IF microscopy on salt-split skin and thus EBA could mistakenly be diagnosed. In contrast to the latter disease, patients with anti-p200 pemphigoid usually well respond to topical or medium-dose oral corticosteroids [1].

The clinical features and immunopathology are summarised in Table 50.2.

Epidemiology
Incidence and prevalence
Anti-p200 pemphigoid is a rare chronic autoimmune disease with an increasing number of published cases [1,2,15]. The actual incidence is considerably higher compared with EBA based on the analysis of 141 consecutive pemphigoid sera with dermal binding by indirect IF microscopy on human salt-split skin received in our routine laboratory from our routine senders. In this cohort, reactivity with p200/laminin γ1 was about sixfold higher compared with reactivity against type VII collagen or laminin 332 [16]. This assumption is in line with the incidence of 0.7/million inhabitants in 2016 retrieved from the autoimmune blistering disease (AIBD) registry in Schleswig Holstein, a state in northern Germany [17]

Age
The mean age of 113 published patients was 65.5 years, ranging from 5 to 94 years [2]. In the so far largest cohort of 245 patients diagnosed in Lübeck, Germany, the mean age was 74 years ranging from 28 to 98 years [18].

Sex
A clear male predominance is apparent with 73% of 113 published patients and 63% of 245 patients in the Lübeck cohort being male [2,18].

Ethnicity
Since the main diagnostic laboratories for anti-p200 pemphigoid are situated in Japan and Central Europe, most published cases originate from these regions. When consecutive sera of patients

from Germany, India and Iran with dermal binding by indirect IF microscopy on salt-split skin were examined in the same laboratory, the frequency of anti-p200 pemphigoid was about 70%, 30% and 5%, respectively [16,19,20]. These data are indicative of different frequencies in different populations.

Associated diseases
Psoriasis was associated in about 30% of the published cases; most were Japanese [1,2,15].

Pathophysiology
The C-termini of laminin β4 and laminin γ1 have been described as an immunodominant region in anti-p200 pemphigoid [3,4,11,12]. Laminins are cross- or T-shaped heterotrimers and composed of three non-identical protein chains, laminin α, β and γ [21]. Laminins are extracellular matrix glycoproteins and major constituents of basement membranes. They interact with nidogen (via the N-terminus), perlecan and integrins (via the C-terminus) [22], for example. Laminin β4 and laminin γ1 are components of various laminins of which laminin 311 (with an α3, β1 and γ1 chain), laminin 321 and laminin 511 are expressed in the DEJ [21,23]. Laminin β4 has previously not been described as a component of the DEJ.

Most autoantibodies belong to the IgG4 subclass. An individual patient with exclusive IgA autoantibodies against the p200 antigen but unreactive with laminin γ1 has been reported [24]. Intermolecular epitope spreading appears to be relatively frequent in anti-p200 pemphigoid. In a cohort of 245 sera, one third reacted with at least one other antigen in addition to p200/laminin γ1, most frequently with BP180, followed by BP230 and more rarely with type VII collagen and laminin 332 [16,18].

To investigate the role of IL-8 in the neutrophil infiltration frequently seen in the patients' upper dermis by histopathology, Iwata *et al*. determined the IL-8 release of cultured human keratinocytes in response to anti-p200 pemphigoid IgG. In contrast to BP IgG, incubation with anti-p200 IgG did not result in the secretion of IL-8 [25]. These results point to different mechanisms of neutrophil accumulation in skin lesions in the two pemphigoid diseases.

Recently, like BP and EBA sera, anti-p200 pemphigoid sera were shown to induce dermal–epidermal separation when employed in an *ex vivo* model using cryosections of human skin incubated with patients' sera or IgG and subsequently, with leukocytes from healthy volunteers [12]. Of note, anti-p200 pemphigoid IgG affinity-purified against various forms of the C-terminus of laminin γ1 as well as the entire laminin γ1 molecule had no effect in this model [12]. Interestingly, patients' sera depleted from laminin γ1 reactivity led to the same extent of dermal–epidermal separation as patients' sera without depletion [12]. In contrast, anti-laminin β4 IgG induced split formation in this *ex vivo* assay (data unpublished). In the same line, we and others were unable to induce clinical disease in mice after transfer of anti-murine laminin γ1 IgG or immunisation of mice with recombinant murine laminin γ1 [12,26]. Since laminin β4 is not expressed in rodents, demonstrating *in vivo* pathogenicity of laminin β4-specific antibodies is challenging. Subsequently, antibodies against the N-terminus of laminin γ1, that are found in about a third of anti-p200 pemphigoid sera, were shown to induce dermal–epidermal separation in the cryosections model [12,27].

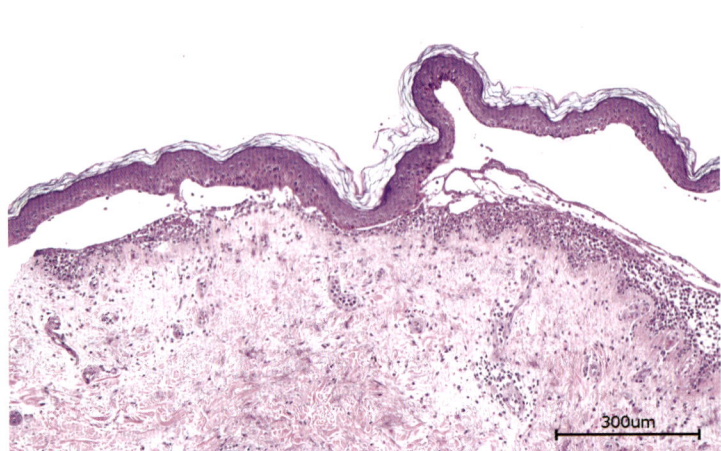

Figure 50.37 Lesional histopathology of anti-p200 pemphigoid. Subepidermal splitting and a dense neutrophilic infiltration below the blister.

Taken together, the *ex vivo* and *in vivo* data indicate that laminin β4 can be regarded as the main autoantigen in anti-p200 pemphigoid. Further experiments addressing the *in vivo* pathogenicity of anti-laminin β4 IgG are being awaited.

Predisposing factors
None described.

Pathology
As for all pemphigoid diseases the histopathological hallmark of a lesional biopsy is the subepidermal split accompanied by the accumulation of eosinophils and neutrophils in the upper dermis [2,28] (Figure 50.37). In some patients, an exclusively lymphocytic infiltrate was found. In other patients, microabscesses at the tips of dermal papillae may develop [2,28]. Importantly, histopathology was shown to not allow the differentiation of anti-p200 pemphigoid from other pemphigoid diseases [28].

As for all pemphigoid disorders, tissue-bound autoantibodies can be visualised by direct IF microscopy of a perilesional biopsy as linear deposits of IgG at the DEJ. Pattern analysis reveals an n-serrated pattern (Figure 50.12). Exclusive IgA deposits were described in a single patient [24].

Genetics
No data available.

Environmental factors
None described.

Clinical features
Presentation
Most patients present with tense blisters on reddish or normal skin resembling BP [1,2,29,30] (Figure 50.38). Palms, plants and head appear as predilection sites (Figure 50.39) [2,31]. As is the case for BP, the clinical picture may vary between different patients

and cases reminiscent of LAD or dermatitis herpetiformis have been described as well as predominant eczematous, urticarial and prurigo-like variants [14,24,31,32]. In about 40% of patients, mucosal surfaces are involved, mostly oral followed by anogenital mucous membranes [2,14,25,31]. Lesions usually heal without scarring; milia formation has been observed in about 15% of patients [1,2].

Clinical variants
None described.

Differential diagnosis
Clinically, BP and LAD are the most relevant differential diagnoses. With involvement of hands and feet, pompholyx may be considered. Because indirect IF microscopy on salt-split skin IgG autoantibodies label the dermal side of the artificial blisters, EBA needs to be excluded by the detection of antibodies against the p200 antigen and/or laminin γ1.

Classification of severity
No scoring system for the quantification of disease activity has been validated in anti-p200 pemphigoid. The BPDAI score, developed for BP, or the ABSIS score may be recorded [33,34].

Complications and co-morbidities
No specific complications and co-morbidities related to the pemphigoid disease have been described. The association with psoriasis has been described earlier.

Disease course and prognosis
The disease typically shows a prompt response to treatment clearly contrasting with patients with EBA. Although clinical studies are lacking, patients appear to respond to lower doses of corticosteroids compared with BP, and most patients remain in remission after tapering of the immunosuppressive medication.

Investigations and diagnosis
Like in all AIBD, diagnosis is based on the combination of the clinical picture, direct IF microscopy and serology. Direct IF microscopy of a perilesional biopsy reveals linear labelling of IgG and/or C3 at the DEJ in an n-serrated pattern, rarely accompanied with linear IgA deposits (Figure 50.12). Like this, EBA, that reveals a u-serrated pattern (Figure 50.33), can be excluded. By indirect IF microscopy on 1 M NaCl-split normal human skin, autoantibodies label the floor of the artificial split (Figure 50.13). The final diagnosis is then made by the demonstration of serum autoantibodies against the p200 antigen by immunoblotting with extract of normal human dermis or epidermis [5,14,31], laminin β4, and/or against laminin γ1 (Figure 50.40). Recently, a standardised indirect IF assay based on the BIOCHIP™ technology using recombinant laminin β4 became widely available. The assay revealed a sensitivity of 99.2 and a specificity of 99.3% analysing 239 anti-p200 pemphigoid and 479 control sera (Figure 50.40).

Management
General principles of management
Due to the rarity of this entity, no randomised controlled studies or case series following a specific treatment regimen are available.

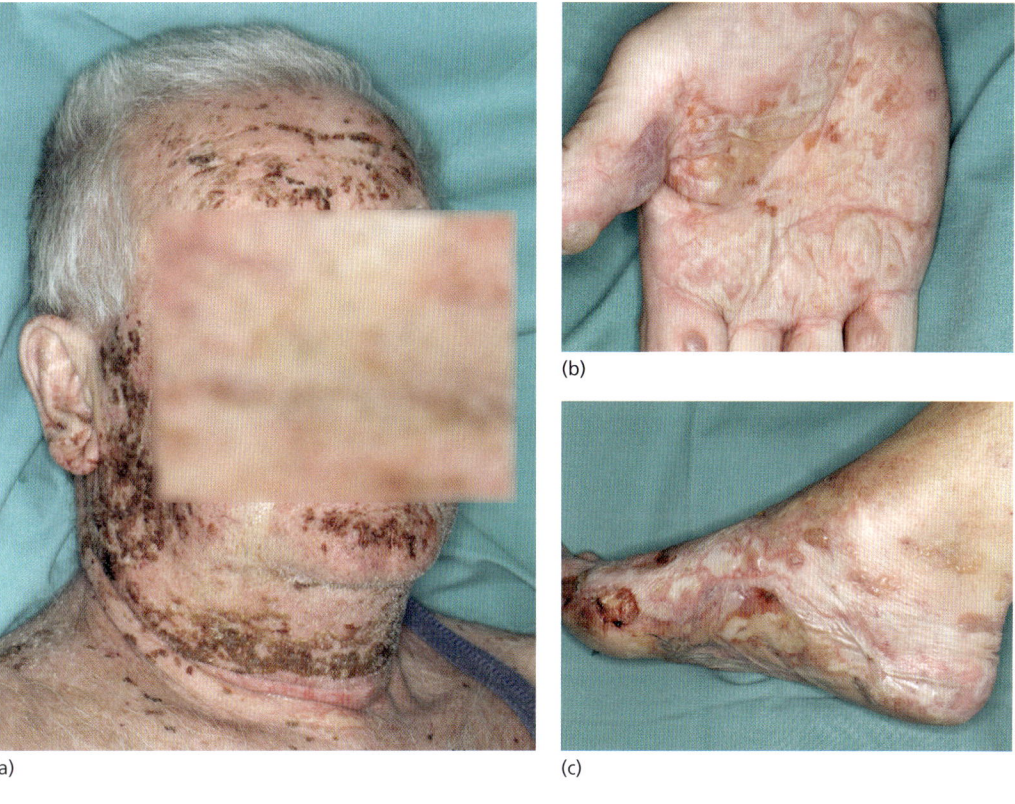

Figure 50.38 Anti-p200 pemphigoid. Erosions, haemorrhagic crusts, and tense blisters on the face (a), palm (b) and foot (c).

(a)   (b)   (c)

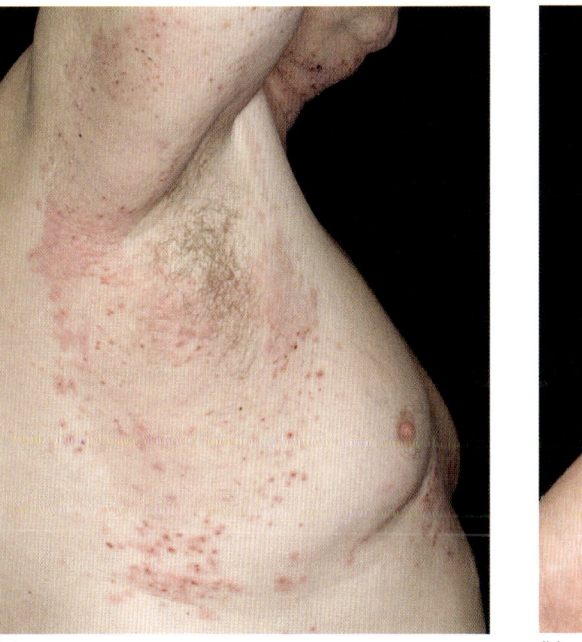
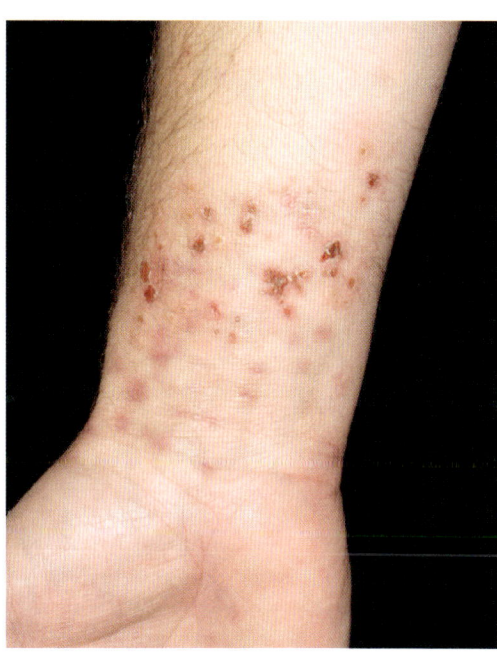

Figure 50.39 Anti-p200 pemphigoid. Erythematous, partly excoriated papules and erythema on the right axilla and vesicles and erythematosus papules on the right wrist in a 52-year-old patient.

(a)   (b)

Therapy of anti-p200 pemphigoid may best follow the established algorithms for BP, although in our experience, patients usually respond faster to topical and oral corticosteroids. To avoid overtreatment, exact diagnosis and differentiation from BP, and more importantly, from EBA is warranted.

Most patients have been treated with tapering doses of prednisolone 0.5 mg/kg/day in combination with an immunomodulant, most frequently by dapsone (in 41% of 113 reviewed cases) followed by tetracyclines (in 20%) and ciclosporin (in 17%). About one third of cases were managed with oral or topical corticosteroids alone [35]. Relapses are not uncommon and were observed in about 40% of 113 reviewed cases, most frequently when topical corticosteroids were used as monotherapy [35]. Individual patients were successfully treated with adjuvant colchicine, azathioprine, mycophenolate, IVIG, rituximab, ustekinumab, plasmapheresis and immunoadsorption [1,30,35–38].

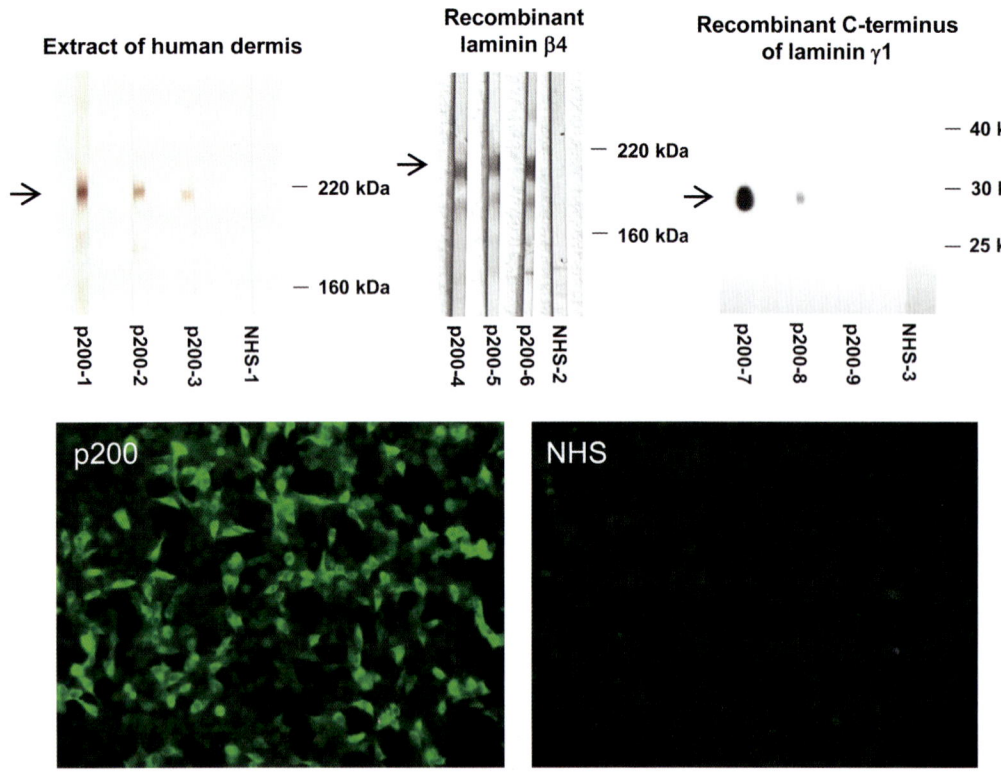

Figure 50.40 Anti-p200 pemphigoid: serum autoantibodies against the p200 antigen, laminin β4 and laminin γ1. By Western blotting with extract of human dermis a 200 kDa protein is recognised in all three patients (p200-1–3) as well as with recombinant laminin γ1 (p200-4–6), while reactivity against recombinant laminin γ1 is only seen in two patients (p200-7–8), but not in patient p200-9 with anti-p200 pemphigoid. The migration positions of molecular weight markers, the p200 antigen (left panel), recombinant laminin β4 (middle panel) and recombinant the C-terminus of laminin γ1 (right panel) are indicated. By indirect immunofluorescence on HEK293 cells recombinantly expressing laminin β4 on their cell surface, IgG reactivity is observed with an anti-p200 pemphigoid (p200) serum but not a normal human serum (NHS). Of note, transfection of cells is suboptimal to provide laminin β4-negative cells as internal negative control.

Treatment ladder

First line
- Very potent topical corticosteroids on the whole body surface 2×/day *or*
- Prednisolone 0.25–0.5 mg/kg/day tapering plus lesional very potent topical corticosteroids 2×/day
- *plus*
- Dapsone 1.0–1.5, mg/kg/day *or*
- Doxycycline 200 mg/day

Second line
- Prednisolone 0.5 mg/kg/day tapering *plus*
- Azathioprine 2.5 mg/kg/day (with normal TPMT activity) *or* mycophenolate (mofetil 2 g/day, gastroresistant mycophenolic acid 1.440 g/day)

Third line
- Addition of IVIG *or* immunoadsorption

Epidermolysis bullosa acquisita

Definition, nomenclature and classification
EBA is a clinically heterogeneous subepidermal AIBD defined by autoantibodies against type VII collagen [1,2]. Here, EBA is classified as pemphigoid disease although originally this term was reserved for AIBD with reactivity against hemidesmosomal proteins, thus excluding EBA. Since this differentiation is rather subtle, EBA is increasingly included in the group of pemphigoid disorders [3]. In patients with predominant IgA anti-type VII collagen antibodies, there is diagnostic overlap with LAD (Figure 50.22). Patients with predominant mucosal involvement and autoimmunity against type VII collagen are classified as MMP [4,5].

Classification links (as appropriate)
- ICD-10: L12.3

Introduction and general description
EBA is a rare pemphigoid disorder with autoantibodies against type VII collagen. Two main clinical subtypes can be differentiated, the so-called classic or mechanobullous form initially described by Roenigk *et al.* resembling hereditary dystrophic epidermolysis bullosa [6] and an inflammatory variant that mimics BP or LAD [7–9].

The first cases of what we now call EBA were most likely described by Elliot in 1895 when reporting two patients with adult onset of skin fragility, erosions and blisters healing with scarring, and milia formation [10]. In 1970, Roenigk *et al.* proposed clinical criteria for EBA including: (i) negative family or personal history for skin blistering; (ii) adult disease onset; (iii) skin lesions that resemble hereditary dystrophic EB; and (iv) the exclusion of all other bullous diseases [6]. Three years later linear deposits of IgG and C3 at the DEJ were noted in an EBA patient by direct IF microscopy [11]. In 1976, direct immunoelectron microscopy localised Ig deposition in EBA in the sublamina densa area differentiating the disease from BP [12]. In 1984, Woodley *et al.* described a 290 kDa protein of the DEJ as target of serum autoantibodies in EBA [13] and, four years later, identified this target antigen as type VII collagen [1].

Diagnosis is made by the detection of autoantibodies against type VII collagen. An ELISA and IF microscopy-based assay for serum anti-type VII collagen antibodies are currently commercially available [14,15]. Importantly, since in only half of the EBA patients circulating autoantibodies can be detected, the visualisation of skin-bound type VII collagen-specific antibodies is paramount. This can be achieved by direct immunoelectron microscopy or, more practically, by serration pattern analysis of a routine direct IF microscopy [2,16]. The pathogenesis of the inflammatory variant of EBA is relatively well understood due to recent advances based on several *in vitro* and *in vivo* models [17,18]. The two mouse models of the inflammatory variant of EBA [19,20] have not only generated novel insights into the pathophysiology of the disease but also allowed the functional preclinical validation of a large variety of anti-inflammatory mediators valuable for future therapeutic use not only in pemphigoid diseases but also in other inflammatory skin disorders. The clinical features and immunopathology of EBA are summarised in Table 50.2.

Epidemiology
Incidence and prevalence
The estimated incidence of EBA lies between 0.2 and 0.5 new cases/million/year in central Europe, Kuwait and Singapore [21–25]. The rarity of the disease in Central Europe is reflected by the lack of a newly diagnosed patient in 2016 in the prospective Schleswig-Holstein (Northern Germany) registry of autoimmune blistering diseases covering a population of 2.86 million. In line with this, the prevalence was calculated to be 2.8/million inhabitants, e.g. a total of 230 patients, in Germany in 2014 [26,27].

Age
The disease occurs at any age with reported mean ages of disease onset of 44, 54 and 57 years in large case series and a mean of 50 years in a review of all reported cases [28,29,**30**,31]. About 5% are children and adolescents, a relatively high rate compared with pemphigus, BP, MMP and anti-p200 pemphigoid [26,**28**,31–38]. In contrast, data of the largest German insurance company with 1.716 million minors based on ICD10 coding revealed only two EBA patients below the age of 18 years in 2016 [39].

Sex
In all larger studies, an about equal sex distribution has been reported [26,31,40].

Ethnicity
In two studies, EBA occurred more frequently in black patients of African descent (66% and 54% of patients, respectively) [41,42]. The incidence may vary between different populations as indicated by the analysis of consecutive sera with dermal binding by indirect IF microscopy on human salt-split skin that showed a relative frequency of 95% and 60% in Iran and Southern India compared with about 12% in Germany [43–45].

Associated diseases
While two case series from the USA and France revealed an association with inflammatory bowel disease, in particular Crohn disease, in 25% and 16% of patients, respectively, this association was not found in 30 Korean patients [29,42,46]. The latter observation is supported by the association with Crohn disease in only 0.9% of all reviewed EBA cases [31]. Two studies detected antibodies to type VII collagen in 6% and 60% of patients with inflammatory bowel disease [46,47]. In line with these findings, expression of type VII collagen was found in the oral cavity, oesophagus, small intestine and colon. In fact, in two murine models of EBA, intestinal inflammatory lesions were seen in about 20% of animals [48].

Associations with numerous systemic diseases, e.g. rheumatoid arthritis, diabetes, cryoglobulinaemia and psoriasis were reported in individual patients [31,49–51]. Recently, an association with haematological malignancies, i.e. lymphoma, was observed in about 8% of EBA patients [52].

Autoantibodies against type VII collagen are also characteristic for bullous systemic lupus erythematosus (see Bullous systemic lupus erythematosus, earlier).

Pathophysiology
The autoantigen of EBA is homotrimeric type VII collagen, a constituent of the anchoring fibrils (Chapter 2) [1,**13**]. Its N-terminal 145 kDa NC1 domain has been identified as the immunodominant region with epitopes spreading across all of this region [1,53–56]. Only rare cases with reactivity against the C-terminal NC2 or the central collagenous domain are reported [34,57,58]. Patients with intermolecular epitope spreading and reactivity with other DEJ antigens, i.e. BP180, BP230, laminin 332 and the p200 antigen, in addition to type VII collagen-specific antibodies, may occasionally been found [**28**,44,59–61].

The pathogenic relevance of autoantibodies in EBA has been shown unequivocally. Serum levels of anti-type VII collagen antibodies correlate with the disease activity in patients and transient neonatal disease was observed following placental transfer of autoantibodies from an affected mother [62,63]. Furthermore, different *in vitro* and *in vivo* models have been established that have resulted in a relatively well understood pathophysiology [19,20,55,64–68]. In these models, patient or rabbit anti-murine type VII collagen IgG was incubated with skin sections leading to dermal–epidermal splitting or injected into mice resulting in a disease phenotype clinically and immunopathologically mimicking human EBA. These models are suitable to explore the process of tissue destruction induced by anti-type VII collagen antibodies. In a further model, immunisation of susceptible mouse strains with the recombinant murine NC1 domain triggered a long-standing autoimmune response resulting in a subepidermal blistering skin disease in 80% of mice [20]. These mouse models, which reproduce the inflammatory variant of EBA, have been vigorously employed to study its pathophysiology [18,69]. In short, CD4 T cells are pivotal for the induction of autoimmunity against type VII collagen with important roles also for B cells, dendritic cells, macrophages T regulatory cells and T follicular helper cells [68,70]. In human EBA, only limited data are available about the role of T cells that were shown to recognise identical regions on the NC1 domain as B lymphocytes [71].

For tissue destruction by anti-type VII collagen antibodies, complement activation in particular of the alternative pathway is crucial, as well as neutrophils recruited and activated via the murine Fcγ receptor IV following interaction with the Fc portion of skin-bound type VII collagen-specific antibodies [19,72–75]. Finally, the release of reactive oxygen species, elastase and matrix metalloproteinase-9 from neutrophils was shown to induce dermal–epidermal splitting [76,77]. In addition, glycosylation of autoantibodies was highlighted to be essential for the interaction of autoantibodies with their Fcγ receptors as well as their interplay with complement activation [70,78,79]. The following inflammatory markers were described as relevant for EBA tissue inflammation: heat-shock protein-90, CARD9, TGFβ, IL-1RA, IL-1β, IL-6, GM-CSF, LTB4, p38 MAPK, ERK1/2, PI3Kb, RORα, flightless 1, G protein-couples receptor 15, phosphodiesterase-4, granzyme B as well as Scr and Syk tyrosine kinases [17,72,80–91].

Furthermore, the mouse models of EBA have been applied to evaluate successfully the anti-inflammatory properties of a variety of agents. Among them are, in addition to drugs already in clinical use for EBA (e.g. methylprednisolone, IVIG and dapsone), calcitriol, etanercept, anakinra, PI3kδ inhibitor, LTB4-C5a inhibitor, soluble CD32, propranolol and dimethylfumarate [72,92–102]. The latter agents now await clinical application not only for EBA but also in other pemphigoid diseases.

Predisposing factors
Penicillin, vancomycin in conjunction with gentamycin, UV-radiation and contact allergy to metals have been implicated as precipitating factors [103–106].

Pathology
As for all pemphigoid diseases, the histopathological hallmark is subepidermal blistering. Depending on the clinical subtype, the inflammatory infiltrate in the dermis is variable, scarce in the mechanobullous variant and dense with predominant neutrophils, eosinophils, monocytes and lymphocytes reminiscent of BP in the inflammatory subtype [50]. The cleavage plane of the blister may be within the lamina densa corresponding to the autoantibody deposits as seen by direct electron microscopy or within the lamina lucida [107–109]. The latter finding may be explained by the lamina lucida as the *locus minoris resistentiae* most susceptible to the proteolytic enzymes secreted within the vicinity of the DEJ.

Tissue-bound autoantibodies can be detected by direct immuno-electron microscopy or direct IF microscopy of a perilesional biopsy as linear deposits of IgG, and/or IgA, and/or C3 at the DEJ. By a 400-fold magnification the linear binding shows a u-serrated pattern with a grass-like appearance of Ig deposits [16] (Figure 50.33). This pattern is unique to EBA and of particular importance since only in about half of patients, can circulating autoantibodies be detected. In all other pemphigoid diseases, an n-serrated pattern is seen (Figure 50.12). By direct immunoelectron microscopy of a perilesional biopsy, a thick band of immune complexes is located below the lamina densa in the anchoring fibril zone. Transmission electron microscopy of a lesional biopsy demonstrates splitting below the lamina densa [2,12,107,108,110,111].

Genetics
EBA is associated with HLA-DR2 (corresponding to HLA-DRB1*15) and DRB1*15:03, an allele found frequently in the general population [41,42]. Korean patients more frequently carried DRB1*13 compared with controls [112]. The relevance of HLA (H2s) and non-HLA genes for disease susceptibility was also described in the immunisation-induced mouse model of EBA [113,114].

Environmental factors
No environmental factors have been discovered so far. For trigger factors see Predisposing factors, earlier.

Clinical features
Presentation
Two main clinical forms can be differentiated, the classical mechanobullous variant, in about a third of patients, and the inflammatory subtype [6,28,29,115,116]. The classical mechanobullous phenotype mimics hereditary dystrophic epidermolysis bullosa when it is severe and porphyria cutanea tarda when it is mild [6]. Clinical characteristics are skin fragility, erosions, blisters, crusts and scars on trauma-prone areas such as hands, knuckles, elbows, knees and toes (Figures 50.41 and 50.42). Scarring alopecia and nail loss may occur [6]. The inflammatory variant resembles other pemphigoid diseases such as BP and LAD [28,29] (Figures 50.43 and 50.44).

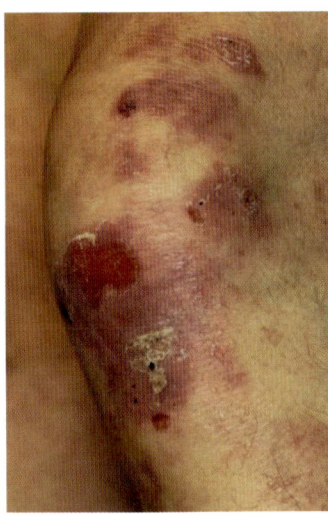

(a)

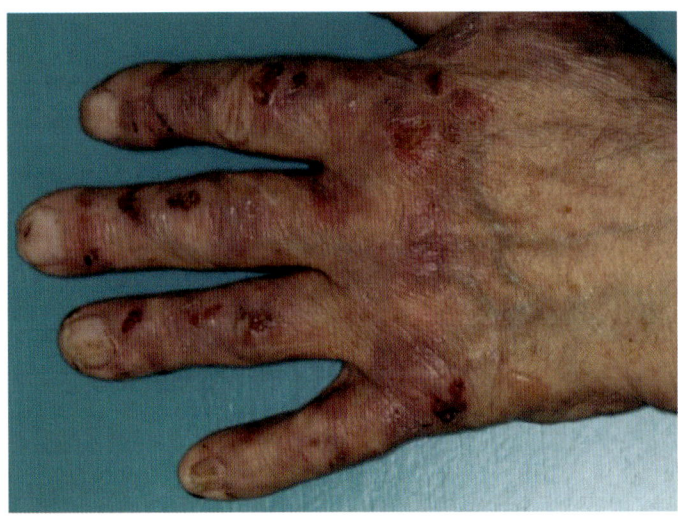

(b)

Figure 50.41 Epidermolysis bullosa acquisita, mechanobullous variant. Erythema, erosions and crusts on the left knee (a) and erythematous plaques, atrophic scars, milia, crusts and a tense blister on trauma-prone extensor surface of the left hand of a 75-year-old man (b).

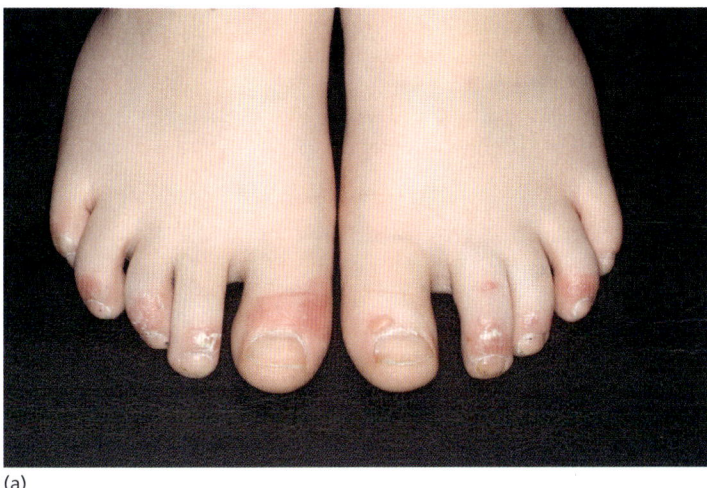

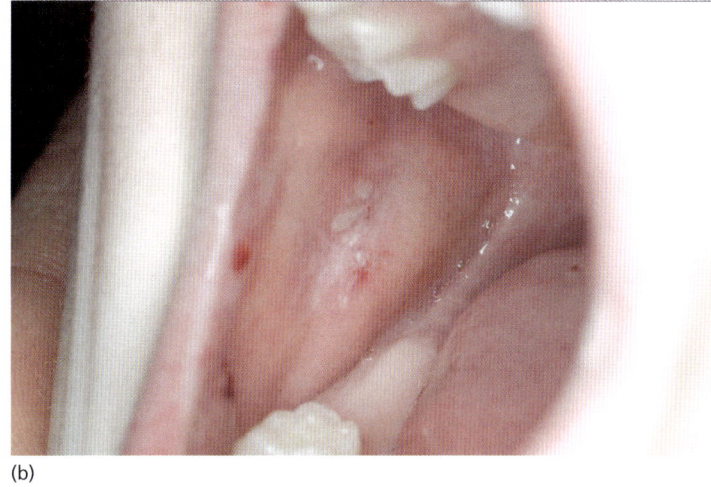

(a)

(b)

Figure 50.42 Childhood epidermolysis bullosa acquisita, mechanobullous variant. Erythema, erosions and tense blisters on the trauma-prone dorsal aspects of the toes (a) and erosions of the buccal mucosa (b) in a 5-year-old boy.

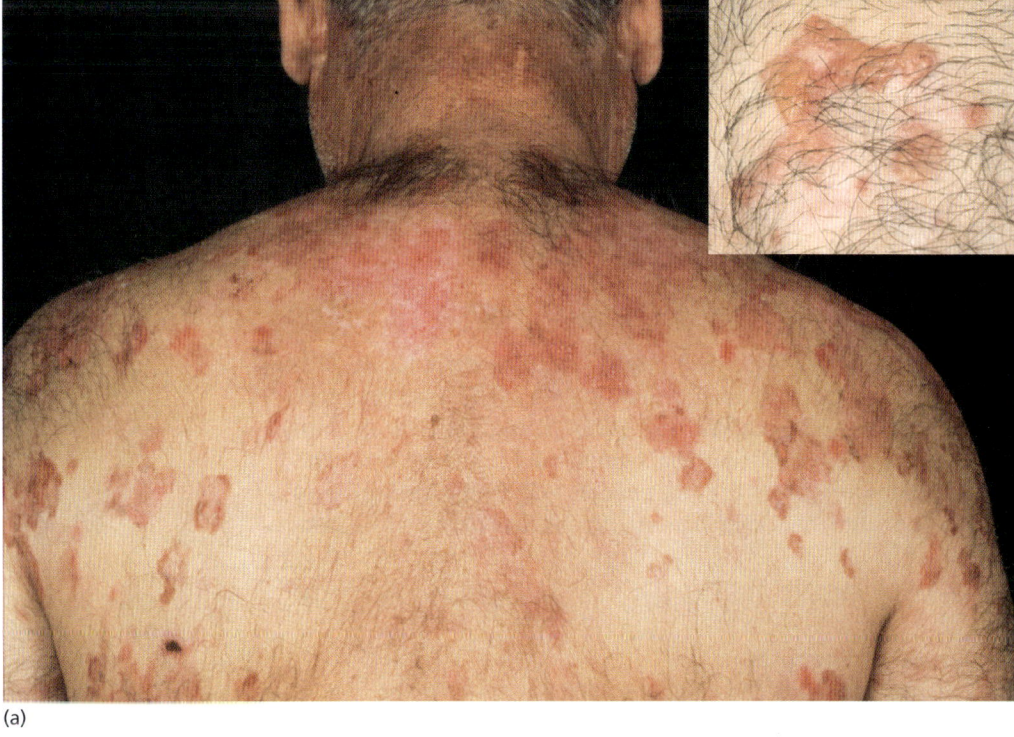

(a)

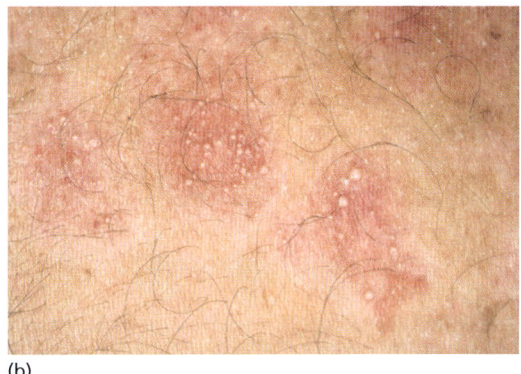

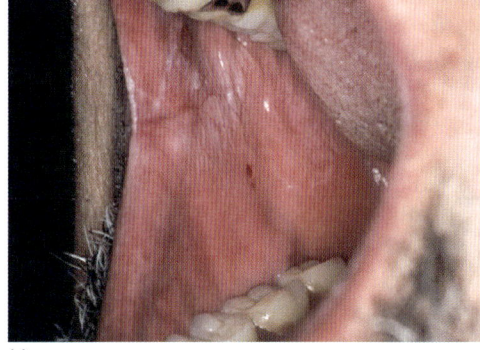

Figure 50.43 Epidermolysis bullosa acquisita, inflammatory variant. Erosions and tense blisters (insert) on the upper back (a), milia (b) and erosions of the buccal mucosa (c).

(b)

(c)

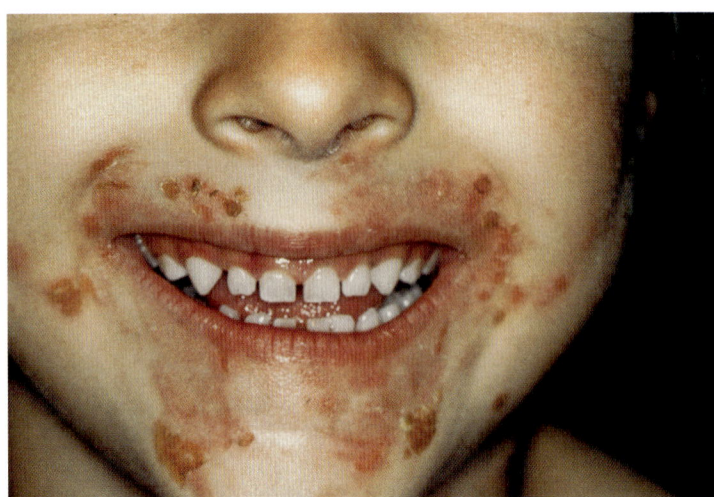

Figure 50.44 Childhood epidermolysis bullosa acquisita, inflammatory variant. Perioral yellowish crusts and erosions.

However, both the classic and the inflammatory form may coexist in the same patient and the clinical presentation of a given EBA patient may change during the disease course [117–119]. Differentiation between the inflammatory subtypes remains somehow arbitrary. Both subtypes may occur in adults (Figures 50.41 and 50.43) and children (Figures 50.42 and 50.44). Mucous membranes are affected in about half of the patients [28,30,40] (Figures 50.42 and 50.43). Patients with predominant mucosal lesions and autoimmunity against type VII collagen are classified as MMP [4,5,120] (Figure 50.22).

Clinical variants

Brunsting and Perry described patients with a subepidermal blistering autoimmune disease and skin lesions of the head and neck region that healed with scarring [121]. These patients are best classified as a variant of cicatricial pemphigoid [120] (see Rare pemphigoid disorders, later). In some patients with the Brunsting–Perry phenotype, autoantibodies against type VII collagen have been described [28,29,122–124]. These patients may also be classified as EBA [28,29,50] (Figure 50.22).

Differential diagnosis

Patients with the mechanobullous subtype need to be distinguished from dystrophic epidermolysis bullosa (manifestation at birth or in childhood, positive family history in dominant inheritance, negative direct IF microscopy) and porphyria cutanea tarda (porphyrins in urine, compatible direct IF microscopy). The inflammatory variants mimic BP (reactivity with BP180) and LAD (predominant IgA autoantibodies). There is a diagnostic overlap with LAD (Figure 50.22). We recommend the diagnosis of EBA in all patients with antibodies to type VII collagen irrespective of the autoantibody isotype, i.e. sub-classifying patients with exclusive or predominant anti-type VII collagen IgA as IgA EBA. This view is based on the comparison of IgA EBA cases with both LAD patients without type VII collagen reactivity (also sub-classified as lamina lucida variant of LAD; see LAD section, earlier) and IgG-EBA patients that showed IgA EBA patients to require more intensive

therapy compared with the LAD patients with the lamina lucida variant, as such resembling IgG EBA more [125].

Classification of severity

No scoring system for the disease activity has been validated in EBA. The BPDAI score, developed for BP, or the ABSIS score may be applied [126,127].

Complications and co-morbidities

No specific complications and co-morbidities related to the pemphigoid disease have been described.

Disease course and prognosis

EBA is a chronic relapsing disease that usually is more difficult to treat compared with other pemphigoid disorders except MMP with ocular, oesophageal and laryngeal involvement [3]. A better overall prognosis was attributed to children with EBA compared with adults [33,37]. No difference with respect to response to treatment was observed between the mechanobullous and the inflammatory variants [29].

Investigations and diagnosis

As is the case for all AIBD, diagnosis is based on the combination of the clinical picture, direct IF microscopy and serology (Figure 50.45). The present diagnostic hallmark is direct IF microscopy including pattern analysis. Pattern analysis, introduced by Vodegel et al. [16], is a major step in the diagnosis of EBA, since serum autoantibodies can be detected in only about half of the patients. The previous diagnostic gold standard, i.e. direct electron microscopy, is currently only performed in a handful of specialised laboratories and has the disadvantage that biopsies need to be processed rapidly and thus cannot be sent to these specialised centres [2].

Pattern analysis of direct IF is based on careful examination of the DEJ that in a 400-fold magnification appears as an undulated rather than linear labelling. When arches are closed at the top, an n-serrated pattern is present (Figure 50.12). When arches are closed at the bottom resembling 'growing grass', a u-serrated pattern is recognised (Figure 50.33). The latter pattern is unique to reactivity with type VII collagen in EBA and the rare cases of type 1 bullous SLE, whereas all other pemphigoid diseases reveal an n-serrated pattern [16]. Serration pattern diagnosis: (i) can be used with snap frozen biopsies or biopsies stored in 0.9% NaCl solution or Michel's medium; (ii) can be performed on routine 6 μm cryosections; (iii) can be evaluated using a normal IF microscopy with a 400-fold magnification (no need for oil); (iv) is easy to learn with an online learning tool available (www.nversusu.umcg.nl); (v) has a high interrater conformity; (vi) can be applied on IgG and IgA deposits; and (vii) allows the recognition of a specific pattern in about 75% of skin samples. Mucosal lesions, however, are not suitable for serration pattern analysis [128,129–132].

In biopsies in which the serration pattern analysis remains inconclusive, more sophisticated alternatives comprise the computer-aided fluorescence overlay antigen mapping (FOAM) [133], the double IF labelling of tissue-bound and defined antigens of the DEJ analysed by laser scanning confocal microscopy [134], and the treatment of biopsies with 1 M NaCl solution to induce an artificial split at the lamina lucida level and subsequent autoantibody detection by indirect IF microscopy on 1 M NaCl-split skin [135].

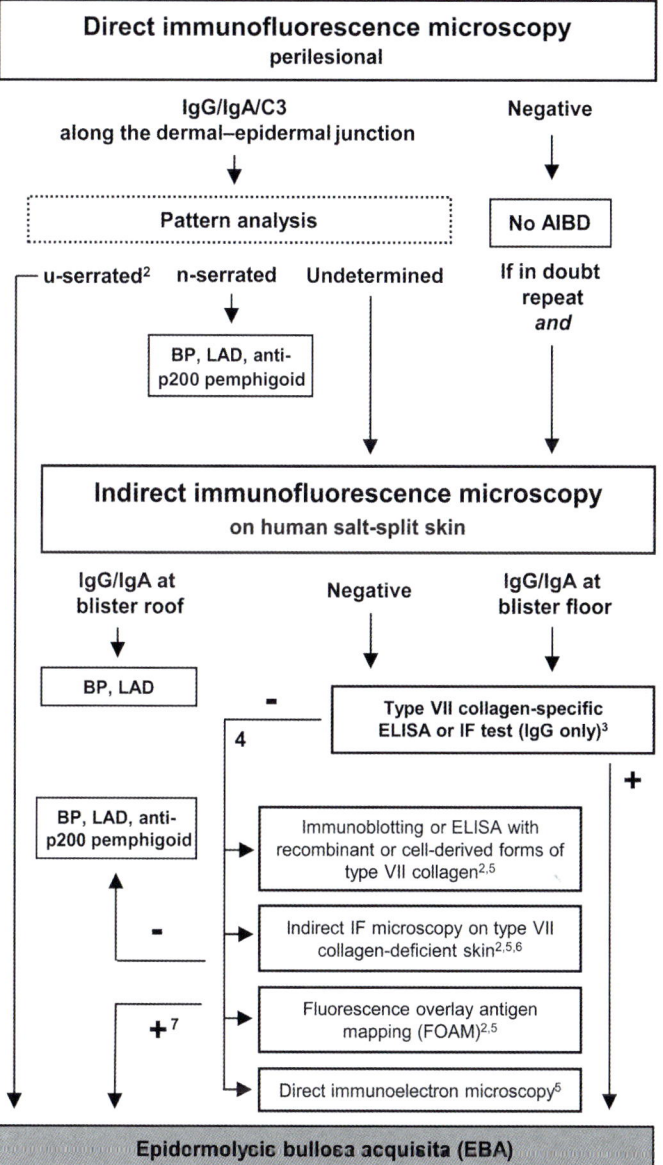

Figure 50.45 Diagnostic pathway for epidermolysis bullosa acquisita (EBA). 1, Patients with predominant mucosal lesions are classified as mucous membrane pemphigoid [4,5]; 2, patients with exclusive or predominant IgA reactivity are best diagnosed as IgA-EBA (detailed in text); 3, commercially available; 4, depending on availability; 5, only available in specialised laboratories; 6, from patients with hereditary dystrophic epidermolysis bullosa; positivity in any of the four assays will allow diagnosis of EBA. AIBD, autoimmune bullous disease; BP, bullous pemphigoid; LAD, linear IgA disease; IF, immunofluorescence.

The latter approach, however, cannot differentiate between EBA and anti-p200 pemphigoid and anti-laminin 332 reactivity.

Exclusive or predominant IgA deposits by direct IF microscopy has been described in several patients [136–139]. In two larger studies, about one third of EBA patients revealed exclusive IgA reactivity [28,125]. As discussed above, these patients may be diagnosed as IgA-EBA rather than as LAD although no general consensus has been reached here (Figure 50.22). Anti-type VII collagen IgE was observed in about a third of EBA sera in patients with both the classical and the inflammatory variant [140]. No patient with exclusive IgE reactivity has been recognised as yet and individual patients with IgM EBA based on direct IF microscopy were described [140–143].

Like in all pemphigoid diseases, indirect IF microscopy on 1 M NaCl-split normal human skin is a useful screening test for serum autoantibodies in EBA with a sensitivity of about 50% [28,29]. In this assay, autoantibodies in EBA label the floor of the artificial split (Figure 50.13). Importantly, testing for IgA antibodies is essential since about a third of EBA sera also contain IgA reactivity [28,144]. In about 15% of EBA patients, exclusive serum IgA reactivity was found. In this subgroup, patients are more likely to have the inflammatory phenotype [28].

Two assays for the detection of serum IgG autoantibodies against type VII collagen are commercially available [14,15]. Both assays are based on recombinant NC-1 domain of type VII collagen [14,15]. Both assays have a very high specificity of >98% and sensitivities between 89% and 100% for the IF test, and 82% and 93% when sera reactive by indirect IF microscopy on human salt-split skin were assayed [14,15,145–147]. Alternative methods for the detection of serum type VII collagen-specific antibodies are immunoblotting with various recombinant forms of type VII collagen, dermal extract, human placental amnion or cultured A431 cells and, elegantly, indirect IF microscopy on hereditary dystrophic epidermolysis bullosa skin, deficient of type VII collagen [148–151]. If serology is negative and pattern analysis of the direct IF microscopy was inconclusive, the visualisation of Ig deposits by direct immunoelectron microscopy is the diagnostic gold standard [107,108,111].

The algorithm proposed for diagnosis of EBA is shown in Figure 50.45.

Management
General principles of management
Treatment of EBA is challenging: disease activity is more difficult to suppress compared with most other pemphigoid diseases and no controlled prospective trials are available [3,49,152–155]. The mainstay is systemic corticosteroids (prednisolone 0.5–2.0 mg/kg/day, depending on disease severity) in combination with colchicine [156–158] and dapsone [152]. For refractory patients or severe forms, ciclosporin, azathioprine, mycophenolate mofetil, cyclophosphamide, extracorporal photophoresis, anti-CD25 therapy (daclizumab, basiliximab) [159,160], plasmapheresis and immunoadsorption [161], IVIG [162], rituximab [163–165], and the combination of IVIG with rituximab [166] have been successfully used (reviewed in [31,153–155,167,168]). In meta-analysis of all reported EBA cases, IVIG and rituximab were significantly associated with complete remission [31].

Most children have been treated with a combination of systemic corticosteroids (prednisolone 1 mg/kg/day) plus dapsone [33,36,37,58].

Treatment recommendation. Treatment recommendations were provided by the French, Japanese and Brazilian Societies of Dermatology, with considerable variations between them with respect to both mild and severe disease [155,169,170]. Gürcan and Ahmed [167] emphasised that the benefit of systemic corticosteroids is low in EBA and proposed the following algorithm: in limited disease or paediatric patients – dapsone, colchicine, dapsone + colchicine + low-dose prednisolone, IVIG and/or rituximab; for moderate or mucocutaneous disease – dapsone, IVIG, rituximab, IVIG + rituximab (without financial restrictions) or <6 weeks of prednisolone, cyclosporine, myophenolates, mycophenolates + immunoadsorption, IVIG and/or rituximab (with financial restrictions) [167].

Treatment ladder

First line
- Prednisolone 0.5–2.0 mg/kg/day (depending on disease severity) *plus*
- Lesional (very) potent topical corticosteroids *plus*
- Colchicine 0.5–3.0 mg/day (the highest dose that does not lead to diarrhoea) *or*
- Dapsone 1.5 mg/kg/day (with normal glucose-6-phosphate dehydrogenase levels)

Second line
- Prednisolone 0.5–2.0 mg/kg/day (depending on disease severity) *plus*
- Lesional (very) potent topical corticosteroids *plus*
- Mycophenolate (mofetil 2 g/day, gastroresistant mycophenolic acid 1.440 g/day) *or*
- Ciclosporin 3–6 mg/kg/day

Third line
- *plus* IVIG 2 g/kg/month *or*
- Rituximab 2× 1 g

Bullous systemic lupus erythematosus

Definition, nomenclature and classification

Bullous systemic lupus erythematosus (BSLE) is an autoimmune subepidermal blistering disease that occurs in patients with SLE [1,2,3]. Blisters and erosions are not restricted to LE lesions, tend to arise in sun-exposed skin and heal without scarring. Most BSLE patients have antibodies against type VII collagen and were designated as type I BSLE. Type II BSLE is characterised by antibodies against other antigens of the DEJ [4,5,6]. As in SLE, BSLE typically affects women with an African background in the third decade. Bullous lesions usually rapidly respond to dapsone [7].

Synonyms and inclusions
- Bullous eruption of SLE
- Vesicobullous SLE

Classification links
- ICD-10: M32.8

Introduction and general description

BSLE is a clinically and immunopathologically distinct subepidermal autoimmune bullous disease that arises in patients with SLE. Diagnostic criteria by Camisa and colleagues from the 1980s comprised: (i) a diagnosis of SLE based on the American Rheumatism Association; (ii) blisters predominantly but not exclusively in sun-exposed areas; (iii) histopathology compatible with dermatitis herpetiformis; (iv) serum reactivity by indirect IF microscopy on salt-split skin; and (v) linear or granular deposits of IgG, and/or IgA, and/or C3 at the DEJ by direct IF microscopy and immune reactants below the basal lamina by direct electron microscopy [1,2,3]. Gammon *et al.* recognised that the majority of BSLE patients have autoantibodies against the same antigen as EBA patients [4] later identified as type VII collagen [8]. In the mid-1990s, Gammon and Briggaman as well as Yell *et al.* proposed a broader definition and subdivided BSLE in type I (with reactivity against type VII collagen) and type II (with anti-DEJ reactivity without anti-type VII collagen antibodies) [5,6]. Meanwhile, autoantibodies against other target antigens of the DEJ including BP180, BP230 and laminin 332 were found in BSLE [9,10] and patients with concomitant SLE and BP, LAD or MMP were reported [5,11,12,13].

The first historical case compatible with BSLE was described in 1889 and a patient with positive direct IF microscopy was reported in 1973 before in 1982, Hall *et al.* assembled the first case series of BSLE and recognised the high efficacy of dapsone [7,14].

Diagnosis is still based on the criteria proposed by Camisa and colleagues [1,2,3]. In addition, serum autoantibodies against constituents of the DEJ may be detected using modern diagnostic assays including immunoblotting and ELISA with cell- or tissue-derived and recombinant forms of the target antigen [15]. Furthermore, serration pattern analysis of direct IF microscopy has been established as a practical tool to differentiate tissue-bound autoantibodies against type VII collagen (u-serrated pattern) from all other anti-DEJ antibodies (n-serrated pattern) [16,17,18]. The clinical features and immunopathology of BSLE are summarised in Table 50.2.

Epidemiology

Incidence and prevalence

The incidence of BSLE was estimated to be 0.22 and 0.26 cases/million/year in France and Singapore, while no cases were found in three epidemiological studies in Germany and Kuwait [19–23]. About 0.5–1.0% of patients with SLE are diagnosed with BSLE [24,25]. However, up to 10% of patients with SLE were reported to develop bullous skin eruptions attributed to acute LE with blistering eruption that needs to be differentiated from BSLE [24,26]. In large cohorts of sera with immunobullous disorders, 1–2% were identified as BSLE [16,23,27].

Age

Most patients are in the second, third or fourth decade of life reflecting the age distribution known for SLE [27]. BSLE may, however, also affect children, and patients in their 60s and 70s were described [27].

Sex

The female preponderance of 90% in BSLE reflects the sex distribution of SLE.

Ethnicity
Although BSLE manifests in all ethnicities, as in SLE, black patients of African descent have a higher risk of developing BSLE [11].

Associated diseases
No particular diseases are associated with BSLE.

Pathophysiology
The target antigen in type I BSLE is type VII collagen [4,8]. Like in EBA, autoantibodies in BSLE predominantly bind to the NC1 domain, in particular the fibronectin-like region [28]. The pathogenic relevance of anti-type VII collagen antibodies has been shown in various *in vitro* and *in vivo* models [29–35] and is detailed earlier (see EBA). In an individual patient with BSLE, anti-type VII collagen serum IgG paralleled skin disease activity [36]. In type II BSLE, either no serum autoantibodies or antibodies against structural proteins of the DEJ other than type VII collagen, such as BP180, BP230 and laminin 332, were reported [5,9–13,37]. The pathogenic effect of autoantibodies against these antigens is discussed in the corresponding chapters.

It may be speculated that, as discussed for lichen planus pemphigoides (see Very rare pemphigoid disorders, later), the interface dermatitis typically present in skin lesions of LE may have triggered an additional autoimmune response against proteins of the DEJ and transglutaminases, resulting in a second autoimmune disease, BSLE. Alternatively, other factors that mediate the increased occurrence of several autoimmune diseases in individual patients may be responsible. Thus, the association of SLE and pemphigus or dermatitis herpetiformis can be explained [5].

Predisposing factors
Precipitating factors have only been described in individual patients and comprise drugs (hydralazine, penicillamine, methimazole) and UVB radiation [38–41].

Pathology
Histopathological findings are relatively uniform and resemble dermatitis herpetiformis with subepidermal splitting, a dense neutrophils-dominated infiltrate in the upper dermis sometimes accumulating in microabscesses of the papillary tips, and dermal oedema [3,6,7,42,43]. In addition, mucin depositions are usually seen in the reticular dermis and sometimes there are signs of leukocytoclastic vasculitis [44]. Basal layer vacuolisation characteristic for cutaneous LE is not present.

Direct IF microscopy of a perilesional skin biopsy shows linear (in about 40% of cases) and granular (in about 60%) staining of the DEJ by IgG. Additional linear or granular labelling of IgM, IgA and/or C3 at the DE is found in about 70–80% of the biopsies [39]. In the major BSLE form (type I), a u-serrated staining pattern is seen [16] (Figure 50.40). By immunoelectron microscopy, immunoreactants were localised beneath the lamina densa as in EBA [6]. The cleavage plane is usually in the area of Ig deposition. However, patients with splitting in the lamina lucida have been described [45]. These discrepancies are best explained by the different autoantibody specificities that have not always been explored in the initial reports.

Genetics
In a North American cohort, the presence of autoantibodies against type VII collagen (in BSLE and EBA) was associated with DRB1 1501 allele [46].

Environmental factors
No environmental factors have been discovered so far. For trigger factors see Predisposing factors, earlier.

Clinical features
History
The disease has an acute onset with usually generalised vesicles and blisters in patients with SLE [27].

Presentation
Primary lesions comprise tense vesicles and bullae with a clear or haemorrhagic content on otherwise normal or reddish skin (Figures 50.46 and 50.47). In addition, reddish plaques in an annular or targetoid configuration may arise in about a third of cases [43]. Lesions are usually generalised with predilection for sun-exposed areas, neck, upper trunk and proximal extremities [27,43]. In contrast to other pemphigoid diseases, the face is relatively often affected and in some patients the only site of manifestation [45,47]. Clinically, BSLE may mimic BP, LAD, dermatitis herpetiformis and EBA. When associated with autoantibodies against type VII collagen (type I BSLE), patients with the classic mechanobullous phenotype and the inflammatory variant known from EBA were described [16,27]. Mucosal lesions are found in about half of patients and healing with scar or milia formation occurred in about 20% of cases [43]. Pruritus is present in about half of patients but usually not intense and a burning sensation may occur instead [43]. Haematological abnormalities were present in nearly all BSLE patients, and renal involvement, mostly class III or IV according to the International Society of Nephrology/Renal Pathology Society classification, also appeared to be high (in 50–90% of patients) [25,43,48]. Interestingly, the onset of the bullous eruption does not necessarily correlate with the activity of the systemic involvement

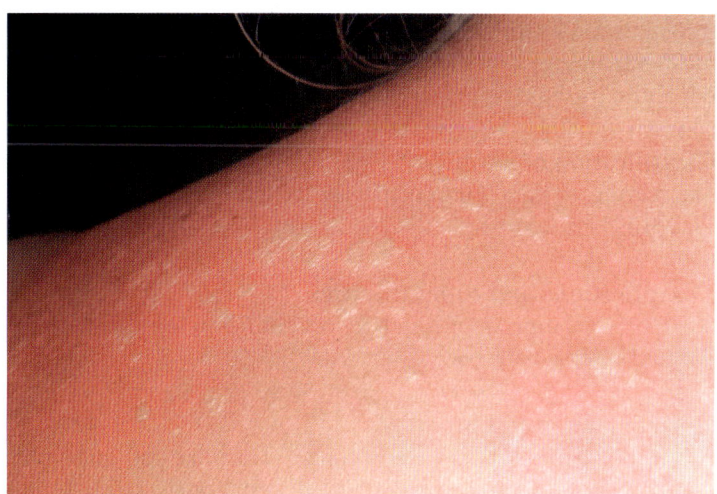

Figure 50.46 Bullous systemic lupus erythematosus. Tense blisters on erythematosus skin.

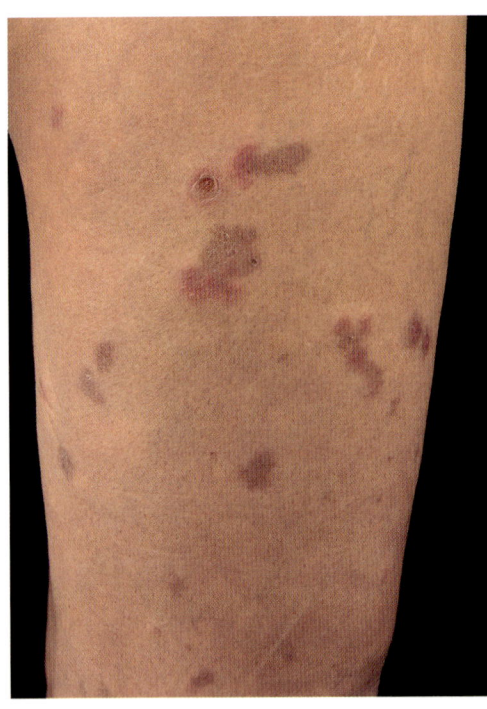

Figure 50.47 Bullous systemic lupus erythematosus. Violaceous maculae and patches and a flaccid blister some days after initiation of systemic corticosteroids. Courtesy of Dr K. Steinbrink, University of Mainz, Mainz, Germany.

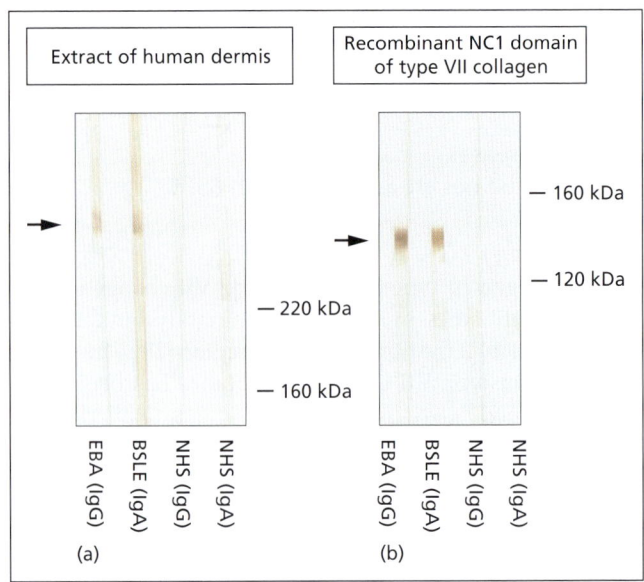

Figure 50.48 Serum autoantibodies in bullous systemic lupus erythematosus type I. IgA autoantibodies label the 290 kDa type VII collagen by immunoblotting with dermal extract (a) and the 140 kDa recombinant NC1 domain of type VII collagen by immunoblotting (b). The clinical picture of this patient is shown in Figure 50.47.

[6,7,27]. In about 40% of patients, BSLE was the first manifestation of SLE [43,48].

Differential diagnosis

Skin lesions of SLE may blister due to the high disease activity of the systemic disease. In these patients, extensive vacuolisation of the DEJ with subepidermal cleavage and a mononuclear cell infiltrate in the upper dermis is seen by histopathology. Alternatively, blisters may arise due to photosensitivity or a hypersensitivity reaction to drugs. By direct IF microscopy, band-like deposits of IgG, IgM and IgA may be present. However, there are no linear or granular Ig depositions [5]. Other pemphigoid diseases, i.e. BP, LAD, EBA, anti-p200 pemphigoid, as well as dermatitis herpetiformis, can be differentiated by the absence of SLE based on the American College of Rheumatology criteria for SLE, the generally good prognosis of BSLE and its rapid response to dapsone.

Classification of severity

No scoring system for the disease activity has been validated for BSLE.

Complications and co-morbidities

No specific complications and co-morbidities related to the pemphigoid disease have been described.

Disease course and prognosis

In most patients, the disease is transient. Unlike the other pemphigoid diseases (except pemphigoid gestationis), BSLE usually completely regresses with no further flares irrespective of the disease activity of the systemic disease [27].

Investigations and diagnosis

Diagnosis is still based on the criteria of Camisa with some modifications with respect to further observations in larger patient cohorts and the development of novel tools for the detection of serum autoantibodies [1,2,3,5,6]. In addition to the vesicobullous eruption, sine qua non conditions for BSLE are a known SLE and linear or granular deposits of IgG, and/or IgA, and/or C3 at the DEJ by direct IF microscopy. By serration pattern analysis, a u-serrated pattern is seen with reactivity against type VII collagen (Figure 50.40) [16]. Histopathology is helpful and typically shows a neutrophil-rich infiltrate in the upper dermis and a subepidermal split formation. Serum autoantibodies are directed against type VII collagen in about 70% of patients (type I BSLE) but reactivity against BP180, BP230 and laminin 332 were also found (in BSLE type II) [5,9,10,12,13,37,43] (Figure 50.48). Serum anti-type VII collagen IgG levels were described to parallel the extent of bullous lesions in two patients with BSLE [36,49].

Management
General principles of management

Dapsone is effective in about 90% of BSLE patients and leads to clinical improvement of the vesicular eruption within days or a few weeks [27,43,50]. In fact, the rapid response to dapsone is one of the characteristics that differentiate BSLE from SLE with concomitant pemphigoid disease. In patients unresponsive to dapsone or in those that do not support the use of dapsone due to haematological involvement of SLE, prednisolone, hydroxychloroquine (mostly combined with dapsone or immunosuppressants), azathioprine and mycophenolate have been advocated [6,43,51–53]. Individual patients effectively treated with methotrexate (10 mg/week), IVIG or rituximab have also been reported [43,54–57].

Treatment ladder for bullous systemic lupus erythematosus

First line
- Dapsone 1.0–1.5 mg/kg/day (exclude glucose-6-phosphate-dehydrogenase deficiency)

Second line
- Prednisolone 0.5–1.0 mg/kg/day (depending on disease severity) *plus*
- Azathioprine 2.5 mg/kg/day (with normal TPMT activity) *or*
- Mycophenolate (mofetil 2 g/day, gastroresistant mycophenolic acid 1.44 g/day) *or*
- Hydroxychloroquine 200–400 mg/day

Rare pemphigoid disorders

Lichen planus pemphigoides

Lichen planus pemphigoides (ICD-10: L43.1) always arises in conjunction with lichen planus and can affect both adults and children [1–3]. At present, fewer than 100 patients have been described in the literature and, as such, no reliable data about its incidence are available. In any case, incidence can be estimated clearly to be below 1/million/year [4]. In contrast to BP, the disease: (i) affects relatively young patients (average disease onset in the forties); (ii) mainly arises on the extremities; (iii) preferentially targets C-terminal epitopes within the immunodominant NC16A domain; and (iv) tends to be less severe [4,5]. For these reasons, lichen planus pemphigoides can also be regarded as a distinct entity within the pemphigoid disorders [6]. Like in bullous systemic lupus erythematosus, it may be speculated that the chronic interface dermatitis may trigger the immune response against BP180. This hypothesis is supported by the notion that lichen planus pemphigoides only remits after lichen planus lesions are sufficiently controlled.

Of note, lichen planus pemphigoides has been reported in association with ACE inhibitors, simvastatin and increasingly with PD-1/PD-L1 inhibitors [4,7–11]. The latter association is intriguing since PD-1/PD-L1 inhibitors were linked to both the development of lichen planus and pemphigoid diseases [12].

Diagnosis is made by the presence of tense blisters also outside of lichen planus lesions (Figure 50.49). In contrast, in bullous lichen planus, blisters are confined to lichen planus lesions. Further diagnostic criteria are the detection of linear deposits of IgG and/or C3 at the DEJ by direct IF microscopy of a perilesional biopsy and serum IgG against BP180 NC16A. Several patients have been diagnosed with oral lichen planus pemphigoides based on the clinical appearance with or without histopathology [13]. These patients may be difficult to differentiate from mucous membrane pemphigoid, since in the latter disease, patients with clinical and histopathological features of oral lichen planus were described [14].

Treatment requires therapy of lichen planus to avoid further stimulation of the anti-DEJ autoimmune process. Otherwise, treatment may follow the same algorithm as in BP. As such, acitretin

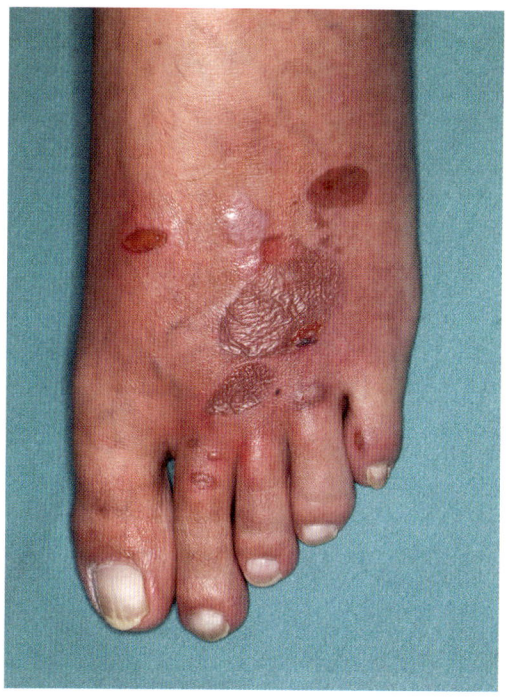

Figure 50.49 Lichen planus pemphigoides. Erosions, red macules, partly ruptured and subsequently desiccated blisters, and a tense vesicle on the left foot. In addition, a lichen planus lesion is seen. Of note, erosions and blisters are separate from the lichen planus lesion.

(20 mg/day) can be combined with very potent topical corticosteroids and in severe or refractory cases, with prednisolone (tapering doses of 0.5 mg/kg/day) with or without dapsone, doxycycline, azathioprine or mycophenoles [4].

Cicatricial pemphigoid

The term cicatricial pemphigoid has previously been used for patients who are now classified as MMP [15]. Following an international expert conference, the term cicatricial pemphigoid is currently only used for the rare clinical variant of a pemphigoid disease in which mucous membranes are not predominantly affected and skin lesions heal with scarring [15]. In case of a u-serrated pattern by direct IF microscopy or serum autoantibodies against type VII collagen, the patient would be classified as EBA (Figures 50.22, 50.50 and 50.51).

Brunsting–Perry pemphigoid is, at present, best regarded as a clinical subtype of cicatricial pemphigoid. Fewer than 100 patients with this phenotype have been reported. In 1957, Brunsting and Perry described a group of patients without mucous membrane involvement who developed subepidermal blisters, erosions, haemorrhagic crusts and atrophic scars on the head and neck [16]. The disease is common in middle-aged and elderly populations. Skin lesions are characteristically confined to the head, neck and upper trunk (Figures 50.52 and 50.53). Mucous membranes can also be involved, however not predominantly [17–19]. Direct IF microscopy shows linear deposits of IgG and/or C3 at the DEJ. Brunsting–Perry pemphigoid probably represents a heterogeneous disorder with several target antigens including type VII collagen, BP180, BP230, laminin 332 and desmoplakin [18–29,**30**]. Type VII collagen is the

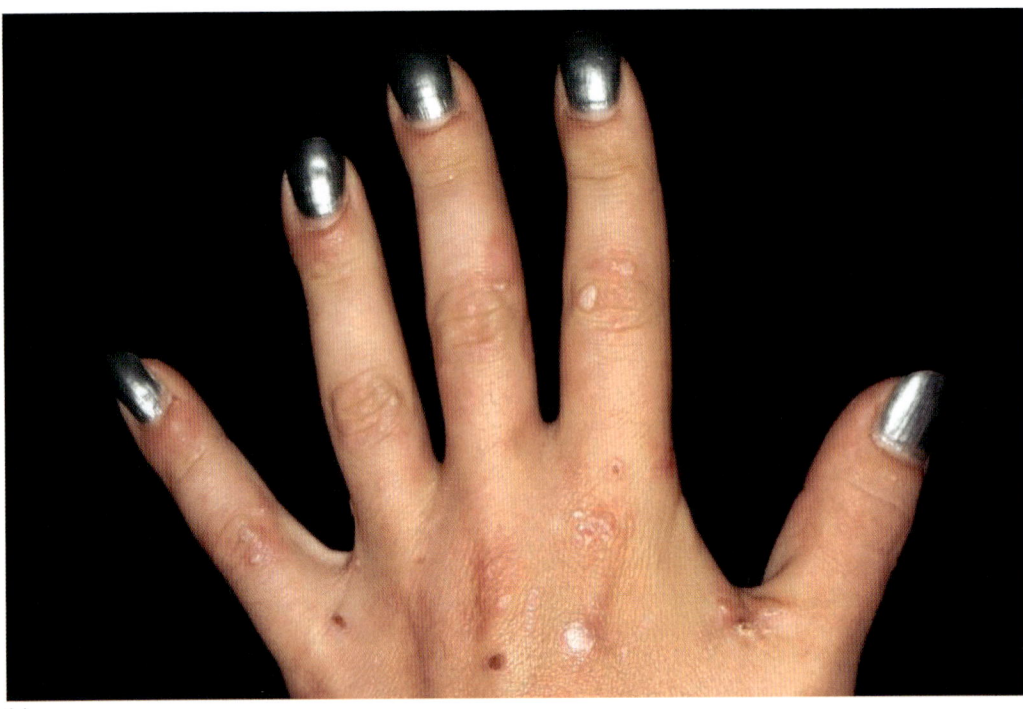

(a)

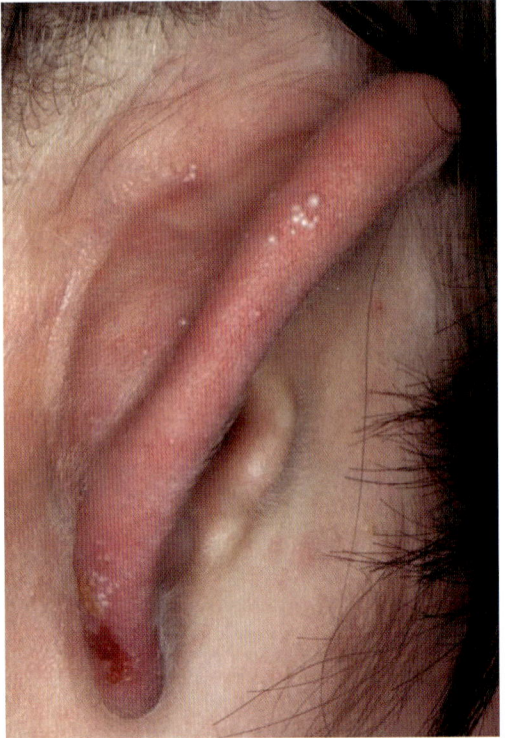

(b)

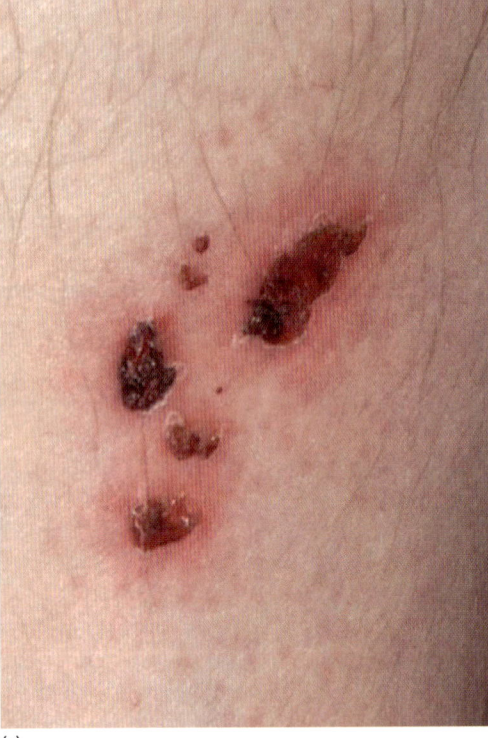

(c)

Figure 50.50 Cicatricial pemphigoid. Thirty-six-year-old woman with tense vesicle between digitus I and II and several atrophic papules and plaques on the dorsum of the left hand (a), milia, crust and erosion on the right ear (b), and crusts on the right thigh (c). Mucous membranes were not involved (not shown). Direct immunofluorescence (IF) microscopy showed linear deposits of IgG and C3 at the DEJ. Serum autoantibodies labelled the epidermal side of human salt-split by indirect IF microscopy but no reactivity with BP180, BP230 and α6 integrin was detected by various ELISA and immunoblotting analyses.

most frequent target antigen, therefore representing a localised form of EBA in these patients [17,18,26,27]. In line with this, in most patients with Brunsting–Perry pemphigoid, electron microscopy revealed split formation below the lamina lucida [31]. In a series of 12 patients, four revealed anti-BP180 and/or BP230 serum reactivity while in the remaining eight, the target antigen was not recognised and pattern analysis of direct IF microscopy was not performed [30]. In individual patients, disease onset was associated with trauma [32], and the combination of frusemide intake and sun exposure [33]. Differential diagnosis includes squamous cell carcinoma, basal cell carcinoma [34], pyoderma, erosive pustulosis of the scalp and dermatitis artefacta.

Treatment usually comprises topical corticosteroids [30]. Good responses to topical tacrolimus, the combination of topical corticosteroids with colchicine or dapsone, as well as dupilumab have also been reported [23,25,35,36].

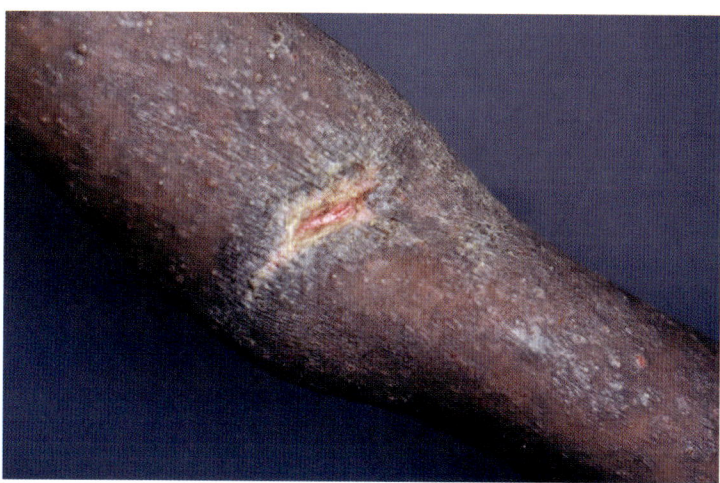

Figure 50.51 Cicatricial pemphigoid. Tense vesicles, erosions, milia and scarring on the right arm of a 24-year-old Ugandan man. Few oral lesions were present without conjunctival involvement. Serum autoantibodies reacted with BP180, BP230 and laminin 332 [72].

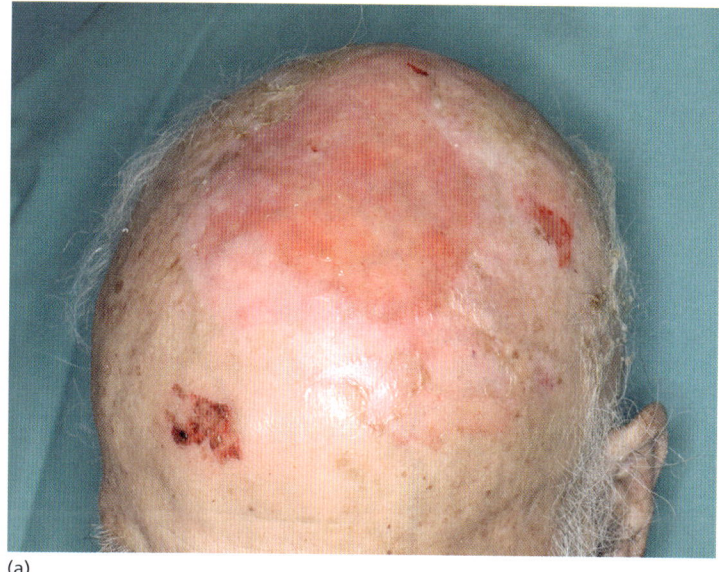

(a)

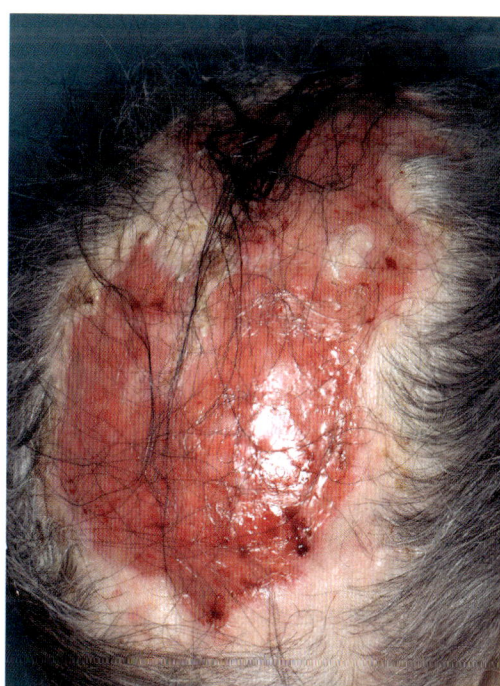

Figure 50.52 Brunsting–Perry pemphigoid. Erosions and some crusts on the scalp of a 76-year-old woman. By direct immunofluorescence microscopy linear deposits of IgG and C3 were seen at the DEJ and serum autoantibodies recognised multiple epitopes on BP180 (NC16A, LAD-1, C-terminus) and BP230.

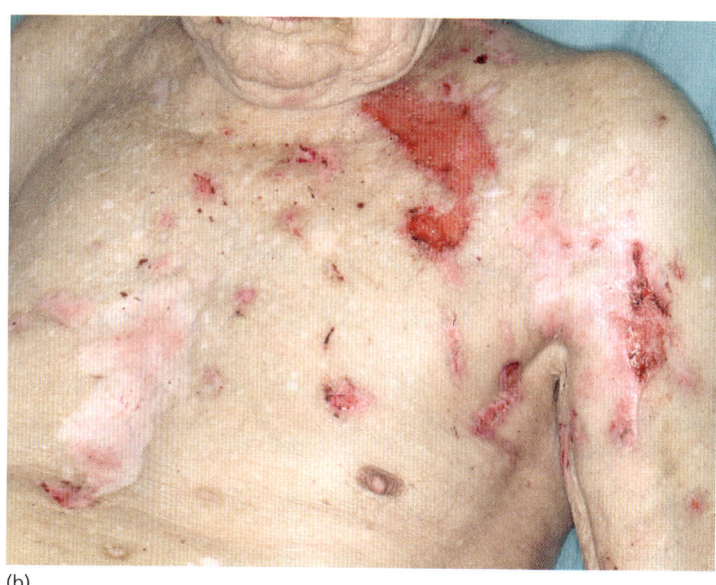

(b)

Figure 50.53 Brunsting–Perry pemphigoid. Erosions on the scalp (a), chest, and upper left arm as well as atrophic scars (b) in a 95-year-old man. Linear staining of IgG and C3 were seen at the DEJ by direct immunofluorescence (IF) microscopy. Serum autoantibodies exclusively labelled the epidermal side by indirect IF microscopy on salt-split skin and reacted with BP180 NC16A.

Anti-type IV collagen pemphigoid

Ghohestani *et al.* reported three patients with generalised blistering and renal insufficiency [37,38]. By lesional histopathology, subepidermal splitting and a dense eosinophilic infiltration of the upper dermis were seen. Direct IF microscopy revealed linear staining of IgG in two patients, of IgA (in one patient) and C3 (in all three patients) at the DEJ. After splitting of the DEJ by 1 M NaCl solution, binding of IgG/IgA at the floor of the artificial blister was seen by direct IF microscopy. Serum autoantibodies reacted with the glomerular basement membrane and the α5 chain of type IV collagen. In one of the three patients, additional reactivity against the α6 chain of type IV collagen was seen [37,38].

IgM pemphigoid

Exclusive labelling of IgM along the DEJ by direct IF is rare with only individual patients being reported [39,40,41–45,46]. In some patients, IgM deposits together with C3 at the DEJ have been described [39,44,47–51], while additional labelling with IgG or IgA is found in 6–18% of pemphigoid patients [52–54]. Some patients with IgM EBA and two with IgM MMP were described and, recently, in three patients with IgM (bullous) pemphigoid, BP180 has been identified as the target antigen [40,42,43,46,55].

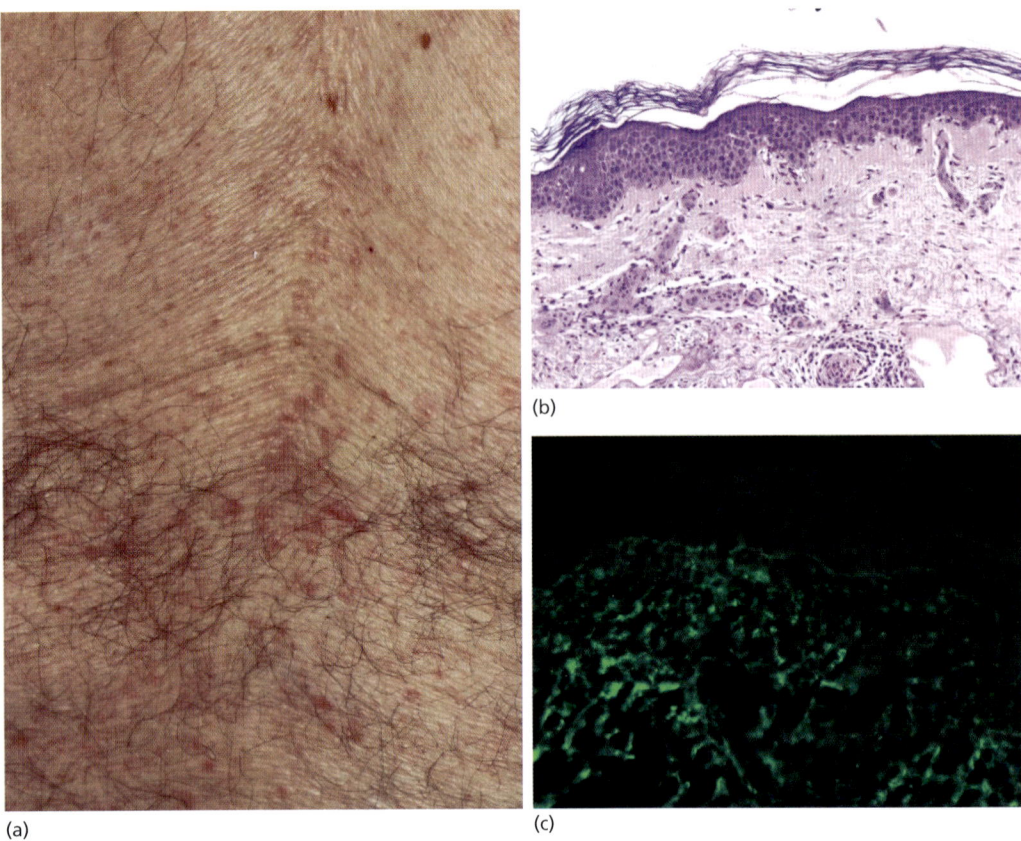

(a)   (b)   (c)

Figure 50.54 IgM pemphigoid. Reddish papules on the abdomen and chest (a). Sparse lymphocytic infiltrate in the upper dermis without subepidermal split formation by lesional histopathology (b) and linear IgM deposits at the dermo-epidermal junction by direct immunofluorescence microscopy (c). The patient is described in more detail as Patient 2 in [46].

Of interest, patients with sole IgM deposits at the DEJ presented with erythema, pruritic papules and plaques without frank blistering (Figure 50.54) [44,45,46]. A similar clinical phenotype was found in patients with exclusive IgM deposition at the DEJ and Waldenström macroglobulinaemia [56–65] and in pregnancy [66,67]. It remains to be elucidated whether a pemphigoid disease with pure IgM deposits at the DEJ is always associated with this distinct non-bullous phenotype and can thus be regarded as a true entity of its own.

Orf-induced pemphigoid

About a dozen patients with immunopathologically confirmed pemphigoid disease following orf have been reported [68,69,70]. Orf, also known as ecthyma contagiosum, is an infection with orf virus, a DNA parapoxvirus of the *Poxviridae* family, that primarily affects sheep and goats. The infection is usually transmitted to humans by caring for infected sheep or goats, classically by bottle-feeding infected orphaned lambs without wearing gloves. In humans, orf presents as a pustule on the hand that develops into a nodule and subsequently ulcerates before healing over several weeks later (Chapter 25). The pemphigoid disorder manifests 2–4 weeks after the orf lesion has appeared with tense blisters, erosions and red macules. Mucosal involvement occurs in about 60% of patients (Figure 50.55). In all patients with mucosal lesions, the oral mucosa was affected [70]. Of note, only a single patient with predominant mucosal lesions was reported [71]. In most patients, the pemphigoid disease resolved over a few weeks with topical corticosteroids or moderate doses of oral prednisolone with or without additional immunomodulants/immunosuppressants

[69,70]. Two patients were described that required more intensive immunosuppressive therapy for up to one year before complete remission without therapy was achieved [68]. In only a few patients, the target antigen has been identified; in all but one patient with reactivity against type VII collagen, IgG1 and/or IGg3 against laminin 332 was found (Figure 50.55) [70,72]. Anti-laminin 332 reactivity is only seen, with the exception of individual patients with additional autoantibodies against other DEJ proteins, in MMP and with predominant IgG4 autoantibodies [73].

Orf-induced pemphigoid appears to be a distinct entity based on: (i) predominant skin involvement with tense blisters and red macules; (ii) a high rate of concomitant mucosal involvement; (iii) relatively young patient age compared with BP and MMP; (iv) limited disease course that requires a less intensive and short therapy; and (v) IgG1 and IgG3 autoantibodies against laminin 332 in the majority of cases.

Dermatitis herpetiformis

Definition, nomenclature and classification

Dermatitis herpetiformis is a chronic, intensely pruritic skin condition associated with gluten sensitive enteropathy. It results in deposition of IgA anti-transglutaminase autoantibodies in the dermal papillae which leads to neutrophil infiltration and blister formation.

Synonyms and inclusions

• Duhring–Brocq disease

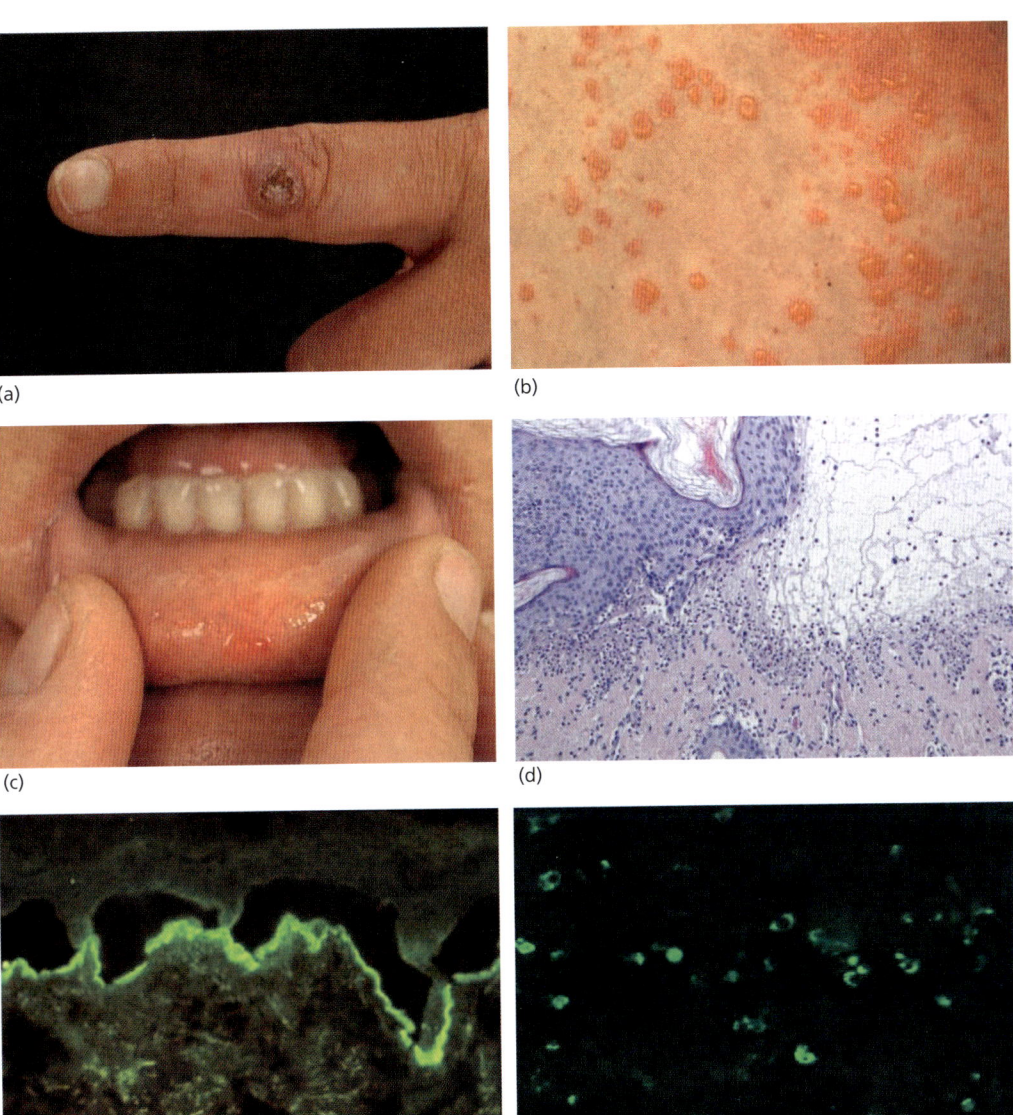

(a)

(b)

(c)

(d)

(e)

(f)

Figure 50.55 Orf-induced pemphigoid. About 5 weeks after the appearance of the orf lesion on the left index finger (a), generalised tense blisters and reddish plaques developed in a 37-year-old female (b). A tense vesicle was present on the lower lip (c) and a few small erosions on the palate (not shown). A lesional histopathology of a blister showed subepidermal splitting and a mixed inflammatory infiltrate including eosinophils in the upper dermis (d). Splitting of a perilesional biopsy by 1 M NaCl solution revealed binding of IgG at the floor of the artificial blisters by direct immunofluorescence (IF) microscopy (e). IgG1 reactivity with recombinant laminin 332 expressed in human HEK293 cells by indirect IF microscopy of the patient's serum (f). No serum antibodies against type VII collagen or the p200 antigen were detectable (not shown) [70].

PART 4: INFLAMMATORY DERMATOSES

Classification links (as appropriate)

- ICD-10: L13.0
- Snomed CT: 111196000
- OMIM: 601230
- Orphanet: ORPHA1656

Introduction and general description

Dermatitis herpetiformis (DH) was first described by Duhring in 1884 [1]. It is a chronic autoimmune blistering disease that results in an intensely pruritic rash that predominantly affects extensor surfaces [2,3,4,5]. The characteristic vesicles are frequently not apparent as they are destroyed by excoriation. DH is closely associated with gluten sensitive enteropathy (GSE [6,7]): both conditions are characterised by the development of IgA autoantibodies against transglutaminases that, in the case of DH, are deposited in the superficial papillary dermis. Therapy of DH involves strict gluten avoidance and the use of sulphonamide drugs such as dapsone [8].

Epidemiology

Incidence and prevalence

DH is most common in people of Northern European descent, where prevalence ranges from 1.2 to 75 per 100 000 people and an incidence range of 0.4–2.6 per 100 000 people/year [9–11]. A large population-based study from the UK suggests that, although the incidence of GSE increased over the period 1990–2011, the incidence of DH fell from 1.8/100 000 to 0.8/100 000 person-years over the same period [12], raising the possibility that improved management of GSE and consequently less pronounced gut inflammation may translate to lower incidence of DH. Interestingly, patients with DH seem to have lower mortality than expected, possibly as a result of the modifications required to their diet as a result of the disease [13].

Age

Onset of DH is most commonly in adult life, typically in the fourth decade, although cases have been reported from childhood to old age [14].

Sex

Several studies have suggested that DH is more common in men than women, with M : F ratios of 1.5–2 : 1 [15].

Ethnicity

DH is largely a condition of people of Northern European descent and is uncommon in Asian and African populations, although occasional cases have been reported [16]. Interestingly, the incidence and prevalence of the disease is similar in North American populations of European descent to those seen in Northern Europe, suggesting that genetic factors are important in disease susceptibility [15]. Asian patients with DH tend to have a distinct fibrillar pattern of IgA deposition in the skin and is only very rarely associated with GSE [17,18].

Associated diseases

The commonest association of DH is with GSE. However, the severity of GSE in DH patients varies hugely, and may be clinically silent or mild [19,20]. Consequently, all patients with DH should be reviewed by a gastroenterologist and investigated accordingly. All patients with DH can be expected to have at least some degree of small bowel inflammation by histopathology. An important consequence of a diagnosis of DH is an increased risk of small bowel lymphoma [21].

Autoimmune diseases tend to associate with one another, presumably because of genetic susceptibility factors, and DH is no different. The commonest association is with autoimmune thyroid disease [22,23], and all patients with DH should be screened for this. Additionally, patients with DH have an increased risk of type-1 diabetes [24], Addison disease [25] and vitiligo [22]. DH and coeliac disease have been suggested to be risk factors for the development of pemphigoid [26], although whether this is due to a predisposition to autoimmunity or whether the relationship is causal remains to be determined.

Pathophysiology
Pathology

The pathology in DH and GSE results from an IgA dominant autoimmune response to transglutaminase molecules [2]. In GSE the principal target is tissue-type transglutaminase 2 (TG2) [27] whereas in DH there is increasing evidence that epidermal transglutaminase 3 (TG3) may be the dominant autoantigen [28]. Both proteins have significant homologies in their enzymatic domains and are expressed in normal epidermis, where TG3 is important in cross-linking and maintenance of the cornified envelope [29].

The series of events that results in inflammation in DH remains to be fully elucidated [30,31], although it is clear that in both GSE and DH, exposure to gluten triggers an autoimmune response against gliadin. One hypothesis is that when gliadin (the alcohol-soluble fraction of gluten) is absorbed, glutamine residues within gliadin are deamidated by TG2, a process that leads to optimal antigen presentation to T cells by HLA-DQ2-positive antigen-presenting cells. Then, IgA antibodies against gliadin, deamidated gliadin, gliadin cross-linked to TG2 and TG2 are generated. By epitope spreading to TG3, IgA reactivity against TG3 develops during the continued exposure to gliadin later in the disease course [30,32].

Subsequent release of TG3 from keratinocytes into the papillary dermis, where it is able to bind circulating IgA antibodies, or deposition of circulating complexes of TG3 and IgA, may lead to the neutrophilic infiltration, inflammation and clefting within the lamina lucida typical of DH.

Observations that the incidence of GSE is rising while that of DH is falling is consistent with this hypothesis: higher awareness and improved diagnostic tools leads to earlier diagnosis of GSE at a time point with less severe gastrointestinal disease and consequently less time for raising an anti-TG3 IgA response by epitope spreading from TG2 [30].

Genetics

Multiple studies have revealed an association between DH and certain HLA types, particularly HLA-DQ2 and, to a lesser extent, HLA DQ8 [33,34], although these associations are less common in Japanese patients [35]. The central role of the MHC in pathogenesis has been confirmed by studies using HLA DQ8 transgenic mice, which develop GSE following gluten challenge [36,37]. Other non-MHC genes have been linked to GSE in genome-wide association studies including myosin IXB, IL12, IL23 and CCR3 [2], although the relevance of these to the pathogenesis of DH (or for that matter GSE) remains unclear.

First-degree relatives of patients with GSE or DH are significantly more likely to be affected by one or other disorder and thus family screening may be indicated [38,39]. Monozygotic twins have a disease concordance rate of over 0.9 [40].

Environmental factors

The principal environmental factor involved in the pathogenesis of GSE and DH is dietary gluten and its constituent gliadin [2]. Interestingly, tTG is responsible for the modification of gliadin into a more immunogenic form capable of better binding to HLA-DQ2 [41]. Other environmental factors relevant to DH include iodine exposure (which can precipitate flares of the disease [42]) and tobacco smoking, which may ameliorate it [43,44].

Clinical features
History

The principal symptom of patients with DH is itch. Patients report a rash, most typically over extensor surfaces of the elbows, knees, buttocks and scalp. There may also be symptoms of associated disorders such as GSE, with bloating, diarrhoea and other gastrointestinal complaints or of other autoimmune diseases including hypothyroidism.

Presentation

The characteristic lesions of DH are grouped reddish papules and vesicles located over extensor sites (Figure 50.56). Because the condition is so pruritic, intact vesicles are rarely seen and the patient may simply present with excoriations [45]. Lesions tend to be symmetrical and heal without scarring. Patients may develop punctate purpura on the palms and soles [46,47]. Mucosal change may occur [48] and dental abnormalities have been reported, particularly enamel pits [49,50]. Interestingly, first-degree relatives of patient with GSE may also show enamel defects [51].

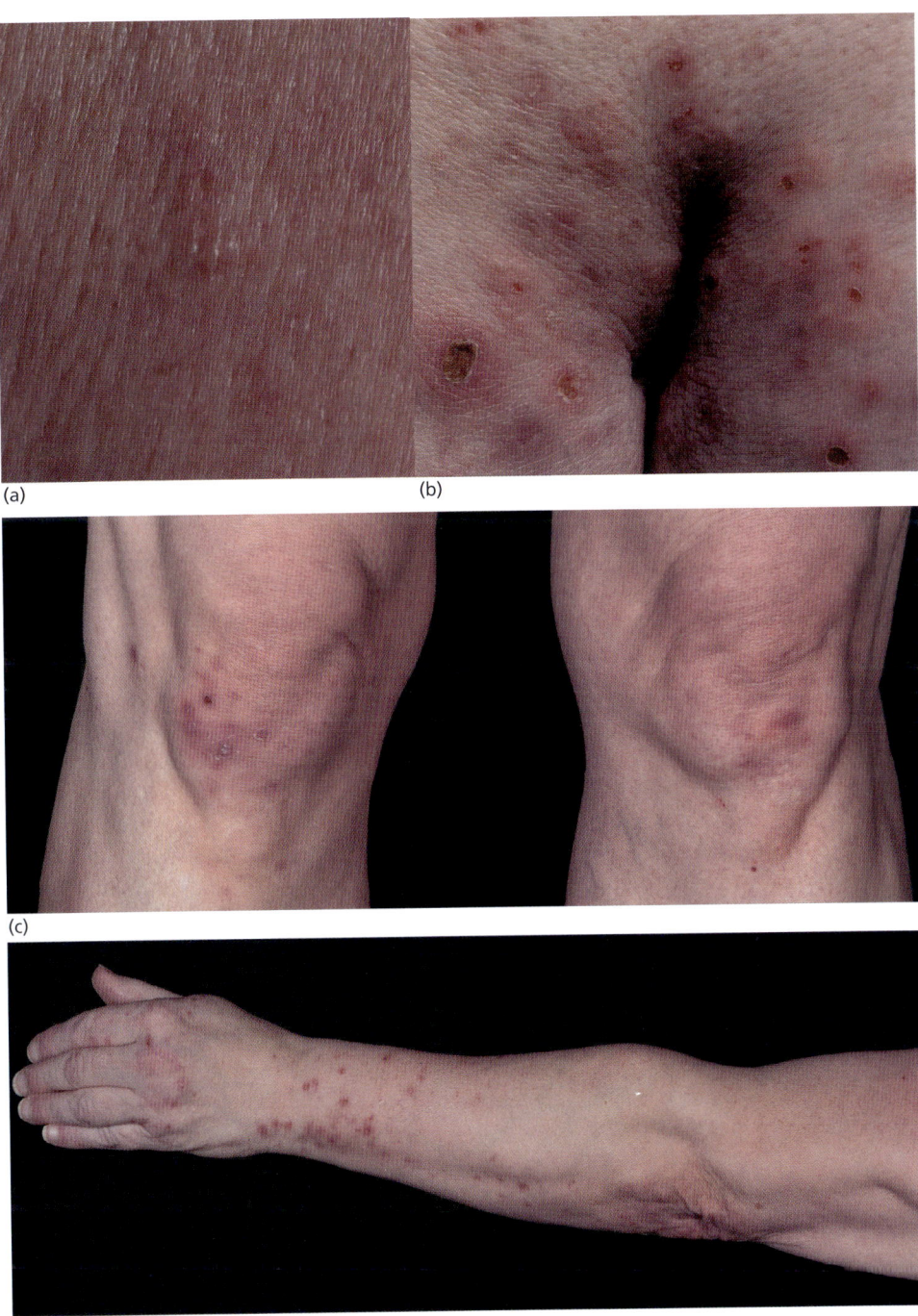

(a)

(b)

(c)

(d)

Figure 50.56 Dermatitis herpetiformis: clinical features. (a) Herpetiform vesicles. (b,c,d) Typical excoriated vesicles on buttocks and extensor surfaces of arms and legs.

Differential diagnosis

The differential diagnosis of DH includes many pruritic and vesiculobullous disorders including linear IgA disease, pemphigoid, eczema and scabies. Because of the often non-specific nature of DH lesions, skin biopsy for direct IF should be considered in the investigation of patients with unexplained or treatment-refractory pruritic rashes.

Complications and co-morbidities

The principal complications and co-morbidities of DH relate to GSE and the associated risk of small bowel lymphoma [52]. GSE may lead to malabsorption resulting in anaemia, weight loss and osteoporosis. In children, short stature is a risk. Rarely, GSE (and consequently DH) may be associated with neurological changes including ataxia and neuropathy [53,54].

Disease course and prognosis

DH is a chronic disease that requires patients to adopt a life-long gluten-free diet. Those that are able to do this, and respond, seem to have excellent long-term survival [13] and are able to decrease or discontinue dapsone treatment. Recent data suggest that patients with GSE who do not respond to a gluten-free diet do poorly [55]. While the disease is a chronic one, remission is recognised and seems to be more common in adult patients over the age of 40 [56].

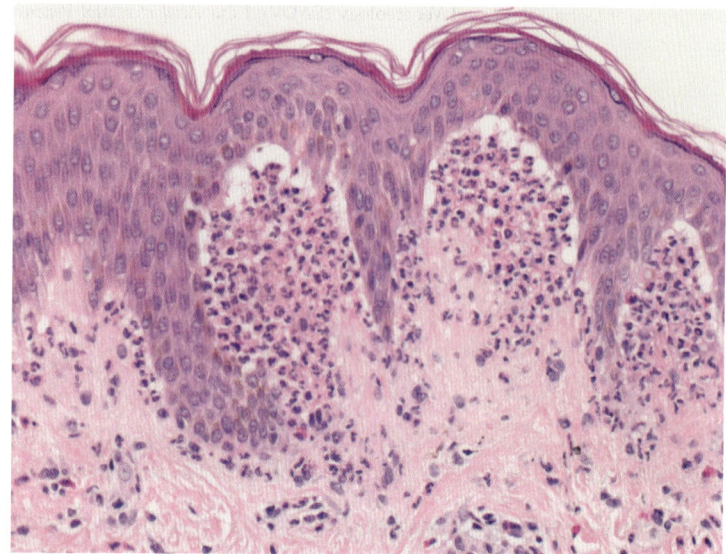

Figure 50.57 Dermatitis herpetiformis: histopathology. There is prominent accumulation of neutrophils in the dermal papillae with clefting and incipient vesicle formation.

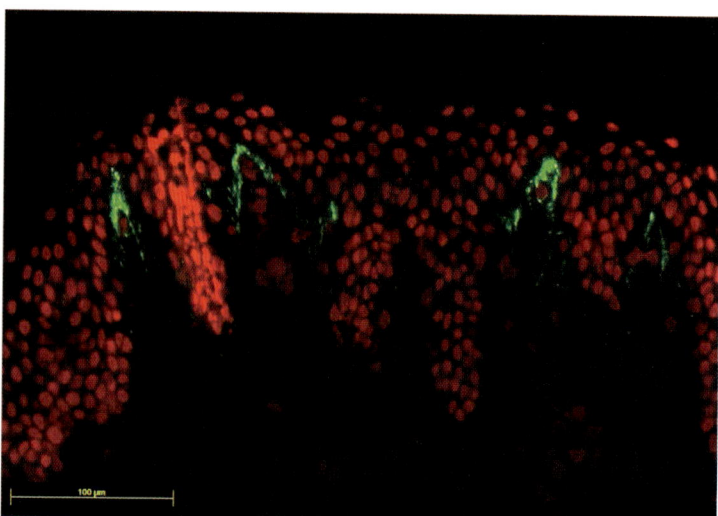

Figure 50.58 Dermatitis herpetiformis: direct immunofluorescence. Note granular IgA deposition in the dermal papillae.

Investigations

The diagnosis of DH is made by the presence of characteristic clinical features, histopathology, direct IF testing and serology [3].

The histopathology of an intact vesicle in DH demonstrates sub-epidermal blister formation with neutrophils located at the tips of the dermal papillae (Figure 50.57). There is frequently an associated perivascular inflammatory cell infiltrate. Because vesicles may not survive the pruritus, clefting may not be seen.

Direct IF samples are best taken from perilesional skin as characteristic changes may be lost in lesional tissue [57,58]. The diagnostic finding is that of deposition of IgA in the papillary dermis (Figure 50.58) in a granular or fibrillar pattern, the fibrillary pattern being particularly associated with DH in Asian patients. Complement 3 may also be found in association with the IgA deposits. Circulating endomysial antibodies may be detected by indirect IF on monkey oesophagus substrate and specific anti-TG2, TG3 and deamidated gliadin antibodies by ELISA.

Management

There are no randomised clinical trials in the management of DH. Therapy is thus based on clinical experience and case series. Pharmacological management is outlined in the Treatment ladder, later.

The cornerstone of long-term DH management is strict adherence to a gluten-free diet [**59,60**,61]. Not only does this improve skin changes over time but it is essential in the management of associated GSE. It should be remembered that the improvement in skin changes can be slow, taking months or years. Patients are best managed in consultation with an experienced dietitian who will be able to provide appropriate support as maintenance of a strict gluten-free diet can be challenging. Pure uncontaminated oats do not cause problems but patients need to avoid all exposure to wheat, barley and rye. Effective gluten avoidance, with resolution of manifest or subclinical GSE, will lead to an increased sense of general well-being and may decrease the long-term risk of lymphoma [62].

Because of the slow response to gluten-free diet, most patients with DH require pharmacological intervention to control their disease in the short to medium term. Dapsone and related sulphonamide drugs have proven highly effective, often suppressing pruritus within days of initiation of treatment. It should be noted that dapsone does not impact on the gastrointestinal aspects of associated GSE.

The mechanism of action of dapsone in DH is through its effects on neutrophil function and recruitment [63] and the drug is typically used at doses of 25–150 mg daily [64]. It is generally well tolerated although haematological side effects may occur including haemolysis [65], methaemoglobinaemia [66] and agranulocytosis [67]. Consequently, patients require regular blood monitoring, particularly in the early stages of treatment (see General principles of management in section on LAD, earlier). Non-haematological adverse effects include a severe drug sensitivity reaction ('dapsone hypersensitivity syndrome' [68]) and a peripheral neuropathy [69]. Patients with glucose-6-phosphatase deficiency (G6PD) are more prone to adverse effects of dapsone [70]) and G6PD activity should be checked before treatment wherever possible. Concurrent administration of cimetidine, via inhibition of cytochrome p-450, has been shown to decrease the adverse effects of dapsone [71–73] and may be helpful in some patients. Dapsone should always be used in combination with a gluten-free diet and with time it may be possible to decrease and potentially withdraw dapsone without relapse, as long as the patient is able to adhere to the diet.

Other sulphonamide drugs have utility in DH including sulphamethoxypyridazine [74], sulphapyridine [75] and sulphasalazine [76]. Their mechanism of action is similar to that of dapsone, and they may be of benefit in patients intolerant of dapsone. At the time of writing, however, sulphamethoxypyridazine is currently unavailable. Systemic steroids are of little benefit, although potent topical steroids may be of use in the short term to lessen pruritus. Colchicine is sometimes considered when other options fail, but evidence supporting benefit is weak [77]. A recent report has suggested that JAK inhibition may also be of benefit [78].

Treatment ladder

All patients should be screened for GSE and follow a gluten-free diet as appropriate.

First line
- Dapsone 25–150 mg daily
- Potent topical corticosteroid

Second line
- Sulphamethoxypyridazine 0.5–1.5 g daily

Third line
- Sulphapyridine 250–750 mg daily
- *or*
- Sulphasalazine 1–2 g daily
- *or*
- Colchicine 500–1500 µg daily

Experimental
- Tofacitinib 5 mg twice daily

Resources

International management guidelines
Pemphigus vulgaris and pemphigus foliaceus

Joly P, Horvath B, Patsatsi A *et al.* Updated S2K guidelines on the management of pemphigus vulgaris and foliaceus initiated by the European Academy of Dermatology and Venereology (EADV). *J Eur Acad Dermatol Venereol* 2020;34:1900–13.

Murrell DF, Peña S, Joly P *et al.* Diagnosis and management of pemphigus: recommendations of an international panel of experts. *J Am Acad Dermatol* 2020;82:575–85.e1.

Paraneoplastic pemphigus

Antiga E, Bech R, Maglie R *et al.* S2k guidelines on the management of paraneoplastic pemphigus/paraneoplastic autoimmune multiorgan syndrome initiated by the European Academy of Dermatology and Venereology (EADV). *J Eur Acad Dermatol Venereol* 2023; 37:1118–34.

Bullous pemphigoid

Borradori L, Van Beek N, Feliciani C *et al.* Updated S2 K guidelines for the management of bullous pemphigoid initiated by the European Academy of Dermatology and Venereology (EADV). *J Eur Acad Dermatol Venereol* 2022;36:1689–704.

Mucous membrane pemphigoid

Rashid H, Lamberts A, Borradori L *et al.* European guidelines (S3) on diagnosis and management of mucous membrane pemphigoid, initiated by the European Academy of Dermatology and Venereology – Part I. *J Eur Acad Dermatol Venereol* 2021;35:1750–64.

Schmidt E, Rashid H, Marzano AV *et al.* European Guidelines (S3) on diagnosis and management of mucous membrane pemphigoid, initiated by the European Academy of Dermatology and Venereology – Part II. *J Eur Acad Dermatol Venereol* 2021;35:1926–48.

Epidermolysis bullosa acquisita

Prost-Squarcioni C, Caux F, Schmidt E *et al.* International Bullous Diseases Group: consensus on diagnostic criteria for epidermolysis bullosa acquisita. *Br J Dermatol* 2018;179:30–41.

Dermatitis herpetiformis and coeliac disease

Görög A, Antiga E, Caproni M *et al.* S2k guidelines (consensus statement) for diagnosis and therapy of dermatitis herpetiformis initiated by the European Academy of Dermatology and Venereology (EADV). *J Eur Acad Dermatol Venereol* 2021;35:1251–77.

Al-Toma A, Volta U, Auricchio R *et al.* European Society for the Study of Coeliac Disease (ESsCD) guideline for coeliac disease and other gluten-related disorders. *United European Gastroenterol J* 2019;7:583–613.

Further information (links to important guidelines)

Guidelines initiated by the European Academy of Dermatology and Venereology: https://www.eadv.org/clinical-guidelines

British Association of Dermatologists' guidelines for the *management of pemphigus* and the *management of bullous pemphigoid*: www.bad.org.uk/healthcare-professionals/clinical-standards/clinical-guidelines

Guidelines of the German Dermatological Society for the diagnosis of pemphigus and bullous pemphigoid and treatment of pemphigus and bullous pemphigoid and mucous membrane pemphigoid: www.awmf.org/leitlinien

French guidelines (protocole national des soins) for the management of pemphigus, management of bullous pemphigoid, management of mucous membrane pemphigoid, management of linear IgA disease, management of epidermolysis bullosa acquisita, and management of dermatitis herpetiformis: www.has-sante.fr

Patient resources
Support groups

Australia: www.blisters.org.au
Canada: www.pemphigus.ca
France: www.pemphigus.asso.fr
Germany: www.pemphigus-pemphigoid-selbsthilfe.de
International Pemphigus and Pemphigoid Foundation: www.pemphigus.org
Italy: www.assoc-apai.org and www.pemfigo.it
Turkey: www.turkdermatoloji.org.tr
UK: www.pemfriends.co.uk and www.pemphigus.org.uk

Patient information

Information leaflets for patients can be found on the webpage of the European Academy of Dermatology and Venereology (EADV; www.eadv.org/patient-corner/patient-leaflets) and the British Association of Dermatologists (www.bad.org.uk/patient-information-leaflets).

Key references

The full list of references can be found in the online version at https://www.wiley.com/rooksdermatology10e

Pemphigus

Bullous pemphigoid

1 Schmidt E, Zillikens D. Pemphigoid diseases. *Lancet* 2013;381:320–32.

29 Persson MSM, Harman KE, Vinogradova Y *et al.* Incidence, prevalence and mortality of bullous pemphigoid in England 1998–2017: a population-based cohort study. *Br J Dermatol* 2021;184:68–77.

35 Liu SD, Chen WT, Chi CC. Association between medication use and bullous pemphigoid: a systematic review and meta-analysis. *JAMA Dermatol* 2020;156:891–900.

59 Schulze F, Neumann K, Recke A, Zillikens D, Linder R, Schmidt E. Malignancies in pemphigus and pemphigoid diseases. *J Invest Dermatol* 2015;135:1445–7.

165 Schmidt E, Sticherling M, Sardy M *et al.* S2k guidelines for the treatment of pemphigus vulgaris/foliaceus and bullous pemphigoid: 2019 update. *J Dtsch Dermatol Ges* 2020;18:516–26.

227 Lamberts A, Meijer JM, Jonkman MF. Nonbullous pemphigoid: a systematic review. *J Am Acad Dermatol* 2018;78:989–95 e982.

236 Murrell DF, Daniel BS, Joly P *et al.* Definitions and outcome measures for bullous pemphigoid: recommendations by an international panel of experts. *J Am Acad Dermatol* 2012;66:479–85.

245 Joly P, Roujeau JC, Benichou J *et al.* A comparison of oral and topical corticosteroids in patients with bullous pemphigoid. *N Engl J Med* 2002;346:321–7.

247 Kridin K, Schwartz N, Cohen AD, Zelber-Sagi S. Mortality in bullous pemphigoid: a systematic review and meta-analysis of standardized mortality ratios. *J Dermatol* 2018;45:1094–100.

258 Williams HC, Wojnarowska F, Kirtschig G *et al*. Doxycycline versus prednisolone as an initial treatment strategy for bullous pemphigoid: a pragmatic, non-inferiority, randomised controlled trial. *Lancet* 2017;389:1630–8.

287 Venning VA, Taghipour K, Mohd Mustapa MF, Highet AS, Kirtschig G. British Association of Dermatologists' guidelines for the management of bullous pemphigoid 2012. *Br J Dermatol* 2012;167:1200–14.

291 Borradori L, Van Beek N, Feliciani C *et al*. Updated S2 K guidelines for the management of bullous pemphigoid initiated by the European Academy of Dermatology and Venereology (EADV). *J Eur Acad Dermatol Venereol* 2022;36:1689–704.

Mucous membrane pemphigoid

3 Rashid H, Lamberts A, Borradori L *et al*. European guidelines (S3) on diagnosis and management of mucous membrane pemphigoid, initiated by the European Academy of Dermatology and Venereology – Part I. *J Eur Acad Dermatol Venereol* 2021;35:1750–64.

4 Schmidt E, Rashid H, Marzano AV *et al*. European Guidelines (S3) on diagnosis and management of mucous membrane pemphigoid, initiated by the European Academy of Dermatology and Venereology – Part II. *J Eur Acad Dermatol Venereol* 2021;35:1926–48.

13 Egan CA, Lazarova Z, Darling TN, Yee C, Cote T, Yancey KB. Anti-epiligrin cicatricial pemphigoid and relative risk for cancer. *Lancet* 2001;357:1850–1.

30 Wojnarowska F, Marsden RA, Bhogal B, Black MM. Chronic bullous disease of childhood, childhood cicatricial pemphigoid, and linear IgA disease of adults. A comparative study demonstrating clinical and immunopathologic overlap. *J Am Acad Dermatol* 1988;19:792–805.

38 Domloge-Hultsch N, Gammon WR, Briggaman RA, Gil SG, Carter WG, Yancey KB. Epiligrin, the major human keratinocyte integrin ligand, is a target in both an acquired autoimmune and an inherited subepidermal blistering skin disease. *J Clin Invest* 1992; 90:1628–33.

46 Balding SD, Prost C, Diaz LA *et al*. Cicatricial pemphigoid autoantibodies react with multiple sites on the BP180 extracellular domain. *J Invest Dermatol* 1996;106:141–6.

57 Setterfield J, Shirlaw PJ, Bhogal BS, Tilling K, Challacombe SJ, Black MM. Cicatricial pemphigoid: serial titres of circulating IgG and IgA antibasement membrane antibodies correlate with disease activity. *Br J Dermatol* 1999;140:645–50.

62 Heppe EN, Tofern S, Schulze FS *et al*. Experimental laminin 332 mucous membrane pemphigoid critically involves C5aR1 and reflects clinical and immunopathological characteristics of the human disease. *J Invest Dermatol* 2017; 137:1709–18.

81 Goletz S, Probst C, Komorowski L *et al*. A sensitive and specific assay for the serological diagnosis of antilaminin 332 mucous membrane pemphigoid. *Br J Dermatol* 2019;180:149–56.

110 Murrell DF, Marinovic B, Caux F *et al*. Definitions and outcome measures for mucous membrane pemphigoid: recommendations of an international panel of experts. *J Am Acad Dermatol* 2015;72:168–74.

145 Lytvyn Y, Rahat S, Mufti A *et al*. Biologic treatment outcomes in mucous membrane pemphigoid: a systematic review. *J Am Acad Dermatol* 2022;87:110–20.

Linear IgA disease

1 Schmidt E, Zillikens D. Pemphigoid diseases. *Lancet* 2013;381:320–32.

2 Hashimoto T, Yamagami J, Zone JJ. History, diagnosis, pathogenesis, and nomenclature in sublamina dense-type linear IgA disease. *JAMA Dermatol* 2021; 157;907–9.

12 Marinkovich MP, Taylor TB, Keene DR, Burgeson RE, Zone JJ. LAD-1, the linear IgA bullous dermatosis autoantigen, is a novel 120-kDa anchoring filament protein synthesized by epidermal cells. *J Invest Dermatol* 1996;106:734–8.

13 Zone JJ, Taylor TB, Kadunce DP, Meyer LJ. Identification of the cutaneous basement membrane zone antigen and isolation of antibody in linear immunoglobulin A bullous dermatosis. *J Clin Invest* 1990;85:812–20.

14 Wojnarowska F, Whitehead P, Leigh IM, Bhogal BS, Black MM. Identification of the target antigen in chronic bullous disease of childhood and linear IgA disease of adults. *Br J Dermatol* 1991;124:157–62.

41 Pas HH, Kloosterhuis GJ, Heeres K, van der Meer JB, Jonkman MF. Bullous pemphigoid and linear IgA dermatosis sera recognize a similar 120-kDa keratinocyte collagenous glycoprotein with antigenic cross-reactivity to BP180. *J Invest Dermatol* 1997;108:423–9.

63 Tsuchisaka A, Ohara K, Ishii N, Nguyen NT, Marinkovich MP, Hashimoto T. Type VII collagen is the major autoantigen for sublamina densa-type linear IgA bullous dermatosis. *J Invest Dermatol* 2015;135:626–9.

71 Garel B, Ingen-Housz-Oro S, Afriat D *et al*. Drug-induced linear immunoglobulin A bullous dermatosis: a French retrospective pharmacovigilance study of 69 cases. *Br J Clin Pharmacol* 2019; 85:570–9.

103 Ng SY, Venning VV. Management of linear IgA disease. *Dermatol Clin* 2011; 29:629–30.

106 Kasperkiewicz M, Meier M, Zillikens D, Schmidt E. Linear IgA disease: successful application of immunoadsorption and review of the literature. *Dermatology* 2010;220:259–63.

Anti-p200 pemphigoid

1 Goletz S, Hashimoto T, Zillikens D, Schmidt E. Anti-p200 pemphigoid. *J Am Acad Dermatol* 2014;71:185–91.

2 Kridin K, Ahmed AR. Anti-p200 pemphigoid: a systematic review. *Front Immunol* 2019;10:2466.

3 Dainichi T, Kurono S, Ohyama B *et al*. Anti-laminin gamma-1 pemphigoid. *Proc Natl Acad Sci U S A* 2009;106:2800–5.

4 Goletz S, Pigors M, Rastegar Lari T *et al*. Laminin β4 is a constituent of the cutaneous basement membrane zone and autoantigen of anti-p200 pemphigoid. *J Am Acad Dermatol*, 2023 in press; doi: 10.1016/j.jaad.2023.11.014.

5 Zillikens D, Kawahara Y, Ishiko A *et al*. A novel subepidermal blistering disease with autoantibodies to a 200-kDa antigen of the basement membrane zone. *J Invest Dermatol* 1996;106:1333–8.

13 Goletz S, Probst C, Komorowski L *et al*. Sensitive and specific assay for the serological diagnosis of anti-p200 pemphigoid based on recombinant laminin β4. *Br J Dermatol*, submitted.

14 Commin MH, Schmidt E, Duvert-Lehembre S *et al*. Clinical and immunological features and outcome of anti-p200 pemphigoid. *Br J Dermatol* 2016;175:776–81.

16 Lau I, Goletz S, Holtsche MM, Zillikens D, Fechner K, Schmidt E. Anti-p200 pemphigoid is the most common pemphigoid disease with serum antibodies against the dermal side by indirect immunofluorescence microscopy on human salt-split skin. *J Am Acad Dermatol* 2019;81:1195–7.

18 Holtsche MM, Goletz S, von Georg A *et al*. Serologic characterization of anti-p200 pemphigoid: epitope spreading as a common phenomenon. *J Am Acad Dermatol* 2021;84:1155–7.

31 Meijer JM, Diercks GF, Schmidt E, Pas HH, Jonkman MF. Laboratory diagnosis and clinical profile of anti-p200 pemphigoid. *JAMA Dermatol* 2016;152:897–904.

Epidermolysis bullosa acquisita

2 Prost-Squarcioni C, Caux F, Schmidt E *et al*. International Bullous Diseases Group: consensus on diagnostic criteria for epidermolysis bullosa acquisita. *Br J Dermatol* 2018;179:30–41.

6 Roenigk HH, Jr, Ryan JG, Bergfeld WF. Epidermolysis bullosa acquisita. Report of three cases and review of all published cases. *Arch Dermatol* 1971;103:1–10.

13 Woodley DT, Briggaman RA, O'Keefe EJ, Inman AO, Queen LL, Gammon WR. Identification of the skin basement-membrane autoantigen in epidermolysis bullosa acquisita. *N Engl J Med* 1984;310:1007–13.

14 Komorowski L, Muller R, Vorobyev A *et al*. Sensitive and specific assays for routine serological diagnosis of epidermolysis bullosa acquisita. *J Am Acad Dermatol* 2012;68:e89–95.

28 Buijsrogge JJ, Diercks GF, Pas HH, Jonkman MF. The many faces of epidermolysis bullosa acquisita after serration pattern analysis by direct immunofluorescence microscopy. *Br J Dermatol* 2011;165:92–8.

30 Hashimoto T, Jin Z, Ishii N. Clinical and immunological studies for 105 Japanese seropositive patients of epidermolysis bullosa acquisita examined at Kurume University. *Expert Rev Clin Immunol* 2016;12:895–902.

125 Becker M, Schumacher N, Schmidt E, Zillikens D, Sadik CD. Evaluation and comparison of clinical and laboratory characteristics of patients with IgA epidermolysis bullosa acquisita, linear IgA bullous dermatosis, and IgG epidermolysis bullosa acquisita. *JAMA Dermatol* 2021;157:917–23.

128 Meijer JM, Atefi I, Diercks GFH *et al*. Serration pattern analysis for differentiating epidermolysis bullosa acquisita from other pemphigoid diseases. *J Am Acad Dermatol* 2018;78:754–9.e756.

145 Holtsche MM, van Beek N, Hashimoto T *et al.* Diagnosis of epidermolysis bullosa acquisita: multicentre comparison of different assays for serum anti-type VII collagen reactivity. *Acta Derm Venereol* 2021;101:adv00420.

168 Kridin K, Kneiber D, Kowalski EH, Valdebran M, Amber KT. Epidermolysis bullosa acquisita: a comprehensive review. *Autoimmun Rev* 2019;18:786–95.

Bullous systemic lupus erythematosus

1 Camisa C, Neff JC, Rossana C, Barrett JL. Bullous lichen planus: diagnosis by indirect immunofluorescence and treatment with dapsone. *J Am Acad Dermatol* 1986;14:464–9.

5 Yell JA, Allen J, Wojnarowska F, Kirtschig G, Burge SM. Bullous systemic lupus erythematosus: revised criteria for diagnosis. *Br J Dermatol* 1995;132:921–8.

6 Gammon WR, Briggaman RA. Bullous SLE: a phenotypically distinctive but immunologically heterogeneous bullous disorder. *J Invest Dermatol* 1993;100:28S–34S.

9 Chan LS, Lapiere JC, Chen M *et al.* Bullous systemic lupus erythematosus with autoantibodies recognizing multiple skin basement membrane components, bullous pemphigoid antigen 1, laminin-5, laminin-6, and type VII collagen. *Arch Dermatol* 1999; 135:569–73.

10 Doebelin B, Dalle S, Balme B, Kanitakis J, Thomas L. Bullous systemic lupus erythematosus with autoantibodies recognizing bullous pemphigoid antigen 1. *Br J Dermatol* 2005;153:232–3.

17 Vodegel RM, Jonkman MF, Pas HH, de Jong MC. U-serrated immunodeposition pattern differentiates type VII collagen targeting bullous diseases from other subepidermal bullous autoimmune diseases. *Br J Dermatol* 2004;151:112–18.

24 Yell JA, Mbuagbaw J, Burge SM. Cutaneous manifestations of systemic lupus erythematosus. *Br J Dermatol* 1996;135:355–62.

25 Pons-Estel GJ, Quintana R, Alarcon GS, Sacnun M, Ugarte-Gil MF, Pons-Estel BA. A 12-year retrospective review of bullous systemic lupus erythematosus in cutaneous and systemic lupus erythematosus patients. *Lupus* 2018;27:1753–4.

43 de Risi-Pugliese T, Cohen Aubart F, Haroche J *et al.* Clinical, histological, immunological presentations and outcomes of bullous systemic lupus erythematosus: 10 new cases and a literature review of 118 cases. *Semin Arthritis Rheum* 2018;48:83–9.

Rare pemphigoid disorders

4 Hubner F, Langan EA, Recke A. Lichen planus pemphigoides: from lichenoid inflammation to autoantibody-mediated blistering. *Front Immunol* 2019;10:1389.

5 Zillikens D, Caux F, Mascaro JM *et al.* Autoantibodies in lichen planus pemphigoides react with a novel epitope within the C-terminal NC16A domain of BP180. *J Invest Dermatol* 1999;113:117–21.

30 Imstepf V, Cazzaniga S, Beltraminelli H, Borradori L, Feldmeyer L. Brunsting-Perry pemphigoid: a retrospective case series of a frequently unrecognized condition. *J Am Acad Dermatol* 2021;85:1324–6.

37 Ghohestani RF, Hudson BG, Claudy A, Uitto J. The alpha 5 chain of type IV collagen is the target of IgG autoantibodies in a novel autoimmune disease with subepidermal blisters and renal insufficiency. *J Biol Chem* 2000;275:16002–6.

39 Baardman R, Horvath B, Bolling MC, Pas HH, Diercks GFH. Immunoglobulin M bullous pemphigoid: an enigma. *JAAD Case Rep* 2020;6:518–20.

40 Suchniak JM, Diaz LA, Lin MS, Fairley JA. IgM-mediated epidermolysis bullosa acquisita. *Arch Dermatol* 2002;138:1385–6.

46 Boch K, Hammers CM, Goletz S *et al.* Immunoglobulin M pemphigoid. *J Am Acad Dermatol* 2021;85:1486–92.

67 Alcalay J, Ingber A, Hazaz B, David M, Sandbank M. Linear IgM dermatosis of pregnancy. *J Am Acad Dermatol* 1988;18:412–15.

68 White KP, Zedek DC, White WL *et al.* Orf-induced immunobullous disease: a distinct autoimmune blistering disorder. *J Am Acad Dermatol* 2008;58:49–55.

70 Yilmaz K, Goletz S, Pas HH *et al.* Laminin 332 is the major target antigen in Orf-induced immunobullous disease. *JAMA Dermatol* 2022;158:670–4.

Dermatitis herpetiformis

1 Duhring LA. Landmark article, Aug 30, 1884: Dermatitis herpetiformis. By Louis A. Duhring. *JAMA* 1983;250:212–16.

4 Reunala T, Hervonen K, Salmi T. Dermatitis herpetiformis: An update on diagnosis and management. *Am J Clin Dermatol* 2021;22:329–38

5 Antiga E, Maglie R, Quintarelli L *et al.* Dermatitis herpetiformis: novel perspectives. *Front Immunol* 2019;10:1290.

6 Lundin KE, Sollid LM. Advances in coeliac disease. *Curr Opin Gastroenterol* 2014;30:154–62.

7 Guandalini S, Assiri A. Celiac disease: a review. *JAMA Pediatr* 2014;168:272–8.

8 Görög A, Antiga E, Caproni M *et al.* S2k guidelines (consensus statement) for diagnosis and therapy of dermatitis herpetiformis initiated by the European Academy of Dermatology and Venereology (EADV). *J Eur Acad Dermatol Venereol* 2021;35:1251–77.

21 Hervonen K, Vornanen M, Kautiainen H, Collin P, Reunala T. Lymphoma in patients with dermatitis herpetiformis and their first-degree relatives. *Br J Dermatol* 2005;152:82–6.

27 Dieterich W, Ehnis T, Bauer M *et al.* Identification of tissue transglutaminase as the autoantigen of celiac disease. *Nat Med* 1997;3:797–801.

28 Sardy M, Karpati S, Merkl B, Paulsson M, Smyth N. Epidermal transglutaminase (TGase 3) is the autoantigen of dermatitis herpetiformis. *J Exp Med.*2002;195:747–57.

38 Hervonen K, Hakanen M, Kaukinen K, Collin P, Reunala T. First-degree relatives are frequently affected in coeliac disease and dermatitis herpetiformis. *Scand J Gastroenterol* 2002;37:51–5.

59 Cardones AR, Hall RP, 3rd. Management of dermatitis herpetiformis. *Immunol Allergy Clin North Am* 2012;32:275–81, vi–vii.

60 Caproni M, Antiga E, Melani L, Fabbri P, Italian Group for Cutaneous I. Guidelines for the diagnosis and treatment of dermatitis herpetiformis. *J Eur Acad Dermatol Venereol* 2009;23:633–8.

CHAPTER 51

Lupus Erythematosus and Antiphospholipid Syndrome

Jan Dutz[1] and Touraj Khosravi-Hafshejani[2]

[1]Skin Care Centre, Vancouver General Hospital, Vancouver; BC Children's Hospital Research Institute, Vancouver, BC, Canada
[2]Department of Dermatology and Skin Science, University of British Columbia, Vancouver, BC, Canada

PART 4: INFLAMMATORY DERMATOSES

Introduction

Systemic lupus erythematosus (SLE) is a complex autoimmune disease characterised by multiorgan involvement and immunological abnormalities. There is a greater prevalence and incidence of SLE in black, Asian and Hispanic population groups, with young females disproportionately affected [1]. Extracutaneous organ systems most commonly affected include the joints, renal system, hematological system, pulmonary system, central nervous system and cardiovascular system. Cutaneous disease is the second most frequently affected organ in SLE and occurs in 80% of patients during their disease course. Skin involvement can be divided into specific and non-specific manifestations depending on the histological presence of an interface dermatitis. The non-specific skin disease of lupus is diverse and includes photosensitivity rash, non-scarring alopecia, bullous lupus erythematosus, neutrophilic dermatoses, vasculitis and vasculopathy. The specific cutaneous manifestations of SLE, all characterised by the histological presence of interface dermatitis, can be subclassified into chronic, subacute and acute cutaneous lupus erythematosus (CLE). CLE can exist as an independent entity or be associated with SLE [2,3]. Collectively, CLE and SLE are forms of lupus erythematosus (LE).

Discoid lupus erythematosus

Definition and nomenclature

Discoid lupus erythematosus (DLE) is a benign inflammatory disorder of the skin, most frequently involving the face and scalp, and characterised by well-defined, red, scaly patches of variable size, which heal with atrophy, scarring and pigmentary changes. The disease may also be more generalised, affecting areas away from the face and scalp. The histology is characteristic. There are haematological and serological changes in approximately half of patients, and these changes, with other evidence, suggest an autoimmune aetiology. The condition forms one end of a spectrum of skin and internal organ disease, ending with SLE [1].

Synonyms and inclusions
- Chronic cutaneous lupus erythematosus (CCLE)
- Chronic discoid lupus erythematosus

Introduction and general description

Discoid lupus erythematosus is one of the forms of cutaneous disease seen within the spectrum of CLE; others are subacute cutaneous lupus erythematosus (SCLE) and acute cutaneous lupus erythematosus (ACLE), the latter seen in patients with the systemic form of the disease, usually in those with severe internal organ disease. DLE is the most common subtype of cutaneous lupus, comprising 80% of all CLE cases [2].

A fourth subtype – lupus tumidus – is also described, but it is unclear where this fits into a lupus classification [3]. In general, the histological hallmark of cutaneous lupus is interface dermatitis, with lymphocytic infiltration, but interface change is absent in lupus tumidus. The same is true of Jessner lymphocytic infiltrate, which is thought by many to be a dermal variant of cutaneous lupus. It can predate classic DLE but has similar genetic predispositions, responds to the same treatments and may occur in patients already known to have DLE [4]. The scarring nature of the classic forms of DLE means that early diagnosis and active treatment are important to avoid irreversible, long-term sequelae.

Epidemiology
Incidence and prevalence

In a large Scandinavian study, the annual incidence of cutaneous lupus was 4/100 000, with 80% being DLE [2]. The prevalence in an American cohort was reported as around 70/100 000 with an annual incidence similar to the Scandinavian study [5]. Overall, the prevalence of CLE without concurrent SLE is similar to the prevalence of SLE.

Age

Peak age of onset is the fourth decade in females, slightly later in males, although it can occur at any age [6]. For example, in a large series, 3% of cases began earlier than 15 years of age and 2.5% after the age of 70 years [7].

Sex

The disease affects twice as many females as males [6,7] with a greater male predilection than in SLE.

Ethnicity

The disease is more common in Asians, African Americans, Afro-Caribbeans and Hispanic Americans than those Americans of European origin, and is more common in those of Asian origin in the UK [6]. It is also more severe in African Americans and Asians compared with white people [7]. Black patients present with more dyspigmentation, scalp and ear involvement and scarring alopecia compared with non-black patients [8].

Associated diseases

Porphyria (including cutanea tarda [9], variegate [10], acute intermittent and erythropoietic protoporphyria [11]), pemphigus, myasthenia gravis and thymoma [12] have all been reported to occur in association with DLE.

Pathophysiology [13]

Cutaneous inflammation in DLE is a process in which interferons (IFNs) – type I and type III – induce Th1-biased inflammation, with a predominantly lymphocytic infiltration (Figure 51.1) [14]. This inflammatory pattern mirrors that of the innate immune system in response to cutaneous viral infection, followed by epidermal damage, basement membrane thickening and a scarring tissue response associated with a loss of follicular stem cells [15]. With CD4 and CD8 T cells, natural IFN-producing plasmacytoid dendritic cells (PDCs) are the predominant cell type, and numbers of granzyme B-positive cells correlate with the extent of scarring [16]. Compared with lichen planopilaris, there is a greater number of PDCs, as well as the presence of PDCs in the dermis, periecrine and dermal–epidermal junction in DLE of the scalp [17]. IFN-α, possibly produced mainly by PDCs [18], and IFN-γ produced by keratinocytes [19] induce the keratinocyte expression of pro-inflammatory chemokines, as well as the apoptosis-inducing TRAIL molecule (tumour necrosis factor-related apoptosis-inducing ligand) and its receptors [20]. A gene expression array study of lesional DLE skin showed a relative enrichment of IFN-γ-associated genes and B-cell-associated genes compared with SCLE or ACLE [21]. Regulatory T cells are reduced in number [22]. The stimuli to this pattern of inflammation include ultraviolet (UV) radiation, acting through molecules such as heat shock proteins, Toll-like receptors and other DAMP (danger-associated molecular pattern) molecules [23].

Treatment failure and progression of disease are common in CLE. This may in part be due to the strong presence of dysregulated tissue resident memory T (Trm) cells, a subset of memory T cells that persist long term and through treatment in diseased inflammatory skin. A higher density of Trm cells has been identified in DLE and SCLE skin lesions compared with ACLE, which may explain the duration of the disease [24]. The survival of Trm cells is mediated by

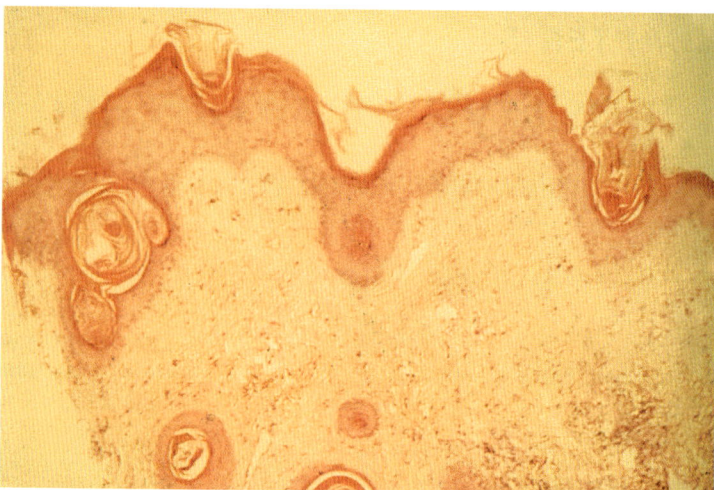

Figure 51.1 Discoid lupus erythematosus showing atrophy of the epidermis, keratotic plugging, liquefaction degeneration of the basal layer, oedema and hyalinisation of the connective tissue below the epidermis and a marked inflammatory infiltrate. Magnification 40×.

interleukin 7 (IL-7) and IL-15 cytokines that result in downstream JAK/STAT (Janus kinase/signal transducers and activators of transcription) signalling. A better understanding of Trm cells in CLE may lead to novel and targeted therapeutic strategies to prevent disease recurrence [25–27].

Predisposing factors

Predisposing factors are shown in Box 51.1 [28–38].

Box 51.1 Predisposing factors to discoid lupus erythematosus (DLE) (percentages of patients affected)

- Trauma (11%) [28], including X-rays [29] and thermal burns [30]
- Stress (12%)
- Ultraviolet exposure (5%) [31], including psoralen with UVA [32] and laser light [33]
- Infection (3%), including herpes zoster and old smallpox vaccination [34]
- Drugs: many drugs are associated with the precipitation or exacerbation of DLE, including isoniazid, penicillamine, griseofulvin and dapsone [35–37]
- Seasonal exacerbation, both in winter (10%) and summer (50%)
- Cold exposure (2%, but 17% of patients reported disease exacerbation due to cold) [38]

Unpublished data from Chapel Allerton Hospital, Leeds, UK unless referenced.

Pathology

The various clinical types of CLE show an essentially similar histological picture (Figure 51.2), and the subsets of CLE cannot be easily distinguished histologically [39]. The salient features are shown in Box 51.2 [40]. In more acute forms there is less hyperkeratosis and dermal infiltration, but more dermal oedema, liquefaction necrosis and atrophy. In tumid lesions the dermal infiltrate can be very dense,

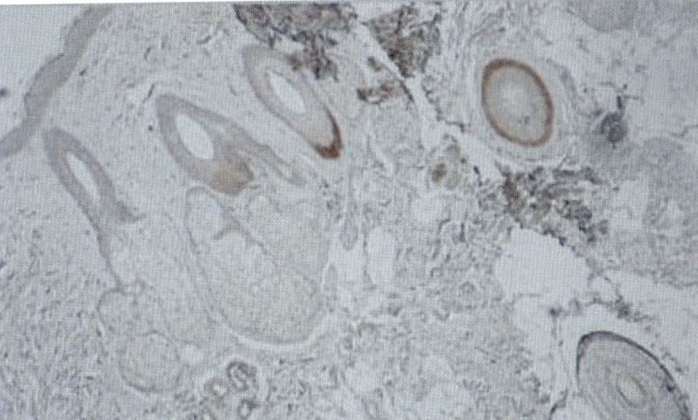

(a)

(b)

Figure 51.2 Discoid lupus erythematosus. (a) The degeneration of the basal layer and predominantly lymphocytic infiltration are well shown. (b) CD8-stained section showing stem cells visible in the bulge region of uninvolved follicles. Magnification 40×.

and sometimes almost granulomatous. Dermal deposits of mucin occur, which may be either diffuse or localised, and form nodular lesions [41,42]. Although keratotic plugs are usually found in the openings of the hair follicles, they may also block the sweat ducts or occur independently of either structure.

Box 51.2 Histological features of cutaneous lupus erythematosus

- Lymphocytic interface dermatitis with basal layer degeneration
- Apoptotic keratinocytes
- Basement membrane thickening (greatest in discoid lupus erythematosus)
- Perivascular and periadnexal lymphohistiocytic infiltrate
- Follicular plugging
- Dermal mucinosis
- Epidermal atrophy

Causative organisms

There are increasing numbers of reports of the involvement of a range of organisms – bacterial and viral – that may be implicated in the onset and exacerbation of lupus, including cutaneous disease. None is confirmed as yet, but the subject has been well reviewed [43,44].

Genetics

A family history was found in 4% of cases [45]; the condition is reported in identical twin sisters and in two or more family members. Recent studies also indicated a striking relationship between polymorphic light eruption (PLE) and DLE, first in twins [46] and then in a large cohort of patients and their relatives, suggesting a common genetic background for these disorders [47]. Differences in the incidence of histocompatibility antigens [48,49] have supported the concept of multiple genotypes. Positive associations with human leukocyte antigen B7 (HLA-B7), -B8, -Cw7, -DR2, -DR3 and -DQw1 are reported, but not always confirmed. The relative risk is increased with certain combinations of antigens: HLA-Cw7, -DR3 and -DQw1 and for HLA-B7, -Cw7 and -DR3. The extended haplotype – HLA*01, B*08, DRB1*0301 – is associated with both SCLE and DLE, and the A*03, B*07, DRB1*15 haplotype has been associated with DLE alone [50]. Patients of either sex who develop skin lesions between the ages of 15 and 39 years have an increased incidence of HLA-B7, and females over the age of 40 years with HLA-B8, compared with controls [48].

Clinical features

The patient usually presents with a rash, but a history of Raynaud phenomenon, chilblains or poor peripheral circulation is often obtained [51]. In 120 patients with DLE seen at Chapel Allerton Hospital, Leeds, UK, 14% had Raynaud phenomenon and 22% had chilblains; a poor peripheral circulation, without a definite story of Raynaud phenomenon, was noted in a further 26% of patients. Joint pains may occur. Most patients have no symptoms of systemic upset, even with widespread cutaneous disease, although fatigue is not uncommon [52].

Presentation

Most patients have disease limited to the head and neck (localised DLE), but a few have much more extensive disease, potentially affecting any area of the skin (disseminated DLE).

Localised disease. The face and scalp are most commonly affected. The circumscribed or discoid form is the most frequent type of disease (Figure 51.3), and occurs particularly on the cheeks, bridge of the nose, ears, side of the neck and scalp. Alopecia occurs in the scalp lesions in approximately one-third of patients [53], and is usually permanent (Figure 51.4). The eyebrows may be sparse, with redness of the eyebrow skin. Usually, lesions occur as well-defined red or pink patches, varying in size from a few millimetres to 10–15 cm. There is adherent scale in many cases, and when this is removed its undersurface shows horny plugs that have occupied dilated pilosebaceous canals. This so-called 'tin-tack' sign can sometimes also be seen in localised pemphigus foliaceus [54]. The surface may present a dirty, brownish yellow appearance that is

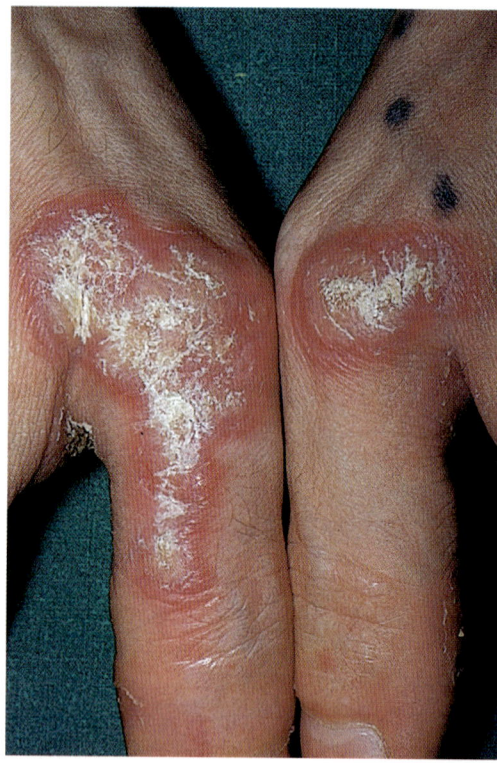

Figure 51.3 Localised discoid lupus erythematosus showing typical scaling on the fingers.

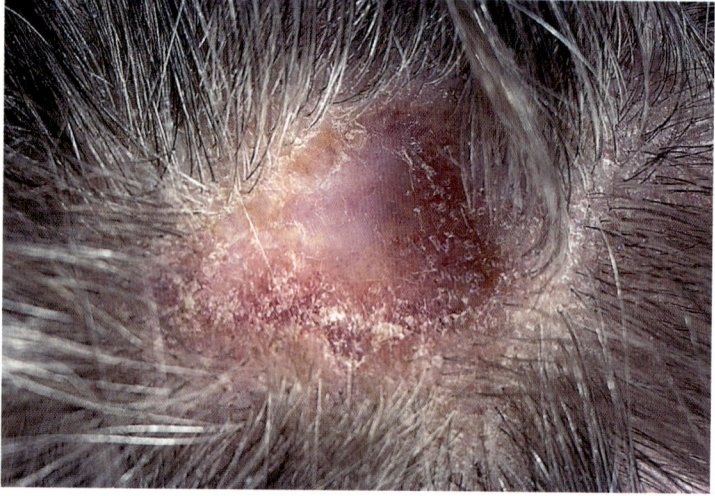

Figure 51.4 Localised discoid lupus erythematosus of the scalp showing follicular plugging.

rough to the touch because of follicular plugging. A hypertrophic or verrucous variant of DLE has also been described, with hallmarks of hyperkeratosis overlying discoid lesions, chronicity and resistance to treatment. These hyperkeratotic and warty indurated plaques of DLE may occur on the face, scalp, extensor forearms and upper trunk but also on the palms and soles and cause difficulty with walking (Figure 51.5) [55–57]. Over the course of some months, particularly if treated, lesions flatten and may clear completely without much scarring. If left untreated, the lesions expand with peripheral inflammation and hyperpigmentation and central depressed

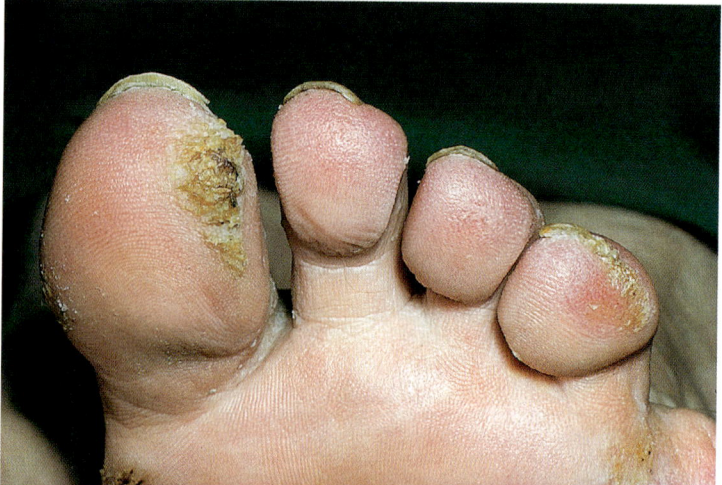

Figure 51.5 Warty lesions of the feet in chronic lupus erythematosus.

atrophy, scarring, telangiectasia and hypopigmentation. More frequently, a thin, white scarred area remains (Figure 51.6a). Localised cribriform scarring occurs, particularly on the face (Figure 51.6b). Wide follicular pits occur mainly in the concha or triangular fossa of the ear (Figure 51.7) in up to one-third of cases of DLE [58]. In approximately 7.5% of patients, the lesions on the face resemble rosacea (Figure 51.8), and differentiation from true rosacea can be difficult. Low-titre antinuclear antibody (ANA) also occurs in rosacea, complicating assessment, but has no clinical relevance [59]. Usually, there are no pustules as in true rosacea. Biopsy may be required to distinguish between LE and rosacea. Tumid lesions may occur, in which the tissues are swollen, brawny, warm and tense (Figure 51.9). This type of lesion may be many centimetres in diameter and involve the whole of one cheek, or even the whole of a limb. Another clinical type of DLE results in annular atrophic plaques [60] on the face, neck and behind the ears. The centre of the plaques is depressed and sclerotic, and lesions resemble morphoea, lichen sclerosus or 'annular atrophic plaques' [10].

Dermoscopic features of non-scalp DLE include follicular keratotic plugs, white perifollicular halo, white scale, speckled brown pigmentation, white structureless areas and arborising vessels [61]. Nearly 60% of patients with DLE will have scalp involvement, in which one-third will lead to scarring alopecia. Trichoscopic features may include follicular red dots, large yellow dots, absent follicular openings, thick arborising vessels, speckled brown or blue-grey dots and discoloration [62].

Scarring. Scarring is common and may be atrophic, hypertrophic, cribriform or acneform [63]. Pigmentary disturbances are common, especially in dark-skinned people (Figure 51.10). Patches of leukoderma may be interspersed with hyperpigmented areas; not all of this is scarring and may be reversible post inflammatory change. Once scarring has occurred, no further inflammation is seen, so that if relapse occurs it usually starts in the reddish zone surrounding the scar. Calcification may occur in plaques [64]. Lesions on the ear lead to considerable atrophy and scarring (Figure 51.11).

Disseminated DLE. Characteristic lesions of DLE may occur in a widespread pattern on the trunk and limbs, or may be localised

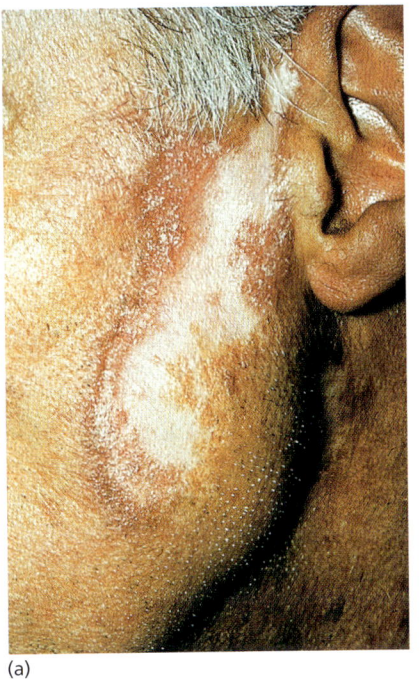

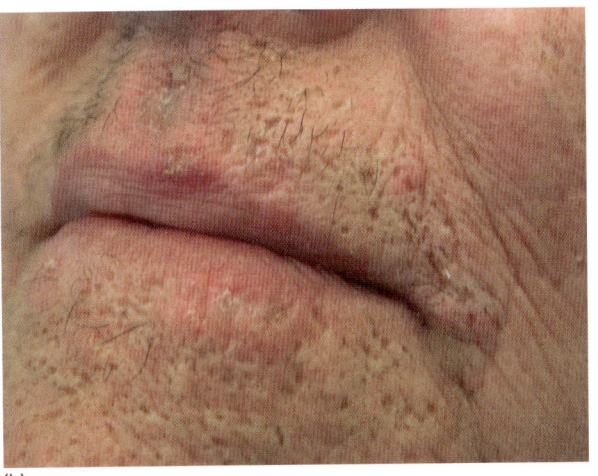

Figure 51.6 Scarring in discoid lupus erythematosus (DLE). (a) Preauricular DLE with pigmentation around the scarred area. (b) Cribriform scarring in DLE.

(a)

(b)

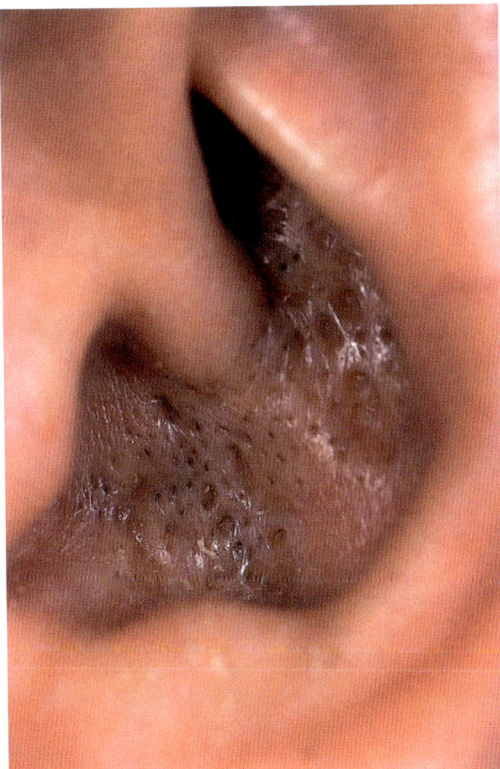

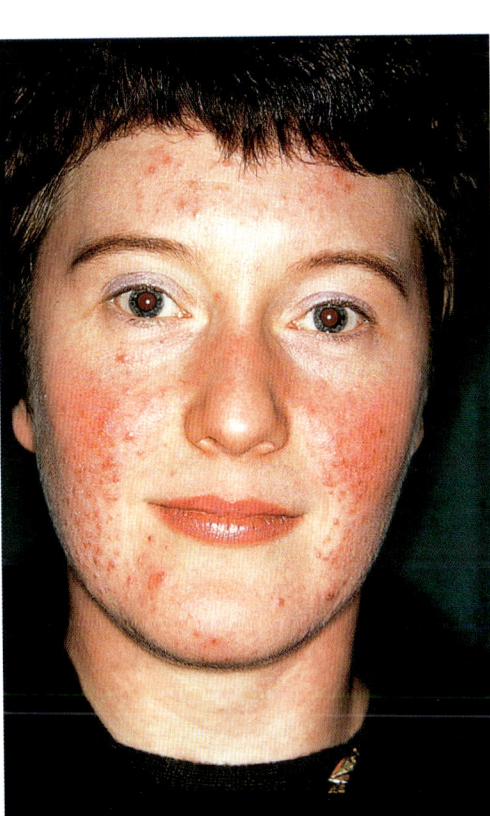

Figure 51.7 Typical lesions in the ear in discoid lupus erythematosus.

Figure 51.8 Rosaceous pattern seen in 7.5% of patients with discoid lupus erythematosus.

to other body sites. This occurs most often in women, and they are usually cigarette smokers. The appearance may be indistinguishable from the papulosquamous type of SCLE, but scarring occurs in most patients. This variety tends to be persistent, resistant to therapy and associated with severe psychological upset. Lesions on the dorsa of the hands (Figure 51.12a), palms [65] or toes (Figure 51.12b)

[66] occurred in 6% of patients at Chapel Allerton Hospital [67]. Purplish plaques may occur on the front of the knees and on the back of the heels. Non-itching, hyperkeratotic, papulonodular lesions on the arms and hands, resembling keratoacanthoma, hypertrophic lichen planus or nodular prurigo, also occur. Sometimes, the appearance resembles psoriasis. In other cases, there may be

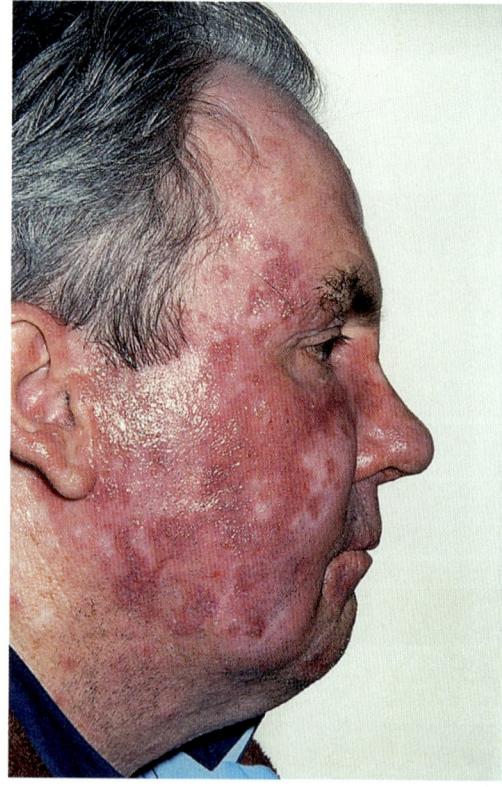

Figure 51.9 Tumid lesions of the face in discoid lupus erythematosus.

very little hyperkeratosis. Another disseminated variety results in a reticulate telangiectasia (Figure 51.13), usually seen on the arms, legs and back of the calves, but potentially widespread. This type of telangiectasia is probably similar to 'lupus erythematosus telangiectoides', first described by Crocker [68]. A further, more annular variant has been called 'lupus erythematosus gyratus repens' and consists of a migratory gyrate annular patch of red skin with the histological features of LE (Figure 51.14), although the lupus band test is negative [69]. There may be an underlying carcinoma. Rarely, bullous lesions may occur [70]. Arteritic lesions resembling those of Degos syndrome or disseminated atrophie blanche occasionally occur, and linear lesions that follow Blaschko lines have been reported [71].

Relationship of DLE to SLE. DLE can be subdivided into a localised form in which lesions are confined to the face above the chin, the scalp and the ears, and a disseminated form in which lesions also occur elsewhere on the body [72,73]. Although haematological and serological abnormalities occur slightly more frequently in the disseminated form, the natural history of the two subgroups is similar, and it is likely that they are subsets of the same disorder. SCLE has been described as a subset intermediate between DLE and SLE [74].

The more controversial point is whether DLE and SLE are variants of the same disease. The evidence in favour of this may be summarised as follows:

- The cutaneous lesions of SLE and DLE may be clinically and histologically indistinguishable.
- Certain clinical features are found in both conditions (Table 51.1).

- Similar haematological, biochemical and immunohistochemical abnormalities can be demonstrated in both conditions (Table 51.1), although the incidence of abnormalities is lower in DLE.
- Patients with DLE occasionally develop evidence of overt SLE.
- Patients with SLE may develop typical lesions of DLE in the chronic phase of their disease [75].
- Conditions such as lupus panniculitis, a recognisable clinical and pathological entity, occur in both DLE and SLE.

This seems to be formidable evidence, but the following observations require explanation:

1 The risk of a patient with DLE developing overt SLE is small. It varies from 1.3% (76) to about 6.5% [67,77]. The risk is higher in patients with disseminated DLE (22%) than in DLE confined to the head and neck (1.2%) [77]. In some series [78], such conversion was not encountered despite follow-up for nearly 30 years. In a retrospective study, progression to SLE was noted in 19% at 20 years with an average time to progression of 8.2 years from diagnosis of cutaneous disease [5].

2 The presence of laboratory abnormalities in DLE does not in itself appear to predispose to the development of SLE [5], although they are common in disseminated DLE [77,79]. The same prognosis was found in a subgroup intermediate between DLE and SLE as in patients with uncomplicated LE [78].

3 Immunoglobulins and complement are present in uninvolved skin of patients with SLE and absent in patients with DLE [80].

4 Most patients with DLE exposed to UV radiation (UVR), stress, trauma, etc. do not develop the systemic disease.

5 The age and sex distribution of SLE [81] is strikingly different from that of DLE [82]. On this basis, it has been proposed [7,67] that genetic predisposition determines the level of risk of developing one or both patterns of disease, and that the risk may be related to one or more genotypes. Genes associated with CLE include *C1QA*, *CSNK2B*, *CTLA4*, *HLA-DRB3*, *HLA-DQA1*, *IL10*, *IRF5*, *ITGAM*, *IZKF*, *MICA*, *MICB*, *MSH5*, *RPP21*, *TRAF3IP2*, *TRIM39* and *TYK2* [83].

At present, it is not possible to determine the genetic pattern of individual patients or to predict accurately the small proportion of patients with DLE-like lesions who will develop SLE, although a link with HLA-B8 and CLE has already been noted [48]. From consideration of the clinical features, the natural history, the age and sex distribution, and studies of histocompatibility antigens, most patients with DLE and haematological and serological abnormalities are not cases of SLE in disguise, but are cases of DLE, which is a separate entity from SLE, and has a different genetic background.

Clinical variants

Chilblain lupus. This may occur in patients with either DLE or SLE [84]. Chilblain lupus is a subtype of chronic CLE characterised by painful or pruritic red to violaceous papules and plaques involving the hands and feet, primarily the fingers and toes. Involvement of the nose and ears may also occur. Secondary sequelae may include ulceration, fissuring and hyperkeratosis [84]. Approximately 6% of patients with cutaneous lupus, predominantly female, develop chilblain-like lesions chiefly on the toes and fingers (Figure 51.15), but occasionally more generally. The lesions are triggered by cold or damp exposure. It can be precipitated by pregnancy [85]. Most

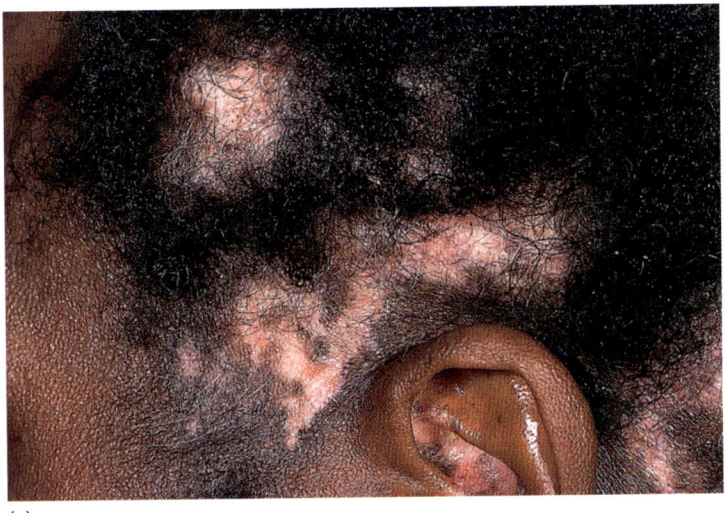

(a)

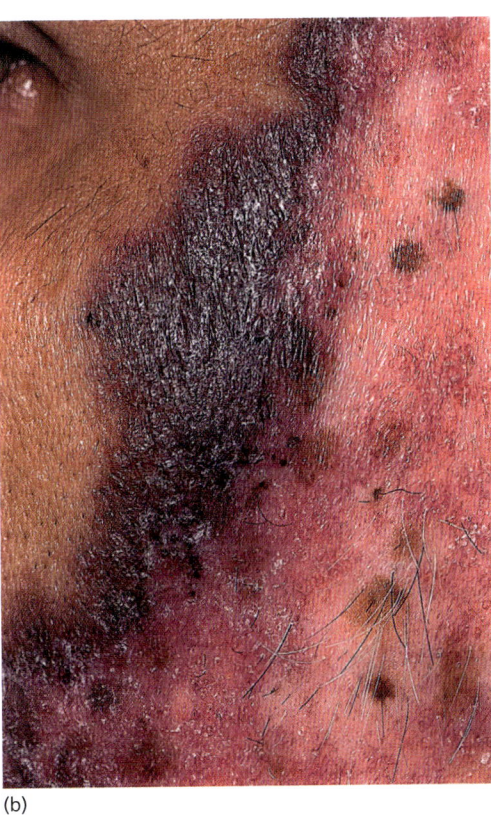

(b)

Figure 51.10 Pigmentary changes in discoid lupus erythematosus (DLE). (a) Patches on the scalp of a black person. (b) DLE in an Asian patient showing marked hyperpigmentation at the border of the affected area.

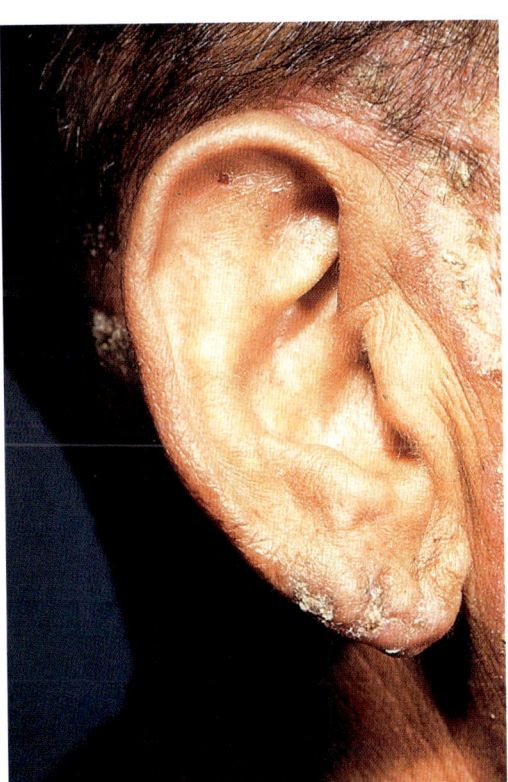

Figure 51.11 Discoid lupus erythematosus of the ear with scarring and atrophy.

patients will have a positive ANA, anti-Ro/SSA or anti-La/SSB [86]. Some patients may have cryo-fibrinogenaemia or cold agglutinins. They are also either smokers or have markedly abnormal peripheral circulation with low resting blood flow. Occasionally, one or more fingers may show a curious atrophic spindling, sometimes with hyperextension of the terminal phalanges and dystrophy of the nails (Figure 51.16). The fingers and toes may become markedly atrophic, with patchy redness and tuft resorption on X-ray. Fifteen per cent of patients develop SLE.

Familial chilblain lupus has been described as the result of autosomal dominant, heterozygous mutations in *TREX1*, *SAMHD1* and *STING* (protein stimulator of interferon) genes with disease manifesting in early childhood. These genes encode intracellular nucleases, and their mutation results in activation of antiviral type I interferons and the development of autoimmunity [87]. Management includes maintaining a warm core and peripheral temperature, and avoiding damp conditions. Topical treatments include high-potency corticosteroids, tacrolimus and pimecrolimus [88,89]. Improvement of skin disease has been observed with the use of oral nifedipine [90], hydroxychloroquine, quinacrine [91], mycophenolate mofetil [92] and JAK inhibitors [93,94].

Lupus erythematosus profundus (panniculitis). Lupus panniculitis is an unusual clinical variety of LE in which the cutaneous infiltrate occurs primarily (but not always exclusively) in deeper portions of the corium (Figure 51.17) [95]. There are only microscopic epidermal changes, giving rise to firm, sharply defined nodules from one to several centimetres in diameter, lying beneath clinically

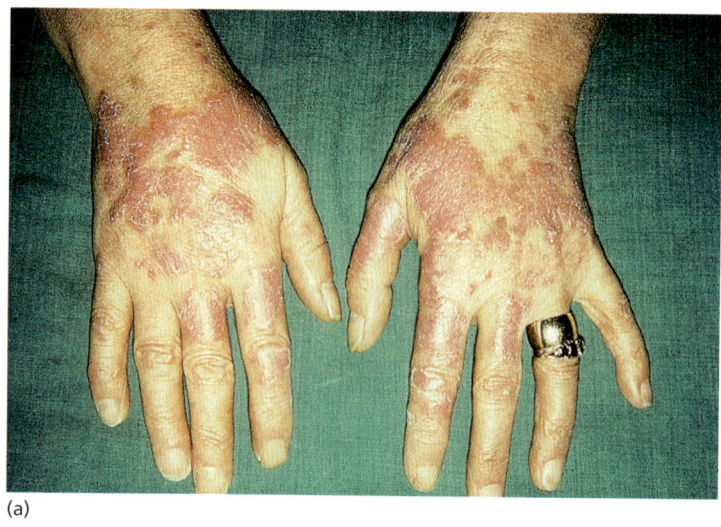

(a)

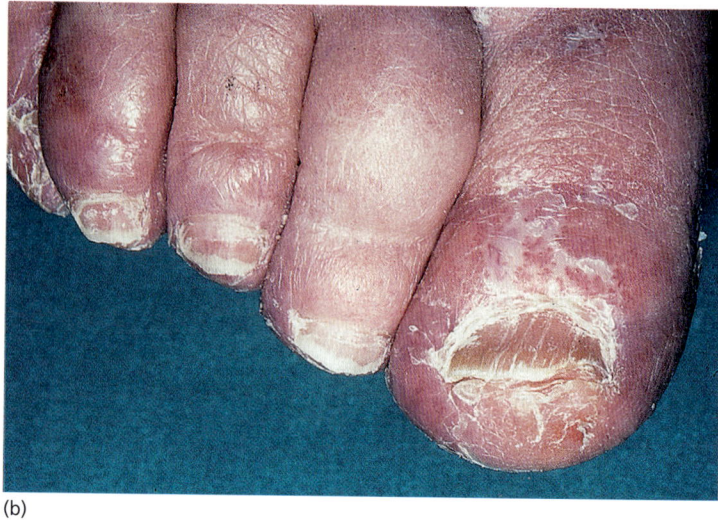

(b)

Figure 51.12 Disseminated discoid lupus erythematosus. (a) Plaques on the back of the hands. (b) Characteristic redness and scaling of the toes. Note the white atrophic scars (atrophie blanche) proximal to the great toenail.

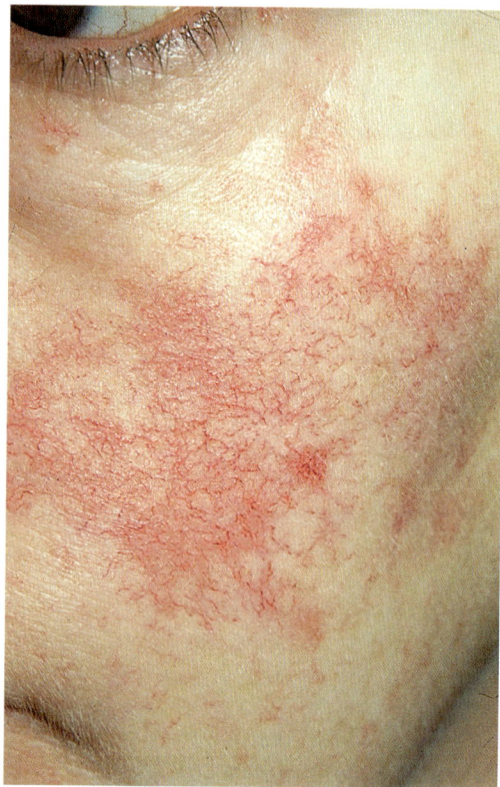

Figure 51.13 Telangiectatic lupus erythematosus of the cheek.

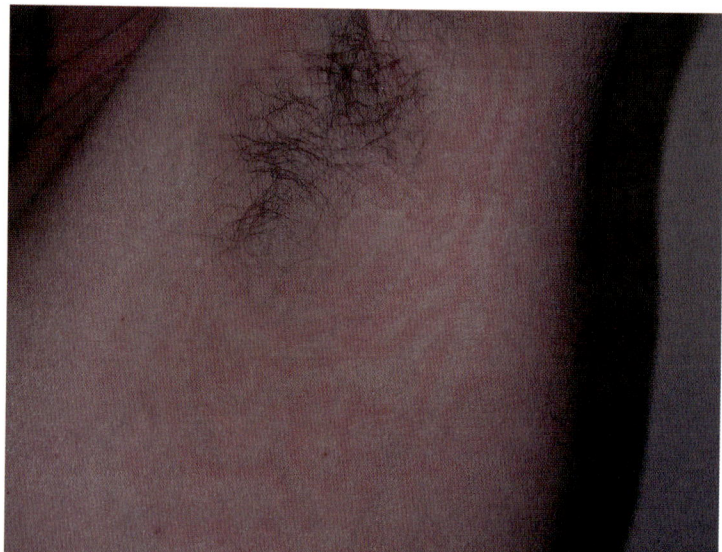

Figure 51.14 Gyrate erythema in lupus erythematosus.

normal skin and followed by atrophy of fat. It disproportionately affects middle-aged women (85%) [96] and presents as chronic and recurring tender, red, indurated subcutaneous nodules or plaques located on fatty areas of the body. Lesions are primarily located on the proximal extremities, face, back and scalp [96]. Long-term sequalae include ulceration, atrophy, calcinosis and disfigurement. Coexistence with an overlying DLE is termed lupus profundus and occurs in more than one-third of patients [96]. Clinical LE profundus occurred in 3–5% of patients with DLE [97], but histological

disease may be found in up to 30% [98]. Kaposi first described subcutaneous nodules in LE in 1883 [99], but Irgang [100] first used the term 'lupus erythematosus profundus' in 1940. Some authors have considered the lesions to be sarcoid [101], but it is now usually accepted as a variant of LE [102], related more to DLE than to SLE [103]. Approximately one-fifth of patients have concurrent SLE.

Histologically LE profundus is characterised by lymphoplasma-cytic lobular or mixed panniculitis with hyalinising fat necrosis and lymphoid follicles. Chronic lesions may display dermal or subcutaneous calcium deposits. Treatment is effective if started early and targeted during the active phase of the disease. Antimalarial medications are first line [104,105]. A short course of systemic corticosteroids may be used initially to reduce active inflammation [106]. Intralesional steroids, dapsone [107], mycophenolate mofetil [108], ciclosporin [109], rituximab [110] and intravenous immunoglobulins (IVIg) [111] have been reported in case reports with variable results.

Table 51.1 Comparison of data on a series of patients with discoid and systemic lupus erythematosus seen at Chapel Allerton Hospital, Leeds, UK.

	Discoid lupus erythematosus (*n* = 120) (%)	Systemic lupus erythematosus (*n* = 40) (%)
Rash	100	80
Joint pains	23	70
Fever	0	40
Raynaud phenomenon	14	35
Chilblains	22	22
Poor peripheral circulation	26	32
ESR >20 mm/h	20	85
Serum globulin >3 g (%)	29	76
LE cells	1.7	83
Antinuclear factor(s):	35	87
Homogeneous	24	74
Speckled	11	26
Nucleolar	0	5.4
Precipitating autoantibodies	4	42
WR positive	5	22
Rheumatoid factor positive	15	37
Direct Coombs test positive	2.5	15
Leukopenia	12.5	37
Thrombocytopenia	5	21

ESR, erythrocyte sedimentation rate; LE, lupus erythematosus; WR, Wassermann reaction.

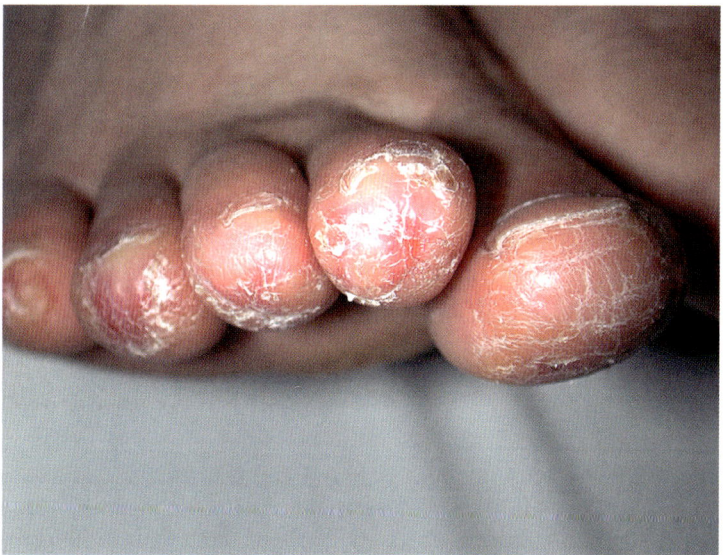

Figure 51.15 'Chilblain' lesions in a patient with Ro-positive systemic lupus erythematosus.

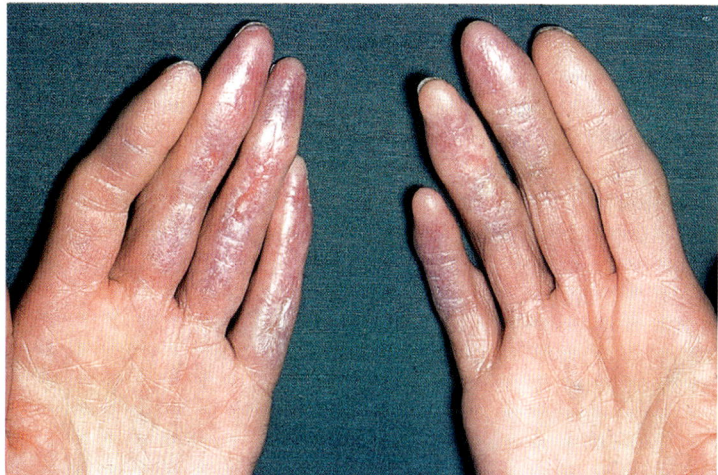

Figure 51.16 Unusual spindling of the fingers and hyperextension of the distal phalanges in discoid lupus erythematosus.

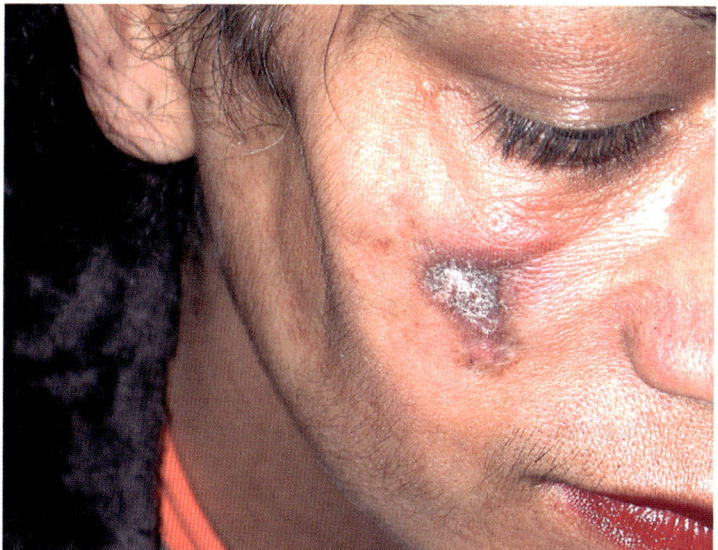

Figure 51.17 Lupus erythematosus profundus.

Tumid lupus erythematosus. Tumid lupus erythematosus (TLE) is a rare subtype of chronic CLE. Due to the small number of patients with ANA positivity and a weak association with SLE, some consider TLE to be a unique subtype of CLE or a separate disease from lupus altogether [112,113]. TLE shares similar histological features with reticular erythematous mucinosis and Jessner lymphocytic infiltrate, and some consider them to be on the same spectrum [114]. Lesions typically present as asymptomatic, annular or urticarial, red, oedematous papules and plaques with minimal or no epidermal change. Lesions are often located on sun-exposed sites including the face, neck and upper trunk and are exacerbated by UV exposure [**115**].

TLE is distinguished histologically by well-demarcated intense periadnexal lymphocytic infiltrates, superficial and mid-dermal perivascular lymphocytic infiltrate and abundant interstitial dermal mucin deposition [116]. There may be focal or minimal vacuolar interface changes, epidermal atrophy and oedema in the papillary dermis [3,117]. Typically, there is no scarring, follicular plugging or dyspigmentation. Differential diagnoses of TLE include DLE, SCLE, Jessner lymphocytic infiltrate, reticular erythematous mucinosis, PLE, pseudolymphoma and leukaemia/lymphoma cutis. Management includes UV protection, antimalarials and high-potency topical steroids. Lesions resolve without scarring, atrophy or hypopigmentation [118,119].

Differential diagnosis

The annular atrophic plaque variety of DLE may resemble morphoea or lichen sclerosus [58]. Jessner lymphocytic infiltration may be confused with the more acute localised oedematous lesions of LE, but the marked histological lymphocytic infiltration in the former should help to distinguish it from the latter, and immunoglobulin deposition does not occur at the dermal–epidermal junction in Jessner lymphocytic infiltration. There is still disagreement on the relationship between DLE and Jessner infiltration. Indeed, some authors believe the latter to be a precursor of classic CLE [4]. Benign lymphocytic infiltration of the skin may be a further form of CLE, as indicated by photo testing [120]. Reticular erythematous mucinosis syndrome (Chapter 57), which can show clinical and histological features similar to DLE, may also be induced by UVR but is a discrete clinical entity [121].

The history and the presence of lesions elsewhere should exclude contact eczema, seborrhoeic eczema and psoriasis. Lupus vulgaris may resemble DLE, but the lesions of the former usually occur at an early age, are rarely symmetrical, may be ulcerated and usually show characteristic 'apple-jelly' nodules on diascopy. Necrobiosis lipoidica can give facial lesions similar to those in DLE. The rosaceous type of LE can usually be differentiated from true rosacea by the absence of pustules and the histology.

Chronic DLE has been found in 12% of patients diagnosed as having scarring alopecia of the pseudopelade type [122]. Lesions on the lips, tongue, scalp and buccal mucosa may be confused with lichen planus, and the skin of some patients may show clinical, histological and immunological features of both diseases [123]. Overlap cases, in addition to LE-like lesions, have lichenoid papules, verrucous lesions, anonychia and oral and vulval lesions resembling lichen planus. Patients with lichen planus do not have features of LE immunopathologically or by HLA typing [124]. Overlap cases either have both diseases or are variants of LE. In favour of the latter, the verrucous lesions show immunofluorescent findings of LE [125].

LE of the legs and feet may resemble chilblains. Plaques of sarcoidosis and lesions of eosinophilic granuloma may cause diagnostic difficulties that can only be resolved histologically. Occasionally, lesions resembling DLE are caused by dermatophytes [126].

The distinction from plaque-type PLE may be difficult, but the absence of both antinuclear factor from the serum and of dermal–epidermal immunoglobulin deposits in PLE may be helpful [127]. PLE may either coexist with or precede DLE by many years. Infants may show sharply marginated, reddish, finely scaling plaques on the cheeks and bridge of the nose, sometimes exacerbated by the sun, or a transitory rash with telangiectases on the face, particularly around the eyes, which clinically and histologically resembles LE [128]. These rashes probably are part of so-called neonatal LE (see separate section later in this chapter). An LE-like rash on the face with sun sensitivity occurs in Bloom syndrome (Chapter 14), which is thought to be caused by an autosomal recessive gene. A congenital telangiectatic area of reddish skin occurs in people with well-proportioned dwarfism, who look similar because of their bird-like facial appearance. The skin changes occur in infancy and may be associated with ectodermal and mesodermal defects [129].

Classification of severity

The accepted system for assessment is the cutaneous lupus erythematosus disease area and severity index (CLASI), which quantifies disease activity and monitors response to treatment and is a useful clinical and research tool [130]. This activity score measures degree of redness, scale, mucous membrane lesions and non-scarring alopecia [130].

Disease course and prognosis

In general, the course of the disease is chronic and relapsing, with exacerbations in spring and summer, but some patients have mild disease that settles spontaneously. Most disease will produce scarring if it is untreated, and the disease will continue episodically for many years. A minority will burn out completely, but may be left with significant and permanent damage to affected areas [67].

Investigations

Patients may require a skin biopsy to confirm the diagnosis, and should have an ANA test, extractable nuclear antigens (ENAs), anti-double-stranded DNA (dsDNA) antibodies and complement 3 and 4 determined to assess the possibility of them having the systemic form of the disease. Routine haematology and biochemistry and urine testing for proteinurea are sensible as baseline investigations. Assessment of visual acuity is also necessary in those needing systemic therapy with antimalarials.

Management

It is important to carry out a complete medical survey of the patient at the first attendance to establish a diagnosis of the subtype of DLE, a likely prognosis and a baseline by which later progress may be judged. Patients should be advised to avoid overwork, mental stress and fatigue, and enquiry should be made for symptoms of depression (often related to facial scarring). Scarred lesions may be camouflaged. Patients should avoid excessive exposure to sunlight and phototoxic medications, and use appropriate sun protection against UVA and UVB. The application of sunscreen should be frequent – preferably every 2–3 h in bright sunlight [131]. Vasodilator drugs, particularly calcium-channel blockers such as nifedipine, are helpful in those with Raynaud phenomenon and chilblain lesions [84]. Patients should have annual assessments for SLE, and regular assessments of disease severity and impact [132]. Guidelines for therapy have been published by several societies [133–135].

First line

Topical therapy can frequently control and sometimes clear lesions without the need for systemic treatment; 0.025% fluocinolone cream or 0.1% betamethasone 17-valerate cream alone can be effective without inducing epidermal atrophy [136]. There are few data supporting the use of one topical corticosteroid over another, although more potent agents appear generally to be more effective. Occlusion may help further. Intralesional corticosteroid injections are helpful in resistant cases [137], even on the lips, mouth and ears. Topical calcineurin inhibitors, such as tacrolimus, provide a useful alternative to corticosteroids in those with localised disease [138].

Second line

For patients with severe, extensive or scarring disease, particularly affecting the scalp, oral prednisolone is often the most helpful initial treatment. A dosage of 0.5 mg/kg, rapidly tapered over 6 weeks, is quickly effective, minimises scarring and allows the slower-acting agents such as antimalarials to work. Long-term therapy with oral corticosteroids is best avoided because of side effects, but may be

Table 51.2 Oral agents useful in the management of chronic discoid lupus erythematosus.

Drug	Daily dosage	Response rate as first line treatment (%)	Response rate as second line treatment (%)	Side effects
Hydroxychloroquine [88,100]	200–400 mg	60–75	20	See Box 51.3
Chloroquine [101]	200–400 mg	60–75	20	See Box 51.3
Acitretin [102]	25–100 mg	50–75	15–20	Dry skin, hair loss, liver or lipid abnormalities, bony ankylosis
Auranofin [103]	3–9 mg	50	15–20	Gastrointestinal upset, haematological, renal or liver abnormality
Dapsone [104]	50–150 mg	25–50	10–20	Rash, haemolysis, dapsone syndrome
Methotrexate [105]	5–30 mg	–	25–50	Gastrointestinal upset, hepatitis, hepatic fibrosis, pulmonary fibrosis
Ciclosporin [106]	2.5–5 mg/kg	–	30–50	Hypertension, renal function abnormalities
Sulfasalazine [107]	1.5 g	–	5–15	
Isotretinoin [108]	20–80 mg	–	15–20	
Thalidomide [93,94]	50–150 mg	80–90	40–50	Drowsiness, constipation, teratogenicity, polyneuropathy
Clofazamine [109]	50–150 mg	40–60	5–15	Orange-pink to brown skin discoloration
Phenytoin [110]	200–300 mg	–	–	
Azathioprine [111]	75–200 mg	–	20–30	Photosensitivity, skin cancer
Cyclophosphamide [95]	50–200 mg	–	–	
Mycophenolate [112]	0.5–3 g	–	40–50	Bone marrow suppression, hepatitis
Mepacrine [113]	100–200 mg	50–60		Hepatitis, yellow skin colour

necessary in a small number of patients resistant to other mainte-nance therapy. In such circumstances, patients should also receive bone protection with vitamin D and calcium supplementation as well as bisphosphonates or related drugs to avoid osteoporosis. Methylprednisolone 500–1000 mg/day for 2 or 3 days, given as an intravenous pulse therapy, may help resistant lesions.

First-line systemic treatment for ongoing use should be with one of the oral antimalarials (Table 51.2). Most would start therapy with hydroxychloroquine, initially at 200 mg twice daily, reducing to 200 mg/day once a response is achieved [139]. Chloroquine phosphate is equally effective, usually at a dosage of 250 mg twice daily, but hydroxychloroquine is used first by most prescribers because side effects, particularly eye toxicity, are less likely provided that the dosage limitations of 5 mg/kg real body weight are adhered to [140,141].

Box 51.3 Side effects of antimalarials

Mild
- Nausea and vomiting
- Abdominal pain

Severe
- Corneal deposits
- Retinopathy
- Pigmentation of the palate, nails and legs
- Bleaching of hair
- Exfoliative dermatitis
- Lichenoid rashes
- Myasthenia
- Extrapyramidal involuntary movements
- Neuropathy
- Psychiatric syndromes
- Myopathy

The comparable safe daily dosage for chloroquine is unclear, but is probably around 4 mg/kg/day of chloroquine base. Cumulative

toxicity is rarely a problem with hydroxychloroquine prior to 10 years of therapy, although it can occur with chloroquine [142]. Mepacrine is also useful, and is safe from an ophthalmological point of view [143], but it is often reserved for later use (because of yellow skin pigmentation). It may be used alone, or as part of a combination of antimalarials, which may be more effective than the equivalent amount of each drug given individually [144]. Monitoring during therapy should include annual ophthalmological screening begin-ning at no more than 5 years after treatment initiation [**145**]. The side effects of antimalarials are listed in Box 51.3.

Third line

For cases not responding to topical corticosteroids, antimalarials and sunscreens, oral thalidomide, lenalidomide [146], methotrex-ate and mycophenolate are the most effective third line agents, although all of the agents listed in Table 51.2 may have a role in individual patients. Thalidomide at a dose of 100 mg/day seems to be as effective as higher doses. If used as initial therapy, response rates of 80–90% may be achieved, but when used as second line treatment the response rate is nearer 50% [147,148]. Short courses are preferable because of the risk of polyneuropathy and its teratogenic effects. The prescription of thalidomide is tightly regulated with a pregnancy prevention programme: patients are allowed only monthly amounts of drug, and all women of fertile potential should be using double contraception and require monthly pregnancy tests.

IVIg may be useful in resistant cases of diffuse disease [149] or panniculitis. Rarely, intravenous pulses of cyclophosphamide may be used, usually at a dosage of 10 mg/kg, at 3–4-weekly intervals. It is usually given in combination with intravenous methylpred-nisolone [150]. Most recently, immunomodulating biologic agents have been used, but an effective agent, efalizumab [151], has been withdrawn from the market because of the occurrence of progressive multifocal leukoencephalopathy.

Rituximab [152] and belimumab [153] have been investigated in the context of SLE and found to be helpful for skin involvement, but personal experience suggests that discoid lesions do not respond well to B-cell antagonists.

PART 4: INFLAMMATORY DERMATOSES

Emerging therapies

Belimumab was approved for the treatment of SLE in 2011 in the USA. Belimumab is a recombinant human immunoglobulin G λ (IgG-λ) monoclonal antibody that inhibits the B-cell-activating factor (BAFF), which is important in the proliferation, differentiation and immunoglobulin secretion of B cells. Inhibition of BAFF targets autoreactive B cells that are active in SLE and results in their apoptosis. A case series and a small open-label study comprising a total of 12 patients with recalcitrant DLE have shown potential in improving disease activity in some patients [154,155].

Apremilast, a phosphodiesterase 4 inhibitor, works to inhibit dendritic cells and leukocyte production of IFN-α and IFN-γ, respectively. In an open-label study of eight patients taking apremilast 20 mg twice daily, four patients had marked reduction in DLE activity at day 85. Scalp lesions also completely regressed in two patients [156].

Fumaric acid esters are small molecules with immunomodulating, anti-inflammatory and antioxidative effects that have been used as a systemic therapy for plaque psoriasis for half a century. An open-label study for their off-label use has shown improvement of longstanding therapy-refractory DLE [157].

There is low to moderate evidence for treatment with pulsed dye laser (585–595 nm) in the treatment of DLE. Not only has there been improvement in symptoms and cosmetic outcomes, but also in disease activity. However, caution is warranted with the use of laser due to the theoretical risk of DLE exacerbation [158–163]. Repairing cosmetic defects in inactive DLE is challenging because they are composed of scarring, hyperpigmentation and telangiectasia. A combination of Q-switched neodymium:yttrium-aluminium-garnet (Nd:YAG) laser and intense pulse light (IPL) may be a treatment to target both dermal melanosomes and superficial telangiectasia, respectively [164]. Caution should be taken when using IPL as it can exacerbate disease and in patients with darker skin types it can further enhance dyspigmentation. Argon lasers have also been shown to improve superficial vascular changes such as redness and telangiectasia in DLE [165]. Erbium:yttrium-aluminium-garnet (Er:YAG) laser has been reported to treat scarring in inactive DLE, without exacerbating disease [166]. In patients with LE panniculitis and lipoatrophy, fat transfer and lipofilling have been the mainstay aesthetic therapy [167–172]. More recently, autologous cell-assisted lipotransfer with the addition of adipose-derived stem cells has shown promising results in improving disfigurement, the survival of grafts and reduction of postoperative atrophy [173]. Dermal fillers using hyaluronic acid [174], poly-L lactic acid [174], polymethylmethacrylate [175] and polyacrylamide [176] have all been reported to establish satisfactory correction of lipoatrophy in patients with LE panniculitis. A common side effect of dermal fillers has been nodularity immediately post-injection. This may improve over time or mitigated by injection of normal saline.

Anifrolumab, JAK inhibitors and a novel humanised IgG1 monoclonal antibody that blocks blood dendritic cell antigen 2 are promising medications on the horizon for the targeted inhibition of type I interferon in DLE [177–179]. Anifrolumab, an antibody to type I interferon receptor subunit 1, has been shown to improve CLASI scores by 50% in 3 months in patients with SLE and CLE [180]. Case series have demonstrated rapid and excellent response of previously drug-resistant DLE to anifrolumab [181–184].

Subacute cutaneous lupus erythematosus

Definition

Subacute cutaneous lupus erythematosus is a specific 'subset' of cutaneous lupus first described by Sontheimer *et al.* in 1979 [1]. Patients exhibit mainly cutaneous disease and usually have a good prognosis. Antibodies to the Ro/SS-A antigen are closely associated with this subgroup.

Introduction and general description

This subgroup of lupus is very characteristic clinically and immunologically, is usually photoaggravated and may be associated with a limited degree of systemic involvement. Approximately 15% of patients fulfil the 2019 European League Against Rheumatism (EULAR)/American College of Rheumatology (ACR) criteria for SLE at the time of diagnosis [2], with arthralgia/arthritis being the most frequent feature. Fever, malaise and central nervous system involvement occur, but renal disease is mild and infrequent. Proteinuria, haematuria and casts may occur [3] but a recent study suggests that only 1.1% of patients develop lupus nephritis [4].

Epidemiology

Incidence and prevalence

The incidence of Ro/SS-A-positive SCLE in Stockholm was estimated to be 0.7 per 100 000 persons per year; the prevalence is estimated to be 6.2–14 per 100 000 persons [5]. In a European database study, patients with SCLE made up 236 of 1002 registered patients with cutaneous LE (23.5%) [6]. Separate nationwide cohort studies in Sweden and Denmark found that approximately 16% and 20% of CLE patients, respectively, were diagnosed with SCLE [7,8].

Age

The disease predominantly affects adults, however there have been increasing reports in children [9–11].

Sex

The disease has a female predominance, with 75–85% of the diagnoses occurring in females [5,6].

Associated diseases

Some patients with SCLE also have Sjögren syndrome [12], rheumatoid arthritis [4], vasculitis [13], Sweet syndrome [14], Crohn disease [15], lichen planus [16], psoriasis [17], hereditary angioedema [18], porphyria cutanea tarda [19], gluten-sensitive enteropathy [20], toxic epidermal necrolysis [21,22], inclusion body myositis [23], calcifying lupus panniculitis [24] or Kikuchi–Fujimoto disease (KFD; necrotising lymphadenitis) [25]. Morphoea [26] and dystrophic calcinosis cutis [27] have sometimes followed the presentation of SCLE. Some patients develop lesions related to mucin deposition [28].

Pathophysiology

Antibodies to the Ro/SS-A antigen are an almost universal finding in this subset of lupus. That these antibodies may be pathogenic was first suggested by LeFeber *et al.* in 1984 [29], who demonstrated that sublethal doses of UVR induced the synthesis and surface expression of Ro/SS-A antigen by cultured human keratinocytes. In 1988, Ro/SS-A antigen was identified in both adult and neonatal epidermis *in vivo* [30]. Subsequent studies have confirmed that UVR increases Ro/SS-A antigen expression on the surface of keratinocytes [29,30] and that this is increased by oestrogen [31]. Thus, it has been postulated that in photosensitive lupus, UVR exposure leads to increased synthesis and subsequent expression of Ro/SS-A antigen on the surface of keratinocytes where it binds antibodies and initiates disease [32]. Further support for this hypothesis comes from a demonstration that photosensitivity and the titre of Ro/SS-A antibodies correlated with the expression of Ro/SS-A in the skin biopsies of patients with LE [33]. Although attractive, this hypothesis does not explain why other patients with Ro/SS-A antibodies (e.g. patients with Sjögren syndrome) do not exhibit photosensitivity and why in the clinical setting Ro/SS-A titres rarely reflect disease activity [34].

Pathogenesis of drug-induced SCLE

Drug-induced SCLE is common, but differs from other drug-induced skin diseases in a number of ways: the onset is often delayed after the introduction of the drug, both on first occurrence and on subsequent exposures, indicating a lack of immune sensitisation. Resolution is also slow after discontinuation of the drug [35]. Antihypertensive agents, such as thiazides and calcium channel blockers, and terbinafine are the commonest causes. Over the last decade, there has been a rise in the association of proton pump inhibitors, statins, non-steroidal anti-inflammatory drugs (NSAIDs), immunomodulators and immune checkpoint inhibitors with SCLE [36,37].

A systematic review of therapeutic monoclonal antibody-associated SCLE found that nearly half of cases were induced by tumour necrosis factor α (TNF-α) inhibitors, with a stark rise in the rates of PD-1 checkpoint inhibitor-induced SCLE, relative to their global use [38]. While the mechanisms of drug-induced SCLE are unclear, they may involve both photoinduction [39] and direct epidermal cytotoxicity of reactive drug metabolites [40].

Autoantibody status

Subacute cutaneous LE was originally labelled ANA-negative lupus, as these patients often exhibited negative autoantibody screens. This was probably because of the use of test substrates that did not contain suitable antigens for the antibodies found in this group of patients. Using human cell lines as substrates, homogeneous ANAs are found in approximately 60% and anti-Ro/SS-A antibodies in approximately 80% of patients [1], rising to higher levels in females [40]. The next common serological associations include rheumatoid factor or anticyclic citrullinated peptide (39%) and anti-La/SSB (38%) [4]. Antihistone and anticardiolipin antibodies occur in approximately 17% and 16% of patients, respectively [4,41]. The prevalence of the autoantibody status outlined is similarly found in patients with drug-induced SCLE [42].

Predisposing factors

A number of drugs have been reported to precipitate or exacerbate SCLE and these are listed in Box 51.4. Up to 65% of cases of SCLE

Box 51.4 Drugs associated with the development of subacute cutaneous lupus erythematosus

Antibiotics
- Doxycycline [122]
- Minocycline [123]
- Nitrofurantoin [125]
- Amoxicillin clavulanate [44]
- Ciprofloxacin [125]
- Norfloxacin [126]
- Rifampicin [127]

Anticoagulants
- Rivaroxaban [128]
- Apixaban [129]

Anticonvulsants
- Carbamazepine [130]
- Oxcarbazepine [44]
- Phenytoin [131]
- Lamotrigine [132]

Antifungals
- Terbinafine [133]
- Griseofulvin [134]

Antihypertensive
- Thiazide diuretics [135]
- Calcium-channel blockers [136,137]
- ACE inhibitors/ARB [138–140]
- Beta-blockers [44,140,141]
- Furosemide [44]

Chemotherapeutics
- Capecitabine [142–144]
- Gemcitabine [145,146]
- Carboplatin [44,147]
- Cisplatin [44]
- Docetaxel [148]
- Paclitaxel [149]
- Doxorubicin [150]
- Systemic 5-fluorouracil [151]
- Tyrosine kinase inhibitors [152–154]

Cholesterol lowering agents
- Simvastatin [155,156]
- Pravastatin [139,157]
- Ezetimibe [44]

Monoclonal antibodies [38,158–160]
- TNF-α inhibitors
- IL-17 inhibitors
- IL-12/23 inhibitors
- PD-1/PDL-1 inhibitors
- Abatacept
- Natalizumab
- Denosumab

Non-steroidal anti-inflammatories [44,161,162]
- Ibuprofen
- Diclofenac
- Naproxen
- Piroxicam
- Acetylsalicylic acid

Proton pump inhibitors [37,163]
- Lansoprazole
- Esomeprazole
- Omeprazole
- Pantoprazole

ACE, angiotensin-converting enzyme; ARB, angiotensin receptor blocker; IL, interleukin; PD-1, programmed cell death protein 1; PD-L1, programmed cell death ligand 1; TNF, tumour necrosis factor.

may be drug-induced [7,42,43]. Drug-induced SCLE varies from idiopathic disease in a number of ways, as well as showing different characteristics. Compared with idiopathic disease, it occurs in older patients (mean age 59 years) and is generally milder, but may involve the face and may show bullous and erythema multiforme-like patterns. A higher number of systemic symptoms such as arthralgias/arthritis and xerostomia has also been reported in drug-induced SCLE [44].

Pathology

Histopathologically, SCLE can be differentiated from DLE by the presence of more epidermal atrophy and less hyperkeratosis, basement-membrane thickening, follicular plugging and inflammatory infiltration [45]. Colloid bodies and epidermal necrosis are present in more than 50% of cases, especially in those with Ro/SS-A antibodies [22]. Immunofluorescence studies have shown that approximately 60% of patients with SCLE demonstrate deposition of IgG and/or complement in a granular pattern at the dermal–epidermal junction [46]. This is more frequent in papulosquamous (88%) than annular (29%) lesions [1]. Dust-like particles of inter- and intracellular IgG in the basement layers of the epidermis may be a specific feature [46]. It has been suggested that pilosebaceous atrophy is the only significant predictor of DLE versus SCLE [22,47]. Excessive basement membrane deposition of laminin and collagen VII is seen in DLE but not SCLE [48]. Studies have shown significant numbers of cells expressing lymphocyte chemokine receptors CCR4 and CXCR3, chemokine ligands CXCL9, CXCL10 and CXCL11 [49] as well as cytotoxic T cells in the basal layers of the epidermis where keratinocytes show apoptotic death [50] and strongly positive staining for TNF-α and IFN-κ in involved skin [51,52]. Additionally, patients with SCLE have high serum levels of TNF-α, IFN-γ, IL-12 and IL-18 [53,54]. Drug-induced SCLE may be differentiated from idiopathic SCLE by distinct histopathological features including the presence of leukocytoclastic vasculitis, reduced dermal mucin deposition and the absence of direct immunofluorescence positivity for granular IgM and C3 deposits at the basement membrane zone [44].

Genetics [55]

Human leukocyte antigen status may have a role in disease susceptibility. The most common haplotype in SCLE is HLA-DR3 and -B8, -DR3 being most commonly associated with the annular phenotype and the expression of Ro/SS-A antibodies [56]. This was determined by classic serological HLA typing, using white-skinned controls. A more recent study has suggested an association with the HLA-A1, -B8, -DR3, -DQ2, -DRw2 and -C4 null haplotype [57].

HLA-DR2 has been associated with an older age of disease onset and papulosquamous lesions [58]. Complement genes are located in the HLA region and patients with SCLE have been reported to have deficiencies in the second, third and fourth components of complement [59]. A single nucleotide polymorphism leading to decreased levels of C1q antigen has been reported in patients with SCLE, the only genetic association of the disease that lies outside the HLA region [55]. Studies have reported an association of SCLE with the TNF-α 308A polymorphism, which may be pathogenic or act as a marker for the HLA-A1, B8, DRB1*0301 haplotype associated with other autoimmune conditions [60].

Environmental factors

As well as the well-known relationship to UV exposure, SCLE may occur in the course of psoralen with UVA (PUVA) treatment of psoriasis [61], radiotherapy [62] and IFN-β-1α therapy [63].

Clinical features

History

Patients may have a history of previous sun-induced skin problems, and often classic polymorphic light eruption. Raynaud phenomenon may occur before the characteristic skin rash, and patients may have mild arthralgia, although frank arthritis is unusual before the onset of the skin rash.

Presentation

This subset presents with either a non-scarring papulosquamous eruption (two-thirds of patients) (Figure 51.18a) or annular polycyclic lesions (one-third of patients) [55]. Lesions usually occur above the waist and particularly around the neck, on the trunk and on the outer aspects of the arms (Figure 51.18b) and have been reported to occur along the lines of Blaschko [64]. The borders may show vesiculation and crusting and occasionally bullae [65], which may be associated with coexistent porphyria cutanea tarda [19,65]. Follicular plugging and hyperkeratosis are not prominent, and the lesions resolve to leave grey-white hypopigmentation and telangiectases. The pigmentary changes usually resolve completely. Diffuse non-scarring alopecia and photosensitivity occur in approximately half of patients, and other features include mouth ulceration (especially of the palate), reticular livedo and periungual telangiectasia. Presentation with pityriasiform lesions [29], erythroderma [66] and poikilodermatous lesions [67] have been described. Dermoscopic features include patchy distributions of scarce white-yellow scales, pink and white structureless areas and a mixed vascular pattern including dotted, linear branching and linear curved vessels [68]. The latter characteristic may be helpful in differentiating between SCLE and its differential diagnoses including nummular dermatitis and psoriasis that demonstrate dotted vessels exclusively [69].

Clinical variants

While these are classic skin eruptions, a chilblain pattern and vasculitis, particularly in those with concomitant Sjögren syndrome, are both described. Occasionally, the annular lesions may resemble the lesions of Rowell syndrome or the gyrate erythema secondary to occult malignancy [70].

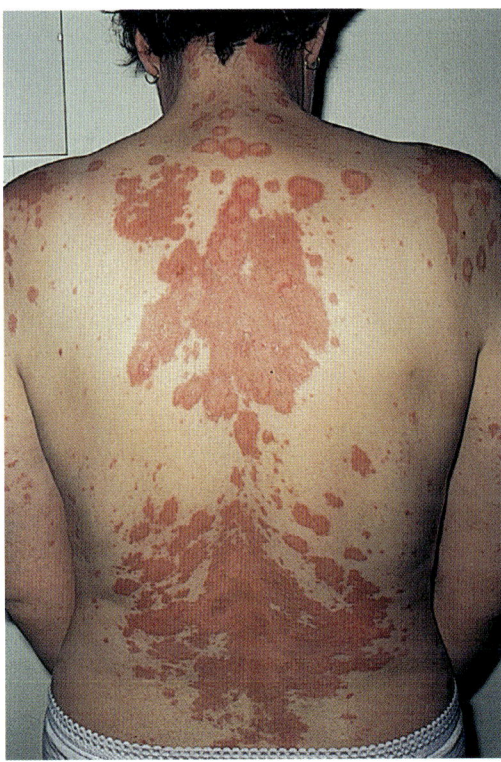

(a)

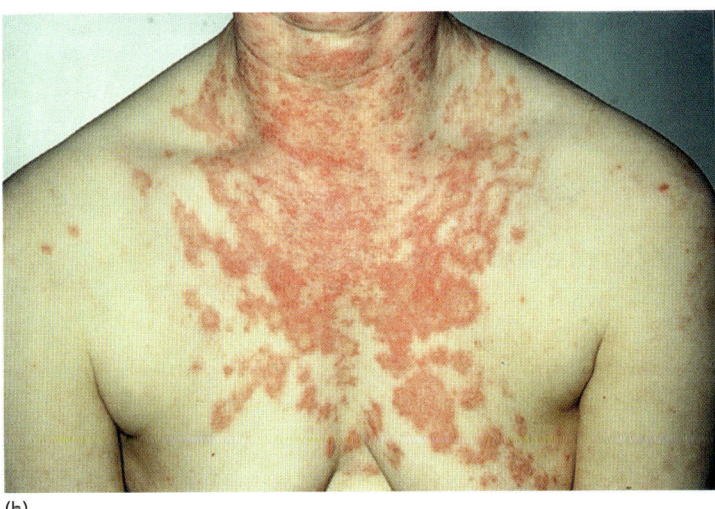

(b)

Figure 51.18 Subacute cutaneous lupus erythematosus. (a) Papulosquamous eruption on the back. (b) Annular polycyclic lesions on the chest.

Differential diagnosis

Box 51.5 shows the most common differential diagnoses.

Complications and co-morbidities

Urticarial vasculitis, chronic interstitial pneumonitis and hypokalaemic tetraparesis have been reported in association with SCLE [71–73]. There have been occasional reports of associations with cancer, namely breast carcinoma [74], meningioma [75], colon cancer [76], gastric adenocarcinoma [77], pancreatic adenocarcinoma [78], hepatocellular carcinoma [79], cholangiocarcinoma [80], non-Hodgkin lymphoma [84], Hodgkin disease [81], lung cancer

---

Box 51.5 Differential diagnoses of subacute cutaneous lupus erythematosus

- Dermatomyositis
- Lupus erythematosus, acute or discoid
- Erythema annulare centrifugum
- Erythema gyratum repens
- Erythema multiforme
- Granuloma annulare
- Lichen planus
- Psoriasis
- Tinea corporis

---

[82], prostate cancer [83], melanoma [85] and squamous carcinoma of the head and neck [86–88]. Occasional patients may develop overt SLE with severe internal organ disease [55,89].

Disease course and prognosis

Subacute CLE often shows a variable exacerbating and remitting course over time, possibly in relation to sun exposure. Studies have shown that over a 3-year period, 17–25% of patients with SCLE developed SLE [7,90]. Worsening CLASI scores over time may be a risk factor to progression to SLE [90]. Median time to SLE diagnosis was 1.65 years in patients with SCLE [8].

Investigations

Due to the possible concurrent diagnosis or eventual development of SLE, patients with SCLE should be screened for internal organ involvement. An initial evaluation includes a thorough history and physical examination including the EULAR/ACL clinical criteria [91]. The initial blood work may include complete blood count with differential, liver enzymes, creatinine and blood urea nitrogen levels, urinalysis, ANA, ENA, dsDNA, complement levels and erythrocyte sedimentation rate or C-reactive protein. Patients with active disease should be followed monthly, whereas patients with stable disease can be seen on a biannual basis [92].

Management

The treatment of SCLE is based upon extrapolation of studies of the treatment of DLE (detailed in section on DLE earlier in this chapter) and upon case reports. Patients should avoid UV exposure, particularly in the spring in the northern latitudes, since they tend to flare rapidly in response to the first significant UV exposure of the year.

First line

The condition in most patients is controlled by sunscreens [93], moderate- to high-potency topical or intralesional corticosteroids [94,95] or the topical macrolides, pimecrolimus [96] and tacrolimus [97].

Second line

In those not responding to first line agents, antimalarial drugs are often helpful [98]. These can be used as either hydroxychloroquine or chloroquine (sulphate or phosphate), although the former is

Table 51.3 Systemic Lupus International Collaborating Clinics classification criteria for systemic lupus erythematosus (SLE), 2012.[a]

Criteria	Definition
Clinical criteria	
1. Acute cutaneous lupus	Including: lupus malar rash (do not include if malar discoid), bullous lupus, toxic epidermal necrolysis variant of SLE, maculopapular rash, photosensitive lupus rash in the absence of dermatomyositis *or* subacutue cutaneous lupus
2. Chronic cutaneous lupus	Including classic discoid rash, hypertrophic (verrucous) lupus, lupus panniculitis (profundus), mucosal lupus, lupus erythematosus tumidus, chilblain lupus, discoid lupus/lichen planus overlap
3. Oral ulcers	Palate, buccal, tongue or nasal ulcers in the absence of other causes
4. Non-scarring alopecia	Diffuse thinning or hair fragility with broken hairs in the absence of other causes
5. Synovitis	Involving two or more joints characterised by effusion or swelling *or* tenderness in two or more joints and at least 30 min of morning stiffness
6. Serositis: pleurisy or pericarditis	More than 1-day duration of pleural/pericaridal effusions or pleural/pericardial rub
7. Renal disorder: persistent proteinuria (>0.5 μg/day) or cellular casts	
8. Neurological disorder	Seizures, psychosis, mononeuritis multiplex, myelitis or acute confusional state in the absence of other causes
9. Haemolytic anaemia	
10. Leukopenia (<4000/mm³ at least once) *or* lymphopenia (<1000/mm³)	
11. Thrombocytopenia (<100 000/mm³ at least once)	
Immunological criteria	
1. ANA above reference laboratory range	
2. Anti-dsDNA antibody above reference laboratory range (or more than twofold the reference range if tested by ELISA)	
3. Anti-Sm: presence of antibody to Sm nuclear antigen	
4. Antiphospholipid antibody positivity	
5. Low complement (low C3, C4 or CH50)	
6. Direct Coombs test in the absence of haemolytic anaemia	

Adapted from Petri *et al.* 2012 [3].

[a] Criteria are cumulative and need not be present concurrently. A patient should be classified as having SLE if they satisfy four of the clinical and immunological criteria, including at least one clinical criterion, *or* if they have biopsy-proven nephritis compatible with SLE in the presence of ANAs or anti-dsDNA antibodies.

ANA, antinuclear antibody; anti-dsDNA, anti-double-stranded DNA; ELISA, enzyme-linked immunosorbent assay.

safer from the ophthalmological point of view and requires less monitoring. However, evidence suggests that long-term use of more than 7 years, or a large cumulative dose, may still be problematic [99]. Hydroxychloroquine should be dosed at no more than 5 mg/kg of real body weight per day. Dosing may need to be adjusted or require discontinuation altogether in patients with significant renal disease, retinal or macular disease or concurrent use of tamoxifen [100]. The antimalarial mepacrine (quinacrine) does not have ocular side effects but does induce a yellow discoloration of the skin. There is evidence that a combination of hydroxychloroquine or chloroquine with mepacrine may be more effective than either alone [101] and that they are less effective in smokers [102].

Third line

Patients not responding to antimalarials may respond to (in order of benefit risk and evidence): oral corticosteroids or methylprednisolone [103], acitretin [104], isotretinoin [105], dapsone [106], oral and subcutaneous methotrexate [107–109], azathioprine [4], mycophenolate mofetil [110], the cereblon inhibitors thalidomide [111,112] or lenalidomide [113], IVIg [114,115], rituximab [116,117] and JAK inhibitors [118–120]. Phototherapy with UVA has also paradoxically been reported to be useful [121].

Systemic lupus erythematosus

Introduction and general description

Systemic LE is a systemic disease characterised by multisystem organ inflammation, most commonly the skin, joints and vasculature, and associated immunological abnormalities. The main clinical features include fever, rashes and arthritis, but renal, pulmonary, cardiac and neurological involvement may occur, with increased mortality. The first classification criteria were developed by the American Rheumatism Association in 1971 and modified in 1982 [1] and in 1997 [2]. The Systemic Lupus International Collaborating Clinics (SLICC) identified 17 criteria that resulted in greater sensitivity but somewhat lower specificity for the diagnosis of SLE than the 1982 ACR criteria [3]. Specifically, terms relating to the cutaneous manifestations of lupus were redefined. According to the 2012 SLICC rules for classification, a patient needed to satisfy at least four criteria, including at least one clinical and one immunological criterion, or the patient must have had biopsy-proven lupus nephritis in the presence of ANAs or anti-dsDNA antibodies. For any individual patient, the SLICC criteria may be used as an aid and guide to diagnosis (Table 51.3). The criteria were further modified in 2019 to improve detection of early SLE and to make a positive

| **Entry criterion** |
| Antinuclear antibodies (ANAs) at a titre of ≥1:80 on HEp-2 cells or an equivalent positive test (ever) |

↓

| If absent, do not classify as SLE |
| If present, apply additive criteria |

↓

Additive criteria
Do not count a criterion if there is a more likely explanation than SLE
Occurrence of a criterion on at least one occasion is sufficient
SLE classification requires at least one clinical criterion and ≥10 points
Criteria need not occur simultaneously
Within each domain, only the highest weighted criterion is counted toward the total score

Clinical domains and criteria	Weight	Immunology domains and criteria	Weight
Constitutional		*Antiphospholipid antibodies*	
Fever	2	Anticardiolipin antibodies OR	
Hematologic		Anti-β2GP1 antibodies OR	
Leukopenia	3	Lupus anticoagulant	2
Thrombocytopenia	4	*Complement proteins*	
Autoimmune haemolysis	4	Low C3 OR low C4	3
Neuropsychiatric		Low C3 AND low C4	4
Delirium	2	*SLE-specific antibodies*	
Psychosis	3	Anti-dsDNA antibody OR	
Seizure	5	Anti-Smith antibody	6
Mucocutaneous			
Non-scarring alopecia	2		
Oral ulcers	2		
Subacute cutaneous OR discoid lupus	4		
Acute cutaneous lupus	6		
Serosal			
Pleural or pericardial effusion	5		
Acute pericarditis	6		
Musculoskeletal			
Joint involvement	6		
Renal			
Proteinuria > 0.5 kg/24 h	4		
Renal biopsy class II or V lupus nephritis	8		
Renal biopsy class III or IV lupus nephritis	10		

Total score:

↓

Classify as systemic lupus erythematosus with a score of 10 or more if entry criterion fulfilled

Figure 51.19 European League Against Rheumatism/American College of Rheumatology criteria for the diagnosis of systemic lupus erythematosus (SLE). Reproduced from Aringer et al. 2019 [4] with permission from John Wiley & Sons.

ANA test an entry criterion [4]. The current EULAR/ACR criteria have a sensitivity of 96% and a specificity of 93%, work well in early disease and across ethnicities, and are becoming the standard in clinical research (Figure 51.19). Nuances in the definitions of SLE may result in reclassification of some cases of SLE as skin-only disease or CLE [5].

Epidemiology
Incidence and prevalence
Systemic LE is an uncommon disease. A study in Birmingham, UK, estimated the prevalence of SLE at 30/100 000 in the white population and 200/100 000 in the Afro-Caribbean population [6], with an incidence estimated at 3.8 per 100 000 per year. In comparison, for every case of SLE there are six cases of pernicious anaemia and 10 of leukemia. In a New Zealand study, SLE was found to be more common in Chinese and in New Zealand Polynesians [7]. The pattern of disease appears to be different in different ethnic subgroups, with black Americans and Hispanics having the highest rate of internal organ damage [8]. Black Americans have an earlier age of diagnosis, more common renal disease and more progression to end-stage renal disease than white Americans [9]. Familial cases are uncommon, but kindreds have an increased incidence of other

autoimmune diseases such as thyroid disease and rheumatoid arthritis [10,11].

Age

The condition tends to occur in early adult life, and the peak age of onset of the first symptom or sign in females is approximately 38 years (35.5 in black women and 40.7 in white women); it is 44.2 years in men [12]. The manifestations of the disease are the same in all age ranges, although serositis and Sjögren syndrome are more common disease manifestations in the elderly [13]. Older individuals, with less severe disease, may have a longer time from symptom onset to diagnosis [14]. Paediatric SLE is uncommon, accounting for approximately 20% of all SLE patients with higher initial disease activity and earlier onset of damage [15].

Sex

The female to male ratio is 7 : 15 [16]. Men with lupus tend to have higher frequencies of renal disease, skin manifestations, cytopenia, serositis, neurological involvement, thrombosis and vasculitis [17].

Pathophysiology
Pathology

The primary lesions of SLE are fibrinoid necrosis, collagen sclerosis, necrosis and basophilic body formation, and vascular endothelial thickening. The basophilic (haematoxylin) bodies are aggregates of homogeneous material staining blue with haematoxylin and staining positively for DNA by the Feulgen technique. This material is similar to that of the homogeneous nuclear material of the LE cell (a neutrophil that has engulfed nuclear material from dying cells) (Figure 51.20).

Box 51.6 lists the main macroscopic and microscopic features of SLE.

Macroscopic appearances. Even in the presence of widespread clinical manifestations and fatal outcome, it is often disappointing to find no macroscopic changes at autopsy. Sometimes, terminal changes and infection obscure the picture. Frequent macroscopic

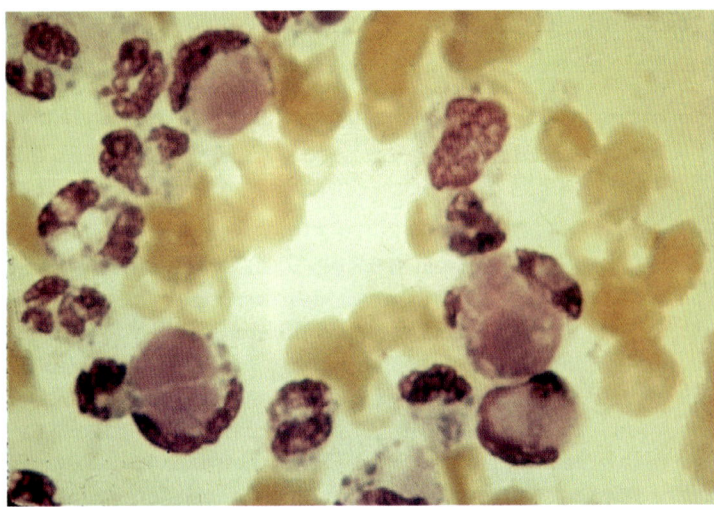

Figure 51.20 Lupus erythematosus cells: the phagocytosed nuclear material is homogeneous and displaces the polymorph nucleus to one side.

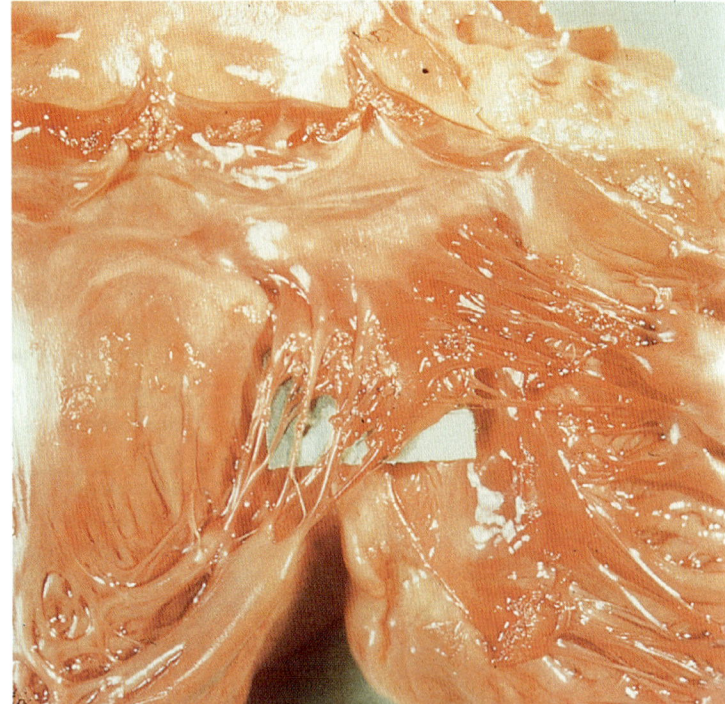

Figure 51.21 Libman–Sacks endocarditis. Note the warty vegetations on the heart valves.

findings include pleurisy with adhesions and effusion, and pericarditis, especially if the patient has died with uraemia. The verrucose vegetations of Libman–Sacks endocarditis are diagnostic (Figure 51.21) [18]. These are small, firm, warty deposits, up to 0.5 cm in diameter, adherent to the valves of both sides of the heart and adjacent endocardium of the ventricles, chordae tendinae and on the papillary muscles. Sometimes, lesions of subacute bacterial endocarditis may be superimposed on the warty lesions.

Box 51.6 Pathological features of systemic lupus erythematosus

Macroscopic features
- Pleurisy
- Pericarditis
- Libman–Sacks endocarditis
- Lymphadenopathy
- Splenomegaly
- May be none

Microscopic features
- Immunoglobulins and complement at the dermal–epidermal junction in skin lesions (90%) and uninvolved skin (60%)
- Haematoxylin bodies in the endocardium, renal glomeruli and elsewhere
- Periarterial fibrosis of the spleen
- Wire-loop lesions in the kidneys

Microscopic appearances. Usually, pathological diagnosis requires histology, but in some cases histological changes can be demonstrated only by immunohistochemistry (Figure 51.22) [19].

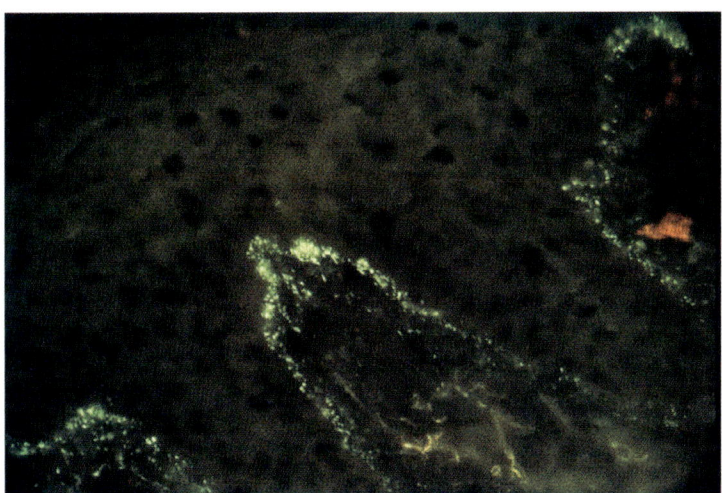

Figure 51.22 Immunoglobulin at the dermal–epidermal junction in systemic lupus erythematosus.

Skin. There is no single diagnostic pathological feature for SLE in the skin, but a combination of features aids diagnosis [20]. The histopathology of the skin is similar in each of the different forms of LE-specific skin disease (ACLE, SCLE and CCLE) and thus can be useful in contributing to the diagnosis of SLE but not in the determination of the clinical subtype of CLE. In ACLE, there is a sparse dermal cellular infiltrate, focal liquefactive degeneration of the basal epidermis and upper dermal oedema [21]. Epidermal necrolysis has been reported [22]. The dermal tissues may be oedematous, and sometimes vesicle formation occurs at the dermal–epidermal junction, with dilatation of the superficial vessels and perivascular lymphocytic infiltration. Mucin may be found in the reticular dermis [23]. Using monoclonal antibodies, the infiltrate is shown to consist of abundant T cells and Ia-positive cells, with rather fewer B cells and macrophages. Helper or inducer T cells and suppressor or cytotoxic T cells occur in equal numbers [24]. All forms of cutaneous lupus have been shown to demonstrate an increase in the expression of type I IFN-related proteins such as MXA [25]. Recent studies demonstrate an increase in the production of type III IFNs by keratinocytes (particularly IFN-κ and IFN-λ) as another common abnormality [26,27]. Neutrophilic infiltrates, with dermal perivascular and interstitial neutrophils, including neutrophilic debris, have been recognised recently to form a cutaneous histological variant that can be indicative of systemic involvement in SLE [28].

Immunohistology. The lupus band test (LBT) was historically used as a diagnostic aid in SLE [29]. The sensitivity of the LBT varies between 10.5% and 78.9% and the specificity between 47.8% and 97.8% depending upon the defining criteria used [29]. Immunoglobulins, predominantly IgG, but less frequently IgM and IgA, together with complement (C1, C3) can be demonstrated at the dermal–epidermal junction by immunofluorescence techniques. Such deposits were first described in skin lesions [30] but are also present in clinically normal skin of SLE subjects [31]. They occur in more than 80% of skin lesions of DLE and SLE, and may be preceded by basement membrane abnormalities in red and purpuric lesions [32]. Deposits occur more frequently in light-exposed areas and are invariably present in acute lesions, although in early and

late stages the test may be negative. If IgG, IgM and IgA are all present, the diagnosis of SLE is likely, and the more common combination of IgG and IgM is also suggestive. The basement-membrane phenomenon can also be demonstrated in the uninvolved skin in three-quarters of active cases of SLE if the biopsy specimens are taken from the exposed skin, preferably from the dorsum of the wrist or forearm. This test is no longer used as a diagnostic criterion in clinical practice and thus is only of historical interest. In addition to dermal–epidermal immune reactant deposition, epidermal nuclear deposits, usually giving a speckled IgG pattern, occur in the basal epidermal nuclei and cells of the lower epidermis in nearly one-third of patients [33].

Internal organs. The characteristic microscopic features in the internal organs include haematoxylin bodies in the heart valves and elsewhere, periarterial fibrosis of the spleen, and the so-called 'wire-loop' lesions in the kidneys. Lymph node enlargement is usually associated with retention of normal architecture, but sometimes necrosis and haematoxylin bodies may be found.

Kidney disease is noted in up to 50% of patients with SLE and is the strongest overall predictor of morbidity and mortality [34]. Decreased levels of C3 and C4 correlate with active SLE and the presence of renal disease. The so-called 'wire-loop' appearance in the kidneys is caused by thickening and hyalinisation of the capillary basement membrane of the glomerular tufts. Although this change may be seen in other diseases such as systemic sclerosis, chronic glomerulonephritis and malignant nephrosclerosis, the changes in SLE are more likely to be localised to one part of the glomerulus. Thickening of the glomerular capillary basement membrane and alterations in reticular tissue in the media of arterioles are associated with deposits of IgG and C3. Lupus nephritis is classified into six types according to location and extent of renal damage as detected by light microscopy, immunofluorescence and electron microscopy using the International Society of Nephrology (ISN) system devised in 2004 [35] and revised in 2018 [36]. In minimal mesangial lupus nephritis (class I), normal glomeruli by light microscopy are found to have mesangial immune deposits by immunofluorescence or electron microscopy. In mesangial proliferative lupus nephritis (class II), mesangial hypercellularity is present. In focal (class III) and diffuse (class IV) proliferative nephritis, there is endocapillary proliferation and inflammation with subendothelial immune deposits. Immunosuppressive therapy is required to manage these types of renal lupus. Membranous nephritis (class V) displays a global thickening of the glomerular capillary walls and is associated with an increased risk of renal vein thrombosis and nephrotic syndrome. Advanced sclerosing nephritis (class VI) is the result of end-stage damage. All patients who develop glomerulonephritis (with active renal sediment) should have a renal biopsy to accurately stage disease and plan therapy (Table 51.4).

Genetic factors

There is considerable evidence to suggest that genetic factors play a part in the pathogenesis [37]. Historically, the condition has been reported in identical twins, with a concordance rate of 65% [38]. However, most individuals with SLE have no family history of the disease. Rare monogenic mutations resulting in deficiencies of the

Table 51.4 International Society of Nephrology classification of lupus nephritis (LN).

Class	Description
I	Minimal mesangial LN: normal glomeruli by light microscope (LM) but mesangial immune deposits by immunoflouorescence
II	Mesangial proliferative LN: mesangial hypercellularity with no subendothelial deposits by LM in 20% of cases; renal failure rare
III	Focal LN: segmental and/or global endocapillary and/or extracapillary glomerulonephritis involving <50% of all glomeruli in 25% of cases; renal failure uncommon
IV	Diffuse LN: glomerulonephritis involving ≥50% of all glomeruli in 40% of cases; renal failure common
V	Membranous LN: global or segmental subendothelial deposits by LM in 10% of cases; renal failure uncommon
VI	Advanced sclerosing LN: ≥90% of glomeruli sclerosed

Table 51.5 Important immunological pathways identified through susceptibility gene analysis.

Pathways	Genes
Innate immune response	
TLR/IFN signalling	*IRF5/7, STAT4, TLR7/8, IRAK1, ACP5, SPP!*
NFκB signalling	*TNFAIP3, TNP1, PRKCB*
Immune complex clearance	
Complement	*C1Q/R/S, C4A&B, C2, C3, CFHR3&1, CR2*
Phagocytosis	*FCGR2A, FCGR3A, FCGR2B, FCGR3B, ITGAM*
DNA degradation	*TREX1, DNASE1*
Adaptive immune response	
Antigen presentation	*HLA-DR2&DR3*, HLA class III genes
T-cell signalling	*PTPN22, TNFSF4, CD$$*
B-cell signalling	*BLK, BANK1, LYN, ETS1, PRDM!, IKZF1*
Cytokine	*IL10, IL21*
Mixed	
Epigenetic modification	
DNA methylation	*MECP2*
Other	
Unknown	*PXK, XKR6* and others

Adapted from Deng and Tsao 2013 [47].

HLA, human leukocyte antigen; IFN, interferon; NFκB, nuclear factor κB; TLR, Toll-like receptor.

classic complement system or defective degradation of DNA invariably result in the development of SLE. Deficiencies of C1q result in SLE-like disease in 93% of individuals. Likewise, a majority of individuals with C1R/C1S deficiency or CD4 deficiency and up to 25% of C2-deficient individuals develop SLE [39]. Mutations in *TREX1* (three prime repair exonuclease 1), a gene encoding an intracellular nuclease, are associated with Aicardi Goutières syndrome, a neurodegenerative disorder with hypocomplementaemia and ANA formation and familial chilblain lupus [40,41]. Mutations in this gene that result in frameshift missense mutations or that alter subcellular protein targeting are also found in up to 2.7% of patients with SLE and are associated with neurological manifestations. In the absence of TREX1, accumulation of endogenous DNA induces IFN-α production eventually leading to autoimmunity [42].

In most cases, disease occurrence does not follow simple Mendelian inheritance. Studies have used linkage analysis within kindreds, candidate gene studies and genome-wide association studies (GWAS) to map and identify genes associated with SLE susceptibility. Over 90 genetic loci, replicated in more than one study, have been identified with most disease-specific genes grouped into four immunological pathways: innate and adaptive immune response, immune complex clearance and mixed (Table 51.5) [43]. Class II HLA molecules are important for the presentation of antigen to CD4 T cells and the promotion of T-cell-dependent antibody responses. Associations between HLA genes and SLE have been studied for over 40 years. The most consistent associations are between HLA-DR2 and HLA-DR3 in white people [44] and these have been recapitulated in African Americans [45]. There is a close association between HLA alleles and autoantibody subsets in patients with SLE, with the strongest association (linkage disequilibrium) between anti-Ro/La antibodies and DR3 and DQ2 [46]. In aggregate, currently identified loci explain about 30% of disease heritability.

The identification of SLE risk loci by GWAS has been recapitulated with the identification of risk loci for other autoimmune diseases. Many autoimmune diseases, including rheumatoid arthritis, systemic sclerosis, type 1 diabetes, inflammatory bowel disease and Behçet disease, share risk loci [48]. Shared genes include HLA class II genes, *PTPN22* and *TNFSF4*, important in controlling the adaptive immune response, and innate immune response genes such as *IRF5*, *STAT4* and *TNFAIP3* [37].

Autoantibodies

Non-organ-specific humoral autoantibodies are the hallmark of SLE [49]. A range of autoantibodies may be present in the disease, although some are more disease-specific (anti-dsDNA and anti-Sm antibodies), and some are much more common (antinuclear and anti-Ro antibodies). Autoantibodies found in SLE are either germline-encoded or the product of somatic hypermutation. The autoantibodies in SLE show characteristics of an antigen-selected response promoted by B- and T-cell interaction. The B cells that make autoantibodies are activated by elevated levels of B lymphocyte stimulator (BLys, also BAFF), a growth factor that is particularly important for the survival of T-cell-dependent B cells that promote autoantibody formation. Belimumab is a monoclonal antibody to BAFF that improves mucocutaneous and arthritis symptoms, as well as lupus nephritis in patients with SLE. This drug was US Food and Drug Administration (FDA) approved for therapy for mucocutaneous and joint symptoms of SLE in 2011 [50] and for active lupus nephritis in 2020 [51]. B-cell-directed therapies continue to be studied for the treatment of lupus nephritis and co-stimulatory molecules remain potential novel targets in the SLE therapeutic armamentarium [52].

In SLE, antigen–antibody complexes containing DNA and RNA products activate the innate immune system through the stimulation of Toll-like receptor 9 (TLR-9) and TLR-7, respectively [53]. Innate immune activation culminates in IFN-α release by dendritic cells and TNF-α release promoting T cells to release IFN-γ, IL-6 and IL-10, all cytokines that promote continued antibody formation [54]. These autoantibody-producing cells are subsequently not adequately downregulated by anti-idiotypic antibodies and regulatory T cells. There is considerable evidence that non-organ-specific autoantibodies, such as anti-DNA and anti-RNA antibodies, are not primarily pathogenic because (i) they are not specific to any disease manifestation; (ii) they are not present in all cases; and (iii) their titres are sometimes independent of the activity of the disease. In contrast, anti-Ro or closely related antibodies are implicated in the development of the rash and heart block found in neonatal LE [55]. Antiphospholipid antibodies, including the so-called lupus anticoagulant, are linked to thrombosis and abortion in patients with SLE. Antiribosomal P proteins have been detected in lupus psychosis [56].

Other immune factors [57]

Patients with SLE have dysregulated production of type I IFNs, principally IFN-α. This results in the dendritic cell activation of autoreactive B and T cells [58]. Using gene-array technology, SLE patients have been stratified into individuals demonstrating high, moderate or weak expression of IFN-α-related genes, suggesting that individuals could be stratified into good and poor responders to IFN-α neutralisation [59]. IFN-α dysregulation also results in activation of the innate immune system and vascular disease, common in SLE. In addition to an increase in memory B cells and circulating plasma cells whose numbers correlate with disease activity [60], there are defects in other cellular immune lineages. For example, there are deficiencies in the function of regulatory T-cell subsets [61]. Cytolytic CD8+ T cells sustain rather than suppress B-cell responses and lymphocyte transformation responses to common antigens [62]. Early signalling events in T cells and B cells are amplified [57]. A recent concept is the role of IL-2 as primary activator of regulatory T cells rather than general T-cell growth factor [63]. In SLE, the production of IL-2 by peripheral blood leukocytes is impaired, thus reducing the inhibitory effects of regulatory T cells upon activated B cells, and the increased longevity of autoreactive T cells [64].

Environmental factors

Environmental factors associated with the onset of SLE include exposure to sunlight and UVR, smoking, infections and medications such as TNF inhibitors [65]. Silica and solvents have also been linked to the onset of SLE [66]. In a Finnish case–control study smoking was significantly, although modestly, associated with SLE [67].

Ultraviolet radiation. Reacting to midday sun with a blistering sunburn or rash has been associated with the onset of SLE [66]. Clinical photosensitivity in the form of polymorphous light reaction and pruritus is associated with more severe systemic disease [68]. Thus UVR may precipitate the onset or exacerbate the course of SLE in up to 60% of patients [69]. Phototesting to UVB and UVA shows reduced minimal erythema doses and the development of skin lesions in patients with LE [70]. The mechanism of action of UVR in exacerbating SLE remains incompletely understood. UV-mediated oxidative DNA damage has been shown to induce resistance to TREX1-mediated degradation resulting in increased local type I IFN production [71].

Infections, stress and hormonal factors. Other factors may precipitate the onset of SLE, and these include bacterial infection, viruses and mental or physical stress. Studies in children suggest that Epstein–Barr virus (EBV) infection may be a trigger

initiating SLE [72]. Oestradiol, prolactin, testosterone and prolactin are thought to modulate the incidence and activity of SLE [73–75]. Oestrogen-containing contraceptive compounds, early menarche and postmenopausal oestrogen use all increase the risk of SLE [73]. Men with Kleinfelter syndrome have a higher incidence of SLE, possibly related to hormonal factors [76]. Prolactin is an immunoregulator: the hormone interferes with B-cell tolerance induction and enhances B-cell proliferative responses to antigens [76]. Prolactin levels are increased in patients with SLE and gonadotropin-releasing hormone (GnRH) is secreted by immunologically active cells, further elevating prolactin levels and suggesting an autocrine effect [75].

Drugs [77]. The precipitation of SLE by drugs [78,79], especially the antihypertensive hydralazine, is well known. However, drug-induced SLE differs from the spontaneous disease: it is uncommon in black people, it occurs in an older age group, renal and central nervous system involvement are infrequent, antihistone antibodies are frequent, anti-DNA antibodies are absent and serum complement is normal [80]. Hydralazine is known to inhibit binding of complement component C4, and this action, with subsequent lack of control of complement activity, may explain the development of lupus-like syndromes [81]. More recent observations have demonstrated that procainamide and hydralazine are potent DNA methylation inhibitors, with procainamide inhibiting DNA methyltransferase 1 [82] and hydralazine inhibiting the extracellular signal-regulated kinases (ERK) pathway [83], both effects ultimately resulting in the increased activation of autoreactive T cells. It has been proposed that drug-mediated alterations in DNA methylation may underlie the initiation of most forms of drug-induced SLE.

Cutaneous involvement in drug-induced SLE may be vasculitic, bullous, erythema multiforme-like or resemble pyoderma gangrenosum. Patients who develop ANAs during drug treatment do not need to have the drug stopped unless they have clinical features of the lupus syndrome [84]. Minocycline-induced SLE is uncommon [85] but use of this drug carries a definite associated risk (odds ratio of 4.23) [86]. It often occurs after 2 years of therapy. Patients who require more than 1 year's therapy should have ANA and liver function tests monitored. Other drugs, particularly certain anticonvulsants, are known to precipitate SLE-like syndromes (Table 51.6). The biologic agents targeting TNF-α are now well known to produce ANA, and occasionally clinical manifestations of lupus [77]. In these patients, arthritis often predominates over cutaneous manifestations and some patients tolerate a switch to a different TNF inhibitor [87].

Clinical features

Clinical features of several series are summarised in Table 51.7. Due to the clinical and serological diversity, the disease may affect almost any organ of the body and can manifest in a broad variety of ways. Large case series have been reported [88] and the subject has been reviewed [89]. Despite the female sex predominance, potential distinguishing features exist in organ involvement and prognosis between sexes. Several authors have reported more damage accrual, particularly renal insufficiency/failure in men [90–92]. In one of the largest cohorts (the Hopkins lupus cohort – John Hopkins Lupus

Table 51.6 Drugs inducing systemic lupus erythematosus-like syndromes.

Drug	High risk	Moderate risk	Low risk	Very low risk	
Antiarrythmics	Procainamide (15–20%)	Quinidine (<1%)		Disopyramide	
				Propafenone	
Antihypertensives	Hydralazine (5–8%)		Methyldopa	Clonidine	Minoxidil
			Captopril	Enalapril	Pindolol
			Acebutol	Labetalol	Prazosin
Antipsychotics			Chlorpromazine	Chlorpothixene	Phenelzine
				Lithium carbonate	
Antibiotics			Isoniazid	Nitrofurantoin	
			Minocyline	Cefepime	
Anticonvulsants			Carbamazepine	Ethosuximide	Phenylbutazone
			Propylthiouracil	Phenytoin	NSAIDs
			D-penicillamine	Primidone	Chlorthalidone
			Sulfasalazine	Trimethadione	Hydrochlorothiazide
Anticholesterolemics				Atorvastatin	Pravastatin
				Fluvastatin	Simvastatin
				Lovastatin	
Proton pump inhibitors				Lanzoprazole	Pantoprazole
				Omeparazole	
Chemotherapeutic agents				Taxane	Fluorouracil
				Cyclophosphamide	Anastozole
				Doxorubicin	Bortezomib
Antiaggregants				Ticlopidine	
Biologics				Etanercept	IL-2
				Infliximab	IFN-α
				Adalimumab	IFN-β

Adapted from Dalle Vedove *et al.* 2012 [77].

IFN, interferon; IL, interleukin; NSAIDs, non-steroidal anti-inflammatory drugs.

Table 51.7 Clinical features of systemic lupus erythematosus (SLE).

Clinical feature	Occurrence in SLE (%)
Fever	90
Arthritis and arthralgia	90
Skin lesions	80
Renal involvement	67
Lymphadenopathy	50
Pleurisy	40
Raynaud phenomenon	35
Pericarditis	25
Hepatomegaly	25
Central nervous system involvement	25
Abdominal symptoms	20
Splenomegaly	15

Center, USA), men were more likely to have haematological and serological manifestations with an increased risk of myocardial infarction, possibly due to an increased frequency of hypertension and positive lupus anticoagulant [92]. Men may also be more liable to seizures and have less skin disease, particularly in white patients [92].

Presentation

The initial manifestations vary [89]. The most commonly observed presenting symptoms are arthralgias followed by cutaneous involvement, with large case series reporting up to 57% of patients presenting with the latter finding [93]. Presentation with serositis and renal abnormalities is less common, however in a large cohort of 1000 patients with early and late manifestations it was found that the majority of manifestations occurred more frequently during the first 5 years of follow-up [93]. In fulminating cases, there is usually marked constitutional disturbance, with fever, weight loss, anorexia, malaise and joint pains; the skin may be involved later, if at all. On the other hand, the evolution can be gradual, starting with localised skin lesions and systemic involvement developing later [94]. The diagnosis in many cases is made only by considering the condition in a patient with an obscure illness. As most cases are females, sex is an important diagnostic point. Constitutional symptoms are common in patients with SLE and fatigue is reported in up to 80% of patients [95]. Similarly, fever is common, particularly during active SLE [89]. Although weight loss is a feature in up to 50% of cases [96], some patients may gain weight, and 18% actually did so in the Leeds series, which included several patients with long histories. Menstruation is irregular in 18% and absent in 75%. Late-onset SLE, defined in the literature as onset >50 years, is uncommon (approximately 12–18%) [97].

Approximately 57–85% of cases have cutaneous findings at some stage [98–100]. The prevalence varies between series. The typical cutaneous findings of a UK population are shown in Figure 51.23 [101]. The classification of LE-related skin disease described by Gilliam is divided between (i) those specific for LE, and showing the characteristic histopathological appearances of interface dermatitis of LE; and (ii) those that are less specific in their origin and not showing histological changes of LE (Table 51.8). Many of

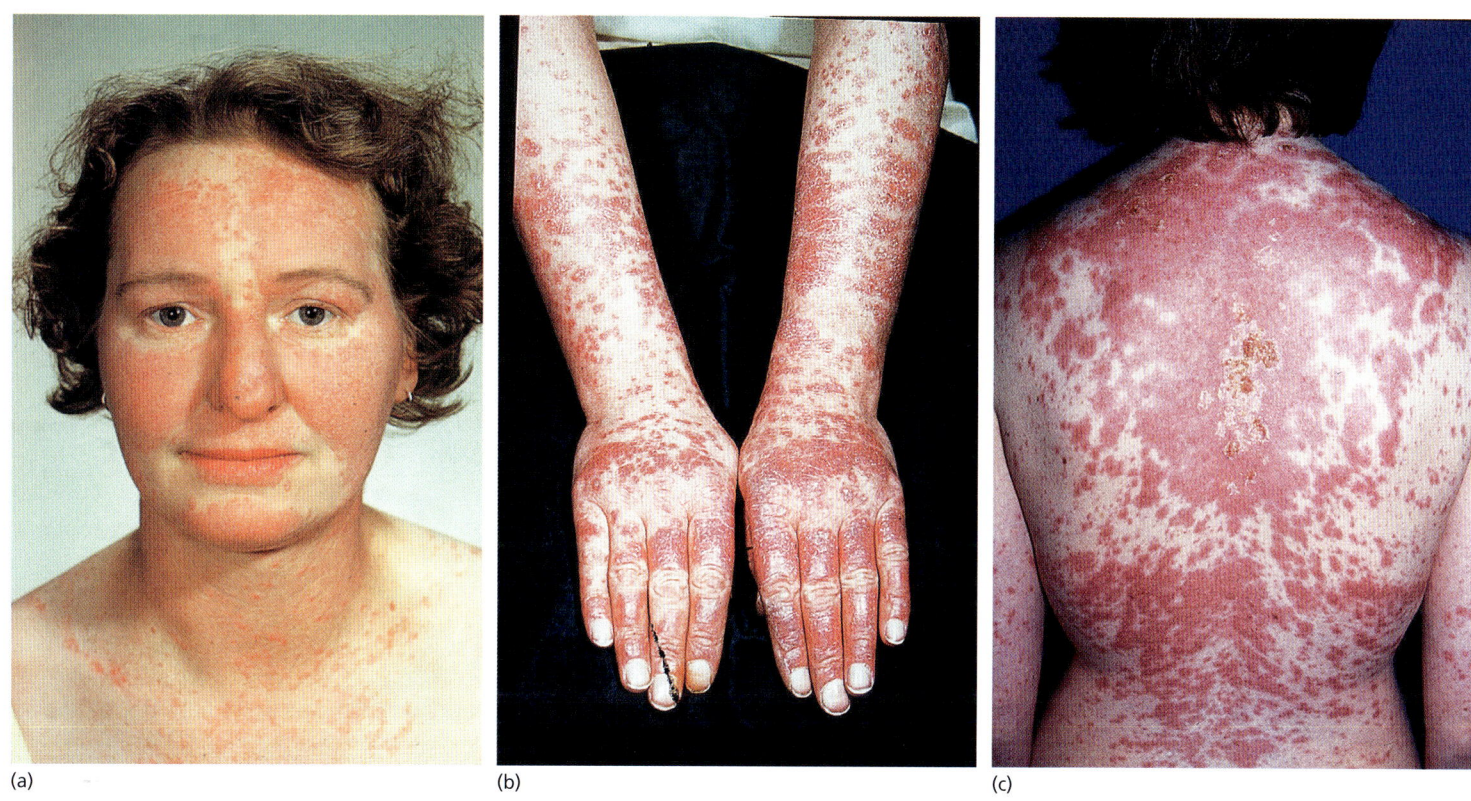

(a)   (b)   (c)

Figure 51.23 Systemic lupus erythematosus. (a) Typical symmetrical, slightly scaling redness of the face and neck. (b) Redness of the dorsa of the hands and forearms. Identical changes may occur in discoid lupus erythematosus. Note the chloroquine pigmentation of the distal part of the nails. (c) Gross involvement of the back.

Table 51.8 Cutaneous features of systemic lupus erythematosus (SLE) in 73 patients.

Cutaneous feature	Occurrence in SLE (%)
Butterfly rash as part of ACLE	51
Chronic DLE	25
Scarring DLE alopecia	14
Subacute cutaneous LE	7
Photosensitivity	63
Raynaud phenomenon	60
Chronic urticaria (>36 h)	44
Non-scarring alopecia	40
Mouth ulceration	31
Chilblain lupus	20
Cutaneous vasculitis	11
Bullous eruptions	8
Facial oedema	4
Livedo reticularis	4
Episcleritis	4
Cheilitis	4

Adapted from Yell *et al*. 1996 [100].
The cutaneous features in the shaded area are considered LE-specific skin changes, with the characteristic histology of cutaneous lupus. The other cutaneous features are considered non-LE-specific cutaneous features.
ACLE, acute cutaneous lupus erythematosus; DLE, discoid lupus erythematosus; LE, lupus erythematosus.

these are also seen in the other connective tissue diseases [101]. Non-specific LE skin diseases are more frequently associated with SLE than LE-specific lesions [102] and are characteristically associated with clinically significant SLE [103].

Lupus-specific changes. The LE-specific cutaneous changes can be divided into three groups based on the amount of time that the skin symptoms typically take to present. These include DLE, SCLE and ACLE. DLE includes localised and generalised DLE, hypertrophic LE, lupus profundus and lupus tumidus. SCLE includes both annular and psoriasiform variants and acute LE both localised and generalised LE and toxic epidermal necrolysis (TEN)-like variants. Patients with any of these LE-specific features may have skin disease alone or SLE if they fulfil the new SLICC or 2019 EULAR/ACR criteria. The risk of SLE with localised versus generalised DLE is 5% versus 20% over time, whereas it is rarely seen with lupus erythematosus tumidus [104]. Lupus panniculitis is reported to occur in approximately 2–3% of patients with SLE [105,106]. Conversely, patients with lupus panniculitis may have up to a 35% chance of preceding, concurrent or subsequent diagnosis of SLE, thus these patients should be followed closely for the development of systemic disease [107–109]. Similarly, although the incidence of SLE in patients with SCLE is approximately 50%, 10–15% have serious organ involvement [110].

ACLE is often associated with active SLE [99], however a small percentage of such patients can experience recurrent ACLE in an isolated fashion over years [111]. Redness is the most common feature, particularly on light-exposed areas (Figure 51.24a). In localised ACLE, a butterfly blush or discrete maculopapular eruption with fine scaling or oedema on the butterfly area of the cheeks is frequently found, typically sparing the naso-labial folds (Figure 51.24b). In generalised LE, a diffuse or papular redness of the face, upper trunk and extremities is described that can resemble a

PART 4: INFLAMMATORY DERMATOSES

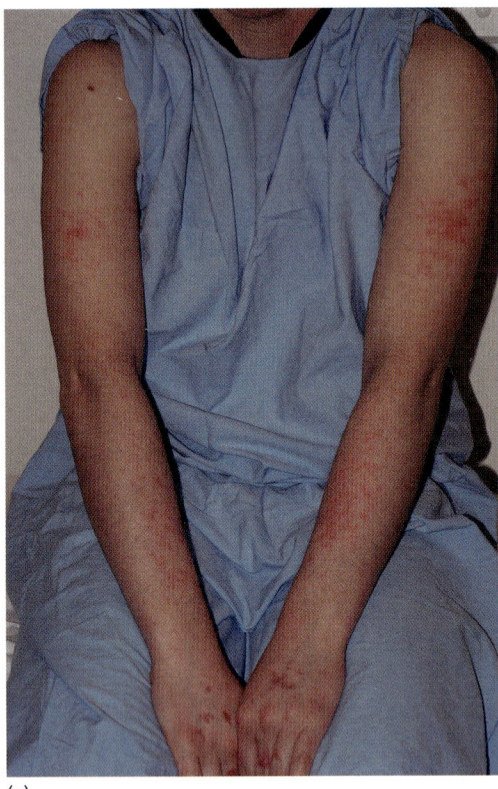

(a)

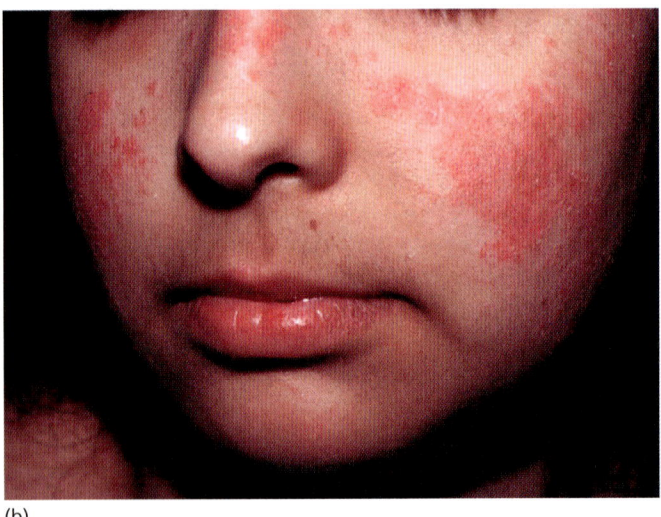

(b)

Figure 51.24 Systemic lupus erythematosus showing acute cutaneous lupus of (a) the arms and (b) the face.

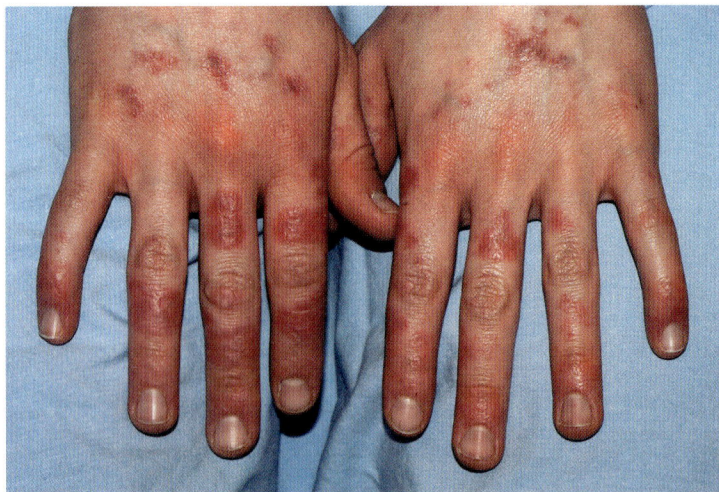

Figure 51.25 Systemic lupus erythematosus showing discoid lesions on the hands characteristically sparring the interphalangeal joints.

systemic disease activity is increased in the 3–6 months following maximal sun exposure [112]. Oedema, especially of the face, may resemble contact dermatitis, seborrhoeic dermatitis, dermatomyositis or erysipelas, and can follow tooth extraction [116]. Occasionally, more acute lesions with bullae may follow exposure to the sun, and bullae may be haemorrhagic. Importantly, the rash in generalised LE and the generalised form of DLE usually spares the distal interphalangeal, proximal interphalangeal and metacarpo-phalangeal joints, an important distinguishing feature from dermatomyositis (Figure 51.25) [99].

Epidermal necrosis or acute syndrome of apoptotic pan-epidermolysis [117] may give an appearance resembling TEN and this must be differentiated from drug-induced TEN in a patient with SLE [118]. Patients with this form of CLE often have significant systemic disease activity such as cerebritis or nephritis. In other cases, lesions are like those of erythema multiforme (Rowell syndrome) (Figure 51.26).

viral exanthema or drug eruption [99]. Photosensitivity is very common and has been observed in 63% in one UK study of 73 patients [100]. Sunlight may either precipitate or aggravate existing disease [112]. UVR from fluorescent lighting [113] and UVA from photocopiers [114] may also cause exacerbations, as can chronic exposure to indoor light sources [115]. Because UV-induced lesions of CLE are characterised by a latency period of up to several weeks, a negative history of photosensitivity does not exclude sensitivity to light as the patient may be unaware of the relationship [104]. In addition, although cutaneous manifestations are more common in the summer months and in days to weeks following UV exposure [104],

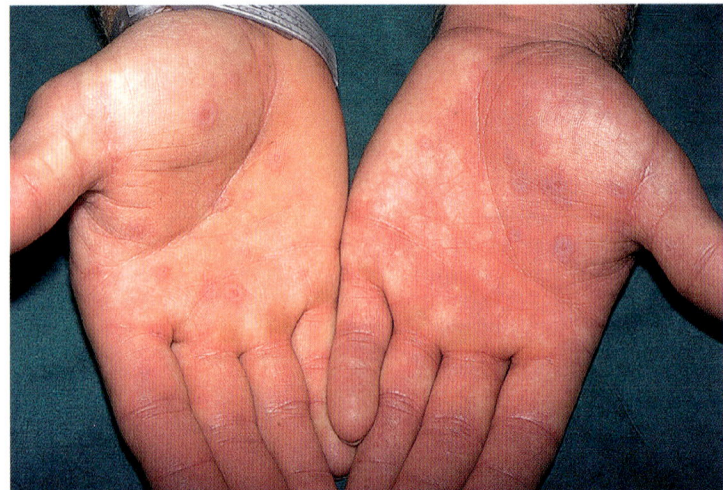

Figure 51.26 Annular lesions of discoid lupus erythematosus resembling erythema multiforme and associated with characteristic immunological abnormalities (Rowell syndrome).

Lesions resembling chronic discoid lesions are initial manifestations in approximately 10% of patients and occur in 20% of patients at some point in the disease course [99,100].

Chilblain LE is an uncommon form of DLE. There is a familial form presenting in childhood, which is autosomal dominant [119], and a sporadic form usually affecting middle-aged females. This is associated with DLE in 50% of cases and persists beyond the cold season in over 30% of cases. Up to 20% of patients with the perniotic lesions of chilblain lupus (see earlier in this chapter) may go on to develop SLE [111]. These lesions may ulcerate, as may the hyperkeratotic kerato-dermatous skin sometimes found [120]. Mutations in TREX1, an intracellular DNAse that digests cytosolic DNA thereby preventing activation of the cell intrinsic type I IFN response pathway, have been described in familial cases of chilblain lupus and SLE [121]. The same mutation is observed in Aicardi–Goutières syndrome, whose clinical phenotype shows chilblain LE-like acral skin disease in addition to progressive neurological disease [122].

Lupus non-specific changes. Sometimes, lesions may be minimal. Redness can be seen over the thenar and hypothenar eminences of the palms and may be confused with palmar erythema of liver disease [104]. Reticulated palmar redness may also be associated with vasculopathy of antiphospholipid syndrome. Non-specific changes in the skin associated with SLE include nail changes, hair changes, urticarial lesions, vasculitis, mucinoses, bullous lesions, mucosal lesions and others. These are detailed here.

Nail changes. A variety of nail changes have been reported in SLE including nail fold erythema, splinter haemorrhages, red lunulae and nail fold hyperkeratosis (Figure 51.27a) [123]. Other nail findings include nail ridging (Figure 51.27b), onycholysis, onychomadesis and punctate or striate leukonychia caused by altered keratinisation of the nail matrix [124]. Blue-black nail pigmentation may also be observed, most commonly in African American patients with SLE, and is thought to occur from increased melanin deposition [125]. This dyschromia may be diffuse or longitudinal and may be caused by medications, most frequently antimalarials (Figure 51.28), but is occasionally associated with methotrexate, cyclophosphamide and gold. Nail fold capillaroscopy (NFC) may reveal glomerulisation of the capillaries [126]. In one series, telangiectasias and erythema of the nail fold were found in 76% of patients with both DLE and SLE, but in no patients with DLE alone, suggesting that this sign is sensitive for systemic disease activity [102]. In addition, although capillary loop drop-out and dilated capillaries are more commonly found in systemic sclerosis and dermatomyositis, this pattern has been found in patients with SLE and appears to be strongly correlated with Raynaud phenomenon and anti-U1 ribonucleoprotein (anti-U1-RNP) antibodies [127]. To date, NFC alone cannot reliably differentiate lupus from dermatomyositis [128] but changes on NFC may be correlated with disease activity [129].

Hair changes. This can be scarring or non-scarring [130]. Non-scarring alopecia remains a diagnostic criterion in the 2019 EULAR/ACR classification criteria for SLE [131]. The most common non-specific skin manifestation of SLE is the diffuse non-scarring alopecia known as telogen effluvium, which occurs in more than

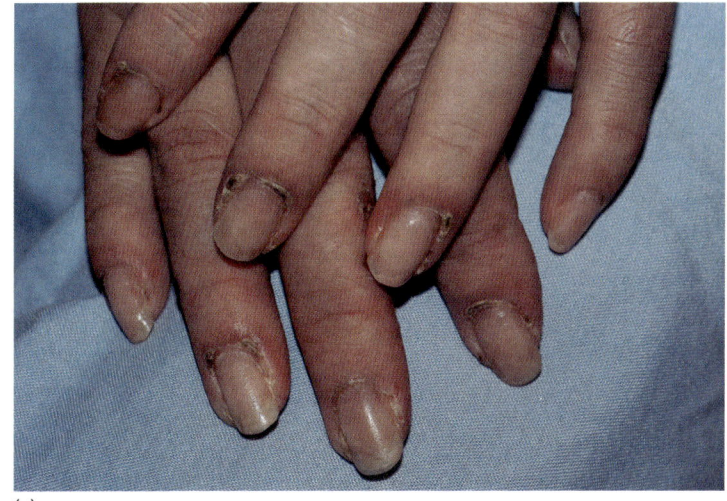

(a)

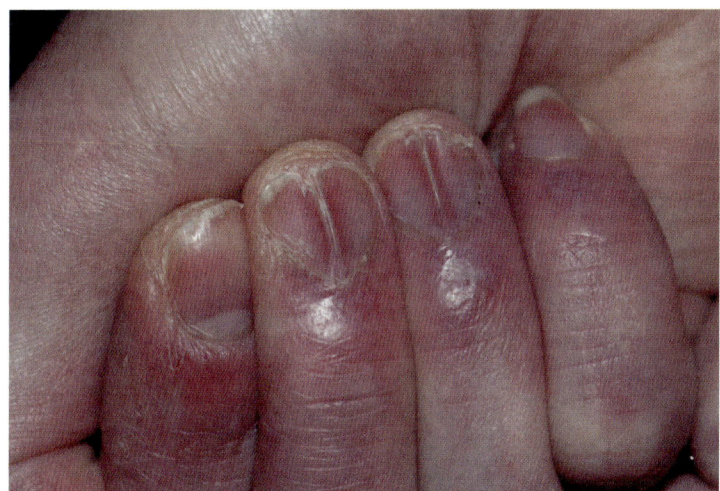

(b)

Figure 51.27 (a) Extensive nail fold necrosis and (b) nail ridging in systemic lupus erythematosus.

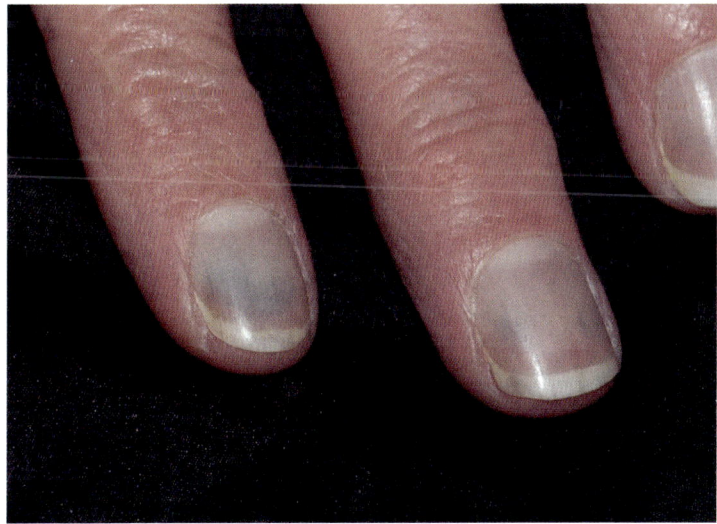

Figure 51.28 Blue nail discoloration as a result of antimalarial therapy.

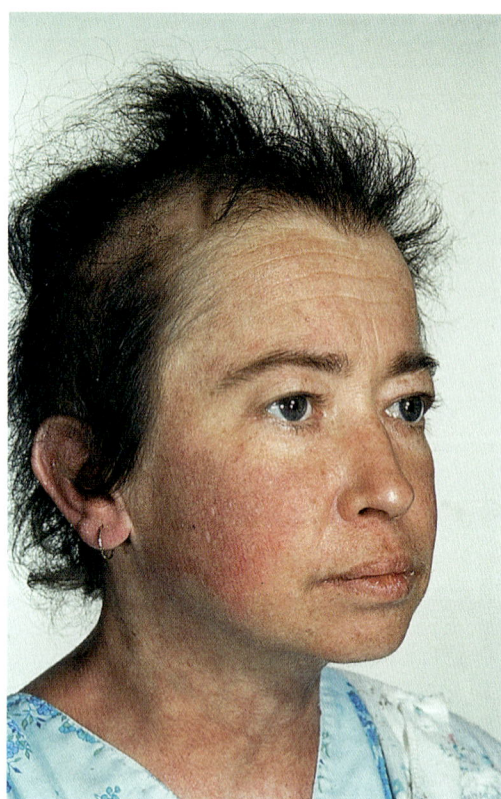

Figure 51.29 Unruly 'lupus hair' with diffuse alopecia.

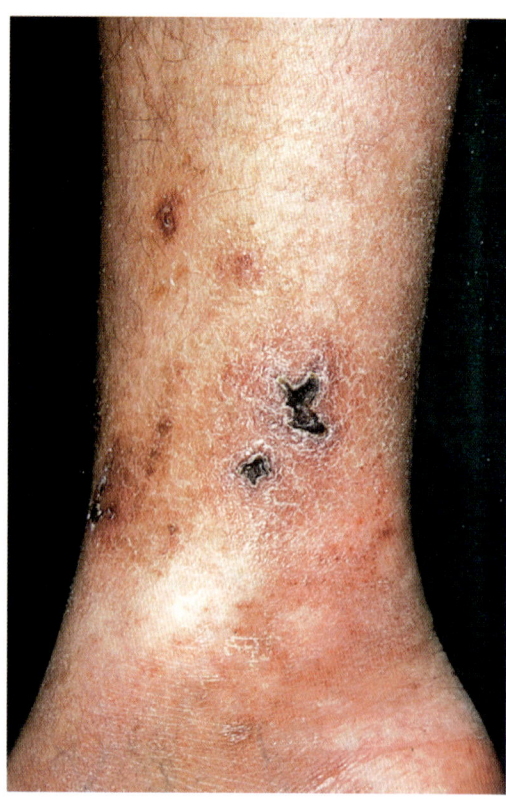

Figure 51.30 Necrotic crusted leg ulcers in systemic lupus erythematosus.

60% of cases either as a transient phenomenon or during increased disease activity [104]. Alternatively, the alopecia can be chronic and associated with disease activity leading to coarse, dry and fragile hair along the peripheral hairline during a systemic flare 2–3 months later, so-called 'lupus hair' (Figure 51.29) [132,133]. Alopecia areata is also more often reported, in approximately 10% of patients with SLE [134]; however recent evidence suggests that non-scarring patchy alopecia in patients with SLE is different from that in alopecia areata [124]. Permanent scarring alopecia is similar to that found in DLE [123]. Frontal fibrosing alopecia is another scarring alopecia that has been associated with autoimmune diseases including SLE [135].

Cutaneous vascular reactions. Vascular reactions are important to recognise in SLE as they frequently indicate underlying vascular pathology [123]. They can be divided into vasculitis or vasculopathy and the distinction between the two conditions is important as their management is distinctly different. Vasculitis is caused by primary inflammation of the vessel walls with secondary occlusion by fibrin, whereas vasculopathy can be defined as narrowing of the vessel walls (i.e. ischaemic) or non-inflammatory vessel lumen occlusion from thromboembolic disease. However, both conditions may present similarly and may coexist.

- **Vasculitis.** Arterioles and venules of the skin are frequently affected in SLE, although any size of blood vessel may be affected – the size of the vessel affected and the intensity of the inflammation determining the appearance. Vasculitis in the context of SLE most commonly affects the skin, and usually presents as a small-vessel leukocytoclastic vasculitis (LCV) with

palpable petechiae or purpura in dependent areas (Figure 51.30) [112,136]. It is seen in 10–30% of patients with SLE [98,136,137]. Vasculitis in SLE is associated with juvenile disease onset, livedo reticularis, Raynaud phenomenon, haematological manifestations and higher disease activity scores at disease onset [137]. Before LCV is attributed to SLE, other causes such as drugs and infection should be excluded. Involvement of medium and/or large vessels may manifest as retiform or stellate purpura with or without necrosis and ulceration or as subcutaneous nodules [99]. Other manifestations include gangrene, periungual infarcts, splinter haemorrhages and urticarial and bullous changes [104]. Gangrene of the fingers and toes [138] may also develop either acutely or insidiously and can occur in patients with both vasculitis and vasculopathy due to thrombosis.

- **Vasculopathy.** Raynaud phenomenon can be seen in 25–60% of patients with SLE and has been observed to be the most common non-specific finding in studies of such patients [98,102]. It is characterised by reversible vasospasm of the fingers and toes, often caused by cold exposure with triphasic colour change: cold-induced pallor, followed by cyanosis pain and numbness, and then red discoloration on rewarming [104]. Predictors associated with LE and Raynaud phenomenon include persistent periungual telangiectasia, involvement of the thumbs, ears, nose and toes, ice-pick or pitted scarring of the pulps and high ANA, anti-RNP and nucleolar antibodies [104]. Raynaud phenomenon in SLE is also associated with migraine [139], pulmonary artery hypertension [140], neurological or neuropsychiatric manifestations and anti-RNP antibodies [141].

Livedo reticularis is seen in up to 35% of SLE patients [142]. It may be seen in patients with SLE both with and without the

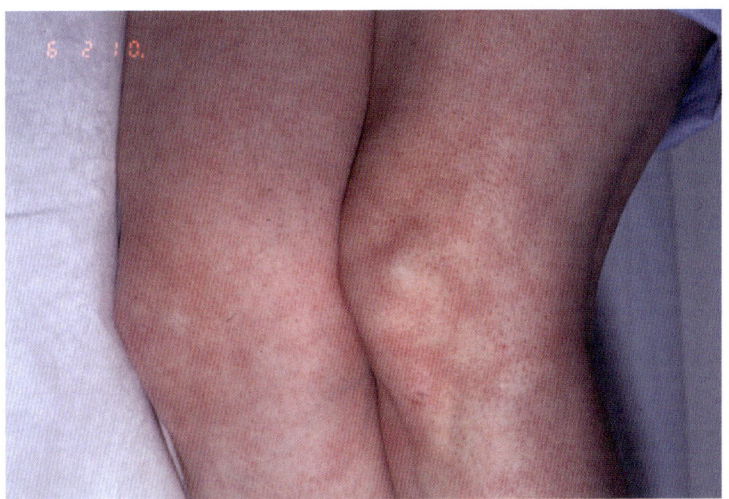

Figure 51.31 Extensive livedo reticularis in the setting of systemic lupus erythematosus.

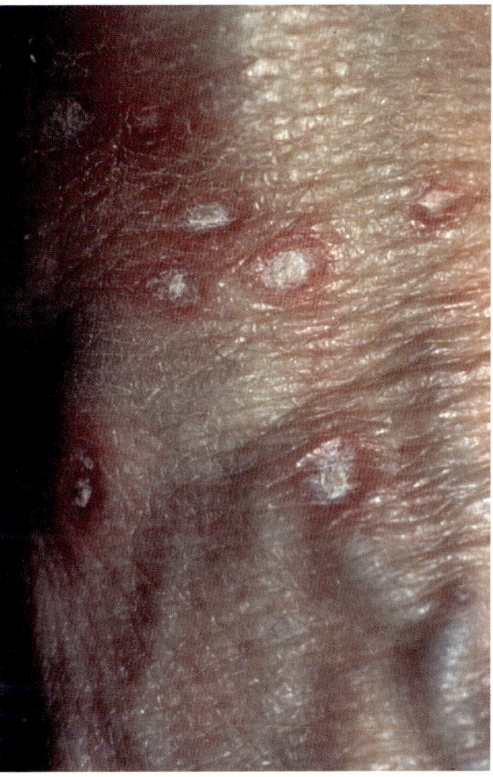

Figure 51.32 Degos-like lesions in a patient with systemic lupus erythematosus.

antipholipid syndrome [99] and presents as a fishnet-like, mottled or bluish red discoloration, which blanches on pressure, most commonly on the buttocks and legs, followed by the outer aspects of the arms and less commonly on the trunk (Figure 51.31) [103]. The net-like discoloration results from hypo-oxygenation due to slow arterial blood flow in dermal arterioles and the collection of the hypo-oxygenated blood in the dermal venules causing the discoloration. Livedo racemosa is distinguished from livedo reticularis based on a 'broken net' type pattern and is thought to be a sign of more severe disease due to the presence of cholesterol and fibrin thrombi and calcification in the vessels [103]. Livedo reticularis in patients with SLE and antiphospholipid syndrome has been associated with central nervous system involvement [143]. In addition to livedo reticularis, patients with both antiphospholipid antibodies (APAbs) and SLE may present with retiform purpuric plaques, which may ulcerate, as well as ecchymoses, purpura, digital gangrene and thrombophlebitis [103]. Lesions are more likely to present at acral locations as smaller blood vessels are more likely to become occluded. Catastrophic antiphospholipid syndrome (CAPS) is rare (<1%), but has a high mortality of approximately 50% [104]. CAPS presents in patients with antiphospholipid syndrome with a disseminated intravascular coagulation-type picture with purpura fulminans [144]. The diagnosis is made on the basis of evidence of thrombosis in at least three organs and histological finding of small-vessel occlusion in at least one organ, a laboratory confirmation of APAbs and the rapid development of clinical manifestations [144].

Atrophie blanche-type lesions (ivory, stellate, painful scars on the lower extremities) with lesions similar to those in Degos disease (malignant atrophic papulosis) – small porcelain-white atrophic macules with peripheral redness and telangiectasia – may also occur in patients with APAbs (Figure 51.32) [145]. In SLE patients with Degos-like lesions, a more benign course without the characteristic visceral involvement (digestive tract or central nervous system) that is commonly described in Degos syndrome is usual. It is thought that because of the broad overlap in clinical and histological findings, cutaneous lesions of Degos disease may represent a common end point to a variety of vascular insults, rather than a specific entity [146]. Lesions of primary anetoderma may also be seen and consist of localised areas of herniated sac-like or flaccid skin as a result of localised elastic loss [147].

- **Other causes of vasculopathy.** Cryoglobulins have been observed in 25–66% of patients with SLE, with the vast majority having type II or III cryoglobulinaemia [148,149]. Type II or mixed cryoglobulinaemia usually presents with palpable purpura of a small-vessel vasculitis, with ulceration and necrosis in severe cases. Hepatitis C virus, rheumatoid factor, low complement and cutaneous vasculitis were more frequent in patients with cryoglobulinaemia than those without in one study [148]. Cholesterol emboli may result from the release of cholesterol crystals during spontaneous break-up of atherosclerotic plaques or intravascular procedures, which travel to smaller vessels and impede blood flow. The presentation in the digital vessels can be similar to SLE vasculitis or antiphospholipid associated vasculopathy with purpuric infarction of the tips of the fingers or toes. Calciphylaxis may also occur in patients with SLE and end-stage renal disease [150]. Erythromelalgia is characterised by burning pain in the hands and feet aggravated by heat and dependence and accompanied by redness and warmth. It can be primary or secondary (e.g. underlying SLE or blood dyscrasias) and is thought to be caused by microvascular arteriovenous shunting [151].

Urticaria. Urticarial lesions occurred in up to 44% of 73 patients with SLE in one series [100]. Hypocomplementaemic urticarial vasculitis [152] can also be seen and consists of painful urticarial lesions lasting 24 h or longer which characteristically leave postinflammatory hyperpigmentation and demonstrate findings of LCV on histology. Anti-inflammatory treatment commonly used to treat SLE may be useful in the management of chronic urticaria [153,154]. However,

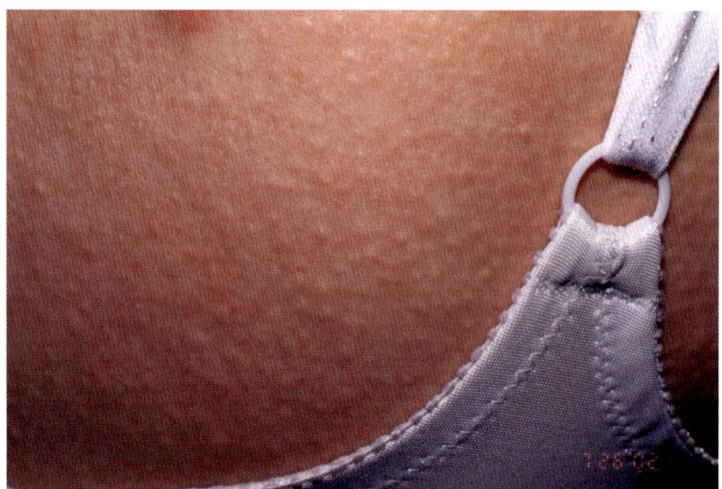

Figure 51.33 Multiple papules on the back due to mucinosis in systemic lupus erythematosus.

antimalarials have been reported to induce aquagenic pruritus and thus an accurate drug history remains paramount [155].

Mucinosis. Although mucin deposits are found frequently on skin biopsy specimens from patients with cutaneous lupus, specific clinical patterns of mucinosis also occur. Papular or nodular lesions resulting from mucinous deposits in the dermis (papulonodular mucinosis) without microscopic features of LE have been reported [156] and form a distinct entity, which may be the presenting feature of LE [157]. It presents as multiple, asymptomatic, flesh-coloured papules, usually on the trunk, arms or head and neck, and can be associated with SLE, SCLE or DLE or can occur alone (Figure 51.33). The differential diagnosis includes TLE, which can be excluded both clinically and histologically. Other differential diagnoses of flesh-coloured papules in this setting include reticular erythematous mucinosis and scleromyxoedema, lichen myxoedematosus and thyroid disease-associated mucinoses.

Other connective tissue changes. Dystrophic calcinosis is rare, and is most often seen in association with lupus panniculitis [158] but can also occur in association with SLE. It occurs most often on the extremities and buttocks as asymptomatic nodules discovered by radiology. Occasionally, the skin overlying the calcinosis can ulcerate leading to the extrusion of chalk-like material. The mechanism underlying calcinosis cutis in SLE is unknown, but may be due to increased calcium concentration in the presence of necrotic and apoptotic cells, secondary to trauma or tissue damage [159]. Subcutaneous nodules occur in approximately 5% of patients [160]. They occur mainly over the backs of the proximal phalangeal joints and wrists, but are also found on the elbows, knees, occiput and flexor aspects of the fingers. They may resemble rheumatoid nodules and can respond to hydroxychloroquine [161]. Some are histologically identical to classic rheumatoid nodules [161].

Pigmentary changes. Pigmentary disturbances are not uncommon and hypopigmentation may result from both SCLE and DLE. In addition, a bluish black pigmentation of the skin may result from antimalarial therapy. In part, this pigmentation is thought to be

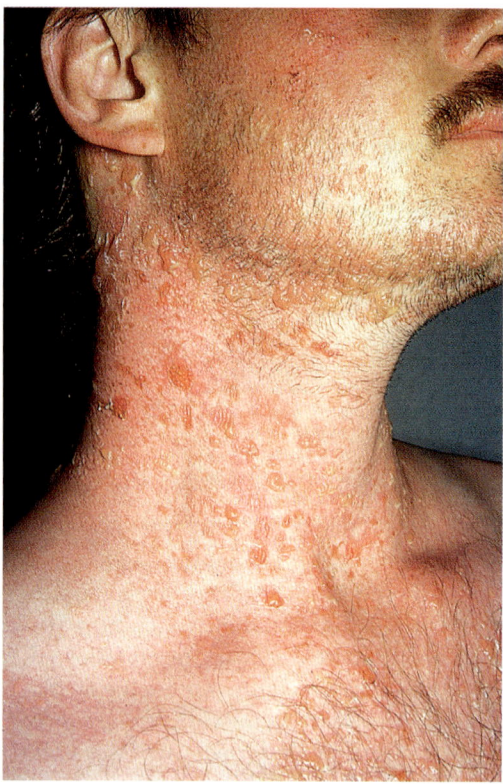

Figure 51.34 Bullous lupus erythematosus of the face and neck.

due to trapped haemosiderin [162]. Yellow discoloration from mepacrine therapy is reversible upon either stopping the drug or modifying the dose.

Bullous lesions in SLE. Blistering is uncommon in SLE and can be divided into three categories:
1 Subepidermal bullae in SCLE and ACLE: these lesions are due to separation of the epidermis and dermis as a result of severe liquefaction degeneration of the basal layer and dermal oedema (TEN-like ACLE and Rowell syndrome) [117].
2 SLE-associated autoimmune bullous disease: this includes dermatitis herpetiformis, pemphigus vulgaris (so-called pemphigus erythematosus), pemphigus foliceous, paraneoplastic pemphigus, bullous pemphigoid, pseudoporphria, epidermolysis bullosa acquisita and IgA disease [104].
3 A separate subset, bullous SLE (BSLE): this is a distinct type of autoantibody-mediated cutaneous SLE that results in a subepidermal blister (Figure 51.34) [163,164].

The diagnosis of BSLE requires (i) SLE; (ii) a vesiculobullous eruption arising but not limited to sun-exposed skin; (iii) a histopathological subepidermal blister and neutrophilic upper dermal infiltrate; and (iv) immunoglobulin and complement deposition at the basement-membrane zone with direct immunofluorescence (DIF) [163,164]. DIF demonstrates linear IgG (± IgA and IgM or C3) deposits at the basement-membrane zone, contrasting with the granular immunostaining seen in LE interface dermatitis. Evidence of antibodies to type VII collagen can be demonstrated by indirect immunofluorescence (IDIF) or DIF on salt split skin, immunoblotting, immunoprecipitation, enzyme-linked immunosorbent assay (ELISA) or immunoelectron microscopy [112].

Clinically, the bullous lesions arise predominantly on normal or red sun-exposed or flexural skin, but may be more widespread, and can heal with milia formation (Figure 51.34). Blistering often parallels systemic flares of SLE, particularly affecting the kidneys [112]. Given that BSLE occurs in the setting of SLE, ANA is generally positive and anti-dsDNA, anti-Sm, anti-Ro, anti-La and anticardiolipin antibodies may also be detected. Low complement, proteinuria or cellular casts on urinalysis as well as haematological abnormalities may also reflect disease activity.

Dapsone either alone or in combination with prednisone is the treatment of choice. The response may be dramatic with cessation of new bullae within 1–2 days. However, rapid recurrence may occur upon withdrawal of dapsone, with remission after reinitiation of therapy. Refractory disease may respond to rituximab [165].

Pemphigus erythematosus combines the immunological features of pemphigus and LE and presents with red, scaly, hyperkeratotic or crusted lesions, sometimes adversely affected by the sun. The lesions occur in a butterfly distribution on the cheeks and in a seborrhoeic distribution on the trunk of patients with Senear–Usher syndrome [166]. DIF demonstrates immunoglobulin and complement in the intercellular substance and at the dermal–epidermal junction of perilesional and, to a lesser extent, of light-exposed and non-exposed skin. Circulating pemphigus-like antibodies and antinuclear factor occur in 80–100%, but anti-DNA and ENA antibodies are not found. Antidesmoglein antibodies 1 and 3 have also been found. The condition occurs spontaneously, but has been induced by penicillamine, propranolol, captopril, pyritinol and thiopronine. Topical corticosteroids alone may control the condition, but systemic corticosteroids, other immunosuppressives or dapsone may be required.

Mucous membrane lesions. Oral ulcers are one of the 2019 EULAR/ACR criteria for identifying patients with SLE and are associated with increased disease activity [167]. These lesions are often non-specific, shallow and tend to occur in crops [168]. LE ulcers are usually non-painful and commonly affect the hard palate (Figure 51.35). Non-LE ulcers such as those in recurrent aphthous stomatitis, which affects up to 20% of the general population, are usually painful and range from a few millimeters in size (minor) to centimetres (major). Recurrent aphthous stomatitis occurs commonly in the setting of SLE; however, in this context, compared with the non-painful ulcers of LE, it is not usually associated with systemic disease activity [169]. Mucous membrane lesions can also occur in the context of DLE, affecting the buccal mucosa most often but also the hard palate and vermilion border of the lower lip [170,171]. Lesions can be of three types – red, discoid or ulcerous – and the three types may coexist [172]. The morphology varies, for example in acute mucosal lesions red macules, red palatal skin, ulcers, blisters or erosions may predominate [173]. Discoid lesions begin as red papules that enlarge into chronic plaques [174], usually appearing as reddish central areas surrounded by well-demarcated irregular white borders and telangiectasia [175]. The appearance can resemble oral lichen planus. Superficial palatal lesions may have a honeycombed appearance. Histologically, a lymphocyte-rich interface mucositis is seen. DIF is similar to that seen in CLE [175]. Cheilitis also occurs in approximately 6%, the lips having a silvery appearance, with redness, scaling and blurring of the vermilion

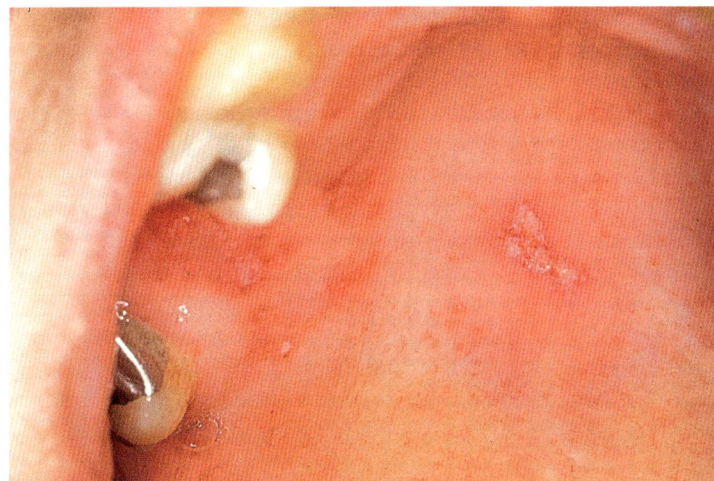

Figure 51.35 Systemic lupus erythematosus involving the palate.

border [176]. Malignant transformation was reported to occur in up to 6.9% in a series of 87 patients, and may be related to increased age (>60 years) [176]. Given the potential risk of transformation to squamous cell carcinoma in these patients, mucosal biopsy should be considered in any non-healing or irregularly ulcerated lesion.

Differential diagnosis [177]

The manifestations of SLE are so varied that the disease is often referred to as the 'great mimicker'. Multiple physician assessments are often required to arrive at a diagnosis. The current EULAR/ACR classification criteria, although not designed for diagnosis, may help in individual patients, and have a sensitivity of 96% and a specificity of 93% [167]. Many patients suspected of having a connective tissue disease may, even after thorough investigation, present problems of categorisation.

The differential diagnosis of SLE includes connective tissue diseases such as rheumatoid arthritis, mixed connective tissue disease, undifferentiated connective tissue disease, KFD, acute viral syndromes (parvovirus, Epstein–Barr virus, infectious mononucleosis and human immunodeficiency virus (HIV)), Behçet disease, familial Mediterranean fever, amyopathic dermatomyositis, drug-induced lupus and others. These differential diagnoses should always be considered when presented with a patient with possible SLE. Coexistent autoimmune diseases such as antiphospholipid antibody syndrome, rheumatoid arthritis, scleroderma, Sjögren syndrome, autoimmune hepatitis, psoriasis, primary biliary sclerosis, thyroid disorders and diabetes may complicate the diagnosis as up to one-third of patients have other autoimmune diseases [178].

Following clinical assessment, if the pre-test probability of SLE is high, ANA testing should be ordered to support the diagnosis. This test is 95–100% sensitive for the diagnosis of SLE [179]. Guidelines for the use of the ANA test are available [179]. Patients may present with a positive ANA as the first criterion of diagnosis and autoantibodies have been noted a mean of 3.3 years prior to diagnosis in a cohort of soldiers who ultimately developed SLE [180]. The terms undifferentiated connective tissue disease or 'latent lupus' may be used in patients with symptoms suggestive of SLE (for example with two or three ACR criteria) but not yet clearly ascribable to SLE [181].

ANA positivity is central to the diagnosis of SLE yet patients may be diagnosed without a positive ANA. The incidence of ANA-negative SLE has been estimated to be 1–5% [182]. The concept of ANA-negative SLE arose prior to the use of modern microscopes and use of the HEp-2 (laryngeal) cell line and was described in patients with photosensitivity and anti-SSA/Ro [183]. Solid phase methods may have increased false negative rates for SLE. In one study comparing autoantibody tests on patients from a single lupus clinic using IDIF and a solid phase method, ANA levels measured by IDIF and anti-dsDNA levels by ELISA were 81% and 47% compared with 76% and 32% by solid phase assay (BioPlex system) [184]. Currently, if an ELISA test or solid phase assay has been used and the clinician's suspicion for SLE is strong, an ANA test with immunofluorescence is recommended.

Complications and co-morbidities

Arthritis [185]. Involvement of the joints occurs at some time in approximately 90% of patients, arthralgia being more common than arthritis. A rheumatoid-like deformity is present in approximately 25% of cases, with marked soft-tissue swelling, especially of the dorsa of the fingers, hands and wrists, although joint erosions on X-ray are not a feature. The deformity is usually less, but the soft-tissue swelling is more marked, than in rheumatoid arthritis. Rarely, erosive symmetrical polyarthritis with rheumatoid arthritis-like deformities, termed rhupus, can occur [186]. These patients may be distinguished from those with lupus arthropathy due to the presence of anticyclic citrullinated peptide antibodies. Jaccoud arthropathy, severe deformity of the hands with ulnar deviation and swan-neck configuration, often with little pain and good function, occurred in 13% and fixed flexion contractures of the elbows in 11% in one series [187,188]. The progressive rheumatoid arthritis-like deformities in this syndrome are due to tenosynovitis rather than synovial inflammation as seen in rheumatoid arthritis. Tendinopathy may result in tendon rupture [189]. The elbows, shoulders, knees and feet may also be involved and soft-tissue nodules may occur, usually indicating calcinosis. Features distinguishing SLE from rheumatoid arthritis are shown in Table 51.9.

Muscle changes. Muscle pain occurs in approximately 50% of patients, and this may be confused with the pain of arthritis. Muscle weakness is a less common feature, and can be related to steroid myopathy or other drug effects. Inflammatory myopathy

Table 51.9 Features distinguishing systemic lupus erythematosus (SLE) from rheumatoid arthritis (RA).

Distinguishing feature	SLE (%)	RA (%)
Deforming arthritis	25	Common
Subcutaneous nodules	5	25
Radiological erosions	Rare	Common
Involvement of kidneys	Common	Rare
Positive LE cell test	80	15
Positive ANA test	90	20
Rheumatoid factor present	40	80

ANA, antinuclear antibody; LE, lupus erythematosus.

occurs in 5–10% of patients and is indistinguishable from idiopathic inflammatory myopathy [190].

Bone changes [191]. Avascular necrosis of the bones occurs in 5–30% of patients with SLE [192,193]. Interruption of blood flow to the bony epiphysis results in bone necrosis and subchondral fractures. Risk factors include the presence of Raynaud phenomenon, vasculitis, antiphospholipid syndrome and glucocorticoid use. Glucocorticoids are thought to promote adipogenesis and fatty infiltration of osteocytes, enhancing apoptosis. Glucocorticoid dose and length of use correlate with risk of avascular necrosis. The femoral head or condyle is most frequently involved [194], but the condition also may involve the knees, ankles, humerus, metatarsals and the carpal bones. It is commonly bilateral, with involvement of multiple joints. The diagnosis should be considered in patients with persistent pain over one or several joints, when there is little activity in other systems. X-rays may be normal, but the diagnosis is often clear on magnetic resonance imaging (MRI) or bone scintigraphy [195]. Surgical management options include core decompression, bone grafting and joint replacement. The condition is thought to be associated with increased pressure in the bone marrow because of altered venous drainage, and core decompression may be successful [196]. Total hip replacement may be required if the hip fails, or in the late stages of disintegration.

Osteoporosis with consequent increased fracture risk is another important bone-related problem in SLE [197]. The prevalence of osteoporosis may attain 50%, with fractures occurring in up to 20% of individuals with SLE. Factors contributing to bone loss include chronic inflammation, glucocorticoid use, renal dysfunction, vitamin D deficiency, ovarian failure and concomitant thyroid disease. Identification of risk factors, regular bone mineral density measurement and appropriate therapy are critical.

Heart [198]. Cardiovascular disease is one of the main prognostic predictors in SLE and is responsible for the increase in late mortality of the disease [199]. Pleurisy and pericarditis have a prevalence of 17% at disease onset and a cumulative incidence of 36%. Patients with pericarditis typically present with tachycardia, substernal chest discomfort and positional pain [198]. Clinically significant valvular dysfunction secondary to Libman–Sacks endocarditis occurs in just 1–2% of patients [200]. The valves on the left side of the heart are commonly involved. Both systolic and diastolic murmurs may be found depending upon the site of the lesion, and bacterial endocarditis can occur on the damaged heart valves.

Coronary artery disease is the most common cause of death in patients with longstanding SLE [201]. A recent meta-analysis ascribed a relative risk of 2.9 for myocardial infarction [202]. The presence of antiphospholipid antibodies may predict the atherosclerosis independently of other risk factors. Young women with SLE are at an increased risk of developing myocardial infarction [203]. Treatment with corticosteroids increases the risk of developing coronary artery disease by contributing to hyperlipidaemia, hypertension and weight gain such that patients on 30 mg of prednisone have a 60% greater 2-year risk of cardiovascular events compared with disease activity-matched patients not taking corticosteroids [204]. The myocardium may also be affected, resulting in cardiac failure, but this is rare [205].

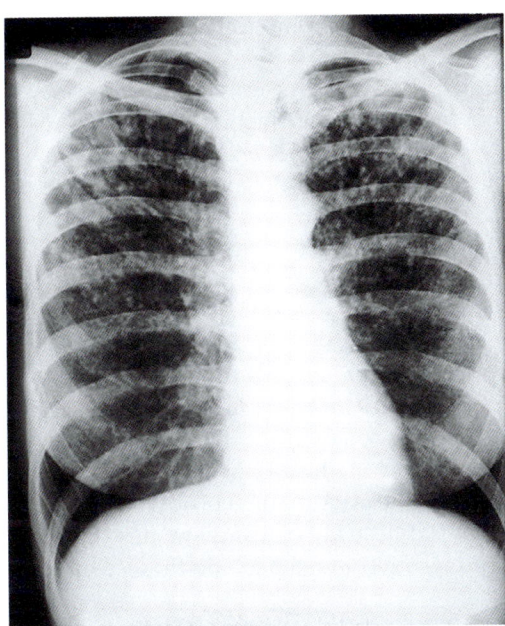

Figure 51.36 Pulmonary infiltration in systemic lupus erythematosus. This cleared in approximately 2 years on treatment with corticosteroids.

Lungs. The incidence of involvement of the pulmonary system varies [206,207]. Transient pleurisy is the most common feature, and in approximately two-thirds of these cases some fluid develops, occasionally haemorrhagic. Pleural thickening can be shown radiographically. Involvement of the lungs is less frequent, and is shown mainly as transient infiltration, sometimes with mottling and reticulation (Figure 51.36). Acute pneumonitis with severe dyspnoea and fever is rare, with an incidence between 1% and 19%, but may be a presenting manifestation of SLE [208]. Chest radiographs show diffuse alveolar infiltrates with a predilection for the bases. Diffuse pulmonary haemorrhage [209] and pulmonary infections must be considered within the differential diagnosis. Shrinking lung syndrome is a condition that is typical of SLE and that consists of a restrictive lung disease without parenchymal changes but with decreased lung volumes associated with elevated hemidiaphragms and basal atelectasis on radiography [201,210]. Diaphragmatic fibrosis has been proposed as a possible mechanism. Pulmonary hypertension occurs rarely compared with systemic sclerosis and is likely multifactorial with factors including vasospasm, vasculitis and thrombotic occlusion.

Renal changes [211]. The renal changes in SLE are very important in assessing the prognosis (see later in this chapter). Renal disease in lupus accounts for 3% of end-stage renal failure, and is an important cause of mortality in SLE [212]. The need for regular screening by urinalysis, blood pressure monitoring, assessment of renal function and early renal biopsy is critical. Usually, renal exacerbations are associated with high titres of antinuclear factor, elevated DNA binding and low serum complement.

The course is variable, and albuminuria and casts may persist for years without marked deterioration in renal function. Kidney damage, if this is going to develop, usually appears early (within the first 3 years) and is more frequent and severe in younger patients [212]. However, renal involvement may appear up to three decades after the diagnosis of SLE [213]. Nephrotic syndrome and renal vein thrombosis have been associated with membranous nephritis (ISN class V). Thus, a renal biopsy in every patient with haematuria, proteinuria or elevation of serum creatinine is advised.

Gastrointestinal tract [214]. Gastrointestinal symptoms occur in about 50% of patients but are usually mild with anorexia, nausea and vomiting being the most frequent. Abdominal pain may be due to mesenteric vasculitis, hepato-biliary disease, pancreatitis or causes unrelated to SLE such as gastroenteritis or appendicitis. In patients with active SLE and abdominal pain, vasculitis may be present in up to 53% [215] and thus comprehensive and aggressive evaluation including complete blood count, amylase, blood chemistry and abdominal radiography is required. Oesophageal dysmotility is common, resulting in heartburn and regurgitation. However, oesophageal dysmotility is not related to activity, duration or therapy of SLE [216]. Pancreatitis is a rare complication of SLE sometimes associated with corticosteroid use [217]. In childhood-onset SLE, pancreatitis has been associated with macrophage activation syndrome [218]. Ascites can occur as a manifestation of nephrotic syndrome, but may be an initial presentation of SLE [219]. Causes can include heart failure, protein-losing enteropathy, constrictive pericarditis or lupus serositis.

Hepatic lesions [220]. Liver disease is present in approximately one-third of patients, but it is usually mild and often asymptomatic. Histology typically shows steatosis (possibly related to glucocorticoid use) or mild hepatitis. Lesions include granulomatous hepatitis, chronic active hepatitis and cirrhosis. There may be a link between antiribosomal P antibody and SLE-associated hepatitis [221]. Autoimmune hepatitis is diagnosed by the presence of interface hepatitis, hypergammaglobulinaemia and the presence of autoantibodies [222]. Type 1 autoimmune hepatitis, previously named 'lupoid hepatitis', involves mainly young women who have antibodies to smooth muscle. Of those with autoimmune hepatitis, only 10% fulfil the criteria for SLE [223].

Thyroid disease. Both hyperthyroidism and hypothyroidism occur in SLE, and there is a high frequency of abnormal thyroid function tests and thyroid autoantibodies in patients without diagnosed thyroid disease [224].

Nervous system. The involvement of the nervous system by SLE results in neurological and psychiatric manifestations [225,226]. To begin to address the diagnostic and therapeutic challenges presented by multiple neuropsychiatric manifestations, the ACR produced a standard nomenclature and case definitions for 19 neuropsychiatric syndromes known to occur in patients with SLE [227]. Using these case definitions, the prevalence of neuropsychiatric disease still varies from 37% to 95%. In decreasing order of frequency these are cognitive dysfunction (55–80%), headache, mood disorders, cerebrovascular disease, seizures, polyneuropathy, anxiety and psychosis (0–8%) [228]. Attribution to SLE has remained difficult. There is no direct correlation between neurological and psychiatric disease and clinical or laboratory indices of disease activity. Primary proposed mechanisms include vascular occlusion or haemorrhage, autoantibody-mediated effects and cytokine

PART 4: INFLAMMATORY DERMATOSES

effects [229]. Neurological and psychiatric events commonly occur within the first year after SLE diagnosis and in the presence of generalised disease activity [226]. Peripheral sensorimotor and autonomic neuropathy occurs, brought about by vasculitis in the vasa nervorum. SLE may also cause psychiatric symptoms, including anxiety, hypomania, emotional lability, memory defects and depression.

Diagnostic work-up should be similar to that in non-SLE patients presenting with the same manifestations. This may include lumbar puncture and cerebrospinal fluid analysis to exclude infection, electroencephalogram, conventional computed tomography scanning and MRI. Although antiribosomal P antibodies have been associated with psychiatric SLE [230], they may have limited diagnostic accuracy [231].

Involvement of the eyes. Ocular changes in SLE are not uncommon [232] and visual loss may be the presenting symptom [233]. The most common ocular manifestation is dry eyes or keratoconjunctivitis sicca (KCS) caused by secondary Sjögren syndrome [234]. Retinal vasculopathy in the form of cotton wool spots is the next most common manifestation and suggests active SLE and lupus cerebritis [235]. Although rare, optic neuropathy is associated with a poor visual prognosis [234]. Ocular manifestations also include episcleritis and scleritis, keratitis secondary to KCS (most often due to poor tear film and secondary changes such as superficial punctate keratopathy), uveitis, orbital inflammation, antimalarial toxicity and APAb retinopathy [234].

Involvement of the ears. Sudden sensorineural hearing loss may occur in patients with SLE and may be associated with the antiphospholipid syndrome. Treatment with anticoagulation may be indicated in these patients [236].

Complications and co-morbidities

SLE in childhood. Approximately 15–20% of SLE has childhood onset [237]. The clinical picture, course and treatment are similar to the disorder in adults, but on the whole, children have more severe disease [237]. A meta-analysis of 16 studies comparing the clinical features of childhood- versus adult-onset SLE demonstrated that malar rash, mucocutaneous involvement, haematological abnormalities, seizures, renal involvement, urinary cellular casts and proteinuria, adenopathy and fever were more common in children [238].

SLE in the elderly [239,240]. The onset of disease over 50 years of age occurs in 12–18% of patients. There is an increased incidence of Raynaud phenomenon, sicca symptoms and pleuritis with increased damage accrual and morbidity despite a reduced incidence of renal disease. Antibodies to Ro and La are frequent and there appears to be an association with HLA-DR3.

SLE in contraception and pregnancy [241]. Fertility is normal if renal function is good. Worsening of SLE is uncommon in pregnancy, especially in those on immunosuppressive therapy [241]. Clinical remission or minimal lupus activity in the 6 months before conception lowers the chances of a significant flare and should indicate an uncomplicated pregnancy and a live birth [241].

There is a higher risk of complicated pregnancies in all patients with SLE, regardless of whether or not SLE is active. Active lupus nephritis poses the greatest risk to pregnancy outcomes in lupus, with a history of lupus nephritis posing a risk of 8–36% of non-elective pregnancy loss [242–244]. Up to 20% will be affected by pre-eclampsia, one-third will have preterm delivery and another third will have a caesarian section [245,246]. Antiphospholipid syndrome, characterised by the presence of APAbs in the setting of either vascular thrombosis or recurrent pregnancy complications, when untreated, may lead to an increased rate of fetal loss in 45–90% of pregnancies [247]. This falls considerably, to less than 30%, if treatment is given [248]. Based on current available evidence and expert opinion, treatment is recommended with prophylactic low-molecular-weight heparin (LMWH) and low-dose aspirin for women with APAbs and a history of pregnancy complications. Similarly for women with APAbs and a history of vascular thrombosis, treatment with full-dose LMWH and low-dose aspirin is indicated, with no treatment recommended for those women with APAbs only [241].

Regarding management of lupus during pregnancy, oral corticosteroids are relatively safe [241]. Side effects include a small absolute risk of cleft lip or palate [249], and as in women who are not pregnant, an increased risk of maternal hypertension and diabetes [250]. Prednisone and prednisolone are recommended, as less than 10% of the dose will cross the maternal–fetal membranes. Steroids may also need to be temporarily increased at the time of delivery and postpartum. If the patient is on azathioprine, this should be continued as there is no evidence of an increase in the rate of malformations. Mycophenolate mofetil is contraindicated and it is recommended that women transfer to an alternate immunosuppression prior to conception, such as azathioprine [251]. Hydroxychloroquine may be continued and there is evidence that it can reduce disease flares and may decrease the risk of recurrent cardiac neonatal lupus and heart block in mothers with anti-Ro antibodies [250].

Although traditionally it was recommended that oestrogen-containing contraceptives should be avoided in women with SLE, clinical trials have now shown that the use of oral contraceptives in women with stable disease does not increase the risk of flare [252]. However, oestrogen-containing contraceptives should be avoided in lupus patients with positive anticardiolipin ± lupus anticoagulant. Conversely, it is recommended that patients with SLE wishing to commence this method of contraception should be screened for these antibodies. The progesterone-only contraceptive Depo-Provera® is an alternative option, however its use for more than 2 years may increase the risk of osteoporosis.

In patients taking azathioprine no adverse events have been reported in breast-fed infants exposed to azathioprine, but a small study showed that the majority of azathioprine is excreted within 4 h of ingestion, prompting the recommendation that feeds be given at least 4 h after the maternal dose [250]. Breastfeeding is probably safe if the patient is on aspirin, low-dose corticosteroids or hydroxychloroquine, but should probably be avoided if other immunosuppressives are used.

Association with other diseases. SLE can occur concurrently with other connective tissue diseases such as rheumatoid arthritis, so-called rhupus as described by Schur [253]. Systemic sclerosis and SLE may occur in the same patient. A subset of patients with scleroderma and antitopoisomerase and anti-U1-RNP antibodies share a high lupus-like IFN gene expression pattern [254]. SLE occurs rarely in association with lichen sclerosus, with 'en coup de sabre' morphoea [255] and linear and plaque morphoea [256]. Secondary Sjögren syndrome can also occur in SLE and is associated with older age, a higher prevalence of Raynaud phenomenon, rheumatoid factor and anti-Ro and anti-La antibodies [256].

Many skin conditions are associated with SLE anecdotally; however, repeated associations with neutrophilic dermatoses, palisaded neutrophilic and granulomatous dermatitis (PNGD), KFD and erythema elevatum dilutinum have been reported. Both pyoderma gangrenosum [257] and Sweet syndrome may be the presenting feature in SLE, with the latter associated with drug-induced and neonatal LE [258]. PNGD, or Churg–Strauss granuloma, is an uncommon condition, most often associated with rheumatoid arthritis [259] but that may occur in the setting of SLE. The clinical presentation varies and may present as asymptomatic papules, nodules or annular plaques which appear symmetrical, often affecting the lateral trunk, abdomen or extensor extremities [260]. Another recently reported entity, amicrobial pustulosis of the folds, is rare and characterised by relapsing pustular lesions involving mainly the cutaneous folds, and typically occurring in the setting of an autoimmune disorder, particularly in young women with SLE [261,262]. It is also classified within the neutrophilic dermatosis spectrum [261].

SLE has been reported with other autoimmune diseases including Hashimoto thyroiditis and pernicious anaemia [263] and may follow primary biliary cirrhosis [264]. Reports also exist of associations with myasthenia gravis, multiple sclerosis and insulin-dependent diabetes [265]. SLE may coexist with psoriasis [266]. Relative risks in individuals with a first-degree relative with SLE for various autoimmune diseases vary from 5.87 for primary Sjögren syndrome, 5.40 for systemic sclerosis, 2.95 for myasthenia gravis, 2.77 for inflammatory myositis, 2.66 for rheumatoid arthritis, 2.58 for multiple sclerosis, 1.68 for type 1 diabetes, 1.39 for inflammatory bowel diseases to 0.86 for vasculitis [267]. An unusual syndrome of breast hypertrophy, or gigantomastia, has been reported [268]. Eruptive dermatofibromas have been reported [269].

Finally, the risk of malignancy has been evaluated in patients with SLE and there is an increased risk of haematopoetic malignancy, particularly non-Hodgkin lymphoma, as well as an elevated risk of lung, hepato-biliary, cervical and vulvo-vaginal cancers but a decreased risk of breast cancer [270].

Kikuchi–Fujimoto disease and SLE. KFD is a benign and usually self-limiting histiocytic necrotising lymphadenitis of unknown aetiology [271,272]. Reported cases are predominantly female, but it can occur in males, and can affect all ages. Clinical features at presentation include tender lymphadenopathy most commonly involving the cervical lymph nodes, associated with fever, weight loss and night sweats in the more severely affected cases. Associations have been reported with SLE, which can present concurrently or follow a diagnosis of KFD. Common features include leukopenia, myalgias and fever. Skin changes have been reported in up to 40% of patients and are usually non-specific and include red papules, patches

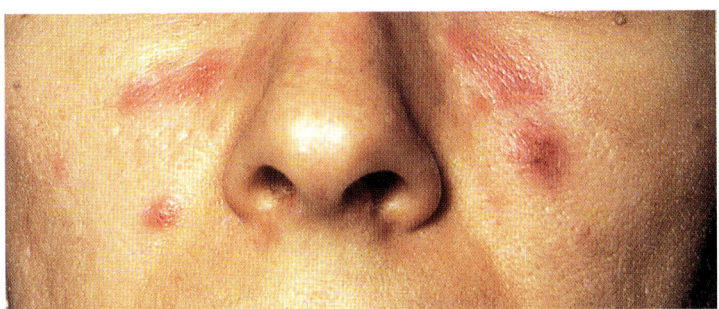

Figure 51.37 Red facial plaques in Kikuchi–Fujimoto disease.

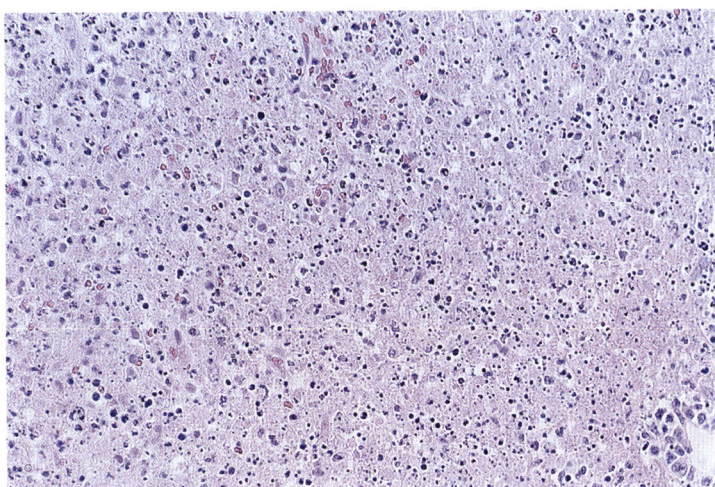

Figure 51.38 Histiocytic necrotising lymphadenitis (Kikuchi–Fujimoto disease) of the lymph node. Courtesy of Dr W. Merchant, Leeds General Infirmary, Leeds, UK.

and plaques and less commonly nodules, bullae and acneform eruptions. In our experience KFD can present concurrently with SLE with a photo-distributed eruption consisting of red, vesicular 'erythema multiforme' like lesions, predominantly on the face, with associated vasculopathic lesions on the fingers, tops and palms (Figure 51.37).

Histology of the skin shows oedema of the papillary dermis, with a patchy perivascular infiltrate in the dermis and subcutaneous fat. The infiltrate consists of histiocytes containing nuclear debris, and small lymphocytes. The nuclei of the histiocytes may be deformed. The lymph nodes show focal or complete loss of follicular architecture, with necrosis of cortical and paracortical areas (Figure 51.38). The extensive infiltrate consists of small lymphocytes, immunoblasts, macrophages and so-called plasmacytoid T cells [273]. Neutrophils are rarely seen, a feature that may help to distinguish this condition from SLE. The disorder can also be accompanied by macrophage activation syndrome. The natural history is for spontaneous healing in a few months but it can be fatal as a result of heart failure brought about by microscopic myocardial necrosis [274]. There was a 3.3% recurrence rate in one series [275]. In most cases no treatment is required, but a course of prednisolone may speed resolution. Various triggers have been incriminated, including the human herpesvirus 6, parvovirus B19, Epstein–Barr virus, dengue virus and infection with *Yersinia enterocolitica*, *Toxoplasma*, cytomegalovirus and HIV [276].

Disease course and prognosis

The course of SLE is very variable. Acute fulminating cases are much less common than subacute cases, which smoulder on for many years. The 5-year survival rate for patients with SLE was as low as 50% in the 1950s, varied between 64% and 87% in the 1980s and reached 95% in the 21st century. In a large, multicentre, international SLE cohort, Bernatsky et al. found decreasing standardised mortality ratios (SMRs) compared with the general population [277]. Survival is related to organ involvement and to frequency of exacerbations [278]. The highest SMRs were seen in female patients, those with younger age, SLE duration <1 year and black/African American populations. Serological as well as clinical remission is uncommon and occurred in 4% of 305 patients [279]. Exacerbations are more frequent in the first 5 years of the disease [278]. Pregnancy does not affect long-term survival. Prolonged survival is associated with an increased risk of atherosclerosis, avascular necrosis and neuropsychiatric dysfunction [280]. In elderly people the presentation is insidious and the clinical course is relatively benign. Renal disease and serological abnormalities are less frequent, and arthritis, with subcutaneous nodules, and pleuropericarditis are more prominent in elderly people [281].

The better prognosis of the more recent series is a result not only of the administration of corticosteroids, but also of earlier diagnosis, the avoidance of stress and drugs such as sulphonamides, and the control of infections by antibiotics. Persistent causes of death include renal disease, severe lupus disease activity, infection and cardiovascular disease. In the SLICC multicenter international cohort study, a lower total cancer mortality risk in SLE was observed with an increased mortality from haematological cancers such as non-Hodgkin lymphoma and lung cancer, but a decreased mortality from breast cancer [277].

Investigations

Because of the varying clinical morphologies, implications of the diagnosis and potential need for systemic therapy, a skin biopsy is often necessary to confirm the diagnosis. Biopsy for DIF is unnecessary if the case is diagnostic and may indeed be false positive if taken from photo-exposed skin [282]. A positive ANA test is required to fulfil the 2019 EULAR/ANA criteria for diagnosis [283]. Thus, laboratory investigations are now necessary to confirm the diagnosis, although even after extensive investigations it may be impossible to be entirely dogmatic in view of the overlap of the manifestations of connective tissue diseases. Most patients with LE will develop anaemia at some point during the disease course. The most prevalent type is anaemia of chronic disease, however iron deficiency, autoimmune haemolytic anaemia, drug-induced myelotoxicity and anaemia of chronic renal disease are less common causes. In autoimmune haemolytic anaemia, a positive direct antiglobulin test (Coombs test) in the context of haemolytic anaemia generally confirms the diagnosis. Both pure red cell aplasia and aplastic anaemia with immune-mediated haematopoietic failure have been reported. Reactive haemophagocytic syndrome can also occur with a reported incidence in SLE of 2.4% [283]. Leukopenia occurs in roughly 50% of patients with SLE [284]. More specifically, lymphopenia has been reported in one study with a cumulative frequency of up to 93% [285]. Leukocytosis may occasionally be found. Thrombocytopenia (platelets <100 000/mm^2) is a common

clinical manifestation in SLE, present in up to 37% of patients [284], and is usually below 40 000/mm^2 in patients presenting with thrombocytopenic purpura. The presence of thrombocytopenia correlates with increased morbidity and cumulative damage accrual [286]. The erythrocyte sedimentation rate is raised at some time in nearly 90% of patients; the C-reactive protein (CRP) is usually normal in the absence of infection, however elevated CRP may also indicate disease activity, therefore these values should be interpreted in context. Polyclonal gammopathy is commonly observed in patients with SLE and is an indication of an autoimmune reaction. Hypoalbuminaemia is also reported in 30–50% of patients [287], and measurement of baseline immunoglobulins may help diagnose primary or secondary immunodeficiencies associated with SLE and treatment, respectively. IgE antibodies may be raised and may correlate with disease activity including nephritis in SLE [287]. Thrombosis occurs with the lupus anticoagulant, but occasionally haemorrhage results from other haematological abnormalities such as disseminated intravascular coagulation or thrombocytopenia, seen in up to 50% of patients with CAPS [288]. The lupus anticoagulant is one of a number of APAbs found in up to 15–34% of patients with SLE, with anticardiolipin antibody found in 12–30% [287].

The LE cell phenomenon, first described by Hargraves et al. [289], is the basis for the LE cell test, which is positive in over 80% of patients. LE cells are neutrophils that have engulfed the nuclear material from degenerate white cells, in the presence of an antibody to deoxyribonucleoprotein (the LE cell factor) (see Figure 51.20) [290]. Sometimes, large masses of nuclear material are found extracellularly and, with surrounding leukocytes, form rosettes. LE cells, if present in large numbers, are highly suggestive of SLE. A positive LE cell test is also a feature of drug-induced LE. The LE cell test has now been superseded by tests for antinuclear factors and anti-DNA antibodies.

One or more ANAs can be detected by fluorescent antibody techniques in over 80% of cases. The incidence depends on the substrate used. Most British laboratories now use human cell lines for antibody testing, particularly Hep-2 cells derived from a human laryngeal cell line. This produces a reduction in the proportion of patients said to be antinuclear factor negative. Previously, the standard substrate was rat or mouse liver. Using rat liver, four staining patterns were historically demonstrated [291] representing four systems of ANAs that are also noted using Hep-2 cells (Figure 51.39):

1 In the *homogeneous pattern*, produced by antinucleohistone, the nuclei are stained all over.
2 The *speckled pattern* shows minute points of fluorescence scattered all over the nucleus, the antigens being saline-soluble proteins.
3 The *nucleolar pattern* shows uniform staining of each nucleolus.
4 Sera containing anti-DNA antibody give rise to the fourth *peripheral or membranous pattern* in which staining occurs at the periphery of the nucleus.

These staining patterns are produced by separate antibodies, but more than one antibody may be present in a single serum, usually in different titres. No particular antibody is specific for any disease. Discrepancies in the incidence between series probably depend on differences in techniques and the substrate used.

Homogeneous antinuclear factor (which is the same factor as the LE cell factor, although the fluorescent antibody test is more

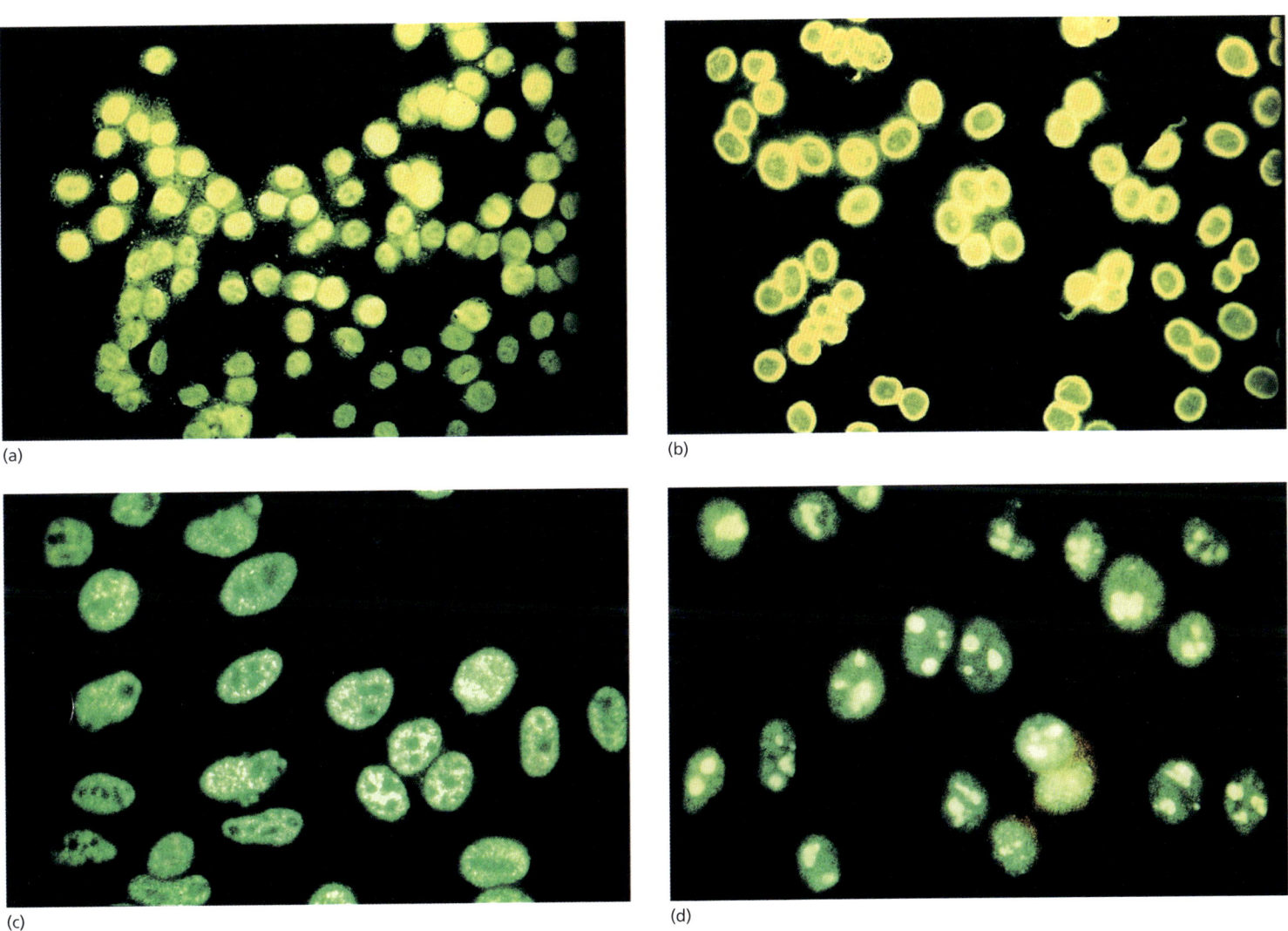

Figure 51.39 Different types of antinuclear factor demonstrated on Hep-2 cells: (a) homogeneous type, (b) peripheral type, (c) speckled type, (d) nucleolar type.

sensitive than the LE cell test) is more than twice as common as the speckled factor, but antinucleolar antibody is only occasionally found. Any person in apparently good health found to have a high titre of antinuclear factor should be followed up for years as there is a considerable likelihood of developing LE or systemic sclerosis. In one retrospective US study of 130 SLE patients, 78% had positive ANA testing at a titre of 1 : 120 or more at an average of 3.3 years prior to diagnosis [192].

When Hep-2 cells are used as substrate, as well as being more sensitive to the presence of ANA, further patterns can be identified [293]. These include centromere staining associated with the CREST syndrome (calcinosis, Raynaud phenomenon, oesophageal dysfunction, sclerodactyly and telangiectasia) and in 6% of patients with SLE, homogeneous, peripheral (specific to SLE), fine and coarse speckles and a ground-glass appearance produced by the Scl-70 antibody found in systemic sclerosis. There are also several patterns of nucleolar staining: homogeneous, speckled and clumpy.

Advances in the technology of immunoassays now permit the rapid and simultaneous detection of multiple autoantibodies and include the use of microarrays, laser beads and nanobarcode particles [294]. Circulating antibodies to DNA are almost always present in active disease. Their demonstration by the Farr radioimmunoassay technique is the most specific aid to diagnosis and is present in approximately 60–70% of patients with SLE at some time during the course of their illness [287]. Levels often correlate with disease activity. The use of serial immunofluorescent ANA testing in SLE patients with known positive ANA is not clinically useful for disease monitoring, however changes in anti-dsDNA antibody titres sometimes correlate with disease activity and lupus nephritis and can be useful in monitoring disease activity [295]. Indeed high (>200 IU/mL) titers of anti-dsDNA have been shown to be an independent predictor of moderate to severe SLE flares [296]. Low C3 has been shown to be an independent predictor of severe lupus flare in a post hoc analysis of belimumab clinical trials [296]. Despite this, a subset of patients with elevated anti-dsDNA titres and hypocomplementaemia did not demonstrate evidence of clinical disease activity when followed up.

Several other antibodies occur in patients with SLE. Anti-Smith (anti-Sm) antibodies are present in approximately 30% of patients with SLE, but are considered specific for the disease and are included in the ACR criteria, although they are not of use in monitoring overall lupus disease activity [287]. The association

PART 4: INFLAMMATORY DERMATOSES

of anti-Sm antibodies and organ involvement is conflicting, but reported to include nephritis, neuropsychiatric lupus, pulmonary fibrosis, serositis and peripheral neuropathy. Antihistone antibodies are associated with drug-induced lupus and are of limited value in the diagnosis or clinical assessment in patients with SLE. Anti-RNP antibodies occur in approximately 23–40% of patients with SLE and are higher in African American patients compared with white populations. The presence of high titres of anti-RNP antibodies is characteristic of mixed connective tissue disease. Among patients with SLE, the presence of anti-RNP antibodies does not predict neuropsychiatric manifestations or lupus nephritis or other manifestations of SLE [297].

Anti-Ro antibody occurs in approximately 30–40% of patients who have an increased tendency to photosensitivity, secondary Sjögren syndrome and interstitial pneumonitis, shrinking lung syndrome and deforming arthropathy, as well as being a marker for neonatal lupus. It is also found in 60–90% of patients with SCLE as well as ANA-negative SLE patients and in lupus-like syndromes with genetic deficiencies of C1q, C2 or C4. Anti-Ro is an antibody to an RNP derived from RNA polymerase III-transcribed Y RNAs with a protein component that appears to be the main target. Two different proteins, one of 60 kDa and another of 52 kDa, react with most positive sera. The 60 kDa protein predominates in SLE, the 52 kDa in Sjögren syndrome [298]. Anti-La, an antibody to another RNP product of RNA polymerase III, is present in 10–15% of patients, often with Sjögren syndrome and with anti-Ro antibody. Anti-Ro and anti-La antibodies should be tested in any female patient with SLE, mixed connective tissue disease, Sjögren syndrome or other systemic rheumatology conditions who is planning a pregnancy because of the increased risk of neonatal lupus syndrome. The concept of ANA-negative lupus was introduced in 1976 [299] with many patients presenting to dermatologists with cutaneous findings similar to SCLE, positive anti-Ro antibodies and photosensitivity [300]. This is a problem in less than 2% if appropriate substrates are used (such as Hep-2 cell or solid-based assays). Rarely, chronic variable immune deficiency and associated conditions may be associated with a loss of autoantibodies in SLE [301].

Inherited deficiencies of the major complement components may occur in SLE. Patients with homozygous deficiencies in C1, C2 and C4 early components of the classic pathway are particularly at risk [302]. The most common is homozygous C2 deficiency in which SLE occurs in approximately 30% of patients [303]. Clinically, the lupus-like syndrome in C2 deficiency shows a low incidence of renal disease, but more cutaneous involvement and arthralgia. Serum ANAs and anti-dsDNA antibodies are often lower in patients with complement deficiency-associated SLE, compared with idiopathic SLE, however anti-Ro antibodies appear more frequent. Isolated C1q deficiency has also been reported, and there is an association between C1-esterase inhibitor deficiency and SLE. In addition to a tendency to SLE, patients with homozygous deficiencies of C1, C2 or C4 often have a high risk of recurrent bacterial infections [303].

Assessment of disease activity [304,305]
In large cohorts, 70% of SLE patients have a course of disease flares and remissions [306]. Due to the multisystem nature of the disease, there is a need for disease activity indices to guide therapy. A number of attempts have been made to devise definitions of disease

activity, accompanied by scoring systems using combinations of clinical and laboratory parameters to allow comparative and longitudinal studies. The following systems are useful in the context of clinical trials in patients with active systemic disease: SELENA (safety of oestrogens in LE national assessment), SLEDAI (SLE disease activity index) [307], SLEDAI-2K [308] and BILAG (British Isles lupus activity grading) [309]. Organ damage, as assessed by the SLICC/ACR damage index [310], has been associated with adverse clinical outcomes. The use of validated activity and damage indices is included in current EULAR management guidelines [311]. However, none of the general activity scores is specifically designed for the assessment of patients who most concern dermatologists, and they do not grade skin disease in any meaningful way. The CLASI has been described for the assessment of cutaneous disease [312] and is increasingly used in clinical trials. A study demonstrated the validity of the CLASI for skin outcomes when compared with the cutaneous domains of the SLEDAI and SDI in individuals with SLE [313]. The CLASI provides a quantitative measure of skin-specific burden of disease allowing for standardised measurements of disease progression. It also distinguishes clearly between activity and damage, which is important for disease management.

Management
General principles of management
The goal of the management of SLE should be to aim for remission of disease activity, to prevent organ damage and to minimise side effects of therapy, all to increase quality of life [**314**]. The management of SLE can be divided into non-pharmacological and pharmacological (Figure 51.40). Although limited data exist, consensus opinion suggests that general measures for SLE patients should include avoidance of sun exposure. Patients should be advised to wear broad-brimmed hats, to cover the 'V' of the neck and the arms and to use a sunscreen with at least a sun protection factor of 30, as patients with photosensitivity may develop fatigue and disease flares following UV light exposure [315]. Sunscreen with avobenzone (blocks UVA1), titanium dioxide or zinc oxide (block UVB and UVA1) are also recommended to block longer UVA wavelengths [316]. Smoking cessation should also be encouraged as cigarette smoking may exacerbate the disease [317]. Furthermore, patients with SLE are at increased risk of accelerated atherosclerosis [318]. Because patients with SLE are advised to avoid UVR, it is important to monitor serum 25-hydroxy vitamin D (25(OH)D) at baseline and treat appropriately to ensure that a recommended minimum serum level of 30 ng/mL (75 mmol/L) is achieved [319]. To correct vitamin D deficiency, 1000 IU per day of oral vitamin D_3 (cholecalciferol) is recommended as this is more effective than vitamin D_2 [320]. In the authors' practice, patients with SLE are advised to take oral vitamin D_3 1000 IU daily PO to supplement dietary vitamin D. Symptomatic therapy for joint pain using NSAIDs is valuable.

Regarding pharmacological therapy, the choice is individualised and depends on the degree of organ involvement and disease severity. It is important to assess the patient's progress considering general well-being and relief of symptoms, and the use of validated damage and activity indices is recommended in the current EULAR guidelines for the management of SLE [**314**]. The erythrocyte sedimentation rate and DNA antibodies are variable and a

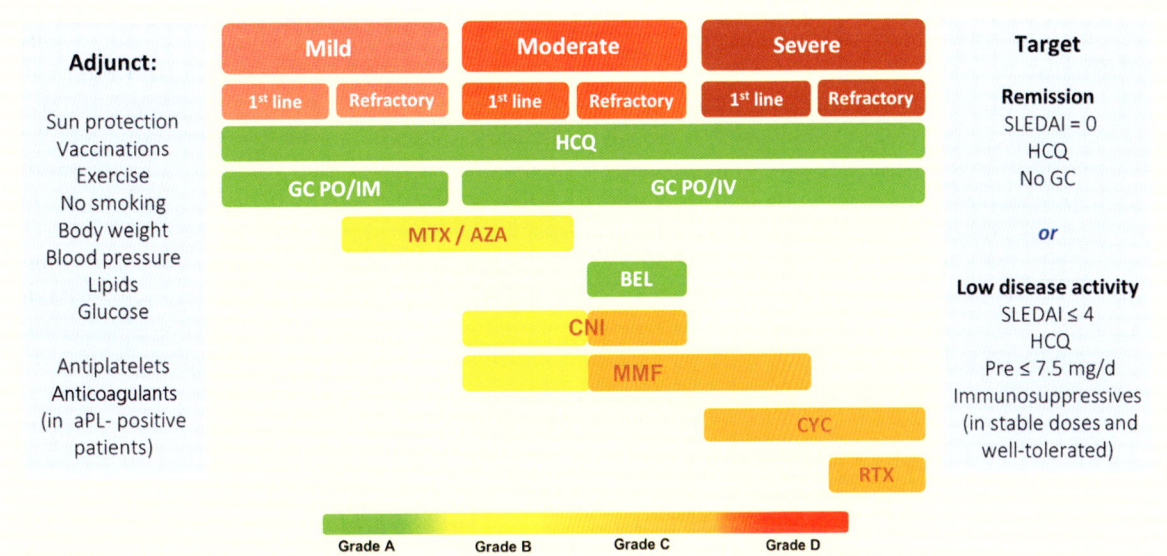

Mild: constitutional symptoms/ mild arthritis/ rash ≤9% BSA/PLTs 50–100 x 10³/mm³; SLEDAI ≤6; BILAG C or ≤1 BILAG B manifestation
Moderate: RA-like arthritis/ rash 9–18% BSA/cutaneous vasculitis ≤18% BSA; PLTs 20–50 x 10³/mm³/serositis; SLEDAI 7–12; ≥2 BILAG B manifestations
Severe: major organ threatening disease (nephritis, cerebritis, myelitis, pneumonitis, mesenteric vasculitis; thrombocytopenia with platelets <20 x 10³/mm³; TTP-like disease or acute haemophagocytic syndrome; SLEDAI >12; ≥1 BILAG A manifestations

Figure 51.40 Treatment of non-renal SLE: recommended drugs with respective grading of recommendation. aPL, antiphospholipid antibodies; AZA, azathioprine; BEL, belimumab; BILAG: British Isles lupus assessment group disease activity index; BSA, body surface area; CNI, calcineurin inhibitor; CYC, cyclophosphamide; GC, glucocorticoids; HCQ, hydroxychloroquine; IM, intramuscular; IV, intravascular; MMF, mycophenolate mofetil; MTX, methotrexate; PLTs, platelets; PO, *per os*; Pre, prednisone; RA, rheumatoid arthritis; RTX, rituximab; SLEDAI, systemic lupus erythematosus disease activity index; TTP, thrombotic thrombocytopenic purpura. Reproduced from Fanouriakis *et al.* 2019 [314] with permission from the British Medical Journal.

poor guide to the adequacy of therapy and the titre of ANAs often persists unchanged despite clinical remission. Anti-dsDNA antibody and serum complement levels may be helpful in predicting exacerbations [314]. Despite this, a subset of patients with elevated anti-dsDNA titres and hypocomplementaemia do not demonstrate evidence of clinical disease activity when followed up [321].

First line

For skin disease alone, topical therapy is an appropriate first line treatment or adjunct for individual lesions. Potency depends on the site, but generally potent fluorinated corticosteroids should only be used for short periods on very inflammatory lesions on the face because of the risk of atrophy and telangiectasia, with 1–2.5% hydrocortisone used subsequently. Alternatively, the calcineurin inhibitors tacrolimus [322] and pimecrolimus [323] may be equally efficacious when compared with clobetasol propionate 0.05% and betamethasone valerate 0.1%, respectively, particularly for TLE. Intralesional triamcinolone acetonide (2.5–5 mg/mL) may also be useful for individual lesions, particularly on the scalp. For patients with extensive or resistant disease, antimalarials are used in regimens as discussed in other chapters.

The use of the antimalarials chloroquine or hydroxychloroquine should also be encouraged, not only in the management of mild disease but in all disease subtypes [324]. A systematic review has shown that antimalarials prevent lupus flares and increase the long-term survival of patients [325]. Antimalarials have also been found to work synergistically with mycophenolate mofetil for the treatment of membranous nephritis and are recommended by the EULAR guidelines for patients with lupus nephritis [326]. Additionally, they have a modest effect on lipid profile, cardiovascular

disease and thrombotic risk, and hydroxychloroquine in particular has been found to decrease lupus activity in pregnancy without harming the baby [325]. Quinacrine is contraindicated in pregnancy as it crosses the placenta. Guidelines provided by ophthalmology address dosing (5.0 mg/kg actual body weight for hydroxychloroquine) and surveillance [327]. There is still debate about the optimal dosing of hydroxychloroquine as doses of 5.0 mg/kg (actual weight) have been associated with an increased rate of flare [328]; in inactive disease, a decreased dose of 200 mg per day is favoured [329].

Corticosteroids are useful, but dosage depends on the degree of organ involvement and disease severity. Low-dose oral prednisolone (0.1–0.2 mg/kg) may be useful in patients with mild SLE and musculoskeletal manifestations resistant to other therapies [330]. High doses of oral prednisolone (1–1.5 mg/kg) or IV methylprednisolone 1 g daily for 3 days (pulse therapy) are used for severe disease with major organ involvement (e.g. renal, systemic vasculitis or neurological involvement) [330]. Once the condition appears to be under control, the dosage may be reduced until a maintenance dose is reached, ideally <6 mg, as the Hopkins lupus cohort have demonstrated that doses of greater than 6 mg increase the risk of organ damage by more than 50% [331]. A single dose daily, given in the morning, produces fewer side effects than split dosing and does not impair the therapeutic response.

Second line

For more severe disease, immunosuppressive drugs are used to minimise the risk of damage and to act as steroid-sparing agents. When considering the choice of immunosuppressant, as well as disease severity, the long-term risk of malignancy must be considered. Cyclophosphamide has been associated with bladder cancer, myelodysplastic syndromes, haematological malignancies, cervical atypia and skin cancers [332]. Mesna may reduce urotoxic side effects, and monthly IV therapy, with adequate hydration, is rarely complicated by bladder injury [332]. Azathioprine is associated with phototoxicity and the generation of carcinogenic DNA adducts [333], as well as a significant increase in the risk of malignancy [334], decreasing our enthusiasm for the use of this drug. Methotrexate is teratogenic and contraindicated in females within 6 months of planned conception. Additionally, mycophenolate mofetil is contraindicated in pregnancy, and in patients wishing to become pregnant a transition from this drug to azathioprine should be made in the preceding months because of the teratogenic risk [332].

Cyclophosphamide is a derivative of mechlorethamine which is metabolised into active metabolites [332]. For induction therapy in lupus nephritis, pulsed IV cyclophosphamide is preferred to oral cyclophosphamide due to reduced toxicity, particularly bladder injury [332], and may be followed by mycophenolate mofetil or azathioprine (the former may be more efficacious as maintenance therapy) [335,336]. However, mycophenolate mofetil may also be used as an alternative for induction treatment of mild to moderate lupus nephritis with similar efficacy to cyclophosphamide [337].

Because of its slower onset of action, azathioprine is often used as a steroid-sparing agent and as a maintenance drug following control of more acute SLE [332]. It has also been reported to be effective in severe cutaneous disease and in the treatment of chronic active hepatitis complicating lupus [338,339]. Azathioprine may be used in pregnancy as there have been no reports of teratogenicity. We prefer to minimise use of this agent due to the recent appreciation of risk of malignancy when compared with other immunosuppressive agents [340].

Mycophenolate mofetil is the morpholinoethyl ester of mycophenolic acid (MPA), which is a non-competitive reversible inhibitor of inosine-5′-monophosphate dehydrogenase, a necessary enzyme in the *de novo* pathway of purine synthesis [332]. This *de novo* synthesis pathway is uniquely essential to activated lymphocytes. Inhibition of both T and B lymphocyte proliferation, inhibition of antibody formation and prevention of leukocyte migration by MPA activity are the result. As well as its efficacy in lupus nephritis (as discussed earlier in this chapter), the Aspreva Lupus Management Study (ALMS) trial showed consistent and similar improvement in assessment of eight organ systems [341]. For patients with significant gastrointestinal side effects, which can occur in up to one-third of patients [342], titrating the dose from 500 mg twice daily to 1–1.5 g twice daily with weekly increases may be useful. In those that are still intolerant, switching to sustained release MPA may be better tolerated and can smooth out blood levels [332].

Methotrexate may be a useful adjunct in patients with mild to moderate SLE and recalcitrant mucocutaneous lesions and musculoskeletal symptoms [343]. A steroid-sparing effect has also been shown by Fortin *et al.*, who compared methotrexate with placebo and found a significantly reduced prednisone dose was given in the methotrexate treated arm [344]. Islam *et al.* demonstrated similar effectiveness of methotrexate 7.5 mg/week compared with chloroquine 150 mg daily over 24 weeks, with

similar articular and cutaneous manifestations of SLE and acceptable toxicity profile [345]. In the authors' experience, following a failure of antimalarials in patients with predominant skin disease, methotrexate at doses of 7.5–15 mg is an effective and quick acting therapy. Patients should be monitored regularly for decline in renal function, and their full blood picture and liver function tests followed. In addition, meticulous contraception is mandatory when used in women at risk of pregnancy.

IVIg may be a useful adjunct in resistant skin disease and is used for haematological disease at 1 g/kg/day for 1–2 days for steroid-refractory thrombocytopenia [330]. A trial of 400 mg/kg/day over 5 days led to a partial or complete remission of skin disease in 63% (10/16) of patients [346]. Ciclosporin has been used in resistant cases of skin disease and for non-renal lupus. One trial of patients with active SLE despite prednisone (>15 mg/day) evaluated ciclosporin (2.5 mg/kg) compared with azathioprine (2 mg/kg) [347]. After 12 months there was no significant difference in the reduction of prednisone or adverse outcomes with no sustained increase in creatinine observed in the ciclosporin group. Voclosporin, a novel calcineurin inhibitor, has shown favourable results when combined with mycophenolate for lupus nephritis [348]. The treatment of lupus-specific cutaneous features (ACCLE, DLE and SCLE) is discussed elsewhere in this chapter, however for patients with non-lupus-specific skin eruptions, dapsone may be useful for the treatment of urticarial lesions [349] and bullous eruptions [350].

Third line

An increasing understanding of the pathophysiology of lupus and the recognition of the multifaceted role that B cells play in lupus have led to the development of the novel biologic drugs to treat the disease, including rituximab (a monoclonal antibody to CD20), belimumab (a BLys inhibitor) and obinutuzumab (a humanised monoclonal antibody to CD20) [330]. In a *post hoc* analysis, two phase III trials (BLISS-52 and BLISS-76) of belimumab have shown improved overall SLE activity, particularly mucocutaneous and musculoskeletal at week 52 and 76, respectively [351]. Belimumab has also shown activity in lupus nephritis [352]. The EULAR supports the use of rituximab in the treatment of refractory nephritis [13]. Potent B-cell depletion with obinutuzumab is effective in lupus nephritis [353] and B-cell depletion with chimeric antigen receptor T-cell therapy can induce remission in refractory disease [354].

It is now known that increased serum concentration of IFN-α is associated with a distinct IFN signature in the peripheral blood and may relate to increased disease activity [355]. Recent studies have confirmed that anifrolumab, an antibody that binds to the type I interferon receptor, improves SLE disease activity [353,356] and may have particular utility for skin disease. The two TULIP (Treatment of Uncontrolled Lupus via the Interferon Pathway) showed an improvement of more than 50% of the CLASI score for skin disease when compared with placebo and a more pronounced effect in those with a high interferon gene signature. The integration of B-cell modulation with belimumab and interferon signalling with anifrolumab into the therapeutic armamentarium provides new options for limiting corticosteroid use and the potential improvement of long-term outcomes.

Neonatal lupus erythematosus

Definition
Neonatal lupus erythematosus (NLE) is a well-recognised subtype of LE and an acquired syndrome of clinical symptoms caused by the transplacental passage of maternal antibodies to SSA or SSB, or both [1]. The most frequent clinical manifestations are cutaneous lesions and congenital heart block (CHB).

Introduction and general description
Congenital heart block was first reported in the children of a mother with Sjögren syndrome in 1928 [2]. McCuiston and Schoch [3] were the first to suggest that NLE may be related to the transplacental transfer of 'a transmittable aetiological agent', reinforced by the fact that NLE skin lesions resolve as maternal antibodies are cleared from the infant's serum [4]. The syndrome has been increasingly investigated, and the role of the antibodies confirmed, the antibody subtypes delineated and treatment options considered and investigated.

Epidemiology
Incidence and prevalence
Congenital heart block occurs in 1–2% of children born to mothers positive for the Ro antibody, while neonatal lupus rash occurs in 8–10% of offspring of these mothers [5]. The risk of CHB in a subsequent pregnancy is 10-fold (20%) if a previous child had NLE [6,7].

Age
Neonates may present up to the age of 12–16 weeks postpartum.

Sex
The condition affects the sexes equally [8].

Associated diseases
The condition occurs in the offspring of women with positive Ro/SSA antibodies and occasionally La/SSB antibodies, which are transmitted across the placenta during pregnancy. Less frequently, anti-U1-RNP antibodies have been found to cause the classic lesions of NLE but not CHB [9,10]. The aforementioned autoantibodies are present in 90% of patients with Sjögren syndrome [11], 20–30% of patients with SLE [12] and 3% of patients with rheumatoid arthritis [13] as well as in SCLE, mixed connective tissue disease or an undifferentiated autoimmune syndrome. However, in 25–60% of cases mothers may not have clinical evidence of an autoimmune disease; half of these asymptomatic mothers will go on to develop an autoimmune disease after 3 years [14]. Up to 1.5% of healthy pregnant women may have the antibodies [15]. Hypothyroidism may also be another associated disease, as women with both hypothyroidism and anti-Ro/SSA were nine times more likely to give birth to children with CHB than women with only anti-Ro/SSA antibodies [16].

Pathophysiology
The presence of the Ro/SSA antibody is strongly associated with NLE, being present in 82–100% of infants and 92–100% of mothers

[17–20]. Studies have suggested that the 52 kDa protein version is more frequently found in CHB [21,22] while the 60 kDa one is more frequently associated with cutaneous disease [23], although this is disputed [24]. The aa200-239 (p200) locus on the 52 kDa R0/SS-A protein may be a more specific predictor of CHB [25] but this is not confirmed [26]. La/SS-B antibodies are less frequent in 50% of NLE infants and 60% of mothers, usually in association with Ro/SS-A antibodies [17]. A further study suggested that 50 kDa La/SS-B antibodies were associated with cutaneous disease [27], while another suggested that anti-idiotype antibodies to La/SS-B antibodies were protective against the development of NLE [28]. U1-RNP antibodies are detected as the only antibody in a limited number of patients with cutaneous NLE [29], but not with CHB.

Lee *et al.* [30] showed that purified Ro antibody bound to human skin that was grafted onto nude mice occurred in a pattern similar to that found in typical LE lesions, and that Ro/SS-A antigen is also present in neonatal skin [31]. Studies have suggested two possible mechanisms for the development of conduction abnormalities in NLE. One hypothesis suggests that fetal autoantigens Ro/SSA and La/SSB translocate to the surface of cardiomyocytes during cellular apoptosis, with the subsequent formation of complexes with maternal antibodies. The complexes are opsonised and phagocytosed by macrophages that release pro-inflammatory cytokines (TNF-α and transforming growth factor β (TGF-β)) leading to atrioventricular node dysfunction and conduction abnormalities [32]. A second hypothesis suggests molecular mimicry, whereby autoantibodies cross-react with cardiac L-type calcium channels, disrupt calcium homeostasis and disrupt potential propagation, leading to arrhythmias [32]. Other workers argue that these antibodies are only indirectly related to disease, the disease process being caused by either (i) the 52 kDa Ro/SS-A antigen showing homology with the 5-hydroxytryptamine-4 serotoninergic receptor, which mediates cardiac damage [21]; (ii) the presence of antibodies to a completely separate 57 kDa protein [33]; (iii) the presence of the TNF-α 308A allele (associated with high TNF-α production), HLA-DRQB1*02, HLA-DRB1*03 and TGF-β polymorphisms [34]; or (iv) via maternal microchimerisms [35]. Differences in clinical features of NLE may depend on the cytokine profile of patients. A report on the cytokine profile of two siblings with NLE showed that although both infants had elevated IL-6, IL-8, IFN-γ and monocyte chemoattractant protein 1, serum levels of IL-12, IL-13 and IL-17 were elevated only in the newborn with skin lesions [36].

Pathology
Following antibody binding, a sequence of opsonisation, apoptosis and fibrosis has been proposed in both skin and the cardiac conducting system [37]. The histopathology in the skin is that of a classic lupus histology.

Genetics
Maternal anti-Ro/SSA antibodies are major risk factors for CHB, however only 12–20% of subsequent pregnancies lead to CHB, despite persisting maternal autoantibodies. Thus additional risk factors are likely involved in fetal CHB susceptibility. The major histocompatibility complex locus has been implicated in autoimmune diseases. Mothers with the HLA-DR3 and HLA-B8 haplotypes, when associated with DQA1 and DQB1, may have offspring more

likely to have NLE and atrioventricular heart blocks [38–41]. Infants with cutaneous disease may carry all three HLA alleles – DRB1*03, DQB1*02 and TNF-α-308A promoter polymorphism – twice as frequently as unaffected children [34]. Additionally, a study performing single nucleotide polymorphism genotyping of individuals in the Swedish Congenital Heart Block study population identified HLA-DRB1*04 and HLA-Cw*05 as fetal HLA allele variants that confer susceptibility to CHB in response to Ro/SSA autoantibody exposure, whereas DRB1*13 and Cw*06 confer protection [42]. Another case series identified the presence of HLA-B*15, HLA-C*02, HLA-DQ5 and HLA-DR10 alleles in a mother and both of her children with NLE [43].

Environmental factors

As in classic SCLE, UV exposure of the neonate may be relevant to the onset of cutaneous disease. UV may increase the expression of antigens on the surface of keratinocytes, thereby increasing interactions with autoantibodies resulting in exacerbation of skin lesions [44]. However, NLE skin lesions may be present at birth or involve UV-protected sites, suggesting that UV exposure may not be necessary for the development of cutaneous disease [45].

Clinical features

Many cases present with either skin or heart problems with no preceding disease in the mother. Others occur in neonates of mothers known to carry the associated antibodies. The presentation may be either cutaneous or cardiac, although rarely other systems may be involved early.

Presentation

Cutaneous features. Approximately half of NLE infants manifest skin lesions [17], which may be present at birth or occur in the first few weeks of life. The most common finding is a red, slightly scaly eruption on the face and periorbital skin (raccoon sign/owl eye/eye mask) (Figure 51.41), with the scalp, trunk, extremities, neck and intertriginous areas involved in decreasing order of frequency [46]. There is resemblance to SCLE on pathology [47]. The eruption can be exacerbated by UV exposure and there are reports of the rash being precipitated by phototherapy for neonatal jaundice [48,49], although the rash is sometimes present at birth [45]. Other manifestations include a vitiligo-like eruption in a black infant [50], morphoea-like lesions [51], atypical targetoid-like lesions [52], cutis marmorata telangiectatica congenita-like lesions [53], transient bullae [54] and papules on the feet [55].

Cardiac features. NLE is typically associated with a structurally normal heart. CHB occurs in approximately 60% of white infants with NLE [17], and may be less common in Japanese patients [56]. Moderate to high levels of maternal anti-Ro/SSA antibody titres appear to be a risk factor for the development of CHB [57]. Associated features may also include pericardial effusions, pleural effusions, ascites, intrauterine growth retardation and hydrops fetalis [58]. Up to 50% of infants with CHB will require pacing in the neonatal period and others will require a pacemaker at a later date [59]. Dilated cardiomyopathy occured in up to 23% with CHB in one Finnish cohort, and has a significant mortality in the first year of life [59].

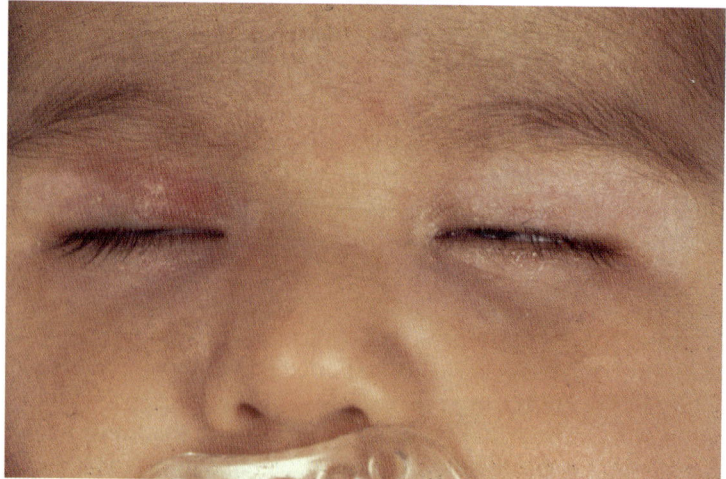

Figure 51.41 Typical 'raccoon' eyelid lesions in neonatal lupus erythematosus.

CHB usually develops between the 18th and 24th gestational weeks. Fetal bradycardia with a ventricular rate of 40–60 beats per minute can be detected prenatally [60]. The CHB is usually complete or third-degree, but first- and second-degree blocks may also occur and resolve completely during the first few months after birth or develop into an irreversible CHB with time [61–63]. Additionally, conduction abnormalities may less frequently result in Wolff–Parkinson–White syndrome, sinoatrial node dysfunction, prolongations of the QT interval and transient sinus bradycardia [62]. Dilated cardiomyopathy is usually detected *in utero* but may develop after birth [9]. Although structural cardiac abnormalities are rare, defects such as patent foramen ovale, ventricular or atrial septal defect, pulmonary stenosis, persistent patent ductus arteriosus and fusion of the chordae tendinae have been reported [64–67].

Haematological features. Approximately 10–20% of infants with NLS develop haematological symptoms such as anaemia (less frequently haemolytic or aplastic anaemia), thrombocytopenia and neutropenia [68]. Cytopenias develop due to immunological suppression of the fetal bone marrow by maternal autoantibodies and to a lesser extent by peripheral destruction of blood components. Other reported haematological manifestations include thrombosis and disseminated intravascular coagulation, microangiopathic haemolytic anaemia and immune thrombocytopenia [69,70].

Hepatic features. The most common hepato-biliary manifestations affecting 10–25% of NLE infants include asymptomatic elevation of aminotransferases, γ-glutamyl transferase, hepatomegaly and splenomegaly [60,71]. Cholestasis and cholestatic hepatitis have been described and hepato-biliary disease was found in 19 of 219 patients with NLE, and in three this was the only finding [72]. Hepato-biliary and haematological manifestations can either be isolated symptoms or accompany cutaneous or cardiac abnormalities [60].

Neurological features. Central nervous system abnormalities are uncommon in NLE and symptomatic neurological expressions are even rarer. The percentage of macrocephaly with or without associated hydrocephalus is higher in infants with NLE compared with the general population, although most cases are asymptomatic [73,74]. Additionally, other structural abnormalities reported include subependymal pseudocysts, subependymal haemorrhage, cerebral haemorrhage, ventriculomegaly, lenticulostriate vasculopathy, vasculitis and calcification of the basal ganglia [75–77]. Symptomatic central nervous system manifestations in NLE are more commonly associated with cutaneous disease than in those with CHB. Reported clinical manifestations include myelopathy, changes in consciousness, focal seizure, spastic paraparesis and neuropsychiatric disorders [75,78–80].

Differential diagnosis

The condition is easily recognised in neonates of at-risk mothers. In those with no known risk, the skin rash may be confused with congenital infections or inherited immune disorders such as the Bloom, Cockayne or Rothmund–Thompson syndromes. Based on morphology, annular erythema of childhood, annular urticaria, tinea faciei/capitis/corporis, seborrhoeic dermatitis, atopic dermatitis, Langerhans cell histiocytosis, congenital rubella and congenital syphilis should also be considered in the differential diagnosis of NLE.

Complications and co-morbidities

Case reports have associated NLE with pneumonitis [18], haemochromatosis [81], aseptic meningitis [82], transient myasthenia gravis [83] and chondrodysplasia punctata [84].

Disease course and prognosis

The rash improves over the first few months of life and has usually resolved without scarring by 12 months of age. Occasional patients exhibit residual telangiectasiae, dyspigmentation or atrophy [46] and atrophic scarring [85]. The heart block, seen in roughly 2% of children born of mothers with anti-Ro antibody, is permanent and requires a permanent pacemaker in roughly 50%.

Infant. Although follow-up data are limited, less than 5% of children go on to develop autoimmune diseases such as juvenile idiopathic arthritis, psoriasis, Hashimoto thyroiditis, nephritic syndrome, iritis and type 1 diabetes [86,87]. Follow-up is therefore advised.

Mother. Although mothers are often asymptomatic at the time of the birth, long-term follow-up studies by several groups have shown that many develop signs and symptoms of autoimmune disease, especially Sjögren syndrome, SLE and undifferentiated connective tissue disease [87]. Follow-up is therefore advised.

Investigations

Although the skin rash is reasonably characteristic, skin biopsy is usually required to confirm the diagnosis; exclusion of infection or the rare inherited syndromes mentioned earlier may be necessary. Antibody testing is required in both the child and mother. Investigations for a complete blood count with differential and liver enzymes should be considered, especially if there are signs of anaemia and/or hepatic dysfunction. Cardiac investigations including an electrocardiogram and echocardiogram are recommended after birth. Mothers with known anti-Ro/SSA and/or anti-La/SSB antibodies should have screening with fetal echocardiography initiated during the pregnancy.

Management

Recognition of the condition in a neonate is important for this and subsequent children, and monitoring of at-risk pregnancies should always occur. Manifestations other than heart block are usually temporary.

Cutaneous lesions

Skin disease is often mild and usually requires no treatment. Sun avoidance should be advised and low-potency topical steroids may be of benefit [17,59]. Antimalarials may be necessary for persistent skin disease. Persistent telangiectasia has been reported to respond to tunable dye laser [88].

Cardiac problems

The mortality rate in neonates with CHB is approximately 20% [65]. A higher risk of mortality is associated with the diagnosis of CHB in <20 weeks' gestational age, hydrops fetalis, low ventricular late (<50 beats per minute), impaired left ventricular function, cardiomegaly, endocardial fibroelastosis, atrioventricular valve regurgitation and low aortic flow velocity [65,89,90]. Up to 50% of infants with CHB may require pacing in the newborn period, and others may require pacemaker insertion at a later date [58].

There has been increasing research addressing whether CHB and its consequences can be prevented or treated *in utero*. Despite initial reports suggesting benefit of fluorinated steroids in the prevention of cardiac abnormalities, recent large cohort studies do not support its use [91,92]. However, in several studies, the maternal intake of hydroxychloroquine has shown to decrease the risk of developing primary CHB, recurrent CHB where there is a prior history of a sibling with CHB, and skin disease. Hydroxychloroquine is used safely in pregnant or breastfeeding mothers with SLE to prevent flares [93–95]. It is proposed that hydroxychloroquine 400 mg daily should be taken between the 6th and 10th gestational weeks [95]. The use of IVIg for both the prevention and treatment of CHB remains of unproven value [96–99]. Plasmapheresis three times weekly with systemic steroids during gestation may have helped to protect an at-risk pregnancy [82].

Haematological and hepatic problems

Most resolve spontaneously without treatment. Symptomatic anaemia and thrombocytopenia may require blood and platelet transfusion, respectively.

Pregnancy

A pregnant patient who is known to have Ro/SS-A or La/SS-B antibodies and her obstetrician should be counselled of the possible problems. The risk of NLE in a Ro/SS-A-positive mother without connective tissue disease or a previous history of NLE is probably low, perhaps about 2%. The risk may or may not be higher for symptomatic Ro/SS-A-positive mothers, but for women who have already had a baby with NLE, the estimated risk of having another affected child ranges widely between studies, but is probably about 25% [87]. Prenatal screening for anti-Ro/SSA and anti-La/SSB antibodies should be undertaken in individuals who are more likely to have these antibodies based upon pre-existing connective tissue diseases. Monitoring of fetal cardiac function in this circumstance is standard practice [39]. It is a safe and non-invasive assessment of heart structure, extranodal disease and conduction abnormalities. Currently, the treatment of first-degree heart block with fluorinated steroids is controversial due to the risks of medication side effects, the spontaneous reversion to normal sinus rhythm without treatment, and the lack of evidence suggesting that untreated first-degree block in the fetus leads to more advanced heart block [100–103]. However, fluorinated steroids may be beneficial for second-degree heart blocks identified *in utero*, as it may decrease inflammation and/or prevent progression to CHB, which is not reversible [101,103]. Weekly screening with pulsed-Doppler fetal echocardiography can be initiated at a 16-week gestational age, and the frequency decreased after 26-week gestational age in the absence of abnormalities, given that less than 20% of CHB cases are detected later on in pregnancy [104]. Observation is a reasonable approach during the first month of life as 2% of reported cases of CHB are diagnosed postnatally [65,103]. Ro/SS-A and La/SS-B antibodies in human breast milk had no pathological consequences [105].

Antiphospholipid antibody syndrome

Definition and nomenclature

The antiphospholipid antibody syndrome (APLS) is an autoimmune disease with clinical features of thrombosis (venous, arterial and microvascular) and pregnancy complications, which include recurrent fetal loss, preterm delivery and placental insufficiency [1]. The condition is associated with a spectrum of autoantibodies directed against the cellular phospholipid component (hence the term 'antiphospholipid antibodies' or APAs); most commonly lupus anticoagulant, anticardiolipin and anti-β_2-glycoprotein I (anti-B2GPI).

Synonyms and inclusions

- APS
- Hughes syndrome
- Familial lupus anticoagulant syndrome

Introduction and general description

Antiphospholipid syndrome was first described by Graham Hughes in 1983, regarding a group of patients with SLE who had lupus anticoagulant and clinical signs of recurrent thrombosis [2]. Thereafter, patients without features of SLE were noted to develop APAs and thus the concept emerged that APLS could exist as a primary syndrome [3,4]. APLS is diagnosed in a patient with thrombosis and/or defined pregnancy morbidity in the presence of persistent APA. The term 'primary APLS' is used when the condition occurs in the absence of any other related disease. The term 'secondary APLS' is used when the condition occurs in the context of other autoimmune diseases, such as SLE.

The most recent criteria for the classification of APLS were developed in 2006. Although classification criteria should not be used for diagnostic purposes, they can serve to guide clinicians in establishing a diagnosis or documenting essential features. According to the revised international APLS classification criteria, a patient is classified as having true APLS when at least one of the two clinical criteria and one of the three laboratory criteria are present. Clinical criteria include the presence of vascular thrombosis or obstetric complications as described later. Laboratory criteria include the presence of anticardiolipin antibodies, anti-B2GPI antibodies and/or lupus anticoagulant on two or more occasions at least 12 weeks apart [5]. However, the classification criteria exclude other clinical, immunological and haematological domains relevant to APLS [6]. An international effort is underway to establish more comprehensive classification criteria to include other clinical manifestations as well as stratification based on both the associated risk factors and APA profile [7].

Epidemiology
Incidence and prevalence
The true prevalence of the syndrome is unclear [8]. In the general population, APA can be detected in about one in five patients who have had a stroke at less than 50 years of age [9]. Approximately half of the patients with APA will develop SLE or another autoimmune disease [10]. Conversely, about 40% of patients with SLE have APA [11]; 26% have lupus anticoagulant, 47% anticardiolipin and 28% anti-B2GPI [12]. In SLE, the lupus anticoagulant is more prevalent in men (40% versus 24.5%) and in white populations compared with African Americans (28% versus 23%) [12,13]. In patients with SLE and lupus anticoagulant, around 40% will eventually develop venous thromboembolism [14]. Approximately one in four patients with a venous thromboembolism, tested for thrombophilia, exhibit APA [15]. Approximately 1 in 10 women with recurrent miscarriage are diagnosed with APLS [16].

Age
The disease is commonest in young to middle-aged adults; however, it also manifests in children and elderly people.

Sex
As with many autoimmune diseases, APLS is more common in women than in men [17]. The apparent female preponderance may be related to the issue that recurrent pregnancy loss is a prominent feature of the disease and that early reported series of patients with APLS were often confined to those with SLE.

Ethnicity
A number of populations have been reported with APLS including white people, Hispanics, Asians, Afro-Caribbeans and native Americans [18].

Associated diseases
Secondary APLS is associated with SLE and other autoimmune diseases such as rheumatoid arthritis, Sjögren syndrome and systemic sclerosis. The development of APAs can occur with syphilis and hepatitis C. Approximately half of the patients with APLS and thrombosis have additional risk factors for thrombosis at the

time of the event, including genetic prothrombotic phenotypes, prolonged immobilisation, surgery, use of oral contraceptives or hormone replacement therapy, pregnancy, nephrotic syndrome, ongoing chronic inflammation and cardiovascular risk factors such as smoking, obesity or diabetes [19].

Approximately 40–80% of patients with Sneddon syndrome have the presence of APAs [20,21]. Some consider Sneddon syndrome to be on a spectrum of APLS. It occurs most commonly in women (80%) with a median age of diagnosis at 40 years. Sneddon syndrome can be inherited in an autosomal dominant fashion with variable penetrance in rare familial cases. Autosomal recessive loss-of-function mutations have recently been identified in a mutation of the cat eye syndrome region, candidate 1 (CERC1), encoding adenosine deaminase 2 [22]. Cutaneous manifestations of Sneddon syndrome include livedo racemose/reticularis, acrocyanosis and Raynaud phenomenon. Neurological manifestations occur in three phases including prodromal symptoms of headache, vertigo and light-headedness in the first phase, followed by recurrent episodes of transient ischaemic attacks and strokes in the second phase and completed by cognitive decline and early-onset dementia in the third phase [23].

Pathophysiology

Lupus anticoagulant is a heterogenous group of autoantibodies, predominantly IgM and IgG but including anticardiolipin and anti-B2GPI antibodies, that target the phospholipid–protein component of the cell membrane. It is a misnomer in that only a minority of patients with lupus anticoagulant are diagnosed with lupus and the 'anticoagulant' demonstrates anticoagulant activity only *in vitro*. Of the three antibody tests, the presence of lupus anticoagulant has the strongest association with thrombosis and pregnancy loss [24]. The positivity of all three tests (lupus anticoagulant, anticardiolipin and anti-B2GPI) – also referred to as 'triple positive' APLS – confers the greatest thrombotic risk [25].

Many mechanisms for thrombosis in APLS have been suggested. The key target of APA is B2GPI, a plasma protein that binds to phospholipid surfaces, particularly when bound and dimerised by anti-B2GPI antibodies. B2GPI (apolipoprotein H) is a cofactor required for APA to bind to cardiolipin [26]. An increase in the risk of thrombosis has not been associated with congenital deficiency in B2GP1. However, the binding of APA to B2GPI on cellular surfaces stimulates endothelial cells, monocytes and platelets resulting in pro-inflammatory and prothrombotic phenotypes such as upregulation of E-selectin and tissue factor [19,27]. Additionally, APA binding to B2GPI downregulates the activity of the tissue factor inhibitor [27], activates complement [28,29], interferes in the protein C anticoagulant pathway [30,31] and inhibits fibrinolysis and annexin V binding to phospholipids [32]. Recent studies suggest that the involvement of neutrophil activation and the release of neutrophil extracellular traps and IL-8 [33–35], as well as the upregulation of mammalian target of rapamycin (mTOR) complex on endothelial cells, contribute to endothelial proliferation and APA-related vasculopathy [36–38]. The mTOR activation also increases expression of tissue factor, TLR-4 and IL-8 [39,40] and leads to B-cell proliferation and T-cell differentiation and activation [41–43].

Genetics

Hudson *et al.* found a possible linkage between the HLA-DRB1*14 allele on chromosome 6p21.3 and familial primary APLS [44]. Ever since, a myriad of DR and DQ alleles have been reported but their association with APLS is difficult to ascertain due to studies with small sample sizes and low statistical power, complexity of the HLA region and differences among ethnicities [45]. In studies of genetic susceptibility outside of non-HLA genes, a meta-analysis showed that the B2GPI Val/Leu(247) polymorphism was associated with susceptibility to APLS and thrombosis and with anti-B2GPI positivity (odds ratio 1.514; 95% confidence interval 1.017–1.253; $P = 0.041$) [46]. Additionally, the genes encoding signal transducer and activator of transcription 4 (STAT4) and B lymphocyte kinase (BLK) are considered common genetic factors for autoimmune diseases such as lupus [47–49], and genetic polymorphisms in both STAT4 and BLK have been associated with primary APLS [50,51].

Clinical features

History

Patients have one or more clinical episodes of arterial, venous or small-vessel thrombosis. Venous thrombosis in APLS is most commonly lower limb deep-vein thrombosis or pulmonary embolism but any part of the venous system may be involved, including superficial, portal, renal, mesenteric and intracranial veins [1]. The most frequent site of arterial thrombosis in APLS is in the cerebral vasculature, resulting in transient cerebral ischaemia/stroke. Myocardial infarction is less common, although subclinical myocardial ischaemia may be underrecognised [52]. In a small number of patients, thrombosis occurs in microvessels of the skin, lungs, kidneys, eyes, heart and other organs. Pregnancy morbidity [1] consists of:

1 One or more unexplained deaths of a normal fetus after the 10th week of gestation.
2 One or more preterm births of a normal fetus before the 34th week of gestation because of (i) eclampsia; or (ii) recognised features of placental insufficiency.
3 Three or more unexplained consecutive spontaneous miscarriages before the 10th week of gestation (with maternal anatomical and parental chromosomal causes excluded).

Presentation in the skin

Cutaneous lesions include thrombophlebitis, purpura and ecchymoses, livedo reticularis/racemosa, livedoid vasculopathy, cutaneous necrosis, gangrene, atrophie blanche, subungual splinter haemorrhages, anetoderma and purpura fulminans as seen in CAPS. Histologically, non-inflammatory thrombosis of small dermal blood vessels can be demonstrated, but necrotising vasculitis is usually not a feature.

Differential diagnosis

Other prothrombotic thrombophilias should be considered. Conditions presenting with thrombocytopenia and thrombosis include heparin-induced thrombocytopenia, thrombotic thrombocytopenic purpura and disseminated intravascular coagulation.

Complications and co-morbidities

In addition to thrombosis and pregnancy morbidity, thrombocytopenia, occult heart valve disease, chorea, cognitive impairment, avascular necrosis, haemolytic anaemia and nephropathy are potential complications of APLS. Transverse myelopathy occurs in SLE and may be more frequent in those with APLS [53]. Of patients with APLS 1% develop CAPS, which is defined as microvascular thrombosis in three or more organs developing within 7 days in a patient with persistently elevated APAs. CAPS confers a high risk of mortality (37%). Organ involvement includes renal dysfunction with hypertension (70%), pulmonary thromboembolism and pulmonary hypertension (70%), cutaneous manifestations including livedo, necrosis, digital gangrene or purpura fulminans (66%), cerebral manifestations including infarcts, seizures, encephalopathy or venous occlusions (60%) and cardiac (53%). Approximately half of the patients with CAPS have an identifying trigger: infection being the most common, followed by trauma, surgery and anticoagulant withdrawal. Co-morbidity with SLE is a poor prognostic factor [54].

Disease course and prognosis

The long-term prognosis of APLS is largely dictated by the risk and effects of recurrent thrombosis and any underlying autoimmune condition in those with secondary APLS. Those with primary APLS have a poor prognosis, with one-third having organ damage and one-fifth unable to perform everyday activities [55]. APLS may contribute to an increased frequency of strokes especially in younger individuals [56]. Strokes may develop secondary to *in situ* thrombosis or embolisation that originates from the valvular lesions of Libman–Sacks (sterile) endocarditis, which may be seen in patients with APLS. Valvular heart disease may be severe enough to require valve replacement. Recurrent pulmonary emboli or thrombosis can lead to life-threatening pulmonary hypertension.

Investigations

When testing for APLS is indicated, testing for lupus anticoagulant and for IgG and/or IgM antibodies to cardiolipin and/or B2GPI (via ELISA assays) should be performed. With regard to antibody testing, titres above 40 units (or above the 99th percentile) are deemed significant positives [1]. Initial positive tests should be repeated to check for persistence at least 12 weeks later. This is to prevent patients with transient positive tests (due to infection, etc.) being diagnosed as having APLS. Testing for IgA antibodies is not recommended [1].

Functional detection of lupus anticoagulant activity requires a multistep procedure of screening, mixing and confirmation steps. The initial step or the 'screening' test involves using a control or limiting phospholipid-containing reagent to measure the time for a plasma sample to clot. When clotting times are prolonged beyond the upper limit of reference with the screening reagent, a 'confirmatory' test is then performed where an excess phospholipid is added to shorten or correct the prolonged coagulation test. Lupus anticoagulant may be present when clotting times are prolonged with the screening reagent and corrected with the excess phospholipid reagent. Thereafter a mixing study is performed where the patient's plasma is mixed with an equal volume of normal plasma. If the clotting time continues to be prolonged then the possibility of a coagulation factor deficiency is eliminated and the presence of an inhibitor is assumed [57]. The activated partial thromboplastin time (aPTT), dilute Russell's viper venom time (dRVVT), kaolin clotting time (KCT), dilute thromboplastin time (dTT) or prothrombin time (using a lupus-sensitive thromboplastin) are the principal functional tests used for the detection of lupus anticoagulant. Lupus anticoagulants are caused by a heterogeneous group of antibodies, thus a combination of two phospholipid-dependent clotting assays is needed as no single test has sufficient sensitivity and specificity [57]. Patients who are on an anticoagulant can have a prolonged aPTT on that basis, making the interpretation of the aPTT or other lupus anticoagulant screening tests difficult.

Other laboratory abnormalities in APLS may include otherwise unexplained thrombocytopenia, anaemia, schistocytes on a peripheral blood smear, or a history of a false positive serological test for syphilis. The presence of an APA in the absence of a thrombotic event or an obstetric complication is not sufficient to make the diagnosis of APLS. APA can be detected in association with infections (e.g. syphilis, Lyme disease, tuberculosis, leprosy, hepatitis A, B and C, HIV, cytomegalovirus, Epstein–Barr virus, SARS-CoV-2 and malaria) [58,59], malignancies (solid and hematological cancers) [60,61] and concurrent intake of medications (e.g. phenytoin, hydralazine, amoxicillin and propranolol) [62].

The type of APA, the presence of a single compared with multiple (double or triple) APA types, their titre and the persistence of APA positivity with repeated measurements define the APA profile. The APA profile allows for evaluation of thrombotic risks and obstetric complications and consequently the intensity of treatment as outlined here [63].

Management

The treatment approach to APLS can be categorised into risk factor modification, primary thromboprophylaxis, secondary thromboprophylaxis, treatment of CAPS, pregnancy prophylaxis and treatment of non-criteria manifestations.

Patients with APA positivity should be encouraged to lead a healthy lifestyle with moderate physical activity. Modifiable risk factors such as hypertension, hyperlipidaemia, diabetes and smoking should be managed, and exogenous oestrogen avoided. The 2019 EULAR recommendations for the pharmacological management of APLS in adults suggest initially identifying major risk factors for thrombotic and obstetric events. Major risk factors include a high-risk APA profile defined as the presence of lupus anticoagulant, the presence of double or triple APA positivity, the presence of a persistently high APA titre, coexistence of other systemic autoimmune diseases such as SLE, a history of thrombotic and/or obstetric APLS and the presence of cardiovascular risk factors [63]. For primary thromboprophylaxis, low-dose aspirin (75–100 mg daily) is recommended in asymptomatic APA carriers, patients with SLE without prior thrombotic or obstetric events and in non-pregnant patients with a history of obstetric complications, all with high-risk APA profiles [63]. Although more robust data are needed, there may be a role for vitamin D supplementation and statins for primary prophylaxis [64]. In APA-positive patients with SLE, hydroxychloroquine may have a protective effect against thrombosis and is thus recommended to be taken concurrently with low-dose aspirin [63,64]. Rituximab may be promising for preventing thromboses in APA-positive patients with SLE refractory to conventional anticoagulant treatment [65].

For secondary thromboprophylaxis, long-term warfarin treatment with a target international normalised ratio (INR) of 2–3 is recommended in patients with APA and a first unprovoked venous thrombosis. In patients with arterial thrombosis, warfarin treatment to a target INR of 2–3 or up to 3–4 can be considered after factoring the patient's thrombosis and bleeding risk. If arterial or venous thrombosis recurs despite warfarin therapy, the INR target can be increased to 3–4, and the addition of low-dose aspirin or change to LMWH can be considered. In general, the use of direct oral anticoagulants is discouraged, in particular in patients with triple positive APA and/or arterial thrombosis due to the high risk of recurrent thrombosis [63]. Sirolimus, an mTOR inhibitor, may be an emerging therapy for APLS, as it has been shown to reduce active vasculopathy [36,66].

Skin changes associated with APLS, including livedoid vasculopathy and cutaneous ulcers, have been reported to be refractory to glucocorticoids; low-dose aspirin, clopidogrel, sildenafil, IVIg, hyperbaric oxygen therapy or a combination of these interventions can be tried. Rituximab or belimumab can be considered in refractory cases [65,67–70].

For pregnant women with APLS and a history of recurrent fetal loss, close liaison with an obstetrician and haematologist is advised. Antenatal administration of heparin combined with low-dose aspirin throughout the pregnancy may be advisable – warfarin is avoided because of teratogenicity. In general, treatment is often begun as soon as pregnancy is confirmed.

Treatment of CAPS includes early diagnosis, as well as management or minimising of any underlying precipitating factors (infections, malignancies, surgical procedures or anticoagulation discontinuation). Patients should receive appropriate multidisciplinary care in the intensive care unit and this may necessitate the use of external ventilation support, inotropes or haemodialysis. Triple therapy, which includes intravenous heparin, high-dose glucocorticoids and IVIg and/or plasmapheresis, is recommended. Rituximab or complement inhibition via eculizumab can be tried for refractory CAPS [71].

Treatment ladder for antiphospholipid antibody syndrome

First line

Primary prophylaxis
- Low-dose aspirin (75–100 mg daily) in asymptomatic carriers and non-pregnant patients with prior history of obstetric complications

Secondary prophylaxis
- Anticoagulation (heparin/warfarin) in the non-pregnant patient
- Heparin and low-dose aspirin to be considered in the pregnant patient

Second line

- Oral direct thrombin and antifactor Xa inhibitors (e.g. rivaroxaban, apixaban) only in venous thrombotic events

with single or double positive APA and contraindication to warfarin
- Combination antiaggregant therapy (low-dose aspirin plus clopidogrel or dipyridamole)
- Low-dose aspirin combined with hydroxychloroquine in those with SLE

Third line

- Immunomodulatory therapies: plasmapheresis, intravenous human IgG and rituximab
- In refractory cases, plasmapheresis

Acknowledgements

We thank Professor Mark Goodfield and Dr Collette McCourt, who prepared the chapter for the previous edition.

Key references

The full list of references can be found in the online version at https://www.wiley.com/rooksdermatology10e

Introduction

1 Barber MRW, Drenkard C, Falasinnu T *et al*. Global epidemiology of systemic lupus erythematosus. *Nat Rev Rheumatol* 2021;17:515–32.
2 Ribero S, Sciascia S, Borradori L, Lipsker D. The cutaneous spectrum of lupus erythematosus. *Clin Rev Allergy Immunol* 2017;53:291–305.
3 Patel J, Borucki R, Werth VP. An update on the pathogenesis of cutaneous lupus erythematosus and its role in clinical practice. *Curr Rheumatol Rep* 2020;22:69.

Discoid lupus erythematosus

2 Gronhagen CM, Fored CM, Granath F, Nyberg F. Cutaneous lupus erythematosus and the association with systemic lupus erythematosus: a population-based cohort of 1088 patients in Sweden. *Br J Dermatol* 2011;164:1335–41.
5 Durosaro O, Davis MD, Reed KB, Rohlinger AL. Incidence of cutaneous lupus erythematosus, 1965–2005: a population-based study. *Arch Dermatol* 2009;145:249–53.
8 Joseph AK, Windsor B, Hynan LS, Chong BF. Discoid lupus erythematosus skin lesion distribution and characteristics in Black patients: a retrospective cohort study. *Lupus Sci Med* 2021;8:e000514.
13 Garelli CJ, Refat MA, Nanaware PP, Ramirez-Ortiz ZG, Rachighi M, Richmond JM. Current insights in cutaneous lupus erythematosus immunopathogenesis. *Front Immunol* 2020;11:1353.
14 Kuhn A, Wenzel J, Weyd H. Photosensitivity, apoptosis, and cytokines in the pathogenesis of lupus erythematosus: a critical review. *Clin Rev Allergy Immunol* 2014;47:148–62.
18 Wenzel J, Worenkamper E, Freutel S *et al*. Enhanced type I interferon signalling promotes Th1-biased inflammation in cutaneous lupus erythematosus. *J Pathol* 2005;205:435–42.
83 Chen HW, Barber G, Chong BF. The genetic landscape of cutaneous lupus erythematosus. *Front Med (Lausanne)* 2022;9:916011.
96 Rangel LK, Villa-Ruiz C, Lo K *et al*. Clinical characteristics of lupus erythematosus panniculitis/profundus: a retrospective review of 61 patients. *JAMA Dermatol* 2020;156:1264–6.
115 Okon LG, Werth VP. Cutaneous lupus erythematosus: diagnosis and treatment. *Best Pract Res Clin Rheumatol* 2013;27:391–404.
117 Rodriguez-Caruncho C, Bielsa I, Fernandez-Figueras MT, Roca J, Carrascosa JM, Ferrandiz C. Lupus erythematosus tumidus: a clinical and histological study of 25 cases. *Lupus* 2015;24:751–5.

130 Klein R, Moghadam-Kia S, LoMonico J et al. Development of the CLASI as a tool to measure disease severity and responsiveness to therapy in cutaneous lupus erythematosus. *Arch Dermatol* 2011;147:203–8.

132 Guo LN, Perez-Chada LM, Borucki R, Nambudiri VE, Werth VP, Merola JF. Development of a working core outcome set for cutaneous lupus erythematosus: a practical approach to an urgent unmet need. *Lupus Sci Med* 2021;8:e000529.

133 Worm M, Zidane M, Eisert L et al. S2k guideline: diagnosis and management of cutaneous lupus erythematosus – part 2: therapy, risk factors and other special topics. *J Dtsch Dermatol Ges* 2021;19:1371–95.

134 O'Kane D, McCourt C, Meggitt S et al. British Association of Dermatologists guidelines for the management of people with cutaneous lupus erythematosus 2021. *Br J Dermatol* 2021;185:1112–23.

135 Lu Q, Long H, Chow S et al. Guideline for the diagnosis, treatment and long-term management of cutaneous lupus erythematosus. *J Autoimmun* 2021;123:102707.

140 Marmor MF, Kellner U, Lai TY, Melles RB, Mieler WF, American Academy of Ophthalmology. Recommendations on screening for chloroquine and hydroxychloroquine retinopathy (2016 revision). *Ophthalmology* 2016;123:1386–94.

141 Fanouriakis A, Kostopoulou M, Alunno A et al. 2019 update of the EULAR recommendations for the management of systemic lupus erythematosus. *Ann Rheum Dis* 2019;78:736–45.

145 Rosenbaum JT, Costenbader KH, Desmarais J et al. American College of Rheumatology, American Academy of Dermatology, Rheumatologic Dermatology Society, and American Academy of Ophthalmology 2020 joint statement on hydroxychloroquine use with respect to retinal toxicity. *Arthritis Rheumatol* 2021;73:908–11.

Subacute cutaneous lupus erythematosus

42 Lowe GC, Henderson CL, Grau RH, Hansen CB, Sontheimer RD. A systematic review of drug-induced subacute cutaneous lupus erythematosus. *Br J Dermatol* 2011;164:465–72.

44 Guicciardi F, Atzori L, Marzano AV et al. Are there distinct clinical and pathological features distinguishing idiopathic from drug-induced subacute cutaneous lupus erythematosus? A European retrospective multicenter study. *J Am Acad Dermatol* 2019;81:403–11.

51 Sarkar MK, Hile GA, Tsoi LC et al. Photosensitivity and type I IFN responses in cutaneous lupus are driven by epidermal-derived interferon kappa. *Ann Rheum Dis* 2018;77:1653–64.

55 Sontheimer RD. Subacute cutaneous lupus erythematosus: 25-year evolution of a prototypic subset (subphenotype) of lupus erythematosus defined by characteristic cutaneous, pathological, immunological, and genetic findings. *Autoimmun Rev* 2005;4:253–63.

Systemic lupus erythematosus

4 Aringer M, Costenbader K, Daikh D et al. 2019 European League Against Rheumatism/American College of Rheumatology classification criteria for systemic lupus erythematosus. *Arthritis Rheumatol* 2019;71:1400–12.

26 Billi AC, Ma F, Plazyo O et al. Nonlesional lupus skin contributes to inflammatory education of myeloid cells and primes for cutaneous inflammation. *Sci Transl Med* 2022;14:eabn2263.

27 Wenzel J. Cutaneous lupus erythematosus: new insights into pathogenesis and therapeutic strategies. *Nat Rev Rheumatol* 2019;15:519–32.

43 Deng Y, Tsao BP. Updates in lupus genetics. *Curr Rheumatol Rep* 2017;19:68.

57 Tsokos GC. Systemic lupus erythematosus. *N Engl J Med* 2011;365:2110–21.

314 Fanouriakis A, Kostopoulou M, Alunno A et al. 2019 update of the EULAR recommendations for the management of systemic lupus erythematosus. *Ann Rheum Dis* 2019;78:736–45.

Neonatal lupus erythematosus

1 Inzinger M, Salmhofer W, Binder B. Neonatal lupus erythematosus and its clinical variability. *J Dtsch Dermatol Ges* 2012;10:407–11.

6 Izmirly PM, Llanos C, Lee LA, Askanase A, Kim MY, Buyon JP. Cutaneous manifestations of neonatal lupus and risk of subsequent congenital heart block. *Arthritis Rheum* 2010;62:1153–7.

30 Lee LA, Gaither KK, Coulter SN, Norris DA, Harley JB. Pattern of cutaneous immunoglobulin G deposition in subacute cutaneous lupus erythematosus is reproduced by infusing purified anti-Ro (SSA) autoantibodies into human skin-grafted mice. *J Clin Invest* 1989;83:1556–62.

32 Izmirly P, Saxena A, Buyon JP. Progress in the pathogenesis and treatment of cardiac manifestations of neonatal lupus. *Curr Opin Rheumatol* 2017;29:467–72.

46 Weston WL, Morelli JG, Lee LA. The clinical spectrum of anti-Ro-positive cutaneous neonatal lupus erythematosus. *J Am Acad Dermatol* 1999;40:675–81.

86 Martin V, Lee LA, Askanase AD, Katholi M, Buyon JP. Long-term followup of children with neonatal lupus and their unaffected siblings. *Arthritis Rheum* 2002;46:2377–83.

93 Izmirly P, Kim M, Friedman DM et al. Hydroxychloroquine to prevent recurrent congenital heart block in fetuses of anti-SSA/Ro-positive mothers. *J Am Coll Cardiol* 2020;76:292–302.

99 Buyon JP, Clancy RM, Friedman DM. Cardiac manifestations of neonatal lupus erythematosus: guidelines to management, integrating clues from the bench and bedside. *Nat Clin Pract Rheumatol* 2009;5:139–48.

104 Donofrio MT, Moon-Grady AJ, Hornberger LK et al. Diagnosis and treatment of fetal cardiac disease: a scientific statement from the American Heart Association. *Circulation* 2014;129:2183–242.

Antiphospholipid antibody syndrome

1 Ruiz-Irastorza G, Crowther M, Branch W, Khamashta MA. Antiphospholipid syndrome. *Lancet* 2010;376:1498–509.

2 Hughes GR. Thrombosis, abortion, cerebral disease, and the lupus anticoagulant. *Br Med J (Clin Res Ed)* 1983;287:1088–9.

8 Biggioggero M, Meroni PL. The geoepidemiology of the antiphospholipid antibody syndrome. *Autoimmun Rev* 2010;9:A299–304.

22 Zhou Q, Yang D, Ombrello AK et al. Early-onset stroke and vasculopathy associated with mutations in ADA2. *N Engl J Med* 2014;370:911–20.

27 Garcia D, Erkan D. Diagnosis and management of the antiphospholipid syndrome. *N Engl J Med* 2018;378:2010–21.

30 Atsumi T, Khamashta MA, Amengual O et al. Binding of anticardiolipin antibodies to protein C via beta2-glycoprotein I (beta2-GPI): a possible mechanism in the inhibitory effect of antiphospholipid antibodies on the protein C system. *Clin Exp Immunol* 1998;112:325–33.

46 Lee YH, Choi SJ, Ji JD, Song GG. Association between the valine/leucine247 polymorphism of beta2-glycoprotein I and susceptibility to anti-phospholipid syndrome: a meta-analysis. *Lupus* 2012;21:865–71.

55 Erkan D, Yazici Y, Sobel R, Lockshin MD. Primary antiphospholipid syndrome: functional outcome after 10 years. *J Rheumatol* 2000;27:2817–21.

56 Sciascia S, Sanna G, Khamashta MA et al. The estimated frequency of antiphospholipid antibodies in young adults with cerebrovascular events: a systematic review. *Ann Rheum Dis* 2015;74:2028–33.

63 Tektonidou MG, Andreoli L, Limper M et al. EULAR recommendations for the management of antiphospholipid syndrome in adults. *Ann Rheum Dis* 2019;78:1296–304.

CHAPTER 52

Dermatomyositis

Patrick Gordon[1] and Daniel Creamer[2]

[1]Department of Rheumatology, King's College Hospital, London, UK
[2]Department of Dermatology, King's College Hospital, London, UK

Dermatomyositis

Definition

Dermatomyositis (DM) is an autoimmune disorder affecting, predominantly, the skin and skeletal muscle. It is classified alongside polymyositis in the idiopathic inflammatory myopathies (IIMs).

The Bohan and Peter classification for dermatomyositis and polymyositis has been in use since 1975 (Table 52.1) [1]. While these classification criteria remain the most cited they do not acknowledge amyopathic DM and fail to distinguish polymyositis from inclusion body myositis. Therefore, the Griggs criteria for inclusion body myositis should be used in addition when this diagnosis is suspected. The Bohan and Peter criteria also perform poorly at discriminating polymyositis from some of its imitators.

In view of the limitations of the Bohan and Peter classification, a new set of criteria encompassing amyopathic DM and inclusion body myositis have been developed, the 2017 European League Against Rheumatism/American College of Rheumatology classification criteria for adult and juvenile idiopathic inflammatory myopathies and their major subgroups [2].

Sontheimer defines amyopathic DM as 'a subset of DM characterized by biopsy-confirmed hallmark cutaneous manifestations of classic DM occurring for 6 months or longer with no clinical evidence of proximal muscle weakness and no serum muscle enzyme abnormalities' [3]. If more extensive muscle testing is carried out, the results should be within normal limits; however, if these investigations are positive or abnormal, the patient can be classified as having hypomyopathic DM. Exclusion criteria for amyopathic DM are (i) treatment with systemic immunosuppressive therapy for two consecutive months or longer within the first 6 months after skin disease onset; and (ii) the use of drugs known to be capable of producing DM-like skin changes (e.g. hydroxyurea) [3]. Clinically amyopathic dermatomyositis (CADM) is a functional designation used to refer to either amyopathic DM or hypomyopathic DM [3].

Introduction and general description

In DM, autoimmune inflammation damages the skin, muscle and, in certain cases, internal organs such as the lungs, joints, oro-pharynx

Table 52.1 The Bohan and Peter classification for polymyositis and dermatomyositis.

Features	Polymyositis	Dermatomyositis
1 Symmetrical proximal muscle weakness	Definite: all of features 1–4	Definite: feature 5 plus any three of 1–4
2 Muscle biopsy evidence of myositis	Probable: any three of features 1–4	Probable: feature 5 plus any two of 1–4
3 Elevation in serum skeletal muscle enzymes	Possible: any two of features 1–4	Possible: feature 5 plus any one of 1–4
4 Characteristic electromyography pattern of myositis		
5 Typical rash of dermatomyositis		

Adapted from Bohan and Peter 1975 [1].

and heart. At one end of the spectrum myopathy predominates, at the other end skin disease is prominent with minimal or absent myositis (amyopathic DM). Interstitial lung disease (ILD) may affect a patient with DM, irrespective of their muscle–skin phenotype. Myositis-specific antibodies can help predict phenotype and internal organ involvement although their availability remains limited.

Mortality is increased in DM; modern IIM series indicate a 10-year survival of up to 90%, with slightly higher mortality in DM than polymyositis [4,5]. Although there is great variability in the precise figures between studies, the main causes of death in IIM are cardiac disease (15–64% of deaths), respiratory disease (5–36% of deaths) and malignancy (10–47% of deaths) [6].

Epidemiology

Incidence and prevalence

The IIMs are rare, with a reported annual incidence varying widely from 0.1 to 6.7 per 100 000 person-years [7,8,9,10]. The highest estimates come from recent epidemiological studies from large administrative claims databases and the lower estimates from studies based on hospital admission data confirmed by chart review.

The prevalence of IIM is in the region of 5.1–22 per 100 000 [7,8,11]. The relative proportion of DM within IIM appears to enlarge with increasing southerly latitude in Europe [12]. Similarly, there was an association between regional ultraviolet (UV) radiation exposure and the proportion of female IIM patients with DM and Mi-2 antibodies in a study in the USA [13]. As such, it would appear that UV radiation may have an influence on the presentation and phenotype of DM.

Age

The peak incidence of DM occurs around 50–60 years of age [14,15]. DM occurs in children although it is much rarer in this age group, with an incidence of around two cases per million children under 16 years old per year, with a median age of onset of 6.8 years [16].

Sex

The incidence of adult DM is approximately twice as high in women [8,9], with some studies suggesting an even greater female predominance in child-bearing years. Although the overall incidence of juvenile DM is much lower than for adults, the female preponderance in children is greater at 5 : 1 [16].

Ethnicity

As with systemic lupus erythematosus, the incidence of DM is greater in African Americans than in white Americans [7].

Associated diseases

There is a strong association between internal malignancy and adult DM. In a large Scandinavian population-based study, 32% of adult DM patients had an associated malignancy, with a standard incident ratio of 3 compared with the general population. However, the reported frequency in the literature varies between 7% and 60% [17,18–20]. Unlike adult DM, juvenile DM is not thought to be associated with an increased risk of malignancy, even though one study did suggest a possible association [21].

The risk of malignancy rises with increasing age, severe skin disease with necrosis, dysphagia, diaphragmatic weakness, lack of extramuscular systemic features (e.g. ILD) and antibodies to antitranscription intermediary factor 1γ (anti-TIF-1γ) or nuclear matrix protein 2 (NXP-2) [22–25].

Neoplasms may be identified in patients before, at or after the onset of DM. In one study, 58% of the malignancies presented after the diagnosis of DM [17]. The risk of cancer is greatest in the first few years after the diagnosis of DM, but there remains an increased, albeit lower, risk more than 5 years after diagnosis [21].

Tumours of many types have been associated with DM although the majority are adenocarcinomas [17]. In a Scandinavian population-based study, carcinomas of the breast and ovary were the commonest malignancies in women, while lung cancer was the leading malignancy both overall and in men [17]. However, in two studies set in the Far East (one in Singapore and the other in Taiwan), naso-pharangeal carcinoma was the commonest myositis-associated malignancy, reflecting the high incidence of naso-pharangeal cancer in this region [18,26].

Pathophysiology

An early histological feature of DM in muscle, which is not found in polymyositis, is the deposition of the membrane attack complex, the terminal complement component C5b-9 within capillaries [27,28]. Human leukocyte antigen (HLA) class I, which is usually absent on the cell membrane of muscle fibres, is diffusely upregulated even in areas apparently unaffected, without inflammatory cell infiltration [29]. Capillary drop-out occurs with a compensatory increase in calibre of the remaining capillaries [28]. In the perifascicular areas muscle fibre atrophy occurs, which has been hypothesised to be a result of hypoxic stress, although models of ischaemic myopathy have not supported this theory [30,31]. The inflammatory infiltrate, which comprises B cells, CD4+ T cells, macrophages and plasmocytoid dendritic cells, is found predominantly in the perivascular and perifascicular areas [32].

These features suggest a humorally mediated microvasculopathy in DM, in contrast to polymyositis where there is evidence of cell-mediated cytotoxicity with CD8+ T cells invading muscle fibres. Consistent with the notion of humoral activation in DM is the recognition that most patients have disease-associated autoantibodies. These may be myositis-specific antibodies (MSAs), such as anti-Mi-2, TIF-1γ, MDA-5 and SUMO-activating enzyme which are only found in myositis patients, or myositis-associated antibodies (MAAs), such as anti-52kD Ro, U1 RNP, PM-Scl and Ku, which also occur in myositis-overlap syndromes and in other diseases [33].

For two of the MSAs, MDA-5 and anti-Jo-1, antibody titres show some correlation with disease activity suggesting a possible pathogenic role [34,35]. Intriguingly, the N-terminal proteolytic fragment of histidyl tRNA synthetase, the target antigen for anti-Jo-1 antibodies, is chemotactic to lymphocytes and activated monocytes [36].

The autoantigens in inflammatory myositis are not organ-specific but are molecules ubiquitous to all human cells. Nonetheless, at least in some cases, they have been found in increased concentrations in target organs. Increased concentrations of the granzyme B-cleavable conformation of histidyl tRNA synthetase (Jo-1) are found in the lung (ILD), the target of antihistidyl tRNA synthetase (Jo-1) disease [37]. Several myositis autoantigens including Mi-2, Ku and the aminoacyl tRNA synthetases are upregulated in diseased muscle due to increased expression in regenerating fibres [38]. Thus, target antigen expression is increased following muscle damage, potentially creating a positive feedback loop. Notably, Mi-2 expression is increased specifically in DM but not in polymyositis, showing disease specificity [38].

Type I interferon-inducible gene expression is increased in DM in both muscle tissue and in the peripheral blood [32,39]. Both anti-Jo-1 and anti-52kD Ro antibodies when combined with necrotic cell material can induce type I interferon production from peripheral blood mononuclear cells [40]. However, pretreatment of the necrotic cell debris with RNAse prevents type I interferon expression, demonstrating that immune complex formation containing RNA is required [40]. Immune complex internalisation via Fc receptors with subsequent stimulation of Toll-like receptors by the ribonucleic acid component of the immune complexes has been proposed as a potential mechanism for this effect [40]. It is notable that other autoantigens in DM, aside from Jo-1 and Ro, bind directly or via macromolecules to nucleic acids and could potentially cause type I interferon induction by similar mechanisms [41].

Pathology

Skin. Despite striking clinical signs in the skin, the dermatopathology of DM is often subtle. A lichenoid tissue reaction with vacuolar

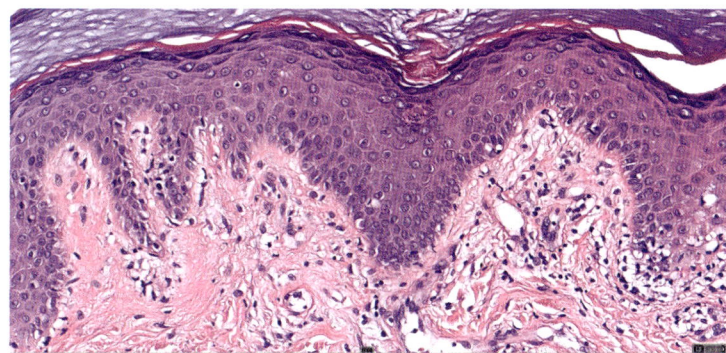

Figure 52.1 Skin histopathology (medium power). There is a mild lichenoid tissue reaction with subtle vacuolar change in the basal layer and occasional Civatte bodies. There is a sparse, superficial, perivascular infiltrate of lymphocytes with upper dermal oedema. Courtesy of Eduardo Calonje.

changes in the basal layer and occasional Civatte bodies is typical (Figure 52.1) [42]. In some cases, there is only a sparse superficial perivascular infiltrate of lymphocytes with upper dermal oedema and mucinous change. The basement membrane may be thickened. In acute DM the changes resemble those of subacute lupus erythematosus, although the dermal oedema may be more extensive and involve all layers of the dermis. In poikilodermatous DM there is epidermal atrophy, dilatation of superficial vessels and melanin incontinence. Hyperkeratosis, acanthosis and mild papillomatosis are seen in a biopsy from a Gottron papule. Unusual skin biopsy findings in DM include subepidermal blistering, dystrophic calcification and lobular panniculitis.

Muscle. Muscle biopsies in DM require specialist staining and should be performed in a specialist neuropathology laboratory experienced in the preparation and reporting of muscle histopathology. Cellular infiltrates containing B cells and CD4+ cells are seen predominantly in the perivascular and perifascicular areas. Muscle fibres show perifascicular atrophy (Figure 52.2a). An early change is C5b-9 deposition on the capillary walls (Figure 52.2b). Capillary drop-out is a common feature and rarely overt muscle infarcts may be seen. Tubuloreticular inclusions are found on electron microscopy within the capillary endothelial cells. HLA class I, which is not usually expressed on muscle fibres, is upregulated and, while myositis is a patchy process, HLA class I upregulation is also found in areas where no inflammatory infiltrates are seen (Figure 52.2c).

Clinical features
History
A dermatosis is the presenting feature in over 50% of DM cases and across the spectrum of clinical presentations skin involvement is a prominent part of the syndrome [43]. Most patients develop a facial rash initially. In some cases this is an acute inflammatory eruption accompanied by oedema; more typically the facial dermatosis begins insidiously and extends over a few weeks. A rash on the hands, extensor surfaces of the limbs and upper torso tends to occur subsequently. In the acute phase, the dermatosis is typically itchy and sore [44]. A proportion of patients give a clear history of photosensitivity [45].

Muscle disease in DM usually becomes clinically apparent in the weeks to months after the onset of skin signs. However, occasionally the dermatosis of DM occurs in isolation, when it is known as amyopathic DM (DM sine myositis). The initial symptoms of myositis are weakness and fatigue. Patients have difficulty in climbing stairs, raising their arms and standing from a sitting position. There may be myalgia but muscle tenderness is relatively rare. If untreated, the weakness will usually progress over a matter of weeks; severe loss of power may result in a patient becoming bed-bound. Respiratory muscle involvement can lead to the development of respiratory failure. Problems with swallowing and aspiration reflect involvement of the pharyngeal and upper oesophageal musculature. Dysphagia occurring early in the disease indicates an aggressive course and is associated with a poor prognosis. Patients should be directly asked whether they have swallowing problems, which may present as a tendency to cough on their food and/or difficulty clearing food from their throats, requiring water and several attempts to swallow a bolus. Other clues for bulbar muscle involvement include recent weight loss, recurrent lower respiratory tract infections and a quiet, nasal voice. As well as involvement of the muscles of ventilation, a proportion of patients develop dyspnoea from interstitial lung disease. It is important to ask about the presence, and extent, of exertional breathlessness and/or cough.

Raynaud phenomenon in DM is particularly associated with the antisynthetase syndrome and mixed connective tissue disease. Joint involvement occurs in approximately one-quarter of cases and presents as generalised arthralgia and morning stiffness.

Presentation
Skin signs. Dermatomyositis is distinguished by a broad spectrum of cutaneous manifestations. Diagnostically, the dermatologist needs to be familiar with the atypical as well as the more common skin signs [43]. Variation in the severity and extent of skin involvement in DM is usual.

Involvement of the face and scalp. The involvement of facial skin is usually a prominent feature of DM. Lilac or violaceous colouring of the skin of the upper eyelids (also termed the 'heliotrope rash') is pathognomonic of DM although this distinctive hue is only appreciable in fair-skinned patients (Figure 52.3). Oedema of the eyelids and periorbital skin also occurs and often reflects activity of the myositis. In most patients extraocular facial skin is affected as well: sometimes the whole face is red, more typically involvement is zonal with certain sites being spared, a variability which may present diagnostic problems. Although usually seen in systemic lupus erythematosus, redness over the bridge of the nose and extending onto the cheeks (butterfly distribution) occurs in some DM patients (Figure 52.4). Involvement of the margins of the face and extending into the scalp is another DM pattern, a configuration which can be mistaken for sebo-psoriasis [46]. There are patients who present with a rosacea-like erythema of the face and those with a photosensitive dermatosis similar to photo-aggravated seborrhoeic dermatitis, drug-induced photosensitivity or chronic actinic dermatitis.

Involvement of the scalp in DM occurs in approximately one-half of DM patients. A lesional scalp is usually intensely itchy, but pain

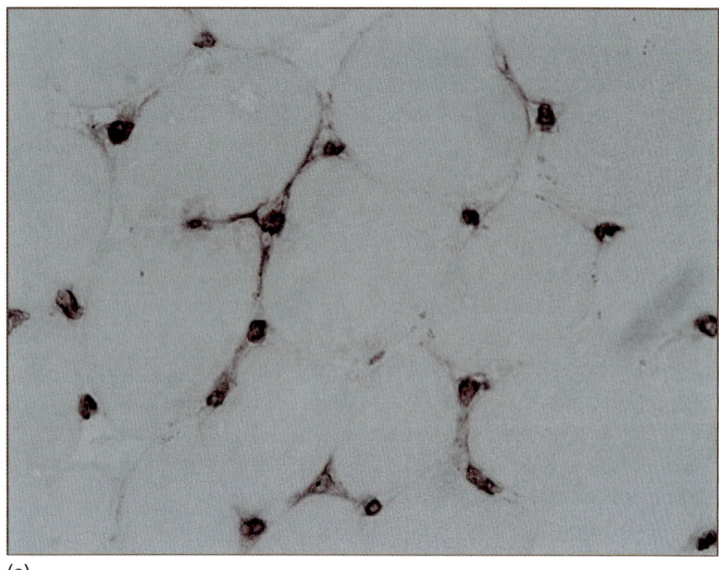

(a)

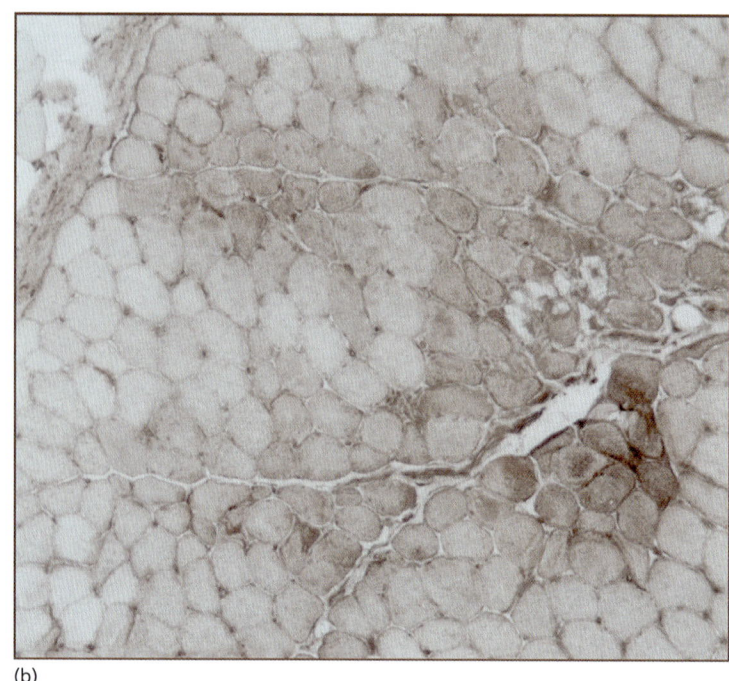

(b)

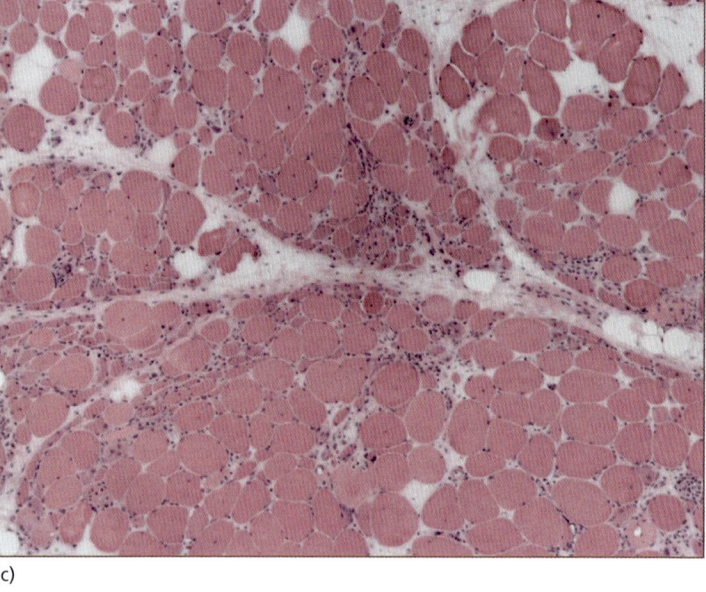

(c)

Figure 52.2 Muscle biopsy. (a) Capillary staining for C5b-9, the membrane attack complex, is an early pathological finding in dermatomyositis. (b) Diffuse upregulation of HLA class I is another early pathological finding in the inflammatory myopathies and can occur in the absence of a cell infiltrate. (c) In dermatomyositis muscle fibre atrophy occurs in a perifascicular distribution. Courtesy of Dr Safa Al-Sarraj, Brain Bank, King's College Hospital, London.

can also be prominent. Symptoms which disturb sleep are not unusual. On examination there is diffuse inflammation of the scalp, most marked at the vertex (Figure 52.5) [47]. Telangiectasis and sclerosis occur in longstanding scalp DM. Milia may accompany severe scalp involvement. Some decreased hair density is usual but this is typically less marked than the alopecia of discoid lupus erythematosus or lichen plano-pilaris.

Involvement of the torso. Almost all DM patients will have redness of the upper torso. Some patients, but not all, are photosensitive in which case the redness of the upper chest has a clear V-shaped demarcation, which in the American literature is known as the 'V-sign'. More often patients have a red patch, which extends in a semicircular distribution over the whole upper anterior chest,

known as the 'bib sign' (Figure 52.6). The 'shawl sign' is a zone of redness which lies across the upper back and commonly extends onto the shoulders (Figure 52.7). When cutaneous DM is active the dermatosis will extend down to the abdomen anteriorly and to the mid/low back posteriorly (Figure 52.8).

In hyperacute DM, blisters or erosions may occur within lesional skin, a presentation which is associated with an aggressive disease phenotype. Flagellate erythema, another sign of acute DM, is characterised by multiple, red, macular streaks occurring on the trunk and proximal limbs. Each flagellate streak is 0.5–1 cm in diameter and may be several centimetres in length. The stripes are aligned diagonally, sometimes in a criss-cross pattern, giving the appearance of a scourging or whipping. A folliculotropic pattern of erythema can be seen in some cases, while hyperkeratotic follicular papules,

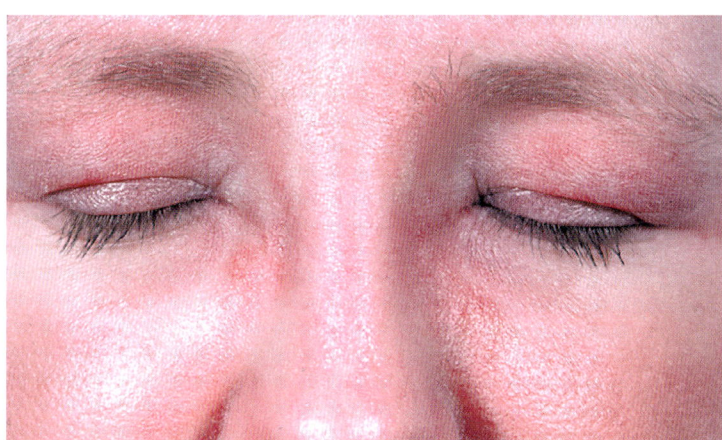

(a)

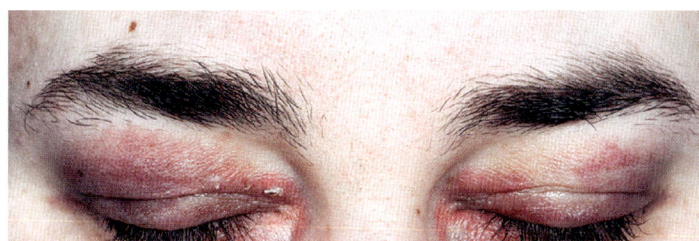

(b)

Figure 52.3 Eyelid involvement in dermatomyositis (DM). (a) There is lilac erythema of the upper eyelids, which are also oedematous. In this patient with DM the facial skin is generally red. (b) Dusky redness affecting both the upper and lower eyelids. The rest of the facial skin is normal.

termed Wong-type DM, can also occur. Poikiloderma (a triad of telangiectatic erythema, epidermal atrophy and dyspigmentation) is an expression of skin damage in longstanding DM and is most clearly observed on the torso in patients with fair skin (Figure 52.9). In darker skin the atrophy and hyper/hypopigmentation of poikiloderma will be apparent but telangiectasis is difficult to discern.

Involvement of the hands and limbs. Gottron papules, which are pathognomonic of DM, are flat or slightly raised lichenoid lesions on the skin overlying the dorsal aspect of the interphalangeal and metacarpophalangeal joints of the fingers (Figure 52.10a). Red linear streaks over the extensor tendons of the hands may accompany Gottron papules (Figure 52.10b). Patients can also develop small inflammatory papules on the palmar surface of the finger creases, termed inverse Gottron papules [48]. Larger lichenoid plaques on the elbows and knees are referred to as the Gottron sign.

A combination of hyperkeratotic inflammation and fissuring on the sides of the fingers, most prominent on the radial border of the index fingers, is known as 'mechanic's' or 'machinist's hands' (Figure 52.11a). These changes are usually seen in the antisynthetase syndrome, a form of DM characterised by the presence of one of the antisynthetase antibodies (e.g. anti-Jo-1). Similar changes can occur

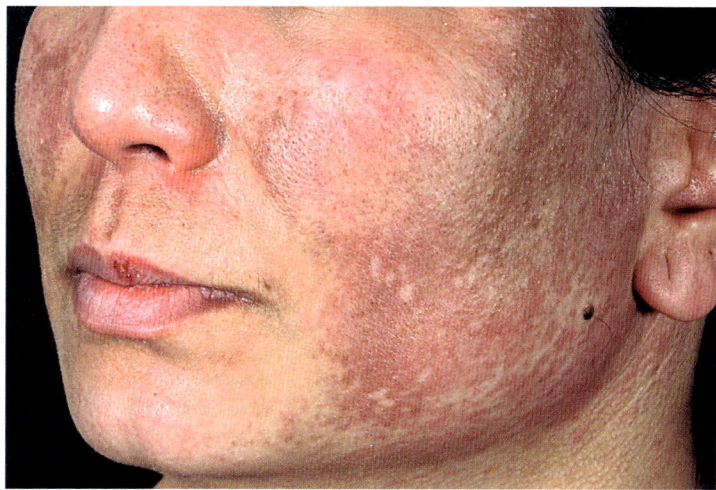

Figure 52.4 Facial involvement in dermatomyositis is often widespread and can mimic many dermatoses, including lupus erythematosus.

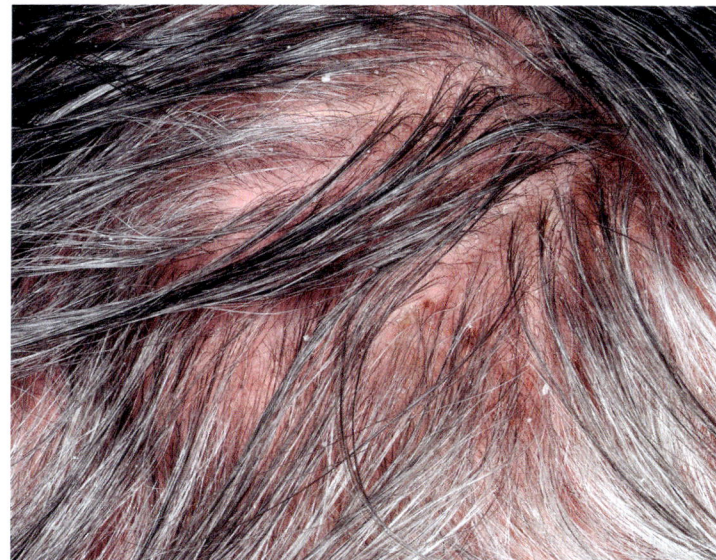

Figure 52.5 A diffuse, non-scarring alopecia is common in dermatomyositis. The scalp is inflamed with violaceous erythema and mild scaling.

on the lateral borders of the feet (Figure 52.11b). Distinctive vasculopathic ulcers, which tend to be punched out and surrounded by a zone of dusky erythema, may occur on the fingers and dorsal aspect of the hands. Ulcerative vasculopathy is seen most commonly in patients carrying the anti-MDA-5 MSA (Figure 52.12) [49].

Erythema of the fingernail folds is almost always present in DM and is accompanied by hypertrophic and ragged cuticles (Figure 52.13). Dermoscopic examination of the nail folds demonstrates microvascular changes similar to those observed in systemic sclerosis, including enlarged capillary loops, loop loss or fall-out, capillary bed disorganisation, budding of capillaries and capillary haemorrhages [50]. On the arms, the rash of DM preferentially affects the extensor surfaces and is characterised by zones of livid erythema with mild scaling (Figure 52.14). The buttocks are often involved in DM; erythema over the hips and lateral thighs has been termed the 'holster sign' (Figure 52.15).

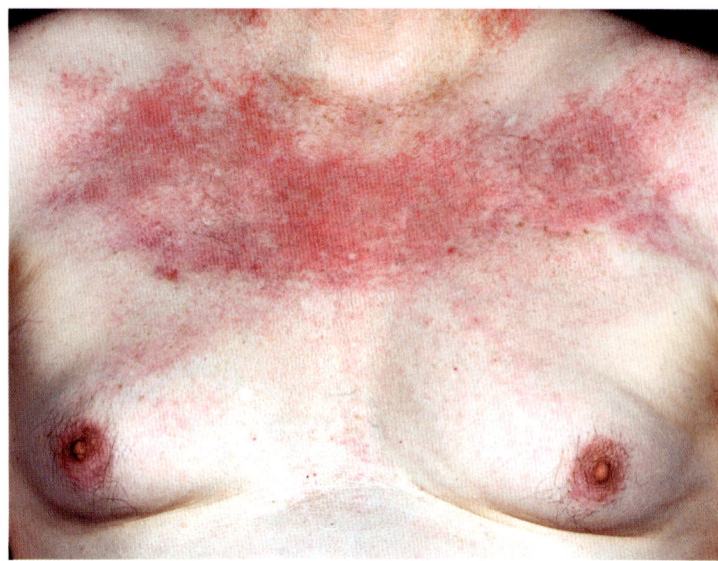

Figure 52.6 The upper torso is a common site of skin involvement in dermatomyositis. A semicircular zone of erythema over the anterior chest is known as the 'bib sign'.

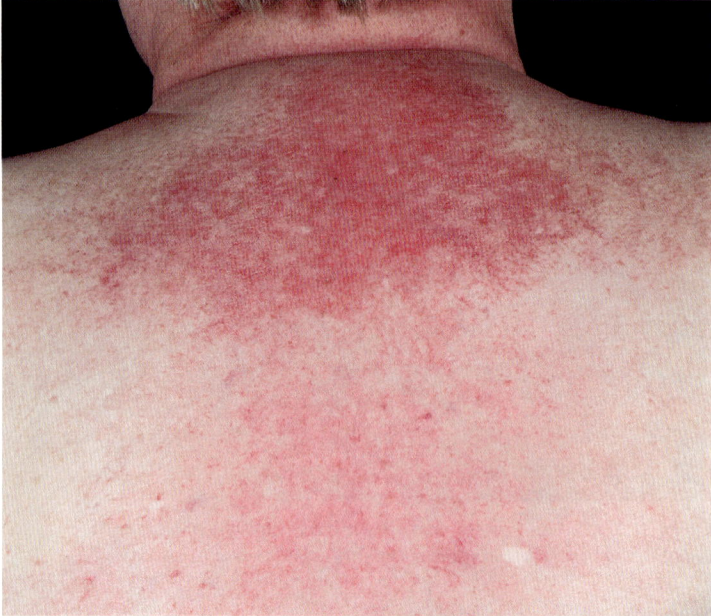

Figure 52.7 Erythema of the upper central back is known as the 'shawl sign'.

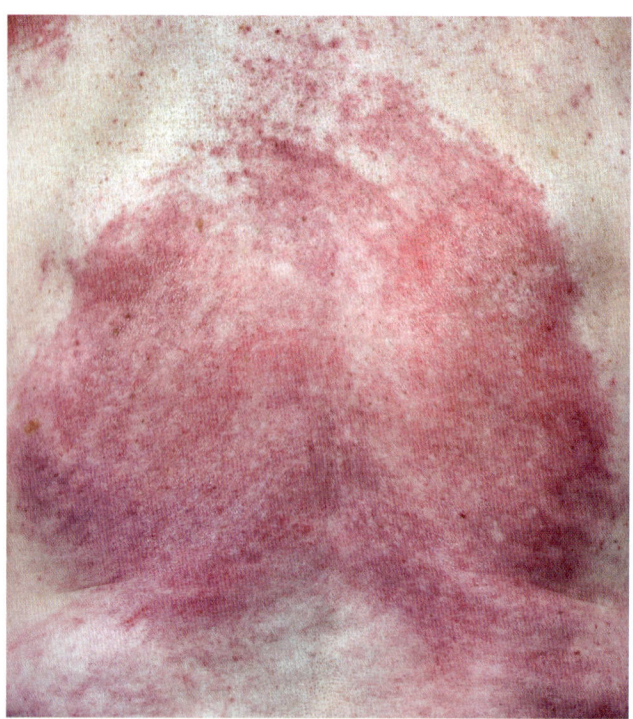

Figure 52.8 In severe dermatomyositis there is skin involvement of the abdomen and low back.

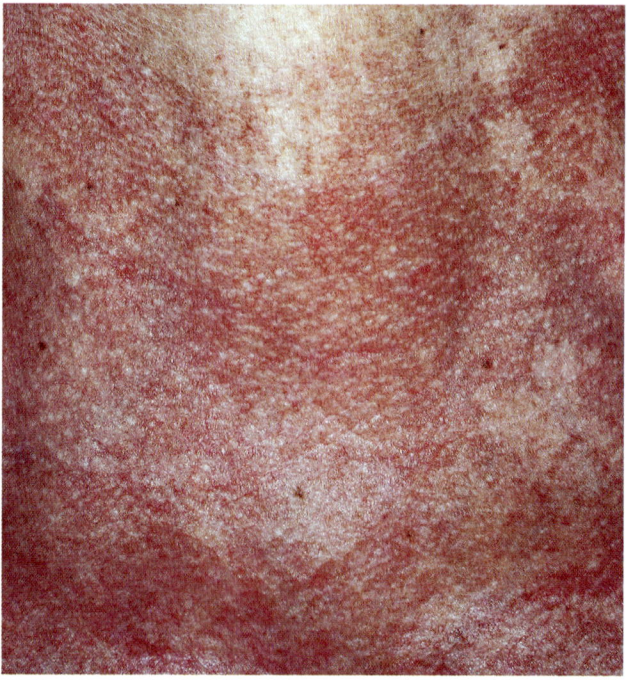

Figure 52.9 Poikiloderma occurs in dermatomyositis; it is composed of telangiectatic erythema, epidermal atrophy and dyspigmentation.

Panniculitis and calcinosis. Panniculitis occurs in a subpopulation of patients and presents with multiple, painful, deep-seated nodules and plaques on the buttocks, upper thighs and upper arms [51]. In contrast to lupus panniculitis, the face is rarely involved in DM. Panniculitis has been widely described in juvenile DM (JDM) and may occur more frequently in patients with anti-MDA-5 antibodies and rapidly progressive interstitial pneumonia. A biopsy of a fresh lesion demonstrates a lobular panniculitis with an infiltrate rich in lymphocytes and plasma cells.

Although more typically recognised as a manifestation of systemic sclerosis, calcinosis occurs quite commonly in DM. It is a frequent complication of JDM and is not uncommon in adult DM: in a large cohort of adult patients the prevalence of calcinosis was approximately 6% [52]. Calcinosis is more common in patients with longer periods of sustained disease activity and digital ulceration. Typical sites of involvement are the pressure areas: the buttocks, thighs and distal limbs. The lesions can be superficial or deep and form nodules, plaques or sheets. The lesions of DM calcinosis are bony-hard and often tender on palpation. Anti-NXP-2 antibody is the MSA most strongly associated with cutaneous calcinosis [53].

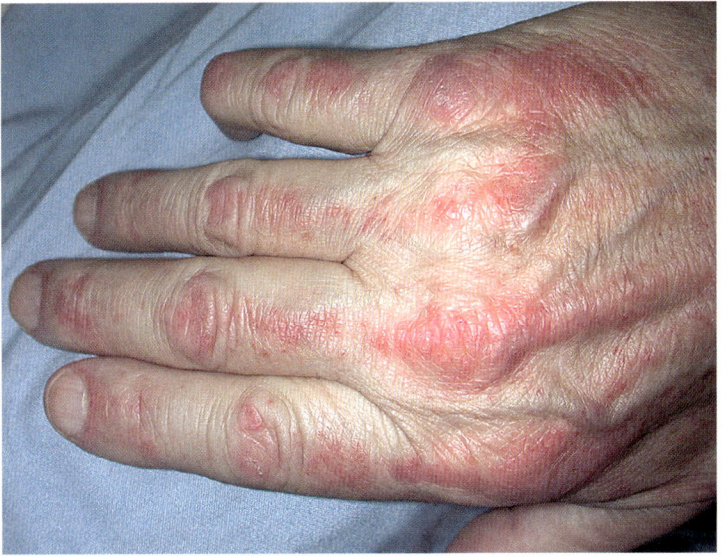 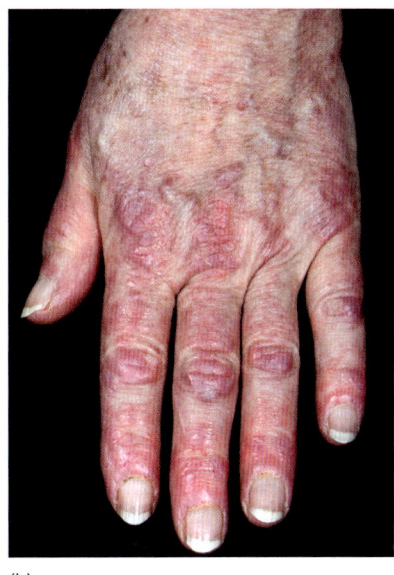

Figure 52.10 Gottron papules. (a) Violaceous, flat-topped, shiny papules on the skin overlying the interphalangeal joints and metacarpophalangeal joints. (b) There are streaks of redness on the dorsal aspects of the fingers, extending onto the backs of the hands.

(a)

(b)

Muscle signs. Dermatomyositis is a proximal myopathy and, as such, patients frequently present with problems climbing stairs, getting out of a chair and performing tasks that require lifting their hands above the head, such as brushing hair. However, since the onset of weakness can be quite insidious, patients may not appreciate that they are weak, particularly if there is associated arthritis or breathlessness. Even in patients who do not complain of weakness, muscle strength should still be assessed by manual muscle testing. A brief screen for muscle involvement can be made by assessing hip flexion, shoulder abduction and elbow extension. If the patient cannot be overcome on these assessments by the examining physician there is unlikely to be demonstrable muscle weakness on formal muscle testing. If there is evidence of weakness, formal manual muscle testing should be performed.

Muscle strength has traditionally been assessed using the Medical Research Council 0–5 grade scale for muscle strength, although the extended 0–10 grade scale may be a more sensitive tool for assessing changes in patients with moderate weakness [54]. The International Myositis Assessment and Clinical Studies (IMACS) group has introduced the MMT8 and MMT26 tools for IIM. These clinical assessment measures grade the strength of specific muscle groups on a scale of 0–10 and produce an overall score which can be compared over time [55]. The MMT8 tool is increasingly being used in research and clinical practice.

Patients with normal muscle strength on manual muscle testing may complain of ongoing weakness with lack of stamina: more subtle changes such as these may be picked up using the Function Index-3 scale which assesses muscle stamina in several muscle groups [56].

Respiratory and other systemic features. Respiratory compromise in DM may be caused by ILD, respiratory muscle weakness or aspiration in patients with dysphagia or immunosuppression. Although estimates vary, ILD is found in around 20–40% of IIM cases [57,58,**59**,60–62] – therefore all patients should be assessed

for this at presentation to allow appropriate therapy and monitoring. Patients usually present with a dry cough and exertional dyspnoea and have fine, late inspiratory crepitations on chest auscultation. However, in mild or early disease these pointers may be absent and in the presence of significant muscle disease can be easily overlooked by both the patient and physician alike. Notably, patients with CADM commonly have coexistent ILD which may be rapidly progressive. As such it is sensible to perform lung function tests and in appropriate cases high-resolution computed tomography (CT) at presentation (see 'Investigations' later in this chapter).

The majority of ILD is non-specific interstitial pneumonitis [60]. Usual interstitial pneumonitis (UIP), cryptogenic-organising pneumonia (COP) and diffuse alveolar damage (DAD) occur less frequently [60]. As its name suggests, COP may be difficult to distinguish from an infective pneumonia. While these are histological subtypes of ILD they have characteristic features on CT, and in the context of dermatomyositis a lung biopsy is rarely required. COP and DAD tend to present the most acutely. Generally, COP has a very good prognosis, responding rapidly to steroids, but in the context of DM a more sinister fibrosing form may occur. DAD is usually a severe disorder and carries a poor prognosis. A presenting carbon monoxide transfer factor (T_{LCO}) of <45%, excess neutrophils on bronchoalveolar lavage fluid, and histology showing DAD or UIP are all associated with poor prognosis [62].

The oro-pharynx and the upper oesophageal sphincter are frequently affected in DM, causing dysphagia. The severity of dysphagia does not correlate well with the severity of limb weakness and patients may not volunteer the symptoms of dysphagia. Proactive screening for the symptoms of dysphagia is necessary; early detection of this complication is important to prevent aspiration.

While mild cardiac abnormalities such as minor rhythm disturbances can frequently be found in DM, clinically overt disease, which generally manifests as cardiac failure, is rare. Cardiac failure due to myocarditis responds to immunosuppression.

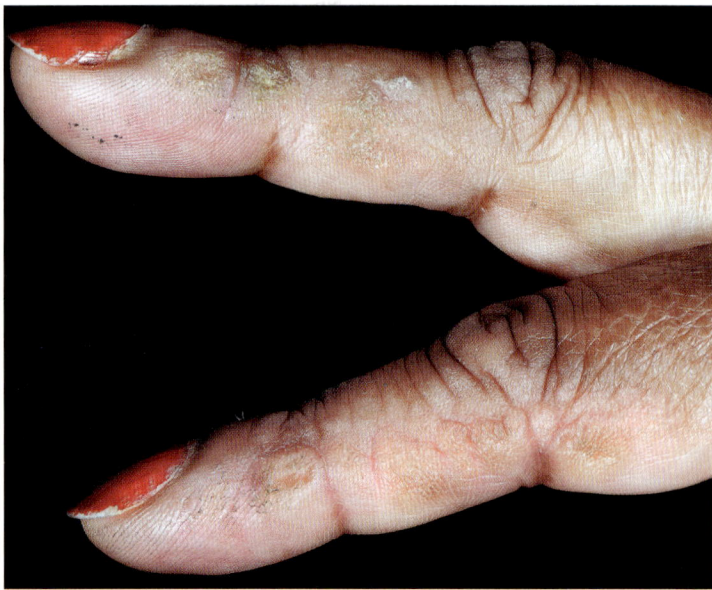

(a)

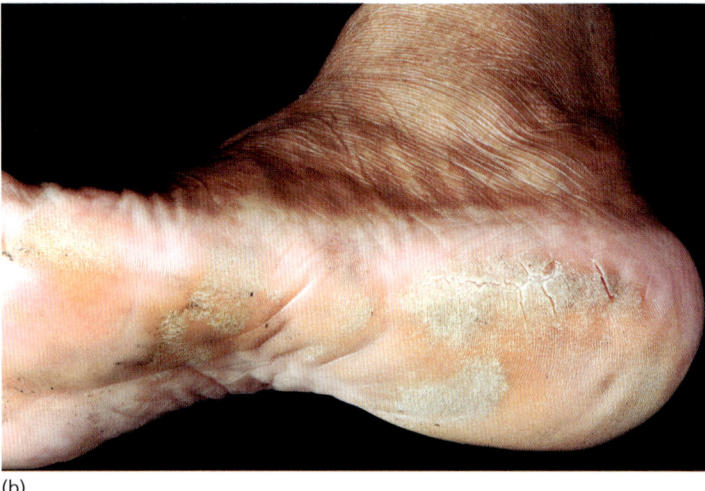

(b)

Figure 52.11 Non-inflammatory hyperkeratosis occurring on (a) the fingers and (b) the feet may be seen in Jo-1-positive dermatomyositis. Involvement of the radial surfaces of the fingers resembles the callosities seen in manual workers, so-called 'mechanic's hands'.

A symmetrical, non-deforming arthritis may develop, usually affecting the small joints of the hands, wrists and ankles. In the antisynthetase syndrome a more aggressive, erosive arthritis may occur and may be the presenting feature in these patients.

Clinical variants

Overlap syndromes. Mixed connective tissue disease is an overlap connective tissue disease characterised by high-titre anti-RNP antibodies, Raynaud phenomenon, sclerodactyly, inflammatory myositis, ILD and pulmonary hypertension.

Antisynthetase syndrome. The antisynthetase syndrome occurs in the presence of antisynthetase antibodies, most commonly anti-histidyl tRNA synthetase (anti-Jo-1) antibody, which is found in 10–20% of DM cases. There are seven other, much rarer,

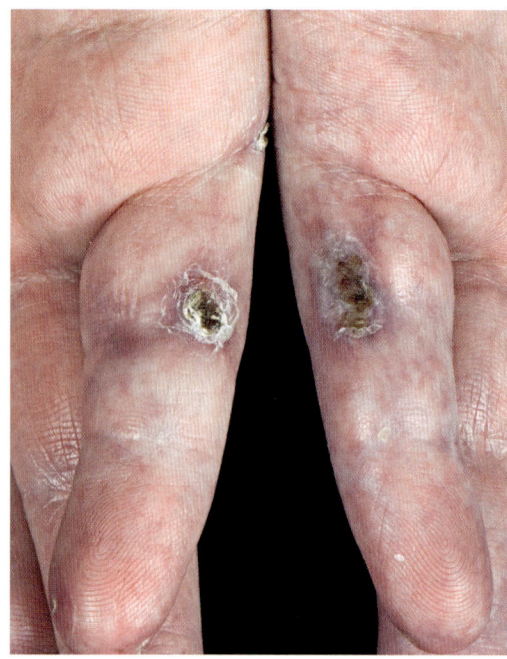

Figure 52.12 Vasculopathic ulcers, which have dusky margins and are 'punched out', may occur in dermatomyositis patients, particularly those who are positive for anti-MDA-5 antibody. The fingers and knuckles are the usual sites of involvement.

antisynthetase antibodies described: threonyl tRNA synthetase (anti-PL-7), alanyl tRNA synthetase (anti-PL-12), glycyl tRNA synthetase (anti-EJ), isoleucyl tRNA synthetase (anti-OJ), asparaginyl tRNA synthetase (anti-KS), tyrosyl tRNA synthetase and phenylalanyl tRNA synthetase (anti-Zo) [63].

The antisynthetase syndrome is characterised by myositis, arthritis, Raynaud phenomenon, ILD, fever and acral skin changes, called 'mechanic's hands' (see 'Presentation' earlier in this chapter). ILD is particularly common, occurring in around 75% of cases [64,65]. The non-anti-Jo-1 patients have a slightly lower frequency of myositis and a slightly higher incidence of ILD than Jo-1-positive patients [65].

Juvenile dermatomyositis. Juvenile dermatomyositis may be superficially considered as DM presenting in childhood. However, there are a few subtle but important distinctions. Unlike adult DM there does not seem to be an increased risk of malignancy in JDM. However, calcinosis, which is relatively rare in adults, is found in 6–50% of children with JDM [66]. Calcinosis is associated with increased disease activity, being commoner in those with a delayed diagnosis and inadequately treated disease. In children four forms of calcinosis occur, a superficial cutaneous or subcutaneous calcinosis, intramuscular tumourous calcification, calcinosis of the myo-facial planes and, in severe cases, an extensive encasing calcinosis or 'exoskeleton'.

Acquired lipodystrophy, a rarely reported feature in adult DM, is a relatively common finding in patients with JDM, occurring in the region of 10% of children [67]. It is associated with insulin-resistant type 2 diabetes and acanthosis nigricans. It may be generalised, partial or focal. In focal disease there may be an associated panniculitis.

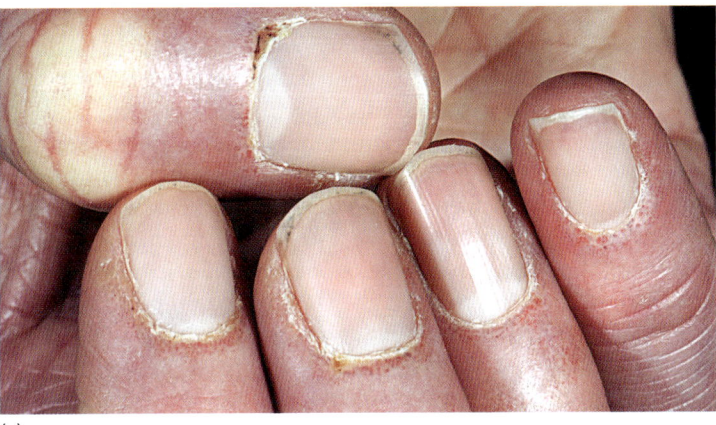

(a)

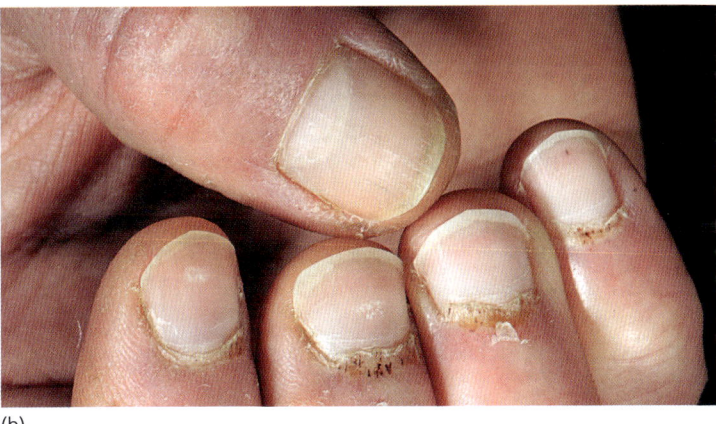

(b)

Figure 52.13 The nail folds and cuticles are usually affected in dermatomyositis. (a) Dilated nail fold capillary loops are visible. (b) The cuticles are hypertrophic and ragged. There are infarcts within the cuticles.

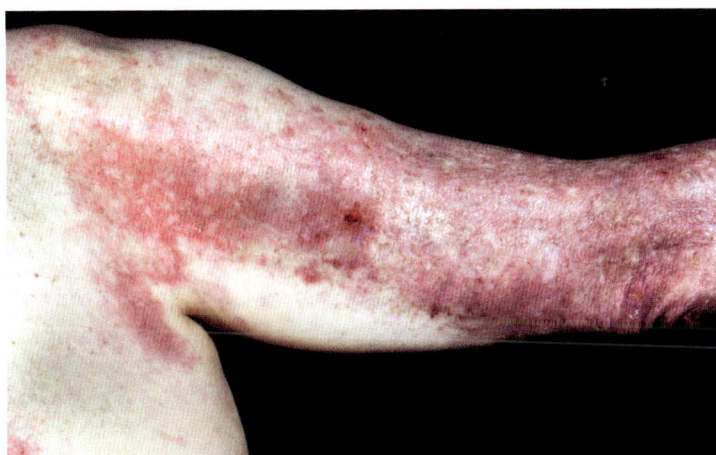

Figure 52.14 Involvement of the extensor surfaces of the arms is typical in dermatomyositis.

Antibody frequency and phenotype association differ somewhat between adult DM and JDM. For example, anti-Jo-1 occurs in around 20% of adult myositis cases but occurs in only a few percent of JDM patients [68]. Anti-TIF-1γ is associated with cancer in adult disease whereas in juvenile disease there is an association with ulcerating skin lesions [69].

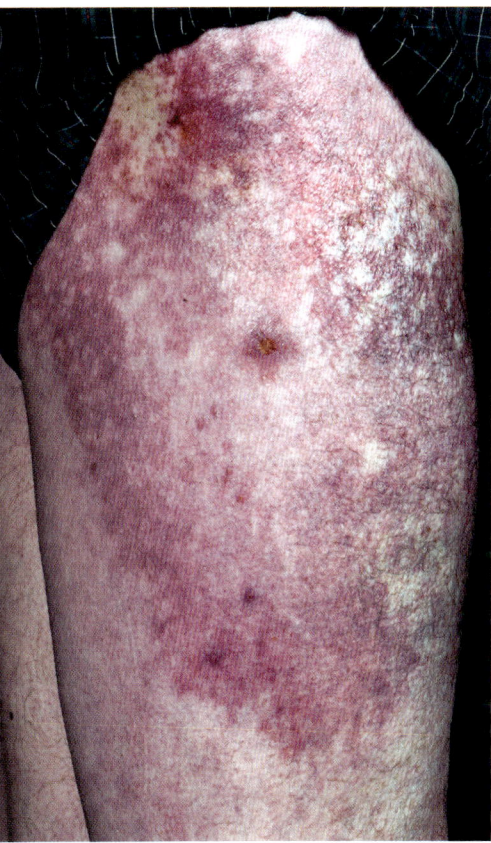

Figure 52.15 The dermatosis of dermatomyositis can affect the gluteal skin and proximal thighs. Involvement of the skin overlying the hips is known as the 'holster sign'.

Clinically amyopathic dermatomyositis. This is characterised by the presence of cutaneous manifestations of DM in the absence of clinical signs of muscle involvement (see 'Classification of severity' later in this chapter). In a series of 103 DM cases from a single centre, eight were diagnosed with CADM; six of these had subclinical myositis and were subsequently classified as having hypomyopathic DM [70]. Despite the lack of myositis, patients with CADM appear to be at risk for developing cancer and ILD. In a number of studies from East Asia, anti-MDA-5 antibodies have been detected at a significantly higher frequency in CADM patients than in DM patients [71]. In Japanese populations a high incidence of rapidly progressive ILD with a mortality of around 50% has been reported in patients with clinically amyopathic disease and anti-MDA-5 antibodies [72]. Consequently, it is important to make a thorough assessment for ILD in patients with amyopathic disease (see 'Investigations').

Drug-induced dermatomyositis. Dermatomyositis has occasionally been attributed to an adverse drug reaction. A review of 70 reported cases of drug-induced DM demonstrated pathognomonic cutaneous findings in three-quarters of patients and compatible skin signs in one-quarter [73]. Hydroxycarbamide was identified as the culprit in 50% of cases. None of the hydroxycarbamide patients had evidence of myositis, whereas myositis was described in 80% of non-hydroxycarbamide cases [73]. Despite many other drugs reported as inducing DM, no other specific agent has the same association as hydroxycarbamide. Clinically, the hydroxycarbamide cases are characterised by a violaceous, lichenoid and scaly eruption on the backs of the fingers and the dorsum of the hands, and the tops of the feet and elbows. The eruption can be atrophic and poikilodermatous. Histologically, there is hydropic degeneration with scattered dyskeratotic cells and a lichenoid lymphocytic infiltrate; telangiectatic vessels occur within the dermis. Although similar to the dermatosis of DM, the features of this reaction are distinct, and it is best described as 'hydroxycarbamide dermopathy' [74]. Most reports occur in patients who have received hydroxycarbamide for many years, the commonest indication being myeloproliferative disorders such as polycythaemia vera [74]. Hydroxycarbamide dermopathy tends to improve within 12 months of drug discontinuation [**73**].

Differential diagnosis

The skin signs in DM can mimic several other dermatoses. When myositis is prominent the diagnosis of DM is usually easily made. However, in amyopathic DM a few differential diagnoses should be considered (Box 52.1).

> ### Box 52.1 Differential diagnosis of the cutaneous signs of dermatomyositis
>
> - Lupus erythematosus
> - Seborrhoeic dermatitis
> - Rosacea
> - Allergic contact dermatitis
> - Psoriasis
> - Lichen planus
> - Lichenoid drug eruption
> - Cutaneous T-cell lymphoma

Classification of severity

Various measures have been developed to assess myositis activity and damage in DM. The DM skin severity index (DSSI), developed by Carroll *et al.*, is calculated from a visual inspection of lesional skin in four main body areas, quantifying redness, induration and scaliness in the same way used for the psoriasis activity and severity index (PASI) [75]. The DSSI has shown significant correlation to the physician's global assessment, assessments of poikiloderma and self-assessment of pruritus [75]. Clinical research studies typically prefer the CDASI (cutaneous dermatomyositis disease area and severity index) as the disease-specific scoring system. Calculation of the CDASI is also increasingly a requirement for the prescription of certain drugs for DM in the UK, notably intravenous immunoglobulin (IVIg).

The IMACS group has also proposed composite measures for the measurement of disease activity in myositis – the MITAX (myositis intention to treat index), the MYOACT (myositis disease activity assessment visual analogue scales) and the MYODAM (myositis damage index) for measuring damage for use in clinical trials [76].

Complications and co-morbidities

Patients with severe muscle weakness may develop hypoventilatory respiratory failure. In the acute setting, monitoring the forced vital capacity (FVC) serially at the bedside is the best way to monitor this, with blood gas measurements to assess for hypoxia and hypercapnia. Another measurement, the sniff nasal inspiratory pressure (SNIP), may be a more accurate predictor of ventilatory failure, with hypercapnic respiratory failure not usually occurring until the ventilatory muscle strength falls below 40% predicted. In contrast, hypercapnia may occur with a FVC >55% predicted. Patients with less critical respiratory muscle weakness and normal daytime blood gases may develop hypercapnia overnight. Thus, in patients with a low SNIP or FVC, overnight pulsoximetry should be performed to assess for nocturnal hypoventilation which may need non-invasive positive pressure ventilation.

Involvement of the oro-pharynx and the upper oesophageal sphincter in DM causes dysphagia. Aspiration pneumonia, exacerbated by respiratory muscle weakness, is the life-threatening complication of oro-pharyngeal involvement. Where dysphagia is prominent patients may present with dramatic weight loss in the absence of an underlying malignancy.

An inflammatory cardiomyopathy may occur in DM. Not surprisingly, cardiac involvement is a poor prognostic factor [77]. As with other autoimmune diseases there is evidence emerging that accelerated atherosclerosis is a cause of late mortality and morbidity [78,79].

Several studies have suggested an increased incidence of cardiovascular disease in patients with DM. As such it is important to minimise modifiable risk factors in these patients such as obesity, hypertension, hypercholesterolaemia, steroid therapy and smoking.

Disease course and prognosis

The disease course is variable, with the majority of patients requiring ongoing long-term immunosuppression. Around 20–35% of surviving myositis patients have a monophasic illness, with around 20–30% following a relapsing, remitting course and the remainder following a chronic, continuous course [4,**80**].

Prognosis relates closely to systemic features, with cancer and ILD being the two major causes of death. In modern series the 10-year survival is in the order of 90% [4,77].

Investigations

Patients with suspected DM should have a full biochemical profile, full blood count, inflammatory markers and muscle enzymes performed. Where available, troponin I should be performed to screen for subclinical myocardial involvement. Troponin T is not cardio-specific and will therefore be raised in parallel with creatine kinase. Where myocarditis is suspected cardiac magnetic resonance imaging (MRI) with T_1 and T_2 mapping should be performed. Inflammatory markers may be normal, as may creatine kinase levels, particularly in clinically amyopathic patients. As an inflammatory myositis may occur in lupus erythematosus and other connective tissue diseases, the following serology tests must be performed: antinuclear antibody (ANA), extractable nuclear antigen (ENA), double-stranded DNA (dsDNA), lupus anticoagulant, complement levels, anticardiolipin antibodies and β_2-glycoprotein 1 antibodies. Approximately 80% of DM patients will have a positive ANA, often at a low titre, which would not generally be considered significant in other clinical scenarios [81]. However, many of the autoantibodies in DM are predominantly cytoplasmic and as such will not cause a positive ANA.

MAAs are antibodies that occur in myositis but are not specific for it. As such they can support the diagnosis, but not confirm it. Anti-52kD Ro antibodies are the commonest MAA, found in 20% of IIM cases, and may be found in conjunction with other myositis antibodies particularly anti-Jo-1 [82]. Anti-Ku, anti-U1-RNP, U3-RNP and PM-Scl antibodies may occur in myositis, usually in the context of overlap syndromes with sclerodermatous features.

The separation of patients into subgroups according to shared traits has developed in parallel with the identification of MSAs [83]. MSAs target either nuclear or cytoplasmic components involved in gene transcription, protein translocation and antiviral responses, and evidence suggests that these autoantigens may be targets in DM pathogenesis. Subsequent studies have demonstrated that clinical phenotypes appear to be aligned to individual MSAs, although the strength of the association varies between different MSAs and between patients (Table 52.2). Interestingly, the MSAs are almost always mutually exclusive: an individual patient with DM will possess only one MSA.

The antisynthetase antibodies are the commonest, occurring in approximately 20% of IIM patients, with anti-Jo-1 being by far the commonest and the other seven antisynthetase antibodies accounting for only a few percent of cases. They delineate a specific phenotype, as discussed earlier, with arthritis, fever, Raynaud phenomenon, ILD, myositis and 'mechanic's hands'. There is a spectrum of disease with some patients having little in the way of skin disease. With some of the rarer antisynthetase antibodies, lung disease may be the predominant clinical feature with clinically amyopathic disease, Raynaud phenomenon and only subtle skin changes. Antisynthetase antibodies are extremely rare in JDM.

Antibodies to MDA-5 were first described in Japan, where they were found in 19–35% of DM patients and were associated with a high incidence of CADM (85–100%) and ILD (92%), with half developing rapidly progressive ILD [72,84]. In western populations MDA-5 antibodies are less frequent, at around 13% of DM patients in an American cohort [85]. In the anti-MDA-5-positive patients there was a high incidence of clinically amyopathic disease (50%) and ILD (67%). Anti-MDA-5 antibodies are associated with a distinctive cutaneous phenotype characterised by vasculopathic ulcers on the fingers, knuckles, elbows and knees (see Figure 52.14) [86]. These ulcers are usually small in diameter but are deep, punched out and surrounded by a dusky violaceous border. Painful red papules on the palmar surfaces of the metacarpophalangeal and interphalangeal joints are also observed with anti-MDA-5 antibodies [86].

Anti-TIF-1γ antibodies are specific to DM and are found in around 15–20% of cases [87]. They are associated with severe skin disease and a high incidence of cancer (50% in one series) [24,87]. As such, these patients should have a thorough screen for malignancy.

Anti-NXP-2 antibodies are frequent in JDM (11–23%) where they are associated with calcinosis [88]. In JDM, patients with anti-NXP-2 appear to have a more severe disease course and worse functional status [88]. Anti-NXP-2 antibodies are rare in adults.

Anti-Mi-2 antibodies are specific to DM and are found in around 10–20% of cases [89]. Patients with this antibody generally have classic cutaneous features of DM with Gottron papules, heliotrope rash, upper chest erythema ('V' sign) and the shawl sign [89]. Muscle disease tends to be mild and ILD rare in patients with anti-Mi-2 antibodies.

Anti-SUMO-activating enzyme antibodies occur in approximately 8% of adult DM patients [90]. Most patients present with skin disease and in one series a high increased frequency of dysphagia was reported [90].

Electromyography can confirm a myopathic process with early recruitment of multiple, small-amplitude, short-duration motor unit action potentials [91]. However, the presence of spontaneous fibrillations, positive sharp waves and bizarre high-frequency discharges is more specific for the inflammatory myopathies. Estimates of the proportion of patients with spontaneous fibrillations vary from 45% to 100% in different studies, possibly relating to the number of muscles sampled [91]. Although relatively specific for myositis, spontaneous fibrillations may also be found in other primary myopathies with muscle fibre degeneration, such as muscular dystrophies and acid maltase deficiency [91].

MRI of the proximal muscles may show oedema suggestive, but not diagnostic, of muscle inflammation. It can be helpful in assessing the extent of disease and guiding where the muscle biopsy should be taken when indicated; normal MRI does not exclude myositis.

In patients with the typical rash of DM a muscle biopsy is not required to confirm the diagnosis. When needed, muscle biopsy should, if possible, be performed prior to the start of systemic

Table 52.2 Clinical associations with myositis-specific antibodies (MSAs) in dermatomyositis.

MSA[a]	Clinical manifestations
Mi-2	Typical cutaneous features
	Mild myositis
TIF-1γ	Severe skin disease
	Malignancy-associated
	Can be associated with CADM
MDA-5	Ulcerative vasculopathy
	Panniculitis
	ILD which may be rapidly progressive with a high mortality, particularly in Far East populations
	Can be associated with CADM
NXP-2	JDM
	Calcinosis
SAE	Severe skin disease
	Malignancy associated
	Myositis/dysphagia may develop later
	ILD uncommon
	Can be associated with CADM
Jo-1, PL-7, PL-12, EJ, OJ, KS, Zo and Ha	'Mechanic's hands'
	Antisynthetase syndrome
	ILD

[a] Myositis-specific antibodies (in order on table): Mi-2, nucleosome deacetylase complex; TIF-1γ, transcription intermediary factor 1-gamma; MDA-5, melanoma differentiation-associated gene 5; NXP-2, nuclear matrix protein 2; SAE, small ubiquitin-like modifier-1 (SUMO-1) activating enzyme; Jo-1, histidyl tRNA synthetase; PL-7, threonyl tRNA synthetase; PL-12, alanyl tRNA synthetase; EJ, glycyl tRNA synthetase; OJ, isoleucyl tRNA synthetase; KS, asparginyl tRNA synthetase; Zo, phenylalanyl tRNA synthetase; Ha, tyrosyl tRNA synthetase.
CADM, clinically amyopathic dermatomyositis; ILD, interstitial lung disease; JDM, juvenile dermatomyositis.

corticosteroid therapy to maximise diagnostic yield. Muscle biopsies should be assessed in an experienced specialist laboratory where immunohistochemistry can be performed on frozen muscle tissue.

Plain radiography is an effective method of detecting and monitoring calcinosis in DM.

ILD is a major cause of mortality in DM and should be actively screened for. Lung function tests should be performed at presentation to include FVC, FEV_1 (forced expiratory volume in 1 s) and T_{LCO}; in ILD these show a restrictive pattern with all of them reduced in equal proportion. If there is concern regarding respiratory muscle weakness, a SNIP or lying and sitting FVC should be performed. A non-contrast CT scan of the chest should be performed if lung function tests show a restrictive pattern. If lung function is normal in patients at high risk of developing ILD, such as those with anti-MDA-5, antisynthetase or anti-RNP antibodies, an initial non-contrast CT of the chest should be considered at presentation and annual lung function tests performed subsequently.

In view of the increased risk of an underlying tumour in DM, screening for malignancy is necessary. There is no agreed protocol on the set of investigations needed. A detailed history and examination should be taken to guide investigations, with one study showing 54% of targeted investigations detecting a malignancy compared with 18% for non-targeted screening investigations [92]. CT scans of the neck, thorax, abdomen and pelvis or a positron-emission tomography CT scan should be performed on all adult patients and will also screen for ILD.

Further investigations should be organised as indicated following a full clinical assessment and risk assessment. Higher rates of malignancy are found with increasing age, severe skin disease, cutaneous ulceration, dysphagia, diaphragmatic weakness and anti-TIF-1γ and NXP-2 antibodies [92]. If there is a high index of suspicion for an underlying malignancy more extensive initial screening and serial screening at 6-monthly intervals for the first 2 years should be considered.

Management

Multidisciplinary care is espoused in the management of patients with DM. A combined treatment programme delineated by specialists in dermatology and rheumatology is necessary in most cases. Clinical input from respiratory medicine and other specialties is often also necessary. Systemic corticosteroid is the primary treatment for DM when both skin and muscles are involved. Oral prednisolone, given at a dose of 0.5–1.0 mg/kg, is usually effective in controlling the symptoms; many patients report improvement in the rash and muscle weakness within 1–2 weeks of starting systemic corticosteroids. If oral prednisolone is lacking in efficacy, or the severity of the muscle disease is life threatening, then pulsed intravenous methylprednisolone can be administered, 0.5–1 g/day for three consecutive days. The chronic nature of DM is such that systemic corticosteroids are usually required for a prolonged period. If the dose is not reduced, then the patient will inevitably be at risk of the side effects of long-term glucocorticosteroid therapy. Several immunosuppressant drugs are used to control the inflammatory process as the dose of prednisolone is slowly tapered [93]. There are very few controlled trials of immunosuppressant use in DM,

however the following have been administered with varying benefit: azathioprine 100–200 mg daily, methotrexate 10–20 mg once per week, mycophenolate mofetil 500–1500 mg twice daily, ciclosporin 3.0–5.0 mg/kg/day and tacrolimus [93].

Intravenous immunoglobulin can be used as a disease-modifying therapy in DM and as a steroid-sparing agent. In 1993 Dalakas *et al.* reported a double-blind, placebo-controlled trial of IVIg in 15 patients with DM [94]. The patients were maintained on prednisolone, at a mean dosage of 25 mg daily, and given either IVIg 2 g/kg body weight or placebo, each delivered monthly for 3 months. The patients who received IVIg demonstrated significant improvement in muscle strength and an observable improvement in skin disease [94]. More recently, a larger double-blind, placebo-controlled trial of IVIg in 95 patients also randomised to IVIg 2 g/kg body weight or placebo monthly showed significant improvement in the ACR/EULAR (American College of Rheumatology/European Alliance of Associations for Rheumatology) response criteria and the manual muscle testing and CDASI score at 16 weeks [95]. However, the evidence for long-term IVIg therapy is based on case series only [96,97].

A few published studies have investigated the role of rituximab in DM. An open-label pilot trial of seven patients studied outcome following 1 g of rituximab administered 2 weeks apart [98]. Three patients had a partial response with a reduction of muscle disease; the dermatosis did not improve. In a multicentre controlled trial, patients were randomised to receive rituximab at either weeks 0 and 1, with placebo at weeks 8 and 9, or placebo at weeks 0 and 1, with rituximab at weeks 8 and 9. Neither the primary nor the secondary end points, based on muscle parameters, were met. However, there was improvement in overall disease activity in both groups with 83% reaching the IMACS definition of improvement [99]. Additionally, in a subsequent *post hoc* analysis, anti-Jo-1 and Mi-2 antibodies strongly predicted clinical improvement [100].

Management of the skin involvement in DM is the prime concern for dermatologists. Systemic corticosteroid in combination with a steroid-sparing immunosuppressant is usually effective, however complete clearance of the dermatosis may take many months of therapy. In amyopathic DM, aggressive systemic immunosuppression may seem inappropriate and therefore topical therapy or milder oral treatment is usually tried. The efficacy of topical corticosteroid, including super-potent steroid, is often disappointing; however, benefit from topical tacrolimus 0.1% ointment has been observed [101]. Uncontrolled studies of hydroxychloroquine, either alone or in combination with mepacrine, have been reported as effective in clearing the cutaneous signs of DM [102]. Methotrexate can also be beneficial in the management of skin disease in DM [103]. Recent case series and case reports have suggested efficacy of Janus kinase (JAK) inhibitors for skin disease, with the largest case series comprising 25 JDM children treated with ruxolitinib or tofacitinib. All showed improvement in their skin disease with 16 (66.7%) showing complete resolution [104].

Calcinosis cutis is a troublesome and symptomatic complication of severe or poorly treated DM. Effective treatment of the underlying DM may lead to an improvement of calcinosis. Various therapeutic modalities have been tried, but studies are lacking to support the unequivocal benefit of any one particular treatment.

Treatment ladder for dermatomyositis

First line

- Pulsed intravenous (IV) methylprednisolone 0.5–1.0 g/day on three consecutive days (for severe life-threatening disease)
- Followed by oral prednisolone 0.5–1 mg/kg/day
- Disease-modifying antirheumatic drug (DMARD) after pulsed methyl prednisolone, such as methotrexate (unless interstitial lung disease (ILD)), azathioprine or ciclosporin
- Consider IV immunoglobulin (IVIg), particularly if the patient has dysphagia

Alternative regimen

- Pulsed IV methylprednisolone 0.5–1.0 g/day on three consecutive days (for severe life-threatening disease)
- Followed by IV cyclophosphamide (for severe life-threatening disease)
- *Plus* prednisolone 1 mg/kg/day
- DMARD after cyclophosphamide, such as methotrexate (unless ILD), azathioprine or ciclosporin
- Consider IVIg, particularly if the patient has dysphagia

Second line

- Mycophenolate mofetil
  or
- Oral tacrolimus

For skin-limited disease

- Potent topical corticosteroid ointment or topical tacrolimus 0.1% ointment
- *Plus* hydroxychloroquine (± mepacrine)

Third line

- Rituximab
- Janus kinase (JAK) inhibitor

Resources

Further information

International Myositis Assessment and Clinical Studies Group: www.niehs.nih.gov/research/resources/imacs.

Myositis UK: www.myositis.org.uk. (Both last accessed May 2022.)

Key references

The full list of references can be found in the online version at https://www.wiley.com/rooksdermatology10e

1 Bohan A, Peter JB. Polymyositis and dermatomyositis. *N Engl J Med* 1975; 292:344–7,403–7.

2 Lundberg IE, Tjarnlund A, Bottai M *et al*. 2017 European League Against Rheumatism/American College of Rheumatology classification criteria for adult and juvenile idiopathic inflammatory myopathies and their major subgroups. *Ann Rheum Dis* 2017;76:1955–64.

3 Sontheimer RD. Would a new name hasten the acceptance of amyopathic dermatomyositis (dermatomyositis siné myositis) as a distinctive subset within the idiopathic inflammatory dermatomyopathies spectrum of clinical illness? *J Am Acad Dermatol* 2002;46:626–36.

8 Cooper GS, Stroehla BC. The epidemiology of autoimmune diseases. *Autoimmun Rev* 2003;2:119–25.

17 Hill CL, Zhang Y, Sigurgeirsson B *et al*. Frequency of specific cancer types in dermatomyositis and polymyositis: a population-based study. *Lancet* 2001;357:96–100.

27 Kissel JT, Mendell JR, Rammohan KW. Microvascular deposition of complement membrane attack complex in dermatomyositis. *N Engl J Med* 1986;314:329–34.

28 Kissel JT, Halterman RK, Rammohan KW, Mendell JR. The relationship of complement-mediated microvasculopathy to the histologic features and clinical duration of disease in dermatomyositis. *Arch Neurol* 1991;48:26–30.

36 Howard OM, Dong HF, Yang D *et al*. Histidyl-tRNA synthetase and asparaginyl-tRNA synthetase, autoantigens in myositis, activate chemokine receptors on T lymphocytes and immature dendritic cells. *J Exp Med* 2002;196:781–91.

43 Connolly A, Gordon PA, Hannah J, Creamer D. The chameleon rash: a review of the polyphenotypic dermatoses of dermatomyositis. *Clin Exp Dermatol* 2021;46:1016–22.

44 Hundley JL, Carroll CL, Lang W *et al*. Cutaneous symptoms of dermatomyositis significantly impact patients' quality of life. *J Am Acad Dermatol* 2006;54:217–20.

49 Daly ML, Gordon PA, Creamer D. Cutaneous features of dermatomyositis associated with myositis-specific antibodies. *Br J Dermatol* 2017;176(6):1662–5.

59 Kang EH, Lee EB, Shin KC *et al*. Interstitial lung disease in patients with polymyositis, dermatomyositis and amyopathic dermatomyositis. *Rheumatology (Oxford)* 2005;44:1282–6.

63 Gunawardena H, Betteridge ZE, McHugh NJ. Myositis-specific autoantibodies: their clinical and pathogenic significance in disease expression. *Rheumatology (Oxford)* 2009;48:607–12.

65 Hervier B, Devilliers H, Stanciu R *et al*. Hierarchical cluster and survival analyses of antisynthetase syndrome: phenotype and outcome are correlated with anti-tRNA synthetase antibody specificity. *Autoimmun Rev* 2012;12:210–17.

71 Cao H, Pan M, Kang Y *et al*. Clinical manifestations of dermatomyositis and clinically amyopathic dermatomyositis patients with positive expression of anti-melanoma differentiation-associated gene 5 antibody. *Arthritis Care Res (Hoboken)* 2012;64:1602–10.

73 Seidler AM, Gottlieb AB. Dermatomyositis induced by drug therapy: a review of case reports. *J Am Acad Dermatol* 2008;59:872–80.

80 Bronner IM, van der Meulen MF, de Visser M *et al*. Long-term outcome in polymyositis and dermatomyositis. *Ann Rheum Dis* 2006;65:1456–61.

93 Gordon PA, Winer JB, Hoogendijk JE, Choy EH. Immunosuppressant and immunomodulatory treatment for dermatomyositis and polymyositis. *Cochrane Database Syst Rev* 2012;Issue 8:CD003643.

94 Dalakas MC, Illa I, Dambrosia JM *et al*. A controlled trial of high-dose intravenous immune globulin infusions as treatment for dermatomyositis. *N Engl J Med* 1993;329:1993–2000.

95 Aggarwal R, Charles-Schoeman C, Schessl J *et al*. Prospective, double-blind, randomized, placebo-controlled phase III study evaluating efficacy and safety of octagam 10% in patients with dermatomyositis ('ProDERM Study'). *Medicine (Baltimore)* 2021;100:e23677.

99 Oddis CV, Reed AM, Aggarwal R *et al*. Rituximab in the treatment of refractory adult and juvenile dermatomyositis and adult polymyositis: a randomized, placebo-phase trial. *Arthritis Rheum* 2013;65:314–24.

104 Ding Y, Huang B, Wang Y *et al*. Janus kinase inhibitor significantly improved rash and muscle strength in juvenile dermatomyositis. *Ann Rheum Dis* 2021;80:543–5.

CHAPTER 53

Undifferentiated and Mixed Connective Tissue Disease and Dermatological Manifestations of Rheumatoid Disease

Philip M. Laws

Department of Dermatology, Chapel Allerton Hospital, Leeds, UK

Undifferentiated connective tissue disease (UCTD) and mixed connective tissue disease (MCTD)

Synonyms and inclusions
- Sharp syndrome

Introduction and general description

Undifferentiated connective tissue disease (UCTD) encompasses a cohort of patients with clinical, serological and pathological features of an autoimmune connective tissue disease (CTD) for which more precise diagnostic classification is not possible [1]. Over time the patient may develop new signs and symptoms which meet classification criteria for a defined CTD, including systemic lupus erythematosus (SLE), rheumatoid arthritis (RA), dermatomyositis/polymyositis and systemic sclerosis (SSc). A diagnosis of UCTD is observed in up to 25% of patients referred to rheumatology clinics and avoids premature classification of a traditional CTD [2,3].

Mixed connective tissue disease (MCTD), first described in 1972, is generally considered a distinct disease with clinical overlap to UCTD but characterised by the presence of U1 ribonucleoprotein antibodies (anti-U1-RNP) [4]. Unlike UCTD, patients with MCTD are not considered to have the potential to progress to a traditional CTD. The overlap of UCTD and MCTD with traditional CTDs has resulted in ongoing debate and difficulty in classification.

Epidemiology

Data on incidence and prevalence of UCTD are limited due to the diagnostic challenges already outlined. Approximately 25% of patients presenting with a CTD could be classified accordingly, highlighting the frequency of this clinical syndrome. In a Scandinavian population, annual incidence of UCTD has been estimated at 13.6/100 000 (9.0–19.6) [5]. Prevalence of MCTD has been reported at 1.9 per 100 000 population in a US population with an average delay of 3.6 years in diagnosis [6]. A Norwegian cohort of 147 patients reported a prevalence of 3.8 (95% confidence interval (CI) 3.2–4.4) per 100 000 adults, with a female to male ratio of 3.3 : 1 and mean age at onset of 37.9 years [7]. Juvenile onset may account for up to a quarter of patients in some studies [8].

Pathophysiology

The pathogenesis of MCTD remains to be clearly elucidated but genetic and environmental factors are important. A hallmark of MCTD that is seen in the majority of patients includes the U1-RNP antibody which binds U1 small nuclear ribonucleoprotein (U1-snRNP) complex, and specifically a 70 kDa motif [8]. The generation of these 70 kDa motifs is associated with cellular apoptosis. Generation of U1-RNP antibodies has been demonstrated through ultraviolet B radiation (UVB) induced cellular injury and suggests a role of photosensitivity in pathogenesis [9].

Autoreactive B and T cells against the U1 snRNP in MCTD have been identified and highlight the broad immune activation associated with disease [10]. Evidence supports the development of epitope spread and may provide some explanation for disease evolution and heterogeneity of clinical phenotype [11,12].

Raynaud phenomenon (RP) is associated with hypertrophy and proliferation of the small- and medium-sized blood vessels [13]. Elevated levels of endostatin, an inhibitor of angiogenesis, have been associated with all-cause mortality and digital ulceration and may be a useful marker for risk of ulceration [13].

Small studies have identified a number of genetic risk factors for MCTD including HLA-DRB1*0401, -DRB4*0101, -DQA1*03, -DQB1*0301 and HLA-B*08 haplotypes [14–16]. Ultraviolet radiation may predispose to a clinical phenotype more in keeping with lupus, although evidence of photosensitivity has been mixed [17,18]. Vitamin D deficiency is common in patients with MCTD, having been observed in 59% of patients in one study [19]. The aetiology of vitamin D deficiency is likely to be multifactorial but may relate to limited UVB exposure due to photosensitivity and impaired ability to get outdoors due to the physical limitations of the primary disease. Vitamin D may also have a role in regulating immune function and therefore be a risk factor for autoimmunity [20].

Rarely, MCTD has been reported to be drug induced and reports include tumour necrosis factor (TNF) inhibitors, vinyl chloride and silica [21–25].

Clinical features
UCTD

A diagnosis of UCTD may be considered in any patient for whom a traditional CTD is being considered but distinct criteria are not met. In a dermatological setting the commonest presentations include:

1 RP in isolation of other symptoms of a CTD. This should be more strongly suspected when serology is positive and nail fold capillary examination is abnormal.
2 Variable rash in a patient with positive serology, other non-diagnostic features of a CTD and skin biopsy which demonstrates vacuolar interface change.

Other presentations more commonly observed in rheumatology services include polyarthritis in a patient not meeting diagnostic criteria for RA or patients with immunological and/or serological abnormalities and multiple non-specific symptoms of an inflammatory diathesis (e.g. fatigue, myalgia, arthralgia).

RP is a common feature of UCTD. Examination of the nail folds for evidence of vascular abnormalities (capillary drop-out, engorged capillary loops, haemorrhage or irregular vessels) is easily assessed with dermoscopy and diagnostically helpful (Figure 53.1) [26].

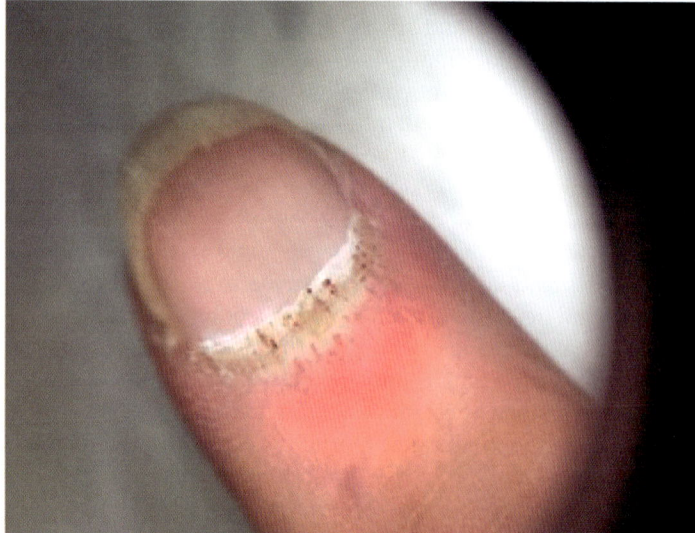

Figure 53.1 Abnormal nail fold in patient with mixed connective tissue disease demonstrating dilated capillary loops, capillary drop-out and thrombosed vessels.

Table 53.1 Diagnostic criteria for mixed connective tissue disease.

	Serology	Clinical	Diagnostic criteria
Alarcon-Segovia's criteria	Anti U1-RNP Titre ≥1 : 1600	1 Swollen hands 2 Synovitis 3 Myositis 4 Raynaud phenomenon 5 Acrosclerosis	Serology and 3 clinical signs (must include myositis or synovitis)
Kahn's criteria	Anti U1-RNP Titre ≥1 : 1200	1 Swollen fingers 2 Synovitis 3 Myositis 4 Raynaud phenomenon	Serology, Raynaud phenomenon and two of remaining clinical features

RNP, ribonucleoprotein. Adapted from Alarcon-Segovia and Cardiel 1989 [39].

Other cutaneous features observed in UCTD are poorly defined but may include dermatitis, photosensitivity, urticaria, unexplained oedema and psoriasis [27]. Non-specific red macules, papules and patches which demonstrate interface change are common and may appear as an annular erythema.

Approximately one-third of patients with a diagnosis of UCTD will subsequently meet diagnostic criteria for a defined CTD, the remaining patients retaining a diagnosis of UCTD [28]. Approximately 10% of patients with UCTD will achieve clinical remission. The risk of disease progression appears highest during the first 2 years after onset. While prognosis in UCTD patients is similar to the background population there is a large impact on quality of life that is comparable to SLE, despite a shorter disease course [29].

MCTD

Patients with MCTD may present after an initial diagnosis of UCTD following a period of diagnostic uncertainty. Diagnostic classification criteria have been proposed (Table 53.1). Other clinical presentations, which overlap with SSc, include RP with oedema and swelling of the hands (puffy hands), sclerodactyly, facial redness, calcinosis cutis, vasculitis of the digits, telangiectasia, livedoid vasculopathy, livedo reticularis (Figure 53.2), oral ulcers (Figure 53.3), urticarial vasculitis, peritendinous or subcutaneous nodules, and dry eyes and mouth [30–34]. Patients may present with atrophie blanche-like lesions associated with vasculopathic changes that may be indistinguishable from lupus on skin biopsy (Figure 53.4). Non-scarring alopecia and facial redness are common clinical problems in patients with CTDs and have both been reported to affect approximately 40% of patients [30,35].

Non-dermatological features are highly variable but include arthritis, myositis, cardiac (13–65%), pulmonary (interstitial lung disease, pulmonary hypertension) and gastrointestinal dysmotility (50%). Renal disease may occur but is typically less severe than that observed in SSc [7,30,36–38]. Prognosis following a diagnosis of MCTD is comparable with the background population with the exception of individuals who develop cardiac or pulmonary disease [6,8,18].

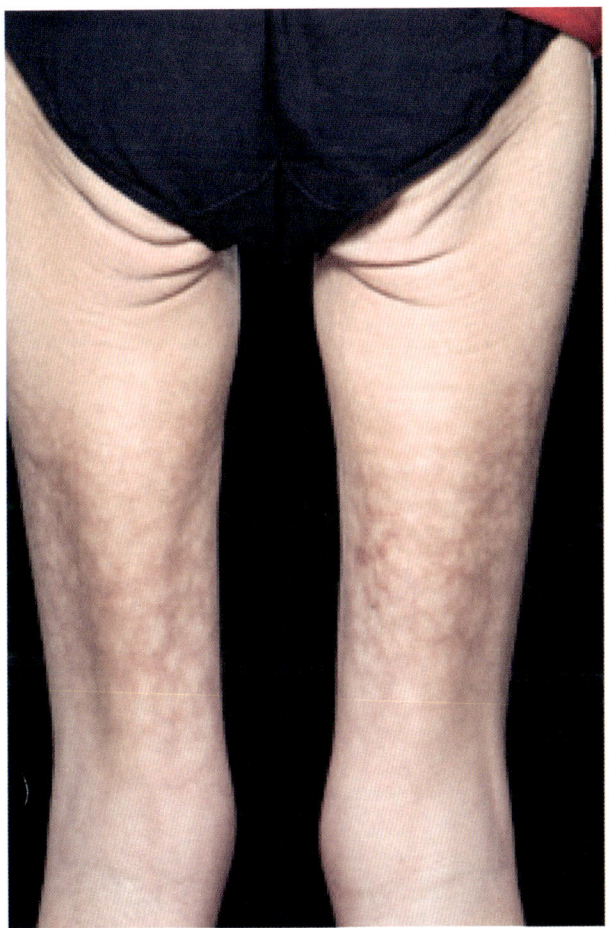

Figure 53.2 Extensive livedo reticularis observed in a patient with mixed connective tissue disease.

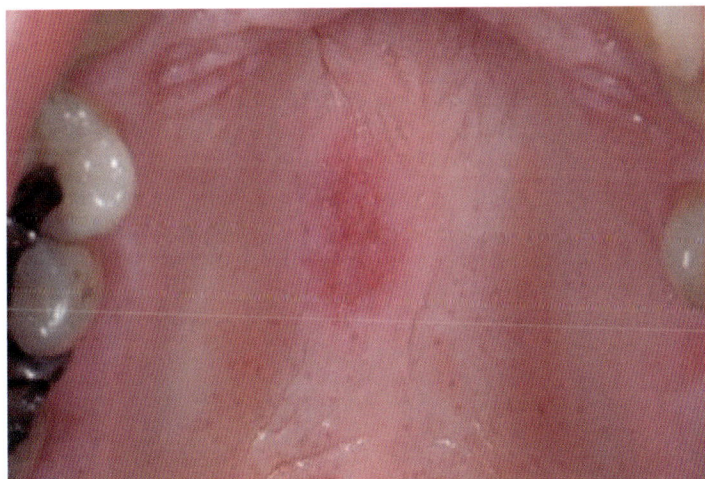

Figure 53.3 Oral erosion on hard palate of patient with mixed connective tissue disease.

The diagnosis of UCTD or MCTD should always be approached with classic CTD differential diagnoses in mind. A broader differential diagnosis may be appropriate according to the constellation of symptoms and clinical findings.

Investigations

Antibody profiles are a key investigation for patients with a suspected CTD but require careful interpretation. Antibodies to U1-RNP are detectable in 75–90% of patients with MCTD but may also be observed in up to 40% of patients with SLE [10,40,41]. This overlap in serology emphasises the importance of clinical classification in addition to serology to ensure accurate diagnosis. Other antibodies observed in UCTD include: Scl-70 1.8%, Ro/SSA 10.8%, La/SSB 4.5%, double-stranded DNA 27%, Sm 3.6%, rheumatoid factor (RF) 22.5%, anticardiolipin 5.4%, lupus anticoagulant 11.7% and Jo-1 1.8% [42]. In patients presenting with RP alone, assessment of antinuclear antibodies (ANA) is required if there is any suggestion that it may be secondary RP as suggested by signs or symptoms of a CTD [43].

Dermatopathology findings will depend on the clinical phenotype and disease expression may be consistent with findings observed in other CTDs [44]. The presence of basement membrane staining with immunoglobulin G (IgG) or IgM helps support a diagnosis of MCTD when trying to distinguish from SSc.

Given the co-morbid disease associated with MCTD, screening at baseline and annually is recommended and should include pulmonary function test (PFT), diffusing capacity of lung for carbon monoxide (DLCO), transthoracic echocardiogram (TTE), B-type natriuretic peptide (NT-pro BNP), urinalysis, blood pressure and electrocardiogram [45]. Consideration of other investigations will be determined by the clinical presentation. Blood abnormalities are common, with approximately 75% of patients having low-grade anaemia and hypergammaglobulinaemia [36,46].

Management

Given the limited evidence for treatment most clinicians recommend managing clinical signs and symptoms according to algorithms associated with traditional CTDs. It is essential to address lifestyle factors that may impact on disease severity and should include smoking cessation and hand and skin care advice, particularly when RP is an issue. Inflammatory lesions including pleurisy, arthritis and pericarditis are considered responsive to corticosteroids at a variable dose of 0.5–1 mg/kg. It is important to consider prompt dose reductions to limit complications of corticosteroids. RP is typically managed with calcium channel blockers, phosphodiesterase inhibitors, prostacyclin analogues (i.e. iloprost) or endothelin receptor antagonist (i.e. bosentan). In patients with an inflammatory disease pattern, antimalarials and methotrexate may be trialled in an attempt to stabilise/reduce corticosteroid requirements. Evidence to support this practice is limited. Other treatment options are likely to be guided by complications of disease and guided in part by cohort studies. Rituximab has been investigated for interstitial lung disease associated with CTDs, including MCTD [47].

Rheumatoid arthritis

Introduction and general description

Rheumatoid arthritis (RA) is an autoimmune disease characterised by an inflammatory polyarthritis, but is best considered a multisystem disease and may be associated with a range of extra-articular features including skin manifestations [48].

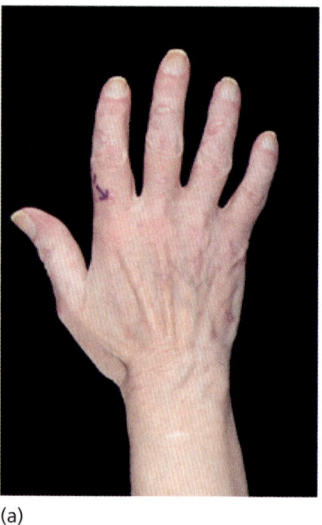
(a)

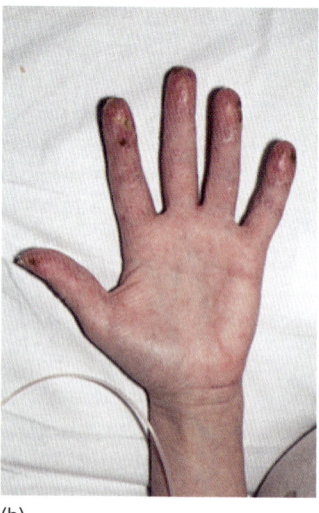
(b)

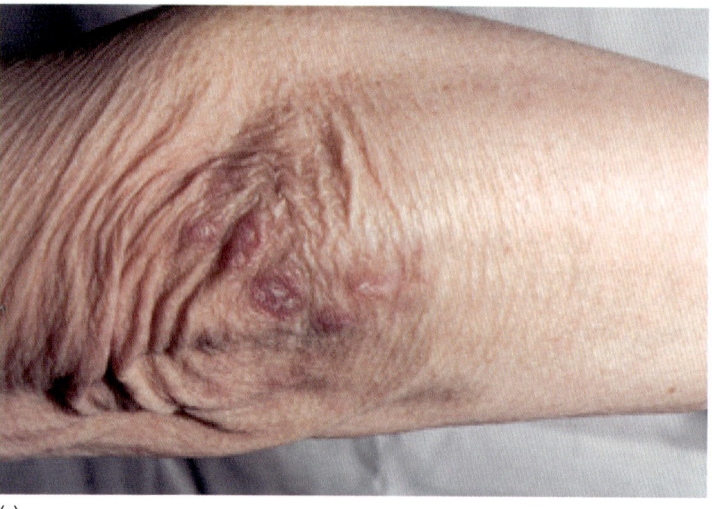
(c)

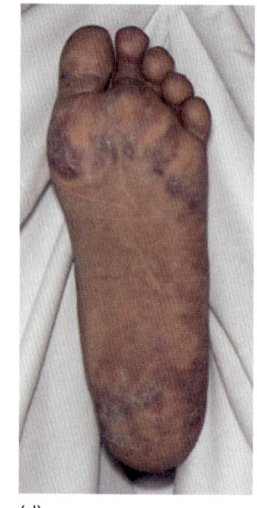
(d)

Figure 53.4 Acral lesions of mixed connective tissue disease (MCTD). (a–c) Atrophie blanche-like changes on hands and elbows of a patient with MCTD. (d) Retiform purpura due to vasculopathy in a patient with MCTD.

Epidemiology

RA affects around 0.25–1% of adults depending on the population being studied [49]. It is common in women with a relative risk of 4–5:1 and a typical age of onset between 30 and 40 years [50]. Concordance between genetically identical twins is approximately 15% and supports an important role for genetic and environmental aetiopathogenesis [51]. Multiple genetic HLA haplotypes have been observed in RA, notably the *0401/0404 genotype [52].

Pathophysiology

RA is characterised by immunological injury of the synovium. Conversion of the amino acid arginine to citrulline is an important early step and may be induced by smoking. Repeat activation of innate immunity with fixing of complement establishes the inflammatory diathesis and promotes neovascularisation. The synovium develops a progressive, destructive inflammatory pathology resulting in progressive joint damage. Cytokines implicated in RA pathogenesis include interleukin (IL)-1, -6, -17A, -18, -23, -27, TNF-α, vascular endothelial growth factor, alarmins, high-mobility group box protein 1 (HMGB1) and chemokines. This broad immune activation and inflammatory milieu result in increased bone turnover, destruction and joint damage. It is increasingly recognised that individuals with RA may respond to different therapeutic targets, suggesting divergent endotypes [53]. This insight provides an opportunity to personalise therapeutic approaches to optimise treatment response. This has been demonstrated in recent clinical studies that identified superior clinical response to tocilizumab (anti-IL-6) compared with rituximab (anti-IL-20) in B-cell-poor RA, as determined by RNA sequencing of synovial biopsies [54].

Clinical features

RA typically presents with joint pain, swelling and stiffness. Extra-articular involvement of RA has been reported in 40–50% of patients, with cutaneous disease affecting one-third of patients [55,56]. Extra-articular manifestations are listed in Box 53.1. It is increasingly clear that the extra-articular manifestations of RA are related to disease severity and the advent of advanced therapies and a treat-to-target approach have seen a reduction in extra-articular manifestations [57,58]. Factors associated with more severe disease include positive ANA, RF and smoking [59].

Box 53.1 Extra-articular manifestations associated with rheumatoid arthritis (RA)

Dermatological manifestations
- Rheumatoid nodules
- Rheumatoid vasculitis
- Pyoderma gangrenosum
- Reactive granulomatous dermatitis
  - Interstitial granulomatous dermatitis
  - Palisaded neutrophilic and granulomatous dermatitis/rheumatoid neutrophilic dermatitis
- Sweet syndrome
- Raynaud phenomenon
- Livedo racemosa
- Livedo reticularis
- Palmar and periungual redness
- Nail abnormalities (longitudinal ridging, nail beading, clubbing, onycholysis, red lunula, pterygium inversum and yellow discoloration)
- Chronic spontaneous urticaria
- Non-melanoma skin cancer (basal cell carcinoma > squamous cell carcinoma)

Non-dermatological manifestations
- Osteopenia
- Ocular disease
  - Episcleritis, uveitis, iritis
- Lung disease
  - Pleuritis, pleural effusion, interstitial fibrosis, pulmonary nodules, bronchiolitis obliterans
- Cardiac disease
  - Pericarditis, myocarditis, ischaemic heart disease, peripheral vascular disease, atrial fibrillation
- Glomerulonephritis
- Anaemia
- Sjögren syndrome
- Felty syndrome – RA with neutropenia, anaemia, splenomegaly, leg ulcers

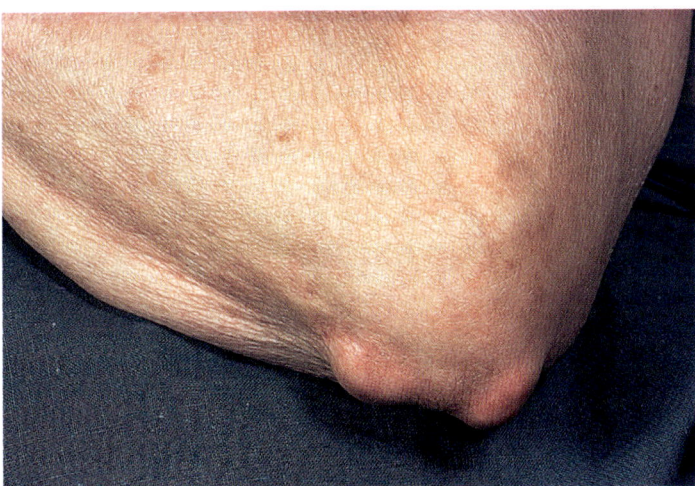

Figure 53.5 Rheumatoid nodules over the elbow.

Rheumatoid nodules

Rheumatoid nodules (RN) are the most common cutaneous manifestation of RA observed in approximately 20% of patients and typically have an indolent course [60]. The most common site is on the ulnar border of the forearm, but they may occur anywhere (Figure 53.5). RN vary in size from 2 mm to several centimetres in diameter, are firm in consistency and may ulcerate with trauma (Figure 53.6). RN may precede typical clinical features of RA by years [60]. Severe and rapidly progressive nodulosis, often over the dorsal hands, may be precipitated by drugs, notably methotrexate, but has been seen with biologic therapies [49,61]. Accelerated rheumatoid nodulosis induced by treatment often improves on drug withdrawal. Risk of developing RN has been linked with homozygosity for HLA-DR4 and DRB1, RF positivity and smoking [62–64].

Histology of rheumatoid nodules includes three zones: a necrotic granuloma containing cellular debris, fibrin and collagen; a middle layer of macrophages palisading this inner zone; and surrounding perivascular granulation tissue with inflammatory cells composed of lymphocytes, plasma cells and histiocytes. Vasculitis may be observed.

Clinical differential diagnoses include subcutaneous granuloma annulare, infectious granuloma, sarcoidal granuloma, xanthoma and foreign body granuloma. The subcutaneous nodules of rheumatic fever can be distinguished histologically from those of RA; there is much fibrinoid material and considerable oedema of the collagen, but relatively little infiltration with fibroblasts, histiocytes or lymphocytes [65]. The nodules with Still disease resemble those seen in rheumatic fever [65].

Reactive granulomatous dermatitis

Reactive granulomatous dermatitis (RGD) includes palisaded and neutrophilic granulomatous dermatitis (PNGD) and interstitial granulomatous dermatitis (IGD). Other diagnostic labels have been proposed but not widely adopted, including linear subcutaneous bands, rheumatoid papules, Churg-Strauss granuloma and cutaneous extravascular necrotising granuloma of Winkelmann. Debate as to whether PNGD and IGD are distinct entities continues, with many supporting that they represent a spectrum of disease. RGD is almost universally associated with an underlying autoimmune disease and most commonly RA (other associations include eosinophilic granulomatosis with polyangiitis, SLE and Behçet disease). The pathogenesis of RGD has not been extensively studied but may relate to immune complex deposition.

Symmetrical red or skin-coloured papules typically coalesce over extensor surfaces. IGD presents on the trunk and may form linear bands (rope sign) (Figure 53.7) [66]. The lesions of PNGD are more typically umbilicated, ulcerate and have a predilection for the limbs (Figure 53.8).

Skin biopsy of IGD demonstrates a CD68 positive histiocytic aggregate in the reticular dermis around degenerate collagen and absence of vasculitis. In contrast, lesions of PNGD are associated with leukocytoclastic debris, fibrin and degenerate collagen. Palisaded granuloma become more prominent in later lesions.

Rheumatoid neutrophilic dermatosis

Rheumatoid neutrophilic dermatosis (RND) is a rare neutrophilic dermatosis associated with RA. Symmetrical red nodules and

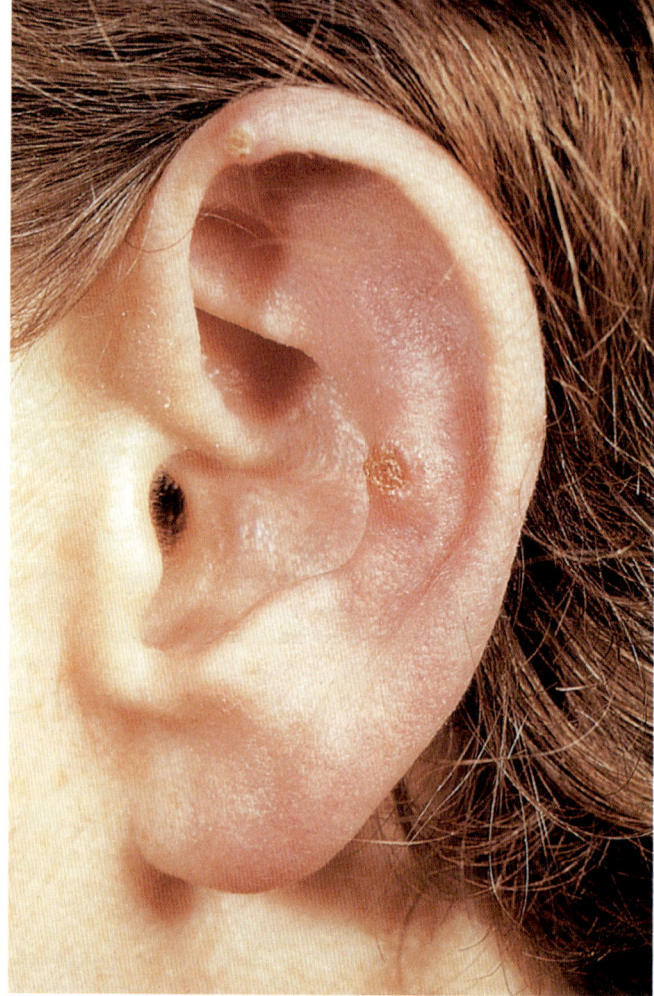

Figure 53.6 Ulcerated rheumatoid nodule on the ear.

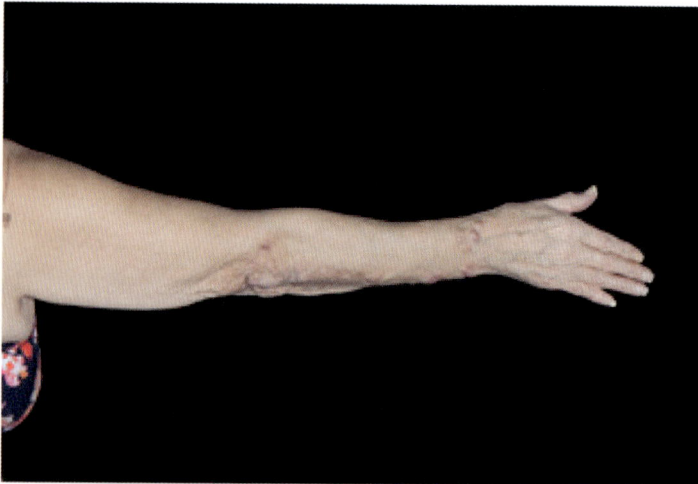

(a)

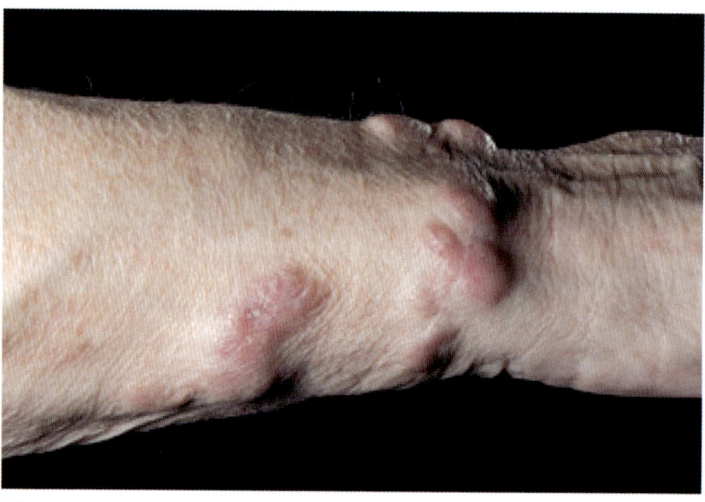

(b)

Figure 53.7 (a,b) Interstitial granulomatous dermatitis in a patient with rheumatoid arthritis.

'urticaria-like' plaques on the dorsa of the hands and arms, extensor aspects of the joints, neck, scalp and trunk are reported in individuals with severe seropositive disease [67]. It should be considered in RA patients who have a biopsy consistent with a dense and diffuse neutrophilic infiltrate in the absence of vasculitis.

The differential diagnosis includes other neutrophilic dermatoses, particularly pyoderma gangrenosum and Sweet syndrome [68–70]. Dapsone, either alone or combined with colchicine, may help rheumatoid vasculitis and neutrophilic dermatosis [71].

Pyoderma gangrenosum
Pyoderma gangrenosum (PG) is a well-established complication of CTDs including RA. The reader is directed to Chapter 49 for a comprehensive review.

Vascular lesions associated with rheumatoid arthritis
RA is associated with a number of vascular pathologies including RP, atherosclerosis, thrombotic risk, vasculitis and leg ulcers [72–74]. RP is associated with numerous autoimmune CTDs, most notably systemic sclerosis and dermatomyositis. Its prevalence is variable in RA but has been reported in 17% [75,76].

Rheumatoid vasculitis
Rheumatoid vasculitis (RV) affects small- and medium-sized vessels and is associated with adverse morbidity and mortality, with studies indicating a 40% mortality at 4 years [77,78]. Incidence of RV appears to be reducing and may reflect improved treatment and reduced smoking rates [55,79]. Anticardiolipin antibodies may be detected, but do not appear to increase risk of thrombotic events [80]. It is hypothesised that immune complex activation, via a type 3 hypersensitivity reaction, results in neutrophil recruitment with endothelial injury [81–83]. Genetic associations have been reported with HLA DRB1*04/04, HLAC03 and KIR2DS2 [59,64,84].

Approximately 90% of patients with RV have cutaneous manifestations and typically high levels of RF and reduced complement levels [85]. Clinical presentation includes livedo reticularis, purpura, atrophie blanche and cutaneous ulcers. Digital lesions are common. The pulps of the fingers show small, painful, purpuric nodules (Bywaters lesions). Initially thought to be a marker for progressive vasculitis, they are now considered benign [86]. Histologically, lesions show leukocytoclastic vasculitis [80]. The

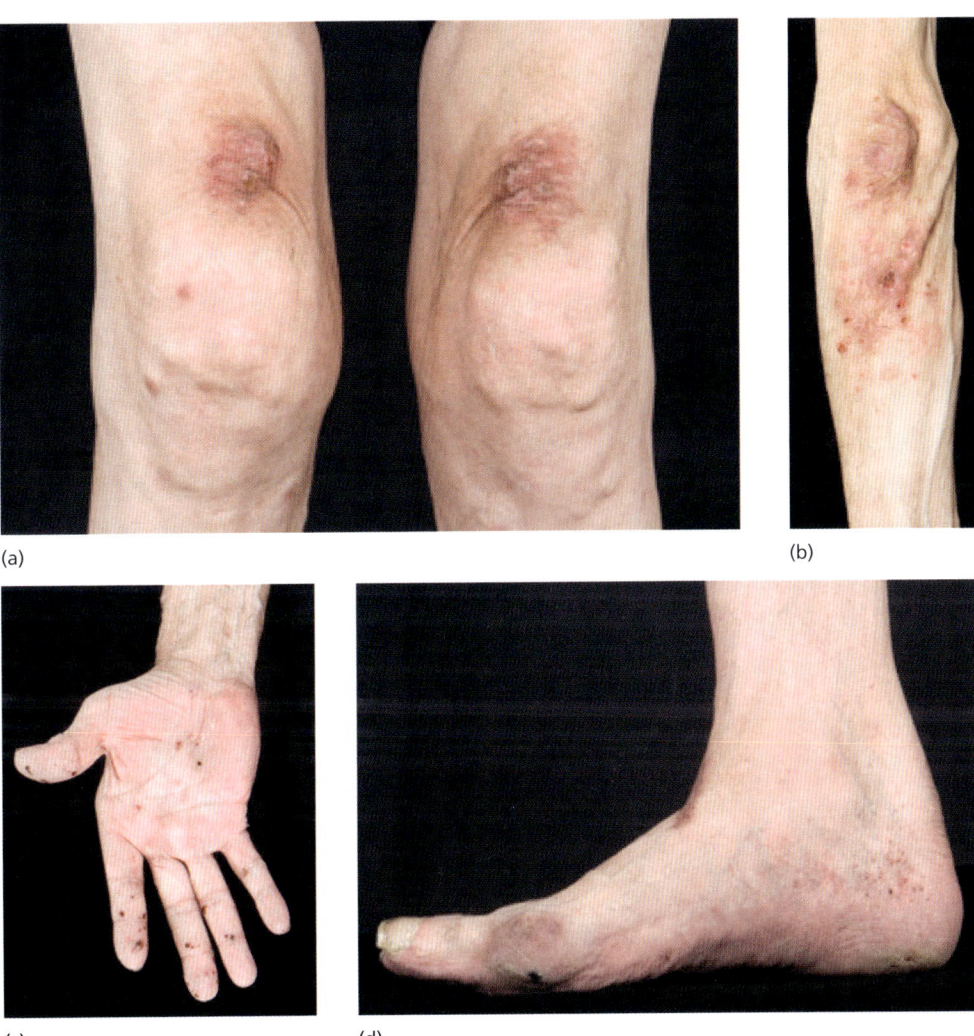

(a)

(b)

(c)

(d)

Figure 53.8 (a–d) Palisaded and neutrophilic granulomatous dermatitis in a patient with rheumatoid arthritis.

occurrence of digital necrosis is closely correlated with the presence of RF and rheumatoid nodules [73,87]. Vasculitis of medium vessels may be indistinguishable from polyarteritis nodosa. The ulcers are well-defined, with a surrounding bluish-red halo, and must be distinguished from pyoderma gangrenosum (Figure 53.9) [88]. Healing occurs with scarring and may be slow [89].

Other manifestations of RV include scleritis, pericarditis, mononeuritis multiplex and gastrointestinal involvement.

Management of RV is difficult due to the lack of clinical trials. Historically, cyclophosphamide was used, although more recently rituximab has developed an established role in management of RA and systemic vasculitides [90].

Leg ulcers

Leg ulcers are a common problem in the elderly and cause significant morbidity with a large financial burden to health care. A single study of 813 patients with RA reported a cumulative incidence of first leg ulcer of 4.8% at 5 years, increasing to 26.2% at 25 years, which was associated with increased mortality, independent of age and sex (HR 2.42; 95%CI 1.71–3.42) [91].

The role of vasculitis in precipitating leg ulceration is complex, in part since clinical overlap with other pathologies is significant [92,93]. Arteritic ulcers are more common in males, particularly

those with subcutaneous nodules and RF. Leg ulcers are more common in Felty syndrome, in which arteritis is associated with splenomegaly, leukopenia, RN and hyperpigmentation [94]. Venous insufficiency, complicated by immobility and postural factors, occurs in nearly half of leg ulcers observed in RA. Other factors include trauma, pressure or arterial insufficiency [92,93,95].

RA-associated leg ulcers are challenging to manage and multidisciplinary input is encouraged. Treatment must ensure adequate dressing support while also considering underlying inflammatory pathologies. Balancing the need for immunosuppression while minimising risk of infection is crucial.

Other dermatological associations of rheumatoid arthritis

Nail changes including ridging (onychorrhexis), clubbing, onycholysis, red lunula and telangiectasia are reported [96]. Palmar erythema has been reported in 18% [97].

Fibroblastic rheumatism

This rare entity, described by Chaouat *et al.* in 1988 [98], occurs at all ages and affects both sexes equally [1,99]. Clinically, it starts suddenly with symmetrical polyarthritis and cutaneous nodules. The nodules are 5–20 cm in diameter and can occur before the onset of arthritis. RP, sclerodactyly, joint effusions and stiffness are

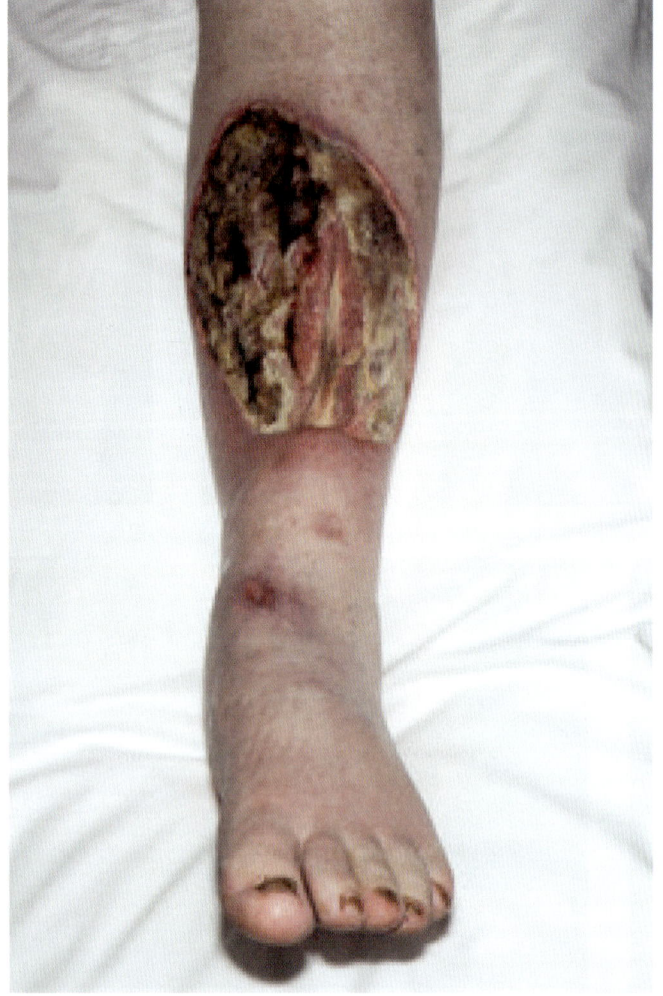

Figure 53.9 Rheumatoid arthritis-associated medium vessel vasculitis. This may be indistinguishable from polyarteritis nodosa on clinical and histological features. Clinical features suggestive of medium vessel vasculitis include the presence of livedo reticularis.

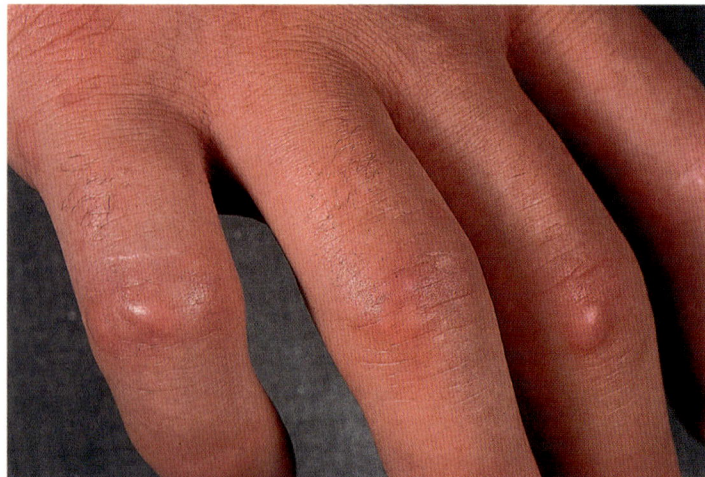

Figure 53.10 Nodules on the dorsa of the interphalangeal joints in fibroblastic rheumatism. Courtesy of Dr M.H.A. Rustin, The Royal Free Hospital, London, UK.

Management

Management of RA is beyond the scope of this chapter, although it is noteworthy that novel therapies have heralded a major advance in disease control and co-morbid disease. A 'treat-to-target' approach to clinical care has resulted in reduced prevalence of typical features of RA and reduction in extra-articular manifestations. Management of vasculitis, PG and leg ulcers overlaps significantly with non-RA manifestations and the reader is directed to the relevant chapter. Evidence supporting treatment of other cutaneous manifestations of RA is limited to case series and often follows treatment of underlying RA disease.

OTHER RHEUMATOID DISEASES

Still disease

Synonyms and inclusions
- Systemic juvenile idiopathic arthritis (SJIA)
- Juvenile rheumatoid arthritis
- Adult-onset Still disease (AOSD)

General description and pathophysiology

Still disease is an inflammatory condition manifest as arthritis associated with daily fevers and rash. Aetiology is unclear, although onset has been linked to various infectious pathogens. In addition to environmental factors, genetic risk has been identified, with a single study reporting association with HLA (HLA)-B17, -B18, -B35 and -DR2 genes [101]. Increasingly it is considered to be part of an autoinflammatory disease spectrum with implicated cytokines including IL-1, -6 and -18 [102].

Clinical features

To consider a diagnosis of Still disease a fever should have been ongoing for a minimum of 2 weeks and arthritis for 6 weeks.

frequent. The nodules occur over the joints including hands, elbows and knees (Figure 53.10). They are smooth, firm and skin coloured. They resolve in 6 months to a few years.

Histology shows a marked proliferation of spindle cells and dermal fibrosis. The hyperplastic cells have the phenotypic features of muscle, suggesting myofibroblastic differentiation [100]. There is a reduction of collagen and non-collagen protein synthesis by the fibroblasts from involved skin, which contrasts markedly with the increase in collagen synthesis in systemic sclerosis. Systemic involvement does not usually occur – all laboratory tests are negative – and spontaneous resolution of the nodules may be expected. Joint erosions may develop and changes tend to persist, despite treatment.

Investigations

Baseline investigations for RA will include serology (including RF and cyclic citrullinated peptide (CCP)), inflammatory markers (erythrocyte sedimentation rate (ESR), C-reactive protein (CRP)) and radiological assessment of the musculoskeletal system. Additional investigations will be guided by clinical presentation.

Table 53.2 Diagnostic criteria for Still disease. Five of the features including at least two major features were >90% specific and sensitive [108].

Diagnostic criteria for Still disease

Major criteria
- Fever
- Arthralgia
- Typical rash
- Leukocytosis

Minor criteria
- Sore throat
- Lymphadenopathy
- Splenomegaly
- Liver dysfunction
- Absence of rheumatoid factor and antinuclear antibodies

The fevers are short lived (<24 hours) and normalise between episodes. There are juvenile (<16 years old) and adult-onset (>16 years old) variants which are increasingly considered part of a disease continuum. Diagnostic criteria are outlined in Table 53.2. Diagnosis may be challenging due to the potential variability in presentation.

Clinical features of SJIA include fever (98%), arthritis (88%) and rash (81%) [103]. Lymphadenopathy is reported in 31%. Constitutional symptoms may be diverse including myalgia, weight loss, pleurisy and pleuritis. Mast cell activation syndrome is reported in approximately 15% of patients with AOSD and can be life threatening [104]. The rash consists of small, non-pruritic salmon-pink macules or papules, with an irregular margin, and is temporally associated with fever. AOSD presents with clinical features similar to those of SJIA with additional features reported including pharyngitis, myalgia and lymphadenopathy [105,106,**107**]. Both sexes are equally affected and the onset is usually in the mid-twenties. Histologically, there is a perivascular dermal infiltrate of lymphocytes and histiocytes. Immunofluorescence is negative. Subcutaneous nodules may occur in Still disease with clinical similarity to RA. The histology resembles that seen in the nodules of rheumatic fever rather than in those of RA [65].

Investigations
Serology is negative. Inflammatory markers are elevated during attacks but often normalise between episodes. This includes ESR, CRP and ferritin. Demonstrating transient elevation in inflammatory markers can be diagnostically helpful. Ferritin levels may be helpful in monitoring activity of disease [109].

Management
Oral corticosteroids (0.5–1 mg/kg/day) are considered first line treatment. Other traditional immunosuppressive therapy such as methotrexate may be considered, although appreciation of Still disease as an autoinflammatory disorder has seen increasing use of targeted therapy including anakinra (anti-IL1RA), canakinumab (anti-IL-1β) and tocilizumab (anti-IL-6) [110–112].

Sjögren syndrome

Synonyms and inclusions
- Gougerot–Houwer–Sjögren syndrome
- Sicca syndrome

Introduction and general description
First described in 1933 by Sjögren, the hallmark feature of this autoimmune disease is dryness of the mucosal surfaces of the eyes (keratoconjunctivitis sicca) and mouth (xerostomia). Inflammation in the salivary, lacrimal and sweat glands may be primary, in which case the exocrine dysfunction occurs alone, or, as secondary Sjögren syndrome (SS), in association with another CTD [113]. In a prospective study of patients presenting with dry eyes 23% had associated CTD [114].

Epidemiology
Incidence of SS has been reported as 7 per 100 000 person-years in a meta-analysis in 2014 [115], although geographic variation may be significant [116,117]. Estimated prevalence is 43 per 100 000 people [115].

The onset occurs most frequently over 40 years old and is rare in childhood [118]. There is a strong female predisposition to disease that varies according to geographic location, with a ratio of 27:1 reported in an Asian study compared with 7:1 in black/African American patients [117].

Pathophysiology
A prominent feature of SS is B-cell hyperactivity with high levels of circulating immunoglobulin. The underlying mechanisms that drive the hyperactivity of B cells remain to be fully defined but environmental factors are considered important. Plasma cells infected by Epstein–Barr virus have been shown to produce Ro and La antibodies [120]. Autoantibodies may be detected 4–6 years before developing symptoms [121]. Innate immune activation of dendritic cells with production of type I interferons promotes immunoglobulin production by B cells, leading to apoptosis of acinar and ductal epithelial cells [122–124]. Recent gene expression profile data from peripheral blood and salivary gland samples demonstrated upregulation of type I interferon-inducible genes and importance of Th17 cells [124–126]. The consequent effect of immune activation through multiple pathways results in cellular injury of glandular tissue with functional impairment.

There is infiltration of salivary and lacrimal glands by lymphocytes and plasma cells with characteristic pathological findings including lymphocyte and plasma cell infiltration, connective tissue proliferation, glandular cell apoptosis, followed by atrophy of glandular structures in affected tissues [122,123].

A genetic predisposition is indicated by the finding of an increased incidence of HLA-B8 and -DR3 in patients with SS [127,128]. Associations with the complement allele C4 AQO and HLA-DRw52 in Japanese patients have been reported [114,128,129]. Recent genome-wide association studies have identified further immune-related loci including L12A, BLK and CXCR5 [130,131].

PART 4: INFLAMMATORY DERMATOSES

Clinical features

The clinical picture is extremely variable although most patients present with a dry mouth and/or dry eyes. A recent study utilising the UK Primary Sjögren's Syndrome Registry (UKPSSR) has reported four clinical subtypes: low symptom burden (LSB), high symptom burden (HSB), dryness dominant with fatigue (DDF) and pain dominant with fatigue (PDF) [132]. This classification recognises the importance of fatigue as a manifestation of SS. Additionally, these clinical and biological subtypes also demonstrated variability in therapeutic response. Other symptoms include a reduction in taste and smell [133]. Lacrimal gland enlargement is unusual in SS and should prompt a search for other differential diagnoses. Manifestations of SS are identified in Box 53.2. The diagnostic criteria, including these features and objective demonstration of exocrine dysfunction, are shown in Table 53.3 [134].

Box 53.2 Manifestations of Sjögren syndrome
[135,136]

- Joint symptoms: arthralgia and arthritis
- Myalgia and myositis
- Sinusitis and hearing problems including deafness
- Tracheal and oesophageal reflux
- Interstitial pneumonitis, pulmonary fibrosis and pulmonary hypertension
- Interstitial nephritis
- Gastrointestinal conditions, including primary biliary cirrhosis
- Fatigue
- Neurological abnormalities: migraine, neuropathies and cerebral vasculitis
- Higher rates of fetal loss

Cutaneous manifestations of Sjögren syndrome
- Xeroderma, pruritus
- Subacute cutaneous lupus erythematosus-like rash
- Annular erythema
- Vasculitis and hypo/hypergammaglobulinaemic purpura
- Raynaud syndrome
- Hyperglobulinaemic purpura and inflammatory vasculitis
- Abnormalities of sweating
- Alopecia – diffuse and generalised
- Erythema nodosum
- Livedo reticularis
- Lichen planus
- Granuloma annulare
- Angular cheilitis

Mucocutaneous features of Sjögren syndrome

The saliva is at first thick and mucoid with salivary volume decreasing through the disease course. The lips and tongue are red, smooth and dry [137]. Dental caries are often severe and chronic candidiasis is common. Recurrent episodes of swelling of one or both parotid glands or, less often, the submaxillary and sublingual glands may be due to inflammation or infection [138]. Mikulicz syndrome, manifest as parotid and lacrimal gland enlargement, may be observed in association with SS. Other causes of Mikulicz syndrome include sarcoid, IgG4-related disease and tuberculosis. Atrophic changes in the mucous membranes of the upper respiratory tract

Table 53.3 Classification criteria for Sjögren syndrome. Adapted from Shiboski *et al.* 2017 [119].

Diagnosis of Sjögren syndrome may be made for an individual who reports symptoms of ocular or oral dryness (Section 1), meets inclusion criteria (Section 2) and does not have any of the alternative diagnoses listed below (Section 3).

Section 1
Questions (1 or more)

1 Have you had daily, persistent, troublesome dry eyes for more than 3 months?
2 Do you have a recurrent sensation of sand or gravel in the eyes?
3 Do you use tear substitutes more than three times a day?
4 Have you had a daily feeling of dry mouth for more than 3 months?
5 Do you frequently drink liquids to aid in swallowing dry food?

Section 2
Inclusion criteria (score of ≥4)   Score

1 Labial salivary gland with focal lymphocytic sialadenitis and focus score of ≥1 foci/4 mm^2 — 3
2 Serology – anti-SSA/Ro positive — 3
3 Ocular staining score ≥5 (or van Bijsterveld score ≥4) in at least one eye — 1
4 Schirmer's test ≤5 mm/5 min in at least one eye — 1
5 Unstimulated whole saliva flow 1 rate ≤0.1 mL/minute — 1

Section 3
Alternative diagnoses

1 Previous head and neck radiation treatment
2 Active hepatitis C infection
3 Acquired immunodeficiency syndrome
4 Sarcoidosis
5 Amyloidosis
6 Graft-versus-host disease
7 IgG4-related disease

---

lead to crusting and dryness, recurrent episodes of infection, hoarseness and/or aphonia [139]. Pulmonary infiltration, atelectasis or fibrosis may occur. Digestive symptoms are attributable to atrophy of the gastric mucous membrane with achlorhydria. Similar changes in the vulva and vagina give rise to pruritus and vaginitis, and dryness of the anal and rectal mucous membranes leads to dyschezia and pruritus.

Skin involvement occurs in 16–67% of patients. The commonest manifestation, often unrecognised, is dry skin, which is reported in two-thirds of patients [140,141]. Other significant features include eyelid dermatitis 42% [142], angular cheilitis 38% [**143**] and pruritus 53% [144]. The xerosis in SS does not appear to be a result of glandular dysfunction but barrier disruption, involving cytokeratins and involucrin [140]. RP is reported in approximately 13% [145].

Annular erythema has been subdivided into three clinical types: (i) Sweet disease-like annular erythema; (ii) subacute cutaneous lupus erythematosus (SCLE)-like [146,147]; and (iii) papular erythema [148]. It may occur in patients with cutaneous lupus or SS and does not appear to be photo aggravated [149]. Recurrent annular erythema is associated with anti-La antibodies [147]. The nail fold capillaries are often abnormal [150].

Purpura and vasculitis are relatively common findings in SS. In a cohort of 558 patients with SS 9.4% (*n* = 52) patients had cutaneous vasculitis [**151**]. Non-thrombocytopenic purpura may occur

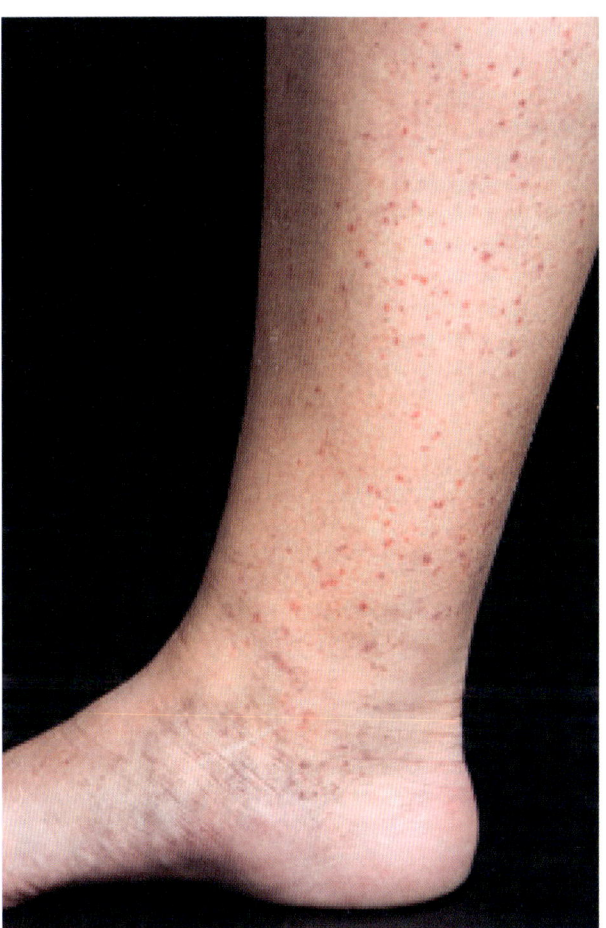

Figure 53.11 Hyperglobulinaemic purpura in a patient with Sjögren syndrome (benign hypergammaglobulinaemic purpura of Waldenstrom).

as recurrent crops of round, pink lesions in dependent areas and typically has a more benign course with negative cryoglobulins. This entity, observed in approximately 50% of patients with vasculitis, has been referred to as benign hypergammaglobulinaemic purpura of Waldenstrom (Figure 53.11) [**151**]. This is thought to be a consequence of B-cell proliferation and may be associated with an elevated ESR, anaemia, leukopenia and polyclonal hypergammaglobulinaemia [152].

Cryoglobulins should be assessed in all patients with SS and vasculitis, which is an independent risk factor for lymphoma and renal involvement. Complement may be normal despite positive cryoglobulins [153].

In patients with ocular or oral dryness the diagnosis is identified early. Infection, salivary stones, tumours of the parotid gland and nasal allergy and inflammation all form part of the potential differential diagnosis. In patients with more insidious onset and varied presentation the diagnosis is frequently not considered.

A number of severity measures have been developed, but the European League Against Rheumatism (EULAR) scoring system is perhaps the best assessed and may be valuable for clinical trial use [154].

The potential complications are many, and include cerebral vasculitis, renal disease and lymphoma, which may occur at any stage and should be suspected in a patient whose symptomatology changes or who becomes generally unwell [155]. Studies suggest the standardised incidence ratio for non-Hodgkin lymphoma in patients is 4.6, 95%CI 3.4–6.0 [156]. Risk factors for lymphoma include IgM kappa monoclonal protein, low complement and cryoglobulins [157].

The disease is chronic, but variably progressive. Some patients have minor persistent sicca symptoms while others will suffer more severe and debilitating disease. Outcome is influenced by any associated CTD, and most significantly by the occurrence of lymphoma [158].

Investigations

Hypergammaglobulinaemia and RF are common, even in patients without arthritis, and serum viscosity is usually raised. ANAs are present in more than 50% of patients. Antibodies to Ro/La have been observed in 53% of patients with SS [113], and along with anti-La/SS-B are an important part of the diagnostic profile of the disease. Anti-Ro antibodies are particularly associated with vasculitis, purpura, lymphadenopathy and haematological and serological abnormalities [133]. Biopsy of the labial salivary glands [148], nasal mucosa [149] and lip may be helpful [146].

Management

It is generally recommended that patients with SS are managed in close collaboration with specialised centres. Evidence-based guidelines have been challenging to develop due to the paucity of clinical trial data, although a recent EULAR task force has provided guidelines for standardisation of care [**159**]. Symptomatic treatment for the dryness of the mucosa and skin is universally required and best managed by lubricating agents (i.e. artificial saliva and tears) and emollients. Additional skin care regimens will be guided by clinical presentation [160]. Lifestyle modification and education are important and should include smoking cessation and avoidance of anticholinergic medications.

Management of systemic disease should be guided by specific symptoms. Oral corticosteroids may be used, generally at a dose of 0.5 mg/kg or less. Treatment with oral corticosteroids should be used cautiously due to the myriad of symptoms associated with long-term use, only for active systemic disease, and should be titrated to 5 mg daily or less where possible. The use of hydroxychloroquine is not currently recommended for symptoms of dryness. Limited data suggest hydroxychloroquine may have a modest role in management of musculoskeletal symptoms associated with SS [161]. With respect to standard immunosuppressive therapies the EULAR task force recommended use of these agents to reduce dependence on corticosteroids with no ability to differentiate leflunomide, methotrexate, azathioprine, mycophenolate mofetil and cyclophosphamide based on available evidence [159]. There is no single therapy that helps hyperglobulinaemic purpura, although graduated compression hosiery may be valuable. While no treatment has so far modified disease progression in SS, B-cell-directed therapies are being investigated [162].

B-cell-directed therapies are increasingly the focus of clinical research with trials including rituximab and ianadumab [163,164]. The current EULAR recommendations are for consideration of rituximab in severe, refractory systemic disease.

Rheumatic fever

Rheumatic fever is a rare systemic inflammatory disease that may occur following untreated streptococcal throat infection. Joint pain, fever and rash may occur 2–4 weeks after infection. Cardiac disease occurs in about half of cases. Erythema marginatum is the characteristic rash of rheumatic fever and occurs in 25% of cases [165]. It appears as evanescent, asymptomatic, pinkish, superficial semicircles and rings, which disappear without scaling or pigmentation in a few days. Histologically, there is a perivascular infiltration of neutrophils in the papillary dermis, and biopsy may help in the early diagnosis of rheumatic fever when the rash precedes arthritis and carditis [166]. Erythema multiforme, petechiae and urticaria may sometimes be seen in rheumatic fever. The overall clinical picture must be distinguished from post-streptococcal reactive arthritis [167].

Subcutaneous nodules occur particularly on the occiput, wrist and the backs of the forearms, and are smaller and more transient than those seen in RA, from which they can be distinguished histologically [168]. Generalised eruptive histiocytomas [169] and erythema elevatum diutinum [169] have also occurred with rheumatic fever.

Key references

The full list of references can be found in the online version at https://www.wiley.com/rooksdermatology10e

1 LeRoy EC, Maricq HR, Kahaleh MB. Undifferentiated connective tissue syndromes. *Arthritis Rheum* 1980;23:341–3.

6 Ungprasert P, Crowson CS, Chowdhary VR, Ernste FC, Moder KG, Matteson EL. Epidemiology of mixed connective tissue disease, 1985–2014: a population-based study. *Arthritis Care Res* 2016;68:1843–8.

7 Gunnarsson R, Molberg O, Gilboe IM, Gran JT, Group PS. The prevalence and incidence of mixed connective tissue disease: a national multicentre survey of Norwegian patients. *Ann Rheum Dis* 2011;70:1047–51.

27 Cheng W, Gilliam AC, Castrovinci A, Pazirandeh M. Anti-thyroid autoantibody-associated interface dermatitis in individuals with undifferentiated connective tissue disease – an unrecognized subset of autoimmune disease? *J Rheumatol* 2007;34:81–8.

48 Yamamoto T. Cutaneous manifestations associated with rheumatoid arthritis. *Rheumatol Int* 2009;29:979–88.

57 Chandrashekara S, Shobha V, Dharmanand BG *et al.* Reduced incidence of extra-articular manifestations of RA through effective disease control: Karnataka Rheumatoid Arthritis Comorbidity (KRAC) study. *Int J Rheum Dis* 2017;20:1694–703.

91 Jebakumar AJ, Udayakumar PD, Crowson CS, Gabriel SE, Matteson EL. Occurrence and effect of lower extremity ulcer in rheumatoid arthritis – a population-based study. *J Rheumatol* 2014;41:437–43.

107 Cozzi A, Papagrigoraki A, Biasi D, Colato C, Girolomoni G. Cutaneous manifestations of adult-onset Still's disease: a case report and review of literature. *Clin Rheumatol* 2016;35:1377–82.

143 Bernacchi E, Amato L, Parodi A *et al.* Sjögren's syndrome: a retrospective review of the cutaneous features of 93 patients by the Italian Group of Immunodermatology. *Clin Exp Rheumatol* 2004;22:55–62.

151 Ramos-Casals M, Anaya JM, Garcia-Carrasco M *et al.* Cutaneous vasculitis in primary Sjögren syndrome: classification and clinical significance of 52 patients. *Medicine* 2004;83:96–106.

159 Ramos-Casals M, Brito-Zeron P, Bombardieri S *et al.* EULAR recommendations for the management of Sjögren's syndrome with topical and systemic therapies. *Ann Rheum Dis* 2020;79:3–18.

CHAPTER 54

Systemic Sclerosis

Catherine H. Orteu[1] and Christopher P. Denton[2]

[1]Department of Dermatology, Royal Free London NHS Foundation Trust, London, UK

[2]Division of Medicine, University College London, London; and Royal Free London NHS Foundation Trust, London, UK

Key references, 54.29

PART 4: INFLAMMATORY DERMATOSES

Definition and nomenclature

Systemic sclerosis is a multisystem autoimmune disease that causes fibrosis in the skin and internal organs with associated vascular and inflammatory manifestations including the Raynaud phenomenon. It has high mortality because of major internal organ complications and substantial morbidity from pain, digital ulceration, calcinosis, telangiectases, and gastrointestinal tract and musculoskeletal involvement [1,2].

Synonyms and inclusions

Systemic sclerosis is one of the scleroderma spectrum disorders and is sometimes referred to as scleroderma. 'Scleroderma' is best kept as an umbrella term for the group of conditions that includes both localised forms (morphoea; Chapter 55) and systemic forms that manifest vascular and internal organ features. Two major subsets of systemic sclerosis, the limited and diffuse forms of the disease, have historically been differentiated based on the extent of cutaneous involvement [3,4]. The term progressive systemic sclerosis is no longer in current usage. In North America the acronym CREST (calcinosis, Raynaud phenomenon, oesophageal dysfunction, sclerodactyly and telangiectasia) is still in use, referring to a subgroup of cases of limited systemic sclerosis (see the section on clinical variants in this chapter). The most generally accepted abbreviation for systemic sclerosis is SSc, with dcSSc and lcSSc used for the diffuse and limited cutaneous forms respectively. The abbreviations lSSc and dSSc have lost favour as more precise subset definitions based on combined skin, antinuclear autoantibody and genetic profiles have been developed (see section on classification). Up to 20% of cases of SSc have features of another autoimmune rheumatic disease and are termed SSc overlap [5–8]. A rare group (2–8%) of SSc cases do not have cutaneous features of skin thickening and are termed SSc *sine* scleroderma [9–12].

Classification

Systemic sclerosis can be reliably defined using validated classification criteria [13]. These criteria provide a weighted score based on specific clinical and immunological features to determine if a patient may be classified as having SSc, but do not define the subset of disease. There is congruity with previous preliminary classification criteria that have been in use for many years [14], but the updated criteria are more sensitive, especially in patients with either early or limited SSc [15]. These criteria take account of better disease assessment and the identification of specific SSc features in investigations such as SSc-specific autoantibodies and/or nail fold capillaroscopy patterns (Table 54.1). Any patient with a score of 9 or more based on the ACR/EULAR 2013 criteria [13] may be classified as definite SSc provided there is no alternative diagnosis that better explains the clinical features (Table 54.1). It should be noted that the classification criteria are weighted for specificity, although operationally they are often used for diagnosis. A diagnosis of SSc could also be made in some cases that do not fulfil the classification criteria, since these have been selected for specificity rather than absolute sensitivity. This is because of their core value to ensure comparable and homogeneous study populations for clinical research.

Subset definition is important and until recently has been based solely upon the extent of skin involvement [3,4]. In lcSSc, which accounts for two-thirds of SSc cases in most series, skin changes occur distally on the limbs, with or without involvement of the head and neck. Involvement of skin areas proximal to the knees or elbows or of the trunk determine dcSSc. In dcSSc, cases have a higher frequency of major internal organ disease, a greater overall mortality and a tendency to maximal activity of the disease within the first 3 years [16]. There is then often greater stability and even improvement of the skin sclerosis. The major features of limited or diffuse subsets are summarised and illustrated in Table 54.2 and Figure 54.1.

One aim of classifying SSc into subsets has been to assist with risk stratification for the development of severe organ-based complications. Increasingly, studies with larger sample sizes have highlighted that there is significant heterogeneity within the cutaneous subsets, and that major complications, such as interstitial lung disease (ILD) can affect up to a third of patients with limited cutaneous disease [18,19]. It has become clear that dividing patients according to cutaneous phenotype alone is not sufficient and alternative models are being sought [17,18]. There are emerging data linking molecular classification from skin biopsy to clinical phenotype in systemic sclerosis [20].

PART 4: INFLAMMATORY DERMATOSES

Table 54.1 Classification criteria for systemic sclerosis.

Item	Subitem	Score
Skin thickening of the fingers of both hands extending proximal to the MCP joints (sufficient criterion)		9
Skin thickening of the fingers (only count the highest score)	Puffy fingers	2
	Thickening (sclerodactyly) distal to MCP but proximal to PIP joints (i.e. whole finger distal to MCP joint)	4
Fingertip lesions (only count the highest score)	Digital tip ulcers	2
	Pitting scars	3
Telangiectasia		2
Abnormal nail fold capillaries		2
Pulmonary arterial hypertension and/or interstitial lung disease		2
Raynaud phenomenon		3
Scleroderma-related antibodies (any of anticentromere, antitopoisomerase-1 (anti-Scl-70) or anti-RNA polymerase III)		3

Total score:
Add the maximum score in each category to calculate total score
Patients having a total score of 9 or more are classified as having definite systemic sclerosis

Adapted from van den Hoogen *et al.* 2013 [**13**]. Reproduced with permission of Wiley. MCP, metacarpophalangeal; PIP proximal interphalangeal.

Table 54.2 Typical features of limited and diffuse cutaneous forms of systemic sclerosis (SSc).

Limited cutaneous SSc	Diffuse cutaneous SSc
ACA+ in >50% of cases	RNAP+ in 25% or ATA+ in >50% of cases
Long history of pre-existing Raynaud phenomenon	Short history or concomitant-onset Raynaud phenomenon
Slower onset and progression of skin sclerosis	Rapid onset and progression skin signs in first 6–18 months Skin disease may plateau and improve in years 2 and 3
Peak skin sclerosis score (MRSS) <14	Peak skin sclerosis score (MRSS) >14
Digital ulcers, calcinosis	Digital ulcers
Lower risk of severe organ-based complications	High-risk of organ-based complications and severe disease
Survival: 88% at 10 years and 61% at 20 years	Survival 72% at 10 years and 40% at 20 years

ACA, anticentromere antibody; ATA, antitopoisomerase; RNAP, anti-RNA polymerase; MRSS, modified Rodnan skin score; Survival data from Nihtyanova *et al.* [**17**].

Autoantibodies are present in 95% of SSc patients at the time of diagnosis, and typically remain unchanged and detectable throughout the course of the disease. Autoantibody patterns in SSc generally include one of the hallmark reactivities including antitopoisomerase-1 antibody (anti-Scl-70 or ATA), anticentromere antibody (ACA), anti-RNA polymerase III antibody (ARA, RNAP or anti-RNApol-III) and others [21–24]. These autoantibody specificities are mutually exclusive of each other in over 99% of patients [17]. They are associated with different risks of complications and appear to cross disease subsets that are based solely on skin (Table 54.3) [25–27]. Thus, while 57% of dcSSc patients are ATA+, this antibody is also present in 20% of cases with limited cutaneous disease. Similarly, >50% of lcSSc patients are ACA+, but this antibody is

also present in up to 10% of patients with dcSSc [19]. This ACA+ dcSSc group has recently been characterised and exhibits an intermediate phenotype between ACA+ lcSSc and non-ACA+ dcSSc [28]. ACA+ patients with dcSSc have a higher incidence of internal organ involvement, ILD, cardiac scleroderma and scleroderma renal crisis (SRC), compared with ACA+ patients with lcSSc. The course of disease in this group was slower than in non-ACA+ dcSSc, with a longer time to peak modified Rodnan skin score (MRSS) and ILD diagnosis, and a comparable overall survival to the ACA+ lcSSc group, confirming a protective role of ACA positivity, even in diffuse cutaneous disease [28]. This highlights the importance of autoantibody specificities in subsetting. Consequently, a more outcome-based classification is now proposed by Nihtyanova *et al.* who have combined autoantibody specificity and extent of skin involvement in a well-defined cohort of 1325 SSc patients and identified seven subsets of patients, allowing more precise risk stratification for organ-based complications and overall mortality (summarised in Table 54.4) [**17**]. This new classification has the advantage of being easy to apply in routine clinical practice.

Another new approach to classification involves using gene expression signatures of skin which are distinct in patients with dcSSc, lcSSc, and normal controls [30]. To date this has shown most promise for the diffuse subset of SSc. Intrinsic gene expression subsets have been identified, including inflammatory, fibroproliferative and normal-like subgroups [30–32]. These subgroups have been used experimentally in clinical trials and correlated with response to immunosuppressive therapies such as mycophenolate, abatacept and nilotinib [33–36]. More recently studies linking SSc autoantibodies (ATA, ARA) with gene expression profiles in skin have identified upregulated pathogenic pathways which differ according to autoantibody subtype and link with cutaneous phenotype, serum markers of fibrosis and progression of disease, particularly in early dcSSc [32,37]. For example, the fibroproliferative subset appears to be enriched for males, African Americans/black individuals and Scl-70 positivity, whereas RNA pol I and III positivity and shorter disease duration appear more likely in the inflammatory subset [20]. The development of a novel and highly accurate, machine-learning based classifier for SSc molecular subsets for individual patient skin samples could now facilitate the targeting of particular therapies to appropriate patient subsets [38].

With improving technologies, signatures based on metabolomics [39–42], radiomics and assessment of the 'exposome' (reviewed in [43]) may in future be combined with cutaneous, autoantibody and genetic profiling, and ultimately integrated using machine learning. These refinements of SSc classification should allow more accurate 'phenome' determination, SSc subsetting, risk assessment and personalisation of SSc care.

Introduction and general description

Systemic sclerosis is rare but important because it has the highest case-specific mortality of any autoimmune rheumatic disease and because it has a major non-lethal burden. Early manifestations are frequently cutaneous and may thus present to dermatology. Awareness of SSc and its cutaneous manifestations is thus paramount for dermatologists, as early diagnosis and treatment leads to markedly improved outcomes. Skin manifestations include thickening or fibrosis, mostly over the extremities and face in

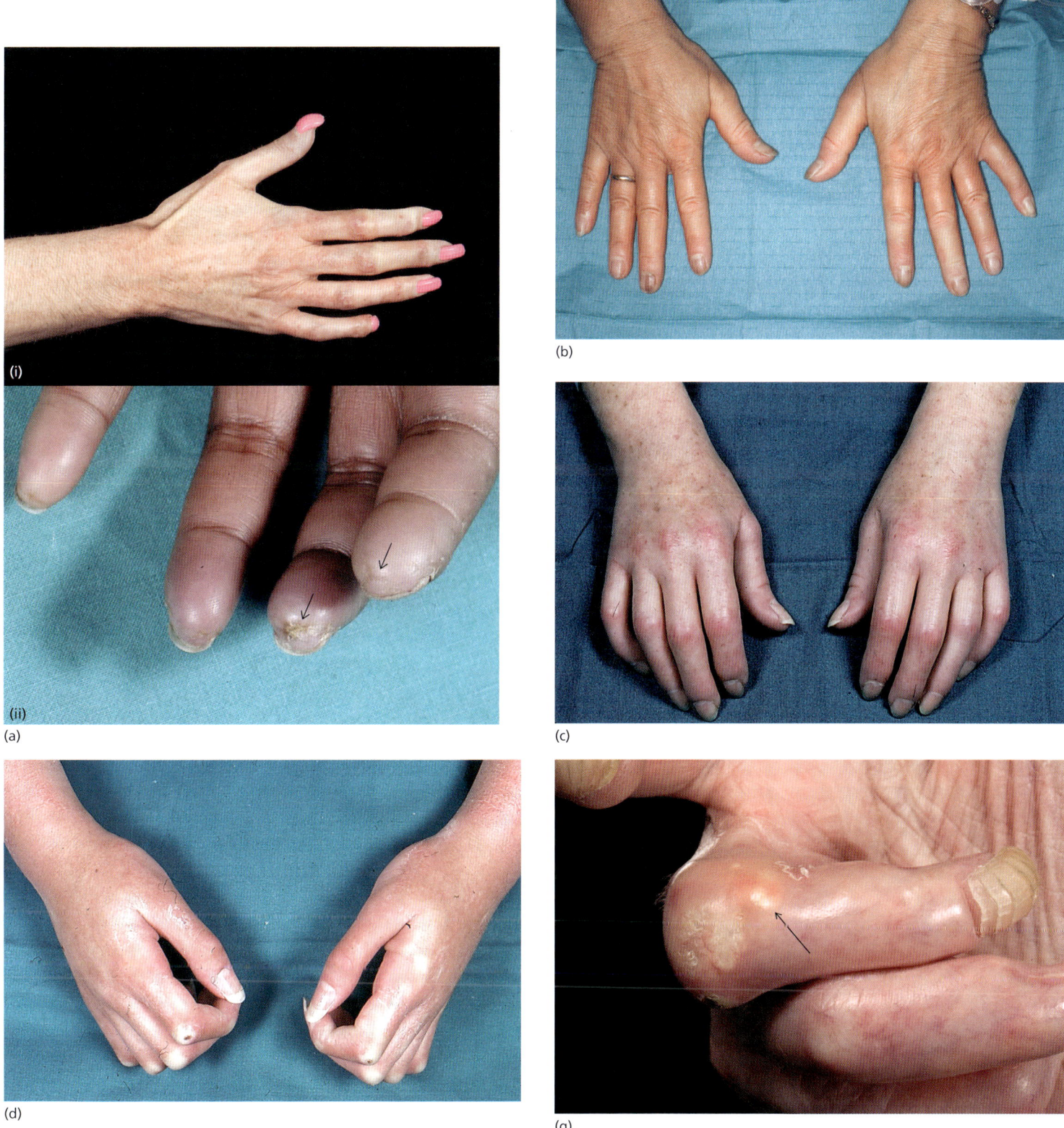

Figure 54.1 Cutaneous features of systemic sclerosis. (a) Raynaud phenomenon showing the typical white discoloration of the fingers caused by vasospasm (i) and bluish discoloration of the fingertips (ring and middle fingers) with digital pitted scars (ii) (arrows). (b) Puffy fingers in early disease. (c) Sclerodactyly and sclerosis extending proximal to the metacarpophalangeal joints. (d) Advanced-stage sclerodactyly with contractures and vasculopathic ulcers over the bony prominences. (e) Loss of fingertip pulps, digital ulceration (*) and pitted scars (arrows). (f) Digital ulceration and necrosis. (g) Advanced disease showing severe flexion contractures and calcinosis (arrow). (h) Typical facial features: note the expressionless facies, mat-like telangiectases, microstomia, perioral furrowing, lip and nasal thinning. (i) Microstomia and sclerosis of the frenulum. (j) Sclerosis of the forearms (i,ii), upper back (iii) and chest (iv) in early progressive antitopoisomerase (Scl-70) positive diffuse disease. (k) Severe sclerosis with contractures and cobblestone appearance (arrow). (l) The abdomen in a white patient with dSSc (diffuse disease) showing mixed hyper- and hypopigmentation. All images courtesy of Dr C.H. Orteu, Royal Free London NHS Foundation Trust.

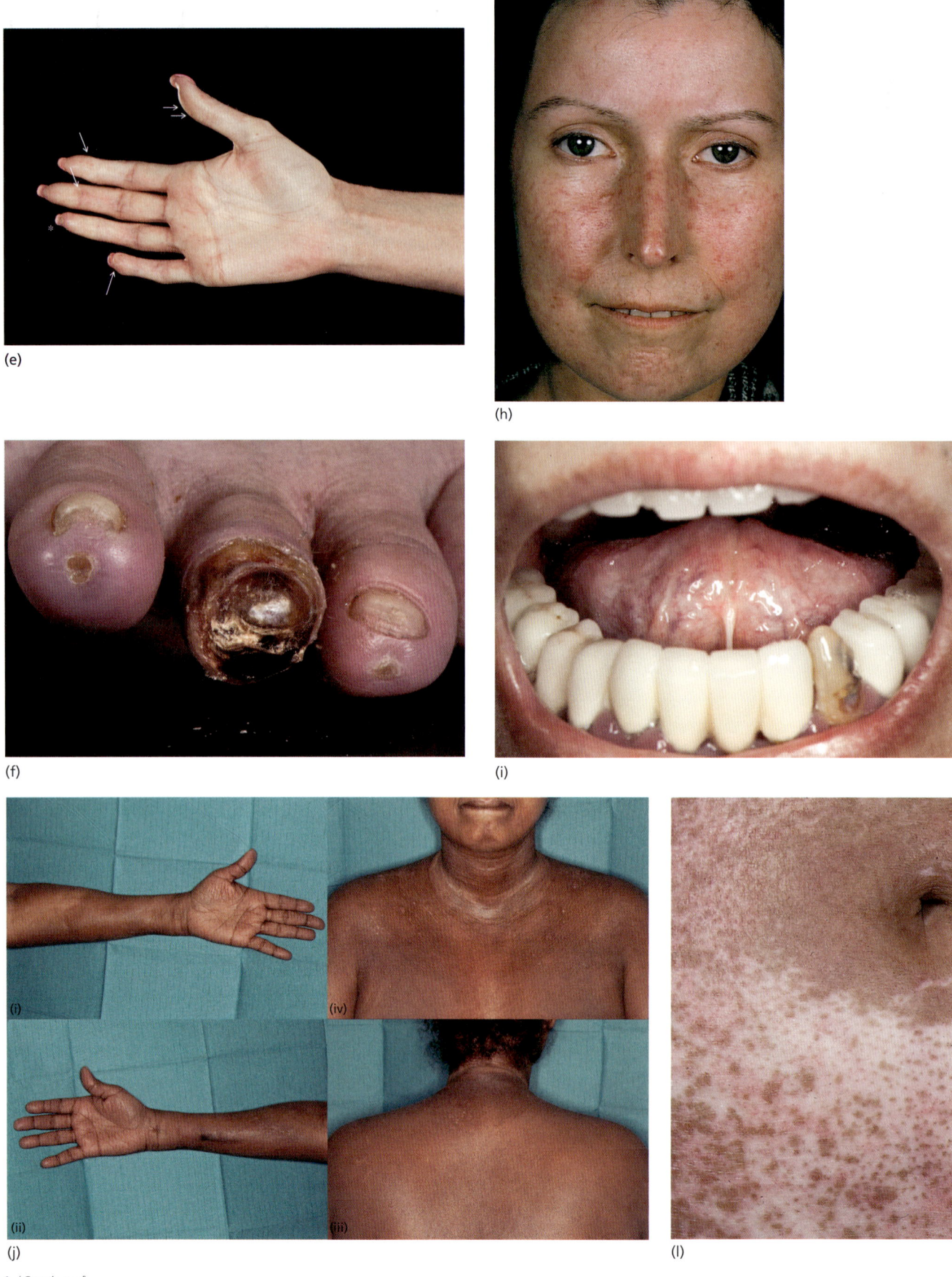

Figure 54.1 (*Continued*)

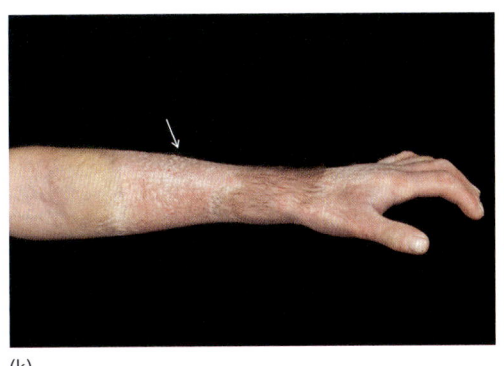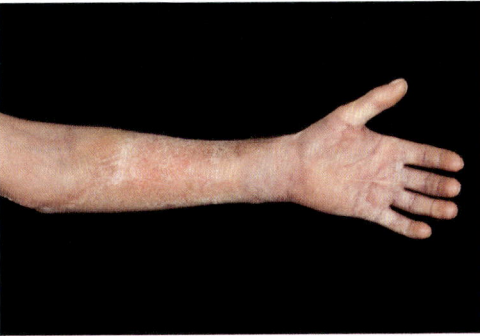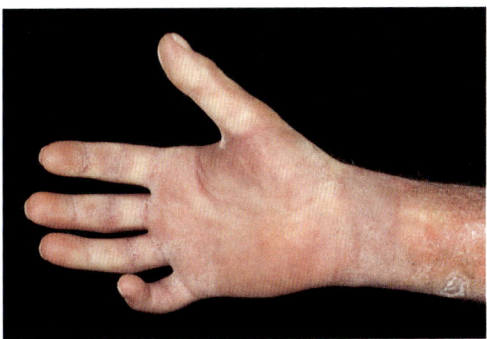

(k)

Figure 54.1 (*Continued*)

Table 54.3 Autoantibodies in systemic sclerosis and their common clinical associations.

Autoantibody	Target antigen	Frequency in SSc cohorts [26]	Skin subset [25]	Clinical features
Antitopoisomerase (ATA, anti-Scl-70)	Topoisomerase-1	9–39%	60–70% are diffuse	Rapid progression of diffuse skin sclerosis High peak skin scores in first 3–5 years Skin may plateau and improve slowly Severe digital vasculopathy/digital ulcers Tendon friction rubs ILD and pulmonary fibrosis ± Severe cardiac disease Secondary pulmonary hypertension Highest overall mortality 80% 10-year, 47% 20-year survival Association with HLA-DQB1*03:01 and DPA1*02:01 Higher prevalence in African Americans
Antiribonucleoprotein (ARA, RNAP)	RNA polymerase III	4–25%	85% are diffuse	Rapidly progressive diffuse skin sclerosis (in first 3 years) Shortest time from first symptom to peak MRSS Highest peak skin scores Skin may plateau and improve over 2–3 years Tendon friction rubs Hypertensive renal crisis (first 3 years) in 14–51% Gastric antral vascular ectasia (watermelon stomach) Risk isolated PAH (late in disease course) Lower risk ILD and cardiac disease High overall mortality 75% 10-year, 47% 20-year survival Association with malignancy (11%) within 36 months of diagnosis Association with HLA-DRB1*11:04 Higher prevalence in white people
Anticentromere (ACA) Two epitopes recognised: centromere A and centromere B	CENP-B protein (centromere protein B)	16–39%	>90% are limited 2.7–7.2% are diffuse [28]	Slow progression of skin sclerosis over years Long history of Raynaud phenomenon (may be >10 years) Frequent digital ulcers Severe gastrointestinal disease +/− malabsorption Isolated PAH in 10–20% (late in disease course) Protective for PF and SRC Lowest overall mortality 89% 10-year, 65% 20-year survival Association with HLA-DRB1*07:01 and DRB1*08:01 Higher prevalence in white people

(*continued*)

PART 4: INFLAMMATORY DERMATOSES

Table 54.3 (continued)

Autoantibody	Target antigen	Frequency in SSc cohorts [26]	Skin subset [25]	Clinical features
Anti-polymyositis-scleroderma (anti-PM-Scl) [29]	PM-Scl-75 and -100	3.6–6%	70% are limited 20–30% are diffuse Found in 33% of patients with SSc/myositis overlap	Overlap syndromes, also found in isolated PM/DM, SLE, Sjögren syndrome and in 9% of patients with isolated inflammatory myopathy Inflammatory myopathy in 60% Gastrointestinal involvement in 63% Pulmonary fibrosis in 57% Inflammatory arthropathy in 38% Calcinosis in 38% Association with malignancy in 20% 96% 10-year, 59% 20-year survival
Antifibrillarin (U3-RNP)	Fibrillarin	1–6%	>50% are diffuse	High peak skin scores Isolated PAH, non-inflammatory myopathy, myositis, gastrointestinal disease and malabsorption, vasculopathy ± Cardiac disease May be rapidly progressive with poor prognosis Younger age at onset Commoner in African Americans – associated with HLA-DRB1*08:04 – and males Higher mortality in first 10 years then stabilises 76% 10-year, 60% 20-year survival
Anti-U1RNP	Directed against the 70 K, A and C proteins associated with U1 RNA	5–35%	80% are limited 20% are diffuse 44% SSc/SLE overlap	Overlap syndromes, arthritis and myositis Occasional but severe PAH and ILD Younger age at onset Commoner in African American and Asian patients 78% 15-year survival Also found in MCTD, SLE, DM/PM and Sjögren syndrome
Th/To directs against subunits of mitochondrial RNA processing and ribonuclease P complexes	Ribonucleoprotein	1–7%	<10% diffuse	Limited skin sclerosis Shorter time from onset Raynaud to puffy fingers compared with ACA+ lcSSc Early PAH (25%) and/or pulmonary fibrosis (45%) Less severe digital vasculopathy Poor prognosis compared with other lcSSc groups Higher prevalence in white people
Anti-U11/U12RNP	Spliceosome components Speckled nuclear staining	1.6–5%	50% are diffuse	Limited data May coexist with anti-U1RNP Pulmonary fibrosis (80%) may be rapidly progressive with high mortality
Anti-Ku	Heterodimer of 70 kD and 80 kD subunits	1–3%	Most are limited	Not specific for SSc (found in other CTDs) Mainly SSc overlap with myositis or SLE features Inflammatory muscle and joint disease Few vascular manifestations Younger age at onset (<40 years)
Anti-RuvBL1/2	Nucleoplasm double hexamer of RuvBL1 and RuvBL2 Speckled nuclear staining	1–2%	Most are diffuse	Mostly males Myositis overlap Occasional cardiac involvement Generally mild internal organ disease

CTD, connective tissue disease; dcSSc, diffuse cutaneous SSc; DM, dermatomyositis; HLA, human leukocyte antigen; ILD, interstitial lung disease; lcSSc, limited cutaneous SSc; MCTD, mixed connective tissue disorders; MRSS, modified Rodnan skin score; PAH, pulmonary arterial hypertension; PF, pulmonary fibrosis; PM, polymyositis; RNP, ribonucleoprotein; SSc, systemic sclerosis; SLE, systemic lupus erythematosus; SRC, scleroderma renal crisis. Data from Bruni *et al*. [29], Caetano *et al*. [28], Steen [25] and Nihtyanova *et al*. [26]. Table courtesy of Dr C.H. Orteu.

Table 54.4 Outcome-based classification of SSc. Combining skin and autoantibody profiles identifies seven subsets and allows improved stratification of risk of complications and mortality in SSc.

Cutaneous subset	SSc-specific autoantibody	Prevalence	Survival at 10 and 20 years	Risk of complication (cumulative incidence at 20 years)			
				Pulmonary fibrosis	**Scleroderma renal crisis**	**Cardiac scleroderma**	**Pulmonary hypertension**
LcSSc	ACA	28.2%	**Highest 89.3%/65.3%**	*Lowest 8.5%*	***Lowest 0.3%***	*Low 4.9%*	Cohort mean* 20.4%
lcSSc	ATA	10.4%	**2nd highest 89.1%/61.8%**	**Highest 86.1%**	*Low 3.8%*	Cohort mean 7%	***Lowest 6.9%***
dcSSc	ATA	11.3%	*Lowest 72%/32.4%*	**2nd highest 84%**	Cohort mean 8.3%	**2nd highest 12.9%**	*Low 15.3%*
dcSSc or lcSSc	Anti-RNAP	11.1%	Cohort mean 76.4%/47.1%	Cohort mean 44.5%	**Highest 28.1%**	*Lowest 2.2%*	Cohort mean 23.3%
dcSSc or lcSSc	Anti-U3RNP	4.2%	Above cohort mean 76%/60.5%	*Low 21.5%*	Cohort mean 11%	**Highest 13.2%**	**Highest 33.8%**
lcSSc	Other	22.3%	Cohort mean 87.1%/56.2%	Cohort mean 53.9%	*Low 2.7%*	*Low 2.4%*	Cohort mean 24.3%
dcSSc	Other	12.5%	*2nd lowest 68.3%/33.6%*	Cohort mean 53.8%	Above cohort mean 15.6%	Above cohort mean 8.4%	Above cohort mean 16.4%

ACA, anticentromere; ATA, anti-topoisomerase; Anti-RNAP, anti-RNA polymerase; ENA, anti-extractable nuclear antigens. 'Other' includes ANA+ENA-, U1RNP, Th/To, SL, Ku, Jo1, Ro, La, XR, PL-7, heterogeneous nuclear RNP and SM antibodies and ANA- patients. 'Cohort mean' signifies 'at or around' the mean level for the whole cohort ($n = 1325$). Table Courtesy of Dr C.H. Orteu adapted from data in Nihtyanova et al. [17].

limited forms of SSc and much more extensively in diffuse cases. Associated features include severe pruritus, digital ulceration, telangiectasia, calcinosis, diffuse hyperpigmentation and 'salt and pepper' dyspigmentation [1] (Figure 54.1). While skin signs will aid diagnosis, SSc is a systemic multisystem disease, thus the main focus of investigation and treatment needs to be on manifestations beyond the skin. Typically, a patient will present with Raynaud phenomenon and symptoms of gastro-oesophageal reflux. This is followed by a phase of non-pitting digital oedema, after which the skin thickens, and sclerodactyly develops. Inflammatory musculoskeletal symptoms may also be present at this stage. These may be the main features, but severe internal organ manifestations such as cardiac, lung or renal complications are a major concern and may already be present at the time of presentation to a specialist. Systematic investigation and treatment of these complications is mandatory for all new cases of SSc and is a cornerstone of modern management.

Epidemiology
Incidence and prevalence
Historically it has been difficult to determine precise or accurate incidence or prevalence figures for SSc. Key factors that have confounded assessment are disease rarity, clinical heterogeneity, case definition and the methodology used to assess frequency [44–46]. This especially reflects whether a population-based or hospital-based approach is used. Subset distribution should also be considered, as it is more likely that diffuse disease will present early and be diagnosed, compared with limited SSc. In the UK, a historical cohort study using data from the GP clinical practice research datalink has estimated the annual incidence of SSc to be 19.4 per million person years between 1994 and 2013. Prevalence was estimated at 307 per million population in 2013 [47,48].

A review of 32 publications from 1969 to 2006 found a range of prevalence from 7 per million to 489 per million, and incidences of 0.6 per million per year to 122 per million per year [46]. A systematic review of 50 publications from 2000 to 2016 found a prevalence of 7.2–33.9 per 100 000 individuals and 13.5–44.3 per 100 000 individuals in Europe and North America respectively. The annual incidence estimates were 0.6–2.3 per 100 000 individuals and 1.4–5.6 per 100 000 individuals in Europe and North America

Table 54.5 Geographical variation in pooled prevalence and incidence rates of systemic sclerosis.

Geographical area	Pooled prevalence rate per 100 000 individuals	Pooled incidence rate per 100 000 person-years
Africa	N/A	0.2
Asia	6.8	0.9
Europe	14.8	1.0
Oceania	23.8	1.6
South America	24.8	1.5
North America	25.9	2.0

Adapted from Bairkdar et al. [44].

respectively [45]. A more recent systematic review of English language literature to October 2020 found an overall global pooled prevalence of 17.6 per 100 000 individuals (range 3.1–144.5) and an overall pooled incidence rate of 1.4 per 100 000 person years [44]. The significant geographical variation identified (Table 54.5) corroborates with previous suggestions that prevalence in Europe is higher than in Japan and other Asian populations, but lower than in the USA [49–52]. The highest rate described has been in Choctaw American Indians and is likely to have a genetic basis [53]. Geographical clustering may equally be influenced by environmental factors as has been suggested for sporadic clusters of increased prevalence seen, for instance, within areas of London, Rome and Ontario [46,54]. In the UK incidence appears to have remained stable over the 20-year period from 1994 to 2013 [48]. Worldwide, however, there seems to be a trend toward an increase in the incidence of SSc over time, but this tendency is unproven because of lack of uniformity in study method and design [44].

Age
Although SSc may occur at any age it is very rare in childhood (the UK incidence rate is 0.27 per million per year [55]) and is most often seen in young and middle-aged adults. There may be two peaks of onset, between 25 and 40 years of age (predominantly in women), and between 45 and 60 years of age. Overall, the mean age of onset of SSc in many cohort studies is estimated at 45–55 years. Men may develop disease on average a little later than this [56].

There appear to be distinct clinical presentations and outcomes in patients with later-onset disease, with those presenting over the age of 60 years of age suffering more frequently from the limited subtype, pulmonary hypertension and cardiovascular disease, and less often with digital ulcers [57–59]. This older age group may, however, exhibit more rapid disease progression and higher mortality [59–62]. Patients with onset in childhood are more likely to have limited or overlap forms of the disease and a better overall survival [63–66]. An exception to this may be children with SSc *sine* scleroderma who seem to have poorer outcomes linked to delayed diagnosis and cardiac involvement [9].

Sex

Overall, there is a four- to five-fold female predominance in SSc [44,48,67,68]. This predominance is most marked in premenopausal women [69,70]. Female reproductive hormones, fetal microchimerism, X-linked genetic factors such as skewed inactivation, X-linked non-coding RNA and X-linked nucleotide polymorphisms, as well as environmental/occupational exposures, may influence the differences in prevalence and outcomes [70]. *In vitro* studies have shown increased cell growth and fibronectin synthesis by scleroderma fibroblasts exposed to female sex hormones [71,72]. Agonist antibodies to oestrogen receptors have been identified in SSc sera and are associated with diffuse disease and nail fold capillary changes [73]. A recent review of the available evidence suggests that oestradiol plays a profibrotic role, but also has a vasodilatory effect at macrovascular level. The proposed protective role of female hormones on the development of pulmonary arterial hypertension (PAH) and the increased prevalence of PAH in males and postmenopausal females are consistent with this [69]. The effects of androgens have been more difficult to elucidate [69]. However, males are more likely to have diffuse disease (50%), anti-topoisomerase antibodies, ILD and a higher mortality [49,61,74,75]. They are at greater risk of developing scleroderma heart disease, SRC, digital vasculopathy, digital ulcers and digital gangrene (reviewed in [76]).

Ethnicity

All ethnic groups can be affected by SSc but there are apparent differences in the clinical features and subgroups that occur in different populations [50,67,77–81]. Some of these differences may correlate with immunogenetic and ANA differences between populations [81–83]. Patients' perception of disease severity and their perceived mental and physical functioning may also vary according to ethnic background [84,85]. A multicentre cohort of 1009 African American SSc cases found a younger age at symptom onset, and higher prevalence of diffuse disease, of scleroderma cardiac disease, pulmonary fibrosis and SRC compared with European cohorts [81]. African American women appear twice as likely as white women to have diffuse disease [86], and African American patients have increased mortality; 43% at 10 years compared with 35% among white patients [87]. These findings have been confirmed by other groups who have shown a higher prevalence of anti-U3-RNP, anti-U1-RNP and ATA antibodies, which are associated with a worse prognosis in African Americans and more ACA antibodies in white people [78,79,87–89]. ATA positivity is also more prevalent in Chinese (59.9%), Korean (62.2%) and Thai (76%) SSc cohorts and

this has been associated with diffuse disease, and with pulmonary fibrosis in cases of Han Chinese descent [90]. Conversely, the frequency of anti-RNA pol III positivity and SRC appears to be less common in Chinese and East Asian populations [49,90,91].

Increasing evidence suggests that ethnicity is associated with specific HLA subtypes and that HLA may determine SSc-specific autoantibody specificities. For example, in North American white and Hispanic subjects, strong positive associations have been found with the DRB1*1104, DQA1*0501, DQB1*0301 haplotypes and DQB1 alleles encoding a non-leucine residue at position 26, while the DRB1*0701, DRB1*1501, DQA1*0201, DQB1*0202 haplotypes appeared protective against the development of SSc. SSc in African American subjects was associated with DRB1*0804, DRB1*11:02 and DQA1*0501, DQB1*0301 alleles [83,92]. HLA-DRB1*15:02 and DRB5*01:02 alleles have been associated with SSc in Thai patients while HLA-DRB1*04 was protective [93]. A systematic review of studies examining the association with HLA-DRB1 allele polymorphisms indicates that DRB1*11:01 and DRB1*13:01 confer a protective effect in white populations, but DRB1*11:04 was associated with a higher risk of SSc, while in Asian populations, DRB1*13:02 was found to be a protective factor [94]. The presence of different scleroderma-specific antibodies (e.g. ATA, ACA and RNAP) has also been linked to different HLA-DR and -DQ haplotypes in particular ethnic groups [92,94,95]. Gourh *et al.* found HLA-DRB1*0804 strongly associated with the antifibrillarin (U3RNP) positive subset of SSc in African Americans and HLA-DPB1*13:01 with the ATA+ subset in African and European Americans, while HLA-DRB1*07:01 was associated with ACA+ subsets in European Americans [83]. Interestingly, there was a direct correlation between SSc prevalence and HLA-DPB1*13:01 frequency in several populations around the world [83,**96**]. Ethnic differences are also seen for associations with non-MHC genes, such as *FBN1* (fibrillin) genes, in Choctaw American Indians and the Japanese, and *SPARC* (osteonectin) in white, Hispanic and Choctaw people [97–99]. These findings support the notion that race is related to distinct immunological and phenotypic profiles in SSc.

Associated diseases

Other autoimmune disease. A systematic review and meta-analysis of 10 studies published between 1960 and 2013, corresponding to a total of 6102 SSc patients, identified a second autoimmune disease in 25% of SSc cases and a third in 4%. The most common associations were autoimmune thyroid disease (AITD, 10.4%), Sjögren syndrome (SjS, 7.7%) and dermatomyositis/polymyositis (5.6%) [100]. Primary biliary cirrhosis, rheumatoid arthritis (RA) and systemic lupus erythematosus (SLE) have also, but less frequently, been associated. The presence of another autoimmune disease was more common in patients with the limited subtype and relatively mild disease [101]. In a study of 719 Canadian and Columbian SSc patients, 36% of patients had first-degree relatives with at least one autoimmune disease, of which the most frequent were RA (18%) and AITD (9%) [102].

Overlap connective tissue disorders. Systemic sclerosis can occur as a component of an overlap connective tissue disorder such as mixed connective tissue disease (MCTD) [15,103–105], and in SSc

Table 54.6 Type and frequency of autoantibodies in 332 patients with systemic sclerosis (SSc) overlap syndromes.

SSc overlap syndromes	Autoantibody	Percentage of patients
All (100%)	ANA	>95%
	Rheumatoid factor	>50%
	ACA	13%
	ATA (Scl-70)	17%
	RNAP	<5%
	U3-RNP	<6.5%
Myositis (43%)	Anti-PmScl	33%
	Jo1	6%
	Anti-Ku	2%
Rheumatoid arthritis (32%)	Anti-CCP	58%
Sjögren syndrome (17%)	ACA	45%
	Ro	30%
SLE (8%)	U1-RNP	44%

Data from Pakozdi et al. 2011 [7].
ACA, anticentromere antibody; ANA, antinuclear antibody; anti-CCP, anticyclic citrullinated peptide antibody; anti-PmScl, antipolymyositis/scleroderma antibody; ATA, antitopoisomerase antibody; RNAP, RNA polymerase; RNP, ribonucleoprotein; SLE, systemic lupus erythematosus.

cohorts 10–20% of cases have features of overlap with another autoimmune rheumatic disease [6–8,81]. Such patients exhibit features of at least two connective tissue diseases (CTDs) concomitantly and present a highly heterogeneous group of disorders with prevailing clinical features of SSc. A diagnosis of SSc overlap syndrome is usually made when manifestations of myositis, arthritis or another autoimmune rheumatic disease are much greater than normally seen in SSc. In a single-centre UK study of 1700 SSc patients, 20% had SSc overlap syndromes – the commonest SSc overlap was with myositis (42.8%), followed by RA (32%), SjS (16.8%) and SLE (8.4%) [6]. The proportion of overlap patients with lcSSc and dcSSc was similar to that seen in the SSc population: 71.7% and 27%, respectively. Patients with myositis overlap, however, were more likely to have dcSSc. Distinct autoantibody profiles appear associated with specific clinical presentations and disease courses (Table 54.6). In the UK study, while ANA was positive in 96.6% overall, myositis overlap patients exhibited antipolymyositis/scleroderma antibody (anti-PmScl) in 33%, anti-Jo1 antibody in 6% and anti-Ku antibody in 2%. In 94% of myositis overlap cases anti-PmScl was the only additional antibody. Anticentromere antibody was absent and antitopoisomerase infrequent in this group. Anticentromere antibodies (45%) and anti-Ro antibodies (30%) were commonest in the Sjögren syndrome overlaps. Anti-U1-RNP was significantly more frequent in SLE overlaps (44%). Rheumatoid factor was unhelpful, being positive in 50% of patients, but anticyclic citrullinated peptide antibody (anti-CCP) was more frequent in patients with RA features [6].

It has been suggested that SSc overlap patients should be considered a distinct subset of the disease, since in addition to their specific autoimmune profiles, they also exhibit differential expression of genes involved in iNOS and toll-like receptor signalling in blood and appear to run a slightly different disease course [106]. In the German SSc registry, which includes 3240 patients from multiple centres, 10% had SSc overlap syndromes and this group of patients developed earlier and more extensive musculoskeletal

disease. Pulmonary fibrosis and heart disease occurred earlier than in lcSSc but later than in dcSSc; oesophageal and renal disease, and pulmonary hypertension, ran a similar course to that in lcSSc [8]. Current evidence suggests that patients with SSc-myositis and SSc-Sjögren syndrome overlaps may have a worse overall prognosis and mortality [5,107], whereas those with SSc-SLE overlap may be younger, have more PAH, but show a tendency towards better median survival [108].

There has been controversy concerning MCTD as a separate entity because of its heterogeneous clinical manifestations and the fact that a subgroup of patients evolve into another CTD during disease progression. It consists of a combination of Raynaud phenomenon, puffy fingers, polyarthritis, oesophageal dysmotility and myositis, in association with anti-U1-RNP antibodies and antibodies against U1-70KD small nuclear ribonucleoprotein (snRNP). PAH and ILD can develop with time and result in increased mortality [103,104]. Up to 10% of patients with MCTD meet the 2013 ACR/EULAR criteria for SSc [15] and in over 20% either SLE or SSc may develop over 10 years. Cluster analysis has revealed three patient groups: one with associated antiendothelial cell and anticardiolipin antibodies who have an increased frequency of PAH, venous thrombosis and cerebrovascular disease; a second with myositis, oesophageal dysmotility and pulmonary fibrosis; and a third with erosive arthropathy, osteoporotic fractures and anti-CCP antibodies [109]. Initial clinical features and autoantibody profiles can be useful for predicting disease evolution [105,109].

Malignancy. Malignancies are reported for between 3.6% and 10.7% of patients diagnosed with SSc [110] and have been associated with older age at SSc onset, male sex and certain SSc-specific autoantibodies (reviewed in [111]). In 2013, three meta-analyses were published examining the incidence of cancer in SSc [112–114]. The conclusions varied according to whether population-based cohort studies, observational studies or all published articles linking SSc to the risk of cancer development were included in the analyses. Overall, an increased risk of cancer in SSc was demonstrated. The pooled standardised incidence rates (SIR) from population-based cohort studies was 1.41 (95% confidence interval (CI) 1.18–1.68) and this was higher in men (1.85 95% CI 1.49–2.31) than women (1.33 95% CI 1.18–1.49) [113]. Interestingly, in this analysis, the pooled SIR increased to 2.79 (95% CI 1.81–4.31) for cancers diagnosed within the first year after SSc diagnosis. An increased risk of lung cancer, non-Hodgkin lymphoma and haematopoietic cancer was confirmed in all three meta-analyses, while an increased risk of bladder (SIR 2.0) and liver cancer (SIR 4.36) was only found in one [113]. The relation with breast cancer, suggested in some previous epidemiological studies, was not confirmed in these meta-analyses. However, in 2014 a large, retrospective, single-centre UK study of 2177 SSc patients identified 7.1% with cancer, the major subtypes being breast (42.2%), haematological (12.3%), gastrointestinal (11.0%) and gynaecological (11.0%) [115]. Other published associations have included oesophageal, oro-pharyngeal and non-melanoma skin cancers [116]. The reason why men with SSc seem to be at greater risk of developing cancer than women is poorly understood and often attributed to cytotoxic therapies or damage from scleroderma [113,117]. Recognition that some patients have a close temporal relationship between cancer diagnosis and clinical onset of SSc has raised the possibility that it may be a paraneoplastic syndrome in a subset of patients [118,119].

Earlier suggestions of increased cancer risk in patients with lcSSc and ACA positivity have not been confirmed [115,120–122]. Indeed, the presence of anticentromere autoantibodies has now been associated with a lower risk of cancer in patients with limited SSc [123]. In contrast, anti-RNA polymerase III (RNAP) antibodies have been associated with cancer in some SSc cohorts, particularly breast cancer in females and in patients presenting within 36 months of SSc diagnosis [115,124–126]. A unique nucleolar RNAP expression pattern has been identified in malignant tissue from some such SSc patients suggesting that autoantigen expression in the cancer and the autoantibody response are associated [127]. This theory is further supported by the presence of missense mutations in the *RPC155/POLR3A* gene in the cancer tissue and mutation-specific T-cell responses in SSc patients with RNAP antibodies, but not in those with ATA or ACA [119]. This has led to the suggestion that malignancy may initiate the SSc-specific immune response and drive disease in this subset of patients. In a different cohort of Canadian patients, ATA and anti-U1RNP, but not anti-RNAP antibodies were associated with increased cancer risk within 2 years of diagnosis [128]. A further group of patients with a similar temporal clustering of SSc and cancer diagnoses has been identified that is ANA positive but negative for the most commonly known SSc autoantibodies (ATA, ACA and RNAP) suggesting that other autoantigens of relevance to the cancer–SSc relationship remain to be defined [123,126]. A recent association with PMScl positivity supports this [29] and suggests a more generic role for tumour directed autoimmunity in SSc aetiopathogenesis. Interestingly, some ANA patterns, including antibodies to the large subunits of RNApol I and III, and to Th/To, appear to be associated with reduced cancer risk and this may have implications for antitumour immune response [129,130].

Pathophysiology

Predisposing factors. The aetiology of SSc is poorly understood. It is likely that the disease occurs in a multistep process, as a consequence of triggering events, in a susceptible individual. Gender, ethnicity and environmental exposures are clearly important. Robust data now support genetic susceptibility factors including a strong HLA association, particularly with DPB1, DRB1 and DQB1 haplotypes, and also altered immune inflammatory genes, especially within the innate immune system (see the section on genetics). The significance of epigenetic modifications is now evident but requires further investigation.

Pathology. The pathology of SSc includes three major facets: vasculopathy; immune-mediated inflammation, involving innate and adaptive immunity; and fibrosis. Exactly how these interact to cause disease is not yet fully understood but there has been significant progress in the last decade and multiple pathogenic mechanisms and different cell types are implicated.

Vasculopathy. The earliest pathological change is microvascular injury with a reduction in capillary density and evidence of endothelial cell (EC) activation [131–133]. Recognised triggers for EC damage include infection, immune-mediated cytotoxicity, antiendothelial autoantibodies, reactive oxygen species and ischaemia-reperfusion injury. Injured ECs may then either undergo apoptosis, endothelial-to-mesenchymal transition (endo-MT) or other forms of activation [134–136]. EC apoptosis results in damage to vessel walls and, because of impaired angiogenesis in SSc, ultimately leads to loss of capillaries with associated tissue ischaemia. EC activation leads to increased endothelin-1 and chemokine production, and impaired nitric oxide and prostacyclin release, resulting in vasospasm. In addition, upregulated expression of cytokines and adhesion molecules facilitates early perivascular infiltration with monocytes/macrophages [137] followed by T and B cells [138,139], dendritic cells [140], and mast cells promoting inflammation [**135**,141]. Vascular injury also activates platelets not only promoting intravascular fibrin deposition and luminal narrowing, but also providing B-cell co-stimulation, platelet-derived growth factor (PDGF), CXCL-4 and TGF-β release [142,143]. Further, thrombin activates Th2 cells, stimulates fibroblast proliferation and myofibroblast transition, also suggesting a role for coagulation in inflammatory and immune responses in SSc [144,145].

Endothelial-to-mesenchymal transition. Endo-MT is a process by which vascular EC transdifferentiate into profibrotic myofibroblasts. Cell–cell junctions and EC markers, such as Von Willebrand factor (vWF), CD31 and vascular endothelial-cadherin (VE-cadherin) are lost, and cells acquire contractile, 'invasive' properties associated with the gain of mesenchymal markers, such as α-smooth muscle actin (α-SMA), smooth muscle 22 (Sm22), and collagen1 (Col1A1). Endo-MT can be triggered by cytokines and growth factors including TGFβ, endothelin-1, IL-1β, tumour necrosis factor α (TNF-α), notch and wnt ligands, IFN, miRNA, caveolin 1 deficiency, hypoxia and oxidative stress [134,146]. In small arteries and arterioles endo-MT results in myofibroblast accumulation in the media and subintima, thickening of the vessel wall and luminal narrowing. This obstructive vasculopathy may ultimately lead to digital ulcers, PAH, SRC and cardiac manifestations of SSc. In thin-walled capillaries, endo-MT results in wall damage because of loss of EC, which migrate out into the perivascular space as myofibroblasts, causing tissue fibrosis and a destructive vasculopathy, as is seen in nail fold capillaries in SSc [147,148]. While their relative contributions are as yet uncertain, pericytes, vascular smooth muscle cells, adipocytes, epithelial cells, macrophages and possibly lymphatic endothelial cells, may also transdifferentiate into myofibroblasts and contribute to fibrosis in SSc [136].

Immune-mediated inflammation. Recent studies have identified monocytes and macrophages as key drivers of inflammation and fibrosis in SSc, highlighting the role of innate immunity [149]. Pro-inflammatory M1 macrophages induced by Th1 cytokines, IFN and TLR4 are prominent in the very early stages of disease. Profibrotic M2 macrophages induced by Th2 cytokines IL-4 and IL-13 are able to secrete TGF-β, FGF, CCN2, PDGF and CCL18 and participate a little later [150,151]. Impaired efferocytosis, that is a reduced ability of macrophages to phagocytose apoptotic debris, may promote chronic inflammation and also drive autoantibody formation through failed clearance of autoantigens exposed on damaged or apoptotic cells [152]. The role of the epidermis has until recently been underestimated [153]. In the early stages of SSc, the epidermis shows a wound healing phenotype, with upregulated expression of keratin 6 and 16, IL-1-α and connective tissue growth factor (CCN2) [154] and with partial epithelial–mesenchymal transition [155]. There is cross-talk between the activated or altered epidermal keratinocytes and dendritic cells, vasculature and fibroblasts. NF-κB upregulation and/or PPAR-g inhibition, and upregulation of IL-6, TNF-α and CCL5 expression in keratinocytes correlate with skin score in SSc [153,156]. Endothelial cell and keratinocyte derived IL-1 can modulate fibroblast properties increasing endothelin-1 and TGF-β production and promoting longevity in myofibroblasts [157,158]. Cytokines, including IL-4,6,8,10,13 and 17, TGF-β, PDGF and endothelin-1 are all overexpressed in skin [**135,159**]. Dermal mast cells, another source of TGF-β, are increased in number in early disease and have been associated with more severe sclerosis and ATA positivity in dSSc [160,161]. Mast cell degranulation and abnormalities of lymphatic drainage may both contribute to the oedema and the pruritus associated with active disease [162]. Lymphatic microangiopathy has been linked to the progression of skin involvement and a progressive disappearance of lymphatic vessels occurs in late SSc [163].

There is some evidence for a functional role of autoantibodies in systemic sclerosis pathogenesis. For the diagnostic ANA patterns, evidence is strongest for anti-topoisomerase-1 and this may account for the poor outcome associated with this reactivity through promotion of fibroblast activation [164] and endothelial damage induced by immune complexes [165]. There is also increasing evidence that antibodies targeting vascular receptors including endothelin and angiotensin may contribute to vascular damage and link adaptive autoimmunity to vascular dysfunction [166].

IL-4, TGF-β and IL-6 are all able to enhance production of collagen and other ECM proteins and are considered to be the main profibrotic cytokines in SSc [160]. TGF-β activates fibroblasts and promotes inflammatory signalling via SMAD, MAPK, p38 and ERK; it may also recruit T cells into skin. IL-6 acts via soluble IL-6R and STAT-3 to enhance collagen production, but also causes EC activation and apoptosis, suggesting it is also important in the early inflammatory stage of SSc. IL-4 can also induce TGF-β production by fibroblasts and macrophages. IL-13 and IL-31 have more recently been identified as important contributors to the fibrotic process [134,167]. Elevated levels of IL-31 have been associated with disease severity and pruritus in atopic eczema, and blockade of the IL-31RA with therapeutic benefit [168,169]. Pruritus in SSc has been associated with more severe skin and gastrointestinal disease suggesting a link between pruritus and fibrosis (see section on pruritus). The identification of raised IL-31 levels in plasma and fibrotic skin and lung lesions in a subset of SSc patients is supportive of this link [170]. The relative contributions of different members of the IL-17 family is still under investigation [171].

The role of dysregulated, activated B cells and elevated BAFF in SSc pathogenesis is now established [172]. B cells produce IL-6 and TGF-β, may directly stimulate fibroblasts by a contact-dependent mechanism and/or through autoantibodies, and may damage vessels through immune complex and antiendothelial cell antibody binding [**135**,173]. DNA and ssRNA released from damaged EC and nucleic acid-containing immune complexes may activate Toll-like receptors, increase the expression of interferon-responsive genes and cause an increased expression of IL-1, IL-6 and TNF-α [174,175]. Polymorphisms in Type I interferon regulatory genes IRF4,5,7 and 8 and STAT4, the finding of excess Type I IFN, CXCL4 and aberrant plasmacytoid dendritic cells in SSc skin and blood, and the correlation of IFN inducible chemokines with disease severity, link Type I IFN activation to pathogenesis in SSc [140,150,176]. Another innate immune pathway thought to be important in mediating fibrosis involves NALP3-mediated inflammasome activation of caspase-1 and the conversion of pro-IL-1 to IL-1. Accordingly, the inhibition of caspase-1 in SSc dermal and lung fibroblasts prevents the secretion of collagens, IL-1β and IL-18 [177].

Fibrosis. Ultimately the profibrotic growth factors and cytokines produced by these various cell types (T and B cells, macrophages, dendritic cells, mast cells and keratinocytes) cause recruitment of circulating fibrocytes, activation and differentiation of resident fibroblasts and mesenchymal transition in other susceptible cell types (see above). The resultant chronically activated, apoptosis resistant α smooth muscle actin expressing myofibroblasts produce excessive extracellular matrix proteins, ROS, tenascin C, fibronectin and DAMPs [**135**]. Proinflammatory and profibrotic pathways are integrated through STAT3 dependent signals and further fibroblast activation is then elicited through biomechanical, integrin and TLR dependent signalling, ultimately leading to a self-sustaining cycle of fibrosis [178,179].

The broad mechanisms involved in the cellular and molecular pathogenesis of SSc are summarised in Figure 54.2. and are reviewed in more detail in [134,136,180].

The histological appearances in SSc are diverse and depend upon the stage and subset of disease and on the affected organ.

In the skin, early vascular injury and EC activation, followed by infiltration of inflammatory cells, occur as described above, although the intensity of the inflammatory infiltrate may be less marked in SSc than is seen in morphoea [131,138,139]. Ultimately, a fibrotic change occurs in the dermis with increased α smooth muscle actin expressing myofibroblasts. The dermis becomes thickened because of increased collagen production, mainly collagen types I and III, without any compensatory increase in collagenase. The process may extend into the fibrous septae of the subcutis. The initially swollen, pale collagen bundles become hyalinised, closely packed and orientated horizontally in parallel to the skin surface. The epidermis may become atrophic with loss of rete ridges. Associated changes such as loss of secondary skin appendages including hair follicles and sweat glands occur [181,182]. In established skin sclerosis a severe reduction in the number of lymphatic capillaries and lymphatic pre-collector vessels occurs that correlates with the risk of developing fingertip ulceration [183]. Interestingly, in those patients who experience resolution of skin disease, some of these cutaneous features can reverse. The typical cutaneous histopathological features are shown in Figure 54.3.

Within the interstitial connective tissue of many internal organs there is increased extracellular matrix deposition, which may be confined to the normal fascial planes. There is often very little evidence of inflammatory change although biopsy material is difficult to obtain. At postmortem there are often increased amounts of connective tissue and collagen rich extracellular matrix, but this

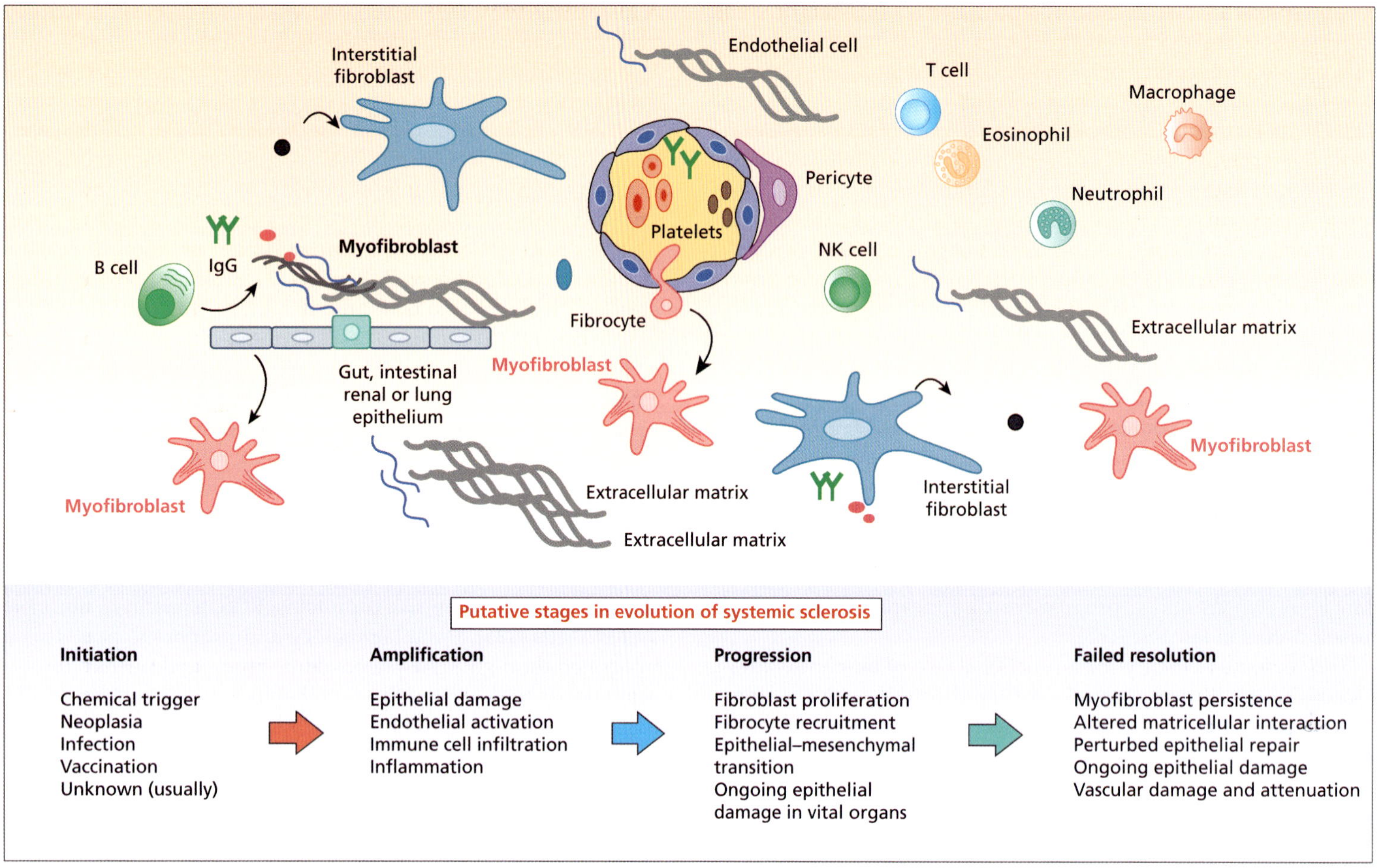

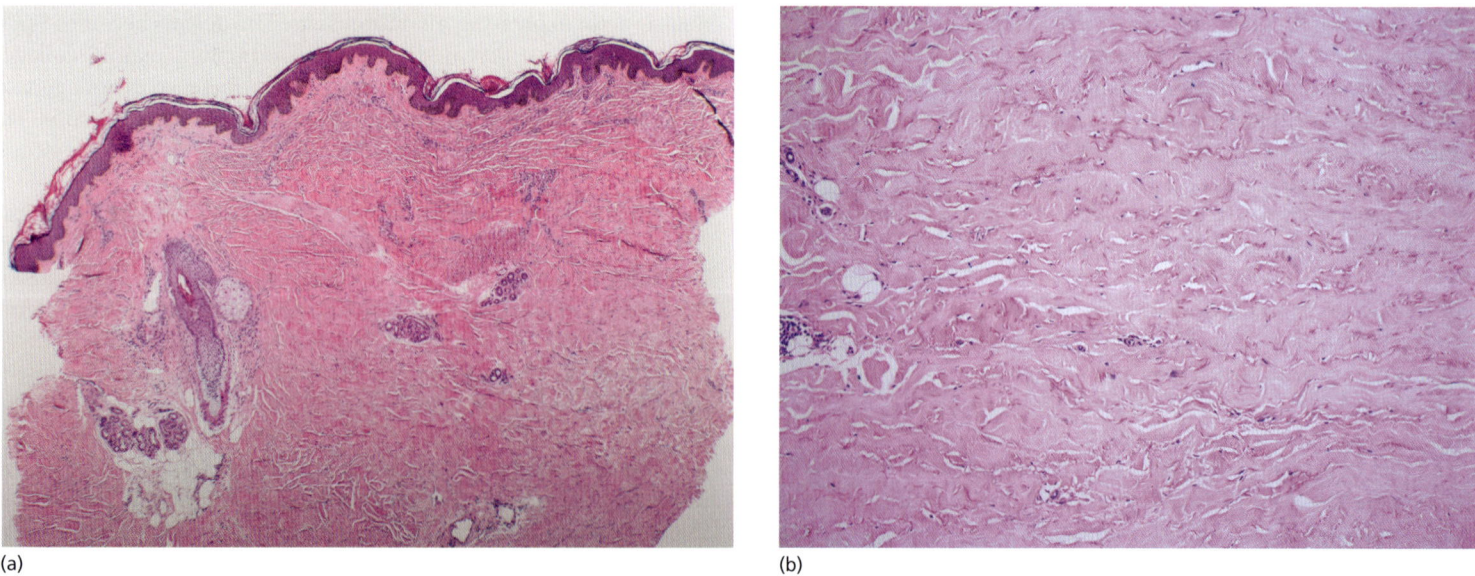

Figure 54.2 The cellular and molecular pathogenesis of systemic sclerosis (SSc): a summary of the complex and multifaceted pathogenesis of SSc that involves cells and mediators of the innate and adaptive immune system, vasculature and mesenchymal compartments as well as epithelial structures and more specialist organotypic cell types. Although the aetiology and triggers are often not known, there is a stereotypical evolution that involves the development and inappropriate persistence of a profibrotic population of active fibroblasts and myofibroblasts. These are likely to arise from at least three lineages: resident fibroblasts, circulating progenitor cells (e.g. fibrocytes) and as a result of transdifferentiation of other specialised cell types such as epithelial or endothelial cells. This transdifferentiation may not be complete or persistent and once fully characterised, the key mediators or factors that regulate these events may be logical targets for therapeutic intervention. ECM, extracellular matrix; IgG, immunoglobulin G; NK cell, natural killer cell.

Figure 54.3 Histopathological features of systemic sclerosis. (a) Low-power view showing 'squared' edges due to thickening of the dermis and extension of fibrosis into the subcutaneous septae. There is a superficial and deep perivascular mononuclear cell infiltrate. Dermal collagen is densely eosinophilic and appears homogenised/'sclerotic' in the lower part of the dermis. Courtesy of Dr Eduardo Calonje. (b) At a higher magnification, collagen bundles are seen to be swollen, eosinophilic and orientated parallel to the epidermis. Courtesy of Dr N. Krassilnik, Department of Pathology, Royal Free London NHS Foundation Trust, UK.

may be spread through relevant organs such as the heart or kidney without necessarily having major functional impact, thus its clinical significance remains uncertain [184].

A key pathological feature of SSc that crosses multiple organ beds is a proliferative vasculopathy with neointimal hyperplasia and luminal narrowing [132]. This is often associated with adventitial fibrosis and, notably in the renal and intrarenal arterial circulation and the pulmonary arterial tree, accompanied by thickening or hypertrophy of the smooth muscle medial layer. The similarities of these vascular histological changes across multiple relevant organ beds suggests that this pathology is as much a hallmark of SSc in internal organs as is fibrosis of the skin. The extent to which it compromises tissue perfusion and leads to other complications is unclear, but it is likely to be especially relevant to the development of digital ischaemia.

Secondary changes leading to other complications are seen in SSc. Thus, lung involvement shows a similarity to other types of lung fibrosis although a non-specific interstitial pneumonia (NSIP) pattern of disease is the most frequent manifestation. NSIP in SSc may have a cellular or fibrotic histological subtype although there is no clear evidence that the histological pattern of lung fibrosis impacts substantially on outcome [185].

The histology of PAH in SSc is broadly similar to that of idiopathic PAH (iPAH), although there is more likely to be associated lung fibrosis [186]. In addition, it has been suggested that the coexistence of features of pulmonary vascular occlusive disease may be relatively common and could contribute to differences in clinical outcome [187]. Some studies suggest that plexiform lesions are less common in SSc-associated PAH, but they are present in autopsy cases and one suggestion has been, that as the SSc cases have a poor outcome and lower long-term survival, they may have less time to develop these hallmark luminal lesions of recanalisation [188]. Key histological features of PAH in SSc include endoluminal proliferation and associated perivascular inflammatory cell infiltrate.

The histological features of SRC overlap with those of related renal pathologies such as pre-eclampsia, accelerated phase hypertension and thrombotic thrombocytopenic purpura [189]. The histological appearances may resemble other forms of thrombotic microangiopathy but are often superimposed upon a greater degree of background fibrotic change and may be associated with intravascular thrombosis. In addition, there is evidence of upregulation of a number of markers of vascular proliferation and damage, including endothelin ligand and receptors, and vascular endothelial growth factor [190]. However, there is a spectrum of severity in terms of vascular damage and proliferative changes and the amount of fibrosis also varies. Interestingly, the severity of acute vascular injury and change appears to correlate with poor long-term outcome and less renal recovery, whereas the extent of scarring or fibrosis, unlike in many chronic renal diseases, seems less important [191,192]. This ability to score biopsies and predict outcome is one justification for renal biopsy in SRC. The other major indication is the presence of clinical or serological features of vasculitis or lupus that may raise the possibility of an alternate renal pathology requiring different treatment.

Causative organisms

It has not been proven that infectious agents have a role in the development of SSc. This may only be relevant in a small proportion of cases or as a co-factor in its complex multistage pathogenesis. Viral-induced autoimmunity can be activated through multiple mechanisms including activation of interferon-inducible genes, molecular mimicry, epitope spreading, bystander activation and immortalisation of infected B cells [193]. Some studies have implicated viruses such as cytomegalovirus, Epstein–Barr virus and parvovirus B19 [194,195] and endogenous retroviruses (reviewed in [196]) in triggering the disease, but there have also been reports of SSc improving dramatically after a severe systemic viral infection perhaps because of immune perturbation [197]. Two cases of SSc after SARS-CoV-2 infection have been reported, with increased NETosis and molecular mimicry proposed as possible mechanisms triggering autoimmunity [198,199]. Interestingly, a recent study which bioinformatically predicted immunodominant peptides of topoisomerase-1, fibrillarin and centromere protein A found that they are homologous to viral protein sequences from the mimiviridae and phycodnaviridae families. This suggests a possible role for infectious triggers in autoantibody generation and pathogenesis in some SSc cases [83]. In most, infection is more relevant because of the risk of opportunistic infection in patients who are immunosuppressed, or through susceptibility to infection of digital ulcers or fibrotic lungs and reduced respiratory reserve. Intestinal tract infection may be relevant; certainly, it contributes to the development of small intestinal bacterial overgrowth, but the intestinal microbiome may also be relevant, thereby explaining the apparent benefit of some antibiotic regimens or approaches such as probiotics for gastrointestinal symptoms [200,201]. Emerging reports have identified unique microbial taxa alterations in the gastrointestinal microbiome of patients with SSc as compared with healthy controls [202,203] and trials of faecal microbiota transplantation are now underway [204].

Genetics

The highest risk factor for developing SSc is having a sibling or first-degree relative with the disease (13–15-fold increased risk) [205]. Early studies identified a genetic predisposition to vasculopathy, Raynaud phenomenon, autoimmune inflammatory diseases (SLE, thyroid disease) and ILD in SSc pedigrees [206,207], and that chromosomal breakage was a feature in familial SSc (reviewed in [208]). Initial candidate gene approaches (reviewed in [209]) have been superseded by genome-wide association studies and Immunochip analyses that have started to dissect both the susceptibility factors and the factors that are associated with the individual subtypes of SSc. This work has confirmed the major role of the HLA region in susceptibility to SSc and in determining autoantibody and clinical features [83,210]. In a large population of European ancestry, Immunochip-based gene mapping identified independent associations for variants of HLA-DPB1, -B and -DOA with SSc per se, for HLA-DRB1, -DQA1 and -DOA with ACA-positive SSc, and for HLA-DRB1 and -DPB1 with ATA-positive SSc. Associations for the non-HLA gene *TAP2* were found with SSc and ACA positivity [210]. These findings have been confirmed and extended in recent studies using imputation analysis of meta-GWAS data from 9095 SSc cases and 17 584 healthy controls [96,211]. These show strong associations between SSc and HLA-DRB1*11:04, HLA-DQB1*02:02, HLA-DPB1*13:01 and interestingly also the class I HLA-B*08:01. Further stratified analysis revealed different HLA-DQA1 haplotype associations in lcSSc and dcSSc, as well as HLA associations exclusive to particular autoantibody subsets (see Table 54.3) [96]. Some of these genes code for products that are involved in the MHC receptor complex (*DPB1*), peptide loading on MHC class II molecules (*DOA*) and antigen presentation (*TAP2*), others are closely linked to the production of ACA (*DRB1*, *DQA1*) and ATA (*DRB1*, *DPB1*).

Multiple susceptibility loci for SSc have also been identified at non-HLA loci [208,211,212]. The most reproducible evidence exists for *STAT4*, *CD247*, *IRF5*, *TNFAIP3* and *DNASE1L3* [213]. Robust evidence also links type I interferon activation to SSc, including polymorphisms in interferon regulatory factor (IRF)5, IRF7 IRF8, tyrosine kinase2 (TK2) and STAT4 and a prominent IFN signature in gene expression studies from peripheral blood and skin (reviewed in [176]). In 2019, the largest meta-GWAS to date, encompassing 14 European cohorts, identified 27 signals at the following non-HLA loci: *ARHGAP31*, *BLK*, *CD247*, *TNIP1*, *CSK*, *STAT4-a*, *STAT4-b*, *DGKQ*, *NUP85-GRB2*, *IL12RB1*, *IL12RB2*, *TNFSF4*, *NAB1**, *FLNB-DNASE1L3-PXK*, *IL12A*, *NFKB1*, *ATG5*, *IRF5-TNPO3*, *RAB2A-CHD7*, *CDHR5-IRF7*, *TSPAN32*, *CD81-AS1*, *DDX6*, *IRF8*, *IKZF3-GSDMB* that were independently associated with SSc [211]. In the first 10 listed, the 95% credibility set comprised one or two SNPs only, with a high probability of causality. Stratified analysis revealed different loci associations for limited and diffuse cutaneous subsets, and for different autoantibody subsets (ACA, ATA, RNAP). In some cases these were stronger than in the global meta-analysis [211]. This study suggested that most of the genetic variations underlying SSc susceptibility are related to transcriptional regulatory mechanisms, including mRNA processing or stability mediated by non-coding-RNAs. Collectively, the results point towards molecular pathways involved in B- and T- cell activation and innate immunity, in inflammatory cytokine-induced collagen production, in VEGF signalling and in transcription, kinase activity, DNA cleavage and repair, apoptosis, pyroptosis, and autophagy. Genomic risk scores are now being established and may eventually translate into an individualised risk assessment for development of SSc [214].

Many of the genetic susceptibility loci identified are shared with other autoimmune diseases such as SLE and RA. One interpretation of this is that innate immune components of SSc are entirely genetically determined, but it is also likely that the factors and processes central to the development of SSc outside the immune component are more complex, with multiple potential interactions at a genetic and epigenome level as well as functionally. Current evidence demonstrates alterations in DNA methylation, histone code modifications, differential expression of regulatory microRNAs and long non-coding mRNAs in SSc cells, mainly in fibroblasts, but also in monocytes, macrophages, dentritic and endothelial cells, some of which are important in TGF-β pathways and downstream signalling cascades (reviewed in [215,216]). Histone modifications regulate expression of genes involved in fibroblast activation to myofibroblasts [217]. TGF-β mediated hypermethylation of DNA in SSc fibroblasts leads to repression of genes responsible for downregulating fibrosis such as SOCS3 [218]. Dysregulated miRNAs in SSc skin and blood are involved in profibrotic pathways as well as impaired angiogenesis and altered immune responses [219]. Epigenetics is thus emerging as a potentially exciting and fruitful approach, especially as it may underlie genetic programmes that are disrupted across multiple loci and may also offer real potential for novel disease-modifying therapeutic strategies [215].

Environmental factors

One of the important aspects to have emerged from epidemiological studies of SSc has been the impact of environmental factors [46,49,196]. This may include infectious agents as discussed above or factors such as vaccination that may trigger immune alteration. It is likely that multiple environmental factors may be important, or that timing and context are critical for environmental triggers to contribute to SSc development.

There are many examples of SSc being triggered by environmental exposures [220]. Silica exposure probably explains the historical association of SSc with mining in the USA and South Africa [221]. Environmental exposure to vinyl chloride and many other organic chemicals have been implicated [49,222]. In a case–control study of 100 SSc cases and 300 controls, occupational exposure – particularly high cumulative exposure to crystalline silica, white spirit, aromatic solvents, chlorinated solvents, trichlorethylene, ketones and welding fumes – was associated with an increased risk of developing SSc. Interestingly, however, no association between SSc and the use of drugs such as anorexigens, pentazocine, bromocriptine, l-tryptophan or hair dyes was found [223]. The possible association between the presence of silicone breast implants and SSc has proved controversial. The case–control study above, and five out of six meta-analyses of previous publications have found no association (reviewed in [220,224]). However, several recent publications have reopened the debate, suggesting an association between ruptured silicone implants, breast cancer and anti-polymerase III antibody positive SSc [224–226]. Smoking does not increase the risk of developing SSc but does appear to impact upon the severity of the disease, particularly in relation to vasculopathy [196,220]. The association between SSc and occupational exposure may vary according to gender. A marked association between SSc and occupational exposure to crystalline silica, chlorinated solvents, trichloroethylene, white spirit, ketones and welding fumes was identified in male patients, and to white spirit, aromatic and other solvents and ketones in female patients [223].

A recent summary of all investigated potential environmental risk factors identified strong level II evidence (>20 observational studies and meta-analyses) for silica and organic solvents, and probable associations with asbestos, epoxy resins and particulate matter (5–10 observational studies each). Insufficient evidence was identified to clearly implicate welding fumes, pesticides and heavy metals. SSc linked to silica and organic solvent exposure was more common in men and associated with higher mortality and morbidity from cutaneous pulmonary and cardiac disease, and cancer [196]. Similarly, a recent Brazilian study found a preponderance of males, shorter disease duration, increased associated myopathy, more severe ILD in lcSSc and lower levels of ANA positivity in dcSSc linked to environmental exposures [222].

Susceptibility to environmental triggers may also be linked to underlying genetic factors, for instance an enhanced profibrotic response to silica has been linked *in vitro* to genetic polymorphisms in TNF-α-induced protein 3 (TNFAIP3) [227].

Clinical features
History
Systemic sclerosis is a clinical diagnosis and good history taking is critical. The clinical diversity of SSc means that a number of stereotypical patterns are observed and this is reflected in the history. Most cases have onset in the adult years and many patients describe Raynaud phenomenon: a change in colour of the fingers and/or toes triggered by exposure to cold or emotional stress both in winter and summer, as the first symptom. Occasionally the ears and nose can be affected. In classic triphasic Raynaud phenomenon the digits become white, then blue (cyanotic) and then red (hyperaemic) and painful on rewarming. In some cases, only biphasic colour changes occur. This may be a new feature, and any case of new-onset Raynaud phenomenon occurring over the age of 40 years is more likely to be associated with an underlying CTD [228]. Another key aspect of Raynaud phenomenon in SSc is that it is more likely to be associated with complications such as pitted digital scars, digital ulceration, paronychia or trophic changes in the finger pulps [229,230]. At its most severe, critical digital ischaemia can lead to gangrene and auto-amputation. Sometimes there is a long history of Raynaud phenomenon from teenage or early adult life and this is more likely to be the case in patients with lcSSc [231]. In cases of dcSSc there is often a less clear pre-existing history of Raynaud phenomenon and in some cases the vascular features may occur simultaneously or even after the onset of other features [232,233].

Another key early symptom is gastro-oesophageal reflux or dysphagia. This may initially be dismissed as a common symptom and treated symptomatically. Often treatment with proton pump inhibitors is very effective, thus a careful history is required.

Swelling and stiffness of the digits is often described in the early stages of SSc and may lead to simple practical problems with jewellery (e.g. rings needing removal or enlargement). More widespread swelling of the extremities may be reported including lower limb oedema, widespread pain or functional limitation in range of movement. Itch is a hallmark of diffuse skin involvement and may be intense during the early or active stages of disease [234]. Skin tightness or thickening depends upon the subset and severity of the SSc. In the most severe cases the oedematous phase of hand and limb swelling quite rapidly develops into skin sclerosis with limited or fixed digits [235]. Associated musculoskeletal pain and skin ulceration as well as vascular insufficiency with Raynaud phenomenon culminate in the very disabling and severe impact of the most severe cases of diffuse SSc. Constitutional symptoms of fatigue and weight loss are common, especially in early diffuse disease [236,237]. The most common cause for weight loss is malnutrition because of reduced appetite, the physical difficulty with eating because of sicca symptoms and dysphagia. In addition, post-prandial bloating, and other gastrointestinal tract symptoms impact on nutrition. However, specific complications of small and large intestinal involvement or ano-rectal disease are generally seen in established SSc. When there are delays in presentation or diagnosis, which is more likely in cases of milder lcSSc or SSc *sine*-scleroderma,

then features of more established SSc may be present at diagnosis or extracted from a careful chronological history. Finally, any of the major internal organ complications of SSc may occasionally be presenting features of the disease, thus breathlessness, chest pain and other cardiovascular symptoms need to be explored. A proportion of cases present with complications such as PAH, lung fibrosis or SRC, as outlined in the next section.

Presentation
The typical presenting features of SSc are Raynaud phenomenon, symptoms of gastro-oesophageal reflux and swelling or discomfort in the extremities. This is followed by specific skin manifestations such as puffiness, tightness, hardening or itching (see section on history). Digital ulcers occur up to 5 years earlier in patients with ATA+ diffuse disease and can be a presenting feature [238]. Telangiectasia and calcinosis tend to occur later in the disease, as do features of internal organ manifestations including cardiorespiratory and more severe gastrointestinal tract involvement. Some cases of SSc will present to rheumatologists, others to dermatologists, and sometimes to organ-based specialists in those cases where a complication of the disease such as lung fibrosis or renal crisis is the first major manifestation. This makes appropriate multidisciplinary care and engagement an important aspect of early management as well as patient education and systematic investigation.

Raynaud phenomenon. The Raynaud phenomenon occurs in >95% of patients with SSc, is usually present at diagnosis and may be the only presenting feature (see section on history also). Tests such as autoantibody profile and nail fold capillaroscopic examination are very helpful in making an early diagnosis and in identifying cases of isolated Raynaud phenomenon that are at risk of progression to CTD [239,240]. Such patients are more likely to have an SSc pattern on nail fold capillaroscopy, sclerodactyly and scleroderma-specific antibodies (ACA, ATA, ARA) [230]. The typical capillaroscopic findings of capillary dilatation, haemorrhages and focal capillary loss (Figure 54.4) can be assessed more easily and with comparable accuracy with a dermatoscope [241,242]. If there is uncertainty with this method, videocapillaroscopy should be performed [243]. Recently, very early diagnosis criteria for SSc (VEDOSS) have been proposed and these appear to predict progression to definite SSc in more than 50% of cases [244]. This is important for risk stratification in patients with Raynaud phenomenon and confirms that the absence of ANA is a strong protective factor identifying patients at very low risk of developing SSc over a 5-year period. Conversely, the presence of one or two VEDOSS criteria, namely ANA positivity, puffy fingers, SSc-specific autoantibodies and abnormal nail fold capillaroscopy, in patients with Raynaud phenomenon confers a progressively higher risk of fulfilling classification criteria for SSc over time [244]. The highest risk of progression at 5 years was in those Raynaud cases with SSc-specific autoantibodies and puffy fingers at baseline. Time from onset of Raynaud phenomenon to the first non-Raynaud symptom in SSc is associated with severity of disease, short intervals being more likely in severe diffuse disease [245].

Cutaneous manifestations.
Skin thickening. The earliest cutaneous manifestations are non-pitting oedema and puffiness, which tend to be seen first in the

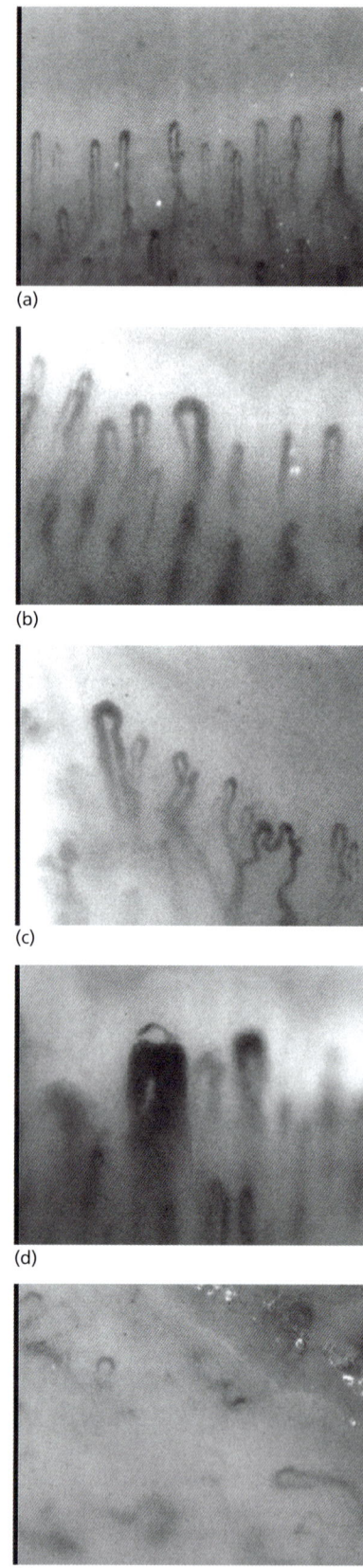

(a)

(b)

(c)

(d)

(e)

Figure 54.4 (a) Normal nail fold capillaroscopy. (b–e) Typical capillaroscopic findings in systemic sclerosis (SSc): changes seen with disease progression. (b) Isolated dilated loops in early disease. (c) Tortuous loops and reducing capillary density in active disease. (d) 'Megacapillaries' and progressive drop-out in active SSc. (e) Few remaining dilated loops, but extensive avascularity in late-stage SSc.

fingers, hands and face. Rapid progression can then occur, usually over 6–12 months particularly in diffuse disease. The skin becomes taught, indurated, thickened and then fixed to deeper structures on the fingers resulting in sclerodactyly with distal tapering. The extension of these changes proximally to the metacarpophalangeal joints is critical to the diagnosis of SSc. Skin sclerosis leads to progressive loss of skin appendages, reduced hair growth, reduced sweating and joint contractures. Mask-like facies develop as the facial skin becomes waxy and wrinkles are diminished. Nasal and lip thinning, radial furrowing of perioral skin, reduced oral aperture and sclerosis of the frenulum may be present. This fibrotic phase may last from 1 to 4 years or longer, and this varies between patients and according to serum autoantibodies. Ultimately, the skin may soften and becomes atrophic, although in rare cases a recurrence of skin thickening may occur. Patients with the most extensive, severe skin thickening in early disease, for example RNAP+ patients, show greater subsequent improvement at 1 and 5 years than ATA+, anti-U3RNP+ and ACA+ patients [17]. Rapidly progressive skin thickening is predictive of internal organ involvement and mortality [246]. In early diffuse disease, changes in skin thickness scores parallel changes in global disease severity [247] and the extent of skin sclerosis is used as a surrogate for disease activity, disease severity and mortality in SSc [248,249]. It can be measured, most commonly employing an MRSS. By this method the degree of skin sclerosis is scored from 0 to 3 by manual palpation at 17 different body sites giving a maximum score of 51 (Table 54.7) [250]. This method has been validated and shown to correlate with skin biopsy thickness, overall disease severity and long-term outcome [248,251]. A number of other methods have been described to monitor skin thickness. These include durometry [252,253], 20 MHz ultrasonography [254,255] and, more recently, optical coherence tomography. The latter has shown a reduction in optical density of the papillary dermis that parallels the increase in dermal fibrosis and MRSS scores [256,257]. A self-assessment skin severity score has recently been described (PASTUL) and is currently being further validated [258] and integrated with the robust SSc skin PRO that measures patient-reported impact of skin disease [259]. These approaches may underpin future clinical assessment to focus on meaningful changes in skin involvement in clinical practice or trials.

Pruritus. Itch is present in 40–60% of SSc cases. It preferentially involves the forearms, scalp and back, but can be generalised. It is associated with xerosis, but thought to be primarily neuropathic in nature [260]. It correlates with the extent of skin sclerosis, MRSS and gastrointestinal symptoms [234]. Interestingly, raised levels of IL-31, a recognised pruritogen, now also implicated in fibrosis, have been found in plasma and fibrotic skin and lung in SSc patients [170]. Although it generally improves over time, itch may be one of the most disabling symptoms of SSc, affecting sleep, overall functioning and quality of life [234,260–262].

Telangiectasia. These may be mat-like or square-shaped and may be large. Telangiectases are most frequently seen on the hands, face and upper trunk, but may also occur on the lower limbs. Histopathology of established telangiectases in patients with LcSSc has shown dilated postcapillary venules located in the papillary and

Table 54.7 The modified Rodnan skin score (MRSS) is used to assess the degree of skin sclerosis in a standardised and reproducible manner [248,250].

Site	Maximum score	
Face	3	
Anterior chest	3	
Abdomen	3	
Subtotal:	**9**	
	Right	**Left**
Upper arm	3	3
Forearm	3	3
Hand	3	3
Fingers	3	3
Thigh	3	3
Leg	3	3
Foot	3	3
Subtotal:	**21**	**21**
Maximum score:	**51**	

The scoring of each skin region is determined by skin thickness and tethering: 0 = normal; 1 = mild skin thickening (easily able to make skin folds between 2 fingers, fine wrinkles acceptable); 2 = moderate skin thickening unable to pinch the skin (difficulty making skin folds and no wrinkles); 3 = severe skin thickening unable to move the skin (which is fixed to deeper tissues) (inability to make skin folds between two fingers). This modified score omits assessment of the neck and back. If these areas are included the maximum score increases to 57.

superficial reticular dermis [263]. They may be a marker for more widespread microvascular disease in SSc and have been associated with more severe nail fold videocapillaroscopy changes and higher rates of digital ulcers, RP and PAH [264,265].

Dyspigmentation. A variety of patterns of dyspigmentation are seen in SSc. Diffuse hyperpigmentation with or without accentuation at sun-exposed sites, and 'salt and pepper' vitiligo-like focal depigmentation occurring over the upper chest and back, on the face at the anterior hairline, at acral sites or in a more generalised distribution are the commonest pigmentary changes seen (Figure 54.1j,l). Dyspigmentation occurs in 37% of SSc cases but is more likely in dcSSc than lcSSc. Diffuse hyperpigmentation in particular has been associated with the presence of digital ulcers [266].

Digital ulcers. Digital ulcers occur in up to 50% of patients with SSc, are associated with nail fold capillary abnormalities, and occur earlier and more frequently in patients with dcSSc and pulmonary disease [232,267]. They occur as complications of ischaemic vasculopathy and/or trauma. Ulcers develop on the hands and feet, on the tips of fingers and toes, over extensor surfaces and bony prominences, and in association with calcinosis. They are frequently complicated by infection and occasionally gangrene. Gangrene occurs in about 9% of SSc patients and is more likely in patients with a past or current history of digital ulcers and diffuse disease [268]. Digital ulcers significantly impact on quality of life because of pain, functional impairment and delayed healing. Removal of necrotic tissue, treatment of infection and maintenance of the correct moisture balance with appropriate dressings are key in promoting ulcer healing [269]. Clinical tools to stratify risk of developing digital ulcers in SSc may allow earlier institution of prophylactic vasoactive therapies [270,271].

Calcinosis. Calcinosis is because of the deposition of hydroxyapatite crystals in the dermis and subcutis. It is determined by physical examination, imaging techniques or a clear history of extruded calcium. It occurs in 25–38% of SSc cases, most often on the hands and particularly the thumbs, causing impaired hand function and pain. It is more common in patients with longer disease duration, ACA positivity, digital ischaemia, digital ulcers and acro-osteolysis [272,273]. The cause is uncertain but abnormalities in mineralisation pathways involving inorganic pyrophosphate, in genes involved in regulation of ectopic calcification and in poly(ADP-ribose) polymerase (PARP) enzymes are currently under investigation [274].

Gastrointestinal manifestations. A majority of SSc patients will develop gastrointestinal manifestations that occur predominantly as a consequence of reduced or abnormal motility. This has been attributed to a combination of myopathic and neuropathic changes [275], but changes to the gut microbiome may also play a role [203,276]. At the level of the oesophagus this occurs in >90% of SSc patients leading to dysphagia and symptoms of gastro-oesophageal reflux disease. Lower gastrointestinal manifestations tend to occur more commonly and more severely in patients with limited SSc. In the stomach, impaired acid secretion, mucosal atrophy and reduced gastric emptying result. When the small bowel is involved, bacterial overgrowth and atonic dilatation result in bloating, malabsorption, malodorous diarrhoea, and episodes of pseudo-obstruction. Involvement of the sigmoid colon and rectum cause constipation and overflow incontinence [277]. Using a validated patient reported outcome measure, the SCTC-UCLA GIT2.0, it has recently been shown that over half of patients with SSc have a moderate or severe gastrointestinal burden despite best current treatment and this represents a major unmet medical need [278,279].

Cardiac and pulmonary vascular manifestations. Cardiopulmonary manifestations vary according to disease subsets as previously described. They include ILD, pulmonary fibrosis, PAH – either isolated or in the context of pulmonary fibrosis – and cardiac myositis and interstitial fibrosis, which lead to cardiomyopathy and cardiac arrhythmias. Interstitial lung disease and PAH are currently the most common causes of disease-related death in SSc [280–283]. The symptoms are largely overlapping and comprise dry cough, breathlessness, palpitations, syncope and peripheral oedema. They require baseline and regular repeat assessments in order to ensure early optimisation of treatment. The gold standard for the diagnosis of PAH is right heart catheterisation showing a mean pulmonary pressure of at least 25 mmHg at rest with a pulmonary capillary wedge pressure of less than 15 mmHg. This is an invasive test and the DETECT study developed an evidence-based detection algorithm for PAH in SSc patients that would minimise the number of missed PAH diagnoses while optimising the use of diagnostic right heart catheterisation [284]. In a two-step process, combined assessments of per cent predicted forced vital capacity (FVC)/diffusing capacity for carbon monoxide (DLCO), past or present telangiectasias, ACA positivity, N-terminal probrain natriuretic peptide and urate levels, and right axis deviation on electrocardiogram lead to a score. If over a threshold level (>300), an echocardiogram is indicated and measurements of tricuspid valve regurgitant velocity and right atrial area then determine the need for cardiac catheterisation to establish whether or not there is PAH [284]. Although all of the current routine treatments for PAH are approved based upon mPAP of at least 25 mmHg the most recent World Symposium for Pulmonary Hypertension has proposed lowering the mPAP to above 20 mmHg. This may broaden the use of treatment and permit intervention at an earlier stage of disease but impact on long-term outcome remains to be determined [285].

Pulmonary manifestations. Although commoner in dcSSc, pulmonary fibrosis occurs in all types of SSc and has emerged as one of the most lethal complications [281]. Of SSc-patients, 50–65% have or will develop ILD during the course of their disease, most within 5 years, and in the most severe cases within 3 years [286,287]. Changes in pulmonary function tests (PFT: including FVC, total lung capacity, DLCO) are a marker of disease severity, but normal values do not rule out early SSc-ILD. It is now recommended that both PFT and high-resolution computed tomography scan (HRCT) should be performed for initial screening and diagnosis. SSc-ILD may be classified into subclinical ILD with no ILD specific symptoms, minimal changes on HRCT and normal PFT; and clinical ILD in those who are symptomatic, have decrements in PFT and/or moderate to extensive disease on HRCT. Risk factors for progression include male sex, Afro-Caribbean ethnicity, being ATA+, ACA−, having progressive diffuse cutaneous disease and raised inflammatory markers (CRP) [281,288]. Biomarkers for diagnosis, severity and ILD progression are being identified [289]. There have been considerable advances in diagnosis [290] and treatments that limit the decline in lung function are now available [291,292] (see section on management). This has resulted in a paradigm shift in approach to management, such that early treatment is recommended in patients with subclinical ILD at high risk of progression [292].

Renal manifestations. A core set of items that characterise SRC has recently been defined and includes blood pressure, acute kidney injury, microangiopathic haemolytic anaemia, target organ dysfunction and renal histopathology [293]. It is still an important complication of SSc occurring in 5–15% of patients, usually within the first 5 years [191,294]. Headaches, fever, malaise, hypertension with associated retinopathy and encephalopathy, pulmonary oedema and acute renal failure may develop suddenly. RNA polymerase III antibodies are present in 59% of patients and confer increased susceptibility. Additional genetic susceptibility in this population of high-risk SSc is also being defined [295]. SRC is rare in patients with anticentromere antibodies. It may be commoner in black SSc cases, in whom it has been associated with anti-Ro antibody positivity rather than RNAP [296]. Most patients have diffuse or rapidly progressive disease. Treatment with oral corticosteroids at doses >10–15 mg/day may increase the risk of developing SRC. Early, aggressive treatment with angiotensin-converting enzyme (ACE) inhibitors in patients with accelerated hypertension in the early stages of SRC has improved the prognosis, such that SRC is no longer the leading cause of death in SSc. Nevertheless, 40% require dialysis 'short term' for up to 3 years, 40% require long-term dialysis and the 5-year survival is 60–70% [294,297]. In addition, it is now recognised that chronic kidney disease is also frequent in SSc and new markers of the process, such as increased urinary levels of

MCP1 and ICAM1, that may permit more accurate detection and allow better future management, are being evaluated [298].

Musculoskeletal manifestations. Tendon friction rubs – a feeling of 'coarse cracking and crepitus' over the finger flexors and extensors, wrists, elbows, knees and ankle joints – occur in approximately 10% of patients at presentation. They have been variably attributed to thickening of the tendon retinacula [299] and to deep connective tissue infiltrates surrounding the tendons [300]. Their presence in early SSc has been associated with diffuse disease and reduced 5- and 10-year survival [301]. They are a marker of active disease and increased risk of systemic organ complications [302,303].

Muscle weakness is a common symptom occurring in some 90% of cases. Two patterns of muscle involvement are recognised: a low-grade myopathy with mild weakness, minimal creatine kinase elevation, minimal electromyographic findings and mild fibrotic changes on histology; and a less common inflammatory myositis, usually in the context of an overlap syndrome and anti-PM-Scl positivity [304]. A Canadian study of >1000 patients found abnormal creatine kinase levels in 5.6% of cases, and a history of myositis/myopathy in 10% [305]. Muscle involvement was associated with male sex, early diffuse disease, ATA or RNAP positivity, ILD and reduced survival.

Clinical variants

Although all cases can be classified into limited or diffuse subsets based on the extent of skin involvement, SSc is a much more heterogeneous disease. Combining the extent of skin sclerosis with autoantibody and gene expression profiles is allowing improved risk stratification and appreciation of further distinct clinical subsets of the disease (see section on classification). It is likely that clinical variants will be defined more precisely as molecular and genetic technologies improve. It is important to identify patients with SSc overlap (see Associated diseases earlier) because the overlap manifestations need to be treated in the context of SSc. For example, it is often important to minimise glucocorticoid exposure as it may be associated with risk of SRC. Also, the overlap features may be more significant for the patient than the features of SSc, and so must be treated effectively and optimally. Roughly 2–8% of SSc cases present with internal organ involvement in the absence of skin sclerosis and have been termed SSc sine-scleroderma (ssSSc) [9–11]. Half of these cases go on to develop sclerotic skin over the following 2 years in an lcSSc distribution [12]. Some authors include patients with non-sclerotic skin manifestations of SSc such as calcinosis, telangiectasia, digital ulcers as a subset of ssSSc, others reserve the term for patients with no skin signs of SSc whatsoever [306]. Demographic characteristics are similar to those of lcSSc cases, but autoantibody profiles vary, and include ACA and ATA in equal measure in some studies [306]. Raynaud phenomenon, abnormal nail fold capillaries, gastrointestinal disease, pulmonary fibrosis, PAH and SSc cardiac disease are frequent but SRC, myositis and SSc overlap disease seem less common in ssSSc [11,12,307].

Differential diagnosis

Establishing a secure diagnosis of SSc depends upon excluding several related, scleroderma-like conditions, as well as appreciating the associations with other autoimmune rheumatic diseases, or causes of clinical conditions that can be a part of SSc but can also occur in other contexts (Box 54.1).

Box 54.1 Scleroderma spectrum disorders

- Inflammatory/autoimmune
  - Systemic sclerosis
  - Morphoea (limited, generalised, pansclerotic, linear and mixed types)
  - Eosinophilic fasciitis
  - Lichen sclerosus et atrophicus
  - Paraneoplastic scleroderma
  - Sclerodermoid chronic graft-versus-host disease
- Scleromucinoses
  - Scleroedema (post infectious, diabetic, paraproteinaemia/ haematological malignancy associated)
  - Scleromyxoedema
- Chemically induced/toxic
  - Nephrogenic systemic fibrosis
  - Toxic oil syndrome
  - Eosinophilia–myalgia syndrome
- Metabolic and endocrine
  - Porphyria cutanea tarda
  - Myxoedema
  - Carcinoid syndrome
  - Amyloidosis
- Sclerodermoid genodermatoses
  - Acrogeria, progeria, Werner disease
  - Stiff skin syndrome
- Acrodermatitis chronica atrophicans (borrelia infection)

Isolated or primary Raynaud phenomenon is very common and is associated with normal nail fold capillaroscopy and negative ANA testing [228,308]. This is the most frequent type of Raynaud phenomenon and occurs in up to 10% of otherwise healthy women, although less commonly in men [309]. Typically, there is a family history and onset of vasospastic symptoms in the teenage years or as a young adult. It is not associated with major complications, trophic changes or digital ulcer disease. Causes of secondary Raynaud phenomenon should be excluded (Table 54.8).

The other major subgroup is morphoea. Localised forms of scleroderma including plaque, nodular and linear morphoea can coexist in patients with established SSc but are not generally a source of diagnostic difficulty [310,311]. Nodular lesions tend to be seen more frequently in diffuse disease, with plaque and linear lesions appearing more often in limited SSc (personal observation). The most likely form of morphoea to be confused with SSc is the pansclerotic subtype of morphoea. Typically, in this variant, rapidly progressive circumferential involvement of the trunk and limbs occurs [312]. Absence of Raynaud phenomenon or any internal organ fibrosis, and relative sparing of the hands and fingers are a clue, but in the early stages it may resemble some cases of diffuse SSc. A positive ANA is seen in a proportion, but SSc-specific autoantibodies such as ACA, ATA, ARA are rarely present (Chapter 55). Nail fold capillaroscopy is usually normal, which provides a robust investigational test to discriminate cases. Cases of fasciitis, especially eosinophilic fasciitis, often present with swelling and limitation

Table 54.8 Causes of Raynaud phenomenon.

Type	Causes and clinical features
Primary Raynaud phenomenon	Familial, onset in adolescence/early adulthood
	Absence of trophic changes or digital ulceration
	Normal capillaroscopy/dermoscopy
	Negative autoantibodies
Secondary Raynaud phenomenon	
CTD-associated	SSc, SLE, APL, Sjögren syndrome, DM, overlap or mixed CTD, undifferentiated CTD, systemic vasculitis, eosinophilic fasciitis, morphoea
Obstructive arterial disease	Atherosclerosis, thromboembolism, Buerger disease, thoracic outflow obstruction
Hyperviscosity	Cryoglobulins, cold agglutinins, paraproteinaemia, thrombocytosis
Mechanical	Vibration white finger, thoracic outflow obstruction
Drugs and toxins	Beta-blockers, ergotamines, oral contraceptives, bleomycin, vinblastine and inadvertent intraarterial injection of many drugs
Neurological disease	Carpal tunnel syndrome, reflex sympathetic dystrophy, hemiplegia, multiple sclerosis, syringomyelia

APL, antiphospholipid syndrome; CTD, connective tissue disease; DM, dermatomyositis; SLE, systemic lupus erythematosus; SSc, systemic sclerosis.

of movement of the extremities [313]. Usually sparing the face and initially more severe in the lower limbs, the condition later spreads to the upper limbs and trunk and can be incapacitating. The woody induration classically spares the hands and feet, and the skin overlying vessels shows typical guttering or the 'groove sign'. Internal organ manifestations are rare but can be present when there is marked and persistent eosinophilia. Eosinophilic myocarditis is a particular concern in such cases but is rare. There is significant overlap between eosinophilic fasciitis and pansclerotic morphoea in adults. The latter may involve deeper tissues including fascia, cause similar 'guttering' and start on distal extremities rather than the trunk (personal observation). In addition, some 30–40% of cases of fasciitis later develop features of morphoea at other body sites [314–316], emphasising that they are likely a spectrum of disease. Widespread skin thickening may also occur as a paraneoplastic phenomenon and phenotypically may resemble either pansclerotic morphoea or systemic sclerosis.

Other important scleroderma-like diseases to be considered include scleromyxoedema, scleroedema, nephrogenic systemic fibrosis, and pretibial and generalised myxoedema. The clinical pattern of skin changes, absence of Raynaud phenomenon and of SSc-specific ANA help discriminate these conditions from SSc (Table 54.9), but in practice a diagnostic skin biopsy, preferably a deep incisional ellipse, may be required. The presence of leonine facies and waxy papules, giving the skin a cobblestone appearance, help to distinguish scleromyxoedema from scleroedema and SSc. However, some patients with scleromyxoedema have a sclerodermiform appearance without papules, and in such cases the more superficial dermal changes and preservation of skin appendages on histology and the presence of a paraprotein may aid diagnosis. Scleroedema occurs in children and adults and typically affects the upper back, neck and face. The skin induration is non-pitting and hard and there is no sharp demarcation between normal and affected skin. Diabetes (typically longstanding and insulin

PART 4: INFLAMMATORY DERMATOSES

Table 54.9 Comparative features of generalised morphoea, eosinophilic fasciitis, scleroedema, scleromyxoedema and nephrogenic systemic fibrosis.

Feature	Pansclerotic morphoea	Eosinophilic fasciitis	Scleroedema	Scleromyxoedema	Nephrogenic systemic fibrosis
Hypercellular dermis (CD34+ fibrocytes)	No	No	No	Yes	Yes
Mucin	+	No	++	++++	++/+++
Depth of skin involvement	Into subcutis fascia and muscle	Fat and deep fascia	Into subcutis (fat replaced by collagen)	To mid-reticular dermis	Into panniculus (thickened septae)
Inflammation	Perivascular lymphocytic with plasma cells in 75% and some histiocytes prominent early in disease course	Yes ± eosinophils	No	Perivascular upper dermis	No/less obvious
Typical site and clinical features	Truncal, proximal limbs, can be generalised; spares fingers, toes and periareolar skin	Extremities (lower limbs especially) but can be generalised; spares fingers and toes; typical 'groove sign'	Back, sides of neck, face; can be generalised; spares hands and feet	Face, neck, hands and forearms (waxy papules, leonine facies); normal hair growth	Extremities, lower trunk (brawny induration, burning sensation)
ANA/ eosinophilia	ANA+/– eosinophilia +/–	ANA+/– eosinophilia +	No	ANA+/–	No
SSc specific ANA	Rare	Very rare	No	No	No
Other associations	Raynaud phenomenon usually absent, normal nail fold capillaries	Polyclonal hypergammaglobulinaemia, morphoea plaques, immune cytopenias, haematological malignancy	Diabetes, infection (especially streptococcal), paraprotein, IgG-κ, IgA, myeloma	Paraprotein IgG-λ	Renal failure, exposure to linear non-ionic forms of gadolinium

ANA, antinuclear antibody; Ig, immunoglobulin; SSc, systemic sclerosis.

dependent), recent infection (particularly streptococcal) and IgG-κ paraproteinaemia are associated. Both scleroedema and scleromyxoedema may be associated with plasma cell dyscrasias, and less commonly with multiple myeloma. Nephrogenic systemic fibrosis involves the extremities and rarely the face. Normal renal function and absence of exposure to less stable linear gadolinium-based contrast media exclude the condition, which is now rarely seen. Normal thyroid function and absent thyroid autoantibodies exclude both generalised and pretibial myxoedema. Associated clinical features and age at presentation should help identify the genodermatoses. Stiff skin syndrome is a rare, scleroderma-like disorder with autosomal dominant inheritance that presents in infancy or early childhood with rock-hard skin, limited joint mobility and mild hypertrichosis. Normally, it occurs in the absence of visceral or muscle involvement. Patients do not present immunological abnormalities or vascular hyperactivity. It is caused by a mutation in the gene for fibrillin-1, which regulates activation of TGF-β. There is a resultant increased collagen microfibril deposition, impaired elastogenesis and increased dermal TGF-β expression [317,318].

A more challenging group of patients are those that demonstrate one of the major internal organ manifestations of SSc but little in the way of other SSc features. Thus, cases of PAH, idiopathic lung fibrosis, primary biliary cirrhosis or severe hypertensive renal failure (such as those presenting with features of thrombotic thrombocytopenic purpura) may also have some laboratory and/or clinical features of SSc. Operationally, the 2013 classification criteria for SSc [13] may be used to help to differentiate these cases as confirmed or definite SSc, but there are always cases that might be considered a *form fruste* of SSc. This is only of major relevance if there are other clinical features that require treatment but generally in these situations the predominant organ-based manifestation takes precedence for management.

Classification of severity

The considerable case-to-case heterogeneity is a challenge in SSc. The important differentiation between limited and diffuse cutaneous disease can generally be made early and certainly within the first 12–18 months of disease. Combining this with subgrouping based on which of the hallmark SSc-specific autoantibodies is present provides an 'outcome-based' classification (summarised in Table 54.4) that has become an important operational aspect of SSc care [17]. The major associations for SSc hallmark ANA patterns are summarised in Table 54.3. These findings have been replicated in a number of different geographical and ethnic groups [26]. While a number of severity scoring systems have been proposed in SSc [319,320], in general, cases associated with diffuse disease or a specific complication such as PAH or lung fibrosis can be regarded as more severe [75,321,322].

An important assessment of severity in all SSc cases is early systematic screening for internal organ disease. This can be protocoled and is important as it permits earlier intervention and greater vigilance for future progression in high-risk cases [323–325]. All patients should have these standard tests within the first 12 months of diagnosis and every 1–2 years in follow up independently of subset (see Investigations later).

Skin scores can be helpful in predicting severity since those patients with the highest MRSS at baseline, even if their skin scores improve, have a worse overall outcome [326]. A weighted 10-point index which includes skin manifestations (patient assessed skin worsening, MRSS, digital ulcers) has been developed and validated to identify patients with active disease [302]. There are now emerging risk scores for other organ-based features that are likely to be useful in clinical practice [324,327,328]. Thus, cases at increased risk of major lung complications may be predicted using a weighted score. There are specific tools now developed and validated for lung fibrosis based upon spirometry and extent of disease on high-resolution computed tomography scan [329,330], and also the composite DETECT tool to assess the risk of PAH in selected at risk cases of SSc (see Cardiopulmonary manifestations earlier) [284,331].

Complications and co-morbidities

Systemic sclerosis is a prototypic multisystem disease and commonly affects many internal organs. Almost all patients will have associated gastrointestinal tract manifestations such as gastro-oesophageal reflux. A proportion will develop more severe gastrointestinal tract involvement and others pulmonary fibrosis, PAH, cardiac disease or SRC. Digital vascular disease is almost universal and, in addition to Raynaud phenomenon, structural vascular damage is associated with ischaemia and digital ulceration. This occurs in up to half of SSc cases in the course of their disease and is a major clinical problem. Inflammatory muscle involvement together with contractural changes in the skin and tendons causes major functional limitations. Myositis, arthritis and the typical cutaneous features of lupus erythematosus or dermatomyositis may occur in cases of SSc overlap. Common co-morbidities include thyroid and other organ-based autoimmune disease. There are also some associated medical conditions such as primary biliary cirrhosis that occur more commonly in SSc than in the general population, although they are not regarded as a part of the SSc disease (see Associated diseases earlier). In addition, common conditions such as macrovascular or coronary atherosclerosis are important especially in the context of the age and treatment profile of patients with SSc.

Disease course and prognosis

As might be predicted based upon the diverse patterns and severity of SSc, there is a large variation in disease course and prognosis. Overall, standardised mortality ratios of 2.72–4.06 are reported [281,322,332]. The average life expectancy of patients with SSc is 16–34 years less than age- and sex-matched population peers [333,334]. The case-specific mortality is high, with up to half of cases diagnosed with SSc ultimately dying from the disease. Between 2000 and 2011, 9.6% of 11 193 SSc cases in the EUSTAR database died. Mean age at time of death was 63.6 ± 13.4 years and mean disease duration was 12.3 ± 12.4 years. Death was considered SSc-related in 57.6%. The main causes of death were ILD (16.8%), PAH (14.7%), cancer (13.1%), primary heart disease (mainly heart failure and arrhythmias) (12.0%) and infection (9.1%). Males and patients <60 years of age had a fourfold and tenfold higher mortality from respiratory disease respectively. SSc cases were five times more likely to die from infection than the general population [75]. Established prognostic factors including male sex, older age, dcSSc, lung and cardiac involvement (including PH and ILD), kidney involvement, and inflammation are now included in the SCOpE score, a robust mortality score to estimate 3-year survival and risk stratify patients [75].

There have been improvements in outcome over the past two decades [323,335]. This reflects better education and awareness of the condition and early systematic assessment of complications that may be more treatable in milder forms than when advanced [323,326]. There has been a major improvement since the 1980s in survival from SRC associated directly with the use of ACE inhibitors [394]. Better treatment of PAH and lung fibrosis is

emerging and there is more robust support for organ-based disease that has certainly also improved survival [292,336,337]. The result of improved survival is that the non-lethal burden of SSc becomes much more important and this appropriately is becoming more of a priority for SSc care.

Investigations

Investigation of SSc is important in diagnosis and also in the classification and clinical stratification of cases. The tests needed depend upon the stage and subset of the disease. There should be a systematic approach to assess risk and/or confirm diagnosis of specific complications such as pulmonary hypertension. Once a significant organ-based complication or co-morbidity has been identified this will require detailed specific assessment that goes beyond the scope of this textbook although the key tests and evaluations that are needed are summarised below.

Diagnosis

This requires careful clinical assessment as outlined above. The most important generic tests are ANA reactivity, nail fold capillaroscopy and investigations to exclude or confirm other autoimmune rheumatic diseases. Recent efforts to diagnose SSc earlier in the course of disease, before significant internal organ damage, have led to the development of criteria for the very early diagnosis of systemic sclerosis (VEDOSS). These are the presence of Raynaud phenomenon, puffy fingers and ANA positivity, abnormal nail fold capillaroscopy with an SSc pattern and SSc-specific autoantibodies. The VEDOSS study has demonstrated a positive predictive value of 88.5% for a diagnosis of SSc, when Raynaud phenomenon is present with ANA positivity and puffy fingers [230,338]. This positive predictive value increases further to 94.1% if SSc-specific autoantibodies are present [244] (see Raynaud phenomenon earlier).

An overwhelming majority of SSc patients have either detectable ANA or Raynaud phenomenon (99.8% in the European League Against Rheumatism (EULAR) Scleroderma Trials and Research Group (EUSTAR) database) [339]. Diagnosis of the Raynaud phenomenon is usually based on history, but thermography if available can be an extremely useful confirmatory tool when there is doubt (Figure 54.5). In their absence, alternative causes of skin sclerosis and the possibility of a paraneoplastic cause should be considered. In addition, there should be routine assessment of biochemical and haematological laboratory tests and assessment for typical organ-based complications (including a baseline assessment of cardiac status by electrocardiogram and echocardiography, and of the lungs by chest radiograph and lung function test) are essential. Any abnormality should lead to assessment by more sophisticated tests such as HRCT, which is helpful in the detection of minor basal or posterior changes of fibrosis; or additional cardiac tests that may include cardiac magnetic resonance, rhythm assessment or stress echocardiography. Some cases may need cardiac catheterisation (see Cardiopulmonary manifestations earlier). It is important to determine all the aspects of the disease that are related to the 2013 EULAR ACR classification criteria (summarised in Table 54.1) as these provide a robust platform to manage and move forward with further assessment and treatment. It should be emphasised that the final diagnosis of SSc is clinical. Skin biopsy is not needed unless there are atypical features or an alternate diagnosis is considered.

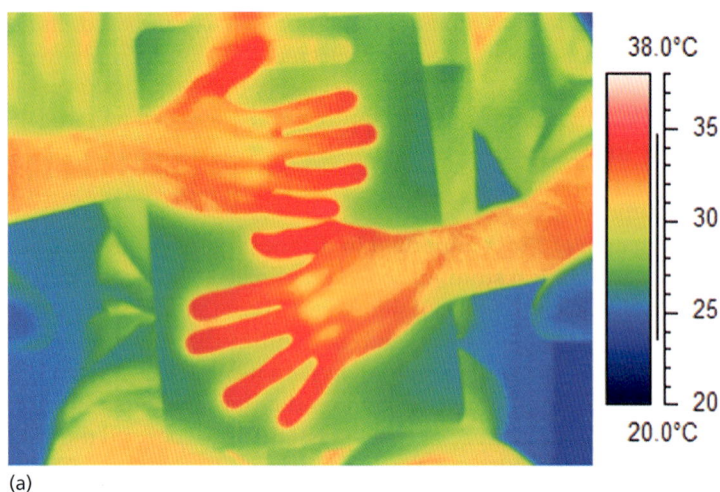

(a)

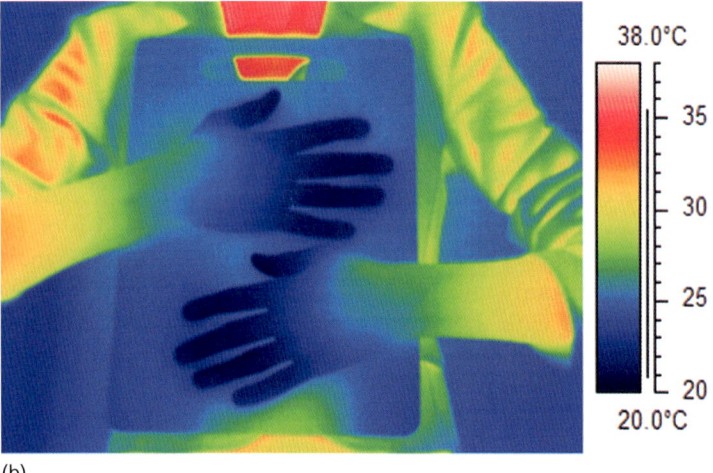

(b)

Figure 54.5 Infrared thermograms recorded 10 min after immersion of the hands in water at 15°C for 1 min for (a) normal fingertip rewarming (temperature 33°C) and (b) fingertip rewarming in a patient with Raynaud phenomenon (temperature 21°C). Courtesy of Dr K Howell, Royal Free London NHS Foundation Trust.

In particular, if deep forms of morphoea or fasciitis are in the differential diagnosis, then a deeper full-thickness fascial biopsy and MRI may be necessary.

Assessment of organ-based disease and systematic follow-up investigations

A cornerstone of the modern management of SSc is the systematic assessment at baseline for involvement of the major internal organs and then systematic or triggered further testing during long-term follow up. At present, annual echocardiography and lung function testing together with systematic symptom assessment is recommended. Other tests may be indicated by clinical developments such as muscle weakness, arthritis or nutritional problems. There are programmes being developed to improve the effectiveness of systematic testing for complications such as PAH, and the DETECT tool may help with this. Risk scores that are weighted composites of multifaceted investigations are being validated and may help to identify cases that are at particular risk to be targeted more effectively [75]. The main regular investigations for major complications of SSc are summarised in Tables 54.10, 54.11 and 54.12.

Management

The management of SSc is complex and depends upon correct diagnosis and appropriate investigation as outlined in previous sections. It is crucial to identify the burden of disease and to attempt to individualise risk so that investigations can be most effective, borderline test results can be interpreted and treatments can be initiated or continued for important aspects of the disease [2,340]. A simple algorithm summarising the broad principles of management of SSc is included in Figure 54.6. This emphasises that some aspects of treatment are generic, especially the use of vasodilators for the Raynaud phenomenon and antacids, especially proton pump inhibitors, for gastro-oesophageal reflux.

A multitude of therapies have been trialled in SSc. Double-blind, randomised placebo-controlled trials (RCTs) have shown no significant benefit in the treatment of skin or systemic manifestations of disease in SSc with N-acetylcysteine [341], chlorambucil [342], interferon α [343], minocycline [344] and recombinant human relaxin [345]. Early controversy as to the effectiveness of d-penicillamine in SSc [346,347], particularly in light of its unfavourable side-effect profile, was resolved in an RCT of high versus very low dose d-penicillamine which showed no difference between treatments or overall [348]. Its use is no longer recommended. Mild beneficial effect on skin scores and disease-associated symptoms, but with variable side effects, was found with interferon γ in one small RCT [349] and several uncontrolled or open label studies [350–352]. In a trial of treatment with oral bovine type I collagen, although the overall findings were not significant, a subgroup analysis showed a reduction in MRSS and suggested possible benefit in patients with late-phase dSSc [353].

Initial findings from non-randomised, open-label or retrospective studies, in just under 100 patients, suggested that UVA1 phototherapy may reduce skin thickness and stiffness (reviewed in [354]). However, a randomised investigator-blinded, controlled study with half-side comparison analysis in nine patients showed improvement overall, but no difference in acrosclerosis between the treated and untreated hand with low-dose UVA1 [355]. Systematic examination of the effect of UVA1 on diffuse skin involvement outside the hands in patients with early inflammatory disease is warranted [356].

A trend towards improvement in skin scores was seen with extracorporeal photopheresis [357,358], and a recently published retrospective study suggests favourable 20-year survival (86.4%) in SSc patients treated with extracorporeal photopheresis [359].

In experimental models of SSc, the tyrosine kinase inhibitors imatinib, nilotinib and dasatinib demonstrated strong antifibrotic effects [360]. Subsequent open-label studies in SSc seemed promising, but two placebo-controlled trials showed only minimal effects on skin and lung fibrosis at the expense of very significant side effects [361–363]. Low-dose treatment in patients with pulmonary fibrosis unresponsive to cyclophosphamide was better tolerated and may remain an option in selected patient groups [361,364].

In a RCT in 63 dcSSc cases, intravenous immunoglobulin at a dose of 400 mg/kg/day for five consecutive days significantly reduced skin scores when two courses of treatment were given, but not after a single course [365]. The benefit disappeared at the end of the study suggesting that, as in dermatomyositis and scleromyxoedema, maintenance therapy may be required. A recent systematic

Table 54.10 Investigation and management of non-cutaneous organ-based complications in systemic sclerosis, with levels of evidence.

Disorder	Investigation	Management	Evidence
Cardiorespiratory			
Pulmonary fibrosis	PFTs (FVC/ DLCO)	*Immunosuppression*	
Cough	HRCT chest	Oral MMF 2–3 g/day	Ia
Dyspnoea	Clinical features (bibasal coarse crepitations)	Nintedanib	Ia
		Rituximab*	Ia
		Tocilizumab*	Ia
		Consider combination therapy, e.g.	
		MMF + nintedanib	
		MMF + tocilizumab	
		Nintedanib + tocilizumab	
		Consider (see text):	
		Cyclophosphamide IV or oral (6–12 months) with MMF (2–3 g/day or if appropriate (see text) Azathioprine (150 mg/day)	Ia
		maintenance	IIa
Palpitations		Prednisolone 10 mg daily	IIa
Syncope		Rigorous antireflux therapy: PPI, H_2-antagonist, prokinetic	IV
		Other interventions:	
		Oxygen – intermittent or long-term low flow	
		Identification and treatment of pulmonary hypertension if present	
PAH	PFTs (FVC/DLCO)	Treatment escalated according to WHO FC stage I–IV	
Cough	ECG	Endothelin receptor blockers:	
Dyspnoea	ACA, troponin T, urate	Ambrisentan, bosentan, macitentan	Ia
Palpitations	6 min walk test	PDE5 inhibitors: sildenafil, tadalafil	Ia
Syncope	Doppler echocardiogram (right atrial area, TR)	Initial combination therapy recommended	Ia
	24 h BP	Guanylate cyclase stimulator: riociguat	Ia [417]
	Right heart catheterisation	Prostacyclin analogues: epoprostenol (continuous) IV, iloprost inhaled or IV, treprostinil oral/SC/IV	Ia
Cardiac dysfunction	Troponin T	*Background therapy*:	All are
Dyspnoea	ECG	Diastolic dysfunction – diuretics	category III
Palpitations	24 h tape and BP	Systolic dysfunction – ACEi ± carvedilol ± selective β-blocker	
Syncope	ECG	*Immunosuppression* (if raised troponin T)	
Hypotension	Cardiac MRI	Cyclophosphamide oral or IV	
Chest pain (pericarditic)	Left heart catheter (if LVEF <50%)	Oral MMF (2 g/day) or azathioprine (150 mg/day) (if TPMT normal)	
ECG abnormality	Endomyocardial biopsy	Prednisolone 10 mg daily	
		Pacemaker/implantable defibrillator (if significant arrhythmia)	
Gastrointestinal			
Reflux/dysphagia	Oesophageal scintigraphy/fluoroscopy/manometry	PPI: omeprazole, lansoprazole	IIa
	Endoscopy	H_2-receptor blocker (famotidine 20–40 mg daily)	III
		Prokinetics (short courses of domperidone/metoclopramide)	III
Diarrhoea/constipation	Barium follow through/MRI/motility studies	Loperamide, opiates	III
	Colonoscopy	Laxatives – non-stimulant	III
Bloating, flatulence, nausea (SIBO)	Hydrogen breath test	Rotating antibiotics/probiotics	III
Faecal incontinence	Colonoscopy, rectal manometry, anal ultrasound/MRI	Bulking agents	III
		Biofeedback therapy	III
		Sacral nerve stimulation	III
Weight loss		*Nutritional support*:	IV
		Oral supplements	
		Naso-jejunal feeding/PEJ feeding	
		Parenteral nutrition	
Upper and lower gastrointestinal		High dose IVIg (2 g/kg/month)	III

(continued)

PART 4: INFLAMMATORY DERMATOSES

PART 4: INFLAMMATORY DERMATOSES

Table 54.10 (continued)

Disorder	Investigation	Management	Evidence
Renal			
Hypertensive renal crisis	Review risk factors Close monitoring of BP	Prompt initiation of ACEi	IIb [191,418]
	U&E, eGFR Proteinuria Renal ultrasound	Additional antihypertensives (ARB, CCB, α-blocker) ACEi, iloprost AVOID HIGH-DOSE STEROIDS (can precipitate SRC)	III III

ª Not currently commissioned for this indication in England.
Grading of evidence:
Ia: systematic review or meta-analysis of randomised controlled trials;
Ib: at least one randomised controlled trial;
IIa: at least one well-designed controlled study without randomisation;
IIb: at least one well-designed quasi-experimental study, such as a cohort study;
III: well-designed non-experimental descriptive studies, such as comparative studies, correlation studies and case–control studies and case series;
IV: expert committee reports or opinions or clinical experience of respected authorities, or both.
ACA, anticentromere antibody; ACEi, angiotensin-converting enzyme inhibitor; ARB, angiotensin receptor blocker; b.d., twice daily; BP, blood pressure; CCB, calcium channel blocker; DLCO, diffusing capacity for carbon monoxide; ECG, electrocardiogram; eGFR, estimated glomerular filtration rate; FVC, forced vital capacity; HRCT, high-resolution computed tomography scan; IV, intravenous; IVIg, intravenous immunoglobulin; LVEF, left ventricular ejection fraction; MMF, mycophenolate mofetil; MRI, magnetic resonance imaging; PAH, pulmonary arterial hypertension; PDE5, phosphodiesterase type 5; PEJ, percutaneous endoscopic jejunostomy; PFT, pulmonary function test; PPI, proton pump inhibitor; SC, subcutaneous; SIBO, small intestinal bacterial overgrowth; SRC, scleroderma renal crisis; TPMT, thiopurine methyl transferase; TR, tricuspid regurgitation; U&E, urea and electrolytes; WHO FC, World Health Organisation functional capacity.

review of 207 cases of SSc treated with intravenous immunoglobulin suggests improvement in skin thickness, gastrointestinal, muscle and joint manifestations. This approach may be particularly beneficial in overlap SSc patients with myositis. The optimum dose (0.4–2 g/kg/month) and duration of treatment remain to be firmly established [366].

In two RCTs, treatment of early diffuse disease with low-dose methotrexate (15–25 mg/week) showed non-significant trends towards improvement in skin scores, DLCO and physician global assessment (PGA) [367,368]. However, when data was re-evaluated using Bayesian methods there was a 96% probability that skin scores and PGA were better on treatment [368,369]. Methotrexate is recommended in early dcSSc, especially in patients with milder (MRSS <25), more slowly progressive skin disease and in patients with SSc-associated inflammatory arthritis [370]. It is usually avoided in patients with ILD or rapidly progressive skin disease.

Azathioprine has shown variable benefit used alone or in combination with cyclophosphamide treatment regimens [371–373]. Current evidence suggests that it is not effective as monotherapy, but may be beneficial for SSc-ILD and skin disease as follow-up maintenance therapy after cyclophosphamide induction [374,**375**]. It may be a useful adjunct in female patients wishing to conceive and in patients intolerant of mycophenolate or methotrexate. Cyclophosphamide has shown benefit in pulmonary fibrosis in randomised, double-blind, placebo-controlled trials [371,376,377], which also showed a significant improvement in skin scores [368,369]. Oral and intravenous treatment regimens may be equally effective for lung and skin disease but further controlled studies are needed [378].

Earlier observational data suggested that mycophenolate was effective in improving or stabilising ILD and skin involvement in SSc (reviewed in [379]). This has now been confirmed in larger clinical trials which demonstrate that oral cyclophosphamide and mycophenolate have similar beneficial effects on lung function and MRSS [380–382]. Patients with the 'inflammatory' gene expression

profile in their skin may be more responsive to mycophenolate mofetil (MMF) therapy and show greater reduction in MRSS [33,383]. Because of its better safety profile, mycophenolate has now become 'standard of care' for early progressive dcSSc and SSc-ILD [384,385].

The last 5 years have seen the introduction of more targeted therapies [**159**]. Nintedanib, a newer intracellular inhibitor of tyrosine kinases, blocks FGF receptor-1, VEGF receptor-2 and PDGF receptor-α. It is well tolerated and is now approved as treatment for SSc-ILD based upon the results of the large SENSCIS randomised clinical trial [**375**] that showed reduced progression of lung fibrosis that was numerically greater in cases that were also receiving background immunosuppression with MMF [386]. Overall, though, no improvement in MRSS was seen with nintedanib in this study. However, the ATA negative patients in SENSCIS showed numerically greater preservation of lung function and improvement of MRSS than the ATA+ group [387].

Tocilizumab, an IL-6 receptor-α inhibitor, has also been approved by the FDA for treatment of SSc-ILD based upon the results of recent randomised clinical trials [388–390] including a Phase 3 trial that demonstrated only a trend of benefit for skin fibrosis [388] but a robust response for lung function [**391**,392]. In a post hoc analysis, a much greater benefit was seen in patients with ATA positivity, disease duration <2 years and CRP >6 g/l [393]. Recent real-world evidence suggests that it is effective in patients with refractory joint and skin involvement, regardless of disease duration or skin subtype, both in adults [394] and in children [395].

Rituximab is a chimeric monoclonal antibody that targets CD20 on B cells, causing depletion of B cells. An observational study of 254 rituximab-treated patients from EUSTAR showed significant improvement in skin fibrosis [396]. A smaller open label RCT found rituximab to be of comparable efficacy to cyclophosphamide for skin and lung manifestations, with a better safety profile [397]. In England, rituximab is available for use in CTD-associated

Table 54.11 Investigation and management of digital vasculopathy in systemic sclerosis, with levels of evidence.

Disorder	Investigation	Management	Evidence[a]
Raynaud phenomenon	Cold challenge/cold provocation test	Warm clothing, gloves, electric handwarmers, avoid cold, stop smoking and stop caffeine. Avoid nasal decongestants, review migraine and ADHD treatments if appropriate	IV
	Nail fold videocapillaroscopy	Topical nitrate preparations (GTN microemulsion (1%, 2%), MQX-503)	Ib [419]
	Nail fold dermatoscopy	Dihydropyridine CCBs: nifedipine 10 mg t.d.s. or sustained release 30–120 mg daily (but lowers oesophageal sphincter tone) or amlodipine 5–10 mg/day (but causes ankle oedema)	Ia [420]
	Serology	Diltiazem extended-release 30–180 mg once-twice/day	IIb [421]
		ARB: losartan 25–100 mg/day	Ib [422]
		PDE5 inhibitor: sildenafil 25–50 mg t.d.s., tadalafil 10 mg alternate daily or 20 mg daily	Ia [423]
		SSRI: fluoxetine 20 mg/day	IIb [424]
		Prostacyclin analogues: IV iloprost (0.5–2 ng/kg/min for 3–5 days) or epoprostenol	Ia [425,426]
		Botulinum toxin injection to interdigital spaces (dorsal approach less painful)	Ib [427,428]
		Statin	III [429]
		Complimentary therapies	
		Vitamins C and E, *Gingko biloba*	IV
		Digital sympathectomy	III
Critical digital ischaemia/ ulceration	Swab, culture, X-ray, MRI	Optimise vasodilatory therapies, prompt assessment and treatment of infection, hydrocolloid occlusion, wound care, pain control	
		PDE5 inhibitor: sildenafil 25–50 mg t.d.s. (healing). Discontinue CCB before starting PDE5 inhibitor	Ia [430,431]
		ERB: bosentan (reduction in new ulcers, improved hand function)	Ia [432,433]
		Parenteral prostacyclin/iloprost or epoprostenol (healing) – further study of oral treprostinil and topical treprostinil delivered via iontophoresis is warranted	Ia [425,426,434]
		Combination of ERB + PDE5 inhibitor +/– ARB	III
		Statin	III
		Antithrombotic therapy:	III
		clopidogrel, aspirin, LMW heparin	III
		Surgical approaches:	III [435]
		Digital injection of adipose-derived stromal vascular fraction	III
		Botulinum toxin injection	III
		Radical microarteriolysis	III
		Sympathectomy	III
		Extracorporeal shock wave therapy	

[a] For categories of evidence see footnote to Table 54.9.
ADHD, attention deficit hyperactivity disorder; ARB, angiotensin receptor blocker; b.d., twice daily; CCB, calcium channel blocker; ERB, endothelin receptor blocker; GTN, glyceryl trinitrate; IV, intravenous; LMW, low molecular weight; MRI, magnetic resonance imaging; PDE5, phosphodiesterase 5; SSRI, selective serotonin reuptake inhibitor; t.d.s., three times daily.

myositis and inflammatory arthritis and may thus be accessed in SSc overlap patients for these indications. Rituximab is now approved in Japan as treatment for SSc based on the recently reported DESIRES randomised controlled trial [398] that demonstrated benefit for skin and lung involvement. Higher CD19 count and MRSS at baseline, and lower B cell counts 2 weeks post-treatment may predict a more favourable response of skin and lung involvement respectively [399,400]. A possible role in treating SSc-PAH and calcinosis have also been proposed [401,402]. Other clinical trial outcomes are awaited, including the RECITAL trial [403] an RCT comparing intravenous cyclophosphamide with rituximab as first line treatment in connective tissue disease associated ILD (including patients with SSc). The optimal timing, duration of treatment and role of combination therapy, e.g. with mycophenolate or autologous haematopoietic stem cell transplantation still needs to be defined.

Other approaches for skin fibrosis have been promising, including targeting IL-4/IL-13 with the bispecific monoclonal antibody romilkimab. IL-4 and IL-13 are elevated in skin biopsies and serum in SSc and have been implicated in fibrosis. In a phase 2A double-blind RCT, romilikimab resulted in a significant reduction of MRSS at 24 weeks. There was also indication of a possible additive effect in patients receiving concomitant immunosuppressive

therapy [404]. This has prompted a study of dupilumab in morphoea (Chapter 56). Abatacept, a recombinant fusion protein binding to CD80 and CD86, prevents CD28 mediated T-cell co-stimulation and has shown clinically meaningful improvements in MRSS and HAQ-DI in the open label extension of the ASSET trial [36,405]. Interestingly, the clinical response to abatacept appears greater in patients with the 'inflammatory' intrinsic gene expression profile in skin [34]. Riociguat, a soluble guanylate cyclase stimulator with effects on vascular remodelling and antifibrotic properties, is approved for the treatment of SSc-PAH [406], but effects on skin and lung manifestations are less clearcut [407]. Prevention of MRSS progression with riociguat was seen in the ARA+ patients but not the ATA+ group in this study. There has also been interest in the antifibrotic effects of cannabinoids. Encouraging results from a phase II RCT of lenabasum in early dcSSc [408] have not been confirmed in the subsequent phase III study [159,409], although subgroup analysis is awaited. The roles of BAFF, JAK, LPA (lysophosphatidic acid) and autotaxin inhibitors and α-MSH agonists, among others, are now under investigation, but require further evaluation (for an excellent recent review see [159]).

For the most severe cases of poor prognosis systemic sclerosis, high dose chemotherapy with immunoablation followed by

Table 54.12 Investigation and management of skin manifestations in systemic sclerosis, with levels of evidence.

	Detection	Management	Evidence[a]
General	Clinical features	Manual lymphatic drainage (Vodder technique)	IV
	MRSS	Physiotherapy and hand stretching exercises	III
Topical therapies	Durometer	At least daily emollient +/− topical antipruritic agent (e.g. lauromacrogols)	IV
	Ultrasound	Topical corticosteroids	III
		Calcineurin inhibitors (evidence in morphoea)	Ib
		Vitamin D analogues (evidence in morphoea)	IIb
		Phototherapy UVA1 PUVA (in SSc)	III (Ib in morphoea)
Diffuse progressive skin sclerosis only		MTX 15–25 mg/week (first line)	IIa
		MMF 2–3 g/day (first line if MRSS >24)	Ia
		IV cyclophosphamide 600 mg/m^2/month for 6 months or 500 mg/m^2 for the first month increasing to 750 mg/m^2	Ia
		Consider UVA1	IV
Diffuse or progressive skin sclerosis *with* lung involvement		MMF 2–3 g/day	Ia
		IV cyclophosphamide 600 mg/m^2/month for 6 months or 500 mg/m^2 for the first month increasing to 750 mg/m^2	Ia
		Oral cyclophosphamide up to 2 mg/kg/day for 1 year	Ia
		Rituximab*	Ia
		Tocilizumab*	Ia
		Romilkimab*	III
Diffuse or progressive skin sclerosis if intolerant of MTX/MMF or trying to conceive		Azathioprine 2–3 mg/kg/day (if TPMT normal)	IIb
Diffuse or progressive skin sclerosis *with* associated myositis or inflammatory arthritis		MTX	IIa
		Rituximab 1 g twice 2 weeks apart	IIa
		Abatacept 125 mg weekly	IIa
		IVIg 2 g/kg over 2–5 days monthly	III
Pruritus		Ketotifen 6 mg/day	Ib
		Lenabasum	Ib
		Naltrexone 2–4.5 mg/day	IV
		Gabapentin/pregabalin/amitriptyline	IV
		Montelukast	IV
		Glucocorticoids	IV
		TLO1/PUVA	IV
Calcinosis	X-ray	Surgery, CO$_2$ laser	IIb
	MRI ^{18}F-NaF PET/CT	CCB: diltiazem	III
	Ultrasound	Intralesional sodium thiosulphate	III
		Extracorporeal shock wave therapy	IV
		Minocycline	III
		Colchicine/rituximab/anakinra	IV
Telangiectasia	Clinical features	Pulsed dye laser: better outcomes	Ib
	Dermatoscopy	IPL: fewer side effects	
		Both are effective (avoid IPL in SLE overlap)	

[a] For categories of evidence see footnote to Table 54.9.
CCB, calcium channel blocker; CO$_2$, carbon dioxide; CT, computed tomography; IPL, intense pulsed light; IVIg, intravenous immunoglobulin; MMF, mycophenolate mofetil; MRI, magnetic resonance imaging; MRSS, modified Rodnan skin score; MTX, methotrexate; PET, positron emission tomography; PUVA, psoralen with UVA; SLE, systemic lupus erythematosus; SSc, systemic sclerosis; UV, ultraviolet; TLO1, narrow-band UVB; TPMT, thiopurine methyl transferase.

autologous stem cell transplantation (SCT) has been shown to be superior to cyclophosphamide in three clinical trials. This includes use of a myeloablative strategy in the SCOT study that had particular benefit on lung function as well as 'event-free survival' [410]. In suitable cases it can lead to excellent short- and longer term outcome [411]. However, case selection for SCT and the morbidity and mortality associated with this form of treatment limit adoption into routine practice, where current standard of care can also give an acceptable event-free survival [412].

A schematic of SSc pathogenesis that highlights the potential targets for disease modifying therapies is reproduced from Campochiaro and Allanore [413] in Figure 54.6. The marked increase in the arsenal of drugs now available for treatment of SSc is encouraging. However, evidence is still lacking as to how to best stratify their use in particular patient subgroups.

The best responses to treatment are seen if given early, in patients with rapidly progressing diffuse disease. In all cases of diffuse skin disease, treatment with immunosuppression should be considered and this should include either methotrexate or mycophenolate [414,415,416]. In patients with milder skin disease or inflammatory arthritis, methotrexate is favoured. In those with higher baseline skin scores (MRSS >24) and/or concomitant ILD, mycophenolate is first line treatment. Rituximab, abatacept or intravenous immunoglobulin may be considered in patients with associated myositis. For refractory or severe skin disease, parenteral cyclophosphamide is currently still recommended. However, as

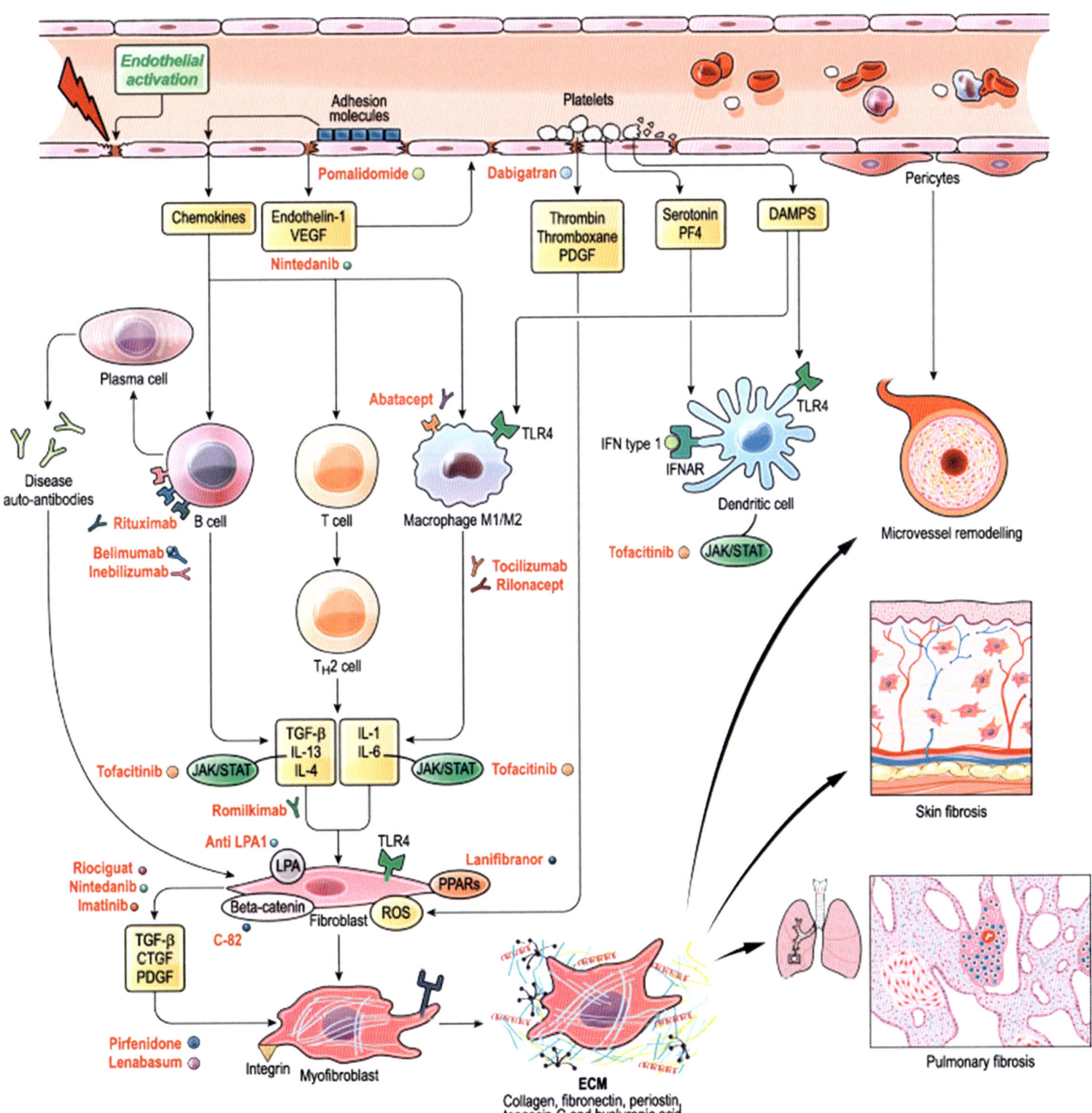

Figure 54.6 Schematic of systemic sclerosis pathogenesis highlighting the potential targets for disease modifying drugs. CTGF, connective tissue growth factor; DAMPS, damage-associated molecular patterns; ECM, extracellular matrix; IFNAR, interferon receptor; JAK, Janus kinase; LPA, lysophosphatidic acid receptor; PDGF, platelet-derived growth factor; PF4, platelet-factor 4; PPAR, peroxisome proliferator-activated receptor; ROS, reactive oxygen species; TGF, tissue growth factor; TLR4, toll-like receptor 4; VEGF, vascular-endothelial growth factor. Reproduced with permission from Campochiaro and Allanore [405].

tocilizumab, romilkimab and rituximab become available for this indication, and in patients with appropriate other organ involvement, their more favourable side-effect profile will place them ahead of cyclophosphamide in the treatment algorithm.

Traditionally, patients with lcSSc have not been treated with immunosuppression. However, increasing appreciation of the prevalence and progression of SSc-ILD and digital ulcers in this group suggests a need for more aggressive therapy [20]. This will be

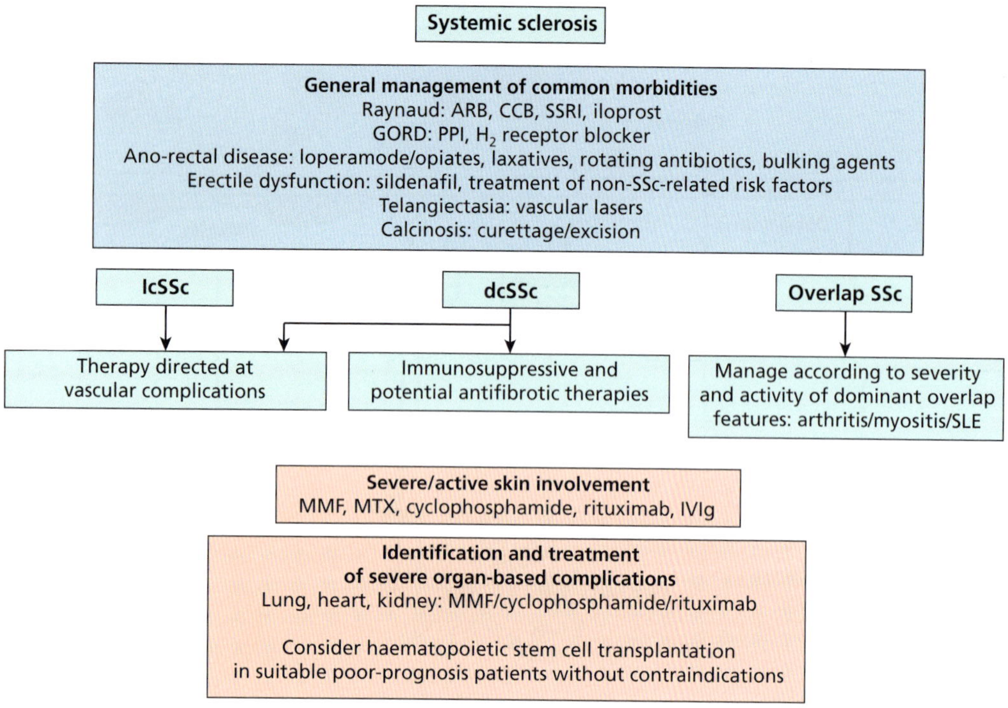

Systemic sclerosis

General management of common morbidities
Raynaud: ARB, CCB, SSRI, iloprost
GORD: PPI, H_2 receptor blocker
Ano-rectal disease: loperamode/opiates, laxatives, rotating antibiotics, bulking agents
Erectile dysfunction: sildenafil, treatment of non-SSc-related risk factors
Telangiectasia: vascular lasers
Calcinosis: curettage/excision

lcSSc

dcSSc

Overlap SSc

Therapy directed at vascular complications

Immunosuppressive and potential antifibrotic therapies

Manage according to severity and activity of dominant overlap features: arthritis/myositis/SLE

Severe/active skin involvement
MMF, MTX, cyclophosphamide, rituximab, IVIg

Identification and treatment of severe organ-based complications
Lung, heart, kidney: MMF/cyclophosphamide/rituximab

Consider haematopoietic stem cell transplantation in suitable poor-prognosis patients without contraindications

Figure 54.7 Management of systemic sclerosis. While a range of supportive therapies may be appropriate for all SSc patients, treatment should be tailored according to individual patients' needs based on the disease subtype, stage and presence of organ-based complications (see Tables 54.9, 54.10 and 54.11). ARB, angiotensin receptor blocker; CCB, calcium channel blocker; dSSc, diffuse SSc; GORD, gastro-oesophageal reflux disease; IVIg, intravenous immunoglobulin; lSSc, limited SSc; MMF, mycophenolate; MTX, methotrexate; PPI, proton pump inhibitor; SLE, systemic lupus erythematosus; SSRI, selective serotonin reuptake inhibitor. Courtesy of Dr C.H. Orteu and Professor C. Denton.

examined in the MINIMISE study (NCT04927390), which will assess benefit of mycophenolate in prevention of disease progression in lcSSc.

There are specific approaches to the management of individual organ-based complications of SSc and these largely follow the management of these manifestations when they occur outside the context of SSc. This is especially the case for PAH. Most patients will be treated with a combination of PDE5 inhibitors and endothelin receptor antagonists. In patients not responding to this combination, addition of a prostacyclin receptor agonist (selexipag) or a prostacyclin analogue (oral/or inhaled treprostinil or intravenous iloprost) or both, should be considered [337,436]. Conversion from a PDE5 inhibitor to riociguat may also be appropriate at this stage [406] and early studies suggest a role for rituximab also [401].

SRC requires early diagnosis, and this may impact greatly on outcome. ACE inhibitors supplemented by other antihypertensives remain the cornerstone of management of SRC [294]. Endothelin-1 is overexpressed in glomeruli and arterioles of patients with SRC [437]; use of endothelin receptor blockade is promising, and may delay onset of SRC, but still requires further investigation [190,438].

It is increasingly clear that the burden of ILD has been underestimated and that there is a window of opportunity for treating this in its early stages before fibrosis develops. Therapeutic strategies are described above as there is marked overlap between treatment for skin and lung involvement in SSc. First line treatment with MMF may be supplemented with nintedanib or cyclophosphamide in England as rituximab and tocilizumab are not yet approved for SSc-ILD. Supportive measures are also critical and include effective treatment of gastro-oesophageal reflux to help prevent ILD progression because of microaspiration at night, identification of associated pulmonary hypertension, management of

infections, and approaches such as cardiopulmonary rehabilitation and supplementary oxygen where appropriate.

Although no RCTs are available, TNF inhibition with infliximab or etanercept may improve the inflammatory arthritis of SSc and may also reduce the risk of cardiopulmonary complications, including PAH [439].

Severe erectile dysfunction affects 70–80% of men with SSc. In a prospective multinational study of the EULAR database, only 18% of 130 males had normal erectile function [440]. It is associated with severe cutaneous, muscular or renal involvement of SSc, elevated pulmonary pressures and restrictive lung disease. While its efficacy is unproven, sildenafil is the most frequently employed treatment [440,441]. No RCTs exist to guide management of calcinosis in SSc. Multiple therapies have been reported in individual cases and small series including warfarin, bisphosphonates, minocycline, ceftriaxone, diltiazem, aluminium hydroxide, probenecid, intralesional corticosteroids, intravenous immunoglobulin, curettage, surgical excision, carbon dioxide laser and extracorporeal shock wave lithotripsy (reviewed in [274]). Based on the association between calcinosis and ischaemia, vasodilators such as diltiazem are commonly used. Intralesional sodium thiosulphate and extracorporeal shock wave therapy may be of benefit in localised deposits, and anti-inflammatories such as minocycline, colchicine and rituximab may be trialled in patients with more widespread involvement [402,442,443].

Although evidence in many areas is still patchy, EULAR and EUSTAR have established recommendations for the treatment of SSc based on a combination of evidence and expert consensus that are widely used, revised and are currently being updated [414,444]. In the UK there are NICE accredited treatment guidelines produced by the British Society for Rheumatology (BSR/BHPR), which also include general and non-pharmacological measures [445]. Specific approaches to the investigation and treatment of individual aspects of SSc are summarised in Tables 54.10, 54.11 and 54.12.

Recent clinical trials have identified differential responses to new treatments according to intrinsic skin gene expression subsets and to autoantibody status. Better understanding of disease biology, improved subsetting and risk stratification, better clinical trial design and outcome assessment will underpin the next stages of progress in managing SSc. There is reason for cautious optimism based upon progress in these areas and emerging data from clinical trials that are starting to better define the potential benefit or toxicity of treatment in particular patient subgroups [340,413].

Resources

Further information

World Scleroderma Foundation: https://worldsclerofound.org/
National Institute for Health and Care Excellence, Evidence reviews: https://www.nice.org.uk/guidance/

Patient resources

Scleroderma and Raynaud's UK (SRUK): https://www.sruk.co.uk/
Federation of European Scleroderma Associations (FESCA): https://fesca-scleroderma.eu/
Manual Lymphatic Drainage UK (MLDUK): http://www.mlduk.org.uk/. (MLDUK promotes awareness and provides contact details for manual lymphatic drainage massage practitioners.)
Versus Arthritis: https://www.versusarthritis.org/about-arthritis/conditions/systemic-sclerosis-scleroderma/

Key references

The full list of references can be found in the online version at https://www.wiley.com/rooksdermatology10e

13 van den Hoogen F, Khanna D, Fransen J et al. 2013 classification criteria for systemic sclerosis: an American College of Rheumatology/European League against Rheumatism collaborative initiative. *Arthritis Rheum* 2013;65:2737–47.

17 Nihtyanova SI, Sari A, Harvey JC et al. Using autoantibodies and cutaneous subset to develop outcome-based disease classification in systemic sclerosis. *Arthritis Rheumatol* 2020;72:465–76.

96 Acosta-Herrera M, Kerick M, López-Isac E et al. Comprehensive analysis of the major histocompatibility complex in systemic sclerosis identifies differential HLA associations by clinical and serological subtypes. *Ann Rheum Dis* 2021;80:1040–7.

135 Varga J, Trojanowska M, Kuwana M. Pathogenesis of systemic sclerosis: recent insights of molecular and cellular mechanisms and therapeutic opportunities. *J Scleroderma Relat Disord* 2017;2:137–52.

159 Lescoat A, Roofeh D, Kuwana M, Lafyatis R, Allanore Y, Khanna D. Therapeutic approaches to systemic sclerosis: recent approvals and future candidate therapies. *Clin Rev Allergy Immunol* 2023;64:239–61.

285 Simonneau G, Montani D, Celermajer DS et al. Haemodynamic definitions and updated clinical classification of pulmonary hypertension. *Eur Respir J* 2019;53:1801913.

375 Distler O, Highland KB, Gahlemann M et al. Nintedanib for systemic sclerosis-associated interstitial lung disease. *N Engl J Med* 2019;380:2518–28.

391 Khanna D, Lin CJF, Furst DE et al. Long-term safety and efficacy of tocilizumab in early systemic sclerosis-interstitial lung disease: open label extension of a phase 3 randomized controlled trial. *Am J Respir Crit Care Med* 2022;205:674–84.

410 Sullivan KM, Goldmuntz EA, Keyes-Elstein L et al. Myeloablative autologous stem-cell transplantation for severe scleroderma. *N Engl J Med* 2018;378:35–47.

414 Kowal-Bielecka O, Fransen J, Avouac J et al. Update of EULAR recommendations for the treatment of systemic sclerosis. *Ann Rheum Dis* 2017;76:1327–39.

PART 4: INFLAMMATORY DERMATOSES

CHAPTER 55

Morphoea and Allied Scarring and Sclerosing Inflammatory Dermatoses

Catherine H. Orteu

Department of Dermatology, Royal Free London NHS Foundation Trust, London, UK

Definition and nomenclature

The term scleroderma derives from the Greek *skleros*, meaning hard, and *derma*, meaning skin. It has been used to encompass a spectrum of disorders (Chapter 54) that include systemic sclerosis (SSc), covered in Chapter 54, and localised forms of the disease. Morphoea, a term used in preference to 'localised scleroderma', encompasses a group of related conditions in which inflammation drives fibrosis and which are characterised by varying degrees of inflammation, fibrosis, sclerosis and atrophy in the skin and subcutaneous tissues, sometimes extending deeply into muscle, bone, eye and brain. Extracutaneous manifestations, most commonly musculoskeletal, occur in 22–75% of cases overall and 46–74% of paediatric onset cases in prospective studies. They may be more prevalent in children than adults. In contrast to SSc, no internal organ fibrosis or vascular changes occur. Antinuclear antibody (ANA) positivity is common but the specific autoantibodies seen in SSc are rarely present. There is no increased mortality, but substantial morbidity may occur as a result of joint contractures, facial and limb asymmetry, extracutaneous manifestations and the psychological impact of the condition [1,2–6].

Synonyms and inclusions
- Localised scleroderma, morphoea
- Circumscribed morphoea, limited plaque morphoea, circumscribed plaque morphoea

- Guttate morphoea
- Atrophoderma of Pasini–Pierini
- Keloidal morphoea, nodular morphoea, nodular scleroderma
- Limited deep morphoea, circumscribed deep morphoea, solitary morphoea profunda
- Deep morphoea, subcutaneous morphoea, morphoea profunda
- Bullous morphoea
- Linear morphoea, linear scleroderma:
  Limb/trunk variant
  Head variant: en coup de sabre, progressive facial hemiatrophy, progressive hemifacial atrophy, Parry–Romberg syndrome
- Linear atrophoderma of Moulin
- Generalised morphoea, generalised localised scleroderma, generalised plaque morphoea, disseminated plaque morphoea
- Pansclerotic morphoea
- Eosinophilic fasciitis, Schulman's syndrome
- Mixed morphoea, mixed localised scleroderma

Terminology

The nomenclature is confusing for patients and doctors. On hearing the term scleroderma, even when it is prefixed by 'localised', many patients assume they have SSc. This is compounded by the results of online searches that frequently find the terms used synonymously and rarely give much information on localised forms of the disease. The terminology can be confusing for doctors too, for instance when terms such as 'limited scleroderma', meaning limited systemic sclerosis, or 'generalised localised scleroderma' meaning widespread morphoea are used. Localised scleroderma is an umbrella term employed in the literature to encompass the various forms of morphoea – namely limited (circumscribed), generalised, linear, pansclerotic and mixed morphoea – which do not usually involve internal organs such as the lungs, heart and kidneys. Linear forms, which are commoner in childhood, are generally referred to in the paediatric and rheumatology literature as linear scleroderma. The term morphoea is preferred by dermatologists for the various subtypes and will be employed throughout this chapter.

Classification

There has been controversy as to which conditions should be included within the morphoea spectrum. This applies particularly to eosinophilic fasciitis and lichen sclerosus, and to atrophic variants, such as atrophoderma of Pasini–Pierini, linear atrophoderma of Moulin and progressive hemifacial atrophy. There has also been debate over whether deep, keloidal and bullous morphoea should be considered as disease modifiers or separate subtypes, and over what, exactly, constitutes generalised morphoea.

Several different classification systems are currently in use (Table 55.1) [7–10]. The most widely used in the literature has been that of Peterson *et al.* [7]. This classification remains controversial, firstly because it includes atrophoderma of Pasini–Pierini, lichen sclerosus and eosinophilic fasciitis, which are not universally agreed to be within the morphoea spectrum, and secondly because it does not include a category for the 2.6–23% of patients who present a 'mixed' subtype (e.g. linear limb with truncal plaque morphoea) [1,11,12]. To address this, the Paediatric Rheumatology European Society proposed the 'Padua' or 'PRES classification' excluding atrophoderma, lichen sclerosus and eosinophilic fasciitis, but including separate pansclerotic and mixed subtypes [8], which appears the most accurate (see later). In 2009 the German Dermatological Society proposed a third classification subdividing morphoea into limited, generalised, linear and deep types, including atrophoderma and eosinophilic fasciitis within the classification, but not lichen sclerosus or the mixed subtype [9]. This classification was later revised by the European Dermatology Forum to include separate subtypes for mixed morphoea and eosinophilic fasciitis [10].

The variation between classification systems has caused confusion and difficulty in interpretation of the published literature on morphoea. For example, there has been a lack of agreement as to what constitutes 'generalised morphoea' with at least three different definitions proposed (see Table 55.1 and the section on generalised subtypes in clinical variants, later). Pansclerotic morphoea has variably been included within deep, generalised or as a separate subtype. Multisite linear morphoea which may fulfil the criteria for generalised morphoea might be included within that subtype, when it is in fact associated with very different risks of damage, extracutaneous involvement and relapse compared with, for instance, isomorphic generalised plaque morphoea. Circumscribed deep morphoea is the only subtype of morphoea ascribed a 'deep variant' in the PRES classification, even though involvement of the deep dermis,

subcutis, fascia and muscle can occur across all morphoea subtypes. In contrast, but equally unsatisfactory, other classifications include a 'deep subtype' which could include patients with deep involvement in linear, circumscribed, generalised or pansclerotic disease all with very different features and complication risks. Similarly, bullous morphoea is a separate subtype in Peterson's classification but can occur in any subtype of morphoea, usually in the context of the active inflammatory phase of the disease.

Two important studies have been published since the last edition of this text which help to better define and classify morphoea subtypes. In the first, the performance of the various morphoea classifications was evaluated in a prospective cohort of 944 patients (444 with adult-onset and 500 with paediatric-onset morphoea) [13]. The PRES criteria [8] performed best and successfully classified 95% of patients into the most relevant disease subtypes with cohesive demographic and clinical features. By comparison, the Peterson's and the European Dermatology Forum (EDF) criteria successfully classified only 56% and 52% of patients respectively [13]. The second study is a cross-sectional study employing the PRES classification subtype criteria, in which computerised skin mapping was undertaken in a cohort of 123 patients with generalised morphoea (a discovery cohort of 73 and validation cohort of 44 patients) and compared with clinical and demographic features. Two lesional distribution patterns, isomorphic and symmetric (see Table 55.2 and section on generalised plaque morphoea, later) encompassed most cases and were associated with distinct demographic and clinical features, allowing much better definition of the 'generalised morphoea' subtype [14].

While there has been significant improvement, there are still issues with classification and terminology, and controversies regarding whether some sclero-atrophic conditions should be included within the morphoea spectrum. The classification employed here is an 'inclusive' one, based on the PRES classification, but which for completeness, incorporates some elements from other classifications which are viewed as controversial (Tables 55.1 and 55.2). It distinguishes limited, generalised, linear, pansclerotic and mixed subtypes as well as a separate morphoea–lichen sclerosus overlap group. The various atrophic variants are included since they frequently overlap with other forms of morphoea, although it is accepted that this remains controversial. The PRES classification definition of generalised morphoea is retained and refined based on Teske *et al.* [14], defining two distinct isomorphic and symmetric patterns of disease, and exclusion of multisite linear disease. The term 'disseminated plaque morphoea' was used in the previous edition of *Rook's Textbook of Dermatology*, and in the author's view this terminology gives a better description of what constitutes 'generalised morphoea' – i.e. plaques at multiple sites which may coalesce – and could be used instead of this term. Alternatively, the term 'generalised plaque morphoea' could be used to clarify that the generalised morphoea subtype represents patients with widespread coalescent plaque disease, in an either isomorphic or symmetric pattern, but *not* widespread linear or circumferential pansclerotic disease. Pansclerotic morphoea, as defined by Kim *et al.* [15] is included as a separate subtype. Eosinophilic fasciitis, another controversial inclusion, can occur in a widespread fashion on trunk and all limbs resembling pansclerotic disease, or in a limited fashion on the lower limbs,

Table 55.1 Classification systems for morphoea.

Peterson *et al.* 1995 [7] 'Mayo'	Laxer and Zulian 2006 [8] 'PRES'	Kreuter *et al.* 2009 [9] 'AWMF'	Knobler *et al.* [10] 'EDF'	Classification and terminology used in this chapter Disease modifiers – see Table 55.2 Depth, bullae, keloids/nodules
Plaque morphoea • Morphoea en plaque • Guttate morphoea • Atrophoderma of Pasini–Pierini • Lichen sclerosus • Keloidal morphoea	*Circumscribed morphoea* • Superficial • Deep	*Limited type* • Morphoea (plaque type) • Guttate morphoea • Atrophoderma of Pasini–Pierini	*Limited type* • Plaque morphoea • Guttate morphoea • Atrophoderma of Pasini-Pierini/superficial morphoea	*Limited morphoea* • Circumscribed plaque morphoea • Guttate morphoea • Atrophoderma of Pasini–Pierini
Generalised morphoea (lesions at three or more of seven anatomical sites)[a]	*Generalised morphoea* Induration of the skin starting as four or more individual plaques which are larger than 3 cm and become confluent, involving at least two of seven anatomical sites[a]	*Generalised type* Lesions at three or more of seven anatomical sites[a] • Generalised localised scleroderma • Disabling pansclerotic morphoea • Eosinophilic fasciitis	*Generalised type* Four or more indurated plaques of more than 3 cm in diameter, involving two or more of seven anatomical sites[a] • Generalised lichen sclerosus morphoea • Disabling pansclerotic morphoea	*Generalised plaque morphoea/disseminated plaque morphoea* Induration of the skin starting as four or more individual plaques that become confluent and involve at least two of seven anatomical sites[a] • Isomorphic pattern • Symmetric pattern
Linear morphoea • Linear morphoea of the limbs or trunk • En coup de sabre morphoea • Progressive hemifacial atrophy/Parry–Romberg syndrome	*Linear morphoea* • Trunk/limb variant • Head variant	*Linear type* • Linear localised scleroderma (usually of the extremities) • Linear localised scleroderma en coup de sabre type • Progressive facial hemiatrophy	*Linear type* • Linear lichen sclerosus /morphoea of the extremities • Linear lichen sclerosus /morphoea en coup de sabre • Progressive facial hemiatrophy/ Parry–Romberg syndrome	*Linear morphoea* Trunk/limb variant • Linear morphoea • Linear atrophoderma of Moulin • Linear deep atrophic morphoea Head/neck variant • Morphoea en coup de sabre • Progressive hemifacial atrophy Multisite linear morphoea
Deep morphoea • Subcutaneous morphoea • Morphoea profunda • Eosinophilic fasciitis • Disabling pansclerotic morphoea	*Pansclerotic morphoea* Circumferential involvement of limbs +/− other areas, affecting the skin subcutaneous tissue, muscle and bone. No internal organ involvement	*Deep type*	*Deep type*	*Pansclerotic morphoea* *Eosinophilic fasciitis*
Bullous morphoea	*Mixed morphoea*		*Mixed type* *Eosinophilic fasciitis*	*Mixed morphoea* *Lichen sclerosus with morphoea*

[a] The seven anatomical sites include the head–neck, right and left upper limbs, right and left lower limbs, anterior trunk and posterior trunk.

when it occurs in association with plaque morphoea elsewhere in 20–40% of cases [16–19]. It is included as a separate subtype but on the understanding that there is significant clinical overlap with pansclerotic disease suggesting that they are part of a spectrum [17–19]. Several recent studies have confirmed that deep involvement can occur in any of the morphoea subtypes and should thus be considered a disease modifier rather than a separate subtype [12,13,20]. Bullous and keloidal lesions may also occur across subgroups and, as suggested by Prasad *et al.* [13] and Abbas *et al.* [2], are also to be considered as disease modifiers.

The above classifications remain based on morphology, extent and distribution of morphoea. More recent transcriptomic data from RNA sequencing in paediatric morphoea skin has shown overlapping gene expression profiles across the different morphoea clinical subtypes and unique profiles for active versus inactive disease [21,22]. 'Inflammatory', 'fibroproliferative' and 'healthy-like' skin cell specific gene expression subsets which correlate with histological inflammatory cell infiltration, disease activity scores and ANA positivity are being characterised [21,22]. Ultimately it is hoped that molecular endotype cross-referencing will help resolve the confusion over clinical classifications.

PART 4: INFLAMMATORY DERMATOSES

Table 55.2 Proposed classification of morphoea and subtype characteristics (based on Laxer and Zulian [8] with modifications as per the text).

Main division	Subtype	Description
Limited morphoea	Circumscribed plaque morphoea	Single or multiple round to oval lesions >1 cm in diameter in up to two anatomical regions.[a] May be oedematous, erythematous to bruise-like, yellowish white, indurated ± a lilac ring, or atrophic and pigmented. Usually involves epidermis and dermis. May involve deeper structures
	Guttate morphoea	Multiple small <1 cm erythematous to yellowish white, round to oval lesions, usually on the trunk. Involves the papillary and superficial dermis
	Atrophoderma of Pasini–Pierini	Multiple, round to oval, non-indurated, sharply demarcated, depressed patches, 'cliff-drop' edge, and usually hyperpigmented. Involves the superficial reticular dermis
Generalised plaque morphoea		Induration of the skin starting as four or more individual plaques that become confluent and involve at least two of seven anatomical sites[a]
	Isomorphic pattern	Plaques coalesce in the inframammary area and bra-line, waistband and around the hips and inguinal regions at sites of repeated minor trauma from clothing. Usually superficial. Frequently coexists with extragenital and genital lichen sclerosus
	Symmetric pattern	Multiple individual plaques are distributed symmetrically about the midline on the trunk and limbs. Frequent 'horseshoe distribution' of plaques across the lower abdomen. Deep involvement is more frequent
Linear morphoea		
Trunk/limb variant	Linear morphoea	Blaschkoid linear induration of the limbs or trunk +/– dyspigmentation, +/– atrophy. May involve the dermis, subcutaneous tissue ± underlying muscle and bone
	Linear atrophoderma of Moulin	Blaschkoid hyperpigmented linear atrophic limb/trunk lesions. Involves superficial dermis
	Linear deep atrophic morphoea	Linear atrophic lesions involving the deep dermis and subcutis
Head/neck variant	Morphoea en coup de sabre	Blaschkoid linear band of induration, +/– dyspigmentation, +/– atrophy affecting the forehead, face and scalp, may involve underlying muscle, bone, eye, oral cavity and brain
	Progressive hemifacial atrophy/Parry–Romberg syndrome	Non-indurated skin, occasional bruise-like pigmentation with associated underlying atrophy on one side of the face. Probable Blaschkoid distribution. May involve the dermis, subcutaneous tissue, muscle, bone, eye, oral cavity and brain
Pansclerotic morphoea		Circumferential involvement of the majority (85%) of body surface areas with sparing of fingers, toes and nipples. Skin is thickened and may be bound down to underlying structures. There may be puckering or a peau d'orange appearance. Affects the dermis and frequently the subcutis, fascia, muscle and/or bone. No internal organ fibrosis
Eosinophilic fasciitis		Symmetrically involves the extremities, but spares the fingers and face, and affects the trunk in one third. Painful, burning erythema and swelling followed by progressive induration and thickening with a peau d'orange appearance and guttering around vessels and tendons. Skin is bound down to underlying structures. Involves deep fascia, tendons and muscle. Dermis may be sclerotic or normal. Concomitant plaque morphoea in 20–40%
Mixed type		A combination of two or more of the above subtypes, most often linear and circumscribed plaque
Morphoea–lichen sclerosus overlap		Most often seen in post-menopausal women with isomorphic generalised plaque morphoea. Extragenital lichen sclerosus lesions may occur at the same site as morphoea or at different sites. Small patches of lichen sclerosus may arise within a larger plaque of morphoea. Usually truncal but may be widespread. Increased prevalence of genital lichen sclerosus
Disease modifiers	Deep	If deep dermis, subcutis and deeper structures involved, lesions may be less well defined, thickened and bound down, sometimes with guttering or a cobblestone or peau d'orange appearance. Overlying skin may appear normal or puckered. Superficial and deep lesions may occur in the same morphoea subtype and in the same patient. Deep involvement associated with more functional impairment and severe disease
	Bullous	Tense subepidermal bullae overlying typical morphoea, usually in patients with active inflammatory often deep disease, most often on lower limbs
	Keloidal/nodular morphoea	Keloid-like or nodular lesions arising from normal or sclerodermatous skin, usually on the trunk, often at keloid prone sites
	Extracutaneous manifestations	Musculoskeletal, neurological, ophthalmic, dental (see later section on extracutaneous manifestations)

[a] The seven anatomical sites include the head–neck, right and left upper limbs, right and left lower limbs, anterior trunk and posterior trunk.

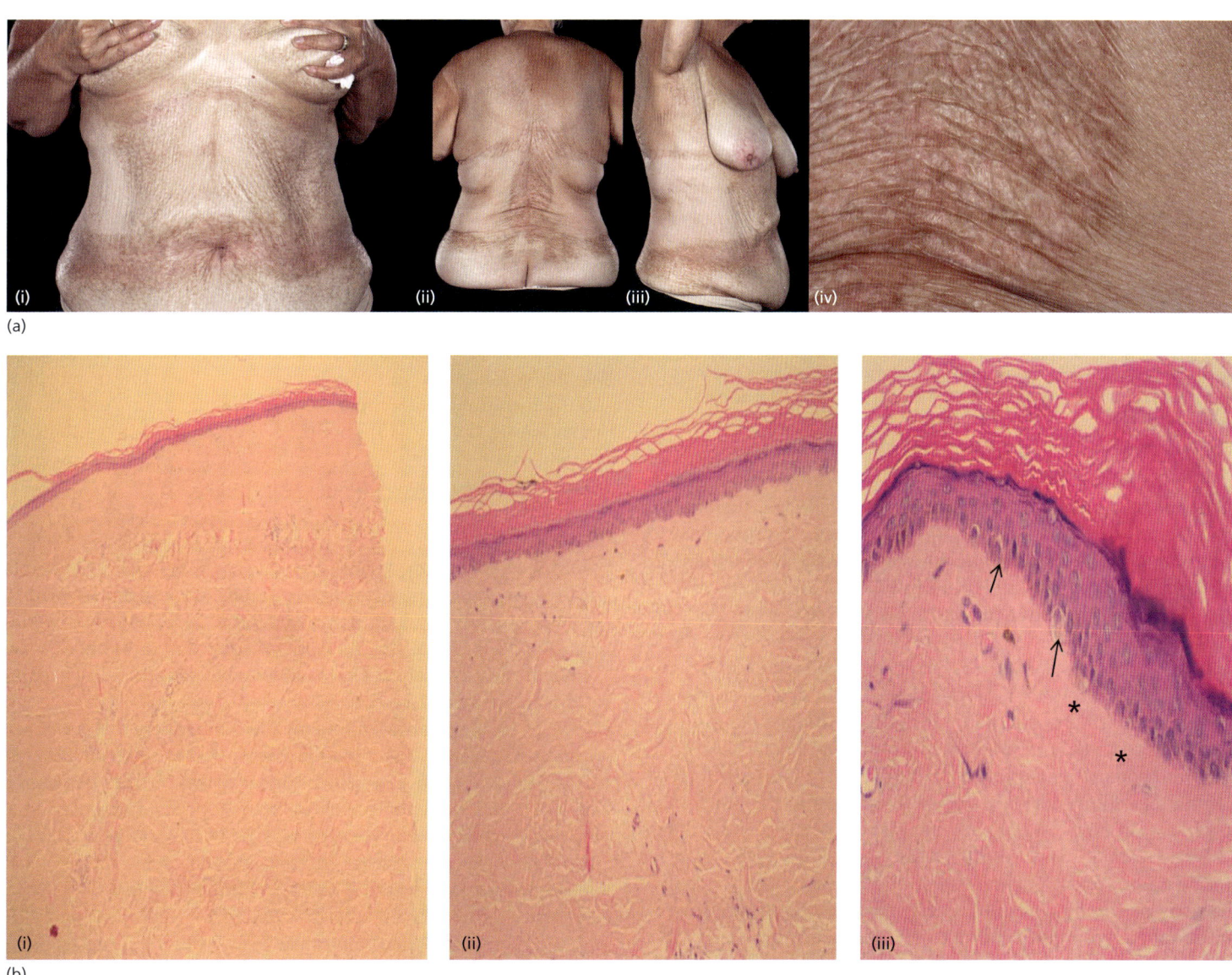

Figure 55.1 (a) Female with widespread, thickened, waxy plaques (i–iii) with a crinkled, hyperkeratotic surface (iv), occurring in an isomorphic pattern, i.e. at sites of pressure from clothing in the waistband, bra-line and inframammary areas (i–iii). (b) Histological appearances confirmed the presence of morphoea at low power (i) and features of lichen sclerosus (orthokeratosis, flattened epidermis, pigmentary incontinence (ii), colloid bodies (arrows) and hyalinisation of papillary dermis (asterisks) (iii)) were seen at a higher power in the same biopsy specimen. Courtesy of Dr V. Swale, Department of Dermatology, Royal Free London NHS Foundation Trust, UK.

Introduction and general description

Morphoea comprises a group of related diseases that share a common underlying pathophysiology of inflammation and increased collagen deposition in an autoimmune setting (Table 55.2). They are largely confined to the skin and subcutaneous tissues, including the underlying fat, fascia, muscle, bone and joints and occasionally with involvement of the mouth, eye and brain [1,3,23,24]. Extracutaneous manifestations, including musculoskeletal, neurological, ocular, oral and dental complications are increasingly well defined and occur in up to 75% of cases. The highest association is in linear and mixed morphoea with onset under the age of 10 years [4,6,12,25–28]. They are 2.5-fold more common in patients with childhood rather than adult-onset linear disease and usually develop after the onset of skin disease [1,5]. ANA is positive in 23–68% of morphoea cases, and appears associated with more severe, deeper disease and an increased risk of relapse after successful treatment [29,30]. Antihistone and anti-ssDNA may also be present, but the SSc-specific autoantibodies such as antitopoisomerase, anticentromere and anti-RNA polymerase are less common [29]. It is distinguished from SSc by the absence of puffy fingers, sclerodactyly and nail fold capillary changes [31] (see also Chapter 54, VEDOSS criteria). The internal organ involvement typical of SSc, namely pulmonary fibrosis and pulmonary hypertension, hypertensive renal crisis, and infiltration and fibrosis of the gastrointestinal tract, do not occur in morphoea. Although previously considered a self-limiting condition, there is now emerging evidence that a protracted, relapsing–remitting course may be common [30,**32**,33,34].

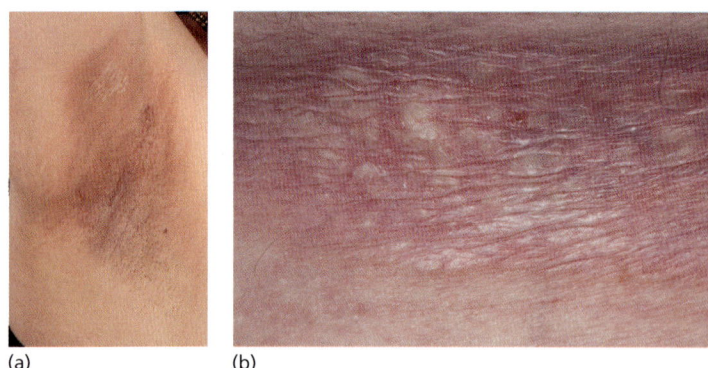

(a)   (b)

Figure 55.2 Varied clinical appearances of lichen sclerosus morphoea overlap: (a) porcelain white plaque with follicular delling overlying a hyperpigmented superficial morphoea plaque. (b) Thickened erythematous plaque with telangiectases, white papules and hyperkeratosis.

If left untreated, lesions may result in significant cosmetic and functional sequelae. In consequence, even though there is no increased mortality, significant morbidity can occur because of facial and limb asymmetry, flexion contractures, extracutaneous manifestations and psychological disability. As in SSc, there is an early, inflammatory, active phase, followed by a sclerotic and then atrophic phase. The key to successful treatment involves initiation during the active inflammatory stage before significant damage has occurred. Factors that have hampered physicians' evaluation and treatment of the condition include its frequently insidious nature, the potential for spontaneous remission and a lack of validated methods to assess disease activity. There has been a recent international effort, not only to better understand the impact that morphoea can have on patients, but also to develop and validate clinical outcome measures [35–39,**40**], consensus best practice [41,42] and treatment guidelines [41–45]. In the future, it is hoped that, as is becoming possible in systemic sclerosis, transcriptomic immunophenotyping will permit better classification and prediction of patients therapeutic responses and allow the development of more personalised medicine (Chapter 54).

Epidemiology

Incidence and prevalence
The overall incidence of morphoea is widely quoted as 4–27 per million per year. However, population-based studies and prevalence data are sparse. In a landmark population-based study in the USA conducted between 1960 and 1993 by Peterson *et al.* [46] and employing her classification system (Table 55.1), an annual age- and sex-adjusted incidence of 27 per million overall and of 5 per million for linear disease were documented. In 2010 a study of UK and Irish children, based on new presentations to appropriate secondary and tertiary care physicians, identified 3.4 cases of morphoea per million children (<16 years) per year and 2.5 per million per year for linear disease [47]. There was no data on prevalence.

Peterson *et al.* estimated prevalence at 5 per 10 000 at age 18 years and at 22 per 10 000 at age 80 years [46]. These prevalence figures are supported by a 2019 US study employing administrative claims data, which estimates the prevalence of morphoea in children (<16

years) to range from 3.2 to 3.6 per 10 000 children (equivalent to 320–360 per million children) [48]. They contrast markedly with UK adult prevalence figures of 2 per million males and 4.7 per million females in the West Midlands obtained based on physician recall in 1988 [49].

Peterson's original population-based study comprised 82 morphoea patients and found that overall, plaque morphoea was the commonest subtype (56% of cases), followed in order of frequency by linear (20%), generalised (13%) and deep (11%) subtypes. Coexisting morphoea subtypes (mixed morphoea) were seen in 11% of cases [46]. More recent data from a cross-sectional study of two prospective cohorts including 944 participants (500 with childhood onset) seen at US tertiary referral centres, identified linear disease as the commonest subtype overall: 50% had linear morphoea, 26% generalised, 15% circumscribed plaque, 4% mixed and 0.3% pansclerotic disease [**13**].This difference likely reflects that more patients with linear disease, at the severe end of the morphoea spectrum, are seen in a tertiary care setting.

Age
Morphoea can occur at any age. Twenty-five cases of congenital morphoea presenting at birth are published, a majority with the linear head subtype [50]. Approximately 35–50% of cases begin in childhood (<16 years) [6,12,**13**,32]. The distribution is bimodal with a mean age at onset of 7–9 years in children and 44–47 years in adults [6,11,**13**,28,**32**,51–53].

The peak age of onset differs for the different clinical subtypes of disease. In general, 75% of plaque disease occurs between the ages of 40 and 50 years, whereas 75% of linear disease occurs between the ages of 2 and 14 years [24]. In Peterson's population-based study, the mean age at onset of disease was 12.2 years in linear, 31.5 years in plaque, 39.9 years in generalised and 45.1 years in deep forms of the disease [46]. In the UK/Irish childhood study, 67% had linear disease (roughly equally distributed between head/neck and limb variants), 29% had non-linear forms and 4% a mixed pattern [47]. In the largest published childhood study to date, Peterson's classification was used in a series of 750 children from 70 centres worldwide. Linear morphoea was again the most frequent childhood subtype (65%), followed by plaque morphoea (26%), generalised morphoea (7%) and deep morphoea (2%) [11]. These data are corroborated by two further large North American studies together covering 503 children. Linear morphoea occurred in 42–54%, followed by plaque in 15–28%, generalised forms in 7–9%, and pansclerotic morphoea/eosinophilic fasciitis in 2.1% [6,53]. In these studies, 19–23% of children had a mixed subtype, and linear–plaque was the most frequent combination (60–85%) [6,11,53].

In adults, circumscribed plaque morphoea is the commonest subtype (44–65% of cases), followed by generalised (20–24%), linear (9–13%) and mixed (4–6%) forms [6,28,**32**,53]. In Prasad's recent large tertiary centre study, of the 53% of participants (500/944) with paediatric onset disease, 70% had linear, 11% circumscribed plaque, 9% generalised and 1% mixed morphoea. Among patients with adult-onset morphoea, 45% had generalised morphoea, 28% linear, 20% circumscribed plaque and <1% mixed morphoea [**13**]. Data collated from 10 paediatric rheumatology and/or dermatology cohorts, including 1997 patients with paediatric onset and 893 with adult onset morphoea confirms that circumscribed plaque morphoea

(61%) and generalised plaque morphoea (22%) are commonest in adult-onset disease, with linear (56%), circumscribed (22%) and mixed (14%) subtypes commonest in patient with childhood-onset morphoea [1]. These studies likely underestimate the numbers of patients with mild circumscribed plaque disease, particularly those with adult-onset disease, who are less likely to access tertiary centres [13].

Sex

Most studies suggest that morphoea is commoner in women. This female preponderance is less marked in children, in congenital morphoea, in linear morphoea [12] and in adult pansclerotic disease [15]. Overall figures from 10 cohort studies give ratios of 2.7 F : M in childhood onset and 3.4 F : M in adult onset morphoea [1]. Reported ratios vary from 7 : 1 to 2.6 : 1 in adults and 3 : 1 to 1.5 : 1 in children [6,11,46,53–55].

Ethnicity

Although it affects all races, between 72.7% and 82% of published cases are in white people and a lower than expected prevalence has been identified in African Americans [6,11,12,13,47,53]. In two US studies from Texas and Illinois the racial distribution in 381 adult and paediatric morphoea subjects was 73–82% white, 12–14% Hispanic, 3–4% African American, 2–3% Asian and 6.5% other (Pacific Islander, American Indian, etc.) [6,27].

Associated diseases
Autoimmune diseases

That morphoea lies within the autoimmune spectrum of disease is supported by the increased prevalence of autoimmune disease described in patients and in their relatives [4,6,53,56]. Disorders reported to occur concomitantly with morphoea include autoimmune thyroid disease, psoriasis, vitiligo, alopecia areata, autoimmune hepatitis, primary biliary cirrhosis, inflammatory bowel disease, type 1 diabetes, polyglandular autoimmune disease type 2, Ménière disease, coeliac disease, multiple sclerosis, systemic lupus erythematosus, rheumatoid arthritis, Sjögren syndrome, antiphospholipid syndrome, Stills disease and mixed connective tissue disease [56–59] and reviewed in [4,6]. A study comprising 123 adults and 122 children from Texas identified concomitant rheumatic or other autoimmune disorders in 18% of patients. These were much commoner in adults (29%) than children (3%) [6]. This association was most marked among adults and children with generalised morphoea, occurring in 49% of this group versus 9% in the other subtypes combined. In this study the prevalence of psoriasis, systemic lupus erythematosus, multiple sclerosis and vitiligo appeared significantly higher in patients with morphoea than in the background population. Sixteen to 25% of patients report a family history of other autoimmune disease ([6,53], see section on genetics, later). In a multicentre worldwide study of 750 children, concomitant autoimmune disease was identified in 1.7% overall, and most frequently included vitiligo, insulin-dependent diabetes, autoimmune thyroid disease and ulcerative colitis [4]. In a retrospective German study of 472 patients (381 adults), the most frequently associated autoimmune diseases were Hashimoto thyroiditis (3.4%), rheumatoid arthritis (1.9%), alopecia areata (1%) and type 1 diabetes (0.8%) [55]. Interestingly, the offspring of parents with

morphoea appear at greater risk of developing rheumatoid arthritis [60]. Furthermore, significant associations with the same group of autoimmune diseases – namely autoimmune thyroid disease, rheumatoid arthritis and systemic lupus erythematosus – have been found in SSc probands and their families, supporting a common pathogenesis (Chapter 54) [61–63].

Other disease associations

While there is evidence of increased risk of cardiovascular disease in many autoimmune diseases, including systemic sclerosis, no association has been identified in patients with morphoea [64].

An association with cancer has been reported anecdotally and been much debated. However, a recent association with pancreatic adenocarcinoma (OR 1.27) was identified in a population-based, nested case–control study [65]. A further US study examined the prevalences of melanoma and non-melanoma skin cancers in adult patients with morphoea compared with the general Johns Hopkins Hospital adult patient population and found odds ratios of 6.6 for melanoma, 12.8 for squamous cell carcinoma and 13.1 for basal cell carcinoma in patients with morphoea [66]. The relative contributions of systemic immunosuppressive therapies, phototherapy and chronic inflammation, as well as the possible impact of an anti-cancer immune response on the development of autoimmunity are yet to be established.

Lichen sclerosus–morphoea overlap

Lichen sclerosus (Chapters 110 and 111) is an autoimmune inflammatory dermatosis with a prevalence estimated at 0.1–3 % [67–69]. It most often affects the anogenital region but can occur at extragenital sites in 11% of women with anogenital disease [68,70]. Anogenital lichen sclerosus may present with pruritus, pain, dysuria or dyspareunia, but extragenital lesions are usually asymptomatic. Lesions may occur anywhere but are frequently at sites of friction and are typically ivory white papules or plaques often with follicular delling. Varying degrees of hyperkeratosis, follicular plugging, eres, and through its binding to a variety of extracellular matrix components including perlecan (a heparin sulphate proteoglycan), type IV collagen, laminin 332, matrix metalloproteinase-9 (MMP-9) and fibulin (a calcium-binding proteoglycan), has a role in the structural organisation of the dermis [103–105]. The gene encoding this protein is mutated in patients with lipoid proteinosis, an inherited disorder characterised clinically by skin and mucosal infiltration and scarring, and histologically by reduplication of basement membranes and hyalinisation of the underlying dermis [104,106]. In both conditions the skin microvasculature is altered with reduplication of vascular basement membranes, loss of papillary dermal capillary loops and enlarged vessels in the deeper dermis [107]. The significance of these changes in the pathogenesis of lichen sclerosus is unclear, but the disruption of ECM-1-mediated control of MMP-9 activity may be important [108]. Antibodies to ECM-1 have not been documented in morphoea, although antibodies to another extracellular matrix microfibrillar protein, fibrillin 1, have been seen and implicated in pathogenesis in patients with linear and plaque morphoea as well as in SSc [109–111]. Upregulated miR-155, TNF and IL-6 may represent further overlaps in pathogenesis of lichen sclerosus and morphoea and potential treatment targets [67].

Pathophysiology

Predisposing factors

The aetiology of morphoea is poorly understood. Trauma, radiation, medications, vaccination and infection have all been proposed to act as triggering events in its development in susceptible individuals [23,24,112]. Evidence for morphoea as an autoimmune disease includes the presence of autoantibodies, HLA associations, and family and personal history of autoimmune disease. The very rare familial cases, the predominance of female gender and Blashkoid nature of linear disease further point to underlying genetic factors. It seems likely that an environmental 'signal', on a background of genetic susceptibility, triggers a sequence of events including vascular activation, inflammation and subsequent fibrosis.

Pathology

Autoimmunity

Autoimmune mechanisms are thought to play an important role in the induction of morphoea and this is supported by the finding of a variety of autoantibodies in all subtypes of the disease [29] and of increased serum levels of B-cell activating factor, a potent B-cell survival factor [113]. The published prevalence of ANA positivity in larger morphoea cohorts varies from 23% to 68% [4,6,11,30,53,55,**114**,115–120]. The prevalence and distribution in a UK childhood incidence cohort was similar at 43% [52]. The role and clinical application of autoantibodies in morphoea is not as clear-cut as in SSc where they predict internal organ complications and prognosis (Chapter 54). In a recent meta-analysis, pooled ANA positivity was 29.9%, but in paediatric-onset disease it ranged from 5.9% to 68%. ANA positivity was more frequent in linear versus non-linear disease but was present across subtypes. In both adults and children it was associated with more severe, more extensive and deeper disease and in children it also associated with extracutaneous manifestations and more disease damage [29,53,116]. In the largest paediatric cohort of 750, ANA positivity was similarly associated with extracutaneous manifestations and those with extracutaneous manifestations also had an increase in other immune activation markers: erythrocyte sedimentation rate (ESR), C-reactive protein (CRP), creatinine kinase (CK), IgG and rheumatoid factor [4]. Further, in a prospective cohort of 77 paediatric morphoea patients, baseline ANA positivity was associated with a 4.8 times greater odds of disease relapse (after successful treatment) at 5 years [30]. Titres of more than or equal to 1/160 were found in 50% and as many as 11% had titres of 1/1520 in this paediatric study. Speckled, homogeneous and nucleolar ANA staining patterns have been identified [116,120,121]. The speckled pattern appears predominant, occurring in 50–81% [116,120]. ANA positivity may also be directed against a variety of recognised extractable nuclear antigens including histones, single-stranded or denatured DNA [116,118,122,123] and topoisomerase II alpha [124]. An increased prevalence of antihistone antibodies (12% versus 2% in controls) [116] has been recorded in morphoea overall and in the linear subtype in particular (32–39%) [116,118]. Like ANA positivity, antihistone antibodies correlated with more extensive disease, higher skin scores and greater functional impairment, suggesting that they may identify a group of patients who require more aggressive therapy. Anti-ssDNA antibodies found in between

7% and 51% of cases have also been associated with more extensive skin involvement, active and deep disease and increased IFN-α2 and IL-33 [116,117,125]. Unlike ANA positivity, neither AHA nor anti-ss-DNA positivity predict increased risk of relapse [30]. Although earlier studies had suggested that titres of ANA and antihistone antibodies may parallel disease activity, this has not been borne out in larger studies [11,116,118].

Antibodies that are usually deemed to be specific markers of SSc, namely anti-topoisomerase antibody (anti-Scl-70 or ATA) and anticentromere antibody (ACA) (Chapter 54), have been identified at lower frequency – for example in 3.2% and 1.7% of 750 children with morphoea, respectively [4,11]. This is comparable to published figures of 0.8–3% for ATAs, although ACA prevalences are more variable 0–12% [6,28,55]. This variability may reflect the use of different assay methods and small numbers in some of the studies. A more recent study evaluated a panel of classic-SSc associated antibodies including ATA, ACA (CENP A), RNApol III in a paediatric morphoea cohort of 69 and found a frequency ranging from 6% to 14%. These three autoantibodies, in particular, were associated with deep tissue involvement, signified by joint contractures, nerve entrapment and muscle involvement, with more skin symptoms of tingling and pain, and skin thickness, but not with specific morphoea subtypes [120].

Other antibodies pathogenically specific to sclerotic skin diseases include antibodies to fibrillin 1, a major component of microfibrils in the extracellular matrix [109], and antibodies to MMP-I, which inhibit collagenase activity [126,127]. Both of these have been identified in patients with linear, plaque and generalised morphoea as well as in SSc.

Antibodies to dsDNA have also been reported in between 2.3% and 14% of cases, but with no clear clinical correlations [4,6,11,55,120].

Rheumatoid factor (RF) was positive in 3–16% of morphoea cohorts [4,11,55,128]. In Zulian's paediatric cohort, 16% of 464 children tested were positive and this correlated with the presence of arthritis [11]. The most recent study of morphoea autoantibody biosignatures from 70 morphoea patients with active inflammatory skin lesions, identified autoantibodies to myelin basin protein (directed against different epitopes to those recognised in multiple sclerosis) in 27% of cases, and this was associated with perineural inflammation and clinical symptoms of pain [129].

A variety of other autoantibodies, including anticardiolipin antibody [11], antimitochondrial antibodies [130] and antibodies to the ribonucleoproteins anti-U1-RNP [131], anti-U3-RNP [132] and anti-Th/To [133] may rarely be present, but are of uncertain significance. It is important to emphasise that the presence of these connective tissue disease associated antibodies has *not* been associated with the development of other connective tissue diseases such as SLE, Sjögren or SSc in morphoea cohorts studied to date. Nevertheless, such patients warrant increased surveillance.

In summary, although their exact roles are as yet incompletely defined, there is evidence for an association between autoantibody profiles and clinical phenotypes in morphoea (Figure 55.3 and for a recent review see [29]). Positive ANA, AHA, anti-ssDNA and RF are prevalent in morphoea cohorts, and significantly correlated with disease severity, depth of involvement and extracutaneous involvement. The association between ANA positivity at baseline and the

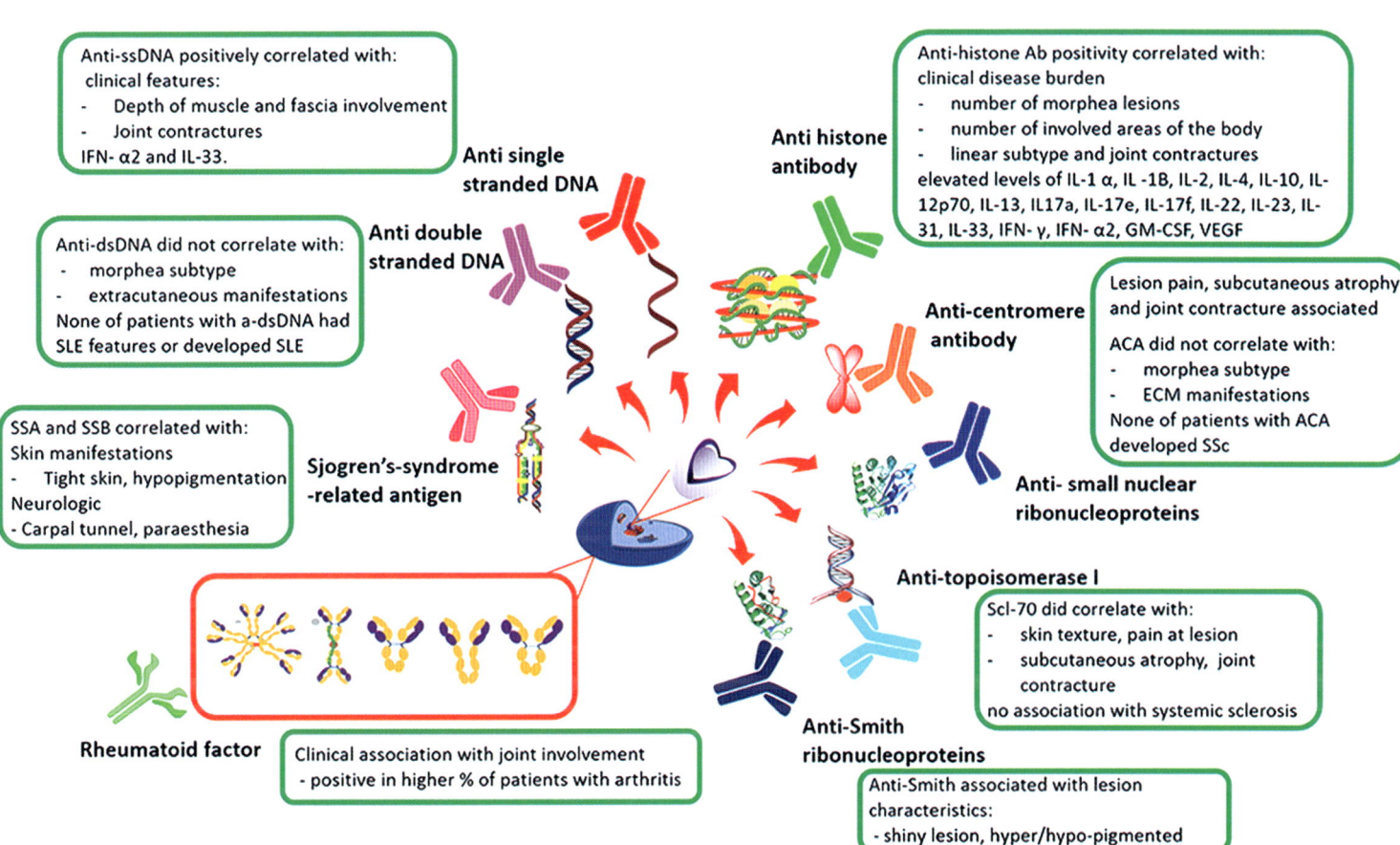

Anti-ssDNA positively correlated with:
  clinical features:
  - Depth of muscle and fascia involvement
  - Joint contractures
IFN- α2 and IL-33.

Anti-dsDNA did not correlate with:
  - morphea subtype
  - extracutaneous manifestations
None of patients with a-dsDNA had
SLE features or developed SLE

SSA and SSB correlated with:
Skin manifestations
  - Tight skin, hypopigmentation
Neurologic
  - Carpal tunnel, paraesthesia

Anti single stranded DNA

Anti double stranded DNA

Sjogren's-syndrome -related antigen

Rheumatoid factor

Clinical association with joint involvement
  - positive in higher % of patients with arthritis

Anti histone antibody

Anti-histone Ab positivity correlated with:
clinical disease burden
  - number of morphea lesions
  - number of involved areas of the body
  - linear subtype and joint contractures
elevated levels of IL-1 α, IL -1B, IL-2, IL-4, IL-10, IL-
12p70, IL-13, IL17a, IL-17e, IL-17f, IL-22, IL-23, IL-
31, IL-33, IFN- γ, IFN- α2, GM-CSF, VEGF

Anti-centromere antibody

Lesion pain, subcutaneous atrophy
and joint contracture associated

ACA did not correlate with:
  - morphea subtype
  - ECM manifestations
None of patients with ACA
developed SSc

Anti- small nuclear ribonucleoproteins

Anti-topoisomerase I

Scl-70 did correlate with:
  - skin texture, pain at lesion
  - subcutaneous atrophy, joint
    contracture
no association with systemic sclerosis

Anti-Smith ribonucleoproteins

Anti-Smith associated with lesion
characteristics:
  - shiny lesion, hyper/hypo-pigmented

Figure 55.3 General overview of morphoea autoantibodies in relation to clinical features. Reproduced from Khatri *et al.* [**29**]/Frontiers Media /CCBY 4.0. Ab, antibody; ACA, anti-centromere antibody; ECM, extracutaneous manifestations; Anti-ssDNA, anti-single stranded DNA; GM-CSF, granulocyte-macrophage colony-stimulating factor; IFNx, interferon; ILx, interleukin; SSA, Sjögren-syndrome-related antigen A; SSB, Sjögren-syndrome-related antigen B; Scl-70, topoisomerase I; SSc, systemic sclerosis; SLE, systemic lupus erythematosus; VEGF, vascular endothelial growth factor.

potential for subsequent disease relapse suggests its possible use as a biomarker [30].

Immunopathology
Vascular activation and damage
Although vascular damage is well recognised to be one of the earliest features involved in the pathogenesis of SSc, it is less well studied in morphoea. Nevertheless, microvascular changes occur, and endothelial cell swelling and apoptosis have been identified in early morphoea lesions, with enlarged vessels, vessel wall reduplication and reduced capillary density in later stages [134–136]. Direct immunofluorescence studies have shown immunoglobulin M (IgM) and C3 staining in the small blood vessels of the papillary dermis [137]. Upregulation of expression of the endothelial cell adhesion molecules vascular cell adhesion molecule 1 (VCAM-1), intercellular adhesion molecule 1 (ICAM-1) and E-selectin [138,139], antiendothelial cell antibody-mediated antibody-dependent cytotoxicity [135] and autologous complement activation [140] have been proposed as mechanisms for endothelial cell injury and activation in morphoea [141]. Direct damage through trauma, infection and radiation may be contributory factors in some cases. Thus, although endothelial–mesenchymal transition contributing to fibrosis has not been documented in morphoea, endothelial cell activation and damage may be an important driving factor in the early inflammatory stages, promoting cytokine release and T-cell recruitment [142].

Epidermal–dermal interaction
The Blaschkoid nature of linear morphoea not only suggests the possibility of genomic mosaicism but also that epidermal keratinocytes may be involved in its pathogenesis. Keratinocytes may affect the extracutaneous manifestations by altering expression of connective tissue growth factor (CTGF), fibronectin or type I collagen. Keratinocytes are known to produce an array of cytokines, growth factors and chemokines including TNF-α, TGF-β, IL-1, IL-6, platelet-derived growth factor (PDGF), FGF, CCL2, endothelin1, fibrillin1, α-MSH and Fli-1 many of which are implicated in fibrosis or wound healing. In addition, epidermal–dermal signalling, involving, for example, Wnt-Beta-catenin, and jagged-notch pathways may not only be important in promoting fibrosis (as suggested by studies in SSc), but may also be a determinant of morphoea patterning through their roles in embryonic development (reviewed in [143]). No primary somatic epidermal mosaicism has been identified in linear morphoea [144]. Nevertheless, further investigation of the role of keratinocytes and the epidermis in driving dermal and subcutaneous inflammation and fibrosis in morphoea is warranted.

Cytokines and cellular signatures

Current evidence suggests that a T helper type 1 (Th1) phenotype, with a strong IFN-γ signature, predominates in the early inflammatory stage of morphoea and later switches to a Th2 predominant profibrotic immunophenotype in the sclerotic and damage phase.

Elevated levels of Th1 and Th2 related cytokines, chemokines and receptors have been found in peripheral blood in morphoea patients. These include Th1 related IL-2, IL-2R, IL-12, TNF-α, TGF-β, MCP-1 and IFN-γ related proteins: CXCL9(MIG), CXCL10 (IP-10), CXCL11 and IFN-γ chemokine receptor (CXCR3), and Th2 related IL-4, IL-6 and IL-13 [119,145–154] (reviewed in Torok *et al.* [155]). More recently, increased levels of CCL18, CXCL13, TNFRII, galectin-9, TIE-1, sVCAM, IL18 and CCL19 have also been identified in sera from 74 morphoea patients (versus 22 healthy controls) [156].

IL-4 stimulates B-cell and fibroblast proliferation, synthesis of extracellular matrix components and immunoglobulin and adhesion molecule production (reviewed in [157]). IL-6 is an inflammatory and profibrotic cytokine, involved in regulation of B cells, fibroblast activation and Th17 cell differentiation. In patients with early stage generalised and linear morphoea, increased serum levels of IL-2, IL2-R and TNF-α were shown to correlate with increased serum IL-4 and IL-6 concentrations, skin scores, anti-ssDNA and antihistone antibodies [146,147]. Elevated IL-1 and IL-6 were found in serum of children with morphoea and disease duration fewer than 24 months, and elevated IL-17 F and IL-22 in disease durations of 24–48 months [119,157]. The latter correlated with ANA, antihistone and ssDNA antibody positivity, and it was suggested that the Th17 signature may reflect more severe or active inflammatory disease. The proposed role of Th17 cells in driving inflammation and early fibrosis [157] has been called into question, however, by the finding of reduced Th17 cells in morphoea skin, despite elevated levels of IL-17A and IL-23 in blood [119,151]. A role for IL1 is suggested in SSc. Endogenous IL-1α from SSc fibroblasts stimulates collagen production by inducing IL-6 and PDGF [158]. Endothelial cell-derived IL-1α and IL-1β and fibroblast growth factor may be produced in response to cellular injury and are also capable of activating SSc fibroblasts [159,160]. Interestingly, although there was no increase in IL-1 family cytokines in morphoea sera at baseline, IL1α levels increased after effective treatment whereas IL-33 levels dropped compared with healthy controls [161].

Increased CD4+ and CD8+ T cells and CD1a+ CD86+ dermal Langerhans cells are known to be present in lesional skin in morphoea [162]. In more recent studies, however, peripheral blood and skin show a marked predominance of CD4+ Th1 cells with reduced functional regulatory T cells [145,163]. Patients with active disease demonstrate larger populations of IFN-γ expressing T cells (CD4+ IFN-γ+ Th1 cells) and NK cells. When comparing active versus inactive disease, CXCL-9, IL-12, MIP-1α, HGF, IL-4 and TNF-α were seen with increased frequency in blood and skin in adults [145], and CXCL9, CXCL10, CXCL11, MIP-3β, IL-9, IL-2 and CCL-1 in paediatric patients [153,155]. Peripheral blood levels of CXCL9 and CXCL10 have been correlated with disease activity measures mLoSSI and PGA-A, underscoring their potential use as serological markers [119,145,152,153]. Gene expression profiling did not reveal a transcriptional IFN signature in blood monocytes, but

immunohistochemistry of affected skin has shown co-localisation of CXCL-9 with CD68+ dermal macrophages in close proximity to CXCR3 expressing CD4+ T cells in dermal perivascular inflammatory cell infiltrates. This suggests potential lymphocyte macrophage interaction via IFN-γ signalling and implicates skin rather than PBMCs as the source of circulating CXCL9 [145,152]. CCL18 is a chemokine produced by dendritic cells, monocytes and macrophages and induced by Th2 cytokines IL-4 and IL-13. It induces Th2 cell chemotaxis and macrophage differentiation to a profibrotic M2 phenotype. CCL18 has recently been shown to be increased in skin from the inflammatory edge of morphoea lesions, but not in unaffected skin. Serum levels of CCL18 may more accurately discriminate between active and inactive disease than CXCL9 and CXCL10 and were shown to mirror mLoSSI and response to effective therapy in morphoea of all subtypes [156].

More recently, RNA sequencing in paediatric morphoea has allowed transcriptomic analysis of the different phases of morphoea. This has revealed a distinct inflammatory response gene signature (IRGS) composed of IFN-γ, IFN-α and TNF-α associated genes in morphoea skin, including interferon inducible chemokines CXCL9, CXCL10, CXCL11 and IFN-γ which are more highly expressed in inflammatory lesions. In contrast, inactive lesions differentially expressed genes encoding for extracellular matrix organisation, collagen and keratinisation, including COL17A1, KRT173, FLG and COL17A. In addition, transcription factors involved in epithelial–mesenchymal interaction, proliferation and extracellular matrix production such as WNT, ERK, PI3K-TBX, FOX, RUNX and SRF were highly expressed [**22**]. Interestingly TGF-β was absent from the morphoea gene signature in this study. When comparing active versus inactive morphoea samples the most significant differences were seen in genes involved in KRAS signalling, epithelial-mesenchymal transition, IL-2 STAT5 signalling, IL6 JAK/STAT3 signalling, and TNF-α signalling via NFKB. The KRAS and JAK/STAT pathways were the most significantly upregulated pathways associated with disease activity suggesting JAK inhibition as a new potential therapeutic option [**22**]. Future studies could usefully be informed by single-cell RNAseq studies and the application of spatial transcriptomics.

Fibroblast activation and sclerosis

Sclerosis involves the production of extracellular matrix components and is thought to result from a combination of increased collagen deposition by fibroblasts and reduced extracellular matrix turnover in morphoea. Th2 related cytokines IL-4 and IL-13 upregulate collagen synthesis, inhibit collagenase activity [164], and are both elevated in morphoea, IL-13 more evidently in later stage disease [146,147,165]. The importance of IL-13 is supported by early gene expression profiling studies in three morphoea patients that suggested robust activation of IL-13 signalling [166]. No TGF-β responsive signature was identified in morphoea biopsies in this study. Linear morphoea fibroblasts have been shown to have a specific cell phenotype which exhibits increased growth, migration and a paradoxically reduced response to TGF-β1. They more often differentiate into myofibroblasts and have a specific, altered cell secretome. Thus, key modulators of the TGF-β superfamily members SOSTDC1 and ADAMTS8 are dysregulated in morphoea and altered SMAD phosphorylation ensues [167].

Enhanced type I and type III collagen mRNA and protein expression have been identified in morphoea fibroblasts and lesional skin [168,169]. Glycosaminoglycan and fibronectin synthesis is also increased. Constitutive overexpression of CTGF combined with increased TGF-β and PDGF production by dermal fibroblasts may contribute to the sustained fibrotic response [170]. CTGF mRNA and protein have been identified in fibroblasts scattered throughout the dermis in morphoea skin sections [171,172]. In contrast to recent transcriptomic studies, skin biopsies and sera of morphoea patients have demonstrated increased TGF-β expression and co-localisation with activated fibroblasts. Upregulation of TGF-β and TGF-β receptors I and II in perivascular lymphocyte-like cells and interstitial fibroblasts have been identified by immunohistochemistry and *in situ* hybridisation in involved skin [173,174]. Increased expression of the matrix-associated tissue inhibitor of metalloproteinase-3 (TIMP-3) in fibroblasts within fibrotic collagen fibres or in the vicinity of inflammatory cells suggests a role for reduced collagenolysis in addition to increased collagen synthesis in the development of fibrosis [175].

Myofibroblasts are the key effector cells in fibrosis. In morphoea patients, enhanced dermal expression of α-SMA, as well as TGF-β1 and fibronectin, all of which are involved in fibrosis, and, at the same time, enhanced expression of Snail1 and reduced expression of E-cadherin, which are involved in epithelial–mesenchymal transition, were observed in the dermal eccrine glands suggesting that epithelial–mesenchymal transition may be involved in the fibrotic process [176]. Fibrocytes are CD34+ cells bone marrow-derived mesenchymal progenitor cells that are recruited from the circulation into sites of injury. During tissue remodelling they lose CD34 expression and gain smooth muscle actin (SMA) expression to become myofibroblasts. Factor XIIIa is a protransglutaminase expressed on a population of dermal dendritic cells now thought to be macrophages, which is involved in cross-linking matrix proteins. CD34 positivity is lost, and factor XIIIa expression is increased in areas of fibrosis in morphoea [177–179]. Together, these findings suggest that a profibrotic wound-healing environment may develop in morphoea as a result of transformation of CD34+ fibrocytes to CD34– myofibroblasts. The increase in factor XIIIa-expressing cells may then function in cross-linking newly formed collagen fibrils and matrix proteins, thereby enhancing the fibrotic process [179].

By these mechanisms, vascular injury leading to recruitment and activation of lymphocytes and mononuclear cells, secretion of pro-inflammatory mediators and fibroblast activation are thought to lead to eventual fibrosis, sclerosis and damage.

Histopathology

There have been few systematic studies of the histopathology of morphoea. However, all subtypes share similar findings of an early active inflammatory phase, in which newer lesions demonstrate a lymphocyte and plasma cell-rich infiltrate. As lesions evolve, the numbers of inflammatory cells reduce as collagen bundles thicken and skin sclerosis increases in the later fibrotic phase. An intermediate picture is frequently found on skin biopsy (Figure 55.4).

The epidermis may be normal, flattened with loss of rete ridges, or slightly acanthotic [180]. In the early inflammatory phase, oedema and a dense predominantly perivascular infiltrate of lymphocytes, plasma cells and macrophages, eosinophils and occasional mast

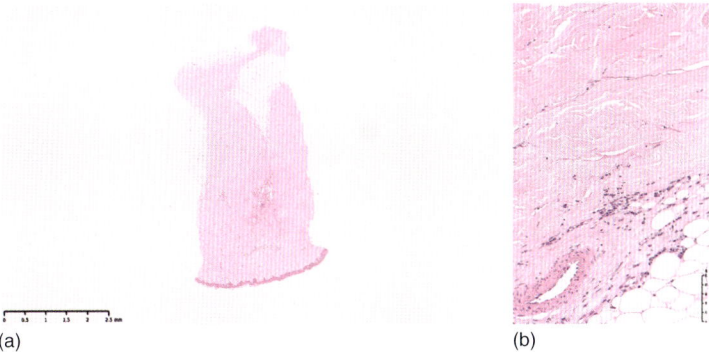

Figure 55.4 Typical histopathological appearances in morphoea. (a) Low power view showing an expanded dermis, superficial and deep perivascular and periadnexal inflammation dense horizontally orientated collagen bundles, loss of adnexal structures and extension into the subcutis. H&E. (b) Higher power view showing broad and thick collagen bundles, scattered aggregates of lymphocytes and plasma cells perivascularly and at the dermal–hypodermal junction. H&E. Courtesy of Dr F. Deroide, Department of Histopathology, Royal Free London NHS Foundation Trust, UK.

cells, is present in the reticular and occasionally the papillary dermis [181–183]. The infiltrate may extend into the lower dermis, around the eccrine glands, into the subcutaneous fat and beyond. The reticular dermis shows swollen collagen bundles running parallel to the skin surface. The subcutaneous fat may be replaced by thickened, wavy fibres of newly formed collagen, rich in type III collagen and fibrillin 1 [184–186]. Vascular changes in the dermis and subcutis consist of endothelial swelling and oedema of the vessel walls. In the sclerotic stage there are few recognisable fibroblasts and little inflammation. Collagen bundles are closely packed, highly eosinophilic and orientated horizontally. The dermal appendages and subcutaneous fat are progressively lost. Reduced numbers of eccrine glands are entrapped by collagen and thus appear higher in the dermis. Fewer blood vessels are seen within the thickened hyalinised collagen; those that are present may show intimal thickening. The fascia and striated muscles underlying the lesions may likewise show fibrosis and sclerosis. Deeper structures including the eye and brain are involved in a significant number of patients with linear morphoea of the face or scalp [187,188]. Brain biopsies performed in some patients with neurological involvement have shown dilated blood vessels, a perivascular lymphocytic infiltrate with features of vasculitis, gliosis and sclerosis of the leptomeninges, and intravascular and intraparenchymal calcification [187–190].

In a recent review of 51 skin biopsies in 40 patients by Chiu *et al.* the most common features were dermal sclerosis (defined as a combination of collagen thickening and homogenisation) in 90%, dermal thickening in 78% and collagen homogenisation in 86%. An inflammatory infiltrate which was composed of lymphocytes and plasma cells was present in all cases, described as moderate to abundant in 73%, with moderate or abundant plasma cell numbers in 55%. Eosinophils were present in only 4/51 biopsies. The inflammatory infiltrate was superficial and deep in 76%, and superficial only in 25%. Fourteen of 51 biopsies showed overlying features of lichen sclerosus. Periadnexal fat loss and/or reduced appendages occurred in 71% and perineural inflammation in 63% [95].

These findings resemble those in the published literature, which describe an inflammatory infiltrate in 84–100%, moderate to abundant plasma cells in 84%, eosinophils in 10–21% and perineural inflammation in between 52% and 84% [183,191,192]. Interestingly, there was no significant difference between active and inactive disease histology in this study. Diagnostic difficulty was encountered in 24/51 biopsies, and the authors suggested that subtle and focal collagen homogenisation and presence of plasma cells may serve as diagnostic clues in such cases [95].

While histopathological changes are similar in all subtypes of morphoea, they do vary in relation to the depth of involvement. In deep forms changes may be confined to the deep dermis and subcutis, or solely involve deeper structures such as the underlying fascia and muscle [193]. In some cases, changes may be entirely superficial and confined to the reticular dermis [178].

In a cross-sectional study of 83 patients (mean age 41 ± 21 years, 91 biopsies) with the range of morphoea subtypes, specific microanatomical locations of sclerosis and inflammation were associated with morphoea subtype and clinical symptoms of pain, skin tightness and functional impairment [194]. The location of sclerosis was defined as a 'top-heavy', 'full-thickness' or 'bottom-heavy' pattern. It mirrored the clinical phenotype, with a top-heavy pattern in isomorphic generalised plaque morphoea and morphoea–lichen sclerosus overlap, and a bottom heavy or full thickness pattern in patients with symmetric generalised plaque morphoea and morphoea profunda (involving the subcutis or deeper). All three patterns were seen in all morphoea variants, supporting the suggestion that depth should be considered a disease modifier rather than a separate subtype of disease. A mild to moderate inflammatory infiltrate was present in 80%, located in the papillary and deep reticular dermis, the dermal–subcutaneous interface, perivascular, periadnexal and perineural areas. It was lymphocyte predominant (91%), but also rich with plasma cells in 75% and eosinophils in 21%. Patient symptoms of pain, tightness and functional impairment were associated with a bottom-heavy pattern of sclerosis and more severe inflammation on the biopsy [194].

In a study of 16 patients, vacuolar degeneration at the dermal–epidermal junction was a common histological feature in morphoea en coup de sabre and a perivascular and/or periappendageal lymphocytic infiltrate and vacuolar degeneration of follicular epithelium were seen in early disease [195] suggesting that there may be an autoimmune attack of basal keratinocytes.

While prior studies implicate a stepwise progression from inflammatory to sclerotic phases [181], the high proportion of cases with concomitant sclerosis and inflammation in this study (46.2%) [194] suggest that ongoing inflammation may continue to drive fibrosis resulting in a more protracted disease course in a significant number of patients.

The cutaneous histopathological findings in morphoea and SSc are similar [196]. Diagnostic difficulties can sometimes arise in patients with the pansclerotic variant. Features that favour morphoea over SSc include more intense inflammation, the presence of perineural inflammation and more diffuse dermal sclerosis, simultaneously involving the papillary and deeper dermis, which is not usually seen in SSc [183,191].

Causative organisms

A putative role for *Borrelia* species in triggering morphoea was initially proposed by Aberer *et al.* in 1985 [197]. It was suggested because of: (i) the clinical and histological similarities between morphoea and acrodermatitis chronica atrophicans, a cutaneous manifestation of late-stage Lyme disease (Chapter 26) [198]; (ii) the finding that lichen sclerosus was observed to coexist with acrodermatitis chronica atrophicans in 12% of cases [199]; and (iii) the response of certain cases of morphoea to antibiotics. Since then, the proposed association has been studied extensively with different outcomes in Europe and North America. It has been suggested that the geographical differences reflect the fact that different subspecies of *Borrelia* predominate in different parts of the world. *Borrelia burgdorferi sensu stricto* is prevalent in the USA and *B. afzelii* and *B. garinii* predominate in Eurasia. High rates of *Borrelia* infection have been documented prior to the onset of morphoea in some European studies, but not in those from the USA [200–204]. In a retrospective review of 90 European morphoea patients, a statistically highly significant association between morphoea, serological evidence of *Borrelia* infection and high-titre ANA positivity was observed when disease onset was in childhood or adolescence, suggesting possible relevance in a subset of morphoea patients [205]. However, a significant number of studies from both sides of the Atlantic have found no association between the two entities [206–212]. The wide range of diagnostic tests used, which include immunoperoxidase, silver stain, focus-floating microscopy, tissue culture, serology and polymerase chain reaction, make it difficult to interpret the data. A literature review identified *Borrelia* DNA in only one of 49 morphoea cases investigated [209]. In summary, there is no conclusive evidence to date that morphoea is caused by *Borrelia* infection. However, immune activation as a result of infection per se could act as a trigger for morphoea in some cases. Possible infectious triggers for morphoea reported in the literature include hepatitis C [213], varicella [214], herpes zoster [215] and SARS-CoV-2 [216].

Genetics

Rare cases of familial morphoea in father and son [217], linear morphoea in sisters [78], first-degree cousins [80] and in monozygotic twins [81,218] are published. A family history of rheumatic or autoimmune disease in first- or second-degree relatives seems more common and was reported in 12% of 750 children [11]. This family history was significantly more likely in patients with generalised morphoea (23.5%) than in those with plaque (12.5%) or linear (9%) disease. Rheumatoid arthritis, systemic lupus erythematosus, psoriasis, vitiligo, lichen sclerosus, autoimmune thyroiditis and insulin-dependent diabetes appear particularly associated [6,11]. A family history of scleroderma was identified in 1.5% of children (although no mention is made whether this was systemic or localised disease) [11]. In a further study, including 123 adults and 122 children, 2% reported a family history of morphoea in a first- or second-degree relative [6]. At 18% overall, the prevalence of familial rheumatic and autoimmune disease was increased fourfold compared with that in the general population [6,46], and was higher in children (22%) than adults (11%). Children with generalised or mixed morphoea and adults with generalised disease had the highest frequencies. Taken together, the increased frequency of personal and familial autoimmunity in the generalised subtype indicates a possible common susceptibility locus for this group of disorders.

There is still a great deal of work to be done to understand the genetic influences underlying morphoea. However, genome-wide gene expression profiling of skin biopsies from three morphoea patients has demonstrated an inflammatory gene expression profile identical to that seen in limited and some diffuse cutaneous SSc patients [166] (Chapter 54). This profile has been linked to T-cell infiltration, early growth response 1 (Egr-1) and IL-13 pathway activation [219] and to CCL2 up-regulation [220]. In a case–control study of peripheral blood of 158 predominantly female and white morphoea patients (adults and children), increased frequencies of class II HLA-DRB1*04:04 (OR 2.3), HLA-DQB1*02:01 (OR 1.89), DRB1*03:01 (OR1.6), DQA1*03:00 (only seen in morphoea cases) and class I HLA-B*37 (OR 3.2), HLA-C*08 (OR 2.6), HLA-C*15 (OR2.7) alleles were demonstrated, with HLA-DRB1*15 particularly associated with the generalised morphoea subtype. The strongest associations were found with HLA-DRB1*04:04 and HLA-B*37 and one risk allele DRB*04:04 in common with SSc was identified [221]. Other HLA-DRB1, -DPB1, -DQB1 and -DQA1 variants are strongly associated with SSc [86] (Chapter 54), and HLA-DRB1 and -DQB variants appear more frequently in patients with lichen sclerosus [67]. Interestingly, HLA-DRB1*04:04 is strongly associated with rheumatoid arthritis, providing further support for a common susceptibility and potential explanation for the high prevalence of rheumatoid factor positivity in morphoea cohorts [60]. RNA transcriptome expression analyses of the skin of 28 children with morphoea has identified 589 differentially expressed genes. Histological skin inflammation scores correlated with the expression levels of genes related to MHC class II antigen presentation and IFN-γ signalling, including HLA-DQB1, HLA-DRB5, HLA-DRB1, HLA-DPB1,HLA-DQA2, HLA-DPA1 and HLA-DQA1, GBP1, GBP2, GBP4, IRF1 and STAT1 [21]. Average dermal collagen thickness correlated with expression of genes involved in IFN-γ signalling and MHC class II antigen presentation and collagen organisation, specifically IFITM3, CD63 and COL12A1. Strong upregulation of the same class II genes HLA-DRB1, -DQB1 and -DQA1, previously identified in blood [221], correlated with both skin inflammatory and fibrosis scoring [21]. In this study, Schutt et al. demonstrated three distinct immunophenotypic clusters: 'inflammatory' associated with strong upregulation of class II-related genes, 'fibroproliferative' associated with FGFR1 amplification, collagen formation and keratinisation pathways, and 'healthy-like' seen in patients in long-term remission. These groups did not correlate with the clinical morphoea subtypes (linear, generalised, circumscribed), but patients in the inflammatory cluster were more likely to have active disease, higher mLoSSI and histological inflammation scores and ANA positivity [21]. Ultimately, as in SSc, it is hoped that identification of these intrinsic skin cell-specific gene expression subsets, potentially linked to differential treatment responses, will allow better tailoring of therapeutics in patients with severe inflammatory morphoea.

Epigenetics has been a recent focus of attention in various fibrotic disorders. MicroRNAs (miRNAs) are small non-coding RNAs that bind to messenger RNAs inhibiting their translation into protein (reviewed in [222]). Downregulated miRNAs, in particular miR-7 [223], miRNA-let-7a [224] and miRNA-196a [225], in the serum and skin of morphoea patients may contribute to the pathogenesis of skin fibrosis by allowing increased type I collagen expression in morphoea fibroblasts. Increased expression of profibrotic miRNA-155 which regulates Akt, Wnt/beta-catenin pathways and endothelial to mesenchymal transition (Chapter 54), and miRNA-483-5p which promotes myofibroblast differentiation

and regulates extracellular matrix has been found in morphoea sera and endothelial cells [222,226]. More recently, increased serum levels of miRNA-181b-5p, miRNA-223-3p, miRNA-21-5p, let-7i-5p, miRNA-29a-3p and miRNA-210-3p have been identified although their significance as yet remains unclear [227]. Levels of let-7i inversely correlated with extent and activity of disease, suggesting its possible future use as a biomarker.

Environmental factors
Trauma and vaccination
A small number of case reports in children specifically document the onset of morphoea at the site of, and in a close temporal relationship to, vaccination for hepatitis B, MMR (measles, mumps and rubella), diphtheria, tetanus, pertussis, pneumococcus, BCG (bacille Calmette-Guérin) [228–234] and, most recently, Covid-19 [235]. The onset of morphoea has also been reported after injection with vitamin B_{12} and K [236–238], interferon-beta1b [239] and enfuvirtide [240]. It has been suggested that morphoea may reflect an immunological response triggered by vascular injury and tissue hypoxia because of trauma at the injection site in susceptible individuals. Others have argued that since multiple vaccines have been implicated, it is the adjuvants in the vaccines that act as the trigger [241]. Newer mRNA vaccines have the potential to trigger innate immunity via TLR activation and generation of type I interferons, a possible mechanism for triggering morphoea [242].

Anecdotal reports and early case series have suggested a potential role for trauma in the development of morphoea and particularly in linear disease [54,117,243]. In large paediatric cohorts comprising 886 children, 13% reported a specific potential triggering event, such as trauma, infection or exposure to a drug, occurring close to the time of morphoea onset [11,27]. Mechanical trauma (including accidental trauma, insect bite reactions and vaccinations) accounted for two-thirds of these cases, infections for a quarter of cases, and drugs and psychological distress for 5% and 3%, respectively. Interestingly children with generalised morphoea had a lower reporting frequency for such events (6%). In contrast, there appeared to be a trend for mechanical factors to act as a trigger in linear and deep morphoea cases [11].

The association of morphoea with skin trauma was systematically investigated in a cohort of 329 adult and childhood cases. Evidence of skin trauma or friction in the distribution of morphoea lesions at the onset of disease was identified in 52 patients (48 adults) (15.8%) [112]. The development of morphoea in the same area as previously healed skin disease or injury, also referred to as Wolf isotopic response [244], occurred in 6%. Skin lesions occurring at sites of repeated current trauma, referred to as the isomorphic response of Koebner [245], were identified in 9% of patients [112]. Isotopic patients were defined as those who had trauma occur at the site of the initial lesion within 6 months of onset of morphoea. Isomorphic patients were those with lesions distributed exclusively in areas of friction in the bra-line, waistband area and inguinal creases. Both groups were female predominant, and the mean age of onset was lower in the isotopic (44.4 years) versus the isomorphic (52.4 years) group. In contrast to the findings in children [11], in this predominantly adult group (48/52 cases), 87% of trauma-induced cases had generalised morphoea (defined in this study as the occurrence of indurated plaques that have become confluent on at least

Table 55.3 Other causes of skin sclerosis.

Disorder	Examples
Autoimmune disorders	Systemic sclerosis, sclerodermoid GVHD
Metabolic disorders	Porphyria cutanea tarda, phenylketonuria, muscle glycogenosis, hypothyroidism, carcinoid syndrome, diabetic cheiroarthropathy with skin thickening
Deposition disorders	Scleroedema, scleromyxoedema, primary systemic amyloidosis
Genetic disorders (see also [359])	GEMSS (glaucoma, lens ectopia, microspherophakia, stiffness of joints, short stature), Werner syndrome, progeria, acrogeria and poikilodermatous epidermolysis bullosa, Moore Federman syndrome (short stature, stiff joints, characteristic facies), stiff skin syndrome, melorheostosis, scleroatrophic Huriez syndrome (scleroatrophy hands and feet, nail hypoplasia, keratoderma hypohidrosis), Myhre syndrome (skin sclerosis, joint contractures, cardiorespiratory and gastrointestinal abnormalities, hearing loss, dysmorphic features)
Occupational causes	Vinyl chloride disease, perchlorethylene, trichloroethylene, organic solvents, pesticides, epoxy resins, silicone
Chemically induced	Eosinophilia myalgia syndrome (L-tryptophan), toxic oil syndrome (ingestion of rapeseed oil contaminated with aniline), nephrogenic systemic fibrosis (gadolinium exposure on a background of renal failure, GFR <30 mL/min)
Drug induced (see section on environmental factors, later)	Bleomycin, pentazocine, progestin, vitamin B_{12}, vitamin K, cocaine, D-penicillamine, peplomycin, interferon β-1a, uracil-tegafur, taxanes (e.g. paclitaxel, docetaxel), methysergide, gemcitabine, bromocriptine, bisoprolol, L-5-hydroxytryptophan with carbidopa, ibuprofen, mitomycin C, balicatib, odanacatib, PD1 inhibitors (e.g. nivolumab, pembrolizumab), etanercept, adalimumab, golimumab, ustekinumab
Associated with haematological disease	POEMS (polyneuropathy, organomegaly, endocrinopathy, monoclonal gammopathy, sclerodermoid skin changes), myeloma

GFR, glomerular filtration rate; GVHD, graft-versus-host disease.

two anatomical sites), compared with 33% of the cohort overall. Isotopic patients also included some cases of linear morphoea and had more severe disease as measured by modified Rodnan skin score (mRSS; Chapter 54) and dermatology life quality index scores [112]. The proposed triggering events in the isotopic group were surgery in 43%, penetrating trauma in 19%, injection in 14%, herpes zoster infection in 10% and radiotherapy, diagnostic X-ray and extreme exercise in 5% each. The majority of lesions occurred on the chest, breasts or abdomen. The underlying mechanism for such trauma-induced morphoea remains uncertain. However, the induction of an aberrant wound healing response with upregulation of endogenous toll-like receptor (TLR) ligands, enhanced innate immune signalling and resultant fibroblast activation may be involved [143,246,247].

Radiation

Most published cases of post-irradiation morphoea have been linked to radiotherapy for breast cancer [248–252]. It is estimated to occur in 1/500 breast cancer patients [252]. More rarely, it has occurred after treatment for gynaecological and head and neck malignancies, subcutaneous lymphoma and metastatic adenocarcinoma [250,251]. Age, radiotherapy parameters and initial post-treatment reaction do not appear to influence the risk of developing post-irradiation morphoea, although a prior diagnosis of SSc may do. Most cases develop within 1–3 years of completing radiotherapy, but rarely delays of 10–32 years are reported [248,251]. In most cases, morphoea develops within the radiotherapy field, but in up to 50% of cases it can extend beyond this [250,251]. The differential diagnosis can be challenging and includes chronic radiation dermatitis, radiation-induced fibrosis, cancer recurrence, post-irradiation recall dermatitis and cellulitis. Histological confirmation is usually necessary to exclude the possibility of cancer recurrence. In terms of pathogenesis, radiation-induced increases in IL-4, IL-5 and TGF-β have been implicated, with resultant fibroblast activation, collagen synthesis and fibrosis [253]. Limited data suggest that patients treated with systemic (rather than topical) agents, most often methotrexate or narrowband ultraviolet-B phototherapy, are more likely to achieve a good clinical response [251]. PDT may

also be an effective therapeutic option since it raises MMP1 and MMP3 RNA and protein levels and reduces collagen I expression in scleroderma fibroblasts *in vitro* and has proven beneficial in case reports [254–256].

Drugs

A variety of drugs have been implicated in the development of morphoea-like lesions usually within 9–12 months of treatment initiation (Table 55.3) [257–261]. A literature review in 2008 identified 15 cases, 7 male, median age 57 years with onset ranging from 1 to 36 months after treatment initiation and in four cases after treatment was stopped [260]. In five cases, typical plaque morphoea occurred at the site of vitamin K, vitamin B12 or pentazocine injections and persisted at 12 months where documented. Two cases of bullous morphoea with eosinophilia were associated with L-5-hydroxytryptophan and carbidopa. Bisoprolol (one case), bleomycin (three cases), peplomycin (one case), D-penicillamine (two cases) and bromocriptine (one case) were reported as possible morphoea triggers, with only partial improvement in four and stable disease in three cases documented 1–12 months after drug cessation in the seven cases for which data were available (reviewed in (260)). New onset morphoea is reported in nine patients (six plaque, one pansclerotic, one linear, one not-specified) on biologic therapies including etanercept, adalimumab, golimumab and ustekinumab with latency periods of 2.8–36 months [262]. Mechanisms suggested include the development of drug-specific lymphocyte responses and autoantibody production causing endothelial damage [263], direct vascular damage, generation of reactive oxygen species and upregulation of IL-1, TNF-α and TGF-β [264]. Toxic effects of the vehicle or preservative at the injection site may also be of relevance in some cases [265].

Further mechanistic insight is suggested by the development of morphoea in patients on high-dose balicatib and odanacatib (both subsequently withdrawn) which inhibit the collagenolytic activity of cathepsin K within lysosomes in skin fibroblasts [265–267]. Lesions consistent with morphoea clinically and histologically developed in 0.16% of 8043 patients treated with odanacatib, versus 0.04% of those on placebo in the 5-year LOFT study [265]. Lesions began from study day 100 to 1300 but improved or resolved on treatment discontinuation in all cases. Similarly, 9/709 (1.27%) patients on balicatib developed morphoea which resolved completely in eight and partially in one over 5–31 months following treatment discontinuation [261]. Truncal involvement, particularly over the chest and abdomen occurred in 19/22 cases in these two studies. Cathepsin K is involved in intracellular collagen degradation. Its expression is upregulated by IL-1α and inhibited by TGF-β1. This suggests a role for failed intracellular degradation of extracellular matrix proteins in the generation of fibrosis and represents a different mechanism to the previously proposed impairment of metalloproteinase-mediated collagen degradation and/or increased collagen production in the extracellular space [267]. Recent increased use of taxanes, including paclitaxel and docetaxel in anticancer therapy has highlighted the variety and high prevalence cutaneous side effects [268]. In a review of taxane-induced scleroderma to April 2022, Ketpueak *et al.* [269] identified 33 cases, 28 of which had sufficient data for analysis. Typical features were onset within 4 months of treatment initiation, with bilateral oedema of the extremities, most often beginning on the lower limbs (in >96%), with associated erythema mimicking cellulitis in 40% and followed by progressive proximal extension and development of skin thickening and sclerosis. ANA positivity and Raynaud phenomenon were occasionally present, but SSc-specific autoantibodies and systemic organ involvement were generally absent. The descriptions in most cases appear very similar to eosinophilic fasciitis or adult pansclerotic morphoea. Skin improvement usually occurred 4–6 months after discontinuing taxanes and in one case recurred after reintroduction of paclitaxel [257]. Increased serum IL-6, reduced dermal fibroblast endothelin1 and Fli1 (a repressor of type I collagen synthesis) and increased versican levels have been suggested as contributory factors in pathogenesis [268]. Scleroderma-like lesions including morphoea plaques, lichen sclerosus, extensive circumferential sclerosis and eosinophilic fasciitis-like presentations are described in around 50 patients on immune checkpoint inhibitors including ipilimumab, nivolumab and pembrolizumab, mostly after 1–6 cycles, with sclerosis appearing most rapidly and extensively with pembrolizumab [270–274]. Relapse of morphoea on nivolumab after a 6-year remission and improvement on cessation of the PD1 inhibitor is supportive of causation [275]. These scleroderma-spectrum anti-PD1 adverse events appear to occur later than autoimmunity involving other organs (thyroid, GI tract, liver) and are often preceded by a significant eosinophilia [271].

The slow or delayed onset of 'drug-induced morphoea' is common and could suggest that onset is coincidental. Other possibilities, however, include that drugs may act as triggers in susceptible individuals, a time-delay may be required to generate autoimmunity, and/or that the rarity and insidious onset of cutaneous lesions may delay diagnosis.

Clinical features

History

The onset and progression of morphoea is usually insidious. Patients may describe changes in skin texture or colour, sometimes with associated itch, burning sensation, pain or numbness. When lesions extend into deeper tissues or across joints, reduced mobility or contractures, and limb girth and length discrepancies may occur. In linear disease of the face and head, asymmetry of facial features, alopecia, indentation or grooves in the skull, ocular pain, altered vision, temporomandibular joint clicking and pain, and oral and dental abnormalities may develop. Headaches and seizures may occur. In generalised subtypes fatigue, myalgia and arthralgia are frequent. Occasionally, patients describe symptoms of gastro-oesophageal reflux. In cases where there is widespread chest wall sclerosis, respiratory symptoms may occur due to a restrictive defect.

Presentation

Individual lesions of morphoea generally begin with an erythematous, oedematous, inflammatory phase, which may be subtle and 'bruise-like' in appearance. The onset is often slow and insidious. Oedematous induration is followed by the development of central sclerosis associated with a change in skin colour and texture to thickened, waxy, yellowish white. There may be loss of hair and absent sweating. This central sclerotic area may be surrounded by an erythematous to violaceous so-called 'lilac ring', reflecting ongoing active disease. Over months or years, lesions become atrophic and hyper- or hypopigmented. In some cases, no sclerotic phase is seen and lesions progress straight to the atrophic hyperpigmented stage. Depending on the depth and type of lesion, changes in the subcutis, muscle, fascia, bone and underlying brain may be present. The average delay between onset of symptoms and diagnosis is 2.9 years in congenital morphoea [50] and ranges from 11 to 24 months in most childhood series [11,52,276]. In North American studies, 63% of 224 patients (129 adults) were given a diagnosis >6 months after onset of disease [51] and 17% of 381 children had a ≥2-year delay from symptom onset to their first paediatric rheumatology appointment [53]. Similar delays occur in the UK [276]. There was a suggestion that the delays in making a diagnosis might be greater in adults than in children and in patients with plaque or generalised morphoea rather than linear disease [51]. In fact delays to diagnosis of head variant linear disease may be even greater with a mean of 8.9 years in one study [277]. Such delays may have a significant impact on outcome, since they delay onset of treatment, which in turn has been shown to impair responses to methotrexate, may result in physicians missing the early 'active' phase of disease that is more amenable to treatment and increase the risk of developing disease-related irreversible damage.

Disease modifiers

Keloidal/nodular morphoea. The terms keloidal and nodular morphoea have been used interchangeably in the literature. Keloid-like nodules are seen in patients with previous or coexistent morphoea or, more often, in fact, in patients with lSSc (Figure 55.5) [278–283]. Clinically, keloidal or nodular lesions arising from sclerodermatous skin may reveal a histological appearance typical of either keloid or morphoea [284]. More rarely histological features of hypertrophic scarring [278,285] or homogenisation and thickening of collagen bundles with an increase in mucin are described. Lesions are most common on the upper body where they may coalesce or occur in a linear pattern [279,285,286]. In some cases, nodules arise from

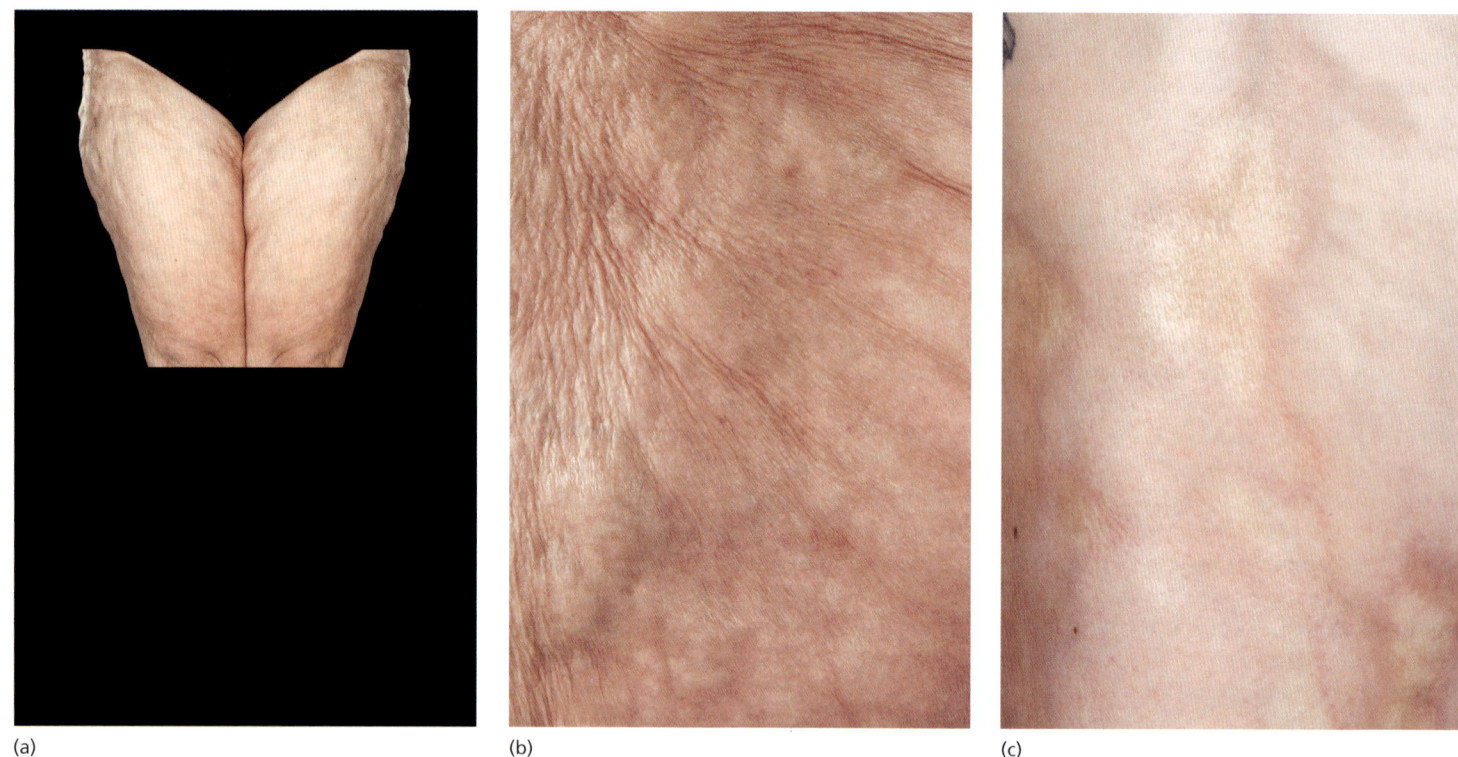

(a)   (b)   (c)

Figure 55.5 (a) Keloidal morphoea in a patient with limited cutaneous systemic sclerosis. Courtesy of Dr C.H. Orteu, Royal Free London NHS Foundation Trust. (b) Low power view showing a thick dermis, dense collagen and reduced adnexal structures. Keloidal changes are just visible (circled). Magnification 40x. H&E. (c) Higher power view showing swollen collagen bundles of the keloidal collagen. Magnification 100x. H&E. Courtesy of Dr F. Deroide, Department of Histopathology, Royal Free London NHS Foundation Trust, UK.

normal skin in patients genetically predisposed to keloid formation [284]. Increased levels of epidermal growth factor and CTGF have been implicated in pathogenesis [287]. In a histological and ultrastructural analysis in a patient with nodular morphoea on a background of diffuse cutaneous systemic sclerosis, Moinzadeh *et al.* found that increased density of immature collagen fibrils and absence of myofibroblasts characterised nodular lesions [288]. There was increased deposition of cartilage oligomeric matrix protein (COMP), collagen XII and fibrillin 1 within nodules in a distribution resembling that seen in keloids rather than normal skin. The authors suggested that COMP may promote fibroblast proliferation and increase production of extracellular matrix as a result of its ability to present TGF-β to fibroblasts and to bind to collagen I and XII. A more recent analysis of keloidal morphoea in patients with background systemic sclerosis reveals a distinct gene expression signature driven by differential expression of fibroblast rather than keratinocyte- or melanocyte-related genes with an even more extreme profibrotic pattern than is seen in diffuse cutaneous SSc [289].

Deep morphoea. The only mention of deep morphoea in the PRES classification is in regard to 'circumscribed deep morphoea'. In other classifications it refers to a separate subtype (see section on classification, earlier). However, the term 'deep morphoea' describes morphoea in which inflammation and sclerosis are found in the deep dermis, panniculus, fascia or muscle (Figure 55.6). Deep involvement has been documented in up to half of morphoea patients in some series [13]. It can occur in all subtypes of morphoea and is best viewed as a disease modifier [2,13] rather than a separate

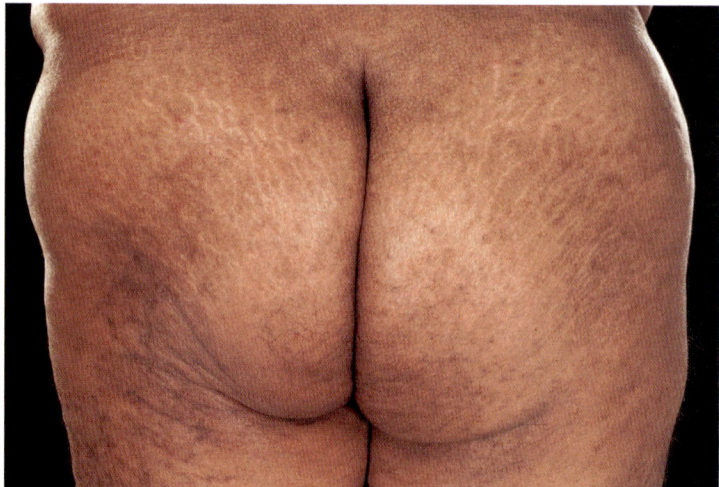

Figure 55.6 Deep involvement in morphoea. The skin is tethered to the underlying involved deep tissues giving a puckered appearance, deep nodularity and bound-down feeling.

subtype. Deep lesions are firm to hard, bound down to underlying structures, edges may be less well defined, the overlying skin may be normal, or puckered, have a cobblestone or peau d'orange appearance, with variable hyperpigmentation. Later, in the damage phase, there is atrophy of the skin, subcutis and underlying tissues, causing significant asymmetry and functional impairment (Figure 55.6c). The characteristics of deep morphoea (synonym morphoea profunda) as described in the literature are included here for completeness. In their original description of morphoea profunda in 23 patients, Person and Su's diagnostic criteria included the presence of diffuse, taut, bound-down, deep cutaneous sclerosis, and of significant hyalinisation and thickening of collagen bundles in the deep dermis, in the septa of subcutaneous fat and in the fascia [193,290]. Although most of the cases they described had widespread, deep involvement, some had individual plaques in keeping with a diagnosis of circumscribed deep morphoea (synonym solitary morphoea profunda). Solitary lesions of deep morphoea were first described by Whittaker et al. in five patients who had solitary, ill-defined, indurated and deeply tethered plaques with a peau d'orange appearance involving the upper trunk [291]. The main histopathological features were sclerosis and hyalinisation of collagen, and a striking accumulation of inflammatory cells in the deep dermis as well as in the subcutaneous tissue, which was predominantly composed of plasma cells and T and B lymphocytes [291]. Involvement below the subcutaneous fat was not identified in Whittaker's five cases, but only one had a deep biopsy. Increased numbers of eosinophils may be present in the skin and circulation [291,292]. Rarely, a plasma cell panniculitis has been described (synonym morphoea panniculitis) [293,294]. The condition has been reported in children and adults [291,295]. Several cases have been documented post-vaccination [229,230,296]. Occasionally, lesions present as non-inflammatory, cupuliform, depressed plaques with no associated induration, pigmentation or texture change, but with excessive dermal collagen deposition and thickened hyalinised collagen bundles in the deep dermis and subcutis on histology [296]. Deep morphoea can thus mimic lipoatrophy clinically and should be considered in patients presenting with asymptomatic atrophic lesions.

Bullous morphoea. Bullous morphoea is characterised by tense subepidermal bullae on a background of typical morphoea. It is rare, with <100 cases reported to date. It represented 1.4% of a Sardinian cohort of 137 morphoea patients seen over 11 years [297] and 7.5% of a cohort of 53 scleroderma cases (morphoea and SSc) [298]. Aetiology is likely multifactorial; bullae may develop as a result of subepidermal oedema induced by lymphangiectasias secondary to dermal sclerosis, and/or from excessive skin trauma or friction at susceptible sites [297,299]. In addition to sclerosis, marked lymphocytic infiltration in the reticular dermis is documented, suggesting it occurs on a background of active inflammatory phase disease [300]. It is best considered as a disease modifier since it has been documented in association with all morphoea subtypes. It occurs most often on the lower legs and, in this author's experience, at sites of chronic friction such as waistband and groins.

Limited morphoea

Circumscribed plaque morphoea. This commonest form of morphoea presents with single or multiple, round to oval lesions >1 cm in diameter, in up to two of seven anatomical regions (head–neck, each limb, anterior trunk, posterior trunk) (Figure 55.7). Histopathological changes are usually limited to the epidermis and dermis (circumscribed superficial plaque morphoea). Sometimes plaques extend more deeply (circumscribed deep plaque morphoea) and involve the subcutis, fascia and underlying muscle (Figure 55.7). There may be puckering or a peau d'orange appearance. Occasionally the primary site of involvement is the subcutis

without involvement of the overlying skin (see section on deep morphoea, earlier and Figures 55.6 and 55.8). Plaques can occur anywhere but are most frequently located on the trunk (41–74%). The breasts are often involved, but the nipples and areolae are uniformly spared. Plaques may occur on the face and neck in 12–13% of patients and need to be distinguished from linear morphoea at these sites as the trajectory and outcomes are different [7,54].

Guttate morphoea. This is a rare variant, similar to plaque morphoea, in which multiple, small (<1 cm), erythematous or yellowish white, mildly indurated lesions develop, most frequently on the trunk. Lesions are superficial and may have a shiny, crinkled surface, clinically resembling extragenital lichen sclerosus. It may be difficult to distinguish guttate morphoea from extragenital lichen sclerosis on clinical and histopathological grounds and some consider guttate morphoea to be a type of lichen sclerosis associated with morphoea [74,301,302]. In contrast to extragenital lichen sclerosus, however, lesions generally resolve leaving hyperpigmentation.

Atrophoderma of Pasini–Pierini. There are divergent opinions as to whether atrophoderma of Pasini–Pierini represents a separate entity or is a primarily superficial and atrophic variant of morphoea [178,303–306] (Figure 55.9). It is a rare condition that represents 0.1% of childhood morphoea cases [11] and that usually occurs in adolescence and young adult life. Three congenital cases are published [307]. Symmetrically distributed truncal lesions are the most common but single lesions and zosteriform distributions are described [304,308,309]. Typically, lesions are non-indurated, blue–grey to brown, hyperpigmented and sharply demarcated depressed patches, with a 'cliff-drop' edge [304,308]. A more recent publication of 16 cases found only 19% to be hyperpigmented, the remainder were either hypopigmented or skin coloured [305]. Histological appearances are variable: they may be normal or show mild lymphocytic infiltration, reduced dermal thickness and normal or sclerotic and hyalinised collagen [303,305]. Elastic stains may also show a spectrum of changes ranging from normal to severe diminution and fragmentation of the elastic fibre network [305]. The inclusion of atrophoderma of Pasini–Pierini within the spectrum of morphoea is supported by the coexistence of areas of induration more typical of morphoea in some patients [303,304]. In a study of 139 patients followed for a mean of 10 years, areas of induration appeared within existing lesions in 17% and plaques of morphoea were found elsewhere on the body in 22% of cases [304].

Generalised plaque morphoea

'Generalised morphoea' has been defined in a variety of ways in the literature (see section on classification, earlier). Falanga suggested five or more lesions, bilateral lesions and evidence of joining together of at least two individual patches [310]. The PRES classification [8] defined generalised morphoea as induration of the skin starting as four or more individual plaques, larger than 3 cm, that become confluent and involve at least two out of seven anatomical sites (head–neck, right upper extremity, left upper extremity, right lower extremity, left lower extremity, anterior trunk, posterior trunk). Peterson et al. [7] and Kreuter et al. [9] define it more simply as plaques involving three or more of these same

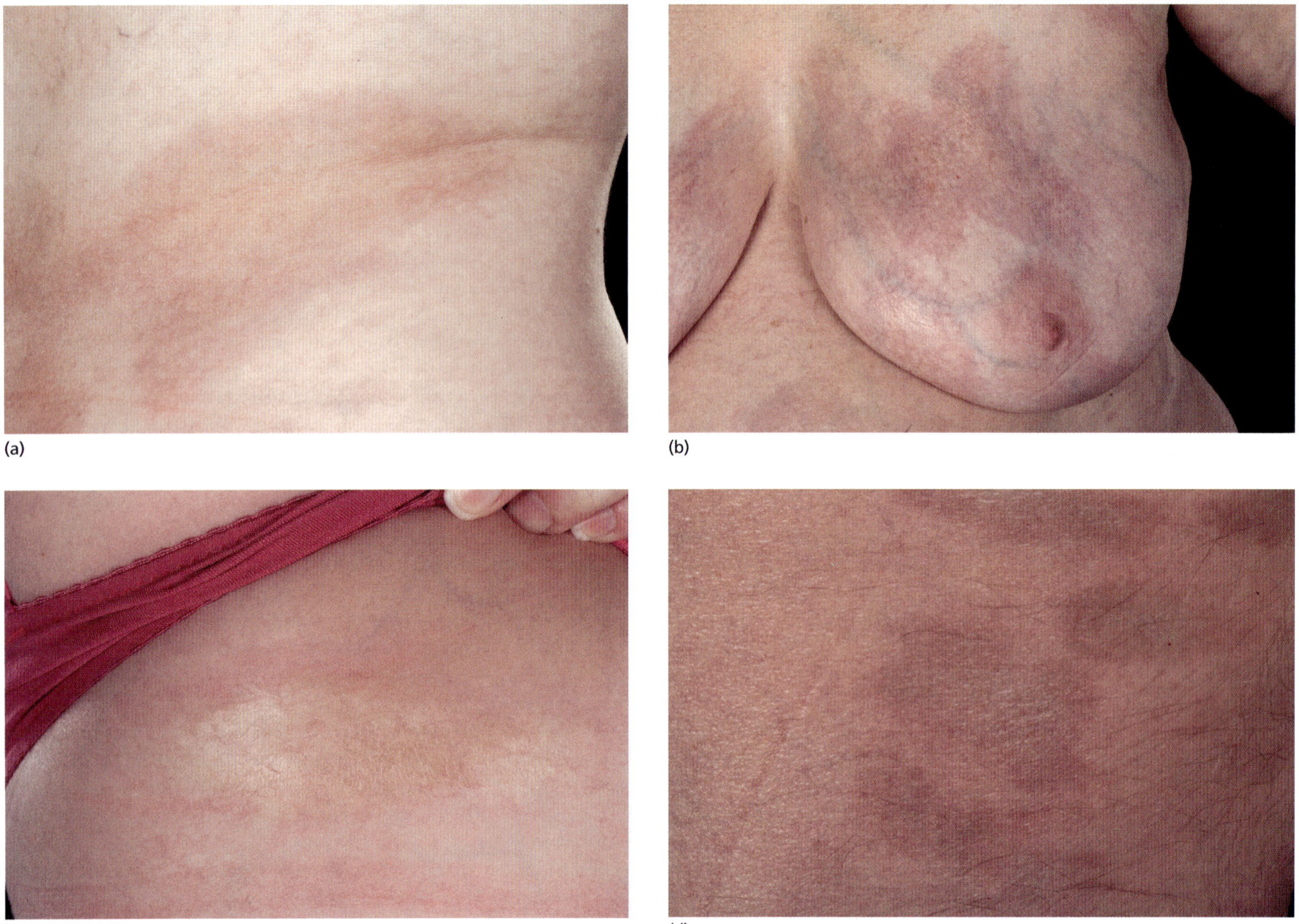

Figure 55.7 (a,b) Early, inflammatory, superficial plaque of morphoea with erythema and bruise-like appearance. (c) Sclerotic centre with inflammatory, peripheral red-lilac ring. (d) Hyperpigmented, atrophic late-stage disease. Courtesy of Dr C.H. Orteu Royal Free London NHS Foundation Trust.

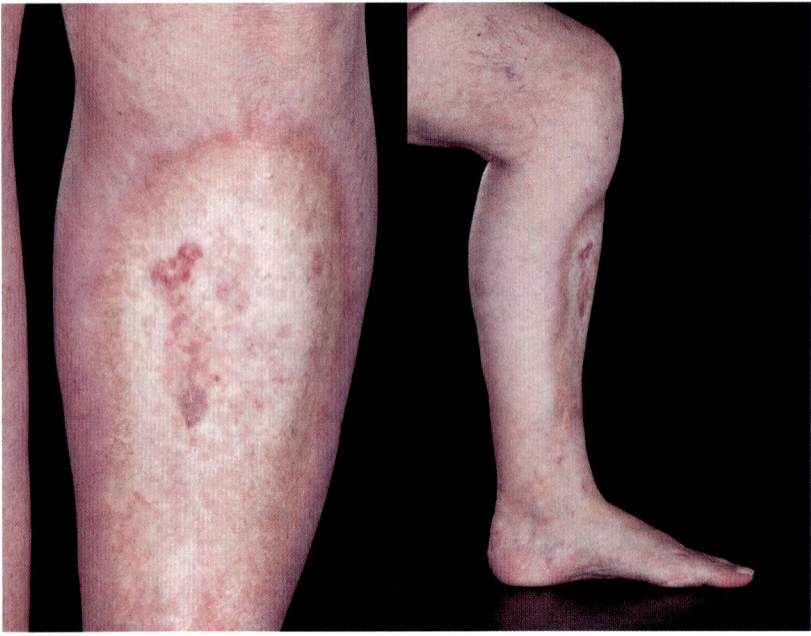

Figure 55.8 Plaque morphoea with deep involvement. Courtesy of Dr C.H. Orteu Royal Free London NHS Foundation Trust.

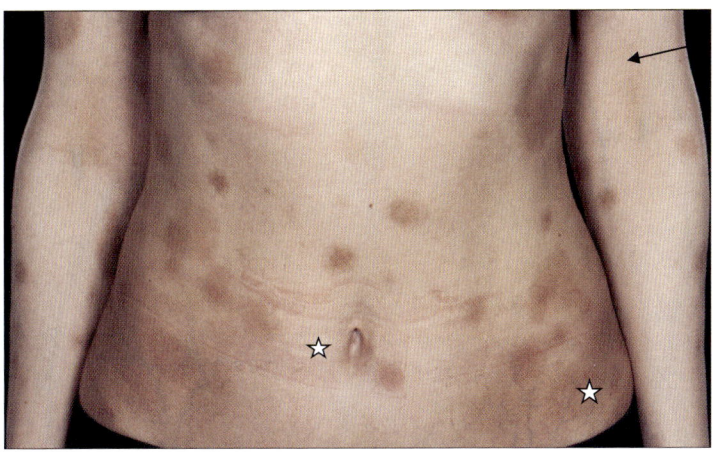

Figure 55.9 Atrophoderma of Pasini and Pierini multiple non-indurated hyperpigmented plaques with visible vessels (stars) and cliff drop edge (arrow). Courtesy of Dr C.H. Orteu Royal Free London NHS Foundation Trust.

seven anatomical sites. Based on these definitions, the literature suggests that generalised morphoea accounts for 7–9% of childhood morphoea cases [11,27,28,53] and between 13% and 52% of adult cases [6,12,**13**,28,46,54]. Plaques gradually develop at multiple sites, enlarge and become confluent. They may occur in different stages of evolution. Both adults and children initially presenting with circumscribed plaque morphoea may, because of ongoing or recurrent disease activity, progress to fulfil the criteria for generalised plaque morphoea [**13**]. Extracutaneous symptoms including myalgia, arthralgia and fatigue are common, and a higher prevalence of concurrent and familial autoimmune disease are documented (see the sections on autoimmunity (earlier), genetics (earlier) and complications and co-morbidities (later)). The term 'generalised plaque morphoea' is preferred to generalised morphoea and is synonymous with 'disseminated plaque morphoea'. Based on the findings of Prasad *et al.* and Teske *et al.* multisite linear disease and pansclerotic morphoea are not included in this subtype [**13**,**14**].

Two subsets of generalised plaque morphoea, 'symmetric' and 'isomorphic', with distinctive demographic and clinical features have now been defined through computerised mapping of the distribution of cutaneous lesions and correlation with demographic variables [**14**]. There is a female preponderance in both subsets, the isomorphic subset being entirely female in this study. The isomorphic subset were older (55.6 ± 12.7 years), and areas of morphoea unique to this subset were the bra-line and waistband. Bilateral inguinal areas and a diamond-shaped region over the mid lower back were also commonly involved (Figure 55.10a,b). The isomorphic pattern has been attributed to koebnerisation of lesions into sites of low-level trauma from clothing [112,311]. Lesions were superficial and overlying lichen sclerosus was commoner (28% vs 18%). In the symmetric subset, morphoea typically affected a butterfly-shaped area on the lower abdomen below the umbilicus, the anterior tibia, popliteal and antecubital fossae, and arcuate areas on the breasts sparing the areolae (Figure 55.10c). Deep involvement occurred more often (23% in symmetric vs 3% in the isomorphic pattern). The symmetric subset was younger (42.2 ± 20 years) with a bimodal distribution, 21% having childhood onset disease [**14**]. Genital lesions in keeping with lichen sclerosus were present in 10.3% of 232 generalised plaque morphoea patients, almost

exclusively in postmenopausal females with isomorphic superficial disease and accompanying extragenital lichen sclerosus [73]. A small retrospective French study of 27 patients with generalised plaque morphoea has confirmed the segregation of patients into isomorphic and symmetric subsets. They found a 56% prevalence of genital lichen sclerosus overall, which was 80% in the isomorphic subset. There was a higher prevalence of associated autoimmunity in the symmetric group (55%) [312].

Pansclerotic morphoea

Pansclerotic morphoea has variably been included within either the generalised [9] or deep [7] subtypes or as a separate subtype of morphoea [8] in published classifications. This is a rarer presentation characterised by extensive, often circumferential involvement of the majority of body surface areas with sparing of the fingers and toes [15] (Figure 55.11). This term has traditionally been used to describe a very rare, widespread and severe progressive disease occurring predominantly in children in which deep fibrosis progresses rapidly to involve muscle, fascia and underlying bone [313,314].

It is mainly referred to as disabling pansclerotic morphoea of childhood in the literature and is frequently complicated by severe joint contractures, chronic ulceration and the development of squamous cell carcinoma [315–318]. Increased serum IgG, a positive ANA and peripheral eosinophilia are documented in some cases [313,317,319,320]. By virtue of the number of body sites involved, this subtype meets the classification criteria for generalised morphoea, but it is a clinically distinct condition, and based on Prasad *et al.*'s evaluation of morphoea classifications, should be viewed as a separate subtype [**13**]. It is unclear whether the particularly severe phenotype described in children occurs as a consequence of growth impairment or because they have a more severe disease pattern than adults.

While the previous descriptions of pansclerotic morphoea in childhood suggest deep tissue involvement, including subcutaneous tissue, muscle and bone in all cases [313,315], the actual definition and frequency of involvement beyond the dermis has been inconsistent [314,321–324]. In a cross-sectional study of the Morphoea in Adults and Children (MAC) cohort, an ongoing prospective registry of patients with morphoea in Texas, USA, the demographic and clinical features of patients with the pansclerotic subtype were described [15]. Because of the relative ambiguity with regard to depth of involvement, in the literature this criterion was removed, and pansclerotic morphoea was defined as the presence of near total body surface area involvement with sparing of the fingers and toes (Table 55.2). The distinction from SSc is made based on the absence of sclerodactyly, nail fold capillary changes and internal organ involvement. Of the 360 patients (97 children, 263 adults) in the MAC cohort at that time, 113 patients with generalised morphoea were identified. Thirteen of these patients, 3.6% of the cohort, met the above criteria for pansclerotic morphoea. A majority had onset of lesions on the trunk with rapid centrifugal spread and abrupt cut-off at the metacarpo- and metatarsophalangeal joints. None had demonstrable bony involvement. They had a more rapidly progressive and severe phenotype than the generalised plaque morphoea group but were distinct from SSc. Interestingly, there were no significant differences between the generalised

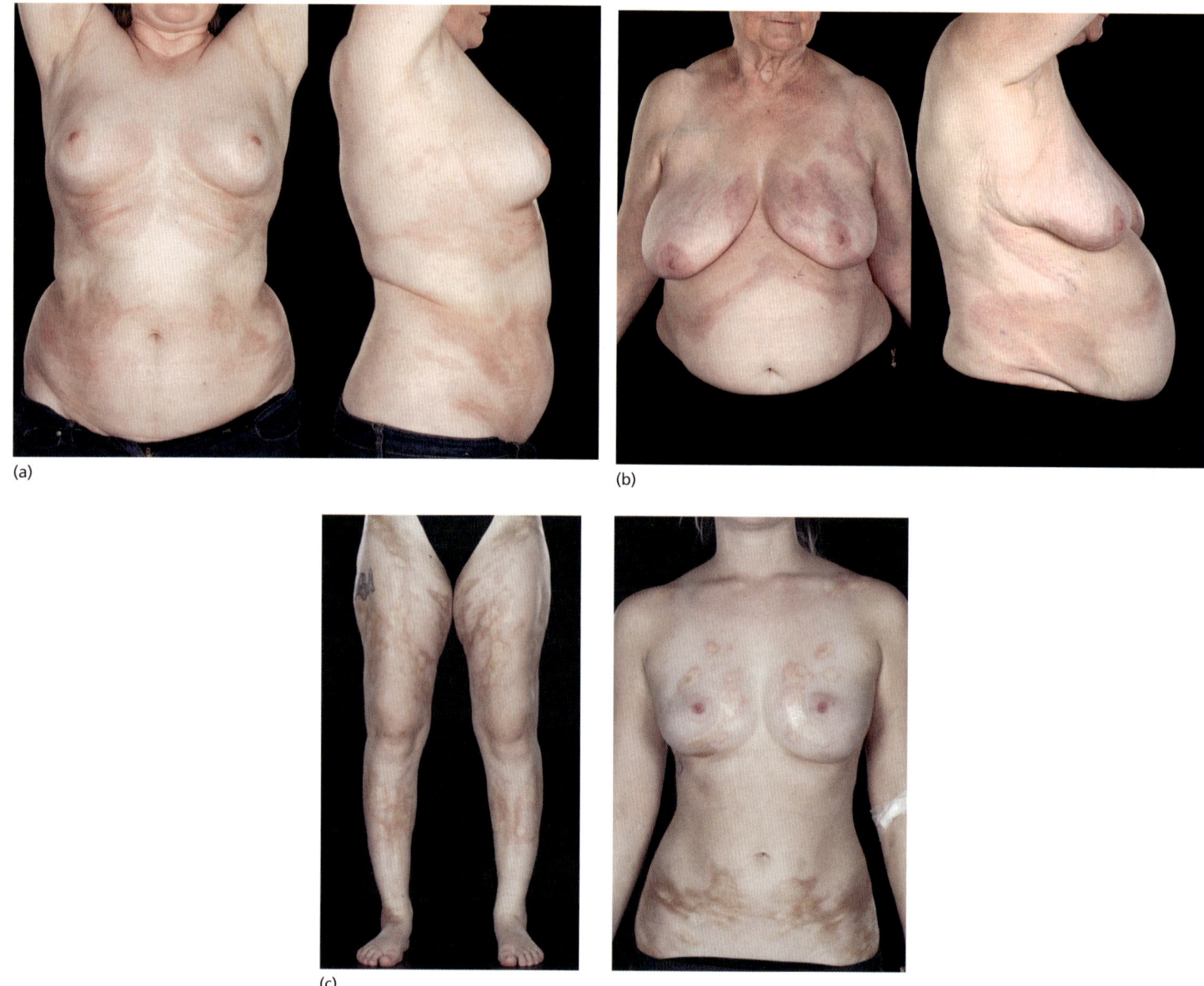

Figure 55.10 Generalised plaque morphoea. (a) Isomorphic pattern: active inflammatory stage with no deep involvement, and an isomorphic pattern of lesions around the bra, waistband area and groins. (b) Isomorphic pattern: early central sclerosis and prominent peripheral inflammatory lilac ring with no deep involvement, and a symmetrical isomorphic pattern involving the inframammary and waistband areas. (c) Symmetric pattern: widespread shiny yellowish and hyperpigmented sclerotic indurated plaques distributed symmetrically on the trunk and limbs. The patient is younger than in (a) and (b) and plaques are deeper, thicker and more tethered. Courtesy of Dr C.H. Orteu, Royal Free London NHS Foundation Trust.

morphoea and pansclerotic groups for age at onset of disease (mean 49 years, standard deviation 19), or prevalence of ANA (29–31%) and antihistone antibodies (7–10%). However, patients with the pansclerotic subtype were more likely to be male (46% versus 6% of generalised morphoea patients) and have a shorter time to diagnosis, higher rates of functional impairment (61% versus 16%) and higher skin sclerosis and damage scores. Even though it was not a defining factor, a high frequency of deep involvement on tissue biopsy (61% versus 17%) was observed. Restrictive defects on pulmonary function tests, dysphagia and/or hand oedema were identified in 4/13 patients and following investigation were attributed to severe, extensive skin sclerosis rather than internal organ involvement *per se* [15].

There is significant clinical overlap between pansclerotic morphoea as defined previously and the various forms of deep morphoea described in the literature. The term subcutaneous morphoea was initially coined by Person and Su in 1979, who described 16 cases with biopsy-proven inflammatory sclerosis of the panniculus or fascia, 13 of whom had extensive, ill-defined, bound-down plaques with a rapid centrifugal progression [290]. Three years later they added seven cases and reviewed the published literature describing patients with deep involvement [193]. On the basis that involvement of the deep dermis, subcutaneous fat, fascia or muscle can be present alone or in any combination, they renamed the condition morphoea profunda, and included eosinophilic fasciitis within its spectrum [193]. The distinction between morphoea

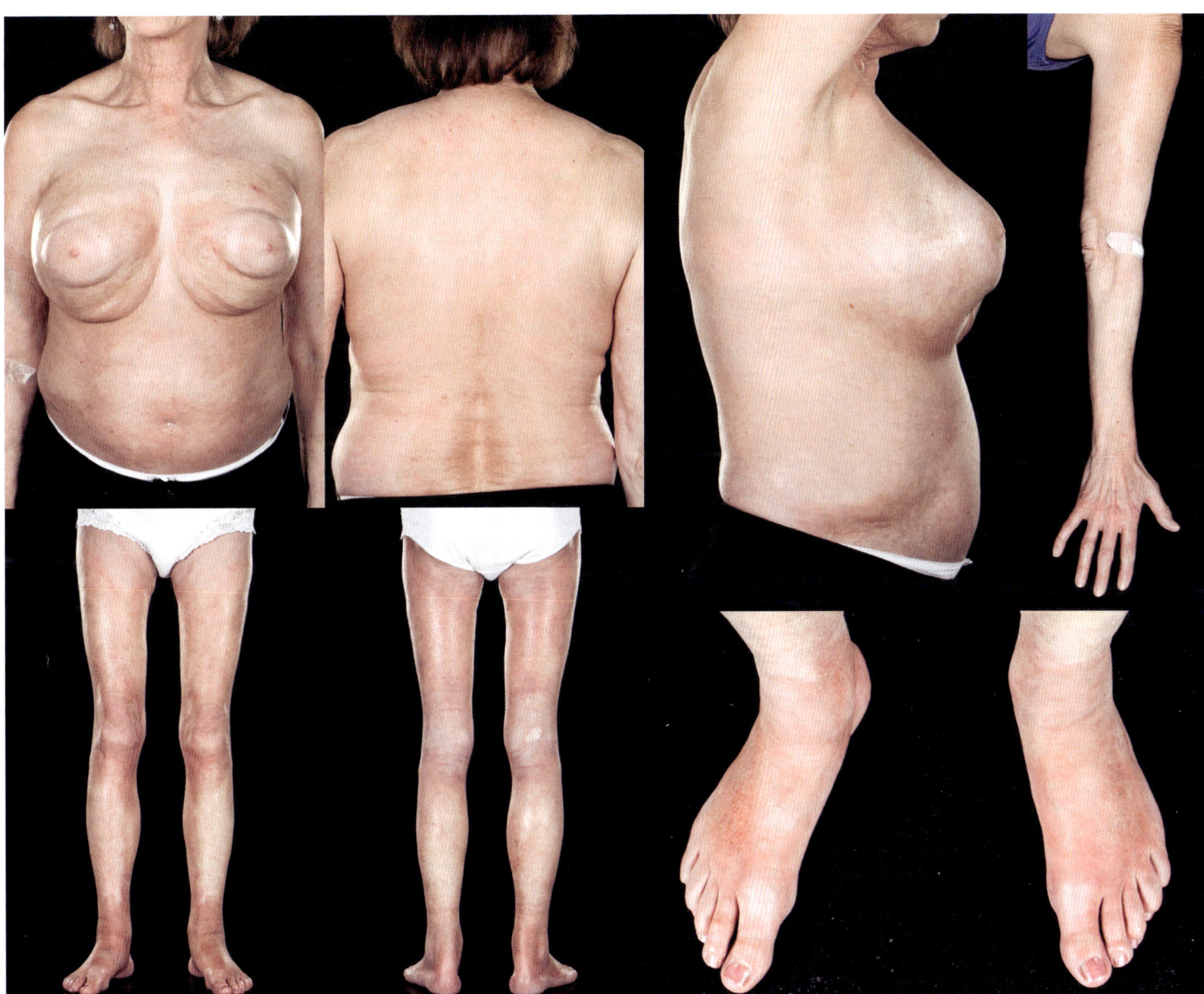

Figure 55.11 Pansclerotic morphoea in one patient showing circumferential involvement of the lower limbs and trunk with sparing of the areolae and hands. Courtesy of Dr C.H. Orteu, Royal Free London NHS Foundation Trust.

profunda, pansclerotic morphoea (as defined previously) and eosinophilic fasciitis remains blurred. The terminology is confusing, as evidenced by the recent use of 'disseminated morphoea profunda' to describe a patient with an isomorphic pattern and deep involvement [325] and of 'generalised deep morphoea' to describe a case with a pansclerotic pattern of disease [326].

Eosinophilic fasciitis

Eosinophilic fasciitis (synonym Shulman syndrome) (Figure 55.12) was first described by Shulman in 1975 [327]. The inclusion of this subtype within the morphoea spectrum is debated but supported by the coexistence of other subtypes of morphoea in 29–41% of cases [16–18,328]. It is usually extensive and involves deep tissues. When included in previous classifications of morphoea it has variably been assigned to the generalised or deep groups.

It symmetrically involves the extremities, particularly the lower limbs, but typically spares the fingers and face [329,330]. Truncal involvement was said not to occur in early reports, but is described in roughly a third, and there is considerable clinical overlap with pansclerotic morphoea in such cases [16,331]. In the early stages there is intense inflammation with painful, burning erythema and marked pitting oedema of the limbs. This is replaced by induration and fibrosis resulting in puckering and a typical peau d'orange appearance, with tethering around vessels producing guttering referred to as the groove sign (Figure 55.12). The sclerotic process involves the fibrous septa of the subcutis and deep fascia and may extend into the underlying muscle. A significant eosinophilic infiltrate in the panniculus and deep fascia may be present in the early stage of disease [16,332,333] but is not invariable [193]. In a recent retrospective observational

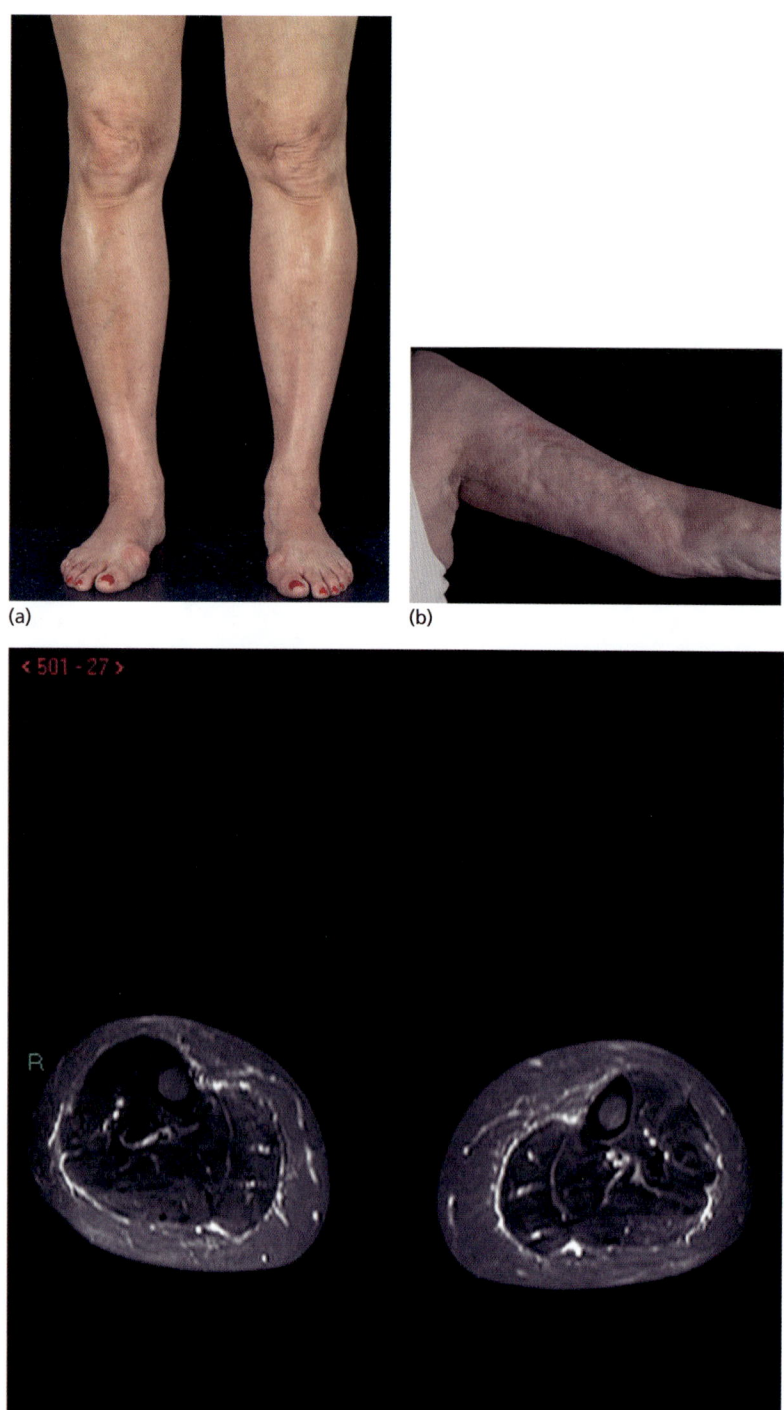

(a)

(b)

(c)

Figure 55.12 Eosinophilic fasciitis. (a) Limited disease involving the lower legs and ankles. The skin appears shiny and taut. (b) Deep involvement, including fascia, with puckering of overlying skin and a groove sign on the forearm. Courtesy of Dr C.H. Orteu. Royal Free London NHS Foundation Trust. (c) T2-weighted MRI image showing bilateral interfascial oedema more marked on the left. Courtesy of Dr Brian Holloway, Consultant Radiologist, Royal Free London NHS Foundation Trust.

study of 70 cases, 59% were male with a mean age of 53.8 years. Prodromal constitutional symptoms were present in one quarter of cases. Skin induration affected all four limbs in 67% and the trunk in 34%. Cutaneous features included hyperpigmentation and erythema in 30%, groove sign in 20% and peau d'orange in 17%. Extracutaneous manifestations included arthritis, joint contractures, myalgia and weakness. Arthralgia was the commonest extracutaneous manifestation and occurred in >50% of cases [17]. Unaccustomed severe exercise may precede the onset of disease

in up to 50% of cases [17,329]. It can result in severe joint contractures and associated morbidity. A high ESR and C-reactive protein (CRP), hypergammaglobulinaemia and peripheral eosinophilia (present in 55–90% of cases) are typical [16–18], but can occur in other morphoea subtypes also. Haematological abnormalities including thrombocytopenia, aplastic anaemia and leukaemia have been associated [16,334]. A deep biopsy of the clinically affected tissue showing inflammation and thickening of deep fascia or an MRI establishing evidence of fasciitis are essential to establish the diagnosis [330] (Figure 55.12c). Multivariate analysis in 128 cases revealed that eosinophilia and fibrosis are predictive of relapse. Of 109 patients followed for >1 year, 45% relapsed and 44% had sequelae, highlighting the potential severity of the condition [19].

Linear morphoea

Linear morphoea accounts for 10–20% of morphoea cases in adults [6,46,54] and 42–67% of cases in children [6,11,27] in published cohorts. Vasquez-Canizares and Li combined the data from 10 paediatric rheumatology and dermatology cohorts, including the largest paediatric cohort [11] and five paediatric and adult onset cohorts [6,28,32,46,55]. Linear morphoea accounted for 1127/1997 (56.4%) of paediatric onset and 87/893 (9.7%) of adult-onset morphoea [1]. Roughly one-third of patients with linear morphoea have adult-onset disease [12]. It may be subdivided into limb/trunk and head variants. In most studies, the limb/trunk variant occurs more often (54–65%) than the head variant (23–41%) [1,11,33]. In contrast, one study of 823 patients with childhood onset disease found a higher frequency of head and neck lesions [25]. Linear head and trunk/limb variants have been found to coexist in 1% of children. It is quite common for the upper and lower limb on the same side to be affected. Although mostly unilateral, bilateral involvement is reported in 2.5–47% of cases [11,12,27,335,336]. Patients with linear morphoea lesions occurring at two or more anatomical body sites potentially fulfil the criteria for inclusion into the generalised morphoea subset. This group exhibit features of the linear subtype and should be referred to as having multisite linear disease, and be excluded from the generalised subset [2,14]. Linear morphoea appears to follow Blaschko lines (Figure 55.13) in the majority of cases suggesting that genetic mosaicism is important in pathogenesis [335,337,338]. Roughly a quarter of patients with linear disease

have another form of morphoea elsewhere (mixed subtype) and most often this is plaque morphoea [1,11].

Head/neck variant

The head variant includes morphoea en coup de sabre (ECDS) and progressive hemifacial atrophy (PHA), which is also known as Parry–Romberg syndrome and progressive facial hemiatrophy (Figure 55.14). In roughly two-thirds of cases disease onset is in the first two decades. Some descriptions suggest that lesions of the forehead and scalp represent morphoea ECDS and that those below the forehead should be considered to be PHA. However, sclerotic lesions can occur on the cheeks, chin and neck and atrophic lesions can occur on the forehead and scalp. ECDS lesions are commoner than PHA, representing 61–73% of head variant lesions overall [1]. In a retrospective cross-sectional study of 96 patients from five German tertiary referral centres, 70 patients had morphoea ECDS, 16 had PHA and 10 had overlap ECDS/PHA [114]. Sclerotic lesions, typical of morphoea ECDS, overlying atrophic areas of PHA are well described and more prevalent in paediatric cases [1,11,277,339]. Cases of typical morphoea ECDS have been reported to evolve into PHA, emphasising the overlap and common pathogenesis [340]. While linear morphoea of the head/neck occasionally has a sudden onset and rapidly progressive course, in many cases the onset of both subtypes of disease is insidious and may progress slowly over many years. While three-quarters of patients experience skin tightening or thickening in the initial stages of disease, some 13% have no clinically obvious inflammatory or sclerotic phase [341]. Concomitant morphoea lesions at other sites, mainly truncal plaque and linear limb lesions, may occur and appear more frequent in PHA (37.5%) and ECDS/PHA overlap (40%) than in ECDS (20%) [11,114]. Head lesions have a higher risk for neurological, oral and eye complications [4,188], particularly if on the superior anterior portion of the head in childhood onset disease [25].

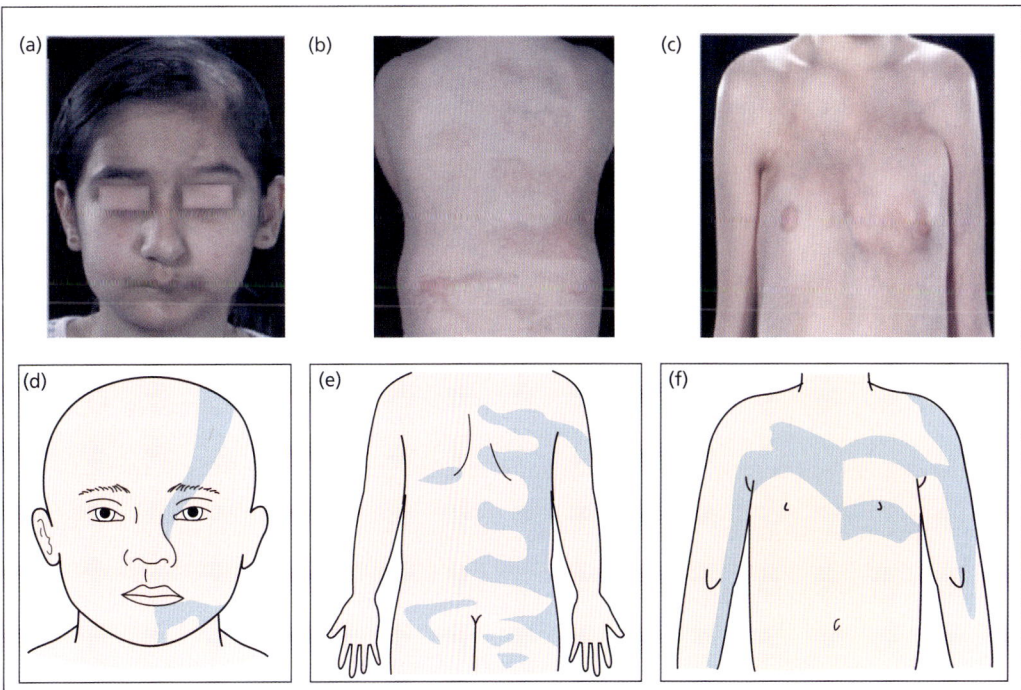

Figure 55.13 Blaschkoid nature of linear morphoea on the face (a, d), back (b, e) and chest (c, f). From Weibel and Harper 2008 [335]. Reproduced with permission of Wiley.

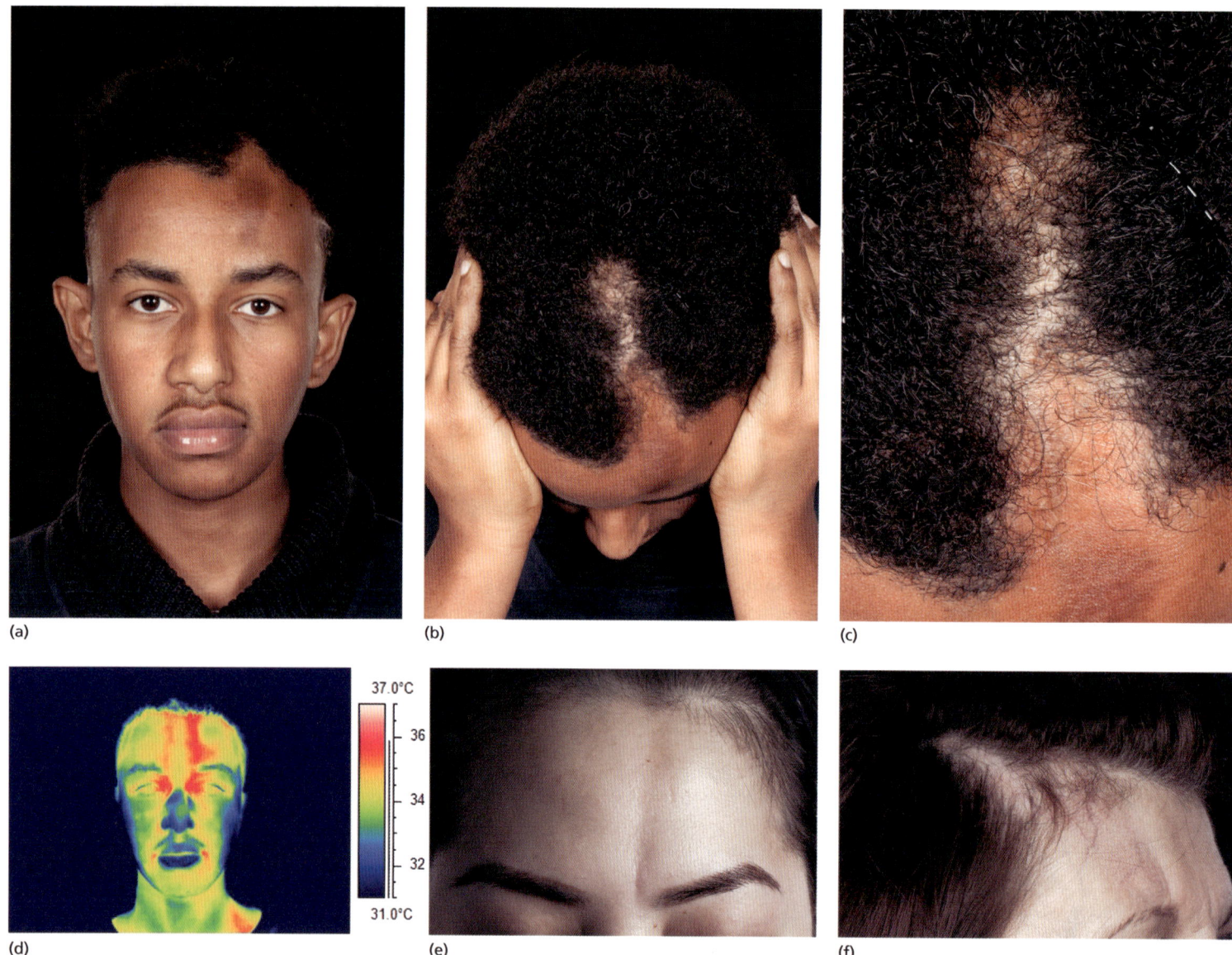

Figure 55.14 Linear morphoea en coup de sabre. (a) Hyperpigmention on the forehead with subcutaneous atrophy and a subtle indentation of bone. (b,c) Alopecia with more sclerotic changes on the scalp. Note the Blaschkoid distribution. (d) Thermographic image of the same patient showing increased temperature of the skin at a site corresponding to disease activity and extension on the left paramedian forehead. (e) Early left paramedian linear depressed narrow groove with normal overlying skin. (f) Longstanding right paramedian linear band of hyperpigmentation and dermal atrophy, with visible vessels and hair loss involving scalp and eyebrow.

Morphoea en coup de sabre. Morphoea ECDS typically presents as a linear band which involves the paramedian forehead and/or the frontoparietal scalp and follows Blaschko lines [335,342] (Figure 55.13). Bilateral and midline lesions occur more rarely [117,336]. Concomitant linear limb/trunk and plaque lesions may occur [114,117]. Sclerosis is thought to involve the skin and subcutis first and then later extend to the underlying fascia and bone. Varying degrees of sclerosis, hyperpigmentation and atrophy may be observed (Figure 55.14). Linear depressions in the skull bones are a common consequence. Alopecia of the eyelashes, eyebrows and scalp occur if they are involved in the band and are generally thought to be irreversible. However, a recent publication described partial resolution of skin sclerosis and regrowth of hair in children treated with corticosteroids and methotrexate [343]. Extracutaneous manifestations are common and neurological, ocular and oral

complications are well recognised [1,4]. A variety of abnormalities are seen on computed tomography (CT) scan and MRI (see the section on extracutaneous manifestations, complications and co-morbidities, later) [187,336].

Progressive hemifacial atrophy. Progressive hemifacial atrophy (synonym Parry–Romberg syndrome, progressive facial hemiatrophy) has traditionally been described as affecting the area supplied by one or multiple branches of the trigeminal nerve [188,344]. More recently it has been suggested that lesions are Blaschkoid, as is the case for other types of linear morphoea [335]. A majority of cases begin in the first decade, but occasional adult onset cases are described [345–347]. It is a unilateral, progressive, primary atrophic disorder of the skin, subcutaneous tissue, muscle and underlying cartilage and bone (Figure 55.15). Overlying skin may

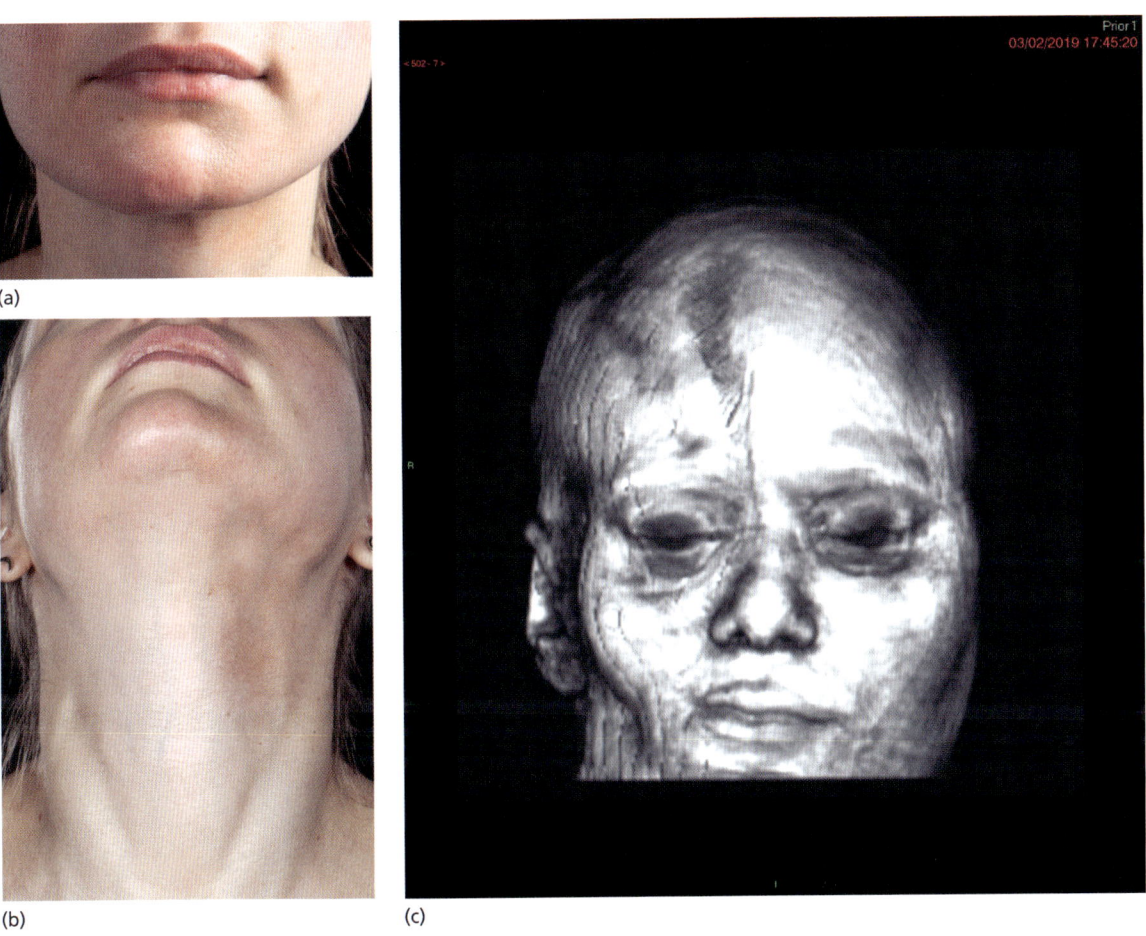

Figure 55.15 (a) Progressive hemifacial atrophy involving the left side of the mandible and chin. (b) Mildly hyperpigmented skin overlies atrophic deeper structures. Note the facial asymmetry, with loss of soft tissue over the chin, jawline and neck. There is frequently a significant delay to diagnosis (5–10 years) in this type of morphoea. (c) MRI-generated 3D reconstruction showing severe combined right-sided linear morphoea en coup de sabre and hemifacial atrophy. Courtesy of Dr G Chow and Dr F Jabeen, Royal Free London NHS Foundation Trust.

appear normal, hyperpigmented, usually a brownish or bruise-like change, but occasionally hypopigmented. Sclerosis is not a feature. A progressive facial asymmetry develops as a result of a gradual loss of fat and muscle, and atrophy of the frontal, maxillary and/or mandibular bones. Temporomandibular joint involvement may cause pain and clicking. The mouth and nose may become deviated towards the affected side while mandibular and intraoral involvement may lead to dental malocclusion and hemiatrophy of the tongue [188,277].

Trunk/limb variant

As in morphoea ECDS, linear bands seem to follow Blaschko lines and may exhibit varying degrees of erythema, sclerosis, atrophy and hyperpigmentation (Figure 55.16) [335,337]. Linear sclerotic bands may appear suddenly or insidiously and then progress. In some cases, small lesions spread widely, but in a piecemeal linear fashion along a limb and then coalesce over time to form a more obvious linear band. Coexistent or preceding plaque morphoea, most often on the trunk (i.e. mixed morphoea), is most common in linear limb disease. A majority of linear lesions are unilateral but bilateral lesions were found in 11% in the largest childhood study [11] and in 5.5–46% of other published series [1,12,27,54,117]. Multisite linear disease (at two or more body sites) may occur in roughly 40% of cases overall

and is more common in paediatric onset disease [1,12,341]. The dermis, subcutis, underlying muscle and bone may be involved. In limb lesions, generalised arthralgias and oedema of the involved extremity can precede the onset of disease [11,54,117]. Myalgia and arthralgias are common, occurring in 24% and 34% respectively in one study [12]. Deep disease occurs in some two-thirds of cases and is associated with limitation of range of motion, and thus with functional limitation [12]. Lesions extending across joints result in flexion contractures or limited range of motion in up to 15% of adults and 30% of children [1]. Myopathic changes, atrophy and weakness of involved and adjacent muscles may occur [348]. In adults, limb girth asymmetry results, and in children growth failure causes additional limb length discrepancies. Joint contractures, muscle atrophy and limb shortening cause pain and significant functional limitations, which in turn lead to a reduction in quality of life and to significant psychological morbidity [4,53,349].

Linear atrophoderma of Moulin. The original 1992 publication described five patients with unilateral, depressed, hyperpigmented Blaschkoid lesions on the trunk and limbs, with onset between 6 and 20 years of age. Histology showed epidermal hyperpigmentation, but a normal dermis and normal collagen on histology [350]. The authors suggested that the impression of skin atrophy might

(a) at presentation   (b) at 6 months   (c) at 42 months

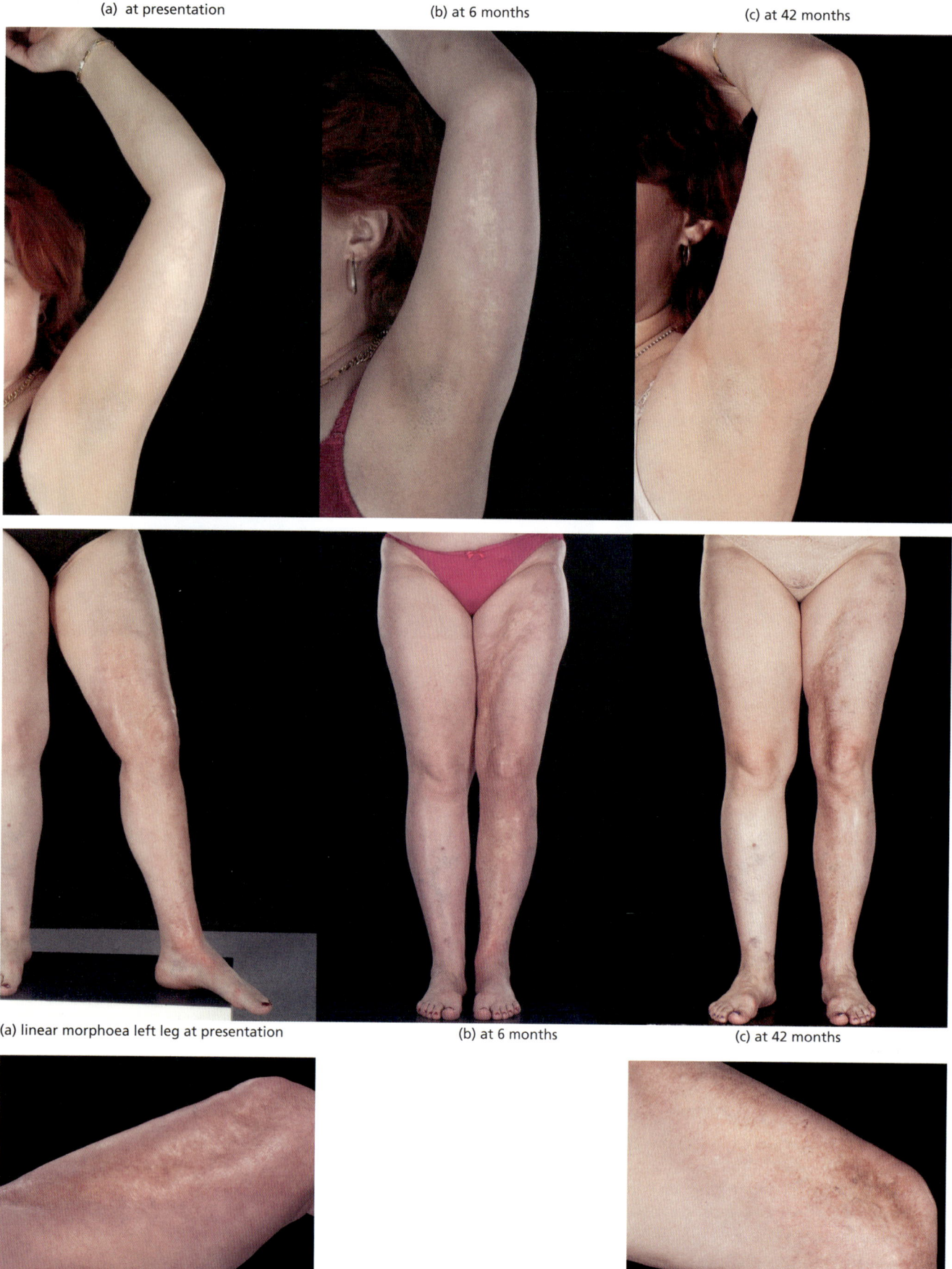

(a) linear morphoea left leg at presentation   (b) at 6 months   (c) at 42 months

Figure 55.16 Linear morphoea of the left arm (top) and leg (below). (a,b) Active inflammatory phase showing (a) the shiny waxy appearance at presentation and (b) a marked increase in sclerosis with peripheral erythema at 6 months. (c) Softened, atrophic, hyperpigmented appearance of late-stage inactive disease after successful treatment with corticosteroids and methotrexate at 42 months.

Table 55.4 Differential diagnosis of the different phases of circumscribed plaque morphoea, pansclerotic morphoea, and eosinophilic fasciitis and linear morphoea.

Circumscribed plaque morphoea			
Early inflammatory phase	**Sclerotic phase**	**Hyperpigmented phase**	**Atrophic phase**
Granuloma annulare	Necrobiosis lipoidica	Postinflammatory hyperpigmentation	Lipodystrophy
Early extragenital lichen sclerosus	Pretibial myxoedema	Actinic lichen planus	Steroid-induced atrophy
Lyme disease –erythema migrans		Café au lait macule	Lupus profundus
Mycosis fungoides		Erythema dyschromicum perstans	Acrodermatitis chronica atrophicans
Cutaneous mastocytosis			Panniculitis (late stage)
Radiation dermatitis			Lichen sclerosus
Fixed drug eruption			
Pansclerotic morphoea and eosinophilic fasciitis		**Linear morphoea**	
Systemic sclerosis			
Sclerodermoid graft-versus-host disease		Linear panniculitis	
Scleroedema		Linear lichen planus	
Scleromyxoedema		Linear lupus erythematosus	
Porphyria cutanea tarda		Linear lichen sclerosus	
Primary systemic amyloidosis		Lipodystrophy	
Nephrogenic systemic fibrosis		Focal dermal hypoplasia	
Carcinoid syndrome		Steroid atrophy	
Drug-induced morphoea			
Chemical and occupational causes of skin sclerosis (Table 55.3)			

therefore be due to atrophy of subcutaneous structures, and this was confirmed in one case by ultrasonography [351]. Subsequently, a variety of pathological findings have been described [352]. In one case, clinical overlap with atrophoderma of Pasini–Pierini and morphoea were seen and, histologically, perivascular inflammation and thickening of collagen fibres in the mid-reticular dermis constituted a significant histopathological overlap [353]. Although it is not universally agreed, linear atrophoderma of Moulin appears to lie within the morphoea spectrum and be akin to a linear Blaschkoid form of atrophoderma of Pasini–Pierini.

Linear deep atrophic morphoea. Three cases of linear primary atrophic morphoea with no preceding clinical inflammation or sclerosis, involving the subcutis and deep dermis, and resembling PHA on a limb, have been reported [354]. Although progressive in nature, they did not result in joint contractures. In one of these and two further cases, linear limb lesions occurred in association with PHA, confirming the relationship between these two presentations [355,356].

Mixed morphoea

Mixed morphoea is the coexistence of more than one subtype of morphoea. The most common combination is linear limb/trunk and plaque morphoea, but any combination can occur. Combining data from 10 large case series suggests that mixed morphoea occurs in 2.6% of patients with adult-onset and 13.6% of patients with childhood-onset morphoea [1].

Differential diagnosis

Skin sclerosis may be seen in a number of conditions that are neither morphoea nor SSc. These include metabolic, deposition and genetic disorders, disease caused by exposure to chemicals, toxins and drugs, graft-versus-host disease and nephrogenic systemic fibrosis (Table 55.3) [357,358]. Increasing knowledge of the genetic basis for monogenic diseases with sclerodermatous features may provide clues to the pathogenesis of autoimmune sclerosing conditions including morphoea and SSc. For further details see the excellent summary table in Jensen *et al.* [359]. The differential diagnosis of morphoea depends on the subtype and stage of disease and is summarised in Table 55.4 (see also Box 54.1 and Table 54.9 in Chapter 54).

Classification and assessment of severity

Severity of disease in morphoea depends largely on the age at onset, extent and depth of disease, and whether there are extracutaneous manifestations, such as bone, joint, central nervous system (CNS), ocular or oral involvement. Measures of severity should assess disease activity, the potential for damage, the degree of irreversible damage caused by previously active disease, associated extracutaneous involvement and the impact on quality of life. The development of composite scores which encompass all of these elements is now underway [36,360]. Until relatively recently there was no uniformly accepted scoring system for assessing disease activity in morphoea. A wide variety of imaging techniques and skin scoring systems have been employed, making it difficult to compare outcomes in different clinical studies and disease registries. The development and validation of the localised scleroderma cutaneous assessment tool or LoSCAT has helped significantly in this regard (see the section on outcome measures in Investigations) [37,39,**40**]. For example, LoSCAT activity (LoSAI) scores of 0–4, –12 and ≥13 were found to correspond with mild, moderate and severe disease activity levels [38].

Severity levels for juvenile localised scleroderma have been proposed by the Childhood Arthritis and Rheumatology Research Alliance (CARRA) [361]. High severity was defined as presentation with generalised or pansclerotic morphoea, craniofacial linear morphoea or another subtype with evidence of high morbidity such as CNS involvement, limb shortening or joint contracture. Moderate severity was defined as circumscribed deep morphoea or linear morphoea of the trunk or limb without evidence of high morbidity. Low severity disease was defined as superficial, circumscribed plaque morphoea. These measures of severity should be equally applicable to adult patients. There is also some evidence that patients with extracutaneous manifestations, particularly children [1,4], appear to have more severe disease, as suggested by greater levels of systemic inflammation and a greater need for systemic immunosuppression [5]. This should prompt a search for evidence of extracutaneous involvement at regular intervals. These can be assigned a score using the recently developed Total Morbidity Score [360] (see section on outcome measures in Investigations, later)

Functional limitation is defined as a clinically appreciable limited range of motion of a joint secondary to contracture or to skin and subcutaneous tissue involvement, but not due to abnormality of the joint itself and/or limb–length discrepancy [116]. This should also be considered a marker of disease severity since it is closely associated with quality-of-life scores and psychological morbidity. The latter should also be assessed as they contribute to severity. A variety of scoring systems are in routine clinical use, most frequently Dermatology Life Quality Index (DLQI), Children's Dermatology Life Quality Index (CDLQI), Health Assessment Questionnaire (HAQ), Children's Health Assessment Questionnaire (CHAQ) and Hospital Anxiety and Depression Score (HADS). The recent development of the Localised Scleroderma Quality of Life Instrument (LoSQI) for children is a positive step towards a more directed assessment of the impact that morphoea has on children [362] (see section on outcome measures, later).

Complications and co-morbidities
Extracutaneous manifestations
Although the classic description of morphoea suggests no internal organ or systemic manifestations, there is now a wealth of evidence to challenge this assumption. Early small series in adults and children identified extracutaneous features in 21–27% of patients [363–365] and described mild degrees of frequently asymptomatic oesophageal dysmotility, mild gas transfer defects, restrictive changes in lung function and myositis. Electrocardiographic abnormalities, particularly incomplete right bundle branch block and echocardiographic abnormalities, and especially involving the mitral valve and left ventricle, were documented in children with varying frequencies [366], but are in fact rare (1–2%) [1,4].

Larger and prospective studies have now confirmed the significant morbidity and high prevalence of extracutaneous manifestations reported in 20–57% of cases in most studies, but up to 75% of children requiring systemic therapy [1,4,5,6,25,44,53]. Children with extracutaneous manifestations have a higher burden of disease, with more extensive cutaneous involvement, a higher number of symptoms, more frequent family history of autoimmunity, ANA and rheumatoid factor positivity, and are less responsive to current standard therapy [4,5,53]. Extracutaneous manifestations are associated with greater functional impairment and lower quality of life scores [53,367]. In a US review of 245 adults and children, patients with generalised morphoea ($n = 35$) had the highest frequencies of arthralgia (24%), dysphagia (14%), dyspnoea (20%) and vascular complaints (mainly Raynaud phenomenon, 8%). In contrast, the linear subtype ($n = 86$) was associated with neurological (31%) and

ophthalmological (8%) complications related to the affected site on the face or scalp [6].

In the largest study in childhood, 22.4% of 750 children had one or more extracutaneous manifestation including arthritis and neurological, ocular, vascular and gastrointestinal complications [4,11]. In this study, symptoms of arthritis were the most common, encountered in 11%, particularly in children with linear disease and rheumatoid factor positivity. Arthritis was unrelated to the site of the morphoea in a quarter of cases, suggesting that a systemic, rather than a local, inflammatory process is involved. Six per cent of children had an oligoarthritis (up to four joints) and 5% a polyarthritis (more than four joints); 30% of the children with arthritis had a positive rheumatoid factor.

Overall, musculoskeletal extracutaneous manifestations are the most common with joint contractures or reduced range of movement in 31% of children and 15% of adults with linear disease [1]. Interestingly, Kunzler et al. have found similar limitations in range of movement and joint contractures in patients with linear and generalised morphoea in 581 patients from the morphoea in adults and children (MAC) cohort, suggesting that adults with generalised morphoea also experience significant functional impairment [12]. In a prospective paediatric study, including a greater range of musculoskeletal involvement such as arthralgia, joint limitation or contracture, muscle spasm, myalgia, myositis, muscle atrophy and bone growth differences, half of the subjects had musculoskeletal involvement and 25% had bony undergrowth/hemiatrophy [5]. This higher prevalence is in line with other prospective paediatric studies [53,368,369] and highlights the impact of morphoea in causing growth impairment, facial hemiatrophy, limb length discrepancies and asymmetry of muscle bulk. Indeed, a study comprising 51 children with linear limb disease identified 51% with orthopaedic complications including joint contractures in 88%, limb atrophy (31%), angular deformity/malalignment (18%) and limb length discrepancies (16%). Fourteen per cent required orthopaedic surgery [369].

Adults and children with head and neck disease have a higher risk of developing neurological, oral, dental and ocular manifestations and this is highest in children with combined ECDS/PHA lesions [5,114] and reviewed in [23]. In a retrospective German study of 96 patients with linear head morphoea, 28% of the cohort had neurological symptoms and/or radiological CNS abnormalities [114]. In a retrospective US study of 73 paediatric patients, neuroimaging was abnormal in 25, mainly identifying ipsilateral white matter lesions. Twelve of 25 had headaches and/or seizures. A majority had stable neuroimaging findings at 1 year [370]. A cross-sectional prospective study of 753 adults and children with morphoea identified neurological symptoms in 55 (7%), a majority (89%) with linear craniofacial disease, independently of morphoea depth and activity [371]. Headache, migraine and epilepsy are the commonest manifestations occurring in 1–5% of subjects overall [1,4,5,114,339,371,372]. Cranial nerve palsies, movement disorders including masticatory spasms, trigeminal and peripheral neuropathy, neuropsychiatric problems, vascular malformations and CNS vasculitis are also documented, but with much lower frequencies [339,371]. Combining data from 10 adult and paediatric cohorts Vasquez-Canizares and Li identified abnormal CNS imaging findings in 42% of paediatric onset and 29% of adult-onset craniofacial linear morphoea [1]. A variety of abnormalities are described, including bone thinning, cerebral atrophy, gliosis, white matter lesions, focal subcortical calcifications and meningocortical changes [372]. Scalp and calvarial abnormalities such as atrophy, T_2-hyperintensities, calcifications and ipsilateral cerebral atrophy are the most commonly reported [187,339,372]. The long-term clinical significance, relationship to activity of skin disease and potential for progression of CNS lesions need further investigation, although current evidence suggests that neurological manifestations are largely unrelated to the activity and severity of cutaneous disease in linear head and neck morphoea [371]. Importantly, while some symptomatic patients have normal imaging, substantial numbers of asymptomatic patients have significant CNS abnormalities on imaging, highlighting the need for screening in patients with disease involving the head and neck [**114**,187,336,339]. Our appreciation of the prevalence and impact of these abnormalities will likely improve with increased prospective screening in patients with head and neck disease.

Oral and dental problems can also occur. In one study of 16 patients these included malocclusion (94%), an overgrowth tendency of the anterior lower third of the face (82%), abnormal mastication (69%), dental anomalies (63%), skeletal asymmetry (56%), bone involvement (50%) and temporomandibular joint involvement (19%) [373]. Abnormalities of the teeth, oral mucosa, salivary glands, tongue, gingivae, jaw and temporomandibular joint may occur and are reviewed by al-Aizari et al. [374].

Ocular complications were seen in 2.1% of 750 children – most frequently episcleritis, anterior uveitis and keratitis, but also glaucoma, xerophthalmia, strabismus, mydriasis and papilloedema [4,375]. In 25% of cases these were unrelated to the site of the skin lesions. Enophthalmos caused by a combination of progressive fat atrophy, shrinkage of the eyeball and thinning of the extraocular muscles [376], xerophthalmiachoroidal and retinal folding, hyperopia, retinal vasculitis, glaucoma and third nerve palsies are also documented and may threaten vision [188,377]. Increased awareness of the risk of silent 'white uveitis' where inflammation occurs without overt symptoms of eye pain or redness, and which occurs in 3.2–8.3% of paediatric morphoea cases has prompted the recommendation that children and adults should have ophthalmology assessment 6 monthly in craniofacial morphoea for the first 4 years [42,336].

There is much less data available with respect to vascular and internal organ manifestations, but these appear to be rare and are not associated with progression to other connective tissue disease such as SSc. Of 750 children, 2.4% had vascular abnormalities. There was one case of cutaneous vasculitis and one of deep-vein thrombosis. The other 2.1% (16 patients) had Raynaud phenomenon which, in a minority, preceded the onset of morphoea. Ten of these patients had a positive ANA but none had any SSc-specific autoantibodies. Nine of the children with Raynaud phenomenon had more than one extracutaneous manifestation, including arthritis, gastro-oesophageal reflux and cardiac arrhythmia. Respiratory (0.7%), cardiac (0.3%) and renal (0.3%) complications were rarer. Four per cent of children had more than one extracutaneous manifestation and again this occurred predominantly in patients with linear disease.

Symptomatic oesophageal involvement, including dysphagia, heartburn and gastro-oesophageal reflux, confirmed on appropriate investigations, was identified in 1.6% of 750 children [4], but also in 8/14 (57%) and 23/56 (41%) of juvenile morphoea cases on smaller studies, up to a third of which were asymptomatic [378,379]. The presence of oesophageal involvement was associated with other extracutaneous involvement

Together these findings suggest a more widespread inflammatory and/or autoimmune process in morphoea, as well as a need for more systematic multiorgan baseline assessments.

Psychological manifestations

Several studies suggest that morphoea has only a mild to moderate impact on quality of life in children and that they have good emotional coping strategies [380–382]. Existing dermatology quality of life measures (CDLQI, DLQI) may not capture important aspects of disease impact in morphoea [383,384]. In a single centre longitudinal study of paediatric cases, the number of extracutaneous manifestations (e.g. joint contracture and hemifacial atrophy) and female sex were more predictive of QoL impact than cutaneous features [367]. A focus group based qualitative approach has recently been used in 11 9–16-year-olds and 16 caregivers and has confirmed that lichen sclerosus affects health-related quality of life across multiple distinct domains, including uncomfortable skin sensations, impacts on body image, bullying and teasing from peers, unwanted intrusive questioning, physical limitations, extracutaneous manifestations and high treatment burden [385].

In adults, increased risk of anxiety and depression was reported in 38% of 74 adult patients, with highest psychological morbidity in those with more severe disease, greater levels of pain and fatigue and a greater impact of disease on daily life and social support [386]. In 277 adults and children, reductions in quality of life correlated with functional impairment and symptoms of active disease such as pain and pruritus, independently of disease subtype, age and sex [349]. Evaluation of QoL in morphoea remains challenging and would benefit from the further development of morphoea-specific assessment tools.

A recent publication employed a novel unbiased statistical approach to explore drivers in QoL in 719 morphoea patients. This identified subsets of patients with morphoea based on shared clinical and QoL themes. One group of patients with linear and generalised disease appeared to have substantial morbidity associated with musculoskeletal involvement and functional limitation, and another group had morbidity driven by somatic complaints (fatigue headaches arthralgia) and depression. Older patients were affected by social isolation and younger ones experienced anger and shame emphasising the difference in impact of morphoea in different age groups [387].

Disease course and prognosis

Early studies indicated that the duration of disease activity, although variable, was usually 3–5 years [54], with plaques generally resolving earlier than other subtypes. In Peterson et al.'s series [46], overall, 50% of the patients had at least 50% softening or resolution by 3.8 years after diagnosis. Fifty per cent resolution occurred on average at 2.7 years in the plaque group, at 5 years in the generalised and linear groups and at 5.5 years in the deep group.

Data on natural history and long-term outcome are difficult to compare due to the heterogeneity of morphoea subtypes, treatments and evaluation methods. There is increasing evidence from retrospective and cross-sectional studies to suggest that in certain types of morphoea permanent remission is not the rule. In a study of 113 adults and 126 children referred over a 20-year period to 2001, mean disease duration of childhood-onset morphoea was twice as long as that for adult-onset disease (13.5 versus 5.8 years). Children with mixed forms of disease were more likely to run a more protracted and complicated course, and relapse was more frequent in generalised, deep and mixed forms [28]. In 52 paediatric patients with linear morphoea seen between 1990 and 2010, although disease stabilised after a mean duration of 5.4 years, 38% had functional limitations. Reactivation of disease was frequent, even after seemingly effective courses of methotrexate and corticosteroids, such that 31% of patients reported active disease after 10 years [33]. A chart review of 344 patients, 119 with childhood-onset disease, identified disease recurrence in 27% of the paediatric-onset group and 17% of the adult-onset group. Relapse was seen in all morphoea subtypes, but the risk was highest in the linear limb variant (36%), irrespective of age at the onset of disease [32]. The median time between disease remission and first relapse was 26 months in paediatric-onset and 27 months in adult-onset disease [32]. Further, in a study of 133 adult patients with linear morphoea, those with childhood-onset disease exhibited more severe cumulative damage, greater functional impairment and had 2.6 times greater odds of active disease [341]. The long-term impact of paediatric-onset morphoea was further highlighted in a group of 27 adult patients (mean age 30.6 years, range 18–78 years, median 26 years) with a mean age at onset of 11.5 years (range 3–17 years, median 13 years) [34]. Seventy-four per cent had linear morphoea and 18.5% had plaque morphoea at disease onset that progressed to meet the criteria for generalised disease over time. Overall, 81% had persistent symptoms of pain, itch or numbness; 89% of patients had persistent disease activity, continuous in 8/27, and with a remitting–relapsing course in 16/27. Seven of 27 (29%) patients described flares of activity triggered by trauma, pregnancy or reduction or discontinuation of systemic therapy. Fifteen of 20 patients with linear disease had permanent sequelae including reduced range of motion and deep atrophy. In 22% there was a 'moderate to very large' impact on quality of life [34]. In a larger study of 133 childhood-onset patients followed between January 1991 and December 2016, disease was still active at >10 years in 12.5%, all with linear morphoea. Twenty-two per cent experienced at least one disease relapse, with first flare most frequently observed 20 months after first treatment discontinuation. Moderate or severe tissue damage was identified in 48.4% and 19.8% presented a functional limitation [388]. Delays in initiation of systemic treatment, even by fewer than 3 months, have been associated with longer disease activity, lower response rates to methotrexate, and higher relapse rates in adults and children [388,389]. Increased risk of relapse, up to 45% at 2 years, in a paediatric cohort has been linked to older age at morphoea onset and ANA positivity. Sixty-eight per cent of relapses occurred between 5 and 37 months after treatment completion. Patients with extracutaneous manifestations were less likely to relapse, possibly due to earlier institution and longer duration of systemic therapy [30]. Further study is needed to better predict those at risk of relapse.

These studies highlight the need for careful counselling of patients and their families on the potentially chronic and often relapsing nature of morphoea and the need for continued vigilance.

There is still uncertainty regarding the relationship between morphoea and SSc. Concomitant morphoea, including plaque, generalised and nodular forms, have been reported in 12/370 (3.2%) [390] and 9/135 (6.7%) [391] of patients with SSc. Increased epidermal IL-1α, dermal mast cell infiltration and degranulation were documented in a small study of nine such cases [392]. Transition from morphoea to SSc is very rare but has been reported in 0.13–1.3% of morphoea cases [54,363,393]. SSc-specific antibodies have been identified in up to 16% of morphoea patients. However, none of these cases have been reported to progress to SSc after 3 or more years of follow-up [4,6,11] and reviewed in [**29**]. Although such patients should be kept under close review, in the absence of VEDOSS criteria (Chapter 54) including SSc-specific nail fold capillary abnormalities, puffy fingers or sclerodactyly, a transition to SSc is extremely unlikely.

Investigations

The diagnosis of morphoea is largely clinical, but an assessment of disease burden and activity are crucial in determining need for therapy (Table 55.5). Accordingly, a number of investigations can be helpful in guiding assessment and management and may be used in conjunction with clinical scores (such as LoSCAT), quality of life measures and patient reported outcome measures (PROMs).

Blood tests. There are no diagnostic blood tests for morphoea. Routine blood investigations are usually normal in circumscribed superficial plaque morphoea. In patients with generalised, pansclerotic, deep or linear disease, consideration should be given to measuring baseline eosinophils, serum immunoglobulins, ESR/CRP, CK, lactase dehydrogenase and/or aldolase, *Borrelia* serology, ANA, rheumatoid factor and thyroid function test at baseline (Table 55.5). An eosinophilia ($>0.5 \times 10^9$/L) is typical in eosinophilic fasciitis, but is also documented in deep and more severe forms of all subtypes of morphoea including generalised, pansclerotic [11,27] and linear, where absolute counts are higher in multisite than single site disease [341]. Raised immunoglobulins and ESR may be a pointer to active, systemic inflammation. Increased levels of creatine kinase and aldolase have been associated with the development of new lesions, muscle atrophy and limb shortening, and may thus suggest deep disease with muscle involvement and possibly disease activity [53]. *Borrelia* serology need only be checked if there is a relevant clinical history or an atypical disease presentation. ANA positivity at baseline has been associated with more severe disease in adults and children, and with increased risk of relapse post-treatment in childhood onset disease [**29**,30] suggesting that this group may require more aggressive systemic therapy and closer long-term follow-up. Rheumatoid factor positivity points to an increased risk of inflammatory arthritis [4]. Other frequently associated autoimmune diseases such as autoimmune thyroid disease should be excluded. If there is concern about the possibility of SSc (e.g. in cases of new or rapidly progressing pansclerotic morphoea or eosinophilic fasciitis) evidence of Raynaud

Table 55.5 Assessment of the patient with morphoea.

Clinical assessment	Investigations
Are lesions symptomatic? Ask about itch, numbness and tingling, burning Are there new or extending lesions?	Measure LoSCAT score (includes mLoSSI, LoSDI, PGA-A, PGA-D DLQI/CDLQI, HAQ/CHAQ, HADS, patient VAS, LoSQI (see outcome measures, later)
Are there extracutaneous manifestations?: musculoskeletal: arthralgia, arthritis, joint contracture, myalgia, myositis, muscle atrophy Headache, migraine, seizures, ocular or oral/orthodontic symptoms, dyspepsia, Raynaud phenomenon, etc.	Photography (3D if available) ± thermography ± ultrasonography ± scanning laser Doppler
Ask about ocular, oral and TMJ symptoms in linear disease of the head	Skin biopsy (if diagnosis or depth in doubt): deep incisional ellipse (through the edge of the lesion, to include fascia and muscle if deep involvement suspected)
Full skin examination to determine extent and activity of lesions	MRI (images brain and depth of extent on limbs), CT (images bony contours) for linear lesions Electroencephalogram (head variant) if symptoms suggestive
Assess for activity: erythema, violaceous colour, tactile warmth, abnormal skin texture Examine for genital lichen sclerosus in isomorphic generalised morphoea	CK, LDH, aldolase (if muscle/deep involvement suspected) Full blood count, eosinophils, immunoglobulins, TFT, ESR, CRP ANA, ENA, rheumatoid factor at baseline/first visit *Borrelia* serology if relevant history Referral to allied specialties as appropriate: ENT, ophthalmology, oral medicine, orthopaedics, plastic surgery, physiotherapy

ANA, antinuclear antibody; CDLQI, Children's Dermatology Life Quality Index; CHAQ, Children's Health Assessment Questionnaire; CK, creatinine kinase; CRP, C-reactive protein; CT, computed tomography; DLQI, Dermatology Life Quality Index; ENA, extractable nuclear antigen; ENT, ear, nose, throat; ESR, erythrocyte sedimentation rate; HADS, Hospital Anxiety and Depression Score; HAQ, Health Assessment Questionnaire; LDH, lactase dehydrogenase; LoSCAT, Localised Scleroderma Cutaneous Assessment Tool; LoSDI, Localised Scleroderma Skin Damage Index; LoSQI, Localised Scleroderma Quality of Life Instrument; mLoSSI, Modified Localised Scleroderma Skin Activity Index; MRI, magnetic resonance imaging; PGA-A, Physician Global Assessment of Activity; PGA-D, Physician Global Assessment of Damage; TMJ, temporo-mandibular joint; TFT, thyroid function test; patient VAS, Visual Analogue Scale.

phenomenon, puffy fingers, sclerodactyly, nail fold capillaroscopic abnormalities and SSc-specific autoantibodies (e.g. anticentromere, anti-topoisomerase and anti-RNA polymerase) should be sought (Chapter 54). CXCL9 and CCL18 have recently been identified as markers of disease activity and may have potential use as biomarkers [145,152,156]. Routine laboratory measurement is not widely available as yet.

Skin biopsy. A biopsy is not usually required, but can be undertaken if the diagnosis or the depth of involvement are in doubt. If a biopsy is performed, an incisional ellipse through the violaceous/inflammatory edge of a lesion, into the sclerotic centre and extending down into the subcutis is preferred, although a punch biopsy may be acceptable. The site should be clearly indicated for the pathologist (e.g. inflammatory edge, sclerotic centre, etc.). If fasciitis is suspected the biopsy should extend into the fascia and underlying muscle and referral to a plastics or general surgeon may be required.

Photography. Regular photographic imaging (e.g. every 6 months) and where available 3D photography are useful adjuncts in monitoring for disease stability or progression.

MRI. MRI (with or without contrast) is a useful tool for assessing the depth and extent of involvement, particularly to assess for fasciitis, tendon and muscle involvement in pansclerotic morphoea/eosinophilic fasciitis and linear limb lesions [394,395] (Figure 55.12c). It identifies clinically occult disease, and is responsive to and a useful measure of change during therapy in linear limb disease [396,397].

In line with recently published minimum standards of care for paediatric morphoea, a contrast-enhanced craniofacial and brain MRI (which may need to include the jaw and neck – depending on the site of the lesion) at baseline is recommended in patients with linear head/neck disease to screen for CNS abnormalities (frequently asymptomatic and unsuspected), and also to assess for disease extent, depth and presence of inflammation [41,398]. This can be used to generate 3D reconstructions which may also aid in assessing for progression of soft tissue loss (Figures 55.15c and 55.17). It is as yet unclear how frequently neuroimaging should be carried out. Up to 20% of CNS lesions may progress and this may occur independently of skin changes [339]. Currently a frequency of every 1–2 years for MRI is suggested [336] and/or if new symptoms develop [42].

CT scan. In some cases, a CT scan can be more helpful than MRI if the extent of bony involvement is in question. Three-D-multidetector CT reconstruction can also be helpful in assessing progression and planning corrective surgery in inactive disease [336].

Other imaging modalities. Multiple imaging modalities are used to evaluate and monitor the skin in morphoea. These have recently been reviewed by Lis-Swiety et al. [399] and compared by Pain et al. [400]. Serial ultrasonography can be used to evaluate skin thickness and loss of muscle and fat [401,402]. Disease activity can be correlated with echogenicity and tissue blood flow measured by colour Doppler [403] and laser Doppler [404,405], ultrasound techniques [406] and infrared thermography [115,400,407], although the latter gives false positive results in patients with atrophy. Ultrasonography is only useful in the hands of a musculoskeletal imaging expert with experience in morphoea. A durometer is a hand-held instrument that measures the depth of skin indentation after the application of a standardised amount of force. Durometry measures skin hardness, a recognised surrogate for skin thickness [408], and has been shown to objectively discriminate affected versus unaffected skin on the trunk and limbs in children with morphoea [409]. Goniometry can be used to assess range of motion across joints.

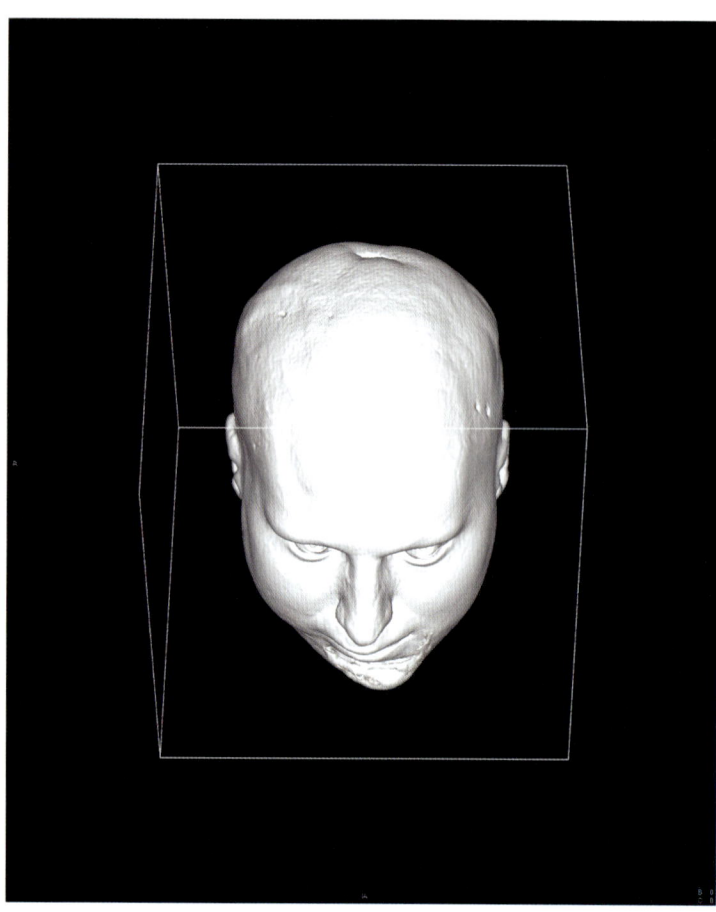

Figure 55.17 Three-D surface rendered image post processed from volumetric isotropic axial T1 MRI imaging of the head showing facial asymmetry involving the right lower hemiface in a patient with progressive hemifacial atrophy. Courtesy of Dr Farrah Jabeen, Royal Free London NHS Foundation Trust.

Referrals to allied specialties such as ophthalmology, ENT and maxillofacial should be considered for patients with head involvement and to orthopaedics and physiotherapy for linear limb disease, particularly in children. Patients with craniofacial morphoea should also have a dental assessment including panoramic radiographs and an assessment of the temporomandibular joint by a rheumatologist at baseline. In children, 6-monthly rheumatology and ophthalmology review is suggested [41]. There are currently insufficient data to make such a recommendation in adults but baseline assessment may be prudent.

Outcome measures

Defining outcome measures in morphoea has proved difficult because morbidity is caused by a combination of cutaneous and subcutaneous damage as well as disease activity. Trying to find accurate measures of disease activity has been a particular challenge. Recent evidence points to ANA positivity and IFN-related pathway chemokines including CCL18 and CXCL9 as promising biomarkers which could in future give simple objective measures of disease activity and response to treatment. In the meantime, a variety of imaging techniques are employed, including serial photography, infrared thermography, Doppler flowmetry, ultrasonography and MRI [399,10], and more recently a computerised

skin scoring method [411]. Of these methods only the computerised skin score, ultrasonography and MRI have been validated. Variable frequency ultrasound (7–15 MHz linear probes) with colour Doppler is a non-invasive technique that reveals details of skin morphology and function. It has shown high specificity and sensitivity for assessing disease activity [403]. The most accurate sonographic signs of activity are increased subcutaneous echogenicity and increased cutaneous blood flow. Laser Doppler imaging measures blood flow within the dermis and is a more accurate reflection of skin inflammation than infrared thermography, which is difficult to interpret when there is soft tissue atrophy. Single-point laser Doppler flowmetry measurements correlate with clinical disease activity [343,404,412]. Scanning laser Doppler imaging had a positive predictive value of 87% and negative predictive value of 94% in a small study evaluating its use in assessing activity and predicting progression [405].

Clinical scoring techniques have the advantage of not requiring expensive or cumbersome equipment. The mRSS, a measure of skin thickness which has been validated in SSc [413], has also been used in morphoea, but is not validated in this condition and does not assess damage. The DIET score (dyspigmentation, induration, erythema, telangiectasia; each scored 0–3, with a maximum score of 12) [414] has the advantage of simplicity, but may not provide an accurate assessment of damage. Four measures of disease activity and damage have recently been combined to develop a morphoea-specific skin scoring system – LoSCAT (Figure 55.18). Initially, two measures of disease activity, the physician global assessment of activity (PGA-A) and the modified localised scleroderma skin index (mLoSSI) were developed and validated in 2009 [37,415]. The PGA-A is graded on a 100 mm analogue scale and includes the following cutaneous variables: the development of new lesions and/or enlargement of existing lesion within the previous month, erythema/violaceous colour and skin thickening/induration at the border of lesions. The mLoSSI includes the sum of three separate scores from the following domains: erythema (none, mild, moderate, severe), skin thickness (none, mild, moderate, severe) and new lesion/lesion extension (present, not present). A patient is classified as having active disease if they have a PGA-A of greater than 0 and a mLoSSI of greater than 0.

Subsequently, two measures of disease damage, the localised scleroderma skin damage index (LoSDI) and the physician global assessment of disease damage (PGA-D), were developed. Disease damage was defined as irreversible or persistent changes of the lesion due to previous active disease or complications of therapy. The LoSDI was calculated by summing three scores for cutaneous features of damage: dermal atrophy, subcutaneous atrophy and dyspigmentation measured at 18 anatomical sites, recording the most severe score from each domain if multiple lesions were present within one anatomical site [39]. The PGA-D is graded on a 100 mm analogue scale and is anchored by 'no damage' at 0 and 'markedly damaged' at 100. Based upon consensus agreement, both cutaneous and extracutaneous manifestations are taken into account when scoring the PGA-D. The cutaneous manifestations include hyper/hypopigmentation and subcutaneous and dermal atrophy. The extracutaneous manifestations include: musculoskeletal involvement (skeletal muscle atrophy, bone atrophy, facial atrophy, limb length discrepancy, physical disability, joint contracture), neurological involvement (CNS symptoms, abnormal brain MRI, eye involvement) and psychosocial quality of life impairment [39].

The LoSCAT was later modified, replacing the mLoSSI with the LoSAI (Localised Scleroderma Activity Index) in which 'skin thickness' is replaced with 'induration (skin swelling at the edge)' and the LoSDI was changed to include 'skin thickness at the

centre' as a further variable. Both versions of LoSCAT are now validated tools to measure both disease activity and damage in morphoea [38,39,**40**,416,417] and both mLoSSI and LoSAI are in current use. The LoSCAT is now being used routinely in clinical practice and as an outcome measure in clinical trials. It can be used to classify patients with morphoea by disease severity and identify

Localised scleroderma cutaneous assessment tool						
	mLoSSI Localised scleroderma skin **activity** index			LoSDI Localised scleroderma skin **damage** index		
Site	New/enlarge (within 1 month) 0 = none 3 = N/E	Erythema 0 = none 1 = pink 2 = red 3 = dark/red violaceous	Skin thickness 0 = none 1 = mild 2 = moderate 3 = marked	Dermal atrophy 0 = none 1 = shiny 2 = visible vessel 3 = obvious 'clifftop'	Subcutaneous atrophy 0 = none 1 = flat 2 = concave 3 = marked atrophy	Dyspigmentation (hypo/ hyperpigmentation) 0 = none 1 = mild 2 = moderate 3 = marked
Scalp/face						
Neck						
Chest						
Abdomen						
Upper back						
Lower back						
RT arm						
forearm						
hand						
thigh						
leg						
foot						
LT arm						
forearm						
hand						
thigh						
leg						
foot						

Total score   mLoSSI (**activity**) _____   LoSDI (**damage**) _____

PLEASE MARK WITH A STRAIGHT LINE:

Physician global assessment of disease **activity**

0 ——————————————————————————————— 100
Inactive   Markedly **active**

Physician global assessment of disease **damage**

0 ——————————————————————————————— 100
No **damage**   Markedly **damaged**
Comment:

Figure 55.18 (a) Localised scleroderma cutaneous assessment tool (LoSCAT) including mLoSSI and LoSDI. From Arkachaisri et al. 2010 [39]. Reproduced with permission of Oxford University Press. (b) Revised modified LoSCAT including LoSAI and modified LoSDI adapted from Teske and Jacobe [38].

PART 4: INFLAMMATORY DERMATOSES

PART 4: INFLAMMATORY DERMATOSES

LoSCAT Localized Scleroderma Cutaneous Assessment Tool	LoSAI (Localized Scleroderma Skin **Activity** Index)			LoSDI (Localized Scleroderma Skin **Damage** Index)			
	New/Enlarged (past month) 0 = none 3 = N / E	Erythema 0 = none 1 = pink 2 = red 3 = dark red /violaceous	Induration (skin swelling at EDGE) 0 = none 1 = mild 2 = moderate 3 = marked	Dermal atrophy 0 = none 1 = shiny 2 = visible vessels 3 = cliff drop	Sub Q / Deep atrophy 0 = none 1 = flat 2 = concave 3 = marked	Dyspigmentation (hyper or hypo) 0 = none 1 = mild 2 = moderate 3 = marked	Skin Thickness (at CENTER) 0 = none 1 = mild 2 = moderate 3 = marked
Scalp/Face							
Neck							
Chest							
Abdomen							
Upper Back							
Lower Back							
R T Arm							
Forearm							
Hand							
Thigh							
Leg							
Foot							
L T Arm							
Forearm							
Hand							
Thigh							
Leg							
Foot							

LoSAI _____   LoSDI _____

PGA-A (Physician Global Assessment of Disease <u>Activity</u>)

_____

(0=inactive)   (100=markedly active)

PGA-D (Physician Global Assessment of Disease <u>Damage</u>)

_____

(0=no damage)   (100=markedly damaged)

Figure 55.18 (*Continued*)

clinically significant improvement in activity [38,418]. Erythema, violaceous colour, tactile warmth, waxy white/yellow change and skin thickening have also been identified as features tracking with disease activity [35]. Based upon these variables the CARRA have developed a further skin activity measure – the Localised Scleroderma Cutaneous Activity Measure (LSCAM) which has also been found to be valid and reliable [419]. LSCAM differs from mLoSSI in including more skin variables and weighing them equally. LSCAM was found to correlate better with PGA-Activity than the mLoSSI in a 1-year prospective study [419]. These measures do not take into account the impact of extracutaneous manifestations and to remedy this the CARRA group also recently developed the Total Morbidity Score (TMS). It includes modules for cutaneous features (i.e. dyspigmentation, subcutaneous atrophy) and extent, musculoskeletal (i.e., arthritis, myositis), growth difference of body (i.e. limb girth or length difference), head/neuro (i.e. facial hemiatrophy, brain involvement), and other organ (i.e. vasculopathy) involvement to give a global assessment of cutaneous damage and morbidity from extracutaneous features, and is thought to provide a more accurate assessment of disease burden [36,360]. More study is needed to further assess the performance of the LSCAM and TMS scores.

Efforts to develop patient reported outcome measures are ongoing for morphoea and some progress has been made within paediatric rheumatology. The CDLQI and CHAQ have been shown in some studies to positively correlate with mLoSSI and the CDLQI with LoSDI [400]. However, although widely used, the CDLQI has suggested only modest effects of morphoea on quality of life (QoL) in children. Further study has shown that although it captures the functional and psychosocial domains of quality of life in morphoea, it includes some items of limited relevance and incompletely explores skin symptoms and treatment burdens [383]. Further exploration employing focus groups has identified areas of impact which include uncomfortable skin symptoms, physical functioning limitations, extracutaneous manifestations, body image, bullying and teasing, unwanted questioning from others, and treatment side effects and burden [385]. This has led to the development of the Localised Scleroderma Quality of Life Instrument (LoSQI) [362], which is currently undergoing validation. A number of patient-reported visual analogue scales have been developed (see examples in Box 55.1) and are under evaluation. Further study is needed to adapt these or develop similar PROMs and morphoea-specific health-related quality of life measures for use in adult morphoea patients.

Box 55.1 Selection of suggested patient reported outcomes included in VAS in paediatric morphoea [362] and adapted from the LoSQI [362], the CHAQ and CARRA jLS pilot consensus treatment plan study [420] with personal communication with Dr Suzanne C Li, Division of Paediatric Rheumatology, Joseph M Sanzari Children's Hospital, Hackensack Meridian School of Medicine, Hackensack, NJ, USA and Dr Clare Pain, Consultant Paediatric Rheumatologist, Honorary Clinical Associate Professor, University of Liverpool, UK

Patient Reported Outcome Measures (PROM) and suggested Visual Analogue Scale (VAS) questions:

- Since my last visit to the doctor, my morphoea is: better/the same/worse
- Considering all the ways that morphoea affects you, rate how you are doing (over the last week) by placing a single mark on the line below (0 very well, 10 very poor)
- How much impact has your disease had on your life in the past month? (0 none, 10 worst possible)
- How much has your morphoea affected you overall in the past month? (0 none, 10 worst possible)
- How itchy and/or scratchy have your lesions felt in the past month? (0 none, 10 worst ever)
- How numb, tingly and/or 'funny' has your skin felt in or around your lesions in the past month? (0 none, 10 worst ever)
- How much pain do you think you had because of your morphoea in the past week? (0 none, 10 worst ever)
- How much worry do you have about long-term problems from your condition? (0 none,10 worst ever)
- How much worry do you have about problems from medications used to treat your condition? (0 none, 10 worst ever)

Management

Morphoea can lead to permanent cosmetic and functional impairment. Early intervention can limit disease progression and its consequences. However, treatment of patients with significant damage but inactive disease exposes them to the potential side effects of the medications, without providing significant benefit. Patient selection and appropriate timing of interventions is paramount. The management of morphoea has been challenging because of a lack of standardised evaluation methods, randomised controlled trials and prospective national/international registries resulting in a dearth of evidence-based treatments. Much of the literature on morphoea treatment is retrospective, uncontrolled and composed of small case series. A Cochrane review examined publications to July 2018 and included only 14 trials, with a total of 429 randomised participants, aged between 3 and 76 years. The studies were heterogeneous such that no meta-analyses were possible. The reviewers concluded that available results were based on low-quality evidence with studies at high risk of performance, detection, attrition and reporting bias [421].

Currently available treatments remain largely untargeted, and none are licensed for use in morphoea. In 2012, Johnson and Jacobe [51] found that the treatment prescribed in morphoea depended more on the specialty of the treating physician than the patient or their type of disease. Thus, from a total of 531 prescriptions for 224 patients (95 children), dermatologists prescribed topical corticosteroids in 41%, other topical treatment in 25%, phototherapy in 16% of cases, systemic corticosteroids in 5% and methotrexate in 4% of cases. Rheumatologists, in contrast, prescribed methotrexate in 34%, systemic corticosteroids in 31% of cases, topical treatments in 10% and phototherapy in only 2% [51]. In this study, 68% of patients with linear morphoea received topical corticosteroids as the mainstay of treatment if they saw a dermatologist (4% received methotrexate), whereas 39% of linear morphoea patients seen by rheumatologists received methotrexate and 8% topical corticosteroids [51]. In a survey of UK dermatologists published in 2014 [422], clinicians were asked which treatment option produced the best outcome in active morphoea based on their experience. There was a wide range of responses: methotrexate with corticosteroids was the most frequent response (37.3%), followed by methotrexate alone (25.4%), phototherapy (18%) and topical steroids (13%). These surveys underscored the need for a joined up multidisciplinary approach to establish effective treatment guidelines and to ensure that patients are not undertreated. As a consequence, in 2017, the European Dermatology Forum developed guidelines for diagnosis and management of sclerosing diseases of the skin applicable to all age groups [10]. In 2018 Constantin *et al.* proposed minimum standards of care for children with morphoea [41] and in 2019 the Paediatric Rheumatology European Society (PRES) developed consensus-based recommendations for the management of morphoea in children [42]. Subsequently, a multicentre audit comparing UK practice with PRES recommendations in 149 paediatric patients identified significant room for improvement since outcome measures such as LoSCAT, MRI of the brain in craniofacial disease and screening for uveitis were still not widely utilised. In contrast, 95% were appropriately treated with methotrexate first line (and mycophenolate second line), 83% received corticosteroids and 34% required two or more disease modifying antirheumatic drugs (DMARDs)/biologics [368]. Current guidelines are largely based on expert opinion and consensus best pactice. It is recommended that the initial evaluation of a patient with morphoea should include an assessment of the type, extent and activity of disease and whether there is extracutaneous involvement (Table 55.5). Treatment can then be based on the subtype, activity, extent and depth of disease, potential for permanent damage/functional impairment, patient symptoms and impact of the morphoea on quality of life [3,10,**423**].

Topical therapies

Circumscribed superficial forms of morphoea can generally be treated topically. The small size and frequently uncontrolled nature of published studies for topical morphoea treatments means that they are at high risk of bias and should be interpreted with caution. Topical steroids remain the most commonly used topical treatment, although there is no direct evidence to support their use. Topical and intralesional corticosteroids are frequently used with good effects, particularly in the early inflammatory stages of disease or if there are pronounced epidermal changes [422]. The EDF guideline recommends that superpotent topical steroids (clobetasol propionate) be used for up to 4 weeks and potent topical steroids (mometasone furoate) for up to 3 months, with intermittent therapy beyond that if needed [10]. Case reports and a prospective open-label study in 13 patients initially suggested a role for topical tacrolimus 0.1% [424–426]. Two small placebo-controlled trials support the use of twice-daily topical tacrolimus 0.1% ointment (10 patients) [427], and daily 5% imiquimod cream (22 patients) [428]. The latter was also found to be safe and beneficial when used 3–7 times weekly, over a 9-month period, in 21 adult and paediatric patients in two small prospective open-label studies [414,429]. Benefit in prospective but uncontrolled studies has been shown for twice-daily application of topical vitamin D analogues (calcipotriol/calcipotriene 0.005%), either alone under occlusion (12 patients) [430] or in combination with topical steroids (six patients) [431] or with low-dose UVA-1 phototherapy (19 children) [432]. Tranilast (N-[3,4-dimethoxycinnamoyl]-anthranilic acid) is approved in Japan and South Korea for the management of allergic and fibrotic disorders. It is thought to act via inhibition of fibroblast proliferation and collagen production and modulation of the kynurenine pathway. There is one small case series comparing 0.1% betamethasone valerate with 0.1% betamethasone valerate and 1% tranilast which showed benefit after daily application for 3 months in three patients with morphoea (two of whom were also on methotrexate) [433]. Pirfenidone is a non-peptide synthetic chemical that inhibits the production of TGF-β1, TNF-α, PDGF, IL-1β, and collagen I and III, all of which have been linked to fibrosis. There is one open phase II study in 12 morphoea patients using 8% pirfenidone gel three times daily for 6 months which suggested improvement based on mLoSSI, durometer and histological assessments [434]. Assessment of topical JAK inhibitors in morphoea is awaited.

Phototherapy

If there is no deep involvement, circumscribed and generalised plaque morphoea – particularly the isomorphic subset – can be treated with phototherapy, preferably UVA-1, but when this is not available topical psoralen and UVA (PUVA), broad-band UVA or narrow-band UVB therapy are alternatives (reviewed in [435]). The rationale for using phototherapy in morphoea is based on the ability of UVA and UVB to induce MMPs such as collagenase [436,437]. UVA wavelengths (320–400 nm) penetrate deeper into the dermis than UVB (280–320 nm). UVA-1 (340–400 nm) is less erythemogenic and penetrates deeper than UVA-2 (320–340 nm). In addition to collagenase, UVA-1 has been shown to upregulate antifibrotic haem oxygenase-1 [438], to cause T-cell apoptosis, to deplete dermal Langerhans and mast cells, to induce interferon-γ (INF-γ), IL-1 and IL-6 production, and to inhibit TGF-β production [439,440]. This latter effect may involve the SMAD family of proteins involved in TGF-β signal transduction [441] and a stimulatory effect on the antifibrotic protein decorin [442,443]. In a mouse model of bleomycin-induced fibrosis, a high-dose of UVA-1 therapy reduced dermal thickness, increased MMP-1 and MMP-3 expression, and reduced expression of collagen types I and III [444]. Although a variety of treatment doses and regimens have been employed, there is consensus that low-dose (10–20 J/cm^2), medium-dose (>20–70 J/cm^2) and high-dose (>70–130 J/cm^2) UVA-1 have all shown efficacy, significantly reducing skin thickness and stiffness in adults and children with all forms of morphoea (reviewed in [440,445,446]). Early inflammatory and sclerotic lesions appear to respond most favourably, and cases with deep involvement

least favourably. Outcome measures recorded in over 90% of cases include variable combinations of clinical examination, skin scores, ultrasound measurement of skin thickness, cutometer measurements and skin biopsies. UVA-1 appeared to be effective in all skin types in a retrospective review of treatment responses in 47 morphoea patients [447]. This is in contrast to Wang *et al.*'s findings that suggested that the antifibrotic effects of UVA-1 were determined by skin type, and that skin darkening as a result of UVA-1 treatment may attenuate its antifibrotic effects [448]. The duration of responses is variable and up to half of the patients may develop recurrence of active morphoea lesions at 2–3 years [449].

Sixty-four patients with morphoea were consecutively included in a prospective, open, randomised controlled three-arm study comparing low (20 J/cm^2) and medium (50 J/cm^2) dose UVA-1 with narrow band UVB five times weekly for 8 weeks. Based on skin scores, visual analogue scales for itch and tightness, histology and 20 MHz ultrasound, significant benefit was noted in all patients who completed the treatment protocol [450]. Based on this study, a Cochrane review concluded that there may be little or no difference between medium- (50 J/cm^2), low-dose UVA-1 (20 J/cm^2) and narrow-band UVB treatment modalities in global improvement of disease activity or damage in adults and children [421]. It has, nevertheless, been suggested that medium-dose UVA-1 may be more effective than low-dose UVA-1 based on ultrasound measurements of skin thickness of individual morphoea plaques [451] and may give better long-term results [452,453]. It is preferred to high doses because of the lower cumulative UV exposure. Although UVA-1 has not been associated with increased skin cancer risk thus far, it has been shown to produce cyclobutane pyrimidine dimers in humans, and so has the potential to be carcinogenic [454].

UVA-1 is not widely available and this has led physicians to investigate the efficacy of other forms of phototherapy in addition to narrow-band UVB. Broad-band UVA has been used at varying doses in a total of 114 patients across three controlled trials, with positive responses documented by clinical examination and skin biopsies [439,455,456]. Bath PUVA resulted in reductions in skin thickness and clinical improvement in 15/19 patients and cream PUVA in 4/4 cases [457–460]. Response rates to UVA therapies are good, ranging from 60% to 80% after a full course of treatment [461], but relapse rates of almost 50% at 3 years follow-up are reported [449].

Corticosteroids, methotrexate and mycophenolate

In patients with progressive disease despite topical agents and/or phototherapy, and in patients with active disease and a moderate to high morbidity risk including linear, deep or disseminated forms of disease (e.g. morphoea en coup de sabre, pansclerotic morphoea or eosinophilic fasciitis), systemic therapy is indicated. There is broad agreement that combinations of pulsed intravenous and/or oral steroids with methotrexate should be used first line.

An open study of 17 patients with severe morphoea (linear/generalised) found that oral corticosteroids (0.5–1 mg/kg/day for 6 weeks then reducing over a mean of 18 months) produced a marked improvement, with reduced inflammation, cessation of new lesion formation and skin softening. A third of patients relapsed on discontinuing therapy [462]. Systemic corticosteroids should be considered in patients with severe, active inflammatory disease and in patients with eosinophilic fasciitis who appear particularly steroid responsive [16,17]. Although effective in the short term, the high rate of relapse on treatment discontinuation necessitates the addition of other agents such as methotrexate.

Methotrexate is a cornerstone of morphoea management [115,128,343,463–468]. Methotrexate is thought to exert its effects at multiple levels [469]. It has been shown to enhance monocyte differentiation [470], reduce peripheral blood mononuclear cell production of IL-8 [471] and stimulate IL-1 receptor antagonist and soluble TNF receptor p75 *in vitro* in rheumatoid arthritis [472]. Reductions in circulating sIL-2R and IL-6 following successful therapy with methotrexate in children and adults with rheumatoid arthritis [473,474] suggest a possible mechanism for its effects in morphoea, since reductions in serum IL-2, -4 and -6 have been found to parallel improvement in cutaneous sclerosis [146]. Furthermore, mast cell numbers and levels of tenascin – an extracellular matrix protein previously shown to be increased in the skin and circulation of morphoea patients [475,476] – are both reduced in lesional skin after methotrexate therapy [477].

Two early uncontrolled case series (17 patients, 9 adults) suggested some improvement in skin lesions with methotrexate alone [277,463]. Four retrospective reviews documented the response to methotrexate alone in 52 cases, and in combination with corticosteroids in 67 cases [465,478–480]. Improvement was described in 79% of cases but was more variable in those treated with methotrexate alone. In three prospective studies, a total of 60 patients (15 adults) were treated with either monthly pulsed intravenous (1 g, 3 days per month for 6 months in the adults and 30 mg/kg, 3 days per month, for 3 months in nine children) or daily oral corticosteroids (2 mg/kg/day (maximum dose 60 mg/day), tapered to 0.25 mg/kg/day for 12 months in 36 children) and methotrexate at doses of 0.3–1 mg/kg/week (maximum dose 25 mg) in children and 15 mg/week in adults [464,467,468]. In these studies, significant improvements were noted based on mLoSSI (mLoSSI score of 0 in 32/36 cases at 36 months) and PGA-A [467] or physician assessment [464] in children. A 50% reduction in skin scores, corroborated by biopsy and ultrasound measurements, was documented in 13/15 adults after a mean treatment duration of 9.8 months [468]. This benefit was then confirmed in a randomised placebo-controlled trial in 70 children with active linear, generalised or mixed morphoea, comparing 12 months of oral methotrexate (15 mg/m^2/week (maximum dose 20 mg/week), $n = 46$) with placebo ($n = 24$) [115]. All patients received a concomitant 3 month course of oral prednisolone (1 mg/kg/day (maximum dose 50 mg)). Response was assessed objectively with infrared thermography, a computerised skin scoring system, by physician global assessment of disease severity and the development of new lesions. Methotrexate was well tolerated, and resulted in a reduction in new lesion formation, computerised skin score and lesion temperature at 12 months. As suggested by a previous study [462], corticosteroid monotherapy resulted in a sustained improvement in approximately 30% of patients at 12 months. However, the likelihood of experiencing a disease flare in the methotrexate-treated group was approximately one-third of that in the corticosteroid-alone-treated placebo group. Over two-thirds of patients were judged to have responded, and in over 50% the clinical improvement persisted long after the discontinuation of methotrexate. Fifteen per cent relapsed at 24 months [115,128]. The open-label extension of this study suggested

that 70% of responders maintained clinical remission off treatment for a mean of 25 months, but that treatment courses of at least 24 months were needed to ensure a sustained remission [128]. Others have suggested that 4 years of treatment may be required to reduce the risk of relapse [481]. The efficacy of methotrexate in achieving disease inactivity and remission of treatment has now been documented via retrospective reviews of large patient cohorts including adults and children [341,389,480,482–484], and in line with the findings of a Cochrane review [421] there is broad agreement that combinations of pulsed intravenous and/or oral corticosteroids with methotrexate should be used first line in patient with moderate to severe, active disease. There remains a lack of consensus regarding the optimum dosing, duration and mode of delivery of corticosteroids in morphoea. Dosing regimens vary for methotrexate, being 15–25 mg/week in adults and 15 mg/m^2/week in the UK and EU and 1 mg/kg/week in the USA for children, with a maximum dose of 25 mg/week in all age groups. The subcutaneous route of administration is recommended for its reduced side effects and superior efficacy. The time course of response to methotrexate is suggested by two studies showing a significant reduction of skin activity scores at 3 months, with most of the response occurring by 6 months of treatment. Thus, if there is worsening of disease at 3 months or disease has not stabilised or become inactive at 6 months, further additional treatment may be needed. Of note, a majority of patients in these studies received corticosteroids for the first 3 months also [343,419]. Relatively high relapse rates have been documented after completion of a full course of systemic treatment, with percentages of 12.5% [**32**], 27% [128], 29% [481], 44% [478] and 41% [30] reported after methotrexate and systemic corticosteroids, and 46% after successful UVA-1 phototherapy [449]. Whether some of this may be linked to the use of short treatment courses or to poor compliance due to limited tolerability is unclear, but these figures suggest a need for alternative therapies [30,44,343]. Thus up to 44% of cases may relapse after successful treatment and require a further course [**32**,466,481,484]. Current data suggest that a second course of methotrexate with corticosteroids is effective in a majority [128,466]. A quarter to a third of patients, however, may not respond to methotrexate therapy. Pansclerotic, and mixed morphoea subtypes, patients with extracutaneous manifestations and greater disease burden appear more likely to relapse or be non-responders [5,44,485]. Delays to treatment initiation, shorter duration of treatment and speed of tapering have also been implicated in methotrexate treatment failure (reviewed in [**423**]). Further work is needed to establish which patient groups are less likely to respond to methotrexate.

The choice of second line agent was prompted by studies in SSc, which showed efficacy of mycophenolate in improving or stabilising interstitial lung disease and skin thickening (reviewed in [486]). This benefit in SSc has been confirmed in larger clinical trials [487,488], which also showed a recurrence of skin thickening after discontinuation or dose reduction of mycophenolate [489]. Patients with SSc and an 'inflammatory' gene expression profile in skin, identical to that seen in morphoea skin samples [490] are more responsive to mycophenolate (Chapter 54) providing a rationale for its use in morphoea. Martini *et al.* initially published 10 cases in 2009 that suggested benefit in morphoea, used alone (one case) or in combination with methotrexate in patients who failed on or were unsuitable for monotherapy [491]. Mertens added seven cases with favourable responses in 2016 [492]. Two further retrospective studies (including 22 children and 77 adults) now support its value for treating morphoea patients who are intolerant of or unresponsive to methotrexate [485,493]. Most of these patients had more severe subtypes (e.g. mixed or pansclerotic morphoea) and many added mycophenolate to methotrexate and corticosteroids. Martini *et al.*'s recent retrospective longitudinal study of paediatric morphoea compared long-term follow-up in 22 mycophenolate-treated methotrexate-resistant patients with 47 methotrexate responsive patients. After a mean 9.4 years of follow-up, 90.9% of patients on mycophenolate and 100% of those on methotrexate had inactive disease. No significant difference in relapse-free survival between the groups was found [485]. Arthur *et al.* documented disease stability in 66/73 patients after 3–6 months of treatment and remission in 35% at 9–12 months [493]. Half of children and a quarter of adults were no longer on mycophenolate at the time of last follow-up [485,493]. Moreno-Arquieta *et al.* reviewed the use of mycophenolate in 29 cases of eosinophilic fasciitis, in combination with corticosteroids. Nineteen had a complete response and six a partial response [494]. Current published evidence is retrospective, involving small numbers of patients and of low quality. Further, randomised, controlled studies on the relative efficacy of and optimum patient selection for mycophenolate versus methotrexate treatment are needed. It is nevertheless recommended as second line therapy by PRES, EDF and CARRA. Dosing regimes suggest gradual escalation to 1 g twice daily in adults and doses of $600 \, mg/m^2$ in children $<1.25 \, m^2$, 750 <mg twice daily in between 1.25 and 1.5 m^2 and 1 g twice daily for patients >1.5 m^2 [10,361]. In 2012, in response to the then lack of consensus on treatment regimens among clinicians caring for patients with morphoea [51,495], the CARRA developed consensus-derived standardised treatment plans for the initial 12 months of therapy for childhood morphoea of moderate or high severity [361]. These plans have established clinical assessment methods and treatment response criteria. They also recommended defined treatment protocols employing methotrexate alone or in combination with oral or intravenous corticosteroids, with mycophenolate mofetil used in addition to or as a replacement for methotrexate according to physician preference. The aim was to reduce the variability in medication and methods of assessment used to facilitate the evaluation of treatment strategies in future comparative effectiveness studies. Results from the initial pilot show efficacy of all three regimens with >75% improvement from baseline. Differences in response were linked to disease subtype and activity at baseline, suggesting that this type of comparative study may ultimately facilitate appropriate patient selection for different treatment regimens [44]. Further, data from one institution shows that the publication of these consensus treatment plans has led to their increased use (from 8% to 78% of patients), which in turn has led to improved patient outcomes, including a reduced need for second line therapy (from 44% of cases to 11.5%) [45]. Similarly, it is hoped that the publication of guidelines for adults [10], and minimum standards of care and consensus-based recommendations for management of children [41,42] will enable a more unified approach, better assessment of extracutaneous manifestations, and better overall care for this rare patient group.

For those patients who are unable to tolerate or fail to respond to the above standard of care there are a number of potential options.

Other DMARDs

A retrospective review of 105 cases seen between 1996 and 2013 at the Mayo clinic treated with hydroxychloroquine monotherapy showed a complete response in 45%, a >50% partial response in 39%, a <50% partial response in 12.4% and no response in 12.4%. The median time to initial response was 5 months, and to maximum response 14 months, suggesting slow but significant improvement in 84% with a low rate of adverse events [496]. A more detailed report of 84 of these same patients identified complete or >50% partial remission in 21/29 linear, 28/29 plaque, 9/14 generalised, 8/10 deep and 2/2 mixed morphoea. Eleven of 36 complete responders relapsed [497]. Although the evidence in this study is low quality, it suggests a possible role for hydroxychloroquine in treating mild–moderate, more superficial disease and warrants further study.

The efficacy of ciclosporin was reported in a single case of childhood linear disease [498] and in two adults with pansclerotic disease [499]. Bali *et al.* identified three other published cases, two of whom improved, and reported 12 cases, four with eosinophilic fasciitis/morphoea overlap, four pansclerotic, two generalised and two linear. Relatively low dose (median 2.4 mg/kg) ciclosporin was used for a median of 14 months. Improvement was reported in nine patients with long-term complete remission in four [500]. These patients all had severe inflammatory disease providing a rationale for use of a T-cell directed therapy. Its side-effect profile precludes prolonged or high dose use, but low dose adjunctive therapy in patients with severe inflammatory morphoea may be beneficial in some cases. There is no evidence to support the use of oral calcitriol [501], INF-γ [502] or D-penicillamine [43].

Finally, ulceration occurring in the context of severe, deep or pansclerotic disease has shown improvement in a small cases series with sildenafil [315]. In one case, improvement of limb ulcers, skin sclerosis and joint mobility was noted with the dual oral endothelin receptor antagonist bosentan [503].

Biologics

Newer T-cell-directed therapies are now being considered and abatacept is commissioned in England for use in patients with severe morphoea unresponsive to standard care (https://www.england.nhs.uk/publication/abatacept-for-treatment-of-severe-treatment-resistant-morphoea-localised-scleroderma/). Abatacept is a cytotoxic T-lymphocyte antigen 4 (CTLA4) IgG1 recombinant fusion protein that selectively inhibits T-cell activation via competitive binding to CD80 or CD86. It has shown clinically significant improvement in SSc skin disease and particularly so in patients with the 'inflammatory' gene signature in skin which was also found in morphoea [504]. Reports on 46 patients (21 adults) with severe extensive or deep morphoea treated with abatacept are now published. Previous treatment with methotrexate, mycophenolate and corticosteroids have failed in the majority. A majority remained on their DMARD and abatacept was added (either intravenous or subcutaneous) [325,505–510]. In the largest childhood series of 18 cases skin activity and PGA-A scores improved at 6 months and by 12 months showed an 83% response rate. This response was

Table 55.6 Consensus-based recommendations for diagnosis, assessment and treatment of paediatric morphoea (juvenile localised scleroderma, jLS) from the European SHARE (Single Hub and Access point for paediatric Rheumatology in Europe) initiative which was set up in 2012 to optimise and disseminate diagnostic and management regimens in Europe for children and young adults with rheumatic diseases. Adapted from Zulian *et al.* [42].

		L	S	Agreement (%)
	Diagnosis and assessment			
	Overarching principle			
	All children with suspected localised scleroderma should be referred to a specialised paediatric rheumatology centre.	4	D	100
1	LoSSI, which is part of LoSCAT, is a good clinical instrument to assess activity and severity in JLS lesions and is highly recommended in clinical practice	3	C	90
2	LoSDI, which is part of LoSCAT, is a good clinical instrument to assess damage in JLS and is highly recommended in clinical practice	3	C	90
3	Infrared thermography can be used to assess activity of the lesions in JLS, but skin atrophy can give false-positive results	4	D	90
4	A specialised US imaging, using standardised assessment and colour Doppler, may be a useful tool for assessing disease activity, extent of JLS and response to treatment	4	D	100
5	All patients with JLS at diagnosis and during follow-up should be carefully evaluated with a complete joint examination, including the temporomandibular joint	2a	C	100
6	MRI can be considered a useful tool to assess musculoskeletal involvement in JLS, especially when the lesion crosses the joint	3	C	100
7	It is highly recommended that all patients with JLS involving face and head, with or without signs of neurological involvement, have an MRI of the head at the time of the diagnosis	3	C	90
8	All patients with JLS involving face and head should undergo an orthodontic and maxillofacial evaluation at diagnosis and during follow-up	2b	B	90
9	Ophthalmological assessment, including screening for uveitis, is recommended at diagnosis for every patient with JLS, especially in those with skin lesions on the face and scalp	2a	C	100
10	Ophthalmological follow-up, including screening for uveitis, should be considered for every patient with JLS, especially in those with skin lesions on the face and scalp	3	C	100
	Treatment			
	Systemic corticosteroids may be useful in the active inflammatory phase of JLS. At the same time as starting systemic corticosteroids, MTX or an alternative DMARD should be started	2b	C	100
	All patients with active, potentially disfiguring or disabling forms of JLS should be treated with oral or subcutaneous MTX at 15 mg/m²/week	1b	A	100
	If acceptable clinical improvement is achieved, MTX should be maintained for at least 12 months before tapering	3	C	100
	Mycophenolate mofetil may be used to treat severe JLS or MTX-refractory or MTX-intolerant patients	2a	B	100
	Medium-dose UVA-1 phototherapy may be used to improve skin softness in isolated (circumscribed) morphoea lesions	1b	A	100
	Topical imiquimod may be used to decrease skin thickening of circumscribed morphoea	3	C	100

DMARD, disease-modifying antirheumatic drug; JLS, juvenile localised scleroderma; L, level of evidence; LoSCAT, Localised Scleroderma Cutaneous Assessment Tool; LoSDI, Localised Scleroderma Skin Damage Index; LoSSI, Localised Scleroderma Skin Severity Index; MTX, methotrexate; S, strength of recommendation; UVA1, ultraviolet A1; US, ultrasound.

maintained in 44% at 24 months [508]. In the largest adult series of 13 patients, significant reductions in activity and damage scores were recorded in 8/13 cases [510]. Musculoskeletal manifestations also improved. These are encouraging results, although more robust data collection is required to assess outcomes fully. With the recent advent of available treatment in England, further data should be forthcoming.

Tocilizumab is an IL-6 receptor-α antagonist with proven benefit in skin fibrosis and lung function in SSc, particularly in ATA positive patients [511]. It has now been used to treat some 25 morphoea cases refractory to other therapies, including 24 children, with some improvement in most [512–521]. In the largest paediatric series, 9/11 cases showed a reduction in mLoSSI on treatment and improvement in joint inflammation (in 3/3) [519].

Both abatacept and tocilizumab appear well tolerated and effective and further study is warranted.

A small case series of five patients have received apremilast, an orally available small-molecule inhibitor of PDE4. PDE4 blockade,

by limiting M2 macrophage differentiation and IL-6 release, may reverse or prevent fibrosis. Four improved within one month, and reductions in LoSCAT scores were reported. One patient discontinued treatment due to nausea [522].

There are eight cases reported of patients with severe morphoea (e.g. pansclerotic/generalised bullous, eosinophilic fasciitis), unresponsive to multiple therapies, treated with JAK inhibitors, including one child [523–525]. A majority were given tofacitinib, one baricitinib and one ruxolitinib. All adults responded positively; time to meaningful improvement ranged from 5 to 9 months. Beneficial effects were also documented in bleomycin treated mice. Inhibition of STAT3 phosphorylation and downregulation of fibroblast COLA1 have been proposed as potential mechanisms. There are no published data on use of topical JAK inhibitors in morphoea, but there is a rationale for their use.

Rituximab is effective in the treatment of SSc, but benefits in morphoea are less certain. There are three cases of morphoea and four of eosinophilic fasciitis, six of whom showed some benefit

PART 4: INFLAMMATORY DERMATOSES

Table 55.7 Morphoea treatments and levels of evidence (in brackets).[a]

Type of disease	First line therapies	Second line therapies	Third line therapies
Circumscribed plaque or superficial disease	Tacrolimus ointment 0.1% b.d. (± occlusion) (IIa) Imiquimod 5% cream (IIa) Topical/intralesional corticosteroids (III)	Calcipotriol–betamethasone (IIb) +/− occlusion Calcipotriol 0.005% b.d. under occlusion (IIb) Calcipotriol +low-dose UVA-1 (IIb)	Phototherapy: UVA-1 (Ib) Psoralen and UVA (bath or cream if available) (III) Broad-band UVA (IIb), narrow-band UVB (Ib)
Superficial generalised plaque disease In addition to topical therapies	UVA-1 phototherapy (medium dose recommended, 3–5 times/week 30–40 treatments) (Ib)	Psoralen and UVA (bath or cream) (IIb) Broad-band UVA (IIb) Narrow-band UVB	Hydroxychloroquine III
Pansclerotic, linear or deep disease (any subtype) or disease unresponsive to other treatments and with significant impact on quality of life	MTX + IV corticosteroids (Ib) MTX + oral corticosteroids (Ib)	MMF (IIb) +/− IV/oral corticosteroids Combination oral medication, e.g. MTX + MMF (III) +/− corticosteroids Abatacept (III)	Ciclosporin (III) Combination oral medication with phototherapy (III) Tocilizumab (III) JAK inhibitor (III) Apremilast (III) Infliximab (III) Extracorporeal photopheresis (III) Ivlg (IV)

IvIG, intravenous immunoglublulin; MTX, methotrexate: MMF, mycophenolate.

[a] Categories of evidence:

Ia: evidence for meta-analysis of randomised controlled trials;

Ib: evidence from at least one randomised controlled trial;

IIa: evidence from at least one controlled study without randomisation;

IIb: evidence from at least one other type of quasi-experimental study;

III: evidence from non-experimental descriptive studies, such as comparative studies, correlation studies and case–control studies;

IV: evidence from expert committee reports or opinions or clinical experience of respected authorities, or both.

[526–530]. Three of these patients had concomitant hypergammaglobulinaemia. Despite the increased evidence of a role for ANA and autoantibodies to myelin basic protein [129] and endothelial cell components [512] in morphoea, the link to pathogenesis and morbidity remains less clear cut than in SSc. Infliximab was reported to induce remission in a case of generalised morphoea with lichen sclerosus overlap unresponsive to conventional therapies [531], an adolescent with mixed morphoea in combination with leflunomide [532] and an adult with generalised morphoea spondylarthritis and primary biliary cholangitis [533]. Imatinib has been used successfully in conjunction with methotrexate and prednisolone in one case but has significant toxicity [534]. Successful therapy with extracorporeal photopheresis has been reported in SSc (reviewed in [535]), and in a small number of morphoea cases including generalised morphoea and eosinophilic fasciitis [326,536–538]. Based on early results in SSc, there may also be some rational for using high-dose intravenous immunoglobulin in resistant cases [539,540].

Improved understanding of the immunopathogenesis of morphoea should help direct future therapies. Appreciation of the role of the Th2 pathway, IL-4 and IL-13 in driving fibrosis has led to investigation in phase II studies of the benefits of bispecific monoclonal antibodies such as romilkimab, associated with a significant reduction in mRSS at 24 weeks in SSc [541] and dupilumab, currently ongoing in morphoea (see https://clinicaltrials.gov/ct2/show/NCT04200755?term=dupilumab&cond=Localised+Scleroderma&draw=2&rank=1). A potential role for STAT3 and STAT4 inhibition,

alpha-MSH analogues, IL-1 blockade and topical PDE4 inhibition, among others, requires further investigation.

The treatments discussed thus far are aimed at switching off active disease and preventing damage. Once damage such as dyspigmentation, atrophy or bony asymmetry has occurred, treatment should aim at improving function and cosmetic appearances, provided that the disease is no longer active. In addition to standard orthopaedic and plastic surgery, various techniques of autologous fat grafting, either alone or in combination with surgery have gained popularity in the treatment of tissue defects of the face and limbs [542,543]. Autologous fat transfer is a safe procedure, useful for reconstructing soft-tissue volumetric defects. Recent research has also demonstrated regenerative and antifibrotic properties, linked to the presence of adipose derived stem cells, and likely through enhanced angiogenesis, inhibition of TGF-β and increased collagenase activity [542,544–546]. Mortality is rare in morphoea, but permanent damage and functional impairment may develop in 20–40% of cases. Outcomes have improved significantly with the increased use of methotrexate therapy since 2000. Earlier disease recognition, increased appreciation of the prevalence, variety and clinical impact of extracutaneous involvement in morphoea, and more widespread use of early aggressive treatment will likely lead to further improvements. The recent introduction of simple effective clinical outcome measures such as the LoSCAT [418], of management guidelines [10], minimum standards of care [41] and consensus treatment plans [42,361] in morphoea is beginning to have an impact, allowing better data collection, better assessment

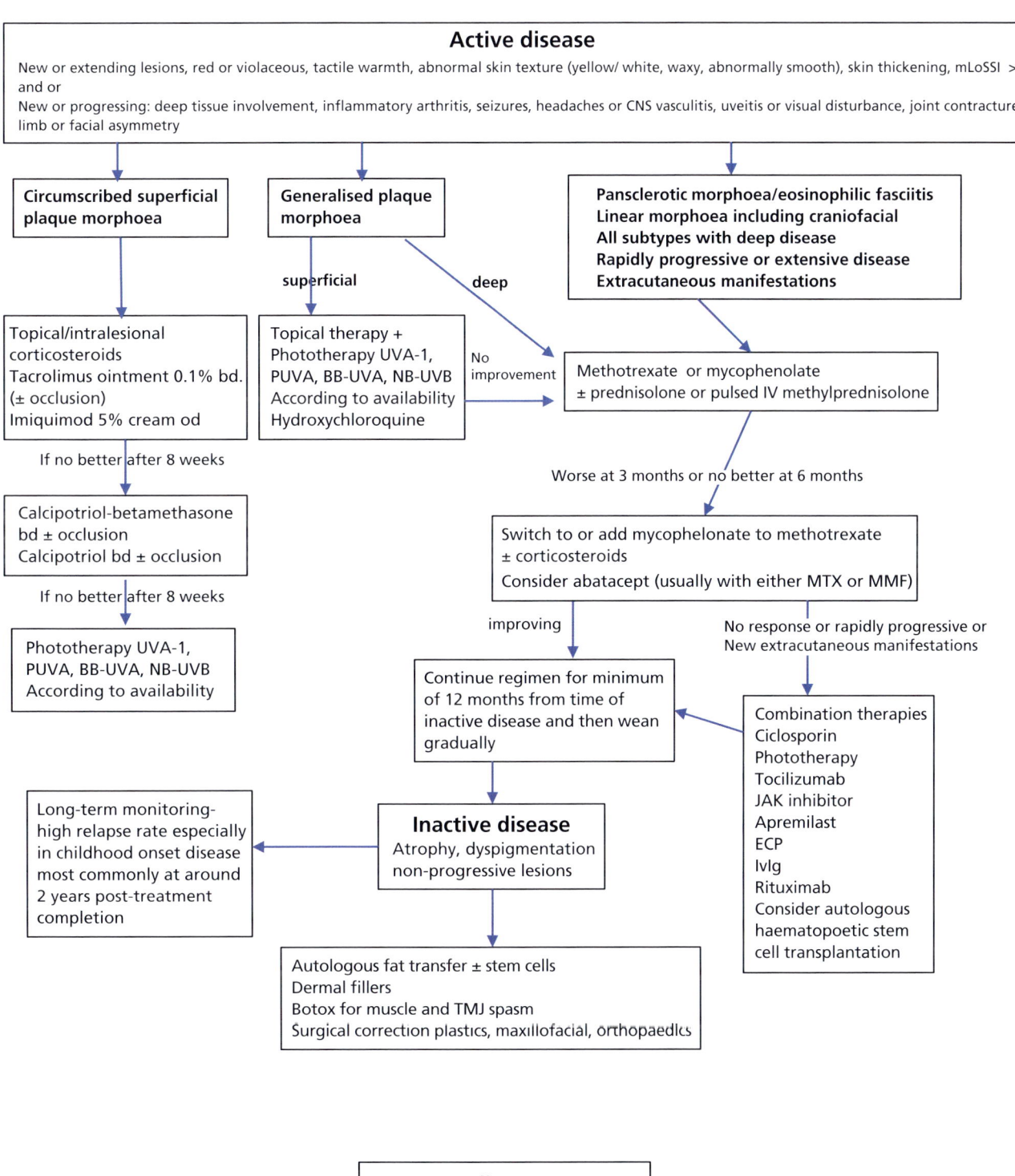

Active disease
New or extending lesions, red or violaceous, tactile warmth, abnormal skin texture (yellow/ white, waxy, abnormally smooth), skin thickening, mLoSSI >0
and or
New or progressing: deep tissue involvement, inflammatory arthritis, seizures, headaches or CNS vasculitis, uveitis or visual disturbance, joint contractures, limb or facial asymmetry

Circumscribed superficial plaque morphoea

Generalised plaque morphoea

Pansclerotic morphoea/eosinophilic fasciitis
Linear morphoea including craniofacial
All subtypes with deep disease
Rapidly progressive or extensive disease
Extracutaneous manifestations

superficial   deep

Topical/intralesional corticosteroids
Tacrolimus ointment 0.1% bd. (± occlusion)
Imiquimod 5% cream od

Topical therapy + Phototherapy UVA-1, PUVA, BB-UVA, NB-UVB According to availability
Hydroxychloroquine

No improvement

Methotrexate or mycophenolate ± prednisolone or pulsed IV methylprednisolone

If no better after 8 weeks

Calcipotriol-betamethasone bd ± occlusion
Calcipotriol bd ± occlusion

Worse at 3 months or no better at 6 months

If no better after 8 weeks

Switch to or add mycophelonate to methotrexate ± corticosteroids
Consider abatacept (usually with either MTX or MMF)

Phototherapy UVA-1, PUVA, BB-UVA, NB-UVB According to availability

improving

No response or rapidly progressive or New extracutaneous manifestations

Continue regimen for minimum of 12 months from time of inactive disease and then wean gradually

Combination therapies
Ciclosporin
Phototherapy
Tocilizumab
JAK inhibitor
Apremilast
ECP
IvIg
Rituximab
Consider autologous haematopoetic stem cell transplantation

Long-term monitoring- high relapse rate especially in childhood onset disease most commonly at around 2 years post-treatment completion

Inactive disease
Atrophy, dyspigmentation non-progressive lesions

Autologous fat transfer ± stem cells
Dermal fillers
Botox for muscle and TMJ spasm
Surgical correction plastics, maxillofacial, orthopaedics

All cases
Physiotherapy, occupational therapy
Psychological and social support
Manual lymphatic drainage massage

Figure 55.19 Therapeutic algorithm for the treatment of morphoea based on existing evidence. BB, broad-band; b.d., twice a day; CNS, central nervous system; ECP extracorporeal photophoresis; IV, intravenous; IvIg, intravenous immunoglobulin; MLD, manual lymphatic drainage; mLoSSI, Modified Localised Scleroderma Skin Activity Index; MMF, mycophenolate; MTX, methotrexate; NB, narrow-band; o.d., once a day; PUVA, psoralen and UVA; s.c., subcutaneous; TMJ, temporo-mandibular joint; UV, ultraviolet.

PART 4: INFLAMMATORY DERMATOSES

of therapeutic efficacy and facilitating management decisions (Table 55.6). Involvement of allied specialists including rheumatologists, orthopaedic surgeons, neurologists, ophthalmologists, orthodontists, physiotherapists and clinical psychologists as part of a multidisciplinary team is crucial to achieving optimum patient outcomes in morphoea and patients with moderate to severe disease should be cared for by doctors experienced in the diagnosis and management of morphoea, with easy access to support from these other specialisms. A therapeutic algorithm and suggested first, second- and third-line therapies are outlined with levels of evidence in Table 55.7 and Figure 55.19.

Resources

Patient resources

Fett NM. Morphea (localised scleroderma). *JAMA Dermatol* 2013;149:1124.
https://www.sruk.co.uk/media/filer_public/00/c0/00c05f90-4962-464b-beb6-823e505af9db/20-19517_sruk-ssc_morphoea_a5_28pp_print.pdf
https://www.rheumaderm-society.org/morphea-information-for-patients/
https://www.osmosis.org/answers/morphea-scleroderma
https://rheumatology.org/patients/localised-scleroderma-juvenile
https://www.england.nhs.uk/publication/abatacept-for-treatment-of-severe-treatment-resistant-morphoea-localised-scleroderma/

Patient support group

Scleroderma & Raynaud's UK, 18-20 Bride Lane, London EC4Y 8EE, UK
Email: info@sruk.co.uk
Web: https://www.sruk.co.uk/
(All last accessed November 2023)

Key references

The full list of references can be found in the online version at https://www.wiley.com/rooksdermatology10e

1   Vasquez-Canizares N, Li SC. Juvenile localised scleroderma: updates and differences from adult-onset disease. *Rheum Dis Clin North Am* 2021;47:737–55.
13 Prasad S, Zhu JL, Schollaert-Fitch K, Torok KS, Jacobe HT. An evaluation of the performance of current morphea subtype classifications. *JAMA Dermatol* 2021;157:1–8.
14 Teske N, Welser J, Jacobe H. Skin mapping for the classification of generalized morphea. *J Am Acad Dermatol* 2018;78:351–7.
22 Mirizio E, Liu C, Yan Q *et al*. Genetic signatures from RNA sequencing of pediatric localised scleroderma skin. *Front Pediatr* 2021;9:669116.
29 Khatri S, Torok KS, Mirizio E, Liu C, Astakhova K. Autoantibodies in morphea: an update. *Front Immunol* 2019;10:1487.
32 Mertens JS, Seyger MM, Kievit W *et al*. Disease recurrence in localised scleroderma: a retrospective analysis of 344 patients with paediatric- or adult-onset disease. *Br J Dermatol* 2015;172:722–8.
40 Kelsey CE, Torok KS. The Localised Scleroderma Cutaneous Assessment Tool: responsiveness to change in a pediatric clinical population. *J Am Acad Dermatol* 2013;69:214–20.
114 Kreuter A, Mitrakos G, Hofmann SC *et al*. Localised scleroderma of the head and face area: a retrospective cross-sectional study of 96 patients from 5 German Tertiary Referral Centres. *Acta Derm Venereol* 2018;98:603–5.
155 Torok KS, Li SC, Jacobe HM *et al*. Immunopathogenesis of pediatric localised scleroderma. *Front Immunol* 2019;10:908.
423 Li SC. Treatment of juvenile localised scleroderma: current recommendations, response factors, and potential alternative treatments. *Curr Opin Rheumatol* 2022;34:245–54.

PART 5

Metabolic and Nutritional Disorders Affecting the Skin

CHAPTER 56

Cutaneous Amyloidoses

Stephan Schreml

Department of Dermatology, University Medical Centre Regensburg, Regensburg, Germany

Introduction

Amyloid means 'starch like' (Latin: *amylum*), a term introduced by Rudolf Virchow, who described extracellular precipitates that turn brown after incubation with iodine [1]. Even though these precipitates are proteins, and not carbohydrates, the terms 'amyloid' and 'amyloidosis' are still used. The key feature of amyloidoses is the extracellular deposition of autologous proteins as morphologically characteristic amyloid fibrils [2–4]. Amyloid proteins show a highly conserved antiparallel β-sheet conformation and form non-branching linear fibrils of variable lengths, with diameters of 7.5–10 nm.

Amyloidoses may be acquired or hereditary. Subclassification differentiates between localised cutaneous amyloidosis and cutaneous amyloidosis due to systemic disease. Amyloid can originate from various precursor proteins. The pathogenetic modification of these precursor proteins may be triggered by chronic inflammation, malignancies, mutations, pro-amyloidogenic peptide sequences and microenvironmental changes.

Cutaneous amyloidoses and cutaneous manifestations of systemic amyloidoses are rare in Europe but far more frequent in South-East Asia, China and South America [5,6]. Even though the clinical presentation varies, particular clinical features may point to amyloidosis. Cutaneous signs are often also the key finding for the initial diagnosis of an underlying systemic amyloidosis. Depending on distribution and amount, amyloid may only lead to localised skin problems or cause progressive and life-threatening organ dysfunction.

Ultrastructure and amyloidogenesis

Amyloid deposits consist of a loose network of unbranched fibrils measuring 7.5–10 nm in diameter [7,8]. The ultrastructural feature of the different amyloid precipitates is a fibrillary antiparallel β-sheet structure. The filaments are composed of protofilaments and filaments aggregate to form fibrils. Fibrils are found in the extracellular space and small amounts are phagocytosed by fibroblasts, sometimes causing a so-called pyknotic degeneration of keratinocytes [7,9]. Fibroblasts may also be involved in the process of amyloid precipitation [10]. The second component of amyloid precipitations is the amyloid P component, which can be detected in almost all deposits amounting to approximately 15% of the total weight of the extracted amyloid [3,4,11]. In contrast to the respective amyloid protein, the amyloid P component is non-fibrillary and shows a pentagonal ultrastructure [11].

The basic pathogenetic principle of amyloidogenesis is extracellular fibrillar protein aggregation. Some experiments suggest the occurrence of various protein conformations with specific biological properties [12]. This may be due to different enzymatic cleavage products of precursor proteins. Two examples include, firstly, a specifically truncated form of β_2-microglobulin (in haemodialysis-associated amyloidosis), obtained from amyloid deposits, which shows amyloidogenic potential, but this cleavage product is absent in the circulation [13]. Secondly, in gelsolin amyloidosis, distinct mutations disrupt Ca^{2+} binding of the protein gelsolin, making it susceptible to abnormal cleavage by furin, a subtilisin-like convertase in the Golgi apparatus [14]. As a consequence, amyloid multimers may be polymorphic and polyfunctional, both also depending on the local microenvironment [12,15]. For instance, it has been shown that heparin enhances β_2-microglobulin amyloidogenesis (haemodialysis patients) in the presence of collagen type I [16]. The amyloid precursor serum amyloid A (SAA) contains a pH-sensitive binding site for heparin and heparan sulphate [17]. Depending on pH, this molecular switch may lead to SAA aggregation, thereby facilitating amyloid A (AA) amyloidosis, for example, in inflammatory microenvironments. Interestingly, glycoaminoglycans such as heparan sulphate are

Rook's Textbook of Dermatology, Tenth Edition. Edited by Christopher Griffiths, Jonathan Barker, Tanya Bleiker, Walayat Hussain and Rosalind Simpson.
© 2024 John Wiley & Sons Ltd. Published 2024 by John Wiley & Sons Ltd.

PART 5: METABOLIC & NUTRITIONAL DISORDERS

ubiquitously present in amyloid deposits [15]. Additionally, it is known that transition metal ions, such as Cu^{2+} and Zn^{2+}, play a crucial role in the formation of Aβ plaques in Alzheimer disease, the most frequent amyloidopathy [18].

Once amyloid has aggregated, serum amyloid P component stabilises the aggregates together with other molecules such as glycoaminoglycans [15] and collagen fibres. In addition, macromolecular crowding reduces the configurational entropy of amyloid proteins, which fosters amyloid aggregation under certain microenvironmental conditions [19,20]. Thus, abnormal cleavage of proteins and microenvironmental factors seem to be common processes involved in amyloidogenesis. Furthermore, specific pro-amyloidogenic peptide sequences of amyloid precursors have been identified [21–28]. A list of relevant pro-amyloidogenic amino acid sequences can be found in the supplement to Schreml *et al.* [29]. One of the best-known pro-amyloidogenic sequences, (G)NNQQNY, was found in yeast prion protein Sup35p [30–32]. Interestingly, molecular chaperones inhibit or alter these amyloid aggregation processes, for example αβ-crystallin and clusterin in haemodialysis-associated amyloidosis [25].

Functional and disease-causing amyloids

It has been found that amyloid proteins also fulfil various biological tasks [33–36], while others lead to serious diseases, such as Alzheimer disease [37]. Therefore, we have to discriminate between functional and disease-causing amyloids, the latter being the focus of this chapter. Functional amyloid not only occurs in mammals, but also in insects, fungi and bacteria [38]. In *Homo sapiens*, Pmel17 serves as a structural scaffold for covalent polymerization of molecules during melanin assembly; chorion S18/S36 is a structural protein of insect egg shells (e.g. *Drosophila melanogaster*); hydrophobins are key components of fungal coats (e.g. *Aspergillus fumigatus*); and bacteria like *Escherichia coli* and *Salmonella typhimurium* need major curlin subunits (csgA) for biofilm formation and host invasion [34,38–43]. Other interesting functional amyloids are specific adhesins for cellular aggregation in yeast cells [44] or type I antifreeze protein (ice-structuring protein preventing ice growth) in winter flounders [45]. These examples show how nature uses the very stable amyloid structure for proteins involved in protection from environmental influences (e.g. Pmel17 in human melanin assembly to prevent UV damage). Additionally, it has been found that peptide and protein hormones in secretory granules of the mammalian endocrine system are sometimes stored in an amyloid-like cross β-sheet-rich conformation [46]. The natural storage of hormones in amyloid-like structures seems not to be toxic for neuronal cells, whereas it is well known that Aβ-polypeptide causes severe neurodegeneration in Alzheimer disease.

Basic classification

Various classification systems for amyloidoses affecting the skin have been proposed. In older classification systems, amyloidoses were mainly classified according to their clinicopathological features. Over the last decades, the proteins involved in the different types of amyloidoses have been characterised, so that there was a tendency to only use biochemical features for classification. However, several different amyloid subtypes may be present in one clinical entity, and the same amyloid precursor may be involved in clinically different amyloidosis subtypes. Therefore, amyloidoses affecting the skin should be distinguished based on both clinical and biochemical investigations.

Amyloidoses are subclassified as primary localised cutaneous amyloidosis (PLCA), secondary localised cutaneous amyloidosis (SLCA), systemic amyloidosis with cutaneous involvement, and secondary cutaneous amyloidosis originating from other systemic diseases [3,4,47].

In PLCA, amyloid precipitates are normally found in the papillary dermis [9]. Nodular PLCA is an exception to the rule, as amyloid is frequently found in the deeper layers of the skin. This is similar to the findings in systemic amyloidosis with cutaneous involvement where subpapillary layers (stratum reticulare, subcutis), dermal appendages and blood vessels may also be involved [**48**].

Clinical presentation

There are varied clinical presentations of the different amyloidoses affecting the skin. Tables 56.1 and 56.2 provide information on clinical presentation, amyloid precursor proteins, associations and variants as well as on extracutaneous findings in systemic amyloidoses. Localised cutaneous amyloidoses often show yellowish or brownish macules, papules or plaques of varying configuration, whereas cutaneous amyloidosis due to systemic disease often initially presents with petechiae, ecchymosis and non-healing ulcers. These differences in clinical presentation are due to the amyloid deposition which in localised cutaneous amyloidoses occurs mainly in the papillary dermis, whereas in systemic amyloidosis, it also affects deeper skin layers. Amyloid precipitation in blood vessel walls makes vessels fragile, eventually causing intracutaneous micro- and macrohaemorrhages. For cutaneous amyloidoses, pruritus is a typical and very common symptom.

Investigations

The most important diagnostic step is a lesional skin biopsy, which should be sent for histology, immunohistochemistry and electron microscopy (Boxes 56.1 and 56.2). In patients with nodular PLCA,

---

Box 56.1 Investigations for cutaneous amyloidoses

- Biopsy and histology
  - Standard stainings: H&E, toluidine blue and alkaline fuchsin
  - Amyloid stainings: Congo red, thioflavin T, uncommon (crystal violet and methyl violet)
- Immunohistochemistry: pancytokeratin-antibodies (AK amyloid), immunoglobulin light chain antibodies (AL amyloid)
- Electron microscopy
  - From skin sample: for all kinds of amyloidoses affecting the skin
  - Abdominal fat or rectum biopsy: for nodular primary localised cutaneous amyloidosis

Table 56.1 Localised cutaneous amyloidoses.

Type of amyloidosis (amyloid subtype)	Amyloid fibril precursor	Cutaneous findings and common distribution (less common in brackets)	Important differentials	Associated diseases and variants
Non-hereditary localised cutaneous amyloidosis = sporadic localised cutaneous amyloidosis				
Papular (lichenoid) PLCA = lichen amyloidosus (AK) (Figure 56.6)	Cytokeratin (predominantly cytokeratin 5)	Soft or hyperkeratotic, partially confluent papules *Distribution*: lower leg, forearm, trunk	Lichen simplex chronicus, hypertrophic lichen planus	*Associations*: MEN2a *Variants*: mixed (syn. biphasic or allotropic) PLCA (= papular and macular), poikilodermatous variant (= lichenoid papules, blisters, poikilodermatous lesions)
Macular PLCA (AK) (Figure 56.7)	Cytokeratin (predominantly cytokeratin 5)	Vaguely demarcated, pigmented plaques; lesions often associated with areas of friction (e.g. scratching due to pruritus; syn. friction or brush amyloidosis) *Distribution*: interscapular region, (extremities, trunk)	Atopic eczema, postinflammatory hyperpigmentation, lichen simplex chronicus, fixed drug eruption, atrophoderma of Pasini and Pierini, anetoderma, morphoea	*Associations*: MEN2a, primary biliary cirrhosis *Variants*: mixed (syn. biphasic or allotropic) PLCA (= papular and macular), poikilodermatous PLCA (macules, blisters, poikilodermatous lesions), anosacral PLCA (predominantly in Japan), amyloidosis cutis dyschromica (hyper- and hypopigmented macules)
Nodular (tumefactive) PLCA (AL) (Figure 56.8)	Immunoglobulin light chains (AL-κ : AL-λ = 1 : 2)	Solitary or multiple, waxy nodules with atrophic epidermis and/or telangiectasia *Distribution*: feet, nose, genitals (legs, head)	Naevus lipomatosus, cutaneous lymphomas	*Associations*: paraproteinaemia, diabetes, Sjögren syndrome, ?CREST syndrome
SLCA (AK)	Cytokeratin (predominantly cytokeratin 5)	See associations	Depends on the clinical presentation (see associations)	*Associations*: skin tumours,[a] discoid lupus erythematosus, PUVA therapy
Hereditary localised cutaneous amyloidosis				
Familial PLCA (AApoE4, AK) (Figure 56.9)	e.g. apolipoprotein E4, cytokeratin	Papules (often tiny and dome-shaped), macules *Distribution*: similar to that in papular or macular PLCA	See differentials under papular (lichenoid)/macular amyloidosis	*Mutations*: oncostatin M receptor β (OSMRβ) mutations (sometimes also found in non-hereditary AK amyloidoses) *Associations*: lipid metabolism disorders

[a] Skin tumours: naevi, sweat gland tumours, pilomatrixomas, actinic keratoses and seborrhoeic keratoses, porokeratosis of Mibelli, Bowen disease, basal cell carcinoma and trichoepithelioma.
AK, amyloid cytokeratin; AL, amyloid from immunoglobulin light chains; AApoE4, amyloid apolipoprotein E4; MEN2a, multiple endocrine neoplasia 2A; PLCA, primary localised cutaneous amyloidosis; PUVA, psoralen and UVA radiation; SLCA, secondary localised cutaneous amyloidosis.

Box 56.2 Investigations for systemic amyloidosis.

- Baseline investigation
  - Creatinine, GFR, proteinuria, full blood count, ECG, coagulation, NT-proBNP, troponin T/I
- Histology
  - Abdominal fat, rectum biopsy or direct tissue biopsy: for all suspected systemic amyloidoses
  - Amyloid stainings: Congo red, thioflavin T
- Immunotyping: immunohistochemistry, immuno electron microscopy or laser capture microscopy with mass spectrometry
- Amyloid subtype-dependent investigations
  - Suspected AL amyloidosis: serum and urine protein electrophoresis and immunofixation, free light chains in serum, bone marrow biopsy, skeletal imaging
  - Suspected cardiac amyloidosis: ECG, cardiac MRI, 99mTcDPD/pyrophosphate scan
  - Suspected hereditary amyloidoses: genetic sequencing
- Whole body amyloid load determination: I-SAP=123-iodine-labelled serum amyloid P component.

Adapted from [49]

it is appropriate to assess for progression to systemic amyloidosis on a regular basis. This assessment should include a full history and physical examination along with an electrocardiogram, complete blood count, serum creatinine level, serum liver-associated enzymes levels, serum protein electrophoresis and urine protein electrophoresis. It has also been suggested that an abdominal fat biopsy (incisional or aspiration, easy access for screening) can be performed to rule out systemic disease [47]. Any indication of systemic disease requires immediate attention as it may be rapidly progressive.

Histology

In papular (lichenoid) and macular PLCA, amyloid is found in the papillary dermis directly below the basal epidermal layer (Figure 56.1). The overlying epidermis often shows acanthosis and hyperkeratosis. Common histological features of biochemically heterogeneous human amyloids are eosinophilia (Figure 56.2), periodic acid–Schiff (PAS) positivity, staining with Congo red [51] and thioflavin T [48], as well as metachromasia after staining with crystal violet or methyl violet. Using Congo red, amyloid exhibits characteristic apple-green birefringence when viewed

Table 56.2 Cutaneous amyloidoses due to systemic disease: typical features of systemic amyloidoses comprise the occurrence of petechiae or haemorrhages (Figures 58.10 and 58.11, often in the periorbital region), mucocutaneous infiltrates (Figures 58.12 and 58.13, especially macroglossia) and sometimes nail dystrophy (Figure 56.15) or bullous manifestations (Figure 56.14).

Type of amyloidosis (amyloid subtype)	Amyloid fibril precursor	Cutaneous findings	Extracutaneous findings	Associated diseases and variants
Non-hereditary systemic amyloidoses with cutaneous involvement				
Primary systemic and myeloma- or plasmocytoma-associated amyloidosis (AL), amyloidosis associated with M. Waldenström (AL and/or AH)	Immunoglobulin light chains Immunoglobulin heavy chains	Petechiae, haemorrhages, nail dystrophy, waxy papules/nodules/plaques, tumourous lesions, scleroderma-like infiltration, purpura, papules, nodules, bullous lesions, alopecia, cutis laxa	Macroglossia, nephropathy, cardiomyopathy, neuropathy, intestinal involvement, CTS	*Associations*: acquired von Willebrand syndrome *Variants*: bullous amyloidosis, oral mucosal bullous amyloidosis
Secondary systemic amyloidosis associated with inflammation/tumour (AA)	SAA	Minor cutaneous involvement, sometimes petechiae, purpura and alopecia	Nephropathy, hepatosplenomegaly, gastrointestinal disorders (bleeding, motility disorders)	*Associations*: chronic infections (e.g. osteomyelitis, bronchiectasis), rheumatoid disease, neoplasia (e.g. thyroid carcinoma, Hodgkin disease)
Secondary haemodialysis-associated systemic amyloidosis (Aβ_2M)	β_2-microglobulin	Soft plaques	CTS, bone cysts, destructive arthropathy	*Associations*: nephropathy, diabetes
Hereditary systemic amyloidoses with cutaneous involvement				
Hereditary transthyretin amyloidosis/familial amyloid polyneuropathy (ATTR)	Transthyretin	Atrophic scars, non-healing ulcers, petechiae	Peripheral and autonomic neuropathy, CTS (especially His 114 variant), cardiomyopathy, nephropathy	*Mutations*: predominantly Val30Met
Hereditary ApoA1 amyloidosis (AApoA1)	Apolipoprotein A1	Maculopapular lesions, petechiae	Cardiomyopathy	
Hereditary lysozyme amyloidosis (AALys)	Lysozyme	Ecchymoses, petechiae	Renal impairment, GI symptoms, sicca syndrome, rarely cardiac invovement	*Mutations*: Trp82Arg, Leu102Ser, Phe57Ile
Hereditary cystatin C amyloidosis (ACys)	Cystatin C	Clinically asymptomatic, but positive histology	Multiple cerebral haemorrhages	
Hereditary gelsolin amyloidosis (Meretoja syndrome) (AGel)	Gelsolin	Cutis laxa, pruritus, petechiae, ecchymoses, hypotrichosis, alopecia	Corneal dystrophy, neuropathy often with cranial nerve involvement, CTS, minor nephropathies	*Variants*: Dutch type (654G→T), Finnish type (654G→A)
Hereditary systemic diseases with secondary cutaneous amyloidosis				
Muckle–Wells syndrome (AA)	SAA	Cold sensitivity, pruritus, cold urticaria-like lesions	Fever, chills, arthralgia, leukocytosis, lancinating limb pain	
TNF receptor 1 associated periodic fever syndrome (TRAPS) (AA)	SAA	Periorbital oedema, migrating cutaneous erythemas, conjunctivitis	Prolonged episodic fever periods, abdominal pain, myalgia	*Mutations*: extracellular domain of TNF receptor 1 (c. 40 distinct mutations)

AA, amyloid SAA; AApoA1, amyloid apolipoprotein A1; Aβ_2M, amyloid β_2-microglobulin; ACys, amyloid cystatin C; AGel, amyloid gelsolin; AH, amyloid from immunoglobulin heavy chains; AL, amyloid from immunoglobulin light chains; ATTR, amyloid transthyretin; CTS, carpal tunnel syndrome; GI, gastrointestinal; SAA, serum amyloid A; TNF, tumour necrosis factor.

under polarised light, a phenomenon called dichroism [52,53]. After staining with thioflavin T, fluorescence microscopy may show the amyloid deposits (Figure 56.3). Blood vessels remain unaffected in lichenoid and macular amyloidoses. In contrast, subcutis and vessels may be diffusely infiltrated in nodular (tumefactive) PLCA [3,54,55].

Immunohistochemistry

For immunohistochemistry, antibodies are available for the subclassification of amyloid precipitates, directed against cytokeratin (papular/macular PLCA or SLCA) or immunoglubulin light chains (systemic AL (amyloid from immunoglobulin light chains)

amyloidosis or nodular PLCA) (see Tables 56.1 and 56.2, Figures 56.3 and 56.4). A cytokeratin profile of PLCA and SLCA has shown positivity for cytokeratin 5 (CK5) in all investigated cases in both formalin-fixed paraffin-embedded tissue sections and frozen tissue sections. CK5 is predominantly found in basal keratinocytes. In descending frequency, other cytokeratins are also present in primary (CK5 > 1 > 14 > 10) and secondary (CK5 > 1 > 10 > 14) cutaneous amyloidoses [56]. Antibodies against CK5 may be used for diagnosing amyloidosis. Also, pan-CK antibodies and, for instance, 34βE12 antibodies are suitable for staining CK5, CK1, CK10 and CK14. Another way of detecting specific amyloid subtypes is to use *in situ* hybridization.

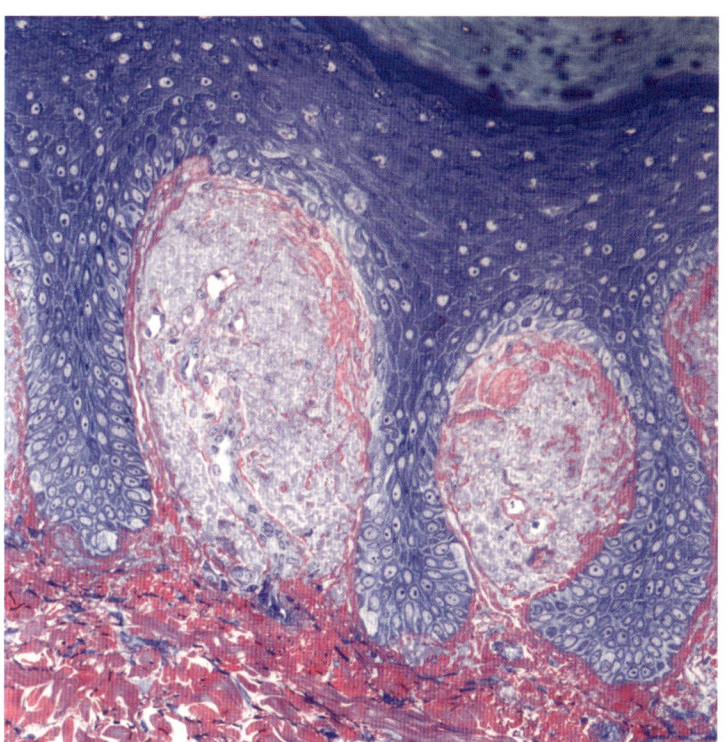

Figure 56.1 Semi-thin tissue section showing amyloid deposition in the papillary dermis. Extensive amyloid deposits are visible as light-blue precipitates within the papillae. Original magnification 20× (plastic-embedded, double staining with toluidine blue and alkaline fuchsin). Reproduced from [47] with permission from John Libbey Eurotext.

Electron microscopy

Definitive confirmation of amyloidosis in tissues can be achieved with electron microscopy, which shows the typical aggregates of amyloid with fibrils 7.5–10 nm in diameter (Figure 56.5). Amyloidoses may even be subclassified according to the different underlying amyloid protein by electron microscopy after

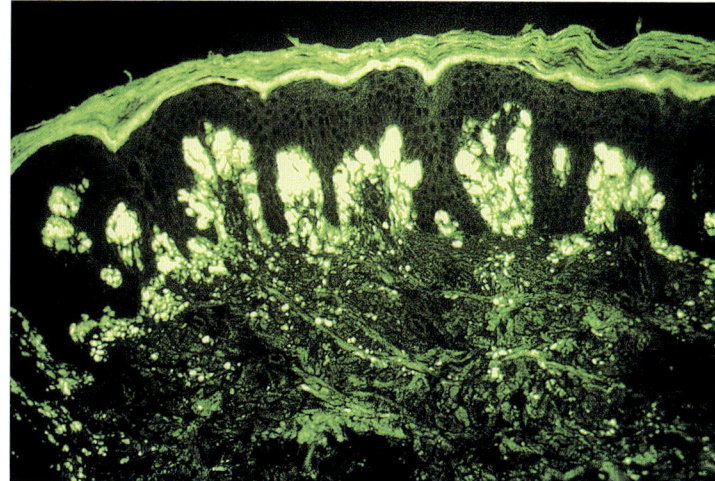

Figure 56.3 Thioflavin staining of primary localised cutaneous amyloidosis viewed under fluorescence microscopy to show the bright yellow to green staining of amyloid. Original magnification 50×.

immunogold labelling [57]. This is especially important in systemic amyloidoses.

Sometimes, differentiation between nodular PLCA and systemic variants may be extremely difficult, and a sophisticated diagnostic approach is needed to diagnose other organ involvement. Apart from organ biopsies, biopsies taken from the rectal submucosa or from abdominal subcutaneous adipose tissue contribute to the diagnosis of systemic amyloidosis. In recent years, abdominal fat pad fine-needle aspiration biopsy has become an important diagnostic tool for diagnosing systemic amyloidosis. This is because of its practicality [58,59] and high sensitivity. Even though only minimal amounts of amyloid are present, a definitive diagnosis of systemic amyloidosis may be achieved by scanning subcutaneous tissue samples or biopsies from the rectal submucosa with an electron microscope.

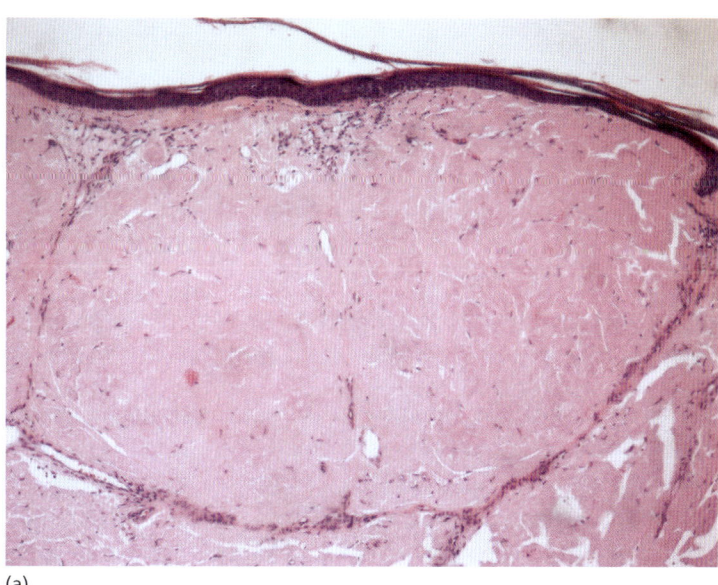

(a)

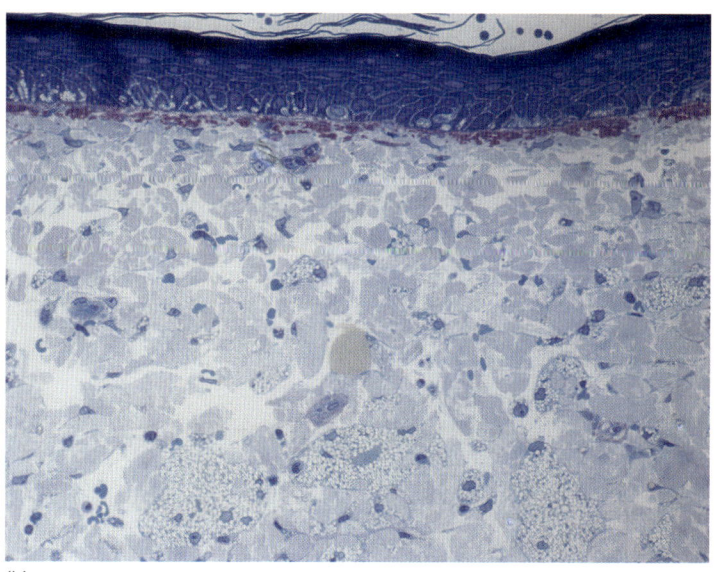

(b)

Figure 56.2 Nodular or tumefactive cutaneous amyloidosis. Amorphous masses of eosinophilic amyloid are present in the entire dermis (a = H&E, b = toluidine blue and alkaline fuchsin). Reproduced from [50] with permission from S. Karger AG.

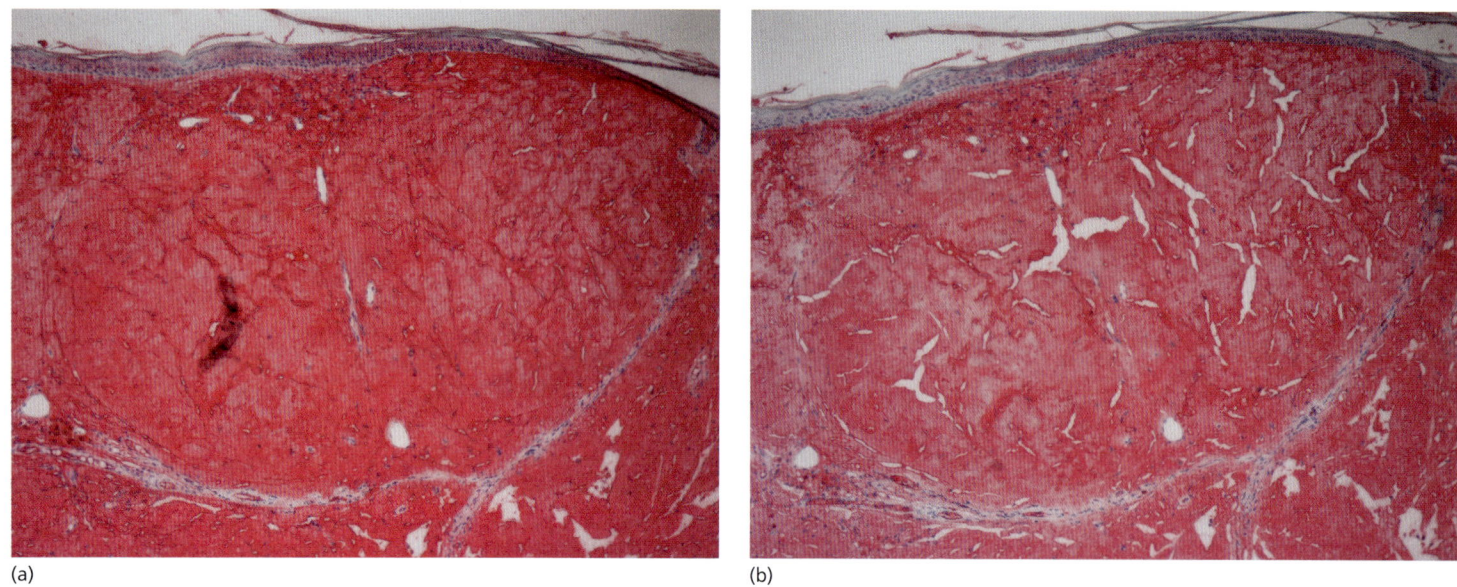

(a)   (b)

Figure 56.4 Immunohistochemistry of nodular amyloidosis. Dermal deposition of (a) κ light chains and (b) λ light chains.

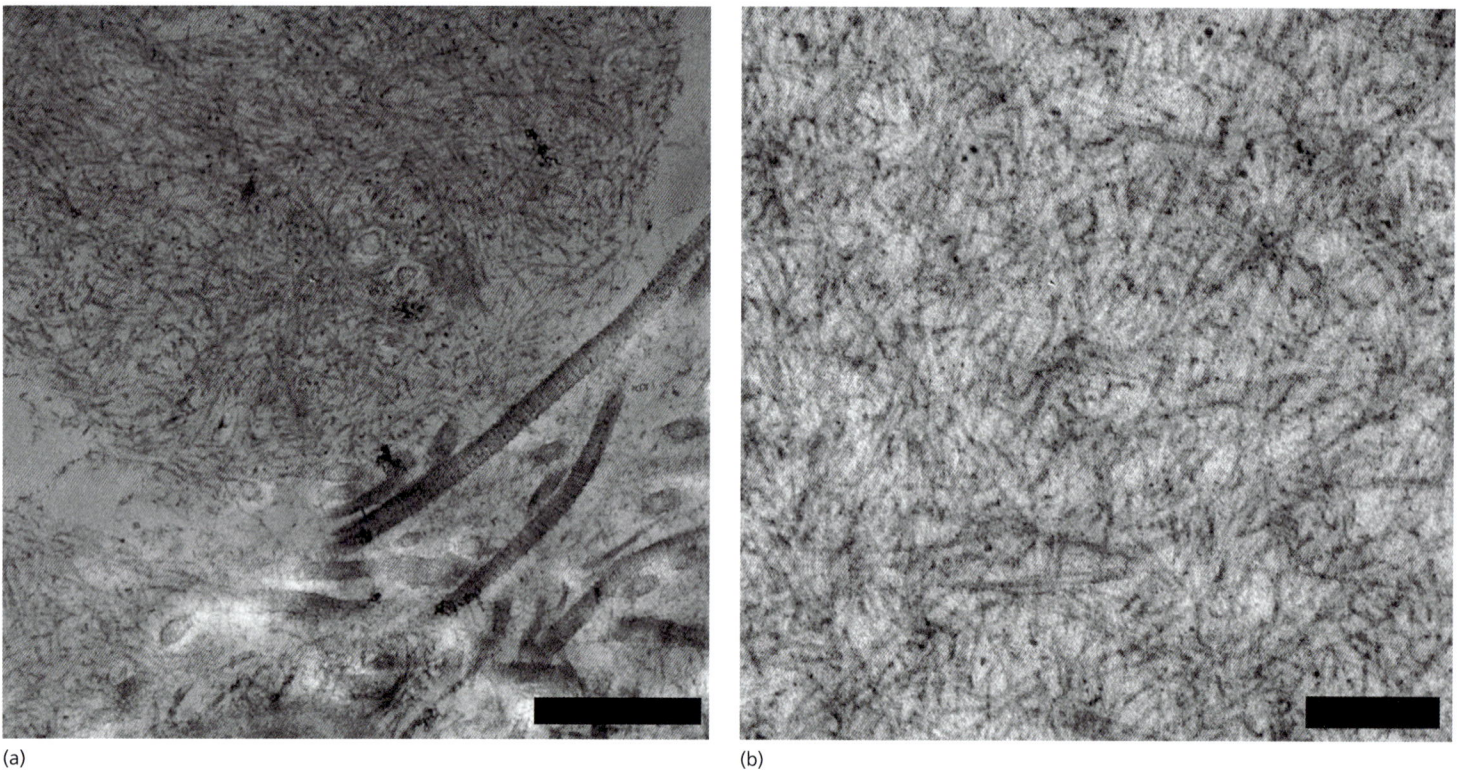

(a)   (b)

Figure 56.5 Electron microscopy of amyloid. (a) Fibrillary extracellular amyloid deposition next to collagen fibres. Bar 500 nm. (b) Amyloid fibrils (thickness 7.5–10 nm). Bar 200 nm. Courtesy of Josef Schröder.

Localised cutaneous amyloidoses

Definition

In localised cutaneous amyloidoses, amyloid precipitates are limited to the skin, mostly to the papillary dermis. Hereditary and non-hereditary types of localised amyloidoses can be differentiated. Primary (PLCA) and secondary (SLCA) forms have been described as subentities of non-hereditary localised cutaneous amyloidoses (Table 56.1).

Introduction and general description

The group of localised cutaneous amyloidoses comprises papular (lichenoid) PLCA (Figure 56.6), macular PLCA (Figure 56.7), nodular (tumefactive) PLCA (Figure 56.8), secondary localised cutaneous amyloidosis (SLCA) and familial PLCA (Figure 56.9). These forms

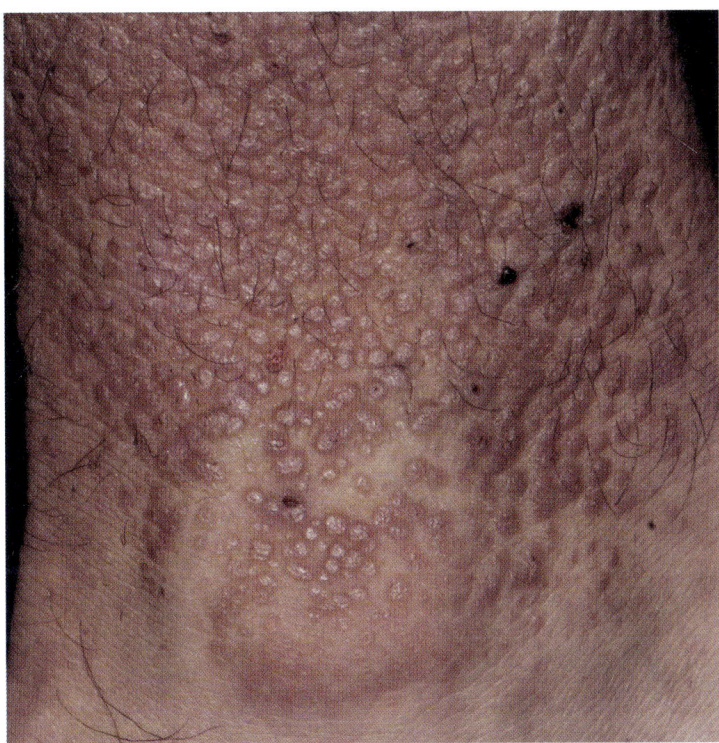

Figure 56.6 Lichenoid primary localised cutaneous amyloidosis on the ankle of a male patient. Reproduced from [47] with permission from John Libbey Eurotext.

are described in detail here. Rare variants are briefly described in the section on clinical variants.

Epidemiology

Incidence and prevalence

Macular ($\approx$ 35%), papular ($\approx$ 35%) and mixed (biphasic, allotropic) maculopapular ($\approx$ 15%) PLCA account for the vast majority of localised cutaneous amyloidoses, whereas nodular (tumefactive) PLCA ($\approx$ 1.5%) is quite rare [5].

Sex

Women seem to be more frequently affected by PLCA than men (female : male = 2–3 : 1) [5]. In contrast to the lichenoid form, macular PLCA occurs more frequently in women.

Ethnicity

It has been reported that in countries nearer to the equator the prevalence of PLCA is higher. The ethnic origin of the patients seems to be of great importance as in Asia, papular PLCA ($\approx$ 75%) is far more frequent than macular PLCA ($\approx$ 10%). Interestingly, mixed maculopapular PLCA is more frequent ($\approx$ 15%) in Asia than the macular type [6].

The most common entity of non-hereditary PLCA is papular (lichenoid) amyloidosis (syn. lichen amyloidosus) (Figure 56.6), which is far more common in South America [5] and Asia [6] than in Europe or the USA. Data on the exact prevalence of these diseases are unreliable but it is known that mixed-race and white patients are the main affected patient groups in South America [5].

The overwhelming majority of localised cutaneous amyloidoses occur sporadically. Case reports on familial PLCA (Figure 56.9)

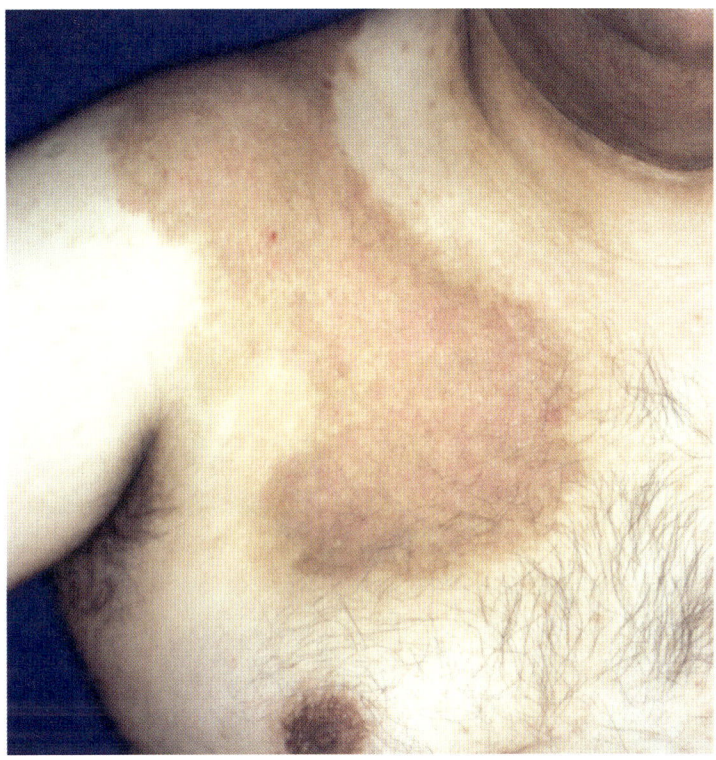

(a)

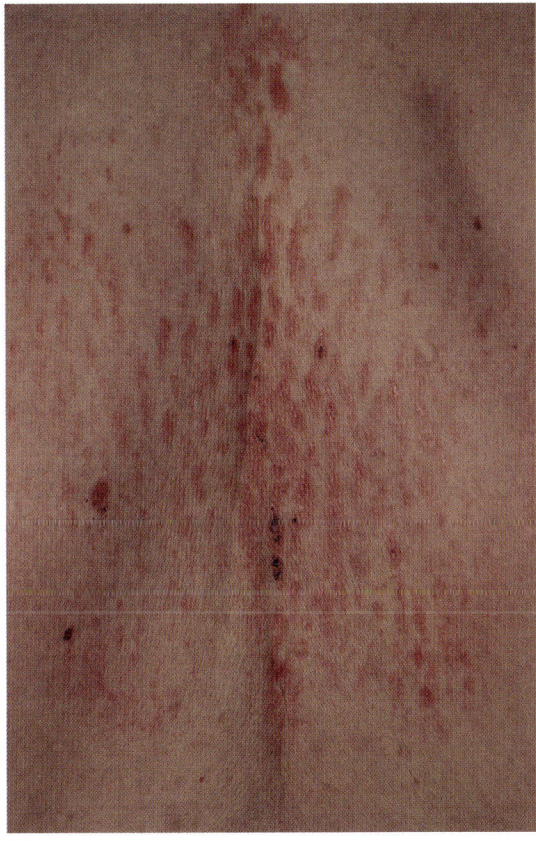

(b)

Figure 56.7 Macular primary localised cutaneous amyloidosis. (a) Macular cutaneous amyloidosis on the chest. Reproduced from [47] with permission from John Libbey Eurotext. (b) Macular cutaneous amyloidosis at the interscapular space. Reproduced from [166] with permission from Springer Nature.

PART 5: METABOLIC & NUTRITIONAL DISORDERS

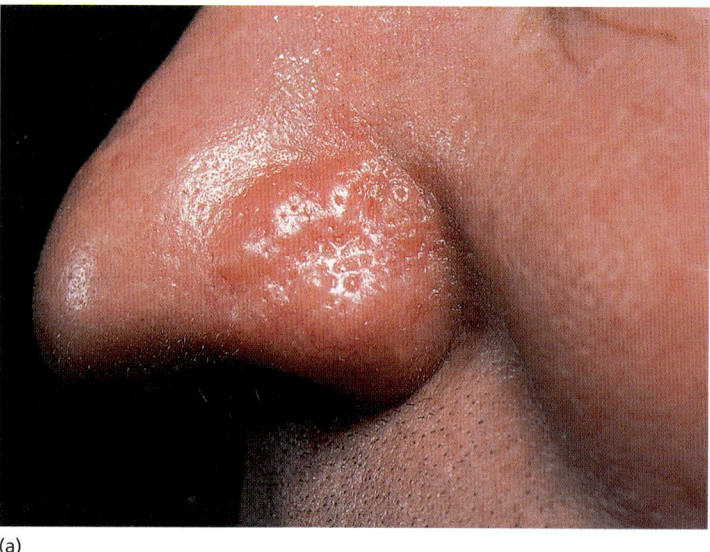

(a)

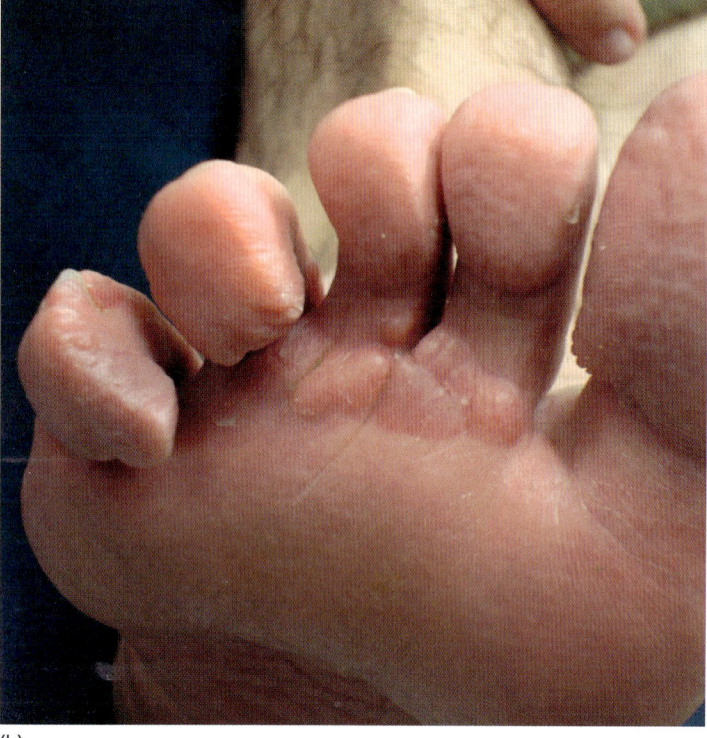

(b)

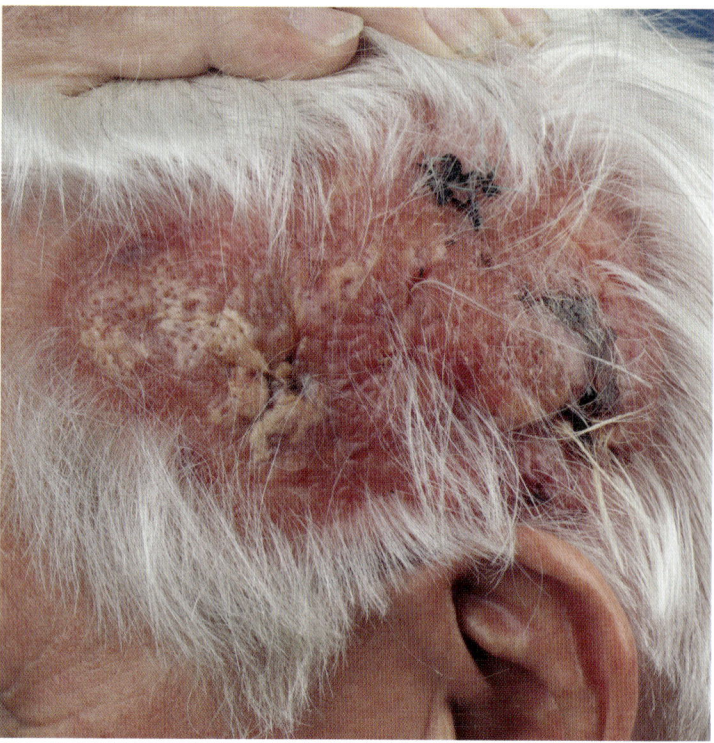

(c)

Figure 56.8 Nodular (tumefactive) primary localised cutaneous amyloidosis. (a) On the side of the nose. Courtesy of St John's Institute of Dermatology. (b) Multiple areas on the toes and sole of the foot. Courtesy of Thomas F. Beachkofsky. (c) Nodular amyloidosis resembling a tumour. Reproduced from [50] with permission from S. Karger AG.

mainly originate from South America, Taiwan and South-East Asia. In white people, hereditary cutaneous amyloidoses are very rare and only a few families have been reported [60,61].

Associated diseases
Associations between papular/macular PLCA and multiple endocrine neoplasia 2a (MEN2a) have been reported [62–65]. A case report has also described a possible association of macular PLCA with primary biliary cirrhosis [63].

Nodular PLCA (Figure 56.8) is the rarest form of the three [50,67,68] and is often found together with diabetes and Sjögren

syndrome [54,55]. One case report has also described the simultaneous appearance of CREST syndrome (calcinosis, Raynaud syndrome, oesophageal involvement, sclerodactyly and telangiectasia) and nodular PLCA [69].

While lichenoid PLCA is the only type that has been specifically associated with the Koebner phenomenon [70], it appears that nodular PLCA can also occur at sites of prior trauma [71,72]. Nodular PLCA shares a feature with macular and lichenoid PLCA, which can be linked to autoimmune diseases such as Sjögren syndrome [54,73–75]. As Sjögren syndrome causes lymphoproliferation, it is possible that this leads to the local clonal plasma cell

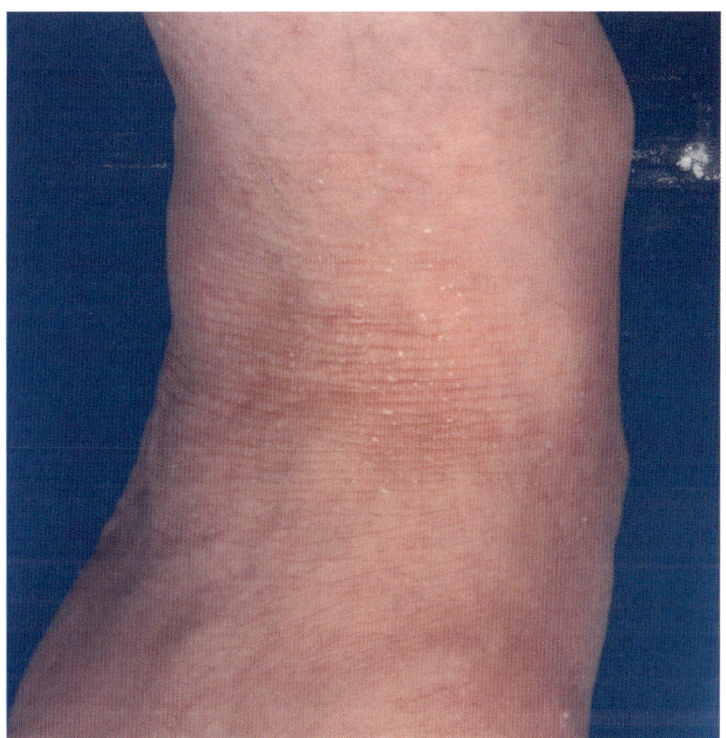

Figure 56.9 Familial primary localised cutaneous amyloidosis showing lichenification and tiny dome-shaped papules on the ventral ankle. Reproduced from [103] with permission from John Wiley & Sons.

expansion seen in nodular PLCA. There have been sparse reports of nodular PLCA being associated with other autoimmune diseases, such as CREST syndrome [69] and primary biliary cirrhosis [74], but currently Sjögren syndrome appears to be the main one frequently reported [54,73,74].

Often, secondary amyloid deposition (SLCA) is found in association with skin tumours (basal cell carcinoma, actinic keratoses, squamous cell carcinoma, skin appendage tumours) and benign lesions (e.g. seborrhoeic warts), solar elastosis, collagenoses (e.g. lupus erythematosus) and after PUVA (psoralen and UVA radiation) therapy [76–81].

Pathophysiology

A commonly accepted theory for papular and macular PLCA is that apoptotic basal keratinocytes release cytokeratins, which are then covered with autoantibodies, phagocytosed by macrophages, and enzymatically degraded to amyloid K (cytokeratin). Cytokeratin 5 (and cytokeratins 1, 10 and 14) is the major constituent of amyloid in papular and macular PLCA. In addition, the lipid transport protein apolipoprotein E4 (ApoE4) has been found to be a component of amyloid precipitates in a study on 14 Japanese patients suffering from either papular or macular PLCA [82,83]. Amyloid K is therefore a key feature of localised cutaneous amyloidoses [3,56,84,85]. The reason for keratinocyte apoptosis in PLCA, however, remains unclear. Some have claimed that a mechanism of apoptosis regulation involving transglutaminase 2 may play a pivotal role in the pathogenesis of PLCA [86,87].

In macular PLCA, friction may play a key pathogenetic role as a mechanical stimulus that may induce apoptosis of basal keratinocytes with subsequent additional cytokeratin (amyloid K precursor) release. In this context, pruritus which provokes scratching of the skin is thought to induce additional amyloid K deposition, which in turn leads to intensified pruritus in a cyclical pattern. However, scratching of intact skin may be the starting point for amyloid K deposition, which is also known as friction or brush amyloidosis. Therefore, friction amyloidosis is sometimes also classified as a form of secondary cutaneous amyloidosis [88,89]. However, there is still controversy regarding friction as a factor in macular PLCA and SLCA. Interestingly, in SLCA, cytokeratin 5 is also the predominant amyloid precursor [56].

The rare form of nodular PLCA is characterised by amyloid that is composed of immunoglobulin light chains (AL amyloid). Plasma cells infiltrating the skin (e.g. in extramedullary plasmocytoma) produce monoclonal immunoglobulin light chains of κ- or λ-type as amyloid precursors. There are two major factors that differentiate nodular amyloidosis from macular and lichenoid amyloidosis. Firstly, nodular amyloid is composed of immunoglobulin light chains derived from a monoclonal expansion of plasma cells [90–92], whereas in papular/macular PLCA amyloid consists of cytokeratins. Secondly, the amyloid of nodular PLCA infiltrates the entire dermis, from the papillary dermis to the subcutis.

In a genome-wide screening of Taiwanese families, evidence for a susceptibility locus on chromosome 5 (5p13.1-q11.2) was found for familial PLCA [93]. Based on this, two distinct mutations of the oncostatin M receptor (*OSMR*) gene (chromosome 5p13.1) in three families with amyloidosis were detected [**94**]. A linkage of familial PLCA to a locus on 1q23 has also been published [95]. Recently, mutations have been discovered in the interleukin 31 (IL-31) receptor A (*IL-31RA*) gene of Taiwanese families with primary familial cutaneous amyloidosis [96]. Interestingly, both *OSMR* and *IL-31RA* are encoded on chromosome 5p, both are cytokine receptors and OSMRβ and IL-31RA can form a heterodimeric receptor. Multiple mutations in the *OSMRβ* gene have been described for familial PLCA [97–**102**]. All mutations affect the extracellular fibronectin type III-like domain of *OSMRβ*, which then fails to heterodimerise and interact with *IL-31RA*. This results in impaired oncostatin M (OSM) and IL-31 signalling, and subsequently in a reduced activation of the JAK/STAT, MAPK and PI3K/Akt pathways [**94**,103]. The associated increase in apoptotic keratinocytes leads to the accumulation of degenerate keratinous material, which may cause pruritus and thereby promote amyloid formation [**94**]. Additionally, *OSMRβ* mutations affect the expression of genes involved in epidermal differentiation and proliferation [98]. These altered gene expression patterns probably account for the lichenification found in patients with familial PLCA.

It has to be noted, however, that *OSMR/IL-31* mutations can also be found in sporadic PLCA [**102**].

Clinical features
Presentation
A characteristic clinical correlate of cutaneous amyloid precipitates is intense pruritus. In papular PLCA, firm papules with pink to brownish lichenoid glossiness (Figure 56.6) are often found on the legs or on the trunk, whereas in macular PLCA, well or vaguely demarcated, hyperpigmented, yellowish to brownish macules (Figure 56.7) often present in the interscapular space or elsewhere on the trunk. Nodular PLCA presents with solitary or multiple, mostly

asymptomatic, brownish to red, firm plaques or nodules, typically on the nose (Figure 56.8a), legs (especially the feet) (Figure 56.8b), genitalia or trunk [69]. However, predilection sites and presentations are quite variable. The clinical presentation of hereditary (familial) PLCA (autosomal dominant) does not significantly differ from non-hereditary papular PLCA. Often lichenification of the skin and tiny dome-shaped papules (Figure 56.9), both predominantly on the ventral body areas, are found.

Clinical variants

A variant of lichenoid and macular amyloidosis is called mixed (biphasic, allotropic) PLCA, in which both lichenoid and macular lesions occur [3,104,105]. In addition, a rare poikilodermatous form of PLCA exists, in which lichenoid or macular lesions occur in combination with blisters and poikilodermatous skin lesions [106]. A familial variant of poikilodermatous PLCA has also been reported [107]. Furthermore, amyloidosis cutis dyschromica is a rare variant with only a few cases reported worldwide [108–110]. The basic clinical features are mottled hyper- and hypopigmented macules with amyloid deposits derived from cytokeratins [108]. Bullous forms of amyloidoses occur both in PLCA and in systemic amyloidoses with cutaneous involvement [111–114].

Differential diagnosis

The differential diagnoses for lichenoid and macular PLCA (see Table 56.1) include xanthomas, perforating dermatoses (collagenoses), nodular PLCA, lichen planus and mycosis fungoides. Differential diagnoses for nodular PLCA include squamous cell carcinoma, verruca vulgaris, adnexal tumours and keloid/hypertrophic scars. The lesions found in different types of PLCA may appear similar to many of the already mentioned diseases, and a diagnostic biopsy is warranted.

Complications and disease course

Data on the disease course of the different forms of PLCA are sparse. While in papular and macular PLCA the aesthetic aspect is often quite problematic and pruritus may be a debilitating symptom, nodular PLCA can even progress to systemic amyloidosis. The rate of progression of nodular PLCA to systemic amyloidosis is controversial [71]: figures between 5% and 50% have been quoted. In 1970, Brownstein and Helwig determined that the risk for this progression was 50% based on a cohort of 10 patients [104]. Woollons and Black looked retrospectively at 15 cases of nodular PLCA and found only one case that progressed to systemic amyloidosis [115]. Northcutt and Vanover determined a progression rate of 15% based on 47 cases of PLCA [116]. However, this study included the original Brownstein and Helwig study, thus adding five patients that may have had systemic amyloidosis to begin with. Because of this, the true rate of progression of the 47 cases researched by Northcutt and Vanover is anywhere between 5% and 15%. Given the data available and the understanding that nodular PLCA appears to be a localised clonal plasmacytoma [3,117,118], it is likely that the true rate of progression is quite low.

Management
See later.

Cutaneous amyloidoses due to systemic disease

Definition
Cutaneous amyloidoses due to systemic disease comprise three groups: (i) non-hereditary systemic amyloidoses with cutaneous involvement; (ii) hereditary systemic amyloidoses with cutaneous involvement; and (iii) hereditary systemic diseases with secondary cutaneous amyloidosis. In the group of non-hereditary systemic amyloidoses with cutaneous involvement, there are primary and myeloma- or plasmocytoma-associated amyloidoses as well as amyloidosis due to Waldenström macroglobulinaemia (amyloid light and/or heavy chains, AL/AH), secondary amyloidoses associated with inflammation or tumours, and haemodialysis-associated forms. The group of hereditary systemic amyloidoses with cutaneous involvement comprises hereditary transthyretin amyloidosis (familial amyloid polyneuropathy), hereditary apolipoprotein A1 amyloidosis, hereditary cystatin C amyloidosis and hereditary gelsolin amyloidosis (Meretoja syndrome). The last group of hereditary systemic diseases with secondary cutaneous amyloid precipitation consists of Muckle–Wells syndrome and tumour necrosis factor (TNF) receptor 1 associated periodic fever syndrome (TRAPS) (Chapter 45). Details are given in Table 56.2.

Introduction and general description
Systemic amyloidoses (Table 56.2) are often characterised by amyloid deposition in mesenchymal structures of the internal organs such as heart muscle, liver and kidneys which may lead to a progressive loss of function and eventually to death. As mentioned, there are also hereditary systemic amyloidoses and systemic diseases with secondary cutaneous involvement. In cutaneous involvement, all skin layers as well as vessel walls may be affected.

Epidemiology
Systemic amyloidoses show cutaneous involvement in about 50% of patients which allows physicians to diagnose the underlying systemic disease at an early stage [119]. An association of acquired von Willebrand syndrome (avWS) and immunoglobulin light chain amyloidosis has been described [120]. For the epidemiology of the different forms of cutaneous amyloidoses due to systemic disease, see Table 56.2 and the full reference list.

Pathophysiology
Most non-hereditary primary systemic amyloidoses are caused by monoclonal plasma cell proliferation. The underlying diseases comprise entities such as multiple myeloma, Waldenström disease, Bence Jones plasmocytoma, heavy chain disease and malignant lymphomas. The common feature of these diseases is the production of monoclonal immunoglobulins [47,121]. Mostly immunoglobulin light chains (isotypes κ and λ) serve as amyloid prescursors (AL = light chain type/Bence Jones amyloid; AL-κ : AL-λ ratio of 1 : 2). However, patients with Waldenström macroglobulinaemia can develop immunoglobulin heavy chain amyloidosis (AH = heavy chain amyloid) and/or immunoglobulin light chain amyloidosis [122]. Despite the clinical variability of AL-type amyloidoses, petechiae and purpura of the face (Figure 56.10) or intertriginous

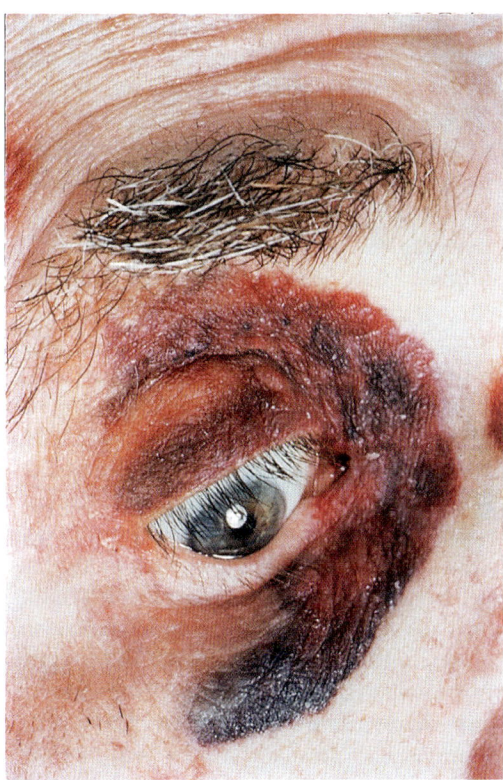

Figure 56.10 Primary systemic amyloidosis with cutaneous involvement showing prominent periorbital bleeding following coughing. Courtesy of St John's Institute of Dermatology.

areas (which may be additionally triggered by friction; Figure 56.11) can be considered as cutaneous features of amyloid. Among the suspected reasons for hemorrhages are that factor X is decreased by binding to amyloid fibrils and that amyloid deposits in the blood vessel walls increase vessel wall fragility.

Amyloid precipitation within the oral cavity mucosa may present as papules in a local deposition (e.g. infiltrates in the lower lip; Figure 56.12) or as macroglossia in a diffuse infiltration (Figure 56.13).

In secondary systemic amyloidoses, a specific underlying disease leads to the deposition of amyloid in different tissues. The disease determines the amyloid precursor structure and hence the type of amyloid, with the most common variant being AA-type amyloidosis. Chronic inflammation (infectious or non-infectious) or neoplastic diseases, as well as sporadic gene defects, lead to enhanced production of SAA, an acute phase protein. Interestingly, experimental cutaneous amyloidosis due to *Leishmania* infection has been described [123]. Hepatic production of SAA is stimulated by IL-1 (and other interleukins), and macrophages degrade SAA to amyloid A. However, skin signs are very rare and manifest as purpura, plaques or nodules. Clinically normal skin may show amyloid A deposition. Secondary amyloidoses of the AA type show a tendency to regress if the underlying disease is treated effectively.

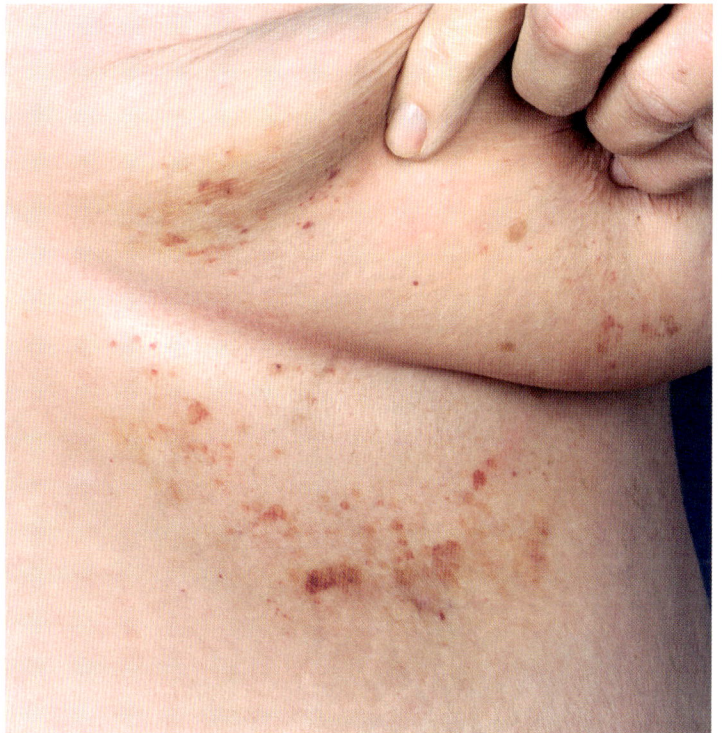

(a)

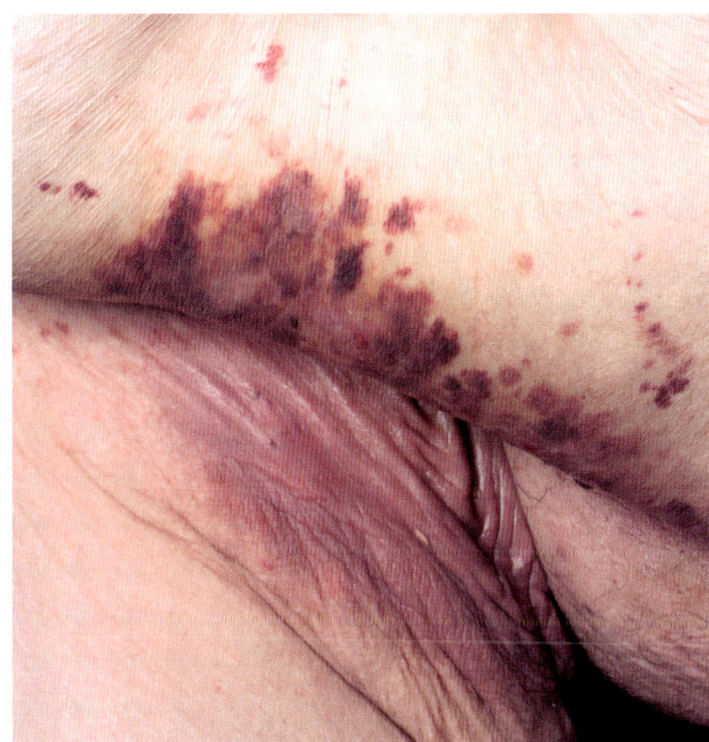

(b)

Figure 56.11 Plasmacytoma-associated systemic amyloidosis with cutaneous involvement: (a) submammary region and (b) inguinal region. From [127]/The Korean Dermatological Association and The Korean Society for Investigative Dermatology.

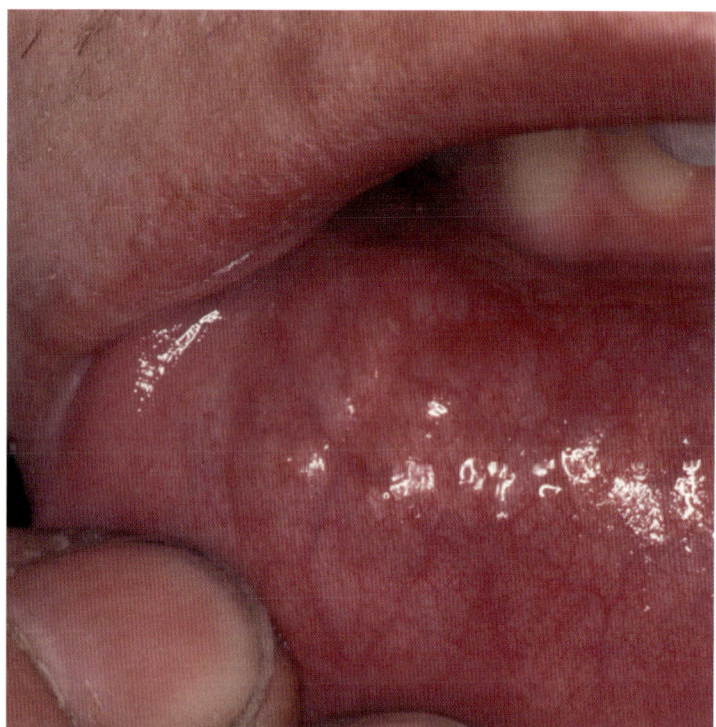

Figure 56.12 Systemic amyloidosis with mucocutaneous involvement showing nodular amyloid infiltrates on the lower lip.

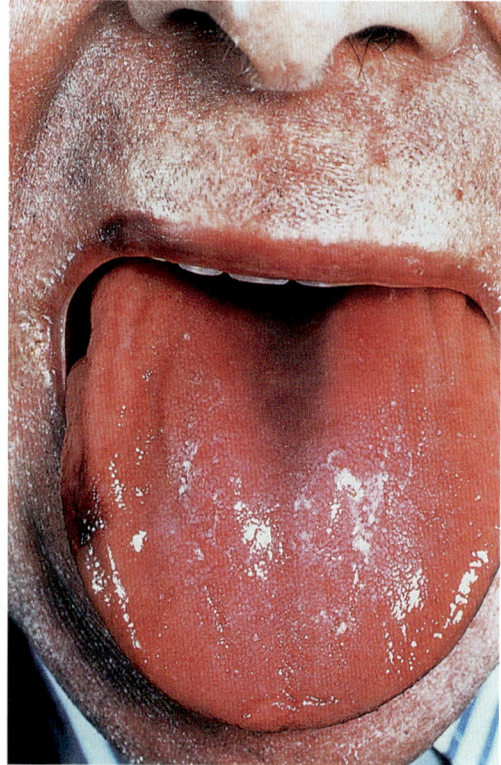

Figure 56.13 Macroglossia in a patient with primary systemic amyloidosis. Courtesy of St John's Institute of Dermatology.

Another variant of secondary systemic amyloidosis with cutaneous involvement occurs in haemodialysis patients with β_2-microglobulin (β-sheet structure) as the amyloid precursor (Table 56.2) [3,124].

In TRAPS, a mutation of the extracellular domain of the TNF receptor 1 leads to inflammatory reactions with subsequent SAA precipitation. Muckle–Wells syndrome is one of the cryopyrin-associated periodic (fever) syndromes (CAPS) and is caused by *NLRP3* mutations. These lead to increased IL-1β signalling, which again triggers hepatic SAA synthesis.

Clinical features

The clinical presentation of cutaneous involvement in systemic amyloidoses is often characterised by petechiae, haemorrhages, ecchymosis and pruritus. Bleeding is often seen in the periorbital (Figure 56.10) or intertriginous (Figure 56.11) regions [125–127] due to the deposition of amyloid in and around vascular structures, a deposition pattern that is rarely seen in localised cutaneous amyloidoses. The only exception to this rule is nodular amyloidosis, in which perivascular amyloid deposition may also be encountered and in which the histology may bear a strong resemblance to systemic amyloidosis with cutaneous involvement.

Typically, amyloid purpura occurs above the nipple line, mostly on the head and neck, especially on the eyelids [47,125]. As purpura may be the first sign of systemic amyloidoses, it is important to bear this sign in mind. The suspected diagnosis of amyloidosis may be the starting point for a multidisciplinary treatment approach as different organs may be involved [128].

As a clinical variant of light chain amyloidoses, bullous cutaneous manifestations (Figure 56.14) [112] (sometimes haemorrhagic [114]) or bullous manifestations of the mucosa [113] may occur.

Confluent white to yellowish, waxy, partially haemorrhagic papules or nodules can be found that predominantly occur on the face, eyelids and scalp. In severe cases, these lesions may lead to ulceration and scarring alopecia. If the dermis is extensively infiltrated by amyloid, scleroderma-like skin changes (especially of the fingers) may occur, known as scleroderma amyloidosum Gottron. Also, blisters and nail dystrophy (Figure 56.15) have been reported as manifestations of myeloma-associated amyloidosis [111]. Bullous forms of amyloidoses occur both in PLCA and in systemic amyloidoses with cutaneous involvement (Figure 56.14) [111–114].

Among the hereditary subtypes, the most common is familial amyloid polyneuropathy due to the deposition of altered transthyretin (a protein of the prealbumin fraction) [129,130]. This form is mainly caused by a Val30Met mutation [131]. Other forms of hereditary amyloidoses are associated with cardiomyopathy (apolipoprotein A1 amyloidosis), multiple cerebral haemorrhages (cystatin C amyloidosis) or carpal tunnel syndrome (familial amyloid polyneuropathy) [132]. In contrast to apolipoprotein A1 amyloidosis, cystatin C amyloidosis is clinically asymptomatic with no skin signs, but histology may show typical amyloid deposition. Massive deforming cutis laxa, extensive petechiae and haemorrhages, as well as hypotrichosis or alopecia, can be seen in gelsolin amyloidosis, also known as Meretoja syndrome [133,134]. Different mutations result in an amino acid exchange [135]. A Dutch (654G-T) and a Finnish (654G-A) variant have been described [136].

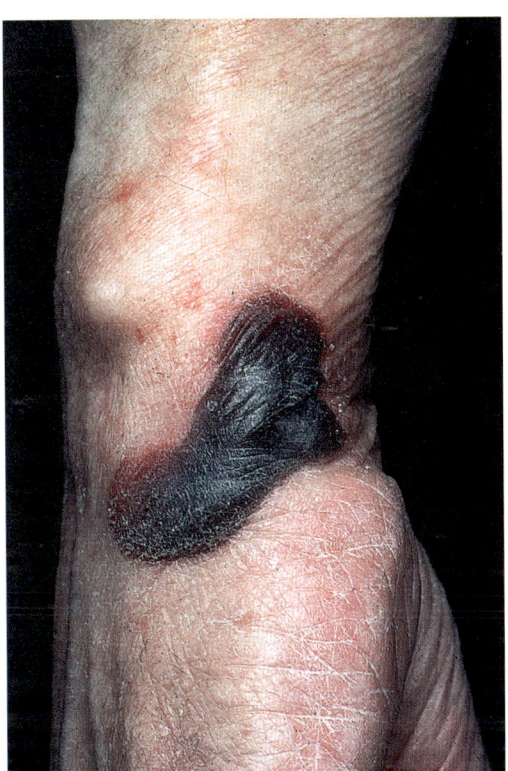

Figure 56.14 Haemorrhagic bulla in primary systemic amyloidosis. Courtesy of St John's Institute of Dermatology.

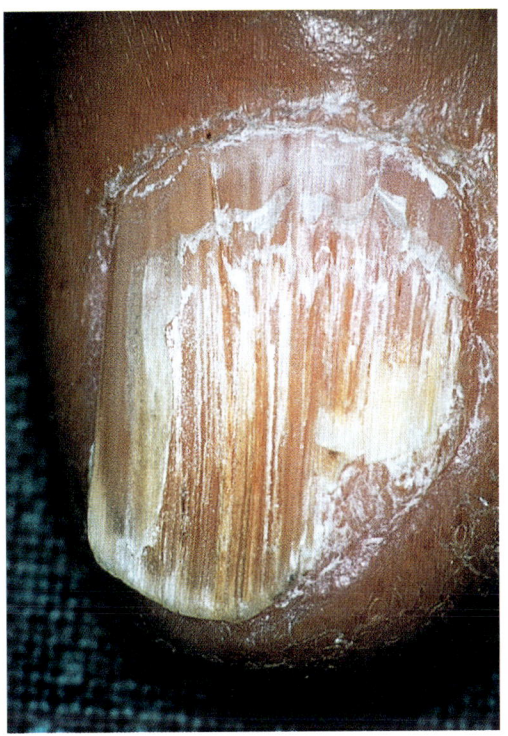

Figure 56.15 Nail dystrophy in a patient with primary systemic amyloidosis. Courtesy of St John's Institute of Dermatology.

The combination of prolonged fever episodes, abdominal pain, myalgia and migrating cutaneous erythemas is characteristic of the rare TRAPS [137,138], which results in secondary cutaneous amyloidosis (presumably amyloid SAA). Another rare syndrome also associated with secondary cutaneous amyloid deposition (presumably amyloid SAA) is Muckle–Wells syndrome, which is characterised by cutaneous amyloid deposition, periodic urticaria-like skin lesions and the development of sensorineural hearing loss [139,140].

Management of cutaneous amyloidoses

The treatment of the different forms of cutaneous amyloidosis remains a challenge for all medical disciplines involved. A multidisciplinary approach should be undertaken, and in cases of systemic amyloidosis the treatment of any underlying disease has the highest priority.

In all types of cutaneous amyloidosis, pruritus is often a major problem leading to further skin irritation, which can cause secondary amyloid precipitation. Therefore, antipruritic treatment should be one component of the treatment regimen. Due to the low number of affected patients, few treatment strategies have been studied in detail, and most of the treatment options are therefore recommended based on studies with small sample sizes or case reports.

Topical treatment should be tried in cases of PLCA (Figure 56.16) with conservative treatment modalities being first line. These options may be followed or combined with laser or surgical

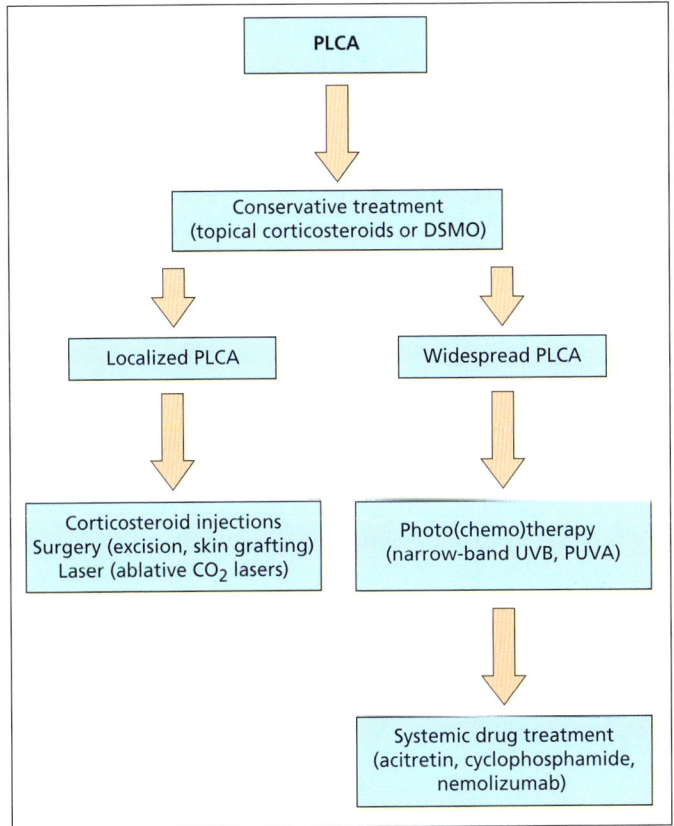

Figure 56.16 Treatment options for primary localised cutaneous amyloidosis (PLCA). DMSO, dimethyl sulfoxide; PUVA, psoralen and UVA radiation; UV, ultraviolet.

PART 5: METABOLIC & NUTRITIONAL DISORDERS

approaches in cases of localised lesions. In contrast, PLCA with widespread lesions may require the additional use of photo(chemo)-therapy and/or systemic drug treatment (dimethyl sulfoxide (DMSO), acitretin, cyclophosphamide). In systemic amyloidoses, the major principle is to treat the underlying disease.

Topical treatment

Topical administration of corticosteroids (with occlusive dressings) or intralesional corticosteroid injections are the classic standard treatments [2]. Others have reported success with phototherapy (narrow-band UVB) and photochemotherapy (PUVA) [141]. Otherwise, DMSO (up to 50%) may be topically applied to relieve pruritus [142]. However, some researchers have not found DMSO to have antipruritic effects or amyloid-dissolving properties [143].

Depending on the clinical presentation, surgical treatment strategies may be helpful when conservative treatments are of limited efficacy (e.g. in nodular PLCA). Efficient surgical treatment strategies involve excision and split-thickness skin grafting [144], dermabrasion [145] and shave excision [75], as well as curettage and cautery [90]. Other modalities such as pulsed dye laser treatments [146] and carbon dioxide laser evaporation [147] have also been successfully used in some cases.

Systemic treatment

Localised amyloidosis. There is one review of case reports discussing the effect of oral retinoids, such as acitretin, in the treatment of lichen amyloidosis [148]. This review shows that oral retinoids administered over about 6 months may lead to a complete remission of papular PLCA (lichen amyloidosis). A case has also been reported regarding the use of oral acitretin in the treatment of mixed (biphasic, allotropic) PLCA. Relief of pruritus, an improvement of the papules and discrete clearance of hyperpigmentation were observed after 4 months' treatment with 0.5 mg/kg body weight of oral acitretin daily [148]. DMSO can be topically applied, but there are also reports on the efficacy of oral DMSO in the treatment of systemic amyloidoses with cutaneous involvement [149]. With respect to papular PLCA, there is one study reporting on significantly reduced pruritus, hyperpigmentation and lesion size after 50 mg per day oral cyclophosphamide over 6 months [150]. Often, the same treatment modalities are used for macular PLCA.

Systemic amyloidosis. In systemic amyloidoses, it is crucial to treat the underlying cause if possible (e.g. multiple myeloma, plasmocytoma, renal insufficiency). Future treatments with siR-NAs or anti-amyloid antibodies are under development [151,152]. The finding of IL-31 as a key player in pruritus has led to the development of an antibody against IL-31 (nemolizumab), which shows great promise in the treatment of atopic dermatitis, prurigo nodularis and potentially cutaneous amyloidosis [153–155]. Interestingly, the role of IL-31 was found to be crucial in familial PLCA (see previously).

Primary systemic amyloidoses or diseases with secondary cutaneous amyloid precipitation should always be treated by a multidisciplinary team. When there is an identifiable underlying disease leading to cutaneous amyloid deposition, all efforts should be made to slow down or stop the progress of the disease [156].

Immunosuppression is a core component in the treatment of systemic amyloidoses secondary to inflammation. For instance, AA amyloidosis resulting from familial Mediterranean fever (FMF) can be improved using colchicine [156]. The addition of anakinra (IL-1 receptor antagonist, IL-1Ra) [157] to colchicine may be beneficial in the treatment of FMF-associated amyloidosis as it tempers the underlying inflammatory reactions. TRAPS-associated amyloidoses may also be treated by TNF blockade and IL-1 antagonists [156]. Muckle–Wells syndrome is one of the cryopyrin-associated periodic (fever) syndromes caused by *NLRP3* mutations. IL-1β is up-regulated in this group of diseases, and therefore treatment options include canakinumab (IL-1β antibody), rilonacept (IL-1-binding protein) and anakinra (IL-1Ra) [158–162]. Other strategies, such as the administration of intravenous immunoglobulins and plasma exchange, have also been successfully used in the treatment of primary systemic amyloidoses [163]. An increasing number of patients with $A\beta_2$ amyloidosis are expected as haemodialysis has enabled the long-term survival of patients with severe chronic renal failure [164,165]. Improvement of renal function so that haemodialysis may be stopped is the key to improving and possibly completely resolving $A\beta_2$ amyloidosis.

Key references

The full list of references can be found in the online version at https://www.wiley.com/rooksdermatology10e

2 Breathnach SM. The cutaneous amyloidoses. Pathogenesis and therapy. *Arch Dermatol* 1985;121:470–5.

3 Breathnach SM. Amyloid and amyloidosis. *J Am Acad Dermatol* 1988;18:1–16.

4 Glenner GG. Amyloid deposits and amyloidosis. The beta-fibrilloses (first of two parts). *N Engl J Med* 1980;302:1283–92.

48 Li WM. Histopathology of primary cutaneous amyloidoses and systemic amyloidosis. *Clin Dermatol* 1990;8:30–5.

49 Wechalekar AD, Gillmore JD, Hawkins PN. Systemic amyloidosis. *Lancet* 2016;387(10038):2641–54.

50 Haverkampf S, Evert K, Schroder J, Schreml S. Nodular cutaneous amyloidosis resembling a giant tumor. *Case Rep Dermatol* 2016;8:22–5.

59 Westermark P, Davey E, Lindbom K, Enqvist S. Subcutaneous fat tissue for diagnosis and studies of systemic amyloidosis. *Acta Histochem* 2006;108:209–13.

94 Arita K, South AP, Hans-Filho G *et al.* Oncostatin M receptor-beta mutations underlie familial primary localized cutaneous amyloidosis. *Am J Hum Genet* 2008;82:73–80.

102 Lu P, Wu FF, Rong ZL *et al.* Clinical and genetic features of Chinese patients with lichen and macular primary localized cutaneous amyloidosis. *Clin Exp Dermatol* 2019;44:e110–17.

104 Brownstein MH, Helwig EB. The cutaneous amyloidoses. I. Localized forms. *Arch Dermatol* 1970;102:8–19.

CHAPTER 57

Cutaneous Mucinoses

Franco Rongioletti

Dermatology Clinic, University Vita-Salute San Raffaele Hospital, Milan, Italy

PART 5: METABOLIC & NUTRITIONAL DISORDERS

Introduction and general description

The cutaneous mucinoses are a heterogeneous group of disorders whose main characteristic is abnormal mucin deposition in the skin [1]. Mucin or protein–hyaluronic acid complex is a normal component of the dermal extracellular matrix produced in small amounts by fibroblasts. It is a jelly-like amorphous mixture of acid glycosaminoglycans (formerly called acid mucopolysaccharides) that are repeating polysaccharides forming a complex carbohydrate. The acid glycosaminoglycans may be fixed on both sides of a protein core (proteoglycan monomer) as in the case of dermatan sulphate or chondroitin-6-sulphate and chondroitin-4-sulphate, or they may be free as in the case of hyaluronic acid, which is the most important component of dermal mucin.

Mucin is capable of absorbing 1000 times its own weight in water, thus playing a major role in maintaining the salt and water balance of the dermis. However, in disease conditions, mucin is increased and since it holds water (hygroscopic), the dermal connective tissue is oedematous. Mucin may be seen on haematoxylin and eosin stains as a light blue-stained material between collagen bundles; however, to highlight these changes special stains are usually needed such as Alcian blue at pH 2.5 (negative at 0.4) or colloidal iron and toluidine blue at pH 4.0. Furthermore, mucin is hyaluronidase sensitive and periodic acid–Schiff (PAS) negative [2].

Mostly for experimental research, monoclonal or polyclonal antibodies have been used to detect heparan sulphate proteoglycans, the three isoforms of hyaluronan synthase and the CD44 surface receptor for hyaluronate [3,4,5]. The pathogenesis of increased mucin deposition in pathological states is unclear. It has been postulated that serum factors such as cytokines and/or immunoglobulins may induce upregulation of glycosaminoglycan synthesis. Cytokines that may play a role in the process include tumour necrosis factor α (TNF-α) and TNF-β, interleukin 1 (IL-1), IL-6 and transforming growth factor β (TGF-β) [1]. A decrease in the catabolic process of mucin degradation could also be involved. Many of the cutaneous mucinoses show increased levels of polyclonal or monoclonal immunoglobulin (e.g. scleromyxoedema, pretibial myxoedema and papulonodular mucinosis of lupus erythematosus).

In Chinese Shar-Pei dogs, known for their distinctive features of deep wrinkles, mucin deposition in the skin is a typical condition and considered to be a consequence of a genetic defect in the metabolism of hyaluronic acid [6].

The cutaneous mucinoses are divided into two groups: primary (idiopathic) cutaneous mucinoses in which the mucin deposit is the main histological feature resulting in clinically distinctive lesions; and secondary mucinoses in which histological mucin deposition is only an additional finding and secondary phenomenon (Box 57.1). Primary mucinoses can be divided into dermal and follicular mucinoses. The former includes lichen myxoedematosus (generalised and localised), reticular erythematous mucinosis, scleroedema, mucinoses in thyroid disease, papular and nodular mucinosis in connective tissue diseases, self-healing cutaneous mucinosis, cutaneous focal mucinosis and myxoid cyst, while the latter include Pinkus follicular mucinosis and urticaria-like follicular mucinosis. Systemic manifestations associated with mucinoses include monoclonal gammopathies in scleromyxoedema and scleroedema, diabetes or infections in scleroedema, hyperthyroidism in pretibial myxoedema, hypothyroidism in generalised myxoedema and lupus erythematosus, and dermatomyositis or scleroderma in papular and nodular mucinosis in connective tissue diseases.

Box 57.1 Classification of cutaneous mucinoses

Primary

Dermal mucinoses

- Lichen myxoedematosus (papular mucinosis):
  - Generalised and sclerodermoid lichen myxoedematosus (scleromyxoedema)
  - Localised lichen myxoedematosus:
    - Acral persistent papular mucinosis
    - Discrete papular lichen myxoedematosus
    - Cutaneous (papular) mucinosis of infancy
    - Nodular lichen myxoedematosus
- Reticular erythematous mucinosis
- Scleroedema
- Myxoedema in thyroid disease:
  - Localised (pretibial) myxoedema
  - Generalised myxoedema
- Papular and nodular mucinosis in connective tissue diseases
- Self-healing (juvenile) cutaneous mucinosis
- Cutaneous focal mucinosis
- Digital myxoid (mucous) cyst

Follicular mucinoses

- Pinkus follicular mucinosis (alopecia mucinosa)
- Urticaria-like follicular mucinosis

Secondary

Epidermal

- Mycosis fungoides
- Keratoacanthoma
- Basal cell carcinoma

Dermal

- Granuloma annulare
- Connective tissue diseases (lupus erythematosus, dermatomyositis)
- Degos disease
- Nephrogenic systemic fibrosis
- Hereditary progressive mucinous histiocytosis
- Obesity-associated lymphoedematous mucinosis
- Hypertrophic scars
- Chronic graft-versus-host disease
- Cutaneous reactions to interferon
- Herpes zoster
- Stasis dermatitis due to venous insufficiency
- Epithelial tumours (basal cell carcinoma)
- Mesenchymal tumours (dermatofibrosarcoma protuberans)
- Neural tumours (neurofibroma)

Follicular

- Haematological malignancies (mycosis fungoides)
- Eczematous dermatoses
- Lupus erythematosus
- Cutaneous drug reactions (imatinib, captopril)
- Insect bites

PRIMARY MUCINOSES

DERMAL MUCINOSES

Lichen myxoedematosus (papular mucinosis)

Definition

Lichen myxoedematosus (LM) is a comprehensive term to define a chronic, idiopathic cutaneous mucinosis characterised by lichenoid papules, nodules and/or plaques due to abnormal dermal mucin deposition and a variable degree of fibrosis and fibroblast proliferation in the absence of thyroid disease. Two clinicopathological subsets are included: (i) a generalised papular and sclerodermoid form (also called scleromyxoedema of Arndt–Gottron) with a monoclonal gammopathy and systemic, sometimes lethal, manifestations; and (ii) a localised papular form which does not have systemic implications. Occasionally, patients with LM have overlapping or atypical features and fall between scleromyxoedema and localised LM (Table 57.1) [1].

Scleromyxoedema

Definition and nomenclature

Scleromyxoedema is the sclerotic variant of LM characterised by a generalised papular eruption on a sclerodermoid background, mucin deposition, increased fibroblast proliferation, fibrosis and monoclonal gammopathy [2]. It has systemic implications.

Synonyms and inclusions
- Generalised papular and sclerodermoid LM
- Arndt–Gottron disease
- Generalised lichenoid papular eruption (Montgomery and Underwood)

Epidemiology

Scleromyxoedema is a rare disease that usually affects adults between the ages of 30 and 80 years. The mean age of patients is 59 years. The illness has no ethnic or sex predominance and has rarely been reported in infants and young children [2].

Pathophysiology

The pathogenesis of scleromyxoedema is unknown. Some cytokines such as TNF-α, TNF-β, IL-1, IL-6 and TGF-β and/or polyclonal and monoclonal immunoglobulins and other unidentified factors in the serum of affected patients may induce upregulation of glycosaminoglycan synthesis from fibroblasts. Although monoclonal paraprotein has been considered pathogenic, the stimulation of fibroblasts occurs even after the removal of the paraprotein

Table 57.1 Classification of lichen myxoedematosus with diagnostic criteria.

Scleromyxoedema	Localised variants of lichen myxoedematosus	Atypical forms of lichen myxoedematosus
Generalised papular eruption and sclerodermoid features	Papular eruption (or nodules and/or plaques due to confluence of papules)	Scleromyxoedema without monoclonal gammopathy
Microscopic triad (mucin deposition, fibroblast proliferation, fibrosis) or interstitial granulomatous pattern	Mucin deposition with variable fibroblast proliferation and absent fibrosis	Localised lichen myxoedematosus with monoclonal gammopathy and/or systemic symptoms
Monoclonal gammopathy	Absence of monoclonal gammopathy	Localised forms with mixed features of the subtypes
Absence of thyroid disorder	Absence of thyroid disorder	Other poorly defined variants
	Subtypes:	
	Discrete papular mucinosis	
	Acral persistent papular mucinosis	
	Papular mucinosis of infancy	
	Nodular form	

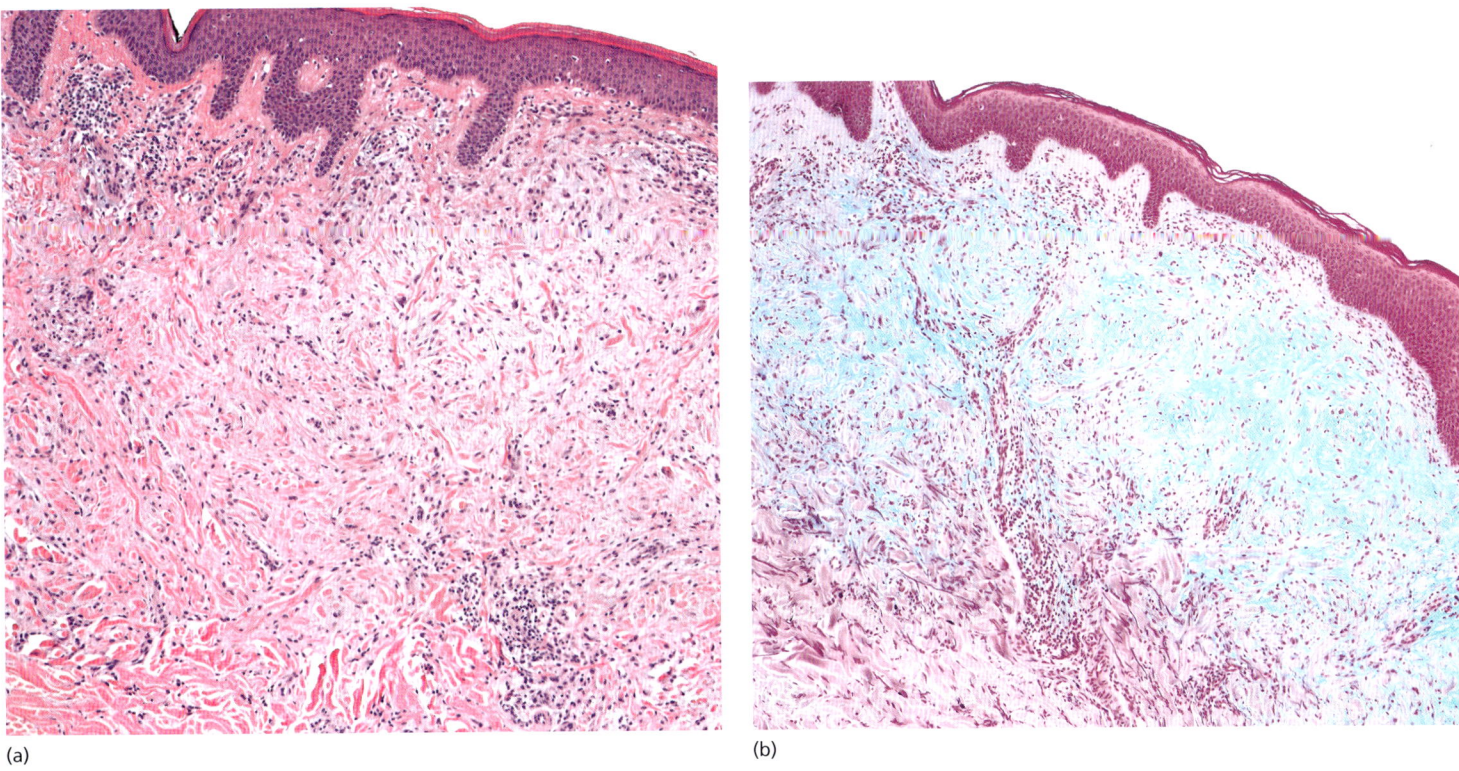

(a)   (b)

Figure 57.1 (a) Scleromyxoedema. The typical triad of microscopic features with diffuse dermal mucin deposition, fibroblast proliferation and fibrotic collagen. (b) Increased dermal mucin stained with Alcian blue at pH 2.5.

[3] In addition, paraprotein levels usually do not correlate with the severity of disease, disease progression or the response to treatment [2]. An abnormally high IL-4 secretion and a profibrotic cytokine have been recently found in the serum of scleromyxoedema patients suggesting a chronic T helper 2 (Th2)-skewed T-cell response against an unknown target antigen [4]. Finally, case reports documenting the development of scleromyxoedema following a cutaneous granulomatous reaction after intradermal hyaluronic gel injections or after breast silicone implantation [5] may suggest a type of autoimmune syndrome induced by adjuvants.

Pathology

Scleromyxoedema is characterised by a triad of microscopic features (Figure 57.1a): (i) a diffuse deposit of mucin composed mostly of hyaluronic acid in the upper and mid-reticular dermis confirmed with an Alcian blue stain at pH 2.5 (Figure 57.1b) or an iron colloidal

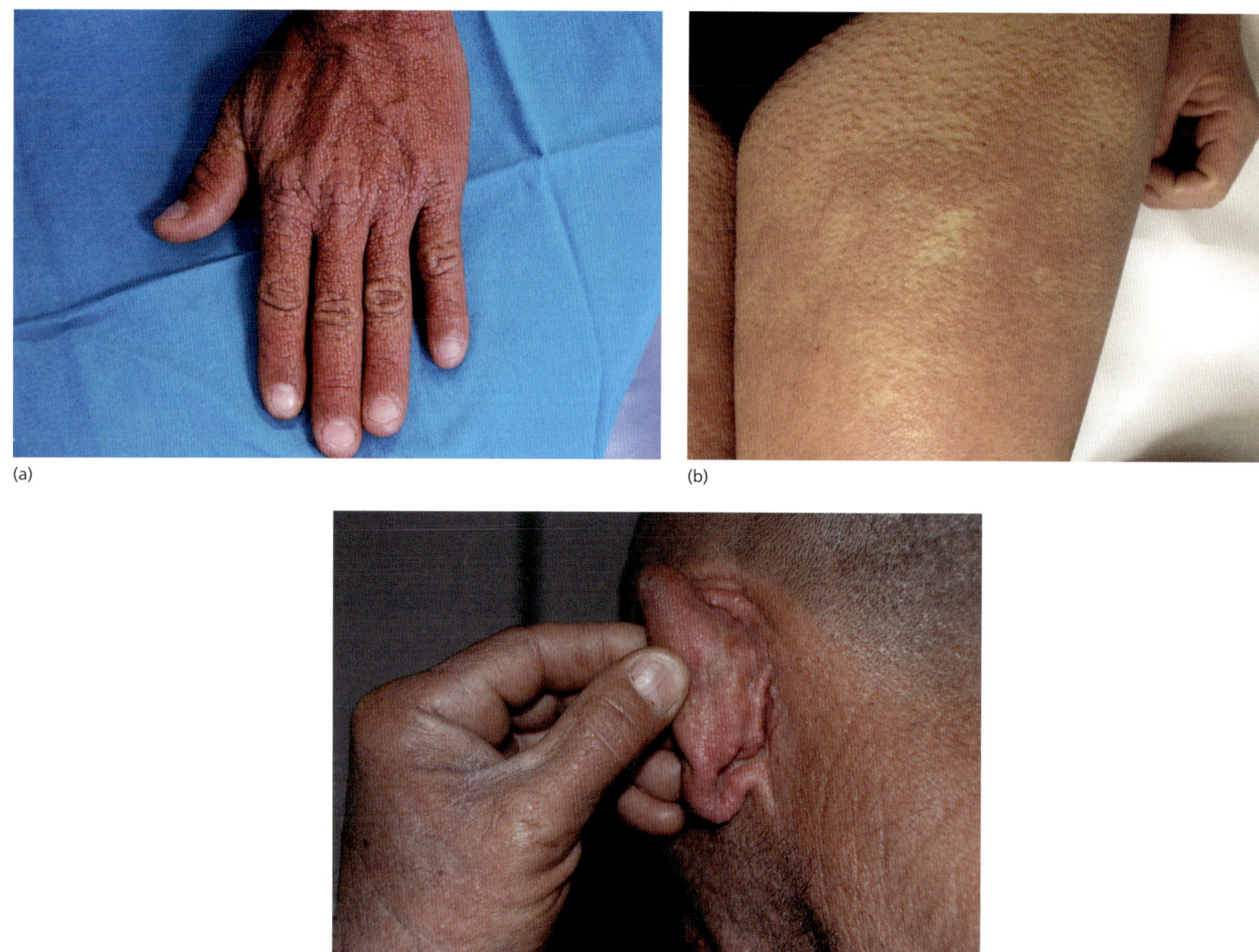

Figure 57.2 Scleromyxoedema. (a) Widespread eruption of closely spaced papules on the back of the hand. (b) Papules on the thigh. (c) Papules behind the ear.

stain and hyaluronidase digestion; (ii) an increase in collagen deposition; and (iii) a proliferation of irregularly arranged fibroblasts [6]. The epidermis may be normal or thinned, the hair follicles may be atrophic and a slight perivascular superficial lymphoplasmacytic infiltrate is often present. The elastic fibres are fragmented and decreased in number. An interstitial granuloma annulare-like pattern with histiocytic CD68+ or CD163+ infiltrate has been described [6,7]. In addition to skin involvement, mucin may fill the endocardium, the walls of myocardial blood vessels as well as the interstitium of the kidney, lungs, pancreas, adrenal glands and nerves. Lymph node involvement may occur [8].

Clinical features

The typical skin features are those of a widespread eruption of 2–3 mm, firm, waxy, closely spaced, dome-shaped or flat-topped papules involving the dorsal aspect of the upper limbs, head and neck region, upper trunk and thighs (Figure 57.2) [1,2]. Papules often are arranged in a strikingly linear pattern; the surrounding skin is shiny and thick (i.e. sclerodermoid in appearance). Rarely,

non-tender nodules may develop. The glabella typically is involved with deep longitudinal folding that gives the appearance of a leonine face (Figure 57.3). Deep furrowing is also evident on the trunk, shoulders and limbs (Shar-Pei sign) giving patients a cutis-laxa like aspect (Figure 57.4). Redness, oedema and a brownish discoloration may be seen in the involved areas, and itching is not uncommon. Eyebrow, axillary and pubic hair may be sparse. Mucosal lesions are absent. As the condition progresses, red and infiltrated plaques develop with skin stiffening, sclerodactyly and reduced mobility of the mouth and the joints of the hands, arms and legs. Over the proximal interphalangeal joints, a central depression surrounded by an elevated rim (due to the skin thickening) is referred to as the 'doughnut sign' (Figure 57.5). Telangiectasia and calcinosis are lacking but Raynaud phenomenon may rarely occur.

Differential diagnosis

These are listed in Table 57.2 [9].

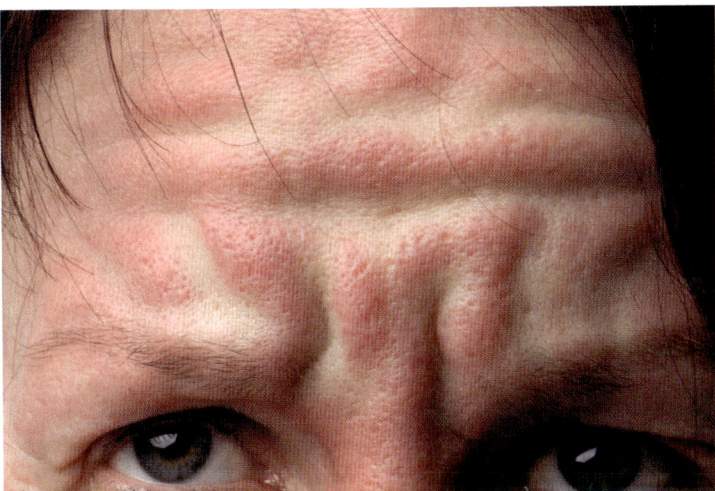

Figure 57.3 Scleromyxoedema. Deep, longitudinal, reddened folding of the skin on the forehead (leonine face). Courtesy of D. Metze, MD, Munster, Germany.

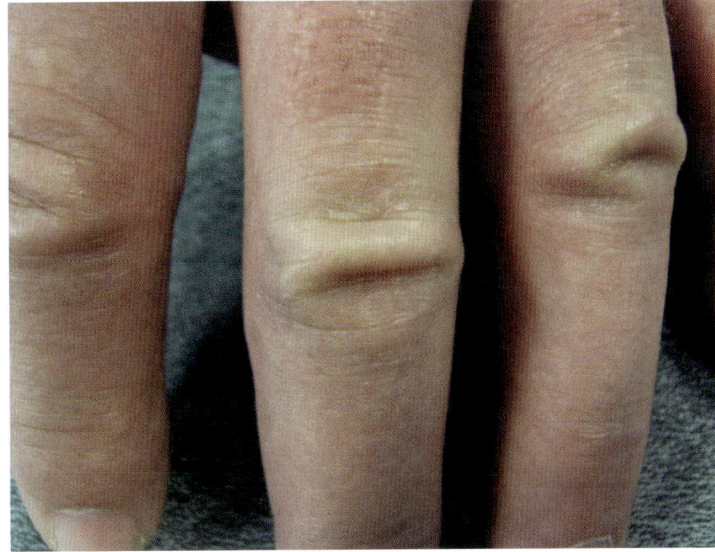

Figure 57.5 Scleromyxoedema. 'Doughnut sign' on the proximal interphalangeal joints.

Table 57.2 Differential diagnoses of scleromyxoedema.

Disease	Differences from scleromyxoedema
Scleroderma (systemic sclerosis)	Absence of papules
	Antinuclear antibodies
	Anticentromere antibody
	AntiScl70 antibody
Scleroedema	Symmetrical non-pitting induration of neck and upper trunk without papules
	Antecedent upper respiratory infection
	Diabetes
Nephrogenic systemic fibrosis	Renal dysfunction and exposure to gadolinium
	Lack of facial involvement and lack of monoclonal gammopathy

Adapted from Ferreli *et al*. [**9**].

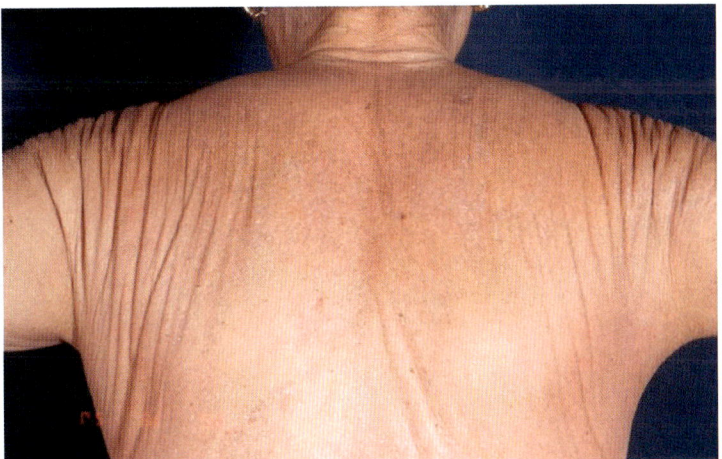

Figure 57.4 Scleromyxoedema. Deep furrowing on the shoulders and back (Shar-Pei sign).

Complications and co-morbidities

Systemic implications are listed in Table 57.3.

Disease course and prognosis

The prognosis of scleromyxoedema is variable. Scleromyxoedema follows a chronic, progressive and sometimes unpredictable course [**2**]. Involvement of the central nervous system, heart, kidney or progression to overt myeloma worsens the prognosis. The main causes of death include dermatoneuro syndrome (scleromyxoedema with concomitant fever, convulsions and coma), cardiovascular complications and haematological malignancies [**2,10**]. Septic complications are mostly linked to melphalan therapy, which is now less commonly used [**1**]. Over the last 30 years, there has been a progressive improvement in the mortality of scleromyxoedema patients decreasing from 35% in 1995, to 23.8% in 2013, and to 3% in a 2020 study that has been partially attributed to the influence of therapy, especially the use of intravenous immunoglobulin [**10**].

Investigations

In addition to skin biopsy, serum electrophoresis with immunofixation is mandatory. Thyroid function test results are normal. Other laboratory tests are usually normal, except in cases of specific extracutaneous symptoms where the internal organs affected should be evaluated. There is little value in imaging studies, although high-resolution cutaneous ultrasonography may become a useful diagnostic and disease activity monitoring tool for skin thickening.

Management

There is no evidence to support any specific definitive treatment for scleromyxoedema because of the rarity of the disorder. There is a limited number of case reports and a lack of randomised controlled trials with incomplete aetiopathogenetic understanding of the disease. In addition, significant toxicity including death, often associated with some therapies such as melphalan, make therapeutic choices more difficult. Intravenous immunoglobulin therapy (alone or in combination with other drugs) has gained widespread acceptance as the first line therapy for both skin involvement and extracutaneous manifestations [**2,9–12**]. Although remissions persisting for a few months and up to 3 years after cessation of

Table 57.3 Systemic implications of scleromyxoedema [2,9,10].

Systemic implications	Type	%
Haematological	Monoclonal gammopathy (> immunoglobulin G lambda)	100 (diagnostic criterion)
	Myeloma, Hodgkin and non-Hodgkin lymphoma, Waldenström macroglobulinaemia, myelomonocytic leukaemia	Rare
Neurological	Carpal tunnel syndrome, peripheral sensory and motor neuropathy, central nervous system symptoms (memory loss, vertigo, gait problems, stroke, seizures, psychosis, dermatoneuro syndrome)	30
Rheumatological	Arthralgias/arthritis, inflammatory myopathy and fibromyalgia	25
Cardiovascular	Congestive heart failure, myocardial ischaemia, heart block and pericardial effusion	5–22
Pulmonary	Obstructive or restrictive lung involvement	17–35
Gastrointestinal	Dysphagia	3–60
Renal	Acute renal failure	Rare

intravenous immunoglobulin infusions have been reported, the response is not permanent and maintenance infusions every 6–8 weeks are required [11]. Thalidomide (or lenalidomide) and/or systemic steroids are considered the second line of treatment, more often in combination with intravenous immunoglobulins than as monotherapy [2,12,13,14]. Autologous peripheral blood stem cell transplantation can be considered as a third line of treatment [2,9,12,15]. In patients with severe or refractory disease (cases with central nervous system or cardiac involvement) and recurrent disease, plasma cell-directed therapies using lenalidomide and/or bortezomib with dexamethasone and intravenous immunoglobulin should be considered [10]. Combined plasmapheresis, intravenous immunoglobulin and high-dose corticosteroids seemed to yield benefit in cases of dermatoneuro syndrome [2,9,16].

Localised lichen myxoedematosus

Introduction and general description
In localised LM, patients have small, firm, waxy papules (or nodules and plaques produced by the confluence of papules) confined to only a few sites. There are no sclerotic features, no paraproteinaemia, no systemic involvement and no association with thyroid disease. Localised LM is classified into four subtypes: (i) acral persistent papular mucinosis; (ii) discrete papular lichen myxoedematosus; (iii) cutaneous (papular) mucinosis of infancy; and (iv) nodular lichen myxoedematosus [1].

Epidemiology
The exact incidence and prevalence rates of the variants of localised LM are unknown as they are rare diseases. Both sexes are equally affected in discrete papular LM. A female predominance (female : male ratio of 3 : 1) has been noted in acral persistent papular mucinosis.

Treatment ladder for scleromyxoedema

First line
- Intravenous immunoglobulin (at a dose of 2 g/kg for 3–5 days for at least 6 months)

Second line
- Thalidomide (lenalidomide) (100–400 mg/day)
- Systemic corticosteroids
  Both commonly used in combination with intravenous immunoglobulin rather than as monotherapy.

Third line
- Autologous peripheral blood stem cell transplantation

Severe, refractory, relapsed disease
- Lenalidomide and/or bortezomib with dexamethasone and intravenous immunoglobulin

Dermatoneuro syndrome
- Combined plasmapheresis, intravenous immunoglobulin and high-dose corticosteroids

Additional therapies

Medical
- Oral retinoids
- Ciclosporin A
- Interferon α
- Hydroxychloroquine
- Chemotherapeutic agents:
  - Melphalan
  - 2-Chlorodeoxyadenosine
  - Cyclophosphamide
  - Methotrexate

Physical
- Plasmapheresis
- Psoralen and ultraviolet A (PUVA), UVA1
- Electron beam
- Extracorporeal photochemotherapy

Pathophysiology
In localised LM, the histological changes are less characteristic than in scleromyxoedema. Mucin accumulates in the upper and mid reticular dermis, fibroblast proliferation is variable and fibrosis is not marked and may even be absent. In acral persistent papular mucinosis, mucin accumulates focally in the upper reticular dermis (sparing a subepidermal zone) and fibroblasts are not increased in number (Figure 57.6). In cutaneous mucinosis of infancy, the mucin may be so superficial as to look as if it were 'enclosed' by epidermis [1] but mucin deposition may also occur in the reticular dermis.

Clinical features
In *acral persistent papular mucinosis*, first described in 1986 [17], multiple ivory to skin-coloured papules develop exclusively on the

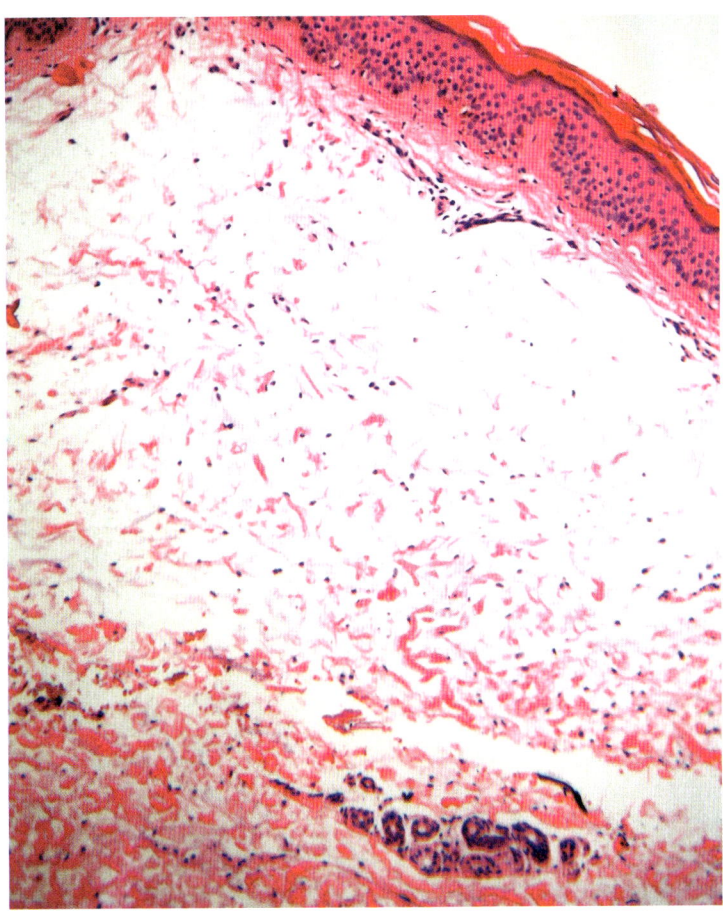

(a)

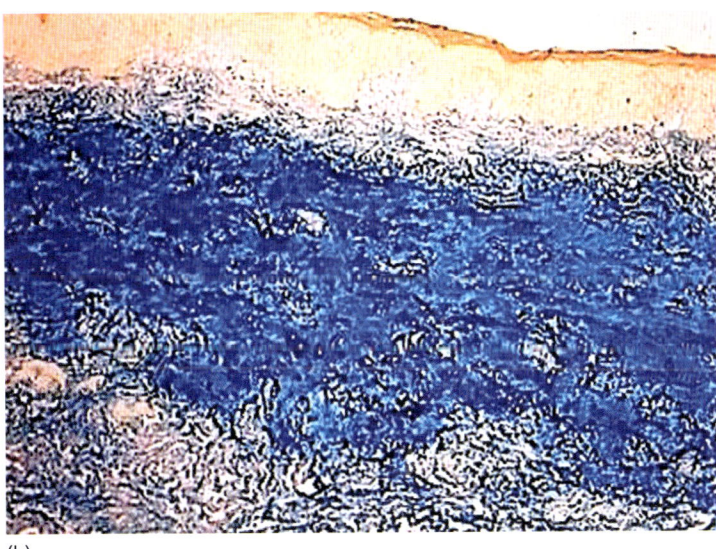

(b)

Figure 57.6 (a) Microscopic features of acral persistent papular mucinosis. Focal mucin accumulation in the upper dermis sparing a grenz zone without fibroblast proliferation. (b) Mucin stained with colloidal iron.

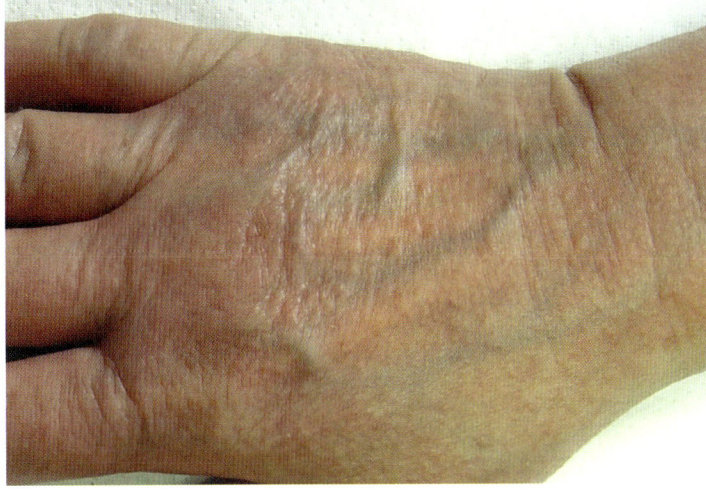

Figure 57.7 Acral persistent papular mucinosis. Multiple skin-coloured papules on the dorsal aspect of the hand.

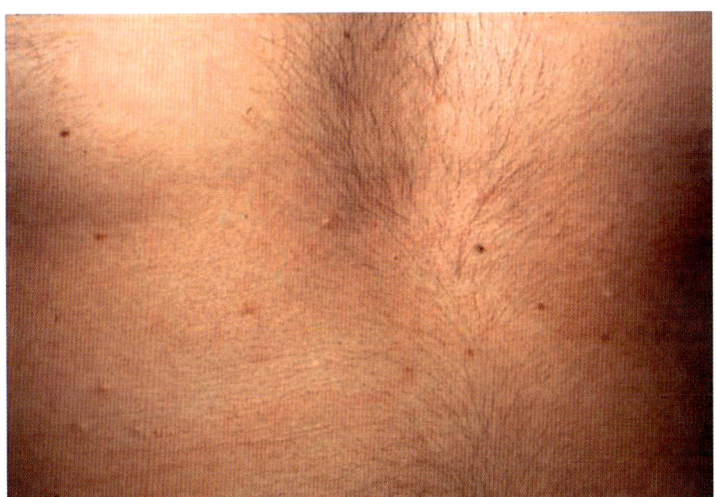

Figure 57.8 Discrete papular lichen myxoedematosus. Mucinous skin-coloured papules on the trunk.

dorsal aspect of the hands and extensor surface of the distal forearms (Figure 57.7) [18]. *Discrete papular LM* presents with reddish or skin-coloured papules, 2–5 mm in size, numbering from just a few to hundreds and affecting the trunk and limbs in a symmetrical pattern (Figure 57.8) [19]. In *cutaneous (papular) mucinosis of infancy*, firm opalescent papules appear on the upper arms, neck and trunk [20]. *Nodular LM* is characterised by multiple nodules on the limbs and trunk, with a mild or absent papular component [20,21].

Localised LM may be observed in association with human immunodeficiency virus (HIV) infection, exposure to toxic oil or L-tryptophan, or hepatitis C virus infection [1,22]. Anecdotal cases of localised cutaneous mucinosis after joint replacement, drug exposure including biologic therapy (anti-TNF-α and anti-IL-12/23) [23] and familial forms of papular mucinosis have also been reported [1]. Whether they are distinct entities or atypical and/or familial forms of localised LM is still unclear.

Differential diagnosis

Histological examination of the skin helps to distinguish localised LM from several papular eruptions that have a similar appearance such as granuloma annulare, lichen amyloidosis, lichen planus and other lichenoid eruptions, and eruptive collagenoma.

Disease course and prognosis

Localised LM in all its variants runs a chronic but benign course in the absence of systemic involvement. Progression to scleromyxoedema has never been proven.

Management

Localised LM is a benign condition that often does not require any therapy (a 'wait and see' approach). Many treatments have been tried including dermabrasion, CO_2 laser, electrocoagulation, topical and intralesional corticosteroids or hyaluronidase injections, oral retinoids and psoralen with ultraviolet A (PUVA) with variable results [1]. Topical calcineurin inhibitors [24] may be of some benefit. However, spontaneous resolution may occur, even in the setting of HIV-associated cases [14].

Reticular erythematous mucinosis

Definition and nomenclature

Reticular erythematous mucinosis (REM) is a rare, chronic, primary cutaneous mucinosis characterised by a persistent reticular macular redness or red papules and plaques in the midline of the back or chest.

Synonyms and inclusions
- Plaque-like cutaneous mucinosis
- Reticular erythematous mucinosis syndrome
- Midline mucinosis

Epidemiology

Reticular erythematous mucinosis is a rare disease that has been described worldwide in patients with different ethnic backgrounds. It affects predominantly middle-aged women, although men and children are not spared [1].

Associated diseases

In general, REM is not related to systemic diseases. However, certain disorders, especially malignancies (e.g. haematological, breast, lung, colon) and thyroid dysfunction have sometimes been associated [1,2]. Autoimmune disorders such as systemic lupus erythematosus, diabetes, idiopathic thrombocytopenic purpura and also HIV infection have been anecdotally reported in patients with REM [2].

Pathophysiology

The aetiopathogenesis is unclear. Viral diseases and immunological disturbances have been implicated. The fibroblasts of patients with REM exhibit an abnormal response to stimulation by exogenous interleukins [3].

Predisposing factors

Although REM has been considered a photoaggravated disorder, the role of sunlight is controversial [1]. Oral contraceptives, pregnancy, menses, heat, X-ray therapy and perspiration have also been implicated in promoting or exacerbating REM [2]. The occurence on traumatic sites such as a mastectomy scar and the relapse after mammary reconstruction suggests a possible link with trauma [4]. Familial cases suggesting a genetic predisposition have been reported [5].

Pathology

Interstitial deposits of mucin are seen in the upper dermis, along with a perivascular and, at times, perifollicular T-cell infiltrate with variable deep perivascular extension. There is slight vascular dilatation. The epidermis is typically normal. Usually direct immunofluorescence is negative but, rarely, granular deposits of immunoglobulin M, immunoglobulin A and C3 have been seen at the dermal–epidermal junction [5].

Clinical features

Reticular erythematous mucinosis is characterised by red macules and indurated papules or plaque-like lesions with a reticular configuration and lack of scale or other surface changes in the midline of the chest (Figure 57.9) or back. Atypical areas such as the arms, abdomen, face and legs are occasionally involved. The lesions are occasionally pruritic.

Differential diagnosis

There may be significant overlap between REM and lupus erythematosus tumidus. Both conditions show clinical and histological similarities, lack immune serological abnormalities, respond well to antimalarials and resolve without residual lesions. However, patients with lupus tumidus who do not exhibit reticulate-patterned lesions on the midline, are strongly photosensitive, have a higher rate of immune reactants on direct immunofluorescence, have a higher tendency to recur and occasionally present with other clinical manifestations of lupus [6]. Seborrhoeic dermatitis and pityriasis versicolor involve the central chest, but they have associated scale and different colour, as has the confluent and reticulated papillomatosis of Gougerot–Carteaud.

Disease course and prognosis

Reticular erythematous mucinosis is a chronic disease which if left untreated has a prolonged duration. The lesions may clear spontaneously, even after 15 years.

Investigations

In general, REM is not associated with abnormal laboratory tests and no extensive work-up is recommended.

Management

Antimalarials (e.g. hydroxychloroquine) are the first line of treatment and they generally result in improvement or healing within

Table 57.4 Types of scleroedema adultorum.

Type	% of total	Characteristics
Diabetic	25–50	Slowly progressive, non-resolving course; occurs in patients with poorly controlled, insulin-dependent diabetes
Non-diabetic	25	Idiopathic
	25–50	With preceding febrile illness (poststreptococcal) and complete resolution in months to 2 years
	10–20	Associated with monoclonal gammopathy including multiple myeloma and slowly progressive, non-resolving course
	Anecdotal	Associated with miscellaneous conditions (e.g. HIV, internal malignancies, autoimmune disorders)

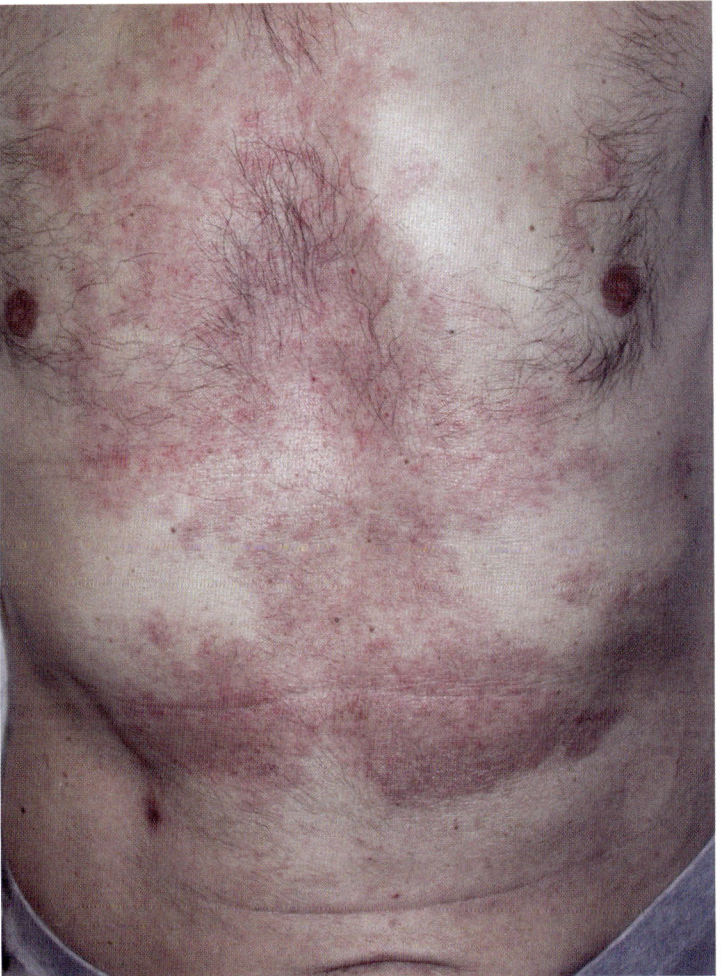

Figure 57.9 Reticular erythematous mucinosis in the midline of the chest and abdomen.

1–2 months [7]. Relapses are not uncommon. The effectiveness of other therapies such as topical and systemic corticosteroids, topical tacrolimus and pimecrolimus, oral antihistamines, tetracyclines, ciclosporin and pulsed dye laser are quite variable [2,8,9]. Despite the potential for an exacerbation of the condition, successful treatment with ultraviolet B (UVB) and UVA1 irradiation have been reported [10,11].

Treatment ladder for reticular erythematous mucinosis

First line
- Antimalarials (e.g. hydroxychloroquine)

Second line
- Topical and systemic corticosteroid
- Topical calcineurin inhibitors

Third line
- Phototherapy (UVA1, UVB)
- Pulsed dye laser

Scleroedema

Definition and nomenclature
Scleroedema is a symmetrical, diffuse, progressive, non-pitting swelling and induration of the upper part of the body caused by a thickened dermis and deposition of mucin. Types of scleroedema adultorum are listed in Table 57.4.

Synonyms and inclusions
- Scleroedema adultorum of Buschke
- Buschke disease
- Scleroedema diabeticorum
- Scleroedema adultorum

Introduction and general description
Scleroedema is a rare condition characterised by a non-pitting induration of the upper part of the body, associated with diabetes or with a history of infection or blood dyscrasia [1].

Epidemiology
Scleroedema is rare and occurs in patients of all ages and ethnic backgrounds. The age distribution varies with the different subtypes. Among patients with diabetes, scleroedema has been diagnosed in 2.5–14%. The form that is associated with diabetes is more prevalent in men (10 . 1), while other forms are seen more commonly in women (2 : 1) [2,3].

Associated diseases
Scleroedema can be divided into diabetic and non-diabetic types (Table 57.1). The former is considered the most common type, accounting for 25–50% of cases. It occurs mainly in obese middle-aged men with poorly controlled insulin-dependent diabetes [1,3]. The non-diabetic form includes (i) an idiopathic type; (ii) a postinfective type with acute onset, usually following a streptococcal upper respiratory infection (and also after influenza, measles, mumps, chickenpox, cytomegalovirus, diphtheria, encephalitis and dental abscesses); and (iii) a monoclonal gammopathy-associated type. Other types described anecdotally are associated with miscellaneous conditions such as autoimmune

disorders (e.g. rheumatoid arthritis, primary biliary cirrhosis, Sjögren syndrome, dermatomyositis, anaphylactoid purpura), internal malignancies (malignant insulinoma, gallbladder carcinoma, carcinoid tumour, pituitary–adrenocortical neoplasms), sclerosing disorders (lichen sclerosus, scleroderma), exposure to organic solvents and HIV infection [2,4,5].

Pathophysiology

The pathogenesis is unknown. An increase of type I collagen synthesis by dysfunctional fibroblasts has been demonstrated in the affected skin. In diabetic scleroedema, the accumulation of collagen may be due to irreversible non-enzymatic glycosylation of collagen and resistance to degradation by collagenase. Alternatively, excess stimulation by insulin, microvascular damage and hypoxia may induce the abnormal synthesis of collagen and mucin. Streptococcal hypersensitivity, injury to lymphatics and paraproteinaemia may also play a role [1].

Pathology

The epidermis is not involved. The dermis is 3–4 times thicker than normal. The collagen fibres appear swollen and are separated by wide spaces. Acid mucopolysaccharides are found in the fenestrated spaces with special stains. However, negative staining does not exclude the diagnosis. The subcutaneous tissue is also involved with fat being replaced by coarse collagen fibres. A slight perivascular lymphocytic infiltrate may be seen but it is uncommon [6]. Fibroblast proliferation is absent. Mucin also accumulates in skeletal muscle and the heart.

Clinical features

Scleroedema is characterised by firm, non-pitting oedema and induration that typically begin on the posterior neck and spreads to the upper back (Figure 57.10), shoulders and scalp. Redness and a peau d'orange appearance of the skin are commonly observed. The hands and feet are characteristically spared. Unusual cases with limited site involvement have been reported [7]. Depending on the involved sites, patients often complain of movement restrictions comprising limited body mobility and facial expressions, or difficulties in mastication and articulation.

Differential diagnosis

In contrast to systemic sclerosis, scleroedema is not associated with sclerodactyly, Raynaud phenomenon, nail fold capillary changes or serum autoantibodies [8]. Additional differential diagnoses include myxoedema, amyloidosis, lymphoedema, cellulitis, dermatomyositis, trichinosis and oedema of cardiac or renal origin.

Complications and co-morbidities

Systemic involvement in scleroedema is not frequent. Extracutaneous complications, in all forms, include serositis, dysarthria, dysphagia, myositis, parotitis, hepatosplenomegaly and ocular and cardiac abnormalities [9].

Disease course and prognosis

Prognosis is largely dependent on the underlying aetiology. Postinfectious scleroedema runs a benign course because it is self-limiting

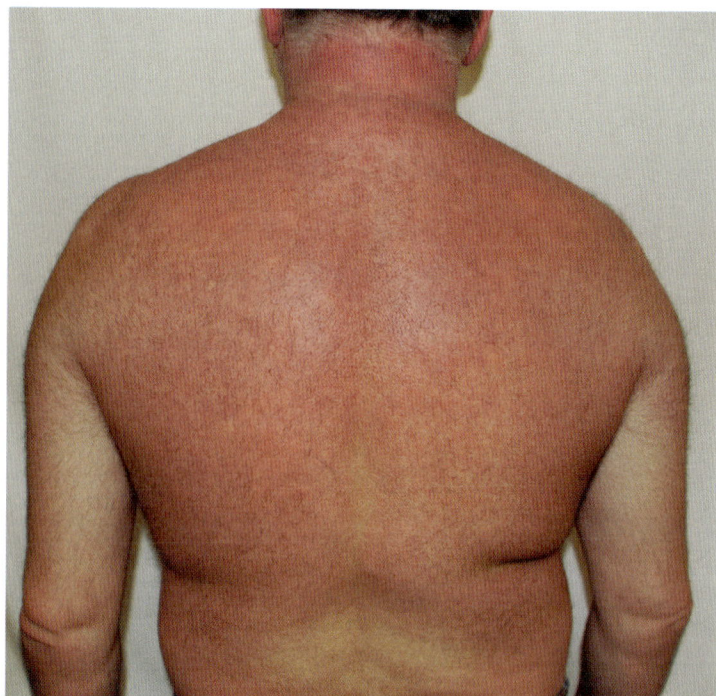

Figure 57.10 Scleroedema in a diabetic patient with firm, non-pitting oedema and induration on the upper back, neck and shoulders on a red background.

in duration and resolves spontaneously within 6 months to 2 years. Scleroedema associated with diabetes or monoclonal gammopathy runs a chronic and disabling course with little tendency to remission. Rarely death may occur when internal organs are involved.

Investigations

Laboratory investigations are useful for detecting an underlying disorder. A recent infection should be excluded (with throat swab culture and antistreptolysin titres). Fasting blood glucose or glycosylated haemoglobin measurements and serum protein electrophoresis and immunofixation should be obtained. Ultrasonography can be performed to evaluate skin thickness at baseline and after treatment while magnetic resonance imaging may be useful for determining the extent of disease progression due to better soft-tissue contrast than ultrasound evaluation [10].

Management

The therapy of scleroedema is quite difficult and has limited success. At present, no effective treatment is known for this disease. For patients with disabling manifestations, initial treatment with phototherapy is suggested as first choice (grade of recommendation is weak). UVA1, PUVA and narrow-band UVB have all been found to be effective [1,11]. Therapy is unnecessary for scleroedema associated with streptococcal infections because it resolves spontaneously. In patients with associated conditions, the disorder can resolve or improve if treatment of the primary disease is successful. In patients with scleroedema-associated multiple myeloma, therapy targeting the plasma cell dyscrasia such as bortezomib may be effective [12]. Some but not all patients with diabetes-associated scleroedema appear to improve with better glucose control.

Other therapies, used in reduced patient numbers and with overall limited success, include immunosuppressive agents such as ciclosporin A and methotrexate, high-dose penicillin, corticosteroids (local, intralesional and systemic), tranilast, tamoxifen and allopurinol [13]. Electron-beam radiotherapy and extracorporeal photopheresis may also give some improvement. Intravenous immunoglobulin seems to be a promising therapy [14]. Patients with motion or respiratory disability should be referred to a physical therapist for musculoskeletal rehabilitation.

Treatment ladder for scleroedema

First line
- Treatment of primary disease
- Phototherapy with UVA1, PUVA or narrow-band UVB
- Physical therapy

Second line
- Electron-beam radiotherapy
- Photopheresis
- Intravenous immunoglobulin

Third line
- Immunosuppresive agents

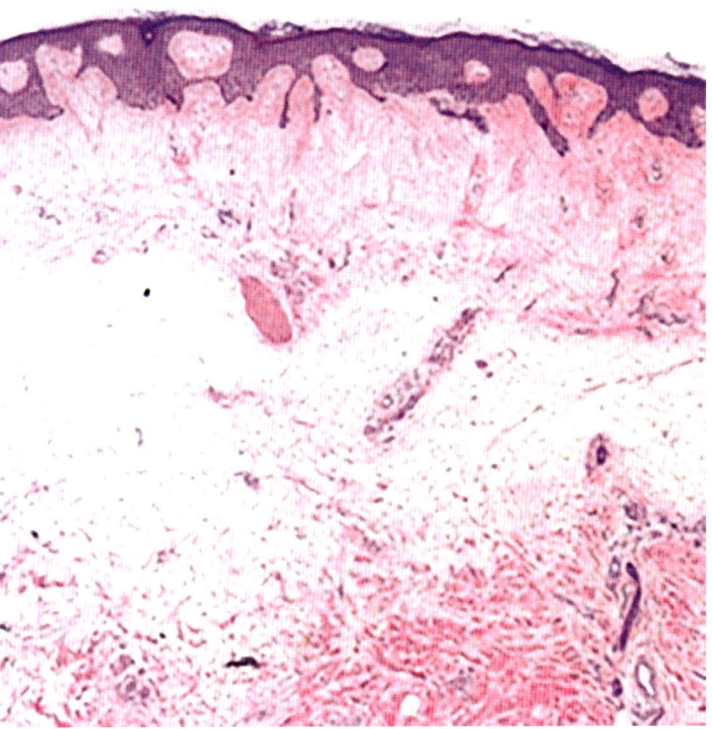

Figure 57.11 Pretibial myxoedema. Hyperkeratosis and irregular acanthosis with collagen fibres in the reticular dermis separated by deposits of mucin with a normal number of fibroblasts.

Myxoedema in thyroid diseases

Localised (pretibial) myxoedema

Definition and nomenclature
Localised (pretibial) myxoedema is an infiltrative dermopathy due to mucin deposition, usually arising on the shins. It is one of the signs of hyperthyroidism, especially of Graves disease [1].

Synonyms and inclusions
- Thyroid dermopathy
- Infiltrative dermopathy

Epidemiology
Localised (pretibial) myxoedema is found in 1–5% of patients with Graves disease, but in up to 25% of patients who have exophthalmus. Women are affected more often than men (3 : 1) with a peak of incidence at age 50–60 years [2].

Pathophysiology
The demonstration of thyroid-stimulating hormone (TSH) receptor protein expression by normal dermal fibroblasts suggests that TSH receptor antibodies may stimulate the production of mucin from these cells. Some cytokines such as TNF-α and γ-interferon secreted by T-helper 1 lymphocytes activated by TSH receptor antigen could also induce glycosaminoglycan synthesis from fibroblasts. Fibroblasts from the dermis of the lower extremities have been found to be more sensitive to this factor than are fibroblasts from other areas of the body [2,3–5]. Insulin-like growth factor 1 receptor antibodies, tyrosine kinase receptor antibodies, trauma, tobacco and lymphatic obstruction may also play a role.

Pathology
Histopathology reveals hyperkeratosis with follicular plugging, acanthosis and sometimes papillomatosis (Figure 57.11). The reticular dermis, particularly the mid to the lower part, shows separation of collagen bundles by large quantities of mucin. A perivascular lymphocytic infiltrate and an increase in mast cells may be found with a normal or increased number of fibroblasts. Elastic fibres are reduced in number [2].

Clinical features
Pretibial myxoedema is one of the signs of Graves disease. Other findings may include goitre, exophthalmus, thyroid acropachy and high levels of long-acting TSH stimulator antibodies. Less commonly, pretibial myxoedema has been described with Hashimoto thyroiditis and in patients with no past or present history of thyroid dysfunction. It is characterised by bilateral thickening and induration of the skin on the shins and dorsa of the feet. There are four main clinical variants: diffuse non-pitting oedema (43%) (Figure 57.12); plaque type (27%); nodular (18%) (Figure 57.13); and elephantiasis (5%) (Figure 57.14) [2,6]. The lesions can vary in colour and may exhibit a characteristic orange peel appearance and texture due to prominent hair follicles. The toes, thighs, upper extremities and face can be involved (Figure 57.15) [7]. Overlying hyperhidrosis

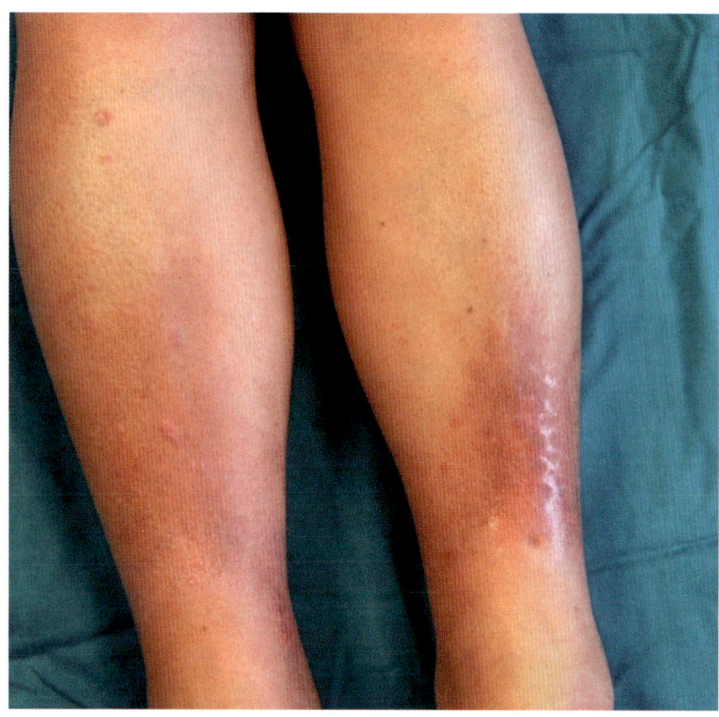

Figure 57.12 Pretibial myxoedema with diffuse non-pitting oedema and plaque-like lesions on the legs.

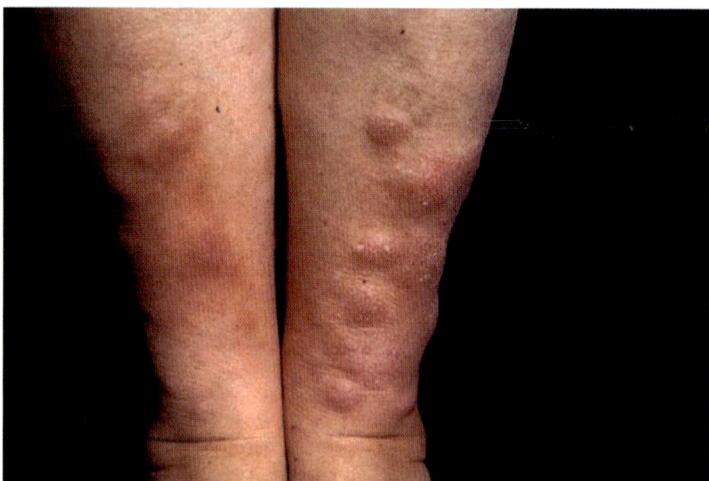

Figure 57.13 Pretibial myxoedema of nodular type.

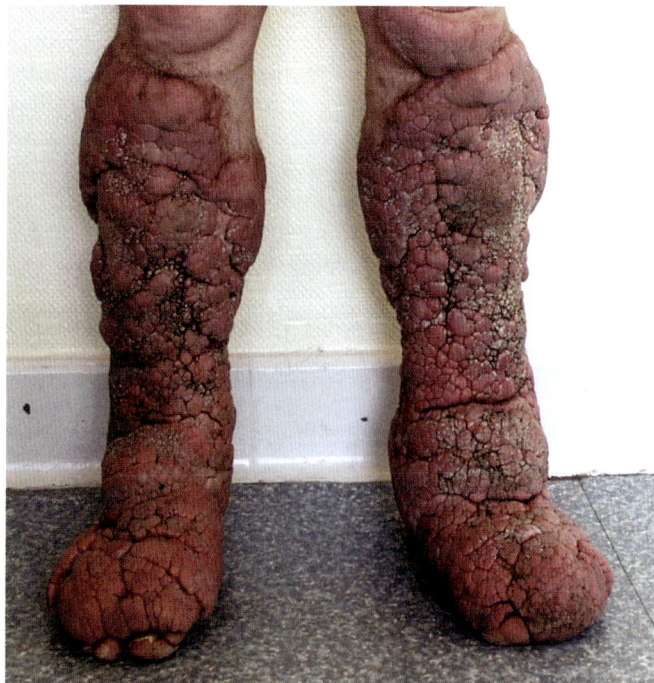

Figure 57.14 Elephantiasic pretibial myxoedema. Courtesy of B. Cribier, MD, Strasbourg, France.

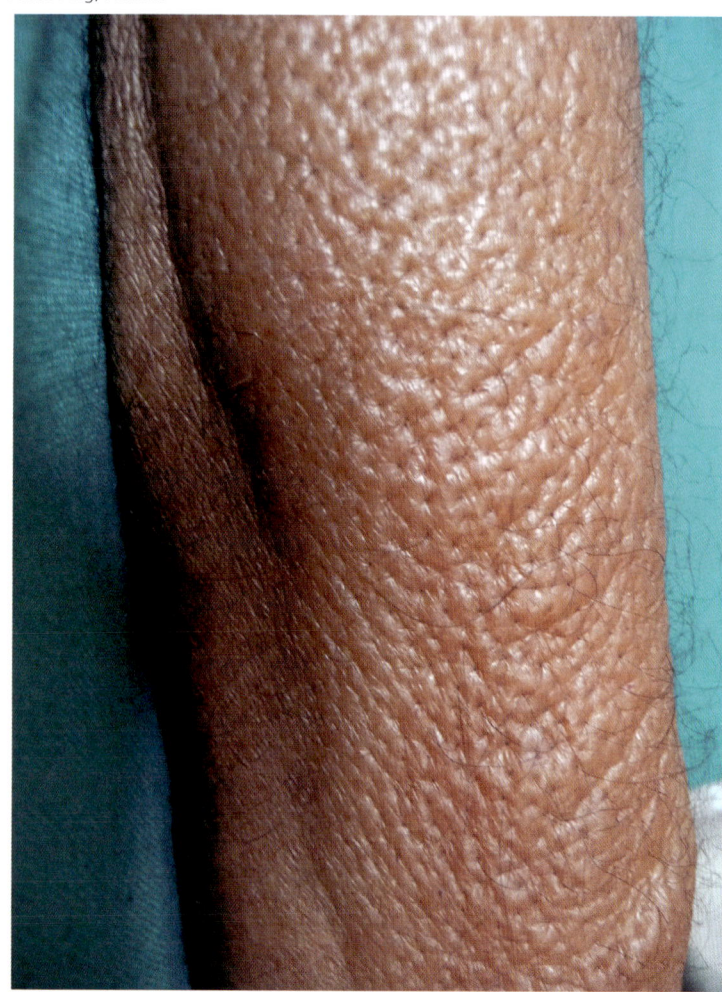

Figure 57.15 Localised myxoedema on the preradial area. Note the orange peel appearance. Courtesy of S. Verma, MD, Vadodara, Gujarat, India.

or hypertrichosis may be associated. In skin of colour, variations of colour are more likely with pigmentary changes of the skin.

Differential diagnosis

In addition to lichen simplex chronicus and hypertrophic lichen planus in which mucin is lacking, pretibial myxoedema should be differentiated from obesity-associated lymphoedematous mucinosis seen in patients without thyroid disease [8].

Disease course and prognosis

Apart from the appearance, associated morbidity is usually not severe, except for patients with elephantiasis who are less likely to have remission. Entrapment of peroneal nerves by mucinous connective tissue may cause foot drop or impaired dorsiflexion.

Investigations

Thyroid-stimulating hormone is abnormally low and long-acting thyroid stimulator antibodies are elevated in 50% of patients with Graves disease.

Management

The initial treatment includes minimising risk factors, such as reducing weight, reducing tobacco use and normalising thyroid function. However, therapy for the associated hyperthyroidism does not improve the cutaneous lesions, and often localised myxoedema develops after treatment has been instituted. Severe myxoedema is most often encountered in patients with longstanding untreated Graves thyroid disease. The first line of pharmacological therapy is medium- to high-potency topical corticosteroids applied under occlusive dressings or delivered by intralesional injection (grade of recommendation is weak) [2,9,10]. Intralesional hyaluronidase or pentoxifylline should be considered in cases refractory to conventional therapy [11].

For the severe elephantiasic form, rituximab, plasmapheresis, intravenous immunoglobulins and octreotide with and without surgical shave removal have been tried with some benefit in uncontrolled case reports [12,13,14]. Usually, skin grafting is followed by relapse. The use of compression stockings and gradient pneumatic compression is useful as it improves lymphoedema. Teprotumumab, a human monoclonal antibody inhibitor of insulin-like growth factor 1 receptor, has been used in patients with severe ophthalmopathy and has been proposed for refractory thyroid dermopathy [15].

Localised myxoedema may also clear spontaneously (on average after 3.5 years) [16].

Treatment ladder for localised (pretibial) myxoedema

First line
- Medium- to high-potency topical corticosteroids applied under occlusive dressings or delivered by intralesional injection
- Compression stockings

Second and third line
- Intralesional hyaluronidase
- For elephantiasic form: rituximab, plasmapheresis, intravenous immunoglobulin and octreotide

---

Papular and nodular mucinosis in connective tissue diseases

Definition

A distinctive cutaneous mucinosis characterised by skin-coloured papules, nodules (Figure 57.16) and plaque-like lesions on the

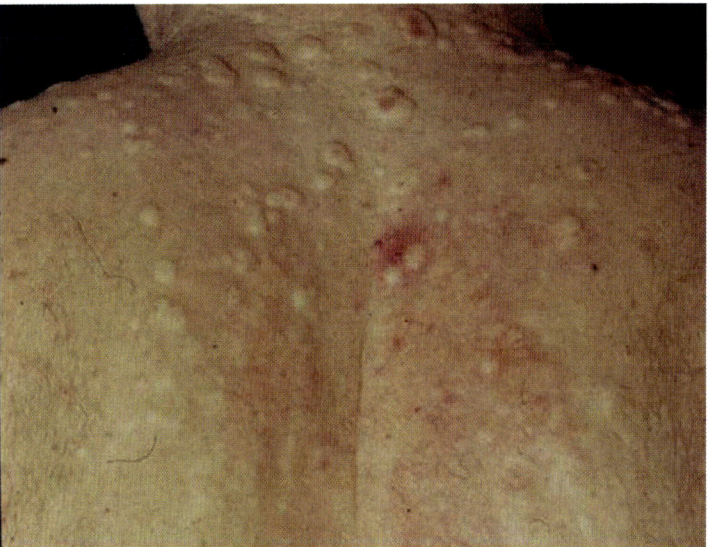

Figure 57.16 Papular and nodular mucinosis in connective tissue disease.

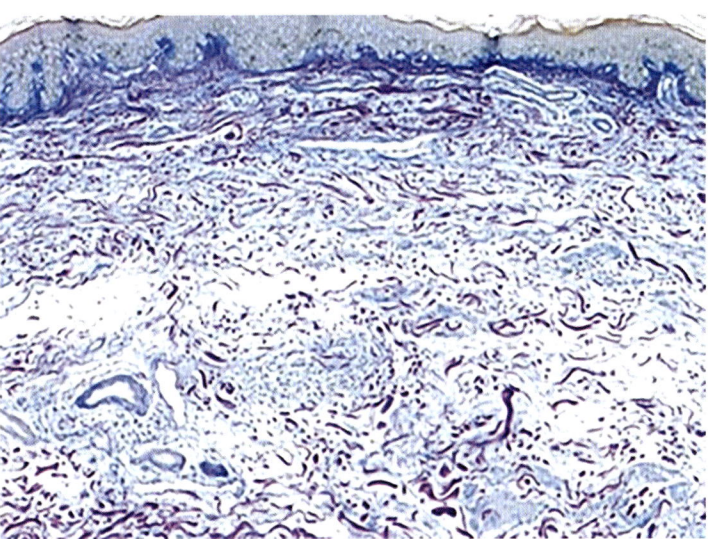

Figure 57.17 Abundant mucin deposition throughout the reticular dermis (colloidal iron stain) in papular and nodular mucinosis in connective tissue disease.

trunk and upper extremities may accompany or even antedate a connective tissue disease, mostly lupus erythematosus (cutaneous lupus mucinosis) and rarely dermatomyositis or scleroderma [1].

Epidemiology

Cutaneous lupus mucinosis occurs in 1.5% of patients with lupus erythematosus in the fourth and fifth decades of life, with a predominance in adult males in East Asian patients and white-skinned females [2].

Pathophysiology

The pathogenesis is unknown but increased glycosaminoglycan production by dermal fibroblasts stimulated by some cytokines or immunoglobulins, or an abnormal immune response linked to human leukocyte antigens HLA-B8 and HLA-DR3 haplotypes have been suggested [1,2].

Pathology

Histologically, mucin is abundant throughout the dermis and sometimes subcutaneous fat (Figure 57.17), occasionally in association with a slight to moderate perivascular lymphocytic infiltrate. The epidermal changes of lupus erythematosus are absent or mild, but a positive lupus band is seen on direct immunofluorescence [1,2].

Clinical features

The clinical course may or may not be related to the underlying connective tissue disease activity. Usually patients with lupus erythematosus who develop papular and nodular mucinosis have systemic disease in about 75% of cases but discoid and subacute cutaneous lupus erythematosus may also be associated with it. Periorbital mucinosis is an unusual presentation [3]. Cutaneous mucinosis in dermatomyositis usually follows the myositis and is characterised by red nodules and plaque-like lesions on the trunk [4]. The development of papular and nodular mucinosis has also been associated with scleroderma in both the systemic and the cutaneous form [5].

Management

Therapy of papular and nodular mucinosis is the same as for the connective tissue disease. However, the evolution of the mucinoses does not always follow the course of the underlying disease. Sunscreens, topical or intralesional corticosteroids and oral antimalarials can be effective in cutaneous lupus mucinosis. Systemic corticosteroids and oral tacrolimus are used for resistant cases [6].

Self-healing cutaneous mucinosis

Definition

A self-healing mucinosis affecting young people with transient cutaneous lesions and mild inflammatory symptoms.

Introduction and general description

Self-healing juvenile cutaneous mucinosis is a rare disease of unknown aetiology occurring in young people (from 13 months to 15 years of age) characterised by transient cutaneous lesions and sometimes mild inflammatory symptoms [1].

Pathophysiology

Abnormal mucin production and fibroblast proliferation are suggested to be secondary to a reactive or reparative response to chronic antigenic stimulation, as can occur in viral infection or inflammation.

Pathology

Histologically, papular lesions show mucin deposition with mild inflammation and a small increase in fibroblasts while nodules show deep mucinous areas associated with bands of fibrosis, multiple capillaries, fibroblastic proliferation and gangliocyte-like giant cells in the subcutis consistent with nodular or proliferative fasciitis [1,2].

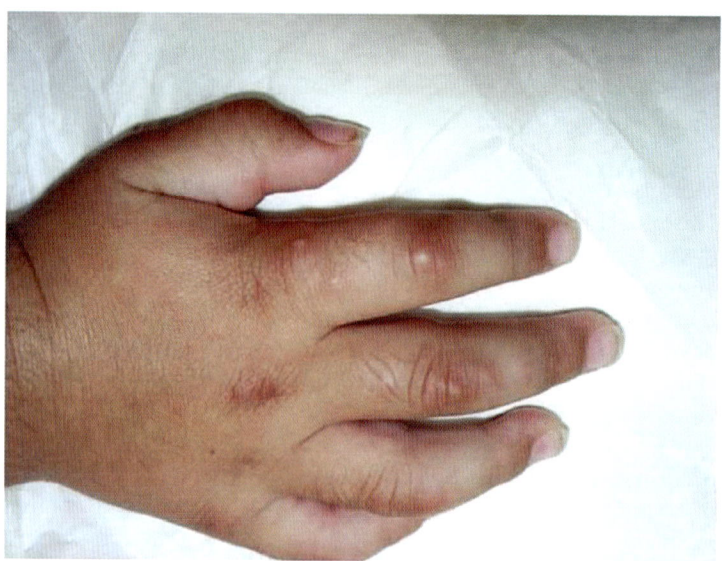

Figure 57.18 Self-healing cutaneous mucinosis. Mucinous subcutaneous nodules and papules on the periarticular areas of the hand in a 6 year-old child.

Clinical features

Self-healing cutaneous mucinosis is characterised by the following criteria: (i) acute eruption of multiple papules, sometimes in linear infiltrated plaques, on the face, neck, scalp, abdomen and thighs; (ii) mucinous subcutaneous nodules on the face with periorbital swelling and on periarticular areas of the limbs which sometimes are the predominant lesions (Figure 57.18); (iii) systemic symptoms such as fever, arthralgias, weakness and muscle tenderness in the absence of paraproteinaemia, bone marrow plasmacytosis and thyroid dysfunction; and (iv) spontaneous resolution in a period ranging from a few weeks to many months (usually from 2 to 8 months) [1,2]. It has also been described in adults [3].

Management

Despite the worrying presentation, the disease heals spontaneously and aggressive therapy should be avoided. Although spontaneous complete regression is expected, the possible development of dermato-rheumatological conditions has been highlighted and hence long-term follow-up could be considered [1].

Cutaneous focal mucinosis

Definition

Cutaneous focal mucinosis is a benign localised form of cutaneous dermal mucinosis.

Epidemiology

Cutaneous focal mucinosis occurs in adults of either sex but it has also been reported in children [1].

Pathophsiology

Cutaneous focal mucinosis is a reactive lesion in which trauma may act as a trigger [1].

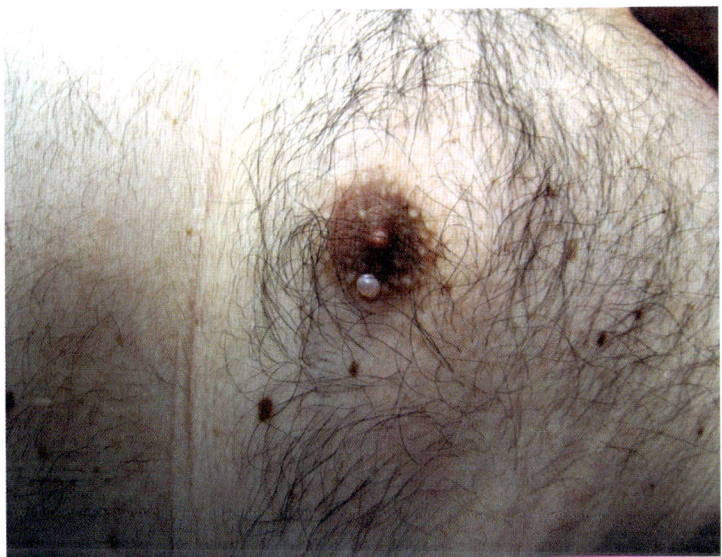

Figure 57.19 Cutaneous focal mucinosis: a solitary whitish papule with cystic appearance.

Pathology

The histology is essential for diagnosis and shows a diffuse, ill-defined dermal accumulation of mucin, sparing subcutaneous tissue, with a normal or slight increase of fibroblasts and absence of inflammation [1,2]. Spindle-shaped fibroblasts are the predominant cell type, with occasional admixed factor XIIIa-positive dendritic cells. The epidermis may be normal or hyperplastic, sometimes forming a collarette. Additionally, the absence of elastic fibres without increased vascularity is seen.

Clinical features

Cutaneous focal mucinosis presents as an asymptomatic, solitary, skin-coloured papule or nodule, sometimes with a cystic appearance, that can occur anywhere on the body (Figure 57.19) or in the oral cavity, but not in proximity to the joints of the hands, wrists or feet [1]. Occasionally, cutaneous focal mucinosis has been reported as a soft fibroma-like polyp or a plaque-like lesion [2,3]. Multiple lesions have been rarely described, sometimes after biologic drugs [4], but they are likely to represent cases of localised lichen myxoedematosus.

Differential diagnosis

The main differential diagnosis is with angiomyxoma, a benign neoplasm which may be associated with the Carney complex. Angiomyxoma, however, is larger (size over 1 cm) and shows subcutaneous involvement by mucin and increased vascularity [5].

Complications and co-morbidities

Contrary to other forms of primary mucinoses, cutaneous focal mucinosis is not usually related to systemic manifestations. Anecdotal associations with hypothyroidism and myxoedema or other forms of mucinoses such as scleromyxoedema and REM and with biological therapy have been described [4,6].

Management

Surgical excision is the treatment of choice and relapse is uncommon.

Digital myxoid (mucous) cyst

Definition

Digital myxoid cyst is a benign ganglion cyst of the digits.

Epidemiology

Women are affected more than twice as often as men.

Pathophysiology

There are two varieties of lesion: the ganglion type derived from joint fluid and synovial cells, which is located over the joints; and the myxomatous type, derived from dermal-based fibroblasts, which is located between the interphalangeal joints [1].

Pathology

There are two types of cysts. The first type is similar to a ganglion, showing a cystic space limited by a fibrous wall with peripheral thickening and sometimes a synovial lining. The second type is similar to cutaneous focal mucinosis, showing a large deposit of mucin-containing stellate fibroblasts with vascular spaces and multiple clefts. The overlying epidermis is acanthotic laterally and more atrophic centrally. Transepidermal elimination of mucoid material may be seen [1].

Clinical features

It is a translucent, dome-shaped, soft or fluctuant 3–10 mm nodule with or without visible semitransparent contents located on the dorsal skin on or near a distal interphalangeal joint of the finger in middle-aged patients (Figure 57.20) [1]. Cysts may also be found on the toes. The surface may be smooth or verrucous. Subungual and multiple forms have been reported [2]. Clinical and radiographic evidence of osteoarthritis is common. Grooving of the nail may be associated with or even precede the cyst itself by up to 6 months [3]. Antecedent trauma has been documented in a small minority of cases. A connection of the ganglion cyst to the underlying joint can be shown by means of magnetic resonance imaging [4]. Puncture or skin biopsy results in drainage of viscous mucin from the cyst. Dermoscopy shows arboriform telangiectasias over white, bluish and reddish orange diffuse background [1].

Management

None of the existing treatments is consistently successful. Digital myxoid cyst can be excised but relapse is not uncommon and many dermatologists recommend more conservative treatments such as multiple needling or aspiration followed by steroid injection, sclerosant injection, cryotherapy, infrared coagulation or CO_2 laser [5].

FOLLICULAR MUCINOSES

Mucin accumulates in the epithelial hair follicle sheaths and sebaceous glands in two primary (idiopathic) distinctive clinical disorders: Pinkus follicular mucinosis and urticaria-like follicular

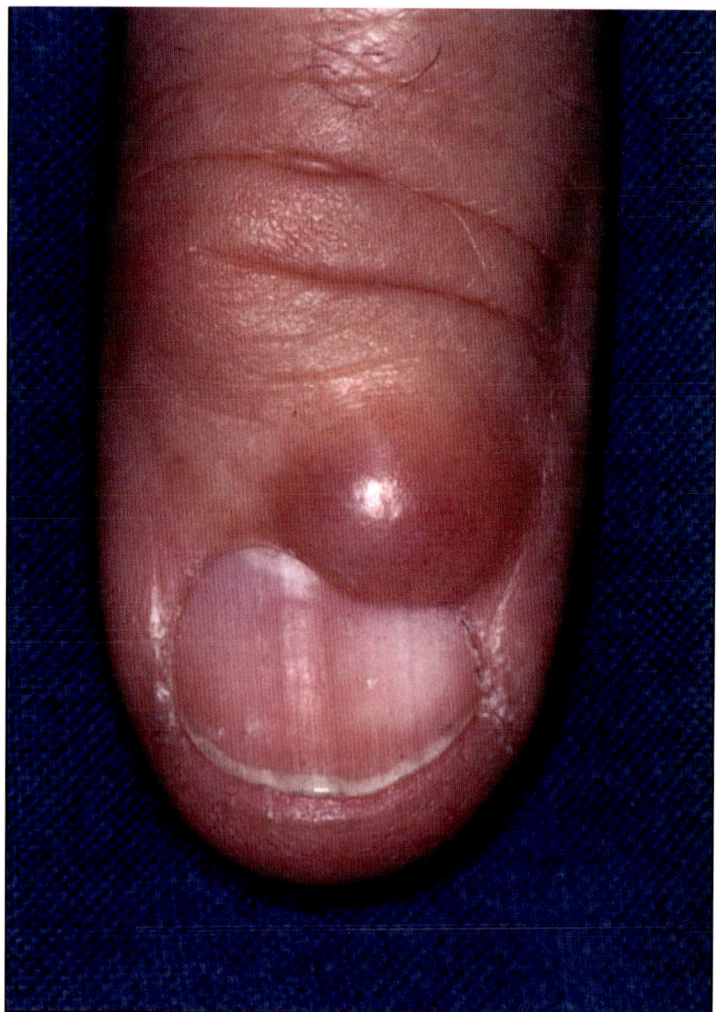

Figure 57.20 Digital myxoid cyst. A translucent dome-shaped nodule on the distal interphalangeal joint of the finger with grooving of the nail.

mucinosis [1]. Follicular mucinosis can also occur as a histological epiphenomenon most often seen in cutaneous T-cell lymphomas (Chapter 139) and other skin diseases [2].

Pinkus follicular mucinosis

Definition and nomenclature

Pinkus follicular mucinosis is an uncommon inflammatory disorder, usually not linked with lymphoma, that has a predilection for children, and young adults aged 11–35 years (mean 20.4 years) [1,2].

Synonyms and inclusions
- Alopecia mucinosa
- Follicular mucinosis
- Mucinosis follicularis

Pathophysiology

It is far from clear why dermal-type mucin is deposited selectively within an epithelial structure. Although follicular keratinocytes have been considered to be the source of the mucin, an aetiological role for cell-mediated immune mechanisms has been proposed. A reaction to persistent antigens such as *Staphylococcus aureus* or *Demodex follicolorum* has also been considered [1]. Familial cases suggest a genetic predisposition [3].

Pathology

Mucin accumulates within the follicular epithelium and sebaceous glands causing keratinocytes to disconnect from each other (Figure 57.21). In more advanced lesions, the follicles are converted into cystic spaces containing mucin, inflammatory cells and altered keratinocytes. A perifollicular infiltrate of lymphocytes, histiocytes and eosinophils is seen. The differentiation between Pinkus follicular mucinosis and mycosis fungoides-associated follicular mucinosis is very difficult and there is no single reliable criterion. Although the existence of primary follicular mucinosis has been questioned, as it has been considered as an 'indolent' localised form of cutaneous T-cell lymphoma, clues in favour of a primary form are the young age of the patient, a solitary lesion on the head or neck and the absence of histological features of epidermotropism or atypical lymphocytes [2,4]. Clonal T-cell rearrangement is not always useful to differentiate the two types. In these cases, clinical follow-up is mandatory.

Clinical features

Pinkus follicular mucinosis presents as an acute or subacute eruption characterised by one or several sharply demarcated pink to red plaques with follicular prominence (Figure 57.22a), scaling and alopecia (Figure 57.22b) [1,4]. Nodules, annular plaques, folliculitis, follicular spines, acneiform eruptions and alopecia areata-like presentation [5] have also been described. A second type which is characterised by a more generalised chronic form in a slightly older age group, with larger and more numerous plaques on the extremities, trunk and face, is probably best regarded as a follicular mucinosis associated with cutaneous T-cell lymphoma rather than a primary condition.

Management

There is no specific treatment for Pinkus follicular mucinosis [1,2]. A wait and see approach should be considered as many cases heal spontaneously in 2–24 months. Topical, intralesional and systemic corticosteroids, topical retinoids, topical calcineurin inhibitors, topical bexarotene, imiquimod, dapsone, antimalarials, indometacin, minocycline, oral isotretinoin, interferon α-2b, photodynamic therapy and UVA1 phototherapy have been reported to be of benefit on an anecdotal basis [6–8].

Urticaria-like follicular mucinosis

Definition

This is a follicular mucinosis presenting with a cyclic eruption of urticaria-like lesions on the face on a 'rosaceiform or seborrhoeic' background.

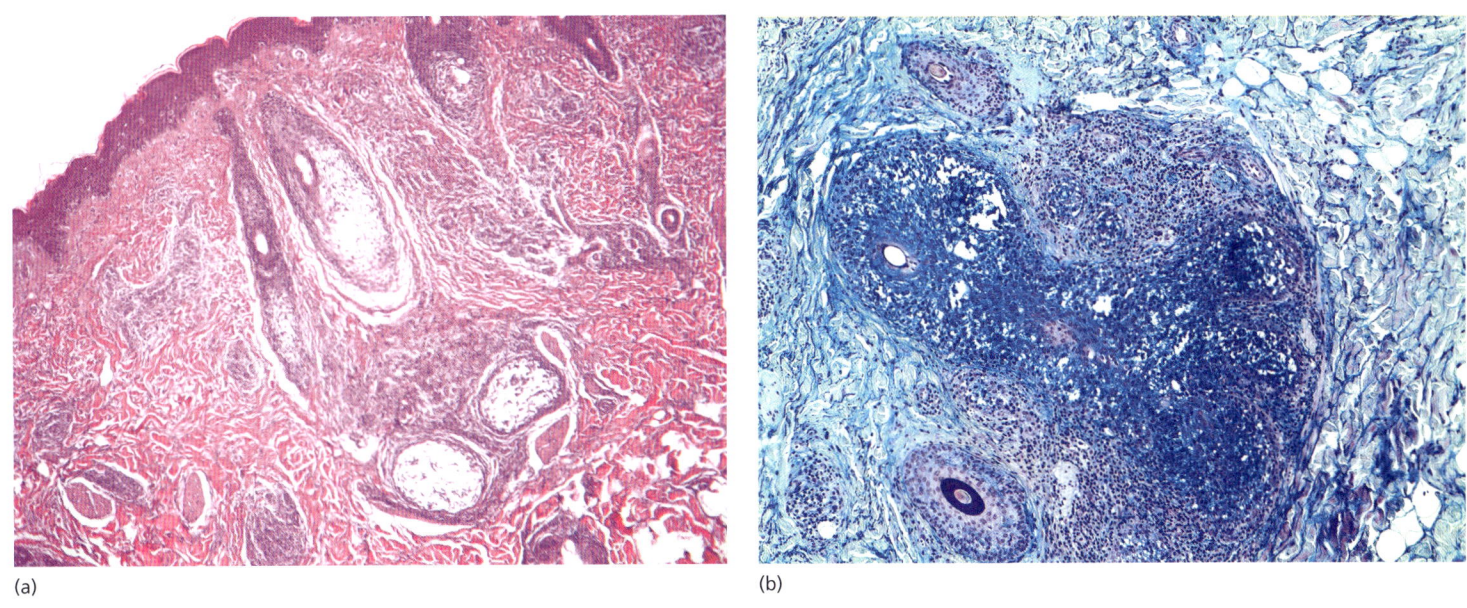

Figure 57.21 Pinkus follicular mucinosis. (a) Mucin accumulates within the follicular epithelium and sebaceous glands causing keratinocytes to disconnect. (b) Follicular mucin stained with Alcian blue.

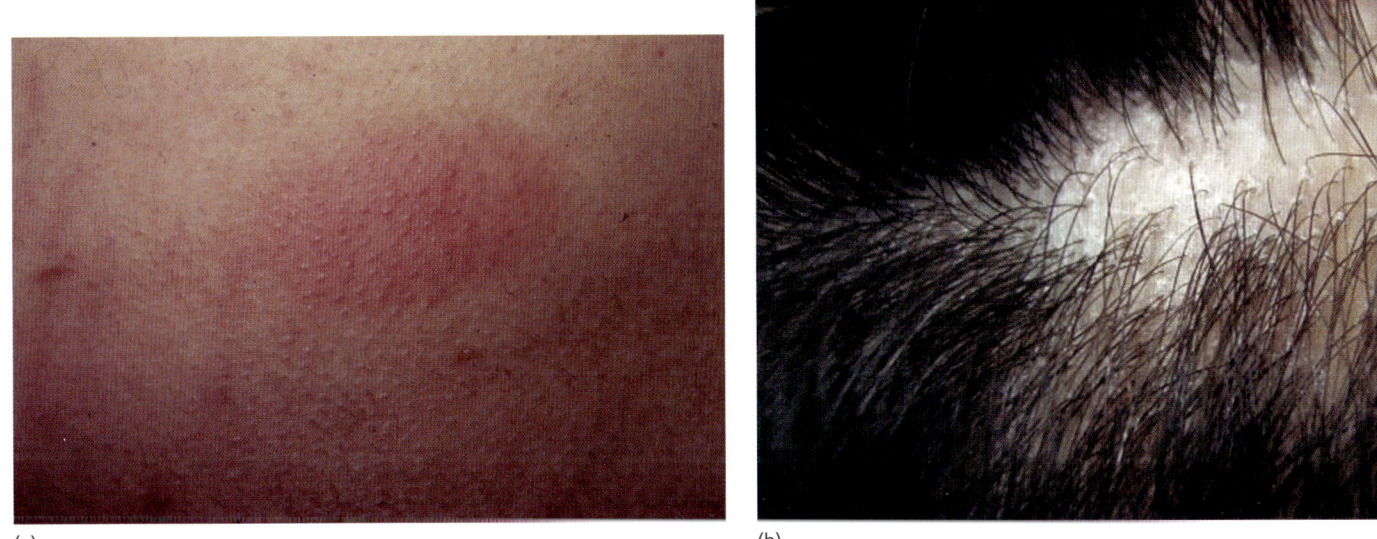

Figure 57.22 Pinkus follicular mucinosis. (a) A sharply demarcated pink to red plaque with follicular prominence. (b) Alopecic plaque in follicular mucinosis.

Introduction and general description

This is a very rare cyclic eruption of urticaria-like lesions that occurs primarily on the head of middle-aged men [1] in the absence of systemic manifestations.

Pathophysiology

On histopathological examination, urticaria-like follicular mucinosis presents with mucin deposition inside the hair follicles associated with a perivascular and perifollicular infiltrate of lymphocytes and eosinophils. Rearrangement of T-cell receptors is more frequently polyclonal and it is not decisive in the differential diagnosis.

Clinical features

Urticaria-like follicular mucinosis presents with recurrent pruritic urticarial papules and plaques of the face and neck on a 'rosaceiform or seborrhoeic' background. As lesions resolve, red macules persist for a few weeks. Hair-bearing regions may be involved, but neither follicular plugging nor alopecia is seen. The diagnosis is usually delayed since the dermatitis is often misinterpreted as urticaria, seborrhoeic dermatitis, rosacea or lupus tumidus before a biopsy is taken.

Management

Urticaria-like follicular mucinosis has a good prognosis although it may last up to 15 years. Therapy is difficult. Antimalarials and dapsone have been reported as beneficial [10].

SECONDARY MUCINOSES

Secondary cutaneous mucinoses include all those entities in which mucin deposition simply represents an additional histological finding and not the main feature (see Box 57.1) [1].

Key references

The full list of references can be found in the online version at https://www.wiley.com/rooksdermatology10e

Introduction and general description
1 Rongioletti F. Mucinoses. In: Rongioletti F, Smoller BR, eds. *Clinical and Pathological Aspects of Skin Diseases in Endocrine, Metabolic, Nutritional and Deposition Disease*. New York: Springer, 2010:139–52.
5 Rongioletti F, Barnhill R. Deposition disorders. In: Barnhill R, Crowson N, Magro C, Piepkorn M, eds. *Dermatopathology*, 4th edn. New York, McGraw, 2020.

Primary mucinoses
Dermal mucinoses
Lichen myxoedematosus (papular mucinosis)
1 Rongioletti F. Localized lichen myxedematosus. In: Callen J, ed. *UpToDate*. Wolters Kluwer, 2021. https://www.uptodate.com/contents/localized-lichen-myxedematosus (last accessed April 2022).
2 Rongioletti F, Merlo G, Cinotti E et al. Scleromyxedema: a multicenter study of characteristics, comorbidities, course, and therapy in 30 patients. *J Am Acad Dermatol* 2013;69:66.
4 Kalli F, Cioni M, Parodi A et al. Increased frequency of interleukin-4 and reduced frequency of interferon-γ and IL-17-producing CD4+ and CD8+ cells in scleromyxedema. *J Eur Acad Dermatol Venereol* 2020;34:1092–7.
7 Rongioletti F, Merlo G, Carli C et al. Histopathologic characteristics of scleromyxedema: a study of a series of 34 cases. *J Am Acad Dermatol* 2016;74:1194–200.
9 Ferreli C, Gasparini G, Parodi A, Cozzani E, Rongioletti F, Atzori L. Cutaneous manifestations of scleroderma and scleroderma-like disorders: a comprehensive review. *Clin Rev Allergy Immunol* 2017;53:306–36.
10 Mahévas T, Arnulf B, Bouaziz JD et al. Plasma cell-directed therapies in monoclonal gammopathy-associated scleromyxedema. *Blood* 2020;135:1101–10.
11 Guarneri A, Cioni M, Rongioletti F. High-dose intravenous immunoglobulin therapy for scleromyxoedema: a prospective open-label clinical trial using an objective score of clinical evaluation system. *J Eur Acad Dermatol Venereol* 2017;31:1157–60.
12 Haber R, Bachour J, El Gemayel M. Scleromyxedema treatment: a systematic review and update. *Int J Dermatol* 2020;59:1191–201.
18 Rongioletti F, Ferreli C, Atzori L. Acral persistent papular mucinosis. *Clin Dermatol* 2021;39:211–14.
20 Rongioletti F. Primary paediatric cutaneous mucinoses. *Br J Dermatol* 2020;182:29–38.
23 Rongioletti F. New and emerging conditions of acquired cutaneous mucinoses in adults. *J Eur Acad Dermatol Venereol* 2022;36:1016–24.

Reticular erythematous mucinosis
1 Rongioletti F, Merlo V, Riva S et al. Reticular erythematous mucinosis: a review of patients characteristics, associated conditions, therapy and outcome in 25 cases. *Br J Dermatol* 2013;169:1207–11.
2 Ocanha-Xavier JP, Cola-Senra CO, Xavier-Junior JCC. Reticular erythematous mucinosis: literature review and case report of a 24-year-old patient with systemic erythematosus lupus. *Lupus* 2021;30:325–35.
6 Cinotti E, Merlo V, Kempf W et al. Reticular erythematous mucinosis: histopathological and immunohistochemical features of 25 patients compared with 25 cases of lupus erythematosus tumidus. *J Eur Acad Dermatol Venereol* 2015;29:689–97.

Scleroedema
1 Rongioletti F, Kaiser F, Cinotti E et al. Scleredema. A multicentre study of characteristics, comorbidities, course and therapy in 44 patients. *J Eur Acad Dermatol Venereol* 2015;29:2399–404.
8 Knobler R, Moinzadeh P, Hunzelmann N et al. European dermatology forum S1-guideline on the diagnosis and treatment of sclerosing diseases of the skin, Part 2: Scleromyxedema, scleredema and nephrogenic systemic fibrosis. *J Eur Acad Dermatol Venereol* 2017;31:1581–94.
11 Miguel D, Schliemann S, Elsner P. Treatment of scleroedema adultorum buschke: a systematic review. *Acta Derm Venereol* 2018;98:305–9.

Localised (pretibial) myxoedema
2 Bartalena L, Fatourechi V. Extrathyroidal manifestations of Graves' disease: a 2014 update. *J Endocrinol Invest* 2014;37:691–700.
8 Ferreli C, Pinna AL, Pilloni L, Corbeddu M, Rongioletti F. Obesity-associated lymphedematous mucinosis: two further cases and review of the literature. *Dermatopathology (Basel)* 2018;5:16–20.
14 Kotwal A, Turcu AF, Sonawane V et al. Clinical experience with rituximab and intravenous immunoglobulin for pretibial myxedema: a case series. *Thyroid* 2019;29:692–9.

Papular and nodular mucinosis in connective tissue diseases
1 Rongioletti F, Smoller BR, eds. *Clinical and Pathological Aspects of Skin Diseases in Endocrine, Metabolic, Nutritional and Deposition Disease*. New York: Springer, 2010:146–7.
2 Dallo C, Lee K, Cragun WC, Lee M. A case of papulonodular mucinosis in a patient with systemic lupus erythematosus. *Am J Dermatopathol* 2020;42:280–2.

Self-healing cutaneous mucinosis
1 Luchsinger I, Coulombe J, Rongioletti F et al. Self-healing juvenile cutaneous mucinosis: clinical and histopathologic findings of 9 patients: the relevance of long-term follow-up. *J Am Acad Dermatol* 2018;78:1164–70.
2 Rongioletti F. Primary paediatric cutaneous mucinoses. *Br J Dermatol* 2020;182:29–38.

Cutaneous focal mucinosis
1 Kempf W, von Stumberg B, Denisjuk N, Bode B, Rongioletti F. Trauma-induced cutaneous focal mucinosis of the mammary areola: an unusual presentation. *Dermatopathology (Basel)* 2014;1:24–8.
2 Kuo KL, Lee LY, Kuo TT. Solitary cutaneous focal mucinosis: a clinicopathological study of 11 cases of soft fibroma-like cutaneous mucinous lesions. *J Dermatol* 2017;44:335–8.

Digital myxoid (mucous) cyst
1 Ferreli C, Caravano M, Fumo G, Rongioletti F. Digital myxoid cysts: 12-year experience from two Italian Dermatology Units. *G Ital Dermatol Venereol* 2018;153:847–54.

Follicular mucinoses
1 Khalil J, Kurban M, Abbas O. Follicular mucinosis: a review. *Int J Dermatol* 2021;60:159–65.

Pinkus follicular mucinosis

1 Khalil J, Kurban M, Abbas O. Follicular mucinosis: a review. *Int J Dermatol* 2021;60:159–65.

4 Rongioletti F, De Lucchi S, Meyes D *et al*. Follicular mucinosis: a clinicopathologic, histochemical, immunohistochemical and molecular study comparing the primary benign form and the mycosis fungoides-associated follicular mucinosis. *J Cutan Pathol* 2010;37:15–19.

Urticaria-like follicular mucinosis

1 Cinotti E, Basso D, Donati P, Parodi A, Rongioletti F. Urticaria-like follicular mucinosis: four new cases of a controversial entity. *J Eur Acad Dermatol Venereol* 2013;27:e435–7.

PART 5: METABOLIC & NUTRITIONAL DISORDERS

CHAPTER 58

Cutaneous Porphyrias

Robert P. E. Sarkany

St John's Institute of Dermatology, Guy's and St Thomas' NHS Foundation Trust, London, UK

PART 5: METABOLIC & NUTRITIONAL DISORDERS

Introduction

The porphyrias are a group of disorders caused by defects in the biosynthesis of haem. Their relevance to the skin arises from the phototoxic properties of the porphyrins, which accumulate in most porphyrias and cause photosensitivity.

The majority of the porphyrias are inherited. Many of them affect other organs as well as the skin. The recognition and management of both the genetic and internal consequences of porphyrias presenting in the skin are a key challenge for the dermatologist.

Clinical management in these disorders is made easier when the clinician understands their theoretical basis. Thus, this chapter is divided into two sections. The first section provides a theoretical basis for understanding the porphyrias, the general principles of clinical management and a clinician's guide to laboratory testing. The second section covers individual porphyrias in detail

Theoretical basis for understanding the porphyrias

Phototoxicity of porphyrins

The phototoxic properties of porphyrins are responsible for the cutaneous features of the porphyrias. Porphyrins are intermediates in the biosynthesis of haem, and consideration of the chemical features of the haem and porphyrin molecules is necessary to understand the cause of porphyrin phototoxicity.

Chemistry of porphyrins and haem

A pyrrole is a ring composed of four carbon atoms and one nitrogen atom. Four pyrroles linked into a ring create a tetrapyrrole, a remarkable and biologically critical molecular structure found in chlorophyll, haem and vitamin B_{12}. A porphyrin is a special type of tetrapyrrole in which four pyrrole rings are linked by methine bridges into a large ring structure [1].

Haem is the molecule created by the insertion of ferrous iron into the centre of the porphyrin molecule protoporphyrin IX (Figure 58.1). Essentially, incorporation of iron into the porphyrin molecule enables it to become biologically useful. Iron's capacity to bind to molecular oxygen and to transfer electrons (by moving between the 2+ and 3+ oxidation states) makes it potentially useful in biological systems, but free iron precipitates in the presence of water. For iron to be useful, it has to be kept soluble by protecting its binding sites against water. In addition, subtle modification of the electronic structure of the iron atom can optimise its ability to transfer electrons and reversibly bind molecular oxygen. Binding of iron to the porphyrin molecule solubilises iron and also optimises its electronic structure. The porphyrin's central cavity is the right size to fit an iron atom, and its four central nitrogen atoms occupy four of the iron's coordination binding sites, leaving only two free. A key feature of the porphyrin structure is that each double bond is adjacent to a single bond, so it is 'aromatic' with 18 of its electrons being delocalised and free to move around the molecule (Figure 58.1). This electron current results in the central nitrogen atoms tending to donate electrons to the iron atom, as well as other

Rook's Textbook of Dermatology, Tenth Edition. Edited by Christopher Griffiths, Jonathan Barker, Tanya Bleiker, Walayat Hussain and Rosalind Simpson.

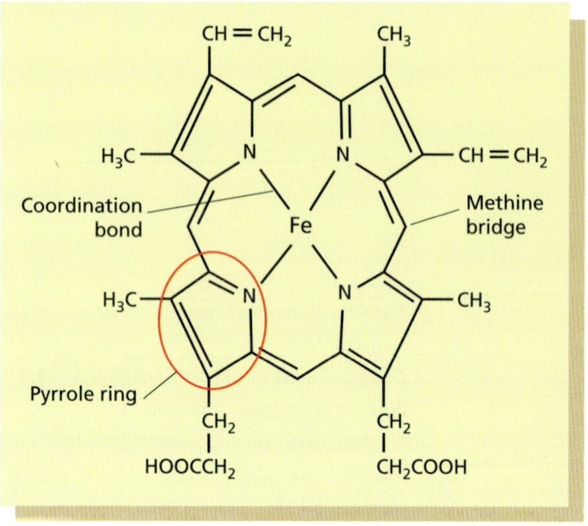

PART 5: METABOLIC &
NUTRITIONAL DISORDERS

Figure 58.1 The haem molecule and its key structural features. The alternation of single and double bonds around the tetrapyrrole ring indicates the aromaticity of the molecule, central to its chemical characteristics. The four coordination bonds between iron and nitrogen atoms are shown. The two remaining bonds between the iron and either molecular oxygen or amino acid residues lie perpendicular to the page.

subtler electronic interactions involving transient changes in the porphyrin's electronic state [2].

Haem can bind to a variety of proteins, and the nature of this interaction reflects the protein's function. In proteins with electron transport functions, such as respiratory cytochromes, amino acids bind to both remaining coordination binding sites on the iron so that haem can transfer electrons through alterations in the iron's oxidation state. In proteins with oxygen-binding functions, such as haemoglobin, an amino acid binds to one of the iron's remaining coordination binding sites, leaving the sixth site free to bind to oxygen. In summary, the aromatic porphyrin structure is well suited to complexing with iron to form haem, rendering the iron useful for electron transfer (respiratory cytochromes), reversible oxygen binding (haemoglobin and myoglobin) and oxidation and reduction reactions (cytochrome P450, catalase), with fine tuning of the iron's functionality being determined by the apoprotein that binds to the haem.

Photochemistry of the porphyrins

The complex electronic structure of the large aromatic porphyrin molecule results in its 18 delocalised electrons having unusual excitation characteristics. These electrons are excited by relatively long wavelength light. The main absorption peak is at 408 nm ('Soret band') [3], and this long wavelength of exciting light predisposes to phototoxic behaviour by the porphyrin. These photons have insufficient energy to chemically alter the porphyrin structure, so that alternative fates for the energy, particularly fluorescence and phosphorescence, become more likely [4]. Thus, following excitation by light around the 408 nm peak, electrons either return to the non-excited ground state by releasing the energy as characteristic red fluorescence, or the porphyrin's excited singlet state transforms (by intersystem crossing) to the longer lived excited triplet state. Transfer of energy from this excited triplet state to neighbouring molecules leads to the phototoxicity responsible for the clinical features of the cutaneous porphyrias. Thus cutaneous disease in

the porphyrias can be thought of as a by-product of the unusual porphyrin structure which enables haem proteins to fulfil their biological functions.

Enzyme deficiencies and the porphyrias

The porphyrias all result from a partial deficiency of one of the enzymes required for the biosynthesis of haem, thus causing accumulation of the enzyme's substrate. The toxicity profile of the accumulated molecule determines the clinical features of the resulting porphyria. A basic understanding of the biosynthetic pathway enables the clinician to interpret laboratory results and to predict the clinical features of each porphyria on the basis of each porphyrin's properties.

Biosynthesis of haem [5,6]

Haem is synthesised from simple biochemicals (glycine and succinyl coenzyme A (CoA)) via an eight-step pathway, each step being catalysed by an enzyme (Figure 58.2). Synthesis of the pyrrole ring (porphobilinogen (PBG)) is followed by assembly of the tetrapyrrole structure (hydroxymethylbilane). One of the pyrrole rings (the 'D' ring) is 'flipped' around to create the III isomer (the alternative I isomer forms in the absence of the cosynthase enzyme). Next, the carboxylic acid side chains of uroporphyrinogen III are progressively decarboxylated via coproporphyrinogen III to protoporphyrinogen, which is then oxidised to protoporphyrin IX. It is likely that the progressive decarboxylation to remove six of the eight electron-withdrawing carboxylate groups increases the flux of electrons onto the molecule's central nitrogens to facilitate coordination with iron. Finally, ferrous iron is chelated into the protoporphyrin's central cavity to form haem. Around 80% of haem is synthesised in erythroid cell precursors in the bone marrow (for haemoglobin production). The decarboxylation of uroporphyrinogen to coproporphyrinogen, and thence to protoporphyrinogen, decreases water solubility, so that uroporphyrinogen is only excreted via the kidneys whereas hydrophobic protoporphyrinogen and protoporphyrin are exclusively excreted into the bile. Coproporphyrinogen is excreted by both routes. Physiological concentrations of porphyrins stay low because of the high efficiency of haem synthesis.

Clinical features of the porphyrias: general considerations

Porphyrias present with either skin disease or acute attacks or both.

Classification of the porphyrias

In any porphyria, a partial enzyme deficiency causes the accumulation of porphyrins [1,2]. The enzyme deficiency associated with each disorder is shown in Figure 58.3. The porphyrias have previously been classified, according to the predominant site of porphyrin accumulation, into the erythropoietic group (congenital erythropoietic porphyria and erythropoietic protoporphyria) and the hepatic group (all the others). This division is not of value clinically. For the clinician, the key division is between porphyrias that cause acute attacks and those that cause skin disease. In this chapter the following classification is used for the six common porphyrias:

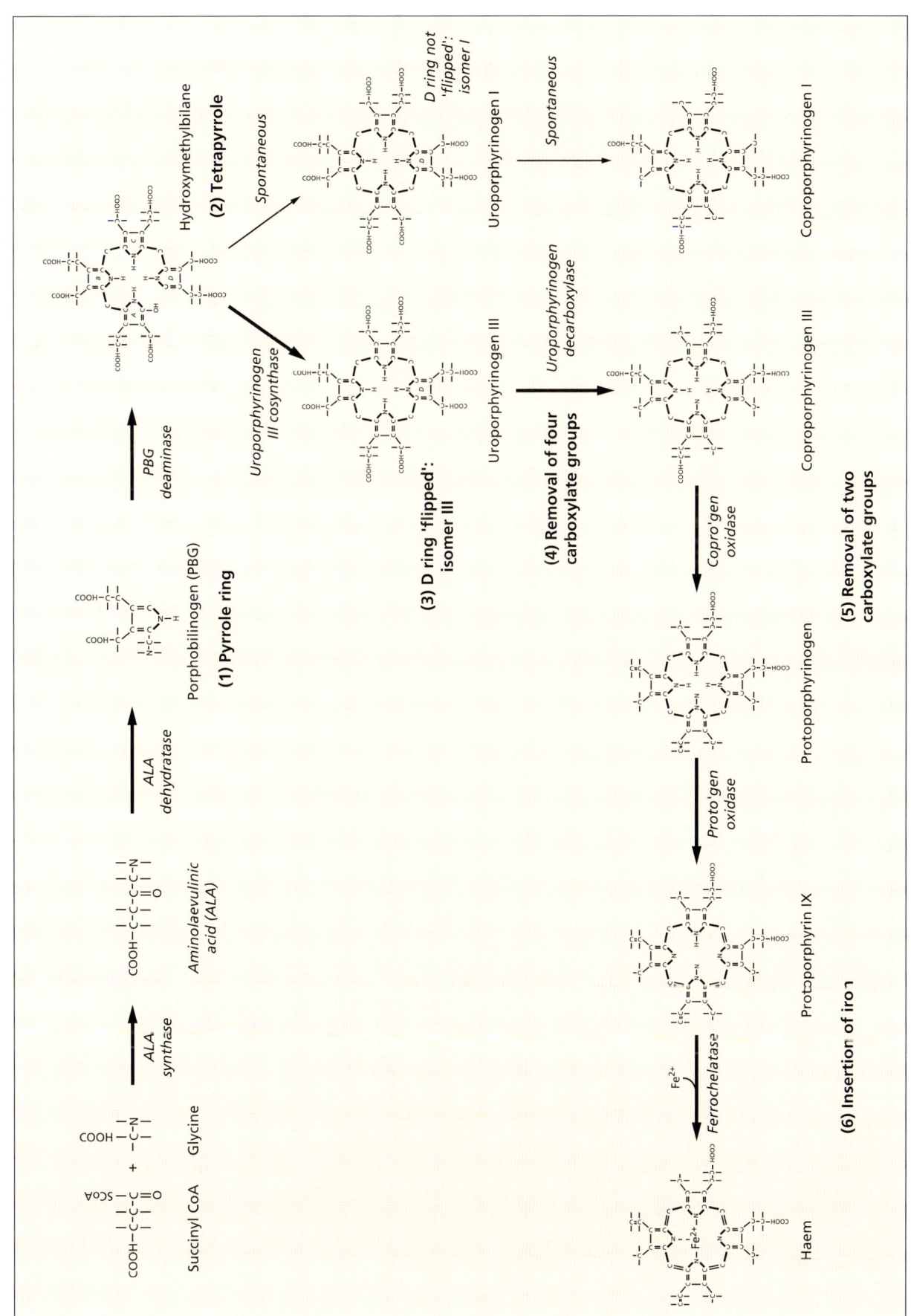

Figure 58.2 The pathway of haem biosynthesis showing the six key structural changes.

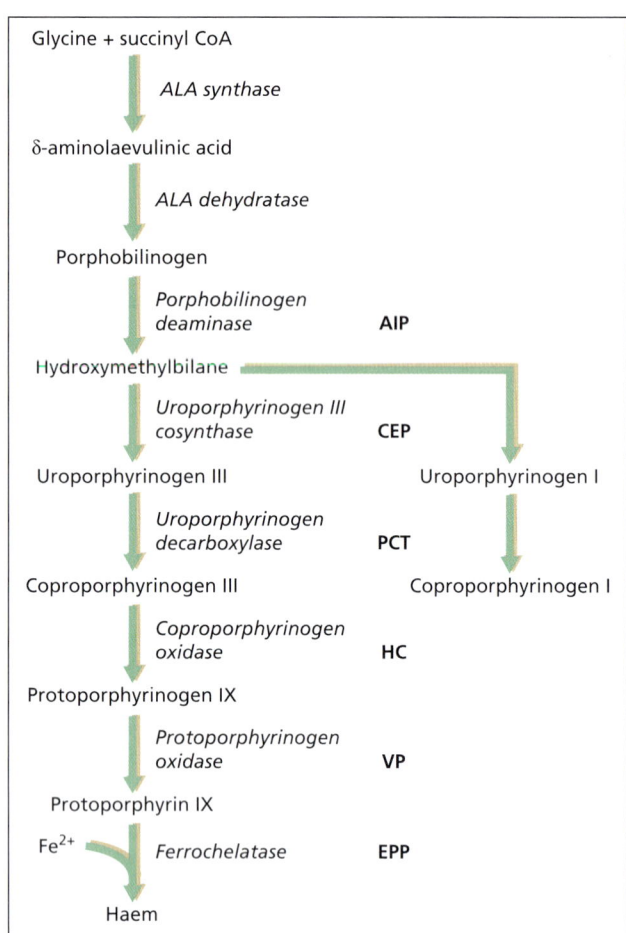

Figure 58.3 The pathway of haem biosynthesis showing the enzyme deficiency associated with each porphyria. AIP, acute intermittent porphyria; ALA, aminolaevulinic acid; CEP, congenital erythropoietic porphyria; CoA, coenzyme A; EPP, erythropoietic protoporphyria; HC, hereditary coproporphyria; PCT, porphyria cutanea tarda; VP, variegate porphyria.

1 Cutaneous disease only:
  • Porphyria cutanea tarda (PCT).
  • Congenital erythropoietic porphyria (CEP).
  • Erythropoietic protoporphyria (EPP).
2 Cutaneous disease and acute attacks:
  • Hereditary coproporphyria (HC).
  • Variegate porphyria (VP).
3 Acute attacks only:
  • Acute intermittent porphyria (AIP).

Porphyria and the skin

The cutaneous porphyrias share many features. Consideration of these underlying similarities is necessary for a logical approach to the clinical management of patients.

All the cutaneous porphyrias, except EPP, present with fragility and blistering of light-exposed skin. The term 'bullous porphyrias' is often used for this group of diseases. Not only can they appear very similar clinically, but the mechanism underlying the skin disease in all cutaneous porphyrias is a local porphyrin phototoxicity reaction. This shared pathogenetic mechanism means that the histopathological appearances in these conditions are also similar. As a result, these disorders can only be reliably differentiated by biochemical analysis. The other important similarity between them is that they

are all caused by Soret wavelength light (408 nm), so the same strategy for photoprotection applies to them all, as detailed here.

Pathophysiology of skin disease in porphyria

Photons of violet light, with a wavelength peak at 408 nm, transform the porphyrin molecule into an excited singlet state (Figure 58.4) [1–3]. This may revert to the unexcited ground state by emission of the characteristic red porphyrin fluorescence. However, intersystem crossing can convert the porphyrin to the excited triplet state which is long lived enough to interact with other molecules, particularly molecular oxygen, converting it to excited singlet oxygen in the process. The singlet oxygen stimulates the production of hydroxyl radicals, which damage tissue directly and also indirectly by stimulating complement activation [4], mast cell degranulation [5] and matrix metalloproteinase activity [6].

The site of this phototoxic reaction in the skin determines the clinical characteristics of the porphyria.

• In *EPP*, lipophilic protoporphyrin tends to localise to membranes including endothelial cell membranes and to remain within erythrocytes. The phototoxic reaction involves the upper dermal blood vessels causing pain.

• In *PCT*, the water-soluble uroporphyrin diffuses easily into surrounding tissues and the phototoxic reaction occurs in the upper dermis. This causes lysis of cells in the superficial dermis with the formation of membrane-limited vacuoles that merge to produce a blister under the basal lamina, producing the characteristic clinical presentation [7].

• In *VP*, copro- and protoporphyrin accumulate (Figure 58.3), but patients suffer from PCT-like upper dermal blisters rather than EPP-like acute pain. This is likely to be because, although hydrophobic porphyrins predominate in the plasma in VP, hydrophilic porphyrins, particularly uroporphyrin, predominate in the skin, probably due to secondary local photoinactivation of uroporphyrinogen decarboxylase (UROD) in the skin by coproporphyrin [2]. In addition, the protoporphyrin in VP is conjugated to a peptide which may reduce its phototoxicity.

There is no simple correlation between the plasma porphyrin concentration and the severity of cutaneous disease in porphyria. This is because of the large number of local variables that can alter the extent of the phototoxic reaction in the skin, and because an increased plasma porphyrin concentration is not always associated with cutaneous disease [8].

Histopathology of the skin in porphyria

In all the cutaneous porphyrias, homogeneous material is seen within the vessel walls of the upper dermal and papillary vascular plexus [9,10]. It is periodic acid–Schiff (PAS) positive and diastase resistant and contains a protein polysaccharide complex, lipids and tryptophan. Immunofluorescence reveals immunoglobulins (mainly IgG) in a similar vascular distribution and IgG at the dermal–epidermal basement membrane zone in involved skin. Electron microscopy shows reduplication of the vascular basal lamina and the presence of masses of fine fibrillar material, mainly around these blood vessels and often also at the dermal–epidermal junction.

In EPP, the vessel wall changes are more pronounced, whereas the basement membrane zone changes predominate in affected skin in PCT and VP. In bullous porphyrias, bullae are subepidermal with

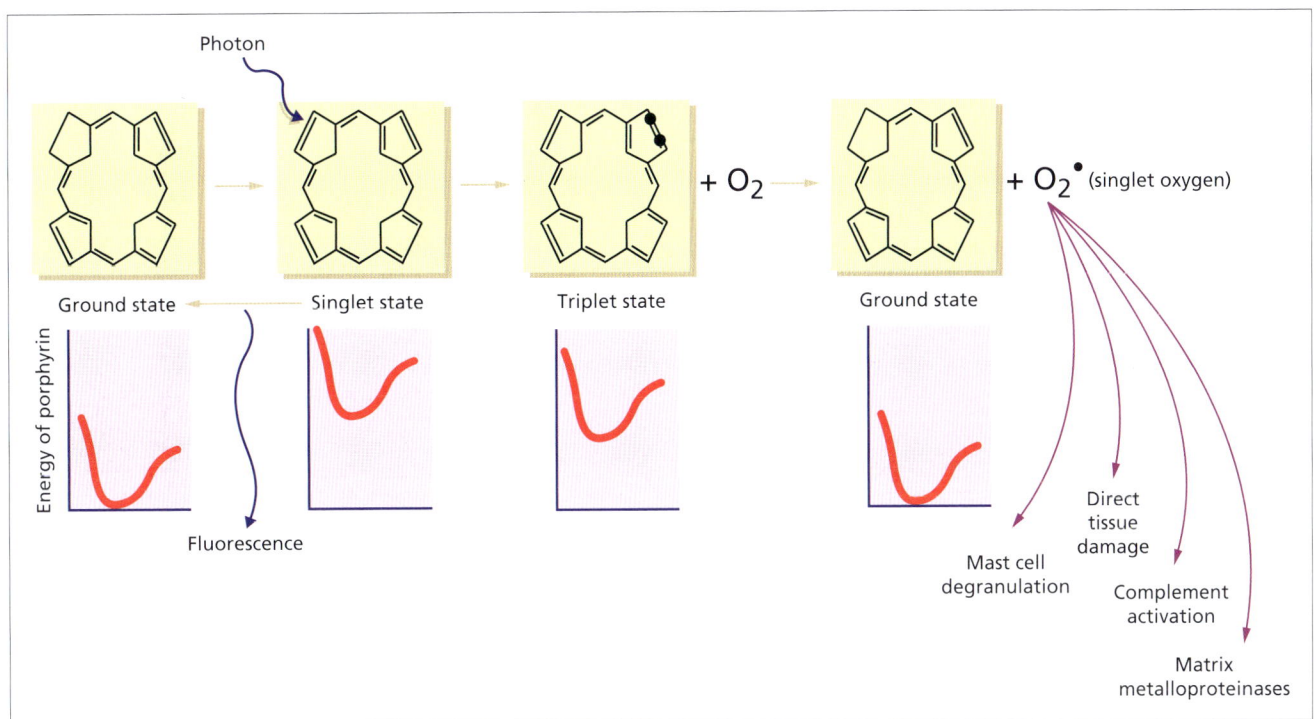

Figure 58.4 The pathogenesis of skin disease in porphyria.

the split occurring in the lamina lucida (Figure 58.5) [11] leaving the dermal papilla protruding into the blister cavity, an appearance called 'festooning' [10]. The findings in bullous porphyrias are indistinguishable from those of pseudoporphyria. In EPP, in the acute phase, there is visible endothelial damage in superficial dermal vessels [12]. Electron microscopy shows the 'amorphous' material seen in vessel walls on light microscopy in light-exposed skin to be a replicated, layered and fragmented basement membrane, with fine fibrillar material permeating the capillary connective tissue sheath and extending beyond the vessel walls, caused by repeated episodes of damage [13,14].

General considerations in the management of skin disease in porphyria

Apart from PCT, and to some extent CEP, where effective specific treatments exist, the management of the skin in the other cutaneous porphyrias is based on preventing violet (Soret wavelength) light penetrating the epidermis. The connection between sun exposure and symptoms is obvious in EPP, but is not obvious to patients with the bullous porphyrias where fragility and blistering are not related to individual episodes of sun exposure. It can therefore be difficult to convince these patients of the importance of photoprotection.

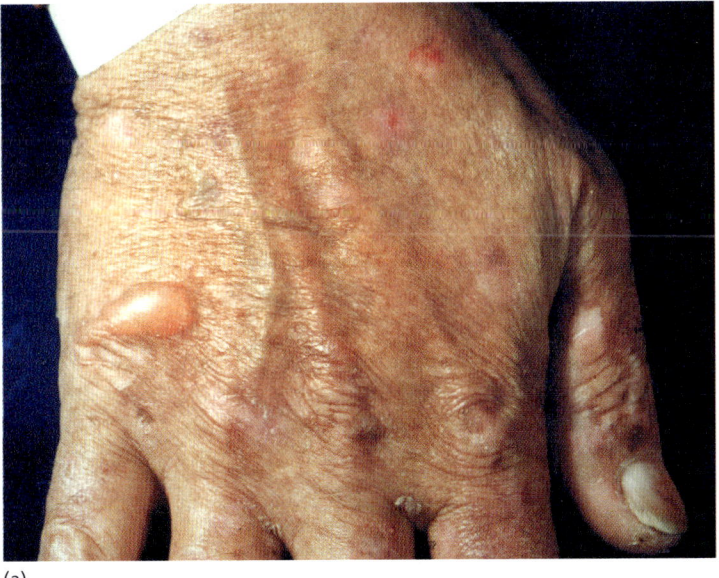

(a)

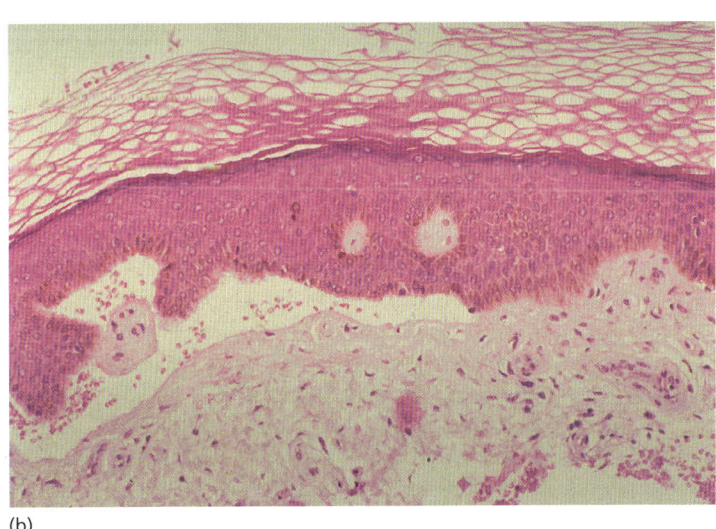

(b)

Figure 58.5 Typical subepidermal bulla in a bullous porphyria: (a) clinical appearance, and (b) histological appearance.

PART 5: METABOLIC & NUTRITIONAL DISORDERS

Basic measures include sun avoidance behaviour, sun protective clothing and hats. Most sunscreens, including ultraviolet (UV) absorbent chemical 'total sunblocks', do not protect against the visible violet Soret wavelength [15]. Any sunscreen providing significant visible light protection will be opaque rather than transparent. Sunscreens containing reflectant particles, particularly large particle size titanium dioxide (pigmentary grade), zinc oxide and iron oxide, can effectively protect against violet light [16]. Cosmetically acceptable sunscreens with reasonable protection up to 430 nm are available commercially, for example Dundee sunscreen (Tayside Pharmaceuticals, Dundee, UK) [15,16]. Dihydroxyacetone paint induces the formation of a light-absorbing brown pigment in the stratum corneum and has been used in some patients with EPP [17]. Some reasonably clear window films can absorb some violet light and are useful on car or home windows particularly in EPP and CEP [18]. In this author's practice two films are currently recommended which are clear and provide reasonable, although not complete, protection against Soret wavelength light (Dermagard film, Bonwyke, Hants, UK; CLS200XSR film, Madico, Tampa Bay, FL, USA). The Madico TA81XSR film is yellower but provides better protection. Films applied to car windows must comply with local legislation which varies considerably in different parts of the world.

Acute attacks of porphyria

Acute intermittent porphyria, HC and VP can all cause acute attacks, and HC and VP may also cause cutaneous disease [1,2]. A rare autosomal recessive acute porphyria, aminolaevulinic acid (ALA) dehydratase porphyria, has also been reported but this does not cause skin disease and will not be discussed further.

Definition

An acute prophyria is a potentially fatal illness frequently triggered by drugs and hormones which are metabolised by cytochrome P450. It is characterised by an acute neurotoxic reaction in many tissues.

Epidemiology

The commonest acute porphyria is AIP, followed by VP. HC is rare. The prevalence of clinically overt acute porphyria in Europe is 1–2 per 100 000 inhabitants, but over 90% of individuals possessing AIP or VP gene defects are asymptomatic, so the enzyme deficiencies are common. PBG deaminase deficiency, which causes AIP, is present in 0.2% of all blood donors [3].

Pathophysiology

Impaired activity of PBG deaminase is associated with acute attacks [4]. The deficiency can be primary (as in AIP) or secondary, the latter being due to inhibition of the enzyme by accumulated coproporphyrinogen and protoporphyrinogen (as in HC and VP) [5]. In the liver, haem is mostly incorporated into cytochrome P450 proteins, whose production is induced by many of the drugs and hormones metabolised by the P450 system. When a drug or hormone induces cytochrome P450, and hence acutely increases the hepatic requirement for haem, the inability of the pathway to respond adequately because of the PBG deaminase deficiency is exposed. This acute hepatic haem deficiency in turn causes secondary accumulation of ALA and increased ALA synthase activity due to loss of end-product negative feedback. The symptoms of the acute attack result from neuronal dysfunction, however the pathogenesis of this is not fully understood. Postulated mechanisms include disturbed metabolism of neurotransmitters (due to reduced activity of haem-containing hepatic tryptophan dioxygenase), direct neurotoxicity of accumulated ALA (which structurally resembles the neurotransmitter γ-aminobutyric acid) and acute haem deficiency within neurons.

Factors that may precipitate an acute attack

The most common precipitants are drugs and the menstrual cycle, with recurrent attacks often occurring in the late luteal phase [1]. Alcohol, cannabis, fasting, stress and infection may also trigger attacks. It is not possible to predict whether a specific drug will provoke an attack in an individual. Drugs should be prescribed only after reference to an up-to-date drug list. Recommended drug lists are available on the Internet from the Welsh Medicines Information Centre [6] or the European Porphyria Initiative [7]. These lists are regularly reviewed and updated by experts, and are lists of drugs, by type, that are known to be safe in acute porphyria. Hence, the lists are designed to answer questions such as 'Which antihypertensive can be safely used in a patient with acute porphyria?' The drug recommendations on these lists are not absolute and are not a substitute for clinical experience and judgement. The risk of a drug provoking an attack is obviously highest where that drug has previously caused an attack in that patient, and in any patients who have previously had symptoms suggestive of an acute attack.

Clinical features

Acute attacks are five times more common in females, and most frequently occur between the ages of 10 and 40 years. They are rare before puberty. The severity of acute attacks varies from mild abdominal pain, sometimes accompanied by vomiting and constipation, through to very severe attacks with bulbar palsy and respiratory paralysis [1,2]. Severe, constant abdominal pain occurs in almost all acute attacks. It can be in any abdominal quadrant or even occur in the back, buttocks and thighs, and may require large amounts of opiate analgesia. There may be guarding but there should be no true peritonism. Vomiting and constipation (due to partial ileus) occur in at least 50% of attacks. The pulse rate and blood pressure are often moderately raised, dehydration is common and hyponatraemia (probably caused by inappropriate secretion of vasopressin) may be severe enough to cause convulsions. The pain, tachycardia, hypertension and partial ileus are all caused by an acute autonomic neuropathy.

Sensory or sympathetic involvement which manifests as severe dysaesthesia or causalgia is rarer. A motor neuropathy occurs in 5–10% of cases, usually heralded by aching pains in the limbs and sometimes by disappearance of the abdominal pain. It may cause a severe acute Guillain–Barré-type syndrome. The motor neuropathy usually occurs when porphyrinogenic drugs have been administered inadvertently during the developing acute attack. Respiratory paralysis is the commonest cause of death. Confusion, abnormal behaviour, agitation and hallucinations occur in up to 50% of attacks. Porphyria is not related to any chronic psychiatric disease except generalised anxiety.

Investigations

The diagnostic finding is of increased urinary PBG excretion. Although qualitative screening tests may be useful in an emergency, their low sensitivity makes it essential to also carry out a quantitative assay [8,9]. Commercially available kits can provide a rapid and reasonably sensitive semiquantitative assay, after which a specific quantitative assay should be carried out (reliable quantitative assay kits are commercially available). A normal urinary PBG concentration excludes an acute porphyric attack (except in ALA dehydratase porphyria). An increased PBG concentration does not necessarily mean that an acute attack is occurring since urinary PBG falls between attacks but does not always return to normal, particularly in AIP. The higher the PBG concentration the more likely an acute attack, but in the presence of an increased urinary PBG, an acute attack can only be diagnosed on clinical grounds. Urinary ALA is also increased during an acute attack but to a lesser extent than PBG and is not as useful diagnostically (the only exception being ALA dehydratase porphyria in which only ALA is increased and urinary PBG is normal).

Management

Long-term management of patients with acute porphyria

Dermatologists may diagnose VP (or less commonly HC) on the basis of cutaneous disease before any acute attack has occurred. Once an acute porphyria has been diagnosed [1,2], the patient should be given a list of drugs with information about their safety in acute porphyria. Many lists exist both of 'safe' drugs and 'unsafe' drugs [6,7]. It is obviously vital for clinicians and patients to be clear about whether they are dealing with a list of safe or unsafe drugs, and there are advantages to using a safe list, as discussed earlier. It is important to recognise that a list of safe drugs is a guide, and that no drug can be guaranteed to be safe in an individual patient. Conversely, drugs which do not appear on a safe list should not be withheld in patients who need them to treat a serious or life-threatening illness; in that situation expert advice should be sought from a specialist centre.

The patient should also be advised to abstain from alcohol, cannabis and prolonged calorie-restricted diets, and to wear an emergency identification bracelet (e.g. MedicAlert) so that medical staff are aware of the diagnosis if the patient is ever found in an unconscious or confused state. Screening of relatives is essential to identify those with clinically latent disease who are also at risk of acute attacks. The choice of test and interpretation of results can be complex and details are covered in the laboratory testing section and under each individual disorder in this chapter. Such testing is ideally carried out in a specialist centre. Relatives diagnosed with an acute porphyria need the same advice as the index case. Conversely, patients with PCT, EPP and CEP can be reassured that acute attacks are not part of their disease.

Treatment of acute attacks

The key to managing an acute attack is early diagnosis [1,2]. Once the diagnosis has been made, the avoidance of acute attack-inducing drugs is essential to prevent exacerbation. Supportive treatment includes analgesia, sedatives and antiemetics (in each case using drugs known to be safe in acute porphyria) and careful management of fluid balance with rehydration and correction of hyponatraemia. The specific treatments are intravenous haematin or haem arginate (Normosang, Recordati Rare Diseases UK Ltd, Bracknell, UK), which have now replaced carbohydrate as the treatment of choice.

These drugs suppress hepatic ALA synthase activity and so reduce ALA and PBG accumulation. Haem arginate is more effective when given earlier during an attack, increasing the importance of early diagnosis. Advice from a specialist centre should be sought when treating an acute attack.

Clinician's guide to laboratory testing in porphyria

Although clinical features may raise the possibility of a porphyria, the cutaneous presentations of several porphyrias are very similar. Precise diagnosis is essential in porphyria because of the differences in clinical management between porphyrias that can be clinically indistinguishable [1–3]. An accurate diagnosis can only be made on the basis of porphyrin analyses carried out in an experienced laboratory. The clinician's role is to suspect the diagnosis of cutaneous porphyria, and then to use laboratory testing to confirm whether this is the diagnosis, and if so to precisely identify the porphyria. For any porphyria characterised by acute attacks, testing for latent porphyria in relatives will then be necessary.

What samples to send

In an adult with suspected bullous porphyria, it is generally sufficient to analyse the urine and either plasma (where fluorimetry is available) or faeces (where it is not) (Table 58.1). However, urine, plasma and faeces all need to be analysed in children because of the increased complexity of the differential diagnosis. Faecal analysis is also necessary in instances when urine and plasma results do not differentiate HC from CEP, and in renal failure, where urine may be unavailable and plasma analysis unhelpful because renal failure increases plasma porphyrins. In suspected EPP, red cells and either plasma or faeces should be analysed.

Handling of samples

Laboratory testing of body fluids measures porphyrins since porphyrinogens are spontaneously oxidised to their respective porphyrins outside the body. PBG has a tendency to polymerise to other molecules but porphyrins are reasonably stable when protected from light and oxidants. Thus, all specimens should be kept at room temperature or at 4°C in the dark and ideally should be analysed within 48 h of collection.

For urine and faecal analysis, fresh random specimens (10–20 mL urine or 5–10 g dry weight faeces) are preferable to 24 h collections. Random specimens yield equally useful results, and 24 h collections delay samples reaching the laboratory. Very dilute urine (creatinine <4 mmol/L) is unsuitable.

Table 58.1 Which samples to send for porphyrin analysis in the cutaneous porphyrias

Clinical presentation	Samples required
Suspected bullous porphyria: adult	Urine plus either plasma or faeces
Suspected bullous porphyria: child	Urine, plasma and faeces
Suspected erythropoietic protoporphyria	Red cells and either plasma or faeces

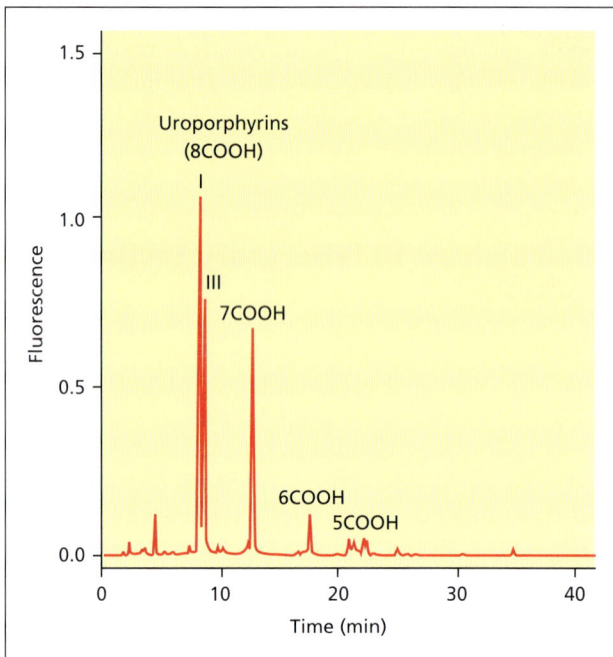

Figure 58.6 High-performance liquid chromatography (HPLC) analysis: the more carboxylate groups it possesses, the faster a porphyrin molecule passes through the column. After passing through the column, porphyrins are detected by fluorimetry. This HPLC trace of urine shows the porphyrin profile typical of porphyria cutanea tarda. Courtesy of Dr A. Deacon, King's College Hospital, London, UK.

Laboratory analysis of porphyrins

Old-fashioned qualitative screening methods for detecting porphyrins in specimens (often involving a Wood light) are insensitive, and negative results from such tests are not of value. Whether testing urine, faeces, red cells or whole blood, quantitative screening using spectrophotometric or fluorimetric techniques is necessary and yields results as a total porphyrin concentration. Whole blood or red cell porphyrin testing measures both the total and free protoporphyrin concentrations. Plasma is analysed by fluorimetric scanning: a diagnostically powerful and simple qualitative technique. In urine and faeces, the finding of an increased porphyrin concentration will lead on to high-performance liquid chromatography (HPLC), which can be used to rapidly identify the accumulated porphyrins (Figure 58.6). For PBG measurement in urine, qualitative tests are insensitive, and quantitative measurement, usually using a kit, is required. Semiquantitative test kits are useful in emergencies where a result is needed quickly.

Interpretation of results [4]

In cutaneous porphyrias, the accumulated porphyrin can usually be detected in plasma as an emission peak on spectrofluorimetry (Table 58.2). Uro- and coproporphyrin are excreted into the urine and copro- and protoporphyrin into the faeces. Protoporphyrin accumulates in red cells in EPP.

1 *Plasma spectrofluorimetry*. In plasma spectrofluorimetry, the sample is excited by 410 nm light, and fluorescent emissions detected. An emission peak at 615–620 nm indicates the presence of uro- or coproporphyrin and suggests a diagnosis of PCT, HC, CEP or hepatoerythropoietic porphyria (HEP) (urine analysis will differentiate PCT and HEP from the other two conditions). A peak at 624–626 nm indicates the presence of a porphyrin–peptide conjugate diagnostic of VP. This 624–626 nm peak is a sensitive indicator of VP and may even persist during periods of clinical remission when faecal excretion becomes normal. It is also positive in most cases of latent VP (in relatives) [5,6]. A peak around 633 nm (it can lie between 626 and 634 nm) is caused by protoporphyrin and suggests EPP, and EPP is an unlikely diagnosis in the absence of this peak. Plasma porphyrin concentrations, particularly uroporphyrin, increase in renal failure and can be as high as those found in patients with PCT.

2 *Whole blood/red cell*. An increased free protoporphyrin concentration is the diagnostic finding in EPP. The total protoporphyrin concentration includes both free and zinc-protoporphyrin. Zinc-protoporphyrin is also increased in iron deficiency, lead poisoning and certain anaemias. In a child with plasma, urine and faecal results typical of PCT, red cell UROD activity needs to be measured to exclude HEP.

3 *Urinary and faecal analysis*. An increased total porphyrin concentration suggests a diagnosis of cutaneous porphyria. The total urinary porphyrin concentration is used to monitor disease activity in PCT. HPLC analysis is used to identify the porphyrins once an increased concentration has been found.

• *In urine*. An increase in uroporphyrin (and other highly carboxylated porphyrins especially heptacarboxyporphyrin) is typical of PCT although this does not exclude VP. Plasma spectrofluorimetry differentiates these two conditions and faecal analysis is required where this is unavailable. When PCT goes into remission and the total urinary porphyrin concentration returns to normal, it may still be possible to diagnose PCT from the characteristic urinary HPLC pattern. Coproporphyrinuria, in the presence of normal faecal porphyrin levels, does not

Table 58.2 The major biochemical findings in the cutaneous porphyrias

Porphyria	Urine	Faeces	Red cell	Plasma fluorimetry
Congenital erythropoietic porphyria	Uroporphyrin I; coproporphyrin I	Coproporphyrin I	Zinc- and free protoporphyrin; uroporphyrin I; coproporphyrin I	Peak at 615–620 nm
Porphyria cutanea tarda	Uroporphyrin III; heptacarboxyporphyrin	Isocoproporphyrin; heptacarboxyporphyrin	Normal	Peak at 615–620 nm
Hereditary coproporphyria	Coproporphyrin III	Coproporphyrin III	Normal	Peak at 615–620 nm
Variegate porphyria	Coproporphyrin III	Protoporphyrin; coproporphyrin III; X-porphyrin	Normal	Peak at 624–627 nm
Erythropoietic protoporphyria	Normal	Protoporphyrin (not diagnostically helpful)	Free protoporphyrin	Peak at 626–634 nm

Adapted from Deacon and Elder 2001 [4].

indicate porphyria and can be caused by certain drugs, lead toxicity and hepatobiliary disease.

- *In urine and faeces.* Increased coproporphyrin suggests VP, but does not exclude HC. Isomer III to isomer I ratios are increased in every porphyria except CEP (where they are decreased). In CEP, excess type I isomers of uro- and coproporphyrin are present in urine and type I coproporphyrin in faeces.
- *In faeces.* In the presence of a plasma spectrofluorimetry peak at 615–620 nm, if urine HPLC does not show the PCT pattern, faecal analysis is required to differentiate HC (increased coproporphyrin III concentration) from CEP (increased coproporphyrin I concentration). Increased faecal isocoproporphyrin is characteristic of PCT. In renal failure, faecal analysis is vital since urine may be unavailable and plasma porphyrins are increased (PCT is the porphyria most commonly associated with renal failure). Increased faecal protoporphyrin is suggestive but not diagnostic of EPP, since it can also derive from bacterial degradation of haem in the gut and may indicate gastrointestinal haemorrhage when porphyrin concentrations are normal elsewhere.

Biochemical diagnosis of an acute attack of porphyria

This is discussed earlier in this chapter. A definitive diagnosis of VP or HC can usually be made on the basis of detailed porphyrin analysis [3,4]. A definitive diagnosis of AIP requires enzyme or genetic tests.

Screening of relatives

In VP and HC, porphyrin levels are normal before puberty. Over the age of 15 years, a plasma fluorimetry scan is a reasonably sensitive biochemical test for latent VP in asymptomatic relatives of patients, picking up most cases. A positive scan is diagnostic of latent VP but a negative result is uninformative [5,6]. Faecal analysis, to measure the ratio of coproporphyrin isomers, will pick up some cases of latent HC after puberty [7]. In VP and HC, a negative porphyrin screening test in a relative needs to be followed by DNA analysis before latent disease can be excluded. The lack of any common mutations in porphyria (apart from South African VP) means that the causative mutation usually has to be identified for each family.

INDIVIDUAL PORPHYRIAS

PORPHYRIAS THAT CAUSE CUTANEOUS DISEASE BUT NOT ACUTE ATTACKS

Congenital erythropoietic porphyria

Definition and nomenclature

This is a severe and rare childhood porphyria causing lifelong mutilating photosensitivity and haematological disease.

Epidemiology

This is a rare disease: the incidence in Europe is 0.007 per year per 10 million population [1], and only about 200 cases have ever been reported worldwide. Rare adult-onset cases of acquired CEP have been reported secondary to myelodysplasia [2].

Pathophysiology

Congenital erythropoietic porphyria is caused by an autosomal recessive inherited deficiency of the uroporphyrinogen III cosynthase enzyme usually due to mutations in the gene encoding that enzyme. Less commonly this enzyme deficiency is caused by mutations in the *GATA1* gene. Since this enzyme is required to form the biologically useful type III porphyrin isomers, its absence results in non-enzymatic reactions producing large amounts of type I isomer porphyrins which cannot participate in haem formation, and which massively accumulate in erythroid cells and then gradually leak into the plasma.

Clinical features
Presentation

Congenital erythropoietic porphyria has a wide spectrum of presentation, from hydrops fetalis through to severe disease starting in infancy and also mild forms presenting later in life. The first sign of CEP is often the child's mother noting brown discoloration of amniotic fluid at the onset of labour, or observing pink or brown porphyrin staining of nappies (which fluoresce red-orange under Wood light).

Severe photosensitivity begins in infancy, often in the neonatal period, with blisters developing in light-exposed skin on minimal light exposure [3,4,5]. Phototherapy for neonatal jaundice may trigger lesions. Most children are so sensitive to the light that they have problems throughout the year. Exposed (and sometimes non-exposed) skin is fragile. The repeated bouts of inflammation with vesicles and bullae, often complicated by secondary infection, cause mutilating scarring, particularly of the face and hands (Figure 58.7). This photomutilation is associated with erosion of the terminal phalanges, onycholysis and destructive changes affecting the pinnae and nose. A diffuse pseudosclerodermatous thickening of exposed skin often gradually develops, with microstomia and sclerodactyly-like changes. Hypertrichosis is found in most patients, particularly on the upper arms, temples and malar region. Patchy hypo- and hyperpigmentation occur even in minimally exposed areas.

A milder late-onset form, presenting at any age from the third decade onward, has been described. This presents in a manner similar to PCT and occurs either as a result of mild inherited gene mutations [6] or as an acquired disease secondary to bone marrow myelodysplasia [2].

The eyes and internal organs are frequently involved [4,5].
- *Eyes.* Keratoconjunctivitis, blepharitis, cataracts, corneal ulcers, scars, cicatricial ectropion and scarring alopecia of eyelashes and eyebrows may all occur. Scleromalacia, pterygium formation,

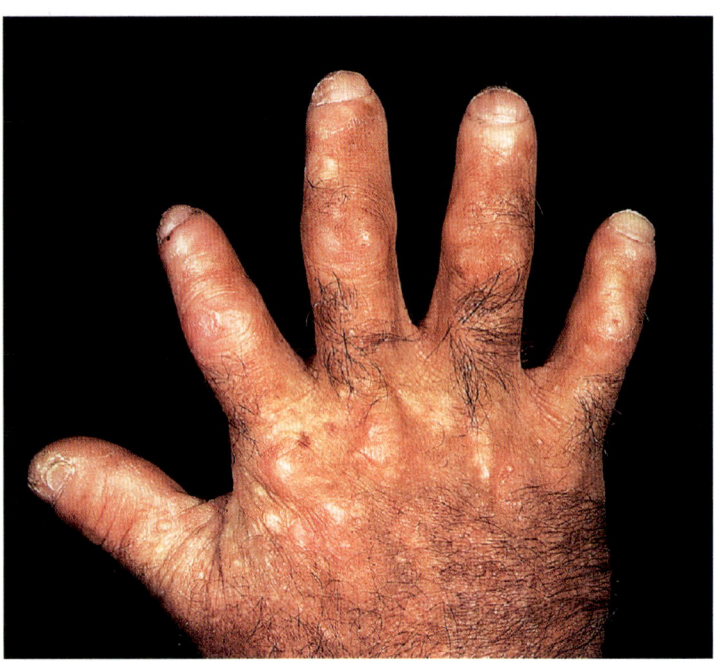

Figure 58.7 Congenital erythropoietic porphyria: scarring of skin with resorption of terminal phalanges. Courtesy of Dr A. du Vivier.

optic atrophy, retinal haemorrhage and scleral necrosis are less common.

- *Bones and teeth.* When teeth emerge, they are almost always stained brown (and fluoresce under Wood light). Decreased bone density, osteopenia and osteolytic lesions secondary to erosion by hyperplastic bone marrow are seen on X-ray and are associated with vertebral compression and collapse and with pathological fractures. In the hands there is resorption of terminal phalanges with acro-osteolysis and cortical bone rarefaction. Occasionally, strict avoidance of the sun may impair vitamin D metabolism.
- *Haematology* [4,5]. The high concentrations of porphyrins in red cells cause haemolytic anaemia, severe enough to induce marrow hyperplasia often with visible expansion of the maxillary bones in the face. Hypersplenism is common. The haemolysis can be fully compensated or may cause a severe anaemia and is occasionally so severe that some patients become transfusion dependent. The severity of the anaemia often fluctuates strikingly over time. Very severe haemolytic anaemia may even cause hydrops fetalis. Bone marrow examination reveals normoblastic hyperplasia. Under violet illumination most normoblasts have persistent red fluorescence localised to their nuclei, with haem-containing inclusion bodies being seen in the nuclei of these fluorescent cells.

Differential diagnosis

The photosensitivity differentiates CEP from other scarring, blistering disorders of childhood including epidermolysis bullosa dystrophica. The cutaneous changes may resemble HEP (the homozygous form of familial PCT) or homozygous VP. The cutaneous disease in late-onset CEP is clinically indistinguishable from PCT or VP.

Disease course and prognosis

In the past, most patients died by the age of 40 years but improvements in supportive care (particularly the use of antibiotics) have improved the prognosis, although the haematological complications may be fatal [7]. Long-term hypertransfusion causes significant problems with iron overload as patients reach adulthood, even when iron chelation has been used. Bone marrow transplantation now holds out the promise of cure for these patients. The key markers of poor prognosis in CEP are early onset of disease (especially in the first year of life) and significant haematological involvement [7].

Investigations

The uroporphyrinogen III cosynthase enzyme deficiency results in the massive accumulation in all tissues of type I isomers of porphyrins, mainly uroporphyrin, along with coproporphyrin and smaller amounts of 7-, 6- and 5-carboxylic acid porphyrins [3]. Red cells and urine contain large amounts of uro- and coproporphyrin (mainly type I) and faeces contain increased concentrations of coproporphyrin (mainly type I). A plasma spectrofluorimetry peak is seen at 615–620 nm. The absence of isocoproporphyrins and the normal level of 5-carboxylic porphyrin excretion in faeces distinguish CEP from HEP. Since GATA1 mutations cause uroporphyrinogen III cosynthase deficiency, the biochemical findings are the same in GATA1-related cases.

Management [7]

Treatment

The photosensitivity is so severe that photoprotection is crucial. Sun avoidance and use of sun protective clothing and hats are essential. Opaque sunscreens containing pigmentary grade titanium dioxide or zinc oxide, possibly with added iron oxide, may be of limited value [8,9]. Amber window films (e.g. Madico TA81XSR) on home or car windows can reduce exposure to Soret wavelength light [10], although more opaque films may be necessary (which are obviously not allowed on car windows).

Prompt treatment of secondary infection is important. Many therapies reduce the porphyrin concentrations by suppressing erythropoiesis. Hypertransfusion with regular blood transfusions to maintain a polycythaemia inhibits endogenous haemoglobin production and decreases porphyrin formation and may reduce haemolysis and cutaneous symptoms in moderately affected patients. However, splenomegaly may increase transfusion requirements and the value of hypertransfusion often decreases at puberty [6]. Hypertransfusion is frequently complicated by iron overload, even when desferrioxamine has been used, and blood-borne infections can be a complication. Intravenous haematin has been tried in late-onset disease [11]. Haemolysis worsens the porphyria by causing anaemia and usually necessitates blood transfusion. Splenectomy may reduce haemolysis although the improvement may be temporary. Lights during surgical procedures may cause phototoxic reactions and filters should be used over the operation lights during any unavoidable surgery, preferably a yellow filter (e.g. Madico TA81XSR). Overall, the results from all systemic therapies in CEP are disappointing [7] and the mainstay of treatment is strict photoprotection and treatment of haemolytic anaemia by hypertransfusion.

Since 1991, allogeneic bone marrow transplantation (bone marrow or umbilical cord blood stem cells) from a human leukocyte antigen-compatible donor has emerged as the treatment of choice in severe CEP. It provides a long-term cure [7,12] although the difficulties of finding a tissue-matched donor, and the dangers of marrow transplantation, mean that it should be reserved for the most severely affected patients and in children with markers of poor prognosis [4,7]. Gene therapy has been successfully used *in vitro*, but no *in vivo* studies have been carried out yet [13].

Recently, phlebotomy has been found to be an unexpectedly effective treatment, leading to improvements in haemolysis, porphyrin levels and photosensitivity [14].

Genetic counselling

Since the usual form of CEP, due to uroporphyrinogen III cosynthase mutations, is autosomal recessive, parents will be unaware of the risk until an affected child has been born and the risk of disease is in further offspring rather than subsequent generations. For parents of an affected child, the chance of each future offspring suffering from the disease is 25%. The diagnosis may be made before birth by measuring the uroporphyrin I concentration in amniotic fluid, which is increased as early as 16 weeks in *utero*. If the mutations in the index case have been identified, or the fetus is homozygous for the common C73R mutation, prenatal diagnosis from chorionic villous biopsy is possible [15]. GATA1 CEP is an X-linked disease affecting males [16].

Porphyria cutanea tarda

Definition

Porphyria cutanea tarda is the commonest of all the porphyrias [1,2]. It is characterised by fragility and blistering of exposed skin. It is usually acquired and is often associated with liver disease. It does not cause acute attacks.

Epidemiology and pathophysiology

Porphyria cutanea tarda results from a deficiency of UROD [3]. This causes an accumulation of uroporphyrin and other highly carboxylated porphyrins. Seventy-five per cent of patients have the *type I* (*sporadic*) form in which the enzyme deficiency is acquired and restricted to hepatocytes, due to inhibition of a normal UROD enzyme [3]. Twenty-five per cent have *type II* (*familial*) disease where the enzyme deficiency is hereditary, present in all tissues and associated with a UROD gene mutation. The penetrance of this autosomal dominant inherited form is so low that a family history is present in less than 7% of cases, and since at least a 75% reduction in enzyme activity is required for clinical expression, some enzyme inhibition in the liver also occurs in familial PCT. Thus, UROD mutations are increasingly considered to be a risk factor for the development of PCT, rather than as representing a completely separate familial form of the disease. Other genetic factors causing susceptibility to the development of PCT are polymorphisms in the cytochrome P450, glutathione-*S*-transferase and glyceronephosphate *O*-acyltransferase genes [4,5]. *Type IIII* disease is rare and

characterised by a hereditary enzyme deficiency localised to the liver. *Toxic porphyria*, in which halogenated aromatic hydrocarbons inhibit the enzyme, is rare and mainly affects workers making herbicides [6]. A major epidemic of toxic porphyria in the 1950s in Turkey was caused by hexachlorobenzene added as a fungicide to seed wheat [7].

In PCT, the UROD enzyme is inactivated by uroporphomethene, a competitive inhibitor of UROD, which is formed by the oxidation of uroporphyrinogen [8]. The inhibitor is generated in the liver by reactive oxygen species in the presence of iron (Figure 58.8) [9]. The accumulated uroporphyrin diffuses from the plasma into the surrounding tissues, causing a phototoxic reaction in the upper dermis in sun-exposed skin. This leads to lysis of cells in the superficial dermis with the formation of membrane-limited vacuoles which merge to produce a blister cavity under the basal lamina [10].

The prevalence varies but in most countries is around 1 in 10 000 [2].

Clinical features [11]
Presentation

Sporadic PCT usually presents in middle age while the familial form can occur at a younger age. Almost all patients notice increased fragility on light-exposed skin, particularly the backs of the hands and forearms, with minor trauma shearing the skin to leave sharply marginated erosions (Figure 58.9). Most patients suffer from bullae which can be over 1 cm in diameter and may be painful. They crust and resolve over a few weeks, leaving atrophic scars, milia and often mottled hyper- or hypopigmentation. Patients rarely associate the development of new lesions with sun exposure but symptoms are generally worse in the summer.

Other common features include patches of scarring alopecia following resolution of bullae on the scalp, hypertrichosis usually on the upper face and forehead (sometimes on the ears or arms [12] and occasionally affecting the whole body) and hyperpigmentation in a melasma-like pattern on the cheeks and around the eyes (or in a diffuse pattern on light-exposed skin or occasionally in a reticulate distribution) [11,12].

Photo-induced onycholysis [13] and accelerated solar elastosis [12] may also occur. Morphoea-like plaques may develop particularly on the head and upper trunk. They are histologically indistinguishable from true scleroderma and mainly occur in long-standing untreated disease. It has been postulated that they arise as a result of the induction of collagen synthesis by uroporphyrin I [14]. These plaques may calcify and may require excision and grafting, if they ulcerate [15].

On the scalp, the morphoea-like change may cause a slowly expanding scarring alopecia starting in the frontoparietal and occipital areas [11,12,16]. Even sclerodactyly or the facial changes of systemic sclerosis have been reported. Rare presentations of PCT include cicatricial conjunctivitis [17] and hair darkening [18].

Clinical variants

The homozygous form of familial PCT, HEP, is associated with over 90% reduction in UROD activity [12,19]. It usually causes a severe disease clinically similar to CEP, with photosensitivity during infancy causing immediate pain on sun exposure, blisters

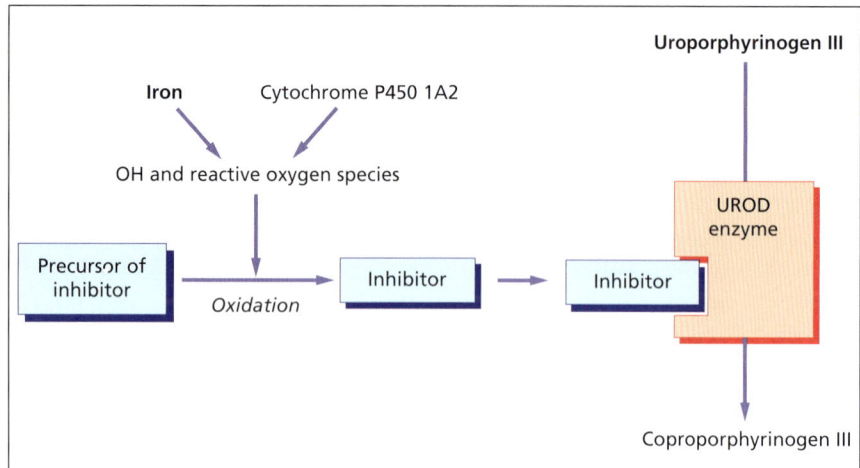

Figure 58.8 Porphyria cutanea tarda is caused by production of an inhibitor of uroporphyrinogen decarboxylase (UROD) in the liver, in the presence of iron. Adapted from Elder 1998 [2].

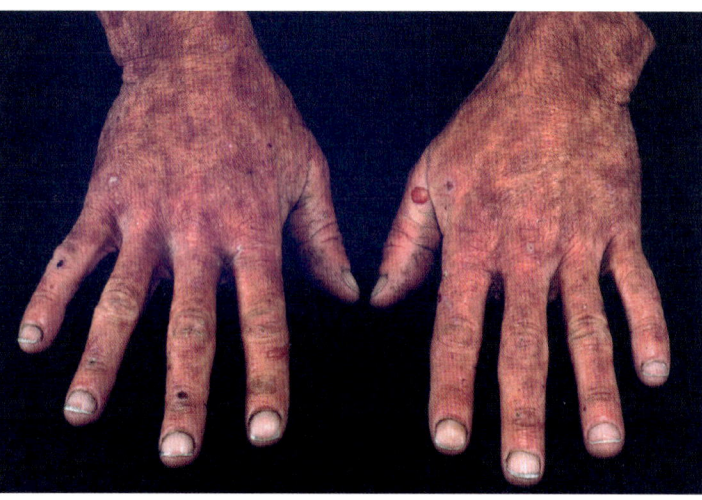

Figure 58.9 Porphyria cutanea tarda: erosions, blisters, pigmentary changes and scarring.

on sun-exposed skin and mutilating scarring of the face and fingers. Prominent hypertrichosis, fluorescent teeth, eye involvement and shortened distal phalanges also occur. Haemolysis is milder than in CEP, and life expectancy is normal. HEP can occasionally present with a milder disease similar to PCT. Since the mutated alleles in HEP have to be associated with some residual enzyme activity to be compatible with life, the UROD gene mutations in HEP patients are different from those found in type II PCT [20].

Differential diagnosis

Porphyria cutanea tarda can be clinically indistinguishable from VP, drug-induced pseudoporphyria, renal pseudoporphyria, HC, late-onset Günther disease or mild HEP. Biochemical analysis is necessary to diagnose PCT and it is particularly important to exclude VP and HC among the differential diagnoses as they can cause acute attacks.

Investigations
Looking for relevant systemic disease

Porphyria cutanea tarda is essentially a liver disorder with secondary effects in the skin. It is crucial to investigate patients thoroughly both regarding other systemic diseases predisposing to the development of PCT and to assess the severity of any liver disease.

Biochemical findings

In PCT, the urinary porphyrin concentration is increased, consisting mainly of uroporphyrin, some heptacarboxylic acid porphyrin, and sometimes also hexa- and pentacarboxylic acid porphyrins [2]. A plasma spectrofluorimetry peak is seen at 615–620 nm. Isocoproporphyrin accumulates in the faeces. Urine analysis alone is insufficient to diagnose PCT, since a few patients with VP have the PCT urine pattern ('dual porphyria') [21]. In patients with renal failure, faecal analysis is essential, since plasma porphyrins are increased by haemodialysis, and urine collection may not be possible. The biochemical marker of disease activity and response to treatment is quantitative urinary porphyrin excretion measured in a random urine sample. In HEP, the findings are as in PCT, but with the additional finding of a raised red cell zinc-protoporphyrin, and lower red cell UROD activity than occurs in type II PCT.

Histopathology

The bullae in PCT are subepidermal with a sparse inflammatory infiltrate and 'festooning' of dermal papillae into the bullae [22]. There is deposition of PAS-positive diastase-resistant fibrillar glycoprotein material in and around the upper dermal blood vessel walls and reduplication of the basement membrane. Immunofluorescence reveals IgG, a little IgM, fibrinogen and complement at the epidermal–dermal junction. Morphoea-like lesions in PCT are histologically indistinguishable from other forms of morphoea.

Risk factors for the development of PCT

The major risk factors for developing PCT are subclinical genetic haemochromatosis, hepatitis C infection, alcohol and oestrogens [**23**]. They all predispose to inhibition of the UROD enzyme in the liver. Since some inhibition of the hepatic enzyme is also required for clinical expression of familial PCT, the same risk factors apply to sporadic and familial PCT. Since most of the risk factors have significant implications both for treatment and for the patient's general health, it is essential to investigate for risk factors in all patients diagnosed with PCT.

- *Haemochromatosis*. As expected in a disorder where hepatic iron plays a key role, almost all patients have increased stainable iron in the liver, and total body iron stores are increased in at least 60% of patients [2,23,24]. In the USA and northern Europe, around 20% of PCT patients have true hereditary haemochromatosis [23,25] with homozygosity for the Cys282Tyr haemochromatosis mutation. Homozygosity for this mutation increases the risk of developing PCT 60-fold [23]. The clinical relevance of heterozygosity for the mutation is unclear. In southern Europe, haemochromatosis is a less important risk factor. The iron overload found in PCT patients who do not have haemochromatosis is milder, and its cause is obscure.

- *Hepatitis C infection*. In southern Europe, 70–90% of all PCT patients are infected with the hepatitis C virus [26,27], compared with around 60% of patients in the USA [23] and 7–36% in northern Europe [28,29].

- *Alcohol*. Between 30% and 90% of PCT patients consume over 40 g of alcohol daily, and 2% of all alcoholics with cirrhosis develop PCT [9].

- *Oestrogens*. Ingested oestrogens, in the oral contraceptive pill or in hormone replacement therapy, are the sole risk factor in over 25% of female patients [23]. Stopping the hormone may be sufficient to induce remission if the duration of therapy has been short [30]. If it is not possible to stop the hormone therapy, transdermal drug delivery is a safer alternative than the oral route [31].

There are other less common risk factors for developing PCT. Haemodialysis predisposes to PCT [32], although PCT is less common in renal failure than pseudoporphyria and faecal porphyrin analysis differentiates these disorders. Human immunodeficiency virus (HIV) infection predisposes to PCT [33], an association mainly due to co-infection with the hepatitis C virus [34]. Non-insulin-dependent diabetes, systemic lupus erythematosus, dermatomyositis, hepatitis A and B infection, haematological malignancy, sideroblastic anaemia, thalassaemia and the drug tamoxifen have also all been reported to be associated with PCT [2,12,35,36].

Most patients possess more than one risk factor for developing PCT, with hepatitis C infection and alcohol being strongly linked in men.

Liver disease in porphyria cutanea tarda

Since PCT is primarily a liver disorder with secondary effects in the skin, liver disease is a major concern [24]. In almost all cases, liver biopsy reveals increased stainable iron, fatty change and intracellular porphyrin crystals. Fifty per cent of patients have more severe changes (lobular necrosis or inflamed fibrotic portal tracts) and cirrhosis occurs in 15% [24]. As expected, the most severe liver disease tends to occur in patients who have alcoholism, hepatitis C infection and iron overload [23]. The accumulated porphyrins are carcinogenic to the liver, so PCT confers an additional risk for developing hepatocellular carcinoma in addition to the risk conferred by the hepatitis C infection present in many patients [37]. In southern Europe, around 3% of PCT patients develop hepatocellular carcinoma during the decade after presentation [38] although the incidence of hepatic malignancy is probably lower than this in countries with lower hepatitis C infection rates. Risk factors for developing hepatocellular carcinoma are thought to be a symptomatic period of more than 10 years prior to treatment, severe changes on hepatic histology at presentation, hepatitis C infection, male sex and age over 50 years at presentation [39,40]. The converse situation, where a primary hepatic tumour secretes porphyrins to cause a PCT-like skin disease, is rare [41]. Hepatic function must be assessed at presentation in all PCT patients, and patients at high risk of hepatic malignancy require regular ultrasound scans and serum α-fetoprotein measurement to detect carcinoma at a treatable stage [39]. PCT should be managed as a liver disorder, and the threshold for referral to a hepatologist should be low.

Management

Photoprotection

Visible light sunscreens containing pigmentary grade titanium dioxide or zinc oxide, sometimes with added iron oxide [42,43], filter films for car and home windows, gloves, hats and clothes play an important role in controlling symptoms during the period of several months before specific therapies take effect.

Elimination of risk factors

The treatment of hepatitis C infection with antivirals results in rapid remission of PCT [44]. Stopping oestrogen therapy [30], if it has not been used for more than 2 years, can induce remission. However, elimination of the underlying cause by abstaining from alcohol does not always induce remission. All patients should be advised to abstain from alcohol or oestrogen therapy to prevent exacerbation of the disease.

Specific treatments

Definitive treatment with venesection or low-dose antimalarials is required in almost all cases. Venesection depletes iron stores and eliminates hepatic iron overload thus restoring normal enzyme activity. Around 500 mL of blood is removed every 1–2 weeks aiming to decrease transferrin saturation to 15%, haemoglobin to 11–12 g/dL and plasma ferritin to below 25 μg/L [45,46]. Blistering usually resolves within 2–3 months, skin fragility within 6–9 months [47], and porphyrin concentrations generally normalise within 13 months [12], at which point treatment should be stopped. Hypertrichosis [12] and sclerodermoid lesions [16] respond more slowly during the years after treatment has stopped. Excision and grafting may be needed for ulcerated sclerodermoid lesions [12].

Desferrioxamine leads to earlier remission than venesection because it rapidly chelates hepatic iron and it may be of value in PCT with renal failure, but it is expensive and requires a subcutaneous pump at night [48,49]. Erythropoietin mobilises hepatic iron into haemoglobin and is the treatment of choice for PCT in renal failure where patients are too anaemic for venesection and cannot excrete chloroquine [50]. PCT in renal failure can improve if the patient is changed from conventional high-flux hemodialysis to haemodiafiltration with ultrafiltrate regeneration by resin adsorption (Supra-HFR) [51].

Low-dose antimalarials are a very effective treatment for PCT. They work by complexing with uroporphyrin and promoting its excretion into the bile [52]. Daily doses of chloroquine cause a potentially dangerous acute hepatitis, but chloroquine at the low dose of 125 mg [53,54] or 250 mg [55,56] taken twice a week is safe and effective. It leads to clinical remission within 6 months and biochemical remission after 6–15 months, at which point treatment is stopped [53,54,55]. Retinopathy does not seem to occur with such low doses of chloroquine [55]. Hydroxychloroquine (100 mg twice weekly) is also effective [57].

Low-dose chloroquine is the treatment of choice except in the following situations in which venesection is preferable: (i) patients who do not respond to chloroquine; (ii) patients with a pathologically high serum ferritin concentration or homozygous for the Cys282Tyr mutation (if genetic analysis is available), who require iron depletion to protect internal organs; and (iii) patients with significant hepatitis C liver disease, who require iron depletion since hepatic siderosis increases their virally induced liver damage [58] and reduces the effectiveness of interferon [59]. Anyway, chloroquine is usually less effective in patients with haemochromatosis [60]. However, chloroquine is not contraindicated in these situations and may be needed when venesection is not possible, particularly in patients with hepatitis C liver disease where venous access is impaired by previous intravenous drug abuse. Remission with low-dose chloroquine generally lasts 17–24 months [53,54]. With venesection, relapse generally occurs around 2.5 years after the end of treatment [11,53]. Long-term follow-up is necessary for all patients to monitor for relapse (by measuring urinary porphyrin excretion) and for the management of coexisting liver disease.

Genetic counselling [61]

Familial and sporadic PCT can be differentiated by measuring red cell UROD activity. Since additional inhibition of the hepatic enzyme is required for clinical expression of disease in familial PCT, UROD mutations can be considered as a risk factor for developing the disease rather than as a different form of PCT. It is difficult to justify family screening in familial PCT in view of the identical management of sporadic and familial PCT, the lack of evidence that identifying latent PCT in relatives alters outcomes and the very low penetrance of familial PCT. It is therefore of little value to measure red cell UROD activity unless one is trying to differentiate HEP from PCT.

Mortality in PCT

Overall, patients with PCT have increased mortality compared with age-matched controls. This is partly due to co-morbidities associated with PCT, and partly due to diseases related to associated lifestyle factors found in PCT patients, such as the high prevalence of smoking [62].

Erythropoietic protoporphyria

Definition

Erythropoietic protoporphyria is a hereditary porphyria characterised by painful, lifelong photosensitivity and occasionally liver disease.

Epidemiology

The incidence of EPP in Europe varies between countries (from 0.03 new cases/million per year in Spain to 0.36 in the UK) [1].

Pathophysiology

Erythropoietic protoporphyria usually results from deficient activity of ferrochelatase, the final enzyme of haem biosynthesis. In a minority of cases, it is caused by gain-of-function mutations in *ALAS2* (the first enzyme in the pathway) [2]. This causes the accumulation of protoporphyrin predominantly in cells of the erythroid series, which causes a phototoxic reaction as the porphyrin-laden cells pass through the small upper dermal blood vessels and are exposed to the Soret wavelength in sunlight. The photoactivated porphyrin from red cells and plasma causes an acute injury to the endothelium mediated by singlet oxygen and the hydroxyl radical [3,4]. Many ferrochelatase gene mutations have been identified in EPP patients and none are particularly common [5]. A few adult-onset cases have been reported that are associated with haematological malignancy and may be associated with chromosomal deletions involving the ferrochelatase gene [6].

Clinical features

Unlike the other cutaneous porphyrias, EPP causes immediate pain on exposure to bright sunlight [7,8]. It presents most commonly in the first year, quite often in babies who usually present with crying in their prams in sunny weather or crying for no obvious reason at night in the summer. Onset later in childhood does occur but onset in adulthood is rare. In spring and summer, with sun exposure lasting from a few minutes up to 1–2 h, patients describe discomfort, tingling or itching in exposed skin, affecting particularly the dorsae of the hands and the face. If exposure continues, severe burning pain follows which can last anywhere from an hour to several days. Children often find partial relief with cold water and wet cloths and this feature may be diagnostically useful. Usually the only physical sign during an attack is oedema which may be subtle (Figure 58.10). Redness is less common and may be more difficult to detect in skin of colour. The lack of physical signs often leads to delay in diagnosis with some patients initially being labelled as malingerers.

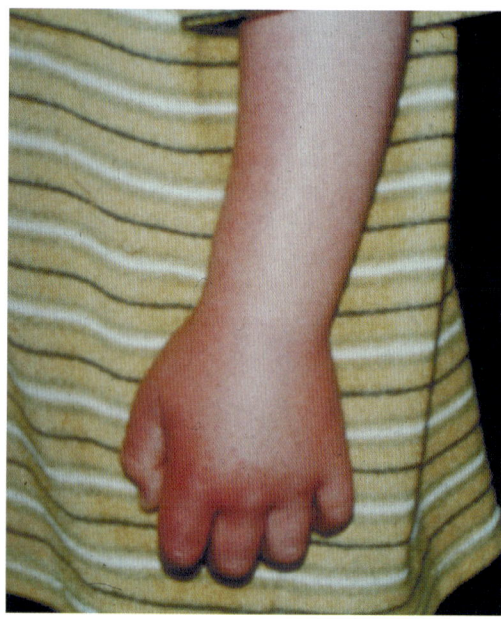

Figure 58.10 Oedema during an acute painful attack in a child with erythropoietic protoporphyria.

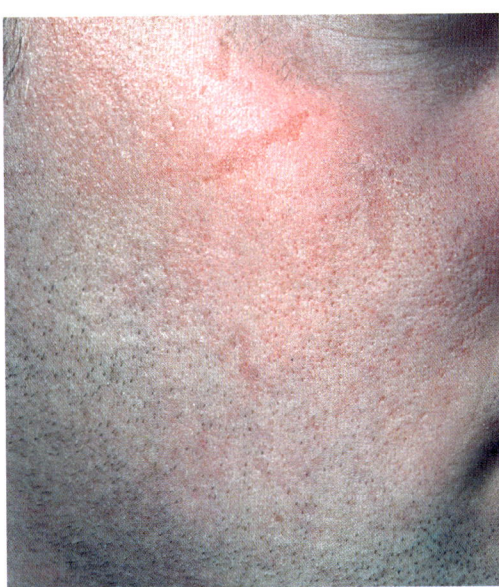

Figure 58.11 Typical scars on the cheeks in erythropoietic protoporphyria.

Many patients experience a 'priming phenomenon' in which sunlight tolerance is reduced on the day after significant sun exposure [9]. In severe attacks, purpuric lesions and crusted erosions or vesicles may occur; these take a week or two to resolve after the attack settles down, and the pain may be severe enough to require hospital admission. Rare cases of EPP have prominent purpura and histological changes resembling a leukocytoclastic vasculitis [10], acute photo-onycholysis [11] or reddish plaques [12] have been described. Solar urticaria can occur in addition to the EPP photosensitive reaction in some patients [13]. Physical signs may develop during childhood with slight thickening of skin over the metacarpophalangeal and interphalangeal joints, superficial vermicular waxy scarring on the nose, shallow linear, punctate or small circular scars on the cheeks and forehead, and radial scars around the lips (Figure 58.11). The skin over the nose, cheeks and forehead can become roughened and 'pebbly' in texture. Fifteen per cent of patients have no physical signs at all [7].

Mild variants of EPP may cause diagnostic confusion because of delayed onset of symptoms, shortened duration of attacks and occasionally absence of pain. Oedema and predilection of the reaction to the face and dorsal hands and feet are diagnostic clues. There is an occasional association between EPP and a seasonal palmar keratoderma. The keratoderma is more commonly seen in autosomal recessive EPP [14].

Children with EPP suffer from social isolation due to difficulty joining friends to play outside, and sensitivity to psychosocial issues is important for clinicians to be aware of. Although EPP is lifelong, childhood and adolescence are frequently the most difficult times because it is potentially easier for adults to organise their lives to reduce sun exposure. Overall, it is not surprising that the disease has such a profound impact on quality of life [7].

Symptoms often improve and porphyrin levels fall during pregnancy [7,15]. Patients may develop a mild hypochromic microcytic or normocytic anaemia which can be associated with decreased serum iron levels and increased serum iron binding capacity [8].

With the exception of patients with EPP liver failure, operating theatre lights do not cause any problems during or after surgery in EPP patients [16]. Anaesthetists can also be reassured that acute attacks do not occur in EPP. In contrast, operating theatre lights can cause a devastating and potentially fatal phototoxic reaction in patients undergoing liver transplantation for protoporphyric liver failure.

Investigations
Biochemical investigation
The diagnostic finding is of an increased red cell-free protoporphyrin concentration [17]. Protoporphyrin is seen as a peak at 633 nm on plasma fluorimetric scanning. Sixty per cent of EPP patients have an increased faecal protoporphyrin concentration, though this is not very useful diagnostically because of its lack of specificity. Urinary porphyrins are normal except in biliary impairment, when coproporphyrinuria develops. Umbilical cord protoporphyrin concentration is not a useful test to identify EPP in newborns [18].

Histopathology [19,20]
In the acute phase, there is visible endothelial damage in superficial dermal vessels [21]. In the chronic phase, in exposed areas of skin, the repeated episodes of damage to small vessels in the upper dermis cause deposition of PAS-positive diastase-resistant hyaline material in the walls of blood vessels of the upper dermal and papillary vascular plexuses. Immunofluorescence shows immunoglobulins (mainly IgG) in a similar distribution. On electron microscopy, the hyaline material can be seen to be a greatly replicated, layered and fragmented basement membrane, with fine fibrillar material permeating the capillary connective tissue sheath and extending beyond the vessel walls [19,22].

Management [7]
Afamelanotide, the α melanocyte stimulating hormone (α-MSH) analogue, is the first effective treatment for EPP, significantly decreasing photosensitivity [23]. No other therapy has ever been proven to be effective in EPP although many have been proposed. Attention to sunlight protection remains the key to management until α-MSH analogues become widely available in clinical practice.

Photoprotection
Basic measures include sun avoidance behaviour, sun protective clothing and hats. It is important to use correct sunscreens [24,25]. Dihydroxyacetone paint has been used in some patients with EPP [26] and window films that absorb violet light can be useful for car or home windows, particularly in severely affected patients. All of these are discussed in detail in the general management section earlier in this chapter.

Acute reactions
For an acute reaction, complete sun avoidance (even through windows) leads to earlier resolution, and fans and cold water provide some pain relief. Antihistamines and most analgesics are of little value. For severe attacks, hospital admission may be necessary for light avoidance and analgesia (usually opiate).

Specific therapies

Until α-MSH analogues are widely available in clinical practice, older treatment options will continue to be relevant. Oral β-carotene has previously been the most widely used treatment, usually at a dose around 180 mg daily in adults (90 mg daily in children) taken throughout the spring and summer. It is postulated to scavenge free radicals involved in the acute phototoxic reaction. Although some patients report that it reduces symptoms, others do not and proof of efficacy from controlled trials is lacking. Patients may need to take it for several months before any effect is observed. The most common adverse effect of β-carotene is reversible skin discoloration.

Controlled trials of *N*-acetylcysteine and colestyramine have been shown to be of no benefit [27,28]. Short courses of a few weeks of psoralen and long-wave UVA radiation (PUVA) [29] and narrow-band UVB [30] used in the early spring may be valuable, particularly in milder cases. These probably increase photoprotection by inducing epidermal thickening and pigmentation. Unlike PUVA, narrow-band UVB does not overlap with the EPP action spectrum and so cannot trigger attacks of pain. Many other systemic treatments with antioxidant or free radical scavenging properties have been used in EPP in an uncontrolled way on small numbers of patients with conflicting and generally unconvincing results.

Bone health

Osteoporosis, often in young adults, is common in EPP [31]. Photoprotection causes vitamin D deficiency and reduced outdoor physical exercise. It is crucial to supplement vitamin D and carry out regular bone density scans.

Genetic counselling

Erythropoietic protoporphyria is generally an autosomal dominant disorder with incomplete penetrance although rare cases of classic autosomal recessive inheritance of two pathogenic mutations have been reported [32,33]. The disease results from co-inheritance of a gene mutation on one ferrochelatase allele with a low expression variant on the other allele. Since the low expression variant is generally considered a common non-pathological polymorphism, the inheritance may be described as 'autosomal dominant disorder with incomplete penetrance' although some geneticists consider this common polymorphic variant as pathological and so describe the inheritance as 'autosomal recessive'. This low expression variant is present in around 10% of the white population and is associated with reduced ferrochelatase mRNA levels resulting from the presence of the polymorphic variant IVS3-48C [34]. This low expression variant is common in Japan and South-East Asia and rare in Africa, which may explain the observed variations between continents [35]. Overall, the probability of each offspring of an EPP patient suffering from the disease is under 10%. Testing for the IVS3-48C polymorphism in a patient's partner is now available and can indicate more precisely whether there is a significant probability of future offspring being affected. This is useful for patients who would not consider having children if there were a significant likelihood of them having the disease. For a disorder that is rarely life-threatening, termination of pregnancy and thus antenatal diagnosis are not relevant.

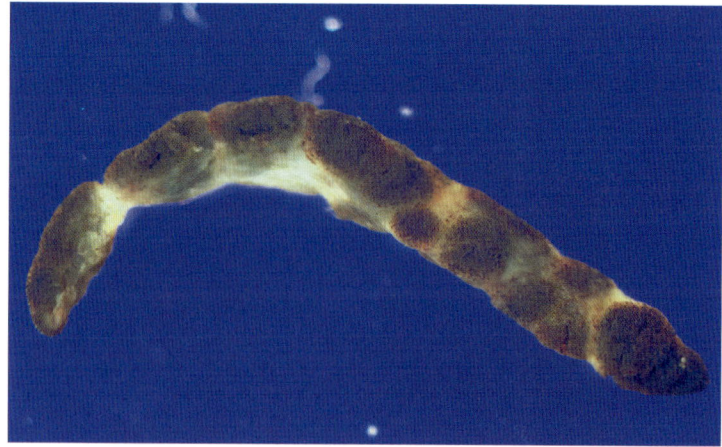

Figure 58.12 Liver biopsy in protoporphyric liver disease showing nodules of cirrhosis and black staining by deposits of protoporphyrin.

Liver disease in EPP

Protoporphyrin is excreted exclusively into the bile. It precipitates to form gallstones in around 12% of patients. It is also hepatotoxic, particularly to bile canaliculi, and severe liver damage occurs in around 1% of patients. EPP liver failure requiring transplantation may occur at almost any age [36]. Usually a patient develops jaundice, worsening photosensitivity and often upper abdominal pain over a period of weeks or months. Investigation shows severe or total cholestasis and a dramatically high red cell protoporphyrin concentration (due to its impaired excretion), which causes the worsening photosensitivity [32].

Liver histology reveals deposition of protoporphyrin in vacuoles within bile canaliculi and hepatocytes, which may be accompanied by cirrhosis (Figure 58.12). Although such acute episodes may resolve spontaneously, the porphyrin-induced cholestasis may become increasingly severe and itself further increase the protoporphyrin concentration in a vicious cycle, in which case the patient will die unless a liver transplant can be performed. Unless filter films are used over operating theatre lights [16], the very high protoporphyrin concentration may result in a severe phototoxic reaction with postoperative burns. A severe and prolonged neuropathy may also occur after liver transplant [36]. Even if these immediate postoperative complications are avoided, protoporphyric liver disease recurs in the graft in 69% of patients over several years which can be severe enough to require retransplantation in a minority. Patients with severe liver disease have been treated by bone marrow transplantation. Although the marrow transplantation does cure the EPP, the dangers of the procedure mean that it is reserved for these rare, life-threatening situations [37]. In severe liver disease, liver transplant followed by hematopoietic stem cell transplantation has been carried out [38].

It is vital to recognise impending protoporphyric liver failure early enough so that arrangements can be made for a liver transplant, if it should become necessary. Thus, all EPP patients should have liver function tests and red cell protoporphyrin concentration checked at least once a year. The appearance of coproporphyrin in the urine has been proposed as an indicator of significant liver disease in EPP [39]. Worsening photosensitivity may be the only clinical indication of the development of severe liver disease. Although protoporphyric liver failure is rare, mild abnormalities of liver function tests are common in EPP [39]. Since the significance of these abnormalities is unclear, it is advisable to monitor them closely in these patients, and to refer the patient to a hepatologist if the abnormality is persistent or deteriorating. In such patients, an ion exchange resin such as cholestyramine may protect the liver against further porphyrin toxicity. The major difficulty for dermatologists is the lack of any means of identifying those EPP patients at risk of liver failure. Since several cases have been described in siblings, patients with a relative who has suffered protoporphyric liver failure should be treated as being at increased risk of developing liver failure themselves. Classic recessive inheritance of EPP may increase the risk of severe hepatic disease, though it is not clear how significant this association is [32].

Iron deficiency anaemia may trigger or exacerbate hepatic disease by increasing porphyrin accumulation [32] and subsequent iron replacement may make the situation temporarily worse by acutely stimulating haem biosynthesis.

PORPHYRIAS THAT CAUSE CUTANEOUS DISEASE AND ACUTE ATTACKS

Hereditary coproporphyria

Definition
This is a rare inherited disease usually characterised by acute attacks that involve the skin as well in a minority of patients.

Clinical features
Like VP, this porphyria presents from puberty onwards. The skin is not affected in most patients suffering from this rare acute porphyria. However, around 10–20% [1] of patients have cutaneous involvement with fragility and blistering in sun-exposed areas, indistinguishable from that seen in PCT or VP. The skin disease may be triggered or exacerbated by intercurrent liver disease [2]. Rare variants include a homozygous form characterised by short stature, acute attacks and skin changes with prominent hypertrichosis and pigmentation [3]. Another rare variant, 'harderoporphyria', causes haemolysis in the neonate or bullae. HC is caused by an autosomal dominant inherited deficiency of coproporphyrinogen oxidase.

Investigations
The biochemical findings are of a 615–620 nm peak on plasma spectrofluorimetry, increased uro- and coproporphyrin concentrations in urine and increased coproporphyrin in faeces. Predominance of the type III isomer in faeces is a sensitive indicator of HC [1].

Variegate porphyria

Definition
This is a rare inherited disease usually characterised by photo-induced skin fragility and blistering that may cause acute attacks.

Epidemiology
In South Africa, VP is common (due to a founder effect [1]) with a prevalence in whites and Afrikaner-descended non-whites of 1 in 200. The incidence of VP in Europe varies between countries, in the range 0.01–0.26 new cases/million/year [2]. Elsewhere the prevalence is around 0.5–1 in 100 000 [2].

Pathophysiology
Variegate porphyria is caused by an autosomal dominant inherited deficiency of protoporphyrinogen oxidase. In addition to causing photosensitisation, accumulated coproporphyrinogen and protoporphyrinogen also inhibit PBG deaminase, the probable mechanism for acute attacks in VP [3]. At least 80% of South African carriers of a pathogenic VP mutation are completely asymptomatic [4].

It is perhaps unexpected that the accumulated copro- and protoporphyrin should cause PCT-like upper dermal blistering rather than EPP-like acute pain. This is likely to be because, although hydrophobic porphyrins predominate in the plasma, hydrophilic porphyrins, especially uroporphyrin, predominate in the skin. This local accumulation is thought to result from secondary local photo-inactivation of UROD in the skin by coproporphyrin [4]. In addition, the protoporphyrin in VP is conjugated to a peptide which may reduce its phototoxicity.

Clinical features [4,5,6]
Skin
Of those patients with symptomatic VP, around 70% of patients have cutaneous involvement, and only around 17% of these patients will ever suffer an acute attack [7]. VP only very rarely presents before puberty and usually the skin disease begins in adolescence or young adulthood. Patients describe skin fragility, usually fairly mild, affecting sun-exposed skin particularly on the backs of the hands [4,5]. The skin disease is generally indistinguishable from PCT, with painful tense bullae occurring in sun-exposed skin, as well as scarring, pigmentary abnormalities, sometimes pseudosclerodermatous changes of the hands and fingers, and occasionally photo-onycholysis. However, a significant number of patients do not describe worsening in the summer and the patients who do describe seasonal variation often have their worst problems in late summer and autumn. In addition, around 50% of patients with VP describe mild, transient, sunlight-related eruptions in the early summer. The examination findings of scarring, patches of hypo- and hyperpigmentation at the sites of blisters, milia and mild hypertrichosis, particularly around the eyes, are indistinguishable from PCT. Intercurrent biliary obstruction exacerbates the cutaneous disease since the accumulated porphyrins are excreted into the bile. Acute photosensitivity can occur in patients with disturbed liver function. Hormonally induced hepatic dysfunction may explain the exacerbations of skin disease seen in females taking oral contraceptives and during pregnancy. VP can sometimes improve in old age with clinical and biochemical remission. Patients with VP have recently been shown to be at increased lifetime risk of hepatocellular carcinoma [8].

Acute attacks [4,5,7,9]
As in other acute porphyrias, women are three times as frequently affected as men and 70% of acute attacks occur between the ages

of 20 and 40 years. Around 17% of patients with cutaneous VP ever suffer an acute attack and the number has declined recently due to improved use of prophylactic measures. The severity of acute attacks varies from mild abdominal pain, sometimes accompanied by vomiting and constipation, through to very severe attacks with bulbar palsy and respiratory paralysis. The presentation, diagnosis and management of acute attacks is covered in the section on acute attacks of porphyria earlier in this chapter.

Clinical variants

In homozygous VP, a mutation on both protoporphyrinogen oxidase alleles results in an enzyme activity less than 20% of normal, compared with the 50% in other VP patients [10]. Fragility, bullae and often hypertrichosis develop in exposed (and sometimes non-exposed) skin in neonates or infants and the skin disease may be severe. Delayed development, epilepsy, sensory neuropathy, nystagmus, various hand deformities and growth retardation also commonly occur. Acute attacks do not occur in these patients. The biochemical findings are the same as in VP except for the lower enzyme activity.

Differential diagnosis

Variegate porphyria cutaneous disease is easily distinguished from non-photosensitive blistering disorders. It can be clinically very similar to PCT, late-onset CEP, HC and pseudoporphyria. Biochemical analysis is required to diagnose VP.

Investigations

A plasma spectrofluorimetry peak around 626 nm (caused by a porphyrin–protein complex) is diagnostic of VP in the absence of a raised free red cell protoporphyrin level and is present in virtually all symptomatic cases of VP. It may persist during periods of clinical remission when faecal excretion becomes normal and is a more sensitive test than measurement of faecal porphyrins [11]. A persistently normal faecal protoporphyrin concentration in adulthood in patients with the VP genetic defect has been proposed as a prognostic marker indicating a greater likelihood of the VP never causing any clinical problems and staying clinically latent [9]. The urine contains increased levels of coproporphyrin and increased concentrations of copro- and protoporphyrin are found in the faeces. In a few patients, the urine shows the typical PCT pattern of uroporphyrin accompanied by hepta- and sometimes hexa- and pentacarboxylic acid porphyrins, a situation known as 'dual porphyria' [12]. Thus, urinary analysis alone can result in the misdiagnosis of VP as PCT, with potentially disastrous consequences. During acute attacks, urinary PBG (and ALA) are raised. The urinary PBG usually falls to normal levels within weeks of the attack resolving but may remain slightly increased outside the context of an acute attack [13].

Management
Treatment

The key to successful management of the skin disease is photoprotection with sun avoidance using clothes, hats and gloves. Opaque sunscreens, containing pigmentary grade titanium dioxide or zinc oxide sometimes with the addition of iron oxide, are protective against Soret wavelength light [14,15]. The skin disease is rarely severe enough to require filter films for car and home windows. As the relationship between sun exposure and skin lesions is not obvious, the role of light in producing the skin lesions should be explained to the patient. β-carotene and canthaxanthin have also been claimed to provide limited protection in some patients and UVB phototherapy may also be of value [4]. If liver function tests indicate biliary obstruction, relief of this will reduce cutaneous symptoms.

The risk of acute attacks is the key issue for the safe management of patients and their families. Patients should be directed to a list of drugs to avoid [16], including those that can induce attacks, and also those known to induce cholestasis, as well as cannabis. They should also be advised to wear an emergency identification bracelet, to avoid low-calorie diets and to avoid all alcohol intake. Liver transplantation has been successfully used to cure variegate porphyria (and acute intermittent porphyria) in cases where acute attacks are frequent, severe and uncontrollable by medical treatment alone [17].

Genetic counselling

It is important to identify relatives who have latent VP because of the risk of acute attacks. The plasma 624–626 nm peak is found in the majority of cases of latent VP but only from teenage years onwards. A positive plasma fluorimetry result is diagnostic of latent VP but a negative result is uninformative [18,19]. The only completely reliable way to identify those carrying the VP gene defect, if the plasma scan is negative, is to identify the protoporphyrinogen oxidase gene mutation in the index case and then assess its presence or absence in relatives. This is labour intensive because, outside South Africa, most families have their own private mutation. Relatives found to have the gene defect are at a low risk (roughly 5–10%) of acute attacks and should take all the precautions taken by any patient diagnosed with an acute porphyria. The risk of a patient passing the mutated gene on to each offspring is 50%, and around 20% of those carrying the mutation will eventually develop symptoms.

MISCELLANEOUS

Pseudoporphyria

Definition

Pseudoporphyria is a non-porphyric dermatosis clinically and histologically indistinguishable from porphyria cutanea tarda. Porphyrin concentrations are entirely normal. Pseudoporphyria is one of the clinical presentations of drug-induced photosensitivity and there are other non-drug-related causes.

Epidemiology and pathophysiology

The causes of pseudoporphyria are photosensitising drugs, haemodialysis and sunbeds [1]. Since pseudoporphyria is one of the presentations of drug photosensitivity, it is unsurprising that the relevant drugs are generally recognised photosensitisers. The most common causes of pseudoporphyria are non-steroidal anti-inflammatory drugs (NSAIDs), especially naproxen and nabumetone. Oxaprozin, ketoprofen, mefenamic acid and diflunisal are also reported causes. NSAID-induced pseudoporphyria is common: in one group of patients treated with naproxen for juvenile rheumatoid arthritis, 12% developed pseudoporphyria [2]. Other drugs reported to induce pseudoporphyria include nalidixic acid, tetracyclines including minocycline, bumetanide, furosemide, isotretinoin, olanzapine, imatinib, dapsone and self-medication with commercially available chlorophyll preparations.

The second group of patients in whom pseudoporphyria is common is those with chronic renal failure undergoing haemodialysis (or less commonly peritoneal dialysis).

The third group of patients are those whose pseudoporphyria is induced by UVA tanning beds. Although some of the reported cases were of patients also taking photosensitising medications, in some patients the use of UVA sunbeds appears to be the sole causative factor [3].

Clinical features
Presentation

The clinical features in the skin are indistinguishable from porphyria cutanea tarda [1] with vesicles, bullae, fragility, milia and scarring on exposed skin, particularly the dorsal hands, but also the face, chest and occasionally other sites. However, hypertrichosis, hyperpigmentation, sclerodermoid changes and dystrophic calcification are much less commonly seen than in PCT. In children, the facial scarring can resemble that seen in EPP but without the painful bouts of photosensitivity seen in that disease. Unlike the porphyrias, pseudoporphyria has no manifestations except in the skin.

Differential diagnosis

The main differential diagnoses are PCT and EPP if there is EPP-type scarring. The diagnosis requires the presence of clinical features of PCT in the skin with normal urine, faecal and plasma porphyrin concentrations reported by an experienced porphyrin laboratory. It is preferable, though not essential, to identify a recognised cause of pseudoporphyria in the patient. Other relevant diseases also need to be excluded such as epidermolysis bullosa acquisita and bullous pemphigoid. The situation is more complex in patients with renal failure. Haemodialysis is associated with increased plasma porphyrin concentrations [4] and urine may be unavailable to test in these patients. The situation is further complicated by the fact that PCT can also be induced by chronic renal failure. Conclusive differentiation of PCT from pseudoporphyria in the context of renal failure and dialysis is not always possible, but can sometimes be achieved on the basis of the degree of increase in porphyrin concentrations in plasma, faeces and (where available) urine. It is important to try to differentiate the two diseases in renal failure because of the implications regarding aetiological factors and treatment options.

Investigations

By definition, the porphyrin concentrations in urine, plasma, red cells and faeces must be normal for a diagnosis of pseudoporphyria to be made. The histopathological and immunofluorescent appearances of affected skin are essentially identical in pseudoporphyria and PCT. Blood vessel thickening and sclerosis of collagen are less common in pseudoporphyria but the two diseases cannot be reliably differentiated with skin biopsies alone [5].

Management

In drug-induced and sunbed-related pseudoporphyria, the key to management is to remove the provoking factor by stopping the relevant drug or sunbed usage. However, symptoms may continue for several months after the discontinuation of a causative drug [6], and scarring may persist. Dialysis-related pseudoporphyria generally persists until renal transplantation removes the need for dialysis. UV light, especially UVA, causes the photosensitive reaction in pseudoporphyria, in contrast to PCT. Hence, broad spectrum UV protection is vital until the disease resolves. As expected, the treatments for PCT such as antimalarials and venesection are not effective in pseudoporphyria.

Key references

The full list of references can be found in the online version at https://www.wiley.com/rooksdermatology10e

Clinical features of the porphyrias: general considerations
Porphyria and the skin

3 Takeshita K, Takajo T, Hirata H *et al*. In vivo oxygen radical generation in the skin of the protoporphyria model mouse with visible light exposure: an L-band ESR study. *J Invest Dermatol* 2004;122:1463–70.

12 Gschnait FG, Wolff K, Konrad K. Erythropoietic protoprophyria – submicroscopic events during the acute photosensitivity flare. *Br J Dermatol* 1975;92:545–57.

Acute attacks of porphyria

7 European Porphyria Network (EPNET). www.porphyria.eu (last accessed October 2022).

Individual porphyrias
Porphyrias that cause cutaneous disease but not acute attacks
Congenital erythropoietic porphyria

2 Sarkany RP, Ibbotson SH, Whatley SD *et al*. Erythropoietic uroporphyria associated with myeloid malignancy is likely distinct from autosomal recessive congenital erythropoietic porphyria. *J Invest Dermatol* 2011;131:1172–5.

4 Katugampola RP, Badminton MN, Finlay AY *et al*. Congenital erythropoietic porphyria: a single-observer clinical study of 29 cases. *Br J Dermatol* 2012;167:901–13.

7 Katugampola RP, Anstey AV, Finlay AY *et al*. A management algorithm for congenital erythropoietic porphyria derived from a study of 29 cases. *Br J Dermatol* 2012;167:888–900.

14 Mirmiran A, Poli A, Ged C *et al*. Phlebotomy as an efficient long-term treatment of congenital erythropoietic porphyria. *Haematologica* 2021;106;913–17.

Porphyria cutanea tarda

1 Sarkany RPE. The management of porphyria cutanea tarda. *Clin Exp Dermatol* 2001;26:225–32.

8 Phillips JD, Bergonia HA, Reilly CA *et al*. A porphomethene inhibitor of uroporphyrinogen decarboxylase causes porphyria cutanea tarda. *Proc Natl Acad Sci* 2007;104:5079–84.

11 Grossman ME, Bickers DR, Poh-Fitzpatrick MB *et al*. Porphyria cutanea tarda: clinical features and laboratory findings in 40 patients. *Am J Med* 1979;67:277–86.

23 Bulaj ZJ, Phillips JD, Ajioka RS *et al*. Hemochromatosis genes and other factors contributing to the pathogenesis of porphyria cutanea tarda. *Blood* 2000;95:1565–71.

38 Gisbert JP, Garcia-Buey L, Alonso A *et al*. Hepatocellular carcinoma risk in patients with porphyria cutanea tarda. *Eur J Gastroenterol Hepatol* 2004;16:689–92.

46 Ratnaike S, Blake D, Campbell D *et al*. Plasma ferritin levels as a guide to the treatment of porphyria cutanea tarda by venesection. *Australas J Dermatol* 1988;29:3–7.

53 Malina L, Chlumsky J. A comparative study of the results of phlebotomy therapy and low-dose chloroquine treatment in porphyria cutanea tarda. *Acta Derm Venereol Suppl (Stockh)* 1981;61:346–50.

57 Singal AK, Kormos-Hallberg C, Lee C *et al*. Low-dose hydroxychloroquine is as effective as phlebotomy in treatment of patients with porphyria cutanea tarda. *Clin Gastroenterol Hepatol* 2012;10:1402–9.

Erythropoietic protoporphyria

2 Whatley SD, Ducamp S, Gouya L *et al*. C-terminal deletions in the ALAS2 gene lead to gain of function and cause X-linked dominant protoporphyria without anemia or iron overload. *Am J Hum Genet* 2008;83:408–14.

4 Takeshita K, Takajo T, Hirata H *et al*. In vivo oxygen radical generation in the skin of the protoporphyria model mouse with visible light exposure: an L-band ESR study. *J Invest Dermatol* 2004;122:1463–70.

7 Holme SA, Anstey AV, Finlay AY *et al*. Erythropoietic protoporphyria in the UK: clinical features and effect on quality of life. *Br J Dermatol* 2006;155:574–81.

16 Wahlin S, Srikanthan N, Hamre B *et al*. Protection from phototoxic injury during surgery and endoscopy in erythropoietic protoporphyria. *Liver Transpl* 2008;14:1340–6.

23 Langendonk JG, Balwani M, Anderson KE *et al*. Afamelanotide for erythropoietic protoporphyria. *N Engl J Med* 2015;373:48–59.

31 Biewenga M, Matawlie RHS, Friesema ECH *et al*. Osteoporosis in patients with erythropoietic protoporphyria. *Br J Dermatol* 2017;177:1693–8.

34 Gouya L, Puy H, Robreau AM *et al*. The penetrance of dominant erythropoietic protoporphyria is modulated by expression of wildtype FECH. *Nat Genet* 2002;30:27–8.

36 Wahlin S, Stal P, Adam R *et al*. Liver transplantation for erythropoietic protoporphyria in Europe. *Liver Transpl* 2011;17:1021–6.

37 Wahlin S, Aschan J, Bjornstedt M *et al*. Curative bone marrow transplantation in erythropoietic protoporphyria after reversal of severe cholestasis. *J Hepatol* 2007;46:174–9.

Porphyrias that cause cutaneous disease and acute attacks
Hereditary coproporphyria

1 Kuhnel A, Gross U, Doss MO. Hereditary coproporphyria in Germany: clinical–biochemical studies in 53 patients. *Clin Biochem* 2000;33:465–73.

Variegate porphyria

6 Timonen K, Niemi KM, Mustajoki P, Tenhunen R. Skin changes in variegate porphyria. Clinical, histopathological, and ultrastructural study. *Arch Dermatol Res* 1990;282:108–14.

16 European Porphyria Network (EPNET). www.porphyria.eu (last accessed October 2022).

18 Long C, Smyth SJ, Woolf J *et al*. Detection of latent variegate porphyria by fluorescence emission spectroscopy of plasma. *Br J Dermatol* 1993;129:9–13.

Miscellaneous
Pseudoporphyria

1 Green JJ, Manders SM. Pseudoporphyria. *J Am Acad Dermatol* 2001;44:100–8.

CHAPTER 59

Calcification of the Skin and Subcutaneous Tissue

Johnny Bourke and Matthew Murphy

South Infirmary-Victoria University Hospital, Cork, Ireland

Dystrophic calcification secondary to inflammatory disease and infections

Definition and nomenclature

This is calcification in the skin and/or subcutaneous tissues resulting from inflammation (without any disturbance of systemic calcium homeostasis).

Synonyms and inclusions
- Cutaneous calcification
- Calcinosis cutis
- Subcutaneous calcification

Introduction and general description

Inflammatory, particularly autoimmune, processes in the skin may result in calcification. Dermatomyositis and scleroderma are the best recognised and most troublesome. CREST (calcinosis, Raynaud phenomenon, oesophageal dysfunction, sclerodactyly and telangiectasia) syndrome is specifically associated. Calcinosis has been described in several variants of lupus erythematosus, particularly lupus panniculitis, and, in contrast, is often asymptomatic. Infections are a relatively rare cause of cutaneous calcification.

Epidemiology
Incidence and prevalence

Cutaneous calcification is thought to occur in 20% of adults with dermatomyositis and approximately 40% of children [1]. In common with autoimmune disease generally, autoimmune-associated calcinosis is also more common in women (male : female 1 : 4 in one series [2]).

Ethnicity

There is no particular predisposition.

Associated diseases

Connective tissue diseases are associated, particularly dermatomyositis and scleroderma, but also all types of lupus. Rarer associations include pancreatitis-induced panniculitis, porphyria cutanea tarda, morphoea and lichen sclerosus. Calcinosis is also seen in association with infection occasionally, most notably onchocerciasis and cysticercosis.

Pathophysiology
Pathology

In addition to the characteristic histopathology of the underlying disorder, calcium deposits stain blue with haematoxylin and eosin (H&E) and black with von Kossa stain [3]. Fine granules are seen in the dermis and large irregular masses occur when the disease involves the subcutis [4]. A chronic lymphohistiocytic infiltrate may be seen at the edge of deposits. Transelimination of calcium is common in dermatomyositis and CREST syndrome. In pancreatic panniculitis, there is fat necrosis with ghost lipocytes and calcification within the cytoplasm.

Causative organisms

Larvae of the filarial *Onchocerca volvulus* and the tapeworm *Taenia solium* may cause calcification. Hepatic, pulmonary and central nervous system calcification is well described following herpetic infection. Cutaneous calcification from intrauterine herpes simplex infection has also been described [5].

Clinical features [6]
History

Cutaneous calcification usually presents many years after the onset of the underlying disease. This is reported to be around

Rook's Textbook of Dermatology, Tenth Edition. Edited by Christopher Griffiths, Jonathan Barker, Tanya Bleiker, Walayat Hussain and Rosalind Simpson.
© 2024 John Wiley & Sons Ltd. Published 2024 by John Wiley & Sons Ltd.

PART 5: METABOLIC & NUTRITIONAL DISORDERS

10 years after onset in scleroderma and adult dermatomyositis, but with a shorter duration of 2–3 years in childhood dermatomyositis [2].

Presentation

In dermatomyositis, calcification develops on the trunk and limbs in both childhood and adult forms of the disease. Yellow-white nodules and plaques frequently ulcerate, discharging chalky material. In its most extensive form involving much of the body, it is sometimes termed calcinosis universalis. Calcification of the underlying muscles with contracture and deformity is also common.

Calcinosis is part of the definition of CREST syndrome, presenting with nodules and plaques that ulcerate and extrude chalky material at sites of trauma, particularly the elbows, knuckles and volar aspects of the fingers. It has also occasionally been described in generalised scleroderma and localised morphoea [7,8].

Cutaneous calcification has been described in association with porphyria cutanea tarda, particularly when associated with pseudoscleroderma. Ulcerating plaques exuding chalky material develop on the head and neck or dorsum of the hands, healing with scarring and causing alopecia on the scalp. Three of 40 patients in one series developed this complication [9].

Cutaneous calcification is a rare complication of systemic lupus erythematosus (SLE); it is often asymptomatic and may be noticed incidentally on radiological examination. Typically, nodules develop in the subcutaneous tissues of the buttocks [10], often at sites of cutaneous involvement by the lupus. Calcification may also develop in lupus panniculitis and has occasionally been described in discoid lupus [11] and subacute lupus [12].

There are occasional case reports of cutaneous calcification in association with overlap connective tissue disease, polymyositis and rheumatoid arthritis [2].

Subcutaneous calcification is seen in panniculitis, particularly when associated with pancreatic disease (pancreatitis or malignancy) but also when it occurs in association with lupus and occasionally other diseases [13]. Cutaneous and subcutaneous calcification is an occasional complication of chronic leg ulcers, irrespective of the cause, and may impair healing. Wollina *et al.* [14] reported calcification in 18% of 212 patients with treatment-resistant ulcers who had been admitted for surgery and grafting.

Subcutaneous fat necrosis of the newborn is seen in premature infants, particularly those treated with whole body hypothermia for perinatal asphyxia. Red well-defined nodules and plaques on the cheeks, back and buttocks usually resolve spontaneously, but may calcify and may be associated with hypercalcaemia. The cause is unknown [15].

Rarely, infections may cause calcification of the skin and/or subcutis. The most commonly cited causes are onchocerciasis and cysticercosis, which may cause calcified nodules of the head, pelvis or pectoral areas. There is one report of cutaneous calcification due to intrauterine herpetic infection.

Differential diagnosis

Other causes of cutaneous calcification are discussed elsewhere in this section.

Complications and co-morbidities

Ulceration with secondary infection is the main complication of cutaneous and subcutaneous infection. When widespread (calcinosis universalis), contracture and deformity may result.

Disease course and prognosis

If untreated, calcification rarely regresses.

Investigations

As well as serological assessment for connective tissue disease, full biochemical assessment is required to exclude any abnormality of systemic calcium homeostasis. This should include serum calcium, phosphate, alkaline phosphatase, vitamin D and parathormone (PTH) estimation. X-ray and/or skin biopsy may help to confirm the diagnosis if there is uncertainty.

Management

Treatment of the underlying connective tissue disease helps to prevent and improve calcinosis [16]. Surgical excision of localised disease, if symptomatic, is the treatment of choice. Surgery may also be appropriate for localised problematic areas in more extensive disease. The plethora of treatments anecdotally reported to be effective is an indication of the therapeutic difficulties that this condition presents [17]. Other treatments for localised disease include intralesional steroids [18], CO_2 laser [19], extracorporeal shockwave lithotripsy [20] and topical and intralesional sodium thiosulphate [21,22]. Systemic agents for more extensive disease are of questionable efficacy and include calcium antagonists [2], bisphosphonates [23], minocycline [24], ceftriaxone [25], aluminium hydroxide [26], probenicid [27], intravenous immunoglobulin [28] and autologous stem cell transplant [29]. Warfarin was reported to be effective in the past [30] but is no longer recommended [17].

Treatment ladder for dystrophic calcification secondary to inflammatory disease and infections

First line

- Treatment of underlying disorder (connective tissue disease, infection) including rituximab, tumour necrosis factor α (TNF-α) blockers and intravenous immunoglobulin (IVIg)
- Surgical excision/wound care/debridement
- Topical sodium thiosulphate (10% solution twice weekly)
- Intralesional sodium thiosulphate (0.1 mL of 25% solution)

Second line

- Diltiazem (up to 480 mg/day)
- Bisphosphonates (oral: alendronate 10 mg/day, etidronate 800 mg/day; IV: palmidronate 1 mg/kg/day for 3 days every 3 months)
- Aluminium hydroxide (up to 2.4 g/day)
- CO_2 laser

- Extracorporeal shockwave lithotripsy
- Intralesional steroid (20 mg/mL every 4–8 weeks)

Third line

- Minocycline (up to 200 mg/day)
- Colchicine
- Ceftriaxone
- Probenicid

Dystrophic calcification secondary to trauma or injection/infusion of calcium-containing materials

Definition and nomenclature

This is calcification in the skin and/or subcutaneous tissues resulting from trauma or injection/infusion of calcium-containing materials.

Synonyms and inclusions
- Heel prick calcinosis
- Iatrogenic calcinosis

Introduction and general description

Calcinosis may develop at the site of trauma, probably as a consequence of cell death, with the release of alkaline phosphatase, intracellular calcium and an alteration of local pH resulting in the precipitation of calcium. Typical examples include heel calcinosis after heel prick testing in infants [1,2–5], calcification of burns [6,7] and keloids after abdominal surgery [8,9]. A leakage of infusions containing calcium salts causes inflammation and cell death, which may initiate calcification. Collagen appears to play an important part in the process, triggering mineralisation [10]. The cause of calcinosis in these cases is usually fairly obvious although clinicians may not have been aware of the presence of calcium in the infusion, such as in heparin or low-molecular-weight heparin.

Epidemiology

Calcinosis from calcium-containing heparin injections is more commonly seen in renal patients with abnormal calcium homeostasis [11,12] but has been described in patients without underlying predisposition [13].

Pathophysiology
Pathology

Trauma-induced calcinosis is characterised by a dermal collection of calcium with variable inflammatory infiltrate and overlying acanthosis and hyperkeratosis of the epidermis. Evidence of transepidermal elimination may also be seen [1]. Extravasation of intravenous (IV) solutions containing calcium [13] results in calcium deposition around collagen bundles. Heparin solutions deposit calcium in septae, lipocytes and fat lobules as well as the media of small dermal and subcutaneous vessels [11,14,15].

Clinical features
History

The history of trauma or recent infusion is usually evident, although calcinosis can occasionally take months or even several years to develop. Heel prick calcinosis was initially reported after multiple heel pricks carried out in the neonatal period, however it may develop after just one test [1].

Presentation

Heel prick calcinosis presents as a firm papule on the heel, which becomes symptomatic if it persists until the infant starts to wear shoes [1]. Calcinosis postinfusion or injection of calcium-containing materials presents with a warm, tender swelling at the site of injection, usually within days to weeks. Ulceration and necrosis may occur. Calcification at the sites of electroencephalography due to the use of calcium electrode paste has also been reported [16].

Disease course and prognosis

Heel prick calcinosis may resolve without treatment [2,3,5], although persistent symptomatic lesions may require excision [1]. Infusion/injection calcinosis tends to resolve once the heparin is stopped, although surgical excision may be needed.

Investigations

It is probably sensible to exclude systemic causes of calcinosis by checking for serum calcium, phosphate, alkaline phosphatase, vitamin D and PTH. X-ray and/or skin biopsy may help to confirm the diagnosis if there is uncertainty.

Management

Conservative management with local wound care of any ulcerated areas is usually all that is needed. Persistent lesions may be excised.

Dystrophic calcification secondary to tumours and genetic disease

Definition

This is calcification in the skin and/or subcutaneous tissues resulting from genetic and neoplastic changes in the skin.

Introduction and general description

Calcification and subsequent ossification of benign and malignant tumours are a relatively common occurrence although often only noted histologically. Hair follicle cysts and tumours are the most common lesions displaying this tendency, most notably pilomatricomas in approximately 75% of cases. A wide variety of other lesions including basal cell carcinomas, epidermoid cysts and vascular and melanocytic lesions may also calcify. Calcification of the skin is seen in genetic disorders of collagen (Ehlers–Danlos disease) and elastin (pseudoxanthoma elasticum (PXE)) as well as Werner syndrome and Rothmund–Thomson syndrome.

Epidemiology
Associated diseases
There are several associated diseases, including benign and malignant tumours of the skin, PXE, Ehlers–Danlos disease, Werner syndrome and Rothmund–Thomson syndrome.

Pathophysiology
Pathology
Pseudoxanthoma elasticum is characterised by fragmented calcified elastic fibres and the accumulation of proteoglycans in the extracellular matrix.

Clinical features
History and presentation
Calcification and ossification of tumours are often asymptomatic and only noticed when removed for histopathological examination. The best recognised tumour is the pilomatricoma which calcifies in 75% of cases and is readily identified as a mobile, hard, subcutaneous papule or nodule [1]. In many other lesions, calcification may go unnoticed. The patient may complain of a hard cutaneous/subcutaneous nodule. Occasionally these become inflamed and tender and may perforate, exuding chalky material. Other hair follicle tumours such as pilar cysts commonly contain foci of calcification, as do epidermoid cysts. Calcification has been reported in a wide variety of benign and malignant tumours [2]. Melanocytic naevi, particularly intradermal ones, occasionally calcify and ossify, as may basal cell carcinomas, pyogenic granulomas, neurilemmomas, seborrhoeic keratoses, atypical fibroxanthomas and melanomas [3,4].

   Calcification of elastic fibres is a central feature of PXE. The first signs are usually evident in the skin as yellow papules on the neck, flexures and abdomen. In Ehlers–Danlos syndrome, calcification may develop at sites of scars or as calcified subcutaneous spheroids. Werner syndrome is characterised by progeria with sclerodermoid changes in the skin. Calcification of the skin, soft tissues, tendons and periarticular areas has been described [5–9].

Investigations
A biopsy may be required to confirm the diagnosis.

Management
Excision of localised areas of calcification/calcified tumours is the only useful treatment.

Idiopathic calcification of the skin and subcutaneous tissues

Definition and nomenclature
This is calcification in the skin and/or subcutaneous tissues with no identifiable cause.

Introduction and general description
There are several clinical presentations of calcinosis cutis without a definite cause: idiopathic scrotal calcinosis [1], subepidermal calcified nodules [2] and tumoral [3] and miliary [4] calcinosis cutis are the most well recognised. Localised calcinosis of the vulva, penis, breast and other areas is also well described. It may be that many of these cases represent dystrophic calcinosis related to benign neoplasms or unrecognised disturbance of systemic calcium homeostasis. Possible causes for several of these entities have been proposed, for example calcification of pre-existing epidermoid or eccrine cysts in scrotal calcinosis [5–7], hyperphosphataemia in tumoral calcinosis [8], calcification of adnexal structures in subepidermal calcified nodules [9] and calcification of syringomas in miliary calcinosis [10].

Epidemiology
Sex
As is self-evident, scrotal calcinosis is exclusive to males. Tumoral calcinosis is twice as common in females [11].

Ethnicity
Tumoral calcinosis [11,12,13] is more commonly seen in Africa (southern, central and eastern) and Papua New Guinea.

Pathophysiology
Calcium deposits will stain blue with H&E and black with von Kossa stain. Fine granules are seen in the dermis and large irregular masses occur when the disease involves the subcutis [11]. A variable, chronic lymphohistiocytic infiltrate may be seen at the edge of deposits. Scrotal calcinosis is characterised by epidermal inclusion cysts (which may rupture), calcified keratin and calcified dermal nodules with surrounding fibrous stroma.

Clinical features [14]
History and presentation
Scrotal calcinosis presents as white, subcutaneous, firm nodules, which are usually multiple (Figure 59.1). Subepidermal calcified nodules present frequently in childhood on the head and extremities with solitary, hard, yellow-white papules/nodules up to 1 cm in diameter (Figure 59.2). Tumoral calcinosis presents with large subcutaneous masses around the major joints and is most usually seen in adolescents. Miliary calcinosis cutis is a rare form of calcification seen most commonly in children with Down syndrome. Idiopathic calcinosis universalis has been described although some of the cases may represent early or amyopathic dermatomyositis.

Investigations
Biopsy and/or radiology can be used to confirm the diagnosis. In extensive disease, assessment of systemic calcium homeostasis may be indicated to exclude other causes.

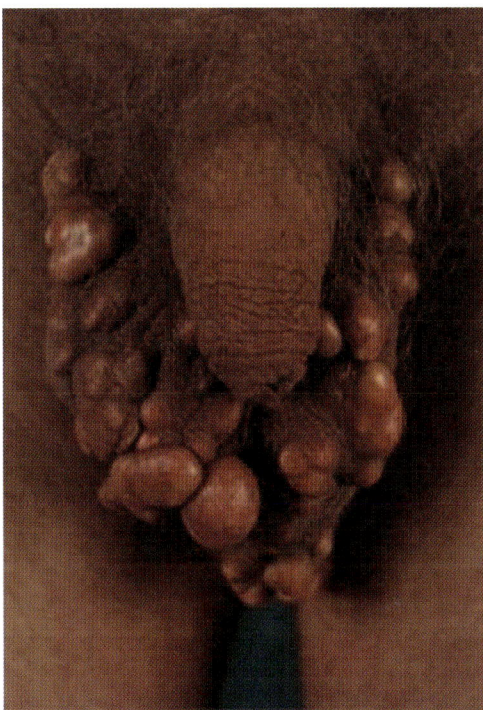

(a)

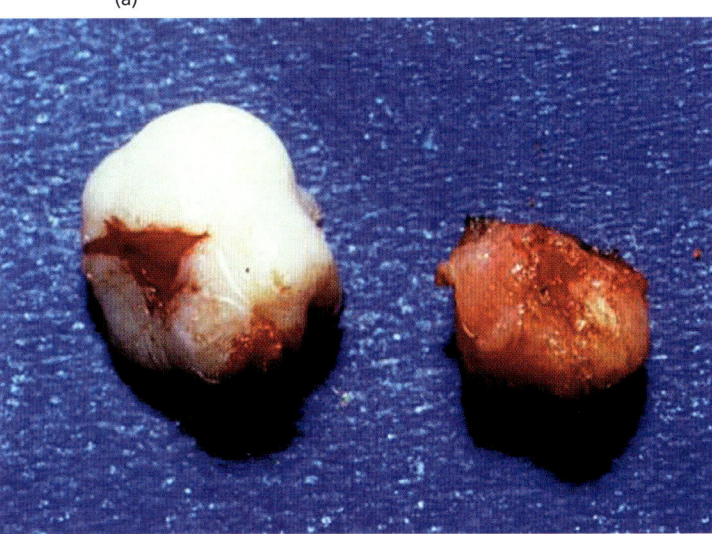

(b)

Figure 59.1 (a) Calcinosis scrotalis. (b) Solitary nodules after removal.

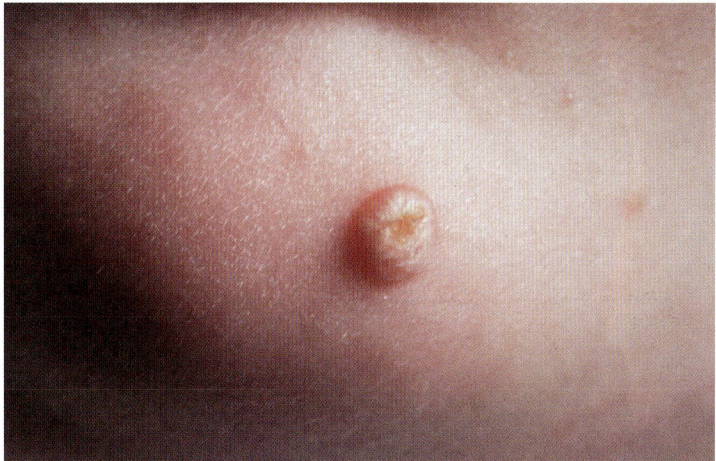

Figure 59.2 Idiopathic calcinosis cutis on the chin of a child.

PART 5: METABOLIC & NUTRITIONAL DISORDERS

Synonyms and inclusions
- Metastatic calcinosis cutis
- Hypervitaminosis D
- Milk alkali syndrome
- Albright hereditary osteodystrophy

Introduction and general description
Metastatic calcification results from an underlying disorder of systemic calcium homeostasis. Cutaneous involvement results most commonly in nodular calcification in a periarticular distribution.

Epidemiology
Incidence and prevalence
The incidence and prevalence of metastatic calcification are unknown.

Age
Metastatic calcification can present at any age.

Associated diseases
Metastatic calcification is seen in hyperparathyroidism, hypervitaminosis D, milk alkali syndrome, sarcoidosis and bone metastases. Hyperphosphataemia and vitamin D deficiency are rarer causes.

Pathophysiology
In metastatic calcification, the precipitation of calcium in tissues results from high circulating levels of calcium and/or phosphate [1].

Predisposing factors
Abnormalities of systemic calcium homeostasis are responsible for metastatic calcification.

Pathology
In metastatic calcification, deposits of calcium which appear blue with H&E and black with von Kossa stains are seen in the dermis and subcutis with variable surrounding inflammatory infiltrate [2].

Management
Excision where practical is the treatment of choice. Spontaneous resolution may occur, particularly in miliary calcinosis.

Metastatic calcification

Definition and nomenclature
Cutaneous metastatic calcification is the deposition of calcium salts resulting from abnormal systemic calcium homeostasis.

PART 5: METABOLIC & NUTRITIONAL DISORDERS

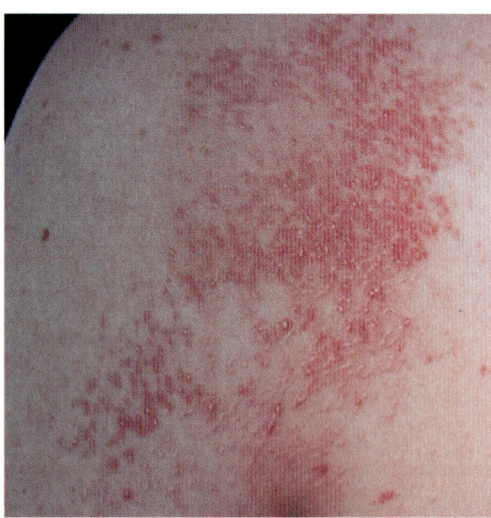

Figure 59.3 Miliary calcinosis cutis.

Clinical features
History
Lesions of metastatic calcification are often asymptomatic.

Presentation
Metastatic calcification presents with predominantly periarticular calcification in addition to signs and symptoms of hypercalcaemia (i.e. abdominal pain, renal failure, cardiac arrhythmias and depression [3]). Extensive miliary calcification (Figure 59.3) has also been reported in hyperparathyroidism resulting from renal failure [4].

Differential diagnosis
Other causes of cutaneous calcification should be considered.

Complications and co-morbidities
These include renal impairment and features of systemic metastatic calcification.

Disease course and prognosis
Metastatic calcification generally resolves once the underlying hypercalcaemia/hyperphosphataemia has been corrected.

Investigations
A full biochemical work-up is needed as well as a clinically directed search for malignancy. In metastatic calcification, radiology and/or biopsy will confirm the diagnosis.

Management
Correction of the underlying hypercalcaemia/phosphataemia is often all that is required in metastatic calcification. Surgical excision may occasionally be needed.

Calciphylaxis

Definition and nomenclature
Calciphylaxis is a life-threatening vasculopathy characterised by calcium deposition in the skin and subcutis both within vessels and in the surrounding tissues.

Synonyms and inclusions
- Calcific uraemic arteriolopathy
- Calcifying panniculitis

Introduction and general description
Calciphylaxis is a serious, life-threatening thrombo-occlusive disorder most commonly seen in the setting of renal failure. The pathophysiology of this condition is poorly understood and there is no universally accepted treatment. Death usually results from either sepsis or systemic thrombosis.

Epidemiology
Incidence and prevalence
Calciphylaxis is estimated to have an incidence of 4.5 per million of the population per year [1]. The prevalence in chronic renal failure is reported to be approximately 1% [2,3] although recent publications suggest that it may be less common, with an annual incidence of 0.04–0.35% [4], and that it occurs in up to 4% of haemodialysis patients [5].

Age
The majority of patients with calciphylaxis are middle-aged or elderly, although it has been reported in infants as young as 6 months [6].

Sex
A female preponderance is generally reported in calciphylaxis (female : male >4 : 1) although Reed and Davis did not find this in their population-based study [1].

Associated diseases
Calciphylaxis is associated with renal failure. It has also been reported in association with hyperparathyroidism, hepatic failure and malignancy [7]. Other reported risk factors include obesity, warfarin and corticosteroid use, diabetes, connective tissue disease and protein S and protein C deficiency [8–10]. McCarthy *et al.* [11], in a case–control retrospective series of 101 patients, confirmed an association with obesity, age, female sex, thrombophilia and warfarin use.

Pathophysiology
The aetiology of calciphylaxis is uncertain. Abnormalities of systemic calcium homeostasis are common but not invariable. Coagulation abnormalities have been recorded but not consistently. It is likely that the pathophysiology is multifactorial. It has been proposed that a final common pathway might be via receptor activator of nuclear factor κB (RANK), RANK ligand and osteoprotogenerin, which appear to regulate extraskeletal mineralisation [12]. Parathyroid hormone, corticosteroids, aluminium (used in dialysis solutions), liver disease and various forms of inflammation can activate this system, which may have a role in calciphylaxis. Matrix Gla protein and fetuin A, which inhibit extraosseous calcification, may also be important [13,14]. A potential role for warfarin could be explained by the inhibition of vitamin K-dependent γ-carboxylation of matrix Gla protein.

Predisposing factors

Renal failure, obesity, abnormalities of systemic calcium homeostasis, hepatobiliary disease and malignancy are recognised predisposing factors for calciphylaxis. Other possible factors include diabetes, warfarin and steroid use and coagulation abnormalities.

Pathology

Medial calcification, intimal fibroplasia and thrombosis of pannicular arterioles with cutaneous necrosis are seen [12]. Extravascular calcium deposition is variable.

Clinical features

History

Painful, often purpuric, areas on the lower abdomen, thighs or lower legs are the hallmarks of calciphylaxis. The severity of pain is often disproportionate to the clinical appearance and may be the first sign of disease progression.

Presentation

The presentation of calciphylaxis is quite variable. The original description by Selye et al. in 1961 in rats [15] was followed in 1968 by a case report typical of calciphylaxis in end-stage renal failure [16]. The patient, an obese woman with acute renal failure, presented with extensive purpuric calcified plaques on the thighs and feet, which subsequently ulcerated. She died 6 months later.

The typical presentation is with purpuric, ulcerating, necrotic, calcified plaques on the lower abdomen or thighs (Figure 59.4). On the lower legs calcification may be less obvious clinically but livedo is characteristic (Figure 59.5). In some cases there is little cutaneous involvement, with more diffuse subcutaneous calcification, which may have a better prognosis. Calciphylaxis has also been reported on the penis [17], breasts [18], tongue [19] and occasionally internal organs [20]. The ulcers are usually irregular, stellate and deep. Surrounding livedo is evidence of the local vascular thrombosis.

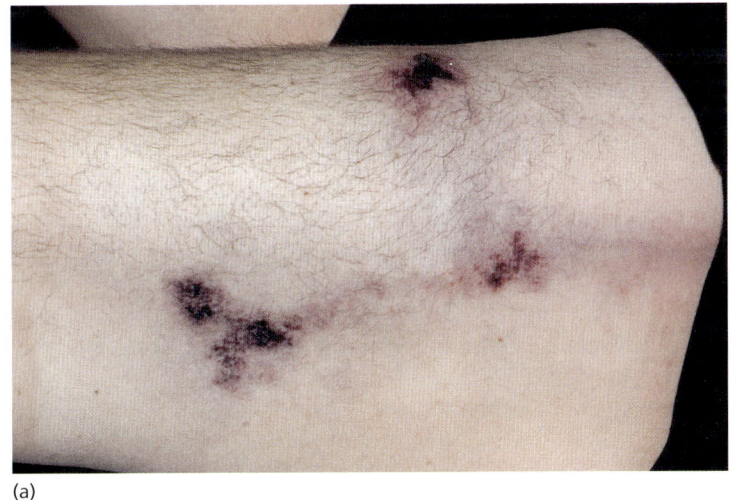
(a)

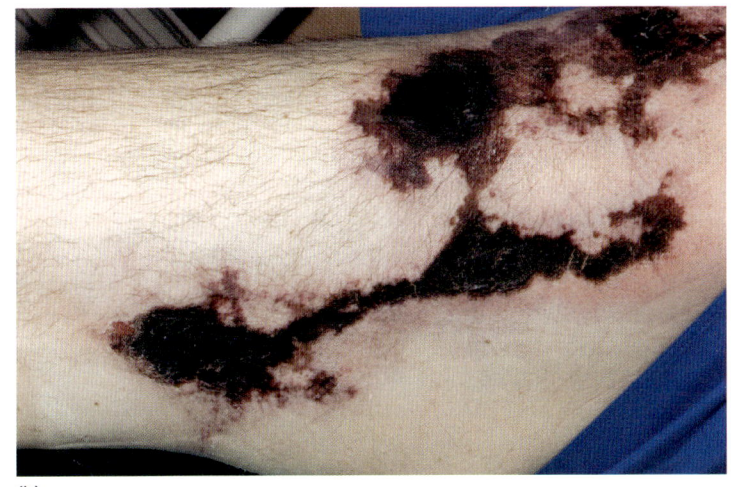
(b)

Figure 59.4 Calciphylaxis with painful purpuric lesions on the thigh in a 53-year-old diabetic patient with renal failure. (a) At presentation. (b) Progressing to gangrenous plaques 3 weeks later.

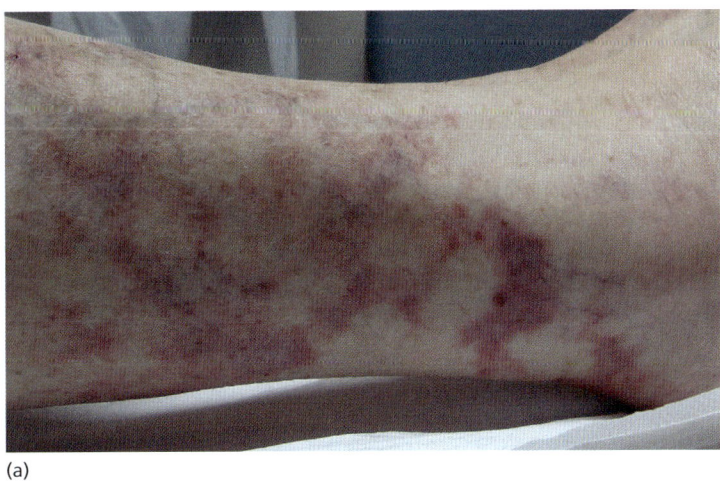
(a)

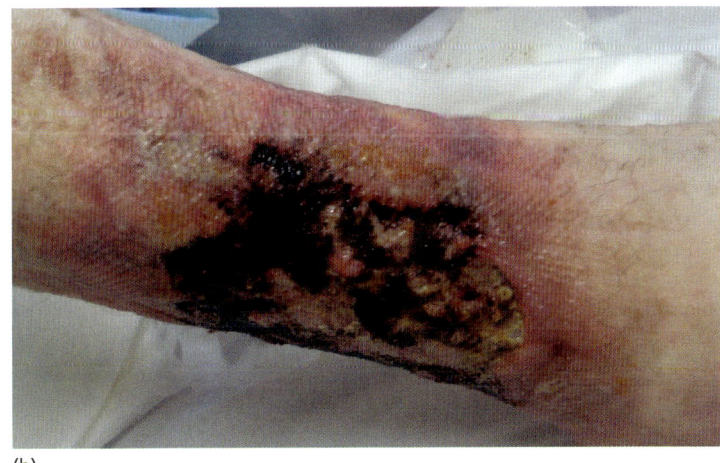
(b)

Figure 59.5 (a) Typical livedo in early calciphylaxis on the lower leg. (b) Progression to ulceration with surrounding livedo.

Table 59.1 Distinguishing features of calciphylaxis and its differential diagnoses.

	Calciphylaxis	Pyoderma gangrenosum	Warfarin necrosis	Hypertensive ulcer (Martorell)
Male : female	1 : 4	4 : 6	1 : 4	1 : 4
Age	>40 years	Any age	>50 years	>55 years
Site	Abdomen, thighs, lower leg	Legs most common	Breast, hip, buttocks, thighs	Lower leg
Pain	Severe	Severe	Moderate	Severe
Edge	Purpuric, livedoid	Purpuric, raised, inflamed	Redness	Purpuric, livedoid
Surrounding tissues	Livedo and firm, subcutaneous, calcified nodules/plaques	Inflamed	–	Livedo
Calcium homeostasis	Often abnormal	–	–	–
Associated diseases	Chronic renal failure, dialysis, hepatic failure, diabetes	Inflammatory bowel disease, rheumatoid arthritis, haematological malignancy	Protein C deficiency	Hypertension
Histology	Medial calcification, extravascular calcium deposition	Non-specific acute inflammation, necrosis and ulceration	Fibrin, thrombi, small veins and venules	Hyaline arteriosclerosis, intimal thickening, luminal narrowing

Differential diagnosis

Other causes of cutaneous calcification should be considered. Calciphylaxis may be mistaken for vasculitis or pyoderma gangrenosum. Warfarin and heparin necrosis may also look similar (Table 59.1).

Some overlap exists between distal calciphylaxis and the rarer hypertensive ulcer of Martorell and treatment of these cases is similar. In its more severe form, necrotising fasciitis may be a consideration although calciphylaxis is rarely as rapidly progressive.

Classification of severity

It is difficult to predict which cases of calciphylaxis will have better outcomes. It has been suggested that those patients with more obvious subcutaneous calcification without livedo or necrosis may have a benign course.

Complications and co-morbidities

The principal complication is septicaemia. Internal organ involvement is rare.

Disease course and prognosis

The rate of progression of calciphylaxis is variable but secondary sepsis is common. Although calcification of cardiac, gastrointestinal and other systemic arteries may be demonstrated, an ischaemic process similar to that found in the skin is not usually seen internally [21]. The mortality is very high (up to 80%) and the median survival is <3 months. Even in those cases where treatment seems to improve the cutaneous features, the mortality is still >60% [22].

Investigations

A full biochemical work-up is needed and a clinically directed search for malignancy. As trauma may aggravate calciphylaxis, several authors suggest that a clinical diagnosis should be made without a biopsy. However, in clinical practice, the need for definitive histology in such a serious condition often outweighs the risk. A single deep biopsy of an indurated plaque is needed to demonstrate calcification of subcutaneous fat and the involvement of vessels (Figure 59.6).

In addition to the assessment of systemic calcium homeostasis, levels of glucose and HbA1c, liver function tests and coagulation screen should also be checked. As secondary septicaemia is common, samples of tissue, swabs and blood should be sent for culture. X-rays of soft tissues may reveal 'net-like' patterns of calcification (Figure 59.7) [23] or diffuse calcification of small to medium-sized arterioles out into the dermis [24]. Bone scintigraphy has been reported to be both sensitive and specific in the diagnosis of calciphylaxis [25]. Computed tomographic radiography, ultrasound and mammography may also be useful.

Management

There is no universally accepted treatment regimen for calciphylaxis [26]. The most promising treatment reported to date is IV sodium thiosulphate. This certainly does seem to improve symptoms quickly (generally within a week) and the short-term outcome appears to be better although the long-term impact is uncertain. Noureddine et al. [27] reported 71% mortality in a cohort of 14 patients treated with IV sodium thiosulphate over a 5-year period. A recent review of the literature is also supportive [28] although controlled studies are lacking. Long-term oral sodium thiosulphate has been reported to be effective at maintaining remission [29]. The correction of abnormal calcium homeostasis is sensible but may not affect outcome. There are several case reports in the literature of successful treatment with cinacalcet [30–33], a calcimimetic agent that reduces PTH levels. It is often used in combination with other agents targeting calcium homeostasis. One paper reported successful treatment of five patients with a combination of sodium thiosulphate, cinacalcet and the phosphate binder sevelamer [34], although other groups report high mortality despite all treatments [35,36]. Parathyroidectomy is of questionable benefit in most cases [11,37] and should be reserved for refractory hyperparathyroidism. Local debridement has been shown to improve survival in one series [11]. General supportive measures including compression if the peripheral circulation is not compromised, treatment of secondary infection and adequate pain control are important as with most atypical ulcers [38]. Anticoagulation is logical but controversial and it is important to exclude warfarin or heparin necrosis before recommending this. Thrombolysis has been proposed as a useful treatment, but a recent retrospective review showed modest benefit, significant morbidity and no significant survival advantage [21]. Hyperbaric oxygen has been reported to be helpful [39].

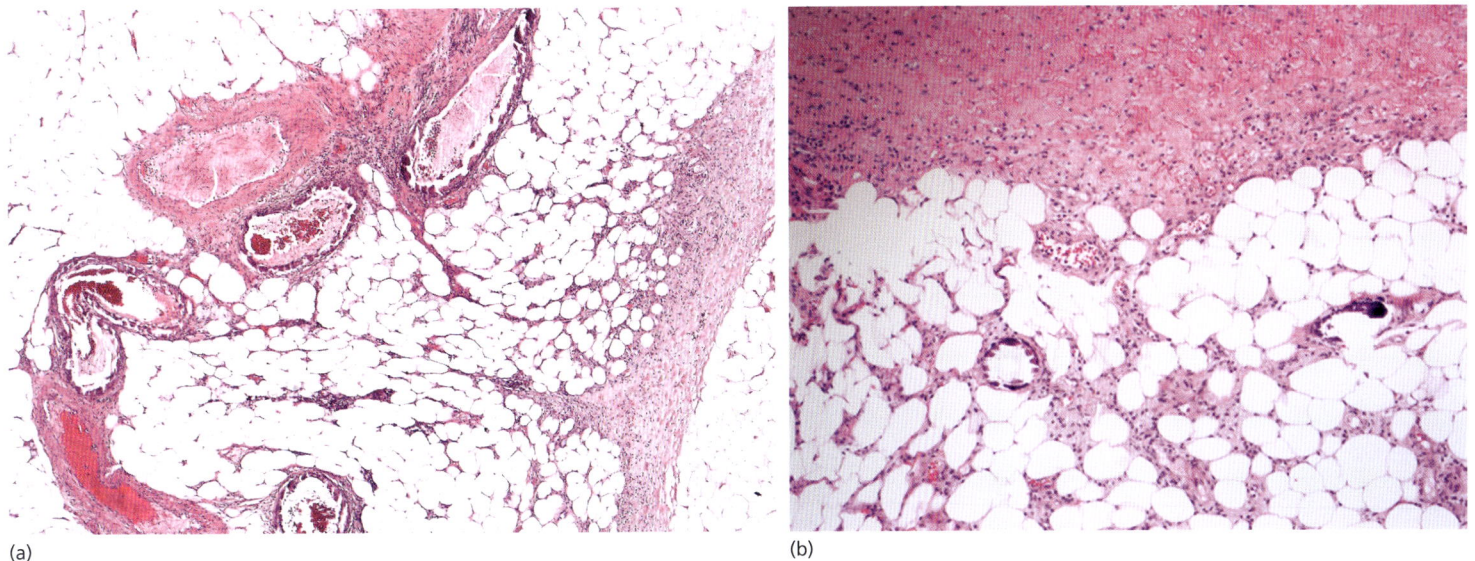

(a)   (b)

Figure 59.6 (a) Calcification of two arterioles. (b) Calcification of small vessels in a background of fat necrosis. (a) Courtesy of Eduardo Calonje. (b) Courtesy of Dr J. Fitzgibbon, Cork University Hospital, Cork, Ireland.

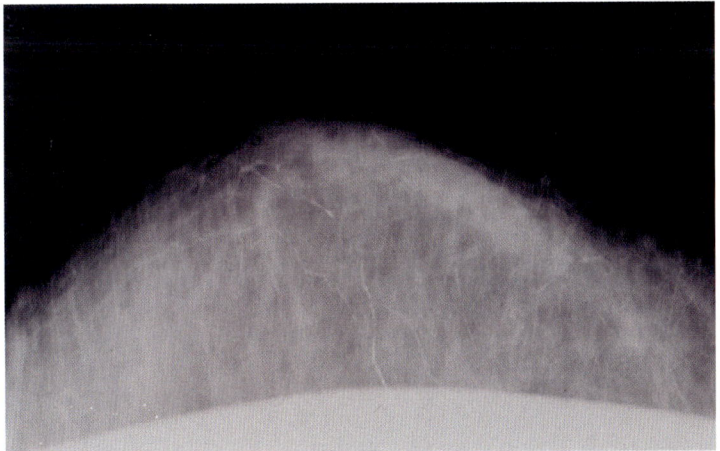

Figure 59.7 Soft tissue radiography showing calcification of vessels of the abdominal wall. Reproduced from Hackett *et al.* 2009 [40] with permission of John Wiley & Sons.

Treatment ladder for calciphylaxis

First line

- Correct abnormalities of systemic calcium homeostasis
- Debride necrotic tissue
- Optimise treatment of underlying renal/hepatic failure or malignancy
- General wound care including treatment of secondary infection, compression if appropriate and adequate pain control
- Intravenous sodium thiosulphate (25 g three times per week)

Second line

- Thrombolysis and anticoagulation
- Parathyroidectomy

Third line

- Hyperbaric oxygen

Key references

The full list of references can be found in the online version at https://www.wiley.com/rooksdermatology10e

Dystrophic calcification secondary to inflammatory disease and infections

3 Brinster B, Calonje E. Degenerative and metabolic diseases. In: Calonje E, Brenn T, Lazaar A, McKee PH, eds. *McKee's Pathology of the Skin*, 4th edn. Amsterdam: Elsevier Saunders, 2012:566–70.
4 Touart DM, Sau P. Cutaneous deposition diseases. Part II. *J Am Acad Dermatol* 1998;39:527–46.
6 Reiter N, El-Shabrawi L, Leinweber B, Berghold A, Aberer E. Calcinosis cutis. Part I. Diagnostic pathway. *J Am Acad Dermatol* 2011;65:1–12.

Dystrophic calcification secondary to trauma or injection/infusion of calcium-containing materials

1 Rho NK, Youn SJ, Park HS, Kim WS, Lee ES. Calcified nodule on the heel of a child following a single heel stick in the neonatal period. *Clin Exp Dermatol* 2003; 28:502–3.

Dystrophic calcification secondary to tumours and genetic disease

1 Walsh JS, Fairley JA. Calcifying disorders of the skin. *J Am Acad Dermatol* 1995;33:693–706.

Idiopathic calcification of the skin and subcutaneous tissues

11 McKee PH, Liomba NG, Hutt MSR. Tumoral calcinosis. A pathological study of 56 cases. *Br J Dermatol* 1982;107:669–74.

Metastatic calcification

1 Touart DM, Sau P. Cutaneous deposition diseases. Part II. *J Am Acad Dermatol* 1998;39:527–46.

PART 5: METABOLIC & NUTRITIONAL DISORDERS

Calciphylaxis

11 McCarthy JT, el-Azhary RA, Patzelt MT *et al.* Survival, risk factors, and effect of treatment in 101 patients with calciphylaxis. *Mayo Clin Proc* 2016;91:1384–94.

28 Peng T, Zhuo L, Wang Y *et al.* Systematic review of sodium thiosulfate in treating calciphylaxis in chronic kidney disease patients. *Nephrology* 2018;23:669–75.

38 Isoherranen K, O'Brien JJ, Barker J *et al.* Atypical wounds. Best clinical practice and challenges. *J Wound Care* 2019;28(Suppl. 6):S1–92.

CHAPTER 60

Xanthomas and Abnormalities of Lipid Metabolism and Storage

Paul D. Flynn

Acute and Metabolic Medicine, Addenbrooke's Hospital, Cambridge; School of Clinical Medicine, University of Cambridge, Cambridge, UK

PART 5: METABOLIC & NUTRITIONAL DISORDERS

Introduction

Disorders of lipid metabolism are heterogeneous. They range from the very rare to the very common including monogenic diseases with high penetrance through to polygenic disorders and those that are paradigms of gene–environment interactions. Some are entirely or partially secondary to diabetes, hypothyroidism, renal failure or liver disease. Dyslipidaemias are associated with an increased risk of atherosclerosis and its complications. They are of particular relevance to dermatologists because they may present with subcutaneous lipid deposits (xanthomas). These may require treatment for the relief of the symptoms they cause, as well as enabling the identification and treatment of a dyslipidaemia before the premature onset of clinical cardiovascular disease.

This chapter includes an overview of the classification of the xanthomas and primary and secondary dyslipidaemias relevant to dermatologists and the overall management of dyslipidaemia. More detailed information on the metabolic non-dermatological issues is available in the third edition of *Hyperlipidaemia: Diagnosis and Management* by P. N. Durrington [1] and the eighth edition of *The Metabolic and Molecular Bases of Inherited Disease* [2].

Classification of dyslipidaemias

There are a number of classifications of disordered lipid and lipoprotein metabolism, none of which is entirely satisfactory.

Table 60.1 World Health Organization classification of hyperlipoproteinaemias.

Type	Lipoprotein abnormality
I	Hyperchylomicronaemia
IIa	Elevated LDL
IIb	Elevated LDL and VLDL
III	Broad β-VLDL
IV	Elevated VLDL
V	Elevated chylomicrons and VLDL

Adapted from Fredrickson *et al.* 1967 [1].
LDL, low-density lipoprotein; VLDL, very low-density lipoprotein.

The most straightforward is the World Health Organization (WHO) classification, usually referred to as the Fredrickson classification [1], based on the class of excess lipoprotein present (Table 60.1). However, this requires plasma ultracentrifugation or lipoprotein electrophoresis, does not include disorders characterised by low levels of high-density lipoprotein (HDL) cholesterol or secondary dyslipidaemias, and is not a diagnostic classification.

For most patients, all that is available is a blood lipid profile comprising total cholesterol, triglycerides and HDL cholesterol measurements with a calculated low-density lipoprotein (LDL) cholesterol. Thus, in practice, patients are classified more broadly as having hypercholesterolaemia, hypertriglyceridaemia, combined (or mixed) dyslipidaemia or other dyslipidaemia, with further characterisation and diagnosis wherever possible based on further tests (Table 60.2).

Table 60.2 Working classification of dyslipidaemias.

	Lipid abnormalities	WHO type	Primary dyslipidaemias	Secondary causes	Cutaneous features
Hypercholesterolaemia	↑ TC ↑ LDL-C Normal Tgs	IIa	Familial hypercholesterolaemia Polygenic hypercholesterolaemia	Hypothyroidism Anorexia Cholestatic liver disease Nephrotic syndrome Acute intermittent porphyria Drugs: thiazide diuretics, corticosteroids	Tendon xanthomas (FH) Xanthelasmas Interdigital plane xanthomas (homozygous FH)

Combined dyslipidaemia	↑ TC
	↑ LDL-C
	↑ Tgs
	± ↓ HDL-C
		III
		IIb
		IV
			Familial dysbetalipoproteinaemia
			Familial combined hyperlipidaemia
				Diabetes
				Metabolic syndrome
				Lipodystrophies
				Hypothyroidism
				Hepatocellular liver disease
				Nephrotic syndrome
				Chronic renal failure
				Paraproteinaemias
				Pregnancy
				Drugs: β-blockers, antiretrovirals,
				  retinoic acid derivatives
					Tuberous xanthomas
					  (in WHO type III)
					Palmar xanthomas
					  (in WHO type III)

Hypertriglyceridaemia	↑↑ Tgs ↑ TC ↓ HDL-C	I IV, V	Lipoprotein lipase deficiency ApoCII deficiency	Diabetes Alcohol excess Chronic renal failure Paraproteinaemias Pregnancy (especially 3rd trimester) Drugs: retinoic acid derivatives, oral contraceptives	Eruptive xanthomas
Other dyslipidaemias	↓ HDL-C only ↑ HDL-C ↓↓ LDL-C ↓ LDL-C		Tangier disease ApoAI Milano Hyperalphalipoproteinaemia Abetalipoproteinaemia Hypobetalipoproteinaemia	Alcohol Anabolic steroids	

FH, familial hypercholesterolaemia; HDL-C, high-density lipoprotein cholesterol; LDL-C, low-density lipoprotein cholesterol; TC, total cholesterol; Tgs, triglycerides; WHO, World Health Organization.

XANTHOMAS

Introduction

The term xanthoma (Greek 'xanthos' meaning yellow) describes a variety of subcutaneous lipid deposits. All xanthomas contain macrophages loaded with cholesterol and cholesterol esters ('foam cells'). There are a number of clinical types, most of which are associated with hyperlipidaemia.

Classification

Xanthomas are divided into those that are secondary to disorders of lipid metabolism (Box 60.1) and those that are classed under histiocytic disorders. Those due to histiocytic disorders are discussed elsewhere (Chapter 135).

Box 60.1 Xanthomas

- Tendon xanthoma
- Tuberous xanthoma:
  - Tuberoeruptive xanthoma
- Eruptive xanthoma
- Dyslipidaemic plane xanthoma:
  - Xanthelasma
  - Plane xanthoma
  - Palmar xanthoma

Tendon xanthoma

Definition and nomenclature
Tendon xanthomas occur as subcutaneous nodules or papules in relation to tendons.

Synonyms and inclusions
- Tendinous xanthoma

Epidemiology
Associated diseases
Tendon xanthomas are most frequently seen in familial hypercholesterolaemia (FH) (see later in this chapter) but are also a feature of the secondary hypercholesterolaemia seen in prolonged cholestasis. They occur in rare lipid disorders such as cerebrotendinous xanthomatosis and sitosterolaemia in which the tendon xanthomas are not associated with raised serum cholesterol levels.

Clinical features

Tendon xanthomas occur most commonly attached to the extensor tendons over the knuckles and in the Achilles tendon, although other tendons can sometimes be affected. In these sites they can usually be moved from side to side. Occasionally they can involve the periosteum at the site of insertion of the patellar tendon where they cannot be moved. As the accumulation of cholesterol is deep within the tendons, the overlying skin does not appear yellow. The xanthomas contain collagen in addition to foamy macrophages and so feel quite hard.

Investigations

Investigations should include a full lipid profile (where an LDL cholesterol level of ≥4.9 mmol/L may indicate FH) and liver function tests.

Management

Tendon xanthomas sometimes improve with cholesterol reduction but do not tend to resolve completely. Where the tendon xanthomas are painful, this symptom usually responds to LDL cholesterol reduction.

Tuberous xanthoma

Definition

Tuberous xanthomas are firm, yellow-red nodules that occur over sites of pressure, commonly the elbows and knees. Where a central tuberous xanthoma is surrounded by several smaller lesions it may be termed a 'tuberoeruptive xanthoma'.

Epidemiology

Associated diseases

Tuberous xanthomas usually indicate the presence of type III hyperlipoproteinaemia (see later in this chapter).

Clinical features

They start as small xanthomas, usually over the extensor aspects of the elbows and knees (Figure 60.1), but can develop into quite exuberant exophytic lesions several centimetres in diameter and height. They can develop over other pressure sites, particularly the heels and plantar surfaces of the feet. They can occasionally occur in the bone marrow. They tend to be painless although they can be itchy and are susceptible to traumatic damage given their position.

Investigations

Initial investigations should include a lipid profile and further investigations could include apolipoprotein E (apoE) genotyping, and lipid electrophoresis or ultracentrifugation.

Management

They respond well to effective treatment of the combined dyslipidaemia with which they are associated.

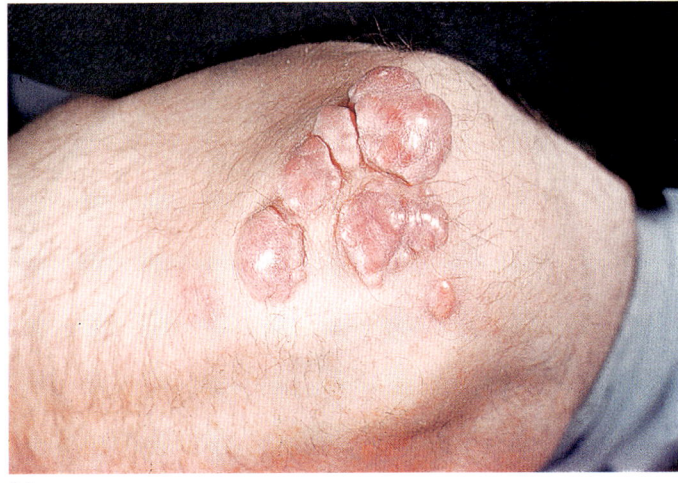

(a)

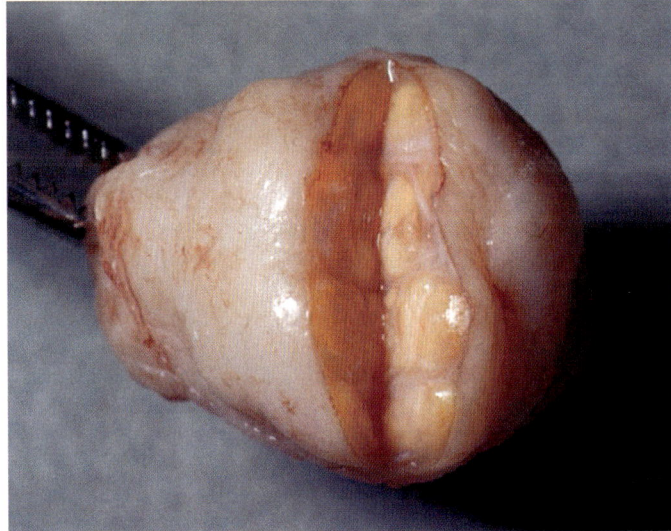

(b)

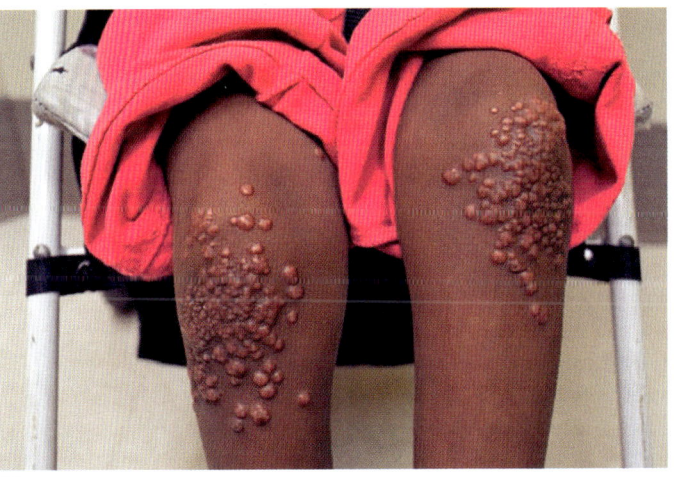

(c)

Figure 60.1 (a) Tuberous xanthomas. (b) Lipid-laden lobules within a tuberoeruptive xanthoma excised from the elbow of a 40-year-old man with familial type III hyperlipidaemia (triglycerides up to 73 mmol/L; cholesterol >24 mmol/L). (c) Tuberoeruptive xanthomas with numerous yellow-red papules and nodules over the knees. (a) Courtesy of Addenbrooke's Hospital. (b, c) Reproduced from Pearson *et al.* 2017 [1] with permission of John Wiley & Sons.

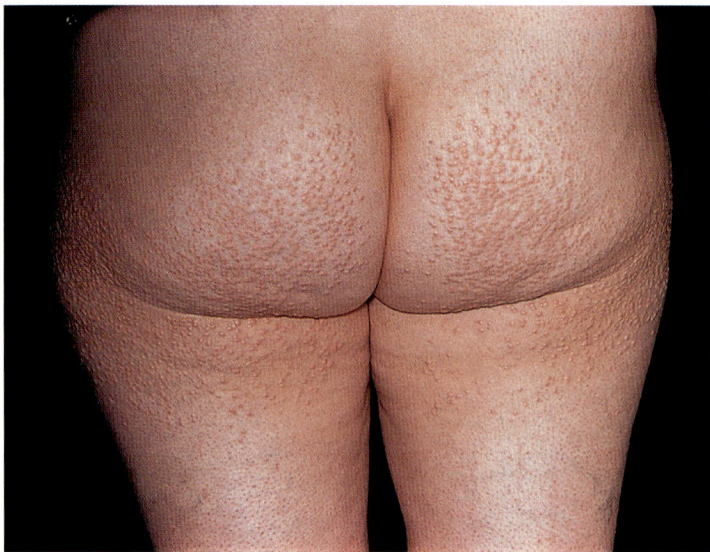

Figure 60.2 Eruptive xanthomas. Courtesy of Addenbrooke's Hospital.

Eruptive xanthoma

Definition

Eruptive xanthomas appear as multiple small papules over extensor surfaces (Figure 60.2).

Epidemiology
Associated diseases

Eruptive xanthomas can be associated with any cause of severe hypertriglyceridaemia.

Clinical features

These small xanthomas consist of yellow papules 2–5 mm in diameter arising on a red base. They usually appear in large numbers over extensor surfaces, particularly the buttocks, back, legs and arms. In extreme cases they are pruritic and are more widely distributed. Their foamy macrophages contain triglycerides as well as cholesterol. Resulting from hypertriglyceridaemia, they are almost always accompanied by lipaemia retinalis, a creamy yellow discoloration of the retinal blood vessels, and a lipaemic appearance of blood or serum samples.

Investigations

Investigations should include fasting lipids (especially triglycerides) and glucose.

Management

Eruptive xanthomas resolve within 2 weeks or so of the normalisation of triglyceride levels.

Dyslipidaemic plane (planar) xanthoma

This group consists of xanthelasmas, plane xanthomas and palmar xanthomas.

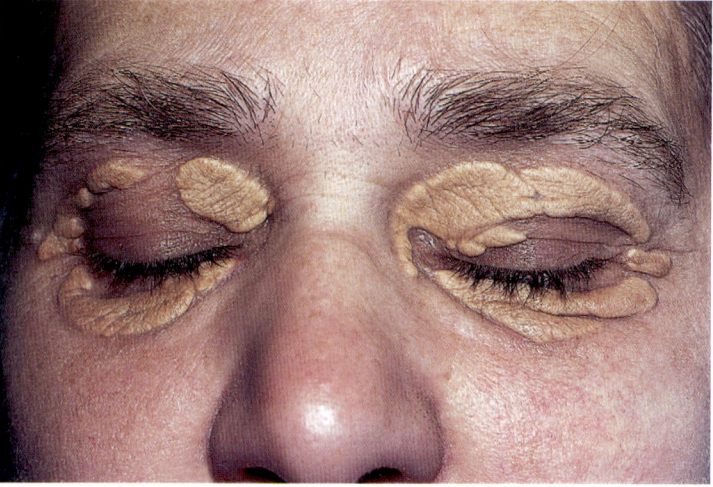

(a)

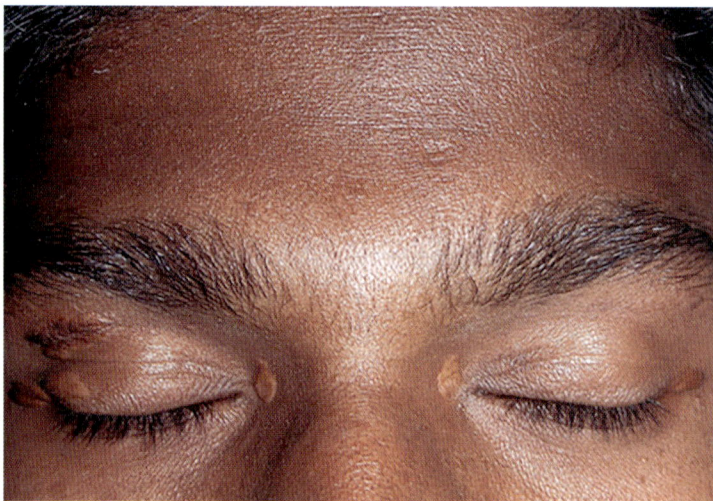

(b)

Figure 60.3 Xanthelasma palpebrarum over bilateral eyelids: (a) extensive and (b) discrete and coalescing lesions. (a) Courtesy of Addenbrooke's Hospital. (b) Reproduced from Pandhi et al. 2012 [1] with permission of BMJ Publishing.

Xanthelasma

Definition and nomenclature

Xanthelasmas are plane xanthomas that develop around the eyes (Figure 60.3).

Synonyms and inclusions
- Xanthelasma palpebrarum

Epidemiology
Associated diseases

Xanthelasmas are seen in FH, type III hyperlipoproteinaemia and chronic cholestasis (especially primary biliary cirrhosis), but are also often seen in people with circulating lipid levels considered normal in the western population.

Clinical features

They most commonly affect the upper eyelids and the area around the medial canthus. They are relatively soft on palpation and range from pale yellow to yellow-orange in colour. In skin of colour, variations of skin pigmentation may be seen.

Complications and co-morbidities

Although previous small studies failed to identify xanthelasma as a risk factor for cardiovascular disease, recent analysis of 12745 participants in the Copenhagen City Heart Study who were followed up for 33 years found xanthelasma to be an independent predictor of coronary heart disease, although not of ischaemic stroke [2].

Investigations

Investigations should include a full lipid profile and liver function tests.

Management

Given their prominent site, xanthelasmas are often a cosmetic problem. Treatments include surgical excision, electrocautery, topical trichloracetic acid, silver nitrate or lasers. However, they often recur after treatment.

If LDL cholesterol levels are high, then treatment to lower the LDL cholesterol (e.g. statins) seems sensible, and anecdotally reduces the risk of recurrence of the xanthelasmas after excision, even if this is not yet confirmed by clinical trial. The statin treatment is often associated with regression of xanthelasmas in hypercholesterolaemic patients without the need for other intervention.

Plane xanthoma

Definition and nomenclature

Plane xanthomas are flat, smear-like lesions that can occur anywhere on the body (Figure 60.4).

Synonyms and inclusions
- Planar xanthoma

Epidemlology
Associated diseases

Plane xanthomas can be a feature of homozygous FH.

Clinical features

These xanthomas are wide-based, flat and macular, although they may develop into raised plaques. They can occur anywhere on the body. Plane xanthomas affecting the interdigital webspace between the first and second fingers are only seen in homozygous FH. Diffuse dyslipidaemic plane xanthoma is less common and more widespread.

Differential diagnosis

Diffuse plane normolipidaemic xanthomatosis (Chapter 135) is a rare form of histiocytosis, often associated with paraproteinaemia

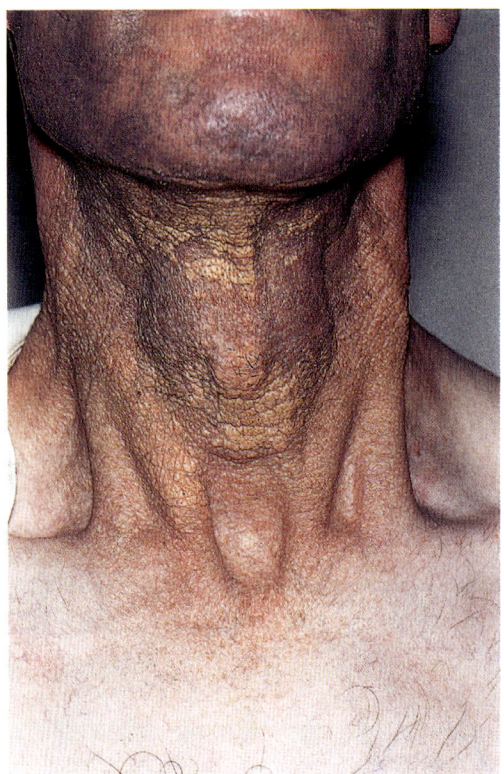

Figure 60.4 Plane xanthomatosis. Courtesy of Addenbrooke's Hospital.

or an underlying systemic disorder, usually of the haematological or lymphoproliferative type. Lipid levels are normal.

Necrobiotic xanthogranuloma (Chapter 135) is a rare, chronic, progressive histiocytosis that is strongly associated with haematological malignant conditions.

Investigations

Familial hypercholesterolaemia and type III hyperlipoproteinaemia may be associated. Initial investigations should include a full lipid profile, serum electrophoresis and autoimmune screen. Further tests could include a skeletal survey and bone marrow examination if necessary.

Management

Like tuberous xanthomas, plane xanthomas respond well to treatment of the dyslipidaemia.

Palmar xanthoma

Definition and nomenclature

Palmar xanthomas run in the palmar creases (Figure 60.5).

Synonyms and inclusions
- Xanthomata striata palmaris

Epidemiology
Associated diseases

They are pathognomonic of type III hyperlipoproteinaemia.

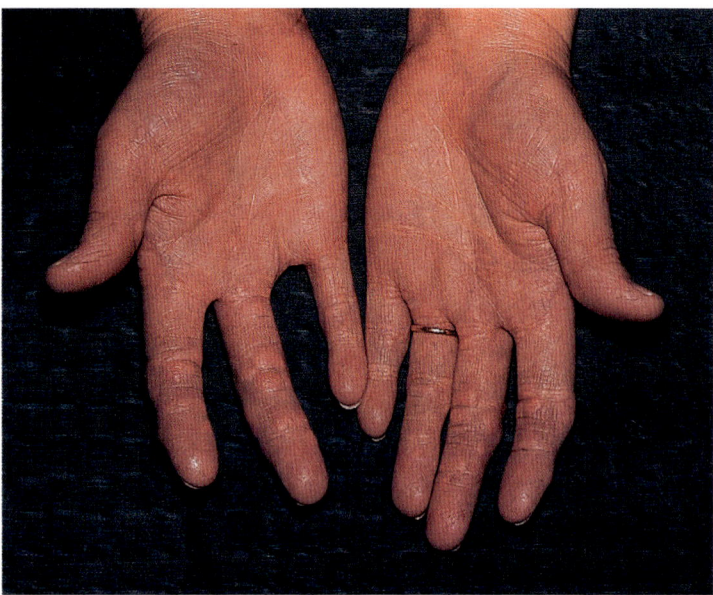

Figure 60.5 Xanthomatosis and yellow palmar creases. Courtesy of Addenbrooke's Hospital.

Clinical features

Linear palmar xanthomas consist of an orange-yellow lipid deposition running along the palmar creases, and occasionally the flexor creases of the wrists.

Investigations

Initial investigations should include a full lipid profile, fasting glucose, urea and electrolytes, liver function tests and thyroid-stimulating hormone levels. Further specialist tests include apoE genotyping, and lipid electrophoresis or ultracentrifugation.

Management

They usually respond well to treatment of the causes of the type III hyperlipoproteinaemia.

PRIMARY DYSLIPIDAEMIAS: HYPERCHOLESTEROLAEMIA

Familial hypercholesterolaemia

Definition

Familial hypercholesterolaemia is an autosomal co-dominant condition characterised by the following:
- High total and LDL cholesterol, slightly low HDL cholesterol and normal triglyceride concentrations.
- Frequent tendon xanthomas (especially of the Achilles tendons).
- Premature onset of cardiovascular disease (CVD).

Epidemiology

Homozygotes number about one in 1×10^6 in white populations. Heterozygotes occur at a frequency of about one in 250–500 in most white populations. However, there is notably higher frequency in certain groups such as Afrikaners and the Lebanese, where there are marked founder gene effects.

Pathophysiology

Genetics

The familial clustering of the three features listed (high total and LDL cholesterol, tendon xanthomas and premature CVD) has been recognised since at least the late 19th century and was the subject of detailed studies in the 1930s [1,2]. In the 1950s, the development of ultracentrifugation for quantifying lipoproteins revealed that the biochemical hallmark of FH is an accumulation of LDL [3], and in 1973 Goldstein and Brown discovered the LDL receptor and showed that its defective functioning was the underlying cause of the condition [4].

The majority of patients with FH have mutations in their LDL receptor associated with a variable degree of loss of function. As a result, there is both defective clearance of very low-density lipoprotein (VLDL) from the circulation with consequent increased conversion to LDL, and impaired clearance of LDL resulting in the significant elevation of LDL cholesterol concentration that accounts for the raised plasma total cholesterol.

Over 1000 disease-associated mutations have so far been described in the LDL receptor gene, which is one of the largest human genes. They have been classified on the basis of the effect they have on the synthesis, expression and processing of the LDL receptor:
- Type 1 mutations prevent receptor synthesis.
- Type 2 mutations impair transport of the receptor from the endoplasmic reticulum to the Golgi apparatus.
- Type 3 mutations affect receptor binding of circulating LDLs.
- Type 4 mutations prevent clathrin-mediated receptor clustering and internalisation.
- Type 5 mutations interfere with receptor recycling from the endosome.

Type 1 mutations tend to result in a complete absence of LDL receptor activity ('receptor negative'), while the other classes of mutations usually cause markedly reduced but not completely absent activity ('receptor defective').

In a small proportion of patients with FH (around 2%), the mutation affects not the LDL receptor but the receptor-binding domain in the LDL apoB100 (familial defective apoB100). This is almost always due to a mutation in codon 3500 (R3500Q) resulting in a substitution of arginine for glutamine. Rarely it is due to a different mutation in codon 3500 (R3500W – in which tryptophan replaces arginine) or in codon 3531. Such patients are phenotypically indistinguishable from those with LDL receptor mutations. A new genetic locus has been found to account for some of the previously mutation negative cases of FH. The gene codes for proprotein convertase subtilisin kexin 9 (PCSK9), a serine protease whose activity appears to decrease LDL receptor expression and LDL clearance and hence increase LDL cholesterol concentrations [5,6]. It has emerged that loss-of-function polymorphisms in the *PCSK9* gene are associated with lower levels of LDL cholesterol and much lower levels of CVD in a wide range of populations. Consequently, methods of inhibiting PCSK9 are now being developed and deployed to reduce cardiovascular risk. Finally, a small group of patients, initially all from Sardinia, have a phenotype similar to homozygous

FH but inherited in a recessive pattern called autosomal recessive hypercholesterolaemia (ARH) [7,8].

Clinical features

The presence of tendon xanthomas (see earlier in this chapter) is the principal cutaneous manifestation of FH and may often be helpful in establishing the diagnosis. They are usually present in childhood in homozygotes and become more common with age in untreated heterozygotes. The prevalence rises from 12.5% in those aged 10–19 years, to 69.2% in those between 20 and 29, and up to 90% by the age of 40 years. This frequency has been reduced significantly by the earlier introduction of effective cholesterol-lowering medication. Plane and tuberous xanthomas may occasionally be seen in FH homozygotes, but not in heterozygotes. Xanthelasmas are not commonly seen in FH.

Differential diagnosis

Very rarely, immunoglobulins directed against the LDL receptor can produce a hypercholesterolaemia with total and LDL cholesterol levels similar to those seen in FH homozygotes but without any tendon xanthomas. This has been referred to as 'pseudo-familial hypercholesterolaemia'.

Complications and co-morbidities

Homozygotes can have total cholesterol levels of 15 mmol/L or higher, be born with tendon xanthomas and suffer from the clinical effects of coronary heart disease as early as their teens. They can also develop a supravalvular aortic stenosis.

Heterozygotes have less marked elevations in their cholesterol than homozygotes (Table 60.3), but 50% of untreated males will have suffered a myocardial infarction and 24% will have died by the age of 50. Heterozygous females have a slightly delayed onset of CVD compared with males but 58% will have had a myocardial infarction and 15% will have died by the age of 60 if not treated [9]. FH thus accounts for a significant proportion of premature CVD and of premature sudden cardiac death. There is a striking preponderance in FH of coronary arterial disease, as opposed to cerebrovascular or peripheral vascular disease.

Investigations

Lipid concentrations in FH are listed in Table 60.3.

Given the genetic heterogeneity underlying FH, diagnosis has largely rested on clinical and biochemical criteria. In the UK, the criteria used by the Simon Broome Register of patients with FH have been widely adopted (Box 60.2) [10]. Other sets of diagnostic criteria have also been developed, such as the Dutch Lipid Clinic

Network Criteria and its UK derivative the FH Wales criteria (www .fhwalescriteria.co.uk; last accessed February 2023), and the Make Early Diagnosis to Prevent Early Disease on Medical Pedigree (MEDPED) system [11,12]. Increasingly, advances in molecular biological techniques are proving helpful in diagnosing FH. This is particularly true where a disease-causing mutation has been identified in one family member. Genetic cascade screening for FH has been adopted in a number of countries and work is underway to develop a systematic approach to this in the UK.

Box 60.2 Simon Broome Register criteria for diagnosing familial hypercholesterolaemia (FH)

Definite FH
- Total cholesterol >6.7 mmol/L or LDL cholesterol >4.0 mmol/L in children under 16 years, or total cholesterol >7.5 mmol/L or LDL cholesterol >4.9 mmol/L in adults

Plus
- Tendon xanthomas in patient or first- or second-degree relative
or
- FH mutation detected

Possible FH
- Total cholesterol >6.7 mmol/L or LDL cholesterol >4.0 mmol/L in children under 16 years, or total cholesterol >7.5 mmol/L or LDL cholesterol >4.9 mmol/L in adults

Plus
- Family history of myocardial infarction <50 years in second-degree relative or <60 years in first-degree relative
or
- Family history of total cholesterol >7.5 mmol/L in first- or second-degree relative

Adapted from Scientific Steering Committee of the Simon Broome Register Group 1991 [10].

Management

Statins have now become the mainstay of treatment and have played a large part in the reduction of cardiovascular mortality seen in recent years in FH. For each 1 mmol/L reduction in LDL cholesterol, there is a 22% reduction in cardiovascular risk, at least up to 3 mmol/L. In comparison with the general population, statins usually have to be started at a much earlier age in patients with FH. To achieve the desired reduction in LDL cholesterol, the National Institute for Health and Care Excellence (NICE) in the UK has advised reducing LDL cholesterol by at least 50%, so higher doses of the more potent statins may have to be used. The same guidance recommends offering statins to those identified as having FH by the age of 10 years. Referral to a specialist lipid clinic is advised to allow counselling of young patients starting life long therapy, especially young women where the specific issue of the potential teratogenicity of the statins and family planning needs to be fully explored. These clinics will have experience of other therapies that can prove helpful including bile acid sequestrants and LDL apheresis.

Table 60.3 Lipid concentrations in familial hypercholesterolaemia.

	Total cholesterol (mmol/L)	LDL cholesterol (mmol/L)	HDL cholesterol (mmol/L)	Triglycerides (mmol/L)
Normal	4.52 ± 0.72	2.84 ± 0.64	1.37 ± 0.33	0.68 ± 0.28
Heterozygotes	7.73 ± 1.63	6.23 ± 1.55	1.11 ± 0.31	0.93 ± 0.58
Homozygotes	17.5 ± 4.39	16.1 ± 4.13	0.88 ± 0.26	1.14 ± 0.58

Data taken from Goldstein and Brown 1973 [**4**].
HDL, high-density lipoprotein; LDL, low-density lipoprotein.

PART 5: METABOLIC & NUTRITIONAL DISORDERS

Ezetimibe reduces intestinal cholesterol absorption mediated by the intestinal sterol transporter NPC1L1 (Niemann–Pick C-1-like protein 1). It is well tolerated and can augment the LDL reduction achieved by statins by a further 20%. Ezetimibe reduces cardiovascular risk in line with the LDL cholesterol reduction achieved [13]. Recently, two monoclonal antibodies directed against PCSK9 (alirocumab and evolocumab) have been licensed for use in treating patients at high cardiovascular risk whose LDL cholesterol remains inadequately controlled despite maximally tolerated statin and ezetimibe [14,15]. In the UK, patients with FH are eligible for this treatment if their LDL cholesterol is greater than 3.5 mmol/L if they have CVD, or if it is greater than 5.0 mmol/L if they do not. Tendon xanthomas and xanthelasmas may respond to the reduction in LDL cholesterol; corneal arcus does not. FH homozygotes must be referred for specialist assessment and treatment. Their cholesterol does not respond well to statins or other drug therapies that work by upregulating LDL receptor expression. Treatments available for these patients include high-dose evolocumab, mipomersen (an antisense oligonucleotide directed against apoB100 mRNA) and lopitamide (an inhibitor of microsomal triacylglycerol transfer protein). The latter two treatments suppress the production of VLDL [16]. FH homozygotes can also require LDL apheresis and occasionally liver transplantation as well as coronary revascularisation and aortic valve surgery.

PRIMARY DYSLIPIDAEMIAS: COMBINED DYSLIPIDAEMIA

Type III hyperlipoproteinaemia

Definition and nomenclature

Type III hyperlipoproteinaemia is associated with combined dyslipidaemia, palmar and tuberous xanthomas and early-onset CVD and peripheral vascular disease.

Synonyms and inclusions
- Broad beta disease
- Dysbetalipoproteinaemia
- Remnant removal disease

Epidemiology

Incidence and prevalence
Estimates of the frequency of type III hyperlipoproteinaemia vary between about 1 and 10 in 10 000.

Pathophysiology
Patients with type III hyperlipoproteinaemia have a characteristic lipoprotein electrophoretic pattern that is the gold standard diagnostic test. There is an increase in small VLDL and intermediate-density lipoprotein and a decrease in LDL. VLDL isolated from type III patients is uncharacteristically enriched with cholesterol esters and gives rise to a broad-β migrating band, rather than the usual pre-β band [1,2]. This results from an accumulation of VLDL remnants and chylomicron remnants and produces a marked increase in plasma total cholesterol and triglycerides.

Genetics
The underlying defect is an abnormal apoE [3], the apolipoprotein in remnant lipoproteins that mediates their binding to the LDL receptor and the LDL receptor-related protein. There are three common isoforms of apoE: apoE2, -E3 and -E4, each differing by one amino acid:

	E2	E3	E4
Residue 112	Cysteine	Cysteine	Arginine
Residue 158	Cysteine	Arginine	Arginine

ApoE2 homozygosity represents the commonest abnormality associated with type III hyperlipoproteinaemia; its cysteine at residue 112 is within the receptor-binding domain of the protein and its cysteine at residue 158 affects salt bridges within the protein and thereby the conformation of the receptor-binding domain. Very occasionally other apoE mutations are associated with type III hyperlipoproteinaemia, many of which severely reduce apoE-mediated receptor binding and can cause the disorder in heterozygotes [4].

Environmental factors
Less than 10% of subjects homozygous for apoE2 develop type III hyperlipoproteinaemia, and most of the rest have lower than average lipid levels. It is clear that a second factor is required for the development of type III hyperlipoproteinaemia, either environmental or genetic. Increased production of chylomicrons or VLDL can be one such factor and may result from excessive caloric intake, increased alcohol consumption, obesity, type 2 diabetes, the metabolic syndrome or from an interplay of multiple genetic influences on lipoprotein metabolism (as presumed to underlie familial combined hyperlipidaemia). Equally, increasing age, hypothyroidism or postmenopausal oestrogen deficiency can further impair apoE-mediated receptor catabolism of lipoproteins and result in the development of the disorder.

Clinical features
The most characteristic skin manifestations are palmar xanthomas (Figure 60.5). Tuberous xanthomas (Figure 62.1) may also be present. Patients with particularly high triglyceride concentrations may also develop lipaemia retinalis and eruptive xanthomas over their buttocks (Figure 62.2).

Complications and co-morbidities
There is evidence of an increased risk of both coronary artery and peripheral arterial disease, especially in those with all the clinical and biochemical features of the disorder – in whom up to 50% have premature CVD [5]. Gout also appears common in this group of patients [6]. Type III hyperlipoproteinaemia has been associated with lipoprotein glomerulopathy, manifesting as proteinuria or the nephrotic syndrome [7]. Renal biopsy shows glomerular foam cells; the condition usually resolves with successful treatment of the abnormal lipid profile.

Management

Identification and treatment of any contributing lifestyle factors or diseases are central to the management of these patients. Patients should be screened for obesity, diabetes and hypothyroidism and treated accordingly. Dietary advice should be given and exercise encouraged as it increases the activity of lipoprotein lipase and thereby increases chylomicron and VLDL remnant clearance. Such measures are often successful in improving the lipid profile on their own; in their absence, drug therapy is usually less effective. Normally both statins and fibrates work well, both in improving the lipid profile and in causing regression of the palmar and tuberous xanthomas [8,9]. Occasionally, combined statin and fibrate therapy may be required.

PRIMARY DYSLIPIDAEMIAS: HYPERTRIGLYCERIDAEMIAS

Type I hyperlipoproteinaemia

Definition

Type I hyperlipoproteinaemia is an autosomal recessive condition in which there is an accumulation of chylomicrons alone due to a deficiency of lipoprotein lipase (LPL).

Epidemiology
Incidence and prevalence

The condition is extremely rare with a frequency of perhaps one per million in most populations but with higher frequency in some populations such as French Canadians due to founder gene effects.

Pathophysiology

It results from a deficiency of LPL and as such shows an autosomal recessive pattern of inheritance. However, there is accumulating evidence that some heterozygotes for LPL deficiency may show a milder degree of hypertriglyceridaemia. An increasing number of mutations in the LPL gene have been described. Some cases result from deficiency of activators of LPL, for example apoCII deficiency. This discovery followed the observation that hyperchylomicronaemia was alleviated in some patients following plasma infusions.

It remains unclear why LPL deficiency can cause an isolated accumulation of chylomicrons, given the role of the enzyme in VLDL catabolism. However, with increasing age there is a progressive shift towards a type V hyperlipoproteinaemic pattern.

Clinical features

The characteristic skin finding in patients with type I hyperlipoproteinaemia is eruptive xanthomas (Figure 62.2).

Complications and co-morbidities

The principal concern in type I hyperlipoproteinaemia is the increased risk of acute pancreatitis with its associated morbidity and mortality. While hypertriglyceridaemia may be a consequence of acute pancreatitis, there is clear evidence it may also be a cause, accounting for up to 10% of cases. The risk increases with increasing triglyceride levels, with a threshold around fasting triglycerides of 10 mmol/L, with the risk rising markedly beyond 20 mmol/L. Other factors must play a part as some patients seem remarkably immune from acute attacks despite grossly elevated triglyceride concentrations. The mortality is further increased because the serum amylase, so often used as a sole diagnostic test for acute pancreatitis, may not be elevated.

Clearance of chylomicrons from the circulation by cells of the reticuloendothelial system can result in hepatomegaly and splenomegaly, with splenic infarcts in some cases.

Investigations

Familial LPL deficiency causes extremely elevated levels of serum triglycerides, often greater than 20 mmol/L. Total cholesterol levels are often substantially elevated as well, reflecting the extreme concentrations of chylomicrons, which contain some cholesterol and cholesterol esters as well as their predominant triglycerides. Blood, serum or plasma from such patients will appear milky and a creamy layer will separate on top of the sample if centrifuged or allowed to stand for some hours. Hyperchylomicronaemia will be present from childhood onwards in homozygous LPL deficiency.

Management

The treatment of severe hypertriglyceridaemia involves strict restriction of all dietary fats to 20–25 g per day to reduce chylomicron production as much as possible. Attention must be paid to any other factors that may increase the production or decrease the clearance of the triglyceride-rich lipoproteins (TRLs). Good control of diabetes, weight reduction where appropriate, alcohol restriction and a review of all other medications are particularly important. Intake of refined carbohydrates should also be limited. Fibrates usually have little effect in genetic LPL deficiency. Nicotinic acid derivatives can be helpful. Bile acid sequestrants are contraindicated as they may increase the triglyceride level. Infusions of fresh frozen plasma are beneficial in those with apoCII deficiency who present with acute pancreatitis. Antioxidant therapy has proved very effective in reducing the frequency of attacks of acute pancreatitis in a number of patients with severe hypertriglyceridaemia. All patients with severe hypertriglyceridaemia should have access to specialist lipid clinics, to be considered for volanesorsen, an antisense oligonucleotide that binds the mRNA for apoCIII. This reduces fasting triglyceride levels by 75% and three-quarters of those treated achieved levels less than 8.5 mmol/L [1].

Eruptive xanthomas respond to lowering of the triglycerides although they tend to last a few days longer than the lipid abnormality.

Type V hyperlipoproteinaemia

Definition

Type V hyperlipoproteinaemia is due to an accumulation of VLDL as well as chylomicrons.

Epidemiology

Incidence and prevalence

Type V hyperlipoproteinaemia affects one in every 5000–10 000.

Pathophysiology

Although it can result from LPL deficiency, this only accounts for a very small proportion of cases. Patients with type V hyperlipoproteinaemia may have relatives with hypertriglyceridaemia, though many of these will have a type IV lipoprotein pattern. This has led to the hypothesis that most type V patients have a reasonably marked defect in the catabolism of TRLs combined with some additional factor that either further decreases catabolism or additionally increases the production of TRLs. Such factors include obesity, poor diabetic control, alcohol consumption, pregnancy, drugs (oral contraceptives, highly active antiretroviral therapy, β-blockers and thiazide diuretics being the main offenders), hypothyroidism, lipodystrophy and renal failure.

Clinical features

Acute pancreatitis, eruptive xanthomas, hepatosplenomegaly, lipaemia retinalis and all the other clinical features of type I hyperlipoproteinaemia may be present. Additionally, hyperuricaemia, glucose intolerance and hepatic steatosis are often seen.

Investigations

Patient samples will demonstrate some milkiness with the separation of a creamy layer (made up of chylomicrons) after standing or centrifugation, but the serum or plasma will be opaque representing the presence of VLDLs. Lipid levels in type V hyperlipoproteinaemia may be as markedly elevated as in type I.

Management

The treatment of type V hyperlipoproteinaemia is exactly as for type I, though fibrates are generally far more effective.

Type IV hyperlipoproteinaemia

Definition

In type IV hyperlipoproteinaemia, VLDLs accumulate but without any increase in chylomicrons.

Pathophysiology

Patients with type IV hyperlipoproteinaemia are heterogeneous and the common abnormality is an increased production of VLDLs by the liver, often accompanied by a partial defect in their catabolism. As with other forms of hypertriglyceridaemia, LDLs tend to be smaller and denser, and this pattern is associated with increased cardiovascular risk.

Clinical features

Apart from those rare type IV patients with marked hypertriglyceridaemia, the clinical features of type I and type V hyperlipoproteinaemia are not present.

Investigations

The degree of hypertriglyceridaemia is usually much less marked than in type I or type V hyperlipoproteinaemia, with many patients having fasting triglycerides of less than 6 mmol/L and most less than 10 mmol/L.

Management

Lifestyle modification along the lines of that advocated for severe hypertriglyceridaemia (see previous section in this chapter) is appropriate for type IV hyperlipoproteinaemia. However, dietary fat restriction does not have to be so marked and can be mainly restricted to saturated fats. The need for drug therapy will largely be guided by estimations of the 10-year CVD risk. Many type IV patients will require such treatment and the first line will often be statins because of their proven efficacy in reducing that risk, even though they do not usually affect hypertriglyceridaemia much.

OTHER PRIMARY DYSLIPIDAEMIAS

Cerebrotendinous xanthomatosis

Definition

Cerebrotendinous xanthomatosis is an autosomal recessive condition and is a rare cause of tendon xanthomas and xanthelasmas.

Epidemiology

Presentation occurs during childhood or early adult life.

Pathophysiology

This condition results from a defect in sterol-27-hydroxylase with consequent increased production of cholestanol and 7-hydroxycholesterol, which accumulate in the plasma and throughout the body.

Clinical features

Cutaneous features include tendon xanthoma and xanthelasma. The accumulation of cholestanol and 7-hydroxycholesterol in the central nervous system causes myelin destruction leading to intellectual disability, seizures, spasticity and ataxia. Peripheral neuropathy results from similar pathology in the peripheral nervous system. Early-onset cataracts, diarrhoea and premature osteoporosis are additional features. Patients have an increased risk of CVD.

Investigations

Plasma cholesterol levels are normal.

Management

Treatment with chenodeoxycholate reduces plasma cholestanol concentrations and improves the neurological manifestations of the disease.

Sitosterolaemia

Definition
Sitosterolaemia is a rare autosomal recessive cause of tendon and tuberous xanthomas.

Pathophysiology
Genetics
This condition results from mutations in the genes *ABCG5* or *ABCG8*, which encode the proteins sterolin-1 and sterolin-2 in enterocytes and hepatocytes. Sterolin-1 and sterolin-2 act together to form a lipid transporter that is thought to facilitate immediate excretion of any plant sterols absorbed across the small intestinal brush border. Defective function thereby allows a much greater absorption of plant sterols into the body, principally β-sitosterol but also sitostanol, campesterol and stigmasterol.

Clinical features
Patients with sitosterolaemia suffer from impaired growth, anaemia, thrombocytopenia and arthritis and are at risk of premature CVD. Cutaneous features include tendon and tuberous xanthomas.

Investigations
Diagnosis is made by measuring serum plant sterol concentrations.

Management
It has recently been shown that ezetimibe reduces plant sterol levels effectively in this condition, suggesting a role for the Niemann–Pick C1-like protein in plant sterol transport in the intestine.

SECONDARY DYSLIPIDAEMIAS

Dyslipidaemias are frequently secondary to or exacerbated by a range of other diseases or medications. The following account is far from exhaustive but will concentrate on those that may produce xanthomas or follow from the use of drugs used by dermatologists.

Secondary dyslipidaemia and diabetes

The commonest cause of secondary dyslipidaemia is likely to be diabetes (Chapter 62). People with type 1 diabetes frequently have quite high HDL cholesterol levels, but they also have a number of abnormalities of their LDLs and VLDLs and they are at high risk of CVD. People with type 2 diabetes have insulin resistance and their typical lipid profile includes relatively normal total and LDL cholesterol levels, but often increased triglyceride and reduced HDL cholesterol concentrations. These quantitative abnormalities are usually accompanied by qualitative changes in the LDLs with a preponderance of highly atherogenic, small, dense LDLs. As a result patients with type 2 diabetes are also at high risk of developing premature CVD.

It is now recommended that statins should be considered for all people with diabetes over the age of 40, and also in younger patients with other CVD risk factors including microalbuminuria. In some patients the development of type 2 diabetes, or worsening of its glycaemic control, can cause marked hypertriglyceridaemia (with type IV or V hyperlipoproteinaemia) with all its clinical features, including eruptive xanthomas, lipaemia retinalis and acute pancreatitis. This is most likely to occur on the background of some mild defect of triglyceride-rich lipoprotein clearance and may be further exacerbated in the concomitant presence of obesity and excess alcohol intake. Diabetes can also precipitate the development of type III hyperlipoproteinaemia in those with the appropriate genetic background (usually homozygosity for apoE2). Such patients may present to a dermatologist with the typical xanthomas of this condition. It follows that in any patient presenting with eruptive, tuberous or plane xanthomas, a fasting glucose and/or HbA1c should be requested along with the lipid profile and other appropriate tests.

Secondary dyslipidaemia and insulin resistance

Patients with insulin resistance but without type 2 diabetes have a similar combined dyslipidaemia. In some, a marked hypertriglyceridaemia can develop which is sufficient to cause eruptive xanthomas. This is seen quite commonly in the lipodystrophies, a group of disorders with either partial or generalised loss of subcutaneous fat. They can be inherited (e.g. Dunnigan–Köbberling syndrome) or acquired. The latter is now most commonly seen in patients with HIV/AIDS treated with protease inhibitors (Chapter 31), especially saquinavir and ritonavir. Management of lipodystrophy-associated dyslipidaemia is likely to require specialist input. The principles are lifestyle change, especially strict dietary fat restriction in hypertriglyceridaemia, optimisation of the drug regimen in HIV, and judicious, monitored use of lipid-modulating drug therapy, given the potential for significant interactions between statins, fibrates and the antiretroviral agents.

Secondary dyslipidaemia due to chronic cholestasis

It has already been noted that xanthelasmas can be a feature of chronic cholestasis. This can occur, for example, in primary biliary cirrhosis, and the presence of xanthelasmas should prompt a request for blood tests including bilirubin and alkaline phosphatase. Longstanding cholestasis is associated with hypercholesterolaemia due to the accumulation of an abnormal lipoprotein (lipoprotein X). It remains unclear whether this dyslipidaemia increases CVD risk but it can cause a wide range of xanthomas as well as xanthelasmas. Both the dyslipidaemia and the xanthomas improve with the relief of biliary obstruction but where this is not possible bile acid sequestrants can be helpful (and may also relieve the cholestasis-associated pruritus). Where necessary, statins must be used cautiously to avoid accumulation and toxicity. Hepatocellular liver disease leads to specific lipoprotein abnormalities, principally abnormal HDL secondary to progressive deficiency of lecithin-cholesterol acyl transferase with mild hypertriglyceridaemia, but these are not usually severe enough to cause xanthomas.

Secondary dyslipidaemia and the nephrotic syndrome

Nephrotic syndrome is complicated by hypercholesterolaemia or a combined dyslipidaemia that can prove difficult to treat. Hypertriglyceridaemia is not usually marked although occasionally a type IV hyperlipoproteinaemia may occur. Xanthomas are not a frequent feature and the dyslipidaemia resolves if the nephrotic syndrome responds to therapy. Chronic renal failure leads to hypertriglyceridaemia, often exacerbated by haemodialysis or peritoneal dialysis, and this can sometimes lead to eruptive xanthomas, especially if other risk factors are present. Lipoprotein(a) levels are elevated and may contribute to the increased CVD risk in this population but do not produce any dermatological signs.

Secondary dyslipidaemia due to drugs

Many drugs can produce dyslipidaemia, with alcohol perhaps being the commonest example and a frequent contributor to marked hypertriglyceridaemia. Prescription drugs used by dermatologists such as corticosteroids, ciclosporin and retinoic acid derivatives should be considered as causes.

Systemic corticosteroids increase total LDL and HDL cholesterol levels. Unless they precipitate diabetes in a susceptible individual they do not cause hypertriglyceridaemia.

Ciclosporin increases LDL cholesterol levels, sometimes quite significantly. It also inhibits cytochrome P450 3A4, the isoforms responsible for the metabolism of fluvastatin, simvastatin and atorvastatin, so patients taking these statins should be advised of the possible interaction and the risk of myalgia. In some patients (e.g. those with hepatic or renal impairment, or taking other drugs that affect CYP450 3A4), it may be appropriate to reduce the statin dose or change to an alternative such as pravastatin or rosuvastatin which are less dependent on CYP450 3A4.

Retinoic acid derivatives often induce hypertriglyceridaemia but this is usually mild and does not necessarily require anything other than dietary modification. Occasionally, however, marked hypertriglyceridaemia with a type IV or V hyperlipoproteinaemic pattern can be provoked, usually in a susceptible individual who may have had evidence of dyslipidaemia prior to treatment. It is therefore sensible to include a full lipid profile on any pre-treatment blood tests and to repeat this several weeks after starting any retinoids.

Key references

The full list of references can be found in the online version at https://www.wiley.com/rooksdermatology10e

Introduction
1 Durrington PN. *Hyperlipidaemia: Diagnosis and Management*, 3rd edn. London: Hodder Arnold, 2007.
2 Scriver CR, Beaudet AL, Sly WS, eds. *The Metabolic and Molecular Bases of Inherited Disease*, 8th edn. New York: McGraw Hill, 2001.

Classification of dyslipidaemias
1 Fredrickson DS, Levy RI, Lees RS. Fat transport in lipoproteins – an integrated approach to mechanisms and disorders. *N Engl J Med* 1967;276:34–42, 94–103, 148–56, 215–52, 273–81.

Xanthomas
Dyslipidaemic plane (planar) xanthoma
Xanthelasma
2 Christoffersen M, Frikke-Schmidt R, Schnohr P et al. Xanthelasmata, arcus corneae, and ischaemic vascular disease and death in general population: prospective cohort study. *BMJ* 2011;343:d5497.

Primary dyslipidaemias: hypercholesterolaemia
Familial hypercholesterolaemia
4 Goldstein JL, Brown MS. Familial hypercholesterolaemia: identification of a defect in the regulation of 3-hydroxy-3-methylglutaryl coenzyme A reductase activity associated with overproduction of cholesterol. *Proc Natl Acad Sci USA* 1973;70:2804–8.
9 Slack J. Risks of ischaemic heart disease in familial hyperlipoproteinaemia states. *Lancet* 1969;ii:1380–2.
16 Marais AD, Blom DJ. Recent advances in the treatment of homozygous familial hypercholesterolaemia. *Curr Opin Lipidol* 2013;24:288–94.

Primary dyslipidaemias: combined dyslipidaemia
Type III hyperlipoproteinaemia
3 Utermann G. Apolipoprotein E polymorphisms in health and disease. *Am Heart J* 1987;113:433–40.

CHAPTER 61

Nutritional Disorders Affecting the Skin

Albert C. Yan and Netravali Michelle Oboite

Children's Hospital of Philadelphia, Pennsylvania, USA

PART 5: METABOLIC & NUTRITIONAL DISORDERS

NUTRITION

Malnutrition

Definition and nomenclature

Malnutrition is defined as the imbalance between the intake of necessary nutrients and physiological needs. Sufficiently prolonged imbalances result in derangements of normal physiological processes.

Protein–energy malnutrition describes the group of conditions characterised by the imbalance between protein and carbohydrate intake and physiological needs leading to characteristic cutaneous and systemic changes. Two phenotypic forms are classically recognised: kwashiorkor and marasmus [1], although variants such as marasmic kwashiorkor have been described [2]. Patients affected by these forms of undernutrition can be identified on the basis of their delayed or decelerated growth parameters, clinical features and underlying aetiology.

Synonyms and inclusions

- Macronutrients: carbohydrates, fat, protein
- Malnutrition: the imbalance between nutrient intake and physiological needs
- Acute malnutrition: <3 months' duration
- Chronic malnutrition: ≥3 months' duration
- Undernutrition: deficient nutrient intake leading to physiological dysfunction
- Stunting: decreased height for age; since height deceleration is often a later indicator of undernutrition, this is often associated as a feature of chronic malnutrition
- Wasting: decreased weight for height; since weight for age is often an early indicator of undernutrition, this is often associated as a feature of acute malnutrition
- Kwashiorkor: a syndrome resulting from deficient protein intake despite sufficient caloric intake leading to wasting; oedema is a prominent feature; also known historically as protein–calorie malnutrition, malignant malnutrition and nutritional oedema syndrome
- Marasmus: a syndrome resulting from global nutrient deficiency leading to stunting; also known historically as athrepsia, baby consumption, decomposition, dietetic marasmus, essential marasmus, infantile atrophy
- Marasmic kwashiorkor: an overlap syndrome with features of both kwashiorkor and marasmus; classically, significant stunting with evidence of oedema

Rook's Textbook of Dermatology, Tenth Edition. Edited by Christopher Griffiths, Jonathan Barker, Tanya Bleiker, Walayat Hussain and Rosalind Simpson.
© 2024 John Wiley & Sons Ltd. Published 2024 by John Wiley & Sons Ltd.

Introduction and general description

Protein–energy malnutrition indicates a state of undernutrition that is caused by imbalances between the deficient intake of protein in relation to carbohydrate, fat and physiological needs.

Macronutrients refer to carbohydrates, fat and proteins, the three major components of our diet.

The classic phenotypic forms include kwashiorkor and marasmus. Kwashiorkor refers to the disease state that arises from the prolonged disproportionate intake of carbohydrate (energy or calories) in excess of other macronutrients, specifically protein. As a result of hypoproteinaemia, affected individuals manifest signs of growth retardation and most notably oedema.

Marasmus, by contrast, refers to the disease state resulting from globally decreased intake of all macronutrients, including carbohydrate, protein and fat. By definition, marasmus patients show growth retardation but do not demonstrate hypoproteinaemia or oedema.

The syndrome referred to as marasmic kwashiorkor describes a variant state in which those affected are not only significantly growth retarded (stunting) as in marasmus but also show evidence of hypoproteinaemia and oedema as in kwashiorkor.

Forms of severe malnutrition can be classified on the basis of specific growth parameters. These have included weight below median weight-for-age [3], ratio of mid-upper arm circumference to head circumference [4] or abnormally low z-scores (standard deviations) below standardised growth parameters such as weight-for-age, height-for-age or body mass index [5–7].

In this context, in 1999 the World Health Organization (WHO) defined paediatric malnutrition utilising z-scores, or numbers of standard deviations below the reference medians established by the US National Center for Health Statistics. A negative number would indicate the number of standard deviations below that median reference. For children 6–60 months of age, moderate malnutrition was defined as having a z-score for weight-for-height between –3 and –2 and severe malnutrition noted when the weight-for-height z-score was <–3 [8]. In 2005, having a mid–upper arm circumference of <115 mm was recommended as an additional screening measure of undernutrition [9].

Malnutrition can also be classified on the basis of the underlying aetiology. These classification schemes have been commonly used in characterising adults with undernutrition, and typically describe three broad categories: malnutrition due to decreased nutrient intake (starvation); malnutrition resulting from acute stress (infectious disease or trauma); and malnutrition secondary to chronic disease with associated end-organ dysfunction, malignancy or rheumatological disease. These last two forms describe disease states related to increased physiological needs outpacing what might otherwise be considered normal nutrient intake [10,11].

Assessing malnutrition in adults with chronic illnesses can be challenging at different states of disease. For example, in patients with liver disease, the presence of oedema and ascites makes traditional anthropometric measurements like body mass index less reliable, whereas tests measuring muscle mass and eliciting muscle function may more accurately reflect risk of malnutrition. Specifically, in one study involving patients with ascites, non-dominant handgrip strength has been found to be a more sensitive and specific predictor of malnutrition compared with body mass index, mid-arm muscle circumference and triceps skin-fold thickness [12].

Epidemiology

Incidence and prevalence

Over the past two decades, there has been a significant improvement in the worldwide burden and prevalence of undernutrition for children under 5 years of age. In 2000, 125 million children were underweight and 197 million were stunted. By 2012, the number of underweight children had decreased to 99 million [13], but as of 2020, the number of stunted children was 149 million [**14**]. These numbers are staggering and further improvements are clearly needed.

Hospitalised patients are at special risk of protein–energy malnutrition. While there has been some variability in the definition of malnutrition in published studies, the prevalence of protein–energy malnutrition among hospitalised children has varied widely and has been estimated at between 4.5% [15] and 34% [16], although there are figures suggesting the rate of children considered at risk for undernutrition to be as high as 62% [17]. Prevalence rates of malnutrition of 17–50% have been reported among hospitalised adults, depending on the population of patients studied [18–20]. The prevalence of protein–energy malnutrition or wasting syndrome among outpatient adult dialysis patients also falls into this range [21]. The prevalence of malnutrition generally tends to be greater among adults with increasing age [22]. In the Philippines, malnutrition among adult patients hospitalised with coronavirus disease (Covid-19) was as high as 71% and strongly associated with co-morbidities of advancing age, chronic kidney disease and pneumonia severity [**23**].

Age

Malnutrition is typically a disease seen among infants and younger children, and is conventionally evaluated in those under 5 years of age. However, protein–energy malnutrition has been well documented among adults, particularly those who are elderly, debilitated with chronic illness or hospitalised [24].

Sex

Sex differences in undernutrition are largely determined by regional and cultural differences. It has been hypothesised that scarce resources may be preferentially provided to male children than to female children resulting in a higher prevalence for undernourished girls, particularly among those with more severe malnutrition. While some studies have documented a greater prevalence of undernutrition among females in Bangladesh (for paediatric patients) [25], the Netherlands [26], Spain [27] and the UK (for geriatric patients) [28], a higher prevalence is noted among males in studies in western Maharashta (India) [29], Ecuadorian Highlands [30], Ethiopia [31] and Guinea-Bissau in West Africa [32]. No sex differences were noted in a study of hospitalised patients in Guangzhou, China [19]. Data are conflicting even within the same country regarding this issue.

Ethnicity

The role of ethnicity is confounded by socioeconomic factors. However, the majority of children with undernutrition live in Asia and Africa. Among those with stunting under the age of 5, 53% lived in

Asia and 41% in Africa. For those with wasting under the age of 5, 70% lived in Asia and 27% in Africa [14].

Associated diseases

Although protein–energy malnutrition is classified as a macronutrient deficiency disorder, it is often a manifestation of globally disordered nutrient intake. As a result, micronutrient deficiencies may also be present, including but not limited to zinc [33,34], selenium and copper [35], ascorbic acid [36], biotin [37,38], iron [39] and folate [40].

Pathophysiology

In kwashiorkor, excess carbohydrate without significant protein intake suppresses insulin production, resulting in the inhibition of protein synthesis [41,42]. Patients with this condition manifest clinically with signs of hypoproteinaemia, including oedema and fatty infiltration of the liver due to deficiencies in lipoproteins. Those chronically affected also demonstrate immune suppression due to decreased production of immune proteins such as immunoglobulins and are therefore at risk for opportunistic infections. Growth retardation is noted but typically falls between 60% and 80% of ideal body weight.

In marasmus, because global macronutrient intake is decreased, the catabolic state leads to fat breakdown and growth retardation which is typically <60% of ideal body weight [43].

Patients with chronic diseases may have physiological needs that exceed available nutritional intake.

Predisposing factors

In paediatric protein–energy malnutrition, factors such as political instability and war, natural disasters, residence in inhospitable environments and economically disenfranchised populations lead to suboptimal and imbalanced diets which may be largely deficient in protein and mostly reliant on carbohydrates such as corn, rice or beans.

Protein–energy malnutrition is significantly less common in industrialised nations. In this setting, this form of malnutrition has been identified in a number of prototypical situations. Altered nutrient intake can result from perceived (real or imagined) food allergies. Several cases of protein–energy malnutrition have been documented from parents switching from milk-based formulas or milk itself to rice beverages due to perceived dietary milk allergies [44–49]. Hypermetabolic (catabolic) states associated with inflammatory or infectious diseases can result in significantly increased physiological needs for protein leading to protein–energy malnutrition. This is exemplified by patients with chronic liver disease [50], AIDS [51] or those undergoing dialysis for chronic renal insufficiency who have what has been termed a 'protein–wasting syndrome' [52]. Decreased absorption of protein from gastrointestinal disorders such as inflammatory bowel disease [53], protein-losing enteropathies (seen in association with systemic lupus erythematosus) [54], cystic fibrosis [55] or following bariatric surgery [56]. Finally, decreased synthesis of protein due to an underlying metabolic disorder has also been suspected as a contributing factor to protein–energy malnutrition in single case reports of glutaric acidaemia [57] and Hartnup disease [58].

Chronic diseases affecting multiple organ systems, like systemic sclerosis, can be associated with both micronutrient deficiencies like selenium and vitamin C [59], as well as global undernutrition and malnutrition [59,60] due to decreased oral intake with microstomia and impaired protein absorption when bowel involvement results in end-organ dysfunction [61].

Pathology

Histologically, skin biopsies from those with protein–energy malnutrition show psoriasiform hyperplasia, hyperkeratosis and epidermal pigmentation; atrophy or rete flattening may be present. Focal dyskeratosis may be observed. If there is accompanying micronutrient deficiency, parakeratosis and epidermal pallor may also be present [62].

Causative organisms

Evidence from mouse models and one study in Malawi suggests that alterations in the gastrointestinal microbiome might also serve as a predisposing factor to protein–energy malnutrition [63]. Depletion of bifidobacteria, anaerobic bacteria found in gastrointestinal tract microbiota, has also been seen in conjunction with severe states of malnutrition [64].

Environmental factors

Environmental factors may contribute to protein–energy malnutrition by creating a lack of access to necessary nutrients. These may include political or economic instability, war, famine, chronic disease and natural disasters.

Clinical features
History

A history should be elicited to determine whether the malnutrition stems from global nutrient deprivation, imbalanced nutrient intake (i.e. carbohydrate intake in excess of available protein intake) or increased catabolism resulting in increased nutrient needs, as might be seen with infections (e.g. HIV disease, malaria, diarrhoeal illness) or underlying chronic disease (chronic renal or hepatic dysfunction). For children who are breastfeeding, an evaluation of maternal diet and breast milk production should be performed if other aetiologies are not apparent. Patients with protein–energy malnutrition are immune suppressed, so special attention should be paid to the possibility of co-morbid opportunistic infections.

Presentation

Children with protein–energy malnutrition show signs of failing to thrive. Their growth velocity is decreased, and weight and eventually length percentiles fall.

Those with marasmus tend to show loss of subcutaneous fat which may result in a wizened or prematurely aged appearance when the buccal fat pads are affected. The loss of perianal fat can result in rectal or anal prolapse. The abdomen may become distended due to hypotonia of the abdominal musculature. The skin is typically wrinkled, loose and dry (Figure 61.1). The hair and nails often grow slowly and may show brittleness. The hair often falls out easily and areas of alopecia may be evident. Lanugo hair may be observed on the face and neck.

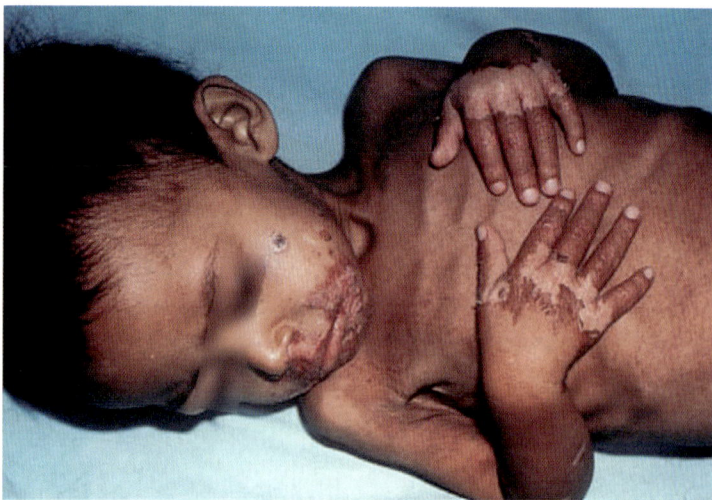

Figure 61.1 Marasmus. Note the loss of subcutaneous tissue, growth stunting, dyspigmentation and desquamative changes. Reproduced from [65] with permission from John Wiley & Sons.

In kwashiorkor, affected individuals may also exhibit loss of subcutaneous fat. Peripheral oedema is a consistent feature due to the associated hypoproteinaemia. Abdominal distention is a feature observed in children and has been attributed to hepatomegaly from increased fatty deposition due to lack of available apolipoproteins. The skin findings are highly characteristic and include a dermatosis (Figure 61.2) that has been likened to 'cracked skin', 'peeling paint', 'enamel paint', 'flaky paint' or 'crazy paving' due to the typical scale and irregular fissuring noted on examination (Figure 61.3). Over time, more defined plaques may arise that may be more concentrated in areas of friction such as the intertriginous areas. As with marasmus, the hair and nails grow slowly and may be brittle. The hair often develops a lustreless, red–brown colour that may show alternation with more normal colour; this so-called 'flag sign' corresponds to alternating periods of significant

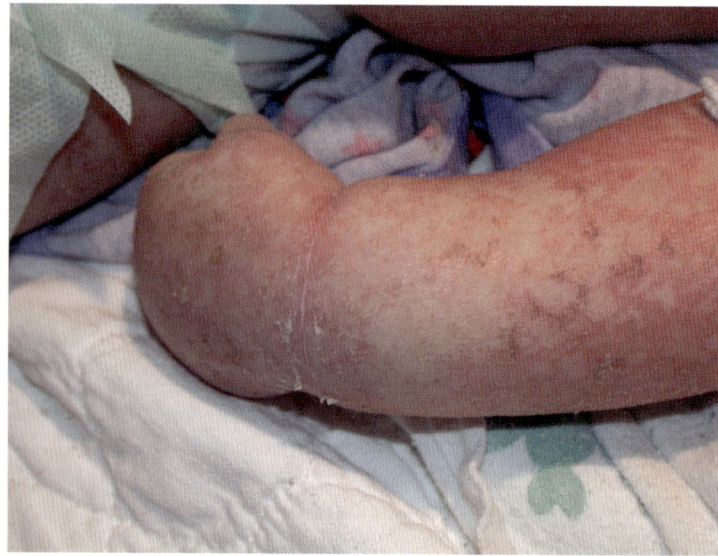

Figure 61.3 Kwashiorkor manifesting as peripheral oedema and a 'flaky paint' dermatitis.

undernutrition and improved nutrition (Figure 61.4). Inflammatory changes of the mucous membranes, such as xerophthalmia, cheilitis, stomatitis and vulvovaginitis, may arise in association with other co-morbid vitamin and mineral micronutrient deficiencies [66].

Those with marasmic kwashiorkor typically have oedema and demonstrate overlapping features of marasmus and kwashiorkor.

Clinical variants
- Marasmus
- Kwashiorkor
- Marasmic kwashiorkor

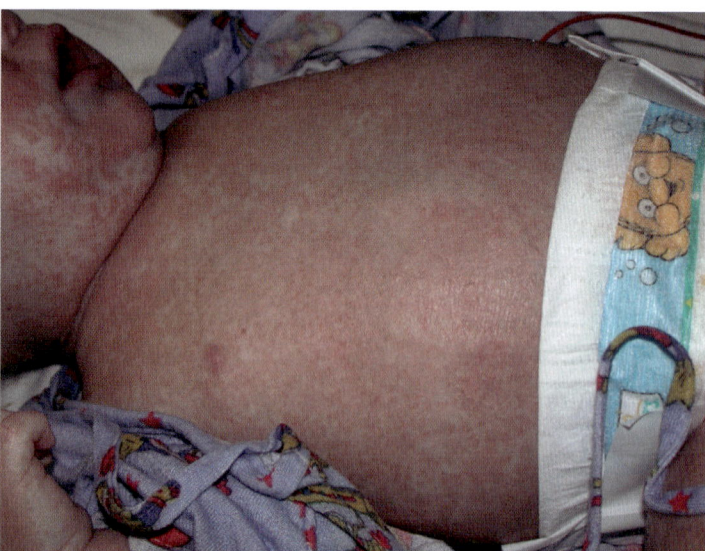

Figure 61.2 Erythrodermic findings in kwashiorkor. This patient was fed rice 'milk' as a primary food source due to parental concerns over presumed food allergies.

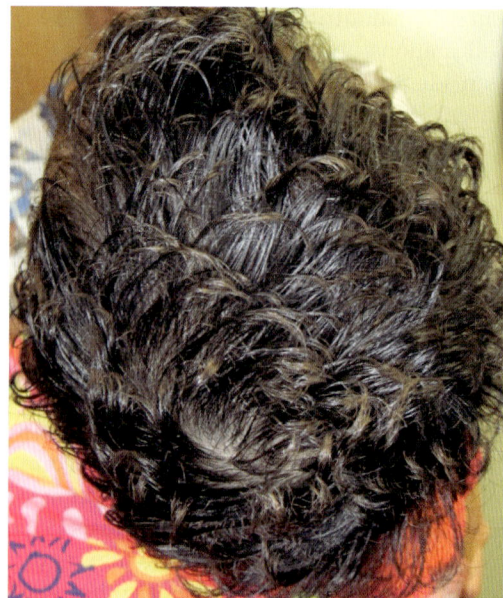

Figure 61.4 Flag sign. The reddening of the hair is associated with periods of protein–energy malnutrition. Note the reddening at the tips of the hair.

Differential diagnosis

There are several important considerations in the differential diagnosis of protein–energy malnutrition (Table 61.1). The diagnosis of protein–energy malnutrition may be challenging, so it is important to maintain an index of suspicion when evaluating patients with rash and oedema. The skin findings are often initially mistaken for atopic eczema, seborrhoeic dermatitis or even contact dermatitis. It is important to note that some patients may have a pre-existing history of atopic eczema prompting the installation of restrictive diets that may result in a superimposed protein–energy malnutrition dermatosis. Heavy metal toxicities related to mercury or selenium can present with erythroderma and oedema. Other nutritional deficiencies may resemble protein–energy malnutrition or may present as co-morbid skin conditions, particularly acrodermatitis enteropathica or acquired zinc deficiency and pellagra.

Classification of severity

Paediatric. The WHO has defined severe acute malnutrition in children below the age of 5 as a weight-for-height z-score of <–3.

Additionally, a mid–upper arm circumference <115 cm (in children 6–60 months) can serve as an independent criterion [67].

For moderate malnutrition, the WHO uses a weight-for-age z-score between –3 and –2, and z-score between –2 and –1 as mild malnutrition. Wasting (weight-for-height) and stunting (height-for-age) are defined as being between 3 and 2 standard deviations below their respective median reference values [67] (Table 61.2).

Table 61.2 Assessing the severity of paediatric malnutrition.

Classification	Z-score values	Weight-for-height (%)	Height-for-age (%)	Weight-for-age (%)
Adequate	–2 < z-score <+2	90–120	95–110	
Mild malnutrition		80–89	90–94	
Moderate malnutrition	–3 < z-score <–2	70–79	85–89	60–80
Severe malnutrition	z-score <–3	<70	<85	<60

Adapted from [67].

Table 61.1 Skin signs of nutritional disease.

Type of skin change	Associated nutritional disorder	Selected differential diagnosis
Skin texture changes		
Erythroderma (exfoliative)	Protein–energy malnutrition (kwashiorkor); essential fatty acid deficiency	Primary skin diseases (atopic eczema, psoriasis, congenital ichthyosis, pityriasis rubra pilaris); drug eruption; malignancy (cutaneous T-cell lymphoma); infection (staphylococcal scalded skin, toxic shock syndrome); immune deficiency syndrome (Omenn)
Phrynoderma	Deficiencies of vitamin A, B-complex, C, E, and essential fatty acids	Keratosis pilaris
Skin colour changes		
Petechiae, purpura	Deficiencies of vitamin A, K Excess intake of vitamin E	Various causes of consumptive coagulopathy (severe infection, malignancy, tissue injury, liver disease, toxic exposures, obstetric complications, vascular tumours, rheumatological disorders), coagulation disorders, thrombocytopenia, vascular fragility syndromes (Ehlers–Danlos syndrome)
Yellow-orange skin changes	Carotenaemia	Jaundice
Darkening of skin (diffuse or macular hyperpigmentation)	Deficiencies of folate or vitamin B_{12}	Addison disease
Photodistributed dermatitis	Pellagra and related disorders (carcinoid syndrome, Hartnup disease); pyridoxine deficiency	Connective tissue disease (systemic lupus erythematosus, dermatomyositis), polymorphous light eruption, solar urticaria; defective DNA-repair syndromes (such as xeroderma pigmentosum)
Seborrhoeic dermatitis-like changes	Deficiencies of B-complex vitamins (riboflavin, pyridoxine, biotin)	Seborrhoeic dermatitis, sebopsoriasis, psoriasis
Mucous membrane changes		
Angular stomatitis	B-complex vitamin deficiencies (riboflavin, pyridoxine)	Angular cheilitis associated with candidal overgrowth
Cheilitis/cheilosis	B-complex vitamin deficiencies (riboflavin, pyridoxine, niacin, B12)	Lip-licking dermatitis
Glossitis	Deficiencies of iron and B-complex vitamins (riboflavin, niacin, pyridoxine, biotin, B12)	Sjögren syndrome; oral contact dermatitis; oral candidiasis; oral lichen planus; syphilis; aphthosis
Napkin dermatitis	Zinc deficiency; B-complex vitamin deficiencies (riboflavin, pyridoxine, biotin)	Napkin dermatitis (irritant, allergic, monilial); seborrhoeic dermatitis; inverse psoriasis; Langerhans cell histiocytosis
Adnexal changes		
Lightening of hair colour	Protein–energy malnutrition; deficiencies of B-complex vitamins (folate, B12); copper deficiency	Poliosis, vitiligo
Corkscrew hairs	Deficiencies of vitamin A and C	
Nail changes	Beau lines: kwashiorkor Koilonychia: iron deficiency Half-and-half: pellagra	Beau lines: severe illness Koilonychia: chronic diabetes Half-and-half: renal disease; psoriasis

Reproduced from [66] with permission from Elsevier.

Table 61.3 Classification of severity of protein–energy malnutrition.

	Paediatric	Adult
Source	World Health Organization	Centers for Disease Control and World Food Programme
Age Definitions	Children 6–60 months of age	Adults
Mild		BMI 17–18.5
Moderate	Weight-for-age z-score between –2 and –3	BMI 16–17
Severe	Weight-for-height z-score <–3 or mid–upper arm circumference <115 cm	BMI <16

Adult. There are a variety of guidelines for assessing the severity of malnutrition in the adult population. These have been based in part on composite scores that include body mass index, dietary intake, unplanned weight loss, serum albumin levels and presence of underlying disease states.

The United States Centers for Disease Control in conjunction with the World Food Programme defines adult malnutrition on the basis of body mass index (Table 61.3). Mild malnutrition is defined as having a body mass index between 17 and 18.5; moderate malnutrition is defined as having a body mass index between 16 and 17; and severe malnutrition is defined as having a body mass index <16 [67].

The Malnutrition Universal Screening Tool (MUST) developed by the Malnutrition Advisory Group of the British Association for Parenteral and Enteral Nutrition is another assessment tool for adults that includes a five-step evaluation process [68]. This tool assigns values to body mass index, degree of unplanned % weight loss during the previous 3–6 months, whether acute illness is present, and whether the lack of nutritional intake is anticipated for more than 5 days. Those with a body mass index between 18.5 and 20 (kg/m^2) are given 1 point, while those with a body mass index <18.5 are given 2 points. If body mass index measurements are difficult due to illness acuity, mid–upper arm circumference can be measured; if the mid–upper arm circumference is <23.5 cm, the body mass index is likely to be <20. Those with unplanned weight loss between 5% and 10% are given 1 point, while those having >10% are given 2 points. If acute illness is present and it is anticipated that there will be or has been no nutritional intake for >5 days, 2 additional points are awarded. Those with a score of 0 are rated at low risk, those with 1 are rated as medium risk, and a score of 2 or greater is a high-risk classification. Monitoring and nutritional interventions vary depending on the degree of risk assessed.

Complications and co-morbidities

Complications of protein–energy malnutrition may arise as a result of treating the disease, or as sequelae of the disease.

Refeeding syndrome is a potentially fatal phenomenon that can arise when a malnourished patient is given nutrients enterally or parenterally after a period of prolonged deprivation. Adaptations during fasting occur in order to prevent protein and muscle catabolism in the malnourished individual. Refeeding provides a glycaemic load that then initiates production of glycogen, fat and protein, requiring vitamin co-factors and electrolytes such as phosphorus and magnesium which can be rapidly depleted during the refeeding process. During this phenomenon, acute electrolyte disturbances can occur leading to hypophosphataemia, hypomagnesaemia and hypokalaemia (the latter induced by the increase in insulin production during refeeding). This can be prevented by a process of slow and graduated refeeding limited to no greater than 50% of the calculated energy requirements, and then gradually increased over a period of up to 4–7 days if refeeding is tolerated [69].

Long-term follow-up of patients with a history of malnutrition has identified a number of associated morbidities including dental caries [70], periodontal disease [71], tooth loss particularly with associated malnutrition in renal disease [72], increased infection risk due to secondary immunosuppression and decreased skin, respiratory and gastrointestinal mucosal barrier integrity [73], personality and mood disturbances [74,75], attention deficit disorder [76], neurodevelopmental abnormalities including cerebellar development and motor coordination [77] and externalising behaviours [78].

Disease course and prognosis

Left untreated, malnourished children have a significantly increased mortality risk. When the weight-for-height is more than 3 standard deviations below the median reference value (severe malnutrition), the risk of death is ninefold greater than those with a weight-for-height above –1 standard deviation. Malnourished children with uncomplicated cases of protein–energy malnutrition have a greater than 88% recovery rate and less than 4% case fatality rate when treated appropriately, while those with underlying co-morbid disease states such as HIV disease have a significantly greater case fatality rate, particularly during the first 4 days of treatment initiation [67].

Among adult haemodialysis patients, the risk of mortality increases with the degree of malnutrition, with those having severe malnutrition showing a statistically significant 1.33 increased relative risk for mortality [79].

Investigations

During the management of the malnourished patient, the following is recommended:

- Monitoring of vital signs.
- Full blood count, to help evaluate for infection and assess the degree of iron deficiency.
- Comprehensive metabolic panel (e.g. electrolytes, renal function, liver function including total protein and albumin), in addition to sodium, potassium, chloride and bicarbonate, calcium, phosphorus and magnesium should be monitored closely.
- Infectious disease evaluation, which may include a blood smear for malaria organisms, blood culture, urine culture, stool for ova and parasites, chest X-ray and testing for tuberculosis and HIV disease.

Management

The goals of management are to replete nutrients and regain homeostasis. Chronic malnutrition creates adaptive metabolic and hormonal mechanisms that result in decreased protein and muscle catabolism. Treatment involves gradual replenishment of nutrients to prevent refeeding syndrome and associated electrolyte and micronutrient depletion, as well as management of coexisting micronutrient deficiencies, immune suppression and co-morbid infections.

The CDC [67] recommends inpatient care for children with evidence of severe oedema and malnutrition, as well as those with mild to moderate oedema and no appetite, or those with associated medical complications. Those without complications and who have an appetite should be managed in the outpatient setting.

The use of antibiotics is recommended for children with moderate to severe malnutrition. Treatment should be directed at identified infections; otherwise, empirical therapy with amoxicillin should be given. Those with mild undernutrition without evidence of an infection should not receive routine antibiotic therapy.

Patients identified as having malnutrition will benefit from a multidisciplinary approach to management, with input provided by the hospital medicine team or critical care specialists, nutrition and infectious disease. Dermatologists often play a role in establishing the diagnosis of protein–energy malnutrition and may help identify associated micronutrient deficiencies such as zinc deficiency.

Resources

Further information

Centers for Disease Control and the World Food Programme. *A Manual: Measuring and Interpreting Malnutrition and Mortality*, 2005. http://www.unhcr.org/45f6abc92.pdf.
World Health Organization. *Guideline: Update on the Management of Acute Malnutrition in Infants and Children*, 2013. http://apps.who.int/iris/bitstream/10665/95584/1/9789241506328_eng.pdf.

Patient resources

American Society for Parenteral and Enteral Nutrition (ASPEN). *Disease-Related Malnutrition and Enteral Nutrition*. http://www.nutritioncare.org/about-aspen/
British Association of Parenteral and Enteral Nutrition (BAPEN). *Introduction to Malnutrition*. http://www.bapen.org.uk/about-malnutrition/introduction-to-malnutrition.
United Nations World Food Programme. *Zero Hunger*. https://www.wfp.org/zero-hunger.
World Health Organization. *Malnutrition*. https://www.who.int/health-topics/malnutrition.
(All last accessed October 2022)

VITAMINS

Vitamin A

Vitamin A is a fat-soluble vitamin that plays a crucial role in keratinisation, epithelial proliferation, vision and development. It is primarily derived from precursors found in dietary plant and animal sources, where it exists as β-carotene and retinyl esters, respectively. Rich sources of vitamin A include dark green leafy vegetables, brightly coloured fruits (e.g. tomato, mango, apricot), egg yolk, animal liver, fish, red palm oil and fortified milk. Dietary carotenes and retinyl esters are converted to retinol, absorbed in the small intestine, then transported via chylomicrons to the liver where they are either stored as retinyl esters, or exported as retinol bound to retinol-binding protein to various tissue sites. Important active metabolites of vitamin A include retinal which functions in rhodopsin generation, and retinoic acid which modulates cell differentiation [1].

Vitamin A deficiency

Definition and nomenclature

A deficiency in vitamin A may result in various ocular complications including blindness, as well as mucocutaneous disease.

Synonyms and inclusions
• Vitamin A: retinol

Epidemiology
Incidence and prevalence

In 2009, the WHO estimated globally that 5.2 million preschool-aged children were affected with night blindness, and that low serum retinol concentrations (<0.70 µmol/L) affected 190 million preschool-aged children. Vitamin A deficiency is considered the most common preventable cause of blindness in children [2]. In addition to children, pregnant and lactating women in low-income countries are also at risk, with 10–20% of pregnant women in developing countries [3] and up to 19 million pregnant women worldwide affected by vitamin A deficiency [4]. Rates of vitamin A deficiency are most prevalent in sub-Saharan Africa and South-East Asia [5].

Age

Vitamin A deficiency can present in all age groups, although children in developing countries appear to be at greatest risk.

Sex

There is no sex predilection for vitamin A deficiency.

Ethnicity

There is no ethnic predilection for vitamin A deficiency.

Associated diseases

Deficiencies in other fat-soluble vitamins (D, E and K) can occur in the setting of fat malabsorption.

Pathophysiology
Predisposing factors

The principal causes of vitamin A deficiency include inadequate dietary intake or malnutrition, fat malabsorption, chronic intestinal inflammation and liver disease. Poor dietary intake can be observed in the setting of eating disorders, restrictive diets (e.g. vegan diet [6]), individuals with autism [7]), chronic illness and poverty. Malabsorption of fat and fat-soluble vitamins can occur secondary to coeliac disease, cystic fibrosis [8], gastric bypass surgery [9], pancreatic insufficiency and biliary duct disease. Chronic intestinal inflammation and diarrhoea associated with inflammatory bowel disease or chronic parasitic infections [10] may result in poor absorption of vitamin A. Finally, liver disease including cirrhosis [11] may lead to defective hepatic storage of vitamin A and subsequent deficiency.

Clinical features

History

The earliest sign of vitamin A deficiency is defective dark vision adaptation and night blindness (nyctalopia), followed by xerophthalmia. Aberrant keratinisation in the oral and nasal mucosa may result in hyposmia (reduced sense of smell) and hypogeusia (reduced taste). Patients also often complain of generalised xerosis.

Presentation

Ocular complications range from night blindness, corneal xerosis and Bitot spots (white keratinised lesions) to corneal ulceration, keratomalacia, corneal perforation, iris prolapse and blindness.

Cutaneous findings include xerosis and scaling, dermomalacia (deep skin fissuring) and phrynoderma (described as 'toad-like appearance'). Phrynoderma is characterised by keratotic follicular papules involving the anterolateral thighs and posterolateral upper arms, and can spread to the extensor extremities, shoulders, posterior neck, back, buttocks and abdomen (Figure 61.5).

Differential diagnosis

Phrynoderma is not specific to vitamin A deficiency and has been described in association with deficiencies in B-complex vitamins, vitamin C, vitamin E and essential fatty acids [12]. More recently, zinc deficiency has also been linked to phrynoderma [13].

Complications and co-morbidities

The most significant complication of severe vitamin A deficiency is blindness.

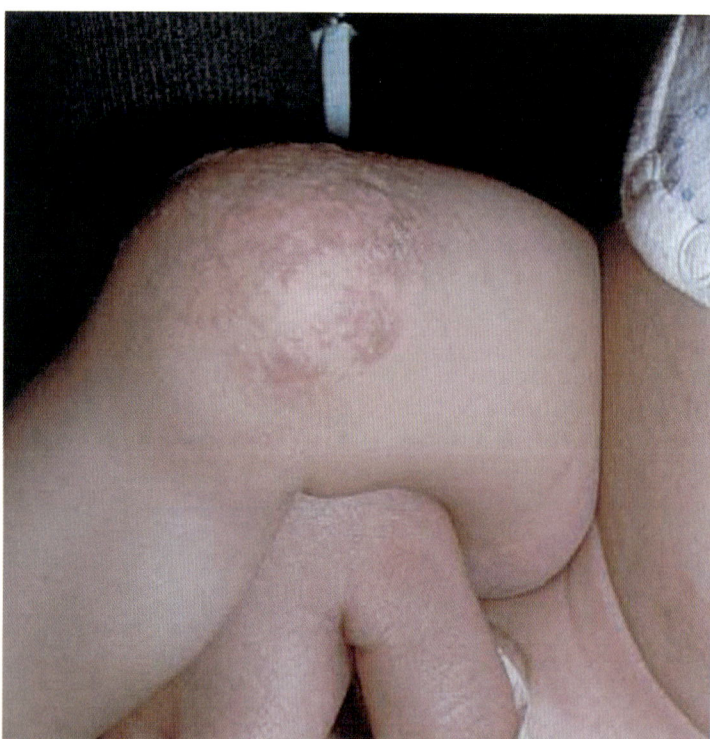

Figure 61.5 Phrynoderma. Reproduced from [12] with permission from John Wiley & Sons.

Disease course and prognosis

Prognosis is generally good but depends on the severity of deficiency and clinical findings. Severe ocular complications are typically irreversible.

Investigations

Diagnosis is confirmed by measurement of serum retinol levels. Normal serum levels range from 20 to 50 µg/dL. One study suggested that testing for the hydrolysis of retinyl glucuronide to retinoic acid could be useful in determining marginal vitamin A deficiency [14].

Management

The recommended daily intake of vitamin A is 1000–5000 IU. Treatment is with 50 000–200 000 IU of daily vitamin A supplementation until clinical signs/symptoms resolve and serum retinol levels normalise. The dose is dependent on age and the treatment period varies with clinical severity [15].

Public health efforts to prevent and treat vitamin A deficiency have included fortifying common food items (such as adding vitamin A in the form of retinyl palmitate to sugar in Guatemala [16]) or agriculture-integrated programmes that invest in harvesting foods rich in β-carotene (such as the orange-fleshed sweet potato in sub-Saharan Africa [17]).

Vitamin A excess

Definition and nomenclature

Excessive intake of vitamin A can lead to acute or chronic vitamin A toxicity and overconsumption of carotenes can manifest with carotenaemia/carotenoderma.

Synonyms and inclusions

• Vitamin A: retinol
• Vitamin A excess: hypervitaminosis A, vitamin A toxicity, carotenaemia, carotenoderma

---

Epidemiology

Age

Vitamin A excess can occur at any age.

Sex

There is no sex predilection for vitamin A excess.

Ethnicity

There is no ethnic predilection for vitamin A excess.

Associated diseases

Studies have suggested that chronic β-carotene supplementation (20–30 mg/day) may be associated with an increased risk of lung and gastric cancer [18,19], as well as an increased risk of aggressive prostate cancer [20] although longer-term follow-up of this supplemented population found no mortality differences between those supplemented and those not [21].

Pathophysiology

Predisposing factors

Vitamin A excess can present as two forms: vitamin A toxicity and carotenaemia.

Vitamin A toxicity can occur as a consequence of an acute overdose over the course of hours to days, or chronic excessive intake over months to years. In general, hypervitaminosis A results from overconsumption of non-prescription nutritional supplements, prescription medications containing vitamin A derivatives [22] and foods high in vitamin A. Ingestion of greater than 20 times the recommended daily allowance (RDA) of vitamin A in a child or greater than 100 times the RDA in an adult may lead to toxicity [23].

Carotenaemia is a benign disorder caused by excessive β-carotene intake. Up to one-third of carotene bypasses conversion to retinol and is directly absorbed in the small intestine. Increased absorption of carotene can be seen in the setting of hypothyroidism, pancreatic lipase and bile acid deficiencies, and with processing of foods (e.g. mashing, pureeing) [24]. Conversely, dietary fibre decreases absorption of carotenes. Individuals with hyperlipidaemia may develop carotenaemia due to a direct relationship and correlation between β-lipoprotein and β-carotene levels. Furthermore, patients with liver disease are predisposed to carotenaemia as a result of impaired conversion of β-carotene to vitamin A. Excessive ingestion of carotenes does not lead to vitamin A toxicity given the slow conversion of carotene to vitamin A in the intestinal mucosa [25].

Clinical features

History

Acute vitamin A toxicity manifests with headaches, vision changes, fatigue, anorexia, nausea, vomiting, myalgias and arthralgias. Weight loss can be observed with chronic intoxication.

In carotenaemia, individuals present with yellow discoloration of the skin.

Presentation

Clinically, individuals with chronic hypervitaminosis A have dry and scaly skin, desquamation, cheilitis, alopecia, follicular hyperkeratosis and hyperpigmentation [26,27]. Associated liver toxicity, pseudotumor cerebri and skeletal changes (premature closure of the epiphyses and pathological bone fractures) may occur [28].

In carotenaemia, carotenes are excreted from sebaceous glands and sweat glands, and ultimately deposit in the stratum corneum. This results in carotenoderma, characterised by prominent yellow-orange pigmentation of the face, palms and soles of the feet (Figure 61.6).

Clinical variants

- Hypervitaminosis A.
- Carotenaemia.

Differential diagnosis

In carotenaemia, carotenoderma can mimic jaundice and medication-induced pigmentation. Unlike jaundice, carotenoderma spares the conjunctiva and other mucous membranes.

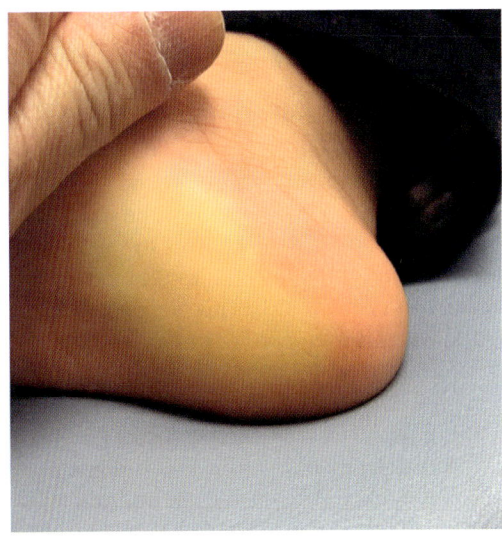

Figure 61.6 Carotenoderma. Note the yellow colour on diascopy of the plantar foot.

Complications and co-morbidities

- Vitamin A toxicity: long-term toxicity can lead to cirrhosis of the liver.
- Carotenaemia: there are no known long-term complications associated with carotenoderma.

Disease course and prognosis

- Vitamin A toxicity: discontinuation of vitamin A leads to resolution of almost all symptoms of vitamin A toxicity, with the exception of cirrhosis and sequelae related to pseudotumor cerebri.
- Carotenaemia: excellent prognosis with no clear long-term adverse effects. Pigmentary changes resolve within weeks to months of decreasing β-carotene intake.

Investigations

- Vitamin A toxicity: measurement of serum vitamin A level will confirm the diagnosis. Associated elevation in calcium and alkaline phosphatase may be observed.
- Carotenaemia: elevated serum carotene level >250 μg/dL.

Management

The recommended daily intake of vitamin A is 1000–5000 IU. Treatment is discontinuation of excess vitamin A and β-carotene intake.

Vitamin D

Vitamin D deficiency

Definition and nomenclature

Vitamin D is a fat-soluble vitamin and hormone essential in the regulation of calcium and phosphorus metabolism.

Synonyms and inclusions
- Vitamin D: calcitriol
- Vitamin D deficiency: hereditary vitamin D-dependent rickets type I and II

Introduction and general description

Vitamin D stimulates intestinal absorption of dietary calcium, activates bone resorption and mobilisation of calcium and phosphorus, and increases renal tubular reabsorption of calcium and phosphate. It is derived from dietary sources (ergocalciferol, vitamin D2), such as fish, fish oils, fortified milk, egg, liver and shiitake mushrooms, as well as endogenous synthesis from the skin (cholecalciferol, vitamin D3). Upon exposure to UV light in the 290–320 nm range, photoisomerisation of 7-dehydrocholesterol occurs in the epidermis, producing previtamin D3. This subsequently undergoes a spontaneous temperature-dependent isomerisation to cholecalciferol. Both vitamin D2 and D3 are hydroxylated in the liver to form 25-hydroxyvitamin D (calcidiol), which then circulates to the kidneys where it is converted to the active form, 1,25-hydroxyvitamin D (calcitriol). A deficiency of vitamin D is defined by most experts as a 25-hydroxyvitamin D level of <20 ng/mL, while a relative insufficiency of vitamin D lies between 21 and 29 ng/mL [29]. Vitamin D deficiency classically results in skeletal abnormalities, as seen in vitamin D-deficient rickets. Of note, there are also two hereditary forms of vitamin D-dependent rickets. The following discussion will focus primarily on acquired vitamin D deficiency.

Epidemiology

Incidence and prevalence

Based on the previous definitions and parameters for vitamin D deficiency, it is estimated that 1 billion people worldwide have vitamin D deficiency or insufficiency. Between 40% and 100% of US and European elderly men and women, not living in nursing homes, are deficient in vitamin D [29]. Geographic latitude may influence the incidence of vitamin D deficiency.

Age

Vitamin D deficiency can affect all ages, although newborns and institutionalised elderly may be at higher risk.

Sex

In the setting of certain cultural or religious practices, women may experience less sun exposure, thus predisposing them to higher rates of vitamin D deficiency.

Ethnicity

Darker-skinned individuals have less cutaneous vitamin D synthesis compared with lighter-skinned individuals with equivalent UV exposure.

Associated diseases

Recent studies suggest that vitamin D sufficiency may be protective against musculoskeletal disease, infection, autoimmune disease, cardiovascular disease, diabetes, neurocognitive dysfunction, various common cancers, infertility and adverse pregnancy/birth outcomes [30,31].

There have been data to suggest an association between low vitamin D levels and coronavirus disease 2019 (Covid-19) infection, severity and morbidity [32], particularly in individuals with profound vitamin D deficiency. Specifically, low serum 25(OH) vitamin D levels were associated with increased pneumonia severity [33], need for invasive mechanical ventilation and death [34].

Nevertheless, the exact protective role of vitamin D in Covid-19 infection still remains to be fully elucidated. It is postulated that vitamin D may regulate the pro-inflammatory cytokine cascade. However, at present, no clear guidelines have been established on supplementation in different populations.

Additionally, vitamin D deficiency has been associated with various congenital ichthyoses [35–39]. It has also been described in the setting of various photosensitivity disorders, including xeroderma pigmentosum and porphyria [40,41].

Pathophysiology

Predisposing factors

Vitamin D deficiency is commonly caused by decreased vitamin D synthesis, malabsorption and poor dietary intake. Decreased endogenous vitamin D synthesis occurs in individuals with increased melanin pigment and/or decreased sun exposure. In some cultures, shielding of the skin with clothing is mandated and therefore prevents adequate UV light exposure. The use of sunscreen can theoretically reduce vitamin D synthesis; however, studies have demonstrated that real-life application of sunscreens does not result in significant vitamin D deficiency [42]. Fat malabsorption states including coeliac disease, cystic fibrosis, pancreatic disease, biliary disease [43] and gastric bypass surgery [44] may predispose individuals to vitamin D deficiency. Liver disease, renal disease and anticonvulsants can also interfere with vitamin D metabolism. Inadequate dietary intake of vitamin D is observed in exclusively breastfed infants [45], preterm infants (due to lower stores and higher demand) and the elderly or disabled.

Genetics

There are two inherited autosomal recessive forms of vitamin D-dependent rickets. Type I involves a defect in vitamin D 1α-hydroxylase of the kidneys, while type II is associated with defects in the vitamin D receptor, resulting in end-organ resistance to physiological amounts of 1,25-hydroxyvitamin D.

Clinical features

History

Patients often present with fractures or dental defects, such as delayed tooth eruption and caries. Acute hypocalcaemia, particularly in infants, can manifest with seizures and tetany. Adolescents may complain of carpopedal spasm and limb pain.

Presentation

Vitamin D deficiency leads to hypocalcaemia, and consequently stimulation of parathyroid hormone secretion and release of calcium from bone. Resultant poor mineralisation of bone accounts for the various skeletal defects, including fraying and widening of the metaphysis, prominent costochondral joints (rachitic rosary), craniotabes, bowing of the lower extremities, frontal bossing, scoliosis and fractures. Dental anomalies and poor enamel may be noted.

The only cutaneous manifestation of acquired vitamin D deficiency is alopecia. Individuals with type II vitamin D-dependent rickets have a clinical phenotype similar to those with generalised atrichia. Although both are born with hair, generalised alopecia with preservation of the eyebrows and eyelashes is observed within a few months. Additionally, small papules and cysts commonly arise on the face and scalp [46,47].

Differential diagnosis
Osteomalacia, osteopenia and/or osteoporosis can be associated with hormonal imbalances, including hyperparathyroidism. Frequent fractures should raise concern for non-accidental trauma.

Complications and co-morbidities
Vitamin D deficiency may result in osteopenia or osteoporosis and their associated co-morbidities.

Disease course and prognosis
Studies suggest that vitamin D-deficient individuals have an increased rate of all-cause mortality compared with those who are vitamin D replete [48]. There are some data to suggest that vitamin D deficiency is also associated with poorer survival in patients with malignant melanoma, although clinical trials are needed to determine if vitamin D supplementation would be beneficial [49].

Investigations
Laboratory abnormalities include low serum 25-hydroxyvitamin D, hypocalcaemia, hypophosphataemia, increased alkaline phosphatase and increased parathyroid hormone.

Management
The recommended daily intake of vitamin D is 200–600 IU, depending on age. Most experts agree that individuals without adequate sun exposure require 800–1000 IU daily.

For patients older than 1 year of age, supplementation with 50 000 IU of vitamin D2 weekly for 8 weeks is a cost-effective method of correcting vitamin D deficiency. Alternatively, taking 1000 IU of vitamin D3 or 3000 IU of vitamin D2 daily may also be effective [29].

For patients under 1 year of age, 1000–5000 IU of vitamin D2 should be given daily until radiological abnormalities normalise. All breastfed infants should be supplemented with 400 IU of vitamin D daily as prophylaxis [50].

Sun exposure and UV light therapy may be useful in correcting vitamin D deficiency [51,52]. D-α-tocopheryl polyethylene glycol-1000 succinate, a vitamin E compound, has been successfully used to treat hepatic rickets [53].

Vitamin E

Vitamin E is a fat-soluble vitamin and potent antioxidant. It is widely available and commonly found in vegetable oils, leafy green vegetables, fortified cereals, nuts and seeds. Natural vitamin E is composed of four tocopherols (α, β, γ, δ) and four tocotrienols (α, β, γ, δ). The most studied is α-tocopherol [54].

Vitamin E deficiency

Definition and nomenclature
Vitamin E deficiency primarily leads to neurological sequelae. Ataxia with vitamin E deficiency (AVED) is a rare inherited disorder caused by mutations in the α-tocopherol transfer protein.

Epidemiology
Incidence and prevalence
Vitamin E deficiency is rarely encountered.

Population restricted studies have shown that the prevalence of AVED is approximately 1 : 1 800 000 in the Alsace region of France, and 3.5 : 1 000 000 in the Padua province of Italy [55,56]. In the USA, less than 0.1% of adults over the age of 20 were found to have vitamin E deficiency [57], despite estimations that >90% of Americans do not consume sufficient dietary vitamin E [58].

Age
Acquired vitamin E deficiency has no age predilection. AVED manifests during late childhood or early teens.

Sex
There is no sex predilection for acquired vitamin E deficiency.

Ethnicity
There is no ethnic predilection for acquired vitamin E deficiency.

Associated diseases
Vitamin E deficiency can be associated with deficiencies in other fat-soluble vitamins.

Pathophysiology
Predisposing factors
Acquired vitamin E deficiency most frequently develops as a result of fat malabsorption. Cystic fibrosis, cholestatic liver disease, short bowel syndrome and abetalipoproteinaemia are examples of disorders with impaired fat absorption.

Genetics
AVED is an autosomal recessively inherited disorder characterised by a defect in the α-tocopherol transfer protein. Consequently, α-tocopherol cannot be incorporated into circulating lipoproteins that distribute the vitamin to non-hepatic tissues, making them vulnerable to oxidative stress [59].

Clinical features
History
Patients with vitamin E deficiency may complain of weakness and blurred vision.

Presentation
Both acquired vitamin E deficiency and AVED can present with devastating neurological manifestations including hyporeflexia, ataxia, weakness, decreased proprioception and vibratory sense, decreased visual acuity, and ultimately dementia, cardiac arrhythmias and blindness [60]. There are no cutaneous manifestations of vitamin E deficiency.

Complications and co-morbidities

Severe vitamin E deficiency can result in significant neurological deficits including blindness.

Disease course and prognosis

Prognosis is good if recognised and treated early.

Investigations

Plasma α-tocopherol concentration can be measured. Genetic testing for AVED is available.

Management

The recommended daily intake of vitamin E is 4–15 mg, depending on age.

AVED is treated with daily supplementation of α-tocopherol 800–1200 mg. Vitamin E deficiency secondary to fat malabsorption may require higher doses of oral supplementation or parenteral supplementation [59].

Vitamin E excess

Definition and nomenclature

Vitamin E excess can result in easy bleeding and bruising.

> **Synonyms and inclusions**
> * Vitamin E: tocopherol, tocotrienol

Epidemiology

Incidence and prevalence

Vitamin E excess is rarely encountered.

Age

Acquired vitamin E excess has no age predilection.

Sex

There is no sex predilection for acquired vitamin E excess.

Ethnicity

There is no ethnic predilection for acquired vitamin E excess.

Pathophysiology

Predisposing factors

Vitamin E excess can arise secondary to oversupplementation.

Clinical features

History

Patients with vitamin E excess may report easy bruising or bleeding.

Presentation

Vitamin E toxicity may predispose patients to develop purpura and haemorrhage due to its inherent antiplatelet effects [61], as well as its ability to augment the effects of anticoagulant medications.

Differential diagnosis

Other causes of haemorrhage should be evaluated, as vitamin E excess is rare.

Disease course and prognosis

Prognosis is good if recognised and treated early.

Investigations

Plasma α-tocopherol concentration can be measured.

Management

The recommended daily intake of vitamin E is 4–15 mg, depending on age.

Hypervitaminosis E is treated by discontinuation of excess intake.

Vitamin K

Vitamin K deficiency

Definition and nomenclature

Vitamin K is a fat-soluble vitamin and necessary co-factor in the synthesis of coagulation factors II, VII, IX and X, and proteins C and S.

> **Synonyms and inclusions**
> * Vitamin K: phytonadione

Introduction and general description

Dietary intake of vitamin K accounts for 50% of the body's daily requirements, while gastrointestinal bacterial synthesis of vitamin K is responsible for the other 50%. Dietary vitamin K (phylloquinone) can be found in green leafy vegetables, Brussels sprouts, lentils, soybeans and beef liver, and is actively absorbed in the small intestine. Vitamin K produced by gastrointestinal flora (menaquinone) is passively absorbed in the small bowel and colon. Vitamin K is crucial in the carboxylation of glutamate residues on coagulation factors II, VII, IX and X, and proteins C and S. A deficiency of vitamin K results in impaired coagulation and haemorrhage, so-called vitamin K deficiency bleeding (VKDB). In the neonatal period, VKDB is classified according to age of onset: early (24 hours after birth), classical (24 hours to 7 days after birth) and late (2–12 weeks after birth) [62].

Epidemiology

Incidence and prevalence

The incidence of early VKDB in neonates varies from 6% to 12% [63,64]. The incidence of classical VKDB in neonates is estimated to be 0.25–1.5% in the older literature [65], and 0–0.44% in more recent reviews [66]. Late VKDB can be seen in every 4.4–7.2 per 100 000 births [67].

Age

Vitamin K deficiency is more frequently encountered in newborns related to both endogenous and exogenous deficiencies.

Sex

There is no sex predilection for vitamin K deficiency.

Ethnicity

There is no ethnic predilection for vitamin K deficiency.

Associated diseases

Deficiencies in other fat-soluble vitamins (A, D and E) can occur in the setting of fat malabsorption.

Pathophysiology

Predisposing factors

Neonates are prone to vitamin K deficiency and VKDB secondary to poor transplacental transfer, lack of gastrointestinal flora to generate vitamin K and often inadequate dietary intake. Early VKDB occurs in infants born to mothers taking medications that interfere with vitamin K metabolism. Classical VKDB is associated with delayed or insufficient feeding. Late-onset VKDB correlates with exclusive breastfeeding without vitamin K prophylaxis, or underlying fat malabsorption diseases [62,68].

Vitamin K deficiency is also observed in the setting of decreased dietary intake, malabsorption, liver disease and various medications. Individuals with limited diets, including alcoholics, anorexics and the elderly, may be at risk for vitamin K deficiency. Impaired fat absorption with resultant vitamin K malabsorption can occur with coeliac disease, biliary and pancreatic disease, α-1 antitrypsin deficiency and cystic fibrosis. Prolonged antibiotic therapy may alter gastrointestinal flora and reduce vitamin K synthesis. A variety of medications can interfere with vitamin K metabolism, including warfarin (inhibits vitamin K epoxide reductase), high-dose salicylates, phenytoin, rifampin, isoniazid, cephalosporins and cholestyramine [69].

Vitamin K deficiency can be seen in adults treated in intensive care units (ICU). It is often present at admission, worsens during the course of ICU stay, and is thought to be secondary to various factors including malnutrition depleting vitamin K stores, prolonged use of medications such as antibiotics and anticoagulants, and pathophysiological changes that may occur after trauma, surgery, septic shock or cardiac arrest [70]. In adults critically ill with Covid-19, it has been postulated that vitamin K deficiency may contribute to the cytokine storm, coagulation abnormalities and the microvascular damage seen [71].

Genetics

Inherited vitamin K-dependent coagulation factor deficiencies secondary to mutations in γ-glutamyl carboxylase and vitamin K epoxide reductase have been reported [62].

Clinical features

History

Bleeding and easy bruising are the primary symptoms. Patients may complain of gingival bleeding, epistaxis, and genitourinary or gastrointestinal bleeding.

Presentation

The clinical presentation of early VKDB is often severe, with cephalic (cephalohaematoma, intracranial), intrathoracic and intra-abdominal bleeding. Classical VKDB is generally milder, and is characterised by umbilical, gastrointestinal, cutaneous and nasal mucosal bleeding. Late VKDB is severe, with intracranial haemorrhage occurring in most patients, often leading to persistent neurological sequelae [72]. Vitamin K deficiency in older children and adults can present with purpura, ecchymoses and gastrointestinal, genitourinary and retroperitoneal haemorrhage.

Clinical variants

- Neonatal vitamin K deficiency: early VKDB, classical VKDB, late VKDB.

Differential diagnosis

Anticoagulation, liver disease, haematological malignancies and inherited coagulopathies (i.e. haemophilia, von Willebrand disease, Wiskott–Aldrich syndrome) may give rise to a bleeding diathesis.

Complications and co-morbidities

Severe intracranial bleeds can result in long-term neurological damage.

Disease course and prognosis

Prognosis is generally good if the condition is recognised early and treated aggressively.

Investigations

Vitamin K deficiency leads to prolonged prothrombin and activated partial thromboplastin times. Serum vitamin K levels may be measured. Proteins induced by vitamin K absence (PIVKA), including des-γ-carboxyprothrombin, can be sensitive markers of vitamin K deficiency [73]. However, PIVKA have also been reported to be elevated in the context of hepatocellular carcinoma and lung cancer [74,75].

Management

The recommended daily intake of vitamin K is 2–120 µg, depending on age and sex.

Neonates should routinely receive a single prophylactic intramuscular dose of 0.5–1.0 mg of vitamin K at birth. Oral vitamin K as an alternative is being evaluated. However, there is currently no consensus on an optimal oral regimen [76].

Vitamin K deficiency is treated with intramuscular or parenteral vitamin K. Children are administered 2 mg, while adults are given 5–10 mg. Acute bleeding is treated with fresh frozen plasma in order to correct deficient coagulation factors.

Vitamin B₁

Vitamin B₁ deficiency

Definition and nomenclature

Vitamin B_1 (thiamine) is a water-soluble B-complex vitamin and a necessary co-enzyme for the metabolism of carbohydrates, lipids and branched chain amino acids, as well as the synthesis of nicotinamide adenine dinucleotide phosphate (NADPH).

Synonyms and inclusions

- Vitamin B_1: thiamine, aneurin
- Vitamin B_1 deficiency: beriberi

Introduction and general description

Thiamine is obtained through dietary sources, such as whole grains, wheat, peas, beans, potatoes and fish. The cooking and processing of these foods, including polishing rice, significantly decrease the thiamine content. Thiamine is largely absorbed in the jejunum of the small intestine. The active phosphorylated form of thiamine is thiamine pyrophosphate (TPP). TPP acts as a co-enzyme for α-ketoglutarate dehydrogenase and pyruvate dehydrogenase, which are involved in the oxidative decarboxylation of carbohydrates and lipids. It also functions as a co-enzyme for transketolase in the pentose phosphate pathway to generate NADPH [77]. Deficiency of thiamine results in beriberi, which encompasses a variety of neurological, cardiovascular and gastrointestinal manifestations. Thiamine excess is extremely rare and will not be addressed in this section. Most cases occur in the setting of intravenous administration of thiamine for suspected thiamine deficiency in alcoholics, with generalised pruritus and anaphylactoid reactions described [78].

Epidemiology
Incidence and prevalence
Thiamine deficiency is rare in developed countries.

Age
Thiamine deficiency can affect all age groups.

Sex
There is no sex predilection for thiamine deficiency.

Ethnicity
There is no ethnic predilection for thiamine deficiency.

Pathophysiology
Predisposing factors
Thiamine deficiency is observed in the context of malnutrition and poor dietary intake, inadequately supplemented parenteral nutrition, gastrointestinal malabsorption and increased metabolic requirements. Individuals with a history of particularly alcoholism, AIDS, malignancy, hyperthyroidism, systemic infection or critical illness are predisposed to thiamine deficiency [77]. Breastfed infants of thiamine-deficient mothers are also at risk for thiamine deficiency.

Clinical features
History
Fatigue, irritability, apathy, restlessness, nausea and vomiting are among the early signs of thiamine deficiency.

Presentation
Wet beriberi has prominent cardiovascular involvement, including cardiomegaly, cardiomyopathy, congestive heart failure, pulmonary hypertension [79], tachycardia, dyspnoea, cyanosis and peripheral oedema. A red burning tongue has also been described.

Dry beriberi has prominent neurological manifestations, including peripheral neuropathy and Wernicke encephalopathy (e.g. ophthalmoplegia, ataxia, nystagmus).

Aphonia, secondary to laryngeal nerve paralysis, is a characteristic feature of infantile beriberi. Cardiac disease has also been described [80]. In 2003, a series of infants in Israel were diagnosed with thiamine deficiency as a result of being fed thiamine-deficient formula. Early symptoms included irritability, lethargy, vomiting, diarrhoea and developmental delay. Neurological disease was also noted, including upbeat nystagmus and ophthalmoplegia [81].

Clinical variants
- Wet beriberi.
- Dry beriberi.

Differential diagnosis
Glossitis may be observed in other vitamin B deficiencies, including riboflavin deficiency, niacin deficiency, pyridoxine deficiency, folate deficiency and cobalamin deficiency. However, beriberi lacks the other cutaneous features that define these syndromes.

Complications and co-morbidities
Late-stage thiamine deficiency can result in Korsakoff syndrome, characterised by anterograde and retrograde amnesia.

Disease course and prognosis
Beriberi can be fatal but prognosis is generally good if disease is caught early. Response to treatment is often dramatic. Significant progression of neurological disease may be irreversible.

Investigations
Detection of elevated thiamine pyrophosphate effect (<15% is normal) confirms the diagnosis of thiamine deficiency. This is calculated by measuring erythrocyte thiamine transketolase before and after thiamine pyrophosphate stimulation [82]. Low blood thiamine levels can also be seen.

Management
Daily requirement of thiamine is 0.5 mg per 1000 kcal. Individuals who ingest a low-calorie diet should maintain a minimum of 1 mg daily [83].

Beriberi is frequently treated with intravenous or intramuscular thiamine, 50–100 mg/day for 7–14 days, then oral supplementation until the condition has resolved.

Vitamin B$_2$

Vitamin B$_2$ deficiency

Definition and nomenclature
Vitamin B$_2$ (riboflavin) is a water-soluble B-complex vitamin. It is an essential co-factor for cellular oxidation-reduction reactions and vitamin B$_6$ metabolism.

Synonyms and inclusions
- Vitamin B$_2$: riboflavin
- Vitamin B$_2$ deficiency: oculo-orogenital syndrome

Introduction and general description

Riboflavin exists as two biologically active forms: flavin mono-nucleotide (FMN) and flavin-adenine dinucleotide (FAD). These co-enzymes, along with a small percentage of free riboflavin, are found in milk, dairy products, meats, fatty fish, eggs, green leafy vegetables, whole grains and enriched breads. Dietary FMN and FAD are both hydrolysed to riboflavin, then actively absorbed in the proximal small intestine [84]. A deficiency in riboflavin can lead to various cutaneous, mucosal and ocular manifestations, the so-called oculo-orogenital syndrome.

Epidemiology
Incidence and prevalence
Riboflavin deficiency is endemic in populations whose diets rely heavily on unenriched cereals or lack dairy products and meats.

Age
Riboflavin deficiency can occur at any age, although it may disproportionately affect school-aged children, adolescents and the elderly.

Sex
There is no sex predilection for riboflavin deficiency.

Ethnicity
There is no ethnic predilection for riboflavin deficiency.

Associated diseases
Studies suggest that riboflavin deficiency may be associated with increased plasma homocysteine levels, impaired iron handling and anaemia, cardiovascular disease, night blindness, developmental abnormalities, peripheral neuropathy and cancer [84].

Pathophysiology
Predisposing factors
Riboflavin deficiency may develop as a result of decreased dietary intake, malabsorption and phototherapy. Adolescents, the elderly, alcoholics and individuals with eating disorders are at risk for inadequate nutritional intake. Breastfed infants of riboflavin-deficient mothers, as well as infants weaned to non-milk products, are also at risk. Impaired absorption of riboflavin has been associated with bariatric surgery and the use of various medications, including chlorpromazine or other tricyclics [85,86]. Borate can complex with riboflavin, increase urinary excretion of riboflavin and inhibit riboflavin-dependent enzymes [87]. In the setting of protein–energy malnutrition, riboflavin deficiency may worsen due to increased renal loss. Finally, phototherapy for neonatal hyperbilirubinaemia causes photodecomposition of riboflavin [88].

Clinical features
History
Acute riboflavin deficiency classically occurs after acute borate ingestion. Chronic riboflavin deficiency presents 3–5 months after initiation of a riboflavin-deficient diet. With chronic deficiency, individuals may complain of photophobia and conjunctivitis.

Presentation
Acute riboflavin deficiency presents with deep red skin (or other variations in skin of colour), epidermal necrolysis and mucositis. The severity of these findings depends on the degree of deficiency [89].

Clinical signs of chronic riboflavin deficiency include angular stomatitis, cheilitis, glossitis, dyssebacia (multiple follicular papules due to sebum in dilated follicular orifices) of the nose and a seborrhoeic dermatitis-like eruption. Angular stomatitis initially presents with small papules at the corners of the mouth, which subsequently extend laterally, macerate, fissure and bleed. Glossitis is characterised by prominent lingual papillae early on, with transition to a smooth magenta-coloured tongue over time. Riboflavin deficiency dermatitis commonly involves the nasolabial folds, nasal ala, nasal bridge, forehead, cheeks and postauricular regions, resembling seborrhoeic dermatitis. It can also affect the flexural extremities, inner thighs and genitalia. It is worse in areas of trauma and chafing, thus making it prominent in the inguinal folds and perineum of infants and in individuals who perform heavy physical activity [89].

Differential diagnosis
Other B-complex vitamin deficiencies may present with stomatitis, cheilitis, glossitis and a seborrhoeic dermatitis-like eruption, including pyridoxine deficiency.

Disease course and prognosis
Riboflavin deficiency carries an excellent prognosis with a striking response after riboflavin supplementation.

Investigations
Diagnosis can be confirmed by measuring erythrocyte glutathione reductase activity. Urinary excretion of riboflavin <40 mg/day can also suggest riboflavin deficiency [90]. A trial of riboflavin supplementation may also be effective.

Management
The recommended daily intake of riboflavin is 0.3–1.6 mg, depending on age and sex.

Treatment is with riboflavin supplementation of 1–2 mg/day in infants and children and 10–20 mg/day in adults.

Vitamin B$_3$

Vitamin B$_3$ deficiency

Definition and nomenclature
Vitamin B$_3$ (niacin) is a water-soluble B-complex vitamin and important component of two co-enzymes, nicotinamide-adenine dinucleotide (NAD) and NADP, which act as hydrogen donors and acceptors in numerous anabolic and catabolic reactions.

Synonyms and inclusions
- Vitamin B$_3$: niacin, nicotinic acid
- Vitamin B$_3$ deficiency: pellagra, Hartnup disease

Introduction and general description

Fifty percent of the body's niacin is obtained from diet, while the other half is synthesised endogenously from the amino acid tryptophan. Niacin exists as NAD and NADP in meats, fish, nuts, eggs, dairy products, dried beans and fortified grains. Corn and maize contain tightly bound niacin, thus preventing intestinal absorption unless the niacin is released by alkaline hydrolysis (i.e. limewater washes). Jowar contains usable niacin but also high levels of leucine which inhibits conversion of tryptophan to niacin. NAD and NADP are hydrolysed to nicotinamide in the intestinal lumen. Intestinal bacteria then convert nicotinamide into nicotinic acid. Both nicotinamide and nicotinic acid are absorbed and transported to the liver, kidneys and intestines, where they are transformed back to NAD and NADP for use in oxidation and reduction reactions. A deficiency of niacin results in pellagra, classically characterised by the four Ds: (1) dermatitis, (2) diarrhoea, (3) dementia and (4) death [91]. Hartnup disease, a rare metabolic disorder, can be associated with niacin deficiency and a pellagra-like presentation. The following discussion will focus primarily on acquired niacin deficiency.

Epidemiology

Incidence and prevalence

Niacin deficiency is endemic in areas with a high grain (unfortified), low meat diet and where corn and maize remain a mainstay, for example South Africa, India and China. Pellagra is rare in developed countries [92].

Age

Niacin deficiency can manifest at any age.

Sex

There is no sex predilection for niacin deficiency.

Ethnicity

There is no ethnic predilection for niacin deficiency.

Associated diseases

Niacin deficiency can be associated with carcinoid syndrome, where excess conversion of tryptophan to serotonin by carcinoid tumours leads to depletion of tryptophan stores and insufficient niacin synthesis [93,94].

Pathophysiology

Predisposing factors

Decreased dietary intake, defective absorption of niacin or tryptophan, and impaired conversion of tryptophan to niacin predispose individuals to the development of niacin deficiency. Individuals with alcoholism, eating disorders and presumed food allergies are at risk for inadequate intake. Restrictive diets from selective eating in children with autism spectrum disorders (ASD) can also lead to pellagra [95]. Malabsorption can occur in the setting of inflammatory bowel disease, gastroenterostomy, subtotal gastrectomy, jejunoileitis and gastric bypass surgery. Hartnup disease results in impaired absorption of tryptophan, a necessary precursor in the synthesis of niacin. Medications, including isoniazid [96], 5-fluorouracil [97] and 6-mercaptopurine, may interfere

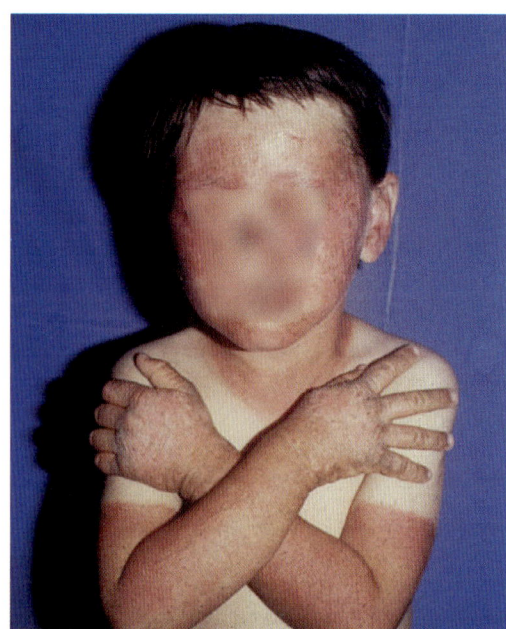

Figure 61.7 Hartnup disease. Reproduced from [101] with permission from John Wiley & Sons.

with the conversion of tryptophan to niacin. Other drugs have been implicated in causing pellagra-like symptoms, such as anticonvulsants [98,99], antidepressants, sulfonamides, azathioprine [100] and chloramphenicol. Carcinoid syndrome also prevents appropriate conversion of tryptophan to niacin by diverting as much as 60% of tryptophan to serotonin production (normally only 1%).

Genetics

Hartnup disease is a rare autosomal recessive disorder characterised by a defective neutral amino acid transport system, resulting in malabsorption of tryptophan, thus giving rise to niacin deficiency. It is caused by mutations in the *SLC6A19* gene, which encodes a neutral amino acid transporter expressed in the intestine and kidneys. Hartnup disease presents with cerebellar ataxia, psychiatric symptoms, aminoaciduria and pellagra [102] (Figure 61.7).

Clinical features

History

Dermatitis, diarrhoea and dementia represent the classic manifestations of pellagra. Gastrointestinal symptoms may present early in the course of the disease, and include abdominal pain, anorexia, nausea, vomiting and diarrhoea. Neurological symptoms, such as headache, anxiety, irritability, fatigue, insomnia, apathy, depression and impaired memory, can ultimately progress to psychosis and dementia [103].

Presentation

Initially, the dermatitis of pellagra is described as intermittent, painful or pruritic redness and oedema in photodistributed areas after sun exposure. Vesicles and bullae may develop in severe cases. Over time, the eruption becomes fixed and is defined by sharply marginated, hyperpigmented and keratotic plaques. The dorsal

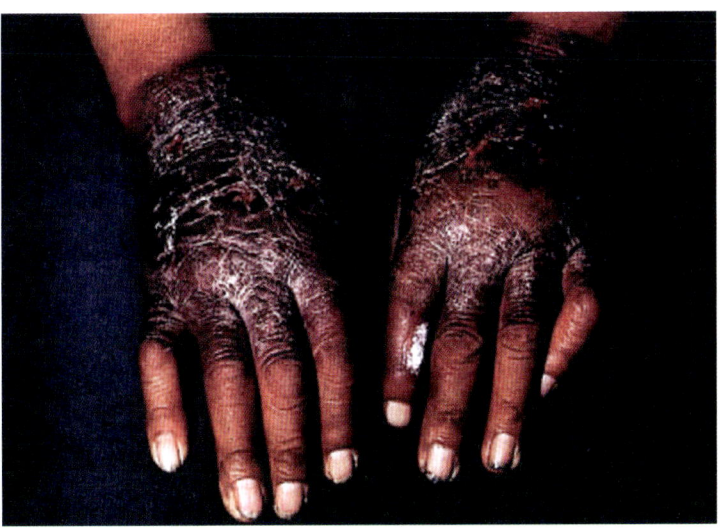

Figure 61.8 Pellagra. Reproduced from [101] with permission from John Wiley & Sons.

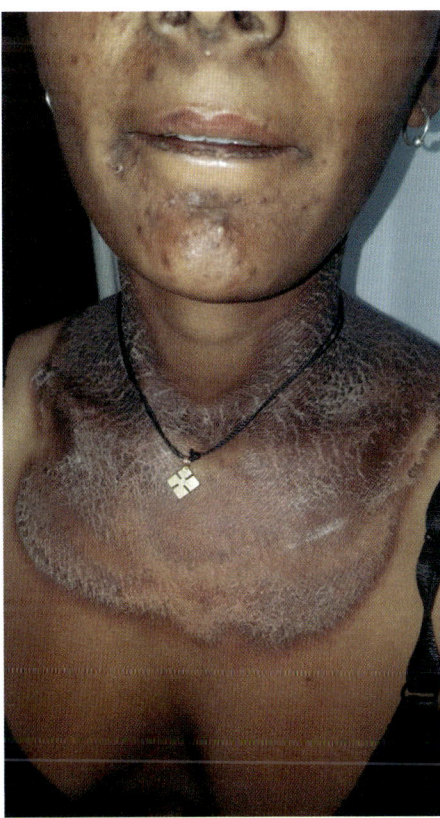

Figure 61.9 Broad hyperpigmented 'collar-like' scaly plaques on the photo-exposed area of the neck and upper chest in a patient with pellagra; often referred to as the Casal necklace. Reproduced from [104] with permission from John Wiley & Sons.

hands are most commonly affected (Figure 61.8). Facial involvement occurs in a symmetrical butterfly distribution. Involvement of the neck and upper chest is frequently referred to as the Casal necklace (Figure 61.9) [104]. Pellagra can also manifest with angular stomatitis, cheilitis, glossitis and oral or perirectal ulcers. Half and half nails have been observed [105].

Differential diagnosis

Pyridoxine deficiency presenting with a pellagra-like dermatitis has been reported. Other photosensitive dermatoses, including porphyrias, polymorphous light eruption, chronic actinic dermatitis, photosensitive drug eruptions and cutaneous lupus, should be excluded.

Complications and co-morbidities

Patients may have severe neurological decompensation, and eventually become stuporous and comatose.

Disease course and prognosis

Pellagra is progressive and can be fatal if not treated. Death can occur within 4–5 years.

Investigations

Pellagra is mainly a clinical diagnosis. Reduced niacin urinary metabolites, such as N-methylnicotinamide and 2-pyridone, and serum nicotinamide and nicotinic acid levels can be helpful in confirming diagnosis.

Management

The recommended daily intake of niacin is 13–20 mg, depending on age and sex.

Treatment includes 500 mg/day of nicotinamide or nicotinic acid over several weeks. Nicotinamide is preferred because nicotinic acid can cause headaches and flushing. Neuropsychiatric symptoms improve within the first 24–48 h of treatment, while cutaneous disease may require weeks to remit [91].

Vitamin B₆

Vitamin B₆ deficiency

Definition and nomenclature

Vitamin B₆ (pyridoxine) is a water-soluble B-complex vitamin and essential co-enzyme for various metabolic processes, including conversion of tryptophan to niacin, fatty acid metabolism, gluconeogenesis, decarboxylation and transamination of amino acids, and prostaglandin and neurotransmitter synthesis.

Synonyms and inclusions
• Vitamin B₆: pyridoxine, pyridoxamine, pyridoxal

Introduction and general description

Pyridoxine, pyridoxamine and pyridoxal represent the three forms of vitamin B₆. They are available in a variety of foods, including meats, vegetables, nuts and whole grains. After dephosphorylation, these molecules are absorbed both actively and passively in the jejunum and ileum, transported to the liver and rephosphorylated to their active forms. A deficiency in vitamin B₆ is uncommon, but can result in cutaneous, neurological and haematological manifestations. Features of vitamin B₆ deficiency may overlap with those of niacin deficiency.

Epidemiology
Incidence and prevalence
The incidence of vitamin B_6 deficiency is not known, as isolated vitamin B_6 deficiency is rare and usually occurs with other B vitamin deficiencies [106].

Age
Vitamin B_6 deficiency can affect all age groups, with the elderly at higher risk.

Sex
There is no sex predilection for vitamin B_6 deficiency.

Ethnicity
There is no ethnic predilection for vitamin B_6 deficiency.

Associated diseases
Vitamin B_6 deficiency can be associated with niacin deficiency.

Pathophysiology
Predisposing factors
Factors contributing to vitamin B_6 deficiency include decreased dietary intake, malabsorption and medications. Alcoholics are particularly prone to poor dietary intake. Individuals with Crohn disease and coeliac disease may suffer from malabsorption [107]. Certain medications bind to vitamin B_6 and act to increase its excretion or decrease its activity, including isoniazid, hydralazine, penicillamine and oral contraceptives [108]. Vitamin B_6 deficiency has also been reported in patients undergoing haemodialysis [109].

Clinical features
History
Individuals may complain of anorexia, nausea and vomiting. Neuropsychiatric symptoms, such as confusion, somnolence, weakness, depression, paraesthesias and peripheral neuropathy, can be prominent.

Presentation
Classically, patients present with a seborrhoeic dermatitis-like eruption involving the face, scalp, neck, shoulders, buttocks and perineum. Angular stomatitis, glossitis and cheilitis are also observed. There can be significant overlap with niacin deficiency and a pellagra-like dermatitis has been reported [110].

Patients can also develop a hypochromic microcytic anaemia.

Differential diagnosis
Both niacin deficiency and pyridoxine deficiency manifest with similar neuropsychiatric and cutaneous symptoms.

Complications and co-morbidities
Pyridoxine deficiency has been associated with refractory seizures [111].

Disease course and prognosis
Prognosis is generally good. Care should be taken when supplementing with pyridoxine as this can be complicated by toxicity, leading to neuropathy and ataxia.

Investigations
Low plasma pyridoxal-5-phosphate is indicative of vitamin B_6 deficiency. Indirect tests, such as a tryptophan load test or measurement of erythrocyte aminotransferase activity, may be useful [112].

Management
The recommended daily intake of vitamin B_6 is 0.1–2 mg, depending on age and sex.

Treatment of vitamin B_6 deficiency includes stopping any triggering medications and supplementation with pyridoxine 100 mg daily. Mucosal lesions resolve within days, while cutaneous and haematological manifestations improve over weeks and neurological sequelae over months.

Vitamin B_9

Vitamin B_9 deficiency

Definition and nomenclature
Vitamin B_9 (folate) is a water-soluble B-complex vitamin and important co-enzyme for amino acid, purine and pyrimidine metabolism.

Synonyms and inclusions
- Vitamin B_9: folate, folic acid

Introduction and general description
Folate is available in most foods, especially leafy green vegetables, dried beans, liver and grains. Tetrahydrofolate is the biologically active co-enzyme form of folate. Folate deficiency manifests with both haematological and mucocutaneous disease.

Epidemiology
Incidence and prevalence
In the USA, data from the National Health and Nutrition Examination Survey (NHANES) reveal that the prevalence of low serum folate decreased from 18.4% in 1988–94, to 0.2% in 2001–02 [113]. This change was attributed to the nationwide dietary folic acid supplementation mandate that was introduced in 1998. Additional NHANES data has shown that this decrease has persisted with the overall prevalence of folate deficiency being <1% from 1999 to 2016 [114].

Age
Folate deficiency can present in all age groups.

Sex
Pregnant women are at higher risk of developing folate deficiency given increased requirements during pregnancy.

Ethnicity
There is no ethnic predilection for folate deficiency

Associated diseases

Studies suggest an association between folate deficiency and elevated homocysteine levels and cardiovascular disease, neuropsychiatric disease and certain cancers [115].

Pathophysiology

Predisposing factors

In the paediatric population, deficient intake of folate can occur in the setting of overly boiled cow's milk or being fed goat's milk exclusively [116]. Alcoholics are at risk of inadequate intake. Malabsorption due to coeliac disease, chronic diarrhoea and gastrectomy has been reported. Antifolate medications, such as methotrexate, trimethoprim, pyrimethamine and oral contraceptive, can cause folate deficiency. Certain antiepileptic medications, including phenobarbital, phenytoin and carbamazepine, induce microsomal hepatic enzymes, thus diminishing folate stores [117,118].

Clinical features

History

Patients may report having anorexia, nausea, vomiting, abdominal pain and diarrhoea. They may also complain of a sore tongue or pain with swallowing.

Presentation

Folate deficiency is characterised primarily by its haematological manifestations, which include a megaloblastic anaemia and hypersegmented neutrophils. Neutropenia and thrombocytopenia can also be noted.

The mucocutaneous manifestations include glossitis with atrophic filiform papillae (Hunter's glossitis), angular cheilitis, mucosal ulceration, perineal seborrhoeic dermatitis, and localised or diffuse hair depigmentation and mucocutaneous hyperpigmentation. Hyperpigmentation is frequently seen in the palmar creases and flexural regions but can also affect the oral mucosa [119,120].

Differential diagnosis

Vitamin B_{12} deficiency can mimic folate deficiency. Unlike vitamin B_{12} deficiency, folate deficiency lacks neurological features.

Complications and co-morbidities

Folate deficiency in women of childbearing age may result in fetal neural tube defects.

Disease course and prognosis

Folic acid supplementation is typically curative of folate deficiency.

Investigations

Diagnosis is made by measurement of serum and red blood cell folate levels [121]. Identifying a megaloblastic anaemia with hypersegmented neutrophils is also helpful.

Management

The recommended daily intake of folate is 65–600 µg/day, depending on age.

Treatment includes addressing any underlying causes of folate deficiency and supplementing with 1–5 mg of folate daily. Concurrent vitamin B_{12} deficiency should be ruled out prior to initiating treatment, as the haematological manifestations of vitamin B_{12} deficiency will respond to folate but the neurological symptoms will not.

Vitamin B_{12}

Vitamin B_{12} deficiency

Definition and nomenclature

Vitamin B_{12} (cobalamin) is a water-soluble B-complex vitamin and critical co-enzyme involved in DNA, protein, lipid and carbohydrate metabolism.

Synonyms and inclusions
- Vitamin B_{12}: cobalamin
- Vitamin B_{12} deficiency: pernicious anaemia

Introduction and general description

Vitamin B_{12} is obtained through dietary sources such as eggs, milk, beef, liver and organ meats. Upon ingestion, gastric acid dissociates vitamin B_{12} from food proteins. After binding to intrinsic factor in the duodenum, vitamin B_{12} is actively taken up by the terminal ileum. About 1–5% of free vitamin B_{12} is absorbed via passive diffusion. In the enterocyte, vitamin B_{12} separates from intrinsic factor, binds to transcobalamin II and is released into the portal circulation for transport to other tissues. The two biologically active forms of cobalamin are methylcobalamin and 5'-adenosylcobalamin. Methylcobalamin is a co-enzyme for methyltransferase, which methylates homocysteine to methionine, while 5'-adenosylcobalamin catalyses methylmalonyl co-enzyme A (CoA) mutase's conversion of methylmalonic acid to succinyl CoA [122]. A deficiency in vitamin B_{12} leads to a clinical profile similar to folate deficiency, with mucocutaneous and haematological manifestations. The distinguishing feature of vitamin B_{12} deficiency is its important neurological findings. Since the body is able to store a large amount of vitamin B_{12}, symptoms of acquired deficiency may take 3–6 years to develop. Vitamin B_{12} deficiency can be associated with both congenital and acquired pernicious anaemia.

Epidemiology

Incidence and prevalence

It is estimated that 3.2% of US adults older than 50 years have a serum vitamin B_{12} level <200 pg/mL [123]. The prevalence of acquired pernicious anaemia ranges from 50 to 4000 cases per 100 000 persons [124].

Age

Acquired vitamin B_{12} deficiency can be observed in all ages. Adult-onset pernicious anaemia usually occurs in people aged 40–70 years.

Sex

There is no sex predilection for vitamin B_{12} deficiency.

Ethnicity

Acquired pernicious anaemia is more common in individuals of European and African ancestry.

Associated diseases

Acquired pernicious anaemia is an autoimmune gastritis characterised by destruction of gastric parietal cells and loss of intrinsic factor. The lack of intrinsic factor prevents adequate absorption of vitamin B_{12} [125]. Autoimmune gastritis can also cause malabsorption of iron and clinical iron deficiency.

Pathophysiology
Predisposing factors

Vitamin B_{12} deficiency results from inadequate intake, malabsorption and inborn errors of transport and metabolism. Populations at risk for poor dietary intake include the elderly, vegans and their breastfed infants, and individuals with psychiatric disease. Defective absorption of vitamin B_{12} can occur secondary to decreased gastric acid production (chronic proton pump inhibitors and H_2 histamine blockers) [126], decreased intrinsic factor (pernicious anaemia, atrophic gastritis, postgastrectomy) and bacterial overgrowth. Other states of impaired absorption include inflammatory bowel disease, coeliac disease, Whipple disease and Zollinger–Ellison syndrome [127].

Genetics

Mutations in the gastric intrinsic factor gene cause a rare disorder of vitamin B_{12} absorption known as congenital pernicious anaemia or congenital intrinsic factor deficiency.

Clinical features
History

Individuals may report symptoms of fatigue, weakness and possibly a sore tongue.

Presentation

Similar to folate deficiency, vitamin B_{12} deficiency is characterised by haematological manifestations, including megaloblastic anaemia and hypersegmented neutrophils, as well as mucocutaneous manifestations such as Hunter glossitis, angular cheilitis, localised or diffuse hair depigmentation and mucocutaneous hyperpigmentation (of the face, nails, palmar creases and flexural surfaces) [129–133] (Figure 61.10). The morphology of the cutaneous hyperpigmentation can present as homogeneous or reticulate 'honeycomb' patterns when diffuse, and accentuation on the joints known as 'knuckle hyperpigmentation' when localised to the dorsal hands and feet. Mucosal pigmentation can include the tongue [134,135]. Hyperpigmentation may be one of the first signs of vitamin B_{12} deficiency and may present prior to anaemia being detected on laboratory investigations [135]. Vitamin B_{12} deficiency is distinguished from folate deficiency by the development of neurological symptoms. Patients normally present with subacute combined degeneration of the dorsal and lateral spinal column, resulting in generalised weakness, paraesthesias, ataxia and symmetrical loss of vibration and proprioception. If left untreated, patients can develop spasticity, paraplegia and incontinence. Other symptoms include somnolence, irritability, apathy, memory loss, dementia and psychosis.

Differential diagnosis

Folate deficiency encompasses similar mucocutaneous and haematological features.

Complications and co-morbidities

Advanced neurological disease may develop, which may be unresponsive to vitamin replacement therapy.

Disease course and prognosis

Prognosis is good with early recognition and treatment. For acquired pernicious anaemia, patients should be monitored for possible development of gastric cancer.

Investigations

Diagnosis is confirmed by detecting a serum cobalamin level <200 pg/mL. A serum cobalamin level of 200–300 pg/mL is borderline low. A megaloblastic anaemia with hypersegmented neutrophils is also observed. The Schilling test, serological antibodies to intrinsic factor and parietal cells, and biopsies of the gastric mucosa provide additional information to secure the diagnosis of acquired pernicious anaemia.

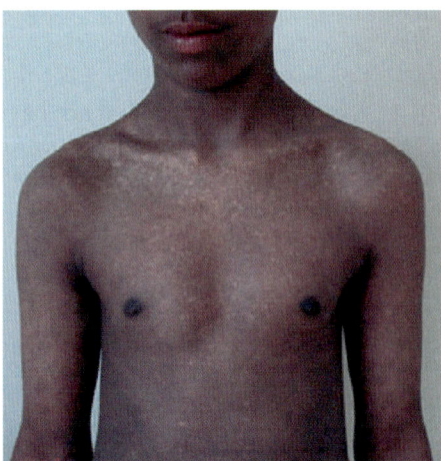
(a)

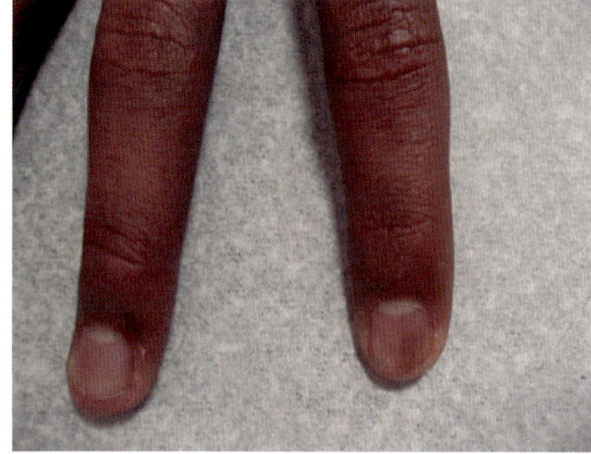
(b)

Figure 61.10 Vitamin B_{12} deficiency with (a) generalised hyperpigmentation and (b) longitudinal hyperpigmented streaks on the fingernails. Reproduced from [128] with permission from John Wiley & Sons.

Management

The recommended daily intake of vitamin B$_{12}$ is 0.4–2.8 µg, depending on age.

Vitamin B$_{12}$ can be administered either parenterally or orally. If given parenterally, it is recommended that patients receive 8–10 loading doses of 1 mg spaced daily to weekly, and then monthly 1 mg injections thereafter. If given orally, 1–2 mg daily is considered to be effective therapy [124].

Vitamin C

Vitamin C deficiency

Definition and nomenclature

Vitamin C is a water-soluble vitamin, antioxidant and essential co-factor for collagen biosynthesis, carnitine and catecholamine metabolism and dietary iron absorption.

> **Synonyms and inclusions**
> * Vitamin C: ascorbic acid
> * Vitamin C deficiency: scurvy

Introduction and general description

Humans are unable to synthesise vitamin C. As such, vitamin C is strictly obtained through dietary intake of fruit and vegetables. Citrus fruits, berries, tomatoes, potatoes and green leafy vegetables are excellent sources of vitamin C. Although most vitamin C is completely absorbed in the small intestine, the percentage of absorbed vitamin C decreases as intraluminal concentrations increase [136]. Vitamin C is required for the hydroxylation of proline residues on procollagen, in turn making it necessary for triple-helix formation of mature collagen. The lack of a stable triple helical structure compromises the integrity of the skin, mucous membranes, blood vessels and bone. Consequently, a deficiency in vitamin C results in scurvy, which is composed of haemorrhage, hyperkeratosis and haematological abnormalities.

Epidemiology

Incidence and prevalence

One of the largest studies of over 24 000 participants, aged 40–72, was performed in England from 1993 to 1997 and showed a vitamin C deficiency prevalence of 1.4% [137]. According to the NHANES (2003–04) study, the overall prevalence of vitamin C deficiency in the USA among children and adults older than 6 years was 7.1% [138]. Within any given population, vitamin C status can be quite variable due to environmental factors (geographic region, season, climate, pollution), demographic factors (age, sex, race, socioeconomic status) and health status (pregnancy, smoking, medical co-morbidities) [139,140].

Age

Vitamin C deficiency can present at any age, although it is uncommon in the neonatal period.

Sex

There is no sex predilection for vitamin C deficiency.

Ethnicity

There is no ethnic predilection for vitamin C deficiency.

Associated diseases

Vitamin C deficiency can be associated with both folate and iron deficiency. Vitamin C decreases urinary folic acid excretion and increases dietary iron absorption.

Pathophysiology

Predisposing factors

Vitamin C deficiency usually arises in the setting of decreased intake or increased requirements or losses. The elderly, alcoholics, food faddists, anorexics, cancer patients, individuals with presumed food allergies, and patients receiving unsupplemented parenteral nutrition or with restricted diets secondary to inflammatory bowel disease, gastrointestinal reflux or Whipple disease, are all at risk for inadequate intake of vitamin C [136]. More recently, numerous case reports of scurvy have arisen among children with autism spectrum disorders, due to their strong food preferences and aversions [**141**]. Increased vitamin C requirements can be observed with tobacco smoking, as well as several medications including aspirin, indomethacin, oral contraceptives, tetracyclines and corticosteroids. Renal failure patients are prone to scurvy due to filtration of water-soluble vitamin C during dialysis [142]. Scurvy has been reported as a complication of interleukin-2 treatment of metastatic renal cell carcinoma and among patients receiving liver transplants [143,144].

Clinical features

History

Scurvy develops 1–3 months after initiating a vitamin C-deficient diet [145]. Individuals may complain of lethargy, fatigue, malaise, emotional lability, arthralgias, weight loss, anorexia and diarrhoea. They may also experience easy bleeding, bruising and poor wound healing.

Presentation

The cutaneous manifestations of scurvy include phrynoderma, corkscrew hairs, perifollicular haemorrhage and purpura, oedema of the lower extremities and splinter haemorrhages [136]. Phrynoderma (enlarged hyperkeratotic hair follicles) initially presents on the posterolateral aspects of the arms. This can subsequently generalise to involve the buttocks, posterior thighs, calves, shins and back. Corkscrew hairs represent fractured and coiled hairs due to impaired keratin cross-links by disulfide bonds. With time, significant vascular congestion occurs, particularly in the lower extremities, leading to perifollicular haemorrhage and oedema (Figure 61.11). This purpura is occasionally palpable, mimicking a cutaneous vasculitis [146]. Blood vessel wall fragility also results in splinter haemorrhages of the nail bed.

Oral disease is prominent among those with pre-existing poor dentition. Individuals may develop a haemorrhagic gingivitis, where the gingiva is initially red, swollen and shiny, and later

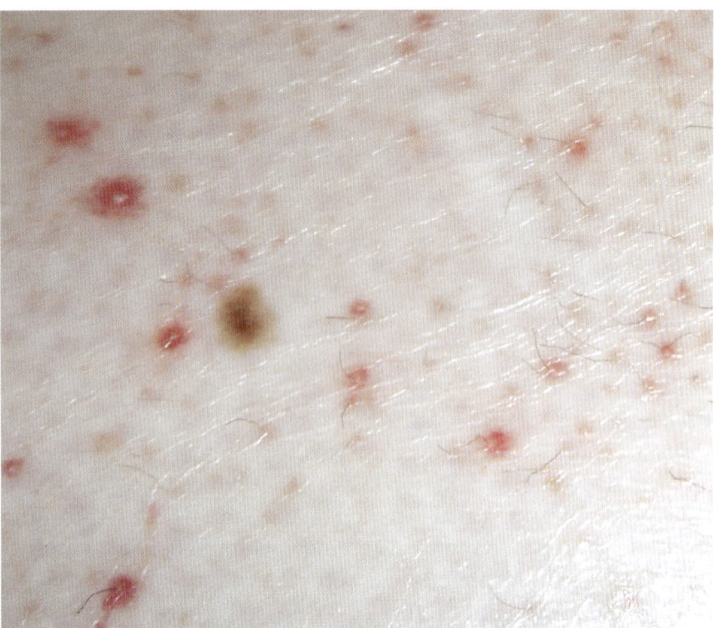

Figure 61.11 Scurvy: note the corkscrew-like hairs and the perifollicular purpura.

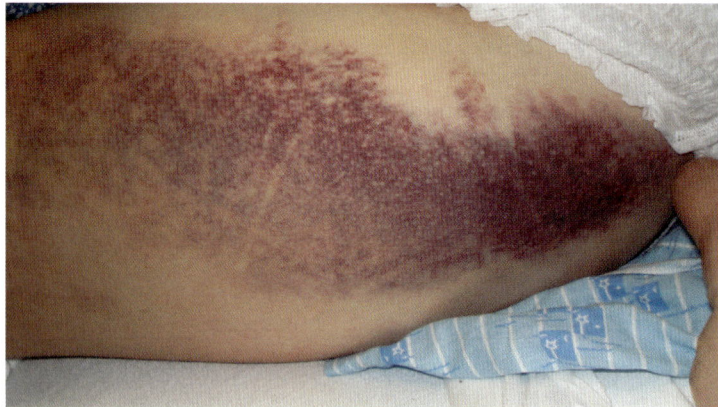

Figure 61.12 Scurvy: note the extensive ecchymoses from minor trauma.

becomes purple, necrotic and prone to bleeding [136]. Additionally, poorly formed soft teeth are prone to infection.

Lack of body hair and dentition may make a diagnosis of vitamin C deficiency challenging without the presence of hair or gingival abnormalities, respectively [147,148]. In these cases, absence of these features should not exclude a diagnosis of vitamin C deficiency if there is a high level of suspicion.

Musculoskeletal disease is frequently seen in children. Haemorrhage can be intramuscular, intra-articular or subperiosteal, leading to pain and pseudoparalysis. Bowing of the long bones, depression of the sternum, and swelling of the costochondral junctions are noted on physical examination. Radiographic findings include a transverse metaphyseal radiolucent band (scurvy line or Trummerfeld zone), widening at the zone of calcification (white line of Frankel), a ring of increased density around the epiphysis (Wimberger ring) and metaphyseal spurs with marginal fractures (Pelkan spurs) [149,150]. Conjunctival, intraocular, intracerebral and gastrointestinal bleeding have been reported.

Differential diagnosis
Trauma, medications, haematological abnormalities, collagen vascular diseases and infections can cause large ecchymoses and be confused with scurvy [151] (Figure 61.12).

Complications and co-morbidities
The major complication associated with scurvy is haemorrhage into various tissue sites, which has the potential to result in permanent functional deficits.

Disease course and prognosis
Scurvy generally carries an excellent prognosis if diagnosed and treated appropriately.

Investigations
Scurvy is largely a clinical diagnosis. Serum ascorbic acid levels may be measured (<11 µmol/L), but this typically reflects recent dietary intake. Measurement of leukocyte ascorbic acid levels tends to be more accurate, but testing is not widely available.

A normochromic normocytic anaemia is common resulting from blood loss, folate deficiency and iron deficiency.

Management
The recommended daily intake of vitamin C is 40–120 mg, depending on age and sex.

Scurvy is treated with ascorbic acid 100–300 mg daily until symptoms remit. Clinical improvement is noted within the first 1–2 weeks, with resolution of fatigue, joint swelling and ecchymoses, and healing of the gingiva. Complete recovery frequently occurs within 3 months [136].

Biotin

Biotin deficiency

Definition and nomenclature
Biotin is an essential co-factor for four carboxylase enzymes involved in fatty acid synthesis and lipogenesis (acetyl-CoA carboxylase), gluconeogenesis (pyruvate carboxylase) and amino acid catabolism (propionyl-CoA carboxylase and 3-methylcrotonyl CoA carboxylase).

Synonyms and inclusions
- Biotin: vitamin B_7
- Biotin deficiency: multiple carboxylase deficiency, holocarboxylase synthetase deficiency, biotinidase deficiency

---

Introduction and general description
Biotin is both synthesised by intestinal bacteria and obtained through dietary sources. As a result, deficiency states are uncommon. Good sources of biotin include eggs, cow's milk, soya beans,

liver, mushrooms, peanuts, hazelnuts and walnuts. Pancreatic biotinidase is required to release biotin from dietary proteins. Biotin diffuses across the gut epithelium, binds to plasma proteins and travels to the liver, where it complexes with various carboxylase enzymes via holocarboxylase synthetase. Endogenous biotin is recycled by biotinidase. Biotin deficiency can be acquired or inherited. The two forms of hereditary multiple carboxylase deficiency are holocarboxylase synthetase deficiency (neonatal, early onset) and biotinidase deficiency (infantile, late onset).

Epidemiology
Incidence and prevalence
The combined incidence of profound and partial biotinidase deficiency is 1 in 60 089 live births [152]. Holocarboxylase synthetase deficiency is extremely rare.

Age
Acquired biotin deficiency can affect all ages. Holocarboxylase synthetase deficiency presents within the first 6 weeks of life. Biotinidase deficiency presents in infancy or early childhood, typically after 3 months of age.

Sex
There is no sex predilection for biotin deficiency.

Ethnicity
There is no ethnic predilection for biotin deficiency.

Pathophysiology
Predisposing factors
Acquired biotin deficiency is often associated with excessive intake of raw egg white [153,154]. Avidin is a glycoprotein found in egg whites which binds to free biotin and prevents its absorption. When eggs are cooked, this bond is broken and biotin may be freely absorbed. Biotin deficiency is also observed in the setting of receiving unsupplemented parenteral nutrition [155,156], unsupplemented infant formula [157], prolonged antibiotic courses and long-term anticonvulsants (e.g. valproic acid, carbamazepine, phenytoin). Anticonvulsants can increase biotin catabolism and disrupt liver function, thus predisposing to biotin deficiency [158–160].

Genetics
Both holocarboxylase synthetase deficiency and biotinidase deficiency are autosomal recessively inherited disorders resulting in altered biotin metabolism.

Clinical features
History
Symptoms of acquired biotin deficiency manifest 3–6 months after initiation of a diet rich in raw egg white.

Presentation
The cutaneous features of acquired biotin deficiency are similar to acrodermatitis enteropathica and essential fatty acid deficiency. It normally consists of a pink to red, scaly periorificial dermatitis around the eyes, nose, mouth and anus. Alopecia, glossitis

and conjunctivitis have also been observed. Patients may complain of lethargy, paraesthesias, myalgias, nausea, anorexia and hypotonia.

Holocarboxylase synthetase deficiency is characterised by several metabolic derangements, including metabolic acidosis (lactic acidosis, ketoacidosis), hyperammonaemia and organic aciduria. Neonates frequently have hypotonia, ataxia, seizures, lethargy and developmental delay. There have been reports of affected individuals presenting with a collodion membrane and subsequent ichthyosis [161]. Classically, patients develop dermatitis in a seborrhoeic, periorificial and intertriginous distribution, with or without associated alopecia.

Similarly, biotinidase deficiency can be associated with metabolic acidosis, organic aciduria, ataxia, hypotonia, seizures, developmental delay, periorificial dermatitis and alopecia. Patients may also develop keratoconjunctivitis, optic nerve atrophy and sensorineural hearing loss. Though metabolic encephalopathy has the potential to be corrected with biotin replacement [162], hearing loss is irreversible [163]. Immune deficiencies have been documented as well [164].

Differential diagnosis
Biotin deficiency, zinc deficiency and essential fatty acid deficiency all have analogous cutaneous manifestations.

Complications and co-morbidities
Patients with multiple carboxylase deficiency may develop permanent neurodevelopmental deficits.

Disease course and prognosis
Prognosis is generally good with early diagnosis and treatment. Morbidity will depend on the extent of delay in treatment and the degree of metabolic stress. Mortality rate is close to 100% with untreated holocarboxylase deficiency.

Investigations
The diagnosis can be confirmed by detecting a low serum biotin level. However, this may not be the most reliable measurement of biotin deficiency; a more sensitive and accurate measurement is urinary levels of biotin and its metabolites [165,166]. Urinary biotin will be decreased and urinary biotin metabolites, including 3-hydroxyisovaleric acid, 3-methylcrotonylglycine, 3-hydroxypropionic acid, methylcitric acid and lactic acid, may be elevated [167]. Checking ammonia, serum amino acids and urine organic acids may be helpful if one suspects an inborn error of metabolism. Decreased biotinidase activity in serum, leukocytes or cultured skin fibroblasts is indicative of biotinidase deficiency. Many states include multicarboxylase deficiency testing as part of newborn screening.

Management
The recommended daily intake of biotin is 5–35 µg, depending on age. Most children and adults meet this requirement through their daily diet, and there is no strong evidence supporting biotin supplementation outside of known inherited or acquired deficiency for hair, nail or skin disorders in healthy individuals [168,169].

Acquired biotin deficiency is treated with 150 μg of biotin daily until symptoms resolve. Biotinidase deficiency often responds well to 5–10 mg of biotin daily, while holocarboxylase synthetase deficiency requires at least 10–40 mg daily, with higher doses frequently needed. Metabolic and cutaneous abnormalities respond rapidly. However, neurological deficits such as hearing loss and vision impairment may be permanent.

Of note, exogenous biotin supplementation has been found to interfere with immunoassays that utilise the streptavidin-biotin interaction causing falsely elevated or decreased laboratory values. Examples of tests that can be affected include free triiodothyronine (fT3), free thyroxine (fT4), thyroid stimulating hormone (TSH), prolactin, creatinine kinase-MB (CK-MB), qualitative β-human chorionic gonadotropin (hCG), alpha fetoprotein (AFP), cortisol and ferritin. In view of this, clinicians should advise patients to withhold biotin supplementation at least 48–72 h prior to blood tests, and if this is not possible, consider enquiring whether different laboratory assays or techniques can be performed for more accurate results [170,171].

MINERALS

Iron

Iron deficiency

Definition
Iron is an essential factor for multiple metabolic pathways, including collagen synthesis, haem synthesis and various oxidation-reduction reactions. It also serves as a co-factor for enzymes such as monoamine oxidase and succinic dehydrogenase.

Introduction and general description
Iron-rich foods include red meat, egg yolk, green leafy vegetables, dried fruits, nuts, dried beans and enriched grain products. Most iron absorption occurs in the duodenum and jejunum via ferrous iron transporter divalent metal ion transporter 1 (DMT-1). Ferric iron is reduced to the ferrous form by ferric reductase along the intestinal brush border to facilitate DMT-1 transport. Intestinal absorption of ferritin and haem is poorly understood. In addition to haematological abnormalities, iron deficiency often manifests with nail, hair and mucous membrane changes.

Epidemiology
Incidence and prevalence
In children between 1 and 4 years of age, 14% are iron deficient; the prevalence decreases to 4% in children aged 3–5 years [1]. Of menstruating females, 9% are iron deficient [1].

Age
Infants are at high risk for developing iron deficiency. In particular, infants transitioning from iron-fortified formula to cow's milk are at risk given higher concentrations of calcium in cow's milk competing with iron for absorption in the gastrointestinal tract.

Sex
Women of childbearing age are at greater risk for iron deficiency as a result of blood loss with menses and iron loss during pregnancy. Iron deficiency anaemia is the most common cause of anaemia in pregnancy [2].

Ethnicity
There is no ethnic predilection for iron deficiency.

Associated diseases
Iron deficiency is seen in approximately 17% of children with cystic fibrosis [3].

Pathophysiology
Predisposing factors
Infants and women of childbearing age are at greatest risk for iron deficiency. Infants are particularly at risk for deficiency as they transition from iron-fortified formula to cow's milk formula due to reduced intestinal absorption in the setting of high calcium concentrations. Menstruation and pregnancy predispose women to iron deficiency. Conditions resulting in chronic bleeding, such as inflammatory bowel disease or gastrointestinal malignancy, may lead to deficiency states. Patients treated with roux-en-Y gastric bypass surgery can present with iron deficiency, likely related to poor gastrointestinal absorption of dietary iron, with the risk increasing over time postoperatively [4].

Causative organisms
Helicobacter pylori infection has been associated with iron deficiency in children and adolescents [5,6].

Clinical features
History
Infants present with iron deficiency within 3–6 months of transitioning from iron-fortified formula to cow's milk. Adults often report fatigue.

Presentation
Nail changes are characteristically observed in iron deficiency. Nails become fragile, longitudinally ridged and brittle with moderate deficiency. As iron deficiency progresses, nails become thin, flat and often spoon shaped (koilonychia). The third and fourth fingernails are most commonly affected.

Mucous membrane changes include absent or atrophic tongue papillae, glossodynia, aphthous stomatitis and angular stomatitis. Hair becomes brittle, dry and lustreless with focally narrow or split hair shafts. The association between iron deficiency and hair loss remains controversial [7,8].

Clinical variants
Plummer–Vinson syndrome is characterised by dysphagia, iron deficiency anaemia and oesophageal webs. It is considered a pre-cancerous condition due to its association with carcinoma of the mouth and upper respiratory tract.

Differential diagnosis
Deficiencies in folate, riboflavin, niacin and vitamin B$_{12}$ can frequently mimic iron deficiency.

Complications and co-morbidities
Severe and chronic iron deficiency can lead to cardiomyopathy and cardiac failure. The mechanism by which anaemia contributes to cardiomyopathy is not fully understood, but a combination of inadequate myocyte perfusion and increased cardiac output to maintain peripheral perfusion is thought to play a role. Cerebral sinovenous thrombosis is another reported complication of iron deficiency [9].

Disease course and prognosis
The mucocutaneous and haematological manifestations of iron deficiency are responsive to iron supplementation.

Investigations
Iron-deficient individuals develop a characteristic microcytic anaemia, with a low haemoglobin, low haematocrit, low mean corpuscular volume (MCV) and low mean corpuscular haemoglobin concentration (MCHC). If a peripheral blood smear is performed, red blood cells appear microcytic and hypochromatic. Low serum iron, low ferritin and high total iron binding capacity (TIBC) are diagnostic of iron deficiency.

Management
The recommended daily intake of iron depends on age and sex: 11 mg/day for infants aged 7–12 months, 7–11 mg/day for children aged 1–13 years, 15 mg/day for adolescent females aged 14–18 years as they begin menstruation, 11 mg/day for adolescent males, 18 mg/day for adult women and 8 mg/day for adult men. Pregnant women should increase iron intake to 27 mg/day.

Treating the underlying cause of iron deficiency is critical. In the case of chronic bleeding, if there is continued blood loss, iron supplementation may not be sufficient to normalise iron levels. Enteral supplementation with ferrous sulphate is recommended. In children, the treatment dose is 1–6 mg/kg/day, depending on the severity of deficiency; 1–2 mg/kg/day dosing can be used to prevent deficiency. Adult treatment of iron deficiency is with 60–65 mg 2–4 times daily, with prophylaxis being 60–65 mg once daily. Common practice has been to encourage concurrent vitamin C intake to facilitate absorption of iron. However, results from a recent randomised clinical trial demonstrated that iron supplementation alone was as effective as iron combined with vitamin C supplementation in the treatment of iron deficiency anaemia [10].

Zinc

Zinc deficiency

Definition and nomenclature
Zinc is an essential mineral that is utilised in over 200 metalloenzymes and plays an important role in many of the body's biochemical processes.

Synonyms and inclusions
- Acrodermatitis enteropathica
- Transient neonatal zinc deficiency

Introduction and general description
Zinc is an essential trace element that is found in most animal products, legumes, whole grains and dairy products. About 10–30% of dietary zinc is absorbed by a transcellular zinc-specific transporter, Zip4, which is found in the small intestine. Zinc deficiency can be inherited (acrodermatitis enteropathica) or acquired. The classic triad of zinc deficiency is diarrhoea, alopecia and a periorificial and acral eruption.

Epidemiology
Incidence and prevalence
About 17% of the world's population is at risk for inadequate dietary zinc intake [11]. The prevalence of acrodermatitis enteropathica is 1–9 per 1 000 000, with a worldwide incidence of 5 per 500 000 children [12].

Age
Acrodermatitis enteropathica and transient neonatal zinc deficiency present in infancy while acquired zinc deficiency can occur at any age.

Sex
There is no sex predilection for zinc deficiency.

Ethnicity
There is no ethnic predilection for zinc deficiency.

Associated diseases
An acrodermatitis enteropathica-like eruption has been described as a presenting sign of cystic fibrosis [13].

Pathophysiology
Predisposing factors
Acquired zinc deficiency is more common than acrodermatitis enteropathica, the inherited form of zinc deficiency. Factors that result in decreased dietary intake, decreased absorption or increased elimination can lead to zinc deficiency. Anorexia nervosa, alcoholism, vegetarianism and inadequately supplemented total parenteral nutrition represent risk factors for decreased dietary intake of zinc. Phytates in grains and legumes bind zinc and inhibit intestinal absorption. As such, diets high in grains and low in meats, notably in South-East Asia, sub-Saharan Africa and rural areas of the Middle East, may result in zinc deficiency. Acquired zinc deficiency has also been seen in a child placed on a liquid ketogenic diet for severe epilepsy [14].

Gastrointestinal disorders such as inflammatory bowel disease, coeliac disease, short bowel syndrome, chronic diarrhoea and gastric bypass surgery can disrupt intestinal zinc absorption. Increased zinc elimination can be observed in the setting of alcoholism, malignancy, burns, infections, pregnancy and renal disease. Medications including diuretics, penicillamine and valproate may decrease serum zinc levels.

Premature infants are at high risk for developing zinc deficiency. Not only do premature infants have higher metabolic demands, they also have inadequate stores since maternal transfer of zinc typically occurs during the last 10 weeks of gestation. Moreover, immature gut epithelium absorbs zinc poorly and premature infants suffer greater urinary, faecal and cutaneous zinc losses compared with full-term infants.

Breastfed infants with acrodermatitis enteropathica present later than formula-fed infants. This is a consequence of superior zinc absorption from human milk over bovine milk. The reason for this difference is unknown; however, it has been postulated that a high molecular weight protein associated with zinc in bovine milk hinders absorption.

Some mothers carry mutations in mammary gland zinc transporters, thus reducing the amount of zinc secreted into breast milk and predisposing infants to zinc deficiency while they are still being breastfed. This presentation has been termed 'transient neonatal zinc deficiency', or more specifically, 'transient zinc deficiency from low maternal breast milk zinc levels' [15].

Genetics

Acrodermatitis enteropathica is an autosomal recessive disorder caused by a mutation in the intestinal zinc transporter gene, *SLC39A4*, found on chromosome 8q24.3. This gene encodes for a ZIP4 transporter on enterocytes.

A maternal mutation in *SLC30A2*, found on chromosome 1p36.11, which encodes for zinc transporter ZnT-2 in epithelial mammary gland cells, results in decreased secretion of zinc into breast milk. Clinicians should provide counselling to families indicating that this condition can occur with subsequent children who are exclusively breastfed by an affected mother.

Clinical features
History

Acrodermatitis enteropathica manifests as breastfeeding infants are weaned from the breast, or between the fourth and tenth weeks of life in formula-fed infants. Infants are often described as listless and apathetic.

Presentation

The classic clinical triad of acrodermatitis enteropathica is diarrhoea, alopecia and a periorificial and acral cutaneous eruption. Children commonly present with symmetrical, eczematous plaques that become vesicular, bullous, pustular or erosive with characteristic crusting at the edges. The perioral eruption usually spares the upper lip, giving it a 'U-shaped' or 'horseshoe-shaped' appearance (Figure 61.13). Superinfection with bacteria (especially *Staphylococcus aureus*) and yeast (*Candida albicans*) can occur because of immune abnormalities. Hair is dry and brittle, and large areas of alopecia may arise. Other cutaneous findings include angular cheilitis, paronychia, delayed wound healing and vitiligo-like hypopigmentation [16].

Infants with transient zinc deficiency from low maternal breast milk can present with similar lesions to those with acrodermatitis enteropathica [17], although unique presentations with annular

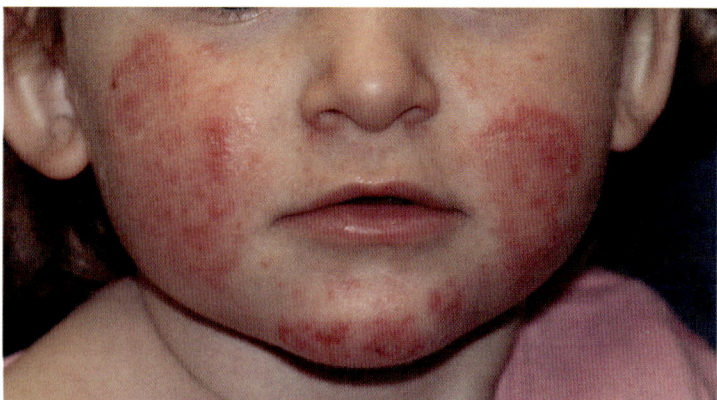

Figure 61.13 Facial eruption of acrodermatitis enteropathica. Note the U-shaped distribution.

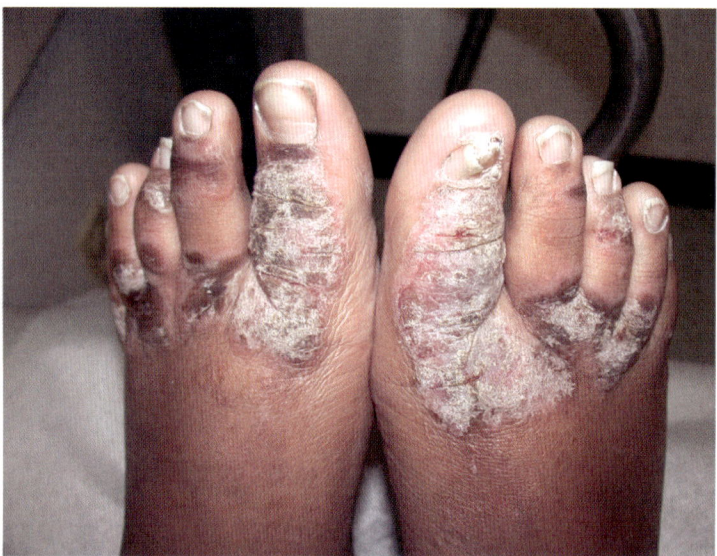

Figure 61.14 Psoriasiform plaques on the extremities of this patient with acquired zinc deficiency associated with nephrotic syndrome.

papulosquamous plaques on the facial cheeks and trunk have been described in the literature [15].

Mild zinc deficiency presents in children and adolescents with a psoriasiform dermatitis on the hands, feet and knees. Growth retardation, hypogonadism in males, abnormal dark adaptation and dysgeusia are also seen.

Clinical variants

A form of zinc deficiency associated with nephrotic syndrome has been reported [18] (Figure 61.14).

Differential diagnosis

The differential diagnosis of acrodermatitis enteropathica or acquired zinc deficiency includes psoriasis, seborrhoeic dermatitis, biotin deficiency, kwashiorkor and irritant dermatitis. Acrodermatitis dysmetabolica is an acrodermatitis enteropathica-like eruption reported in association with methylmalonic aciduria, propionic aciduria, maple syrup urine disease, citrullinaemia, ornithine transcarbamylase deficiency and glutaric aciduria type I [19].

Complications and co-morbidities
Zinc deficiency can be complicated by infection and may be fatal if untreated.

The *SLC30A2* gene implicated in transient zinc deficiency from low maternal breast milk zinc levels is present in highest concentration in placental tissue; low zinc levels in placental tissue and amniotic fluid are correlated with oligohydramnios, suggesting a possible link between both conditions in affected children [20].

Disease course and prognosis
Rapid clinical improvement within 24–48 h is expected with zinc supplementation. If untreated, zinc deficiency ultimately can be fatal.

Investigations
Diagnosis is confirmed by a combination of clinical and laboratory findings. Low zinc levels (<70 µg/dL fasting or <65 g/dL non-fasting) are diagnostic, but obtaining an accurate level can be challenging. Zinc levels can vary with inflammation, stress, trauma, time of day and phlebotomy method. It should be measured in the morning, and care should be taken to ensure the needles, catheters, rubber stoppers and collection tubes do not contain zinc, and that the sample is not haemolysed. Hypoalbuminaemia may contribute to a low zinc level and therefore serum albumin should be measured. Measurement of alkaline phosphatase, a zinc-dependent enzyme, can be helpful.

To confirm the diagnosis of transient zinc deficiency from low maternal breast milk levels, both the mother's serum and breast milk zinc levels should be obtained, in addition to the infant's serum zinc levels.

Skin biopsies are not diagnostic, but often show psoriasiform hyperplasia with confluent parakeratosis, spongiosis, pallor of the upper epidermis and focal dyskeratosis.

Management
The recommended dietary intake of zinc is 2–3 mg/day for children up to 3 years of age, 5 mg/day for children 4–8 years of age and 8 mg/day for children 9–14 years of age. Adolescents and adults require 8–13 mg/day.

Zinc deficiency is managed with enteral supplementation (zinc sulphate or zinc gluconate) or parenteral supplementation (zinc chloride). Patients with acrodermatitis enteropathica require lifelong supplementation with 3 mg/kg/day of elemental zinc (50 mg elemental zinc per 220 mg zinc sulphate; 50 mg elemental zinc per 50 mg zinc gluconate). It is important to differentiate acrodermatitis enteropathica from transient zinc deficiency from low maternal breast milk zinc levels, since the latter requires zinc supplementation only for the duration of breastfeeding. Supplementation for acquired zinc deficiency ranges from 0.5 to 1.0 mg/kg/day of elemental zinc for children and up to 15–30 mg elemental zinc per day for adults. If deficiency is secondary to intestinal malabsorption, higher doses may be necessary.

Copper

Copper deficiency

Definition and nomenclature
Copper is an essential co-factor for several metalloenzymes in the human body, including tyrosinase and lysyl oxidase.

Synonyms and inclusions
- Menkes disease
- Menkes syndrome
- Menkes kinky hair syndrome
- Kinky hair disease
- Steely hair disease
- Copper transport disease
- Tricholipodystrophy

Introduction and general description
Copper-rich foods include chocolate, dark leafy greens, eggs, beef and pork liver, whole grains, fish and oysters. Absorption of copper occurs through the intestinal copper transporter ATP7A. Deficiency states result from decreased absorption or decreased dietary intake, and are characterised by various neurological, dermatological and musculoskeletal abnormalities. Copper deficiency in Menkes disease is related to a congenital defect in copper transport.

Epidemiology
Incidence and prevalence
The birth incidence of Menkes disease is 1 per 300 000 in Europe and 1 per 360 000 in Japan [21,22]. The prevalence and incidence of acquired copper deficiency after roux-en-Y gastric bypass is 9.6% and 18.8%, respectively [23].

Age
Menkes disease presents at 2–3 months of age. Acquired copper deficiency can manifest at any age if predisposing factors are present.

Sex
Menkes disease is an X-linked recessively inherited disorder affecting males. Females are unaffected carriers.

Ethnicity
There is no ethnic predilection for either inherited or acquired copper deficiency.

Pathophysiology
Predisposing factors
Decreased dietary intake from malnutrition or chronic unsupplemented parenteral nutrition can lead to acquired copper deficiency. Individuals with excessive intake of iron, zinc, antacids or vitamin C can develop copper deficiency due to inhibition of intestinal copper absorption. Gastric bypass surgery, short gut syndrome, cystic fibrosis and coeliac disease also place individuals at risk for impaired copper absorption.

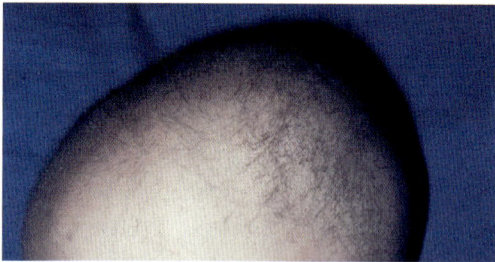

Figure 61.15 Menkes syndrome: pale skin and kinky hair. Reproduced from [28] with permission from John Wiley & Sons.

Genetics
Menkes disease is an X-linked recessive disorder caused by a mutation in *ATP7A*, which encodes for a copper transporting ATPase-polypeptide.

Clinical features
History
Preterm labour, large cephalic haematomas, hypothermia, hypoglycaemia, fractures and prolonged neonatal jaundice can be early signs of Menkes disease. A case of neonatal erythroderma has been reported in Menkes disease [24]. Classic symptoms usually present at 2–3 months of age. Adults with acquired copper deficiency tend to have a history of predisposing factors, but onset of clinical symptoms of deficiency may take months to years.

Presentation
The primary manifestation of acquired copper deficiency is a myeloneuropathy that affects both sensory and motor nerves. Patients experience progressive symmetrical sensory loss in addition to weakness of the upper and lower extremities [25,26]. Progression to optic neuropathy, with possible permanent vision loss, can occur if the deficiency is left untreated [27]. Other symptoms include hypopigmentation of the hair and skin, and bony abnormalities, such as osteoporosis, fractures and flaring of the anterior ribs.

At 2–3 months of age, children with Menkes disease present with loss of developmental milestones, hypotonia, seizures and failure to thrive. These infants have a characteristic cherubic appearance with a depressed nasal bridge, pudgy cheeks, 'Cupid's bow' upper lip and doughy skin. The skin is depigmented and feels soft and inelastic, especially at the nape of the neck, axillae and trunk (Figure 61.15). Hair changes can be the first sign of disease at 1–2 months of age. Scalp and eyebrow hair resemble steel wool, appearing short, sparse, lustreless, tangled and depigmented. Pili torti (Chapter 66) is the classic finding on trichogram (Figure 61.16), but monilethrix (Chapter 66) can also be seen. A high arched palate with delayed tooth eruption may be observed on oral examination. Osteoporosis, scalloping of the posterior aspects of the vertebral bodies, subperiosteal new bone formation, ossification of sutures, diaphyseal periosteal reaction, metaphyseal widening and lateral spur formation are frequent bone findings, most often affecting the long bones and the skull. Subdural haematomas, metaphyseal widening and frequent bony fractures can mimic child abuse. Hydronephrosis, hydroureter and bladder diverticula are common renal abnormalities.

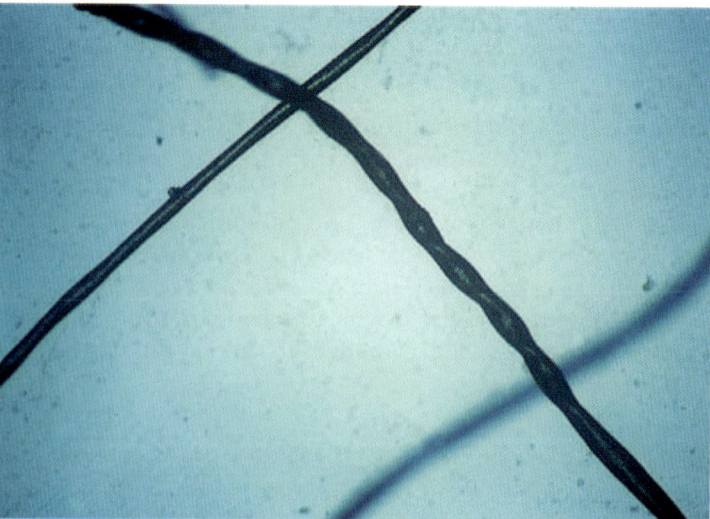

Figure 61.16 Menkes syndrome: pili torti of patient in Figure 61.15. Reproduced from [28] with permission from John Wiley & Sons.

As in acquired copper deficiency, neurological deficits are a prominent feature of Menkes disease. Infants have severe truncal hypotonia with poor head control but increased tone in the extremities. Deep tendon reflexes are increased. Severe developmental delay occurs, with children only able to smile and babble. Visual fixation and tracking are impaired and optic discs are pale on examination. Hearing, suck and cry remain normal. Seizures can be difficult to treat. Death occurs around 3–4 years of age secondary to elongation and tortuosity of large blood vessels and resultant vascular complications.

Differential diagnosis
The anaemia and neutropenia of acquired copper deficiency should be distinguished from myelodysplastic syndrome. Cutis laxa, child abuse, osteogenesis imperfecta and Ehlers–Danlos syndrome may mimic Menkes syndrome clinically.

Complications and co-morbidities
Neurological manifestations are prominent in both acquired copper deficiency and Menkes disease. Sensory and motor myeloneuropathy occurs in acquired copper deficiency. Infants with Menkes disease have severe truncal hypotonia, increased deep tendon reflexes and significant developmental delay. Seizures are also common in Menkes disease.

Disease course and prognosis
Copper supplementation in acquired copper deficiency can prevent further neurological degeneration but does not guarantee recovery of lost function. Vision loss from optic neuropathy can be permanent [27].

For Menkes disease, if treatment is initiated during the neonatal period or early infancy, neurological deterioration can be mitigated. However, once disease is present, it may not be reversed [29,30].

Investigations
In acquired copper deficiency, normocytic or macrocytic anaemia and neutropenia are prominent findings [31]. Hypocupraemia and hypoceruloplasminaemia may also be noted.

Diagnosis of Menkes disease is made by a combination of clinical, laboratory and genetic testing. Hypocupraemia and hypoceruloplasminaemia are seen. Copper and ceruloplasmin can be low in healthy neonates. Dopamine β-hydroxylase is a copper-dependent enzyme and measurement of the ratio of plasma dihydroxyphenylalanine (DOPA) to dihydroxyphenylglycol may be useful in diagnosing Menkes disease [32]. Testing for mutations in *ATP7A* can confirm the diagnosis of Menkes disease.

Management
The recommended daily intake of copper for infants up to 12 months of age is 200–220 µg/day. Children 1–13 years of age require 340–700 µg/day, with the recommended intake increasing with age. Adolescents and adults require 890–900 µg/day.

Treatment of copper deficiency includes copper supplementation and addressing the underlying cause. Children with Menkes disease require lifelong supplementation with parenteral copper, usually cupric chloride, in order to bypass impaired intestinal absorption. Vitamin C has been reported to prevent binding of copper to metallothionein, theoretically increasing the availability of copper for absorption. The evidence for use of vitamin C in Menkes disease is limited [33]. In acquired copper deficiency, intravenous copper can be used to correct deficiency rapidly and copper gluconate can be used for long-term enteral supplementation.

Selenium

Selenium is a necessary component of several proteins, known as selenoproteins, including glutathione peroxidase, thioredoxin reductase and iodothyronine diodinase. Selenium is obtained through dietary intake of selenium-rich foods such as seafood, red meat, egg yolks, grains, Brazil nuts and chicken. The amount of selenium in plant-based food correlates with the amount found in the soil from which it was grown. Selenium exists in either organic or inorganic forms. The inorganic form of selenium or selenite is well absorbed, but not as well retained in the body as the organic forms, selenomethionine or selenocystine.

Selenium deficiency

Definition and nomenclature
Selenium deficiency, also known as Keshan disease, is caused by inadequate intake, defective absorption or increased losses.

Synonyms and inclusions
- Keshan disease
- Kashin–Beck disease

Epidemiology
Incidence and prevalence
Selenium deficiency is uncommon. The highest incidence is reported in parts of China where the soil is selenium deficient.

Age
Children are more likely to be affected by Keshan disease.

Sex
Women of childbearing age are more likely to be affected by Keshan disease.

Ethnicity
There is no ethnic predilection for selenium deficiency.

Associated diseases
Selenium deficiency has been associated with the development of dilated cardiomyopathy in patients with recessive dystrophic epidermolysis bullosa. Although no causative link has been identified, selenium deficiency likely represents one of multiple factors that predispose these patients to cardiomyopathy [34]. Primary heart disease in systemic sclerosis is associated with selenium deficiency and selenium testing is recommended when cardiac involvement is suspected [35].

Pathophysiology
Predisposing factors
Patients receiving total parenteral nutrition require selenium supplementation and deficiency may result if there is inadequate parenteral selenium [36]. Protein-restrictive diets can increase the risk of developing selenium deficiency. Gastrointestinal diseases may lead to decreased selenium absorption or increased selenium excretion [37]. In a prospective observational study of 50 children and young adults with congenital ichthyoses from Spain, selenium was the most common micronutrient deficiency (seen in 34%) followed by iron, vitamin D and zinc [38].

Environmental factors
If soil is selenium deficient, then the grains grown in the soil may also be selenium deficient. Certain regions of China including Keshan and Tibet have documented low soil selenium levels, and selenium deficiency is endemic in these regions. Heavy erosion of surface soil can lead to selenium-deficient soil because of trace mineral depletion [39].

Clinical features
History
Patients with selenium deficiency will commonly present with a history of a predisposing factor for deficiency. It is important to elicit whether a patient has lived in or travelled to a selenium deficiency endemic region. Keshan disease and Kashin–Beck disease have only been described in endemic areas of Asia.

Presentation
Keshan disease is characterised by a multifocal myocarditis that can progress to a fatal cardiomyopathy. Acute or chronic cardiac dysfunction, cardiomegaly, arrhythmias and electrocardiographic abnormalities have been described. Extracardiac findings include muscle pain or weakness, erythrocyte macrocytosis without anaemia, pancreatic exocrine dysfunction, hepatic congestion and mesenteric lymphadenosis. Cutaneous manifestations of Keshan disease are non-specific and include Terry nails-like white nail beds and hypopigmentation of the skin and hair.

Kashin–Beck disease describes selenium deficiency with predominantly bony disease. This osteoarthropathy affects the epiphyseal and articular cartilage and the epiphyseal growth plates. Enlarged joints and shortened fingers and toes may be noted.

Clinical variants
- Keshan disease.
- Kashin–Beck disease.

Differential diagnosis
The differential diagnosis for Keshan disease includes hepatic cirrhosis and kwashiorkor. Kashin–Beck disease should be distinguished from rickets.

Complications and co-morbidities
Myocarditis from Keshan disease can lead to long-term cardiac dysfunction and cardiomyopathy.

Disease course and prognosis
If diagnosed and treated early, the long-term prognosis for selenium deficiency is good and cutaneous findings respond well to supplementation. If left undiagnosed or untreated, permanent cardiac damage and cardiomyopathy may result.

Investigations
Measurement of plasma selenium levels and glutathione peroxidase activity confirms the diagnosis of selenium deficiency.

Management
For children less than 3 years of age, the recommended daily intake of selenium is 15–20 μg/day. Children 3–13 years of age require 20–40 μg/day. The recommended intake for adolescents and adults is 55 μg/day, but women who are pregnant or breastfeeding should increase to 60 and 70 μg/day, respectively.

Treatment is with selenium supplementation enterally or parenterally. Enteral selenium is available as selenomethionine, selenium-enriched yeast or sodium selenite. Parenteral selenium supplementation of 5–7 μg/kg/day can be used for acute correction of selenium deficiency [40].

Selenium excess

Definition
Selenium toxicity results from excess ingestion of selenium, whether intentional or unintentional.

Epidemiology
Incidence and prevalence
Selenium toxicity is not common. With the exception of occurrences in endemic areas such as Hubei in China, sporadic outbreaks have been reported from increased dietary intake.

Age
There is no age predilection for selenium excess.

Sex
There is no sex predilection for selenium excess.

Ethnicity
There is no ethnic predilection for selenium excess.

Pathophysiology
Predisposing factors
Selenium toxicity has been reported as a consequence of excess supplement ingestion [41,42]. Other documented causes include ingestion of glass blue used in the manufacturing of stained glass [43], selenite broth used to isolate *Salmonella* and gun blueing agent used for finishing firearms [44].

Environmental factors
Endemic selenium toxicity was described in Enshi County in Hubei, China, in the 1960s as a result of selenium-contaminated soil. Selenium-containing coal was used to fertilise the soil in that region [45].

Clinical features
History
A thorough history, including use of nutritional supplements, occupation history and hobbies, can reveal where exposure may have occurred.

Presentation
White horizontal streaks appear on the surface of nails and as the nails become increasingly brittle, breakage eventually leads to nail loss. New nail growth is also fragile, although the nails can be thickened with a rough surface. Hair is brittle and may be associated with an exfoliative dermatitis on the scalp. Teeth, hair and nails can develop a reddish hue. The neck and extremities become red and swollen and develop blisters and slow-healing ulcerations.

Acute selenium toxicity can be fatal. Neurological signs include peripheral paraesthesias, hyperreflexia, numbness, seizures and paralysis. Acute tubular necrosis leading to acute renal failure requiring dialysis has been reported [46]. Nausea, vomiting, diarrhoea, hypersalivation, garlic or sour-milk smelling breath and severe corrosive gastritis with resultant deep gastric ulcers can occur.

Complications and co-morbidities
Acute selenium toxicity is complicated primarily by neurological deficits, including peripheral anaesthesia, seizures and paralysis.

Disease course and prognosis
The cutaneous findings of selenium toxicity are reversible once the source of excess selenium is removed. Renal and neurological dysfunction can be permanent if irreversible organ damage has occurred.

Investigations
Plasma selenium levels are diagnostic of selenium toxicity.

Management
For children less than 3 years of age, the recommended daily intake of selenium is 15–20 μg/day. Children 3–13 years of age require 20–40 μg/day. The recommended intake for adolescents and adults is 55 μg/day, but women who are pregnant or breastfeeding should increase to 60 and 70 μg/day, respectively.

Treatment involves supportive management of the complications of toxicity such as gastric ulcers and acute renal failure. Removing the source of excess selenium is essential.

Manganese

Manganese deficiency and excess

Definition and nomenclature
Manganese functions as an important co-factor for pyruvate carboxylase and superoxide dismutase and activates glycosyl-transferases necessary for glycoprotein and glycosaminoglycan synthesis.

Synonyms and inclusions
• Manganese excess: manganism

Introduction and general description
Manganese is found in nuts, leafy greens, legumes, whole grains and tea. Humans absorb about 5% of dietary manganese but the mechanism is poorly understood. Iron, magnesium and calcium may reduce manganese absorption. Manganese deficiency results from inadequate dietary intake, while manganese excess is due to excessive consumption. Both manganese deficiency and excess are uncommon.

Epidemiology
Incidence and prevalence
Manganese deficiency and excess are extremely uncommon.

Age
There is no age predilection for either manganese deficiency or excess.

Sex
There is no sex predilection for either manganese deficiency or excess.

Ethnicity
There is no ethnic predilection for either manganese deficiency or excess.

Pathophysiology
Predisposing factors
Long-term parenteral nutrition predisposes individuals to an imbalance in manganese through either inadequate or excess supplementation. Manganese toxicity has been reported after ingestion of well water with toxic levels of manganese [47,48], with abuse of a combination of ephedrine, acetylsalicylic acid and potassium permanganate, also known as 'Russian Cocktail' [49], and with ingestion of incorrectly manufactured Epsom salts [50]. Selenium may be protective against manganese toxicity, specifically in neonates at risk for manganese neurotoxicity from prenatal exposure [51].

Clinical features
History
The cause of manganese deficiency or excess may be elicited by history but this may not be apparent initially. Patients with manganese deficiency may present with nausea, vomiting and weight loss.

Presentation
The cutaneous manifestations of manganese deficiency are non-specific and include mild dermatitis, lightening of hair colour, miliaria crystallina and slowed hair and nail growth.

There are no characteristic cutaneous changes associated with manganism. Neurological symptoms predominate, ranging from hyperactivity and oppositional behaviour [52] to Parkinson-like symptoms [53].

Complications and co-morbidities
Manganism can result in neurological symptoms that mimic Parkinson disease.

Disease course and prognosis
The symptoms of manganese deficiency are reversible with supplementation. Removing the source of manganese toxicity may lead to resolution of symptoms, but disease can sometimes progress even without further exposure [54].

Investigations
Blood manganese levels are used to diagnose manganese deficiency or manganism.

Management
Adequate intake of manganese for children is 1.2–1.5 mg/day. Adolescents require 1.6–1.8 mg/day, while adults require 1.8–2.3 mg/day.

Manganese deficiency is treated with supplementation. Calcium disodium ethylenediamine tetra-acetate (CaEDTA) increases urinary excretion of manganese by 3.8 times and can be used as chelation therapy in manganism [55]. Eliminating the source of excess manganese is essential.

ESSENTIAL FATTY ACIDS

Essential fatty acid deficiency

Definition and nomenclature

Synonyms and inclusions
• Essential fatty acid: EFA
• Linoleic acid (18:2n-6): LA
• α-linolenic acid (18:3n-3): ALA

Introduction and general description
Fatty acids are composed of variable-length hydrocarbon chains that have methyl and carboxyl groups at either end. They may be unsaturated (with at least one double bond) or saturated (without

double bonds) in the acyl chain. The human body can make most fatty acids or can obtain them from the diet. However, two polyunsaturated fatty acids, linoleic acid (LA; 18:2n-6, an n-6 fatty acid) and α-linolenic acid (ALA: 18:3n-3, an n-3 fatty acid) cannot be synthesised because humans lack the desaturase enzymes that insert double bonds into the n-6 and n-3 positions of the hydrocarbon chains. These fatty acids are instead obtained solely from the diet and are therefore deemed essential fatty acids (EFAs) [1,2].

The EFAs, LA and ALA are desaturated and elongated into longer-chain fatty acids, with LA specifically converted to arachidonic acid (AA; 20:4n-6) and ALA converted to docosahexaenoic acid (DHA; 22:6n-3) and eicosapentaenoic acid (EPA; 20:5n-3) [1,3]. It is from these longer-chain fatty acids that eicosanoids (e.g. prostaglandins, thromboxanes and leukotrienes), which behave as inflammatory mediators and growth factors, are generated [1,4]. The n-6 eicosanoids derived from AA are pro-inflammatory, whereas the n-3 eicosanoids generated from EFA are anti-inflammatory [5]. EFAs are also critical bioactive and structural components of phospholipid membranes that ensure normal physiological function of virtually every tissue including the epidermal barrier. It is therefore not surprising that prolonged EFA deficiency (EFAD) is characterised by a wide variety of clinical manifestations [1,2] including a characteristic dry scaly rash, alopecia, impaired wound healing, liver dysfunction related to mitochondrial dysfunction and diminished adenosine triphosphate synthesis, and increased susceptibility to infections. In infants and children it causes reduced growth rates as well as altered neural and retinal development.

Epidemiology
Incidence and prevalence
EFAD is rarely diagnosed in healthy adults or children in the 21st century, especially when fat intake as part of a regular diet is unrestricted. This is uncommon because close to 10% of adipose tissue is composed of LA, which can be mobilised in patients with adequate fat stores to prevent EFAD when exogenous fat is insufficient [6]. However, it has been demonstrated to occur in individuals ingesting low-fat diets, on restricted or fat-free parenteral nutrition, or with severe fat malabsorption [7]. There is very little reported in the literature on prevalence of EFAD given infrequent testing and previous lack of sensitive detection methods, but in a study of 47 patients with chronic intestinal disease (25 with Crohn's disease, 11 with ulcerative colitis, 7 with short bowel syndrome, 4 with coeliac disease), >25% had laboratory evidence of EFAD [8]. Strandvik *et al.* evaluated 110 cystic fibrosis patients on a normal diet and found that those with severe mutations in *CFTR* had significantly lower concentrations of LA and DHA regardless of pancreatic function [9]. Finally, it has been reported that up to 60% of infants who receive lipid-restricted parenteral nutrition may develop EFAD [**10**,11].

Age
There is no reported age predilection for acquired EFAD, although infants, who do not efficiently convert lipid precursors into EFAs, are particularly susceptible, with preterm infants having an even higher risk secondary to limited fat stores [**10**,11–13].

Sex
There is no sex predilection for acquired EFAD.

Ethnicity
There is no ethnic predilection for acquired EFAD.

Associated diseases
Please see 'Predisposing factors' later for a broad description of associated diseases. In addition, recent studies suggest that an aetiological basis of neuropsychiatric disorders is the dysregulation of phospholipid metabolism. The literature suggests the clinical signs and symptoms of EFAD occur more frequently in children with attention deficit hyperactivity disorder (ADHD) and autism spectrum disorder (ASD) [14–16].

Pathophysiology
Predisposing factors
Acquired or secondary causes of EFAD include chronic malnutrition, gastrointestinal disorders that lead to fat malabsorption, and lipid-restricted parenteral nutrition. Any gastrointestinal condition that interferes with digestion, absorption and/or metabolism of EFAs may lead to EFAD. This includes but is not limited to bowel resection, especially involving the distal jejunum and ileum, bariatric procedures, inflammatory bowel disease, short bowel syndrome, coeliac disease, cholestatic liver disease, cystic fibrosis and pancreatic insufficiency [17]. Lipid-restricted parenteral nutrition is proactively prescribed in patients with significant hypertriglyceridemia to decrease the risk of pancreatitis and to prevent the development of intestinal failure-associated liver disease (ILFAD). The latter is often seen with long-term use of lipid injectable emulsion (ILE) made primarily from soybeans in those receiving long-term parenteral nutrition [17,18]. A recently recognised risk factor for the development of EFAD is related to the increasing incidence of ILE product shortages [19].

Genetics
In addition to secondary aetiologies, clinical manifestations of EFAD are also seen in genetic deficiencies in elongase and desaturase enzymes that metabolise LA and ALA into AA and DHA end-products. Typical examples include Sjögren–Larsson syndrome and certain forms of acrodermatitis enteropathica, in which patients develop intellectual disability, extensive ichthyosis and altered prostaglandin metabolism despite sufficient intake of EFAs [20].

In addition, there is genetic variability among two key enzymes in EFA metabolism, delta 6 desaturase (FADS2) and delta 5 desaturase (FADS1), with two commonly occurring haplotypes that differ significantly in their ability to convert LA and ALA to AA, DHA and EPA [21]. They are associated with variability of serum concentrations of fatty acids, but whether either of these is preferentially linked to EFAD is unknown [22].

Clinical features
History
EFAD can be avoided if at least 2–4% of total caloric intake is from LA and 0.25–0.5% is from ALA, and it is not difficult for healthy individuals to meet these requirements [23–25]. Given the low incidence of EFAD, a high degree of suspicion is warranted, especially since biochemical abnormalities often precede the development of obvious clinical signs. Physicians should consider this diagnosis in patients with a dry and scaly rash with severely limited intake,

digestion, absorption and/or metabolism of fat, as in the clinical conditions described previously. Special attention should also be paid to preterm infants and chronically malnourished individuals who have a propensity towards inadequate fat stores, and therefore greater reliance on exogenous fat. In infants receiving parenteral nutrition without fat, EFAD becomes clinically apparent within 1 week. In adults, it may present as early as within 10 days but may be delayed for up to 4–6 weeks [26–29]. Patients with chyle leaks who are maintained on very low-fat diets for at least 3 weeks are also at risk of EFAD [30–32]. Detection of physical signs suspicious of deficiency should prompt laboratory evaluation.

Presentation

In the initial description of EFAD, Burr and Burr reported in 1929 that rats on a fat-free diet had poor weight gain versus normally fed controls despite equivalent caloric intake, and developed excessive thirst and a scaly, dandruff-like rash on their paws and tails, followed by alopecia; these symptoms were reversible only with addition of LA [33]. In humans, Holt et al. first demonstrated in 1935 that infants on diets containing <0.1% calories from LA developed EFAD characterised by a dry, leathery and eczematous eruption, along with superficial erosions in the intertriginous zones [34].

Since these early investigations, a flurry of case reports towards the end of the 20th century, in infant and adult patients, established that EFAD may affect every organ system and manifest with a diverse set of clinical findings. The skin is the most frequently affected tissue and hallmark findings include a dry, thick, scaly and often eczematous dermatitis with flexural accentuation in a background of generalised, desquamating redness, coarse, sparse hair with the development of alopecia, brittle nails and poor wound healing. Hepatomegaly secondary to fatty infiltration of the liver is also common. Neurological deficits including weakness, reduced sensation and blurry vision occur infrequently. EFAD in infants and children is often associated with poor growth and increased susceptibility to infection [7,17,35,36].

Differential diagnosis

It is important to realise that EFAD may occur with many other nutritional deficiencies including the B vitamins, vitamin C and zinc. Many of these other deficiencies may present with similar findings [17].

Disease course and prognosis

With effective repletion, clinical and laboratory abnormalities of EFAD can reverse relatively quickly [7,17,36].

Investigations

There are no universally defined criteria for at-risk screening for EFAD, although some suggest baseline screening in selected patients who are receiving fat-free parenteral nutrition for >4 weeks and up to every 3–4 months. Regardless, it is important to note that laboratory findings associated with EFAD appear before clinical signs and symptoms are apparent [17,36]. These include decreased plasma levels of LA and ALA and an elevated triene:tetraene (T:T) ratio, the latter indicating biochemical evidence of EFAD. Triene and tetraenes are hydrocarbons with 3 and 4 double bonds between carbon atoms, respectively. As noted earlier, desaturases

that catalyse formation of these double bonds and elongases that extend hydrocarbon chains act on LA to yield AA and on ALA to yield DHA and EPA [1,3]. When levels of LA and ALA are inadequate, the non-essential n-9 fatty acid oleic acid (18:1n-9) becomes the substrate for these enzymes, driving production of Mead acid (20:3n-9), a triene. Taken together with the decreased production of AA (tetraene) from LA, the result is an elevated T:T ratio [7,36]. Traditionally, a T:T ratio >0.2 is considered to be diagnostic of EFAD and will manifest before any other laboratory anomalies or clinical symptoms [37]. More recent assays are using thresholds an order of magnitude lower than 0.2, based on improved methods of measuring EFA levels, and are reporting reference ranges for the T:T ratio reflective of typical values and EFA intake of a given population [38,39]. Importantly, the T:T ratio does not account for ALA levels and may be affected by the EFA profile of the specific ILE that a patient is receiving. Some suggest that a complete fatty acid profile be obtained when evaluating for EFAD [7,39,40].

In addition to the T:T ratio, non-specific biochemical abnormalities are seen in EFAD. These include elevated liver enzymes, hyperlipidemia, thrombocytopenia and aberrant platelet aggregation [17]. Notably, these may also occur as a consequence of ILE administration [41].

While the T:T ratio is the gold standard diagnostic test for EFAD, a non-invasive, observational test known as the Fatty Acid Deficiency score (FAD) has been developed recently. The FAD correlates with laboratory findings of EFAD and measures seven clinically perceptible signs of EFAD including excessive thirst, frequent urination, dry skin, dry hair, soft or brittle nails, dandruff and rough, dry, bumpy skin [15,16].

Management

Patients with EFAD may be treated with parenteral nutrition formulations with ILE containing LA and ALA. It is recommended to provide at least 10% of total energy from polyunsaturated fat and 2–4% of total calories should be derived from LA [17,23–25]. For example, for patients treated with standard, soybean oil-based ILE that contains 50% LA, the minimum amount of fat to prevent EFAD is 100 g (i.e. 500 mL of 20% ILE) per week [42]. Greater amounts may be needed to treat pre-existing EFAD, although dosing guidelines regarding how much more ILE to administer are lacking [17]. Newer ILE formulations are blends of soybean oil and additional lipid components and thus have lower percentages of LA. These include Smoflipid® (Fresenius Kabi, Lake Zurich, IL, USA) that has 21.4% LA as well as medium-chain triglycerides, olive oil and fish oil; ClinOleic 20% (Baxter Corporation, Mississauga, ON, Canada) has 18.5% LA and also contains olive oil. To ensure adequate replacement, the clinician needs to calculate the amount of LA delivered based on the composition of the administered ILE [17,41]. Some recommend cycling parenteral nutrition to help meet EFA requirements. This approach takes advantage of the fact that human adipose tissue is 10% LA and therefore a substantial source of EFAs. With cycling, insulin secretion and lipogenesis are relatively suppressed when parenteral nutrition is hypocaloric or 'off', enabling release of LA from fat stores [6,7].

For patients receiving parenteral nutrition who cannot receive ILE, such as those with high risk of hypertriglyceridaemia or an allergy to ILE, oral and topical preparations with EFAs are alternative treatment options [17,36]. Richardson and Sgoutas reported that in 2 of 4 patients with EFAD receiving fat-free parenteral nutrition, oral LA supplementation in the form of safflower oil reversed the EFAD [43]. Oral EFA preparations are likely to be at least partially effective in patients with sufficient intestinal absorption. These patients should also be encouraged to consume foods rich in EFAs such as condiments containing corn, sesame, safflower, soybean or sunflower oils as well as fatty fish or omega-3 fatty acid supplements [17].

Data regarding the topical administration of LA containing oils have been mixed and some studies suggest that topical application has no impact on infant or adult EFAD [17,36]. However, in one study, topical application of sunflower seed oil was associated with rapid reversal of both clinical and laboratory findings of EFAD in two infants receiving fat-free parenteral nutrition. In another study, EFAD patients received topical sunflower or olive oil applied to the right or left arm, respectively, with resolution of the scaly rash and higher levels of LA in the right arm [35,44]. In another report, topical application of safflower oil in three infants on fat-free parenteral nutrition improved their scaly dermatitis but did not normalise their elevated T : T ratios [45].

Regardless of the method of EFA repletion, consensus guidelines for monitoring EFA status are lacking [17]. Some suggest evaluating T : T ratios and EFA levels every 2–4 weeks until normalisation, but the selected approach should be tailored based on clinical judgement.

Key references

The full list of references can be found in the online version at https://www.wiley.com/rooksdermatology10e

Nutrition

12 Sharma P, Rauf A, Matin A, Agarwal R, Tyagi P, Arora A. Handgrip strength as an important bed side tool to assess malnutrition in patient with liver disease. *J Clin Exp Hepatol* 2017;7:16–22.

14 United Nations Children's Fund (UNICEF), World Health Organization (WHO), International Bank for Reconstruction and Development/The World Bank. Levels and trends in child malnutrition: key findings of the 2021 edition of the joint child malnutrition estimates [Internet]. Geneva: WHO, 2021. https://data .unicef.org/resources/jme-report-2023/#:~:text=The%20UNICEF%2DWHO %2DWB%20Joint,2022%20for%20stunting%20and%20overweight (last accessed October 2022).

23 Larrazabal RB, Jr, Perez BMB, Masamayor EMI, Chiu HHC, Palileo-Villanueva LAM. The prevalence of malnutrition and analysis of related factors among adult patients with the Coronavirus Disease 2019 (COVID 19) in a tertiary government hospital: the MalnutriCoV study. *Clin Nutr ESPEN* 2021;42:98–104.

59 Dupont R, Longué M, Galinier A et al. Impact of micronutrient deficiency and malnutrition in systemic sclerosis: cohort study and literature review. *Autoimmun Rev* 2018;17:1081–9.

60 Rosato E, Gigante A, Gasperini ML, Proietti L, Muscaritoli M. Assessing malnutrition in systemic sclerosis with Global Leadership Initiative on Malnutrition and European Society of Clinical Nutrition and Metabolism Criteria. *J Parenter Enteral Nutr* 2021;45:618–24.

61 Türk İ, Cüzdan N, Çiftçi V, Arslan D, Doğan MC, Unal İ. Malnutrition, associated clinical factors, and depression in systemic sclerosis: a cross-sectional study. *Clin Rheumatol* 2020;39:57–67.

64 Million M, Diallo A, Raoult D. Gut microbiota and malnutrition. *Microb Pathog* 2017;106:127–38.

73 Bhutta ZA, Berkley JA, Bandsma RH, Kerac M, Trehan I, Briend A. Severe childhood malnutrition. *Nat Rev Dis Primers* 2017;3:1–18.

Vitamins

3 Bailey RL, West KP, Jr, Black RE. The epidemiology of global micronutrient deficiencies. *Ann Nutr Metab* 2015;66(Suppl. 2):22–33.

4 World Health Organization. Global prevalence of vitamin A deficiency in populations at risk 1995–2005: WHO global database on vitamin A deficiency. Geneva: WHO, 2009. http://apps.who.int/iris/bitstream/handle/10665/44110/9789241598019_eng.pdf;jsessionid=5E5FB253AD3D71F9C35343106FA2A145?sequence=1 (last accessed October 2022).

5 UNICEF. Vitamin A deficiency [Internet]. New York: UNICEF, 2019. https://data .unicef.org/topic/nutrition/vitamin-a-deficiency/ (last accessed October 2022).

13 Monshi B, Stockinger T, Vigl K, Richter L, Weihsengruber F, Rappersberger K. Phrynoderma and acquired acrodermatitis enteropathica in breastfeeding women after bariatric surgery. *J Dtsch Dermatol Ges* 2015;13:1147–54.

16 Arroyave G, Mejia LA, Aguilar JR. The effect of vitamin A fortification of sugar on the serum vitamin A levels of preschool Guatemalan children: a longitudinal evaluation. *Am J Clin Nutr* 1981;34:41–9.

17 Low JW, Mwanga ROM, Andrade M, Carey E, Ball A. Tackling vitamin A deficiency with biofortified sweetpotato in sub-Saharan Africa. *Glob Food Sec* 2017;14:23–30.

21 Virtamo J, Taylor PR, Kontto J et al. Effects of α-tocopherol and β-carotene supplementation on cancer incidence and mortality: 18-year post-intervention follow-up of the Alpha-Tocopherol, Beta-Carotene Cancer Prevention (ATBC) Study. *Int J Cancer* 2014;135:178–85.

32 Kazemi A, Mohammadi V, Aghababaee SK, Golzarand M, Clark CC, Babajafari S. Association of Vitamin D status with SARS-CoV-2 infection or COVID-19 severity: a systematic review and meta-analysis. *Adv Nutr* 2021;12:1636–58.

33 De Smet D, De Smet K, Herroelen P, Gryspeerdt S, Martens GA. Serum 25 (OH) D level on hospital admission associated with COVID-19 stage and mortality. *Am J Clin Path* 2021;155:381–8.

34 Radujkovic A, Hippchen T, Tiwari-Heckler S, Dreher S, Boxberger M, Merle U. Vitamin D deficiency and outcome of COVID-19 patients. *Nutrients* 2020;12:2757.

57 Kemnic TR, Coleman M. Vitamin E deficiency. *StatPearls [Internet]*. Treasure Island, FL: StatPearls Publishing, 2020. https://www.ncbi.nlm.nih.gov/books/NBK519051 (last accessed October 2022).

58 Traber MG. Vitamin E inadequacy in humans: causes and consequences. *Adv Nutr* 2014;5:503–14.

70 Dahlberg S, Schurgers L, Schött U, Kander T. Vitamin K deficiency in critical ill patients; a prospective observational study. *J Crit Care* 2019;49:105–9.

71 Anastasi E, Ialongo C, Labriola R, Ferraguti G, Lucarelli M, Angeloni A. Vitamin K deficiency and covid-19. *Scand J Clin Lab Invest* 2020;80:525–7.

90 Gibson RS. Principles of Nutritional Assessment. Third Edition. https://nutritionalassessment.org/ Email: Rosalind.Gibson@Otago.AC.NZ. Licensed under CC-BY-SA-4.0. Chapter on thiamine authored by KC Whitfield and chapter on riboflavin authored by K Pentieva. Last accessed July 2, 2023.

95 Zaenglein A, Martin A, Carlson L, Williams KE. Pellagra secondary to selective eating in a child with autism. *Pediatr Dermatol* 2020;37:698–700.

106 Brown MJ, Ameer MA, Beier K. Vitamin B6 deficiency. *StatPearls [Internet]*. Treasure Island, FL: StatPearls Publishing, 2020. https://europepmc.org/books/n/statpearls/article-31220/?extid=31985953&src=med (last accessed October 2022).

114 Pfeiffer CM, Sternberg MR, Zhang M et al. Folate status in the US population 20 y after the introduction of folic acid fortification. *Am J Clin Nutr* 2019;110:1088–97.

134 Kaur S, Goraya JS. Dermatologic findings of vitamin B12 deficiency in infants. *Pediatr Dermatol* 2018;35:796–9.

135 Verma VK, Vijayavarman V. A case report on hyperpigmentation in vitamin B12 deficiency. *Int J Res Med Sci* 2019;7:1944.

137 Rowe S, Carr AC. Global vitamin C status and prevalence of deficiency: a cause for concern? *Nutrients* 2020;12:2008.

139 Carr AC, Rowe S. Factors affecting vitamin C status and prevalence of deficiency: a global health perspective. *Nutrients* 2020;12:1961.

140 Carr AC, Lykkesfeldt J. Discrepancies in global vitamin C recommendations: a review of RDA criteria and underlying health perspectives. *Crit Rev Food Sci Nutr* 2021;61:742–55.

141 Yule S, Wanik J, Holm EM et al. Nutritional deficiency disease secondary to ARFID symptoms associated with autism and the broad autism phenotype: a qualitative systematic review of case reports and case series. *J Acad Nutr Diet* 2021;121:467–92.

147 Deirawan H, Fakhoury JW, Zarka M, Bluth MH, Moossavi M. Revisiting the pathobiology of scurvy: a review of the literature in the context of a challenging case. *Int J Dermatol* 2020;59:1450–7.

148 Day W, Gyurjyan-Bunch A, Van Voorhees A. Severe scurvy in an adult male without clear risk factors for nutritional deficiency. *JAAD Case Rep* 2019;5:309–11.

165 Zempleni J, Mock D. Biotin biochemistry and human requirements. *J Nutr Biochem* 1999;10:128–38.

166 Mock DM. Biotin status: which are valid indicators and how do we know? *J Nutr* 1999;129:498S–503S.

168 Patel DP, Swink SM, Castelo-Soccio L. A review of the use of biotin for hair loss. *Skin Appendage Disord* 2017;3:166–9.

169 Lipner SR. Rethinking biotin therapy for hair, nail, and skin disorders. *J Am Acad Dermatol* 2018;78:1236–8.

170 Ali M, Rajapakshe D, Cao L, Devaraj S. Discordant analytical results caused by biotin interference on diagnostic immunoassays in a pediatric hospital. *Ann Clin Lab Sci* 2017;47:638–40.

171 Trambas C, Lu Z, Yen T, Sikaris K. Depletion of biotin using streptavidin-coated microparticles: a validated solution to the problem of biotin interference in streptavidin–biotin immunoassays. *Ann Clin Biochem* 2018;55:216–26.

Minerals

10 Li N, Zhao G, Wu W *et al*. The efficacy and safety of vitamin C for iron supplementation in adult patients with iron deficiency anemia: a randomized clinical trial. *J Am Med Ass Netw Open* 2020;3:e2023644.

14 Osmani S, Smidt AC, Phan CM, Johnson DW. Acquired acrodermatitis enteropathica from a ketogenic diet. *J Am Acad Dermatol Case Rep* 2021;9:75.

15 Tang T, Lam JM. Unique presentation of transient zinc deficiency from low maternal breast milk zinc levels. *Pediatr Dermatol* 2018;35:255–6.

17 Vashist S, Rana A, Mahajan VK. Transient symptomatic zinc deficiency in a breast-fed infant associated with low zinc levels in maternal serum and breast milk improving after zinc supplementation: an uncommon phenotype? *Indian Dermatol Online J* 2020;11:623.

20 Mason M, Leitenberger S. Transient neonatal zinc deficiency: a review of two pediatric cases. *J Am Acad Dermatol* 2016;74(5s1):AB218.

36 Dupont R, Longué M, Galinier A *et al*. Impact of micronutrient deficiency and malnutrition in systemic sclerosis: cohort study and literature review. *Autoimmun Rev* 2018;17:1081–9.

39 Rodríguez-Manchón S, Pedrón-Giner C, Cañedo-Villarroya E, Muñoz-Codoceo RA, Hernández-Martín Á. Malnutrition in children with ichthyosis: recommendations for monitoring from a multidisciplinary clinic experience. *J Am Acad Dermatol* 2020;85:144–51.

52 Yang X, Bao Y, Fu H, Li L, Ren T, Yu X. Selenium protects neonates against neurotoxicity from prenatal exposure to manganese. *PloS One* 2014;9:e86611.

Essential fatty acids

10 Carey AN, Rudie C, Mitchell PD *et al*. Essential fatty acid status in surgical infants receiving parenteral nutrition with a composite lipid emulsion: a case series. *J Parenter Enteral Nutr* 2019;43:305–10.

36 Gramlich L, Ireton-Jones C, Miles JM. Essential fatty acids requirements and intravenous lipid emulsions. *J Parenter Enteral Nutr* 2019;43:607–707.

PART 5: METABOLIC & NUTRITIONAL DISORDERS

CHAPTER 62

Skin Disorders in Diabetes Mellitus

Johnny Bourke and Matthew Murphy

South Infirmary-Victoria University Hospital, Cork, Ireland

PART 5: METABOLIC & NUTRITIONAL DISORDERS

Introduction

Diabetes is classified loosely into four types:

1 Type 1: insulin dependent; usually juvenile onset, associated with human leukocyte antigen (HLA) -DR3, -DQB1*0201 and -DR4 and diabetes-associated autoantibodies, and prone to ketoacidosis.
2 Type 2: generally non-insulin dependent; usually adult onset and associated with other features of the metabolic syndrome such as obesity.
3 Secondary diabetes: iatrogenic or associated with pancreatic, hormonal and genetic disease.
4 Gestational diabetes: associated with pregnancy.

However, there is considerable overlap between these groups [1]. Diabetes is linked to a considerable number of skin disorders [2–8]. These are grouped below on a pathophysiological basis.

Vascular damage

Several processes are involved in diabetic vascular damage. Accumulation of advanced glycation end-products (AGEs) due to hyperglycaemia and oxidative stress is thought to be pivotal [9]. AGE deposits can be demonstrated non-invasively by autofluorescence in the skin and are a measure of local and systemic damage from diabetes [10]. Hyperglycaemia also increases flux through the polyol and hexosamine pathways with activation of protein kinase C, nuclear factor κB (NFκB), mitogen-activated protein kinase (MAPK) and other intracellular messengers [11]. The resulting cascade of metabolic events leads to endothelial proliferation, thickened basement membrane with deposits of periodic acid–Schiff (PAS) stain-positive material, and narrowing of arterioles, capillaries and venules [12,13]. Microangiopathy is responsible for the retinopathy, nephropathy and probably also neuropathy and diabetic dermopathy. Larger vessel disease manifests as atherosclerosis leading to peripheral vascular disease, ischaemic heart disease and cerebrovascular accidents. Doppler waveform measurement may be a more accurate method of assessment of peripheral vascular disease in diabetics rather than ankle brachial pressure index, which may be falsely elevated due to stiffer calcified vessels [14].

Leg ulceration

Ulceration of the leg and foot may be due to vascular and/or neurological damage involving a range of cellular and humoral processes. There is both structural impairment of cutaneous blood flow due to vascular damage and functional impairment, probably resulting predominantly from autonomic neuropathy [15]. Functional impairment is characterised by altered vascular resistance and failure of the normal hyperaemic response to stresses such as trauma and infection. These lead to chronic inflammation, impairment of circulation on a macrovascular and microvascular level, localised tissue hypoxia, autonomic and sensory neuropathy and impaired paracrine signalling. Elevated tissue glucose levels further compound matters by impairing healing interfering with the key cellular processes of haemostasis, inflammation, cellular proliferation and remodelling [16]. The main principles of ulceration management are wound debridement, pressure off-loading, revascularisation and antimicrobial therapy when infection is present.

Rook's Textbook of Dermatology, Tenth Edition. Edited by Christopher Griffiths, Jonathan Barker, Tanya Bleiker, Walayat Hussain and Rosalind Simpson.
© 2024 John Wiley & Sons Ltd. Published 2024 by John Wiley & Sons Ltd.

Wet gangrene of the foot

In someone suffering from diabetes, a sudden loss of perfusion to the already compromised cutaneous microcirculation (e.g. due to local infection or heart failure) may result in a wet necrotic area. This differs from the dry peripheral gangrene seen in arteriopathies. It is a late manifestation of diabetic microangiopathy [3].

Erysipelas-like reaction

Well-defined red skin on the legs and feet of elderly diabetic patients may be related to diabetic vascular disease [13]. Similar changes on the feet may herald the onset of Charcot arthropathy (see the section on the diabetic foot later in this chapter).

Diabetic dermopathy

Asymptomatic, oval, dull-red papules 0.5–1 cm in diameter evolve slowly on the shins, forearms, thighs and over bony prominences (Figure 62.1), producing a superficial scale and, ultimately, atrophic brown scars. It is common (approximately 10% of diabetic cases) and is a marker for complications of diabetes such as retinopathy, nephropathy and neuropathy [17,18]. Pathologically, there is hyperpigmentation of the epidermal basal layer, deposition of haemosiderin and melanin in the dermis and arteriolar basement membrane thickening [19].

Rubeosis

This peculiar rosy reddening of the face, and sometimes of the hands and feet, in longstanding diabetes has been attributed to microangiopathy or decreased vascular tone. Recent surveys [17,20] suggest a prevalence of less than 10% in contrast to 50–60% found in previous studies [21,22].

Neurological damage

Approximately 50% of those with diabetes develop a chronic, symmetrical, length-dependent sensorimotor polyneuropathy [23], probably due to damaged endoneurial microvessels. It is closely related to poor glycaemic control and AGE deposition with resultant inflammation also plays a role here [24]. Autonomic dysfunction and neuropathic pain are later features. Patients complain of numbness, tingling, aching and burning of the legs, which intensifies in bed at night. Autonomic neuropathy impairs sweating of the legs with compensatory sweating elsewhere and oedema, redness and atrophy in advanced cases [3].

Diabetic foot

Diabetic Charcot arthropathy [25] typically presents as a warm, swollen and red foot and ankle, which may mimic cellulitis. It is principally due to a combination of motor, sensory and autonomic neuropathy leading to a painless, degenerative and progressive destruction of the architecture of one or more joints in the ankle and/or foot. Circulatory abnormalities, unprotected trauma and abnormal pressure points lead to dislocation and the fusion of joints, fracture and resorption of bone. The foot becomes deformed with distally displaced plantar fat pads, depressed metatarsal heads, hammer toes and pes cavus. Proper foot care is essential to prevent the formation of indolent perforating ulcers ('mal perforans').

Diabetic foot ulcer

The lifetime risk for a patient with diabetes of developing a foot ulcer is estimated to be 15% although it may be higher [26]. A painless and slowly penetrating ulcer of the sole and of other pressure sites is suggestive of diabetic neuropathy. The ulcer is circular and punched out in shape, occurring in the middle of a callosity (Figure 62.2). An initial subepidermal haemorrhagic bulla may give rise to discoloration of the surrounding skin [4]. The principal risk factors for diabetic foot ulceration are duration of diabetes, poor control of HbA1c level and peripheral neuropathy [27]. Vascular disease, secondary trauma and maceration with infection also

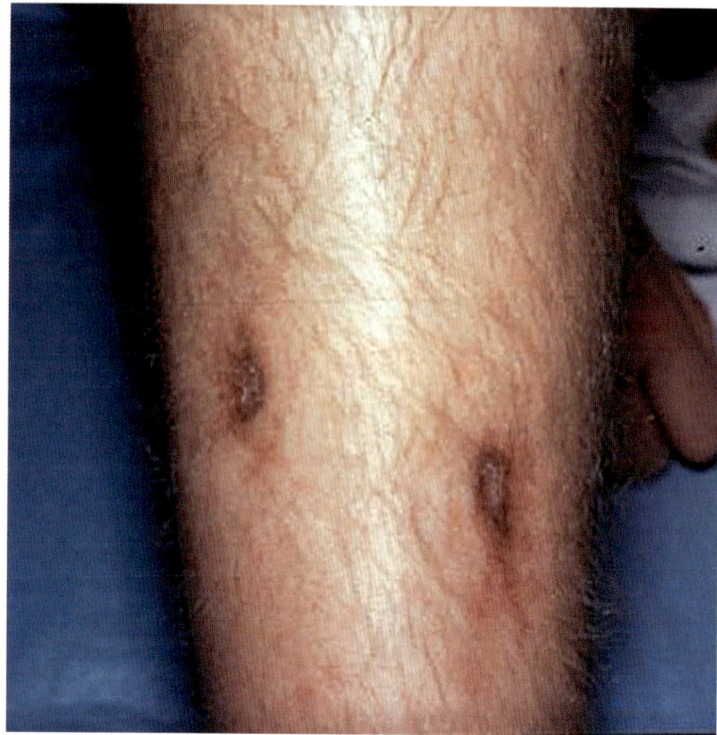

Figure 62.1 Diabetic dermopathy on both shins.

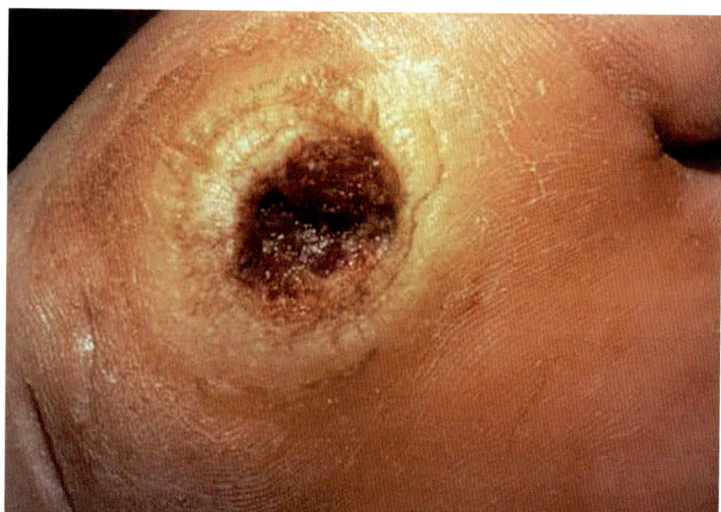

Figure 62.2 Diabetic foot with neurotrophic ulceration and necrosis ('mal perforans').

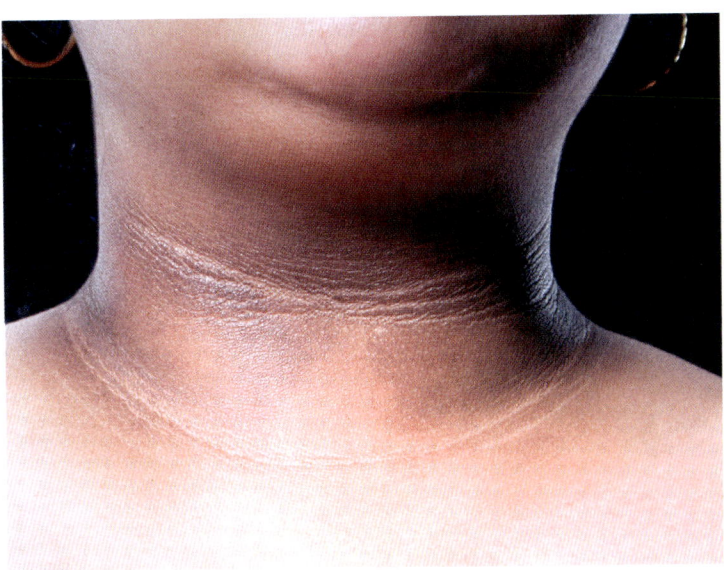

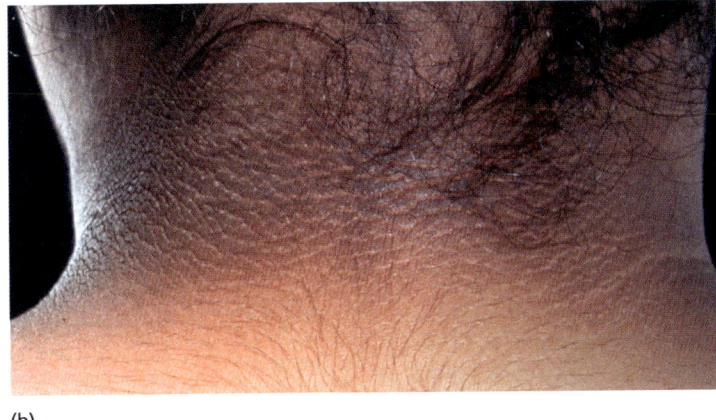

(b)

(a)

Figure 62.3 Velvety warty hyperpigmentation on the front (a) and back (b) of the neck in acanthosis nigricans. Courtesy of Dr Robin A. C. Graham-Brown.

contribute. Digital thermography has been proposed as a way of preventing diabetic ulceration by early detection of raised foot temperature in Charcot arthropathy and/or cellulitis [28].

Multidisciplinary management should address the need for revascularisation, offloading pressure by appropriate footwear, crutches and occasionally surgery (arthroplasty, ulcer excision and grafting). The multidisciplinary team should include access to an endocrinologist, neurologist, podiatrist, orthotics, orthopaedic surgeon, vascular surgeon, plastics and reconstructive surgeon, infectious disease specialist and diabetic foot nurse as needed. Local treatment includes debridement, pressure off-loading, treatment of infection and dressings [29]. There is little evidence that newer dressings are more effective [30–33].

Infections

Infections may be a presenting feature of diabetes, particularly type 2. Although case–control studies have largely not shown diabetes to be a risk factor for cellulitis and dermatophyte infection of the feet [34,35], population-based studies do appear to demonstrate an increased risk of skin and soft tissue bacterial and fungal infections [36–38] and recurrent erysipelas is more common in diabetics [39]. *Candida* of the mucous membranes, nail folds and flexures, and balanitis, and consequent phimosis, are more common particularly in poorly controlled diabetes [40–42]. Certain rare infections are particularly associated with diabetes. Fournier gangrene and melioidosis are two such examples [43,44]. There are also reports of a possible link between Fournier gangrene and sodium glucose co-transporter 2 (SGLT2) inhibitors [45]. *Pseudomonas* infection of the ear can cause serious infection due to local invasion of the surrounding bone, nerves and arteries, with significant mortality [46,47].

Obesity, hyperlipidaemia and the metabolic syndrome

Acanthosis nigricans (Chapter 85)

Smooth, velvety, hyperkeratotic, hyperpigmented skin (Figure 62.3) predominantly affecting the flexures is most commonly seen in obese type 2 diabetic patients. Skin tags are also commonly present. It is also seen in malignancy where it may be much more extensive and occurs in a variety of syndromes associated with insulin resistance (leprechaunism, Rabson–Mendenhall, Berardinelli–Seip, Dunnigan, Alstrom, Laurence–Moon–Bardet–Biedel and Prader–Willi syndromes, and congenital lipodystrophy) as well as Cushing syndrome and acromegaly. The final common pathway is probably via stimulation of tyrosine kinase growth factor receptors in the epidermis [48]. In the setting of insulin resistance, the relevant receptor is insulin-like growth factor 1 receptor, which is present on fibroblasts and keratinocytes in the skin.

Skin tags

Skin tags are small, soft, pedunculated lesions occurring on the eyelids, neck and axillae, often associated with obesity. They appear to be a marker for diabetes, independent of obesity and acanthosis nigricans (most studies have been hospital-based [49–53]). Among 216 patients with skin tags, 57 (26%) had diabetes of the non-insulin-dependent type, of whom only about 25% were classified as obese [54].

Eruptive xanthomas of the skin

Eruptive xanthomas may develop quite dramatically in diabetic patients with hyperlipidaemia, resulting in a significant risk of pancreatitis (Figure 62.4) [55]. The lesions slowly resolve when the diabetes and hyperlipidaemia are properly managed.

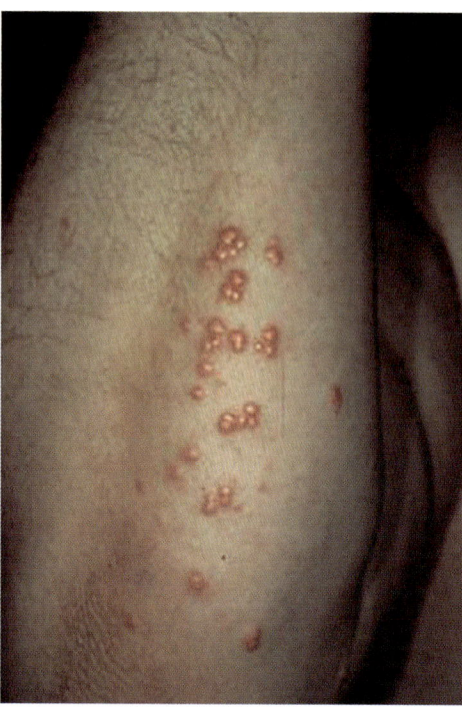

Figure 62.4 Eruptive xanthomas in a diabetic patient with hyperlipidaemia.

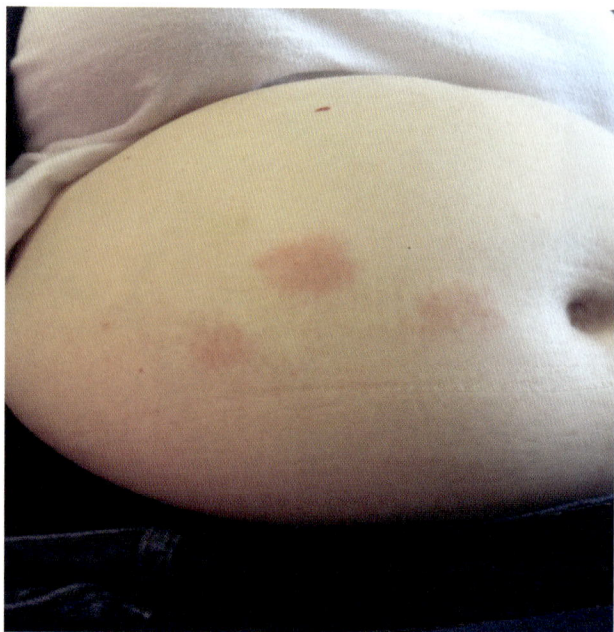

Figure 62.5 Urticarial reaction to insulin.

The metabolic syndrome

The metabolic syndrome was first used in 1977 by Herman Heller to describe a constellation of risk factors associated with atherosclerosis. These are hypertension, insulin resistance, hyperinsulinaemia, glucose intolerance and/or obesity. There has been increasing recognition of the relationship between various skin diseases and the metabolic syndrome and thus with type 2 diabetes. Links associating the metabolic syndrome with both psoriasis and hidradenitis are well documented [56,57]. Association with other diseases is less clear [58].

Treatment-related skin manifestations

Insulin lipodystrophy

Both atrophy and hypertrophy may occur even with newer synthetic insulins and analogues. Lipohypertrophy affected almost two-thirds of patients in one survey [59]. It is more common in patients who do not rotate the site of injection of insulin and can lead to impaired insulin absorption and poorer diabetic control. Lipoatrophy appears to be an immunological reaction [60]. The introduction of synthetic insulin has made it much less common (in 1–2% of cases).

Allergic reactions to insulin and glucose monitors

Localised allergic reactions to insulin including newer insulin analogues and its excipients include urticaria, painful nodules and granulomas (Figure 62.5) [61]. The use of continuous subcutaneous insulin pumps may help, but contact dermatitis from the presence of acrylates, epoxy resin, glue components and nickel needles has been reported [62–66]. Percutaneous glucose monitors have become much more widely used in recent times and allergic reactions to acrylates, particularly isobornyl acrylate, have caused significant problems with some models [67].

Allergic reactions to oral hypoglycaemic drugs

A wide range of drug reactions to diabetic medications has been described. Sulphonylureas are the most common culprits, particularly a disulfiram-like reaction to chlorpropamide. Photosensitivity, pruritus, erythema multiforme, erythema nodosum, urticaria and lichenoid and morbilliform eruptions have all been described [3,68].

Disease associations and genetic syndromes

Reactive perforating collagenosis (folliculitis)

This has been reported in patients with diabetes with and without renal insufficiency (Figure 62.6). It is attributed to glycation of collagen and minor injuries such as pressure or scratching [8,69].

Autoimmune disease

Genetic risk for several autoimmune diseases overlaps, resulting in greater frequency of other autoimmune disorders in patients with type 1 diabetes [70,71]. These include thyroid disease (occurring in 15–30% of patients; more commonly hypothyroidism), coeliac disease (4–9%), vitiligo (4.5%) and Addison disease (0.5%), and the associated dermatological manifestations of those diseases (dermatitis herpetiformis and pretibial myxoedema). The association with alopecia areata is less clear [72,73].

Genetic and other systemic diseases

Diabetes is a feature of several genetic diseases [3,74] including Werner syndrome, lipoid proteinosis and autoimmune polyendocrine syndrome. It is also seen in many systemic diseases including haemochromatosis, Cushing syndrome, acromegaly and

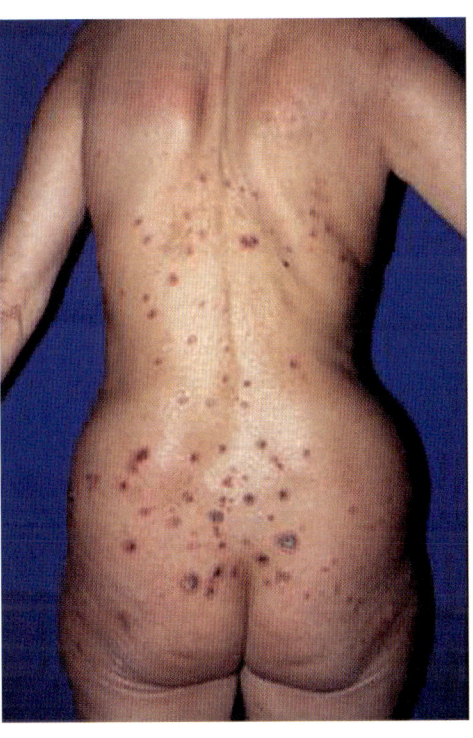

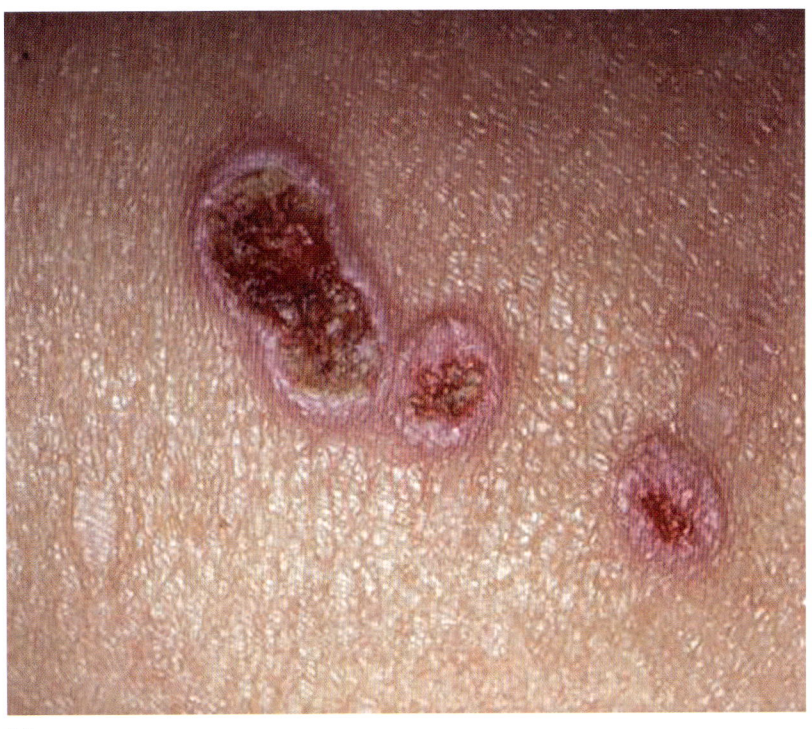

(a)   (b)

Figure 62.6 (a) Perforating collagenosis on the back of a 64-year-old woman with diabetic retinopathy. (b) Close-up view.

the lipodystrophies (familial partial lipodystrophy, acquired partial lipoatrophy and human immunodeficiency virus (HIV) associated lipodystrophy). A reduced risk of atopy has been reported in diabetes [75].

Miscellaneous disorders

Granulomatous disorders (Chapter 95)
Necrobiosis lipoidica (NLD) is probably the most widely recognised diabetic skin disorder (Figure 62.7). The lifetime risk of diabetes in patients with NLD may not be as high as the 65% previously indicated. One recent study found that only 22% of NLD patients developed diabetes or impaired glucose tolerance over a 15-year follow-up [76]. NLD is uncommon in the diabetic population as a whole (0.3–1.2%) although it may be seen in 2–3% of type 1 diabetes [77–79].

Granuloma annulare (Figure 62.8) is probably not associated with diabetes [8]. Retrospective case series [80,81] suggest a link with generalised granuloma annulare (21% in one series of 100 patients) but there are no case–control studies confirming these figures.

Annular elastolytic giant cell granuloma is a rare disorder of connective tissue affecting the head and neck areas that is most commonly associated with diabetes in up to 40% of cases. It is described in detail in Chapter 94.

Stiff skin and joints
Skin thickening and stiff joints are also attributed to irreversible cross-linking of collagen and other proteins in the skin and accumulation of AGEs such as carboxymethyl lysine and pentosidane [8].

Receptors for AGE products (RAGEs) have been described that stimulate several inflammatory and fibrogenic growth factors and cytokines via protein kinase C. There is no definitive treatment for any of the following conditions. Improved diabetic control is likely to be helpful. Aspirin reduces glycoxidative damage but the effect is slow. Physiotherapy may help to maintain mobility. Other treatments, of uncertain benefit, include phototherapy, photophoresis, radiotherapy, prostacyclin, high-dose penicillin, ciclosporin, factor XIII and sorbinol. Research into agents blocking cross-linking of proteins or interfering with AGE–RAGE interaction is at an early stage with some encouraging animal studies [8].

Cheiroarthropathy
This is characterised by waxy tight skin on the backs of the hands (Figure 62.9) and limited joint mobility ('prayer sign'). Originally reported in patients with type 1 diabetes, it has also been found in type 2 diabetes [82]. It is an index of underlying microvascular changes [83], neuropathy, retinopathy and also of stiff cervical joints, which may cause difficulties with intubation in anaesthesia [84].

'Finger pebbles'
These are multiple, grouped, minute papules on the extensor surface of the fingers in or near the knuckle pads or periungual region. They are more common in, but not exclusive to, those with diabetes [85]. They are distinct from knuckle pads and may be seen with or without acanthosis nigricans.

Scleroedema diabeticorum
There is uncertainty as to whether scleroedema associated with diabetes is a separate form of the condition or not [86,87]. It is

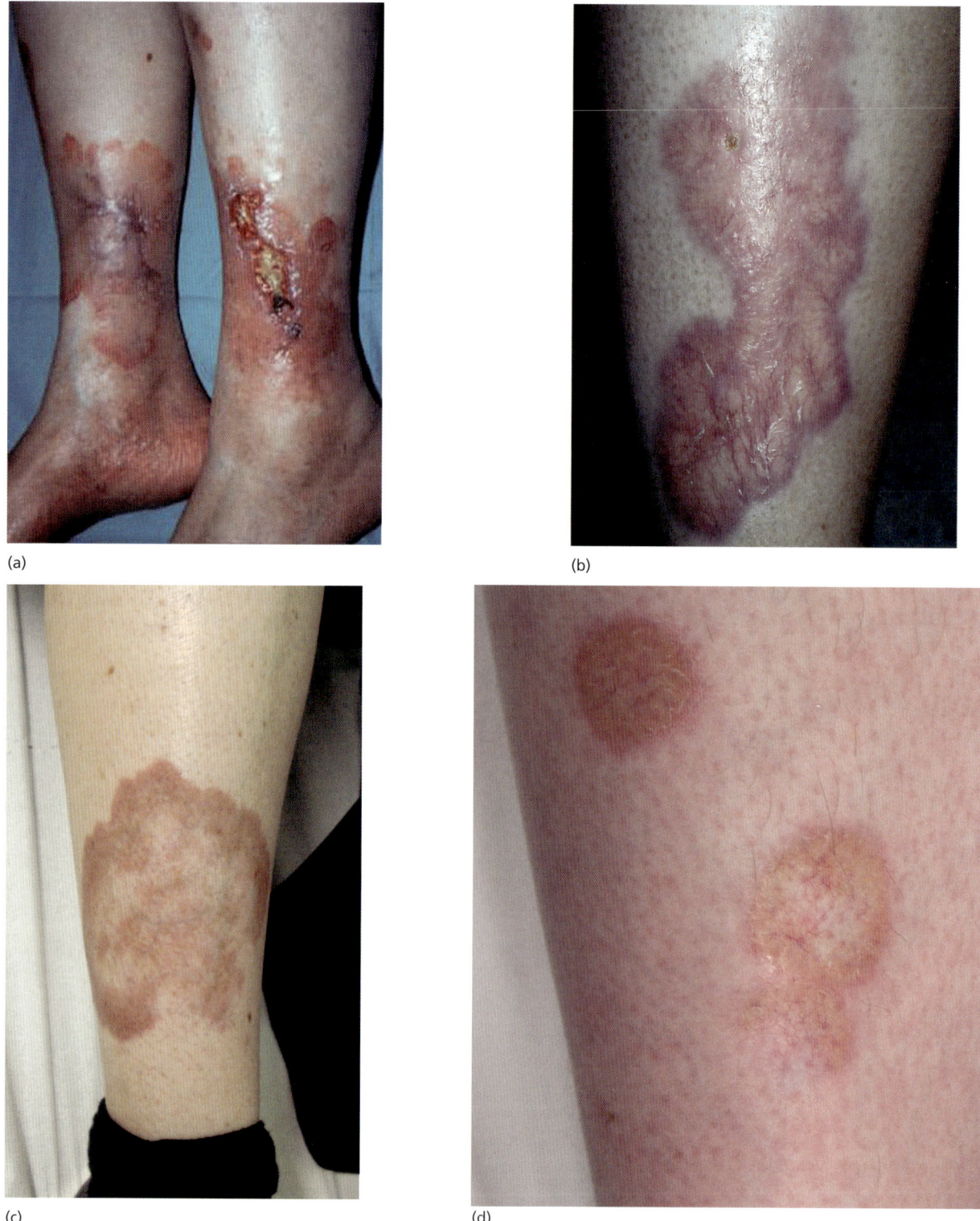

(a)

(b)

(c)

(d)

Figure 62.7 (a–d) Necrobiosis lipoidica with ulcerations on the shins at various stages of evolution.

characterised by ill-defined induration of the skin, most commonly on the neck and upper back (Figure 62.10). The condition is mainly seen in overweight adults with type 2 diabetes. It is essentially permanent and does not respond to treatment, but is painless and usually causes little morbidity.

Pruritus

Although some textbooks report an association with diabetes, there are few detailed studies. A recent paper from Japan reported an increased prevalence of truncal pruritus compared with controls (11.3% versus 2.9%) and detected an association with autonomic

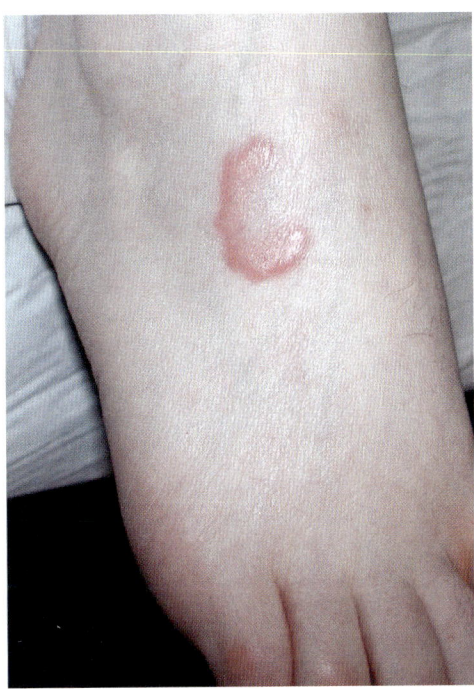

Figure 62.8 Granuloma annulare of the foot.

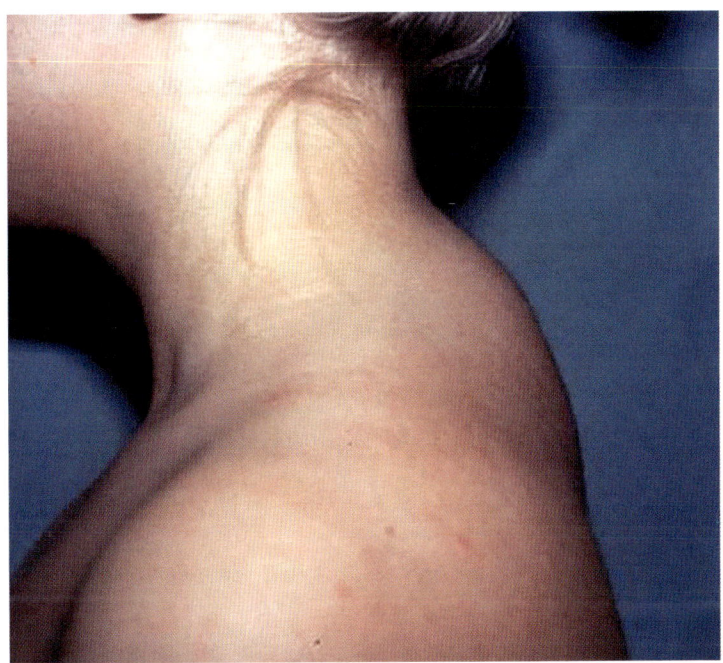

Figure 62.10 Scleroedema diabeticorum with a 'buffalo hump' in a young woman with diabetes.

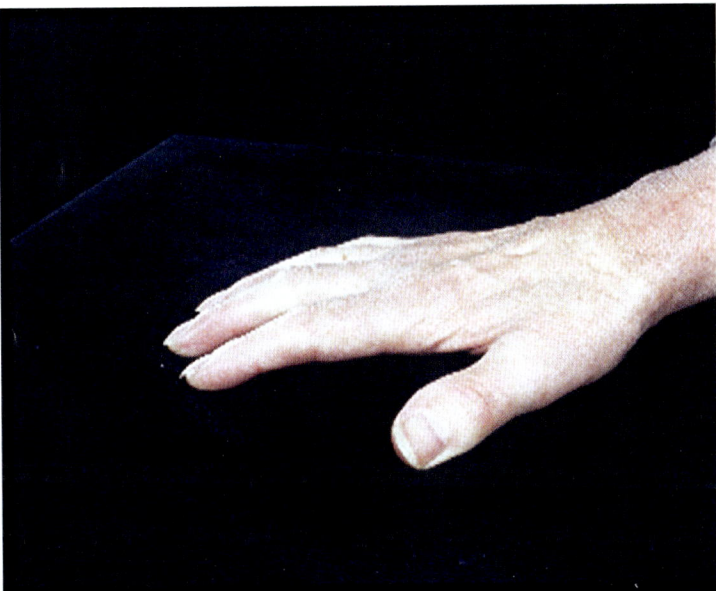

Figure 62.9 Cheiroarthropathy of the hands. Courtesy of Dr Robin A. C. Graham-Brown.

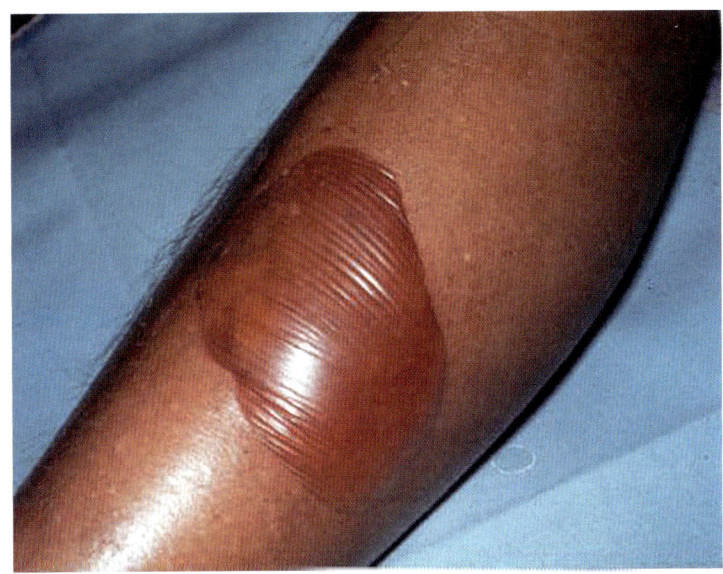

Figure 62.11 A large diabetic bulla on the shin of a patient with diabetes.

neuropathy [88]. Ano-genital pruritus may be due to secondary infection with candidiasis or β-haemolytic streptococci [3].

Diabetic bullae

Non-scarring subepidermal bullae up to several centimetres in diameter on a non-inflamed base may affect the lower legs and feet, and occasionally the hands and fingers (Figure 62.11) [89,90]. They are uncommon but believed to be a distinct marker for diabetes. They heal over several weeks.

Other associations

There are indirect associations between diabetes and both calciphylaxis and nephrogenic fibrosing dermopathy related to diabetic nephropathy, although a recent review of the literature called the link with the latter into question [91,92]. Yellow skin and nails have been reported to be more frequent in patients with diabetes with a questionable relationship to carotene [3]. The evidence for a link with lichen planus is conflicting [93–95].

Key references

The full list of references can be found in the online version at https://www.wiley.com/rooksdermatology10e

3 Huntley AC. The cutaneous manifestations of diabetes. *J Am Acad Dermatol* 1982;7:427–55.

8 Cox NH. Diabetes and the skin: an update for dermatologists. *Expert Rev Dermatol* 2007;2:305–16.

23 Tesfaye S, Boulton AJM, Dyck PJ *et al.* Diabetic neuropathies: update on definitions, diagnostic criteria, estimation of severity, and treatments. *Diabetes Care* 2010;33:2285–93.

25 Wukich DK, Sung W. Charcot arthropathy of the foot and ankle: modern concepts and management review. *J Diabetes Complicat* 2009;23:409–26.

27 Crawford F, Inkster M, Kleijnen J, Fahey T. Predicting foot ulcers in patients with diabetes: a systematic review and meta-analysis. *Q J Med* 2007;100:65–86.

48 Torley D, Bellus GA, Munro CS. Genes, growth factors and acanthosis nigricans. *Br J Dermatol* 2002;147:1096–101.

68 Litt JZ. *Litt's Drug Eruptions and Reactions Manual*, 19th edn. Boca Raton, FL: CRC Press.

71 Barker JM. Clinical review: type 1 diabetes-associated autoimmunity: natural history, genetic associations, and screening. *J Clin Endocrinol Metab* 2006;91:1210–17.

76 O'Toole EA, Kennedy U, Nolan JJ *et al.* Necrobiosis lipoidica: only a minority of patients have diabetes mellitus. *Br J Dermatol* 1999;140:283–6.

88 Yamaoka H, Sasaki H, Yamasaki H *et al.* Truncal pruritus of unknown origin may be a symptom of diabetic polyneuropathy. *Diabetes Care* 2010;33:150–5.

PART 6
Genetic Disorders Involving the Skin

CHAPTER 63
Inherited Disorders of Cornification

Vinzenz Oji[1,2], *Kira Süßmuth*[1], *Dieter Metze*[1], *Angela Hernandez Martin*[3] *and Heiko Traupe*[1]

[1]Department of Dermatology, University Hospital Münster, Münster, Germany
[2]Hautarztpraxis am Buddenturm, Münster, Germany
[3]Dermatología, Hospital Infantil Universitario Niño Jesús, Madrid, Spain

Rook's Textbook of Dermatology, Tenth Edition. Edited by Christopher Griffiths, Jonathan Barker, Tanya Bleiker, Walayat Hussain and Rosalind Simpson.
© 2024 John Wiley & Sons Ltd. Published 2024 by John Wiley & Sons Ltd.

Introduction

This chapter deals with ichthyoses, palmoplantar keratodermas (PPKs) and miscellaneous inherited or acquired cornification disorders. The majority of keratinisation disorders are nowadays referred to as Mendelian disorders of cornification (MeDOCs) [1]. This is a very broad group that is clinically characterised by hyperkeratosis or visible scaling or both. The term 'Mendelian' implicates that these diseases are genetically determined in nature. In many of them distinct genetic defects can be elucidated revealing quite a few mechanisms, and sometimes even pathways (for example the hepoxilin pathway [2]), that underlie their pathology. The work of the group of Peter Elias [3] and of Masashi Akiyama [4] has made it clear that numerous genes defective in different types of ichthyosis such as *ABCA12*, *ALOXE3*, *ALOX12B*, *CPY4F22*, *CERS3*, *ABHD5* and *ELOVL4* are essential for the formation of the corneocyte lipid envelope and that this is a key structure for skin barrier function and ichthyosis pathogenesis. From a molecular perspective, it would therefore be tempting to provide a classification based on molecular grounds, sorting out for instance keratinopathies relating to mutations in keratin genes from diseases relating to defects in corneocyte lipid envelope formation or cholesterol biosynthesis. However, mutations, for instance in keratin genes, can cause very variable clinical phenotypes ranging from bullous diseases as in epidermolysis bullosa simplex (*KRT5* and *KRT14*) [5] to ichthyosis Curth Macklin (*KRT1*) [6], not to mention pigmentation disorders like Galli–Galli or Dowling–Degos disease caused by *KRT5* mutations [7]. Since this textbook is aimed primarily at dermatologists and physician scientists who have the task of making a clinical diagnosis and providing adequate management for the patients they care for, this chapter uses a classification scheme that is based upon clinicogenetic and morphological features. These clinical diagnoses are then discussed with their molecular pathology.

From a 'classic dermatological' perspective, we distinguish today among the many MeDOC ichthyoses, PPKs and a remaining group of miscellaneous keratinisation disorders, such as the various forms of porokeratosis. Darier disease is dealt with elsewhere in this textbook (Chapter 64). It should be noted that at the First Ichthyosis Consensus Conference it was decided to no longer make a distinction between erythrokeratodermas and ichthyoses, but rather to group them together [1]. In PPK, unlike ichthyosis, the cornification disorder is not widespread, but almost exclusively affects the hands and feet.

There are entities that could be regarded as either belonging to the ichthyosis or the PPK group. One such example is loricrin keratoderma [8,9]. Still, for the clinician the distinction between ichthyosis and PPK is diagnostically valuable and helpful. It dates back more than 100 years and was first introduced by Peukert in 1899 [10]. This chapter will also cover cornification disorders that do not have a genetic basis, but are acquired or of unknown etiology, for example acquired ichthyoses or pityriasis rotunda.

ICHTHYOSES

The term 'ichthyosis' was first introduced more than 200 years ago by Willan in his textbook on cutaneous diseases [1]. The word ichthyosis is derived from the Greek word 'ichthys', which means fish. It was coined at a time when characteristics of human diseases were compared with those occurring in the animal kingdom. The literal translation 'scaly fish disease' is embarrassing and should be avoided. As a technical term it is deeply entrenched in the medical literature and today refers to those MeDOCs that share a conspicuous scaling which is generalised and affects the whole integument [2,3].

An important advance of the First Ichthyosis Consensus Conference [4] was that we now differentiate between non-syndromic (Table 63.1) and syndromic (Table 63.2) forms of ichthyoses – a distinction already proposed by other authors [2,5,6]. In contrast, onset of the disease – namely the distinction between congenital and non-congenital onset – is no longer used as a major criterion, since some diseases such as recessive X-linked ichthyosis manifest at birth in some patients and after several months in others. Instead, it is suggested to distinguish between common and rare forms of the diseases. Common forms include ichthyosis vulgaris (IV) and X-linked ichthyosis (XLI). However, one should keep in mind that XLI has a prevalence of 1 : 2000–3000 in European populations and would be considered a rare disease according to the criteria of the European Union [7].

In order to avoid redundancy, the pathophysiology of the ichthyoses is not discussed in a special chapter of its own, but covered here with the respective entities. All types of ichthyoses result in abnormal differentiation and/or abnormal desquamation showing, for example, impaired corneocyte shedding (retention hyperkeratosis) or accelerated keratinocyte production (epidermal hyperplasia/hyperproliferative hyperkeratosis). The development of hyperkeratosis in these diseases may be understood as a homeostatic repair response aimed at compensating for an abnormal epidermal barrier [3,4].

Table 63.1 Clinicogenetic classification of inherited ichthyoses: non-syndromic forms.

Disease	Mode of inheritance	Genes
Common ichthyoses		
Ichthyosis vulgaris (IV)	Semidominant	*FLG*
Non-syndromic (recessive) X-linked ichthyosis (XLI)	XR	*STS*
Autosomal recessive congenital ichthyosis (ARCI)		
Harlequin ichthyosis (HI)	AR	*ABCA12*
Lamellar ichthyosis (LI)	AR	*TGM1, NIPAL4, ALOX12B, ABCA12, PNPLA1, CERS3, LIPH*[a]
Congenital ichthyosiform erythroderma (CIE)	AR	*ALOXE3, ALOX12B, ABCA12, CYP4F22, NIPAL4, TGM1, PNPLA1, CERS3, LIPH*[a]
Self-healing collodion baby (SHCB)	AR	*TGM1*
Self-improving congenital ichthyosis (SICI)	AR	*ALOXE3, ALOX12B, PNPLA1, CYP4F22*
Acral self-healing collodion baby	AR	*TGM1*
Bathing suit ichthyosis (BSI)	AR	*TGM1*
Keratinopathic ichthyosis (KPI)		
Epidermolytic ichthyosis (EI)	AD	*KRT1, KRT10*
Superficial epidermolytic ichthyosis (SEI)	AD	*KRT2*
Congenital reticular ichthyosiform erythroderma (CRIE)	AD	*KRT1, KRT10*
Annular epidermolytic ichthyosis (AEI)	AD	*KRT1, KRT10*
Ichthyosis Curth–Macklin (ICM)	AD	*KRT1, KRT10*
Autosomal recessive epidermolytic ichthyosis (AREI)	AR	*KRT10*
Epidermolytic naevi or systematised mosaic presentations[b]	Somatic mutations	*KRT1, KRT10, KRT2*
Other non-syndromic forms		
Loricrin keratoderma (LK)	AD	*LOR*
Erythrokeratodermia variabilis (EKV)	AD	*GJB3, GJB4*
Recessive progressive symmetrical erythrokeratoderma (RPSE)	AR	*KRT83*
Autosomal dominant lamellar ichthyosis (ADLI)	AD	*ASPRV1*
Peeling skin syndrome type B	AR	*CDSN*
Exfoliative ichthyosis (EXI)	AR	*CSTA, SERPINB8*
Peeling skin syndrome type A	AR	*FLG2*
Keratosis linearis–ichthyosis congenita–keratoderma (KLICK)	AR	*POMP*

Adapted from Oji *et al.* 2010 [4].

[a] ARCI of late onset.

[b] May indicate a gonadal mosaicism, which can cause generalised EI in the offspring generation.

AD, autosomal dominant; AR, autosomal recessive; XR, X-linked recessive.

Table 63.2 Clinicogenetic classification of inherited ichthyoses: syndromic forms.

Disease	Mode of inheritance	Genes
X-linked ichthyosis syndromes		
X-linked ichthyosis (XLI)[a]	XR	*STS* (and others[a])
Ichthyosis follicularis alopecia photophobia (IFAP)[b]	XR	*MBTPS2*
Conradi–Hünermann–Happle syndrome (CDPX2)	XD	*EBP*
Autosomal ichthyosis syndromes with prominent hair abnormalities		
Netherton syndrome (NS)	AR	*SPINK5*
Ichthyosis with hypotrichosis[c]	AR	*ST14*
Neonatal ichthyosis–sclerosing cholangitis (NISCH)[d]	AR	*CLDN1*
Autosomal ichthyosis syndromes with prominent neurological signs		
Refsum syndrome (HMSN4)	AR	*PHYH, PEX7*
Multiple sulphatase deficiency (MSD)	AR	*SUMF1*
Gaucher syndrome type 2	AR	*GBA*
Sjögren–Larsson syndrome (SLS)	AR	*ALDH3A2*
Neutral lipid storage disease (NLSD) with ichthyosis	AR	*ABHD5*
Trichothiodystrophy (TTD)	AR	*C7ORF11, ERCC2, XPD, ERCC3, XPB, GTF2H5, TTDA*
Cerebral dysgenesis–neuropathy–ichthyosis–palmoplantar keratoderma (CEDNIK)	AR	*SNAP29*
Arthrogryposis–renal dysfunction–cholestasis (ARC)	AR	*VPS33B*
Stormorken syndrome	AR	*STIM1, ORA1*
Coloboma–heart defect–ichthyosiform dermatosis–mental retardation–ear anomalies (CHIME) syndrome	AR	*PIGL*
Neu–Laxova syndrome (NLS)	AR	*PHGDH, PSAT1, PSPH*
Autosomal ichthyosis syndromes with deafness		
Keratitis–ichthyosis–deafness (KID)	AD	*GJB2 (GJB6)*
Desmons syndrome (DS)[e]	AR	*AP1B1*
Mental retardation–enteropathy–deafness–neuropathy–ichthyosis–keratodermia (MEDNIK) syndrome	AR	*AP1S1*
ELOVL4 deficiency	AR	*ELOVL4*
Autosomal ichthyosis syndromes with potential systemic distress		
Ichthyosis–prematurity syndrome (IPS)	AR	*SLC27A4*
Severe wasting–multiple allergies–metabolic wasting syndrome (SAM)	AR	*DSG1*

Adapted from Oji *et al.* 2010 [4].

[a] In the context of a contiguous gene syndrome.

[b] Genetically and clinically different from autosomal dominant IFAP syndrome (IFAP2)

[c] Allelic variant: congenital ichthyosis–follicular atrophoderma–hypotrichosis–hypohidrosis (IFAH).

[d] Also known as ichthyosis–leukocyte vacuoles–alopecia–sclerosing cholangitis (ILVASC).

[e] Also published as MEDNIK-like syndrome or autosomal recessive KID syndrome.

AD, autosomal dominant; AR, autosomal recessive; CDPX2, chondrodysplasia punctata type 2; HMSN4, hereditary motor and sensory neuropathy type 4.

COMMON ICHTHYOSES

Ichthyosis vulgaris

Definition and nomenclature

Ichthyosis vulgaris is a mild scaling disorder with a prevalence in Europe of 1 : 100 according to data from a population study in northern England [1].

Pathophysiology

Ichthyosis vulgaris is due to mutations in filaggrin (*FLG*), which are inherited as an autosomal semidominant trait [2,3]. Only a

Table 63.3 Keratinopathic ichthyoses.

Features	Epidermolytic ichthyosis (EI)	Superficial epidermolytic ichthyosis (SEI)	Ichthyosis Curth–Macklin (ICM)	Congenital reticular ichthyosiform erythroderma (CRIE)[a]
MIM number	113800	146800	146600	609165
Mode of inheritance	AD (rarely AR in *KRT10*)	AD	AD	AD
	Systematised mosaic presentations possible	Systematised mosaic presentations possible		
Gene	*KRT1* or *KRT10*	*KRT2*	*KRT1* or *KRT10*	*KRT10* or *KRT1*
Onset	At birth	At birth	Early childhood	At birth
Initial clinical presentation	Large erosions, mild scaling, erythroderma at birth	Erythroderma, widespread blistering	Spiky diffuse PPK	Exfoliative CIE, larger areas forming a reticular pattern predominantly on the extremities
Disease course	Resolution of erosions replaced by hyperkeratosis in the first months. Annular type: development of numerous annular polycyclic red scaly plaques on the trunk and extremities that enlarge slowly, and then resolve (intermittent presentations of EI)	Within weeks development of hyperkeratosis particularly over extensor sides of joints	Progressive worsening of PPK and development of hyperkeratotic plaques over joints and/or hyperkeratotic papules on the trunk and extremities	During childhood and puberty a characteristic patchy pattern starts to evolve
Cutaneous findings:				
Distribution of scaling	Generalised, or predilection of friction areas over joints	Friction areas	Palms and soles, large joints, rarely extremities and/or trunk	Generalised, later reticular ichthyosiform pattern
Scaling type	Adherent, moderate	Adherent, fine to moderate	Thick spiky hyperkeratosis	Fine
Scaling colour	White-brown	Brown ('moulting')	Yellow-brown hyperkeratoses	Yellow-brown
Skin redness	Frequent	Initially, fades	Erythroderma possible	Pronounced
Palmoplantar involvement	*KRT1*: epidermolytic PPK. *KRT10*: palms and soles are spared (exceptions possible)	Usually no	Massive PPK leading to deep, bleeding and painful fissures, flexural contractures, constriction bands	Yes
Hypohidrosis	Possible	Possible	None	–
Scalp abnormalities	Scaling	–	None	Scaling
Other skin findings	Pruritus, blisters after minor trauma, proneness to skin infections/impetigo	Pruritus, bullae may occur after minor mechanical trauma, hypertrichosis	–	–
Extracutaneous involvement	Growth failure with some severe phenotypes	–	Gangrene and loss of digits	Growth failure with some severe phenotypes
Risk of death	Elevated during neonatal period	–	–	Elevated during neonatal period
Skin ultrastructure	EHK, aggregations and clumping of keratin filaments in suprabasal cells; partly cytolysis, lamellar body accumulation	Superficial EHK, cytolysis in granular cells of affected body areas; no keratin clumping	Binuclear cells, particular concentric perinuclear 'shells' of aberrant – putatively – keratin material	Vacuolisation of superficial granular cells and filamentous material in vacuolated cells

Adapted from Oji *et al.* 2010 [12].

[a] Also known as ichthyosis variegata and ichthyosis en confetti.

AD, autosomal dominant; AR, autosomal recessive; CIE, congenital ichthyosiform erythroderma; EHK, epidermolytic hyperkeratosis; PPK, palmoplantar keratoderma.

minority of those individuals who harbour only one *FLG* mutation develop clinically obvious ichthyosis, although they do exhibit accentuated palmar and plantar creases and may have somewhat dry skin. About two-thirds of IV patients have two *FLG* mutations and present with a clear-cut clinical phenotype. In one-third of the patients who have only one *FLG* mutation, disease expression is much milder [4]. This clinical difference relating to the mutation load is reflected by functional studies concerning, for example, skin hydration, transepidermal water loss [5,6] and/or different gene expression in the epidermis [7]. *FLG* mutations result in impaired epidermal barrier formation and a marked reduction of natural moisturising factors which play a critical role in hydration of the stratum corneum. Irrespective of the presence of IV, *FLG* mutations predispose to atopic eczema (AE), allergic rhinitis, asthma, food allergies, hand eczema, nickel sensitisation and eczema

herpeticatum in AE [1,8,9]. Of note, *FLG* mutations are prevalent in the healthy population (up to approximately 10%) [7].

Clinical features

Ichthyosis vulgaris is not present at birth. It usually develops during the first months of life. Wells and Kerr [10] found demonstrable scaling in 40% of their patients at the age of 3 months. Even careful parents may have difficulties in reporting the exact time of disease onset and it should be noted that scaling may disappear or be reduced markedly in the summertime due to seasonal variation and increased humidity. IV patients present with light grey scales covering mainly the extensor surfaces of the extremities and the trunk (Figure 63.1a). The scales tend to be smaller than in XLI, and the groin and larger flexures are always spared. Almost all IV patients exhibit accentuated palmar creases (Figure 63.1b), and

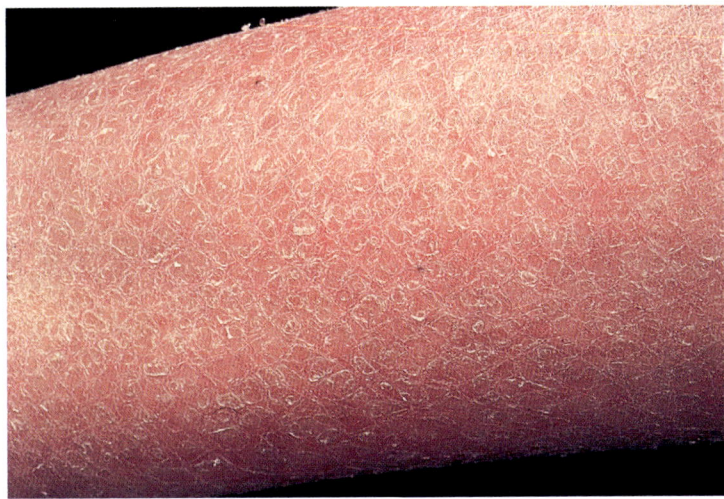

(a)

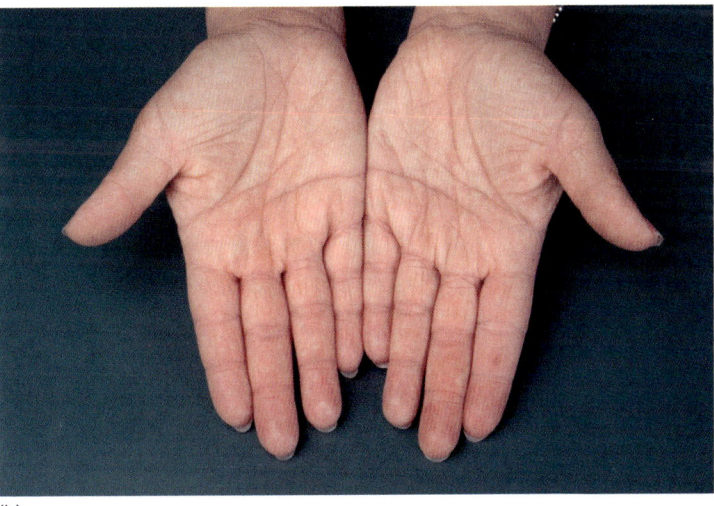

(b)

Figure 63.1 Ichthyosis vulgaris. (a) Fine scaling and (b) accentuated palmar creases. (a) Courtesy of Dr M. Judge, Salford Royal NHS Trust, UK. (b) Courtesy of the Department of Dermatology, University Hospital Münster, Münster, Germany.

this clinical feature is not influenced by factors such as season or humidity. A considerable number of patients indicate that they suffer from hypohidrosis and cannot perspire well [4]. Other frequent features of the disease are keratosis follicularis and mostly mild concomitant AE, and allergic rhinitis [1,4,8]. Recently, there has been described a mild autosomal recessive inherited ichthyosis that is due to mutations in the *CASP14* gene, encoding caspase 14 (CASP14), which should be considered as a differential diagnosis of IV and mild forms of autosomal recessive congenital ichthyoses (ARCI). CASP14 is involved in the degradation of filaggrin [11].

Investigations

Histology reveals orthohyperkeratosis with a diminished or absent granular layer. Immunohistochemical studies show an absent or markedly reduced filaggrin signal. Ultrastructure reveals scarce and crumbly keratohyalin granules. The ultrastructural and immunohistological defects correlate very well with the number of *FLG* mutations in their severity [4,6,12].

Management

Ichthyosis vulgaris patients benefit from ointments that hydrate the stratum corneum [13], and from creams containing glycerol [14]. In those patients without concomitant AE, urea-containing creams (up to 10%) or creams containing lactic acid (up to 12%) also work well. In contrast to ARCI, excessive bathing procedures are not necessary, but showering and subsequent application of ointments are advisable. In the future, topical protein substitution therapy may become a promising approach [15].

Recessive X-linked ichthyosis

Definition and nomenclature

Recessive X-linked ichthyosis is a rather mild scaling disorder. Based on systematic screening of pregnancies for steroid sulphatase deficiency, a prevalence in males of 1 : 1500 has been determined [1].

Synonyms and inclusions
- Steroid sulphatase deficiency
- Placental sulphatase deficiency
- XLI
- Arylsulphatase C deficiency

Pathophysiology

Recessive X-linked ichthyosis is caused by mutations in the *STS* gene encoding steroid sulphatase [2]. Around 90% of cases are caused by deletions which in 75% span the whole gene sequence [3]. These deletions can extend to adjacent genes which may occasionally result in more complex phenotypes such as XLI occurring together with Kallmann syndrome, with the recessive form of X-linked chondrodysplasia punctata or with brain abnormalities including intellectual disability, unilateral polymicrogyria and retinitis pigmentosa [4]. Disease severity may be enhanced by a concomitant filaggrin mutation [5,6] as well as by a further, still unidentified, modifier. As a result of enzyme deficiency, cholesterol sulphate accumulates in the epidermis. High concentrations of cholesterol sulphate inhibit proteases such as kallikrein 5 and kallikrein 7 that are pivotal for normal degradation of corneodesmosomes. Indeed, in XLI skin, serine protease activity was found to be markedly reduced [7]. This in turn leads to decreased desquamation, and as a consequence to hyperkeratosis. XLI can thus be considered as a prototypic example of a retention hyperkeratosis. Measurements of transepidermal water loss have revealed a clear-cut increase of transepidermal water loss that is even more pronounced than, for example, in IV patients, while skin surface pH was not significantly altered [8].

Clinical features

The disease affects almost exclusively boys although female patients have been documented [9]. The mothers of affected children frequently report birth complications relating to the presence of the enzyme defect in the placenta. Insufficient cervical dilatation is often found in pregnant women with placental sulphatase deficiency and may cause prolonged delivery necessitating caesarean section or

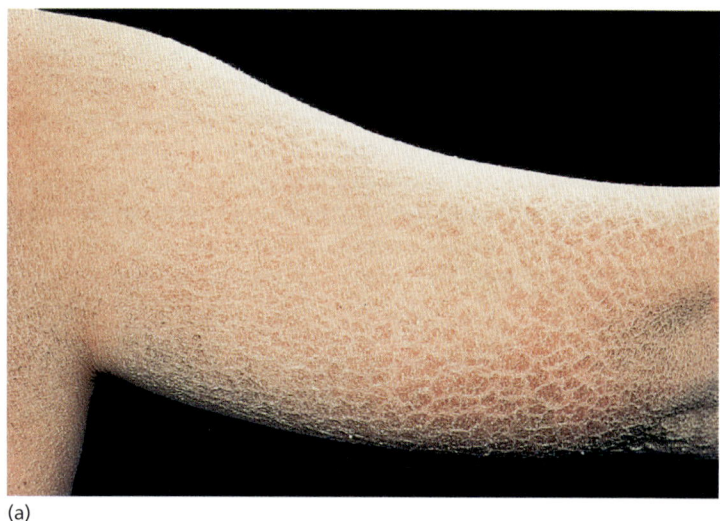

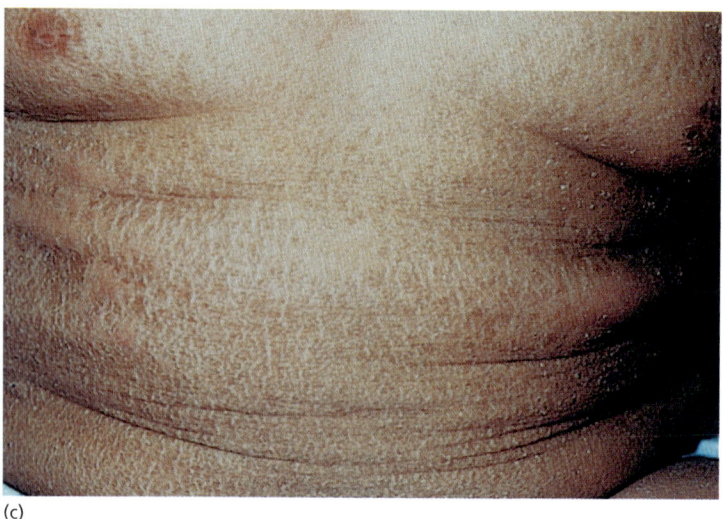

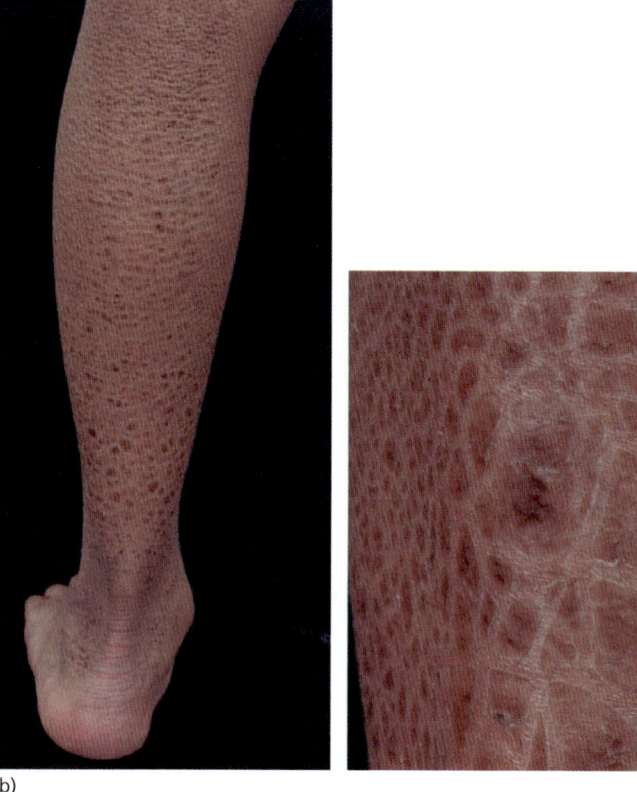

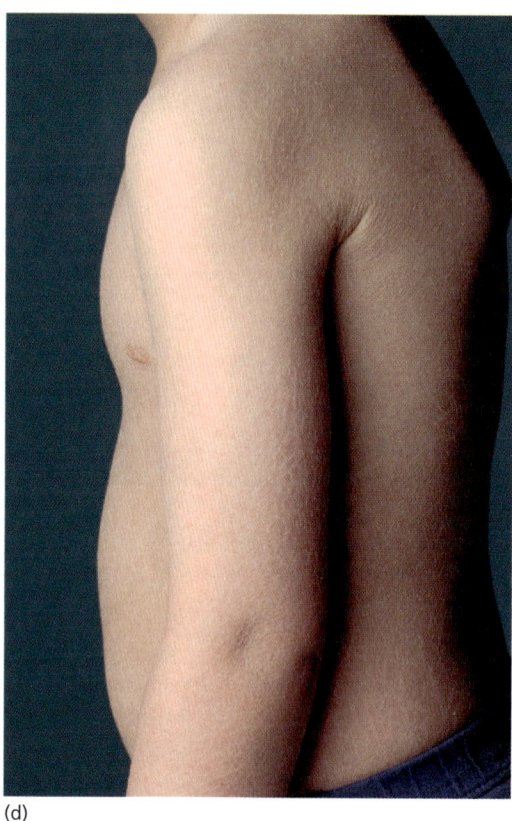

Figure 63.2 Recessive X-linked ichthyosis. (a) Scaling on the arm, (b) on the legs, (c) on the trunk and (d) patient with light grey scaling. (a–c) Courtesy of Dr M. Judge, Salford Royal NHS Trust, UK. (d) Courtesy of the Department of Dermatology, University Hospital Münster, Münster, Germany.

forceps delivery. About 15–20% of patients show manifestations at birth [10]. Typically, patients develop large, thick, dark brown to yellow-brown hyperkeratoses covering the trunk, the extremities and the neck at an age of 2–6 months (Figure 63.2). The antecubital folds and the popliteal folds are usually spared as in IV. The palms of the hands and the soles remain unaffected. In around 30% of patients, the colour of the scale is light grey (Figure 63.2d). These patients are often misdiagnosed as having IV. Dark hyperkeratosis giving the lateral aspects of the trunk and the back of the neck a 'dirty look' is a further feature which is typical of XLI and is usually

not present in IV. Recently, a high prevalence of *FLG* mutations was found in a European cohort with XLI. Patients with additional *FLG* mutations tend to show a more severe phenotype. XLI with and without additional *FLG* mutations was associated with atopic manifestations [11].

Deep stromal corneal opacity is a frequent finding if patients undergo an expert ophthalmological examination, but it usually does not affect visual acuity. XLI may be associated with cryptorchidism in up to 20% [12], with attention-deficit hyperactivity disorder (ADHD) in up to 40% or with autism in around

25% [13]. It is of note that steroid sulphatase-deficient mice carrying a deletion of the *STS* gene exhibit behavioural abnormalities relevant to ADHD such as inattention and hyperactivity. Moreover, these mice display altered serotonergic function that may account for their abnormal behaviour [14]. Of note, there is a high prevalence of epilepsy in patients with XLI [15]. Itch is common in XLI but less prevalent than in other subtypes of ichthyosis [16].

Investigations

If multiple family members are affected, careful scrutiny of the pedigree tree is instrumental in establishing the mode of inheritance of the disease. The existence of an affected grandfather or of affected uncles on the maternal side is suggestive of the diagnosis of XLI in a patient with ichthyosis.

Histology shows orthohyperkeratosis and a well-maintained, often thickened stratum granulosum. Marked follicular plugging can be noted in around 30% of patients although clinically there is no obvious keratosis follicularis. Ultrastructurally, a marked increase of persistent corneodesmosomes typical for retention hyperkeratosis can be seen.

Analysis making use of fluorescent *in situ* hybridisation (FISH) or comparative genomic hybridisation/comparative microarray analysis (CMA) allows rapid diagnosis in those cases with large deletions [17], but will miss around 10% of cases. Standard sequencing techniques are used to identify point mutations. Likewise it is possible to measure steroid sulphatase activity biochemically, for instance in fibroblasts or in plasma. Also, lipoprotein electrophoresis is a simple but useful tool revealing increased mobility of β-lipoproteins. Analysis of plasma levels for cholesterol sulphate by quantitative high-performance liquid chromatography (HPLC)/mass spectrometry is a very elegant method, but unfortunately currently available only for research purposes.

Management

Recessive X-linked ichthyosis patients benefit from the same therapeutic strategy that is applied for IV, namely the use of moisturisers. Again, excellent results can be achieved with a glycerol-containing cream. In the summertime, often spontaneous marked improvement can be observed, while in winter the skin condition becomes worse. It is of note that treatment with moisturisers does not normalise the transepidermal water loss but rather tends to further increase it, whereas skin dryness does improve [8]. Systemic retinoids may be given at low dosage during periods of disease exacerbations or for patients with severe manifestations [18].

NON-SYNDROMIC CONGENITAL ICHTHYOSES

See Table 63.1.

AUTOSOMAL RECESSIVE CONGENITAL ICHTHYOSIS

Definition and nomenclature

Unlike for example IV or XLI, the term ARCI does not denote a single MeDOC, but rather is an umbrella term that includes all non-syndromic autosomal recessive congenital forms of ichthyosis without a tendency towards blistering [1]. Thus the spectrum includes harlequin ichthyosis (HI), bathing suit ichthyosis (BSI), lamellar ichthyosis (LI), congenital ichthyosiform erythroderma (CIE), self-improving congenital ichthyosis (SICI), as well as transient manifestations such as collodion baby [2,3]. These diseases and their diverse genetic defects will be discussed separately.

> **Synonyms and inclusions**
> - Ichthyosis congenita
> - Terms like LI or CIE describe extreme ends of the clinical spectrum, but are used in older textbooks as synonyms

Epidemiology
Prevalence
Registry-based data from Spain [4] and Germany [5] show that the prevalence of ARCI in Europe is in the range of 1.6 per 100 000.

Pathophysiology
Autosomal recessive congenital ichthyosis is associated with mutations in a plethora of genes (see Table 63.1), which encode proteins involved in lipid transport, such as *ABCA12* [6], in lipid biosynthesis such as *CERS3* [7] and in fatty acid metabolism or have a role in assembling suprastructures such as the cornified envelope. A definite 'unified field theory' explaining how these various proteins interact with each other and result in a barrier defect and in hyperkeratosis is still lacking, but it seems that the corneocyte lipid envelope provides a bidirectional scaffold required for both lamellar membrane formation and generation of a replete, underlying cornified envelope [8].

Genotype–phenotype correlations have been reported for some of these disorders. This is best illustrated by the *ABCA12* gene. Missense mutations in this gene cause either LI [9] or CIE [10] whereas nonsense or frameshift mutations result in life-threatening HI [6]. The combination of the two types of mutations results in an intermediate phenotype [12]. Similarly, BSI has been associated with distinct temperature-sensitive mutations in *TGM1* [13]. The numerous remaining ARCI types resolve into clinical phenotypes like LI, CIE or SICI, all of which can be caused by mutations in a number of different genes with no clear genotype–phenotype relationships. Around 10–20% of ARCI cases cannot be attributed to known genes [14].

Clinical features
See the relevant sections in the following ARCI disease types.

Mangement
See 'Management of congenital ichthyoses' later in this chapter.

Harlequin ichthyosis

Definition
Harlequin ichthyosis is the most devastating type of ARCI. It is still often lethal in around 44% of cases [1]. Based on preliminary

data from the Network for Ichthyoses and Related Keratinization Disorders (NIRK) registry in Germany, the prevalence of HI is estimated to be in the region of 1 in 2 million. It appears to be roughly 10 times lower than transglutaminase 1 (TG1)-deficient ARCI.

Pathophysiology

It has already been pointed out that peculiar nonsense and/or frameshift mutations in the *ABCA12* gene cause HI [2,3]. These types of mutations usually result in mRNA decay and loss of expression of the protein [4,5]. Heterozygous mutations have a survival advantage over homozygotes [1].

ABCA12 transfers lipids such as glucosylceramides, which are essential for epidermal barrier formation, into lamellar bodies. It plays an essential role in the formation of lamellar bodies that also transport proteases such as kallikrein 5, 7 and 14 and secrete these proteins into the intercellular space in the stratum corneum [6]. These proteases play an important role in desquamation by degrading corneodesmosomes [7], thus leading to retention hyperkeratosis [8].

Clinical features

Neonates are born with armour-like skin (truncal plates with fissuring) (Figure 63.3a) which can considerably impair movement and the ability to drink and breathe. Bilateral ectropion and eclabium are present and hyperkeratotic skin may result in ears lacking retroaural folds. Around 10% of children develop autoamputation of digits [1]. A major problem in early infancy is a proneness to infection of the skin, as well as other organs such as the lungs. Respiratory problems are the major cause of death in neonates. Data from an animal model seem to implicate that HI is not only a skin disease, but can also affect lung function causing alveolar collapse [9]. In those children who survive the critical initial phase of the disease, the thickening of the stratum corneum improves somewhat and large lamellar scales, accompanied by marked ichthyosiform erythroderma, develop (Figure 63.3b, c). In later life persistent ectropion is a frequent major problem, and often these patients have problems achieving and maintaining normal body weight despite high-calorie supplementation. Vitamin D deficiency causing rickets and osteomalacia can occur [1].

Investigations

Harlequin ichthyosis has a striking histology showing enormous thickness of the stratum corneum. There is parakeratosis and hypergranulosis and non-polar lipids are reduced, while expression of proteases like kallekrein 5 and cathepsin D is dramatically reduced [10]. Electron microscopy reveals numerous abnormal lamellar bodies in the stratum granulosum and accumulation of extruded irregular lamellar bodies as vesicular structures between the epidermal cornified cells. This defect of lamellar bodies is highly pathognomic for HI allowing its diagnosis (Figure 63.4).

Management

Management requires an interdisciplinary approach and will be discussed in detail in the later section on the management of a collodion baby; see also the reviews by Rajpopat and co-workers [1] and Glick and co-workers [11].

Collodion baby and self-improving congenital ichthyosis

Definition

The term collodion baby describes a transient condition in newborns. Except for HI, most ARCI patients present at birth as 'collodion babies' [1], but it should also be noted that several syndromic types of congenital ichthyosis such as trichothiodystrophy (TTD) or Gaucher syndrome type 2 typically present as collodion baby.

Pathophysiology

See the relevant sections in BSI, LI and CIE.

Clinical features

The neonate is encased in a shiny parchment-like membrane, which cracks within a few days after birth (Figure 63.5) and usually peels off within the first 4 weeks of life. Initially, the clinical presentation can be quite severe and often includes ectropion and everted lips of different degrees. Afterwards for a brief time healthy skin becomes visible. In other cases, the collodion membrane is very mild and needs to be differentiated from physiological desquamation [2]. Collodion babies look very much alike at birth, but later take different clinical courses. In around 80% of cases, collodion baby is then followed by the onset of an ARCI subtype. The clinical presentations may evolve into BSI or into the phenotypes of LI (e.g. in severe TG1 deficiency) or CIE (e.g. in lipoxygenase deficiency). However, around 10–20% of cases develop into SICI [3] or self-healing collodion baby (SHCB) [4]. It is possible that in some cases specific mutations particularly sensitive to average hydrostatic water pressure during pregnancy may underlie the dynamic phenotype of SHCB. Patients with SICI have very mild involvement but most of them have facial reddening, thickened skin on the dorsal hands and feet and thickened palms and soles with hyperlinearity but without hyperkeratosis (Figure 63.6) [5].

Differential diagnosis

Ichthyosis prematurity syndrome (IPS) (see later in this chapter) is an important differential diagnosis of SICI and SHCB.

Management

See 'Management of congenital ichthyoses' later in this chapter.

Bathing suit ichthyosis

Definition

Bathing suit ichthyosis is a peculiar type of ARCI first recognised in South African Bantu of the Nguni ethnic group [1]. While children are born as collodion babies, they later develop a lamellar type of ichthyosis that spares the face and the extremities and follows the distribution pattern of bathing suits.

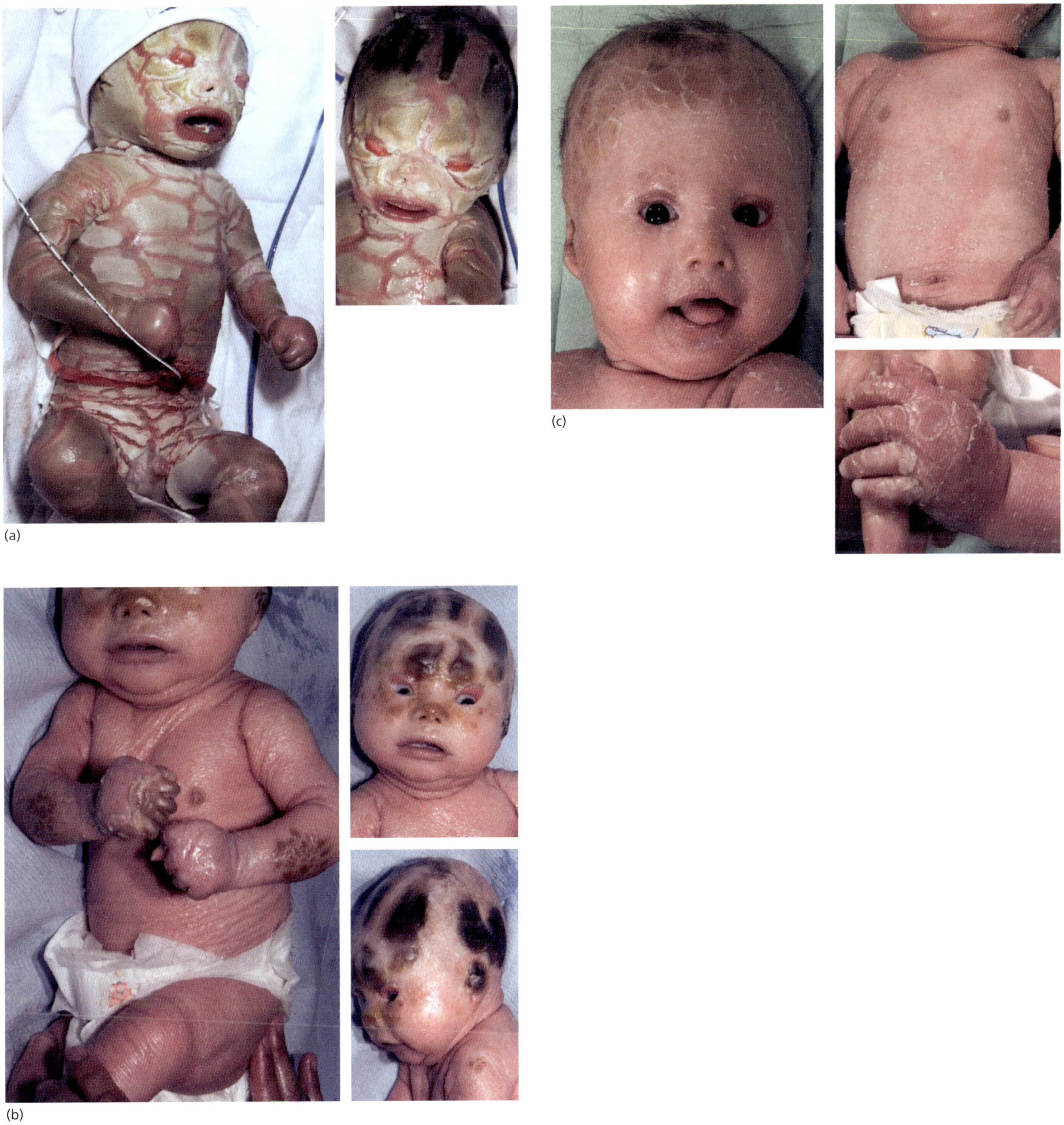

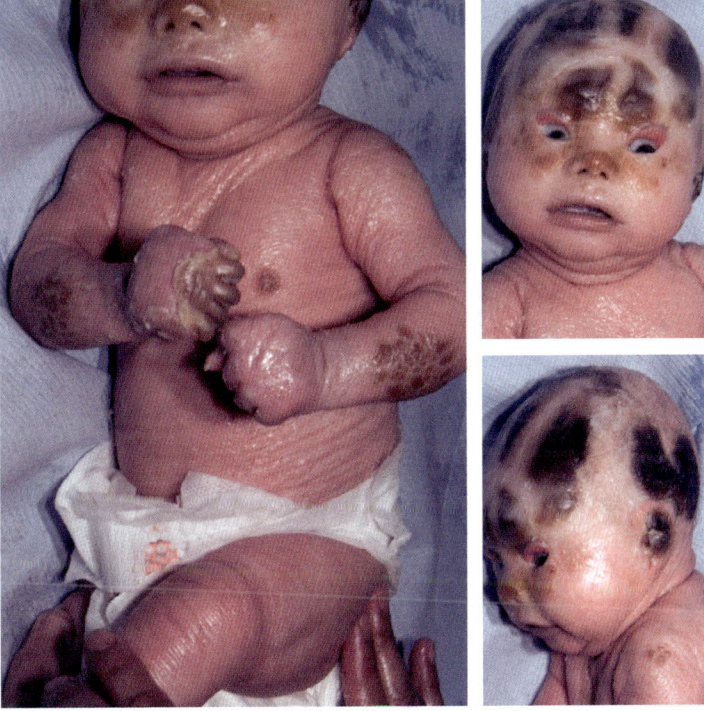

(a)

(b)

(c)

Figure 63.3 Harlequin ichthyosis. (a) Neonate, (b) aged 6 weeks on retinoid therapy and (c) aged 6 months. Courtesy of Dr M. Judge, Salford Royal NHS Trust, UK.

Pathophysiology

Bathing suit ichthyosis was found to be due to peculiar missense mutations in *TGM1* that render the enzyme TG1 temperature sensitive [2,3]. Recombinant expression of the *TGM1* mutations in BSI showed that they exhibit a marked shift in temperature optimum from 37°C to 31°C. Deficient activity of BSI mutants could be rescued and even reconstituted by decreasing the temperature to below 33°C. All BSI mutations showed an activity above 10% at their temperature optimum at 31°C and a dramatic decrease at 37°C [4]. It is of note that the vast majority of BSI-causing mutations

PART 6: GENETIC DISORDERS

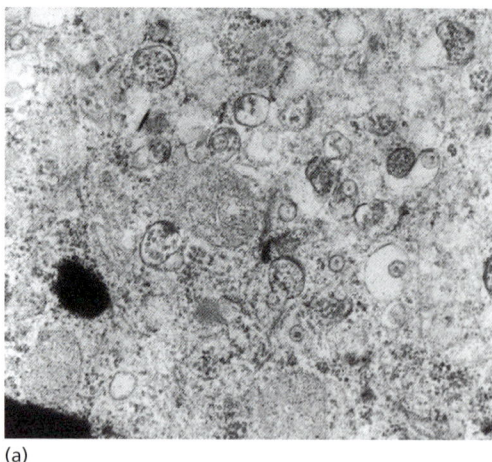

(a)

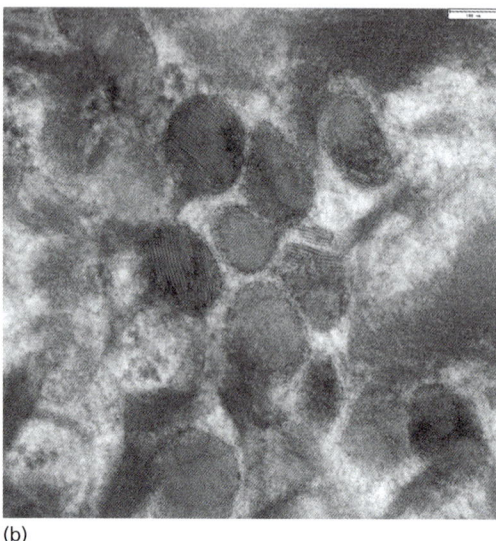

(b)

Figure 63.4 Ultrastructural diagnosis of harlequin ichthyosis. (a) Abnormal lamellar bodies in ABCA12 deficiency. (b) Morphology of normal lamellar bodies in granular layer cells with their diverse cargos: mostly lamellated, but also homogeneous areas (higher magnification). Courtesy of Dr I. Hausser, Heidelberg, Germany.

affect arginine residues (e.g. p.Arg315His) and often affect exons 5, 6 or 7 [5–8]. A few of these patients eventually heal completely and could also be regarded as examples of SICI [5,8].

Clinical features

The most striking aspect is the dynamic of the phenotype. Children are born as collodion babies involving the entire skin. Shedding of the collodion membrane is followed by the development of large, dark grey/brownish scales affecting the trunk and the scalp, but sparing the face and extremities (Figure 63.7). The palms and soles are dry and diffusely mildly hyperkeratotic. Digital thermography has validated a striking correlation between warmer body areas and the presence of scaling in patients [2]. The disease tends to become worse in the summer months and to improve in winter [9]. Hypohydrosis as is often seen in ARCI may play a crucial role in local heat accumulation that results in an additional reduction of TG1 activity [10]. In the authors' experience, hyperkeratoses can develop in the ear canal affecting the ability to hear.

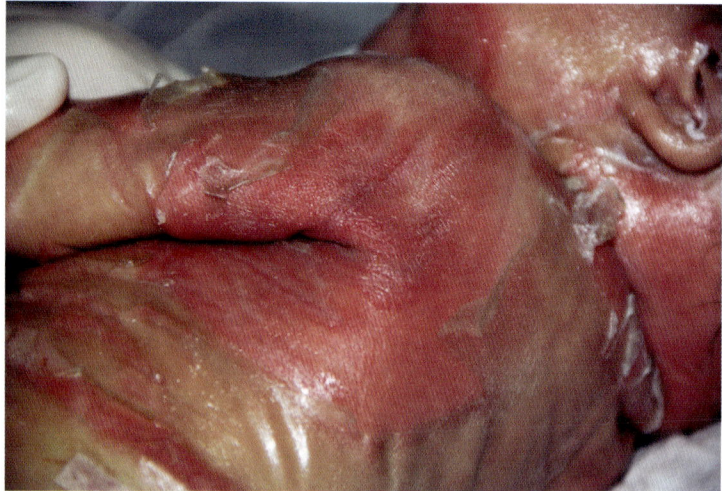

Figure 63.5 Autosomal recessive congenital ichthyosis. Sheddding of collodion membranes after 1 week.

Investigations

In situ assessment of TG1 activity reveals a deficiency only in affected skin, with sufficient activity in unaffected healthy-appearing skin [2]. Likewise, ultrastructural analysis reveals a massively thickened stratum corneum displaying multiple cholesterol clefts which are typical for TG1 deficiency, while the stratum corneum is of normal thickness in healthy skin and shows no cholesterol clefts [2].

Management

Management corresponds to that of LI, but special attention should be given to the ears and to removing keratotic material from the ear canal.

Lamellar ichthyosis and congenital ichthyosiform erythroderma

Definition

When the term 'lamellar ichthyosis' was coined by the American dermatologist Phillip Frost in the 1960s [1], it was used to denote a type of ARCI that is characterised by large, plate-like, dark-brown hyperkeratoses covering the entire body, but usually presenting rather mild palmoplantar involvement (Figure 63.8a). At the other end of the clinical spectrum, ARCI patients may present with very marked erythroderma and mostly fine often whitish or grey scales. These patients often have pronounced palmoplantar keratosis and have been referred to as having CIE (Figure 63.8b).

Epidemiology

Prevalence

Deficiency of TG1 as the most frequent cause of ARCI is responsible for 32% of ARCI cases in Germany, while in the USA it has been found in up to 55% of the cases studied [2]. In Europe, mutations in *ALOX12B* account for 12% of ARCI, and *ALOXE3* mutations are responsible for a further 5% of cases. *NIPAL4* mutations account for 16% of ARCI and are thus a frequent cause. Around 8% of ARCI cases are due to mutations in the *CYP4F22* gene [3,4].

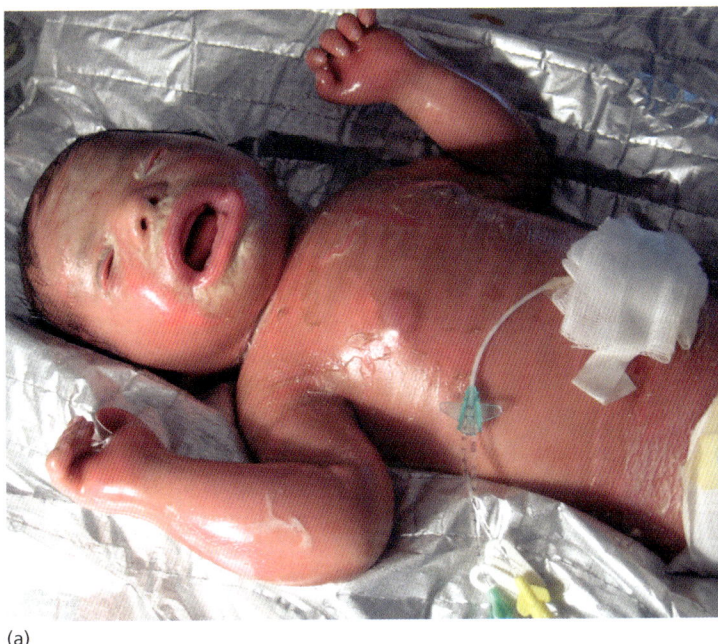
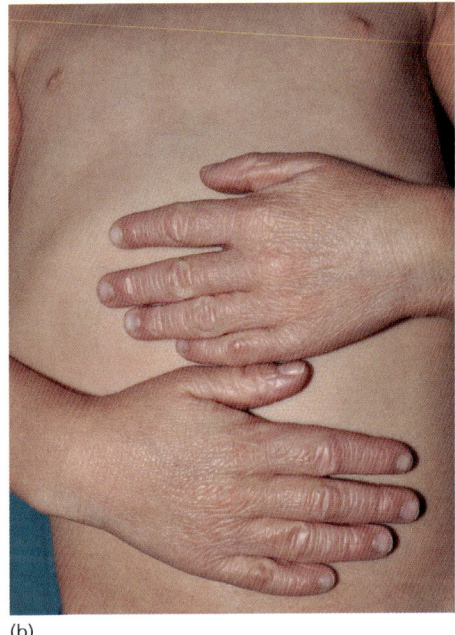

Figure 63.6 Self-improving congenital ichthyosis. (a) Collodion baby at birth. (b) Mild ichthyosis and lichenification of the skin of the hand.

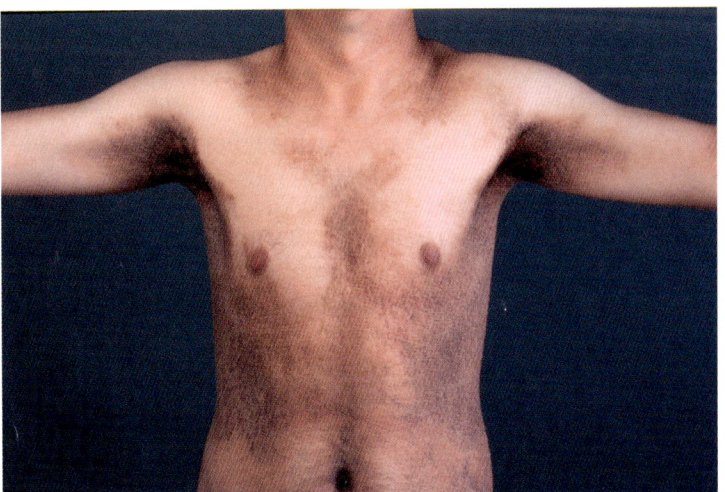

Figure 63.7 Bathing suit ichthyosis. Lamellar scaling on areas with a high skin temperature. Courtesy of the Department of Dermatology, University Hospital Münster, Münster, Germany.

Pathophysiology

Cell kinetic studies in the 1980s seemed to discriminate between the phenotypes of LI and CIE [5], which at that time were considered to represent distinct entities. However, genetic studies disclosed that the LI phenotype as well as the CIE phenotype is by no means specific for a certain gene, but mutations in the same gene may be associated with both phenotypes [6]. The specific pathogenesis may concern a malfunction of the following proteins.

- Transglutaminase-1 critically contributes to the assembly of the cornified envelope by catalysing calcium-dependent cross-linking of proteins, such as involucrin-, loricrin- and proline-rich proteins, and by binding Ω-hydroxy ceramides to proteins such as involucrin, thus connecting the lipid envelope with the cornified envelope [7,8].

- The epidermal lipoxygenases E3 and 12B act on adjacent steps in the hepoxilin pathway and are believed to play a role in the secretion of lamellar bodies so that mutations in the genes encoding these enzymes result in impaired secretion of lipids and formation of the intercellular lipids in the stratum corneum [9–12].

- The *NIPAL4* gene encodes for the protein ichthyin. Patients having a *NIPAL4* mutation show a markedly increased expression of epidermal lipoxigenases and TG1 in their skin, indicating a common metabolic pathway essential for skin barrier homeostasis [13,14]. The precise function of this protein is not entirely understood. It appears to localise to desmosomes and keratins [15] and to interact with fatty acid transporter protein 4 [16], which is defective in IPS.

- The gene *CYP4F2* encodes a cytochrome P450 polypeptide that is a homologue of a leukotriene B4 Ω-hydroxylase. The actual function of this gene for the epidermal barrier has not been established, but it has been hypothesised that it participates in the hepoxilin pathway by catalysing the conversion of trioxilin A3 to 20 hydroxy-(R) trioxilin [17].

- Mutations in the *CERS3* gene encoding ceramide synthase 3 are a rare cause of ARCI [18,19]. Inactivating mutations in this gene are associated with a loss of very long acyl chains from C26 up to C34 in terminally differentiating keratinocytes of affected patients and thus impairing epidermal barrier formation.

- *LIPN* encodes an acid lipase that is involved in triglyceride metabolism in mammals and is expressed exclusively in the epidermis. A 2 bp deletion in *LIPN* was found to be associated with a mild form of CIE showing diffuse ichthyosis [20].

- *SDR9C7* belongs to the short-chain dehydrogenase/reductase family and has been identified as the causative gene in several Lebanese families [21]. *SDR9C7* seems to be involved in vitamin A metabolism and to have a potential role in epidermal differentiation.

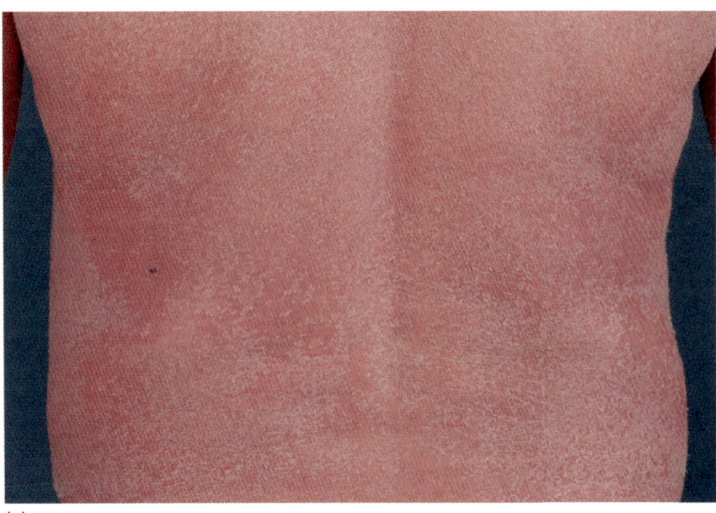

(a)

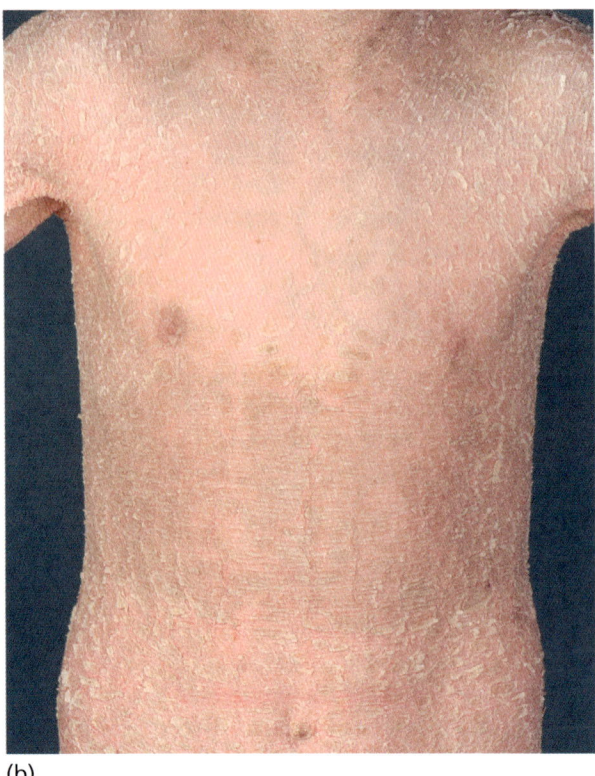

(b)

Figure 63.8 (a) Lamellar ichthyosis. (b) Congenital ichthyosiform erythroderma. Courtesy of the Department of Dermatology, University Hospital Münster, Münster, Germany.

- Mutations in *SULT2B1* have been reported in three independent families [22]. *SULT2B1* is a member of the large cytosolic sulfotransferase superfamily that is engaged in the synthesis and metabolism of steroids in humans. It is specifically expressed in the stratum corneum/granulosum, suggesting a function in late keratinocyte differentiation and epidermal homeostasis.
- *PNPLA1* belongs to the patatin-like phospholipase family and is related to *PNPLA2*, which causes neutral lipid storage disease with myopathy but without ichthyosis. *PNPLA1* mutations were

first identified as a cause of ichthyosis in golden retriever dogs and afterwards in humans, who feature fine white scales and moderate erythroderma and PPK and a pseudosyndactyly of the second and third toes [23].

Clinical features

A definite genotype–phenotype relationship for LI and CIE has not yet been achieved, but in the authors' experience there are clinical clues in ARCI that tend to be indicative for certain genes. The majority of patients having *TGM1* mutations present with classic LI (see earlier definition), often having complaints such as ectropion or alopecia ichthyotica. There is no obvious erythroderma, but beneath the thick scales some erythema can be present. Ears are often deformed and small. As indicated earlier, specific temperature-sensitive mutations in *TGM1* are associated with BSI. Moreover, there is a group of patients who initially present as collodion babies, progress to mild CIE and later may present with very mild or even absent scaling. This phenotype is referred to as SICI (see Figure 63.6) [6,24]. *TGM1* patients who carry premature termination codon mutations (e.g. nonsense or frameshift mutations) are more likely to report sweating abnormalities such as hypohidrosis and overheating than those who have missense mutations [2].

Neonates with lipoxygenase mutations are often born with a mild type of collodion and in later life mostly present with the CIE phenotype, although some also present brownish scales. Typically, they show a striking palmoplantar hyperlinearity (Figure 63.9), which is reminiscent of the accentuated creases in IV [10]. However, mild keratotic lichenifications of the elbow fossa or of the dorsum of the hands help to rule out this differential diagnosis. Patients may progress to SICI [24]. Those with *ALOX12B* mutations more often exhibit pronounced palmoplantar keratosis than patients with *ALOXE3* mutations [10]. Many of these patients report reduced or completely absent sweating ability [25], and many complain of pruritus.

Patients with a *NIPAL4* mutation often present with a CIE/LI overlapping phenotype, ectropion, clubbing of the nails and a pronounced and diffuse yellowish keratoderma on the palms and soles (Figure 63.10a, b) [26]. This may be reminiscent of classic PPKs such as a focal non-epidermolytic type. Scaling may be reticulate on the trunk (Figure 63.10c).

Most patients with *CYP4F2* mutations present with a CIE or mild collodion baby phenotype at birth [27]. As the children grow older, they develop whitish-grey scales which are more pronounced in the periumbilical region [17]. Palms and soles show pronounced hyperlinearity or even PPK.

Patients with mutations in *CERS3* are born as collodion babies and then progress to CIE often with improvement of the ichthyosis phenotype in the summertime. Also, patients have marked plantar hyperlinearity (Figure 63.11) and may experience pruritus and recurrent uncomplicated bacterial and *Pityrosporum* infections [18].

LIPN mutations cause a late-onset form of ichthyosis at the age of 5 years, but have been linked to the ARCI spectrum [20].

Reported patients with *SDR9C7* mutations present with congenital ichthyosiform erythroderma and have suffered persistent

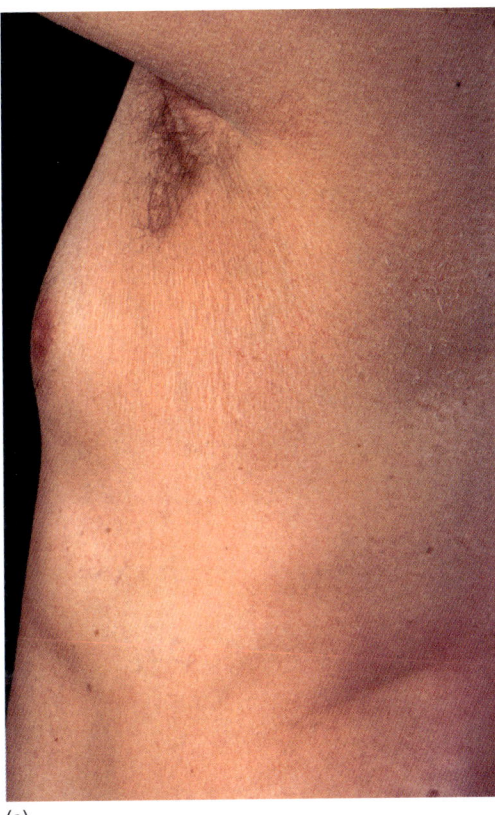

(a)

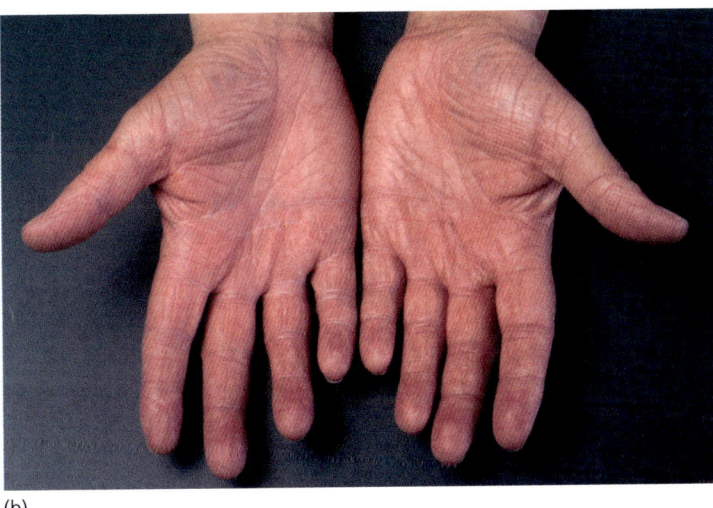

(b)

Figure 63.9 (a, b) Clinical phenotype of *ALOXE3* mutations. Note palmoplantar hyperlinearity resembling accentuated creases in ichthyosis vulgaris (b). Courtesy of the Department of Dermatology, University Hospital Münster, Münster, Germany.

fungal cutaneous infections since the first decade. Severity decreases with age [21].

Individuals with *SULT2B1* mutations are born as collodion babies and show a variable degree of red skin and hyperkeratosis with mild or no involvement of the axilla, face, popliteal fossa and back [22].

Investigations

Diagnosis of TG1 deficiency can be made by sequencing [2,3,8] or by measuring *in situ* TG1 activity in cryostat sections [28].

Ultrastructural investigations reveal so-called cholesterol clefts in the stratum corneum (Figure 63.12) [29]. *NIPAL4* mutations may correlate with the ultrastructure of abnormal lamellar bodies and elongated membranes in the stratum granulosum classified as ARCI electron microscopy type III [30]. Direct sequencing is necessary for the diagnosis of lipoxygenase deficiency and other ARCI subtypes (*CERS3, CYP4F2, LIPN, SDR9C7, PNPLA1* or *SULT2B1*) that lack specific ultrastructural markers. Biochemical measurements of lipoxygenase activity is feasible but is currently available only in specialised research laboratories [31]. The same applies for ultrastructural methods with frozen sections or osmium tetroxide and ruthenium tetroxide postfixation that may enable advanced electron microscopic diagnostics of all ARCI subtypes [32].

KERATINOPATHIC ICHTHYOSES

Definition

Keratinopathic ichthyoses (KPIs) are a group of very severe, ultra-rare cornification disorders (Tables 63.1 and 63.3). In Denmark they have a prevalence of 1 in 350 000 [1]. Patients often present at birth with erythroderma, scales and erosions. The term 'keratinopathic' was coined at the Sorèze Consensus Conference as an umbrella term for all types of ichthyoses that are caused by mutations in one of the keratin genes [2].

Pathophysiology

Epidermal keratins are intermediate filaments that contribute to the formation of the keratinocyte cell cytoskeleton. This cytoskeleton extends from the nucleus of the keratinocyte to the cell membrane where keratins attach either to desmosomes or hemidesmosomes [3]. Mutations in keratin genes like *KRT1, KRT10* or *KRT2* are usually associated with epidermolytic hyperkeratosis (EHK) on histology (Figure 63.13) and with the occurrence of cytoplasmic keratin aggregates (keratin clumps) or perinuclear shell formation, which can be seen only with electron microscopy [4,5].

These keratin aggregates can be induced by trauma or environmental conditions, such as high temperature, fever or skin infections, that are known modulators of disease severity. The keratin aggregates are reminiscent of those in classic protein folding disorders such as neurodegenerative diseases like Huntington disease [6]. Cells expressing mutant keratin aggregates have increased sensitivity to hyperosmotic stress which can be reduced, for example, by the chemical chaperone trimethylamine-*N*-oxide [7]. Likewise, it has been shown that retinoids reduce the formation of keratin aggregates in heat-stressed keratinocytes from an epidermolytic ichthyosis (EI) patient with a *KRT10* mutation [8]. Keratin aggregates have been shown to interact with activated mitogen-activated protein kinase (MAP) kinases, molecular chaperones such as Hsp70 and components of the ubiquitin–proteasome system and may contribute to inflammatory changes seen in the disease [9]. Moreover, *KRT1* knock-out mice release large amounts of the pro-inflammatory interleukin 18 (IL-18); depletion of IL-18 partially rescued Krt1–/– mice [10], suggesting novel approaches to therapy.

Although KPIs have been traditionally considered as autosomal dominant disorders [11], recessive and semidominant

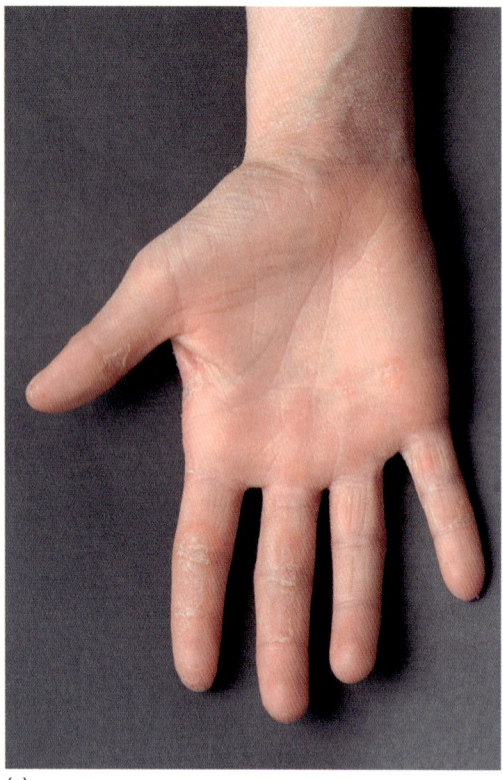

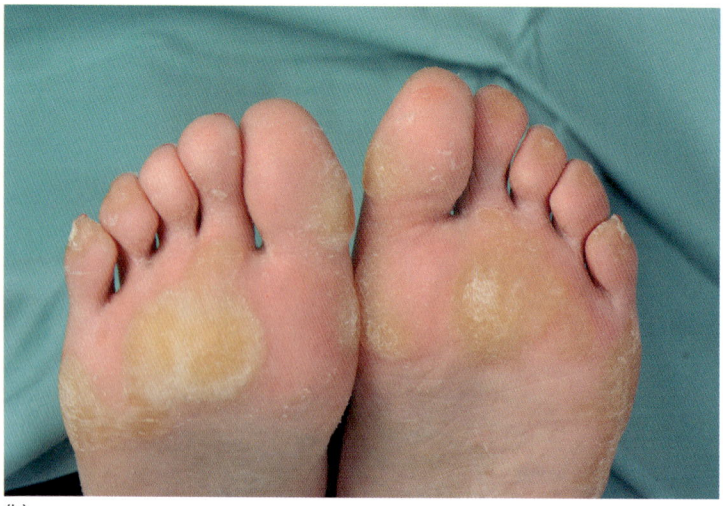

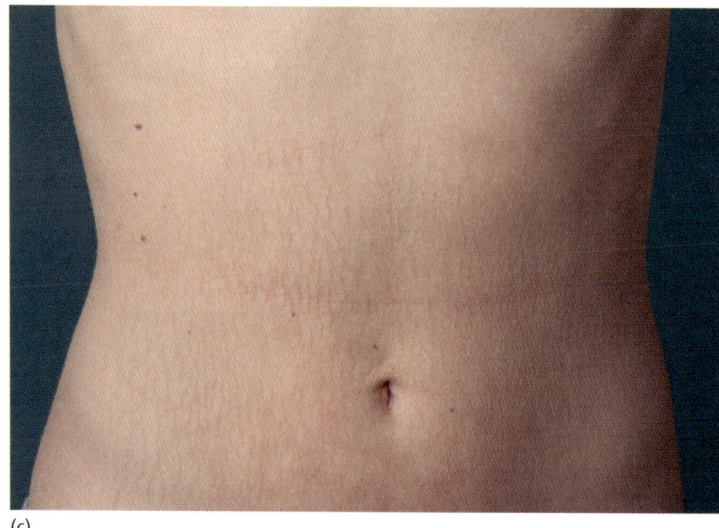

Figure 63.10 Clinical phenotype of *NIPAL4* mutations. (a, b) Diffuse yellowish keratoderma on the palms and soles. (c) Reticulate scaling on the trunk. Courtesy of the Department of Dermatology, University Hospital Münster, Münster, Germany.

inheritance of *KRT10* [12] and *KRT1* [13] mutations has been reported, respectively. Gene therapy would have to address the dominant negative effect of the mutations to restored filament stability [14].

The vast majority of mutations in KPIs consist of heterozygous single-point mutations that are found in the highly conserved helix boundary motives of *KRT1* and *KRT10* that play a crucial role in filament formation [15–17]. Up to 75% of KPI-causing mutations are *de novo* mutations [18,19].

Epidermolytic epidermal naevus results from somatic mutations in *KRT1* or *KRT10*. Germ-line mosaicism in these cases, which may be associated with a small epidermolytic naevus in a patient (Figure 63.14a), can result in full-blown disease in his or her offspring [20,21]. Occasionally, forms of EI can be seen where many Blaschko linear stripes of the skin are affected by widespread hyperkeratosis representing multiple epidermolytic naevi, resulting from extensive postzygotic mosaicism [22,23].

Epidermolytic ichthyosis

Synonyms and inclusions
- EHK
- Bullous CIE
- Ichthyosis type Brocq

Clinical features [1–6]
At birth, the presentation usually consists of CIE often associated with marked blistering. In the classic French literature, this presentation was referred to as 'burned child/enfant brûlé' (Figure 63.14b). In neonates, the differential diagnosis therefore often includes epidermolysis bullosa. In the first months of life, the blistering resolves and hyperkeratosis develops instead. However, fragility of the skin remains and when patients suffer from fever or skin

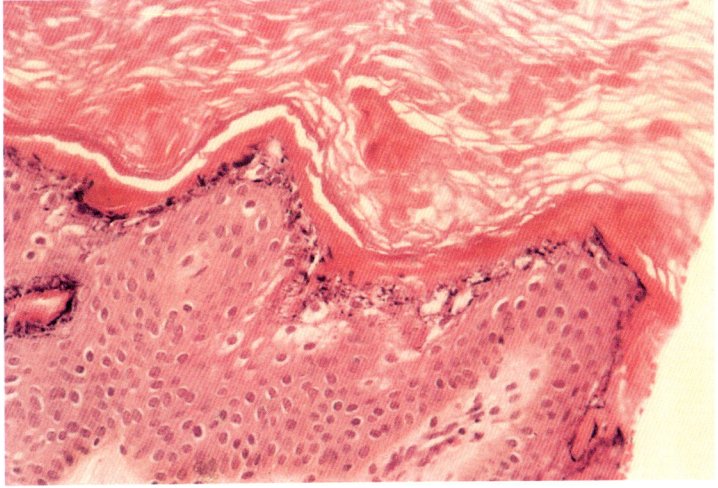

Figure 63.13 Histological diagnosis of epidermolytic hyperkeratosis.

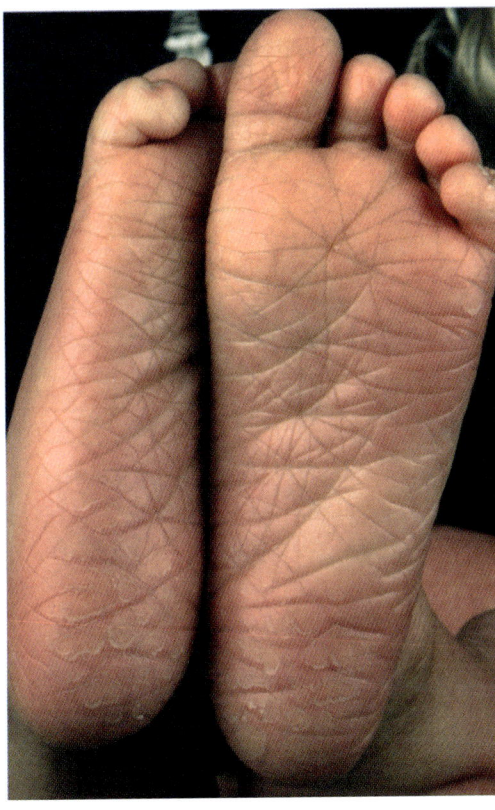

Figure 63.11 Clinical phenotype of *CERS3* deficiency showing mild plantar keratoderma with hyperlinearity. Courtesy of the Department of Dermatology, University Hospital Münster, Münster, Germany.

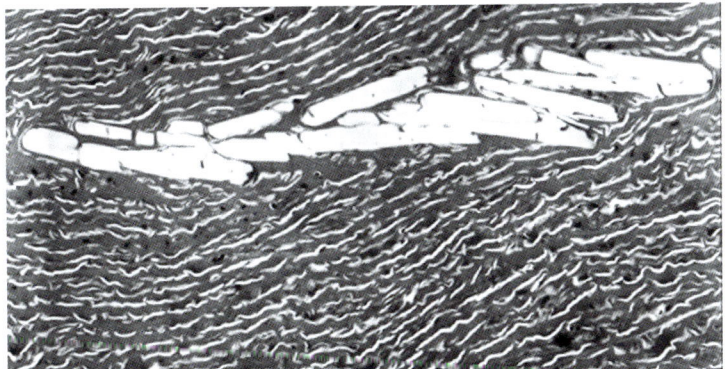

Figure 63.12 Ultrastructure of transglutaminase 1-deficient skin with typical cholesterol clefts in the stratum corneum. Courtesy of Dr I. Hausser, Heidelberg, Germany.

infections or are exposed in the summer to high ambient temperature or mechanical friction, bouts of blistering can occur. The older child and adult patients usually present with marked keratotic lichenification, meaning rippled keratotic ridges, in particular in the axilla, the elbows and the flexural aspects of the knees. It is striking that this severe involvement correlates with skin regions where the body temperature is somewhat elevated and thus this aggravation may be induced by differences in body temperature. On the knees and lower legs, patients sometimes present with spiny hyperkeratosis (Figure 63.15a–c). In patients harbouring *KRT10* mutations, the palms and soles are usually spared (Figure 63.15d) [1], and they

tend to respond well to moderate dosages of systemic retinoids (see 'Management of congenital ichthyoses' later in this chapter), while patients having *KRT1* mutations usually have severe involvement of the palms and soles which can significantly impair walking so that some patients actually require a wheelchair. Itch is a co-morbidity frequently observed in EI [7]. Urticaria may trigger blister formation in EI, and resolution of symptoms after treatment with omalizumab has been reported [8].

Investigations [9,10]

The types of KPI mentioned earlier share a striking histology, namely EHK. In superficial EI, this finding is less marked and expressed mainly in the stratum granulosum and upper epidermis, and it may be important to take a biopsy from a site of maximal clinical involvement, for instance from the knees. Similar considerations apply for annular EI. As mentioned, the ultrastructure of these diseases is characterised by collapsed keratin aggregates (tonofilaments). These aggregates often form around the cell nucleus, have lost their connection to the desmosomes and therefore promote intraepidermal blistering. As already discussed, the presence of keratin aggregate links the pathology to that of protein folding diseases [11].

Superficial epidermolytic ichthyosis

Synonyms and inclusions
- Ichthyosis bullosa Siemens

Clinical features [1–9]

The clinical presentation of superficial epidermolytic ichthyosis (SEI) resembles that of EI. However, the course of the disease is milder and more localised, meaning that large parts of the body are clear. Typically, the keratosis is limited to the region around the navel and on the dorsal aspects of the hands and feet or the arm

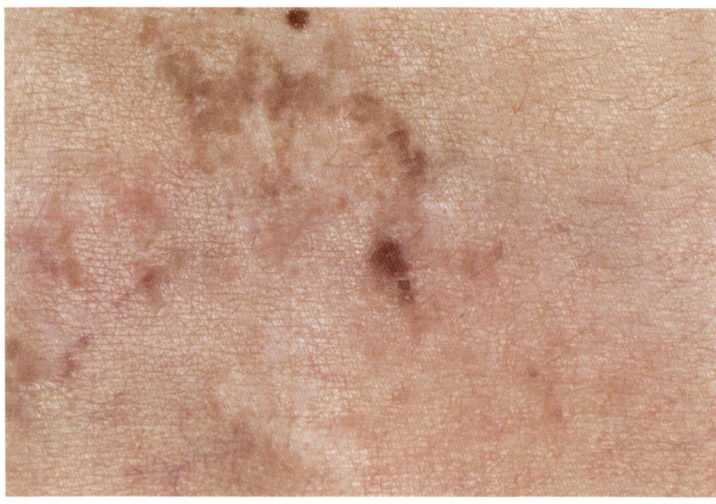

(a)

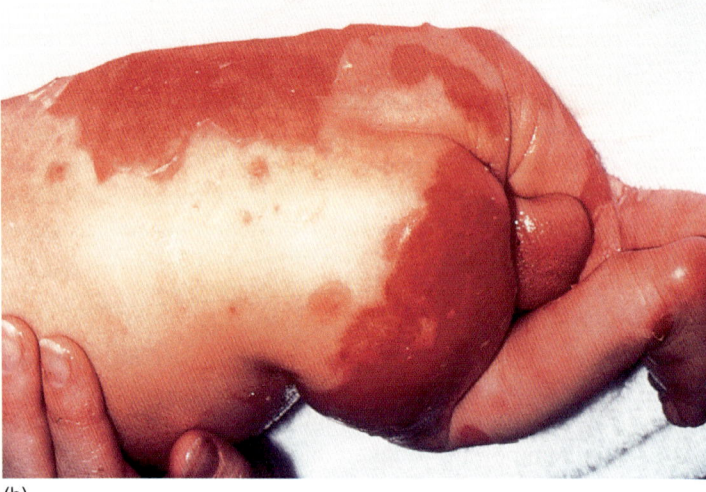

(b)

Figure 63.14 Special genetic aspect in keratinopathic ichthyosis. (a) Epidermolytic naevus in a father of an affected boy with generalised epidermolytic ichthyosis due to keratin 10. (b) Neonatal presentation of epidermolytic ichthyosis ('enfant brulé'). (b) Courtesy of Dr M. Judge, Salford Royal NHS Trust, UK.

and the axillary region (Figure 63.16). A phenomenon that is quite typical is the presence of superficially denuded areas, for instance on the back of the hand (Figure 63.17) [2]. For this phenomenon Siemens, who first described the disease in 1937, coined the German term 'Mauserung' (moulting) [1]. Co-occurrence of hypertrichosis of the extremities has often been reported in SEI [10].

Annular epidermolytic ichthyosis

Synonyms and inclusions
- Cyclic epidermolytic ichthyosis

Clinical features
Annular epidermolytic ichthyosis (AEI) is a rather mild variant of EI [1,2], which shares a similar onset at birth, but later greatly improves and can feature bouts of disease activity associated with the development of numerous annular and polycyclic hyperkeratotic lesions especially on the trunk and extremities [1]. Outbreak of disease flares can be associated with high temperature in the summer, fever or pregnancy [3]. It has been suggested that AEI may be regarded as a mild phenotype of EI rather than as a true subtype [4,5].

Congenital reticular ichthyosiform erythroderma

Synonyms and inclusions
- Ichthyosis variegata
- Ichthyosis en confetti

Pathophysiology
Congenital reticular ichthyosiform erythroderma (CRIE) is due to particular *KRT10* or *KRT1* mutations [1,2]. Patients initially display generalised redness and scaling with subsequent localised spontaneous healing which manifests with small pale white spots. The revertant phenotype is due to multiple recombination events in the *KRT10* gene [1], which can be considered as a kind of natural gene therapy.

Clinical features
This disease was described independently in 1984 by a German group [3] and by a Swiss group [4], who coined the term 'confetti ichthyosis'. It is characterised by very severe CIE and from the age of 3 years by the gradual onset of hundreds of pale normal-appearing confetti-like spots which can grow up to 2 cm in size (Figure 63.18). Many of these patients are severely ill and fail to thrive. Further clinical features include prominent PPK, hypertrichosis of dorsal limbs, extropion, short stature, and contraction neck deformity [5–8].

Investigations
Histology and ultrastructure differ from typical EI showing, for example, binuclear cells and perinuclear vacuolisation, and probably not the typical keratin aggregates [6].

Ichthyosis Curth–Macklin

Synonyms and inclusions
- Ichthyosis hystrix Curth–Macklin

Pathophysiology
Pathogenic mutations in *KRT1* affect the variable tail domain (V2) of keratin 1 and result in a profoundly different abnormality of the cytoskeletal architecture than in EI [1,2]. For keratin 10, a deletion at the end of the 2B domain of the protein has been reported [3].

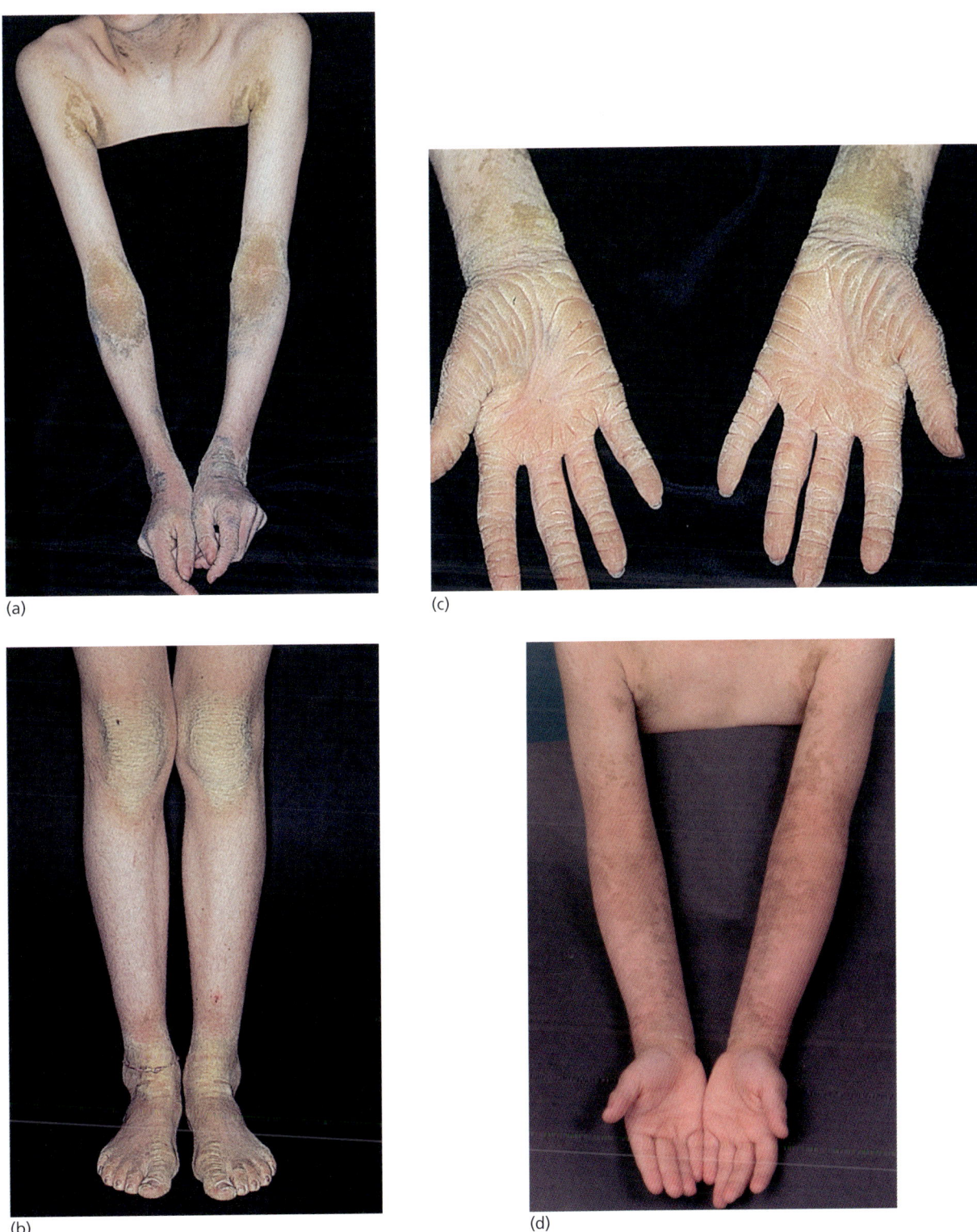

Figure 63.15 Epidermolytic ichthyosis without mosaicism. (a) Arms, (b) legs, and (c) palms indicative of *KRT1* mutations and (d) palms indicative of *KRT10* mutations. (a–c) Courtesy of Dr M. Judge, Salford Royal NHS Trust, UK.

Clinical features

The skin of patients with ichthyosis Curth–Macklin (ICM) is characterised by extensive spiny hyperkeratosis ('hystrix' like) covering the entire body and involving the palms and soles (Figure 63.19) [4].

Investigations

Histology reveals perinuclear vacuolisation and the formation of binucleated cells, without keratin aggregates, while ultrastructural studies usually reveal a shell-like perinuclear arrangement of keratins [5,6].

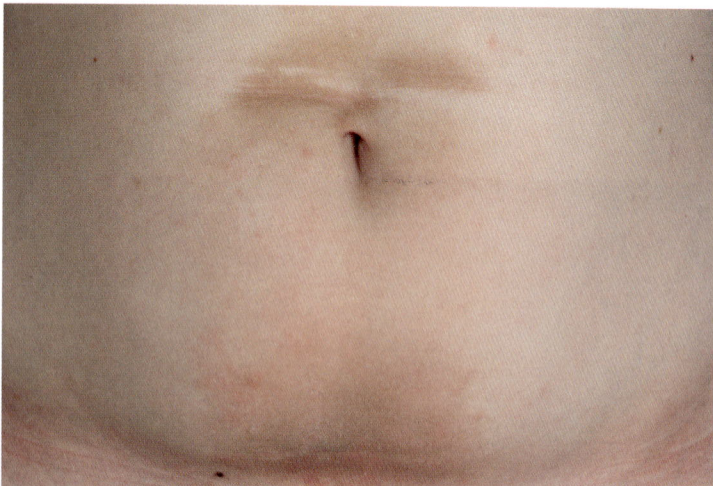

Figure 63.16 Superficial epidermolytic ichthyosis, showing involvement around the navel. Courtesy of the Department of Dermatology, University Hospital Münster, Münster, Germany.

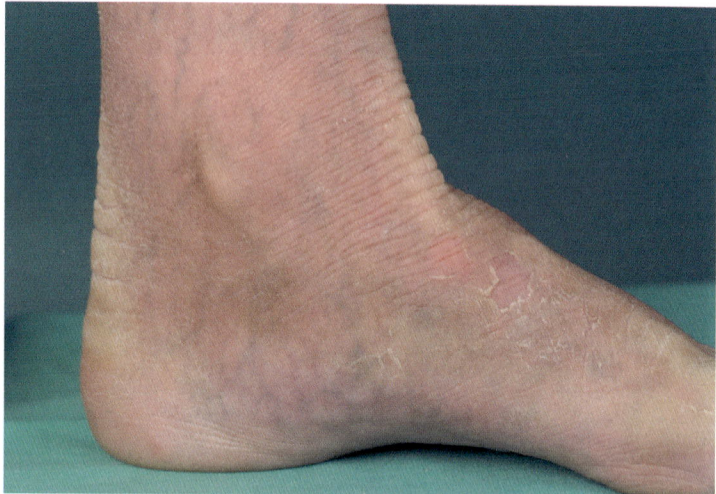

Figure 63.17 Moulting ('Mauserung') phenomenon in superficial epidermolytic ichthyosis. Courtesy of the Department of Dermatology, University Hospital Münster, Münster, Germany.

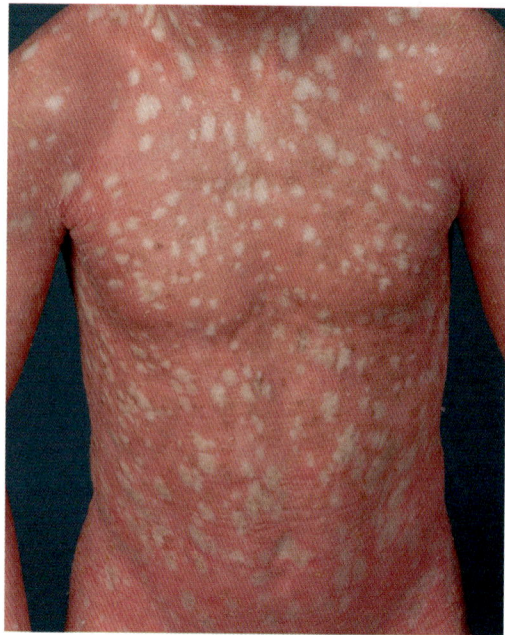

Figure 63.18 Congenital reticular ichthyosiform erythroderma. Note the pale confetti-like spots representing localised spontaneous healing. Courtesy of the Department of Dermatology, University Hospital Münster, Münster, Germany.

ERYTHROKERATODERMA

In the past, it was common to distinguish between 'true' ichthyosis involving the entire body and more localised ichthyosiform conditions. When these localised conditions were characterised by red skin and hyperkeratosis they were called erythrokeratoderma or erythrokeratodermia [1–3]. At the Sorèze Consensus Conference, it was decided that the various conditions that still carry the name erythrokeratoderma should also be considered as 'ichthyosis' [4]. Clinical expression of molecular defects can be quite variable as is seen for instance in SEI, which likewise would qualify as 'erythrokeratoderma'. Moreover, some syndromic types of erythrokeratoderma such as the keratitis–ichthyosis–deafness (KID) syndrome have traditionally been regarded by most authors as an ichthyosis.

Erythrokeratoderma variabilis

Definition and nomenclature

Erythrokeratoderma variabilis (EKV) is a rare disease characterised by migrating polycyclic red lesions accompanied by hyperkeratosis.

Synonyms and inclusions
- Mendes da Costa syndrome
- Erythrokeratodermia variabilis

Pathophysiology

Inheritance of EKV is usually autosomal dominant. In many but certainly not all families, dominant negative mutations in *GJB3* encoding connexin 31 or *GJB4* encoding connexin 30.3 have been found [1–4]. Autosomal recessive mutations in *GJB3* have likewise been reported [5]. Connexins form gap junctions, which are aqueous intercellular channels that are found in all tissues of the human body, including the skin, nervous tissue, heart and muscle [2,6]. Additional genes have been associated with other forms of EKV or EKV-like phenotypes including *GJA1* [7], *PERP* [8], *TRPM4* [9] and *KDSR* [10].

Clinical features [11,12]

Onset is usually in infancy. The manifestations vary within a family and within the individual. There are two types of lesions: (i) relatively fixed, well-demarcated keratotic and red plaques, often bizarrely shaped, which show a predilection for extensor surfaces, the lateral trunk and buttocks and extend and regress in area, thickness and degree of red skin; and (ii) transient, red, polycyclic or comma-shaped macular lesions occurring at any site (Figure 63.20).

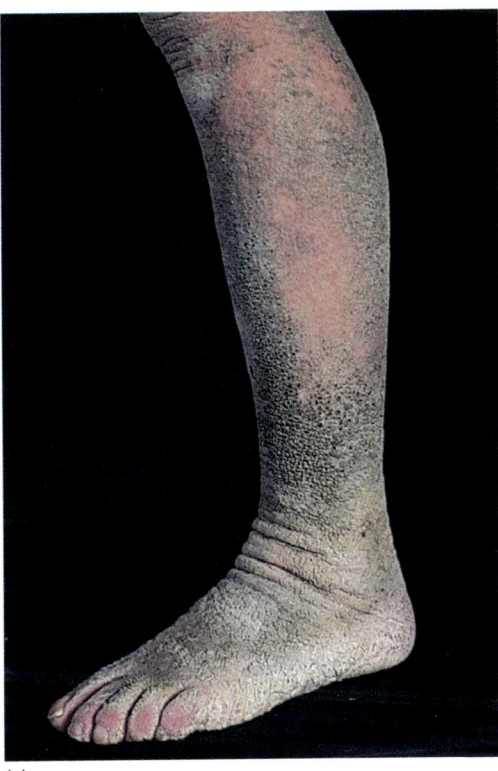

(a)

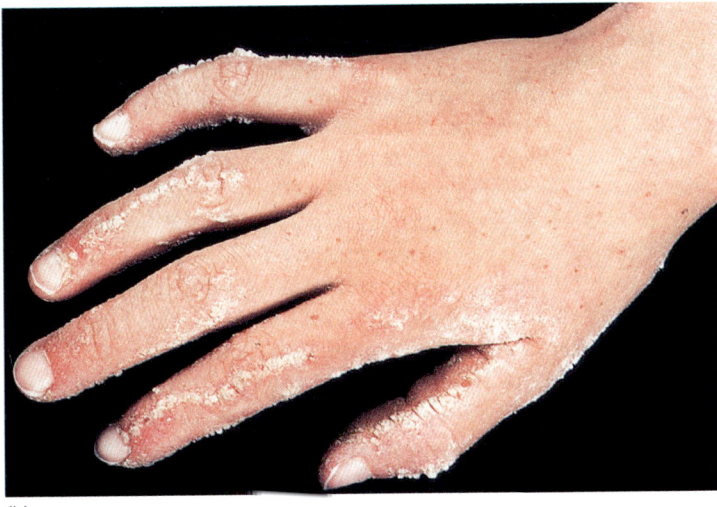

(b)

Figure 63.19 (a, b) Ichthyosis. Hystrix with striate lesions on the hand (b). Courtesy of Dr M. Judge, Salford Royal NHS Trust, UK.

Management

Acitretin treatment is the treatment of choice [13]. Likewise, the beneficial effect of low-dose isotretinoin has been reported [14],

Progressive symmetrical erythrokeratoderma

Definition and nomenclature

Progressive symmetrical erythrokeratoderma (PSEK) is a rare clinical variant of erythrokeratoderma with striking symmetrical

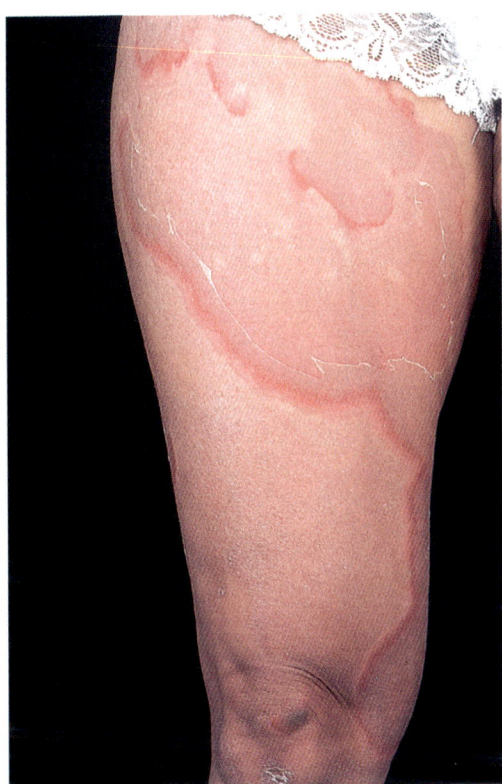

Figure 63.20 Erythrokeratoderma variabilis, showing migrating polycyclic red lesions.

appearance [1]. It is unclear whether this type of erythrokeratoderma deserves the status of a distinct clinicogenetic entity or rather represents a manifestation of EKV. The umbrella term 'erythrokeratoderma variabilis progressiva' has been suggested [2].

Synonyms and inclusions
- Gottron syndrome

Pathophysiology

From a genetic point of view, this clinical presentation is most likely also caused by the same connexin genes that underlie EKV. Actually, the same mutation G12D in the gene *GJB4* has been identified in unrelated Dutch patients, some of whom presented as having EKV [3], while others were diagnosed as having PSEK [4]. The occurrence of both types of erythrokeratoderma sharing the same ultrastructure has been reported in siblings [5]. Moreover, a homozygous loss-of-function mutation of *KRT83* has been described for a recessive form of PSEK. This disease would be allelic with dominant monilethrix [6].

Clinical features

The skin is usually normal at birth. Large geographical but symmetrical, fine scaly plaques with an orange-red skin appear in infancy (Figure 63.21). There is little pruritus and the lesions are non-migratory in nature, as opposed to classic EKV. The shoulder girdle, cheeks and buttocks are most often affected. Keratoderma may be present.

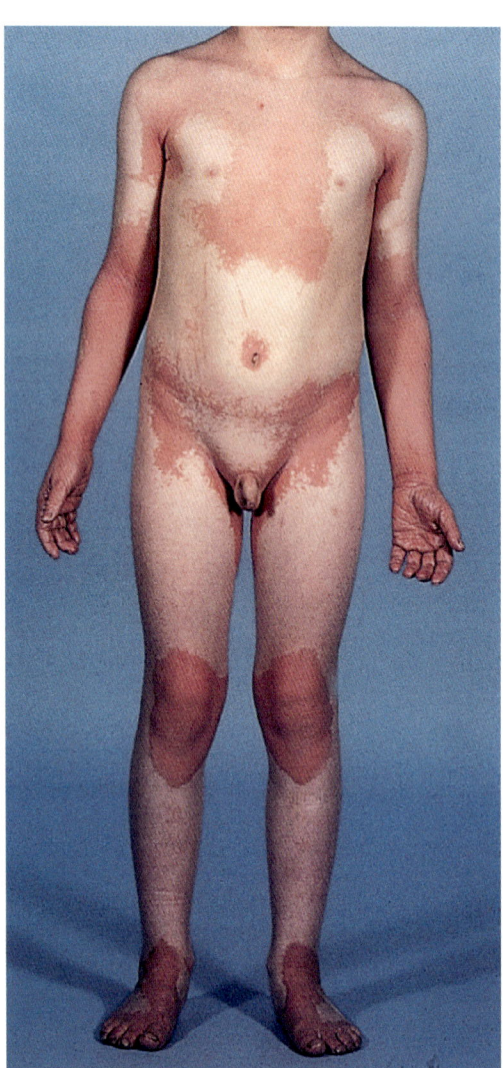

Figure 63.21 Symmetrical progressive erythrokeratoderma. Courtesy of Dr A. G. Smith, North Staffordshire Hospital, Stoke-on-Trent, UK.

Management
Topical calcipotriol may be of benefit [7].

Symmetrical acrokeratoderma

Clinical features
A Chinese group reported a study concerning 34 cases of symmetrical acrokeratoderma. Here, brown to black hyperkeratotic plaques were symmetrically distributed over the acral regions with marked worsening of the condition in the summer and improvement during winter. No genetic studies have been done so far and a relationship to IV has been suggested [1]. Clinically, there is whitish hyperkeratosis on the back of both hands and fingers, and the wrists in particular, after 5 minutes of water immersion reminiscent of aquagenic keratoderma. However, the authors emphasised that their patients did not suffer from palmoplantar involvement that could be typical for cystatin A deficiency [2].

OTHER NON-SYNDROMIC FORMS OF ICHTHYOSIS

There are some distinct generalised cornification disorders that are very much characterised by a palmoplantar phenotype. One example – loricrin keratoderma – is discussed in the section 'Non-syndromic palmoplantar keratoderma' later in this chapter, others are described here.

Autosomal dominant lamellar ichthyosis

Definition
This MeDOC form is a classic non-syndromic type of congenital ichthyosis that follows an autosomal dominant inheritance pattern. It was first delineated by Traupe et al. in 1984, who described three consecutive generations of a family, in whom affected members exhibited non-bullous congenital ichthyosis corresponding to a mild variant of lamellar ichthyosis [1].

Pathophysiology
A normal keratin pattern and only a limited number of lipid inclusions were found in the stratum corneum and this permitted a clear-cut ultrastructural distinction from ARCI [2]. Lipid chemical investigations of plantar scales of the same German family revealed an abnormal scale lipid pattern characterised by excessive amounts of free fatty acids, triglycerides, elevated n-alkanes, reduced free sterol and decreased total ceramides [3].

Soon after its first delineation in 1984, a Spanish group reported in 1986 a second family comprising five affected family members [4]. Then it took 24 years before Boyden et al. in 2020 reported three further families and elucidated mutations in ASPRV1 as the molecular cause of autosomal dominant lamellar ichthyosis (ADLI) [5]. All affected members of the families including the first German family had heterozygous missense mutations of ASPRV1 which segregated with the disease and disrupted protein residues within close proximity to autocatalytic cleavage sites, resulting in altered autocleavage and filaggrin processing. ASPRV1 encodes aspartic peptidase retroviral-like 1, a protein that acts as skin aspartic protease, and shows a strong localisation in the granular layer of the epidermis and the inner root sheath of hair follicles. ASPRV1 has an important role in regulating stratum corneum hydration as it cleaves profilaggrin, and in hairless mice a deficiency of this enzyme results in dry skin, a thicker and less hydrated stratum corneum, an accumulation of aberrantly processed profilaggrin accompanied by a marked decrease of filaggrin [6]. ASPRV1 undergoes an autoactivation process at pH5 generating a 14 kDa protein. Autoactivation of ASPRV1 could be inhibited by site-directed mutagenesis and it is of note that the protease inhibitor indinavir, used as a human immunodeficiency virus (HIV) drug, likewise inhibits autoactivation [7]. In the hairless skin aspartic protease (SASPase) deficient mouse model, prominent corneocyte surface protrusions were noted but the levels of natural moisturising factors were not reduced [8]. It is of interest that a mutation affecting a conserved residue close to the autoprocessing cleavage site in ASPRV1 has been described as the cause of ichthyosis in a German shepherd dog [9].

Clinical features [1,4,5]

Patients with ADLI exhibit large, translucent scales covering the entire body including the flexural folds, palms and soles. On the back of the feet often a marked keratotic lichenification is noted. There are no signs of erythroderma or blistering, but patients can suffer from considerable pruritus. The palms may show obvious keratoderma or marked hyperlinearity, while the feet usually show marked plantar keratoderma. As in most types of congenital ichthyosis, sweating is impaired in ADLI.

Investigations

Histological examination reveals orthohyperkeratosis and a marked and partly increased granular layer. A distinct histological finding was that some areas of the biopsies taken showed parakeratosis associated with the presence of a marked granular layer, which is quite unusual. Because of this peculiar histological pattern in conjunction with the autosomal dominant inheritance, ADLI was considered a distinct skin disorder. An ultrastructural investigation showed that a prominent transforming zone was found between the granular and horny layers [1].

Keratosis linearis–ichthyosis congenita–sclerosing keratoderma

Definition, nomenclature and classification

This MeDOC form belongs to the group of ichthyoses, but like loricrin keratoderma, it is dominated by keratoderma [1].

Synonyms and inclusions
- KLICK syndrome

Classification links
- MIM: 601952

Pathophysiology

The ultrastructural phenotype of the skin pointed to a disorder of keratohyaline granules [2]. There is orthohyperkeratosis with occasionally a parakeratotic stratum corneum reminiscent of the findings in ADLI [2]. Surprisingly, all affected individuals reported so far are carriers of a specific homozygous 1 bp deletion located upstream to the coding region of the *POMP* gene [3]. Immunohistochemical staining revealed an altered distribution of the proteasome subunits. Proteasome insufficiency results in impaired protein degradation and in the accumulation of undegraded ubiquitinylated protein, thus generating reactive oxygen species, and may lead to increased stress of the endoplasmic reticulum (ER). The so-called ER stress interferes with epidermal differentiation, as has been shown in connexin disorders [4]. Moreover, *POMP* is known to be the causative gene for proteasome-associated autoinflammatory syndrome 2 (PRAAS2), which shows that keratosis linearis–ichthyosis congenita–sclerosing keratoderma (KLICK) may be regarded an autoinflammatory keratinisation disease [5].

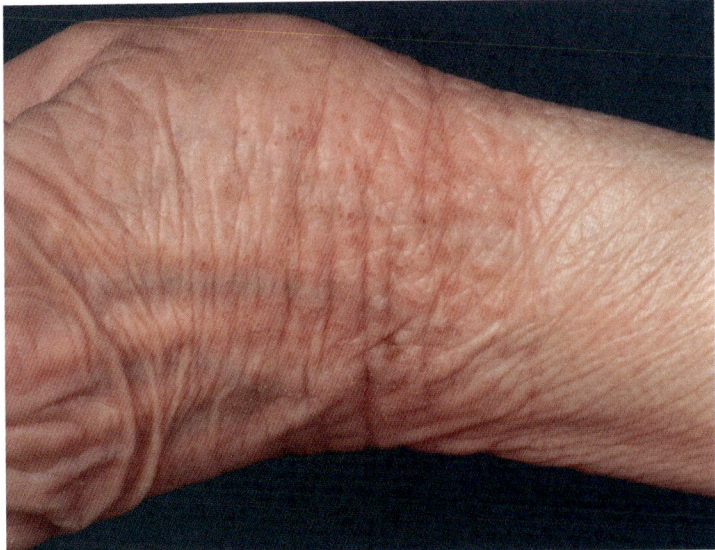

Figure 63.22 Keratosis linearis–ichthyosis congenita–sclerosing keratoderma (KLICK). Note the linear distribution of the keratotic papules.

Clinical features [1,2,6,7]

Clinically, the disorder manifests as a more sclerosing variant of loricrin PPK associated with mild congenital ichthyosis. In contrast to loricrin keratoderma, it is inherited in an autosomal recessive fashion. Affected individuals demonstrate keratotic punctuate plugs or papules that are distributed in a linear pattern and are found on the flexural areas of the extremities – a distinct and probably pathognomonic phenotype (Figure 63.22). However, this distinctive clinical finding is not present at birth, but seems to appear at the age of 10 years. In younger patients, the KLICK syndrome may resemble classic types of erythrokeratoderma [8]. There are no associated features, but there is a report of secondary squamous cell carcinoma [9].

Investigations

Ultrastructure confirms the histological finding of hypergranulosis and shows abnormally big keratohyaline granules.

Exfoliative ichthyosis

Synonyms and inclusions
- Peeling skin syndrome 4 or 5

Pathophysiology

Loss-of-function mutations in the *CSTA* gene encoding the protease inhibitor cystatin A are the cause of this autosomal recessive disease [1]. Functional and ultrastructural data show that the defect manifests mainly within the basal and suprabasal layers of the epidermis characterised by expression of keratin 14. Immunostaining reveals that the disease is characterised by the absence of epidermal cystatin A and shows no degradation of corneodesmosomes [2]. Another gene, which was confirmed for exfoliative ichthyosis, is *SERPINB8* [3].

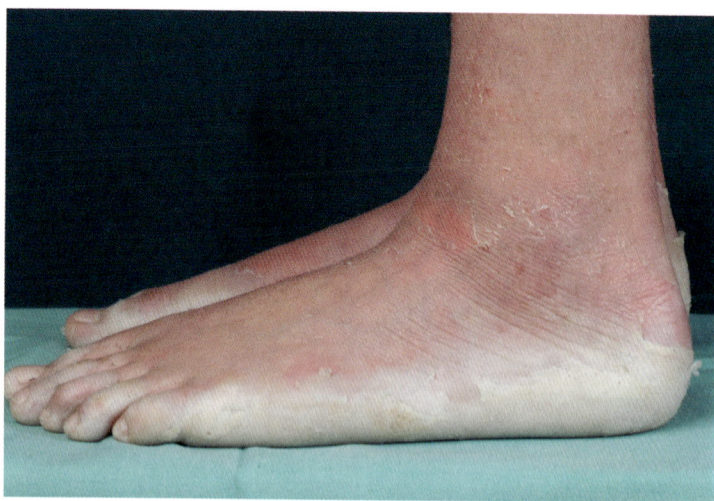

Figure 63.23 Exfoliative ichthyosis with pronounced plantar keratoderma. Courtesy of the Department of Dermatology, University Hospital Münster, Münster, Germany.

Clinical features [3,4]

Exfoliative ichthyosis (EXI) is characterised by pronounced PPK (Figure 63.23), which tends to be sensible to sweat and water exposure, similar to acral peeling skin syndrome [4], the Bothnia type of non-epidermolytic PPK, or transient aquagenic keratoderma. Exfoliative ichthyosis affects the entire integument, showing mild, dry and scaly skin, and as such fulfils the criteria of a non-syndromic form of congenital ichthyosis. Skin peeling may occur, easily elicited by moisture or minor trauma, and resembles the 'moulting' phenomenon in SEI. Differential diagnosis also includes acral peeling skin syndrome, which is not always due to *TGM5* mutations, but can also be caused by *CSTA* mutations [5,6]. It is of note that cystatin A has an additional role as a protease inhibitor in the superficial epidermis and has been associated with atopic eczema and house dust mite allergy in acral peeling skin syndrome [6].

Management

Efficient symptomatic treatment options seem to be lacking because local therapy tends to increase humidity-associated sensibility.

SYNDROMIC CONGENITAL ICHTHYOSES

See Tables 63.2, 63.4 and 63.6.

X-LINKED SYNDROMES CONCERNING DISTAL CHOLESTEROL BIOSYNTHESIS

Conradi–Hünermann–Happle syndrome

Definition and nomenclature

Conradi–Hünermann–Happle syndrome (CHHS) is an ultra-rare X-linked dominant skin disorder that usually affects only females and is lethal in males. Clinical hallmarks of CHHS are a mosaic presentation of linear ichthyosis, chondrodysplasia punctata,

asymmetrically shortened limbs, unilateral sometimes sectorial cataracts and short stature.

Synonyms and inclusions
- Happle syndrome
- Conradi syndrome
- X-linked dominant chondrodysplasia type II
- X-linked dominant ichthyosis

Pathophysiology

The mouse model tattered is due to a mutation in the gene for emopamil-binding protein (EBP) that functions as a delta8-delta7 sterol isomerase in the late steps of cholesterol biosynthesis [1]. Mutations in the same gene were found to underlie CHHS mutations in humans [1–3]. The genetic defect is associated with metabolic alterations in the serum, namely markedly elevated levels of 8-dehydrocholesterol and of cholest-8(9)-en3-β-ol, that can help to identify somatic mosaicism even in clinically unaffected males. However, the extent of the metabolic alterations detected in the serum does not allow prediction of the severity of the clinical phenotype [3]. The process of X-inactivation underlies the Blaschkoid pattern of distribution of skin lesions in CHHS. X-inactivation patterns of the patients showed no skewing, thus supporting the assumption that inactivation of the *EBP* gene occurs at random [4]. Mosaicism in the parent generation has been reported several times [3–5]. The disease is characterised by anticipation, namely worsening of disease severity in subsequent generations [6]. Pathogenic splicing variants of *EBP* may cause extreme variability of the disease [7]. It is of note that focal dermal hypoplasia can be associated with large submicroscopic deletions of the X-linked *PORCN* gene that also includes the adjacent *EBP* locus, although these patients with focal dermal hypoplasia did not exhibit features of CHHS [8]. It is believed that the accumulation of 8-dehydrocholesterol and other cholesterol precursors interferes with sonic hedgehog signalling and thus explains the developmental abnormalities in CHHS, such as facial dysmorphism, chondrodysplasia punctata or kyphoscoliosis [9,10]. The ichthyosis in CHHS is difficult to explain. It has been shown that lamellar bodies lack their normal lamellar structure [11].

Clinical features

Affected babies are typically female, premature and born with either partial collodion membrane or generalised ichthyosiform erythroderma. Within the first year, generalised linear and swirling patterns of erythroderma and scaling, following the lines of Blaschko, are established (Figure 63.24). Intervening areas of skin are unaffected. Palmoplantar hyperkeratosis and nail dystrophy may occur. Recurrent infections especially in the flexures can be troublesome, and scalp and eyebrow hair is sparse and lustreless. The ichthyosis improves in early childhood and the residual signs are often so subtle in adult life that an affected mother may be missed. Signs to be sought in older children and adults include swirls of fine scales, linear pigmentary change, patchy atrophy, follicular atrophoderma mainly on the limbs and dorsal hands, and a striate cicatricial alopecia, all in a Blaschkoid pattern.

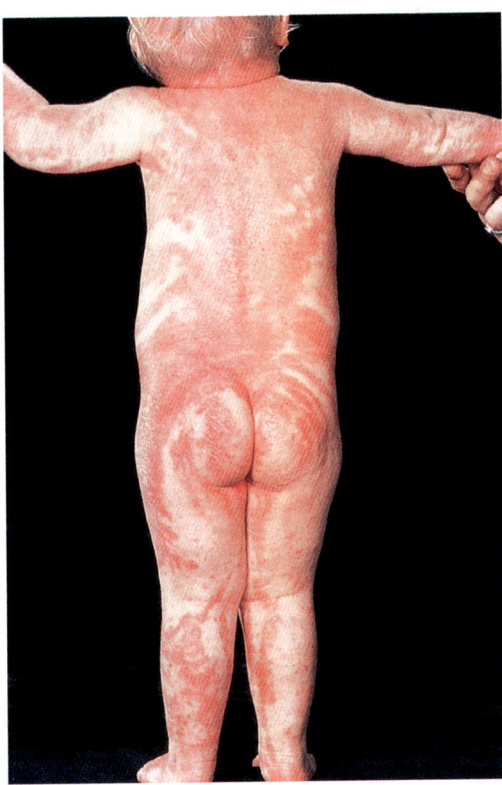

Figure 63.24 Conradi–Hünermann–Happle syndrome. Courtesy of Dr D. J. Atherton, London, UK.

Other variable features include rounded or asymmetrical facies with frontal bossing and hypertelorism, a broad flat nasal bridge, congenital asymmetrical cataracts in 60% of patients, short stature, asymmetrical or, rarely, symmetrical shortening of limbs, kyphoscoliosis, supernumerary digits and other skeletal defects. Stippled calcification (asymmetrical) of the long-bone epiphyses, vertebrae, pelvis, carpus and tarsus, and cartilage, including the trachea, is a characteristic but not universal radiological finding in the neonatal period, and usually resolves by adulthood. Patients have normal or mildly impaired intellectual development and neural hearing loss has been reported. It is of note that a lack of segmental fusion of the liver has been observed in a male patient [12].

Differential diagnosis
Milunsky and co-workers reported on a non-mosaic male with a mutation in *EBP* that presented a much milder phenotype characterised by failure to thrive, crossed renal ectopia and stenotic ear canals, but lacking chondrodysplasia punctata [13]. This unusual case was later discussed as a separate and novel clinicogenetic entity due to a hypomorphic mutation in *EBP*, a situation reminiscent of different phenotypes generated by hypomorphic *NEMO* mutations [13]. In the meantime several such cases have been recorded and the term MEND syndrome (male *EBP* disorder with neurological defects) has been proposed for this distinct entity [14]. It is of note that MEND is inherited as an X-linked recessive trait with extreme behavioral symptoms, and female carriers of the hypomorphic *EBP* mutation seem to be unaffected [15,16]. This situation is reminiscent of the so-called CK syndrome (MIM: 300831), named for the initials of the original proband, which is caused by hypomorphic temperature-sensitive mutations in *NSDHL* [17], while classic *NSDHL* mutations are associated with the X-linked dominant congenital hemidysplasia–ichthyosiform naevus–limb defect (CHILD) syndrome [18].

Management
Urea-containing emollients are helpful in controlling ichthyosis, but additional antimicrobial therapy may be needed for skin infections in infancy. The effect of retinoids is unknown, and the need for treatment diminishes with age. Continued orthopaedic surveillance and appropriate procedures may be indicated for skeletal anormalies. Cataracts usually do not affect vision.

Congenital hemidysplasia–ichthyosiform naevus–limb defect syndrome

Definition
The CHILD syndrome is a very rare, X-linked dominant, male-lethal disorder with distal cholesterol biosynthesis, featuring as a clinical hallmark the CHILD naevus.

Pathophysiology
The CHILD syndrome also represents a disorder of distal cholesterol biosynthesis (see earlier section) and is sometimes confused with the CHH syndrome. It was fully delineated in 1980 as an X-linked dominant trait that is lethal in males by the German dermatologist Happle [1]. In the initial report, the cutaneous phenotype was categorised as ichthyosis, but later the Happle group described it as an inflammatory naevus [2] showing a strikingly unilateral arrangement and differentiated the CHILD naevus from other epidermal naevi such as inflammatory linear verrucous epidermal naevus (ILVEN). In 2000, the same group established that the CHILD syndrome is due to mutations in the *NSDHL* gene encoding a 3β-hydroxysteroid dehydrogenase [3]. This enzyme is a decarboxylase that together with the enzymes C4 methyloxidase and 3-ketosterol reductase forms the C4 demythelase complex, which has an important role in cholesterol biosynthesis. Two mouse X-linked dominant male-lethal traits, bare patches (Bpa) and striated (Str), had previously been associated with mutations in *Nsdhl* and serve as animal models for this disease [4]. These mouse models reveal that Nsdhl deficiency has a deleterious effect on hedgehog signalling in early placental development, since male embryos for several mutant *Nsdhl* alleles die in mid-gestation with a thin and poorly vascularised placenta [5,6]. It is of interest that hypomorphic *NSDHL* mutations cause a X-linked recessive disease in males that has been termed the CK syndrome (see also the section on CHHS). CK patients have no cutaneous phenotype, and features in these patients have been attributed to the accumulation of toxic sterol metabolic intermediates rather than cholesterol deficiency.

Clinical features
The hallmark of the CHILD syndrome is the CHILD naevus, which is a peculiar inflammatory epidermal naevus having a unique

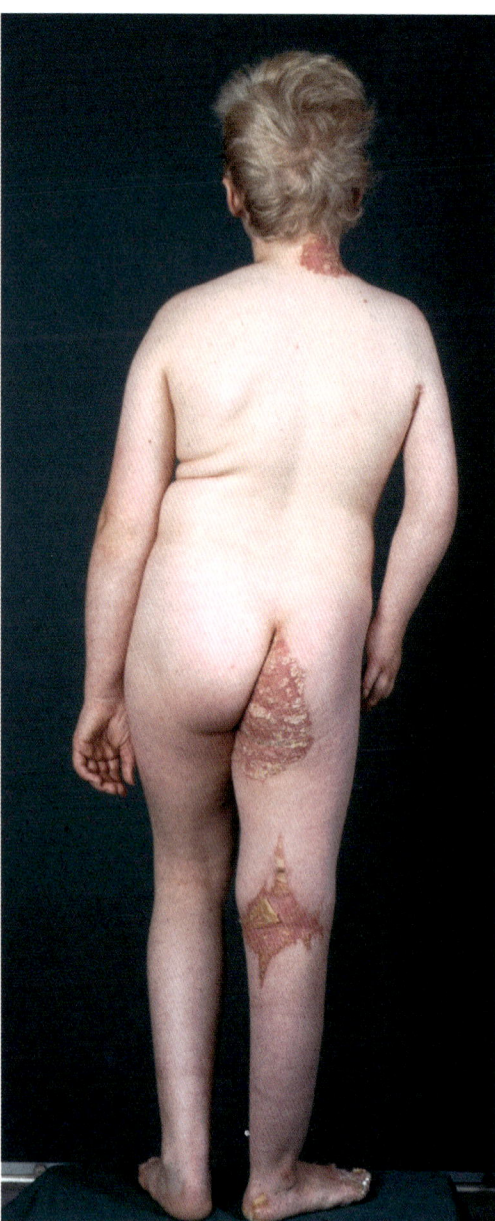

Figure 63.25 Congenital hemidysplasia–ichthyosiform naevus–limb defect (CHILD) naevus with yellowish keratosis and ipsilateral limb defect. Courtesy of the Department of Dermatology, University Hospital Münster, Münster, Germany.

lateralisation pattern with a strict midline demarcation and ptychotropism (affinity to body folds) (Figure 63.25). This naevus shows hyperkeratosis, which has a typical yellow, wax-like scaling that is quite different from that seen in CHHS and allows the paediatric dermatologist to make the proper diagnosis easily. However, an important misdiagnosis of actual CHILD naevi can be ILVEN (personal experience of H.T.). Associated ipsilateral extracutaneous defects in the form of hypoplasia or aplasia may involve the limbs and other skeletal structures as well as internal organs such as the lung, heart and kidney [1]. Although most reports deal with sporadic cases – around 60 cases had been reported in 2006 – this may be an underestimation of familial occurrence. Thus the molecular work-up of a large family revealed segregation of the causative *NSDHL* mutation through three generations affecting five patients

of whom four presented with very mild or minimal skin lesions such as periungual hyperkeratosis and onychodystrophy of the left index finger which may reflect extreme lyonisation occurring at random [7]. It is of note that the majority of cases affect the right side of the body, but left-sided cases have also been reported [8].

Management

The cutaneous phenotype usually improves in the first years of life a great deal, however the large lesions that remain constitute a serious burden due to itching and oozing. Simple dermabrasion has been shown to fail and to be associated with recurrence of the naevus [9]. In contrast, dermabrasion followed by immediate covering with split-skin grafts from the unaffected contralateral side has been effective for long-term therapy and has been interpreted as 'donor dominance' that cures the CHILD naevus [10]. Recently, a pathogenesis-based topical therapy aiming at suppression of epidermal cholesterol biosynthesis and simultaneous application of topical cholesterol in a cream has been reported with excellent clinical response [11]. This elegant therapeutic approach prevents the accumulation of toxic sterol metabolites by a statin treatment and at the same time addresses the deficiency of cholesterol. Instead of lovastatin it is also possible to use simvastatin [12] and permeation of the 2% cholesterol–2% lovastatin cream may be enhanced by adding glycolic acid [13]. It is of note that this pathogenesis-directed therapy is likewise beneficial in porokeratosis, reflecting a block in early cholesterol biosynthesis [14].

Ichthyosis follicularis–atrichia–photophobia syndrome

Definition

Ichthyosis follicularis–atrichia–photophobia (IFAP) syndrome is a rare X-linked recessive trait featuring ichthyosis follicularis, atrichia, photophobia and severe retardation of growth and psychomotor development. It has a clinical and molecular overlap with BRESEK/BRESHEK syndrome (brain anomalies, retardation, ectodermal dysplasia, skeletal malformations, Hirschsprung disease, ear/eye anomalies, cleft palate/cryptorchidism and kidney dysplasia/hypoplasia) [1] as well as X-linked keratosis follicularis spinosa decalvans (KFSD) [2]. The autosomal dominant IFAP variant IFAP2 is identical with mucoepithelial dysplasia.

Pathophysiology

X-linked recessive inheritance of this condition was already suggested in 1991 [3] and was firmly established by the observation of functional cutaneous mosaicism showing Blaschko linear lesions reflecting lyonisation in women heterozygous for the IFAP syndrome [4]. Histologically there is a mild acanthokeratosis and hyperkeratosis of the follicular openings and a well-preserved granular layer and an absence of sebaceous glands [3]. This histology differs greatly from hereditary mucoepithelial dysplasia. Causative missense mutations were eventually identified in the

X-linked gene *MBTPS2* encoding membrane-bound transcription factor protease, site 2 [5]. Shortly afterwards, it was shown that KFSD likewise is caused by different mutations affecting other sites in the *MBTPS2* gene [2] and that the so-called BRESEK/BRESHEK syndrome is also due to specific mutations in *MBTPS2* [1,6]. Finally, even an X-linked variant of Olmsted syndrome has been linked to a mutation in *MBTPS2* [7].

Membrane-bound transcription factor protease site 2 is a zinc metalloprotease essential for cholesterol homeostasis as well as ER stress response [5,6]. In cultured cells of IFAP patients, residual enzyme activity was only about one-third of wild-type activity and survival in cholesterol-depleted media was below 10%. It is of note that only missense mutations and intron mutations partially affecting transcription [8] are known so far. Most likely total loss of *MBTPS2* is not tolerated by male embryos and a residual enzyme activity is required for survival [6].

Clinical features

The full-blown spectrum of the IFAP syndrome is variable and seen only in males. All patients have the triad of follicular ichthyosis, congenital atrichia of the scalp (absence of hair) and photophobia. Children can be born as collodion babies. In particular, as neonates, they present with generalised follicular keratosis over the entire body including the scalp. Follicular involvement can be very prominent, for instance over the knees. It can improve markedly in early childhood. The most striking abnormality is the congenital alopecia (atrichia) (Figure 63.26). A non-cicatricial complete body alopecia is almost a classic feature. Psoriasiform plaques, angular cheilitis, periungual inflammation, dystrophic nails, hypohidrosis and atopic eczema can be present [9]. In contrast dental development is normal. Superficial corneal ulceration and vascularisation lead to progressive corneal scarring and underlie photophobia, the third cardinal feature [9]. Neurological features

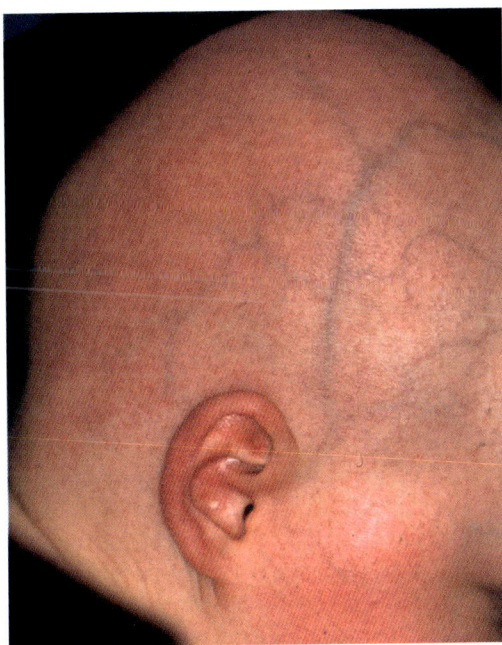

Figure 63.26 Ichthyosis follicularis–alopecia–photophobia (IFAP) syndrome. Courtesy of Dr A. S. Paller, Department of Dermatology and Pediatrics, Chicago, USA.

include intellectual disability and seizures as well as olivocerebellar atrophy, malformation of the temporal lobes, mild inner cerebral atrophy and hypoplasia of the corpus callllosum [10,11]. The syndrome overlaps with the BRESEK and BRESHEK syndromes [3]. Female carriers can present with much milder symptoms such as cutaneous hyperkeratotic lesions that follow the lines of Blaschko or asymmetrical distribution of body hair or Blaschko-linear presentation of hypohidrosis that can be visualised by testing, but otherwise goes unnoticed [4,11].

Differential diagnosis

In the past, several cases of hereditary mucoepithelial dysplasia (HMD) have been diagnosed as IFAP syndrome [12]. HMD can also feature photophobia and keratosis pilaris, and there is a clinical and molecular overlap with the autosomal dominant type of IFAP syndrome.

Management

A moderate response to low-dose acitretin has been reported [13]. Emollients are helpful. Intensive lubrication of the ocular surface remains the mainstay of therapy for photophobia.

Autosomal dominant IFAP2 syndrome and hereditary mucoepithelial dysplasia

Definition

The IFAP syndrome is heterogeneous, and recently a distinct autosomal dominant form of IFAP syndrome has been described [1]. This autosomal dominant IFAP syndrome forms a clinical and molecular spectrum with hereditary mucoepithelial dysplasia and is due to *SREBF1* variants encoding a protein that promotes the transcription of several lipogenes [2,3]. Hereditary mucoepithelial dysplasia exhibits a psoriasiform histology that clearly differentiates this disease from X-linked IFAP syndrome.

Pathophysiology

Following the elucidation of the *MBTPS2* mutation as the molecular cause of X-linked IFAP syndrome it was noted that in some cases this mutation could not be found, and that two cases diagnosed as IFAP syndrome had been observed in a mother and daughter which would not be compatible with classic X-linked IFAP syndrome [3]. Molecular analyses in 11 families revealed heterozygous mutations in the gene *SREBF1* which encodes a sterol regulatory element-binding protein promoting the transcription of lipogenes involved in the biosynthesis of fatty acids and cholesterol. This transcription requires the cleavage of a site 1 protease. It is of note that in the X-linked IFAP syndrome *MBTPS2* affects a site 2 protease of the sterol metabolism in a similar manner [1]. There are some histological differences to the X-linked IFAP syndrome. The autosomal dominant variant has a clinical and molecular overlap with autosomal dominant hereditary mucoepithelial dysplasia and shows a psoriasiform histology in addition to dyskeratotic features and cytoplasmic vacuoles [4].

Clinical features

From a clinical point of view the overlap with hereditary mucoepithelial dysplasia is obvious: cases exhibit in addition to photophobia and alopecia, in particular, periorificial redness, angular cheilitis and psoriasis-like plaques with a psoriasiform histology and the presence of dyskeratotic cells can be noted [5,6].

EXFOLIATIVE DISORDERS OF CORNIFICATION

Comèl–Netherton syndrome

Definition and nomenclature

Comèl–Netherton syndrome (CNS) is a rare autosomal recessive disorder characterised by the triad of congenital ichthyosis, hair shaft anomalies and severe atopic diathesis. At birth, patients often display CIE, which in around 90% of cases gradually evolves into a milder phenotype with polycyclic migrating plaques known as ichthyosis linearis circumflexa (ILC). The disease features associated symptoms such as life-threatening neonatal hypernatraemic dehydration, failure to thrive and recurrent infections [1–3].

> **Synonyms and inclusions**
> - Netherton syndrome
> - Ichthyosiform erythroderma with hypotrichosis and hyper-IgE

Epidemiology

Worldwide prevalence is estimated at 1 in 50 000–200 000. CNS may account for up to 18% of all cases of infantile erythroderma; however, diagnosis is often delayed [4].

Pathophysiology

The disease is caused by recessive mutations in *SPINK5* (serine protease inhibitor Kazal-type 5) [5], which encodes the multidomain serine protease inhibitor LEKTI (lymphoepithelial Kazal-type-related inhibitor) expressed in the epidermis, thymus and oral and vaginal mucosa [6]. The protein is organised into 15 potential inhibitory domains with a four/six-cysteine residue pattern (Kazal-type like/Kazal-type). Subtilisin-like proprotein convertases like furin proteolytically cleave the LEKTI full-length protein. Subsequent processing creates several inhibitors with different target specificities [7,8], for example domains 5 and 6 exhibit trypsin-inhibiting activity. Hence, LEKTI controls serine proteases that are part of the kallikrein network of the epidermis, for example kallikrein 5 (KLK5) and KLK7 are responsible for the processing of corneodesmosin [9–12]. Loss of control within the cascade of kallikreins [13] leads to overdesquamation of corneocytes and degradation of desmosomal proteins (corneodesmosin and desmoglein 1), interferes with the *Staphylococcus aureus*/*S. epidermidis* skin homeostasis [14] and induces changes of stratum corneum ceramides [15] of the pro-inflammatory skin response. The system involves PAR-2 (protease-activated receptor 2) [16] as well as thymic stromal lymphopoietin as a biological marker, which

correlates with disease activity [17–19]. Another target of LEKTI is caspase 14 (involved in filaggrin processing) [20,21].

Finally, the immunological profile of Netherton syndrome is of great interest considering the therapeutic option of repurposing biologics [22]. Aberrations in lymphocyte subpopulations have been described [23], but primarily Netherton syndrome is regarded as a severe local skin barrier defect in the absence of an underlying systemic immunodeficiency [24]. The molecular fingerprint shows a great T-cell activation and a broad immune phenotype with T_H1/interferon γ, and skewing of T_H2/IL-4 receptor/IL-5 [25]. Of note, ablation of KLK5 and KLK7 or induction of the secretory leukocyte protease inhibitor (Slpi) that controls KLK5 and KLK7 fully rescues lethality or reduces the phenotype of Netherton syndrome in mice, respectively [26,27]. For example, a specific therapy for Netherton syndrome may be based on KLK5 inhibitors [28]. So far, it is unclear whether *ex vivo* lentiviral gene therapy [29–31] might offer a specific therapy to patients in the future.

Clinical features [1,2,32–36]

Clinical diagnosis requires a combination of congenital erythroderma, neonatal failure to thrive and early development of atopy with high levels of immunoglobulin E (IgE) and hypereosinophilia. The hair shaft anomaly of trichorrhexis invaginata ('bamboo hair') confirms the diagnosis (Figure 63.27a) [3].

Skin symptoms. Collodion membrane is not a common feature, and erythroderma may also develop a few days after birth (Figure 63.27b). A typical ILC lesion is a red, exfoliating or scaly, annular or polycyclic patch with an incomplete advancing double edge of peeling scale (Figure 63.27c). ILC is episodic, with lesions migrating often in a cephalocaudal direction, over several days. Lesions without the double-edged scaly margin are commonly seen.

Hair. Although trichorrhexis invaginata is typical of CNS, other anomalies such as pili torti may also be seen. Hair, eyebrows and eyelashes can be present, sparse or absent at birth. Children may develop rare, thin, spiky and fragile hair of slow growth, but interindividual differences are striking.

Atopy. Recurrent urticaria and facial angioedema, triggered by certain foods, are common complications, although the incidence varies [37]. The most common food allergens are nuts and fish. Reports exist on eosinophilic oesophagitis and colonic mucosal eosinophilia [38]. Food allergy can manifest in childhood or even in infancy. Most important, pruritus has an extreme influence on disease burden [39].

Growth retardation. Infants are usually born at term with average birth weight, but often develop failure to thrive, which might be explained by a frequent 'dermopathic enteropathy' and/or high energy loss through skin inflammation and hyperproliferation [38,40,41]. Nasogastric tube feeding might be required in severe cases in early life. However, most of these infants begin to gain weight in their second year, although they generally remain below the 25th centile for height and weight. One probably often unrecognised clinical feature is growth hormone deficiency [42] that may show good response to growth hormone therapy [26].

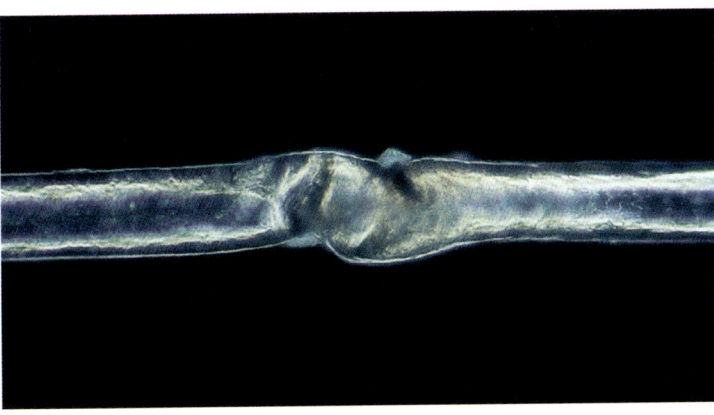

(a)

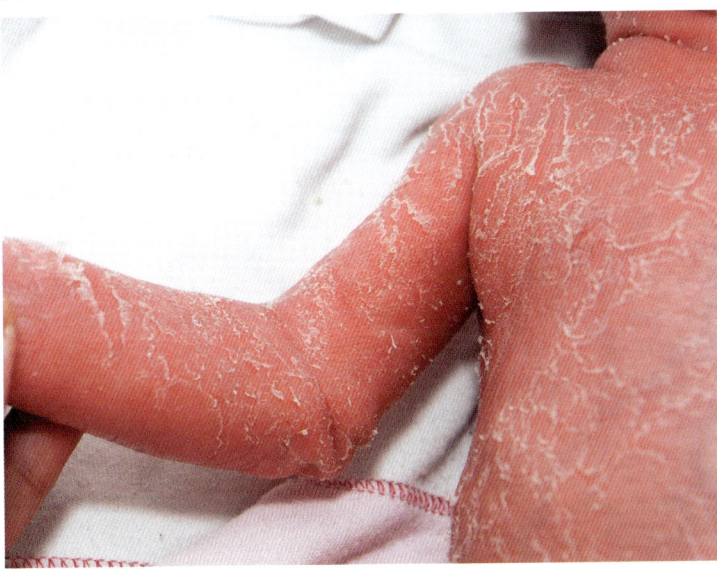

(b)

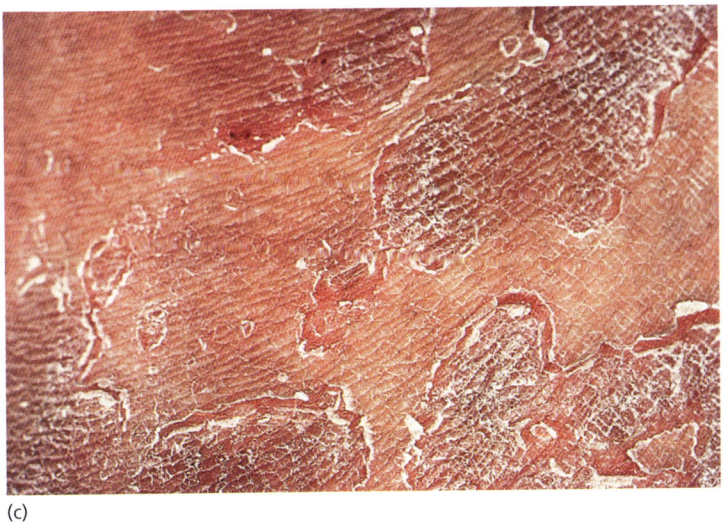

(c)

Figure 63.27 Comèl–Netherton syndrome. (a) Trichorrexis invaginata. (b) Congenital ichthyosiform erythroderma with failure to thrive. (c) Ichthyosis linearis circumflexa. (a,c) Courtesy of Dr M. Judge, Salford Royal NHS Trust, UK.

Differential diagnosis

Erythrodermic forms of ARCI are important differential diagnoses, considering that atopy and hair shaft anomalies in CNS may not be present during the first months of life. Extreme eosinophilia could be diagnostic for Omenn syndrome (MIM: 603554). Moreover, ectodermal dysplasia with eczema, inflammatory peeling skin disease and severe dermatitis–multiple allergies–metabolic wasting (SAM) syndrome need to be considered (see later in this chapter).

Complications [43–48]

Perinatal complications include hypernatraemic dehydration, severe infections and malnutrition due to high calorie consumption and enteropathy. Later in life, bacterial (*S. aureus*) and yeast colonisation of the skin and human papillomavirus (HPV)-associated viral warts (in older patients) are common. Severe complications include HPV-associated papillomatous skin lesions of the groin and perineal regions, spinous cell carcinoma and giant condyloma of Buschke–Löwenstein [49]. Unexpected complications include arterial hypertension or cardiac disease such as pulmonary artery stenosis [50,51].

Investigations

Loss of detection of the LEKTI antigen in the epidermis is a useful diagnostic feature [8,52,53]. On histology, psoriasiform dermatitis with parakeratosis, acanthosis and a peculiar eosinophilic material just below the stratum corneum are often observed [54]. Often disregarded as artefactual, subcorneal or intracorneal separation can consistently be found and is a diagnostically useful hint [55]. Microscopic examination of the hairs usually leads to a rapid diagnosis: trichorrhexis invaginata refers to the protrusion of the distal part of the hair shaft into the cup shape of its proximal part [2]. Of note, this feature may not be apparent before 1 year of age. In addition, it is most likely to be found in eyebrow hair [56]. Also, at the ultrastructural level, the epidermis in CNS displays features such as altered lamellar body secretion and loss of corneocyte adhesion [57]. In around 90% of the cases, diagnosis can be confirmed by *SPINK5* sequence analysis [21], which might be important for prenatal diagnosis of siblings [58,59].

Management [3,60]

The impaired epidermal barrier is a major clinical problem, including the risk of systemic toxicity from topically applied agents [61,62]. Newborns are prone to hypernatraemic dehydration and/or systemic sepsis, and may need intensive medical care immediately after birth. The application of amnion membrane allografts has been described as helpful in a critically ill infant [63]. Recurrent infections require antibiotic treatment. Consequent strengthening of the skin barrier relies on regular bathing, emollients and ointments (paraffin-based ointments, such as 50/50 white soft and liquid paraffin). Antiseptics might be added. Topical steroids should be avoided as far as possible or only used for a short period [61,62,64]; topical anti-inflammatory immunomodulators (pimecrolimus 1% or tacrolimus 0.05–0.1%) may be offered as an alternative, but systemic absorption is a concern [65–67]. Topical calcipotriol [68] and ultraviolet A (UVA) therapy can be tried [69,70]. The application of 0.33% brimonidine gel for facial redness may have a good effect for 6–7 h [71].

PART 6: GENETIC DISORDERS

Type I hypersensitivity reactions, in particular food allergies to fish and nuts, should be prevented by dietary restrictions or may be treated specifically [72]. Hypotrichosis tends to improve after puberty; however, girls in particular may profit from wearing a wig. Older patients with Netherton syndrome must be checked for HPV-induced skin cancers. Surgery, CO_2 laser, cryotherapy and/or imiquimad may be an option for vegetative lesions of the inguinal region considering the need for close and intense postoperative management [73,74].

Systemic therapy

Intravenous immunoglobulin (IVIg) therapy (0.4 g/kg/month) has demonstrated impressive results – especially in children with initial failure to thrive [75–78]. Improvement has been reported with antitumour necrosis factor α (anti-TNF-α) monoclonal antibodies (infliximab) in severe forms of CNS [79–81]. Blocking of IL-4 and IL-13 (dupilumab) is effective against itch and is possibly safer [82–85], although recent case reports show mostly temporary improvement of eczematous lesions [86]. An improvement of allergic skin manifestations has been described in a single case report on omalizumab (anti-IgE-antibody) [87]. Treatment with ustekinumab (anti-IL-12/IL-23 antibody) showed a relapse-free period for the time of observation of 1 year [88] and appears as a safe treatment option also for children. Targeting the IL-17 pathway as suggested by Paller *et al.* [**89**] using secukinumab [90,91] or ixekizumab [92] showed good effects on ichthyosis severity score, quality of life and pruritus. So far, no severe side effects have been reported on therapies with biologics in CNS.

Severe dermatitis–multiple allergies–metabolic wasting syndrome

Definition

The acronym SAM recently introduced by Samuelov *et al.* (2013) refers to severe dermatitis, multiple allergies and metabolic wasting [1].

Pathophysiology [1,2]

The disorder results from deficient membrane expression of desmoglein 1, which is also involved in the pathogenesis of pemphigus foliaceus and impetigo and is degraded in the absence of LEKTI in CNS [3,4]. Loss-of-function mutations in *DSG1* encoding desmoglein 1 (*DSG1*) that cause the SAM syndrome are inherited in a semidominant fashion; heterozygous carriers of *DSG1* mutations show focal PPK (see 'Striate (and focal) palmoplantar keratoderma' later in this chapter).

Clinical features

This autosomal recessive disease is clinically reminiscent of ARCI, Netherton syndrome or peeling skin syndrome 1 [1,5]. The phenotype encompasses a broad spectrum [6]. Interestingly, while classic SAM syndrome was initially considered to always represent a life-threatening condition, several patients have now been described with no or little systemic involvement despite having biallelic *DSG1* mutations [6].

Investigations

At the histological level SAM syndrome shows psoriasiform dermatitis and demonstrates subcorneal separation and acantholysis within the stratum spinosum and granulosum. At the ultrastructural level half-split desmosomes may be seen [1].

Management

Above all, Carvajal-Huerta syndrome needs to be differentiated (see later in this chapter). Patients with clinical features consistent with severe skin dermatitis, multiple allergies and metabolic wasting were reported to carry pathogenic mutations in desmoplakin (*DSP*), and a very favourable therapeutic response to ustekinumab has been reported [7].

Peeling skin syndromes

Peeling skin syndromes (PSSs) refer to a heterogeneous group of generalised and/or palmoplantar disorders and overlap with other exfoliative forms of ichthyosis [1]. Clinical, ultrastructural, genetic and pathophysiological aspects demonstrate a fascinating relation between LEKTI deficiency (Netherton syndrome), desmoglein 1 deficiency (SAM syndrome) and corneodesmosin deficiency (inflammatory peeling skin disease) [2,3].

Peeling skin syndrome type B

Definition and nomenclature

The term 'peeling skin syndrome' was introduced by Levy and Goldsmith in 1982 [1]. Traupe differentiated PSS type A and B [2]. Inflammatory peeling skin disease initially described by Wile in 1924 [3] refers to PSS type B and is an ichthyosiform erythroderma characterised by lifelong patchy peeling of the skin with accompanying pruritus.

> **Synonyms and inclusions**
> * Peeling skin syndrome type 1 (PSS1)
> * Inflammatory peeling skin disease

Pathophysiology

Peeling skin syndrome type B is due to autosomal recessive loss-of-function mutations in *CDSN* encoding corneodesmosin [4]. This finding has been independently confirmed by several groups [5–10]. CDSN is a secreted protein expressed in cornified epithelia and hair follicles [11]. It is specific to corneodesmosomes, cell–cell junction structures responsible for the stratum corneum cohesion [12]. Corneodesmosin adhesive properties are attributable to glycine-rich domains, which undergo sequential proteolysis leading to desquamation of corneocytes [13]. The essential role of CDSN for maintaining the integrity of the epidermis and hair follicles is demonstrated in mice [14]. Inactivation of the gene induces a lethal

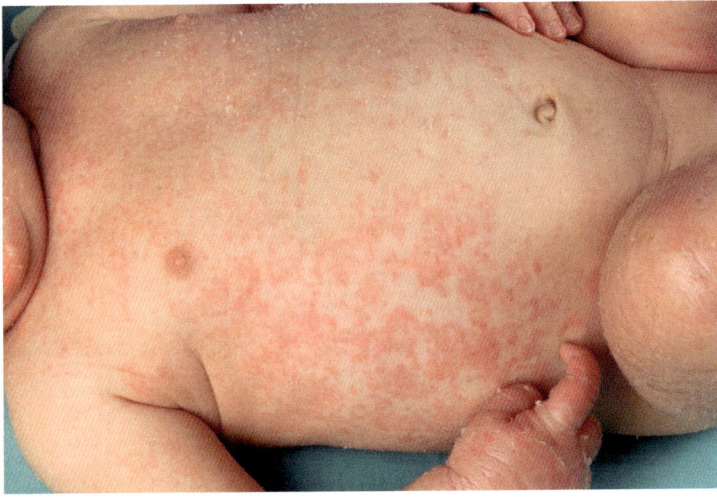

(a)

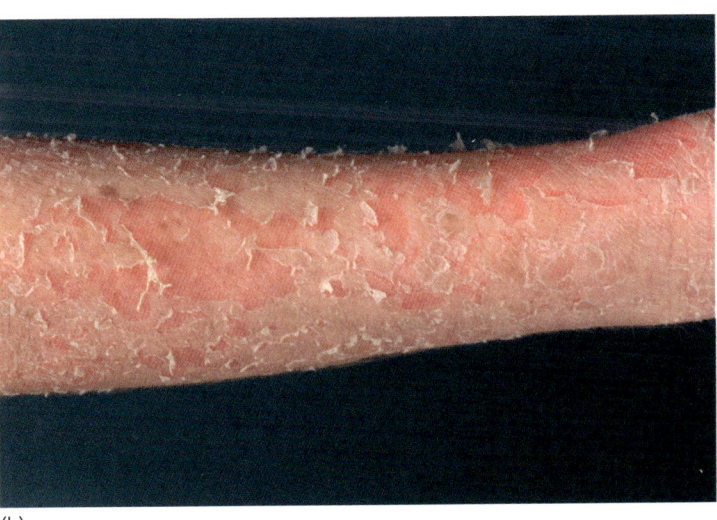

(b)

Figure 63.28 Inflammatory peeling skin disease (peeling skin syndrome type B). Courtesy of the Department of Dermatology, University Hospital Münster, Münster, Germany.

epidermal barrier disruption and hair follicle degeneration [15]. Interestingly, dominant nonsense mutations in *CDSN*, leading to the synthesis of an abnormal protein, cause hypotrichosis simplex due to the accumulation and toxic effect of abnormal corneodesmosin in the hair follicles [16,17] (Chapter 66).

Clinical features [1–4,18–23]

Inflammatory peeling skin disease presents at birth or a few days later. Infants develop ichthyosiform erythroderma with skin abnormalities consisting of spontaneous patchy peeling affecting the entire skin (Figure 63.28). Depending on mechanical stress and environmental factors (e.g. low humidity or temperature changes), patients experience recurrent episodes of peeling with severe pruritus. The presentation might be reminiscent of Netherton syndrome [24,25], however individuals do not show 'bamboo hairs' or hypotrichosis, and do not develop ichthyosis linearis circumflexa. The disease persists throughout life and is often accompanied by significant atopic manifestations.

Differential diagnosis

Hypotrichosis and failure to thrive seem unusual or less severe than in Netherton syndrome [4]. Other exfoliative inflammatory phenotypes should be distinguished including SAM syndrome and EXI.

Investigations

Histopathology reveals subcorneal splitting and/or enhanced detachment of corneocytes. As such, Netherton syndrome and PSS type B appear similar at the histological and ultrastructural levels [4,22,26]. Immunostaining for corneodesmosin and LEKTI may help to distinguish between these two disorders [4,21].

Management

There is no effective treatment. Episodes of skin peeling are accompanied by severe and refractory pruritus. Allergies need to be prevented; tacalcitol cream [27], emollients with dexpanthenol and antiseptics or the use of thermal water spray can be tried. Protein replacement therapy might be the sole option for a future effective therapy [28].

Acral peeling skin syndrome

Definition and nomenclature

Acral peeling skin syndrome (APSS) [1] is typically confused with epidermolysis bullosa simplex of localised type [2] and was recently reclassified as a type of epidermolysis bullosa [3].

> **Synonyms and inclusions**
> • Peeling skin syndromes 2 and 4

Pathophysiology

This autosomal recessive condition [1] is caused by missense mutations in *TGM5* encoding transglutaminase 5 [4] and rarely by pathogenic variants in *CSTA* encoding cystatin A [5].

Clinical features [1,2,5,6]

The disease is characterised by superficial painless peeling of the skin, predominantly on the dorsal aspects of the hands and feet. In infants, it frequently manifests with blistering on the palms and soles and is aggravated by mechanical factors and by humid warm environments. Distinction from epidermolysis bullosa simplex [2,7] or EXI [8] may be difficult, but it is clearly different from generalised peeling skin diseases. Interestingly, downregulation of *ALOXE3*, which is associated with ichthyosis, suppresses the phenotype of APSS; and this effect might be explained by an increase of corneodesmosin [9].

Differential diagnosis

Acral peeling skin syndrome should also be distinguished from keratolysis exfoliativa [10,11]. This apparently common but underdiagnosed condition affects young adults, usually in the summer months, and may be related to sweating. Lesions appear as tiny white rings or 'air bubbles', which soon rupture and peel off ('ringed keratolysis') (Figure 63.29). Attempts to identify a specific fungal or bacterial agent prove negative.

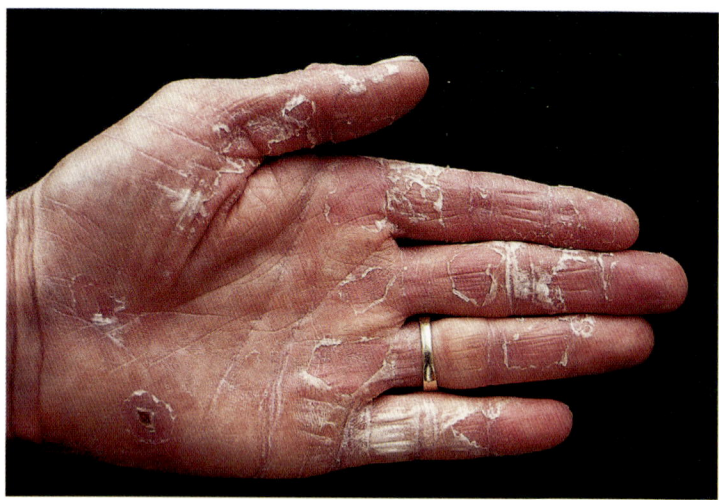

Figure 63.29 Keratolysis exfoliativa of the palms.

Peeling skin syndrome type A

Definition and nomenclature

Fox reported the first case of generalised, non-inflammatory and asymptomatic skin shedding called 'keratolysis exfoliativa congenita' [1]. Other cases have been described as 'familial continual skin shedding' [2,3] or 'decidious skin' [4].

> **Synonyms and inclusions**
> • Peeling skin syndromes 3 and 6

Pathophysiology

A single recessive missense mutation in *CHST8* has been described in a large consanguineous kindred with generalised PSS type A, but its pathogenic consequences are not well understood so far [5]. It appears that the main gene of the non-inflammatory variant of peeling skin syndrome is *FLG2* [6–8]. Filaggrin 2 is expressed throughout the stratum corneum. It might be essential for cell–cell adhesion, and its absence leads to a decrease of corneodesmosin [8].

Clinical features [5,9–11]

Non-inflammatory PSS type A usually starts between 3 and 6 years of age and is characterised by asymptomatic, generalised skin peeling with areas of hyperpigmentation, without skin blistering or redness. There are no associated disorders.

NEURO-ICHTHYOTIC SYNDROMES

The combination of neurological manifestations and ichthyosis can be found in at least 16 distinct genetic disorders (reviewed in [1]). In mildly affected patients, cutaneous symptoms may not be apparent, or the ichthyosis may have a late onset, as in in Refsum syndrome. There is no effective therapy for the neurological symptoms of the diseases; however, special dietary restriction in Refsum syndrome and zinc acetate therapy in the mental retardation–enteropathy–deafness–neuropathy–ichthyosis–keratodermia (MEDNIK) syndrome [2] are striking examples of successful pathogenesis-based

treatment. In the realm of bone dysplasias, a novel neuro-ichthyosis has been proposed featuring lamellar ichthyosis with acrodysostosis-like skeletal dysplasia and cerebellar atrophy, but further case studies need to be reported, and no distinct gene defect has been identified so far [3].

Gaucher disease type II, ARC syndrome and MEDNIK syndrome

Gaucher disease type II represents a classic neuro-ichthyosis presenting at birth with collodion membranes [1,2]. Other diseases in the list of ultra-rare neuro-ichthyoses are the arthrogryposis–renal dysfunction–cholestasis (ARC) syndrome [3–8] and the MEDNIK syndrome (Table 63.4) [9,10].

CEDNIK syndrome

Pathophysiology (Table 63.4)

The mouse model for cerebral dysgenesis–neuropathy–ichthyosis–palmoplantar keratoderma (CEDNIK) syndrome established the pivotal role of *SNAP29* in epidermal differentiation [1]; a zebrafish model highlights its role for neuromotor development [2].

Clinical features

Patients with CEDNIK syndrome exhibit ichthyosis and/or PPK and hypotonia as well as significant developmental delay [3–5]. Moreover, hypomyelination, seizures and early puberty emerged as previously underrecognised features [6].

Stormorken syndrome

Pathophysiology

This autosomal dominant disorder belongs to the group of channelopathies affecting calcium homeostasis in various tissues. The phenotype overlaps with tubular aggregate myopathy and is due to dominant gain-of-function mutations in *STIM1* or *ORA1*, which induce excessive extracellular Ca^{2+} entry and result in a multisystemic disease [1].

Clinical features

Stormorken syndrome [2] is characterised by muscle weakness, miosis, thrombocytopenia, bleeding, ichthyosis, migraine, dyslexia and short stature [3,4].

Refsum disease

Definition and nomenclature

Refsum disease (RD) is an ultra-rare, autosomal recessive, neurocutaneous lipid storage disorder featuring deteriorating vision and hearing, ataxia, neuropathy and usually mild ichthyosis.

Table 63.4 Neuro-ichthyosis syndromes.

Features	Gaucher syndrome type 2	MEDNIK	CEDNIK	ARC
MIM number	230900	609313	609528	208085
Mode of inheritance	AR	AR	AR	AR
Gene	*GBA*	*AP1S1*	*SNAP29*	*VPS33B*
Onset	At birth, or later	At birth or within first weeks of life	After 5–11 months	At birth, can sometimes be late
Initial clinical presentation	CIE or less frequently mild collodion membrane	Inflammatory rashes, similar to EKV	Until up to 1 year of age, normal skin; thereafter LI type	Xerosis and scaling within a few days of birth
Disease course	Ranging from mild to moderate	Progressive	Fatal	Fatal
Cutaneous findings: Distribution of scaling:	Generalised	Generalised	Generalised with sparing of skin folds	Generalised with sparing of skin folds
Scaling type	Fine or moderate; scaling may resolve after neonatal period	EKV-like	Coarse and large (plate-like)	Fine or plate-like (extensor sites)
Scaling colour	White or grey or brown	EKV-like	Whitish	White or brownish
Skin redness	Unusual	EKV-like	Absent	Absent
Palmoplantar involvement	–	Not specifically	Yes	Spared
Scalp abnormalities	–	Not specifically	Fine sparse hair	Mild scarring alopecia
Other skin findings	–	Nail thickening, mucous membrane affected	None	Ectropion
Extracutaneous involvement	Hydrops fetalis; progressive neurological deterioration; hepatosplenomegaly, hypotonia, respiratory distress, arthrogryposis, facial anomalies	Congenital sensorineural deafness, peripheral neuropathy, psychomotor and growth retardation, chronic diarrhoea, intellectual disability	Sensorineural deafness; cerebral dysgenesis; neuropathy; microcephaly; neurogenic muscle atrophy; optic nerve atrophy; cachexia	Arthrogryposis (wrist, knee or hip); intrahepatic bile duct hypoplasia with cholestasis; renal tubular degeneration; metabolic acidosis; abnormal platelet function; cerebral malformation
Risk of death	Death often by 2 years of age	Life-threatening congenital diarrhoea	Lethal within the first decade	Lethal within first year of life
Skin ultrastructure	Lamellar/non-lamellar phase separations in SC	Histology: hyperkeratosis with hypergranulosis	Impaired lipid loading onto LB and defective LB secretion	Defective LB secretion
Special analyses	Liver function tests; decreased β-glucocerebrosidase activity (leukocytes); Gaucher cells (bone marrow); increased acid phosphatase (serum)	Elevation of VLCFAs (blood), treatable by zinc acetate therapy	Absent SNAP29 protein on immunohistochemistry, magnetic resonance imaging	Liver and renal biopsy

Adapted from Oji *et al.* 2010 [10].

AR, autosomal recessive; ARC, arthrogryposis–renal dysfunction–cholestasis; CEDNIK, cerebral dysgenesis–neuropathy–ichthyosis–palmoplantar keratoderma; CIE, congenital ichthyosiform erythroderma; EKV, erythrokeratodermia variabilis; LB, lamellar body; LI, lamellar ichthyosis; MEDNIK, mental retardation–enteropathy–deafness–neuropathy–ichthyosis–keratodermia (erythrokeratodermia variabilis 3, Kamouraska type); SC, stratum corneum; VLCFAs, very long-chain fatty acids.

Synonyms and inclusions
- Heredopathia atactica polyneuritiformis

Pathophysiology

In the early 1960s, accumulation of a storage product identified as a branched-chain 20-carbon fatty acid (phytanic acid) in the plasma and tissues of patients with RD was reported [1]. Phytanic acid is derived from plant chlorophyll and cannot be synthesised by human tissues. In normal circumstances it is barely detectable in the serum, but in RD it accounts for 5–30% of serum lipids. It replaces other fatty acids in lipid-rich tissues thus interfering with membrane structure and function. RD was found to be caused by inactivating mutations in *PHYH* encoding a human phytanoyl-CoA hydroxylase which is responsible for alpha oxidation of phytanic acid [2]. Mutations in *PEX7*, encoding peroxin 7, were found to cause adult RD [3,4]. This gene functions as a receptor for the PHYH protein and incorporates it into peroxisomes [5]. It is of note that accumulation of phytanic acid does not occur exclusively in

RD, but can also be found in other diseases like Zellweger syndrome and in children with dysmorphic features, hepatomegaly, retinitis pigmentosa and hearing loss [6,7]. For some time this latter condition was called 'infantile Refsum disease' because of the phytanic acid accumulation. However, in the meantime it was shown that 'infantile RD' is actually a hepatic peroxisome disorder and the designation 'infantile RD' has been abandoned [5].

Clinical features

The age of onset usually is in late childhood. Diagnosis is often delayed until early adult life. Progressive retinitis pigmentosa initially causes night blindness and, later, failing vision and constricted visual fields. Neurological features develop in adolescence or in the early twenties. Anosmia and impaired taste is a frequent finding. Sensorineural deafness with tinnitus develops in more than 50%. A mixed sensorimotor polyneuropathy (type IV) with hypertrophied peripheral nerves and elevated cerebrospinal fluid protein are characteristic findings. Cerebellar ataxia causes increasing disability. Around 30% of patients show deformities of the hands or feet such as the presence of shortened metacarpal and fourth metatarsal bones early in life. Ichthyosis occurs in around 25% of RD patients and coincides with or postdates the onset of neurological signs. It resembles ichthyosis vulgaris. On histological examination, many of the basal cells are vacuolated and special lipid stains such as oil red O stain will reveal numerous fat globules within the basal cell layer and other keratinocytes [8]. Ultrastructural studies of the barrier lipid organisation of the stratum corneum in RD have revealed a detachment or complete absence of the corneocyte lipid envelope [9].

Management

Early diagnosis is key to proper management of these patients [10]. Exclusion of sources of chlorophyll in the diet is mandatory in the treatment of RD. The major dietary exclusions are green vegetables (phytanic acids) and animal fat (phytol) and the aim of the dietary treatment is to reduce daily intake from the usual level of 50 mg/day to less than 5 mg/day. Rapid weight loss should be avoided as it mobilises tissue phytanic acid, which can lead to acute clinical manifestations. Nowadays, lipid apheresis (that is the extracorporeal elimination of lipoprotein–phytanic acid complexes) is often used in initial treatment [11], followed by a phytanic acid-poor diet [10].

Multiple sulphatase deficiency

Definition and nomenclature

Multiple sulphatase deficiency (MSD) is an exceedingly rare, autosomal recessive, lysosomal storage disorder.

Synonyms and inclusions
- Mucosulfatidosis

Pathophysiology

All known sulphatases are deficient and result in the accumulation of glycosaminoglycans and sulphated lipids [1]. The responsible gene *SUMF1* encodes a protein which is responsible for post-translational modification of sulphatases and catalyses the conversion of a conserved cysteine within the catalytic domain of various sulphatases into a C-alpha formyl glycine [2].

Clinical features

The enzyme deficiency can present as a very severe neonatal MSD [3,4], as a severe late-infantile MSD with onset in the first year of life, or as a mild late-infantile MSD with symptoms occurring between the age of 2 and 4 years, and also as juvenile MSD presenting usually only a few of the symptoms such as intellectual disability and ichthyosis. The disease is typically characterised by developmental delay and failure to thrive and features of Hurler syndrome. A mild ichthyosis and progressive neurological degeneration evolve in the second or third year, but the phenotype varies according to the reduction in the enzyme activity [5]. A first neurological sign is often that children can no longer sit unsupported and lose their communication skills. Around 80% of children demonstrate motor delay and 60% have a language delay [6]. Speech development can be further complicated by hearing loss in 65% of affected patients [6].

Management

No specific therapy is available. Children with predominant mucopolysaccharidosis (MPS) II or MPS VI-like features may be candidates for enzyme replacement therapy.

Sjögren–Larsson syndrome

Definition

Sjögren–Larsson syndrome (SLS) is a rare autosomal recessive neurocutaneous condition featuring congenital ichthyotic hyperkeratosis, spastic diplegia and mild to moderate intellectual disability. In the UK prevalence is estimated to be 1 : 300 000, while in Sweden it is 1 : 100 000 and in the Province of Västerbotten in the north of the country it is even higher at 1 : 10 000.

Pathophysiology

Microsomal fatty aldehyde dehydrogenase (FALDH) deficiency underlies SLS [1]. FALDH catalyses the oxidation of many different medium- and long-chain fatty aldehydes into fatty acids. Its deficiency results in the accumulation of fatty aldehydes and fatty alcohols in various tissues. FALDH has also been implicated in omega oxidation of the eicasanoid LTB4 [2]. SLS patients excrete large amounts of LTB4 in their urine. It is believed that accumulation of LTB4 explains the marked pruritus in the disease. Further supporting this possibility, oral zileuton, which inhibits LTB4 synthesis, improves the pruritus in SLS but has no effect on ichthyosis or neurological disease [3]. The pathogenesis of SLS-associated ichthyosis has been linked to the hepoxilin pathway [4]. The neurological defect results from an abnormal lipid composition of the myelin. The gene that codes for FALDH is nowadays called *ALDH3A2*. More than 90 *ALDH3A2* mutations have been reported in SLS [5,6].

Clinical features

Preterm birth is common and has been attributed to abnormal LTB4 inactivation [2]. Children are usually not born as collodion babies, but the skin is dry and mildly reddened at birth and scaling develops within the first 3 months of life. Thereafter, a mild erythroderma persists and a variable degree of scaling develops consisting of diffuse peeling on the trunk and more pigmented, lamellar-type ichthyosis on the lower limbs (Figure 63.30). Keratotic lichenification is often seen around the flexures, neck and mid-abdomen. The face is usually spared. Severe and persistent pruritus is a notable feature of SLS; scratch marks and dermographism are often seen on the trunk, but skin infections are rare. Neurological symptoms and signs appear during the first 2 years of life and consist of delay in reaching motor milestones due to spastic diplegia, or much less commonly of spastic tetraplegia. Seizures occur in up to 40% of patients. Delayed speech and dysarthria are common. Distinctive ophthalmological findings are so-called glistening white dots surrounding the fovea that are due to crystalline inclusions [7]. Abnormal neurological findings are associated with white matter signal changes on magnetic resonance imaging (MRI) revealing a leukoencephalopathy [8].

With early physiotherapy, most patients learn to walk unaided or with crutches in childhood. Increased muscle tone leads to altered posture and movement which predisposes to contractures (ankles, knees, hips), kyphoscoliosis and dislocated hips. Patchy leukodystrophy and myelination defects have been reported on computed tomography and MRI scanning studies in these patients.

Management

Dietary approaches with supplementation of medium-chain fatty acids have not been successful so far. Inhibition of LTB4 synthesis by zileuton improves pruritus in some patients, but not ichthyosis [3]. Retinoid therapy (etretinate, acitretin) has proven effective in relieving scaling and disabling keratotic lichenification, but less successful in controlling itching [9]. In contrast, IL-13-blocking agents represent an effective therapy for pruritus in SLS (based on the personal experience of V.O.). Intensive physiotherapy [10] and skills learning in early childhood clearly improve motor and social development in SLS. Bezafibrate, a lipid-lowering agent, was shown to induce FALDH activity in fibroblasts in patients with residual enzyme activity, but clinical studies have not been carried out so far [11].

Keratitis–ichthyosis–deafness syndrome

Definition

Keratitis–ichthyosis–deafness (KID) syndrome and hystrix-like ichthyosis and deafness (HID) syndrome are clinically distinct types of congenital ichthyosis featuring severe sensorineural deafness. Despite their heterogeneous phenotypic manifestations, both conditions are related to mutations in *GJB2* encoding connexin 26. Other diseases like Vohwinkel syndrome, as well as focal PPK with deafness and porokeratotic eccrine ostial duct naevus (PEN) – a unique type of epidermal naevus – likewise relate to *GJB2* mutations (Table 63.5).

Pathophysiology

Connexins are universal membrane proteins that form inter- and intracellular channels for ion and molecule transfer, which is the basis of all cellular communication. Mutant connexin expression leads to abnormal cellular and calcium homeostasis and, in some cases, immune responses which cause cell dysfunction, lysis and death. Mutations in genes encoding gap junction proteins, namely connexins, have been reported in various epidermal diseases including hidrotic ectodermal dysplasia (connexin 30), erythrokeratoderma variabilis with and without deafness (connexin 31 and 30.3), Vohwinkel syndrome (connexin 26), KID syndrome (connexin 26), HID syndrome (connexin 26) and in PEN [1–6].

Recurrent and novel *GJB2* mutations have been recorded in a significant number of patients [7,8]. It is of note that the hearing deficiencies are often due to recessive mutations, whereas KID and HID syndromes are normally transmitted as autosomal dominant traits. In contrast, PEN results from mosaicism for *GJB2* mutations, and therefore a mother affected by PEN may give birth to a child affected by KID syndrome [5], a situation reminiscent of mosaicism in EI.

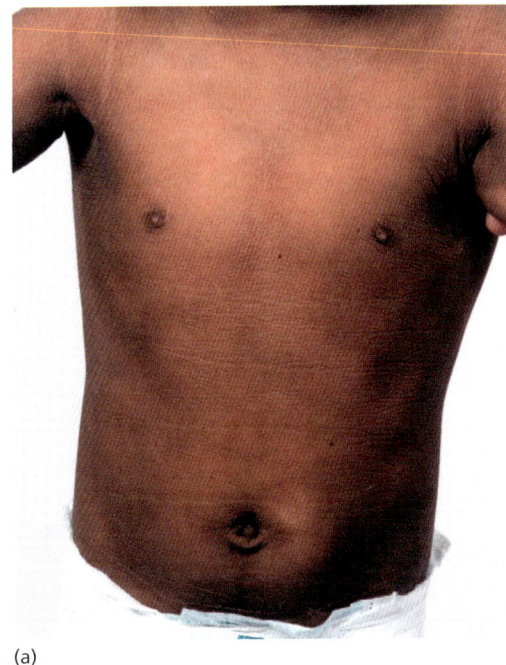

(a)

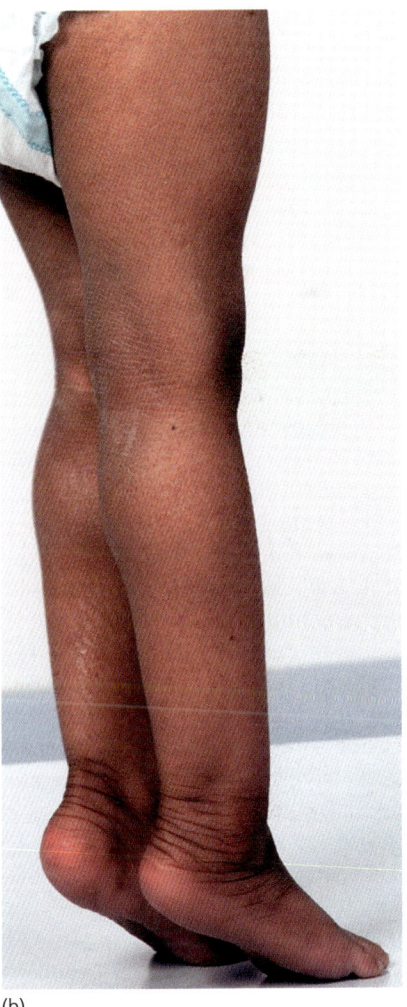

(b)

Figure 63.30 Sjögren–Larsson syndrome. A 3-year-old girl with (a) keratotic lichenification and (b) spastic diplegia. Courtesy of Dr M. Judge, Salford Royal NHS Trust, UK.

Table 63.5 Disorders associated with mutations in *GJB2* (connexin 26).

Disease	MIM number	Mode of inheritance	Mutation in *GJB2*
Keratitis–ichthyosis–deafness (KID)	148210	AD	G12R, N14Y, S17F, G45E, D50N, D50Y
		AR	N176D, G12Vfs*2
Hystrix-like ichthyosis–deafness (HID)	602540	AD	D50N
Bart–Pumphrey syndrome	149200	AD	N54H, N54K, G59S
Palmoplantar keratoderma–deafness	148350	AD	G59R, G59A, R75W, R75Q, E42, G130V
Vohwinkel syndrome	124500	AD (AR)	Y65H, D66H, G130V
Mucositis–deafness		AD	F142L
Hypotrichosis–deafness		AD	N14K
Vohwinkel-like papular palmoplantar keratoderma–deafness		AD	H73R
Deafness	220290	AR (AD)	M34T, 35delG, 167delT, 235delC, etc.
	220290	AD	R75W, R75Q, etc.

Adapted from de Zwart-Storm *et al.* 2008 [4].
AD, autosomal dominant; AR, autosomal recessive.

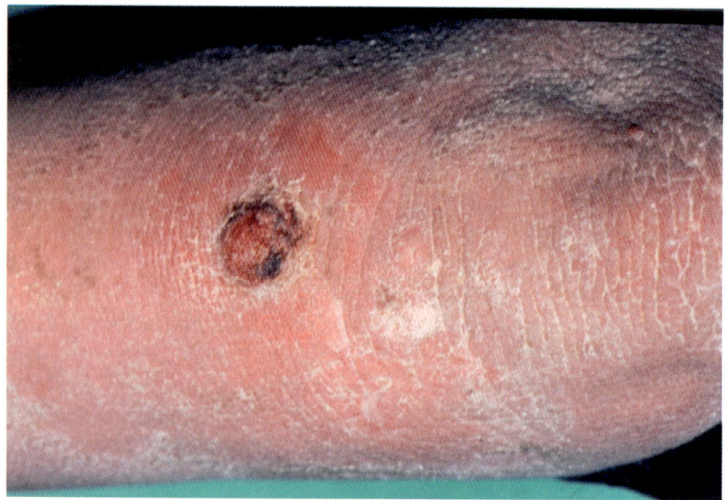

Figure 63.31 Keratitis–ichthyosis–deafness syndrome. Adult with squamous cell carcinoma on the arm. Courtesy of Dr D. J. Atherton, Great Ormond Street Hospital for Children, London, UK.

Some mutations are closely associated with KID syndrome such as the p.D50N mutation, which was detected in 12 of 14 patients in one report [8]. Functional studies have highlighted that at least two *GJB2* mutations, namely p.D50A and p.A88V, do not simply inhibit channel formation, but rather result in high-conductance hemichannels at the cell surface. Such gain of function due to *GJB2* mutation thus creates channels that can result in toxicity by accelerating cell death in low extracellular calcium solutions [9]. Infant mortality in KID syndrome with the *GJB2* mutation p.A88V or p.G45G is very high, but death in KID syndrome caused by other *GJB2* mutations is rare [10].

Clinical features

Many affected neonates have generalised red skin and some have diffuse scaling and a leathery skin. They may resemble those with ichthyosis prematurity syndrome [11]. But in KID infants develop linear and spiny hyperkeratosis around the flexures, elbows and knees, and hystrix-like scaling on the limbs. Scattered follicular hyperkeratosis appears on the trunk. Typical features are the evolution of symmetrical, well-demarcated hyperkeratotic and warty plaques on the scalp, ears and face and occasionally on the trunk and limbs. Some patients develop thick perioral rugae, and an aged or leonine facies. Keratotic, hyperplastic and inflammatory nodules may develop on the scalp, face, trunk and lower legs, and *in situ* and invasive squamous cell carcinomas arising within these dysplastic lesions have been reported in several KID patients in adult life (Figure 63.31). A 37-year-old man died of metastatic squamous carcinoma of the skin; his daughter also has KID syndrome [12]. Likewise squamous cell carcinoma of the tongue has occurred in three young patients [13–15] and a 28-year-old patient had a fatal malignant fibrous histiocytoma [16]. Multiple hair follicle tumours (including malignant progression to tricholemmal tumours) occurred in an adult with KID syndrome [17] and two further adult patients developed metastatic malignant pilar tumours [18].

Most patients have extensive scarring alopecia of the scalp and loss of the eyebrows, eyelashes and body hair resulting from follicular hyperkeratosis and atrophy. IFAP syndrome needs to be considered as a differential diagnosis (see earlier in this chapter). A reticulate PPK resembling grained leather is a characteristic feature, and progressive nail dystrophy and shedding may occur. Acneform eruptions and cysts on the upper trunk are common, and chronic deep abscesses and discharging sinuses (follicular occlusion triad) are a distressing late complication in some patients. Chronic cutaneous, granulomatous fungal and *Candida* infections may develop and contribute to the alopecia, nail dystrophy and body odour. Death in infancy from overwhelming infection (viral, bacterial and mycotic) has been reported in at least four patients with KID syndrome. Premature caries, oral leukoplakia, short stature, breast hypoplasia and cryptorchidism are occasional complications.

Congenital severe sensorineural deafness is evident during infancy in most patients. In typical KID syndrome, progressive corneal vascularisation occurs in early childhood, often after a febrile illness, and leads to photophobia and blindness by adolescence in 75% of patients. A progressive peripheral neuropathy has occurred in several adults with KID.

The HID syndrome in contrast to KID shows full-blown CIE with hystrix-like keratosis in particular on the trunk and on the extremities and the entire body is affected, while in KID syndrome hyperkeratosis is usually confined to sites of predilection and the trunk is usually spared in later life.

Of note, the clinical appearance of PEN – caused by mosaic *GJB2* mutations – can resemble that of KID syndrome, showing a hyperkeratotic verrucous, hard, epidermal naevus that features a peculiar histopathology including ortho- or parakeratotic plaques protruding from eccrine ducts [19].

Recently, a novel autosomal recessive *GJB2*-associated disorder was delineated featuring true ichthyosis follicularis, and as might be expected in *GJB2* mutations, bilateral sensorineural hearing loss and punctate PPK [20].

Management

Early and frequent audiological and ophthamological assessment of patients with KID and HID syndrome is necessary to enable appropriate treatments such as hearing aids, cochlear implants and speech therapy to be instituted in a timely manner [21]. The ocular lesions are treated topically with lubricants, antibiotics, steroids or ciclosporin drops as indicated. Surgical procedures and corneal transplant to treat advanced keratitis of the eye have usually failed [22], but ocular surface stem cell transplantation [23] or gas-permeable lenses may be an option [24].

Ocular antiseptic baths and cleansers, intermittent antibiotic and antiviral therapy and prolonged systemic antifungal agents play an important role in controlling skin infections and odour [25]. Cleansing, debridement, dressing, excision of hyperplastic lesions and grafting may become necessary to reduce the potential for malignant transformation. Systemic retinoids like acitretin are helpful in controlling the disease, including visual symptoms [26], but isotretinoin may exacerbate corneal neovascularisation [27]. Teatment with alitretinoin resulted in marked improvement of an extremely severe case of dissecting cellulitis of the scalp [28].

Desmons syndrome

Definition and nomenclature

Desmons syndrome is new in the list of ichthyosis syndromes and is characterised by neonatal onset of ichthyosis, erythroderma and deafness accompanied by failure to thrive and developmental delay [1,2].

Synonyms and inclusions
- Ichthyosis deafness photophobia syndrome
- Ichthyosiform erythroderma, corneal involvement and deafness
- MEDNIK-like syndrome
- AP1B1 deficiency

Pathophysiology

The neurocutaneous disorder results from recessive loss-of-function mutations in the gene *AP1B1*, which encodes the adaptor-related protein complex 1 beta 1 (AP1B1) subunit [3,4]. Similar to MEDNIK syndrome [5], which is due to mutations in *AP1S1*, Desmons syndrome has been linked to those with mutations in adaptor protein and other genes central to vesicular function, and is considered a copper-related metabolic disease [6]. However, a lack of copper toxicity may reflect a fundamental difference in the clinical presentation and pathogenesis of Desmons disease and MEDNIK syndrome [4].

Clinical features

At birth, Desmons disease might present like an inflammatory form of autosomal recessive congenital ichthyosis with ectropion (Figure 63.32) [1,3,4]. Considering the profound sensorineural deafness and vascularising keratitis the disease might be reminiscent of KID syndrome [7], but the clinical course of the skin phenotype is different. At the same time, there is an enteropathy, hepatopathy

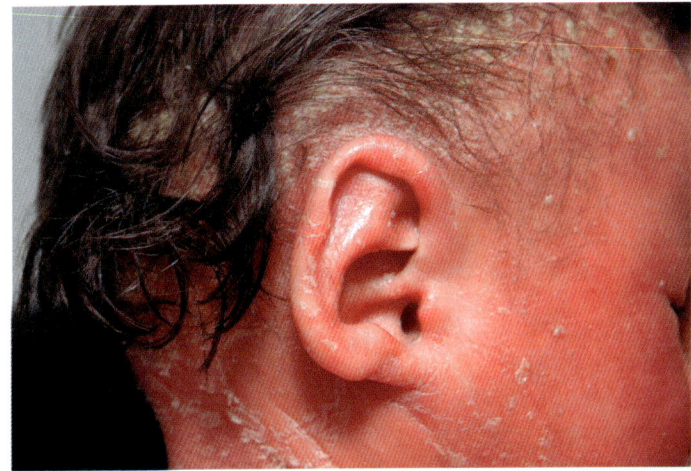

Figure 63.32 Girl at the age of 1 year suffering from severe erythroderma due to Desmons syndrome (AP1B1 deficiency).

and mild hair phenotype similar to MEDNIK syndrome [5]. Severe failure to thrive and developmental delay within the first month of life seem to be compensated in later childhood [2].

Investigations

Histopathology of the skin presents epidermal thickening, hyperkeratosis [2] and an abnormally high number of basophilic vesicles within the proliferative layers of the epidermis [3]. These vesicles are also observed via transmission electron microscopy [3].

Management

Management of the disease requires a multidisciplinary approach. The inflammatory skin phenotype may show a dramatic response to biologics such as ustekinumab (unpublished data).

ELOVL4 deficiency

ELOVL4 deficiency [1,2] has been regarded as an erythrokeratoderma with sensorineural deafness [3] – clinically reminiscent of KID syndrome. In a five-generation Canadian pedigree, erythrokeratoderma appearing in infancy and clearing in later life was associated with late-onset ataxia and neuropathy [4].

Neutral lipid storage disease with ichthyosis

Definition and nomenclature

Neutral lipid storage disease with ichthyosis (NLSDI) is a rare type of syndromic, autosomal recessive, congenital ichthyosis featuring congenital ichthyosiform erythroderma and lipid droplets in various tissues. Most patients originate from Mediterranean countries.

Synonyms and inclusions
- Chanarin Dorfman syndrome

Pathophysiology

The disease is due to mutations in *ABHD5* (previously known as *CGI-58*) [1]. Another type of neutral lipid storage disease without ichthyosis, but with myopathy, has been designated NLSDM and is caused by mutations in the *PNPLA2* gene [2]. *ABHD5* is widely expressed in tissues such as skin, muscle, liver and brain, but also lymphocytes [3], and localises to the surface of cytoplasmic lipid droplets [4]. The genetic defect leads to acyl-ceramide deficiency, likely contributing to the pathogenesis of ichthyosis [5]. For diagnostic purposes, it is useful to search for lipid droplets in leukocytes (Jordan anomaly) (Figure 63.33a) [6]. It is important to note that the characteristic lipid inclusions have to be specifically looked for in both affected patients and possible gene carriers. If an automated blood cell count is done, a 'normal' result will be handed out erroneously. Lipid deposition results in a combination of skin, hepatic, muscle and ocular abnormalities.

It is of note that the *PNPLA2* gene – associated with NLSDM – encodes adipose triglyceride lipase which is necessary for lipolysis of cellular fat stores in non-cutaneous tissues [2]. Adipose triglyceride lipase requires the *ABHD5* gene product as a cofactor, which explains the fact that NLSDI and NLSDM share common features in non-cutaneous tissues and also suggests the existence of an epidermal lipase also utilising ABHD5 as a cofactor [7].

Clinical features

This is a multisystem disorder, but the clinical features are variable [8,9]. Affected newborns are either collodion babies or erythrodermic. The pattern of skin disease thereafter resembles mild to moderate CIE with fine white scales on a reddish background and a lamellar scaling on the trunk and legs (Figure 36.33b). Scaling may diminish in warm weather and with advancing age. Pruritus is often troublesome and hypohidrosis may occur. Mild ectropion, flexural and neck lichenification and palmoplantar hyperkeratosis are common. Nail dystrophy and scalp alopecia have rarely been reported.

Muscle involvement ranges from an asymptomatic or subclinical myopathy with elevated muscle enzymes in most patients to marked proximal myopathy in a few cases. Hepatomegaly, abnormal liver enzymes and fatty infiltration of the liver are common, even in childhood, and liver involvement is observed in more than 80% of patients. Cirrhosis may evolve rapidly, even in childhood. An Italian cohort study recently reported that two out of six patients died of hepatic failure [10]. Liver biopsy is more sensitive than biochemical markers in detecting the degree of involvement. Spenomegaly and malabsorption, resulting from intestinal mucosal lipid deposition, are occasional features. Cataracts of the nuclear type (subcapsular) may be detected from infancy in over 50% of cases, but rarely affect vision. Nystagmus may occur. Short stature, retinal disease, nerve deafness, ataxia, microcephaly, spasticity, neuropathy and developmental delay have been reported, but most patients are intellectually normal. Fetal renal complications occurred in an infant with NLSDI. Prognosis depends on the pattern and degree of organ involvement. Unlike NLSDM patients, NLSDI patients do not develop cardiomyopathy [11].

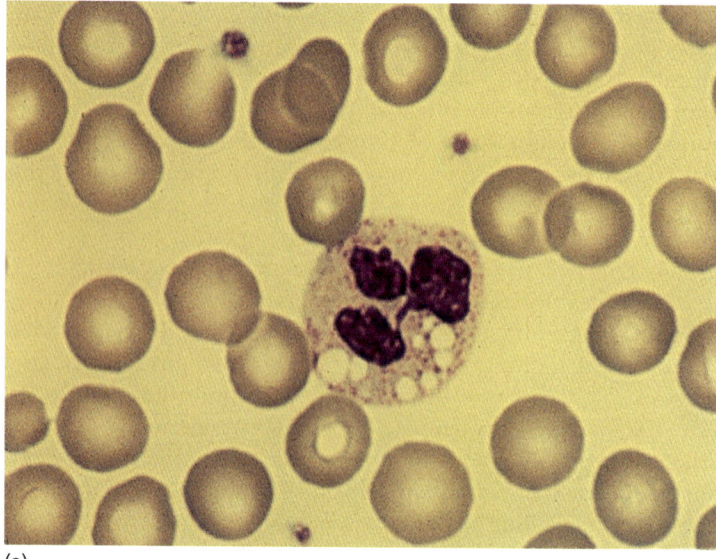

(a)

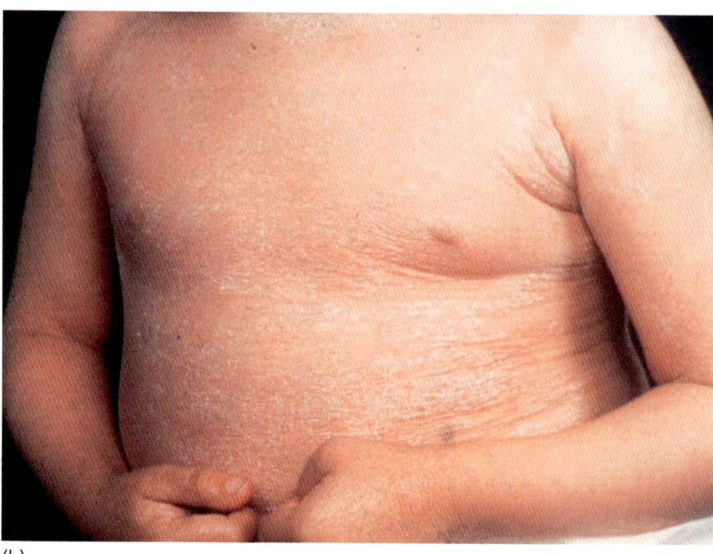

(b)

Figure 63.33 Neutral lipid storage disease with ichthyosis. (a) Lipid vacuoles (Jordan anomaly). (b) Ichthyosiform erythroderma. Courtesy of Dr M. Judge, Salford Royal NHS Trust, UK.

Management

Emollients are helpful and although liver function tests usually show abnormalities in these patients, the administration of acitretin has been beneficial even in the presence of compromised liver function [12]. The effect of dietary approaches is doubtful [13].

Trichothiodystrophy

Definition and nomenclature

Trichothiodystrophy is a rare and heterogeneous group of neurocutaneous genodermatoses that have in common a hair defect termed TTD or sulphur-deficient brittle hair.

Synonyms and inclusions

- Tay syndrome
- IBIDS syndrome (ichthyosis, brittle hair and nails, intellectual impairment and short stature)
- PIBIDS syndrome (photosensitivity, ichthyosis, brittle hair and nails, intellectual impairment and short stature)
- Amish brittle hair syndrome

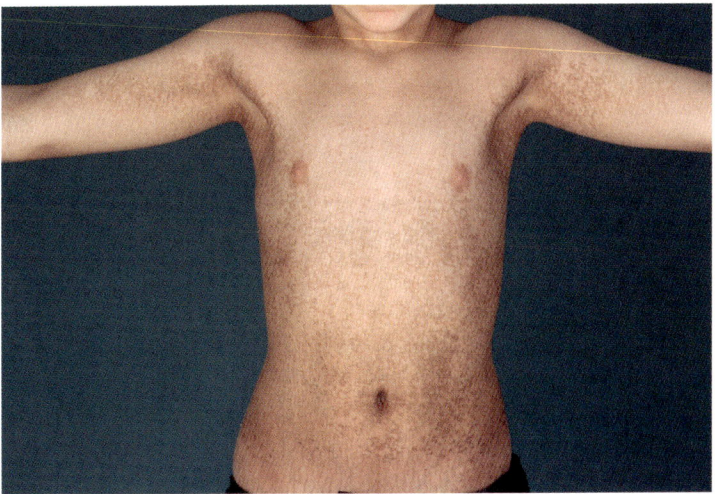

Figure 63.34 Trichothiodystrophy showing lamellar scaling similar to bathing suit ichthyosis.

Pathophysiology

All types of TTD are autosomal recessive traits. From a genetic point of view, one can distinguish a photosensitive TTD group with (i) DNA repair anomalies involving various subunits of the transcription factor TFIIH; (ii) a non-photosensitive group without a DNA repair defect that features mutations in the *C7ORF11* gene coding for TTDN1 protein; and (iii) a group without a DNA repair defect and with still unclear underlying genetic defects [1,2]. Since little is known about the function of the *C7ORF11* gene that encodes the protein for non-photosensitive TTD (TTDN1), pathophysiological investigations have focused on the photosensitive group, in which mutations in *ERCC2* (XPD), *ERCC3* (XPB) and *GTF2H5* (TTDA) – all of which are subunits of the transcription/DNA repair factor IIH (TFIIH) – have been identified [2]. TFIIH is a complex of 10 proteins that are essential for both nucleotide excision repair and transcription [3]. Mutations in TTD-associated genes destabilise the superstructure of TFIIH and result in a low concentration of TFIIH, which in turn limits the level of transcription of a variety of target genes – in particular deregulation of thyroid hormone target genes in the brain occurs. In this way, the TTD phenotype is explained [4]. In contrast, TTDN1 is a nuclear protein that is not involved in DNA repair, but has several phosphorylation sites and is considered a regulator of mitosis [5]. Dysregulation of the liver X receptor (LXR) responsive genes such as *ABCA12* may contribute to the phenotype of ichthyosis in the disorders [6].

Clinical features

Patients affected with the photosensitive forms of TTD are often born prematurely and typically present with a collodion membrane or with a CIE-like phenotype [3,5]. Pregnancies of TTD neonates have to be considered as high-risk pregnancies and are frequently complicated by pre-eclampsia, decreased fetal movement, haemolysis, elevated liver enzymes and low platelets (HELLP syndrome) [7]. TTD neonates often have a low birth weight, are small for gestational age and require admission to a neonatal intensive care unit [7]. In infancy, they have an increased risk of early death from sepsis and recurrent infections with chronic neutropenia [2,8].

Congenital ichthyosis (collodion baby) – when present – often progresses to only mild ichthyosis, for instance predominantly on the trunk (Figure 63.34), histologically showing a thin granular layer and thus resembling IV in later life [1]. It has been pointed out that the frequency of congenital ichthyosis with initial presentation as collodion baby is significantly higher in patients carrying mutations in genes encoding components of the TFIIH complex, while in contrast hypogonadism is significantly more frequent in the non-photosensitive group [1]. Scalp and eyebrow hair is fragile, sparse, short and unruly, but may improve with age. Associated features are eczema, palmoplantar hyperkeratosis, pulp atrophy, digital flexion contractures, fragile small nails and hypoplastic aural cartilage [9]. An elfin-like and aged (progeric) face resulting from fat atrophy might be seen.

Photosensitivity and photophobia occur in most patients having TFIIH-related mutations, but this feature can improve with age. In contrast to xeroderma pigmentosum, a highly increased risk of malignancy is not regarded as a feature of photosensitive TTD [10], but cumulative sun exposure has an effect on the DNA repair defect [11]. A temperature-dependent deterioration in hair (e.g. sudden loss of all hair) and worsening of skin and neurological features have been observed in several patients at the time of febrile illness [12] and have been attributed to increased instability in the TFIIH complex [13].

Mild to moderate intellectual impairment is the rule and hypogonadism may lead to delayed puberty and infertility in adult patients. A friendly disposition and cuddlesome behaviour may be typical for TTD [14,15]. Important further characteristics of TTD are cataracts, otosclerosis, dental anomalies and neurological signs such as microcephaly, spasticity, cerebellar dysfunction, seizures and autism [16].

Investigations

On polarising microscopy the typical 'tiger-tail pattern' can be noted that relates to a low content of the amino acid cysteine in the hair. If polarised light microscopy is not available, trichoscopy may be applied, which shows alterations such as a wavy contour of the hair shaft, short broken hair, glomerule-like curls and twists of broken hair [17]. Most important in early infancy, patients should be checked for immunological abnormalities (haematology, immunoglobulins) [8].

Management

Infants with TTD need close surveillance for recurrent infections, hypogammaglobulinaemia and/or neutropenia. Supplemental immunoglobulins or granulocyte colony-stimulating factor might be required [8]. Emollients are helpful in skin comfort. The effect of retinoids on ichthyosis has been disappointing. Strict sun avoidance, protective measures and sunscreens are recommended for the photosensitive patients [11]. Advice on avoidance of physical hair treatment is helpful in reducing fur.

Neu–Laxova syndrome

Definition and nomenclature

This is an lethal, autosomal recessive, malformation syndrome in which the cutaneous features (congenital ichthyosis) have never been studied adequately. The tight skin described in several reports is reminiscent of restrictive dermopathy [1–3].

> **Synonyms and inclusions**
> • Phosphoglycerate dehydrogenase deficiency

Pathophysiology

Neu–Laxova syndrome (NLS) is heterogeneous and inherited as an autosomal recessive trait. It is caused by mutations in the *PHGDH* gene that lead to phosphoglycerate dehydrogenase deficiency [4]. This enzyme is involved in the first and limiting step of L-serine biosynthesis. Recently, it has been shown that mutations in *PSAT1* and *PSPH* encoding two other enzymes of the L-serine biosynthesis pathway may lead into NLS [5]. The phenotype, albeit showing substantial variation in severity, may therefore represent the severe end of serine-deficiency disorders [5]. Histology of the skin reveals focal parakeratosis. No systematic analysis of the cutaneous phenotype with immunofluorescence studies or ultrastructure is available.

Clinical features

Neu–Laxova syndrome is characterised by congenital ichthyosis, marked intrauterine growth retardation, microcephaly, short neck, central nervous system anomalies, limb deformities, hypoplastic lungs, oedema and abnormal facial features including severe proptosis with ectropion, hypertelorism, micrognathia, flattened nose and malformed ears [1–3]. Prenatal ultrasound findings of marked ocular proptosis in a growth-restricted, oedematous fetus are suggestive of the diagnosis [3,6]. A polyhydramion is typical and most likely the result of the congenital ichthyosis as polyhydramion can also be seen in harlequin ichthyosis and ichthyosis prematurity syndrome. Several cases diagnosed by exome sequencing as having mutations in the *PHGDH* gene showed prenatal skin oedema but no obvious ichthyosis [7].

Diffential diagnosis

From a dermatological point of view, restrictive dermopathy is the most relevant differential diagnosis. Similar to NLS it is characterised by intrauterine growth retardation, thin, tightly adherent, translucent skin, typical facial dysmorphology with a mouth forming an O, generalised joint contractures, fetal akinesia and polyhydramion. Most cases are due to mutations in the *ZMPSTE24* gene, while a few seem to be due to mutations in *LMNA* [8,9].

Management

All reported cases have been lethal so far. Considering the metabolic basis of the disorder and similar to other serine deficiency therapies, NLS might be a treatable condition when recognised and treated early enough [5,9]. A supplement therapy may be provided for pregnant women who previously had a child affected by NLS [4], which underscores the need for accurate diagnosis of neonates with congenital ichthyosis and for an understanding of its lethal course [10].

CHIME syndrome

Definition and nomenclature

Coloboma–heart defect–ichthyosiform dermatosis–mental retardation–ear anomalies (CHIME) syndrome is an exceedingly rare, autosomal recessive, neurocutaneous condition.

> **Synonyms and inclusions**
> • Zunich neuroectodermal syndrome

Pathophysiology

The CHIME syndrome is due to mutations in the gene *PIGL* which encodes the de-N-acetylase required for glycosyl phosphatidyl inositol (GPI) anchor formation [1]. Large deletions in *PIGL* seem to be a common mutational mechanism [2]. *PIGL* is an ER-localised enzyme that catalyses the second step of GPI biosynthesis. It thus is a congenital disorder of glycosylation. Glycosylation is the biosynthetic process of adding glycans to proteins and lipids and is an important modification of secretory and membrane-bound proteins [3]. Defects within the *N*-glycosylation or *O*-glycosylation biosynthesis pathway result in congenital disorders of glycosylation [4]. GPI biosynthesis plays a role in the anchorage of more than 150 cell surface proteins including receptors, enzymes and adhesion molecules [2]. Patients often present elevated alkaline phosphatase (ALP) levels, as ALP is a GPI-anchored enzyme [2].

Clinical features

In 1983, Zunich and Kaye [5] reported a child with migratory CIE, retinal colobomas, neurological disease, fine sparse hair and dental abnormalities. Further cases featuring in addition cardiac abnormalities have been described [5–8]. Generalised pruritus, skin redness and scaling develop within the first month, and figurate, red, scaly and itchy patches migrate on the head and body from early childhood. The palms and soles are thickened; the scalp hair is fine, sparse and hypopigmented. Cranial defects, alopecia, hypertelorism, a broad nasal bridge, wide mouth, full lips and wide-spaced teeth contribute to a characteristic facial appearance. Neurological features include hearing loss, seizures, developmental delay and outbursts of violent behaviour. A 4-year-old with CHIME syndrome developed leukaemia. The disease is considered to be a cancer-prone genodermatosis [9].

Table 63.6 Selected syndromic ichthyoses with hair abnormalities and gastrointestinal or respiratory symptoms.

Features	Ichthyosis with hypotrichosis (IH)[a]	Neonatal ichthyosis–sclerosing cholangitis (NISCH)[b]	Ichthyosis–prematurity syndrome (IPS)
MIM number	602400	607626	608649
Mode of inheritance	AR	AR	AR
Gene	*ST14*	*CLDN1*	*FATP4*
Onset	At birth	At birth (or shortly after)	At birth (polyhydramnion, prematurity, >6 weeks)
Initial clinical presentation	Lamellar ichthyosis, severe hypotrichosis, absent eyebrows and eyelashes	Mild scaling, neonatal jaundice with hepatomegaly; frontal alopecia in early childhood	Respiratory distress, generalised skin hyperkeratosis with focal accentuation on scalp and eyebrows
Disease course	Over time, scalp hair growth and appearance/colour may improve	Mild ichthyosis, liver involvement variable	Severe at birth, spontaneous improvement
Cutaneous findings: Distribution of scaling	Generalised, including the scalp; face may be unaffected	Predominant on trunk	Focal accentuation (see above)
Scaling type	Coarse, plate-like, adherent	Fine to polygonal, thin	Caseous (vernix caseosa-like)
Scaling colour	Brown to dark	Normal	Whitish
Skin redness	Unusual	Unusual	Mild to moderate
Palmoplantar involvement	No	No	Yes, initially
Hypohidrosis	Yes	No	No
Scalp abnormalities	Hypotrichosis in youth; sparse, unruly hair in adolescence; recessing frontal hair line in adults	Major criterion: coarse thick hair, frontotemporal scarring alopecia; hypotrichosis, curly/woolly hair	Extensive at birth
Other skin findings	Follicular atrophoderma	–	Follicular keratosis ('toad skin'), atopic eczema, asthma, eosinophilia
Extracutaneous involvement	Sparse and curly eyebrows; occasionally photophobia and pingueculum	Major criterion: sclerosing cholangitis or congenital paucity of bile ducts	Pulmonary involvement and asphyxia at birth; later on atopic asthma, eosinophilia and occasionally hyper IgE
Risk of death	Normal	Not observed, but theoretically possible from liver involvement	Perinatally potentially fatal due to respiratory asphyxia; otherwise normal
Skin ultrastructure	High presence of intact corneodesmosomes in the upper SC, residues of membranous structures in the SC	Splitting of desmosomal anchoring plaques in the SG	Deposits of trilamellar membranous curved lamellae in swollen corneocytes and perinuclearly in oedematous granular cells
Special analyses	Hair microscopy may reveal dysplastic hair, pili torti or pili bifurcate	Liver function tests, cholangiography, liver biopsy	Blood cell count (eosinophilia)

Adapted from Oji *et al*. 2010 [1].
[a] Allelic variant: congenital ichthyosis–follicular atrophoderma–hypotrichosis–hypohidrosis (IFAH).
[b] Also known as ichthyosis–leukocyte vacuoles–alopecia–sclerosing cholangitis (ILVASC).
AR, autosomal recessive; IgE, immunoglobulin E; SC, stratum corneum, SG, stratum granulosum.

PART 6: GENETIC DISORDERS

Management

Emollients (moisturisers) have been recommended for the ichthyosis [6].

MISCELLANEOUS SYNDROMIC ICHTHYOSES

Table 63.6 describes some syndromic ichthyoses with hair abnormalities and gastrointestinal or respiratory symptoms.

Ichthyosis–prematurity syndrome

Clinical features

The disease is characterised prenatally by polyhydramnion and increased echogenic signals of amniotic fluid [1]. Affected neonates are often born between the 30th and 35th gestational weeks, and suffer from transient, potentially life-threating asphyxia, which is the result of reduced lung function and bronchial obstruction from keratin plugs [2–4]. One neonate has been described who developed a compartment syndrome on one hand [5]. The neonatal erythroderma (Figure 63.35a) evolves into a mild ichthyosis reminiscent of CICI (Figure 63.35b) [6], but patients are prone to pruritus and atopic manifestations [4].

Pathophysiology

Ichthyosis–prematurity syndrome (IPS) is caused by recessive mutations in the *FATP4* gene [1,2], which encodes a fatty acid transporter and acyl coenzyme A synthetase expressed in the suprabasal layers of the epidermis [3]. Reduced function leads to disturbance of the intercellular lipid layer of the stratum corneum [4,5]. It can be concluded from the mouse model that FATP4 might be more important for the generation of the epidermal barrier than for its maintenance, which may explain the transient character of the disease [6,7]. In addition deletions of *FATP4* may interfere with the enzyme synthesis of the visual cycle, but clinical symptoms have not been reported [8].

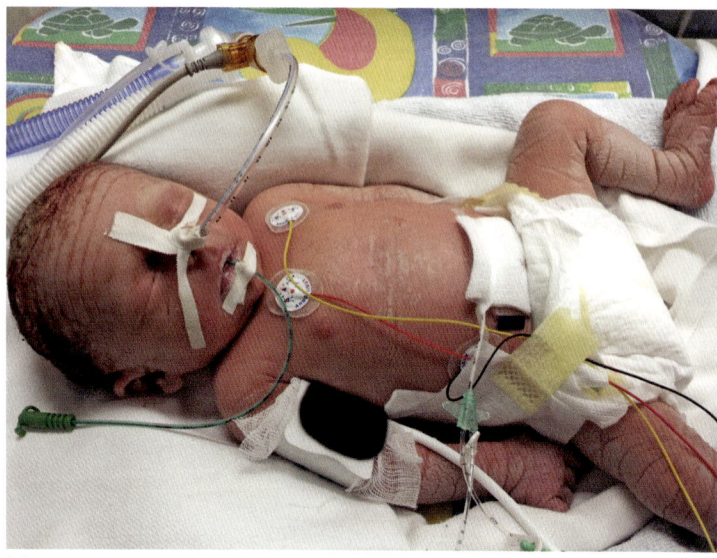

(a)

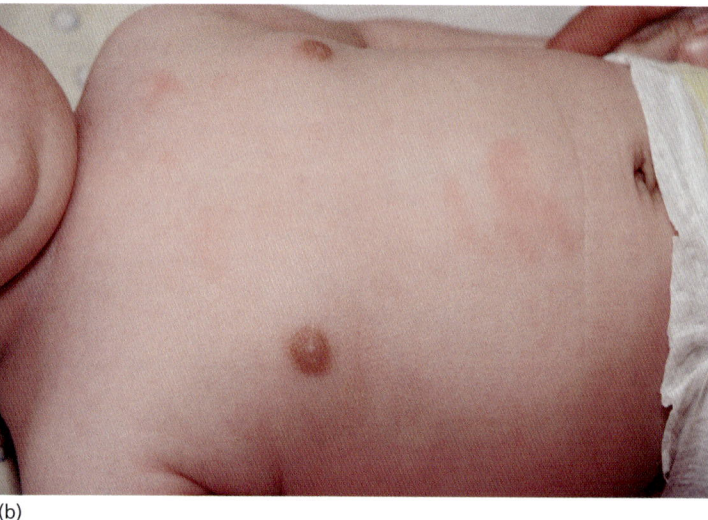

(b)

Figure 63.35 Ichthyosis prematurity syndrome. (a) Neonatal presentation. (b) The same patient after 3 months. Note the mild velvet-like skin texture. Courtesy of the Department of Dermatology, University Hospital Münster, Münster, Germany.

Investigations

Ultrastructure reveals the distinct phenotype of so-called 'ichthyosis congenita type IV', which is characterised by irregular lentiform depositions of membrane-like material in granular cells and horny scales [9].

Management

Considering the similar skin phenotype at birth, KID syndrome should be excluded [10]. Information about the risk of IPS, for instance for subsequent pregnancies of parents who have previously had a child affected by IPS, may decide between a benign or unfavourable course of the condition as treatment can start early. Optimal treatment with adequate bronchial suction, if initiated early enough, and optimal perinatal care will avoid life-threatening hypoxaemia and/or complications such as infantile cerebral paresis [6].

Further syndromic ichthyoses with prominent hair abnormalities

Netherton syndrome or neuro-ichthyoses such as trichothiodystrophy or MEDNIK syndrome feature a distinct hair phenotype (see earlier in this chapter). Moreover, the group of ichthyoses with prominent hair abnormalities includes the ichthyosis with hypothrichosis (IH) and neonatal ichthyosis–sclerosing cholangitis (NISCH) syndromes [1,2].

Ichthyosis with hypotrichosis

Definition and nomenclature
The ichthyosis presents at birth, but without collodion membranes. Two allelic variants have been described.
1 Autosomal recessive ichthyosis with hypotrichosis (ARIH) features ichthyosis and whole-body hypotrichosis, but no atrophoderma [1,2].
2 Congenital ichthyosis–follicular atrophoderma–hypotrichosis–hypohidrosis (IFAH) refers to a very similar phenotype associated in addition with follicular atrophoderma (e.g. follicular pitting on the dorsal aspects of the hands and fingers) [3,4].

Synonyms and inclusions
• Ichthyosis and follicular atrophoderma with hypotrichosis and hypohidrosis

Pathophysiology
Both phenotypes are associated with autosomal recessive mutations in the *ST14* gene [1,2], which encodes matriptase, a novel key player of the epidermal protease network [5,6]. The transmembrane serine protease is an efficient activator of epidermal prokallikreins. Matriptase deficiency leads to a decrease of filaggrin processing [7]. An elegant LEKTI-deficient mouse model showed that corneodesmosome integrity was restored when matriptase was ablated [8]. As such, ST14 deficiency might be seen as the functional counterpart to LEKTI deficiency, which leads to an increase of epidermal kallikrein activity [6,9]. Clinical heterogeneity may be caused by different types of *ST14* mutations [1,4,9–13]. The hair phenotype can be explained by the fact that matriptase is expressed in the cortex cells and shaft of the anagen hair [14].

Neonatal ichthyosis–sclerosing cholangitis

Synonyms and inclusions
• Ichthyosis–leukocyte vacuoles–alopecia–sclerosing cholangitis
• Ichthyosis–hypotrichosis–sclerosing cholangitis–claudin 1 deficiency

Pathophysiology
Neonatal ichthyosis–sclerosing cholangitis belongs to the disorders of tight junctions due to autosomal recessive mutations in *CLDN1* encoding claudin 1 [1–3]. Claudin 1 is part of the epidermal tight junctions, but is also expressed in human cholangiocytes and hepatocytes [4]. The primary lack of claudin 1 leads to increased

paracellular permeability between epithelial cells, which may explain the phenotype of hypercholanaemia or epidermal barrier defect [1]. In mice, homozygous deletion of *CLDN1* leads to neonatal lethality because of transepidermal loss of water and desiccation. In humans, other tight junction components may partially compensate for claudin 1 deficiency [2].

Clinical features

Sclerosing cholangitis is a severe, chronic condition characterised by inflammation and obliterative fibrosis of the intra- and extrahepatic bile ducts. NISCH syndrome is characterised by scalp hypotrichosis with scarring alopecia and ichthyosis, and shows a primary sclerosing cholangitis of variable severity [5–9]. Hence, infantile jaundice and ichthyosis may be an important clinical symptom of the disease, but early molecular analysis is recommended as the disease also presents without signs of liver disease [10]. Histology of the skin reveals normal epidermis with a compact, mildly orthohyperkeratotic stratum corneum. The amount of keratohyalin is described as reduced, and ultrastructural features show a large number of corneodesmosomes [7].

Management of congenital ichthyoses

Inherited ichthyoses require lifelong management based on the establishment of the correct molecular diagnosis (Figure 63.36). This section focuses on autosomal recessive congenital ichthyoses as well as keratinopathic ichthyoses; however, it may be applicable to other forms of hereditary ichthyosis.

General aspects of therapy

Congenital ichthyoses are hereditary, non-curable diseases, in which currently only symptomatic relief can be provided. Their variable degrees of scaling, hyperkeratosis and skin inflammation require different approaches. Ocular and ear complications are common in neonates and infants – in both syndromic and non-syndromic ichthyoses; and children often suffer from pruritus, fissuring, sweating impairment (hypohidrosis) and superinfections that need individualised care. Although some types of congenital ichthyoses may show spontaneous and seasonal variations, most patients will require daily therapy throughout life. In infancy and childhood almost all cases need to be managed with topical therapy/balneotherapy, while systemic treatment options – namely oral retinoids – are limited for most severe cases.

Since the ichthyoses are chronic lifelong diseases, there is a need for well-tolerated, safe and effective treatments. However, the degree of scientific evidence on the benefits and risks of the available treatments is low. A recent review of clinical trials of treatment for congenital ichthyoses revealed only six trials that met the criteria of the methodology of the Cochrane Collaboration [1] and therefore most of what is stated here cannot be considered to be evidence based. The small number of patients included in the studies, the high risk of bias and the short follow-up of patients require careful evaluation of the results. The difficulties that are encountered when carrying out randomised, double-blind, multinational, placebo-controlled studies in these ultra-rare diseases are highlighted by a recent report on treatment with liarozol for moderate and severe LI. This retinoic acid metabolism-blocking agent resulted in good clinical improvement and was well tolerated, but the study failed to meet the end points, possibly owing to the small sample size following premature termination [2]. National guidelines for the management of ichthyoses are available in Germany. In 2019 the first European guidelines of care for the management of congenital ichthyoses were published [3,4]. Given that there are no studies focused on long-term adverse effects, on optimal management of particular forms of ichthyoses such as collodion baby, or about ocular and auditory complications, most recommendations in these guidelines are therefore mainly based on experts' recommendations, patients' and caregivers' experience, and an exchange with patient organisations such as the German SI e.V. (Selbsthilfe Ichthyose e.V.) or the European Network for Ichthyosis (ENI) [5].

Non-specific measures are primarily needed to alleviate symptoms [6], and one has to keep in mind that ichthyosis (hyperkeratosis) develops as a repair response to an inherent defect of the epidermal barrier. In a skin humanised mouse model of TG1 deficiency, topical enzyme replacement therapy restored TG1 activity and showed a healing of the ichthyosis [7]. However, as long as no targeted therapy is available for patients, most treatments have the goal of reducing scaling, but will enhance the barrier defect to some degree [8]. Thus transepidermal water loss increases after successful treatment of ARCI with either systemic retinoids [8] or topical keratolytics [9].

Topical treatment options. Topical therapy is aimed at restoring the epidermal barrier, facilitating desquamation and improving the overall cutaneous appearance. It is the mainstay of treatment in all types of congenital ichthyosis, regardless of type and severity. A variety of topical products including emollients, topical keratolytics and epidermal proliferation modulators have been assayed with variable efficacy (Table 63.7) [3] but, in practice, choice will depend on patients' and clinicians' own experience and personal preferences. Also, local availability can vary depending on the country. Thus, in Germany and France, ointments with higher water content are preferred for the treatment of ichthyoses, while in other countries petrolatum-like ointments requiring bandages seem popular – often not allowing the direct wearing of normal cloth. The therapeutic outcome of topical therapy is largely limited by non-adherence, as treatments are not only time consuming and include greasy products but often show disappointing results.

Emollients. Emollients include both moisturisers and lubricants. Moisturisers increase the ability of the stratum corneum to incorporate water while lubricants are occlusive substances with a high content of lipids that form a layer on the skin, preventing water loss. Moisturisers are used in creams and contain mainly sodium chloride, urea and glycerol. Petrolatum and paraffin are common lubricating agents; however, although safe and inexpensive, they are greasy, may impair sweating and are cosmetically unacceptable for some patients. Emollients are usually safe and can be applied on all body surfaces. The frequency of application depends on the ichthyosis severity and patient's choice, but most individuals need topical therapy at least twice a day.

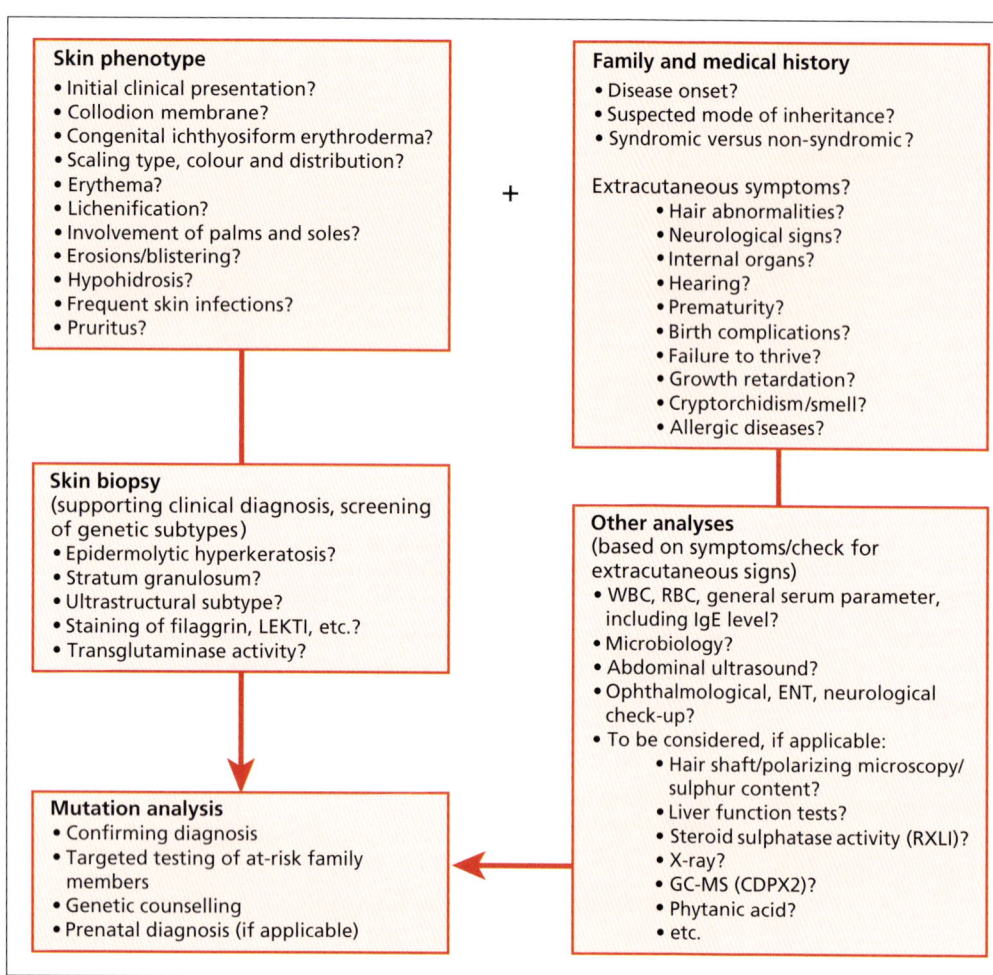

Skin phenotype
- Initial clinical presentation?
- Collodion membrane?
- Congenital ichthyosiform erythroderma?
- Scaling type, colour and distribution?
- Erythema?
- Lichenification?
- Involvement of palms and soles?
- Erosions/blistering?
- Hypohidrosis?
- Frequent skin infections?
- Pruritus?

+

Family and medical history
- Disease onset?
- Suspected mode of inheritance?
- Syndromic versus non-syndromic?

Extracutaneous symptoms?
- Hair abnormalities?
- Neurological signs?
- Internal organs?
- Hearing?
- Prematurity?
- Birth complications?
- Failure to thrive?
- Growth retardation?
- Cryptorchidism/smell?
- Allergic diseases?

Skin biopsy
(supporting clinical diagnosis, screening of genetic subtypes)
- Epidermolytic hyperkeratosis?
- Stratum granulosum?
- Ultrastructural subtype?
- Staining of filaggrin, LEKTI, etc.?
- Transglutaminase activity?

Other analyses
(based on symptoms/check for extracutaneous signs)
- WBC, RBC, general serum parameter, including IgE level?
- Microbiology?
- Abdominal ultrasound?
- Ophthalmological, ENT, neurological check-up?
- To be considered, if applicable:
  - Hair shaft/polarizing microscopy/sulphur content?
  - Liver function tests?
  - Steroid sulphatase activity (RXLI)?
  - X-ray?
  - GC-MS (CDPX2)?
  - Phytanic acid?
  - etc.

Mutation analysis
- Confirming diagnosis
- Targeted testing of at-risk family members
- Genetic counselling
- Prenatal diagnosis (if applicable)

Figure 63.36 Diagnostic management and clinical monitoring in ichthyosis. CDPX2, chondrodysplasia punctata type 2; ENT, ear, nose and throat; GC-MS, gas chromatography–mass spectrometry; IgE, immunoglobulin E; LEKTI, lymphoepithelial Kazal-type related inhibitor; RBC, red blood cell; RXLI, recessive X-linked ichthyosis; WBC, white blood cell.

Keratolytics. Randomised controlled trials (RCTs) assessing the best keratolytic agents are scarce and only include small numbers of patients with each ichthyosis type, preventing any definite conclusion regarding the best keratolytic agent. Different options are shown in Table 63.7. The patient's age, ichthyosis type and severity, as well as extent and location of the lesions must be taken into consideration before prescribing keratolytic agents. Children have a thinner skin and a higher skin surface area : body mass ratio, and therefore are at higher risk of systemic absorption. In particular, all kinds of keratolytics should be avoided in newborns and young infants, in particular salicylic acid. The frequency of application is variable, and can be tapered depending on the clinical response. Side effects are usually mild and include itching, a burning sensation and irritation. In areas such as the face or the folds, less potent keratolytics are recommended to prevent irritation, and in areas of fissuring they should be avoided. Systemic toxicity due to cutaneous absorption of salicylic and lactic acid is a rare but worrisome event.

Salicylic acid may cause life-threatening poisoning in neonates and long-term toxicity in older patients. Systemic toxicity or salicylism develops when blood concentrations of salicylates exceed 35 mg/dL and it is characterised by nausea, vomiting, confusion, stupor, coma and eventually death. Acidosis and hypoglycaemia in children and hyperglycaemia in adults may occur as well. Several cases of salicylism in patients with ichthyosis have been reported, including some babies extensively treated with concentrations of salicylic acid as low as 1% [10]. The potency and toxicity of salicylic acid formulations depend on their concentrations, but also on the vehicle (mineral oil or petrolatum versus solution) and the status of the epidermal barrier. In general, preparations for ichthyosis treatment should contain concentrations lower than 5% of salicylic acid. N-acetylcysteine (NAC) is a thiol derivative used as a mucolytic agent that inhibits both keratinocyte and fibroblast proliferation by reversibly blocking the cell cycle in the G1 phase [11]. Its effectiveness and tolerance have been reported in a series of five patients with lamellar ichthyosis [12] and in a number of isolated case reports. No significant side effects have been recorded except for mild and transient burning. An important disadvantage of NAC is the unpleasant sulphuric smell ('rotten eggs'). Importantly, the compound needs buffering because the final formula may have a pH as low as 2; however, excessive buffering may inactivate NAC. Topical retinoids modulate keratinocyte proliferation and differentiation. Tazarotene and adapalen have been tried with variable results [3]. An RCT with trifarotene, a novel third-generation retinoid, is currently in progress in patients with moderate to severe ARCI.

Table 63.7 Emollients and keratolytics commonly used for topical therapy of ichthyoses.

Group	Agent	Concentration (%)	Comment
Lubricating agents	Petrolatum/vaseline Paraffin		
Hydrating agents	Urea	<5	Better avoided during first year of life because of possible systemic absorption
	Lactic acid		Alternative to urea. Commercial preparations are often optimised by buffering.
	Sodium chloride	3–10	Ointments often have adverse effects, e.g. irritation/stinging; possible as bath additive
	Dexpanthenol	5–10	Supporting normal epidermal differentiation
	Macrogol 400	20–30	Moisturiser and keratolytic
	Propylene glycol	15–20	Moisturiser and keratolytic
	Vitamin E acetate	5	Moisturiser
	Glycerol	10–15	Moisturiser
	Urea	>5	Humectant and keratolytic
Keratolytic agents	Propyleneglycol	>20	
	α-Hydroxy acids (glycolic acid)		Critical in children
	Tretinoin, tazarotene, adapalene		Frequent stinging/risk of absorption and teratogenicity in women of child-bearing age
Keratolytic agents with effects on epidermal differentiation	N-acetylcysteine		
	Calcipotriol, tacalcitol		High risk of systemic absorption; treat less than 10% of body surface
	Dexpanthenol		Supporting normal epidermal differentiation

Warning: salicylic acid might cause life-threatening poisoning in neonates and long-term toxicity in older patients.

Hydrotherapy. Patients with ARCI or KPI generally need to bath at least once a day. Bathing helps to mechanically remove the scales and reduces discomfort. However, it is time consuming, lasting approximately 30–60 min daily or twice daily. Additives such as salt, oil or sodium bicarbonate can be added to provide additional hydration and promote exfoliation. The benefit of sodium bicarbonate (commonly known as baking powder) was established by the work of the late dermatologist Wolfgang Küster, who treated more than 300 in-patients with these diseases by this manner [13]. The mechanism behind the effectiveness of sodium bicarbonate is still unclear, but it has been pointed out that the addition of two handfuls of baking soda to a bath tub raises the pH from 5.5 to 7.9 [14]. Normal desquamation requires the enzymatic dissolution of corneodesmosomes by serin proteases such as kallikrein 5 and kallikrein 7, which have alkaline pH optima. Interestingly, most fresh water or lake water has a pH of around 5, while sea water, which many patients also report to be beneficial, usually has a pH above 8.1. Mild non-allergenic soaps and syndets are necessary to remove residual fat-soluble substances. After soaking the skin for around 20–30 min, a sponge, microfibre cloth, silk glove or even pumice stone can be used to rub the skin and facilitate mechanical scale removal. This can take additional 20–30 min. Drying with a towel and the immediate application of large amounts of ointment onto the still 'hydrated' skin are beneficial to help retain hydration. Bathing is also recommended for hygienic reasons. Antiseptics such as triclosan (contained in a number of soaps), chlorhexidine (dilution 5/1000 to 5/10 000), octenidine 0.1%, polihexanide 0.1% and potassium permanganate (dilution 1/10 000) can be used to target bacterial colonisation and infections. Also, diluted bleach baths (0.005%) may lessen microbial overgrowth and odour. Hydrotherapy with thermal water has proved useful in an open-label prospective study [15].

Management of collodion baby
Collodion baby as well as HI should be regarded as dermatological emergencies and require an interdisciplinary approach [1,2]. Infants suffering from collodion baby as well as from HI [3,4] have a profoundly disturbed epidermal barrier which is associated with increased transepidermal water loss [5] and may result in hypothermia and/or hypernatraemic dehydration. Further problems are proneness to infection, ectropion, poor sucking, restricted pulmonary ventilation and occasionally digital vascular constriction [6,7]. These neonates are best taken care of in a neonatal intensive care unit [1,6,7]. A disease severity score may help to monitor response to treatment [8].

Neonates should be transferred to a neonatal intensive care unit and placed in a high-humidity incubator with close monitoring of body temperature. Typically, it is recommended to start with humidity in the range of 60–80%, and to decrease every 3–4 days in order to reach normal humidity conditions, so that the children can be transferred to an open crib. In the authors' experience, it is sufficient to use bland ointments (e.g. a dexpanthenol-containing ointment) two to four times a day. A report from the Netherlands casts doubt on the value of emollients, arguing that particular occlusive emollients, such as petrolatum or lanolin, predispose to skin infections. However, in most institutions, water-in-oil emollients are applied at least twice daily. Percutaneous absorption is very high and substances typically used in older children with ichthyosis, such as urea or lactic acid, should be avoided in the first year of life. In particular, *the use of salicylic acid is strictly forbidden*, as its use can result in metabolic acidosis within 72 h even when used in very low concentrations [9].

Conventional systemic treatment options

Systemic retinoids (SRs) are synthetic analogues of all-*trans* retinoic acid, a vitamin A derivative, that bind to retinoid acid receptors (RARs) and retinoid X receptors (RXRs) regulating the transcription of genes involved in keratins, growth factors and cytokines expression [1]. In ichthyotic skin, oral retinoids seem to promote a reduction of hyperkeratosis, a tendency to normalisation of keratinocyte proliferation and differentiation, and a lessening of coexisting inflammation. Different SRs have been used in ichthyosis therapy, including etretinate (which is no longer available in most European countries), acitretin, isotretinoin and alitretinoin [2]. Acitretin, a second-generation retinoid, is the first choice in the treatment of ichthyoses because of numerous published studies, however there are no studies comparing its efficacy and tolerability profile to isotretinoin.

SRs improve scaling, hyperkeratosis, hair regrowth, hypohidrosis and ectropion. However, they tend to increase skin fragility and are only effective for as long as they are used. Although SRs have been largely used, especially in ARCI and keratinopathic ichthyosis, there are no RCTs assessing the minimum starting age and optimal dose. In general, daily doses of up to 0.5 mg/kg adequately control the disease, but lower maintenance doses are often sufficient. SRs have a slow turnover in the body and the clinical effects last for days or even weeks; therefore, they can be administered once daily or even every second day, and an interruption of therapy is not reflected in clinical changes immediately [3]. Thus, some patients may benefit from discontinuous therapy ('therapy holidays') particularly those with CIE during warm weather. The clinical response is observed after 2–4 weeks of treatment initiation. Although SRs have numerous and feared potential side effects, they are usually mild and reversible. Acute and chronic toxicities must be discussed before starting therapy. Acute mucocutaneous toxicity including xerosis, cheilitis, dry nose and conjunctiva irritation are common. Analytical abnormalities can be observed in liver enzymes, lipids and blood cell counts. Chronic toxicity mainly affects the skeletal system and consists of diffuse skeletal hyperostosis, that is, spurs and calcifications along the spine (usually the anterior spinal ligament) and at tendon and ligamentous insertions around the joints [4]. Side effects are usually mild and reversible except teratogenicity and bone changes. Patients need analytical assessment (blood cell count, biochemistry panel and human chorionic gonadotropin in female adolescents) before starting treatment and periodic follow-up during therapy. Blood tests should be performed every 2–4 weeks at the beginning of treatment and every 3–6 months in long-term therapy, or more often if there are laboratory abnormalities or pregnancy issues. The optimal periodicity of skeletal surveys is controversial in children. Baseline radiographs can be obtained but frequency of the follow-up is not well established.

SRs are teratogens and this issue requires thorough discussion and adequate contraception in female adolescents. SRs are lipophilic drugs that are slowly eliminated from the body [5]; in particular, acitretin has the potential to persist in the body because of its conversion to etretinate, and therefore pregnancy must be avoided for 3 years following acitretin therapy [6]. The shorter teratogenicity period of isotretinoin makes it a good therapeutic alternative for female adolescents [7].

Acitretin therapy noticeably improves symptoms in the majority of patients with ARCI. Patients with CIE may respond less well to systemic retinoids – some even can get worse – and also they tolerate moisturisers such as lactic acid or urea less well, and may require lower doses [8]. While the effect of acitretin on ARCI phenotypes seems not to be related to the genetic abnormality, KPI shows a clear correlation between the mutated keratin gene and the response to SRs. In superficial KPI, caused by *KRT2* mutation, a silencing of this gene by retinoid therapy will be beneficial, while in KPI caused by *KRT1* mutation, downregulation of *KRT2* will be deleterious because wild-type keratin 2 partially compensates for mutated keratin 1 in the dimerisation process with keratin 10. Therefore, the response to acitretin will be better in superficial KPI than in *KRT10*-deficient KPI but the latter is still better than in KPI due to *KRT1* deficiency [9]. In KPI, red skin and blistering are commonly exacerbated after starting SR therapy, particularly in hot and humid climates. To avoid this, it is recommended to start with a low dose, followed by a slow increasing of the dose.

SRs have been used with some success in a few syndromic forms of congenital ichthyoses including KID syndrome, SLS, IFAP syndrome, Chanarin–Dorfman syndrome (CDS), NISCH syndrome and CNS [10]. However, they should be used with caution in forms with liver involvement or biliary disease such as CDS or NISCH, and in congenital ichthyoses with bone anomalies such as CHHS.

Dermatologists who want to start a patient on a systemic retinoid should be aware of the relevant side effects, such as teratogenicity or hepatotoxicity, to name but a couple. There is an excellent set of guidelines on the efficacy and use of acitretin in dermatology from the British Association of Dermatologists [11]. More recently, consensus recommendations for its use in children and adolescents have been published by a panel of US experts [12]. The attitude of physicians in the UK towards the use of acitretin is shared in most European countries [13]. In Germany, there is a reluctance to use long-term retinoid therapy in children mostly because of fear of interference with bone development, such as premature closure of the epiphyseal growth lines. Patients with ichthyosis may be treated when they are over the age of 16 or have stopped growing significantly. Only a detailed survey on a larger cohort of patients from several countries could provide definite data to answer satisfactorily whether there is a significant risk of bone growth toxicity for children [**14**].

In women of child-bearing age, a major advantage of isotretinoin over acitretin may be its short half-life. While isotretinoin is cleared within several months, acitretin can persist in the body for up to 2 years because of conversion to etretinate, in particular when taken with alcohol [15]. 'Drug holidays' are an option, in particular when using isotretinoin.

There is very limited experience in congenital ichthyosis with oral alitretion, a drug used for hand eczema. Alitretion is rapidly cleared and, in contrast to acitretin and isotretinoin, binds to both types of nuclear retinoid receptors (i.e. RARs and RXRs). In a recent clinical trial, two of four patients who had previously been on acitretin preferred to continue with alitretinoin. A side effect of alitretinoin therapy may be hypothyroidism that can cause tiredness, and it seems to be advisable to monitor thyroid-stimulating hormone levels in these patients [16]. A dramatic improvement of dissecting cellulitis of the scalp has been reported in a patient with KID syndrome who had not responded to previous acitretin therapy [17].

Immunophenotyping and target therapy

The immune abnormalities underlying the ichthyoses are poorly understood [1]. In recent years, studies on immunophenotyping have aimed to determine a target therapy based on molecular pathogenesis [2]. Histopathological and immunological data show that patients with ichthyoses resemble patients with atopic dermatitis and/or psoriasis [3]. O'Shaughnessy et al. published an improvement of hyperkeratosis in an in vitro model of lamellar ichthyosis after treatment with an IL-1 receptor antagonist [4]. Immunological fingerprinting show an IL-17-dominant profile in patients with inherited ichthyoses, suggesting that IL-17/IL-36-targeted medication may be beneficial [5].

Remarkably, significant numbers of case reports have been published on therapeutic attempts with biologics. Results for Netherton syndrome are particularly promising (see earlier in this chapter). The efficacy of secukinumab in ABCA12 deficiency has been described [6]. Omalizumab has been successfully used in a specific case of epidermolytic ichthyosis, and apremilast seems efficient in the intermediate types of ARCI associated with ABCA12 [7]. Ustekinumab showed a prompt effect in a patient with autosomal recessive congenital ichthyosis due to *NIPAL4* mutations [8] or with SAM-like syndrome (see 'Carvajal-Huerta syndrome' later in this chapter) [2].

A better understanding of the molecular basis of inflammation in MeDOCs may lead to novel targeted therapies that are more beneficial than retinoids or broad immunosuppressants; as such, the gap between autoinflammatory diseases and inflammatory MeDOCs seems to become smaller [9,10]. So far, therapy with biologics appears to be well tolerated and helpful for specific presentations of ichthyoses. Hence, the discussion has been opened to distinguish between the innate immunophenotype of MeDOCs addressed by 'drug repurposing' and those addressed by 'in label' treatment of co-morbidity'.

In any case, even though the inflammation should be successfully mitigated in ichthyosis, clinicians should be aware of the primary barrier defect, which has to be treated continuously. With regard to safety and long-term effects, clinical trials and case series with longer treatment periods are required.

Special aspects of treatment

Most ichthyoses – syndromic or not – require a multidisciplinary approach that clearly extends beyond topical and systemic therapy.

Eye. Eye problems are common in all types of ichthyosis. Scales on the eyelashes, blepharoconjunctivitis, madarosis, lagophthalmos and ectropion may eventually lead to corneal damage [1–3]. The main goal of eye care is maintaining the ocular surface integrity, so careful prophylactic ocular lubrication is strongly recommended. In patients who require frequent eye drop administration, preservative-free topical medication is preferred [4,5]. In addition to ocular lubrication, room humidifiers may also improve

the corneal hydration status. Intensive treatment with eyelid emollients and massage may improve eyelid retraction, ectropion and lagophthalmos. Although surgical techniques may be required in severe cases, therapy with topical retinoids, N-acetylcsteine and hyaluronic acid fillers has proved useful [6–8] and may prevent or postpone the need for surgery in cases with mild ectropion. Patients with chronic corneal involvement, persistent corneal epithelial defects or ectropion and eyelid retraction require specialised ophthalmic care and should be followed up regularly. Severe ectropion has to be addressed to avoid complications such as corneal perforation [9–11]. For severe cases, there are different methods for surgical corrective treatment of chronic ectropion [12–14], including repeated hyaluronic acid gel filler injections aimed at delaying invasive surgical procedures [15]. Basal cell carcinoma may be masquerading as chronic ectropion in LI [16].

Ear. Patients with ichthyosis have a significant prevalence of oto-rhino-laryngological symptoms. Excessive desquamation within the external auditory canal promotes ear plugging and predisposes to outer ear infections and conduction deafness [17]. In a recent prospective study of 76 children and young adults with ichthosis, 10.5% of them had both obstructive clusters and abnormal tympanic membranes [18]. Children with severe involvement were most commonly affected. Patients with BSI have also been shown to have the same issue [9]. Since hearing loss in children can harm their intellectual development, early comprehensive assessment and periodic follow-up by an ear, nose and throat (ENT) specialist are needed to prevent irreversible hearing loss. Ear pruritus and ear pain are also important complaints in congenital ichthyoses in all age groups [19]. Therefore, involvement of ENT specialists in the management of patients with congenital ichthyoses is crucial to ensure the application of the best therapeutic and preventative measures [19,20].

Hair. Scalp desquamation is a common issue in all types of ichthyosis. It ranges from fine scaling, such as in IV and XLI, to adherent scales and thick crusts in severe types. Although early treatment of scalp desquamation is believed to help prevent cicatricial alopecia, no solid evidence exists supporting this theory. Mechanical removal of the scales with brushes and combs is advised to avoid excessive thickening of the scales and potential microbial superinfection. In general, lotions, solutions and shampoos are more cosmetically acceptable than greasy products; however, in some instances oil-in-water creams may be needed to remove thick adherent scales, with or without occlusion. Keratolytics may also be useful but attention must be paid to increased absorption through the scalp. Brushing and scalp care must be particularly careful in ichthyosis with brittle hair such as Netherton syndrome and trichothiodystrophy [21].

Pruritus. Itch is a major concern in patients with ichthyosis and has a significant impact on daily life, being present in up to 93% of all patients [22]. Patients with Netherton syndrome are the most severely affected, while those with XLI had a lower itch profile. Weather changes, hot environment and stressful situations seem to worsen itch. The most significant consequences of itching were lesions from scratching, difficulties in falling asleep, bad mood and loss of concentration. Regular topical skincare, such as wet wrappings with emollients, helps to reduce itch. Antihistamines and antidepressants are of little value in improving pruritus.

Hypohydrosis and lifestyle recommendations. Sweating impairment is a major problem in congenital ichthyoses, in particular in the summer time [23], even in patients with a mild phenotype such as SICI. Patients are at risk of overheating, heat exhaustion and heat stroke. Physical activity must be limited, particularly in warm and humid weather, and natural fibre clothing is preferred over synthetic fabrics. Children should stay in a fresh environment with air conditioning, fans or other cooling devices. Sun exposure has pros and cons; although it improves some types of ichthyosis (IV and XLI) and may prevent rickets, it may worsen heat intolerance and sun protection may be difficult. Interestingly, oral retinoid treatment can normalise sweat gland function and markedly improve the quality of life in ARCI patients [23].

Musculoskeletal system. In many cases, in particular in infants and small children, physiotherapy is of enormous value (e.g. to treat flexural contractions).

Nutritional issues and growth. Impairment of the epidermal barrier and increased transepidermal water loss have been proven to play a central role in congenital ichthyosis-associated growth failure [24]. Additionally, increased epidermal turnover, chronic skin inflammation and cutaneous protein losses, especially in congenital ichthyosis patients with erythroderma, contribute to increased resting energy expenditure [25]. A recent prospective observational study of 50 children with ichthyosis emphasised the risk of undernutrition in this age group, particularly in the most severely affected patients and in the youngest ones [26]. Micronutrient deficiencies were found in 60% of patients, including deficiencies of selenium (34%), iron (28%), vitamin D (22%) and zinc (4%). Vitamin D deficiency has been reported in up to 41% of children with congenital ichthyosis [27], particularly in those with darker phenotypes and suffering from ARCI or KPI. Scale thickness, low sun exposure and low vitamin D intake have been the advocated causes. In one French study [28], ichthyosis severity, dark skin and winter/spring seasons were identified as independent risk factors for vitamin D deficiency [29]. Also, the possible causative effect of SR in vitamin D-deficiency rickets has been pointed out [30]. Recently, dramatic improvement of congenital ichthyosis with vitamin D supplements has been reported [31], supporting the role of vitamin D as a regulator of genes involved in epidermal differentiation [32]. Consequently, regular monitoring for clinical, biochemical, hormonal and nutritional parameters is strongly recommended to provide adequate vitamin D and micronutrient supplementation according to the degree of deficiency. Special attention should also be paid to signs of delayed puberty in older school children and adolescents.

Superinfections. Epidermal barrier disturbance significantly modifies the cutaneous microbiome and promotes bacterial and fungal colonisation. These changes are illustrated for many forms of congenital ichthyoses, in which patients develop a characteristic and sometimes unpleasant smell. The exact frequency and type of cutaneous infections are unknown, but some ichthyoses such as forms of ARCI or KID syndrome seem to be associated with a higher incidence of dermatophytosis [33,34] (*Trichophyton rubrum* infection may even mimic EI if patients have not been seen before; authors' own experience). KPI, KID syndrome, peeling skin disease and Netherton syndrome can be complicated by bacterial superinfections, often caused by *Staphylococcus aureus* [35,36]. A thorough periodic physical examination for signs of infections is needed at regular intervals. Microbiological samplings should be performed if an infection is suspected. Clinically obvious skin infections require specific therapy with topical or systemic agents [37].

Psychosocial aspects. Congenital ichthyoses are characterised by visible clinical signs and distressing symptoms such as pruritus, pain or heat intolerance that can disturb patients' personal well-being and social relationships. In addition, the topical treatment is time consuming and expensive and interferes in daily life and budgets. It has been shown not only that congenital ichthyoses impact negatively the quality of life of both the patient and their relatives [38], but that the economic impact of the disease is considerable when there is no reimbursement possibility [39]. It is not clear when the ideal moment is to offer specialised psychological support. New parents can be devastated in the early stages but may need some time to adapt before seeking psychological support. Children may need help to cope with bullying issues, particularly when transitioning to adolescence. Dermatologists in charge of the patients must address this issue and direct patients and caregivers to receive psychological support when needed.

Patient organisations and other resources

Patient organisations for ichthyoses are non-profit organisations that inform, educate and support patients and their families, often in collaboration with health professionals (Table 63.8). They organise meetings where members can meet others in the same situation and share experiences, uncertainties and advice. Considering the disease severity in ichthyoses, membership in a patient organisation can be extremely helpful for the patients and their families and should be recommended. There are active patient associations in many European countries. At the European level these national self-support groups have formed the European Network for Ichthyosis (ENI; www.ichthyose.eu). In the USA, the Foundation for Ichthyosis and Related Skin Types (FIRST) has been active since 1981 and has the aims of educating, inspiring and connecting all those touched by ichthyosis and related disorders. Sources for general information on the disease are, for example, the homepage of the German network for ichthyoses, NIRK (www.netzwerk-ichthyose.de), or the network of FIRST (www.firstskinfoundation.org). Genetic analysis can be done in expert centres throughout Europe; detailed information is provided at www.orpha.net. Finally, social media such as Facebook, Twitter and Instagram allow an easy and quick connection of worldwide patients, caregivers and all interested individuals in the field.

ACQUIRED ICHTHYOSES

Acquired or late-onset ichthyosis presents with features similar to IV and must be distinguished from xerosis, eczema, IV, XLI and RD, in which scaling develops in early adult life [1].

Table 63.8 Resources and further information.

Websites	
Patient organisations for ichthyosis	
Austria	www.selbsthilfe-tirol.at
Belgium	https://ichthyosis.be/nl
Denmark	www.iktyosis.dk
Finland	www.iholiitto.fi
France	https://ichtyose.fr
Germany	www.ichthyose.de
Italy	www.ittiosi.it
Spain	www.ictiosis.org
Sweden	https://iktyos.se
Switzerland	www.ichthyose.ch
UK	www.ichthyosis.org.uk
USA	www.firstskinfoundation.org
Other databases and internet links	
Website hosted at National Center for Biotechnology Information (NCBI)	www.genetests.org
Orphanet (portal for rare diseases and orphan drugs)	www.orpha.net
Human Intermediate Filament Database	www.interfil.org
German guidelines for ichthyoses	https://www.awmf.org

All websites in table and accompanying text last accessed June 2022.

Pathophysiology

Differential diagnoses of the underlying cause include malignancies and autoimmune, nutritional, metabolic, infectious and neurological diseases as well as medications [2].

Clinical features

Scaling is usually not associated with inflammation and ranges from pityriasiform to lamellar; it might be more obvious on the extensor aspects of the limbs.

Malignancies. Increased expression of transforming growth factor α (TGF-α) or epidermal growth factor receptors (EGFRs) mediated by a tumour may cause hyperproliferative paraneoplastic cutaneous conditions. The most common ichthyosis-associated malignancy is Hodgkin disease, and the skin changes may occur simultaneously, postdate or rarely precede the diagnosis [3–5]. The fine scaling affects the trunk and limbs, usually spares the flexures and histologically resembles IV with orthohyperkeratosis and a reduced or absent granular layer. It clears with effective anticancer treatment and can be an early marker of subsequent recurrence. It may be associated with pruritus, an independent symptom of lymphoma. Reduced dermal lipogenesis, measured by radio-labelled carbon uptake, paralleled the severity of the ichthyosis and contrasted with results in IV in one study [6].

Acquired ichthyosis has also been reported in association with non-Hodgkin lymphoma [5,7,8], cutaneous T-cell lymphoma (Figure 63.37a) [8,9], lymphomatoid papulosis [10,11], multiple myeloma [12], breast, lung, cervix, renal cell or liver carcinoma [13,14], leiomyosarcoma [15], rhabdomyosarcoma [16] and Kaposi sarcoma [17]. It has been the presenting sign of myelodysplasia [18],

has followed on from bone marrow transplant [19] or has occurred with graft-versus-host disease [20].

Metabolic and distinct internal diseases. Disturbances of lipid and vitamin absorption may cause those ichthyoses that develop with chronic metabolic derangement such as malnutrition or malabsorption (including coeliac disease and Crohn disease) [1,2], essential fatty deficiency [21] and Shwachman syndrome (pancreatic insufficiency) [22]. Ichthyosis may be a presenting feature of inborn errors of metabolism, such as methylmalonic acidaemia [23] and holocarboxylase and biotinidase deficiencies [24]. It may complicate renal failure with or without secondary hyperparathyroidism [25], primary hyperparathyroidism [26], autoimmune thyroiditis [27] and diabetes, where it affects the shins [28]. Ichthyosis may rarely occur with connective tissue diseases such as systemic lupus erythematosus [29], sarcoidosis (Figure 63.37b) [34], dermatomyositis without associated malignancy [30], systemic sclerosis/lupus overlap [31], so-called Haber syndrome [32] and eosinophilic fasciitis [33].

Infections. Ichthyosis has been noted in patients with leprosy [35], HIV infection with or without malignancies [2,36,37] and human T-cell lymphotropic virus type 1 (HTLV-1)-associated myelopathy [38].

Drugs. The cholesterol-lowering drugs, triparanol and nicotinic acid, induce ichthyosis in a proportion of patients [39,40]. Triparanol also causes poliosis and alopecia. Normal desquamation depends on the conversion of cholesterol sulphate (which maintains the structure of intercellular lipid lamellae in the subcorneal layers) to cholesterol, by cholesterol sulphatase, located on keratinocyte cell membranes. This enzyme is unaffected by hypocholesterolaemic agents. Keratinocytes lack low-density lipoprotein receptors, which may explain why so few treated patients show this complication. Hydroxymethylglutaryl coenzyme A (HMG-CoA) reductase inhibitors are also a rare cause of ichthyosis [41]. Ichthyosis and variable effects on hair have been attributed to certain butyrophenones, the phenothiazine dixyrazine, maprotiline [42], cimetidine (an antiandrogen) [43], allopurinol, hydroxyurea [44], clofazamine [45] and of course acitretin [46].

Pityriasis rotunda

Definition

Pityriasis rotunda describes a rare, persistent, sharply defined, circular patch of ichthyosiform scaling with no inflammatory changes. This name is preferred to pityriasis circinata, reported by Toyama in 1906, and to acquired pseudo-ichthyosis [1,2].

Epidemiology

Pityriasis rotunda is relatively common in the Far East, especially Japan, where it accounts for some 0.2% of dermatological cases [2]. It has been reported also in South African Bantus [3], in an Egyptian [4], in Afro-Caribbeans living in London [5] and an African Canadian woman [6]. It has been described in a Mediterranean woman [7] and in two cohorts from Sardinia [8,9]. Its true

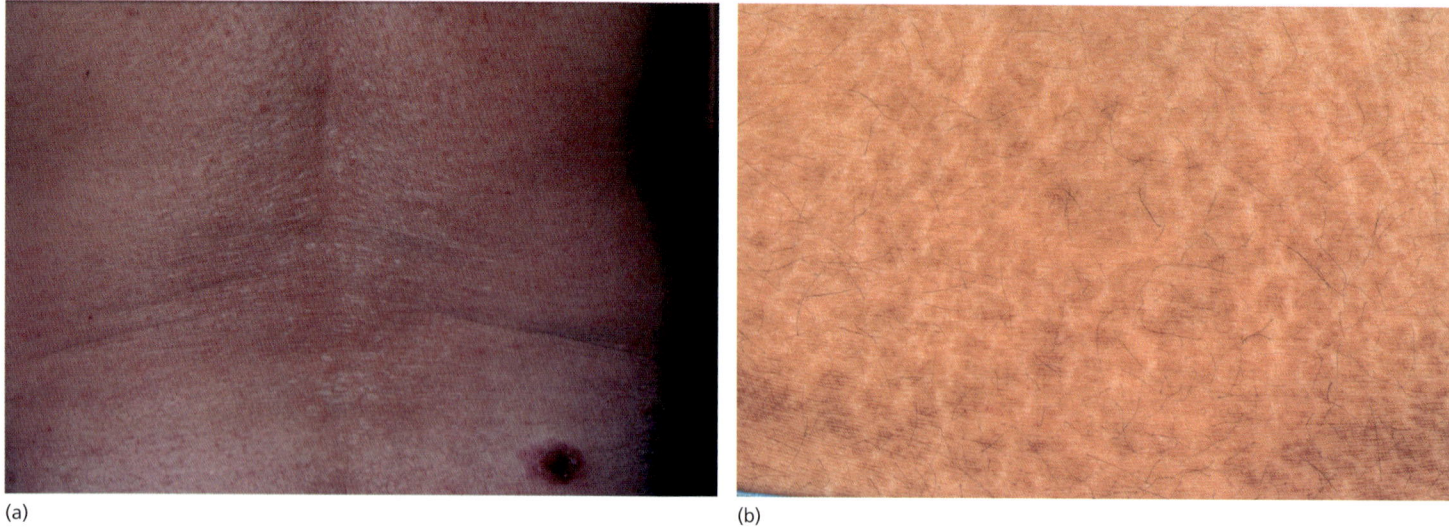

(a)   (b)

Figure 63.37 Acquired ichthyosis. (a) Man with cutaneous T-cell lymphoma. (b) Asian man with multisystem sarcoidosis. (b) Courtesy of Dr M. Judge, Salford Royal NHS Trust, UK.

incidence and geographical distribution are unknown. It is possible that genetic factors are involved and familial occurrence has been observed [8–12]. A familial association with IV has also been noted [2,9,12].

Pathophysiology
Systemic illnesses, particularly tuberculosis and malnutrition, coexist in up to 50% of South African patients [2,3,13]. It may rarely be an acquired cutaneous marker of malignancy [14–16]. Pityriasis rotunda was observed in 16% of 63 South African black patients with hepatocellular carcinoma and nearly 5% of those with tuberculosis in one report [17]. Other reports mention association with hepatitis C [18]. However, cases reported from Sardinia had no associated systemic disorders and pityriasis rotunda tended to occur at a younger age [8,9].

Clinical features
Typical lesions of pityriasis rotunda are circular, sharply defined, hyperpigmented patches of dry skin with ichthyosiform scaling, usually 2–3 cm in diameter but sometimes much larger, up to 14 cm (Figure 63.38). Lesion numbers range from 4 to 200. They rarely itch, but slowly enlarge and coalesce. A hypopigmented halo has been described in some patients, and sometimes the entire lesion can be hypopigmented. Onset in childhood carries a better prognosis, with remission seen in later childhood in almost 50% [8,9]. Lesions are commonly situated on the buttocks, thighs, abdomen, back or upper arms, and may be solitary or multiple. They most often develop between the ages of 20 and 45 years (2 and 76 years are the reported extremes) and may remain unchanged throughout life.

Investigations
The age of onset, distribution, strikingly circular outline and absence of pruritus and inflammatory change should suggest the diagnosis. The histological changes resemble those of IV, with compact orthohyperkeratosis and a reduced granular layer. There may be loss of the epidermal ridge pattern, pigmentary incontinence and mild perivascular lymphocytic infiltrate. Immunohistochemical

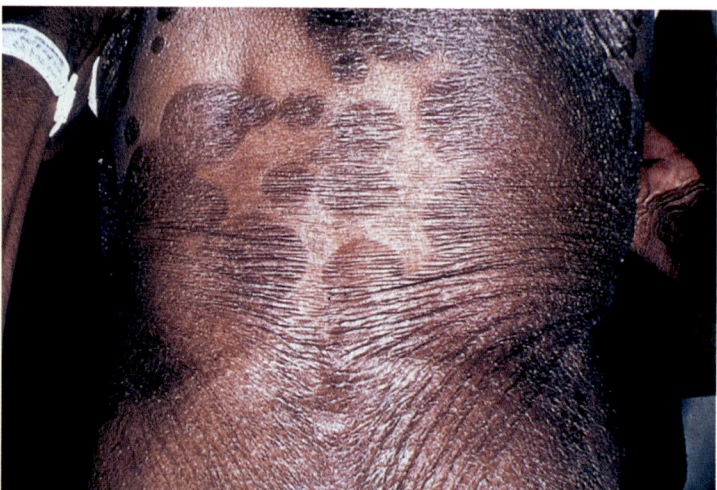

Figure 63.38 Pityriasis rotunda. Courtesy of Dr M. Judge, Salford Royal NHS Trust, UK.

studies have shown a marked reduction in loricrin and filaggrin expression in lesional skin [18], the latter caused by loss of the profilaggrin N-terminal domain [19]. Electron microscopy in one case revealed epidermal lipid vacuoles and other changes [8].

Management
Investigations for an underlying cause may be indicated. In pre-lymphomatous eruptions the lesions show atrophy and telangiectasia. Dermatophytosis and pityriasis versicolor can be excluded based on negative mycological studies (microscopy and culture). Emollients, urea compounds and topical keratolytics may help. Topical tretinoin cream or systemic retinoids in more extensive disease can be useful to some extent but topical steroid and antifungal agents are not. Where malnutrition, infection or malignancy is the underlying cause, appropriate therapy should clear the lesions.

PALMOPLANTAR KERATODERMAS

Definition and diagnostic approach

Palmoplantar keratodermas form a heterogeneous group of hereditary or acquired disorders defined by excessive *epidermal thickening of the palms and soles* (see Tables 63.9, 63.11, 63.13, 63.14 and 63.15 below) [1,2]. This clinical finding is observed as an isolated symptom and non-syndromic entity, but can also be part of a more complex (syndromic) phenotype, for instance in PPK with cardiomyopathy. Of note, many generalised MeDOC forms manifest with PPK [3], for example palmoplantar hyperkeratosis in ARCI is a 'key feature' of ichthyosis due to *NIPAL4* mutations [4,5]. This section focuses on inherited 'classic PPKs' that are characterised by prominent or predominant palmoplantar involvement. A number of classifications of keratodermas have been published [1,2,6–11], but none unites satisfactorily the clinical presentation, pathology and molecular pathogenesis. However, syndromic and non-syndromic hereditary forms may be distinguished (Table 63.9) and differentiated from acquired PPKs. Finally, there are various other monogenetic diseases that may have a palmoplantar phenotype with features of hyperkeratosis (Table 63.10).

Clinical features

The 'clinical pattern' is sometimes helpful. Diffuse, focal/areate, striate or punctate patterns can be distinguished, but there are no absolute boundaries between these groupings. In diffuse keratodermas, the whole of the palmar or plantar epidermis, usually including the centripalmar skin and the instep, is uniformly thickened. In focal, areate or nummular keratodermas, the areas of palmoplantar skin under most pressure are disproportionately thickened. Striate keratoderma overlaps clinically with focal keratoderma, but the lesions are conspicuously longitudinal, particularly on the fingers, where keratoderma overlies the flexor tendons. Punctate, papular or disseminated keratoderma consists of multiple scattered discrete round lesions. Transgredient keratoderma extends beyond palmoplantar skin, contiguously or as callosities on pressure points on the fingers or knuckles, or elsewhere. Confluent hyperkeratosis may extend around whole digits. Cicatrising keratodermas ('mutilating') are those in which constricting bands appear around the digits. Such pseudo-ainhum is found in many severe transgredient keratodermas, and is not diagnostic of any one syndrome.

General diagnostic aspects and morphology

Associated hyperhidrosis or fungal infections are common clinical symptoms, as many keratodermas, particularly on the feet, are spongy and malodorous. Water retention by abnormally keratotic and porous stratum corneum contributes to maceration and microbial overgrowth. Sometimes minor extrapalmoplantar signs such as insulated hyperkeratosis can be found. Therefore, the overall integument including mucous membranes, nails, hair, ability to sweat, etc. needs to be examined. Diagnosis of suspected extracutaneous symptoms may require a multidisciplinary approach, and a thorough family history is mandatory. Skin biopsy for histology and/or

Table 63.9 Palmoplantar keratodermas (PPKs).

Disease	Mode of inheritance	Genes
Non-syndromic forms		
Epidermolytic palmoplantar keratoderma (EPPK)	AD	KRT9
Pachyonychia congenita (PC):		
PC6a	AD	KRT6A
PC16	AD	KRT16
PC6b	AD	KRT6B
PC17	AD	KRT17
PC6c	AD	KRT6c
Non-epidermolytic palmoplantar keratoderma (NEPPK):		
Mal de Meleda	AR	SLURP1
Type Gamborg-Nielson	AR	SLURP1 (variant)
Type Nagashima	AR	SERPINB7
Autosomal recessive	AR	SERPINA12
Type Bothnia	AD	AQP5
Type Kimonis	AD	KRT1 (V1 domain)
Loricrin keratoderma (LK)	AD	LOR
Striate (and focal) palmoplantar keratoderma (SPPK):		
SPPK1	AD	DSG1
SPPK2	AD	DSP
SPPK3	AD	KRT1 (V2 domain)
Punctate palmoplantar keratoderma (PPPK)	AD	AAGAB, COL14A1
Spiny keratoderma (SK)	AD?	Unknown
Marginal papular keratoderma (MPK):		
Acrokeratoelastoidosis (AKE)	AD?	Unknown
Focal acral hyperkeratosis (FAH)	AD?	Unknown
Cole disease (CD)	AD/AR	ENPP1
Transient aquagenic keratoderma (TAK)	AD/AR?	Unknown
Syndromic forms		
Palmoplantar keratoderma and cardiomyopathy:		
Naxos syndrome	AR (or AD)	JUP
Carvajal-Huerta syndrome	AR (or AD)	DSP
Palmoplantar keratoderma and hearing impairment:		
Vohwinkel syndrome	AD	GJB2
Bart–Pumphrey syndrome	AD	GJB2
Keratitis–ichthyosis–deafness (KID)	AD	GJB2
Other GJB2-associated diseases	AD/AR	GJB2 (see Table 63.5),
Mitochondrial PPK with hearing impairment	Maternal	MT-TS1
Palmoplantar keratoderma and cancer:		
Huriez syndrome (HS)	AD	SMARCAD1
Tylosis with oesophageal cancer (TOC)	AD	RHBDF2
PPK, sex reversal and cancer	AR	RSPO1
Palmoplantar keratoderma in ectodermal dysplasia and related diseases:		
Clouston syndrome	AR	GJB6
Schopf–Schulz–Passarge syndrome	AR	WNT10A
Papillon–Léfèvre syndrome	AR	CTSC
Haim–Munk syndrome	AR	CTSC
Olmsted syndrome (OLS)	AD	TRPV3
	XR	MBTPS2
Palmoplantar keratoderma and ophthalmic manifestations:		
Oculocutaneous tyrosinaemia	AR	TAT
Palmoplantar keratoderma and neurological manifestations:		
See neuro-ichthyotic syndromes (CEDNIK, SLS, NLSDI, TTD)		

AD, autosomal dominant; AR, autosomal recessive; CEDNIK, cerebral dysgenesis–neuropathy–ichthyosis–palmoplantar keratoderma; NLSDI, neutral lipid storage disease with ichthyosis; SLS, Sjögren–Larsson syndrome; TTD, trichothiodystrophy; XR, X-linked recessive.

PART 6: GENETIC DISORDERS

Table 63.10 Other inherited diseases with a palmoplantar phenotype.

Disease	Genes	Cross-reference
Ichthyoses:[a]		
ARCI (*NIPAL4*, *TGM1*, *CERS3*, *ALOXB12*)	See Table 63.1	
EI	See Table 63.1	
SEI	See Table 63.1	
CRIE	See Table 63.1	
EKV	See Table 63.1	
LK	See Table 63.1	
KLICK	See Table 63.1	
EXI	See Table 63.1	
IFAP	See Table 63.2	
SAM	See Table 63.2	
CEDNIK	See Table 63.2	
SLS	See Table 63.2	
KID	See Table 63.2	
NLSD with ichthyosis	See Table 63.2	
TTD	See Table 63.2	
Naegeli–Franchescetti–Jadassohn syndrome	*KRT14*	Chapter 68
Epidermolysis bullosa simplex	*KRT5*, *KRT14*	Chapter 69
Kindler syndrome	*KIND1*	Chapter 69
Hypohidrotic ectodermal dysplasia	*EDA*	Chapter 65
Autosomal recessive ectodermal dysplasia	*GRHL2*	Chapter 65
Ectodermal dysplasia–skin fragility syndrome	*PKP1*	Chapter 65
Dyskeratosis congenita	*DKC1*, *TERC*, *TERT*, *TINF2*, *NOLA2*, *NOLA3*, *TCAB1*, *RTEL*	Chapter 68
Darier disease	*ATP2A2*	Chapter 64
Pityriasis rubra pilaris	*CARD14*	Chapter 36
Rapp–Hodgkin syndrome	*TP63*	Chapter 65
Hay–Wells syndrome	*TP63*	Chapter 65
Acro-dermato-ungual–lacrimal–tooth (ADULT) syndrome	*TP63*	Chapter 65
Cowden syndrome	*PTEN*	Chapter 78
Hypertrophic osteoarthropathy/ pachydermoperiostosis	*HPGD*, *SLCO2A1*	Chapter 70

[a] See Tables 63.1 and 63.2 for abbreviations.

ultrastructure still plays a critical role in the diagnosis of keratodermas as it can provide essential clues for further genetic analyses [11], for instance distinguishing between epidermolytic and non-epidermolytic hyperkeratosis or demonstrating signs of disadhesion.

NON-SYNDROMIC PALMOPLANTAR KERATODERMAS

Epidermolytic palmoplantar keratoderma

Definition and nomenclature

Palmoplantar keratoderma is associated with epidermolytic changes on histology and is due to mutations localised to a hotspot region of *KRT9* or infrequently to specific domains of *KRT1*. Voerner

described diffuse PPK with autosomal dominant inheritance, clinically indistinguishable from that described by Thost and Unna but with histological features of EHK in affected palms and soles [1]. Thost's original family in fact was apparently also affected with epidermolytic palmoplantar keratoderma (EPPK).

> **Synonyms and inclusions**
> - Epidermolytic PPK with knuckle pads, keratosis and palmoplantaris diffusa
> - Voerner–Unna–Thost keratoderma
> - Unna–Thost disease
> - Voerner disease

Epidemiology

Epidermolytic palmoplantar keratoderma is probably the most common form of diffuse keratoderma [2,3]. A prevalence of 4.4/100 000 was found in Northern Ireland [4].

Pathophysiology

Epidermolytic palmoplantar keratoderma was initially found to map to the type 1 keratin gene cluster on chromosome 17 and was subsequently shown to result from rare mutations in *KRT1* and more common mutations in *KRT9* [5–8], which is preferentially expressed in palmoplantar skin [9,10]. The disruption of intermediate filament integrity due to these mutations is predicted to reduce the resilience of the cytoskeleton to minor external trauma, leading to blistering and hyperkeratosis as well as epidermolysis with tonofilament clumping. Most mutations identified to date affect the helix initiation peptide, but a 3 bp insertion in the helix termination motif has also been identified [11]. Infrequently, keratin 1 is involved: *KRT1* gene mutations affecting the 2B domain, in the helix termination peptide, and splice site mutations have been described [12–15]. EPPK with unusual 'tonotubular' filaments on electron microscopy [16] is due to mutations altering the 1B rod domain of keratin 1 [17,18].

Clinical features [1,19]

Diffuse keratoderma develops in infancy. In adults, there is confluent keratoderma (Figure 63.39), sparing the dorsal surfaces, with a sharp demarcation and red edge (Figure 63.40). Blistering is not a major feature, but a history of blisters or fissuring of the palms may hint at reduced structural strength. The hair, teeth and nails are normal, but knuckle pads [20] and nail changes were found in several patients [1], many of whom have *KRT9* mutations. Disabling pain especially on the palms might indicate the subtype of 'tonotubular' PPK [18]. Moreover, limited transgredient lesions (e.g. at the dorsum of the Achilles tendon, often referred to as Greither keratoderma) may indicate an EPPK form associated with *KRT1* mutations. Clinically, pure EPPK can be distinguished from epidermolytic ichthyoses which often involve the palms, soles and flexural areas [12].

Investigations

Histologically, EPPK shows epidermolytic change in suprabasal keratinocytes. Round or ovoid eosinophilic inclusions may be detected [21], with large tonofilament aggregates visible on electron

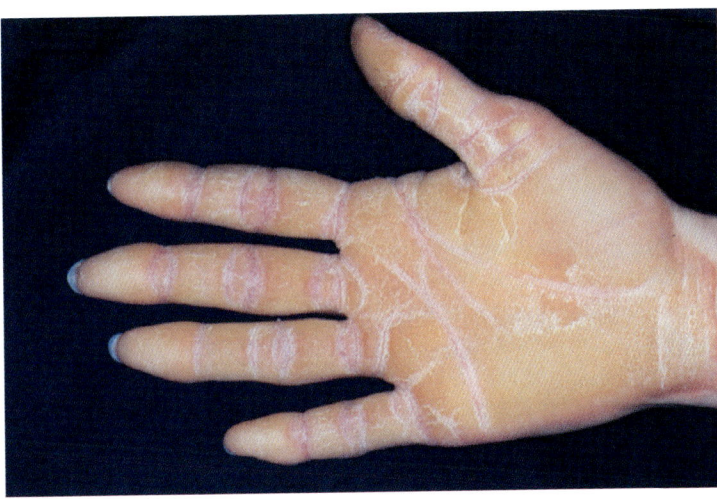

Figure 63.39 Epidermolytic palmoplantar keratoderma caused by a mutation in *KRT9* encoding keratin 9.

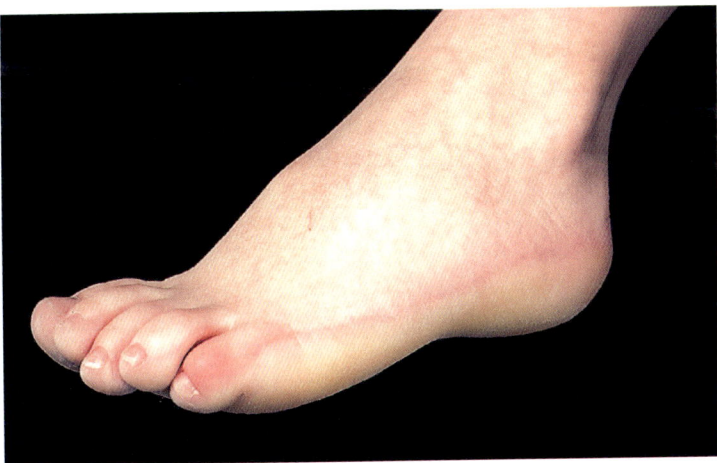

Figure 63.40 Voerner–Unna–Thost keratoderma: even yellow hyperkeratosis of the sole with red border.

microscopy [22,23]. Moreover, the ultrastructure may reveal the peculiar finding of whorls of keratins containing tubular structures observed in transverse and longitudinal sections ('tonotubules') [16–18]. It may be advisable to take biopsies from different palmoplantar sites because focal EHK may escape diagnosis in mild forms [15].

Management
The mainstay is mechanical debridement, followed by mild keratolytic relubrication to help avoid fissures. Oral retinoids can be tried at a low dose, but excessive peeling may be a problem [24]. Topical calcipotriol has reportedly been helpful [25].

Pachyonychia congenita

Definition and nomenclature
Pachyonychia congenita (PC) is a group of autosomal dominant keratinisation disorders caused by a mutation in one of five keratin genes *KRT6A*, *KRT16*, *KRT6B*, *KRT6C* or *KRT17*. The variable clinical findings affect a number of ectodermal structures, including the nail bed, oral mucosae, palmoplantar skin, teeth and pilosebaceous unit [1–3].

Synonyms and inclusions
- PC-6a, PC-6b, PC-6c, PC-16, PC-17
- PC type 1 (Jadassohn–Lewandowsky)
- PC type 2 (Jackson–Lawler)

Epidemiology
Hypertrophic nail dystrophy gave rise to the name of PC [4]; however, the most problematic manifestation of the disease is focal plantar keratoderma with severe and often profoundly incapacitating pain [1]. Historically, PC has been classified under two major categories: PC type 1 (Jadassohn–Lewandowsky) and PC type 2 (Jackson–Lawler) [5–10], caused by mutations in genes encoding two pairs of dimerising keratins, *KRT6A*/*KRT16* and *KRT6B*/*KRT17*, respectively. PC type 1 was thought to be associated with PPK and oral leukokeratosis while PC type 2 was thought to be associated with pilosebaceous cysts and neonatal teeth [11]. A large-scale genotype/phenotype analysis of hundreds of patients did not confirm these associations [1,12,13], which led to a novel classification system that specifically relies on the causative keratin mutation, for example PC-6a, PC-6b, PC-6c, PC-16 and PC-17 [11,14–17]. Extensive clinicogenetic information on the diseases is provided by the International PC Consortium (IPCC).

Pathophysiology
Similar to several other keratin disorders, the majority of causative mutations in PC-related keratins are heterozygous missense mutations or small insertions/deletion mutations that disrupt cytoskeletal function via dominant negative interference leading to cell fragility [14]. The variable distribution of lesions in PC corresponds to different expression patterns of the mutant keratins [11,15–17]. For example, mutations in the prominent nail keratin K6a additionally affect oral mucosae [18]. In contrast, K17 is constitutively expressed in the pilosebaceous unit with lesser expression in palmoplantar skin and mucosae [18–20].

Clinical features [1,3,14]
A comprehensive analysis of clinical symptoms has been published [13]. Three clinical features are reported in more than 90% of patients across all mutation subtypes. *toenail dystrophy*, *plantar keratoderma* and *plantar pain* which in patients older than 3 years are highly diagnostic for PC (Figure 63.41).

Thickened toenails, that is hyperkeratosis of the nail bed, appear within the first to ninth years of life. *KRT6A* mutation carriers show an early age of onset. Of note, in many cases not all 20 nails are involved.

Plantar keratoderma variably manifest as calluses, fissures and thickened skin. Thick yellow keratoses are found on sites of pressure. Frictional blisters may occur, especially in hot weather in childhood. Plantar pain is a very common symptom of PC and has an important impact on the quality of life. Around a quarter of

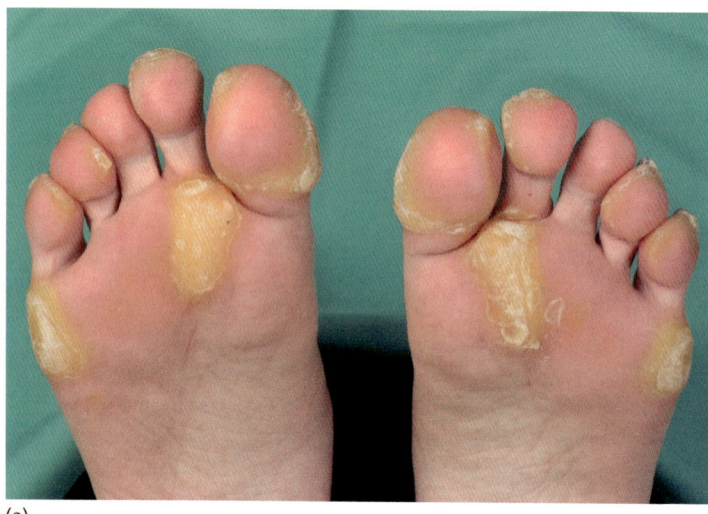

(a)

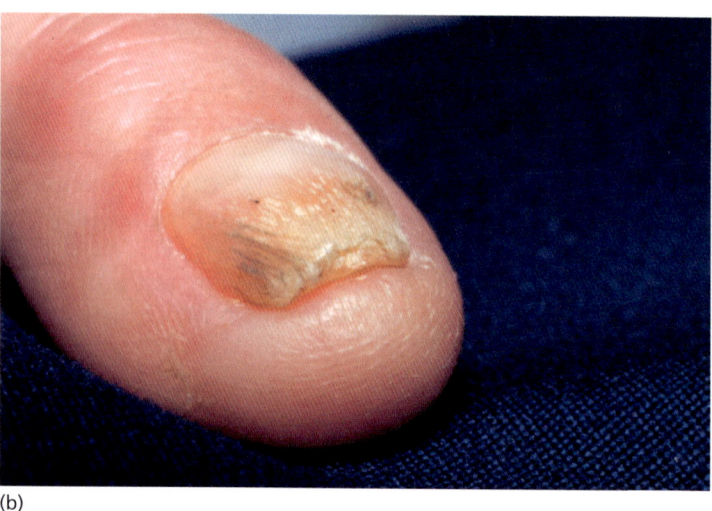

(b)

Figure 63.41 Pachyonychia congenita: (a) focal keratoderma on mechanically stressed areas; and (b) a typical wedge-shaped nail.

patients with PC regularly require analgesic medication and many are confined to wheelchairs. The source of this exceptional pain is still a matter of debate but may be related to the conspicuous presence of blisters underneath the plantar calluses [21].

Additional diagnostic findings include follicular hyperkeratoses on the knees and elbows, oral leukokeratosis, palmoplantar hyperhidrosis, cysts and natal teeth [22–26]. Patchy, white, thickened areas are seen on the tongue and oral mucosa. Severe oral lesions resemble candidiasis [27]. Laryngeal involvement may produce hoarseness and in infancy even fatal respiratory obstruction [28]. Some individuals – particularly if carrying *KRT17* mutations – develop cysts in the form of steatocystomas and/or pilosebaceous cysts. The phenomenon of erupted teeth present at birth has primarily been reported in *KRT17* mutation carriers [13,29]. Axillary cysts may mimic hidradenitis suppurativa [30].

A recent analysis of 815 individuals with PC registered with the International PC Research Registry (IPCRR) revealed further genotype–phenotype correlations and predictive genetic variants. Distinct *KRT16* mutations were associated with a milder phenotype

whereas an increased number of involved fingernails was found in a *KRT17* mutation [31]. Mutations in K6c seem to be more associated with a mild focal keratoderma when compared with any other type of PC [32].

Investigations

Tonofilament aggregates seen on electron microscopy demonstrate the intermediate filament disorder [14,22]. On histology, the palmoplantar epidermis shows gross hyperkeratosis with alternating ortho- and parakeratosis. Acanthosis is present with patchy hypergranulosis, in which large and malformed keratohyalin granules are present, but there is no gross epidermolysis [33,34]. Cysts may be keratinous epidermoid cysts, eruptive vellus hair cysts or true steatocysts.

Mutational analysis of the keratin genes may be provided by the IPCC. Molecular differential diagnosis includes the frizzled 6 gene (*FZD6*), which is associated with autosomal recessive twenty nail dystrophy [35]. Heterozygous missense mutations in the connexin 30 gene, normally associated with Clouston syndrome, have been identified in a number of families with pachyonychia-like nail changes and no other phenotype [36].

Management

Mechanical reduction of hyperkeratosis and of nails, by filing, cutting, grinding and soaking supported by medical professional treatment, produces symptomatic benefit; attention to footwear and orthotics may reduce blistering and callosities. The treatment for patients with cysts is surgical removal/incision and drainage. Emollients and keratolytics may only help in milder cases of keratoderma [37,38]. Systemic retinoid treatment is often unsatisfactory due to increased tenderness [37,39]. The treatment of hyperhidrosis may reduce blistering [40]. Botulinum toxin injection has been found to be remarkably effective at restoring functionality as well as attenuating pain [41,42]. Because of a dependence of the constitutive *KRT6A* promoter activity on STAT1, statins are effective in the treatment of PC. They can thus reduce the expression of distinct keratin genes (*KRT6A* and *KRT17*). A successful treatment with rosuvastatin has been described, however topical treatment with statins was not effective [43].

Resources

International PC Consortium (IPCC): www.pachyonychia.org (last accessed June 2022). (Patients or clinicians may contact the IPCC via email or register online. Detailed information on disease expression (including photographs for each type of PC), diagnostics and updates on clinical studies are provided.)

Painful hereditary callosities

The term painful hereditary callosities most probably encompasses many different aetiological entities. In fact, plantar callosities of sufficient size are inevitably painful. Reported cases with blisters and tonofilament clumping are likely to correspond to an epidermolytic or keratinopathic disorder [1–4]. 'Painful callosity' is a clinical feature seen in PC; a novel minor variant has been described

Table 63.11 Isolated non-epidermolytic palmoplantar keratoderma (NEPPK).

Features	Mal de Meleda[a]	NEPPK type Nagashima	AR PPK	NEPPK type Bothnia	NEPPK type Kimonis	'Greither keratoderma'[b]
Synonyms	Keratosis palmoplantaris transgrediens of Siemens	Keratosis palmoplantaris Nagashima	–	Non-epidermolytic palmoplantar tylosis	Non-epidermolytic keratinopathic PPK	Keratosis extremitatum hereditaria progrediens
MIM number	248300	603357	–	600231	600962	144200
Inheritance	AR	AR	AR	AD	AD	AD
Gene	SLURP1	SERPINB7	SERPINA12	AQP5	KRT1 (V1 domain)	E.g. KRT1 and others
Age of onset	Before 2 years, mainly under 20 years	At birth or in early infancy, mild and non-progressive	Early infancy	During childhood	At birth or in early infancy	After 2 years, may disappear in later life
Palmoplantar key features	Transgredient massive PPK, malodorous maceration, functional handicap with reduced mobility of hands and feet, nail involvement, asymmetrical presentations, hyperhidrosis, dermatophyte superinfection	Well-demarcated reddish and diffuse palmoplantar hyperkeratosis extending to the dorsal surfaces of the hands, feet, inner wrists and ankles, water sensitivity, hyperhidrosis	Well-demarcated palmoplantar yellowish diffuse hyperkeratosis	Diffuse hyperkeratosis with yellowish tint over the whole of the palms and soles, sometimes transgredient, white spongy appearance upon exposure to water, distinct margin between affected and normal skin, sometimes with papular border, hyperhidrosis, superinfection	Diffuse palmoplantar hyperkeratosis, discrete papules on the dorsa of fingers, hyperkeratotic pads over knuckles, red halo separating hyperkeratotic from healthy skin, superinfection	Transgredient and progressive PPK, hyperkeratosis on ventral aspect of wrists, papules on the dorsa of fingers and knuckle pads, red border separating hyperkeratotic from healthy skin, hyperhidrosis
Other clinical findings	Perioral redness, insulated keratotic skin lesions particularly over the joints, amputation of digits possible	Achilles tendon, ankles, elbows and knees can be involved	Extending to the Achilles tendon and associated with slight peeling of skin	–	Extending to skin over the Achilles tendon, hyperkeratosis of the umbilicus and nipple areolae, very mild keratosis and dryness of the knees and elbows	Extending to skin over the Achilles tendon, flexural areas, elbows and knees, amputation of digits or blistering described
Histology and ultrastructure	Orthohyperkeratosis and papillomatosis, acanthosis without cytolysis, dermatophyte infection[c]	Orthohyperkeratosis, acanthosis without cytolysis	Hyperorthokeratosis, acanthosis and widening of intercellular spaces in one individual	Orthohyperkeratosis without cytolysis, dermatophyte infection[c]	Orthohyperkeratosis without cytolysis	Unspecific and ill defined, keratin intermediate filament aberrations possible
Remarks	1/100 000 in general population	High frequency in Japan and China (1.2–3.1/10 000)	Worsens with exposure to water	Improvement after oral erythromycin	Similar to Unna–Thost keratoderma	If woolly hair is present exclude Carvajal-Huerta syndrome

[a] Keratoderma of Gamborg-Nielsen (MIM: 244850) represents a clinical variant of mal de Meleda.
[b] Greither keratoderma is not considered a clearly defined entity.
[c] Histology may show the presence of spongiosis, vesiculation and neutrophils.
AD, autosomal dominant; AR, autosomal recessive; PPK, palmoplantar keratoderma.

(PC-6c) [5]. Painful keratoderma may also refer to desmosomal diseases [6], to oculocutaneous tyrosinaemia (type II) [7] or may be associated with othopaedic diseases such as hallux valgus [8].

Non-epidermolytic palmoplantar keratoderma

Definition
Non-epidermolytic palmoplantar keratoderma (NEPPK) refers to a heterogeneous group of non-syndromic forms of diffuse keratoderma that histologically do not show cytolysis in the upper spinous or granular layers (Table 63.11).

Historically, the eponym Thost–Unna keratoderma referred to NEPPK characterised by diffuse, thick, yellow hyperkeratosis [1,2]. Meanwhile, the original Thost family was found to have EPPK [3]. Considering mal de Meleda (MDM) as an important differential diagnosis, at least three different NEPPK entities can be distinguished: the Bothnia type [4–6], the Kimonis type [7] and the Nagashima type [8,9]. Greither described an autosomal dominant PPK with gradual onset and a tendency to improve in the fifth decade [10]. This eponym now lacks a clear definition [11,12] and it is likely to be genetically heterogeneous [13,14], either belonging to the EPPK group or overlapping with erythrokeratoderma [15].

Pathophysiology

Studies of a family from Bothnia in northern Sweden and three English pedigrees showed linkage centromeric to the type 2 keratin gene cluster on chromosome 12 [16–18]. Using linkage data and exome sequencing it has now been shown that this form of NEPPK is caused by dominant missense mutations in the *AQP5* gene [19], encoding aquaporin 5 (AQP5). Aquaporins are a family of cell membrane proteins that allow the osmotic movement of water across the cell membrane. AQP5 is localised to the plasma membrane of the keratinocytes of the stratum granulosum. The causative mutations exert a gain-of-function effect leading to increased keratinocyte water uptake rather than transepidermal water loss [19]. Another autosomal dominant NEPPK entity has been described by Kimonis *et al.*, found in one family to be due to a mutation occurring in a highly conserved lysine residue in the V1 domain of keratin 1 [7]. In contrast, the Nagashima PPK is an autosomal recessive disorder almost exclusively observed in Asia and caused by nonsense mutations in the *SERPINB7* gene. *SERPINB7* codes for a serine protease inhibitor, whose target protease in the skin still needs to be identified [20]. More recently, a novel form of autosomal recessive PPK was found to result from loss-of-function mutations in *SERPINA12*, encoding another serine protease inhibitor [21]. Decreased SERPINA12 activity was found to result in reduced inhibition of kallikrein 7 activity as well as decreased levels of desmoglein 1 and corneodesmosin, two known kallikrein 7 substrates, which are required for normal epidermal differentiation.

Clinical features [5,7,8,10,22,23]

Non-epidermolytic PPK may present in the first few months of life and is usually obvious after 2 years of age. An even, variably thick, often yellow hyperkeratosis occurs over the whole surface of the foot, starting on the heel and anterior arch, spreading later to the palms (Figure 63.42). NEPPK can be transgredient and is characterised by a well-defined red border. Hyperhidrosis is usual, and dermatophyte infections and pitted keratolysis are frequent. The nails, hair and teeth are normal.

Differential diagnosis

Mal de Meleda as well as EXI and aquagenic PPK are important differential diagnoses.

Non-epidermolytic keratoderma reported by Sybert *et al.* [22] resembled mal de Meleda, including autoamputation of the toes, but dominant inheritance was suggested. The description of recessive non-epidermolytic keratoderma reported by Gamborg-Nielsen [6] also sounds similar to mal de Meleda.

Investigations

A biopsy serves mainly to exclude epidermolytic keratoderma. Because of the variable findings in EHK, detailed light and/or electron microscopic studies are useful in most cases of diffuse PPK [3]. Otherwise, histological changes are non-specific: orthokeratotic hyperkeratosis, hypergranulosis or normogranulosis and moderate acanthosis are often seen. Spongiosis due to dermatophyte infection may be a source of confusion. Genetic analyses can help to confirm the diagnosis.

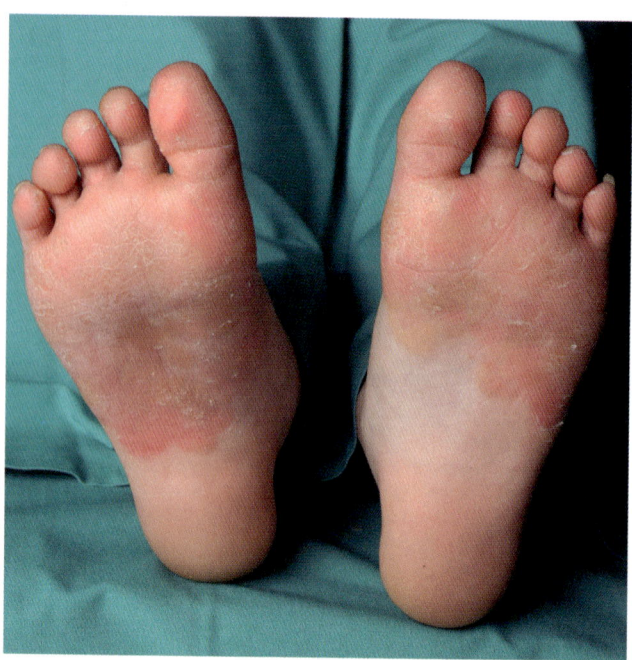

Figure 63.42 Girl with a non-epidermolytic palmoplantar keratoderma due to an *AQP5* mutation, who additionally suffered from *Trichophyton rubrum* superinfection. Courtesy of the Department of Dermatology, University Hospital Münster, Münster, Germany.

Management

Keratolytic therapy, such as 5–10% salicylic acid in white soft paraffin, or a gel of 5–6% salicylic acid in 70% propylene glycol, may be used. Occlusion with polythene for a few nights enhances the efficacy of the keratolytics. Low-dose systemic acitretin (0.2–0.5 mg/kg) may be tried – especially in patients with functional impairment. Importantly, fungal superinfection and bacterial overgrowth should be treated. Response to erythromycin has been described in NEPPK Bothnia type [23], and topical tacrolimus has been reported to be of benefit in NEPPK Nagashima type [24].

Mal de Meleda

Definition and nomenclature

Mal de Meleda is a rare autosomal recessive transgredient keratoderma named after the Croatian island of Meleda (Mljet) where it was first identified [1,2]. The disease has been reported widely in the Mediterranean littoral.

Synonyms and inclusions

- Keratoderma palmoplantaris transgrediens
- Acroerythrokeratoderma
- Meleda disease

Pathophysiology

Mal de Meleda is caused by biallelic mutations in *SLURP1* (secreted Ly-6/PLAUR related protein 1) [3–6]. Almost all cases occur in consanguineous pedigrees, and families from Croatia (including Meleda), Algeria, Israel and Tunisia share very few ancestral haplotypes, indicating founder mutations [3–8]. Haplotype analysis in western European patients with the disease showed a founder effect for the W15R mutation [9]. SLURP1 represents an auto- and paracrine ligand of the α7 nicotinic acetylcholine receptor (nAChR) involved in the fine tuning of physiological cell activation and adhesion, for instance by upregulated expression of transglutaminase 1, K10, p21 and caspase 3 [10]. The gene is expressed late in epidermal differentiation, in the granular layer, and particularly in association with the acrosyringium [3,11].

Clinical features [2,12–15]

Onset is in early childhood, and the development of hyperkeratosis is preceded by red skin changes. Patches of waxy, ivory-yellow hyperkeratosis extend across the whole surface of the palms and soles (Figure 63.43), and on to the dorsal surfaces of the hands and feet ('glove-and-socks' distribution). Insular lesions of the knees and elbows represent a key feature of this PPK. The reddened component often persists in the central palms and soles, typically with hyperhidrotic maceration and malodour. Fungal superinfection is common (Figure 63.44) [16]. Circumferential hyperkeratosis of the fingers may lead to sclerodactyly and digital constrictions (pseudo-ainhum) (Box 63.1); nail changes include hypercurvature, thickening and koilonychia [14,15]. Angular cheilitis and lip involvement are possible [17]. Hyperpigmented spots [18], melanoma arising within the affected skin [19,20] and Bowen disease of the sole have been reported [21]. Heterozygous female carriers may have a mild clinical phenotype [22]; also pseudodominant inheritance has been reported [23].

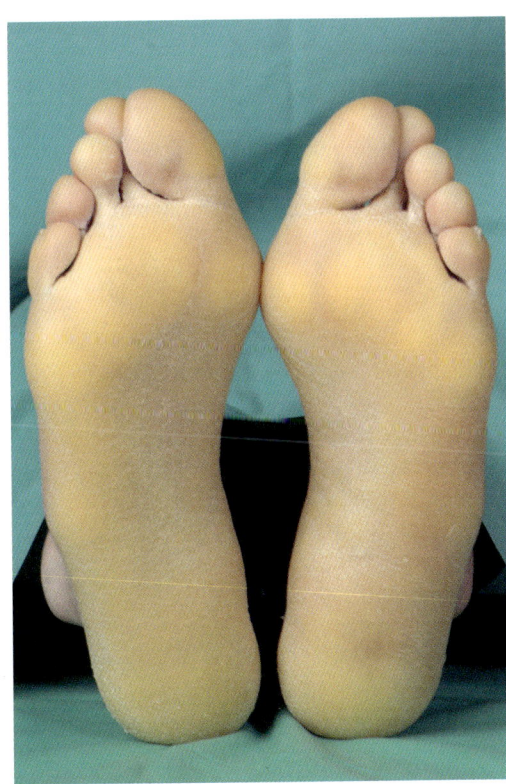

Figure 63.43 Mal de Meleda. Plantar phenotype without superinfection. Courtesy of the Department of Dermatology, University Hospital Münster, Münster, Germany.

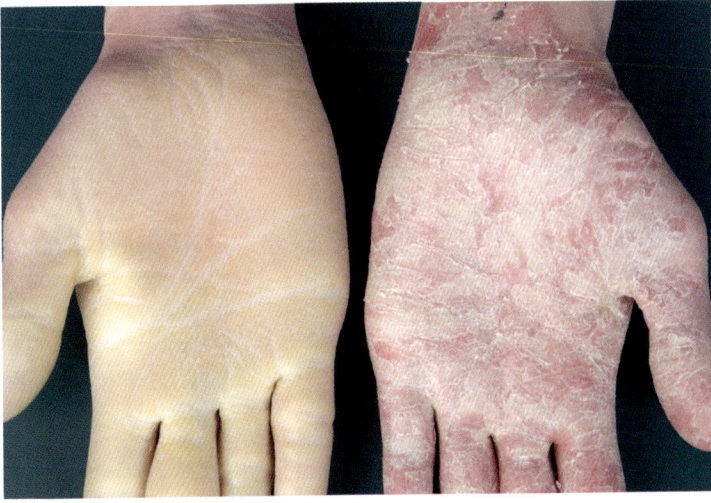

Figure 63.44 Mal de Meleda. *Trichophyton rubrum* superinfection of the left hand. Courtesy of the Department of Dermatology, University Hospital Münster, Münster, Germany.

Box 63.1 Inherited skin diseases and pseudo-ainhum

Keratodermas
- Vohwinkel syndrome (and Bart–Pumphrey syndrome)
- Clouston syndrome
- Mal de Meleda
- Papillon–Léfèvre syndrome
- Olmsted syndrome
- Loricrin keratoderma or KLICK (less common and severe than in Vohwinkel syndrome)

Generalised MeDOCs
- Lamellar ichthyosis
- Erythrokeratodermia variabilis

Inherited epidermolysis bullosae
- Chronic epidermolysis bullosae
- Kindler syndrome

Others
- Tuberous sclerosis
- Erythropoietic protoporphyria

KLICK, keratosis linearis ichthyosis congenita–sclerosing keratoderma; MeDOCs, Mendelian disorders of cornification.

Differential diagnosis

See the other NEPPKs described in Table 63.11. Keratoderma of Gamborg-Nielsen (MIM: 244850) represents a clinical variant of mal de Meleda. Keratoderma described by Sybert *et al.* [24] also resembles mal de Meleda.

Investigations

There is a greatly thickened corneal layer and an increased stratum lucidum, with marked acanthosis but without cytolysis [12]. The association of papillomatosis is a typical finding (authors' experience). A prominent perivascular lymphohistiocytic infiltrate may be seen, and sweat glands may be enlarged. Electron microscopy indicates a less abrupt transition from granular to cornified layers [18].

Management

Oral retinoids are effective but the hyperkeratosis may respond better than the inflammation of the skin [25–29]. The excision of keratoses and split-thickness skin grafts can be an option in order to relieve functional impairment. Long-term follow-up in one patient demonstrated no recurrence of keratosis on surgically treated areas [30]. Patients with a long history of mal de Meleda should be regularly seen for secondary malignancies [21]. Fungal superinfections should be treated.

Loricrin keratoderma

Definition and nomenclature

In two related pedigrees, Camisa and Rossana *et al.* delineated a diffuse transgredient honeycomb keratoderma with annular constrictions around the digits, accompanied by a mild ichthyosis [1–3]. In true Vohwinkel syndrome, there is impaired hearing but no generalised ichthyosis [4].

> **Synonyms and inclusions**
> - Variant Vohwinkel syndrome
> - Mutilating keratoderma with ichthyosis
> - Camisa syndrome

Pathophysiology

Loricrin keratoderma is caused by mutations in the *LOR* gene encoding loricrin, a glycine-rich cornified envelope protein [3,4]. Several different single nucleotide insertions have been identified in this gene, which uniformly result in frameshift and lead to expression of an abnormal protein with an abnormal, arginine-rich C-terminal peptide containing nuclear recognition signals [3–11]. The mutant protein is transported to the nucleus, where it is thought to interfere with the regulation of cornification [12]. Direct or indirect consequences include moderate alterations on the cornified envelope, increased corneocyte fragility and abnormal epidermal barrier function with accelerated repair kinetics [13]. Transgenic mice in whom loricrin has been knocked out are largely asymptomatic [14], but mice expressing a pathogenic loricrin mutation showed generalised scaling, thickened footpads and a constricting band causing autoamputation of the tail [15,16]. Progressive symmetrical erythrokeratoderma has been attributed in one case to a mutation in *LOR* [17], although these findings have not been reproduced [18] and are still debated.

Clinical features [4–11]

Generalised desquamation may be noted at birth, and collodion babies are reported [6,7,10]. However, the ichthyosis is generally mild and may pass unnoticed. A rugose keratoderma develops

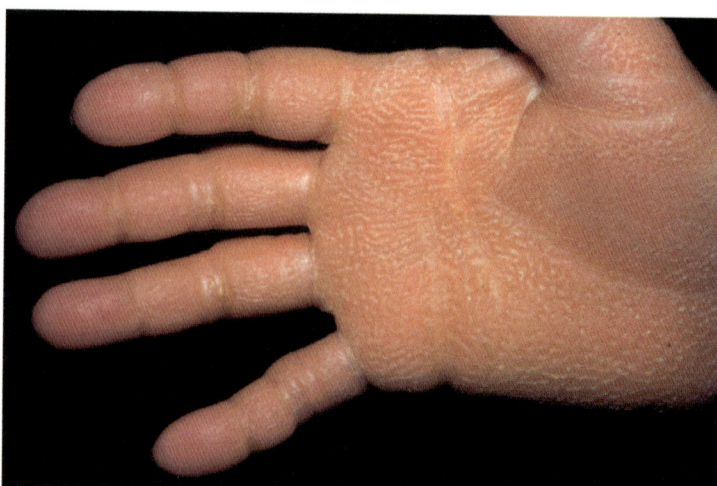

Figure 63.45 Loricrin keratoderma.

during childhood, gradually extending to a confluent honeycomb pattern (Figure 63.45). Cases with PPK but without typical honeycomb-like appearance have been described [19]. The edges of the keratoderma are diffuse (in contrast to true Vohwinkel syndrome) and cicatricial bands (pseudo-ainhum) may develop around the digits. Knuckle pads and warty keratoses have been reported, but are not a prominent feature. Hence, the combination of honeycomb keratoderma with mild non-syndromic ichthyosis is typical [7], but in sporadic cases autosomal recessive KLICK syndrome (see earlier in this chapter) should be considered an important differential diagnosis.

Investigations

In addition to hyperkeratosis, histological features include hypergranulosis and parakeratosis, that is, nuclei may be retained in the stratum corneum [1,7]. Electron microscopy shows dense intranuclear granules in granular cells, and a thin cornified cell envelope in the lower cornified layers with abnormal extracellular lamellae [13]. Immunoelectron microscopy shows the presence of loricrin in these nuclei [3,4].

Management

A beneficial use of isotretinoin, with effects on constructional bands and thus prevention of autoamputation, has been described [1,20]. Results from a mutant loricrin HaCaT model demonstrate increased vascular endothelial growth factor (VEGF) release that may be the cause of pathogenic keratinocytic proliferation. Inhibitors of VEGF receptor 2 might be attractive to treat loricrin keratoderma [21].

Striate (and focal) palmoplantar keratoderma

Definition and nomenclature

Isolated striate palmoplantar keratoderma (SPPK) is usually transmitted as an autosomal dominant trait and is caused by defects in at

Table 63.12 Isolated or syndromic palmoplantar keratoderma (PPK) associated with keratinocytic disadhesion.

Features	Striate palmoplantar keratodermas (SPPK)			Naxos syndrome	Carvajal-Huerta syndrome
Synonyms	SPPK1	SPPK2	SPPK3	PPK with arrhythmogenic cardiomyopathy	PPK with left ventricular cardiomyopathy
MIM number	148700	612908	607654	601214	605676
Inheritance	AD	AD	AD	AR (or AD)	AR (or AD)
Gene	DSG1 (Desmoglein 1)	DSP (Desmoplakin)	KRT1 (V1 domain of K1)	JUP (Plakoglobin)	DSP (Desmoplakin)
Age of onset	First or second decade of life	First or second decade of life	Early childhood	Early childhood, adolescence cardiomyopathy	Early childhood, childhood cardiomyopathy
Palmoplantar key features	Striate hyperkeratosis on the flexure site of fingers and palms, more diffuse and focal changes on the soles; triggered by manual work/mechanical stress			Striate or focal keratoderma	Striate or focal keratoderma, can spread over the Achilles tendon
Other clinical findings	Hyperhidrosis and pain	Woolly hair without cardiomyopathy is possible	–	Woolly hair, dilated cardiomyopathy	Woolly hair, possibly short, keratoses on knees/elbows, right/biventricular cardiomyopathy
Histology and ultrastructure	Disadhesion of keratinocytes and widening of the intercellular spaces, possibly less pronounced than in DSP mutations	Disadhesion of keratinocytes and widening of the intercellular spaces, cytoplasmic densities	Less electron-dense KIF within the SP, normal desmosomes, their insertion with KIF network seems attenuated	Disadhesion of keratinocytes and widening of the intercellular spaces, clumping of desmosomes and KIF	Wide intercellular spaces, clustering of desmosomes, ultrastructural signs for KIF disruption
Remarks	Same gene as for severe dermatitis–multiple allergies–metabolic wasting (SAM) syndrome	Same gene as for Carvajal-Huerta syndrome, skin fragility, woolly hair and lethal acantholytic EB	Similar mutation as in ichthyosis Curth–Macklin	Same gene as for acantholytic EB	Same gene as for SPPK2, skin fragility, woolly hair, acantholytic EB

AD, autosomal dominant; AR, autosomal recessive; EB, epidermolysis bullosa; KIF, keratin intermediate filament; SP, stratum spinosum.

least three different genes (Table 63.12) [1–3]. It is associated with a spectrum of Mendelian diseases of the desmosomes [4]. Most important, keratoderma with cardiomyopathy should be excluded.

Synonyms and inclusions
- Brunauer–Fuhs–Siemens syndrome
- Keratosis palmoplantaris varians of Wachters
- Striate PPK
- Keratosis palmoplantaris areata et striata

Introduction and general description

Historically, the occurrence of both insular and striate keratodermas within one family led Wachters [5] to suggest a single entity, keratoderma varians. Today, several distinct keratodermas with striate and/or focal pattern are recognised; moreover, some of them may be associated with a syndromic entity. Considering the influence of environmental factors such as mechanical stress, the recognition of predominantly striate and/or focal presentations may, however, still serve as a clinical clue for diagnosis: striate hyperkeratosis is particularly but not uniquely associated with 'keratinocytic disadhesion'. This histological clue may support the diagnosis of a desmosomal defect.

Pathophysiology

Initially, autosomal dominant striate keratoderma was mapped to the desmosomal cadherin cluster on 18q12.1 [6]. SPPK has been shown to result from haploinsufficiency for desmoglein 1 due to heterozygous mutations in DSG1 [1,2,7–11]. Heterozygous mutations in DSG1 are not exclusively associated with a striate pattern of hyperkeratosis as they have also been found to cause focal and diffuse PPK [12,13]. Moreover, since carriers of heterozygous mutations in DSG1 display PPK only while the offspring of two such heterozygous carriers can be affected by a life-threatening condition known as SAM syndrome (see earlier in this chapter), DSG1 mutations are actually inherited in a semidominant fashion [12,14].

The second SPPK locus on 6p21 is linked to dominant nonsense mutations in the desmoplakin gene (DSP) also leading to haploinsufficiency [15,16]. The majority of genetic reports on isolated striate keratoderma show dominant DSG1 mutations [1], whereas there are several reports on striate or focal keratoderma with cardiac involvement due to recessive (or dominant) DSP mutations (see 'Carvajal-Huerta syndrome' later in this chapter) [17,18]. Finally, there is one report on a frameshift mutation in the V2 tail domain of keratin 1 [19]. The mutation is similar to those being reported for ichthyosis Curth–Macklin [20,21].

Clinical features

As the name implies, there is a linear pattern of skin thickening on the palms and flexor aspects of the fingers [21–23]. However, lesions on the soles may be more areate or confluent (Figure 63.46), and striate lesions can be seen in affected members of pedigrees in which other patterns of keratoderma predominate. Mechanical stress is important; pain, hyperhidrosis and mild hyperkeratosis of the knees have been reported [1]. The presence of other features, especially woolly hair, should be specifically sought, and the possibility of cardiac disease considered. In summary, striate keratoderma is a striking key feature but not a specific one.

PART 6: GENETIC DISORDERS

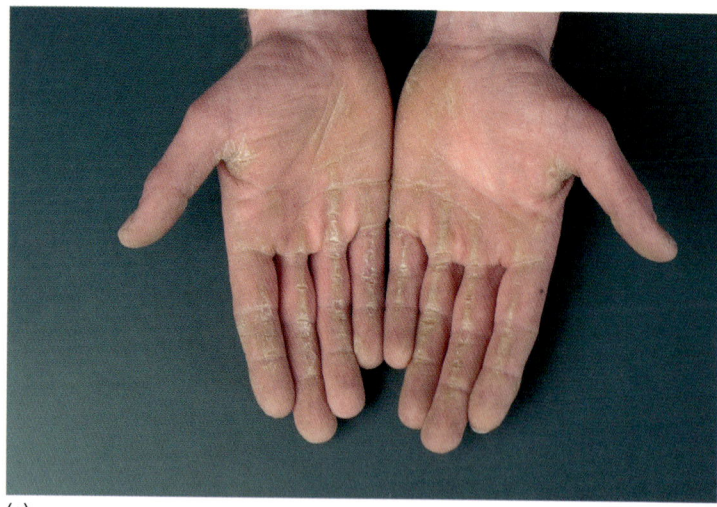

(a)

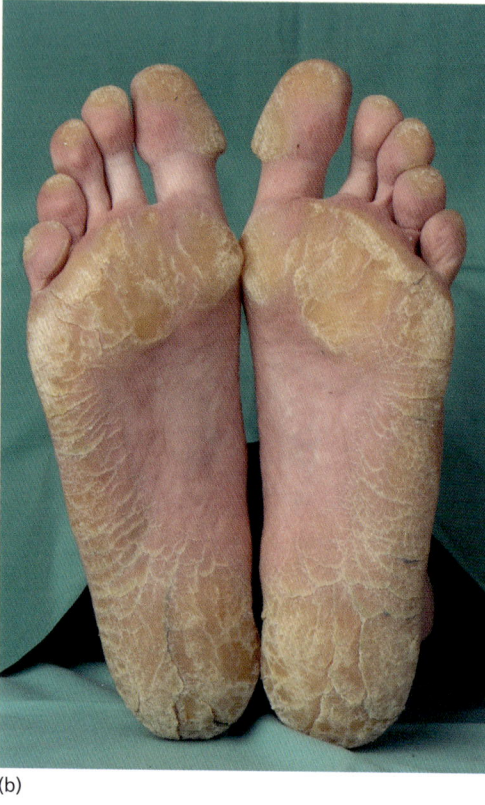

(b)

Figure 63.46 Striate and focal palmoplantar keratoderma of the (a) hands and (b) feet in the same patient. Courtesy of the Department of Dermatology, University Hospital Münster, Münster, Germany.

Differential diagnosis

In addition to EPPKs, connexinopathies [24] and other syndromic diseases [25,26] as well as acquired keratodermas [27] have to be considered. Importantly, Howel-Evans syndrome should be considered if focal and nummular keratoderma predominate and histology is unspecific (see 'Tylosis with oesophageal cancer/Howel-Evans syndrome' later in this chapter).

Investigations

Disadhesion of keratinocytes with widening of the intercellular spaces is an important histological clue for these cell–cell junction diseases [28]. Moreover, electron microscopy of keratoderma associated with *DSP* mutations shows abnormal keratin filaments with loss of desmosome connections. Desmosome size seems reduced in *DSG1*, and perinuclear aggregation of keratin filaments seems more marked in *DSP*-associated disease [29].

Management

Several reports point to a good response to systemic acitretin treatment and/or application of high-percentage urea creams [30–32].

Palmoplantar keratoderma punctata

Definition and nomenclature

This autosomal dominant keratoderma is clinically characterised by small rounded papular lesions on the palms and soles that tend to coalesce over pressure points [1–3].

Synonyms and inclusions
• Keratosis punctata palmoplantaris type Buschke–Fischer–Brauer
• Palmoplantar keratoderma punctata type 1 (PPKP1)
• Keratoma dissipatum
• Disseminated clavus
• Papulotranslucent acrokeratoderma

Epidemiology
Prevalence

The incidence of palmoplantar keratoderma punctata (PPKP) is estimated as 1.17/100 000 individuals in Croatia [4].

Pathophysiology

The disorder has been mapped to two chromosomal regions, 15q22 [5–7] and 8q24.13–8q24.21 [8]. The first locus harbours the *AAGAB* gene in which mutations have been found in patients with PPKP1 [9,10]. *AAGAB* encodes the α- and γ-adaptin-binding protein p34 [9–16]; p34 deficiency results in increased epidermal growth factor signalling which in turn may drive keratinocyte proliferation [13]. The second locus on 8q was found to be associated with one missense mutation in the gene *COL14A1* in a Chinese family [17], which needs to be confirmed for other families [15].

Clinical features [1–4]

This autosomal dominant condition often has a later onset with lesions appearing in early adolescence but also up to the sixth decade of life [1]. Pinpoint keratotic papules, initially translucent and with a depression in the centre but later opaque and warty, appear on the palms and soles (Figure 63.47). Interfamilial variable severity is typical [13]. Enviromental factors and personal skincare regimes may affect the degree of hyperkeratosis [18]. In many families, small and large lesions coexist, including broader focal plantar callosities. Lesions are more florid in manual workers. There is no involvement of the dorsa of the hands or legs, nor of the knees or elbows. Hyperhidrosis and fungal infections are unusual [1]. It is not fully understand if PPKP is truly associated with an excess of

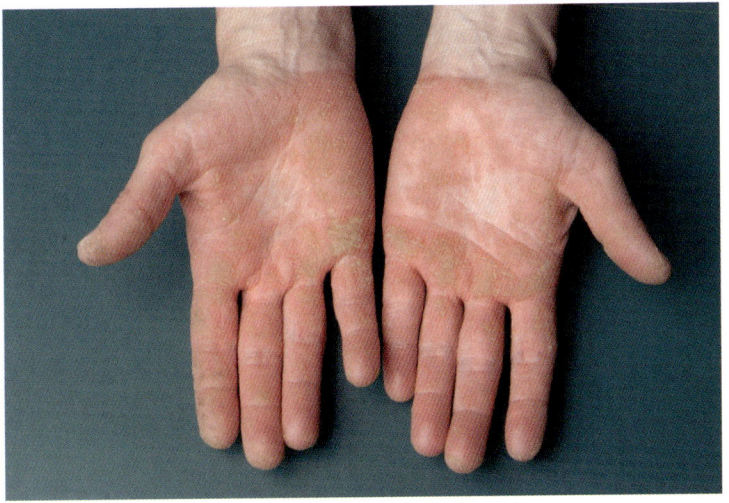

(a)

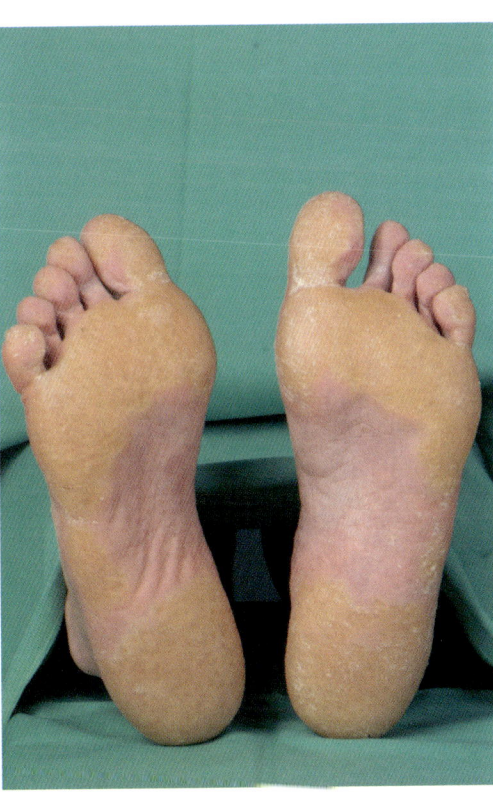

(b)

Figure 63.47 Punctate palmoplantar keratoderma. (a) Small, even keratotic papules on the palms and (b) confluent hyperkeratosis on the feet of the same patient. Courtesy of the Department of Dermatology, University Hospital Münster, Münster, Germany.

malignancies, however an increased prevalence of malignancies in patients with PPKP has been described [13,19].

Differential diagnosis

Most importantly, focal keratoderma associated with malignancies such as breast and colonic adenocarcinoma [20,21] should be differentiated (see 'Tylosis with oesophageal cancer/Howel-Evans syndrome' later in this chapter). Autosomal dominant punctate porokeratosis (also referred to as PPKP2) may present with similar clinical features [22]. In acrokeratoelastoidosis (referred to as PPKP3) disorganised elastic fibres are a histopathological hallmark [23].

Investigations

Punctate lesions are orthohyperkeratotic on histology with compact acanthosis and hypergranulosis with a depression in the centre of the lesion, but may also show hypogranulosis and (focal) parakeratosis [1].

Management

Careful choice of footwear and regular use of a pumice stone are useful in alleviating discomfort. Literature reports indicate no major beneficial effects of keratolytic ointments, topical retinoids or topical calcipotriol on the keratoses [1,24,25]. Systemic treatment with oral retinoids may yield a small effect depending on the dosage (0.5–1.0 mg/kg/day) [1,3,26]. Receptor tyrosine kinase inhibitors that are involved in p34 signalling are under development and of potential relevance for future treatment [9,27].

Spiny keratoderma

Definition and nomenclature

Spiny keratoderma is a rare condition of unknown aetiology and exists as a hereditary/benign or idiopathic form [1–3]. Importantly, aquired digitate keratoses [4] need to be excluded. Brown [1] described the first case as 'punctuate keratotic projections' ('punctate keratoderma'), and since then the disease has been described under a variety of terms, of which 'porokeratosis' is a misleading misnomer.

> **Synonyms and inclusions**
> - Music box spiny keratoderma
> - PPKP2 [5]
> - Punctate porokeratotic keratoderma [2,6,7]
> - (Multiple minute palmoplantar digitate hyperkeratosis [4])
> - (Filiform hyperkeratosis [8])

Clinical features

Fine 1–2 mm papules that project from the palmoplantar surface are described as filiform, spiked, prickly, minute digitate or music box-like spines (Figure 63.48). Unilateral presentations have been reported [9]. Spiny keratoderma may be inherited as an autosomal dominant trait. The lesions may start in early childhood and gradually increase in number; they appear in the first up to the fifth decade [1–3]. Discomfort can be caused by a tendency to catch on clothing and other objects [9].

Differential diagnosis

Darier disease [10,11], epidermodysplasia verruciformis [12], arsenic keratosis [4], multiple filiform verrucae, paraneoplastic follicular hyperkeratosis [13] and/or multiple minute digitate hyperkeratosis (reviewed in [4]) should be differentiated.

Investigations

Histology demonstrates dense columns of parakeratosis above a hypogranular epidermis [2,3,9,14]. The absence of dyskeratosis

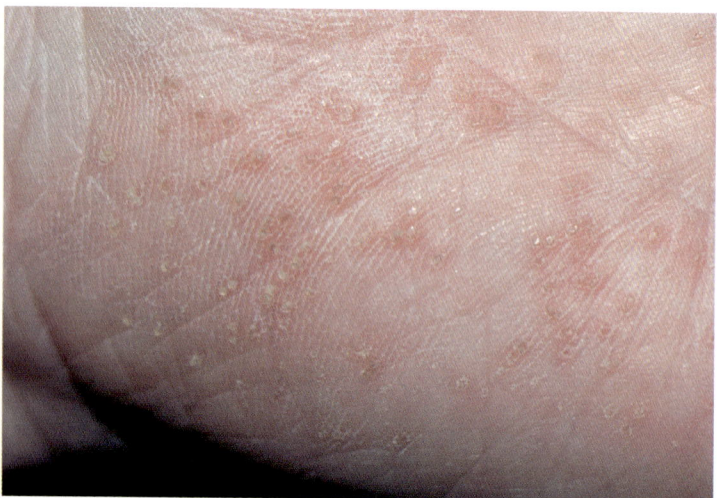

Figure 63.48 Spiny keratoderma that have been present since the age of 20 on the palms and soles. Their son and daughter are also affected.

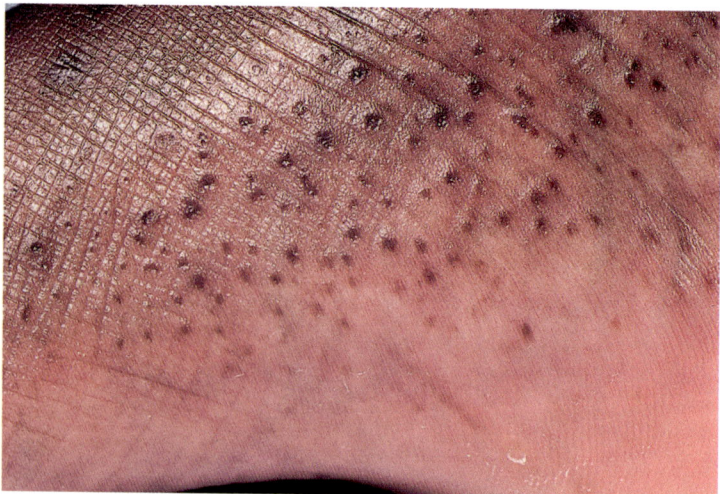

Figure 63.49 Marginal papular keratoderma (acrokeratoelastoidosis, punctate palmoplantar keratoderma type 3): crateriform punctate keratosis at the margin of the sole (Wallace line).

and vacuolated keratinocytes below the parakeratotic columns differentiates the disease from porokeratosis [3,15]. Autoimmune screen, blood investigations for a full blood count, renal/liver function and radiological tests are necessary to exclude an associated condition such as polycystic kidneys and liver [16], renal failure [17], tuberculosis [18], hyperlipidaemia [19], malignancy such as multiple myeloma [8,20–23] or HIV-associated type 6 pityriasis rubra pilaris [24].

Management
Mechanical debridement (e.g. dermabrasion) may be more effective than topical keratolytics [9]. Etretinate or actitretin has a temporary effect [8,12,25]. Topical 5-fluorouracil ointment has been tried with differing results [14,16].

Marginal papular keratoderma

Definition and nomenclature
Marginal papular keratoderma (MPK) is heterogeneous and refers to acrokeratoelastoidosis as well as focal acral hyperkeratosis, which are both characterised by papules, plaques and nodules located at the junction between the palmar and dorsal skin of the hands or feet along the thenar and hypothenar eminences (Figure 63.49) [1,2].

Synonyms and inclusions
• Acrokeratoelastoidosis
• Focal acral hyperkeratosis
• PPKP3 [3]

Pathophysiology
Autosomal dominant inheritance with linkage to chromosome 2p or sporadic occurrence has been described [4].

Clinical features
Costa [5,6] reported 13 cases with cornified and umbilicated papules distributed along the borders of the hands and feet. He noted fragmentation and rarefaction of elastic fibres in the dermis, and introduced the term acrokeratoelastoidosis. Fiallo *et al*. [7] argued that the primary defect is in the elastic tissue. However, Dowd *et al*. [8] reported 15 cases, several familial, with similar oval or polygonal crateriform papules along the borders of the hands and feet in whom there was no solar damage or elastorrhexis. To distinguish this entity, it was termed focal acral hyperkeratosis. However, eight of Costa's 13 patients appeared identical [5]. Rongioletti *et al*. [1] suggested unifying the marginal papular keratodermas with a pragmatic division into the hereditary type with elastorrhexis (acrokeratoelastoidosis), or without it (focal acral hyperkeratosis).

Differential diagnosis
The following entities may be differentiated from marginal papular keratodermas.

Punctate keratosis of the palmar creases. This condition most commonly occurs in Afro-Caribbean or black individuals, may be transmitted in an autosomal dominant fashion and may be associated with AE and/or manual labour [9–14]. It clinically shows sharply defined 1–4 mm hyperkeratoses – hard warty lesions – confined to the palmar creases [15]. This location is possible but unusual for punctuate keratoderma [16]. Around one-third of black but rarely white individuals may show hyperkeratotic pits involving the flexural creases of the palms [17,18].

Keratoelastoidosis marginalis. This is an acquired condition also known as digital papular calcific elastosis [19,20]. It presents with degenerative collagenous plaques that are firm, sometimes concave, forming a linear band principally around the web of the thumb and index finger at the margin of the volar and dorsal surfaces. There is histological evidence of solar damage [21–23].

Mosaic acral keratosis. Mosaic acral keratosis [24], reported in African patients with widespread polygonal papular lesions over the ankles and shins, may present with marginal keratoderma [25].

Investigations
Histology shows focal orthohyperkeratosis. The key microscopic finding in acrokeratoelastoidosis is the presence of massive elastosis, whereas no elastic fibre changes are present in focal acral hyperkeratosis [1,13].

Cole disease

Definition and nomenclature
This genodermatosis features punctuate keratoderma and pigmentary anomaly. Cole disease is characterised by congenital or early-onset punctate keratoderma with irregularly shaped hypopigmented macules of the extremities [1–4].

> **Synonyms and inclusions**
> - Guttate hypopigmentation
> - Punctate PPK with or without ectopic calcification

Pathophysiology
Ultrastructural analyses suggest a defective melanosome transfer from melanocyte to keratinocyte, as melanocytes show numerous melanosomes in the cytosol and dendritic extensions, whereas neighbouring keratinocytes are almost devoid of melanin [2]. Eytan *et al.* [4] demonstrated that specific missense mutations in the gene *ENPP1* underlie the disorder. The gene product ENPP1 is a cell surface protein that catalyses the hydrolysis of adenosine triphosphate (ATP) to adenosine monophosphate and generates extracellular inorganic pyrophosphate, which is a major inhibitor of mineralisation. While recessive mutations in *ENPP1* cause a range of inherited forms of ectopic calcifications, dominant mutations in this gene cause Cole disease. Cole disease-causing mutations affect a specific domain of *ENPP1* which regulates insulin signalling. The fact that insulin signalling impacts on epidermal growth factor signalling suggests a pathophysiological link between Cole disease and punctate keratoderma due to *AAGAB* mutation [5]. In addition, there are recessive mutations that cause a clinical spectrum of dyschromatosis and a more severe form of Cole disease [6]

Clinical features
The disease manifests during the first year of life. Affected individuals present with a relatively mild focal or punctuate keratoderma (Figure 63.50). In addition, they develop sharply demarcated, irregular macules with varying degrees of hypopigmentation, mainly located over the extremities [1–3]. There might be an early-onset calcific tendinopathy or calcinosis cutis [4].

Differential diagnosis
Epidermolysis bullosa simplex with mottled pigmentation and Naegeli–Franceschetti–Jadassohn syndrome (Chapter 68) may be confused with Cole disease.

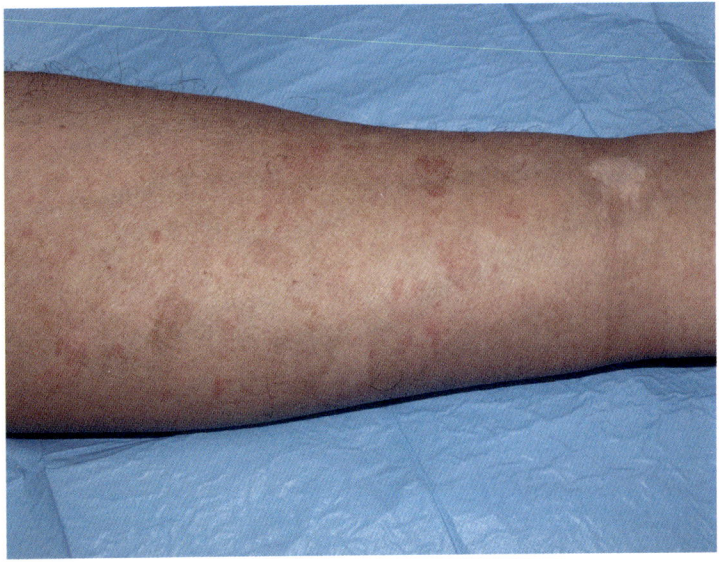
(a)

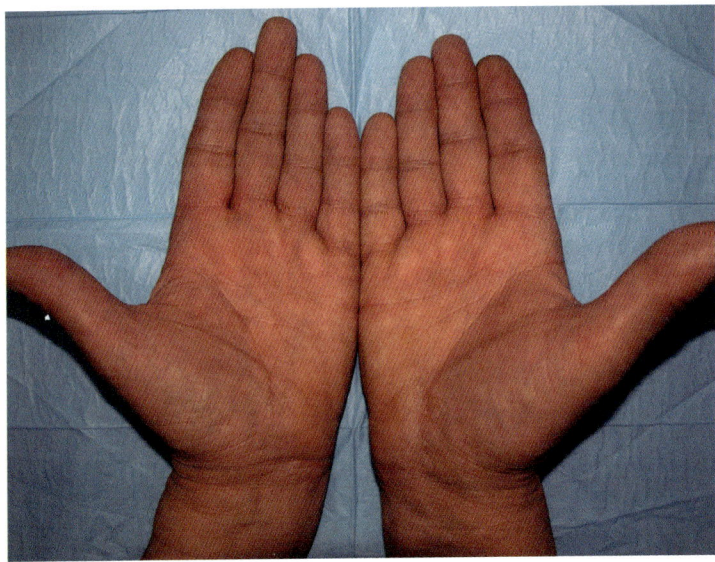
(b)

Figure 63.50 Cole disease. (a) Forearm with hypopigmentation and (b) mild keratoderma in the same patient. Courtesy of Dr Y. Gilaberte, Hospital San Jorge, Huesca, Spain.

Investigations
Histology shows hyperorthokeratosis, hypergranulosis and acanthosis. Ultrastructure confirms a reduction of the melanin content of keratinocytes with disproportionately large melanosomes of melanocytes. The number of melanocytes is normal.

Transient aquagenic keratoderma

Definition and nomenclature
This peculiar, mainly palmar, disorder represents a mild keratoderma that is triggered or exacerbated by contact with water or sweat [1].

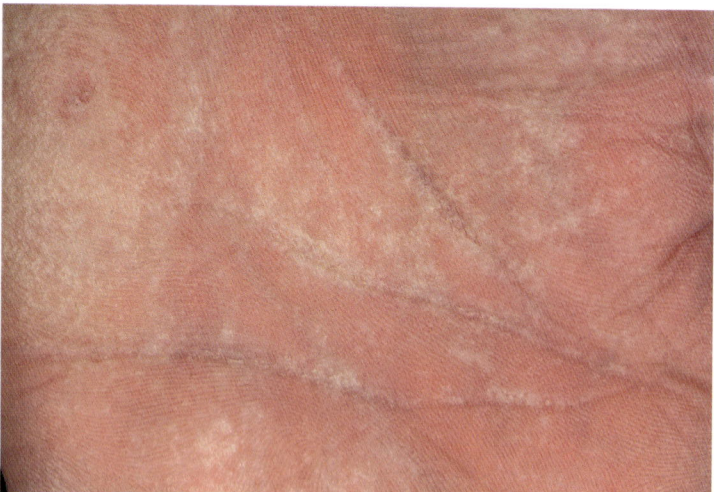

Figure 63.51 Transient aquagenic keratoderma showing whitish maceration of the palmar skin following immersion. Courtesy of Dr G. Kavanagh, Royal Infirmary of Edinburgh, UK.

Synonyms and inclusions
- Transient reactive papulotranslucent acrokeratoderma
- Aquagenic syringeal acrokeratoderma

Pathophysiology

Most cases of transient aquagenic keratoderma (TAK) appear to be acquired, but autosomal recessive [1] or dominant [2] cases have been described. The disease may be associated with the use of cyclo-oxygenase 2 inhibitors [3]. The relationship with other diseases such as asthma is unknown [4]. It may be differentiated from *hereditary papulotranslucent acrokeratoderma* (MIM: 101840), in which lesions are persistent once they appear [5,6].

Clinical features [1–4,6–13]

Affected individuals aged 6–45 years, more often women, typically show a subtle keratoderma appearing after a few minutes of immersion of their hands in water or after sweating (Figure 63.51). Only in some patients are the soles affected. One characteristic sign might be that patients bring with them a vessel to immerse their hands in water ('hands in the bucket' sign) [13]. The painful, burning or itching, whitish papular lesions are associated with dilated acrosyringeal ostia, which can be seen by dermoscopy [14]. Lesions subside shortly after drying the hands, leaving minimal hyperkeratosis in the centre of the palms.

Differential diagnosis

Transient aquagenic keratoderma should be differentiated from other keratodermas that are sensitive to exposure to water, for example Bothnia type NEPPK [15,16]. Importantly, aquagenic wrinkling of the palms (Figure 63.52) is associated with cystic fibrosis (in about 50% of affected patients) and can be observed in up to 10% of heterozygous *CFTR* gene mutation carriers [17–21].

Investigations

Histology might reveal hyperplasia of the eccrine sweat glands, with slight dilatation of the lumen [4].

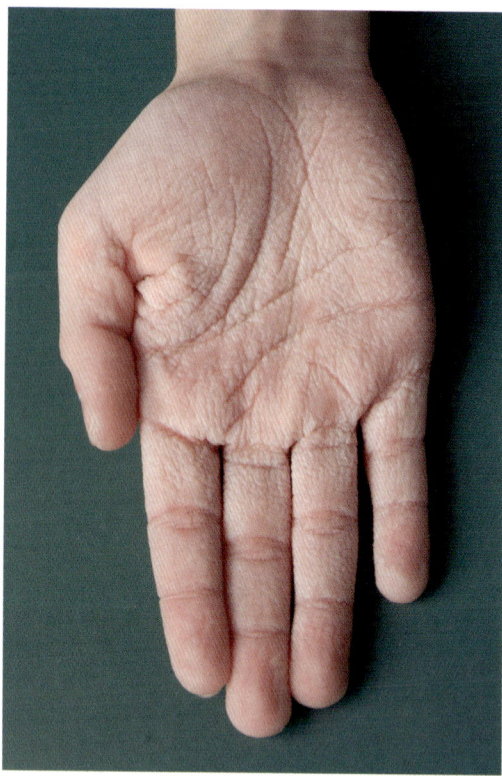

Figure 63.52 Aquagenic palmar wrinkling in cystic fibrosis.

Management

Treatment with 20% aluminium chloride hexahydrate followed by urea cream [4,11] or botulinum toxin [22] may lead to significant improvement.

SYNDROMIC KERATODERMAS

PALMOPLANTAR KERATODERMA AND CARDIOMYOPATHY

Whenever woolly hair is associated with any kind of PPK, especially in striate keratoderma, a search for possible cardiac abnormalities is recommended [1,2]. Like isolated striate keratoderma (type I/II), the following syndromic disorders are histologically characterised by keratinocytic disadhesion [3].

Naxos syndrome

Definition

The disease is associated with arrhythmogenic right ventricular cardiomyopathy/cardiomyopathy [1] and is accompanied by PPK and woolly hair (see Table 63.12) [2,3].

Pathophysiology

The first reported seven pedigrees from the Greek islands of Naxos and Milos have been found to share a 2 bp deletion within the

JUP gene encoding plakoglobin [4], a cell junction protein found in desmosomes in the epidermis and cardiac muscle. As can be seen in other desmosomal genodermatoses [5], different mutations of *JUP* show a large phenotypic spectrum, for example mutations allowing expression of altered plakoglobin may show mild skin fragility, keratoderma and woolly hair only [6]. Of note, autosomal dominant *JUP* mutations underlie isolated arrhythmogenic right ventricular cardiomyopathy [7] and a Naxos variant with leukonychia and oligodontia [8]. Finally, complete loss of plakoglobin due to homozygous nonsense mutations may lead to acantholytic epidermolysis bullosa [9].

Carvajal-Huerta syndrome

Definition
The disease represents a cardiocutaneous syndrome with NEPPK, woolly hair and dilated cardiomyopathy (see Table 63.12) [1].

Pathophysiology
Recessive desmoplakin (*DSP*) mutations producing a premature stop codon and leading to a truncated protein cause this disorder [2]. Other genetic defects in *DSP* have been found to generate a wide range of phenotypes. A 10 amino acid insertion in *DSP* exerting a dominant negative effect on desmosomal assembly has been found to be associated with cardiomyopathy and mild hyperkeratosis of the elbows and knees [3]. Heterozygous carriers of the missense mutation p.S299R showed isolated arrhythmogenic right ventricular cardiomyopathy without cutaneous phenotype [4]. Complete loss of the tail domain of desmoplakin presents as acantholytic epidermolysis bullosa [5]. Hence, dosage of desmoplakin is critical in maintaining epidermal integrity, as illustrated by compound heterozygote patients carrying one null allele and one missense mutation, who developed pronounced skin fragility and alopecia without cardiac anomalies [6].

Of note, a novel entity combining woolly hair, hypotrichosis and PPK but no cardiac abnormalities was recently reported. The disease was found to be caused in one report by a mutation in *KANK2* [7].

Clinical features
The three Equadorian pedigrees initially described by Carvajal-Huerta displayed recessive inheritance of a striate keratoderma with woolly hair and associated cardiomyopathy developing in the teenage years [1]. As such, the syndrome resembles Naxos disease, but it presents at a younger age with bilateral predominantly left ventricular involvement leading to early heart failure with cardiac enlargement and disrupted cardiac contraction [8,9]. Moreover, patients have been described showing an ichthyosis similar to SAM syndrome [10].

Investigations
Histological studies demonstrate large intercellular spaces of suprabasal keratinocytes (keratinocytic disadhesion). Ultrastructure may reveal clumping of desmosomes [2,11] or signs for intermediate filament disruption such as perinuclear localisation of keratin in suprabasal keratinocytes [1]. On resting electrocardiogram, affected patients exhibit repolarisation and/or depolarisation abnormalities; structural/functional abnormalities of the ventricle(s) will be found on echocardiography or cardiac MRI [3,12].

Management
Cardiac function in patients with striate keratoderma should be investigated as early diagnosis and intervention may improve outcome. Depending on the myocardial symptoms, implantation of an automatic cardioverter defibrillator with/without anti-arrhythmic drugs or, at the end stages, heart transplantation are options [7]. Screening of possibly affected family members should be initiated considering dominant as well as recessive inheritance [3,13,14]. Desmoplakin deficiency showing a SAM syndrome-like presentation may well respond on therapy with ustekinumab [10].

PALMOPLANTAR KERATODERMA AND HEARING IMPAIRMENT

The association of hereditary keratoderma with hearing loss is most commonly caused by defective connexin function [1,2], whereby premature termination codons in the gap junction beta 2 (*GJB2*) gene encoding connexin 26 are the most common cause of non-syndromic *autosomal recessive* deafness [3–5]. In several pedigrees with diffuse or transgredient autosomal dominant keratoderma and varying degrees of prelingual deafness, missense mutations in connexin 26 have been found (MIM: 148350) [6–10].

Notwithstanding, in 'palmoplantar keratoderma with hearing impairment' establishment of a thorough family history is crucial considering that maternal inheritance possibly points to a rare *mitochondrial* type of keratoderma [11].

Vohwinkel syndrome and Bart–Pumphrey syndrome

Definition and nomenclature
Vohwinkel [1] and Wigley [2] independently reported honeycomb-like keratoderma associated with stellate keratoses on the knuckles and the formation of circumferential bands around digits (pseudo-ainhum). Vohwinkel's family had moderate sensorineural deafness [3], and subsequent cases have confirmed autosomal dominant inheritance [4–7].

Synonyms and inclusions
- Keratoma hereditarum mutilans
- Cicatrising keratoderma with hearing impairment
- Keratoderma with sensorineural deafness

Pathophysiology

In three unrelated English, Spanish and Italian pedigrees with 'classic' Vohwinkel syndrome, Maestrini et al. [8] found the same mutation, p.D66H, in *GJB2* encoding connexin 26, a gene also implicated in Bart–Pumphrey syndrome [9] as well as KID syndrome [10]. The phenotypic variants related to mutations in *GJB2* are reviewed in Table 63.5. A full list of dominant and recessive mutations in *GJB2* can be found on the connexin-deafness homepage [11].

Connexin 26 is expressed in the cochlea where it may permit the recycling of potassium to endolymph [12,13]. In skin, the protein is found in palmoplantar epidermis and sweat glands, and is upregulated in conditions such as psoriasis [14,15]. Patients homozygous for mutations preventing any expression of connexin 26 have no discernible skin phenotype, indicating that dominant negative or gain-of-function effects may be involved in the pathogenesis of cutaneous manifestations of mutations in *GJB2*.

There are various mechanisms which may underlie the phenotypic effects of connexin gene mutations [16,17]: mutant proteins are sometimes unable to form functional gap junction channels; in other cases, aberrant trafficking of mutant proteins may prevent some of them reaching the cell surface membrane and lead to their accumulation in organelles triggering the ER stress response [18]; finally, mutant proteins may exert deleterious effects on other connexins' function (e.g. c.del42E has been shown to exert a dominant negative effect on the wild-type connexin 43) [19].

Clinical features [1–7,20]

Palmoplantar keratoderma begins in childhood as shiny or translucent papular hyperkeratosis, gradually becoming confluent on the hands and feet. Striate lesions may be seen. Warty papules on the knuckles and other extensor sites coalesce into the pathognomonic 'starfish' keratoses. The edge of the keratoderma at the wrists and Achilles tendon consists of spiky, digitate, hyperkeratotic projections onto normal skin. This contrasts with the diffuse edge seen in loricrin keratoderma [21]. Multiple keratoses on the digits produce circumferential hyperkeratosis, which predisposes to the formation of cicatricial bands and autoamputation (Figure 63.53). The little finger and fifth toe are commonly affected. A high-tone sensorineural hearing loss [6] is probably present from birth, but may escape detection unless tested. It does not appear to be progressive. Focal epilepsy has been described in Vohwinkel syndrome [22].

Bart–Pumphrey syndrome

The allelic condition (MIM: 149200) is characterised by knuckle pads (similar to the focal keratoses of Vohwinkel syndrome), keratoderma, leukonychia and mixed sensorineural and conductive deafness [9,23–25].

Investigations

Histology may be non-specific, showing papillomatosis with prominent orthohyperkeratosis.

Management

Vohwinkel syndrome has been successfully treated by etretinate [7] and acitretin [26] and the cicatricial bands released surgically

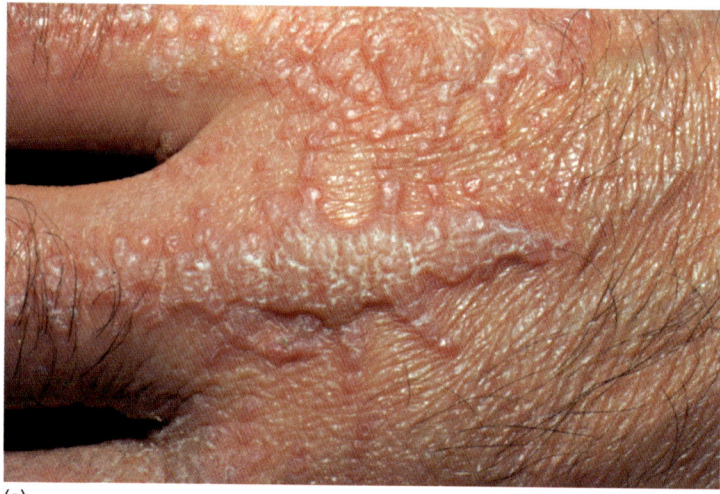

(a)

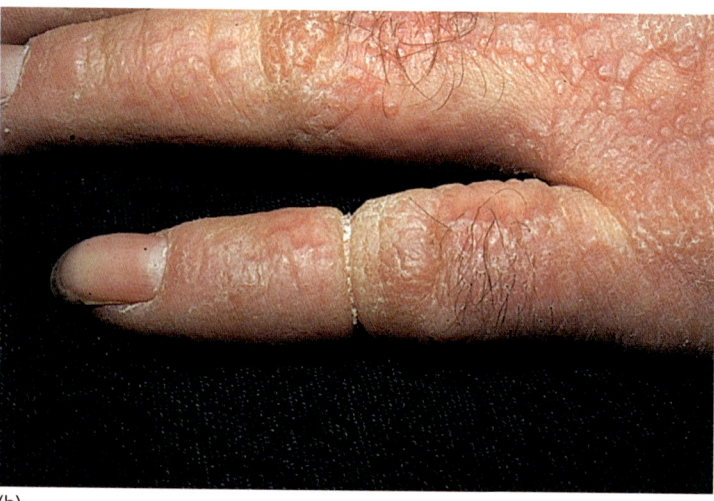

(b)

Figure 63.53 Vohwinkel syndrome: (a) 'starfish' lesions and (b) pseudo-ainhum.

[27–29]. Early screening for hearing impairments and appropriate rehabilitation (hearing aids, speech therapy, language training, cochlear implantation, educational programmes) for the hearing loss are important to achieve auditory speech recognition effectively [30].

Mitochondrial palmoplantar keratoderma and hearing impairment

In a Scottish family, Reid et al. [1] reported familial progressive post-lingual deafness with variable plantar keratoderma (Figure 63.54) caused by a specific mutation in mitochondrial DNA (mtDNA), encoding both a serine transfer RNA and the first subunit of cytochrome oxidase [2].

The same point mutation, namely m.7445A>G, was identified in a New Zealand family, in Japanese patients [3,4] and other pedigrees [2,5,6], who demonstrated PPK, mainly plantar, and sensorineural deafness (Table 63.13). Among those patients with clinical and audiological features of hearing loss due to

Table 63.13 Palmoplantar keratoderma (PPK) in ectodermal dysplasias and mitochondrial diseases.

Features	Clouston syndrome	Odonto-onycho-dermal dysplasia	Papillon–Léfèvre syndrome	Mitochondrial PPK
Synonyms	Hidrotic ectodermal dysplasia 2 (HED2)	PPK with cystic eyelids, hypodontia and hypotrichosis, eccrine tumours with ectodermal dysplasia, Schöpf–Schulz–Passarge syndrome	Keratoderma with periodontitis	Mitochondrial sensorineural hearing loss with PPK
MIM number	129500	224750, 257980	245000	590080
Inheritance	AD	AR (minor symptoms if heterozygous)	AR	Maternal
Gene	GJB6	WNT10A	CTSC	MT-TS1 (A7445G, mtDNA)
	Connexin 30	Wingless-type MMTV integration site family, member 10A	Cathepsin C	Mitochondrial tRNA serine 1
Age of onset	Early life	Early life	Before second year of life	Early childhood
Palmoplantar key features	Combination of nail dystrophy, hypotrichosis and PPK (papillomatous, fissured and transgredient), pseudo-ainhum possible	Macerated PPK with late onset, acral hyperhidrosis	Transgredient PPK, preceded by red skin, hyperhidrosis, pseudo-ainhum possible	PPK with early honeycomb appearance, mainly plantar, focal or diffuse, alongside the fingers, callus on the heels and toes, with or without red border
Other clinical findings	Dystrophic nails, often small and thickened, with clubbing, pale and fine hair with (progressive) hypotrichosis, eyebrows sparse or absent, hyperpigmentation over the joints	Cysts of the eyelids (not necessarily in early age), reduced primary and/or lack of secondary dentition, nail dystrophy, hypotrichosis, smooth tongue, follicular and other adnexal tumours occur in older patients	Periodontosis, severe gingivitis, loss of deciduous teeth by the age of 4–5 years, psoriasiform plaques on the knees and elbows, tendency to pyogenic infection, hair may be sparse *Haim–Munk syndrome* (MIM: 245010) + onychogryphosis, arachnodactyly and acro-osteolysis	Progressive sensorineural hearing loss with onset during childhood, variable severity, coincidence with warty linear epidermal naevus, ichthyosis vulgaris and/or cholesteatoma are described
Histology and ultrastructure	Targeted mutation analysis, exclude pachyonychia congenita	Histology of hidrocystomas	Hyperkeratosis with irregular parakeratosis and a moderate perivascular infiltrate, ultrastructural lipid-like vacuoles in granulocytes and corneocytes, tonofilament reduction, irregular keratohyalin granules	Increased granular layer, moderate acanthosis without epidermolytic changes
Remarks	Special hair care, wigs, artificial nails, keratolytics	Different manifestations may be regarded as allelic disorders	Good response to retinoids, combination with antibiotics and dental care lessening the gingival inflammation and saving the teeth	Targeted mutation analysis, hearing aids, cochlear implantation, speech therapy, educational programmes

AD, autosomal dominant; AR, autosomal recessive; MMTV, mouse mammary tumour virus.

PART 6: GENETIC DISORDERS

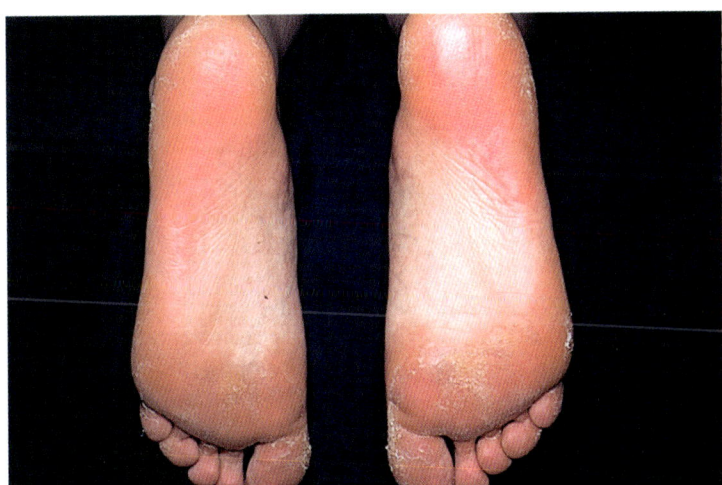

Figure 63.54 Mitochondrial keratoderma with deafness.

mitochondrial mutations, around one-quarter may have the A7445G substitution [7]. Individual differences in the mitochondrial contents of wild-type and mutant DNA ('heteroplasmy') affect the resulting phenotype including the severity of hearing loss, keratoderma and age of onset. Of note, mtDNA mutations may be responsible for ~3.5% of patients with hereditary deafness; but other mutations (e.g. m.1555A>G) are not associated with keratoderma [8].

PALMOPLANTAR KERATODERMA AND CANCER

Skin malignancies arising from PPK skin have been observed in mutilating keratoderma [1], porokeratosis [2] and Clouston syndrome [3] as well as non-syndromic focal or diffuse PPKs [4,5]. Melanoma of the affected skin has been reported in various keratodermas (Table 63.14) [6–12]. It may be more common in Japanese patients, because of the higher incidence of acral melanoma in this population [13]. The reported association between EPPK and breast/ovarian cancer [14,15] is not a general feature of the disease. Reports on punctate/focal keratoderma with malignancies [16–18] may include cases of Howel-Evans syndrome and should be differentiated from punctate PPK due to an *AAGAB* mutation, which is not clearly associated with malignancies (see 'Palmoplantar keratoderma syndrome' earlier in this chapter).

PART 6: GENETIC DISORDERS

Table 63.14 Palmoplantar keratoderma (PPK) associated with cancer.

Features	Huriez syndrome	Tylosis with oesophageal cancer (TOC)	Palmoplantar keratoderma, sex reversal and cancer
Synonyms	Scleroatrophic and keratotic dermatosis of limbs	Howel-Evans syndrome	Palmoplantar hyperkeratosis with SSC and 46, XX sex reversal, true hermaphroditism with PPK
MIM number	181600	148500	610644
Inheritance	AD	AD	AR
Gene	*SMARCAD1*	*RHBDF2* (iRhom2)	*RSPO1* (R-spondin protein 1)
Age of onset	Early infancy	Puberty	Infancy (?)
Palmoplantar key features	Accentuated scleroatrophy on the palms and fingers, hyperkeratosis and dry skin, soles less often affected, dermatoglyphics often absent	Focal non-epidermolytic PPK	Mild PPK with sclerodactyly, nail hypoplasia, hyperhidrosis
Other clinical findings	Malignant degeneration of the affected skin at a young age with a 100× higher risk of SCC	Oral leukokeratosis, follicular hyperkeratosis, high life-time risk of squamous oesophageal cancer (95% by age of 65)	Male patient: hypospadia, hypogenitalism, gynaecomastia. Female patient: true hermaphroditism (clitorial enlargement, ambiguous external genitalia, ovotesticular gonads). Premature loss of permanent teeth due to chronic periodontal disease, predisposition to SCC and laryngeal carcinoma
Histology and ultrastructure	Hypergranulosis and acanthosis, reduced numbers of Langerhans cells	Non-epidermolytic hyperkeratosis, abnormal cytoplasmic staining of iRhom2 in the epidermis	Non-epidermolytic hyperkeratosis, karyogram, shares features of Huriez syndrome
Remarks	Acitretin may reduce painful hyperkeratosis and incidence of skin cancer	Genetic counselling, screening of mutation carriers and preventative endoscopy	Karyogram in male or female patient: 46, XX (SRY–)

AD, autosomal dominant; AR, autosomal recessive; SCC, squamous cell carcinoma.

Huriez syndrome

Introduction and general description

This syndrome represents a prototypic form of a cancer-prone keratoderma [1,2], in which the risk of squamous cell carcinoma of the affected skin is increased by around 100-fold [3,4]. The disease is characterised by a triad of diffuse scleroatrophy of the hand, mild PPK and hypoplastic nail changes (Figure 63.55) [5,6]. Kindler disease and cryptic forms of junctional epidermolysis bullosa as well as dyskeratosis congenita must be differentiated.

Pathophysiology

SMARCAD1, the gene associated with Huriez syndrome, codes an ATP-dependent chromatin remodeller of the Snf2 ATPase family. The disease is caused by haploinsufficiency of a mutated *SMARCAD1* isoform that affects the homologous recombination repair of DNA double-strand breaks [7,8]. Mutations affecting the same *SMARCAD1* splice site are linked to adermatoglyphia [9] and Basan syndrome [10], two autosomal dominant genodermatoses that share adermatoglyphia, hypohydrosis and nail abnormalities with Huriez syndrome. Whereas the development of squamous cell carcinoma has only been observed in Huriez syndrome, skin blistering and facial milia were only reported in Basan syndrome. Thus, Huriez syndrome, adermatoglyphia and Basan syndrome are allelic disorders with variable expressivity [7].

Tylosis with oesophageal cancer/Howel-Evans syndrome

Pathophysiology

The disorder maps to a 42.5 kb segment of chromosome 17q23 [1–3]. The region is commonly deleted in oesophageal carcinomas [4]. Missense mutations in *RHBDF2* (rhomboid 5 homologue 2) encoding an intramembrane protease underlie the disease as first shown by Blaydon *et al*. [5] and then confirmed [6,7]. The RHBDF2 protease regulates the maturation of TNF-α convertase (TACE) in the skin [8,9]. Functional data suggest that mutant RHBDF2 increases signalling through EGFR resulting in hyperproliferation and dysregulation of wound repair, which might stimulate the subsequent development of precancerous lesions [5].

Clinical features

Howel-Evans described two families with autosomal dominant keratoderma associated with later development of oesophageal cancer [10]. Pressure points of the sole are predominantly affected, and less so the palms (Figure 63.56) [11]. There is variable oral leukokeratosis and follicular accentuation. Thirty-seven per cent of the original affected family members developed oesophageal cancer. A further, extensive German American family has been reported, with an increased (38-fold) risk of oesophageal cancer [1]. The disorder can be distinguished from PC by the absence of nail changes [12].

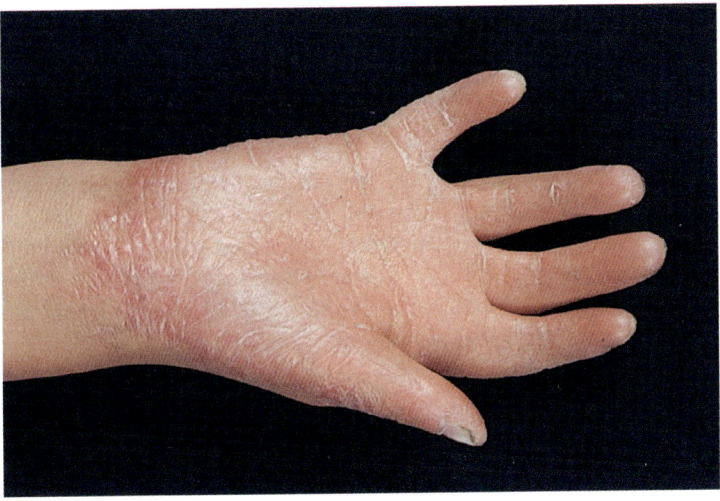

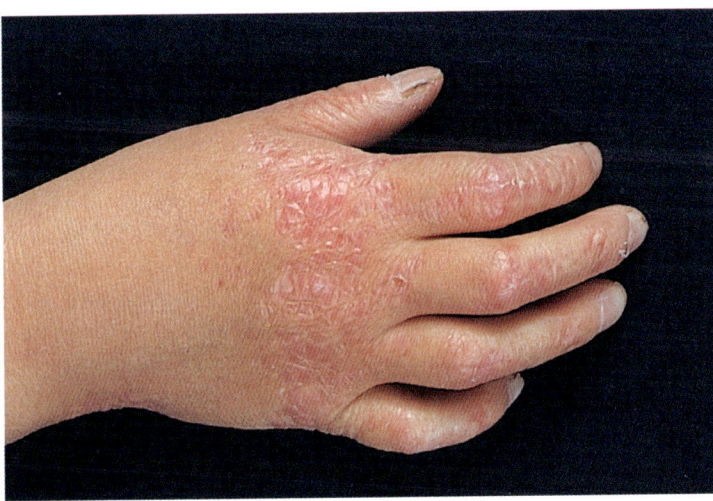

Figure 63.55 Huriez syndrome showing (a) keratoderma and (b) atrophic skin over the dorsa of the hand and sclerodactyly. Courtesy of Dr M. van Steensel, Department of Dermatology, University of Maastricht, the Netherlands.

Palmoplantar keratoderma, sex reversal and cancer

Introduction and general description

This form of PPK entity is inherited in an autosomal recessive fashion and is characterised by female-to-male sex reversal in females. Consequently, most affected individuals with this keratoderma present as male individuals with or without signs of hypogenitalism. (This is in contrast with true hermaphroditism which is characterised by the coexistence of male and female gonadal structures.) Sex reversal is most often due to translocation of the *SRY* gene encoding the testis-determining factor (XX males SRY+) [1]. In PPK with sex reversal and cancer, male patients carry a normal female chromosome set *without* the *SRY* gene (XX male, SRY–) [2], but also XY males without sex reversal may display the keratoderma. Inter-

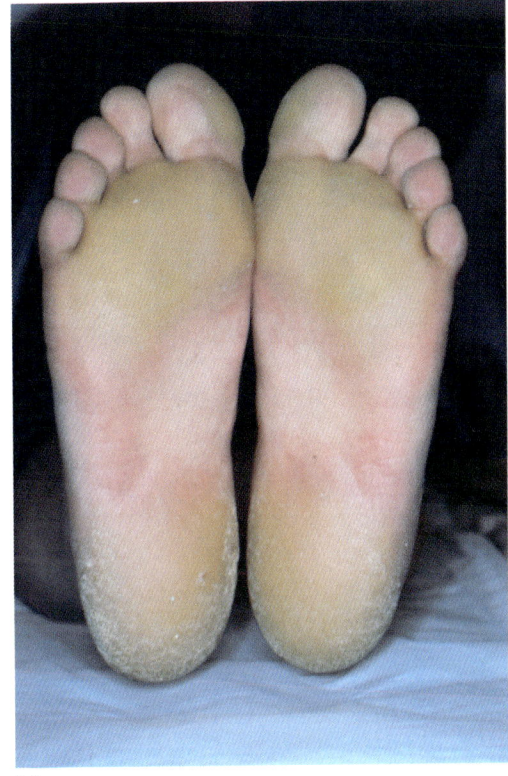

(a)

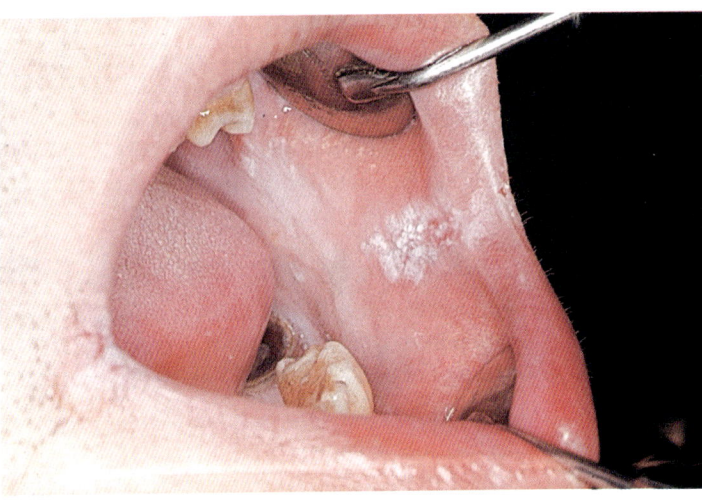

(b)

Figure 63.56 Tylosis with oesophageal cancer (Howel Evans syndrome). (a) Keratoderma and (b) oral mucosal lesions. Courtesy of Professor W. R. Tyldesley, Liverpool University School of Dentistry, Liverpool, UK and Dr M. S. Lewis-Jones, Ninewells Hospital, Dundee, UK.

estingly, the skin phenotype is reminiscent of Huriez syndrome; affected patients have a predisposition to squamous cell carcinoma [2–5].

Pathophysiology

Homozygous loss-of-function mutations in *RSPO1*, encoding respondin 1, were shown to cause scleratrophic PPK associated with either female-to-male sex reversal and squamous cell carcinoma [6] or true hermaphroditism, congenital bilateral corneal opacities, onychodystrophy and hearing impairment [7]. R-spondins are a small family of growth factors interacting with the so-called FZD–LRP receptor complexes [8]. Mutations in *RSPO1* were shown to be associated with larger intercellular spaces suggesting that the *RSPO1* defect impairs desmosomal junctions [6]. Disruption of R-spondin 1 remarkably illustrates the fact that mutations in a single gene, namely *RSPO1*, can lead to complete female-to-male sex reversal even in the absence of the testis-determining factor (*SRY*) [8]. Of note, the pedigree of the affected families may show a recessive mode of inheritance, in which only males seem to be affected due to the female-to-male sex reversal phenotype.

PALMOPLANTAR KERATODERMA IN ECTODERMAL DYSPLASIA AND RELATED DISEASES

Table 63.13 gives some details of these keratoderma diseases.

Clouston syndrome (hidrotic ectodermal dysplasia type 2)

Introduction and general description

The combination of small dystrophic nails developing in early infancy with hypotrichosis and brittle hair in conjunction with papillomatous and fissured transgredient keratoderma [1–3] is suggestive [4], but the presentation may resemble PC [5]. Recently, there have been reported patients with Clouston syndrome and absence of PPK [6].

Pathophysiology

This autosomal dominant ectodermal dysplasia is caused by mutations in the gap junction β-6 (*GJB6*) gene encoding connexin 30 [7,8], which is a potential target of p63 [9].

Odonto-onycho-dermal dysplasia

Synonyms and inclusions
- Schöpf–Schulz–Passarge syndrome
- PPK with cystic eyelids, hypodontia and hypotrichosis
- Eccrine tumours with ectodermal dysplasia

Introduction and general description

This term encompasses a large and heterogeneous group of autosomal recessive disorders that are allelic, sharing various common dental anomalies in association with PPK and nail dystrophy [1–3]. Several specific subtypes have been recognised based on specific clinical manifestations such as Schöpf–Schulz–Passarge syndrome. This presentation is characterised by hypotrichosis, nail fragility, early loss of deciduous teeth, hydrocystomas of the eyelids or other

follicular and adnexal tumours occurring in older patients [4–7]. The diffuse PPK may develop due to multiple palmoplantar eccrine syringofibroadenoma [8].

Pathophysiology

The diseases are caused by mutations in the *WNT10A* gene encoding a signalling molecule expressed in skin critical for the development of ectodermal appendages [1,2]. Phenotypic heterogeneity is the rule with mutations in *WNT10A* causing disorders ranging from monosymptomatic severe oligodontia to Schöpf–Schulz–Passarge syndrome. Of interest, heterozygotes (mostly males) can also display clinical features such as tooth and nail anomalies [2].

Papillon–Léfèvre and Haim–Munk syndrome

Introduction and general description

In Papillon–Léfèvre syndrome, redness and thickening of the palms and soles are associated with periodontitis and frequent bacterial skin infections (Figure 63.57). Hyperkeratotic lesions can also affect the elbows and knees, and pseudo-ainhum (see Box 63.1) has been described in this syndrome. Dural and choroid plexus calcifications have also been reported. The prevalence has been estimated as 1–4 in 1 million [1–9]. The first symptoms usually appear between 1 and 4 years [10]. Haim–Munk syndrome is allelic with Papillon–Léfèvre syndrome, combining its features with onychogryphosis, arachnodactyly and acro-osteolysis [11–13]; this latter condition has been reported mostly in a single Jewish family of South Indian origin (so-called 'Cochin Jews') [14]. Retinoids have been shown to be of benefit to patients, including in the treatment of oral disease and the prevention of autoamputation [15,16].

Pathophysiology

The conditions are both caused by homozygous mutations in the *CTSC* gene encoding the lysosomal protease cathepsin C [13,17,18]. Cathepsin C is expressed in various tissues, that is, cells of the immune system such as nuclear leukocytes, in the lung, kidney and other epithelial tissues. Its main functions are protein degradation and proenzyme activation. Thus, the activity of several critical proteases is decreased in Papillon–Léfèvre syndrome [19]. Neutrophil phagocytosis and reactivity to T- and B-cell mitogens are impaired [20–22] explaining the predisposition to pyogenic infection, which may also involve internal organs [23–25]. High levels of oxidative stress markers, the role of mitochondrial dysfunction and a deficiency of coenzyme Q10 have been described [26,27]. Natural killer cell cytotoxicity seems to be impaired [28]. Severe gingivitis and periodontitis affect both deciduous and permanent dentition leading to loss of teeth unless treated [5–7,29,30]. Virulent Gram-negative organisms invade the alveolar socket, usually including *Actinobacillus actinomycetemcomitans* [31–33]. Moreover, there are some reports on melanoma and/or squamous cell carcinoma associated with cathepsin C deficiency [34–36].

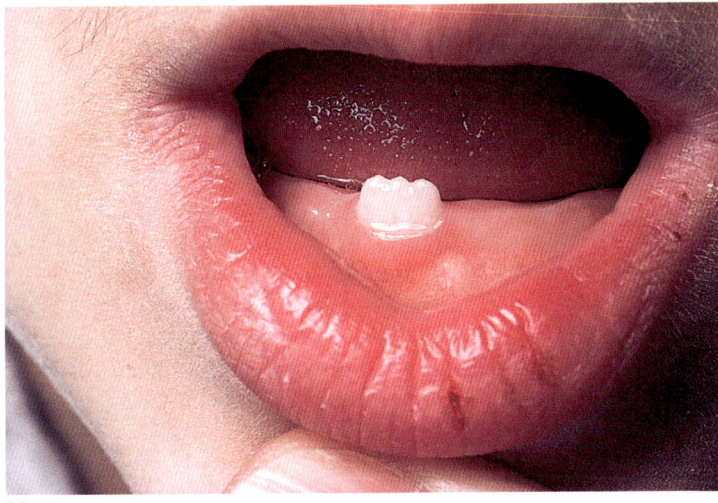

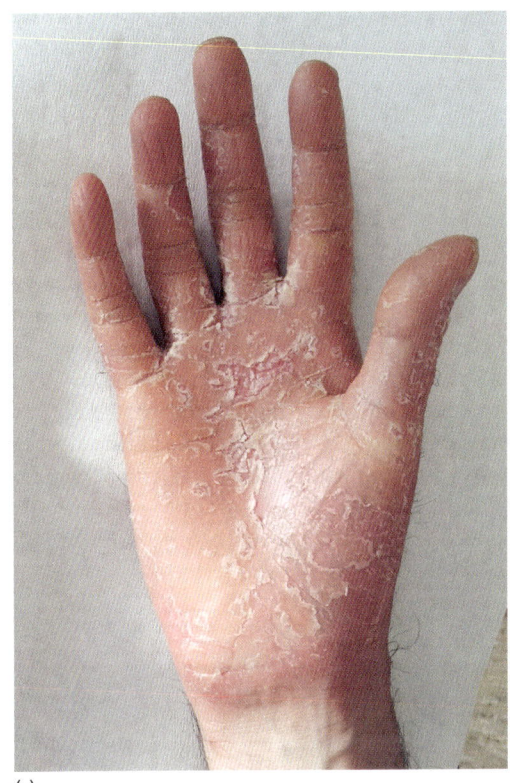

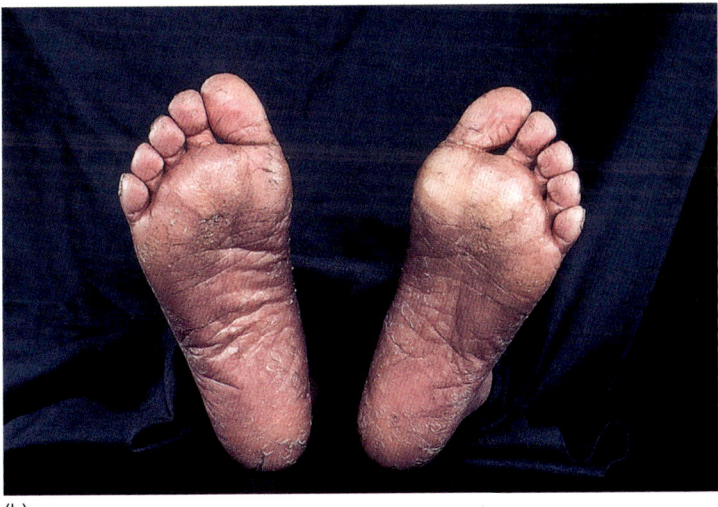

Figure 63.57 Papillon–Léfèvre syndrome: (a) Loss of dentition. (b) Diffuse plantar hyperkeratosis. (c) Psoriasiform palmar phenotype.

Olmsted syndrome

Definition and nomenclature

The disease often presents sporadically, and is clinically characterised by severe, mutilating, transgredient keratoderma with prominent periorificial hyperkeratosis. Recently, autosomal dominant, autosomal recessive and X-linked recessive forms have been confirmed and the responsible genes identified [1–6].

Synonyms and inclusions
• Mutilating PPK with periorificial keratotic plaques

Epidemiology

A total of 65 cases have been reported worldwide, of which only 16 cases were familial with different modes of inheritance [4–8].

Pathophysiology

The disease may be added to the list of skin channelopathies: gain-of-function mutations in the transient receptor potential vanilloid 3 (*TRPV3*) gene were identified as a cause for autosomal dominant Olmsted syndrome [4]. Sporadic cases are caused by *de novo* dominant mutations [8]. Autosomal recessive inheritance of mutations in the same gene has also been reported [6]. *TRPV3* encodes a critical element for a member of the TRP cation selective ion channels that are involved in the regulation of skin barrier formation, hair growth, epidermal differentiation (through TGF-α/EGFR signalling), skin inflammation, pain and pruritus [9,10].

In contrast, patients suffering from an X-linked recessive variant with alopecia universalis and severe nail dystrophy were shown to carry specific mutations in *MBTPS2*, the same gene that is associated with IFAP, KFSD and BRESEK/BRESHEK syndrome [5,11–13] (see 'Ichthyosis follicularis–atrichia–photophobia syndrome' earlier in this chapter). It was shown that there are a number of mutation-specific phenotypes due to this gene defect, as predicted by Oeffner *et al.* [11]. *MBTPS2* encodes a zinc metalloprotease essential for cholesterol homeostasis and the ER stress response [11].

Clinical features

Onset is in the first year of life, with symmetrical, sharply defined palmar and plantar keratoderma surrounded by red skin, and flexion deformities, constriction or spontaneous amputation of the digits (Figure 63.58) [1]. The disease tends to have a slow but progressive course. The keratotic lesions are pruritic and mildly painful with pressure [3,14,15]. Periorificial plaques present with skin inflammation and warty hyperkeratosis involving the mouth and perianal regions. Massive hyperkeratosis and/or fissuring of the gluteal cleft may cause pain and considerable discomfort. Keratoses extending to the flexor sites of the forearms or knees may show a follicular and striate aspect [14,16]. Alopecia, nail and tooth anomalies, joint laxity and corneal dystrophy have been observed

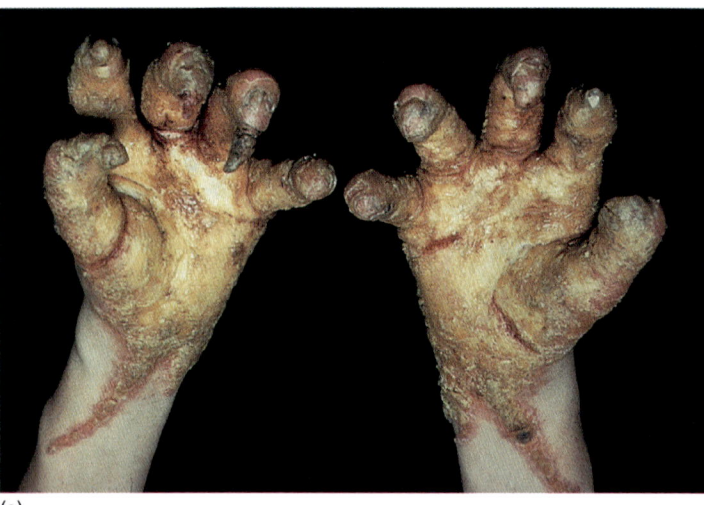

(a)

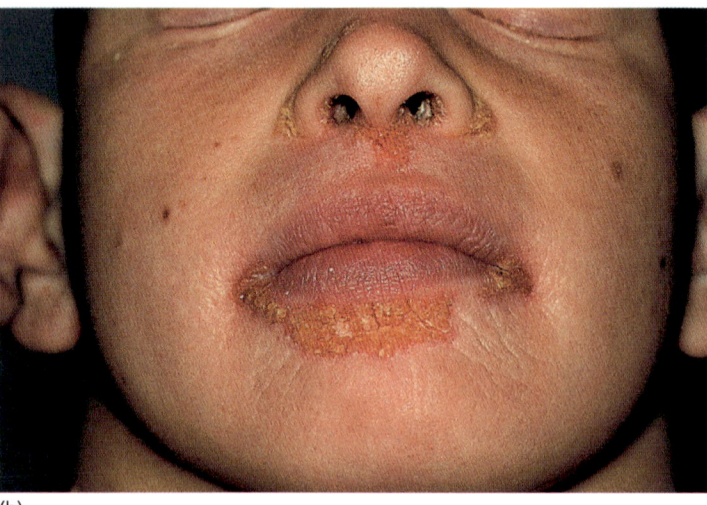

(b)

Figure 63.58 Olmsted syndrome: (a) gross keratoderma with striate features and (b) periorificial hyperkeratosis. Courtesy of Professor R. K. Winkelmann, Mayo Clinic, Scottsdale, AZ, USA.

[3,17]. Recurrent skin infections [18] and the development of squamous cell carcinoma or malignant melanoma have been reported in a considerable number of cases of Olmsted syndrome [3,4,19,20]. High IgE levels with eosinophilia, erythromelalgia and deafness have been rarely observed in association with *TRPV3* mutations [21–24].

Differential diagnosis

Palmoplantar keratodermas with periorificial lesions and digital constrictions may be reminiscent of mal de Meleda, acrodermatitis enteropathica, mucocutaneous candidiasis, psoriasis inversa, hidrotic ectodermal dysplasia (Clouston syndrome), PC, Papillon–Léfèvre syndrome and Vohwinkel keratoderma [3,25,26].

Investigations

Histopathology reveals psoriasiform hyperplasia, orthohyperkeratosis and parakeratosis with perivascular inflammatory infiltration including increased numbers of mast cells [4,27]. Cytochemical staining indicates hyperproliferation of the epidermis [24,28].

Management

Treatment of the disorder is problematic. Variable improvement has been seen with etretinate [29,30] or acitretin [8,15]. Topical keratolytics, emollients and corticosteroid as well as calcineurin inhibitors may offer temporary relief of hyperkeratosis, pain or itching [3,21,31]. Excision and skin grafting of severe keratoderma showed favourable long-term clinical results in some patients [32]. Erlotinib (an EGFR inhibitior) led to thinning of keratoderma, reduction of pain and pruritus and resolution of perioral plaques within 3 weeks to 3 months [33–35]. Improvement of quality of life has been reported too [34]. The initial significant response was not fully maintained over the years in one publication [33].

Resources

Ectodermal Dysplasia Society: www.ectodermaldysplasia.org.
National Foundation for Ectodermal Dysplasias (NFED): www.nfed.org.
   (Both last accessed June 2022.)

PALMOPLANTAR KERATODERMA AND OPHTHALMIC MANIFESTATIONS

Oculocutaneous tyrosinaemia (tyrosinaemia type II)

Definition and nomenclature

Tyrosine aminotransferase deficiency causes herpetiform corneal ulcers and painful palmoplantar keratoses with progressive mental impairment [1,2].

Synonyms and inclusions
- Tyrosine transaminase deficiency
- Richner–Hanhart syndrome

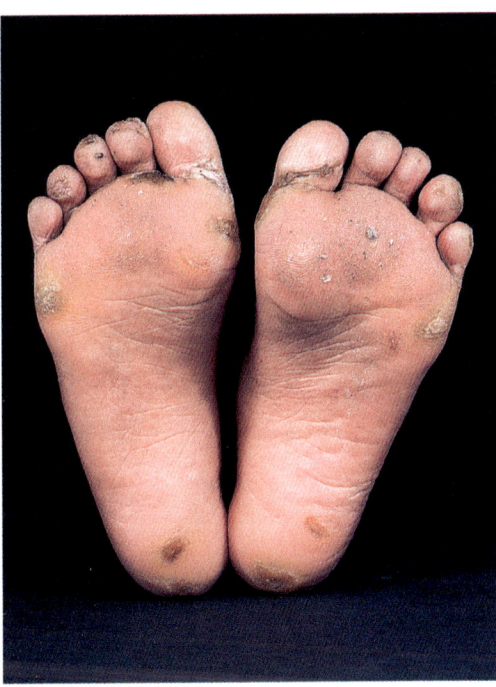

Figure 63.59 Oculocutaneous tyrosinaemia (Richner–Hanhart syndrome) with callosity-like hyperkeratoses.

Pathophysiology

This autosomal recessive condition is caused by biallelic mutations in *TAT* encoding tyrosine aminotransferase [3]. Tyrosine aminotransferase deficiency impacts on the degradation pathway of tyrosine and phenylalanine [4–6]. The keratinocytic ultrastructure reveals clumped tonofilaments with adherent globoid keratohyalin granules, suggesting enhanced microfilament aggregation due to an excessive amount of intracellular tyrosine [7].

Clinical features

In the first year of life, photophobia and corneal ulcers occur. A year or two later, red crusts appear on the pressure-bearing areas of the soles (Figure 63.59), followed by painful circumscribed hyperkeratosis [1,2], typically making the child walk on their toes. The keratoses vary from gross keratoderma to patchy hyperkeratotic yellow-white papules. Bullous lesions and hyperhidrosis are sometimes seen. In incomplete forms, keratoderma may be the presenting feature [8], although conversely keratoderma may be delayed until the second decade [9]. Unless correctly treated, behavioural problems arise within a few years and progressively worsen, ending in inanition or death [10].

Investigations

Elevated tyrosine levels in newborn screening by tandem mass spectrometry and analysis of the tyrosine aminotransferase gene can confirm the diagnosis. In urine, high levels of tyrosine and its metabolites are present [11]. Slit lamp examination may reveal tyrosine crystals in ocular lesions [12]. Histology shows acanthosis with hyperkeratosis with thickening of the granular layer [7].

Management

In general, reduction of plasma tyrosine can be achieved by restricting the intake of natural protein. To avoid deficiency of essential amino acids, a phenylalanine- and tyrosine-free amino-acid formula is used (plasma tyrosine level below 600 μmol/L). Early initiation of diet causes prompt resolution of the ocular and cutaneous symptoms and prevents the development of mental manifestations [11,13–15].

PALMOPLANTAR KERATODERMA AND NEUROLOGICAL MANIFESTATIONS

This category largely overlaps with the neuro-ichthyotic syndromes, for example CEDNIK, SLS and Chanarin–Dorfmann syndromes as well as TTD (see Tables 63.2 and 63.4). It seems that there are only a few genetic diseases in which pure PPK manifests together with neurological symptoms. Some reports associate neuropathy or spastic paralysis with keratoderma. These include striate keratoderma with spastic paraplegia, pes cavus and intellectual disability in four brothers [1]; autosomal dominant punctate keratoderma and spastic paralysis [2]; autosomal dominant focal keratoderma with nail dystrophy and motor and sensory neuropathy [3]; and Charcot–Marie–Tooth disease [4]. Atypical erythrokeratoderma with deafness has also been associated with peripheral neuropathy [5].

As an example of a differential diagnosis, acro-osteolysis with keratoderma (Bureau–Barrière syndrome) [6,7] may show diffuse keratoderma with osteolysis in the forefoot area, polyneuropathy of the lower legs and painless ulcers of the feet. The disease is non-familial and often subsumed under the concept of neurotrophic ulcers [8].

ACQUIRED KERATODERMAS

This disease group refers to numerous underlying causes summarised and reviewed by Patel *et al.* [1]. Callosities or more extensive thickening of plantar epidermis commonly accompanies obesity and occurs with increasing age or orthopaedic problems [2].

Keratoderma climactericum (Haxthausen disease) [3,4]. The specificity of this entity described in women over the age of 45 is uncertain. For more than 30 years no new reports were available. A strong association with obesity and hypertension has been noted, with pressure areas of the heel and the forefoot involved first (Figure 63.60). Skin inflammation and heavy hyperkeratosis with fissuring make walking painful. The hyperkeratotic areas slowly extend to become confluent. Later, the central palms may be affected. Symptoms may be worse in winter. Deschamps *et al.* [4] excluded endocrine dysfunction, contact dermatitis and fungal infection, and found normal serum vitamin A levels. However, Wachtel [5] described three young women in whom an identical condition arising following bilateral oophorectomy was reversed by oestrogen replacement. Laurent *et al.* [6] implicated keratinisation of the acrosyringium by the finding of composite keratohyaline granules in the granular cells of the interductal granular cells, believed to serve as a marker for acrosyringeal differentiation [7]. In one report, topical 0.05% oestradiol in a water-in-oil base was successful

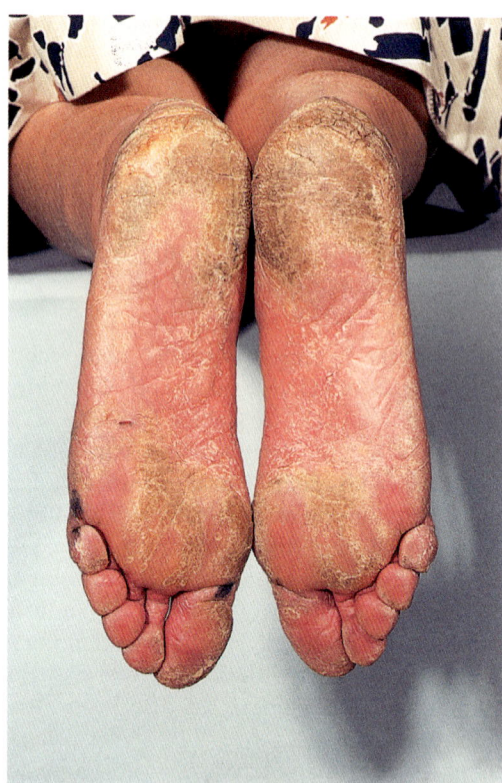

Figure 63.60 Keratoderma climactericum.

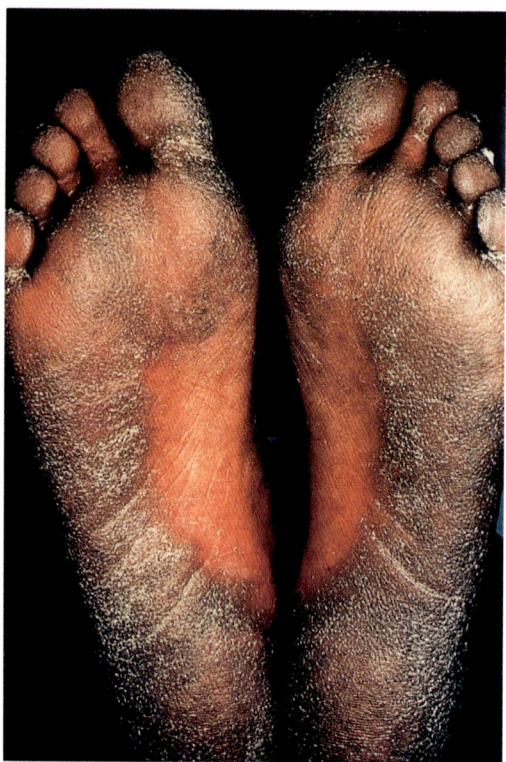

Figure 63.61 Keratoderma associated with lupus erythematosus. Courtesy of Dr I. Sarkany, Royal Free Hospital, London, UK.

where keratolytics and emollients had failed [8]. Given the success of etretinate, acitretine may be the treatment of choice [1].

Inflammatory dermatoses. In psoriasis, both diffuse gross and centripalmar hyperkeratosis are seen. A scalloped margin ('festonné'), Caro–Senear lesions (depressed plaques) on the sides of the fingers and involvement of the knuckles may suggest the diagnosis. The lesions of reactive arthritis are compact, heaped up and resemble the heads of nails (keratoderma blenorrhagica). Extensive hyperkeratotic eczema may be difficult to distinguish on clinical and histological grounds but marked itching may indicate eczema. The even orange hyperkeratosis of pityriasis rubra pilaris is associated with an acute follicular eruption in adults and by lesions on the knees and elbows in children. Lupus erythematosus may show dry and atrophic [9], hypertrophic (Figure 63.61) [10] or ulcerative [11] palmar lesions. Keratoderma is also reported in association with acrocyanosis and livedo reticularis [12]. Antidesmocollin 3 antibodies were found in a patient with an immunobullous disorder and acquired diffuse PPK [13]. In lichen planus, warty lesions may be mistaken for viral warts; lichen planus and other lichenoid eruptions such as lichen nitidus may mimic punctate keratoderma [14].

Infections. Trichophytosis, especially resulting from *Trichophyton rubrum*, may be unilateral and lacking inflammatory signs. Keratoderma may be seen in crusted scabies (Figure 63.62). The tendency of secondary syphilis lesions to involve the palms is well known, and hyperkeratotic late syphilides may be warty or focal [15]. Tropical diseases such as late yaws may be complicated by keratoderma. In immunocompromised patients, viral warts may be confluent on the palms or soles.

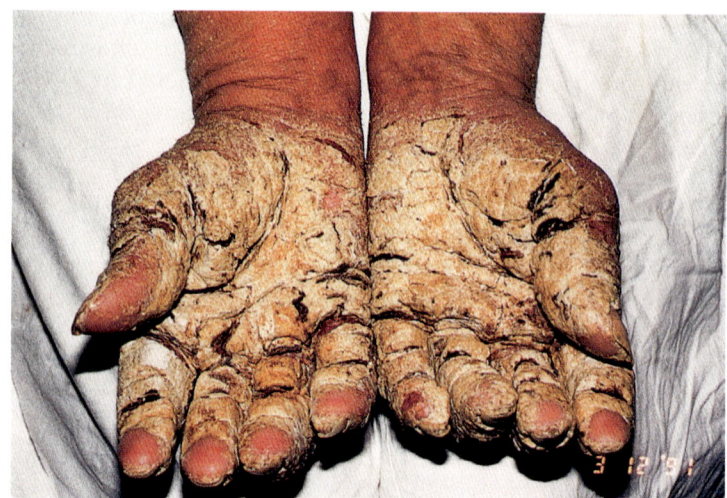

Figure 63.62 Norwegian scabies manifesting with keratoderma. Courtesy of Dr. N. Walker, Oxford Radcliffe Hospital, Oxford, UK.

Myxoedema and lymphoedema. Palmoplantar hyperkeratosis with myxoedema, improving with treatment, has been reported on several occasions [16,17]. As such, hypothyroidism must be suspected in patients with acquired PPK [18]. In chronic lymphoedema, the skin overlying the lymphoedematous area first becomes diffusely thickened, and then develops into a velvety papillomatous surface, which is ultimately covered by large irregular warty projections (lymphostatic verrucosis or mossy foot) [19–21]. The condition may simulate chromoblastomycosis. Lymphoedematous keratoderma occurs most characteristically in filariasis, but may develop in the context of chronic lymphoedema of any origin. Histologically, there is hyperkeratosis, acanthosis and papillomatosis. The dermis is oedematous with dilated lymphatics, conspicuous new-vessel formation, some sclerosis and a variable infiltrate of inflammatory cells. Both the hyperkeratotic component and the lymphoedema improved in three cases given etretinate 0.6 mg/kg/day [19].

Malignancy. In addition to 'tripe palms' (Chapter 148) and Bazex acrokeratosis paraneoplastica (Chapter 148), acquired diffuse PPK has been observed with cancer of the bronchus [22,23], and filiform PPK has been reported with cancer of the breast, colon and kidney [24–26]. As for acquired ichthyoses, mycosis fungoides is an important differential diagnosis for acquired PPK [27]. Carcinogens, of which the best documented example is arsenic, may produce both keratoderma and internal malignancy [28,29]. One survey showed that palmar keratoses occur four to five times more frequently in patients with cancer than in controls [30]. An increased incidence of keratoses in patients with lung or bladder cancer has been debated [31–33]. Smoking [31] and papillomavirus infection [32] are suggested culprits. Keratoses associated with cancer are histologically distinct from arsenical keratoses [34].

Drugs. Keratoderma may be seen as a result of hypersensitivity to drugs such as iodine. Keratoderma may result from tegafur, glucan, lithium and halogenated weed-killers, and dioxin intoxication [35–39]. Arsenical-induced irregular warty keratoses, or more even glassy lesions, are still occasionally seen [40]. Agents used in cancer treatment commonly cause palmoplantar redness (hand–foot syndrome) and may cause keratoderma [35,41,42].

MISCELLANEOUS DISORDERS OF KERATINISATION

Keratolytic winter erythema

Definition and nomenclature

This rare epidermal disorder, characterised by recurrent skin peeling, palmoplantar erythema and seasonal variation, was originally described as erythrokeratolysis hiemalis in 1977.

Synonyms and inclusions
- Oudtshoorn disease
- Erythrokeratolysis hiemalis

Epidemiology

It has been observed in at least 35 South African families of European descent originating from the Oudtshoorn district of Cape Provence [1,2]. The incidence in this population is 1/7000. Cases have since been identified in several other countries, and a familial link to the Oudtshoorn cluster is evident in most.

Pathophysiology

This an autosomal dominant disorder with variable penetrance and linkage to chromosome 8p22–p23 has been reported in five South African and one German kindreds [3]. No pathogenic mutations were initially found in candidate genes within the disease region, cathepsin B (*CTSB*) and farnesyl-diphosphate farnesyltransferase 1 (*FDFT1*) [4,5]. However, a duplication of an intergenic enhancer element upstream of the cathepsin B gene on chromosome 8 has been identified that leads to upregulation of cathepsin B in the stratum granulosum and subsequent detachment of the epidermis [6]. The genetic alteration may have originated in a French immigrant in the late 1700s. Over 400 descendants are affected. A Norwegian family with four affected members did not show linkage to chromosome 8p22–p23, suggesting genetic heterogeneity [7]. A frequent precipitant is cold dry weather and, although in South Africa it is most active in the winter months, it may be perennial in temperate climates. Other triggers include febrile illness, surgery, stress and menstruation, and it improves in pregnancy and with age. The father of an affected toddler was unaffected but paternal aunts and other family members had similar palmoplantar eruptions and her paternal great-great-grandmother originated from Oudtshoorn [8], suggestive of partial penetrance.

Of note, a point mutation in the *CTSB* gene was found to result in increased cathepsin B proteolytic activity and PPK, with no apparent season-related fluctuation in disease activity [9].

Clinical features

Symmetrical keratolysis of the hands and feet may begin at any age from infancy to early adult life but it is not usually present at birth. Cyclical centrifugal peeling (sometimes preceded by erythema multiforme-like papules) at several sites on the palms (Figure 63.63a) and soles is a constant feature, and may spread to the dorsal hands and feet, and the interdigital spaces. Episodes may be preceded by itch and hyperhidrosis and associated with pustulation. Palmoplantar inflammation develops, and is followed by the evolution of painless, superficial, opaque, dry blebs, which peel or can be pulled away, leaving a red base with intact markings. A second wave may begin at the centre of a lesion, resulting in gyrate and polycyclic annular erythema, which eventually resolves. Cycles repeat every few weeks and the palms and soles appear normal between attacks. Similar rosette lesions may arise on the lower legs, knees and rarely the thighs (Figure 63.63b), upper arms and shoulders. Truncal lesions were reported in one patient [2], and facial involvement in another [10].

Differential diagnosis

This includes familial peeling skin syndromes, pustular bacterids, annular erythema, erythema multiforme, Hailey–Hailey disease, erythrokeratoderma and localised epidermolysis bullosa simplex. A similar phenotype affecting the palms, more active in summertime, was reported in two siblings (British) who had atypical autosomal recessive erythropoietic protoporphyria [11].

Investigations

A biopsy of the advancing edge of a lesion shows hyperplasia, spongiosis and, in the upper stratum spinosum, keratinocytes with pale

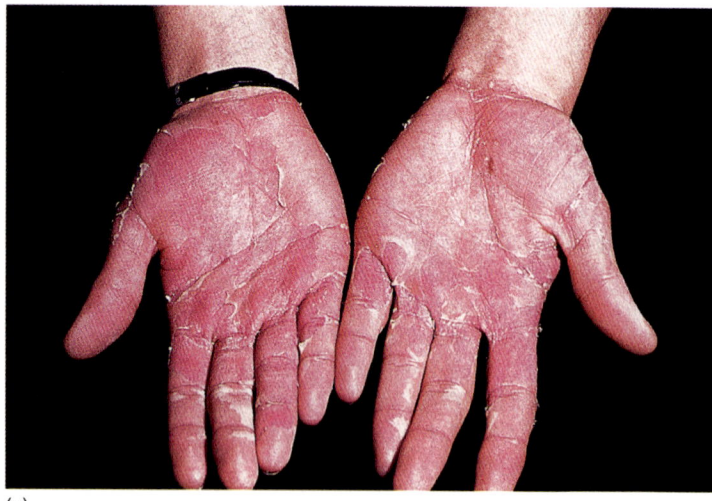

(a)

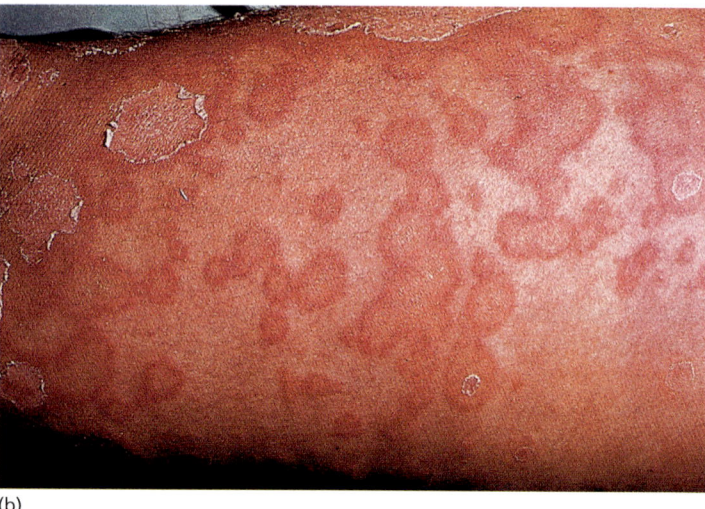

(b)

Figure 63.63 Oudtshoorn disease: (a) palmar lesions, and (b) truncal lesions.

cytoplasm, perinuclear vacuolisation and pycnotic nuclei. In the abscence of a granular layer, the epidermis forms a parakeratotic wedge, which becomes sandwiched within the hyperkeratotic stratum corneum and is shed [2]. During regeneration, undifferentiated keratinocytes are not confined to the basal layer but appear in the lower half of the epidermis [12]. Skin histology in the Norwegian family was non-specific [6].

Management

There is no effective treatment, and topical keratolytics, retinoids and steroids may aggravate the condition. Urea and tar compounds, antiperspirants, oral retinoids and photodynamic therapy have been tried [13].

Porokeratoses

Definition and nomenclature

Porokeratoses refer to a heterogeneous group of keratinisation disorders, in which the presence of a so-called 'cornoid lamella' in a

lesion can be seen. Clinical distinction between the various forms of disseminated porokeratosis may not be justified [1].

The disorders are characterised by marginate keratotic lesions, histologically showing a column of parakeratotic keratinocytes (the cornoid lamella). Various forms are recognised, but terminology and classification are still debated [2,3]. Some forms appear to be premalignant [4].

> **Synonyms and inclusions**
> - Parakeratosis centrifugata atrophicans
> - Parakeratosis Mibelli

Pathophysiology

Disseminated superficial (actinic) porokeratosis (DSAP) has been mapped in Chinese pedigrees to 12q [5], 15q [6], 18p [7] and 16q [8]. Loss of heterozygosity at 12q and sequence variations in genes at this locus have been reported, but the significance of these findings is uncertain [9–13]. More recently, heterozygous germline mutations in the mevalonate pathway genes have been reported in familial and sporadic porokeratosis of Mibelli and in DSAP [14–20]. Second-hit somatic mutations were detected in linear porokeratosis [21,22]. The mevalonate pathway regulates keratinocyte growth and differentiation, cytoskeleton assembly and intracellular signalling. Of note, biallelic mutations in *MVK* are associated with a neurological disorder called mevalonic aciduria. It is still unclear why no cutaneous phenotype is seen in the parents of children with mevalonic aciduria, who are obligatory carriers of *MVK* mutations.

The centrifugal progress of individual lesions is thought to reflect the migration of a clone of abnormal cells [23]. There is keratinocyte dysplasia, and Otsuka *et al.* [24,25] have reported aneuploidy and chromosomal abnormalities in lesional keratinocytes. The tumour suppressor protein p53 is overexpressed in the cornoid lamella [26–29], but D'Errico *et al.* [29] found no evidence of p53 mutations or radiation hypersensitivity in DSAP-derived keratinocytes and fibroblasts. Cytogenetic anomalies in fibroblasts, particularly chromosome 3, are also recorded [30]. An association with immunosuppression [2] suggests impaired immunity is permissive, perhaps by reduced immune surveillance of dysplasia, but the possibility of an infective aetiology [31] remains. Esser *et al.* [32] found evidence of HPV types 66 and 14, respectively, in two patients with porokeratosis of Mibelli.

Clinical features
Clinical variants
Disseminated superficial actinic porokeratosis. This form is the most common presentation, with multiple lesions of up to 10 mm predominantly found in sun-exposed sites in middle-aged individuals, in particular on the extremities of women, especially those with sun-sensitive skin (Figure 63.64). The papules are surrounded by a keratotic ridge albeit finer than in Mibelli porokeratosis. They are easily mistaken for actinic keratoses, with which they may coexist. Lesions are not induced by artificial light exposure [33], but have been provoked by photochemotherapy [34]. Radiotherapy has also been shown to exacerbate the disease. No evidence that skin

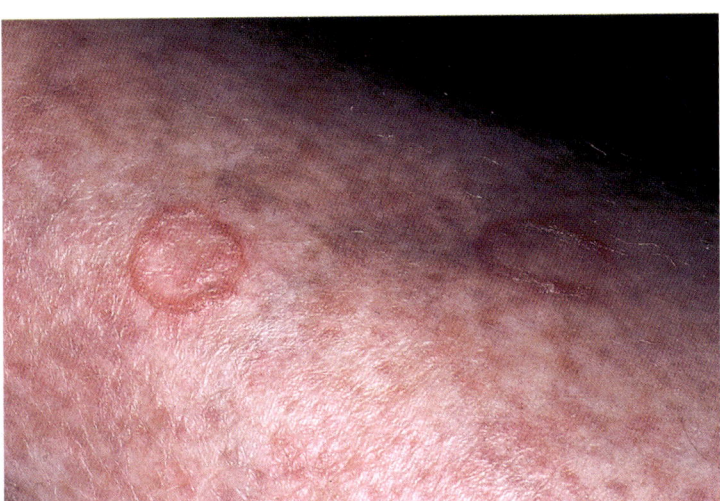

Figure 63.64 Disseminated superficial actinic porokeratoses: annular keratotic lesions with a raised margin.

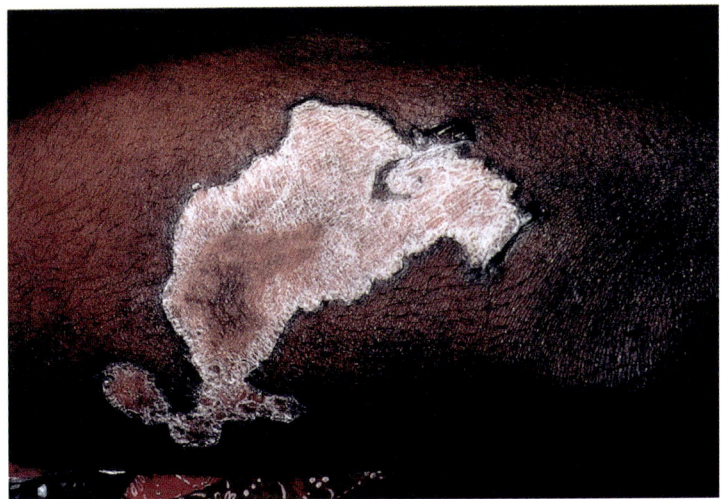

Figure 63.65 Porokeratosis of Mibelli.

cancer arises in the porokeratotic lesions was found in a study of 29 patients [35].

Disseminated superficial porokeratoses of immunosuppression. This variant has been reported after renal, hepatic, cardiac and bone marrow transplantation, and in AIDS [2]. The distribution of the lesions is similar to DSAP, but a history of sun exposure is less likely [36].

Disseminated superficial porokeratosis of childhood. The condition may be inherited as an autosomal dominant disorder, but sporadic cases are seen. Widely disseminated flat lesions usually begin in childhood, the majority appear between the ages of 5 and 10 years, but they may be present at birth or may first appear at puberty or later. Palmoplantar lesions may be associated (porokeratosis palmaris et plantaris disseminata) [37]. Widespread lesions appeared first at the age of 1 month in a male infant with craniosynostosis and other congenital abnormalities [38].

Porokeratosis of Mibelli [39,40]. The eponym Mibelli is sometimes used generically for porokeratoses, but usually refers only to the form with single or scanty and larger lesions. These develop as annular dry plaques (Figure 63.65) surrounded by a raised, fine, keratotic, elevated border with a central groove. Lesions are most common on the limbs and by centrifugal spread may achieve several centimetres in diameter. The centre is usually atrophic but may be hyperkeratotic [41]. The face, scalp, nails, genitalia, oral mucosa and cornea may also be affected. The condition may be familial, inherited as an autosomal dominant trait with onset in childhood (MIM: 175800), or sporadic and of later onset.

Giant porokeratoses. These are up to 20 cm in diameter with a surrounding elevated edge of 1 cm. They are very rare [42], and are most often found on the foot. Large lesions are said to have the highest potential for malignant transformation [4,42,43].

Palmoplantar porokeratosis (of Mantoux). Parakeratotic hyperkeratosis histologically reminiscent of the cornoid lamella occurs in some punctate keratodermas, but the absence of marginate lesions distinguishes this entity from true porokeratosis [44]. Nonetheless, annular lesions of the palms and soles with a cornoid lamella are recognised [32,45].

Linear porokeratosis [43,46,47]. Linear porokeratoses showing typical cornoid lamellae and following the lines of Blaschko usually appear in childhood. These lesions probably result from a predisposition to porokeratosis in an abnormal clone of epidermal precursors. Malignant degeneration and metastasis have been reported in this variant [43,48]. Linear accentuation of disseminated actinic porokeratosis has also been reported [49–51].

Porokeratosis ptychotropica [52–54]. This rare type of porokeratosis is confined to body folds ('ptyche', Greek for a fold). Brownish to reddish macules or plaques usually develop symmetrically on the perianal region, and, as reported in one patient, on the scrotum. The typical presence of multiple cornoid lamellae as seen histologically (punctate type of porokeratosis) explains the keratotic or verrucous appearance and expansile papular growth. The highly pruritic disease is mostly confined to men ranging from 6 to 84 years of age. Linear porokeratoses or DSAP may coexist.

Investigations

The characteristic histopathology is seen on the edge of the lesion when cut at right angles. The stratum corneum is hyperkeratotic, and at the raised border a column of poorly staining parakeratotic stratum corneum cells, the cornoid lamella, is seen running obliquely through the surrounding normal-staining cells. The underlying keratinocytes are large, vacuolated, with some of them dyskeratotic and pleomorphic. The granular layer is absent beneath the parakeratotic column. Beneath, a variably dense lichenoid lymphocytic infiltrate, less frequently colloid bodies and amyloid material, may be present [55,56]. These changes can also affect the hair follicles or acrosyringia. The involvement of the sweat pores explains the term 'poro' keratosis. The central area of a lesion is usually atrophic, but may occasionally show gross hyperkeratosis.

The papillary dermis is fibrotic and contains melanophages [57]. Cornoid lamellae may also be found in other conditions, such as viral warts, some ichthyoses and naevoid hyperkeratoses, but the characteristic changes of the underlying keratinocytes are absent.

Management

Treatment of disseminated superficial porokeratoses is usually unnecessary. Photoprotection should be recommended. Keratolytics offer little relief. Topical tacalcitol [58], topical retinoids, 5-fluorouracil ointment [59,60], imiquimod cream [61] and oral etretinate [62] have been effective. Diclofenac gel was disappointing [63]. Cryotherapy, carbon dioxide, pulsed dye laser therapy and photodynamic treatment have all been used with variable results [64–66]. Deep dermabrasion by a dermatome is useful in porokeratosis ptychotropica [67]. Only recently, a pathogenesis-directed therapy was shown to improve various forms of porokeratosis in a case series with five patients [68]. Topical application of cholesterol, an essential mevalonate pathway end-product, together with lovastatin, seems to effectively block the accumulation of mevalonate pathway toxic metabolites.

Perforating keratotic disorders

The nature of perforating (epidermal elimination) disorders is uncertain [1]. They present as keratotic papules, but as epidermal involvement may be secondary to dermal disease they are probably not true disorders of keratinisation. The unifying term 'acquired perforating dermatosis' and a subclassification have been proposed [2,3]. Many patients suffer from chronic pruritus and can be diagnosed as having an umbilicated type of prurigo [4].

Pathophysiology

The concept of a genuine perforation is increasingly disputed [5]. Trauma from scratching is thought to initiate the lesions. An umbilicated type of prurigo shares many clinical and histological features with acquired reactive perforating dermatosis. A reduced wound healing capacity due to underlying systemic disorders, particularly diabetes mellitus and uraemia, has been assumed for the development of umbilicated skin lesions with a perforating aspect [6]. Familial occurrence, with ocular involvement, is reported (MIM: 149500) [7,8].

Clinical features

Follicular or non-follicular keratotic papules or nodules up to 1 cm in diameter are seen mainly on the limbs (Figure 63.66). Some of the lesions show a central depression containing an adherent necrotic plug. It is most often seen with diabetes or before, during or after dialysis for renal failure [9]. Eleven per cent of 72 British patients on renal dialysis developed a perforating dermatosis [10]. Many individual reports of association with malignancy, infection or inflammatory conditions have been published, but often also with renal failure or diabetes [6,11]. A patient who developed a perforating folliculitis with two anti-TNF agents improved on withdrawal [12].

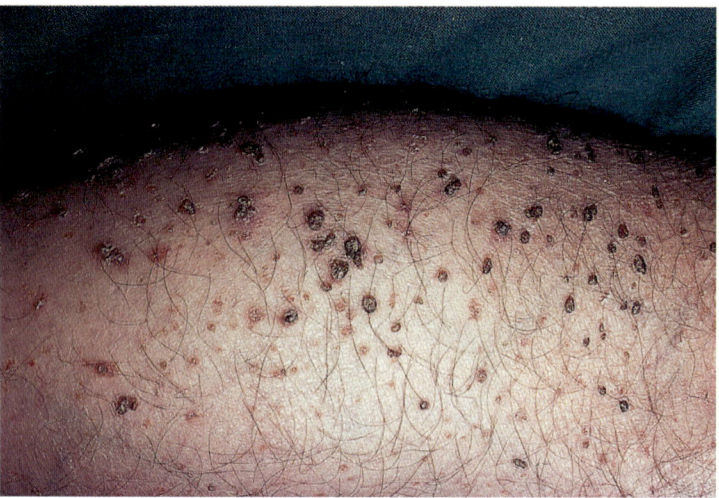

Figure 63.66 Kyrle disease/acquired perforating dermatosis: large keratinous plugs on the thigh.

Clinical variants

Necrotising infundibular crystalline folliculitis. Lucke *et al.* [13] reported two cases of a disorder characterised by transepidermal elimination of negatively birefringent, needle-shaped crystals similar to monosodium urate. Kossard *et al.* [14] reported a similar case and suggested that the disorder was due to the initiation of crystal formation around microorganisms from follicular lipids at critical concentrations. Clinically, multiple waxy papules develop with a predilection for the forehead, neck and back. A dermatomal distribution on the chest and back has been described following an episode of herpes zoster in a patient on PD-1 immune checkpoint inhibitor therapy [15]. Histology reveals necrosis of the follicular epithelium and sometimes a perifollicular neutrophilic infiltrate. Crystalline deposits with yeasts and Gram-positive bacteria are found in the follicular ostia and are enclosed by parakeratotic columns [16]. In addition, these histological changes can also be found as a coincidental finding in the vicinity of epithelial skin neoplasms [16]. Resolution of the lesions after topical or systemic antimycotic treatment suggests a microbial pathogenesis [16].

Elastosis perforans serpiginosa (Chapter 94). This presents as grouped arcuate or serpiginous keratotic papules and is associated with Down syndrome, disorders of connective tissue and penicillamine treatment. Histologically, amorphous masses that bind elastic tissue stains can be seen traversing the epidermis [17].

Reactive perforating collagenosis (Chapter 94). This mainly affects children, with the formation of 2–5 mm papules, usually on the limbs. Lesions in all stages of eruption and resolution are present at any one time [18].

Investigations

Histology of acquired perforating dermatoses may show follicular and non-follicular lesions with broad or narrow ulcer craters [11]. Degenerate collagen, elastic tissue and keratin are seen mixed with an unidentified clear material, which has been regarded by some as an accumulation of a metabolite [2]. Changes diagnosed as perforating folliculitis, reactive perforating collagenosis or *Kyrle disease* (hyperkeratosis follicularis et parafollicularis in cutem penetrans) may all be found [19–21].

Management

In most cases of acquired perforating dermatosis, lesions can be cleared by treatment with potent topical or intralesional steroids and antipruritic therapy [22]. Success with conventional or narrow-band ultraviolet B phototherapy has also been recorded [23–25]. Topical tretinoin may reduce the lesions. Other agents reported to be effective include allopurinol [26] and doxycycline [27].

Multiple minute digitate hyperkeratoses

Definition and nomenclature

A number of entities have been described using names including *minute* and *filiform keratoses, disseminated spiked hyperkeratosis, minute aggregate keratosis* or *digitate keratosis* [1–4]. An inclusive approach to classification has been proposed under the name 'multiple minute digitate hyperkeratoses' [5]; and a useful algorithm is given in Caccetta *et al.* [6].

Clinical features

Cases may be sporadic [3] or familial with probable autosomal dominant inheritance [2,7,8], early or late onset, transient or persistent. Non-follicular spiky keratoses develop on the trunk and limbs (Figure 63.67) [6]. Reported associations include drugs, malignancy, especially haematological, and X-irradiation [4,5,8–13]. Hyperkeratotic spicules on the face, particularly on the nose, are follicular and often associated with paraproteinaemia, multiple myeloma and croyglobulinaemia, but may be also idiopathic [10,11]. One case associated with carcinoma of the larynx cleared following surgery [14]. Filiform keratoses occur with a pityriasis rubra pilaris-like eruption and acne conglobata in association with HIV infection [15]. A familial form of filiform keratosis has

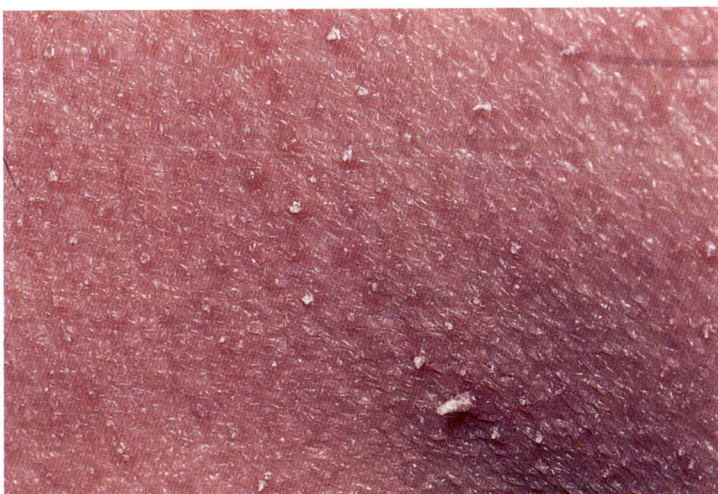

Figure 63.67 Digitate hyperkeratosis. Courtesy of Dr F. A. Ive, Dryburn Hospital, Durham, UK.

been described to be associated with thickened nails, plantar hyperkeratosis, joint laxity and long fingers [16].

Differential diagnosis

Spiny palmoplantar keratosis [17,18] is recognised as a particular type of PPK (see 'Spiny keratoderma' earlier in this chapter).

Investigations

Histologically, there are focal areas of compact orthohyperkeratotic spicules mostly arising from a pointed epidermal elevation. The stratum granulosum usually is prominent [6,19]. Parakeratosis may be present [16,20] but use of the term porokeratosis is misleading [5,6]. Hyperkeratotic spicules associated with paraproteinaemia reveal eosinophilic inclusions in the hyperkeratotic columns that represent immunoglobulin deposits [10].

Management

Treatment including keratolytics and retinoids is often unsuccessful [6].

Flegel disease

Definition and nomenclature

Flegel disease is a rare and benign cornification disorder of older individuals characterised by multiple, reddish-brown, keratotic papules affecting the extremities [1,2].

Synonyms and inclusions
- Hyperkeratosis lenticularis perstans

Pathophysiology

This is inherited as an autosomal dominant condition [3]. Despite the strong genetic component in the disorder, no reports identifying a candidate gene have appeared to date. A low proliferation rate of keratinocytes together with downregulation of filaggrin, loricrin and high-molecular-weight keratins and loss of the keratin pattern in the horny layer suggest a retention hyperkeratosis and complex dysregulation of the epidermal differentiation [4].

Clinical features

Keratotic red-brown papules 2 3 mm in diameter with discrete irregular margins ('cornflake sign') appear over the dorsa of the feet and on the lower parts of the legs, after the third or fourth decade. Dermoscopy may support the diagnosis by showing white scales, a brownish background and sparse brown dots [5]. The lesions may spread to the upper part of the legs and thighs, also disseminating over the arms and trunk or concha of the ear. Fine points may appear on the palms and soles (Figure 63.68) [1,6]. Some patients complain of pruritus. The keratotic scale can be removed, leaving a non-exudative, red bleeding base.

Investigations

Histologically, there is hyperkeratosis with a focal parakeratosis overlying a thinned flat epidermis with a loss of keratohyalin granules. In the periphery of the lesions, the epidermis is acanthotic

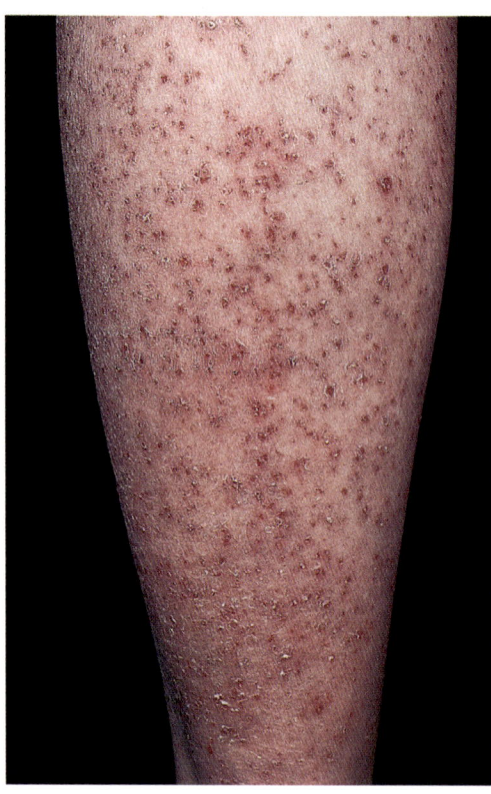

Figure 63.68 Flegel disease: polygonal keratotic lesions on the legs.

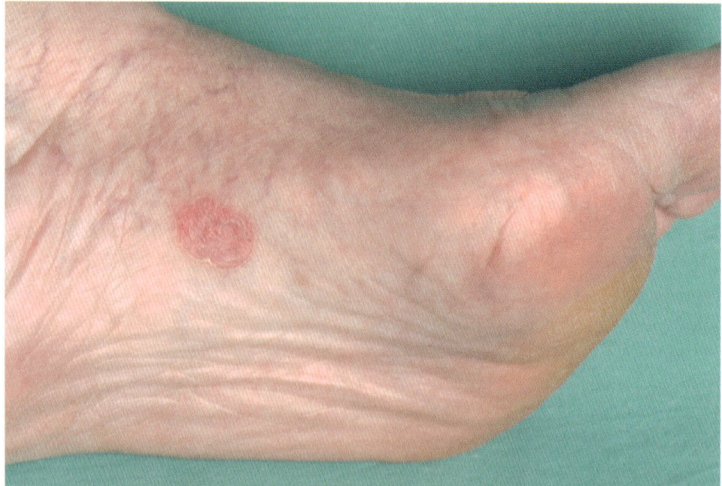

Figure 63.69 Circumscribed hypokeratosis on the inner part of the forefoot of a female patient. Courtesy of Dr F. Schedel, Department of Dermatology, University Hospital Münster, Münster, Germany.

with collarette-like elongated rete ridges. A lymphocytic lichenoid infiltrate can be found in early lesions. Upon electron microscopy, membrane-coated granules (Odland bodies) appear reduced and malformed at least in evolving lesions [1,3,4,7,8].

Management

Treatment remains difficult and many modalities have been recommended, including cryotherapy, topical corticosteroids, topical and systemic retinoids, calcipotriol, psoralen and UVA (PUVA) and 5-fluorouracil, albeit with variable efficacy [2,4,9].

Circumscribed palmoplantar hypokeratosis

Definition and nomenclature

Circumscribed palmoplantar hypokeratosis presents with well-demarcated, depressed patches of reddened skin on the palms or soles.

Synonyms and inclusions
- Circumscribed acral hypokeratosis
- Circumscribed hypokeratosis of the hand

Pathophysiology

This condition is considered a localised keratinisation disorder of an expanding clone of keratinocytes [1]. Acanthosis, dilated tortuous

capillaries and coarse keratohyalin granules are also suggestive of a viral origin. Molecular studies failed to detect HPV apart from one report that found HPV-4-specific DNA [2].

Clinical features

Circumscribed hypokeratosis of the palms and soles is characterised by a solitary, red, sharply circumscribed depression on the thenar or hypothenar region of the palms or on the soles (Figure 63.69). Only rarely more than one lesion appears. Most patients are women between the ages of 42 and 84 years [3,4]. Congenital cases are exceptional [5]. Sometimes there is a history of prior trauma or burn at the site [6]. Circumscribed acral hypokeratosis is considered to be a benign process; however one case each of actinic keratosis and Bowen disease have been described in association with circumscribed acral hypokeratosis [7]. Alternatively, the features of circumscribed acral hypokeratosis may occure secondary to an underlying squamous cell carcinoma *in situ* [8].

Investigations

Histologically, an abrupt thinning of the stratum corneum over a diminished granular layer forms a sharp stair between normal and involved skin [6]. Some histological features suggest a traumatic genesis [9]. Malignant transformation is unlikely although susceptibility to photocarcinogenesis has been assumed [7,10].

Management

Topical calcipotriol [11], cryotherapy [12], photodynamic therapy [13] or fluorouracil cream [14] can be tried. However, total excision of the lesion is the definite treatment.

Waxy keratoses of childhood

Definition and nomenclature

This condition appears typically in children presenting with asymptomatic small hyperkeratotic papules, for instance on the trunk or proximal limbs. The aetiology is unknown, and only a few cases have been reported so far [1].

> **Synonyms and inclusions**
> • Kerinokeratosis papulosa

Clinical features

Three children in two families showed generalised, discrete, domed keratotic papules, which were flesh coloured or yellowish [2]. Dermatoscopy reveals a cribriform pattern [3]. Two young patients reported earlier with 'disseminated hypopigmented keratoses' appeared to be identical [4]. Late manifestation in an adult has been observed [5]. The disorder has been reported in a linear form [6] and as a linear exacerbation in generalised disease [7], further supporting the notion that it could be a genodermatosis. The pattern resembles confluent and reticulated papillomatosis (Gougerot–Carteaud syndrome), but waxy keratosis shows more hyperkeratosis. Differential diagnosis includes the leukodermic macules in Darier disease in dark skin [8]. Larger papules with a mosaic pattern and acral distribution have been diagnosed as mosaic acral keratosis (see also 'Marginal papular keratoderma' earlier in this chapter) [9].

Investigations

Histological findings are marked orthokeratotic hyperkeratosis, tenting and papillomatosis of the epidermis, and mild acanthosis. The detection of HPV-57 might hint at an etiological role of HPV [3].

Hyperkeratosis of the nipple

Definition

This condition is defined by progressive diffuse hyperkeratotic thickening of both areolas, with a predominance in women.

Pathophysiology

The occurrence and aggravation around puberty, pregnancy or systemic hormone treatment suggest a hormonal influence [1].

Clinical features

The lesions are bilateral and involve predominantly the top of the nipple. Lesions may cause tenderness or discomfort, pruritus, sensitivity to touch or discomfort with breastfeeding [2]. Naevoid hyperkeratosis of the nipple and areola may either appear isolated or associated with an epidermal naevus and other dermatoses such as acanthosis nigricans, Darier disease, chronic eczema, chronic mucocutaneous candidiasis or cutaneous T-cell lymphoma [3,4].

Differential diagnosis

The most important differential diagnosis is Paget disease.

Investigations

Histologically, papillomatosis, acanthosis and hyperkeratosis of the epidermis can be found. The rete ridges are filiform and anastomising and the basal layer appears hyperpigmented. A sparse lymphocytic infiltrate and intraepidermal collections of lymphocytes must not be confused with T-cell lymphoma.

Management

Treatment includes topical agents (keratolytics, steroid, retinoic acid, calcipotriol) [5,6] and ablative modalities (cryotherapy, carbon dioxide laser, radiofrequency, shave excision) [7–9].

Key references

The full list of references can be found in the online version at https://www.wiley.com/rooksdermatology10e

Ichthyoses
2 Traupe H. *The Ichthyoses. A Guide to Clinical Diagnosis, Genetic Counseling, and Therapy.* Berlin: Springer-Verlag, 1989.
3 Elias PM, Williams ML, Crumrine D, Schmuth M. *Ichthyoses: Clinical Biochemical, Pathogenic and Diagnostic Assessment.* Basel: Karger Verlag, 2010.

Exfoliative disorders of cornification
Comèl–Netherton syndrome
89 Paller AS, Renert-Yuval Y, Suprun M *et al.* An IL-17-dominant immune profile is shared across the major orphan forms of ichthyosis. *J Allergy Clin Immunol* 2017;139:152–65.

Management of congenital ichthyoses
General aspects of therapy
3 Mazereeuw-Hautier J, Vahlquist A, Traupe H *et al.* Management of congenital ichthyoses: European guidelines of care, part one. *Br J Dermatol* 2019;180:272–81.
4 Mazereeuw-Hautier J, Hernández-Martín A, O'Toole EA *et al.* Management of congenital ichthyoses: European guidelines of care, part two. *Br J Dermatol* 2019;180:484–95.
6 Vahlquist A, Gånemo A, Virtanen M. Congenital ichthyosis: an overview of current and emerging therapies. *Acta Derm Venereol* 2008;88:4–14.

Conventional systemic treatment options
14 Oji V, Preil ML, Kleinow B *et al.* S1 guidelines for the diagnosis and treatment of ichthyoses – update. *J Dtsch Dermatol Ges* 2017;15:1053–65.

Palmoplantar keratodermas
1 Greither A. Erbliche Palmoplantarkeratosen. *Hautarzt* 1977;28:395–403.
2 Thomas BR, O'Toole EA. Diagnosis and management of inherited palmoplantar keratodermas. *Acta Derm Venereol.* 2020;100:adv00094.
3 Oji V, Tadini G, Akiyama M *et al.* Revised nomenclature and classification of inherited ichthyoses: results of the First Ichthyosis Consensus Conference in Sorèze 2009. *J Am Acad Dermatol* 2010;63:607–41.

CHAPTER 64

Inherited Acantholytic Disorders

Mozheh Zamiri

Department of Dermatology, Queen Elizabeth University Hospital, Glasgow, UK

DARIER DISEASE

Definition, nomenclature and classification

Darier disease (DD) is an autosomal dominant genodermatosis characterised by a chronic eruption of keratotic papules, the histology of which shows acantholysis and dyskeratosis.

Synonyms and inclusions
- Darier–White disease
- Keratosis follicularis

Classification links
- MIM: 124200

Introduction and general description

Darier disease was first described independently by Darier and White in 1889 [1,2]. It is characterised by chronic and recurrent focal and aggregated keratotic papules, generally of teenage or adult onset, predominantly in seborrhoeic areas. Other lesions include distinctive nail and palmoplantar abnormalities [3,4,5] and mucosal involvement. Histology of the keratotic lesions shows suprabasal acantholysis with overlying dyskeratosis [3]. The disorder is inherited in an autosomal dominant manner [4] but new mutations are relatively common and the eruption may present in a naevoid distribution. Although DD has no consistent extracutaneous associations, an increased frequency of neuropsychiatric disease has been noted [6–9]. It is generally managed with topical antimicrobials and corticosteroids, but oral retinoids are the mainstay of management in severe cases.

Epidemiology

Darier disease has a worldwide distribution; prevalence is estimated at 1 : 30 000–55 000 [3,4,7,10–12]. Men and women are equally often affected, with the rash usually first appearing in early teenage years, but patients may present in childhood or not until their sixth or seventh decade [3]. Penetrance is complete in adults [4], although phenotypic expression may be variable with some patients featuring

nail changes only [5]. In some families, plane wart-like keratoses, known as acrokeratosis verruciformis, predominate [10,13,14].

Pathophysiology

Histologically, DD shows disordered cell adhesion (acantholysis) and differentiation (Figure 64.1), and lesions are not only perifollicular [15]. Lacunae appear suprabasally in the earliest lesions, and extend irregularly throughout the Malpighian layer [3,5]. In the overlying epidermis, rounded dyskeratotic cells with eosinophilic cytoplasm ('corps ronds') give rise to small cells with shrunken cytoplasm ('grains') and the stratum corneum is hyperkeratotic. Immunohistochemistry shows desmosomal components diffusely distributed in the cytoplasm of acantholytic cells, and their intra- and extracellular domains are dissociated [16–18]. Ultrastructurally, tonofilaments separate from the desmosomes with aggregation of keratin filaments around the cell nucleus [19].

DD and also Hailey–Hailey disease (HHD) are due to mutations in the intracellular calcium pumps, members of an evolutionarily ancient family of P-type cation transport adenosine triphosphatases (ATPases) [20]. In DD mutations are found in *ATP2A2* [21,22–25,26], a gene at chromosome locus 12q24.1 [27,28], encoding sarco/endoplasmic reticulum Ca^{2+}-ATPase type 2 (SERCA2) [21] located in the endoplasmic reticulum (ER). SERCAs are transmembrane channels that pump Ca^{2+} against a calcium gradient [29]. When ATP phosphorylates the channel, the resultant conformational change causes the release of the Ca^{2+} ions into the ER lumen [30]. The pump is then dephosphorylated and the cycle can recommence. The *ATP2A2* gene has 20 or 21 exons depending on the isoform and encodes a 4.4 kb transcript with four isoforms due to alternative splicing [30]. SERCA2a is expressed in slow-twitch skeletal and cardiac muscle [29,31–33]; SERCA2b and SERCA2c are more widely expressed. SERCA2d exists in muscle [32]. SERCA2b is the major isoform in the epidermis [12,34].

Over 280 different pathogenic mutations in *ATP2A2* have now been reported in patients with DD [21,22–25,26,35–44] (see also LOVD, www.lovd.nl/, last accessed February 2022), which include missense, nonsense and frameshift mutations, and in-frame deletions, splicing or insertions scattered throughout the sequence of *ATP2A2*. At least 75% are unique mutations to the family affected [44] but in 12–40% of patients no mutations are found [12]. Many

PART 6: GENETIC DISORDERS

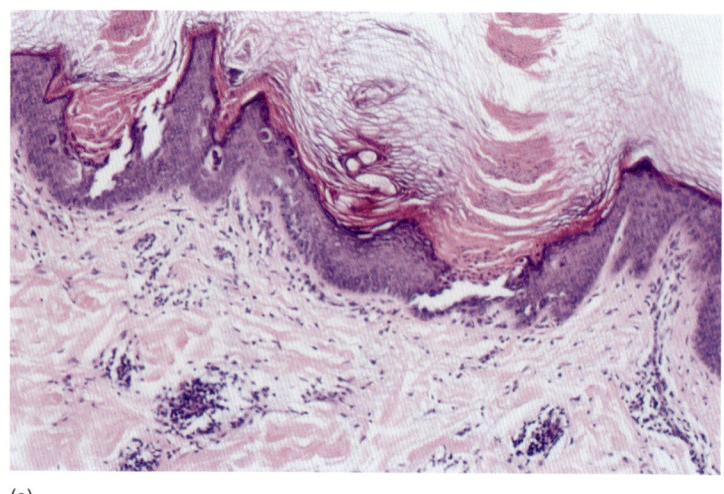

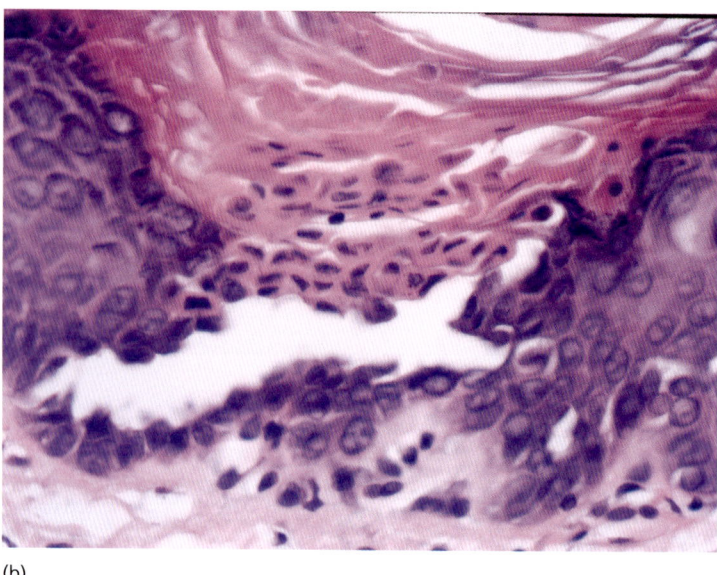

(a)

(b)

Figure 64.1 Histology of Darier disease demonstrating (a) acantholysis with suprabasal clefting; and (b) in close-up, rounded dyskeratotic cells with eosinophilic cytoplasm (corps ronds) and hyperkeratosis with pyknotic retained nuclei (grains).

are predicted to produce haploinsufficiency in SERCA2, with consequent reduction in function, but the mechanisms are not fully understood [45]. Epidermal keratinocyte differentiation and adhesion are dependent on high concentrations of Ca^{2+} [46]. Functional studies have shown most variants cause normal to reduced Ca^{2+} ATPase activity, and/or reduced levels of Ca^{2+} transport rate and/or reduced levels of phosphorylation at the catalytic site independent of mutation type and location [26,35,45,47,48]. This is predicted to result in increased cytoplasmic and reduced ER calcium levels. At elevated temperatures, specific missense mutations have also been shown to permit leakage of Ca^{2+} back to the cytoplasm [49], offering a mechanism for exacerbation by heat. It has been suggested that missense mutations are associated with more severe disease [23], possibly due to a dominant negative effect on the normal allele [45]. Some studies have suggested a correlation between specific mutation types and neuropsychiatric disease [50]. However, clear genotype–phenotype correlation has not been clearly established [21,23,26,44] and phenotypic variability within families suggests that other genetic, epigenetic or environmental factors also modify the phenotype.

In DD, the normal increase of epidermal Ca^{2+} gradient from basal to superficial layers is disrupted [51,52]. ER calcium stores are necessary firstly for intracellular calcium-dependent signalling, which, amongst other roles, regulates the transport of adhesion proteins to the cell membrane [53]. On receipt of purinergic signals, mediated by G-protein-coupled cell membrane receptors and inositol trisphosphate (IP3), ER calcium is rapidly discharged into the cytoplasm. Increasing cytoplasmic calcium in turn causes the cell-membrane-store-operated channel TRPC1 (transient receptor potential cationic 1) to admit extracellular calcium, increasing the calcium flux [30]. Compromised SERCA2 function in DD is associated with upregulation of TRPC1, which augments cell proliferation and restricts apoptosis [54]. A second SERCA2-dependent signalling pathway in keratinocytes is mediated by sphingolipids [55]. Reduced

ER Ca^{2+} interferes with correct protein folding, sorting and post-translational modification by the molecular chaperones calreticulin and calnexin [56,57]. Cultured DD keratinocytes [58] or SERCA2-deficient cells [58] show impaired trafficking of the adhesion molecule desmoplakin to the cell membrane. Ca^{2+} depletion-induced ER stress impairs the formation of both adherens junctions and desmosomes [59], with desmosomal loss permitting invasion of herpes simplex virus 1 (HSV-1) with suppression of interferon β (IFN-β) and the antiviral factor ISG14 [60].

SERCA2 is sensitive to ER stress, resulting in insolubility and aggregation. Pathogenic missense mutants in SERCA2 are more prone to aggregate and are resistant to proteasome degradation [61]. Conversely, nonsense mutations and frameshift deletions were subject to increased proteasomal degradation [45]. Reduced expression of antiapoptotic proteins of the *Bcl-2* gene family, although possibly secondary to other changes, may contribute to apoptosis [62–64].

Nevertheless, *ATP2A2* is widely expressed, yet the phenotype is primarily cutaneous. Mice haploinsufficient in SERCA2 have impaired cardiac function and develop squamous cell carcinomas [65–68], features not seen in DD. Cutaneous localisation may be explained by the absence of compensatory mechanisms such as SERCA3 in the epidermis [34,69]. However, onset is relatively late, only part of the skin is affected, and the lesions are focal and not limited to adnexal structures.

Clinical features
History
The peak age of onset is between 6 and 20 years but disease may present in infants or old age [3]. Minor nail or palmar changes or acrokeratoses may be detected before the rash appears [4]. The disease usually runs a chronic relapsing course although spontaneous remissions can occur. Aggravating factors include friction, heat, sweating and sunlight or ultraviolet B (UVB) [3,4].

Presentation

Discrete or confluent rough, greasy, skin-coloured or yellowish brown papules are commonest on the seborrhoeic areas of the trunk, face, scalp margins, temples, ears, scalp, neck and flexures: the perineum, axillae and groin (Figure 64.2). Hair growth is unaffected. The disease often begins with small groups of keratotic papules on sun-exposed sites such as the neck. Isolated nipple hyperkeratosis may precede other signs of disease [70]. Coalescing papules, particularly in the axillae, perineum, groin and natal cleft, may form irregular, warty, fissured plaques (Figure 64.3), sometimes becoming vegetating and malodorous [3]. Scattered papules may be present on the limbs, but in some cases confluent hyperkeratotic plaques on the limbs are the major site of disease [23,71].

Acrokeratosis verruciformis (AKV), plane wart-like lesions best seen by transverse illumination, are commonest on the dorsal hands but can be detected in other sites (Figure 64.4). Hands including nails may show the earliest signs of disease [3,4]. Nail fragility, painful longitudinal splits or distinctive red and white longitudinal bands terminating in V-shaped nicks are typical (Figure 64.5). Over time nails may become severely dystrophic. Focal palmoplantar lesions, pits (Figure 64.6) or keratoses are common, occasionally causing a more diffuse keratoderma. Filiform keratoses have been noted [72,73]. Mucosal involvement presents with white umbilicate or cobblestone papules (Figure 64.7). Oral, oesophageal, cervical and rectal mucosa may be affected [74–82]; diagnosis in these cases will require pathological examination (Figure 64.8). Oral lesions are most common on the palate [74,83–87]. Confluent buccal lesions may resemble leukoplakia. Salivary duct occlusion and recurrent sialadenitis are recognised [86,88–90].

Ocular manifestations include hyperkeratotic plaques and seborrhoeic debris at the eyelid margin with typical histological changes [91,92]. The chronic blepharitis is associated with dry eye syndrome and corneal erosions [93] and endophthalmitis following cataract surgery has been reported [94,95]. A variety of corneal abnormalities may occur [96,97].

Extensive, malodorous and painful skin in DD impacts on social interaction, work or school [98]. The extent of skin area affected and clinical severity have a negative impact on health-related quality of life [99].

Clinical variants

There is considerable variation in severity of disease, even within families, from subtle palmar or nail changes to widespread involvement. Reported variants include erosive or vesiculobullous disease, especially in flexures [100,102–104], and eroded or hyperkeratotic plaques (Figure 64.9a), particularly of distal limbs [23,71,105–108]. Patients may have multiple comedones or nodulocystic acne with typical DD histology, causing deeply pitted scars (Figure 64.9b) [109–112]. Palmoplantar haemorrhagic macules with irregular margins (Figure 64.9c) [23,113–117] occur consistently within families and may be due to specific mutations [23,118]. Pigmented papular lesions of the trunk resembling Grover disease have been described [119]. In type IV/V skin, focal lesions also produce guttate leukoderma – confetti-like hypopigmented macules and papules (Figure 64.10a) [120–125]; similar lesions in type II/III skin are sometimes detectable (Figure 64.10b). It is possible that DD in

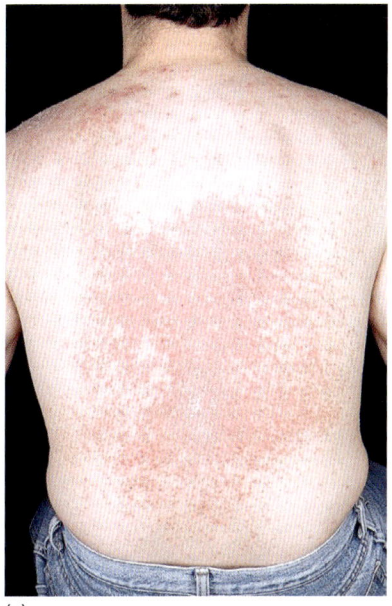

(a)

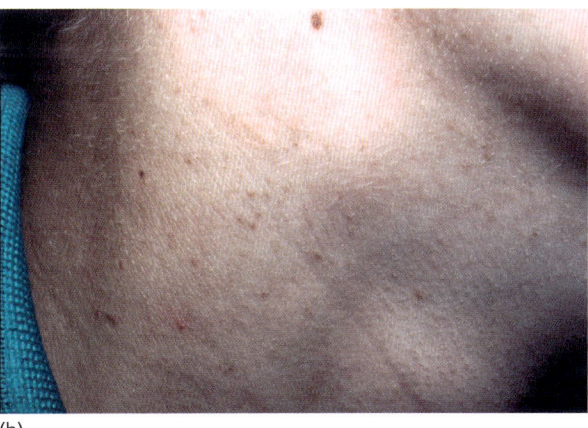

(b)

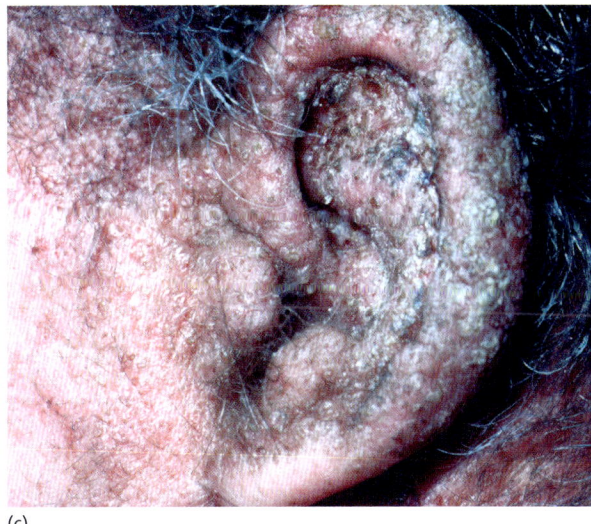

(c)

Figure 64.2 Lesions of Darier disease: (a) profuse keratotic papules in the seborrhoeic areas; (b) early keratotic papules developing on the sun-exposed skin of the neck of a 9-year-old girl; and (c) confluent lesions on the ear of a 57-year-old man.

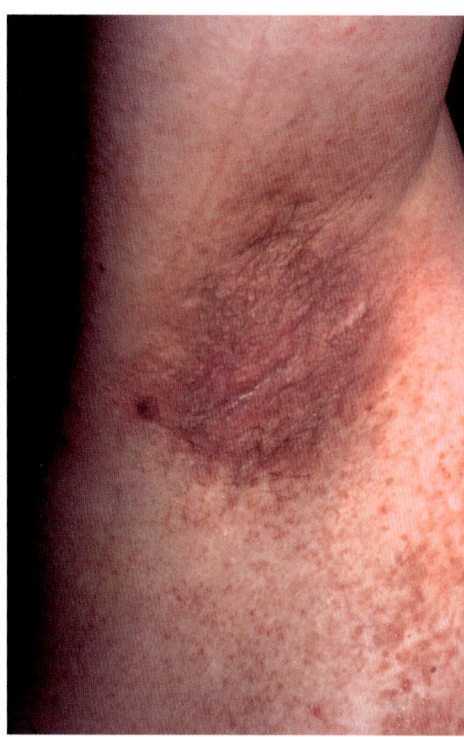

(a)

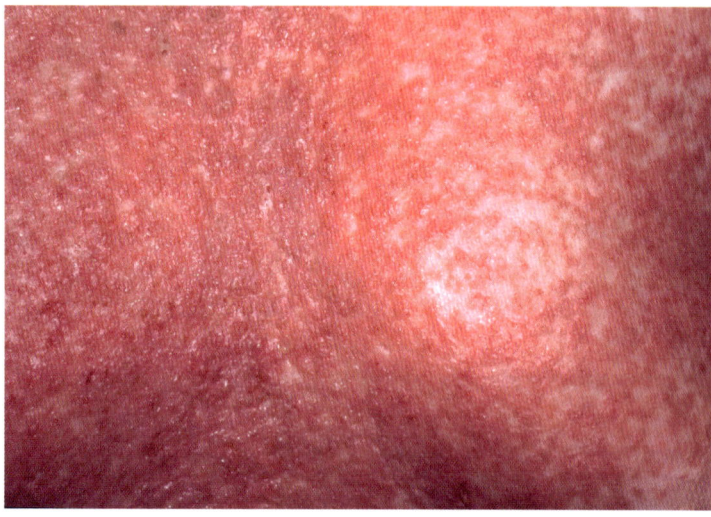

(b)

Figure 64.3 Darier disease: (a) confluent papules forming irregular, warty, fissured plaques in the axilla; and (b) confluent inflamed and eroded lesions of the chest.

type V skin may have a mitigated course, and thus be underdiagnosed [126].

Differential diagnosis

Darier disease may resemble seborrhoeic dermatitis, particularly in the scalp, or acne, and nail and hand signs may help to distinguish these. Erosive, bullous or hypertrophic lesions of the flexures clinically and histologically overlap with HHD, but other cutaneous evidence of DD is often present elsewhere; HHD usually presents later [127]. Dowling–Degos disease and acanthosis nigricans present with pigmented flexural lesions and confluent reticulate papillomatosis

with flat lesions mainly limited to the upper trunk. Erosive or bullous flexural DD may suggest pemphigus vulgaris/vegetans or pyoderma vegetans. Acral papules can resemble plane warts or AKV, which may be allelic to DD [128]. Papular acantholysis of the vulva may in some cases be an expression of DD or HHD [78,129,130].

Acantholysis is an incidental feature of many other epidermal disorders. DD is often suggested by pathologists in cases of transient or persistent acantholytic dermatoses (Grover disease) [131,132], but the clinical presentation and absence of family history or supportive signs may help to distinguish this. *ATPA2* mutations are not found [133]. Galli–Galli disease, which presents with acantholytic flexural papulovesicules or freckles, is an allelic variant of Dowling–Degos disease (MIM: 179850) due to mutation in *KRT5* encoding keratin 5 [134–137].

In AKV of Hopf (MIM: 101900), multiple flesh-coloured or lightly pigmented papules are seen on the dorsa of the hands, feet and other sites [138]. The lesions are clinically identical to those seen in DD [128,139,140]. Histology shows a 'church spire' pattern of hyperkeratosis (see Figure 64.4b), but acantholysis is not usually found. In some but not all pedigrees, AKV of Hopf has been found to be allelic to DD [**26**,128,141–145].

Localised or segmental epidermal naevi following the lines of Blaschko, which have the clinical features and acantholytic dyskeratotic histology of DD (Figure 64.11), are frequently reported [146–149]. In view of late onset, photoaggravation and occasional associated signs, such naevi have been thought to be a mosaic form of DD. Type 1 somatic mosaicism for *ATP2A2* mutations has been confirmed in some such naevi, but not in all those studied [**150**,151–153], and may present later [154]. In theory, an individual mosaic for *ATP2A2* mutations could transmit DD to a child if the mutation was also present in the gonads [152], but this has not as yet been reported.

In rare cases, a severely affected linear eruption of DD is superimposed on generalised disease. This is suggested to be due to type 2 mosaicism in which a heterozygous individual suffers a postzygotic loss of heterozygosity causing localised homozygosity or hemizygosity for the underlying mutation [152,155,156]. A localised acantholytic lesion in an infant from a family with DD may have a similar explanation [157].

Classification of severity

The following grades are proposed:

- *Grade 0*: subclinical; the typical rash is absent or subtle and asymptomatic but associated features such as acrokeratoses or nail dystrophy are present. This grade is usually only recognised in the context of a family history.
- *Grade I*: mild; localised keratotic papules occupy up to 10% of affected areas (e.g. trunk or flexures) and may give rise to pruritus or mild irritation. Many cases of naevoid DD fall into this group.
- *Grade II*: moderate; extensive papular and subconfluent lesions with crusting or secondary infection affect 10–30% of the affected area, or there is extensive and symptomatic papular flexural involvement.
- *Grade III*: severe; widespread confluent, crusted, eroded or bullous rash affects >30% of the trunk or confluent, eroded or hyperkeratotic disease of the limbs or flexures.

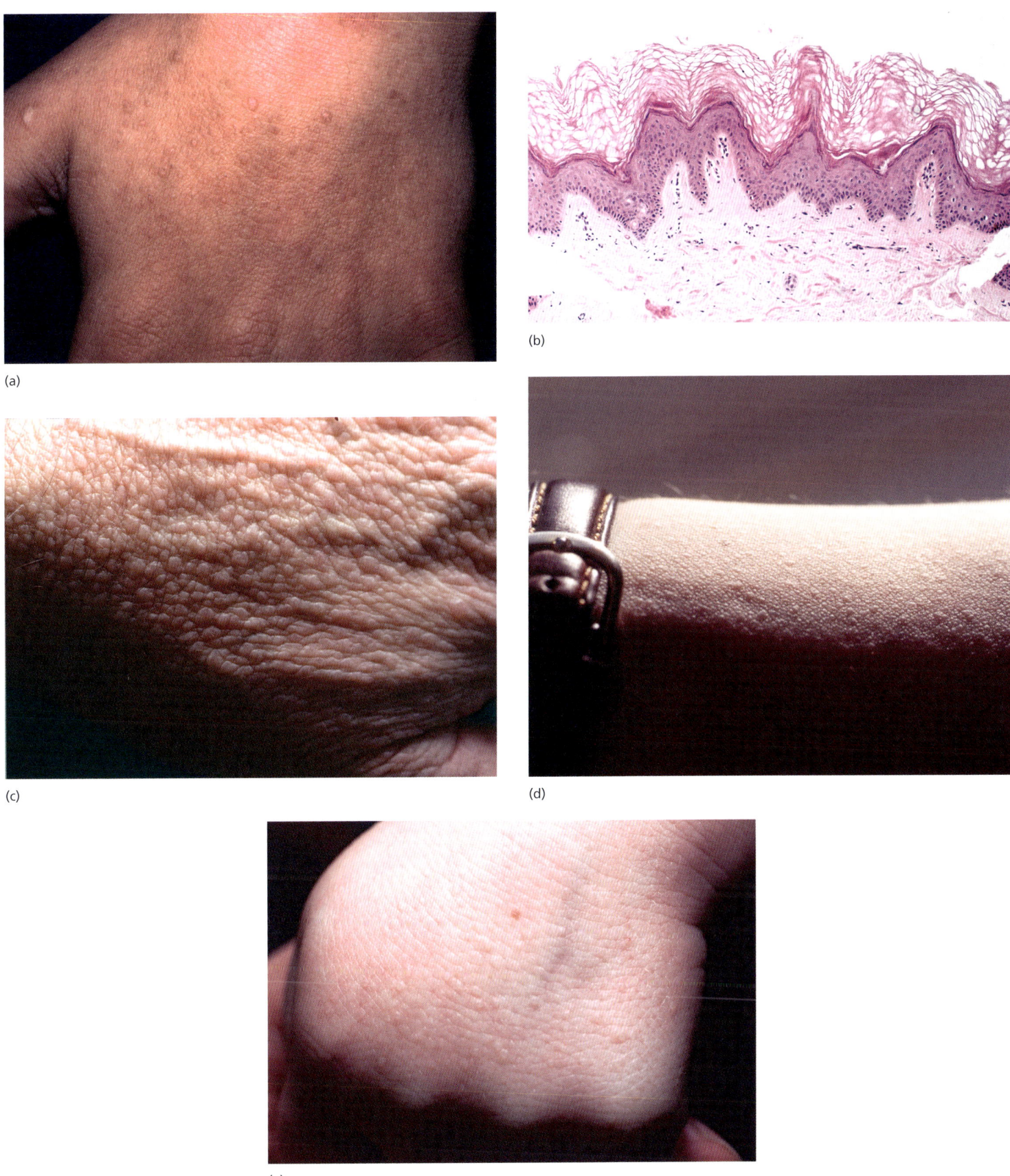

Figure 64.4 Acrokeratosis verruciformis (AKV) in Darier disease: (a) plane wart-like lesions on the dorsal hands in a 15-year-old boy; (b) 'church spire' pattern of hyperkeratosis in biopsy; (c) multiple AKV lesions best detected with oblique illumination in a 45-year-old man; (d) similar lesions on the forearm of a 31-year-old woman; and (e) the hand of a 4-year-old boy with molecularly confirmed Darier disease.

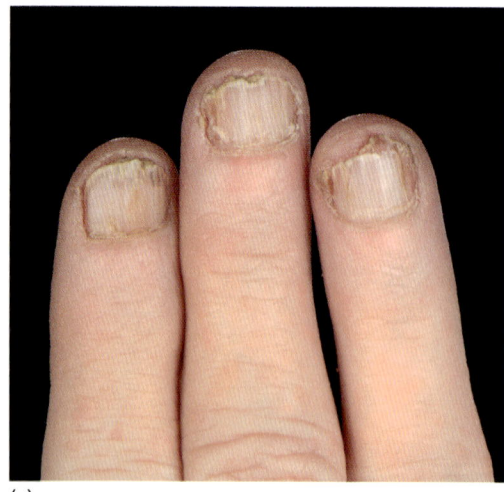

(a)

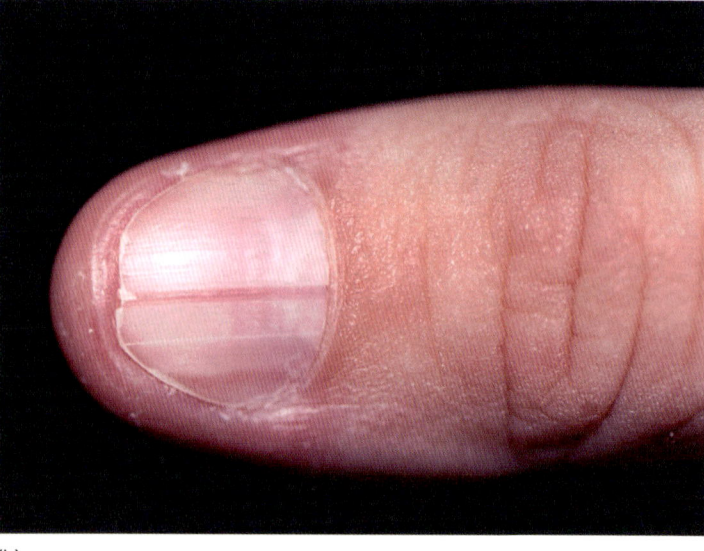

(b)

Figure 64.5 Nail dystrophy of Darier disease: (a) fragile nails with longitudinal splitting and terminal notching; and (b) early nail changes in a 28-year-old woman showing a fine white band and a longitudinal red band terminating in a notch.

Any assessment of clinical severity used to guide treatment decisions should also take into account variation over time and the effect of the disease on the patient and their quality of life.

Complications and co-morbidities

Impetiginisation and eczematisation are common, and patients have an increased susceptibility to infection with herpes simplex (Figure 64.12), herpes zoster or cowpox; severe infections may be disseminated or fatal [158–166]. There is conflicting evidence regarding cell-mediated immunity defects in DD [167–170] and there may be an increased risk of chronic pyogenic infection [171]. There are reports of squamous cell carcinomas of the skin or mucosa [172–177] and mammary Paget disease [178], but the true incidence is not known. Bone and renal cysts have been recorded [179–182]. Despite the importance of SERCA2a in the heart, there is no evidence of a general cardiac dysfunction in DD [183,184].

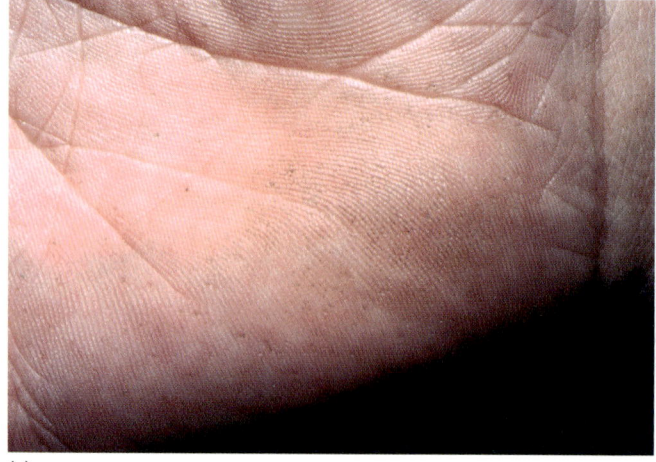

(a)

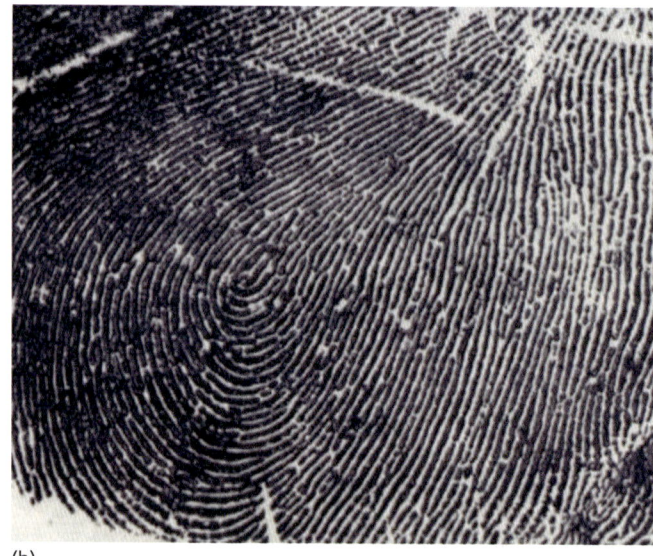

(b)

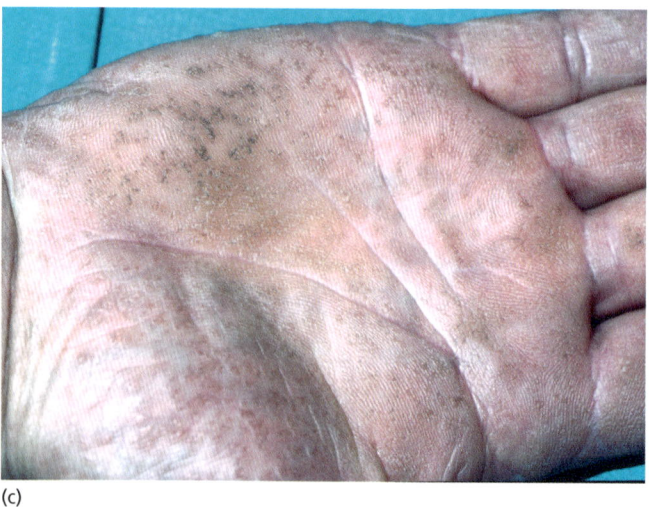

(c)

Figure 64.6 Palmoplantar lesions of Darier disease: (a) pitting in a 15-year-old boy; (b) palm print demonstrating interruptions to the print pattern; and (c) keratotic and pitted lesions in a 57-year-old man.

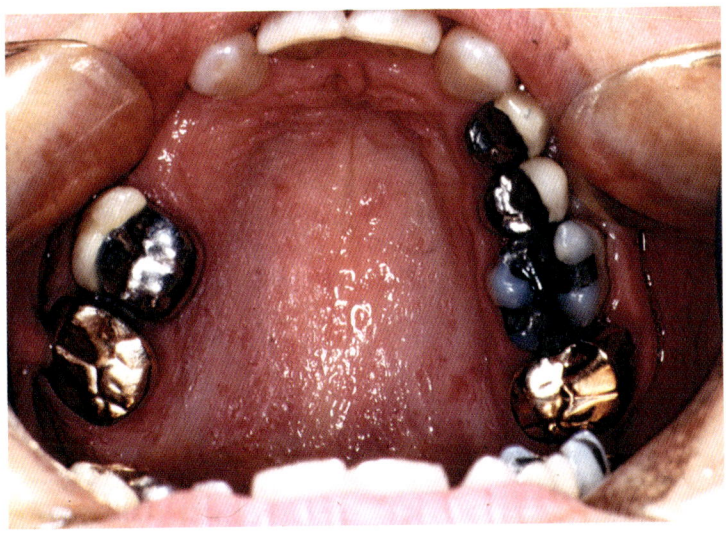

(a)

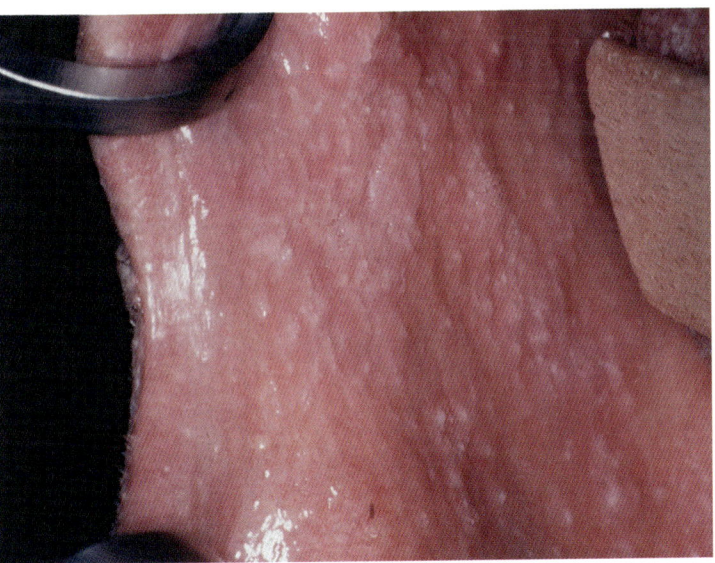

(b)

Figure 64.7 Oral mucosal involvement in Darier disease: (a) umbilicated and cobblestone papules in a 31-year-old woman, and (b) confluent buccal lesions in a 51-year-old man. (a) Courtesy of Dr R. I. Macleod, Royal Victoria Infirmary, Newcastle upon Tyne.

Neuropsychiatric features, including depression, bipolar disorder, epilepsy, intellectual disability, subclinical impairment in cognitive ability and attempted suicide, have been reported in association with DD [6–9,43,185–187]. It has been suggested that the accumulation of mutant protein aggregates in neurons could provide a mechanism for these features [58]. *ATP2A2* has been excluded as a common susceptibility gene for bipolar disorder, but co-segregation of closely linked loci may explain families in whom the disorders are associated [188–193]. Lithium may exacerbate cutaneous disease, possibly by suppressing levels of epidermal SERCA2 [194–197].

Disease course and prognosis
Darier disease has a chronic, relapsing course, with unpredictable severity. It can both improve and deteriorate in old age [3].

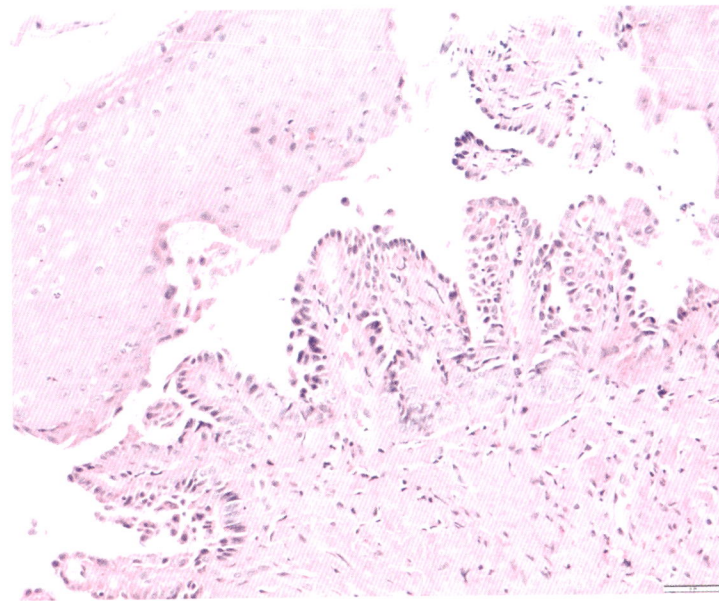

Figure 64.8 Oesophageal biopsy demonstrating suprabasal clefting and dermal villi, associated with dyskeratotic cells (corps ronds). Magnification 400× (H&E). Courtesy of Dr H. Telfah, University Hospital Crosshouse, Kilmarnock.

Investigations
The disorder is usually diagnosed clinically, with histological confirmation. No specific systemic features need be sought in the absence of symptoms. Commercial *ATP2A2* gene sequencing is available, but is not generally needed for genetic counselling, and molecular diagnosis in presymptomatic children has no specific implications for care. In symptomatic or overtly infected lesions, specimens should be taken for bacteriological culture, and virological or fungal investigations should be considered in exacerbations or treatment-resistant disease. A high index of suspicion of herpes simplex superinfection should be maintained, even in the absence of apparent vesicle formation.

Management
There are no large controlled studies of treatment for DD [198]. Isolated reports of successful approaches may be unrepresentative. Mild disease may only require emollients, including those with urea or lactic acid to minimise hyperkeratosis, simple hygiene to prevent secondary infection and avoidance of excessive heat or sun [199]. Topical antiseptics such as chlorhexidine skin cleanser or potassium permanganate baths, and topical antibiotics and antifungals, may be used to prevent or treat secondary infection, with improvement in malodour [200]. Long-term oral antibiotics are not generally recommended.

In acute, symptomatic and inflammatory disease, topical corticosteroids are commonly used. In general, potent or even highly potent steroids are necessary and are often combined with topical antimicrobials. Chronic use of potent topical corticosteroids should be avoided, especially in the flexures. Infected exacerbations are most commonly due to staphylococcal infection and short courses of appropriate oral antibiotics may be necessary. In view of the risk of multiresistant *Staphylococcus aureus* and terbinafine-resistant *Trichophyton rubrum* [201] microbiological investigations are recommended. Herpes simplex infection complicating DD needs urgent oral or parenteral antiviral agents such as aciclovir [160]. Cidofovir has been used in cutaneous cowpox infection [164].

A variety of topical retinoids have been reported as effective [202–207]. Topical tacalcitol helped one case, but calcipotriol irritated 8 of 12 patients [208]. Many topical agents prove to be irritant, but success with tazarotene in aqueous dilution to 0.01% [205] with intermittent use has been suggested [**198**]. The topical immunosuppressive agents tacrolimus and pimecrolimus have been used [209–211] but herpesvirus infection must first be excluded. Topical 5-fluorouracil was effective in a few patients [212–216], and both diclofenac sodium 1% gel [217] and topical glypyrronium have been reported [218].

Oral retinoids are the mainstay of treatment of severe disease. Acitretin 0.25–0.5 mg/kg/day or isotretinoin 0.5 mg/kg/day reduce hyperkeratosis and malodour with safe long-term data emerging [219–224]. Oral alitretinoin provides an alternative, although benefits can be short-lived [225], and may be useful in women of child-bearing potential [226–231]. Ciclosporin has no effect in chronic stable disease but has been reported to be effective in severe inflammatory or eczematised episodes [232–235] and vulval disease [235]. UVB phototherapy or psoralens and UVA are probably ineffective and risk exacerbating the disease but have been successfully used [236]. Four of six patients benefited from photodynamic

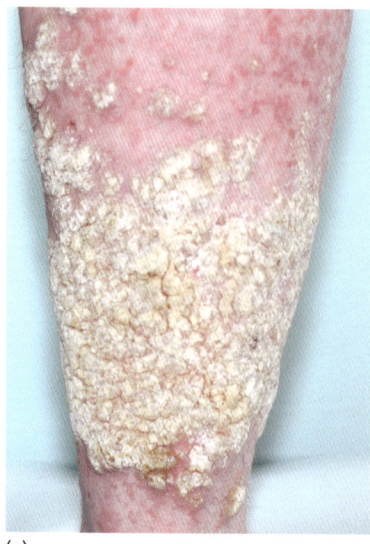

(a)

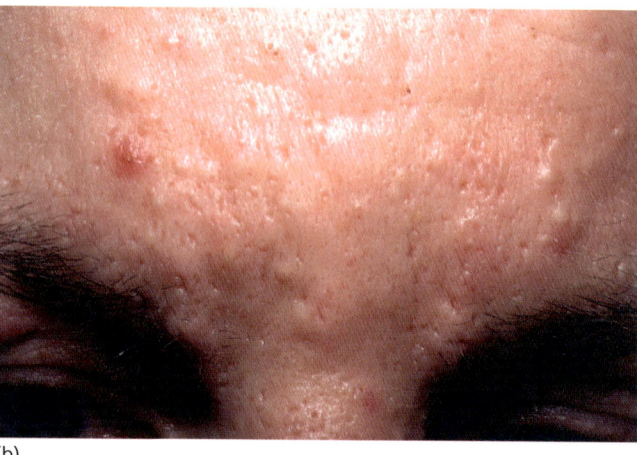

(b)

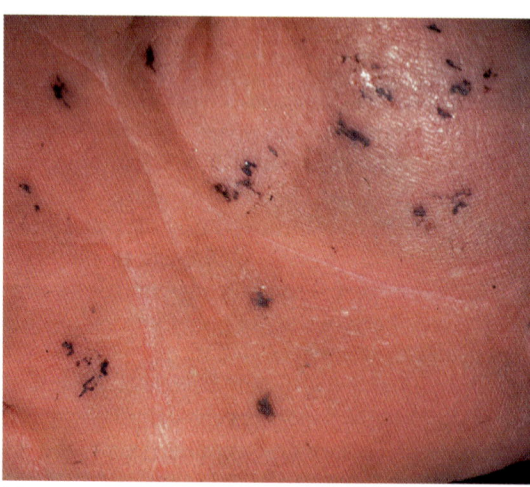

(c)

Figure 64.9 Variant forms of Darier disease: (a) cornifying plaques on the lower legs; (b) multiple comedones and deep pitted scars; and (c) haemorrhage into palmoplantar lesions of Darier disease is found with specific *ATP2A2* mutations. Reproduced from Ruiz-Perez *et al.* 1999 [24] with permission of Oxford University Press.

Treatment ladder of Darier disease

First line
- Emollients and topical antiseptics
- Avoid excess heat or UVB

Second line
- Moderately potent/potent topical combination corticosteroids with antifungals/antibiotics
- Topical retinoids (consider dilution or intermittent use)
- Exacerbations:
  - Oral antibiotics (subject to bacteriology)
  - Antifungal agents for proven infection
  - Oral antivirals, e.g. aciclovir
  - Chronic disease: oral acitretin 0.25–0.5 mg/kg/day, isotretinoin 0.5 mg/kg/day

Third line
- Topical 5-fluorouracil cream
- Topical tacrolimus
- Topical tacalcitol
- Topical diclofenac gel 1%
- Oral alitretinoin
- Low-dose naltrexone
- Photodynamic therapy
- Intravenous immunoglobulin
- Surgical or physical therapies
- Inflammatory disease: oral ciclosporin 2.5 mg/kg/day; exclude infection
- Flexural disease:
  - Botulinum toxin
  - Breast reduction

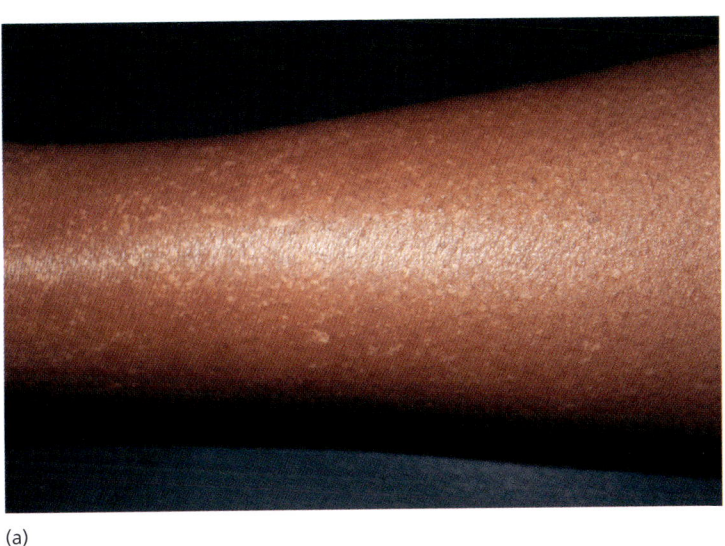 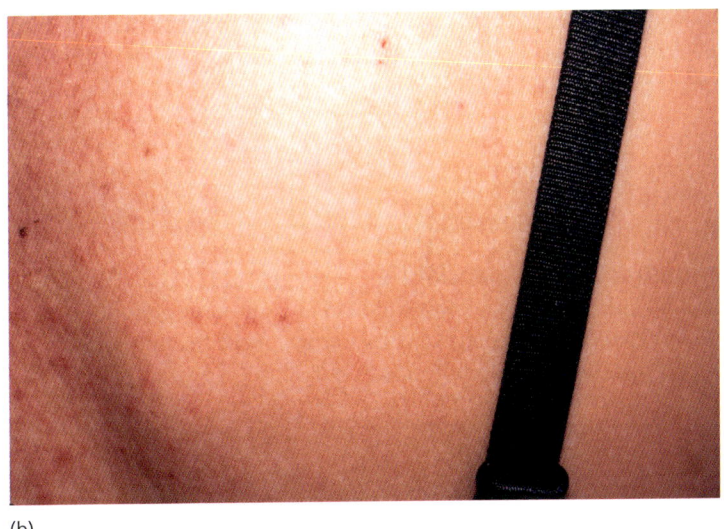

(a)   (b)

Figure 64.10 Guttate leukoderma: (a) hypopigmented macules and papules in pigmented skin, and (b) similar lesions on the back of a 31-year-old white woman. (a) Courtesy of Dr Yoseph Legesse, University of Addis Ababa, Ethiopia.

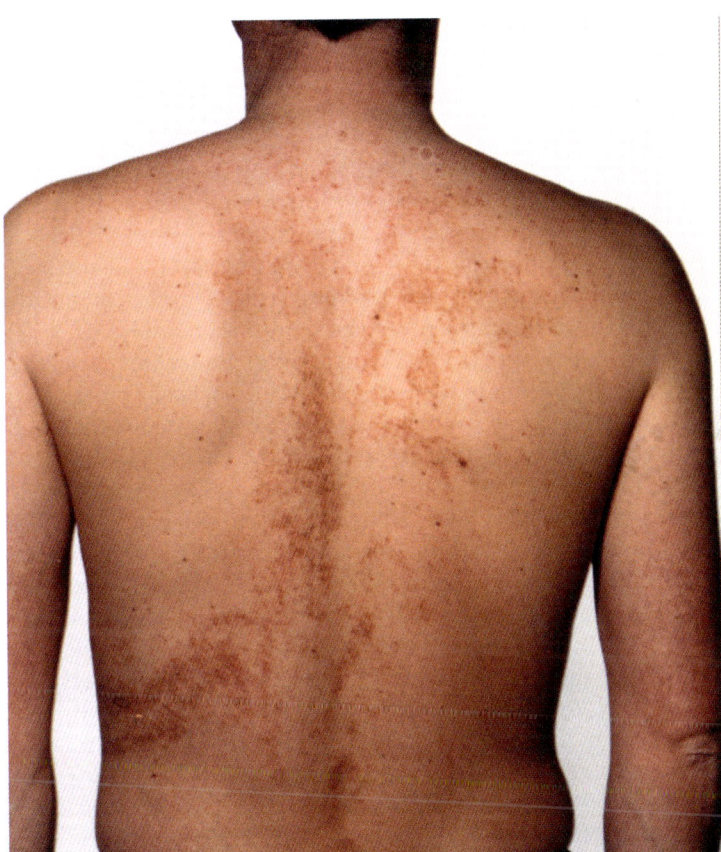

Figure 64.11 Epidermal naevus following the lines of Blaschko; the clinical and histological appearances are those of Darier disease.

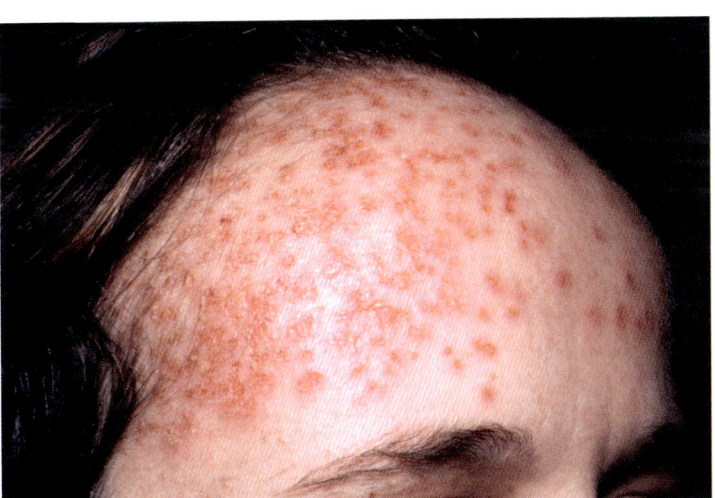

(a)

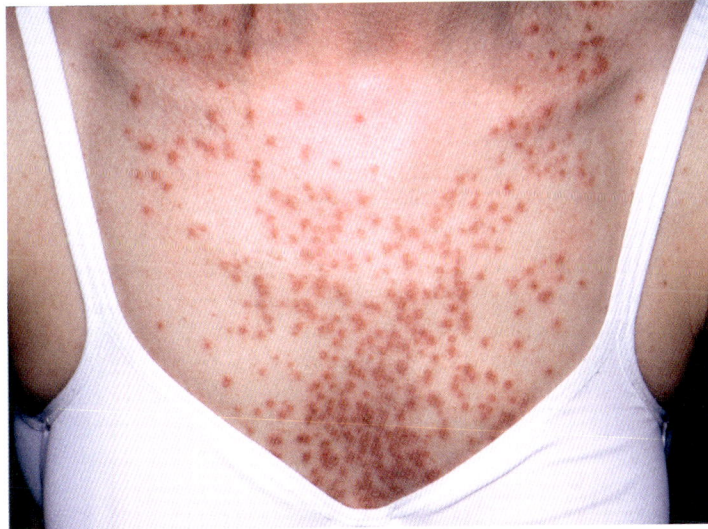

(b)

Figure 64.12 (a, b) Herpes simplex superinfection of skin lesions in a patient with Darier disease.

therapy [237,238], but this provoked a flare in another case [239]. Low-dose intravenous immunoglobulin has been used for recalcitrant disease [240], and variable responses to low-dose naltrexone 3–5 mg, with/without oral magnesium supplements, have been reported [241,242]. Physical therapies used to treat localised disease include excision and grafting, electrodessication, dermabrasion and ablative laser and radiation therapy [104,**198**,217–254]. Botulinum toxin can be considered to reduce maceration in flexural or lumbosacral disease, sometimes proving effective rapidly [255–260], and breast reduction has been used for inframammary disease [261].

HAILEY–HAILEY DISEASE

Definition and nomenclature

Hailey–Hailey disease is an autosomal dominant genodermatosis characterised by erosions and blistering, most prominently in the flexures and sites of friction or trauma.

Synonyms and inclusions
• Familial benign chronic pemphigus

Introduction and general description

The disorder, first described by the Hailey brothers in 1939, typically presents as erosions and blistering, maceration and commonly secondary infection, affecting flexures and sites of friction [1,2]. Histology of lesions shows widespread acantholysis with minimal dyskeratosis. A family history is often obtained, but the disorder is not fully penetrant and in mild cases may never be diagnosed. HHD follows a chronically relapsing course. It is generally managed with a combination of simple measures, topical and oral antimicrobials, topical corticosteroids and oral retinoids.

Epidemiology

Incidence and prevalence

An incidence of 1 in 50 000 has been reported, although HHD is probably underrecognised [1].

Pathophysiology

Hailey–Hailey disease is a disorder of keratinocyte adhesion [3]. Histological analysis of lesional skin from HHD demonstrates widespread partial loss of cohesion between suprabasal keratinocytes, or acantholysis, said to resemble a 'dilapidated brick wall' (Figure 64.13). Acantholytic clefts and bullae form suprabasally, and may contain floating clusters of loosely adherent cells. Adherens junctions may allow keratinocytes to continue to adhere [4]. Mild dyskeratosis may be present.

HHD is due to mutations in *ATP2C1*, a gene at chromosome 3q21-24, which encodes human secretory pathway Ca^{2+}/Mn^{2+} ATPase isoform 1 (SPCA1) [5,6,7,8], a calcium pump of the Golgi apparatus membrane. It is analogous in structure and function to the SERCA pumps in the ER, although only one Ca^{2+} or Mn^{2+} is transported per cycle. Over 190 missense, nonsense and other mutations throughout the *ATP2C1* gene have been described [6,9,10–26]. The disease is likely to be due to haploinsufficiency: most mutations are predicted to result in reduced or absent expression of SPCA1 or to affect highly conserved, functionally critical domains. There appears to be no consistent genotype–phenotype correlation [9,12,27].

SPCA1 is found in the membrane of the Golgi complex, but its distribution is limited to tubular parts of the trans-Golgi network [28]. *ATP2C1* is most highly expressed in the basal layer of

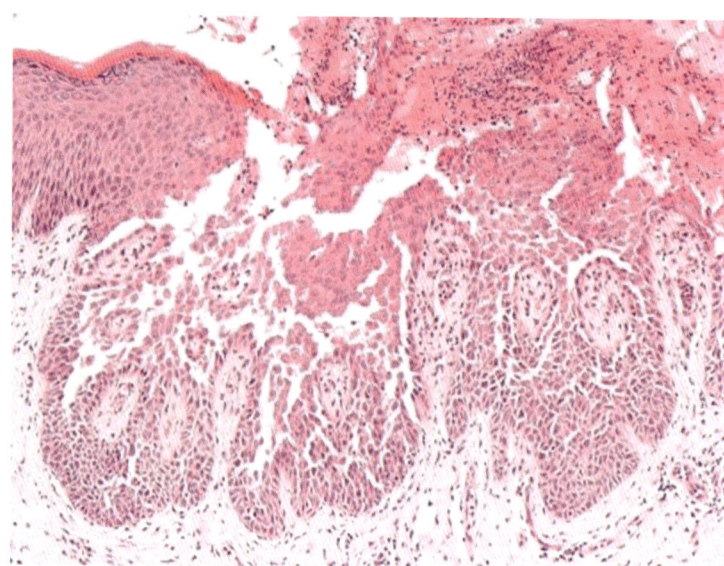

Figure 64.13 Lesional skin in Hailey–Hailey disease showing prominent acantholysis throughout the spinous layer, giving a so-called 'dilapidated brick wall' appearance. There is overlying scale and crust, but little dyskeratosis. Courtesy of Professor R. A. J. Eady, St John's Institute of Dermatology, London, UK.

epidermis [29], but it is also present in suprabasal keratinocytes [5]. Calcium sequestration into the Golgi is reduced in HHD keratinocytes [30]. SPCA1 is less important than SERCA2 for the regulation of cytoplasmic calcium, and reported effects of pathogenic mutations in *ATP2C1* on resting cytosolic calcium levels vary [6,31]. However, small interfering RNA (siRNA) inactivation of *ATP2C1* expression increased resting cytosolic Ca^{2+} [32]. Transient release of Ca^{2+} from the Golgi lumen to the cytosol stimulates the fusion of membranes containing cargo proteins and Golgi cisternae, and is crucial for the secretion and progression of newly synthesised proteins through the Golgi apparatus [33]. The restoration of cytoplasmic calcium to basal levels by SPCA1 is necessary for delivery to their targets [33]. In yeast, loss of PMR1, the homologue of SPCA1, causes defects in protein processing and trafficking and defective degradation of misfolded ER proteins [5]. In HHD keratinocytes, trafficking of desmoplakin and desmoglein 3 to the cell membrane is reduced [34]. SPCA1 deficiency also renders keratinocytes more vulnerable to the ER stress response [35,36]. *In vitro* effects of downregulation of *ATP2C1* expression also reduced actin reorganisation [37]. Mice haploinsufficient in SPCA1 did not show cutaneous changes, but had an increased incidence of squamous papillomas and carcinomas of skin and oesophagus [38].

As with Darier disease and SERCA2, the gene for SPCA1 is widely expressed, so that it is unclear why the loss of one allele of *ATP2C1* leads to a phenotype confined to the skin [5,39–41]. A lack of compensatory mechanisms in keratinocytes may be responsible [5,42]. Additional factors such as heat, friction or infection are clearly required to trigger the clinical disorder, as presentation is late and localised. *In vitro* studies suggest that pro-inflammatory cytokines such as interleukin 6 (IL-6) and IL-8 may regulate *ATP2C1* gene expression, and triggers such as UVB may reduce SPCA1 to critical levels [43–45]. The reduction of *ATP2C1* mRNA expression by UVB irradiation in keratinocytes was prevented by

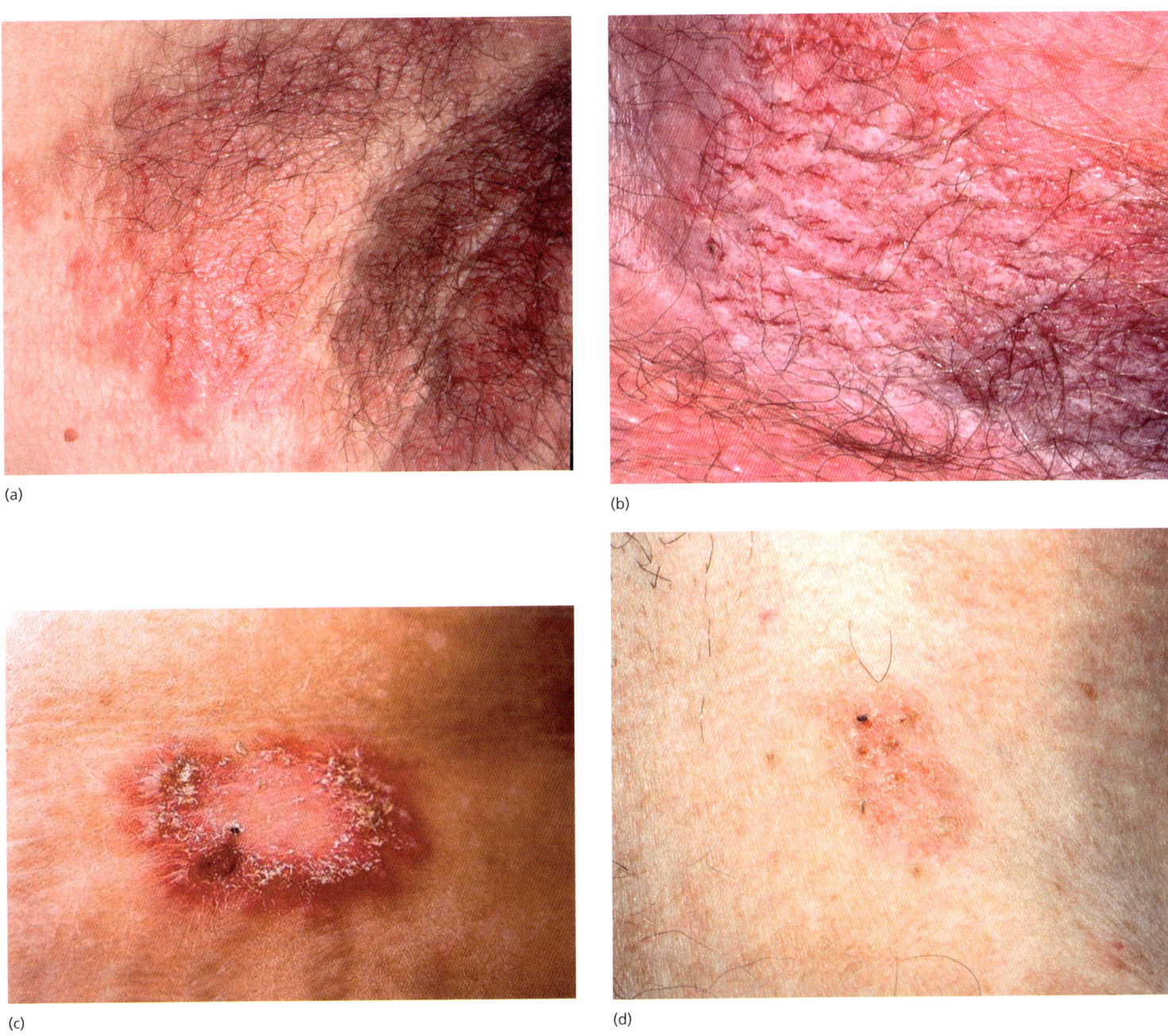

(a)

(b)

(c)

(d)

Figure 64.14 Lesions of Hailey–Hailey disease: (a) typical fissured plaque in the axilla; (b) inflamed, macerated and fissured lesions of the groin in a 40-year-old man; (c) annular plaque with a crusted rim; and (d) indeterminate lesion resembling discoid eczema. (a–c) Courtesy of Professor R. A. J. Eady, St John's Institute of Dermatology, London, UK.

retinoids, corticosteroids, ciclosporin, tacrolimus and vitamin D$_3$ [44,45].

Clinical features

History

Hailey–Hailey disease typically presents between the second and fourth decades [3] with painful, pruritic and often malodorous lesions of flexures or other sites of friction (Figure 64.14a, b). HHD may be localised or generalised, occasionally causing erythroderma [46–48]. In the axilla, inframammary or abdominal folds, groin or perineum, lesions show fissuring and erosion with macerated epidermis progressing in more severe cases to vegetations. Less occluded areas, such as truncal or neck lesions, are more likely to show vesicopustules or flaccid bullae, but may simply be crusted

erosions resembling discoid eczema, or annular plaques with peripheral scales (Figure 64.14c, d), often with postinflammatory hyperpigmentation. Common precipitating factors include heat, sweating, friction and infection. Other reported triggers include contact allergy, adhesive dressings or electrocardiogram electrodes, UV irradiation and scabies [1,3,49–55]. Lesions may localise at the sites of inflammatory dermatoses such as psoriasis, seborrhoeic dermatitis or drug eruptions [50,56,57]. Linear white bands (longitudinal leukonychia) are present in the nails of some patients (Figure 64.15a), but without the nail fragility of DD [1,58–62]. Oral (Figure 64.15b), conjunctival, oesophago-gastric or vaginal involvement is rarely described, usually in association with trauma or infection [1,63–68]. Even mild disease has been shown to reduce

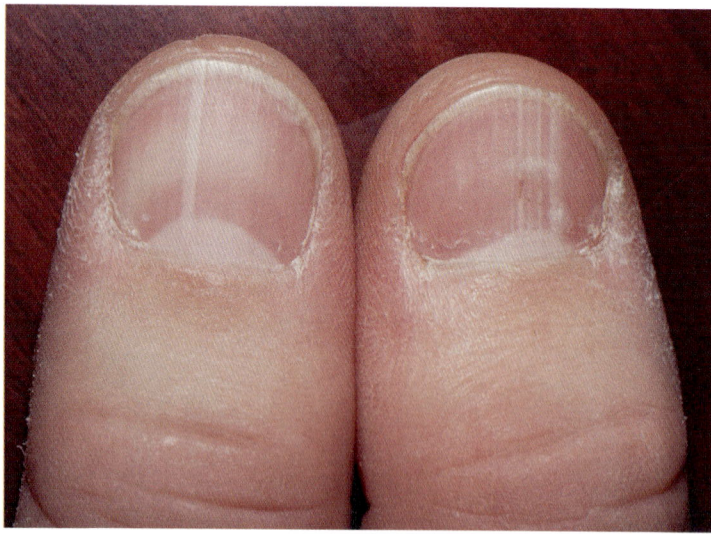

(a)

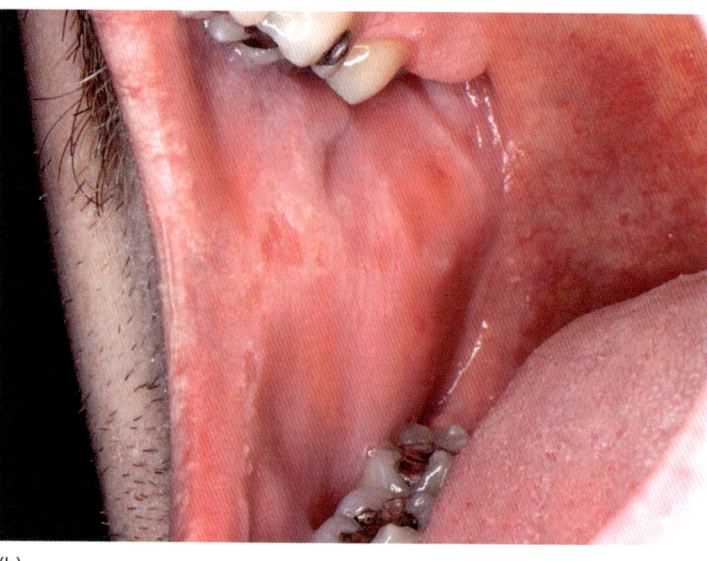

(b)

Figure 64.15 Extraepidermal lesions in patients with Hailey–Hailey disease: (a) linear white bands in the nails; terminal notches of Darier disease are not found; and (b) painless oral erosions; biopsy confirmation was not possible.

quality of life, and flexural or groin involvement can be particularly disabling [69].

Clinical variants

Papular acantholytic dermatosis of the genito-crural area without other features of HHD [70–72] is in some cases allelic to HHD [73–75].

Reports of relapsing linear acantholytic dermatoses with histopathological and ultrastructural features of HHD [76] suggest disease due to type 1 mosaicism, with some cases presenting in childhood [77,78], and one associated with familial HHD [79]. Mosaic variants in *ATP2C1* have been confirmed [80,81].

Differential diagnosis

The diagnosis of HHD is often delayed or missed [1,49,82]. Isolated intertriginous erosions suggest flexural seborrhoeic eczema

or psoriasis, with bacterial or fungal superinfection, which may indeed be present, but the existence of fissures may be a clue. In non-occluded areas, lesions resemble tinea corporis or discoid eczema, or autoimmune pemphigus. HHD vesicles may mimic herpes simplex, which may also complicate the disorder [83–88]. Apparent response to antibacterials and/or topical corticosteroids can further delay diagnosis. Severe bullous and erosive lesions can suggest erythema multiforme or even toxic epidermal necrolysis [54]. Hypertrophic or vegetating flexural HHD overlaps clinically and histologically with flexural DD. Typical papular or nail lesions of DD elsewhere may help to differentiate the disorders. Similarly, in pemphigus vegetans, the presence of oral lesions may aid distinction. Hypertrophic vulval HHD may mimic viral warts [71,89] or vulval intraepithelial neoplasia [1,90]. Reported reactions to adhesive dressing mimicking contact allergy may be due to HHD [53]. Clinically, the presence of longitudinal leukonychia may help to diagnose HHD [1,57,58]. Histology, including immunofluorescence, may be necessary to exclude autoimmune pemphigus. DD typically shows less marked acantholysis and more dyskeratosis, but the distinction may not be easy in the presence of florid and superinfected flexural disease.

Classification of severity

The following are proposed:
- *Grade 0*: subclinical; an obligate carrier in a family, with no apparent disease or nail lesions only.
- *Grade I*: mild disease; localised (e.g. perineal or axillary) and intermittent lesions responding to simple topical therapies.
- *Grade II*: moderate; chronic lesions at two or more body sites (e.g. axillary and groins) or locally severe and refractory to topical treatment.
- *Grade III*: severe; extensive or chronically disabling disease despite topical and systemic treatment.

In Burge's study [1], although criteria were not defined, 20 of 58 patients had mild, 36 moderate, and 2 severe disease.

Complications and co-morbidities

Secondary bacterial and candidal infections are common [82,91], and unrecognised tinea may be present. Herpes simplex should be suspected, especially for painful or disseminated exacerbations [84], and scabies infection may exacerbate HHD [55]. Human papillomavirus (HPV) may be present in verrucous perineal lesions [92,93]. Squamous cell carcinoma reported in association with HHD may be related to HPV carriage [94–97], but HPV was not detected in a case associated with the use of topical tacrolimus [98]. Bullous pemphigoid following HHD is also reported [99]. As with any chronic dermatosis, the possibility of allergic contact dermatitis should be considered [100,101]. Affective disorder has been found to co-segregate in three families with HHD [102–104].

Disease course and prognosis

Hailey–Hailey disease pursues a chronic relapsing and remitting course but may improve in old age [1].

Investigations

Skin biopsy demonstrates the characteristic features described earlier. Swabs for bacterial, fungal and viral culture or other investigation should be taken to exclude complicating infection. Sequencing of the responsible gene, *ATP2C1*, is not generally needed for diagnosis or genetic counselling, but is available commercially.

Management

Basic measures include loose clothing, absorbent pads in flexures and, where appropriate, weight loss. Emollients and antimicrobial agents may in theory prevent exacerbations [1,49,105].

Potent or highly potent topical corticosteroids can be effective, especially combined with antibacterial/antifungal agents. Their prompt and early use for exacerbations is recommended [1], but extended treatment should be avoided because of the risk of cutaneous atrophy, especially in the flexures [106]. Topical antimicrobial agents used have included tetracyclines, aminoglycosides, fusidic acid and imidazoles. Broad spectrum agents such as oral flucloxacillin, erythromycin or tetracyclines may be helpful, but skin swabs for bacterial, fungal and yeast culture, and viral polymerase chain reaction (PCR), are important in guiding treatment. Painful, recalcitrant disease may indicate superinfection by herpes simplex and systemic antiviral treatment should be considered if PCR results are not promptly available. Analgesia, even oral morphine in severe disease, is necessary.

Successful topical use of tacrolimus has been reported [107–111], although it may be an irritant [112]. Herpes simplex and other infections should be excluded, and one patient treated with topical tacrolimus developed a vulval squamous cell carcinoma [98]. Other topical agents reported to help include calcitriol, tacalcitol, Castellani paint [113–116] and, in a single case, 5-fluorouracil [117]. The ability of gentamicin to induce readthrough of nonsense mutations in *ATP2C1* has been demonstrated *in vitro* but its relevance to patient care is unproven [118].

The evidence base for systemic agents is also limited, but systemic corticosteroids are useful for acute severe inflammatory disease [46,49,119]. Oral acitretin [91,120–123] or alitretinoin [124], ciclosporin [22,125–129], methotrexate [130,131], azathioprine [132], dapsone [133–135], calcitriol [136] and oral glycopyrrolate [137] have all been reported as beneficial. It is recommended that systemic agents be withdrawn when control is achieved. Long-term oral doxycycline [138], minocycline [139–141] and sustained remission following oral terbinafine have been reported [142]. Low-dose naltrexone with/without oral magnesium has been used in both widespread and limited vulval disease [143–147] but response to apremilast has been variable [148–150]. Oral magnesium chloride [151,152], vitamin D [153,154] and the melanocortin analogue afamelanotide [155] are emerging. The biologic agents etanercept [156] and alefacept [157], and oral thalidomide [158], have been used with success in single cases.

Physical interventions reported include ablative treatments such as cryosurgery [46], dermabrasion [159–163], electrodessication [164], various forms of laser therapy [165–172] and argon plasma coagulation [173]. A novel treatment, cold atmospheric argon plasma, may also be effective [174]. Surgical excision of flexural disease, with or without grafting [175–178], and breast reduction for inframammary disease [179,180] have been reported. Superficial radiotherapy has had mixed results [181,182], and electron beam therapy [183,184] has also been advocated. Axillary or inframammary use of botulinum toxin can reduce sweating [5,162,185–192].

UVB phototherapy with/without acitretin, and excimer light, have controlled HHD in single case reports [193–196], despite UV light usually exacerbating HHD [197]. Photodynamic therapy can be painful and has variable outcomes [198–201].

Treatment ladder of Hailey–Hailey disease

First line
- Reduce heat, friction and sweating
- Weight loss
- Emollients and topical antiseptics

Second line
- Moderately potent/potent topical combination corticosteroids with antifungals/antibiotics
- Oral antibiotics and/or antivirals for secondary infection
- Oral prednisolone 20–30 mg/day; short course in acute flares

Third line
- Topical tacrolimus
- Low-dose long-term antibiotics, e.g. doxycycline/minocyline
- Oral ciclosporin or methotrexate
- Oral retinoids
- Oral naltrexone
- Oral vitamin D/magnesium chloride
- Flexural disease:
  - Surgical ablation or excision
  - Breast reduction
  - Botulinum toxin

Key references

The full list of references can be found in the online version at https://www.wiley.com/rooksdermatology10e

Darier disease

3 Burge SM, Wilkinson JD. Darier-White disease: a review of the clinical features in 163 patients. *J Am Acad Dermatol* 1992;27:40–50.

4 Munro CS. The phenotype of Darier's disease: penetrance and expressivity in adults and children. *Br J Dermatol* 1992;127:126–30.

21 Sakuntabhai A, Ruiz-Perez V, Carter S *et al*. Mutations in ATP2A2, encoding a Ca2+ pump, cause Darier disease. *Nat Genet* 1999;21:271–7.

26 Nellen RG, Steijlen PM, van Steensel MA *et al*. Mendelian disorders of cornification caused by defects in intracellular calcium pumps: mutation update and database for variants in ATP2AA and ATP2C1 associated with Darier disease and Hailey-Hailey disease. *Hum Mutation* 2017;38:343–56.

30 Hovnanian A. SERCA pumps and human diseases. *Subcell Biochem* 2007;45:337–63.

127 Burge SM. Hailey-Hailey disease: the clinical features, response to treatment and prognosis. *Br J Dermatol* 1992;126:275–82.

150 Sakuntabhai A, Dhitavat J, Burge S *et al*. Mosaicism for ATP2A2 mutations causes segmental Darier's disease. *J Invest Dermatol* 2000;115:1144–7.

198 Cooper SM, Burge SM. Darier's disease: epidemiology, pathophysiology, and management. *Am J Clin Dermatol* 2003;4:97–105.

PART 6: GENETIC DISORDERS

HH disease

1 Burge SM. Hailey-Hailey disease: the clinical features, response to treatment and prognosis. *Br J Dermatol* 1992;126:275–82.

3 Burge SM, Millard PR, Wojnarowska F. Hailey-Hailey disease: a widespread abnormality of cell adhesion. *Br J Dermatol* 1991;124:329–32.

6 Hu Z, Bonifas JM, Beech J *et al*. Mutations in ATP2C1, encoding a calcium pump, cause Hailey-Hailey disease. *Nat Genet* 2000;24:61–5.

9 Nellen RG, Steijlen PM, van Steensel MA *et al*. Mendelian disorders of cornification caused by defects in intracellular calcium pumps: mutation update and database for variants in ATP2AA and ATP2C1 associated with Darier disease and Hailey-Hailey disease. *Hum Mutation* 2017;38:343–56.

CHAPTER 65

Ectodermal Dysplasias

Peter Itin

Department of Dermatology, University Hospital of Basel, Basel, Switzerland

Ectodermal dysplasias

Definition and nomenclature

Ectodermal dysplasias, a large group of heterogeneous heritable conditions, are characterised by congenital defects in two or more ectodermal structures, one of which at least involves the hair (trichodysplasia), teeth (dental defects), nails (onychodysplasia) or sweat glands (dyshidrosis) [1]. Mesodermal and occasionally endodermal disturbances of development may coexist. Mutations in genes that are involved in development or homeostasis of ectodermal structures are causatives [2]. The molecular basis of more than 100 out of approximately 220 known ectodermal dysplasias has been deciphered.

Traditional classification schemes based on purely clinical criteria lack practicality as, when applied strictly, they encompass many groups of diseases (e.g. keratodermas with additional skin or nail or hair alterations or ichthyoses with associated features) [3], leading to endless lists of disorders of little use to the clinician. Recent evidence implicates genetic defects in different key pathways orchestrating ectodermal organogenesis. It is likely that with the increasing number of disorders of known aetiology, a better understanding of the pathogenesis of ectodermal dysplasia will lead to their reclassification based on a combination of clinical and molecular defining features [2].

Synonyms and inclusions
- Congenital ectodermal defects
- Hereditary ectodermal defects

Introduction and general description

Ectodermal dysplasias form a complex and highly diverse group of heritable disorders. Although several syndromes have very specific features, many of them have common clinical characteristics. By some authors' estimations, the broader definition of ectodermal dysplasias encompasses some 200–220 individual conditions [4]. Any approach to summarising current knowledge about this group of conditions presents several challenges [5]. Firstly, and most importantly, how is an ectodermal dysplasia defined, and which distinct entities should be labelled under this broad term? The first well-documented patients with what we now call ectodermal dysplasia were described by Danz in 1793 [6]. He reported on two Jewish boys with congenital absence of hair and teeth. In 1875 Charles Darwin reported on a Hindu family with hypodontia and malformed teeth: 'The men thus affected have very little hair on the body and become bald early in life. They also suffer much during hot weather from excessive dryness of the skin'. This family would now be recognised as having X-linked hypohidrotic ectodermal dysplasia, but the term 'ectodermal dysplasia' did not appear until 1929 [7]. Prior to this report, a small series of cases with hypotrichosis, hypodontia, onychodysplasia and anhidrosis had been described under various names such as 'dystrophy of hair and nails', 'imperfect development of skin, hair and teeth' and 'congenital ectodermal defect'. The designation outlined by Weech specified three essential aspects of ectodermal dysplasias: (i) most of the disturbances must affect tissues of ectodermal origin; (ii) these disturbances must be developmental; and (iii) heredity plays a causal role. Weech had in mind the X-linked anhidrotic form of ectodermal dysplasia (Christ–Siemens–Touraine syndrome (CST) or hypohidrotic ectodermal dysplasia (HED); MIM: 305100)

PART 6: GENETIC DISORDERS

Rook's Textbook of Dermatology, Tenth Edition. Edited by Christopher Griffiths, Jonathan Barker, Tanya Bleiker, Walayat Hussain and Rosalind Simpson.
© 2024 John Wiley & Sons Ltd. Published 2024 by John Wiley & Sons Ltd.

in males but noted that it had also been reported in females. He also noted that this pattern of involvement was occasionally inherited as a non-sex-linked trait [7]. For some authors and clinicians, the term ectodermal dysplasia is still used specifically with reference to the CST syndrome and the autosomal dominant and recessive forms of HED. As more clinical reports of patients with similar but subtly distinct patterns of anomalies were recorded, the term 'ectodermal dysplasia' became extended to include many different genetic entities. In an attempt to encapsulate this heterogeneity and diversity of symptoms seen, Touraine suggested the expression 'ectodermal polydysplasia'. Attempts at more formal classification soon followed; initially conditions were classified as hidrotic or anhidrotic, but this simple classification failed to reflect the complexity of nail, hair and dental anomalies associated with the various forms of ectodermal dysplasias.

Currently, the most widely accepted and used definition of the ectodermal dysplasias is of a group of inherited disorders that share in common developmental abnormalities of two or more of the following: skin, hair (Figure 65.1), teeth (Figure 65.2), nails (Figure 65.3), sweat and sebaceous glands and other ectodermal structures. Additional organs derived from embryonic ectoderm include the mammary gland, central nervous system, external ear, melanocytes, cornea, conjunctiva, lacrimal gland and lacrimal duct. There are advantages and disadvantages of this approach to ectodermal dysplasia definition. One definite benefit is that the problems encountered by many patients and families are similar regardless of the specific subtype of ectodermal dysplasia; parents and children can benefit by being part of large support networks, exemplified by the UK Ectodermal Dysplasia Society (http://www.ectodermaldysplasia.org) and the US National Foundation for Ectodermal Dysplasias (http://www.nfed.org). Although a broader definition has the benefit of inclusivity, many conditions encompassed by this definition are not usually considered as primarily ectodermal dysplasias. For example, inherited

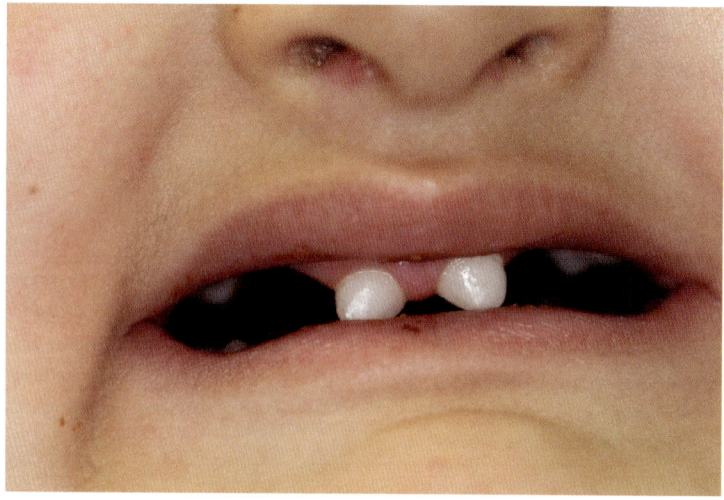

Figure 65.2 Hypodontia and dental malformations in ectodermal dysplasia.

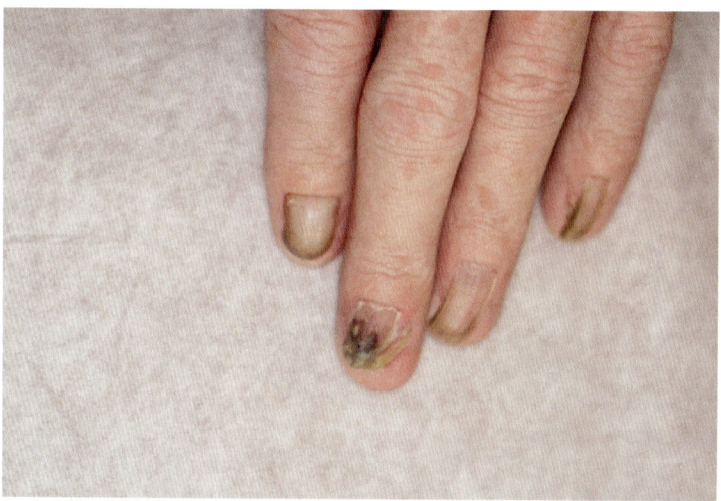

(a)

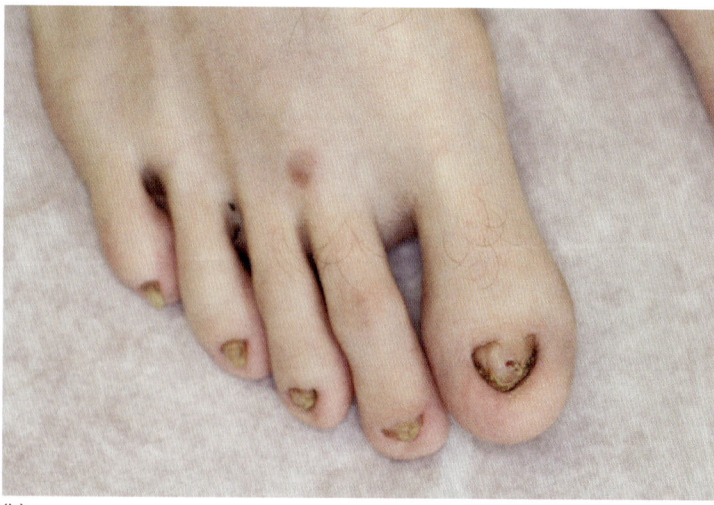

(b)

Figure 65.3 Nail dysplasia of the fingers (a) and toes (b) can be a marker of ectodermal dysplasia.

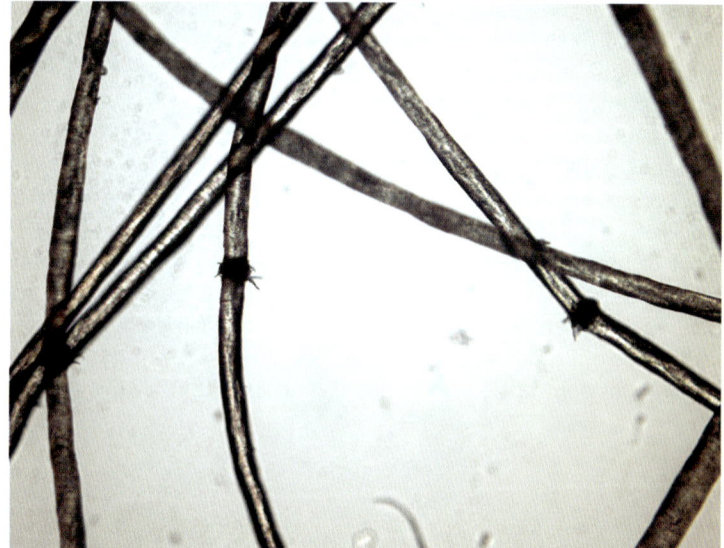

Figure 65.1 Hair shaft abnormalities such as trichorrhexis nodosa in ectodermal dysplasia.

Table 65.1 Classification of ectodermal dysplasias.

Ectodermal dysplasia (ED)	MIM	Inheritance
Subgroup hair–teeth–nails–sweat glands		
1 Acro-renal field defect–ED–lipoatrophic diabetes (AREDYLD)	207780	AR
2 Alopecia–contractures–dwarfism–mental retardation syndrome	20355	AR
3 Ankyloblepharon–ectodermal defects–cleft lip/palate (AEC)	106260	AD
4 Anonychia with flexural pigmentation	106750	AD
5 Arthrogryposis and ED	601701	AR
6 Cleft lip/palate–ED (CLPED1) syndrome (Zlotogora–Ogur syndrome; Margarita Island syndrome)	225060	AR
7 Curly hair–acral keratoderma–caries syndrome (Van Steensel *et al.* 2001 [60])	607656	AD
8 Dyskeratosis congenita, AD (dyskeratosis congenita; Scoggins type)	127550	AD
9 Dyskeratosis congenita, AR	224230	AR
10 Dyskeratosis congenita, X-linked (Zinsser–Cole–Engman syndrome)	305000	XR
11 Ectrodactyly–ED–cleft lip/palate syndrome 1 (EEC1)	129900	AD
12 Ectrodactyly–ED–cleft lip/palate syndrome 3 (EEC3)	604292	AD
13 Hypohidrotic ED with acanthosis nigricans (Lelis syndrome)	608290	?
14 ED with natal teeth, Turnpenny type	601345	AD
15 Hypohidrotic ED with hypothyroidism and agenesis corpus callosum	225040	AD? AR? X-linked, contiguous gene syndrome?
16 Focal dermal hypoplasia (FDH)	305600	XD
17 Hypohidrotic ED, AD (ADHED)	129490	AD
18 Hypohidrotic ED, AR (ARHED)	224900	AR
19 Hypohidrotic ED, X-linked (XLHED; Christ–Siemens–Touraine syndrome)	305100	XR
20 Hypohidrotic ED with immunodeficiency	300291	XD
21 Hypohidrotic ED with immunodeficiency, osteopetrosis and lymphoedema (OLEDAID) syndrome	300301	XD
22 Hypomelanosis of Ito (HMI; incontinentia pigmenti type I (IP1))	300337	XD
23 Keratitis–ichthyosis–deafness (KID) syndrome, AD	148210	AD
24 Keratitis–ichthyosis–deafness (KID) syndrome, AR	242150	AR
25 Naegeli–Franceschetti–Jadassohn syndrome (NFJS)	161000	AD
26 Odonto-onycho-dermal dysplasia (OODD)	257980	AR
27 Odonto-trichomelic syndrome	273400	AR
28 Pachyonychia congenita, type 1 (PC1)	167200	AD
29 Pachyonychia congenita, type 2 (PC2)	167210	AD
30 Papillon–Lefevre syndrome	245000	AR
31 Rosselli–Gulienetti syndrome	225000	AR
32 Scalp–ear–nipple syndrome (Finlay–Marks syndrome; ED with adrenal cyst)	181270; 129550	AD
Subgroup hair–teeth–nails		
33 Ackerman syndrome	200970	AR
34 Acro-dermato-ungual–lacrimal–tooth (ADULT) syndrome	103285	AD
35 Arthrogryposis–ED–cleft lip/palate–developmental delay	301815	XR
36 Cardio-facio-cutaneous (CFC) syndrome	115150	AD
37 Clouston syndrome	129500	AD
38 Coffin–Siris syndrome	135900	AD? AR? XD?
39 Costello syndrome	218040	AD
40 Cranio-ectodermal dysplasia (Sensenbrenner syndrome)	218330	AR
41 Dermo-odontodysplasia	125640	AD
42 ED syndrome with distinctive facial appearance and preaxial polydactyly of feet (single case)	129540	AD?
43 ED, tricho-odonto-onychial type	129510	AD
44 Ellis–van Creveld (EvC) syndrome	225500	AR
45 GOMBO syndrome	233270	AR
46 Growth retardation–alopecia–pseudo-anodontia–optic atrophy (GAPO) syndrome	230740	AR
47 Hidrotic ED, AR (Fried tooth and nail syndrome)	602401	AR
48 Incontinentia pigmenti 2 (IP2)	308300	XD
49 Oculo-trichodysplasia (OTD)	257960	AR
50 Odonto-tricho-ungual–digital–palmar syndrome	601957	AD? XD?
51 Pineal hyperplasia–insulin-resistant diabetes	262190	AR
52 Rothmund–Thomson syndrome (RTS)	268400	AR
53 Schinzel–Giedion midface–retraction syndrome	269150	AR? AD?
54 Schoepf–Schulz–Passarge syndrome	224750	AR
55 Sener syndrome	606156	?
56 Thumb deformity and alopecia	188150	AD
57 Tricho-dento-osseus (TDO) syndrome	190320	AD
58 Tricho-odonto-onychial dysplasia	275450	AR?
59 Tricho-rhino-phalangeal syndrome, type 1 (TRPS1)	190350	AD
60 Tricho-thio-dystrophy, photosensitive (TTDP)	601675	AR
61 Witkop syndrome	189500	AD

(continued)

Table 65.1 (*continued*)

Ectodermal dysplasia (ED)	MIM	Inheritance
Subgroup hair–teeth–sweat glands		
62 Böök syndrome	112300	AD
63 Ichthyosis follicularis–atrichia–photophobia (IFAP) syndrome	308205	XR
64 Johnson neuroectodermal syndrome	147770	AD
65 Leukomelanoderma–infantilism–retardation–hypodontia–hypotrichosis	246500	AR
66 Ulnar–mammary syndrome (UMS)	181450	AD
67 Hypohidrotic ED with hypothyroidism and ciliary dyskinesia (HEDH syndrome)	225050	AR
68 ED/skin fragility syndrome	604536	AR
Subgroup teeth–nails–sweat glands		
69 Amelo-onycho-hypohidrotic syndrome	104570	AD
70 Limb–mammary syndrome (LMS)	603543	AD
Subgroup hair–teeth		
71 Barber–Say syndrome	209885	AR? AD? XD?
72 Blepharo-cheilodontic syndrome	119580	AD
73 Brachymetapody–anodontia–hypotrichosis–albinoidism	211370	AR
74 Cataract–hypertrichosis–mental retardation (CAHMR) syndrome	211770	AR
75 Cerebellar ataxia–ED	212835	AR
76 Dubowitz syndrome	223370	AR
77 ED–neurosensory deafness	224800	AR
78 ED–ectrodactyly–macular dystrophy (EEM) syndrome	225280	AR
79 Gingival fibromatosis with hypertrichosis	135400	AD
80 Gorlin–Chaudhry–Moss syndrome	233500	AR
81 Hallermann–Streiff syndrome (HSS)	234100	AR
82 Hypertrichosis universalis	145700	AD
83 Johanson–Blizzard syndrome (JBS)	243800	AR
84 Oculo-dento-osseous dysplasia, AR	257850	AR
85 Oculo-dento-digital dysplasia (ODDD)	164200	AD
86 Oro-facio-digital syndrome 1 (OFD1)	311200	XD
87 Pili torti	261900	AR
88 Pilodental dysplasia with refractive errors	262020	AR
89 Progeroid short stature with pigmented naevi (Mulvihill–Smith syndrome)	176690	AD
90 Rodrigues blindness (microphthalmia, microcornea and sclerocornea with short stature and hair and dental abnormalities)	268320	AR
91 Trichodental dysplasia	601453	AD
92 Uncombable hair–retinal pigmentary dystrophy–dental anomalies–brachydactyly	191482	AD
93 Zunich neuroectodermal syndrome	280000	AR
Subgroup hair–nails		
94 Alopecia congenita with keratosis palmoplantaris	104100	AD
95 Anonychia-onychodystrophy with hypoplasia or absence of distal phalanges (Cooks syndrome)	106995	AD
96 Cartilage–hair hypoplasia (CHH)	250250	AR
97 Curly hair–ankyloblepharon–nail dysplasia syndrome (CHANDS)	214350	AR
98 Hidrotic ED, Christianson–Fourie type	601375	AD
99 ED, 'pure' hair–nail type	602032	AD?
100 Hairy elbows (hypertrichosis cubiti)	139600	AD
101 Ichthyosis and male hypogonadism	308200	XR?
102 Ichthyosis with alopecia, eclabion, ectropion and mental retardation	242510	AR
103 Lymphoedema–hypoparathyroidism syndrome	247410	AR? XR?
104 Monilethrix	158000	AD
105 Onycho-trichodysplasia and neutropenia	258360	AR
106 Polyposis–skin pigmentation–alopecia–fingernail changes	175500	?
107 Popliteal pterygium syndrome, lethal type	263650	AR
108 T-cell immunodeficiency–congenital alopecia–nail dystrophy	601705	AR?
109 Trichomegaly with mental retardation, dwarfism and pigmentary degeneration of retina	275400	AR
110 Tricho-thio-dystrophy, non-photosensitive 1 (TTDN1)	234050	AR
Subgroup hair–sweat glands		
111 Focal facial dermal dysplasia types I–IV	136500; 227260	AD, AR
112 Tetra-amelia–ED–lacrimal duct abnormalities (single case)	273390	AR
Subgroup teeth–nails		
113 Corneo-dermato-osseous (CDO) syndrome	122440	AD
114 Deafness, congenital, and onychodystrophy, AD	124480	AD
115 Deafness–onychodystrophy–osteodystrophy–mental retardation (DOOR) syndrome	220500	AR? AD?
116 Dermato-osteolysis, Kirghizian type	221810	AR
117 Haim–Munk syndrome (HMS)	245010	AR
118 Hearing loss, sensorineural, with enamel hypoplasia and nail defects (Heimler syndrome)	234580	AR

Table 65.1 (*continued*)

Ectodermal dysplasia (ED)	MIM	Inheritance
119 Lacrimo-auriculo-dento-digital syndrome (LADD)	149730	AD
120 Odonto-micronychial dysplasia	601319	AR
121 Oto-palato-digital syndrome, type 1 (OPD1)	311300	XD
122 Pycnodysostosis	265800	AR
123 Weyers acrofacial dysostosis	193530	AD
124 Williams–Beuren syndrome (WBS)	194050	AD
Subgroup teeth–sweat glands		
125 Kohlschutter–Tonz syndrome (epilepsy–dementia–amelogenesis imperfecta)	226750	AR? XR?
126 Marshall syndrome I	154780	AD
Subgroup nails–sweat glands		
127 ED–absent dermatoglyphic pattern–changes in nails–simian crease	129200	AD

Adapted from Visinoni *et al.* 2009 [3].

AD, autosomal dominant; AR, autosomal recessive; XD, X-linked dominant; XR, X-linked recessive.

conditions as diverse as incontinentia pigmenti, dyskeratosis congenita, trichothiodystrophies, cardiofaciocutaneous syndrome, pachyonychia congenita and Goltz syndrome by this definition are ectodermal dysplasias, but common practice has been to consider many of these as separate entities.

Classification: clinical approaches

The second challenge presented by this group of conditions is that of designing a meaningful and functional classification system. Until the end of the 20th century, classification systems for ectodermal dysplasias were based on clinical manifestations. Several authors addressed the issue of delineating nosological groups of conditions linked by shared phenotypical traits. The most comprehensive accounts of clinical phenotypes and inheritance patterns of ectodermal dysplasia were produced by Pinheiro and Freire-Maia in their classic monograph and in subsequent writings [8]. Their classification designated conditions by groups depending on the presence of hair, nail, tooth or sweat gland abnormalities, and assigned conditions to groups using a '1-2-3-4 system' to collate conditions that had involvement of hair (1) (89%), teeth (2) (78%), nails (3) (73.5%) or sweat glands (4) (38%) (Figures 65.1, 65.2 and 65.3). This classification was a comprehensive attempt to bring order to an unwieldy group of conditions but was difficult to use and grouped together disparate clinical entities such as Goltz syndrome and pachyonychia congenita. In common with any other classification of ectodermal dysplasias based on clinical findings, this system is confounded by the subtleties of inheritance such as incomplete penetrance and variable expressivity of phenotype. This is especially true in the ectodermal dysplasias, in which sweating is often not formally measured and tooth or nail anomalies may be mild. A comprehensive contemporaneous consideration of the breadth of ectodermal dysplasia conditions in the tradition of Freire-Maia and Pinheiro is given by Visinoni *et al.* (Table 65.1) [3]. Clinical classifications now need to become more focused and better integrated with phenotype, genotype and molecular pathways [2]. Difficult decisions will need to be made to balance inclusiveness (of every possible ectodermal dysplasia) with accessibility and practicality of usage. In addition, the new classification should allow the inclusion of oligosymptomatic or even monosymptomatic variants of ectodermal dysplasia, which will be only possible by integrating clinical and molecular data.

Classification: molecular approaches

The last two decades have seen several important insights into the molecular basis of a number of the ectodermal dysplasias [1]. In some cases the molecular data have confirmed clinical impressions, for example the Hay–Wells syndrome and ectrodactyly–ectodermal dysplasia–cleft lip/palate (EEC) syndrome have ectodermal dysplasia and clefting of the palate and lip in common and these conditions are now known to be allelic [9]. Prompted by the great advances in molecular knowledge, several authors have proposed new molecular-based classification systems [1,2,3,10]. These approaches classify conditions based on the class of molecule responsible for the disorder, for example categorising together those with mutations in structural or developmental molecules (Box 65.1). This approach has many advantages, especially for the characterisation of defects in preparation for molecular diagnostics and, hopefully, molecular therapy. These systems, however, need to be integrated with clinical findings and need to be accessible to all clinicians involved in the care of these patients. Importantly, it has to be realised that currently it is not possible to provide a molecular diagnosis for all patients, even in those with classic clinical features of conditions well characterised at a molecular level. In addition, access to and the affordability of molecular diagnostics often represent an obstacle to molecular characterisation.

Box 65.1 Molecular pathways that are important in ectodermal dysplasias

- Hedgehog signalling pathway
- Wingless signalling pathway
- TNF-α signalling pathway
- NF-κB signalling pathway
- ED signalling pathway
- p63 signalling pathway
- Gap junctions–connexin pathway
- Axin pathway
- Bone morphogenic protein
- Fibroblast growth factor
- Notch pathway

Epidemiology

Incidence and prevalence

A study by Nguyen-Nielsen *et al.* [11] documented an occurrence of 1.6 hypohidrotic ectodermal dysplasia patients in 100 000 people in Denmark when only molecularly confirmed X-linked hypohidrotic ectodermal dysplasia were taken into account. Therefore the prevalence rate of all ectodermal dysplasias must be higher. Ectodermal dysplasias are observed globally.

Age

The diagnosis of ectodermal dysplasias is made within the first years of life, often after complications such as hyperthermia or pneumonia have occurred.

Sex

As all inheritance patterns occur, males and females are affected. In conditions inherited in an X-linked fashion, females often have less severe disease but are not free of manifestations.

Ethnicity

Ectodermal dysplasias have been observed in all parts of the world and in all races.

Associated diseases

Often atopic eczema, allergic asthma, rhinitis and food allergies are associated.

Pathophysiology

The skin and its appendages are mainly composed of ectodermal structures but the development of appendages is orchestrated by signals from the mesoderm with the help of ectodermal placodes. A rather complicated network of signalling pathways coordinates the formation and function of ectodermal structures [2]. In recent years much has been learned about the molecular mechanisms of ectodermal embryogenesis and this has allowed the establishment of a more rational basis for the classification of ectodermal dysplasias. Interestingly, not only full-blown ectodermal syndromes but also mono- or oligosymptomatic ectodermal malformations may result from a mutation in an ectodermal key gene. Embryogenesis occurs in distinct tissue organisational fields and specific interactions among the germ layers may lead to a wide range of ectodermal dysplasias.

The skin is the product of ectodermal and mesodermal stem cell differentiation [12]. However, according to the Spemann organiser theory, even the endoderm has a role in all organ formations including the skin [13]. Orchestrated skin development is only possible by intensive information exchange, especially between the mesoderm and ectoderm. Mesodermal signalling pathways such as wingless (Wnt) are crucial for the induction of appendages of the skin. Wnt signalling, for example, has influences on mesenchymal cells and on epithelial cells [14]. The same is true for the ectodysplasin cascade [14]. Whereas the mesoderm induces the placodes through Wnt signalling, the ectoderm evolves into epidermis through activation of the ectodysplasin and sonic hedgehog pathways [15]. There is a cross-talk of several signalling cascades, such as the ectodysplasin and p53 signalling pathways. Genetic defects in signalling pathways, which disturb the interaction between the ectoderm and mesoderm, lead to ectodermal dysplasia. Dickkopf expression leads to the positioning and orientation of the placode and the sonic hedgehog cascade is responsible for the formation of hair germ. Ripply, which is a retinoic acid-inducible repressor, is required for setting the borders of the pre-placodal ectoderm [16]. Work by Mikkola and co-workers shows that numerous genes and gene pathways such as the tumour necrosis factor (TNF), NF-κB (nuclear factor 'kappa light chain enhancer' of activated B-cells) and Wnt pathway, transforming growth factor β (TGF-β) pathway, fibroblast growth factor pathway and chemokine pathway are involved in hair development [17]. Embryo development network analysis revealed a relationship between disease genes and embryo development-associated genes [18]. A similar transcription factor and microRNA profile is found during embryonic and disease development in numerous organs including the skin.

Ectodermal dysplasias manifest mainly in ectodermal structures and often involve a key gene affecting embryogenesis of the skin, such as ectodysplasin, wingless, *p63* or *sonic hedgehog* (*SHH*) [1,19]. The ectodysplasin A (EDA) pathway plays a conserved role in fine-tuning the size, spacing and position (and probably thereby shape) of ectodermal organs in vertebrates. EDA has a dual role in ectodermal organogenesis: inhibition of bone morphogenetic protein (BMP) activity and induction of *SHH* expression [20]. The Wnt pathway regulates both EDA and ectodysplasin A receptor (EDAR), and the activin and BMP pathways also regulate EDAR [19]. The role of Wnt in physiology and disease is well documented in numerous papers [21]. In the skin, Wnt signalling is important for the establishment of the dermatome architecture, dermis, skin regions with individual appendages, axial determination and intra-appendage regions [22]. Focal dermal hypoplasia, a multiorgan developmental disorder, underscores the importance of Wnt proteins in ectodermal–mesodermal communication as causative mutations were found in *PORCN* encoding a member of the Wnt cascade. *WNT10A* mutations are frequent causes of a broad spectrum of ectodermal dysplasias with teeth, nail, skin and hair abnormalities. Also the rare syndrome of odonto-onycho-dermal dysplasia is caused by mutations in the same gene. Schöpf–Schulz–Passarge syndrome is a consequence of a homozygous nonsense mutation in *WNT10A* [23]. The fact that isolated hypodontia can also be found in 50% of patients with *WNT10A* mutation underscores the fact that ectodermal dysplasias are often clinically heterogeneous [24].

It has been shown that pathogenic variants in only four genes (*EDA1*, *EDAR*, *EDARAAD* and *WNT10A*) account for 90% of hypohidrotic/anhidrotic ectodermal dysplasia cases [1,25]. p63 plays a crucial role in the maturation of the epidermis; it is important for barrier formation, terminal differentiation of keratinocytes, adhesion and proliferation as well as for basement membrane formation [26]. Non-syndromic cleft lip has been observed with mutations in *p63* [27], which underlines the fact that monosymptomatic ectodermal malformations may result from a mutation in an ectodermal key gene. Fibroblasts from healthy donors and two EEC syndrome patients carrying two different point mutations in the DNA-binding domain of p63 were reprogrammed into induced pluripotent stem cell (iPSC) lines [28]. EEC syndrome iPSC from both patients showed early ectodermal commitment into K18(+) cells but failed to further differentiate into K14(+) cells (epidermis/limbus) or K3/K12(+) cells (corneal epithelium). APR-246

(PRIMA-1(MET)), a small compound that restores functionality of mutant p53 in human tumour cells, was able to revert corneal epithelial lineage commitment and reinstate a normal p63-related signalling pathway. This study shows a possible avenue for future therapy.

Signalling pathways in human skeletal dysplasias often also have an impact on the skin. They include TGF-β, Wnt, hedgehog, Notch, BMP, fibroblast growth factor (FGF) and others. Mutations in genes encoding FGF receptors cause Crouzon syndrome, Apert syndrome, Beare–Stevenson syndrome and numerous other syndromes that show cutaneous involvement. Sclerosteosis or Van Buchem disease also features nail alterations and the responsible gene is *SOST* (sclerostin) [29]. *AXIN2* mutations can lead to tooth agenesis as well as to ectodermal dysplasia with malignant tumours [30]. *Patched gene* (*PTCH*) mutations or *SHH* mutations can lead to basal cell naevus syndrome and other malformations mainly in ectodermal structures. Numerous mutations in genes that encode for adhesion molecules can lead to ectodermal dysplasia, including mutations in connexin genes causing keratitis–ichthyosis–deafness syndrome, oculo-dento-digital dysplasias, Clouston syndrome, Vohwinkel syndrome, Bart–Pumphrey syndrome and others. However, mutations in the structural components of desmosomes can also lead to isolated heart diseases, which have no relation to ectodermal dysplasia. In addition, mutations in desmosome-forming genes can also lead to combined skin and cardiac problems. There are numerous diseases with mutations in genes important for cell to cell adhesion that are placed within the ectodermal dysplasias but without clear systematics [31].

The following section reviews some of the commoner ectodermal dysplasias, classified according to the signalling pathway most prominently associated with their pathogenesis.

Ectodermal dysplasias due to mutations in TNF-like/NF-κB signalling pathways.
The transcription factor NF-κB regulates the expression of multiple genes encoding important mediators of immune and stress responses, cell adhesion, protection against apoptosis and inflammatory reactions [32]. In addition, this transcription factor plays critical roles in the development and homeostasis of the epidermis and the proper function of lymphatic vessels [33]. NF-κB is composed of homo- or heterodimers of five proteins belonging to the Rel family. NF-κB is usually maintained in an inactive state within the cytoplasm when bound to inhibitory proteins of the IκB family: IκBα, IκBβ and IκBε. IκB molecules are phosphorylated on two critical serine residues in response to multiple stimuli such as cytokines, various stress signals and viral and bacterial infections. Phosphorylation at these sites enables recognition of IκB molecules by a ubiquitation complex. Following polyubiquitation, IκBs are degraded by the proteasome, thus releasing free NF-κB which then enters the nucleus and activates target genes [34]. The kinase that phosphorylates IκB has been designated IκK (for IκB kinase) and has been shown to consist of two catalytic subunits (IκKα/IκK1 and IκKβ/IκK2) and a third component IκKγ (more usually known as NEMO) that plays a structural and regulatory function within the complex. Cell lines lacking NEMO are unable to activate NF-κB in response to most stimuli. Extensive work with mouse models has confirmed the centrality of the NF-κB pathway in apoptosis, inflammatory and immune functions. A complete absence of NF-κB leads to prenatal death due to massive TNF-induced liver apoptosis, and more subtle knock-outs that alter NF-κB activity all lead to immune defects. The NF-κB pathway has been found to be defective in a number of ectodermal dysplasias. In many cases these predominantly phenotype-driven, mouse–human comparison studies have yielded significant new insights into molecular pathways. One of the best characterised NF-κB-related systems is the ectodysplasin pathway, which serves as an upstream activator of NF-κB. Since 1997, defects in this pathway have been demonstrated in the X-linked, autosomal dominant and recessive subtypes of HED. Subsequently, mutations in downstream components of the pathway have been shown to underlie familial incontinentia pigmenti and HED associated with immunodeficiency and/or osteopetrosis.

The X-linked HED gene, *EDA*, which maps to Xq12-13.1 and is also mutated in the mouse orthologue *tabby*, was first described in 1996 [35]. *EDA* encodes two isoforms of a transmembrane protein, ectodysplasin A, that has homology to the TNF family [36]. The extracellular domain of EDA has a collagen-like repeat and a furin cleavage site, unique among TNF proteins. Cleavage is necessary to enable solubility and functionality of EDA. The two longest isoforms, EDA-A1 and EDA-A2, bind to two different receptors: EDA-A1 binds to the EDAR protein and EDA-A2 binds to another X-linked receptor, XEDAR [**19**]. Mutations have been identified in all domains of EDA in patients with HED, and many of these mutations are thought to have an effect on solubility or cleavage of EDA, rendering it non-functional. The physiological role of EDA in hair follicle morphogenesis was demonstrated with the isolation of the gene for autosomal dominant/recessive HED. Patients with autosomal dominant or recessive HED are phenotypically identical to those with X-linked HED. The *EDAR* gene carrying mutations in this disorder is homologous to the *downless* (*DL*) mouse gene and encodes a member of the tumour necrosis factor receptor (TNFR) superfamily which functions as an ectodysplasin receptor, EDAR. Loss-of-function mutations in *EDAR* have been reported in autosomal recessive HED while dominant negative mutations affecting the death domain of EDAR cause autosomal dominant HED [37].

The EDA/EDAR pathway was further refined when the molecular basis of a third mouse homologue was identified. The *crinkled* (*cr*) is a spontaneous mouse mutant with a phenotype identical to *downless* and *tabby* [**19**]. Using positional cloning techniques, the causative gene was found to encode an adapter protein termed EDARADD (EDAR-associated death domain) for the EDA/EDAR complex. Mutations in the human homologue of this gene, named *EDARADD*, were identified as a cause for autosomal recessive HED [38]. The EDARADD interacts with the intracellular death domain of EDAR, linking it to downstream signals, leading to NF-kB activation [39]. EDARADD associates with TRAF 1, 2 and 3. NF-κB activation by the EDAR pathway is NEMO dependent [39], and the relevance of this interaction to human ectodermal dysplasias became clearer when loss-of-function mutations were identified in the X-linked *IKBKG* gene (more usually known as *NEMO*) in incontinentia pigmenti [39]. Mutations in this gene are usually lethal in males. However, less severe (hypomorphic) mutations in *IKBKG* have been described in several male patients with an unusual phenotype of HED associated with immune deficiency

(EDA-ID) [40]. Mutations in the coding region are associated with the EDA-ID phenotype, while specific mutations affecting the stop codon of *IKBKG* cause a more severe syndrome of osteopetrosis and/or lymphoedema associated with EDA-ID [41].

Two other EDAR-related members of the TNFR superfamily, XEDAR and TROY/TAJ, have been reported [**19**]. Signals from each of these receptors were shown to activate NF-κB, providing further candidate genes and candidate signalling systems for human HED. The TNFR-associated factor 6 (TRAF-6) is a cytoplasmic adapter protein that links signals from members of the TNFR superfamily to activation of transcription factors such as NF-κB through IKK (inhibitor of κB kinase) complex activation. TRAF-6 −/− mice display HED, revealing yet more complexity to these signalling systems. HED can result from mutations in *TRAF-6* [42].

TP63-related phenotypes: overview of the molecular pathway.

p63 plays a crucial role during the formation of the epidermis [43]. p63 is important for barrier formation, terminal differentiation of keratinocytes, adhesion and proliferation as well as for basement membrane assembly [26]; it is also involved in cleft palate. p63 has numerous target genes including *EDAR*, *NOTCH*, *BMP*, *CTNNB1* and *FAS*. Because p63 is linked with many other signalling pathways, the clinical features of p63-related diseases are rather heterogeneous and broad [44]. p63 regulates human keratinocyte proliferation via the MYC–gene network [45]. The expression of numerous genes is altered in the absence of a fully functional p63. Accordingly, mutations in *TP63* encoding p63 have been found in ankyloblepharon–ectodermal defects–cleft lip/palate (AEC) syndrome skin to disrupt several signalling pathways [46]. Epigenetic modifications have been shown to affect p63 regulation of terminal differentiation genes. p63 mutations can lead to altered stability and transcriptional activity in distinct ectodermal dysplasias [47]. Non-syndromic cleft lip has been observed with mutations in *TP63* [**27**] which underlines the fact that monosymptomatic ectodermal malformations may result from a mutation in an ectodermal key gene. The E3 ligase itch mediates the degradation of p63, providing another level of regulation and thus suggesting novel therapeutic strategies for ectodermal dysplasia [48].

The p53 gene family comprises key regulators of the cell cycle, which are mutated in more than 50% of human cancers. p63 regulates human keratinocyte proliferation via a MYC-regulated gene network and differentiation commitment through a cell adhesion-related gene network [45]. p63 and p73 are related molecules that share high amino acid identity with p53. p63 and p53 are critical regulators of gene expression during embryogenesis. They regulate the development of facial prominence and limb buds, and are essential for cranial closure and development of the lens. Limb defects are best explained by a failure of the apical ectodermal ridge to develop [49]. The role of p63 and p73 in human cancers has been extensively studied. Whereas p53 has an important role in tumorigenesis, this is not as prominent in p63. The *TP63* and *TP73* genes also differ from *TP53* in that they each encode several different isoforms by utilising two different transcription initiation sites (for a review see [50]).

Mutations in *p63* have now been identified in five distinct human phenotypes, all of which have ectodermal dysplasia as a key feature

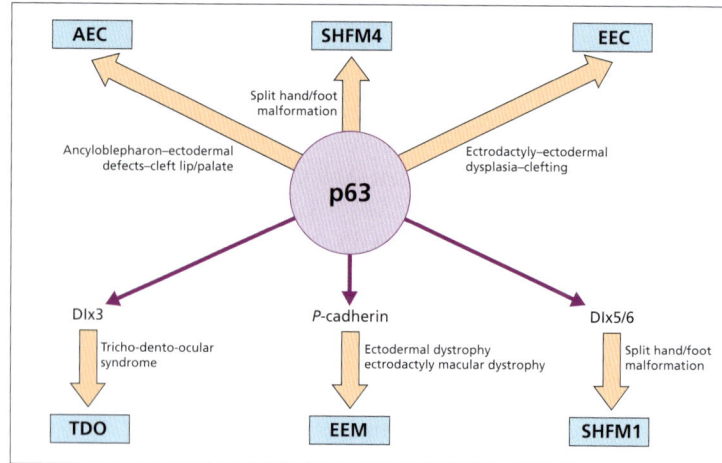

Figure 65.4 The central role of p63 in ectodermal dysplasia. Adapted from Koster 2010 [26].

(Figure 65.4) [26,44]. Some genotype–phenotype correlations have been identified (for a review see [50]).

- *EEC syndrome.* TP63 mutations account for most cases of EEC syndrome. Van Bokhoven *et al.* [**51**] were able to demonstrate mutations in 40 out of 43 families with EEC. All but one of these mutations were sited within the DNA-binding domain, and sequence alterations affecting five amino acid residues accounted for 75% of all mutations.
- *AEC syndrome.* In the AEC syndrome (also known as Hay–Wells syndrome), where the limb abnormalities are absent or minimal, mutations have been exclusively detected within the sterile alpha motif (SAM) domain-encoding region of the *TP63* gene and are associated with complex gain-of-function as well as loss- and change-of-function effects [**51**].
- *Limb mammary syndrome (LMS).* This autosomal dominant syndrome was first reported in a Dutch family with a constellation of features that had not previously been reported, including hand and foot anomalies and mammary gland aplasia/hypoplasia. The skin and hair were normal in all affected individuals, but some had lacrimal duct atresia, nail dysplasia, hypohidrosis, hypodontia or cleft palate [50]. In addition, internal female genital dysplasias have been observed [52]. LMS is distinguished from EEC syndrome by the consistent finding of mammary anomalies in LMS (infrequent in EEC), and the much more frequent finding of skin, nail and tooth anomalies in EEC syndrome. The clefting in LMS is of the palate only, whereas in EEC syndrome the lip and palate are affected. In LMS, *TP63* frameshift mutations leading to truncations of p63 protein have been reported in exon 13 in two unrelated patients [**51**], and an N-terminal mutation in a further family [26].
- *ADULT syndrome.* Mutations in the acro-dermato-ungual–lacrimal–tooth (ADULT) syndrome have yielded interesting insights in that the first mutation was identified in exon 3′, which is only expressed in the transactivating isotypes of p63 and causes an amino acid substitution outside the DNA-binding domain [53]. A subsequent report has demonstrated a mutation that confers significant transactivation activity on ΔN-p63γ, an otherwise inert isoform of p63 [50].

- *Non-syndromic split-hand–split-foot malformation (SHFM) syndrome.*
  This condition has no dermatological features and therefore is
  not discussed in detail here. However, the molecular basis of the
  isolated SHFM syndrome is also a mutation in p63 [45]. SHFM
  syndrome is a genetically heterogeneous group of conditions, but
  some cases (possibly around 10%) are attributable to *TP63* mutations [51]. Some of these mutations seem specific for SHFM but
  others underlie both EEC and SHFM [50].

Defects in transcription factors other than p63. In addition to the
p63 pathway, several other ectodermal dysplasias have now been
attributed to defects in transcription factors that control the expression of several target genes important in ectodermal morphogenesis [54]. In many cases, positional cloning studies have yielded the
primary mutation in a specific gene but the detailed molecular signalling pathways have yet to be delineated.

Ellis–van Creveld (EvC) syndrome is a recessive ectodermal dysplasia that is characterised by a skeletal dysplasia with short limbs,
short ribs, postaxial polydactyly and congenital heart defects.
The gene has been identified [55]. There is evidence that the
two ciliary proteins, Evc and Evc2, the products of human disease genes associated with the EvC syndrome, act downstream
of smoothened to transduce sonic hedgehog signalling. Loss of
Evc/Evc2 does not affect sonic hedgehog-induced smoothened
phosphorylation and ciliary localisation but impedes sonic hedgehog pathway activation mediated by constitutively active forms of
smoothened [56].

Witkop syndrome (MIM: 189500) is an autosomal dominant
ectodermal dysplasia with primary manifestation in the teeth (taurodontia and partial or complete anodontia) and nails (koilonychia,
longitudinal ridging and nail pits) [57]. Mutations have been identified in the *MSX1* gene, a member of the homeobox gene family and
an important regulator of transcription.

Of the ectodermal dysplasias more likely to be seen by a dermatologist, tricho-dento-osseous (TDO) syndrome and tricho-rhino-
phalangeal syndrome (TRPS) are both caused by mutations in genes
coding for important transcription factors. The causative gene for
TDO syndrome is *DLX3*, encoding a homeodomain transcription
factor that is developmentally expressed in many structures derived
from epithelial–mesenchymal interactions, such as the teeth, hair
follicles and limb buds. A dominant mutation responsible for TDO
syndrome was found to impair the ability of DLX3 to downregulate δNp63α [58]. TRPS types I and III are caused by mutations in
TRPS1 which is important in the development and differentiation
of bone, kidney and hair follicles [59]; a microdeletion syndrome
(8q42.11 to 8q24.1), that includes *TRPS1* and *EXT1*, underlies TRPS
type II.

Genetics
As ectodermal dysplasias are such a heterogeneous group of diseases, autosomal recessive, autosomal dominant, X-linked and mitochondrial inheritance have been described.

Environmental factors
Epigenetic factors seem to be important for the phenotypical expression of the disease.

Resources

Further information

Canadian Ectodermal Dysplasia Syndromes Association: http://ectodermaldys
  plasia.ca/.
Ectodermal Dysplasia Society: http://www.ectodermaldysplasia.org/.
Ectodermal Dysplasias International Network: https://edinetwork.org/.
National Foundation for Ectodermal Dysplasias: http://nfed.org/.
(All last accessed February 2022.)

X-linked hypohidrotic ectodermal dysplasia with immunodeficiency

Definition, nomenclature and classification
X-linked hypohidrotic ectodermal dysplasia with immunodeficiency (EDA-ID) is a rare disease with the clinical hallmarks of
hypohidrosis, delayed teeth eruption, coarse hair and immunodeficiency complicated by frequent bacterial infections. Causative
mutations have been identified in the *IKBKG* gene, which codes
for the inhibitor of κ light polypeptide gene enhancer in B-cell
kinase-γ, better known as NF-κB essential modulator (NEMO).
NEMO phosphorylates and degrades IκB to activate NF-κB. NEMO
dysfunction leads to an impaired antimicrobial response to polysaccharides, impaired NK-cell activity, hyper immunoglobulin M (IgM)
syndrome and hypogammaglobulinaemia. Often patients have
co-morbidity with inflammatory bowel disease and rheumatoid
arthritis.

Synonyms and inclusions
- Hypohidrotic ectodermal dysplasia with immunodeficiency, osteopetrosis and
  lymphoedema

Classification links
- ICD-10: D82.8
- MIM: 300291, 612132
- Orphanet: ORPHA98813

Introduction and general description
The observation of unusually severe recurrent infections in a
small subset of patients with otherwise typical HED features led
to the suggestion that there may be a specific syndrome of HED
and immunodeficiency (EDA-ID) [1]. The EDA-ID syndrome was
first reported in a boy with miliary tuberculosis, and the second
reported case had recurrent life-threatening infections caused by
Pseudomonas aeruginosa, *Mycobacterium avium* and cytomegalovirus.
A third child had a milder phenotype with repeated infections due
to *Staphylococcus aureus* and *Streptococcus pneumoniae*, and three
further siblings from a different kindred had recurrent severe infections with *S. pneumoniae*, with impaired response to polysaccharide
antigens. All of these cases were males, suggesting X-linked inheritance. Since these original reports, the disease phenotypic spectrum
has been delineated and includes severe life-threatening or recurrent bacterial infections in the lower respiratory tract, skin, soft

PART 6: GENETIC DISORDERS

tissues, bones and gastrointestinal tract, as well as meningitis and septicaemia in early childhood. Overall, the causative pathogens have most often been Gram-positive bacteria (*S. pneumoniae* and *S. aureus*), followed by Gram-negative bacteria (*Pseudomonas* spp. and *Haemophilus influenzae*) and mycobacteria. Most patients have severe hypogammaglobulinaemia, with low serum IgG levels and varied levels of other immunoglobulin isotypes (IgA, IgM and IgE). Some patients have massively elevated IgM levels, and an impaired antibody response to polysaccharides is the most consistent feature of this condition.

Hypomorphic mutations in the X-linked *IKBKG* gene or somatic mutations in this gene result in various forms of anhidrotic ectodermal dysplasia with immunodeficiency [2]. Missense mutations in the gene encoding NEMO are associated with reduced signal-induced nuclear translocation of NF-κB proteins, resulting in defective expression of NF-κB target genes [3,4]. It has been shown that the pathogenic mutation preferentially impairs the interaction with K63 and M1-linked di-Ub, which correlates with its ubiquitin-binding defect *in vivo* [5]. Impaired NK cell activity is reported in some, but not all, patients with EDA-ID; the degree and range of immunological abnormalities seen may relate to the type of *NEMO* mutation involved.

Epidemiology
Incidence and prevalence
Prevalence is not known in any detail. The incidence has been assumed to be approximately 1 in 250 000 live male births for the X-linked form.

Age
Typical signs and symptoms may develop early. Sparse hair with hypotrichosis or complete alopecia, abnormal teeth with conical shape or missing teeth and sweating impairment, combined with recurrent infections, are the leading clinical findings to make an early diagnosis. The disease can be associated with lymphoedema and osteopetrosis.

Sex
Transmission is X-linked recessive in patients with mutations in the coding regions of NEMO. This means that the disease usually occurs in males.

Ethnicity
There is no ethnic preponderance.

Associated diseases
Twenty-five per cent of patients have inflammatory bowel disease and rheumatoid arthritis. There is a variant associated with osteopetrosis and lymphoedema. Recurrent bacterial infections are common [1].

Pathophysiology
Genetics
The disease is usually inherited in an X-linked recessive fashion. Somatic mosaicism is also frequently observed. Fewer than 10 patients have been reported with an autosomal dominant form of the disease due to mutations in the *NFKBIA* gene encoding the NF-κB, subunit 1, which is related to the NF-κB signalling pathway as well.

Environmental factors
Absent or decreased sweating leads to heat intolerance.

Clinical features
History
The lack of normal hair growth is typical. Many patients fail to thrive. Fever of unknown origin as a child and later heat intolerance are typical manifestations. Missing teeth or malformed teeth are also characteristic and a clue for diagnosis in children. Mutations in *IKBKG* should be considered in male infants with recalcitrant seborrhoeic or atopic eczema-like eruptions and intertrigo, especially when features of ectodermal dysplasia are present [6].

Differential diagnosis
Apart from recurrent bacterial infections, the clinical manifestations, differential diagnosis and natural course are very similar to those in patients with classic HED. The ectodermal dysplasia-related signs and symptoms, however, are less pronounced than in the classic form and osteopetrosis and lymphoedema are features uniquely found in X-linked EDA-ID.

Hypohidrotic ectodermal dysplasia

Definition, nomenclature and classification
X-linked hypohidrotic ectodermal dysplasia (Freire-Maia 1-2-3-4) is the most common of the ectodermal dysplasias. However, autosomal dominant and autosomal recessive forms have been described. The disorder is characterised by hypotrichosis with fine, slow-growing scalp and body hair, sparse eyebrows, hypohidrosis, nail anomalies and hypodontia. Peg-shaped primary and secondary teeth are typical. Decreased sweating leads to heat intolerance and enhances dryness of the skin. X-linked hypohidrotic ectodermal dysplasia (ECTD1, HED/EDA) is caused by a mutation in the *EDA* gene, which encodes ectodysplasin. In addition, autosomal recessive forms (ECTD10B, ECTD11B) and autosomal dominant forms (ECTD10A, ECTD11A) of HED are caused by mutation in the *EDAR* and *EDARADD* genes, respectively. About 90% of hypohidrotic ectodermal dysplasias are caused by mutations in four genes (*EDA1, EDAR, EDARADD* and *WNT10A*). These genes are important in two signalling pathways which are involved in early steps of ectodermal placode formation: ectodysplasin/NF-κB and Wnt/β catenin. Treatment needs a multidisciplinary approach. Early diagnosis is imperative to avoid life-threatening complications induced by hyperthermia and infections.

Synonyms and inclusions
- Ectodermal dysplasia 1
- X-linked hypohidrotic/hair/tooth-type ectodermal dysplasia
- X-linked anhidrotic ectodermal dysplasia
- Christ–Siemens–Touraine syndrome

Introduction and general description

X-linked HED was first described by Danz in 1792 and then by Charles Darwin in 1875. HED is a monogenic disorder inherited in an X-linked fashion, but autosomal dominant and recessive inheritance types have been described too. A fourth and rare type with immunodeficiency also exists. Hypohidrotic or anhidrotic ectodermal dysplasia is the most prevalent type within the spectrum of ectodermal dysplasias. Clinical hallmarks are hypotrichosis on the scalp but also of the eyebrows and eyelashes, hyperpigmentation around the eyes, dry skin and peg-shaped primary and secondary teeth with hypodontia (Table 65.2). Teeth abnormalities occur in 79% of all cases. Frontal bossing and a saddle-bridged nose may occur. The most important finding is anhidrosis or hypohidrosis. Affected individuals show heat intolerance with episodes of hyperpyrexia, which may result in seizures and neurological damage [1].

Epidemiology

Incidence and prevalence

In a study by Nguyen-Nielsen *et al.*, the population-based prevalence was 21.9 per 100 000 [2], as recently confirmed [3].

Age

The most frequent age at time of X-linked HED diagnosis occurs between the ages of 11 and 18 years.

Sex

Females with X-linked HED show less prominent findings, often displaying patchy lesions arranged along the lines of Blaschko, as opposed to the generalised presentation seen in males.

Ethnicity

There is no ethnic dominance.

Associated diseases

Immunodeficiency, sometimes associated with osteopetrosis and lymphoedema, may occur together in several subtypes of HED. Breast hypoplasia or aplasia might be an additional finding [4].

Table 65.2 Clinical features in patients with autosomal dominant hypohidrotic ectodermal dysplasia.

Complication	Occurrence (%)
Smooth, dry skin	78
Sparse hair	89
Sparse eyebrows	100
Sparse body hair	62
Decreased sweating	85
Heat intolerance	50
Onychodysplasia	39
Dental anomalies	100

Adapted from Aswegan *et al.* 1997 [11].

Pathophysiology

Hypohidrotic ectodermal dysplasia results from mutations in genes encoding members of the ectodysplasin/NF-κB pathway [5]. In 50% of cases, mutations in *EDA* encoding the epithelial morphogen ectodysplasin A of the TNF family, cause X-linked HED. Mutations in *EDAR*, which encodes the ectodysplasin A receptor, or EDARADD, encoding the EDARADD protein, cause both autosomal recessive and autosomal dominant HED. NEMO (also known as inhibitor of NF-κB kinase subunit γ (IKK-γ)) is a protein that in humans is encoded by the *IKBKG* gene located on Xq28. *IKBKG* mutations cause HED with immunodeficiency. Other forms of HED have been shown to result from mutations in: (i) *WNT10A* encoding wingless 10A; (ii) *TRAF6* encoding TNFR-associated factor 6; (iii) *NFKBIA* encoding the nuclear factor of κ light polypeptide gene enhancer in B-cell inhibitor α; and (iv) *EDA2R* (also known as *XEDAR*) encoding the ectodysplasin 2A receptor.

Pathology

Histology shows missing or reduced sweat glands and also reduced sebaceous glands. The epidermis is thin with flattening of the rete ridges. Hair follicles and their sebaceous glands are variably reduced in number. Apocrine glands may be absent, sparse or even normal. Mucous glands of the upper respiratory tract may be sparse or absent. Hair shaft abnormalities are variable and include longitudinal clefts or grooves and transverse fissuring. Radiographs of the jaws may reveal dental hypoplasia or aplasia [1].

Genetics

X-linked, autosomal dominant and autosomal recessive traits exist.

Environmental factors

Patients should avoid hot places and extensive physical activity without cooling devices and special clothes. Patients should drink cool liquids in warm environments. Wearing a hat in sunny climates is obligatory.

Clinical features [5]

History

A history of heat intolerance is characteristic but not obligatory. Sometimes other family members have been affected in the pedigree. Missing or malformed teeth can lead to the diagnosis.

Presentation (Table 65.2)

- *Hair* In a recent review, hypotrichosis was reported in 88.1% for males and in 61.6% for females [3]. The hair is sparse (76%) and mostly straight, dry and lustreless with a heterogeneous hair colour (Figure 65.5a). Decreased hair density is most prominent at the temporal and occipital regions. There is a marked increase of single hair follicular units. The bar code appearance on hair microscopy that mirrors a microscopic artefact is often seen in patients with HED. There are parallel dark bands of different lengths running across the full width of the shaft. Scanning electron microscopy studies have shown follicular distortion, follicular ridging and distorted bulbs but these findings are non-specific. Eyebrows are scanty or absent (Figure 65.5b); occasionally just the outer two-thirds are missing. The eyelashes may

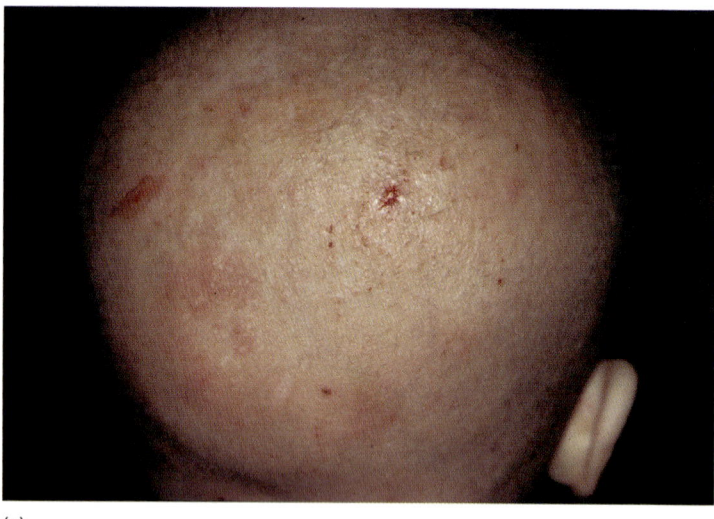

(a)

(b)

Figure 65.5 (a) Hypotrichosis and (b) reduced eyebrows and cilia in hypohidrotic ectodermal dysplasia.

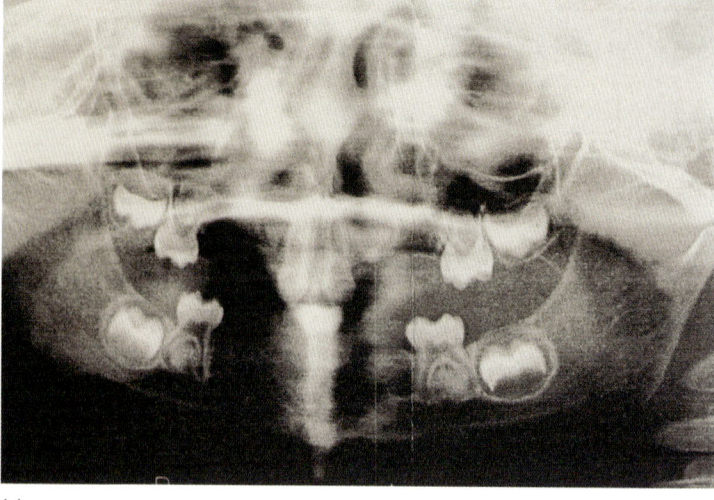

(a)

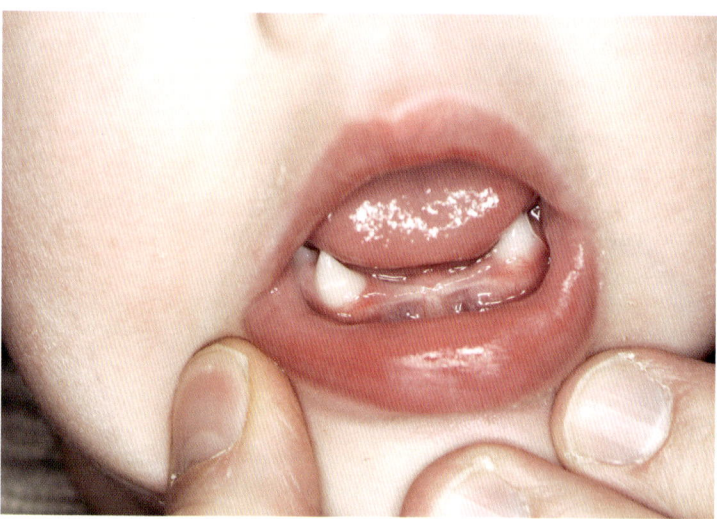

(b)

Figure 65.6 (a) Hypodontia and (b) conical teeth and hypodontia in hypohidrotic ectodermal dysplasia.

be normal, sparse or completely absent. Secondary sexual hair in the beard, pubic and axillary regions is variably present and may be normal. Hair on the torso and extremities is usually absent. Approximately 70% of obligate female carriers of X-linked HED describe their hair as being sparse or fine. Light and electron microscopy shows variable hair shaft defects and diameter, including twisting, trichoptilosis, pili canaliculi and trichorrhexis nodosa [1].

- *Teeth*. In several studies a prevalence of more than 95% for hypodontia is given [3]. A wide range of dental abnormalities may be associated, ranging from a complete absence of teeth (anodontia) to sparse, abnormally shaped teeth (Figure 65.6). Studies reveal a mean of 24 missing teeth, out of a total of 28, in affected males. Dentition is delayed and the erupted teeth tend to be small, widely spaced and frequently conical or peg shaped. Both deciduous and permanent teeth are affected. The alveolar ridges are hypoplastic, which gives rise to full, everted lips. About 80% of obligate female carriers of X-linked HED have distinct dental abnormalities including absent permanent teeth and small or peg-shaped teeth.
- *Nails*. Onychodysplasia has been reported in 39% of cases.
- *Sweat glands*. Reduced or absent sweating was found in 95.7% in males and 71.6% in females [3]. Sweating is often severely diminished or absent due to a paucity or absence of eccrine glands. An absence of sweating leads to an inability to thermoregulate by evaporative cooling, and hyperthermia can occur with physical exertion or in a warm environment. Due to a lower body surface area ratio, thermoregulation is most problematic in infants and young children who may experience recurrent bouts of fever as high as 42°C. Heatstroke is the most common cause of death in patients with anhidrotic ectodermal dysplasia within the first years of life. Heat intolerance does occur in older children and adults, but is less problematic as they are better able to control their body temperature by drinking cold liquids, wetting their skin or clothing and seeking out cool surroundings. Up to 25% of

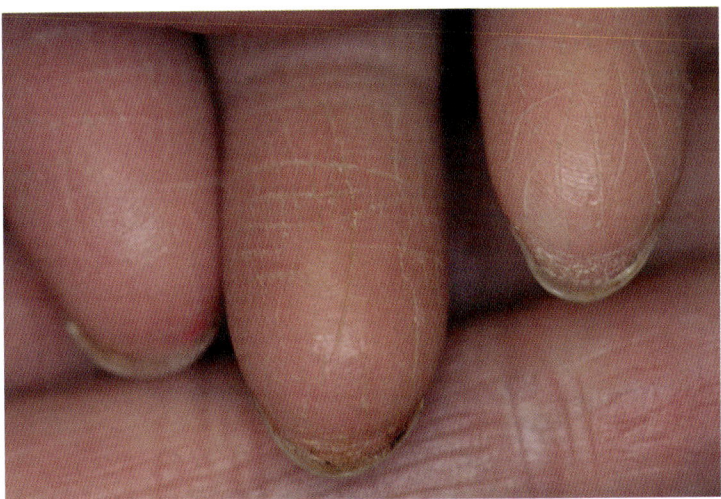

Figure 65.7 Rudimentary dermatoglyphics in hypohidrotic ectodermal dysplasia.

heterozygous females experience heat intolerance and almost half notice their ability to sweat is reduced. The hypohidrotic areas of skin in female carriers of X-linked HED occur in defined linear patterns corresponding to the lines of Blaschko.
- *Skin.* At birth, affected males may demonstrate marked scaling or peeling of their skin which may be mistaken for a collodion membrane. In children and adults, the skin is fine, smooth and dry. Periorbital hyperpigmentation and fine wrinkling around the eyes are characteristic features of the disorder. Eczema is common and is prominent in the flexural areas. Small milia-like papules may be found on the face. Dermatoglyphics are often reduced or even absent (Figure 65.7). Lower lips are often rather prominent and ears show a characteristic deformation ('Spock ears') (Figure 65.8).

Clinical variants
Clinical manifestations are highly variable between individuals. Some have only slight, subjective heat intolerance although reduced to missing sweat glands are almost always identifiable.

Differential diagnosis
Differential diagnosis of HED includes other forms of HEDs including ectodermal dysplasia with immunodeficiency or deafness. In addition, Sjögren syndrome with symptomatic sicca syndrome should be ruled out in oligosymptomatic patients.

Classification of severity
Inter- and intrafamilial clinical heterogeneity has been observed in X-linked HED, suggesting that additional genetic factors may influence the severity of this condition. It has been shown that the *EDAR* 370A allele attenuates the severity of HED caused by *EDA* gene mutations.

Complications and co-morbidities
Anhidrotic ectodermal dysplasia is associated with mortality rates as high as 21%. Severe non-fatal illness was reported in 14 of 49 documented cases within the first year and total episodes of severe illness were observed in 43% [6]. More recent studies documented a

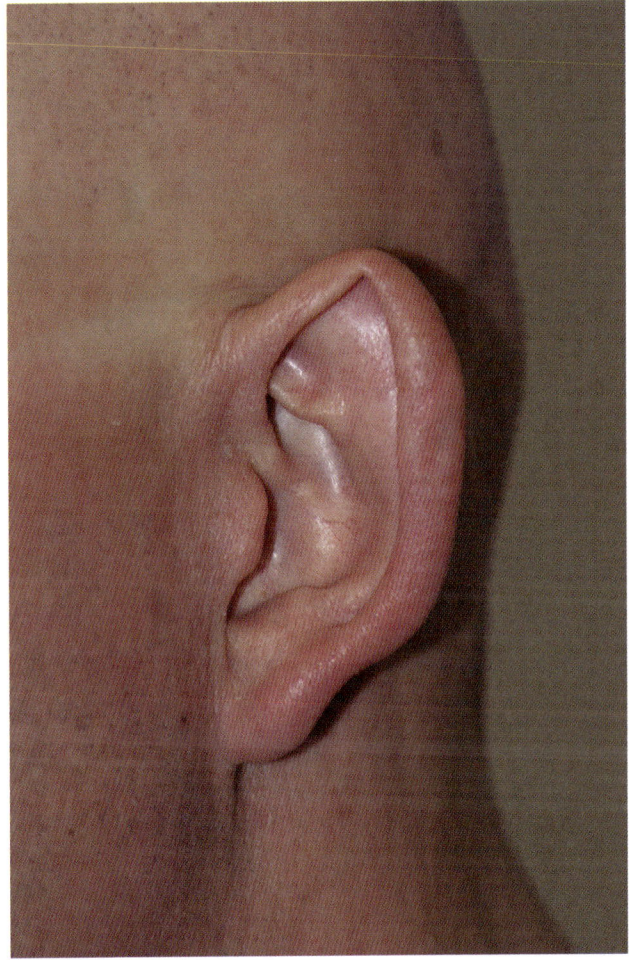

Figure 65.8 'Spock ears' in hypohidrotic ectodermal dysplasia.

much more favorable natural course within the first 5 years of life [7]. Other complications in survivors were eczema in 71%, asthma and recurring wheezing in 65%, nasal crusting in 79%, recurring upper respiratory tract infections in 44% and feeding problems in infancy in 68% (Table 65.3).

Disease course and prognosis
Early diagnosis is imperative to avoid life-threatening complications induced by hyperthermia and infections [7]. Avoiding heat and physical overexertion is the most important preventative measure to recommend. Cooling the body with wet clothing and cool drinks is the only efficient way of treating hyperthermia. Orthodontic intervention is necessary, particularly for language development. Meticulous dental hygiene should be taught to the children as caries develop early.

Investigations
Gaide and Schneider [8] showed that treatment of pregnant Tabby mice, a mouse model for anhidrotic ectodermal dysplasia with a recombinant form of EDA1, engineered to cross the placental barrier, permanently rescued the Tabby phenotype in the offspring. Notably, sweat glands can also be induced by EDA1 after birth. The same group showed that in dogs postpartum treatment induced

Table 65.3 Complications of hypohidrotic ectodermal dysplasia at different ages.

Complication	Rate of occurrence
First year	
Mortality	9/43 (21%)
Severe non-fatal illness	14/49 (29%)
Total episodes of severe illness	25/58 (43%)
Years 0–3	
Mortality	12/43 (28%)
Severe non-fatal illness	18/51 (49%)
Total with episodes of severe illness	32/65 (49%)
Other complications in survivors	
Eczema	39/55 (71%)
Asthma or recurring wheezing	35/54 (65%)
Nasal crusting	42/53 (79%)
Recurrent fevers in infancy	27/50 (54%)
Recurrent upper respiratory tract infections in childhood	21/47 (44%)
Feeding problems in infancy	32/47 (68%)
Specific allergies	14/53 (26%)

Reproduced from Clarke *et al.* 1987 [6] with permission of BMJ Publishing Group.

PART 6: GENETIC DISORDERS

tooth growth. The first successful human study was published recently by Schneider *et al.* [9].

Management

Exposure to heat must be monitored. Strict monitoring of body temperature is necessary for babies in an incubator. Older children should learn to handle heat and heat-generating activities with physical cooling measures, such as frequent drinking of cool liquids, wetting the clothes or wearing special cooling vests and caps. Early dental management may lead to restoring function and improving the appearance of the teeth. Orthodontic treatment often includes bone grafting or sinus-lift procedures followed by the placement of dental implants supporting dental prostheses. HED with immunodeficiency requires immune-based therapies plus aggressive management of infections or haematopoietic stem cell transplantation.

The high prevalence of asthma-like symptoms in X-linked HED patients as young as 6 years and a similar prevalence of dry eye problems indicate that screening evaluation, regular monitoring and consideration of therapeutic intervention should begin in early childhood.

Hypohidrotic ectodermal dysplasia with severe atopic dermatitis was successfully treated with tofacitinib [10]. Twice daily 3% minoxidil 1 mL was applied with success in a patient with HED. After 1 month the patient showed growth of vellus hair and after 1 year dramatic hair growth was observed.

Resources

Further information
National Center for Biotechnology Information, GeneReviews fact sheet: http://www.ncbi.nlm.nih.gov/books/NBK1112/.
National Foundation for Ectodermal Dysplasias, fact sheet: http://nfed.org/index.php/about_ed/types_of_ectodermal_dysplasias.
National Organization for Rare Diseases, fact sheet: http://www.rarediseases.org/rare-disease-information/rare-diseases/byID/804/viewAbstract.
Online Mendelian Inheritance in Man, fact sheet: http://omim.org/entry/305100. (All last accessed February 2022.)

Ankyloblepharon–ectodermal defects–cleft lip/palate syndrome

Definition, nomenclature and classification

Ankyloblepharon–ectodermal defects–cleft lip/palate (AEC) syndrome is the result of missense mutations in *TP63* affecting the p63 SAM of the gene, which is a protein–protein interaction domain. AEC syndrome is inherited in an autosomal dominant fashion. The syndrome is characterised by cleft lip/palate, severe scalp erosions and abnormalities of the epidermal appendages, including hypotrichosis, hypodontia, absent or dystrophic nails and mild hypohidrosis (Box 65.2). One distinctive feature is ankyloblepharon filiforme adnatum – partial thickness fusion of the eyelid margins.

Synonyms and inclusions
- AEC syndrome
- Hay–Wells syndrome
- Ankyloblepharon filiforme adnatum–ectodermal dysplasia–cleft palate syndrome

Classification links
- ICD-10: Q82.4
- MIM: 106260
- Orphanet: ORPHA1071

Box 65.2 Clinical features of the AEC syndrome

Main clinical features
- Craniofacial anomalies: midfacial hypoplasia with high forehead, small mouth, narrow nose, short philtrum and short vermillon border of the upper lip
- Severe erosive scalp dermatitis with secondary infections
- Cleft lip or palate
- Hypoplasia of the uvula
- Poor dentition: hypodontia and conically shaped teeth
- Poor hair growth: sparseness of eyebrows and eyelashes, pili torti and pili canaliculi
- Dystrophic nails: hypertrophy, brittleness, narrow shape and chromonychia
- Hypohidrosis
- Hypospadias in boys

Other clinical features reported
- Erythroderma and scaling skin at birth
- Short stature
- Low intellectual capacity
- Depapillated tongue
- Conductive hearing loss
- Hypoplastic maxilla
- Atretic ear canal
- Dysplastic eustachian orifices
- Ophthalmological complications: bilateral punctal atresia, underdevelopment of lacrimal ducts and corneal scarring

Adapted from Camacho *et al.* 1993 [11].

Introduction and general description

In 1976, Hay and Wells described a syndrome inherited in an autosomal dominant fashion with ankyloblepharon, ectodermal defects and clefting of the lip and palate [1]. The disorder is today considered to be identical with Rapp–Hodgkin syndrome (MIM: 129400) [2].

Epidemiology

Incidence and prevalence

The AEC syndrome is rare and its precise incidence and prevalence are not known.

Age

The AEC syndrome manifests at birth with eroded scalp dermatitis and collodion membrane.

Sex

Both sexes are equally affected as the syndrome is inherited in an autosomal dominant pattern.

Ethnicity

No ethnic predominance is known.

Associated diseases

There are no associated disorders in the AEC syndrome.

Pathophysiology

The AEC syndrome belongs to the TP63-related phenotypes (see overview of molecular pathology earlier in this chapter).

Predisposing factors

If one parent has the syndrome, the chance of disease transmission to the next generation is 50%.

Pathology

Histopathology of lesional skin shows mild atrophy, focal orthokeratosis and mild superficial perivascular lymphocytic infiltrates. Melanophages reflect postinflammatory changes. Examination of the hair shafts reveals thin hair and loss of melanin pigment in some patients. In addition, structural abnormalities include pili torti, pili trianguli et canaliculi and irregular indentation and shallow grooves [3]. Scanning electron microscopy of the affected hair shaft shows various defects, including fractures of the cuticle and pili torti, none of which is specific for the disorder. Nails may be hyperconvex and thickened, dystrophic or absent. Skin biopsy of involved scalp tissue shows a thin granular layer and stratum corneum. Hair follicles are reduced in size and arrector pili muscles appear hypertrophic. Sweat stimulation tests reveal a patchy loss of sweat glands over most of the body.

Genetics

The AEC syndrome follows an autosomal dominant mode of transmission. About 70% of cases are caused by a *de novo* mutation in *TP63*.

Clinical features (Box 65.2)

History and presentation

At birth about 90% of patients feature a collodion-like picture. In one series, 75% of patients had eroded skin at birth and 63% of patients continued to suffer from chronic scalp erosions and recurrent scalp infections [4]. Three of the seven initial patients had scalp infections or folliculitis of the scalp in association with hair loss. The scalp is commonly involved with severe and erosive dermatitis with secondary crusting and superinfection. Scalp hair is sparse in 89%, wiry in 100% and rather fair in 89% [5]. Focal or diffuse alopecia is common. Patients have rudimentary eyelashes and the eyebrows are also often affected. Absent fingernails occur in 39% and absent toenails in 11%. Dystrophic nails were found in 18 out of 18 patients. Ankyloblepharon refers to fusion of the eyelids, and in its mildest variant there is a partial thickness fusion of the central portion of the eyelid margins with sparing of the canthi (ankyloblepharon filiforme adnatum). Conjunctivitis and blepharitis may result from eye abnormalities. The original family featured partial or complete hair loss, absent or dystrophic nails, widely spaced teeth and partial anhidrosis. Decreased sweat production was found in 16 out of 16 patients although a recent study suggested a lower prevalence of this complication [5,6]. Additional anomalies may include lacrimal duct atresia, supernumerary nipples, syndactyly and auricular deformities. Ichthyosiform scaling is found in 17% and hyperkeratosis in 39%. Pigment changes occurred in all patients with AEC syndrome.

Clinical variants

CHAND syndrome – which stands for curly hair, ankyloblepharon and nail disease – is most likely identical with AEC syndrome [7]. McGrath *et al.* [8] have shown that the syndrome is caused by heterozygous missense mutations in the SAM domain of p63. Mutations in *TP63* have highly pleiotropic effects, as they can cause several allelic disorders including the EEC and ADULT syndromes, LMS and SHFM type 4. Rapp–Hodgkin syndrome is no longer considered as a separate entity, but is a clinical variant of AEC syndrome. Interestingly, in AEC syndrome the mutations give rise to amino acid substitutions in the SAM domain. However, in EEC syndrome mutations were found to result in amino acid substitutions in the DNA-binding domain. A newborn with overlapping features of AEC and EEC syndrome has been reported [9].

Differential diagnosis

Differential diagnosis includes epidermolysis bullosa simplex and hypohidrotic ectodermal dysplasia.

Complications and co-morbidities

Palate clefting and teeth abnormalities interfere with eating and talking, so that early surgery is necessary to prevent long-term complications. Abnormalities of the external ear canals and palate frequently cause problems with chronic otitis media and secondary hearing loss. Atresia of the lacrimal duct can lead to epiphora, chronic conjunctivitis and photophobia. Scalp erosions and chronic scalp infections may be severe enough to warrant surgical intervention with skin grafting [10].

PART 6: GENETIC DISORDERS

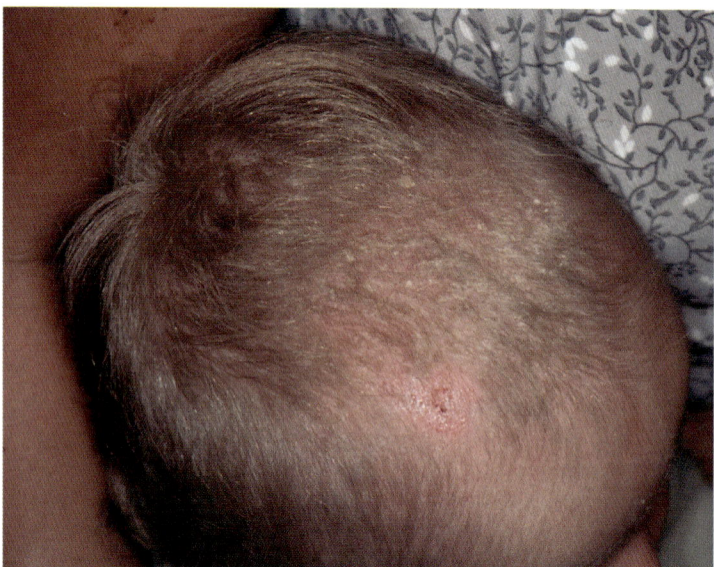

Figure 65.9 After erosive dermatitis on the vertex, marked hypotrichosis remains in the frontal part of the scalp. A mutation in p63 was documented in this patient.

Disease course and prognosis

At birth, over three-quarters of affected newborns have red, eroded, peeling skin resembling a collodion membrane. This resolves over the first few weeks and the underlying skin is dry (Figure 65.9). Over two-thirds of individuals have chronic problems with severe, recurrent scalp erosions and scalp infections with eventual scarring which is a major feature of AEC syndrome. Palmoplantar keratoderma was reported in four of the original seven patients described by Hay and Wells and later palmoplantar changes were found in 18 out of 18 patients [5].

Management

Emollients are appropriate for the collodion-like membrane in the newborn. Neonates with AEC often have marked skin fragility and they should be handled with extreme care. Neonatal intensive care nursing protocols such as those existing for neonates with epidermolysis bullosa should be used. Ankyloblepharon filiforme adnatum may require surgical correction or may lyse spontaneously. Lacrimal duct atresia is surgically correctable. The scalp requires aggressive wound care and treatment with topical or systemic antibiotics as warranted. Other abnormalities such as cleft lip/palate, hypospadias and maxillary hypoplasia need to be surgically corrected. Teeth preservation and restoration is imperative.

Resources

Further information

Ectodermal Dysplasia Society: http://www.ectodermaldysplasia.org/.
Genetic and Rare Diseases Information Center, fact sheet: http://rarediseases.info.nih.gov/gard/2076/eec-syndrome/resources/.
National Foundation for Ectodermal Dysplasias: http://www.nfed.org/.
(All last accessed February 2022.)

Ectrodactyly–ectodermal dysplasia–cleft lip/palate syndrome

Definition, nomeclature and classification

The main features of the EEC syndrome are ectrodactyly (split-hand or -foot deformity), cleft lip/palate, tear duct anomalies and abnormalities of the epidermal appendages including hypotrichosis, hypodontia, dystrophic nails and occasional hypohidrosis.

Synonyms and inclusions
- Ectrodactyly–ectodermal dysplasia–clefting syndrome
- Ectrodactyly–ectodermal dysplasia–orofacial clefts
- EEC syndrome

Classification links
- ICD-10: Q82.4
- MIM: 129900, 604292
- Orphanet: ORPHA1896

Introduction and general description

The EEC syndrome was initially described by Eckholdt and Matens in 1804 and since then the clinical spectrum has been further delineated. Rosselli and Gulienetti described in 1961 a patient with typical features of the EEC syndrome. In 1970 Rüdiger *et al.* suggested the designation EEC for the syndrome. In more than 90% of cases, the syndrome is caused by mutations in the *TP63* gene. The EEC syndrome is inherited in an autosomal dominant manner. It can be phenotypically highly variable with subtle limb and cranio-facial involvement even with apparently classic EEC mutations [1]. Management typically needs the cooperation of various specialists.

Epidemiology

Incidence and prevalence

The EEC syndrome is very rare and only about 300 cases have been reported. Out of 312 cases with oro-facial clefts included in the French registry between 1995 and 2006, only two patients with EEC syndrome were included [2].

Age

Normally the disease manifests at birth or at a very young age.

Sex

Both sexes are affected equally as the syndrome is inherited as an autosomal dominant trait.

Ethnicity

There is no specific ethnicity affected.

Associated diseases

Associated diseases include malformations of the genito-urinary system with renal agenesis, urethral atresia or hydronephrosis, conductive or sensorineural hearing loss, choanal atresia, mammary gland/nipple hypoplasia, several ophthalmological pathologies such as lacrimal duct alterations with atresia or hypoplasia of the lacrimal duct (which are seen in over 90% of affected individuals), photophobia, corneal ulcerations, keratitis, blepharitis, entropion and endocrine pathologies (hypoplastic thymus, hypopituitarism, growth hormone deficiency).

Pathophysiology

In about 90% of cases, EEC is the result of missense mutations in the *TP63* gene (3q27) encoding the p63 transcription factor. This transcription factor is crucial for the development of the ectoderm and limbs. A complex series of genetic experiments revealed that the presence or absence of one variant type of the p63 protein, called TAp63, determines whether or not a child with a *TP63* mutation will develop EEC. It has been reported recently that clefting and skin defects are caused by a loss of p63 function, and limb anomalies are due to gain- and/or dominant-negative mutations [3]. TAp63 is a strong modifier of EEC-associated phenotypes with regard to both penetrance and expressivity [3].

Pathology

Radiographs of hand or foot deformities show missing or hypoplastic metacarpals and metatarsals. Scanning electron microscopic studies of the hair shafts of affected individuals show longitudinal grooves, distorted bulbs and cuticular defects. These findings can be seen in a number of other ectodermal dysplasias and are not specific to the EEC syndrome.

Genetics

The disease is inherited in an autosomal dominant fashion with incomplete penetrance and variable expression. Five hotspot mutations are responsible for almost 90% of all cases of EEC [4].

Environmental factors

As a reduction or absence of sweat glands may occur, hot and dry environments can be dangerous and lead to heat stroke, epilepsy or even death.

Clinical features

History

Often a positive family history is given.

Presentation

Patients present with the major signs of the syndrome: ectrodactylia (Figure 65.10), syndactylia of the hands and feet and clefting of the lips and palate (Box 65.3). In addition, numerous alterations in the ectoderm may be present such as hypopigmented dry skin, hypotrichosis with fine hairs of the scalp and eyebrows (Figure 65.11), small, malformed or missing teeth and nail dystrophies. Often sweat and sebaceous glands are missing or reduced. The clinical presentation can be highly variable and oligosymptomatic cases are common [5,6]. Common associated findings include malformations of the uro-genital system, deafness, choanal atresia, hypoplasia of

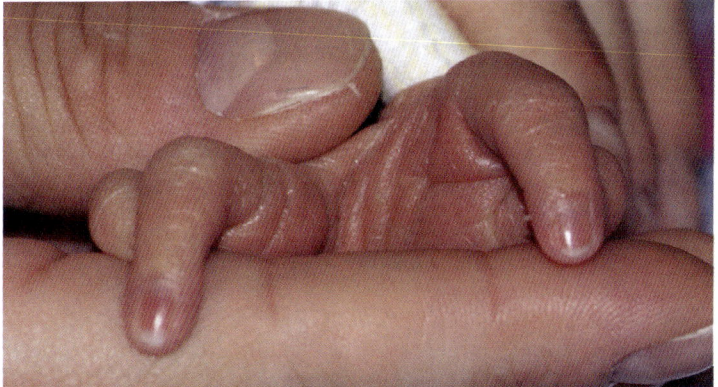

Figure 65.10 Ectrodactyly in the ectrodactyly–ectodermal dysplasia–cleft lip/palate syndrome.

the breast or nipples, ophthalmological pathologies with abnormalities of the lacrimal ducts, photophobia, ulcerations of the cornea, keratitis, blepharitis and ectropion, and hormonal dysregulations. Prenatal diagnosis of the EEC syndrome based on the identification of the 'lobster claw' anomaly is possible by three-dimensional ultrasound [7].

Box 65.3 Criteria used in the diagnosis of the EEC syndrome

Major criteria
- Ectodermal dysplasia
- Ectrodactyly
- Cleft lip/palate
- Lacrimal duct anomalies

Minor criteria
- Renal anomalies
- Deafness
- Mental retardation
- Choanal atresia

Differential diagnosis

Differential diagnosis includes the whole spectrum of p63 syndromes including the AEC and ADULT syndromes, LMS and non-syndromic SHFM [4]. In addition, EvC syndrome has to be separated from the EEC syndrome [8]. Finally, van der Woude syndrome features cleft lip and cleft palate as with p63 syndrome [9]. Hypodontia and lower lip pits are typical. This syndrome was found to be caused by mutations in *IRF6* [10], which is under the regulation of p63, explaining the phenotypic overlap. Of interest, lower lip pits were also recently reported in association with a *TP63* mutation [11].

Classification of severity

There is a genotype–phenotype association of severity.

Complications and co-morbidities

Malformations of the kidneys with dilated ureters or urethral atresia, double ureters, hydronephrosis, multiple renal cysts and renal agenesia or dysplasia may coexist. Endocrine abnormalities

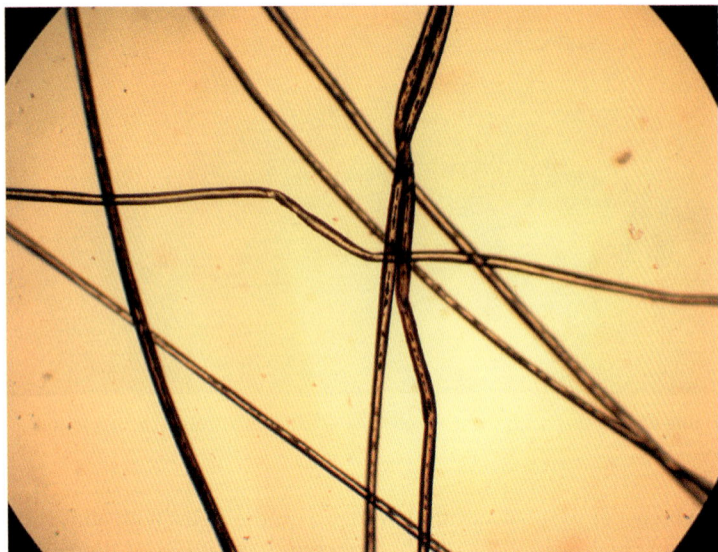

Figure 65.11 Hair shaft alterations in the ectrodactyly–ectodermal dysplasia–cleft lip/palate syndrome.

include absent thymus, hypopituitarism, isolated growth hormone deficiency and pituitary diabetes insipidus.

Investigations

In patients with the typical signs and symptoms of EEC, the diagnosis is straightforward. However, molecular genetic confirmation by documentation of a *TP63* mutation is recommended.

Management

Management is mainly symptomatic [12]. However, molecular genetic research slowly improves gene therapy possibilities as mentioned earlier [13].

Resources

Further information

Ectodermal Dysplasia Society: http://www.ectodermaldysplasia.org/.

Genetic and Rare Diseases Information Center, fact sheet: http://rarediseases.info.nih.gov/gard/2076/eec-syndrome/resources/.

National Foundation for Ectodermal Dysplasias: http://www.nfed.org/.

(All last accessed February 2022.)

Tricho-dento-osseous syndrome

Definition, nomenclature and classification

Tricho-dento-osseous syndrome is a rare autosomal dominant disease characterised by curly hair, enamel dysplasia with pitted teeth, enamel hypomineralisation, precocious dentition and sclerotic bones [1,2]. In addition, cranio-facial morphology is highly variable. Lichtenstein *et al*. [3] defined the features of this disorder in 107 individuals and proposed the name tricho-dento-osseous (TDO) syndrome.

Synonyms and inclusions

• TDO

Classification links
• ICD-10: Q82.4
• MIM: 190320
• Orphanet: ORPHA3352

Introduction and general description

Tricho-dento-osseous syndrome is a very rare ectodermal dysplasia with dense bones, especially in the skull.

Epidemiology

Incidence and prevalence

The disease is very rare and no epidemiological data exist.

Age

The disease manifests at birth with thick and kinky or curly hair on the scalp. The hair may straighten in later life.

Sex

It is an autosomal dominant disorder and therefore both sexes are equally affected.

Ethnicity

There is no ethnic predilection.

Associated diseases

Clinodactyly is rarely seen.

Pathophysiology

Pathology

On dental radiographs, unerupted teeth and taurodontia (increased size of the tooth pulp chamber) are found [1,2]. Scanning electron microscopic analysis of affected teeth shows pits and depressions in the tooth enamel, uniformly thin tooth enamel and an abnormal collagenous membrane around the open apices. Radiographs of the skull reveal sclerosis and sometimes thickening of the calvarium. The long bones may also be sclerotic.

Genetics

Mutations in the distal-less homeobox 3 (*DLX3*) gene are causative for the syndrome [2]. This gene is important for enamel mineralisation and bone formation [4].

Clinical features

History

Often there is a positive family history for the disease. Unruly hair at birth is typical.

Presentation

Patients have kinky hair at birth but, with age, show increasingly less uncombable hair. There are several dental malformations, including enamel hypoplasia, which lead to pitted teeth, taurodontism and caries [1,2]. Fingernails are thin, brittle and peel readily. Toenails may be thickened or normal. Sweat and sebaceous glands are normal and the skin is unremarkable. There is frontal bossing, the jaw is square and the head is elongated. Partial premature fusion of the cranial sutures occurs in three-quarters of affected individuals. The bones of the skull are radiographically dense and may be thick. This is not problematic for the patient and may be found incidentally when radiographs of the skull are obtained for unrelated reasons.

Clinical variants
Cranio-facial variations in the tricho-dento-osseous syndrome are well documented.

Differential diagnosis
Curly hair and nail dysplasia are also seen in CHAND (curly hair, ankyloblepharon and nail dysplasia) syndrome, but ankyloblepharon makes this disorder distinct. Witkop syndrome (tooth and nail syndrome) lacks kinky or curly hair.

Disease course and prognosis
Hair alterations can ameliorate over time. Affected individuals are healthy, but lose most of their teeth by the age of 30 years.

Investigations
Confirmation of the clinical diagnosis can be made by mutation analysis.

Management
Treatment includes appropriate dental care and restoration.

Tricho-rhino-phalangeal syndrome

Definition, nomenclature and classification
Tricho-rhino-phalangeal syndrome is an ectodermal dysplasia characterised by malformations of the hair and nail combined with facial abnormalities and cone-shaped epiphyses of the middle phalanges of some fingers and toes.

Synonyms and inclusions
- TRPS I–III
- Tricho-rhino-phalangeal syndrome types I–III
- Langer–Giedion syndrome (type II)

Classification links
- ICD-10: Q87.1, Q87.8
- MIM: 190350, 190351, 150230
- Orphanet: ORPHA77258, 502

Introduction and general description
This syndrome was first described by Giedion in 1966 [1]. Three subtypes of TRPS with considerable clinical overlap can be distinguished.

Epidemiology
Incidence and prevalence
This syndrome is very rare and no prevalence and incidence numbers exist.

Age
Hypotrichosis, bulboid nose and short fingers may be obvious very early after birth depending on the severity of the phenotype.

Sex
Both sexes are equally affected in this autosomal dominant genodermatosis.

Pathophysiology
Genetics
Tricho-rhino-phalangeal syndrome I is an autosomal dominant disorder caused by mutations in the *TRPS1* gene which encodes a GATA-type transcription factor that has nine zinc-finger motif [2]. Thus TRPS is today classified within the spectrum of ectodermal dysplasias as a transcription factor disease [3]. TRPS1 is a transcriptional repressor that mediates cell differentiation in several tissues [4,5] including the chondrocyte and perichondrium [6]. TRPS II (Langer–Giedion syndrome) represents a continuous gene deletion syndrome including the loss of the *TRPS1* and *EXT1* genes. Patients with more severe shortening of phalanges and metacarpals and marked growth retardation (TRPS III) have missense mutations in the GATA-type DNA-binding zinc finger domain [7].

Clinical features
Clinically, the syndrome is characterised by growth retardation, cranio-facial abnormalities, brachydactyly of the hands and feet, sparse and slow-growing hair, a pear-shaped nose, elongated philtrum and thin upper lip (Box 65.4) [8]. Typical radiological findings include cone-shaped epiphyses, shortening of the metacarpals and phalanges, hip malformations and short stature. Nails have been described as dystrophic, hypoplastic, brittle, slow growing, koilonychotic and leukonychotic. In addition, longitudinal striation is often observed.

Three subtypes of TRPS with considerable clinical overlap can be distinguished (Table 65.4). Type I may feature, in addition to the above mentioned characteristics, moderate postnatal growth retardation, rarely intellectual disability and moderate brachydactyly with shortened phalanges and metacarpals. Eyebrows are generally sparse or may be medially thick and laterally thin.

Type II is usually called the Langer–Giedion syndrome. TRPS II is characterised by the presence of multiple cartilaginous exostoses which clearly distinguishes it from TRPS I and III [9]. Intellectual disability and microcephaly are typical features of TRPS II. Eyebrows are generally thick, broad and bushy. Redundant and loose skin in infancy, disappearing during childhood, has been reported in TRPS II. Growth retardation is only moderate and mild brachydactyly may be present. Most cases are sporadic. It has been shown that Langer–Giedion syndrome is a true contiguous gene syndrome due to the loss of functional copies of at least two genes, *TRPS1* and *EXT1*, encoding exostosin glycosyltransferase 1, which is also involved in the pathogenesis of hereditary multiple exostoses [10].

Type III, also known as Sugio–Kajii syndrome, is the rarest form [11,12]. It is characterised by marked short stature, severe brachydactyly due to shortening of the phalanges and metacarpals and pronounced cone-shaped epiphyses. The eyebrows are normal; exostoses and mental deficiency are absent. Inheritance is autosomal dominant. Sporadic cases have been reported. Lüdecke *et al.* [13] performed extensive mutation analysis and concluded that TRPS III is at the severe end of the TRPS spectrum and that it is caused by missense mutations in the GATA-type DNA-binding zinc finger domain.

Box 65.4 Clinical findings in patients with tricho-rhino-phalangeal syndrome (TRPS) types I–III

Skin appendages
- Fine, sparse, slowly growing scalp hair
- Flattening of hair shafts
- Sparse eyebrows and eyelashes
- Sparse body hair
- Brittle, slow-growing nails

Cranio-facial abnormalities
- Pear-shaped and bulbous nose
- Elongated philtrum
- Thin upper lip and bulge under the lower lip
- Hypoplastic mandible and midfacial hypoplasia
- Microcephaly
- Retrognathia
- High-arched palate
- Small and supernumerary teeth
- Large, laterally protruding ears

Skeletal abnormalities
- Short metacarpals and phalanges
- Bulbous ends of metacarpals
- Cone-shaped epiphyses
- Winged scapulae and lax joints
- Perthes-like changes in the hips and laterally placed patellae
- Exostoses

Other abnormalities
- Melanocytic naevi
- Growth retardation
- Intellectual disability

Reproduced from Itin *et al.* 1996 [12] with permission of Karger Publishers.

Resources

Patient resources
TRPS Support Group UK: http://trpsuk.org/ (last accessed February 2022).

Hidrotic ectodermal dysplasia

Definition, nomenclature and classification

Hidrotic ectodermal dysplasia is a rare genodermatosis within the spectrum of ectodermal dysplasias [1]. The disorder affects the skin, nails and hair but sweating is normal in affected patients. Mutations in a connexin gene lead to the symptom complex characterised by hypotrichosis and brittle hair, dystrophic nails and clubbing with prominent dermal ridges on the finger pulps and variable keratoderma. Hyperpigmentation especially over the joints is common [2].

Synonyms and inclusions
- Clouston disease
- Ectodermal dysplasia 2 (formerly)

Classification links
- ICD-10: Q82.8
- MIM: 129500
- Orphanet: ORPHA189

Introduction and general description

Hidrotic ectodermal dysplasia or Clouston disease is an autosomal dominant inherited disorder and is characterised by the clinical occurrence of nail dystrophy, alopecia and keratoderma.

Epidemiology
Incidence and prevalence

The prevalence of hidrotic ectodermal dysplasia is given at 1–9 per 100 000 although no exact epidemiological studies exist [3,4].

Age

Sparse hair and dystrophic nails are seen in early life. Continuous hair loss may lead to partial or total alopecia until puberty. Hair is

---

Table 65.4 Clinical findings in the major forms of tricho-rhino-phalangeal syndrome (TRPS).

	TRPS I	TRPS II	TRPS III
Inheritance	Autosomal dominant	Mostly sporadic	Autosomal dominant
Exostoses	–	+++	–
Eyebrows	Normal or sparse	Normal or bushy	Normal
Loose skin	–	+	–
Intellectual disability	– (described in single cases)	Often present	–
Microcephaly	–	+	–
Growth retardation	(+)	–	+++
Brachydactyly	+	+	+++
Abnormalities of metacarpals and phalanges	+	+	+++
Genetic defect	Nonsense mutation in *TRPS1* gene	Deletion in 8q24.11-13	Missense mutation in *TRPS1* gene

Adapted from Itin *et al.* 1996 [12].

sparse and brittle from early childhood. Palmoplantar keratoderma begins in childhood but aggravates with age. There is marked variability in the phenotype expression even within the same family.

Sex
As the disease has an autosomal dominant inheritance pattern, both sexes are equally affected.

Ethnicity
Initially, most cases were described in French Canadian families. Later, a family of Chinese Malay and individuals of African, Spanish and Irish descent have been described so that the disease seems to occur globally.

Associated diseases
Secondary conjunctivitis and blepharitis are due to sparse or absent eyelashes. Strabismus and cataract have been reported sporadically. Photophobia, conjunctivitis, blepharitis and sparse eyelashes and eyebrows are often present. Thickened skull bones without functional consequences may be observed. In single cases Clouston syndrome has been reported with mild sensorineural deafness and photophobia.

Pathophysiology
Mutations in *GJB6*, which is located on chromosome 13q12 and codes for connexin 30 (Cx30), are responsible for the disorder. This is an autosomal dominant inherited disorder due to a mutation in Cx30 [5]. Several cases of eccrine syringofibroadenomas have been described in hidrotic ectodermal dysplasia. Immunostaining in normal human skin sections demonstrates a predominant expression of Cx30 in the hair follicles, nails and palmoplantar epidermis, which partially overlaps with p63 expression. In addition, the coexpression of Cx30 and p63 in developing mouse hair follicles and nail units has been documented. In cultured cells, Cx30 protein expression was significantly upregulated by the ΔNp63α isoform. Further *in vitro* analyses suggested that ΔNp63α regulates Cx30 expression via binding to sequences in intron 1 of the Cx30 gene [6].

Pathology
Conventional histology of palms and soles shows orthohyperkeratosis with a normal granular layer. Under electron microscopy an increased number of desmosomes can be seen in the stratum corneum.

Clinical features
History
A positive family history may be present in this autosomal dominant disorder. As the clinical manifestations are highly variable, the history is not straightforward. About one-third of patients have nail dystrophy only. Hypotrichosis can be diffuse or patchy. Paronychial infections are rather common and persistent.

Presentation
Patients present with partial or total alopecia (Figure 65.12). There are sparse scalp hairs and in infancy hairs are twisted, brittle and pale. Hair loss may lead to total alopecia by puberty. Eyelashes are

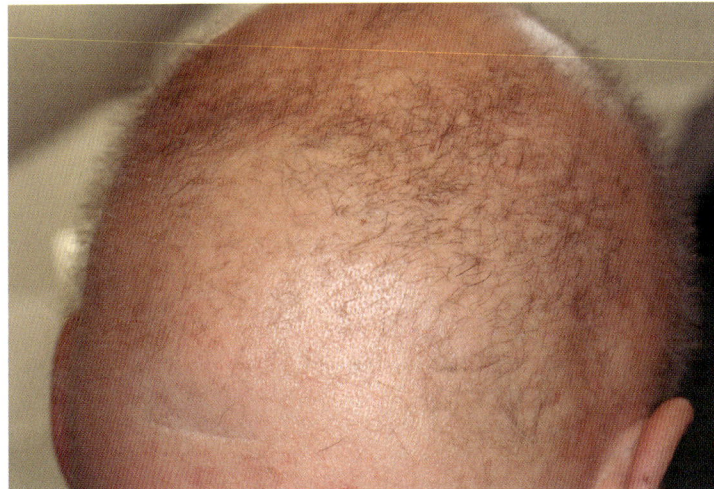

Figure 65.12 Hypotrichosis in hidrotic ectodermal dysplasia.

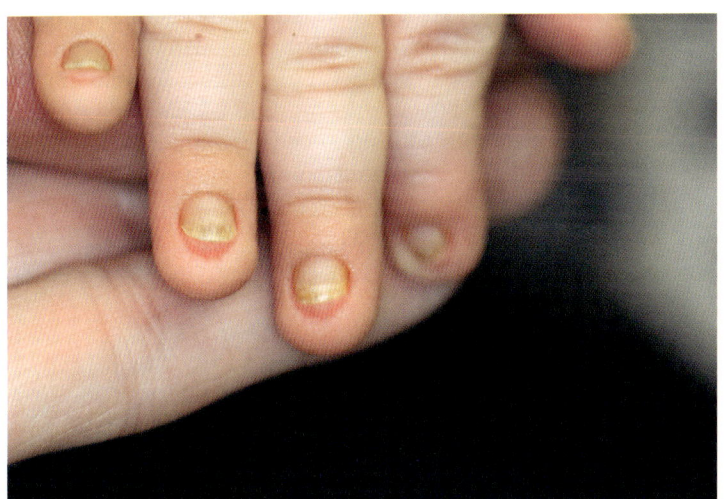

Figure 65.13 Hidrotic ectodermal dysplasia with micronychia, yellowish-coloured nail plates and pronounced dermatoglyphics.

short and sparse and eyebrows as well as axillary and pubic hair are also sparse or absent. The nails may be whitish in early childhood and then have a tendency to thicken. The nails are slow growing and often have striations and thickening and distal onycholysis. Affected nails are a very constant finding. The nails may be malformed and also small and short. A variable expression of palmoplantar keratoderma is known, and pronounced dermatoglyphics may exist on the finger tips (Figure 65.13). Hyperpigmentation especially over joints is common.

Clinical variants
Phenotypic expression is highly variable.

Differential diagnosis
Differential diagnosis includes pachyonychia congenita and pure hair–nail ectodermal dysplasia. In 1996, an African family with six affected people over three generations was described with short and sparse scalp hair and eyelashes. The nails were dystrophic and thickened but sweating, skin and teeth were normal.

Classification of severity

Mono- or oligosymptomatic expression of the disease is quite common. One-third of all patients with hidrotic ectodermal dysplasia have nail dystrophy as the only manifestation. The severity of the disease is highly variable, even in the same family.

Disease course and prognosis

The clinical features increase over time but the expected lifetime is normal.

Investigations

To confirm the clinical diagnosis mutation analysis for Cx30 is mandatory.

Management

There is no causal or specific treatment for this syndrome. Keratolytics and emollients should be used for palmoplantar keratoderma and, in severe cases of alopecia, wigs can be helpful. Professional pedicures and manicures can help to reduce the obvious aspects of nail dystrophy. It has been reported that tretinoin – which enhances the absorption of minoxidil and acts by enlarging the miniaturised hair follicles – can be effective in hidrotic ectodermal dysplasia [7]. In mutant mice with Clouston syndrome a potent antagonist antibody targeting connexin hemichannels alleviated the clinical symptoms [8].

Resources

Further information

GeneReviews. Hidrotic ectodermal dysplasia 2: http://www.ncbi.nlm.nih.gov/books/NBK1200/ (last accessed February 2022).

Focal dermal hypoplasia

Definition, nomenclature and classification

Focal dermal hypoplasia (FDH) is a rare genodermatosis that affects tissues of ectodermal and mesodermal origin. Clinically the syndrome is characterised by cutaneous, skeletal, dental, ocular and soft tissue defects. FDH has been associated with a mutation in the *PORCN* gene on the X chromosome that encodes a protein involved in the WNT signalling pathway. An X-linked dominant inheritance pattern is documented in numerous pedigrees with lethal effects in males which survive only in the case of mosaicism. Recently, Happle pointed out that non-syndromic anophthalmia/microphthalmia caused by a novel *PORCN* mutation indicated that PORCN mutations can occur as hypomorphic alleles, giving rise to survival of male non-mosaic patients [1].

Synonyms and inclusions
- Goltz syndrome
- Goltz–Gorlin syndrome

Classification links
- ICD-10: Q82.8
- MIM: 305600
- Orphanet: ORPHA2092

Introduction and general description

In 1962 Goltz and co-workers defined a syndrome now known as FDH with numerous ectodermal and mesodermal malformations [2]. Only 200–300 cases have been described in the literature so far. Clinical key features are linear enamel hypoplasia according to the Blaschko linear pattern, periorificial papillomas, fat herniations and linear telangiectasias and pigmentation anomalies along the Blaschko lines [3].

Epidemiology

Focal dermal hypoplasia is very rare and the prevalence is estimated at less than 1 in 1 000 000; 90% of affected patients are females. Mosaicism for mutations in *PORCN* or chromosomal anomalies underlie FDH in about 10% of affected males [4].

Age

Patients are born with multiple malformations and diagnosis is possible at birth.

Sex

Of affected patients, 90% are female.

Ethnicity

No ethnical predisposition is known.

Associated diseases

It is an ectodermal–mesodermal malformation disease with numerous organs involved.

Pathophysiology

Focal dermal hypoplasia is inherited as an X-linked dominant trait, with 90% of affected individuals being female; 95% of the mutations are new. FDH is caused by mutations in the *PORCN* gene encoding an important element of the WNT signalling pathway. WNT proteins play important roles in embryo development, tissue homeostasis and stem cell maintenance. Consistent with the female-specific inheritance pattern of FDH, *PORCN* hemizygous *Drosophila* male embryos show growth arrest during early embryogenesis and fail to generate mesoderm, a phenotype previously associated with loss of Wnt activity and similar to the human homologue.

Pathology

Skin biopsies from the reddish lesions show acanthosis and slight hyperkeratosis of the epidermis, sometimes with subepidermal cleft formation. In atrophic lesions the epidermis shows atrophy and hyperpigmentation of the basal cell layer. A wedge-shaped area of scar formation composed of hyaline collagen bundles in parallel arrangement and numerous fibroblasts often is found beneath the epidermis. The fatty tissue almost reaches the epidermis because collagen fibres of dermal tissue are scarce. This phenomenon has been described as heterotopic fat [5]. Blood vessels with prominent endothelial cells are found in large numbers within and at the periphery of lesional tissue. Some blood vessels may be densely filled with erythrocytes, and extravasations of red blood cells with small areas of haemorrhage can be seen. Small islands of adipose tissue are common in close vicinity to the fibrous tissue in the lower reticular dermis. A positive immunohistochemical reaction for vimentin, fibronectin and collagen type III is observed in the scar tissue. No collagen type IV is detected in the basement membrane zone of the epidermis covering the lesion [6].

Genetics
An X-chromosomal dominant inheritance pattern with lethality in males is typical in FDH [7]. Mutations in the *PORCN* gene lead to changes in the WNT cascade, which is very important during embryogenesis.

Clinical features
History
The clinical spectrum of FDH includes abnormalities of the skin and various defects of the eyes, bones, teeth, nails, oral structures and soft tissue [4]. The most prominent clinical features of the cutaneous disease are reddish or red-yellow cribriform atrophic skin lesions. Hyperpigmentation or hypopigmentation is common in atrophic sites. Telangiectases in atrophic skin is a common finding (Figure 65.14). A Blaschko linear distribution pattern is typical and the areas involved are usually the trunk and extremities but the lesions may be found on any part of the body. Linear enamel hypoplasia is an important key feature (Figure 65.15). Numerous oral alterations have been described including hypodontia, jaw cysts, clefting, hemihypoglossia of the tongue and papillomatosis. Other cutaneous abnormalities include lipomatous nodules and papillomatous lesions. Ocular abnormalities occur in about 40% and include coloboma, strabism, microphthalmia and nystagmus. Skeletal changes include syndactyly (Figure 65.16), polydactyly, lobster claw deformation and osteopathia striata. Additional features associated with FDH include facial dysmorphism, supernumerary nipple or nipple hypoplasia, hernias, abnormal genito-urinary development, and occasionally structural brain abnormalities.

Differential diagnosis
Differential diagnoses include the group of focal facial dermal dysplasias types 1–4 and MIDAS syndrome (see following section).

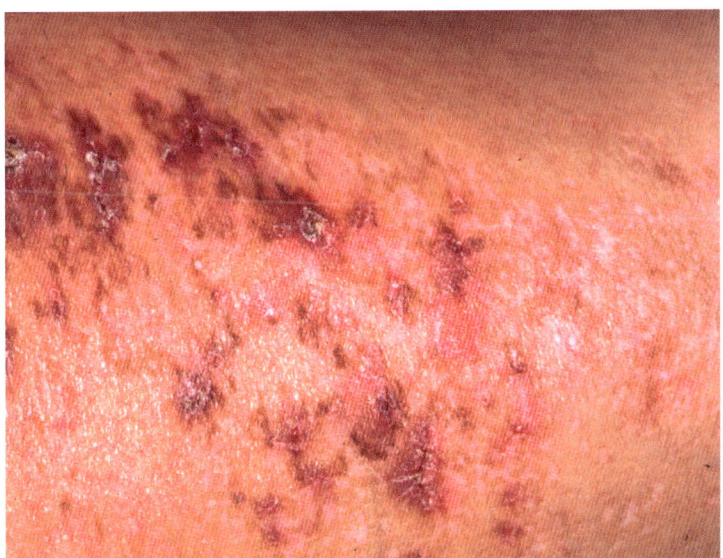
Figure 65.14 Striate atrophic and telangiectatic lesions in focal dermal hypoplasia.

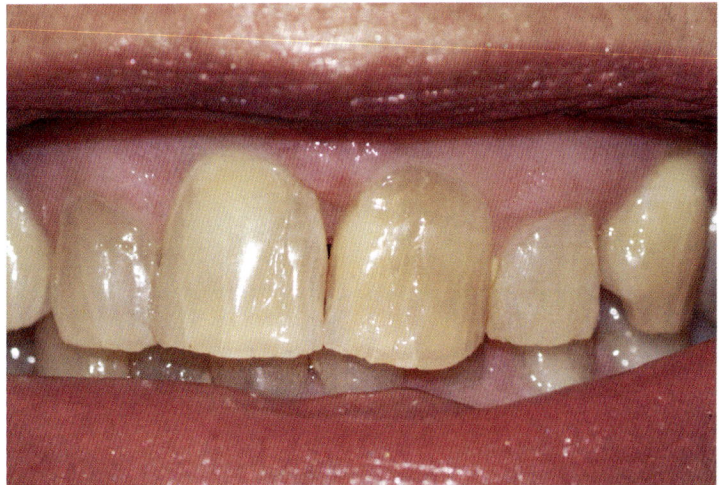
Figure 65.15 Blaschko linear enamel hypoplasia in focal dermal hypoplasia.

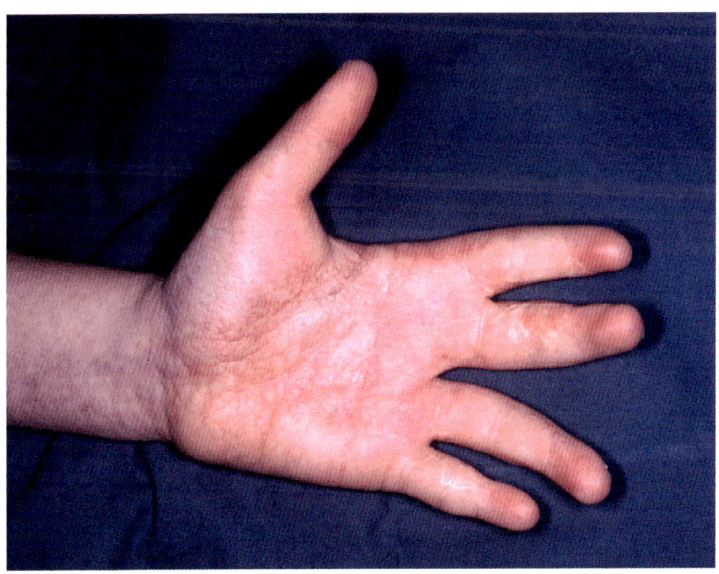
Figure 65.16 Operated syndactyly in focal dermal hypoplasia.

Management
Interdisciplinary clinical management of patients with FDH should be organised. Children should be presented to the dentist and ophthalmologist as soon as possible. Orthopaedic specialists are also important in the treatment of affected patients. In addition, psychological and behavioural management is necessary.

Resources
Patient resources
National Center for Advancing Translational Sciences, overview of organisations supporting patients with FDH: http://rarediseases.info.nih.gov/gard/6457/focal-dermal-hypoplasia/cases/54865 (last accessed February 2022).

MIDAS syndrome

Definition, nomenclature and classification
MIDAS syndrome (microphthalmia, dermal aplasia and sclerocornea), coined by Happle, is also named microphthalmia with

linear skin defects syndrome. It is an X-linked dominant disorder with male lethality characterised by unilateral or bilateral microphthalmia with linear skin defects limited to the face and neck. It is a very rare disease with less than 1 in 1 000 000 affected.

A related form of congenital linear skin defects with microcephaly, facial dysmorphism and additional malformations exists and is caused by a mutation in the *COX7B* gene on chromosome Xq21.

Synonyms and inclusions
- MIDAS syndrome
- Microphthalmia with linear skin defects
- Microphthalmia
- Dermal aplasia
- Sclerocornea

Classification links
- ICD-10: Q11.2
- MIM: 300887, 300952, 309801
- Orphanet: ORPHA2556

Introduction and general description

MIDAS syndrome is a rare X-linked male-lethal disorder with microphthalmia and other ocular malformations and linear aplastic skin lesions which are usually limited to the face and neck and develop hyperpigmented skin alterations in healed aplastic skin with age. In addition, microcephaly, intellectual disabilities, agenesis of corpus callosum and cardiac malformations may occur. Most patients have a cytogenetically visible deletion or unbalanced translocation leading to Xp22 monosomy. Heterozygous intragenic mutations in *HCCS* have been shown to be responsible for the disease [1]. *HCCS* encodes the holocytochrome c-type synthase, which catalyses the incorporation of heme moieties into cytochrome c and cytochrome c1. Cytochrome c plays a crucial role in oxidative phosphorylation, but also has been shown to regulate apoptosis. Cells lacking *HCCS* activity may therefore be prone to undergo apoptosis, which in turn may affect tissue formation. Further supporting a role for mitochondrial enzymes in the pathogenesis of MIDAS syndrome, mutations in another gene, *COX7B* on Xq21.1, encoding a structural subunit of cytochrome c oxidase, have been found in females with the MIDAS phenotype [2].

Epidemiology

Incidence and prevalence

The disease is very rare with fewer than 1 : 1 000 000 cases.

Age

Clinical manifestations are partially apparent at birth and internal malformations or intellectual impairment become evident within the first years of life.

Sex

It is an X-linked dominant disorder with lethality in males.

Ethnicity

No racial predilection has been reported.

Associated diseases

The syndrome may be complicated by cardiac malformations (18%), hypoplastic corpus callosum and abnormal myelination, microcephaly, mild to severe intellectual disability (25%), hearing loss, diaphragmatic hernia, anterior-placed anus or imperforate anus and genito-urinary malformations.

Clinical features

History

Family history may reveal a mother to daughter transmission.

Presentation

The most consistent clinical features are microphthalmia/anophthalmia (93%) and sclerocornea/corneal opacity and congenital linear skin defects in a Blaschko-line pattern on the head and neck (95%) (Box 65.5) [3]. Additional manifestations are various ocular anomalies, cardiac defects, brain imaging abnormalities, microcephaly, postnatal growth retardation and facial dysmorphism. Nail dystrophies may occur.

Box 65.5 Criteria used in the diagnosis of the MIDAS syndrome [3]

Major criteria
- Linear skin defects (dermal aplasia)
- Microphthalmia

Minor criteria
- Other ocular abnormalities
- Central nervous system involvement
- Developmental delay
- Congenital heart defects
- Diaphragmatic hernia
- Nail dystrophy
- Preauricular pits and hearing loss
- Genito-urinary malformations

Clinical variants

A related form of congenital linear skin defects with microcephaly, facial dysmorphism and additional malformations exists and is caused by a mutation in the *COX7B* gene on chromosome Xq21.

Differential diagnosis

Differential diagnoses include focal dermal hypoplasia, incontinentia pigmenti (Bloch–Sulzberger disease), oculocerebrocutaneous syndrome and Aicardi syndrome.

Investigations

Ophthalmological and dermatological examinations, brain magnetic resonance imaging with and without contrast, hearing evaluation and cardiac evaluation are indicated. Clinically suggestive constellations for MIDAS syndrome should be confirmed by chromosome analyses and molecular genetic analyses which document a mutation in *HCCS* or *COX7B*.

Management

Eye and skin problems should be managed by specialists. Patients with MIDAS syndrome should be checked for cardiac, uro-genital and central nervous malformations. Learning disability should be evaluated early on.

Focal facial dermal dysplasia

Definition, nomenclature and classification

Focal facial dermal dysplasia (FFDD) represents a heterogeneous group of rare disorders with bilateral facial developmental defects. The lesional skin resembles aplasia cutis congenita. There are four types of FFDD [1]. Type 1 is also called Brauer syndrome and is inherited in an autosomal dominant pattern; the skin abnormalities in the bitemporal area resemble forceps marks. In addition, sparse lateral eyebrows, a flattened nasal tip and distichiasis can be observed. Type 2 is also called Brauer–Setleis syndrome. The clinical features are very similar compared with type 1 but the periorbital skin is also affected with atrophic and wrinkling skin. Inheritance is also autosomal dominant. Type 3 is called Setleis syndrome and has the same clinical characteristics as type 2 but inheritance is autosomal recessive. Causative mutations have been identified in the *TWIST2* gene [2]. Type 4 shows isolated preauricular skin lesions and the inheritance pattern can be autosomal recessive or dominant [3]. It is caused by mutations in the *CYP26C1* gene [4].

Synonyms and inclusions

FFDD type 1
- Brauer syndrome
- Hereditary symmetrical aplastic naevi of temples
- Bitemporal aplasia cutis congenita

FFDD type 2
- Brauer–Setleis syndrome

FFDD type 3
- Setleis syndrome

FFDD type 4
- Focal preauricular dermal dysplasia

Classification links
- ICD-10: Q82.8
- MIM: 136500, 227260, 614973, 614974
- Orphanet: ORPHA398166

Epidemiology

Focal facial dermal dysplasia is a very rare disease group with an incidence of less than 1 in 1 000 000.

Clinical features

The common denominator in all types in FFDD is atrophic skin changes in the bitemporal region.

Key references

The full list of references can be found in the online version at https://www.wiley.com/rooksdermatology10e

Ectodermal dysplasias

1 Itin PH. Ectodermal dysplasia: thoughts and practical concepts concerning disease classification – the role of functional pathways in the molecular genetic diagnosis. *Dermatology* 2013;226:111–14.

2 Wright JT, Fete M, Schneider H et al. Ectodermal dysplasias: classification and organization by phenotype, genotype and molecular pathway. *Am J Med Genet* 2019;179A:442–7.

9 Guo S, Chen R, Xu Y, Mu Y, Chen L. Ankyloblepharon–ectodermal defects–cleft lip/palate syndrome. *J Craniofac Surg* 2017;28:e349–51.

11 Nguyen-Nielsen M, Skovbo S, Svaneby D, Pedersen L, Fryzek J. The prevalence of X-linked hypohidrotic ectodermal dysplasia (XLHED) in Denmark, 1995–2010. *Eur J Med Genet* 2013;56:236–42.

19 Trzeciak WH, Koczorowski R. Molecular basis of hypohidrotic ectodermal dysplasia: an update. *J Appl Genetics* 2016;57:51–61.

25 Cluzeau C, Hadj-Rabia S, Jambou M et al. Only four genes (EDA1, EDAR, EDARADD, and WNT10A) account for 90% of hypohidrotic/anhidrotic ectodermal dysplasia cases. *Hum Mut* 2011;32:70–2.

27 Maillard A, Alby C, Gabison E et al. P63-related disorders: dermatological characteristics in 22 patients. *Exp Dermatol* 2019;28:1190–5.

51 Van Bokhoven H, Hamel BCJ, Bamshad M et al. p63 gene mutations in EEC syndrome, limb-mammary syndrome, and isolated split hand-split foot malformation suggest a genotype–phenotype correlation. *Am J Hum Genet* 2001;69:481–92.

X-linked hypohidrotic ectodermal dysplasia with immunodeficiency

1 Kawai T, Nishikomori R, Heike T. Diagnosis and treatment in anhidrotic ectodermal dysplasia with immunodeficiency. *Allergol Int* 2012;61:207–17.

2 Fusco F, Pescatore A, Conte MI et al. EDA-ID and IP, two faces of the same coin: how the same IKBGK/NEMO mutation affecting the NF-κB pathway can cause immunodeficiency and/or inflammation. *Int Rev Immunol* 2015;34:445–9.

Hypohidrotic ectodermal dysplasia

1 Peña-Romero AG, Sáez-de-Ocariz M, Toussaint-Caire S et al. Clinical, trichoscopy, and light microscopic findings in hypohidrotic ectodermal dysplasia: report of 21 patients and a review of the literature. *Pediatr Dermatol* 2020;38:442–8.

3 Anbouba GM, Carmany EP, Natoli JL. The characterization of hypodontia, hypohidrosis, and hypotrichosis associated with X-linked hypohidrotic ectodermal dysplasia: a systematic review. *Am J Med Genet* 2020;18A:831–41.

5 Itin PH. Etiology and pathogenesis of ectodermal dysplasia. *Am J Med Genet A* 2014;164A:2472–7.

7 Wohlfart S, Meiller R, Hammersen J et al. Natural history of X-linked hypohidrotic ectodermal dysplasia: a 5-year follow-up study. *Orphanet J Rare Dis* 2020;15:3–11.

9 Schneider H, Faschingbauer F, Schuepbach-Mallepell S et al. Prenatal correction of X-linked hypohidrotic ectodermal dysplasia. *N Engl J Med* 2018;378:1604–10.

10 Li X, Wu X, Elston DM, Zhang J, Zhou C. Hypohidrotic ectodermal dysplasia with c.28delG mutation in ectodysplasin A gene and severe atopic dermatitis treated successfully with tofacitinib. *Acta Derm Venereol* 2020;101:adv00352.

Ankyloblepharon–ectodermal defects–cleft lip/palate syndrome

2 Guo S, Chen R, Xu I, Mu Y, Chen L. Ankyloblepharon–ectodermal defects–cleft lip/palate syndrome. *J Craniofac Surg* 2017;28:e349–51.

3 Dishop MK, Bree AF, Hicks MJ. Pathologic changes of skin and hair in ankyloblepharon–ectodermal defects–cleft lip/palate (AEC) syndrome. *Am J Med Genet* 2009;149A:1935–41.

5 Julapalli MR, Scher RK, Sybert VP, Siegfried EC, Bree AF. Dermatologic findings of ankyloblepharon–ectodermal defects–cleft lip/palate (AEC) syndrome. *Am J Med Genet* 2009;149A:1900–6.

6 Ferstl P, Wohlfart S, Schneider H. Sweating ability of patients with p63-associated syndromes. *Eur J Pediatr* 2018;177:1727–31.

10 Cole P, Hatef DA, Kaufman Y *et al*. Facial clefting and oroauditory pathway manifestations in ankyloblepharon–ectodermal defects–cleft lip/palate (AEC) syndrome. *Am J Med Genet* 2009;149A:1910–15.

Ectrodactyly–ectodermal dysplasia–cleft lip/palate syndrome

1 Maclean K, Holme SA, Gilmour E *et al*. EEC syndrome, Arg227Gln TP63 mutation and micturition difficulties: is there a genotype–phenotype correlation? *Am J Med Genet* 2007;143A:1114–19.
2 Doray B, Badila-Timbolschi D, Schaefer E *et al*. Epidemiology of orofacial clefts (1995–2006) in France (Congenital Malformations of Alsace Registry). *Arch Pediatr* 2012;19:1021–9.
5 Zheng J, Liu H, Zahn Y *et al*. Tooth defects of EEC and AEC syndrome caused by heterozygous TP63 mutations in three Chinese families and genotype–phenotype correlation analyses of TP63-related disorders. *Mol Genet Genomic Med* 2019;7:e704.
6 Wenger T, Li D, Harr HM *et al*. Expanding the phenotypic spectrum of TP63-related disorders including the first set of monozygotic twins. *Am J Med. Genet* 2018;176A:75–81.
10 Kondo S, Schutte BC, Richardson RJ *et al*. Mutations in IRF6 cause Van der Woude and popliteal pterygium syndromes. *Nature Genet* 2002;32:285–9.
12 Elhamouly Y, Dowidar K. Dental management of a child with ectrodactyly ectodermal dysplasia cleft lip/palate syndrome: a case report. *Spec Care Dentist* 2019;39:236–40.

Tricho-dento-osseous syndrome

1 Whitehouse LLE, Smith CEL, Poulter JA *et al*. Novel DLX3 variants in amelogenesis imperfecta with attenuated tricho-dento-osseous syndrome. *Oral Dis* 2019;25:182–91.
2 Li Y, Zhang H, Liu H *et al*. Morphological analyses and a novel de novo DLX3 mutation associated with tricho-dento-osseous syndrome in a Chinese family. *Eur J Oral Sci* 2015;123:228–34.

Tricho-rhino-phalangeal syndrome

4 Momeni P, Glöckner G, Schmidt O *et al*. Mutations in a new gene, encoding a zinc-finger protein, cause tricho-rhino-phalangeal syndrome type I. *Nature Genet* 2000;24:71–4.
6 Napierla D, Sam K, Morello R *et al*. Uncoupling of chondrocyte differentiation and perichondrial mineralization underlies the skeletal dysplasia in trichorhino-phalangeal syndrome. *Hum Mol Genet* 2008;17:2244–54.
7 Wang C, Xu Y, Qing Y *et al*. TRSP1 mutation detection in Chinese patients with tricho-rhino-phalangeal syndrome and identification of four novel mutations. *Mol Genet Genomic Med* 2020;8:e1417–26.

12 Itin PH, Bohn S, Mathys D, Guggenheim R, Richard G. Trichorhinophalangeal syndrome type III. *Dermatology* 1996;193:349–52.
13 Lüdecke HJ, Schaper J, Meinecke P *et al*. Genotypic and phenotypic spectrum in tricho-rhino-phalangeal syndrome types I and III. *Am J Hum Genet* 2001;68:81–91.

Hidrotic ectodermal dysplasia

1 Fraser FC, Der Kaloustian VM. A man, a syndrome, a gene: Clouston's hidrotic ectodermal dysplasia (HED). *Am J Med Genet* 2001;100:164–8.
4 Ando Y, Tanaka T, Horiguchi Y, Ikai K, Tomono H. Hidrotic ectodermal dysplasia: a clinical and ultrastructural observation. *Dermatologica* 1988;176:205–11.
5 Cammarata-Scalisi F, Rinelli M, Pisaneschi E *et al*. Novel clinical features associated with Clouston syndrome. *Int J Dermatol* 2019;58:e143–6.
8 Kuang Y, Zorci V, Buratto D *et al*. A potent antagonist antibody targeting connexin hemichannels alleviates Clouston syndrome symptoms in mutant mice. *EBioMedicine* 2020;57:1–13.

Focal dermal hypoplasia

1 Happle R. The PORCN non-Goltz spectrum (PONGOS): a new group of genetic disorders. *Am J Med Genet* 2021;185A:13–14.
3 Itin P. Alterations in nails and teeth as a clue for genodermatoses. *Hautarzt* 2014;65:513–19.
4 Wang L, Jin X, Liu D *et al*. Focal dermal hypoplasia: updates. *Oral Dis* 2014;20:17–24.
7 Heinz L, Bourrat E, Vabres P *et al*. Mosaicism due to postzygotic mutations in women with focal dermal hypoplasia. *Br J Dermatol* 2019; 180:657–61.

MIDAS syndrome

1 Wimplinger I, Morelo M, Rosenberger G *et al*. Mutations of the mitochondrial holocytochrome c-type synthase in X-linked dominant microphthalmia with linear skin defects syndrome. *Am J Hum Genet* 2006;79:878–89.
2 Indrieri A, van Rahden VA, Tiranti V *et al*. Mutations in COX7B cause microphthalmia with linear skin lesions, an unconventional mitochondrial disease. *Am J Hum Genet* 2012;91:942–9.
3 Durack A, Mehta SG, Allen LE, Ozanic Bulic S, Burrows NP. Linear skin defects and microphthalmia. *Clin Exp Dermatol* 2018;43:860–2.

Focal facial dermal dysplasia

1 Kowalski DC, Fenske NA. The focal facial dermal dysplasias: report of a kindred and a proposed new classification. *J Am Acad Dermatol* 1992;27:575–82.
3 Mertens SH, Shankar S. A case of focal facial dermal dysplasia type 4. *Pediatr Dermatol* 2019;36:e58–9.

CHAPTER 66

Inherited Hair Disorders

Eli Sprecher

Division of Dermatology, Tel Aviv Sourasky Medical Center, Tel Aviv, Israel

PART 6: GENETIC DISORDERS

Definition

Congenital and inherited disorders of hair growth and differentiation, also known as genotrichoses, can be subdivided into conditions associated with either excessive hair growth, known as *hypertrichoses*, or defective hair development, termed *alopecias* [1]. Diseases in which hair is absent from the entire surface of the skin are known as *atrichias* whereas disorders featuring hair paucity are named *hypotrichoses*. Some of these disorders are associated with *structural abnormalities of the hair shafts*. For example, patients featuring woolly hair often display hypotrichosis as well [2]. Finally, inherited disorders of the hair follicle unit can present in isolation or as part of more complex clinical entities in which case they are known as syndromic genotrichoses. In the following sections, the clinical and pathogenetic features of representative genotrichoses are provided. A list of all major disorders associated with hypertrichoses and alopecias is provided in Tables 66.1, 66.2 and 66.3.

Introduction and general description

The past two decades have witnessed dramatic developments in the field of hair research and the number of inherited hair disorders whose molecular basis has been discovered has grown exponentially [3]. Two major reasons underlie this recent trend. First, the hair follicle is regarded today as a unique model for the study of complex developmental and regulatory interactions between epithelial and mesenchymal tissues [4,5,6,7]. Second, hair disorders are known to be the source of considerable morbidity. Absence (*alopecia*) or excess (*hirsutism*) of hair is obviously compatible with normal lifespan; yet individuals affected with these conditions often experience aberrant hair growth as a significantly detrimental event, affecting many aspects of their personal and social life [8–12].

Because most of these disorders are exceedingly rare, epidemiological data are mostly non-existent.

HYPERTRICHOSES

GENERALISED HYPERTRICHOSES

This group of very rare disorders manifests generally at birth with generalised hypertrichosis (Figure 66.1). The various forms of generalised hypertrichosis are recognised on the basis of the presence of specific extracutaneous manifestations. Unfortunately, because the molecular basis of many of these diseases is still elusive, it is often not clear whether they are distinct entities or represent different clinical manifestations of common underlying genetic defects (see Table 66.1).

Table 66.1 Hypertrichoses.

Disease name	MIM	Inheritance	Gene or genetic defect	Cutaneous features	Extracutaneous features
A *Hypertrichosis as main disease feature*					
Cantu syndrome	239850	AD	*ABCC9* *KCNJ8 (?)*	Hypertrichosis	Macrosomia Facial dysmorphism Gingival hyperplasia Bone abnormalities Cardiac defects Mild intellectual disability
Congenital generalised hypertrichosis	307150	RXL	Insertions on chromosome Xq27.1/possible involvement of *FGF13*	Congenital generalised hypertrichosis in males; patchy hypertrichosis in females	Scoliosis Dental/palate anomalies Deafness
Generalised hypertrichosis terminalis	135400	AD	CNV variations on chromosome 17/possible involvement of *SOX9* or *ABCA5* (autosomal recessive hypertrichosis also described in association with a loss-of-function mutation in *ABCA5*)	Excessive terminal hair growth involving face and body	Facial dysmorphism Gingival hyperplasia
Histiocytosis and lymphadenopathy syndrome (H syndrome)	602782	AR	*SLC29A3*	Hyperpigmentation, localised hypertrichosis	Hepatosplenomegaly, heart anomalies, hearing loss, hypogonadism, short stature, hyperglycaemia
Hypertrichosis universalis	145700	AD	Unknown	Excessive lanugo-type hair growth Double eyebrows	–
Hypertrichosis universalis congenital, Ambras type	145701	AD	Complex rearrangements on chromosome 8/possible involvement of *TRPS1*	Excessive vellus hair growth involving entire body surface	Facial dysmorphism Skeletal abnormalities
Trichomegaly	190330	AR	*FGF5*	Long eyelashes Hypertrichosis of eyebrows, cheeks and forehead	–
B *Hypertrichosis as minor disease feature*					
Barber–Say syndrome	209885	AD	*TWIST2*	Hypertrichosis Lax and atrophic skin	Facial dysmorphism including prognathism, abnormal ears, bulbous nose, macrostomia and thin lips Hypoplastic nipples Abnormal external genitalia
Coffin–Siris syndrome	135900	AR	*ARID1A, ARID1B, ARID2, DPF2, SMARCD1, SMARCC2, SMARCE1, SMARCA4, SMARCB1, SOX11, SOX4*	Generalised hypertrichosis with scalp hypotrichosis Nail dysplasia Cutis marmorata	Short stature Psychomotor developmental delay Agenesis of the corpus callosum Coarse facial features Skeletal dysplasia Cardiac defects Kidney defects Gastrointestinal complications
Congenital generalised lipodystrophy (Berardinelli–Seip syndrome)	608594 269700 612526 613327	AR	*AGPAT2* *BSCL2* *CAV1* *PTRF*	Hypertrichosis Acanthosis nigricans	Decreased adipose tissue Diabetes Hypertriglyceridaemia Hepatic steatosis
Cornelia de Lange	122470 300590 610759 614701 300882	AD RXL AD AD RXL	*NIPBL* *SMC1A* *SMC3* *RAD21* *HDAC8*	Low posterior hairline Hypertrichosis Exuberant eyebrow growth Curly eyelashes Cutis marmorata Single transverse palmar crease	Short stature, hearing loss, microcephaly, facial dysmorphism, cleft lip/palate, cardiac defects, kidney defects, intellectual disability

(continued)

Table 66.1 (*continued*)

Disease name	MIM	Inheritance	Gene or genetic defect	Cutaneous features	Extracutaneous features
Craniofacial dysmorphism, skeletal anomalies and mental retardation syndrome	614132	AR	TMCO1	Hypertrichosis Low hairline Gingival hyperplasia	Facial dysmorphism including wide nasal bridge with small nose, bushy eyebrows, flat face, low-set ears and macrocephaly Cleft lip/palate Skeletal dysplasia Neuropsychiatric manifestations
Donohue syndrome (leprechaunism)	246200	AR	INSR	Hypertrichosis/hirsutism Acanthosis nigricans Dysplastic nails Keratoderma Loose and wrinkled skin due to loss of adipose tissue	Severe failure to thrive Elfin facies Abdominal protuberance Oversized penis/clitoris Polycystic ovaries Gingival hyperplasia Large hands and feet Premature breast and nipple enlargement
FHEIG syndrome	618381	AD	KCNK4	Generalised hypertrichosis	Neurological and skeletal abnormalities Facial dysmorphism
Hurler syndrome	607014	AR	IDUA	Hypertrichosis since early infancy or childhood Prominent over the eyebrows Dermal melanocytosis	Short stature, coarse face, gingival hyperplasia, abnormal dentition, macroglossia, eye problems, cardiac, gastroenterological, skeletal and neurological defects
KINSSHIP syndrome	619297	AD	AFF3	Abnormalities of teeth and gums and hypertrichosis (limbs)	Horseshoe kidney, Nievergelt/Savarirayan type of mesomelic dysplasia, seizures, intellectual disability, respiratory distress, bulbous nasal tip, wide mouth often with a square upper lip
Leigh syndrome	256000	AR	Mutations in genes encoding the various components of the mitochondrial respiratory chain complexes I–V	Generalised hypertrichosis	Progressive neurological deterioration, ophthalmoplegia, lactic acidosis
Lymphoedema–distichiasis syndrome	153400	AD	FOXC2	Growth of extra row of eyelashes	Lymphoedema
Schinzel–Giedion midface retraction syndrome	269150	AD	SETBP1	Hypertrichosis Facial haemangioma Hypoplastic dermal ridges Clubbing	Failure to thrive Facial dysmorphism with proptosis due to shallow orbits, prominent forehead and macroglossia Genito-urinary abnormalities Skeletal dysplasia Neurological defects and mental disability
Trisomy 18	–	–	–	Generalised hypertrichosis	See Chapter 74
Wiedemann–Steiner syndrome	605130	AD	KMT2A	Thick eyebrows Hairy elbows Generalised hypertrichosis (in some patients)	Facial dysmorphism Skeletal abnormalities Short stature, FTT Delayed psychomotor development
Zimmerman–Laband syndrome	135500	AD	KCNH1 KCNN3 ATP6V1B2	Generalised hypertrichosis Gingival fibromatosis Nail dysplasia	Facial dysmorphism including bulbous soft nose, thick lips and thick floppy ears Skeletal dysplasia and joint hyperextensibility Hepatosplenomegaly Cardiovascular defects Intellectual disability

AD, autosomal dominant; AR, autosomal recessive; CNV, copy number variations; FHEIG, facial dysmorphism, hypertrichosis, epilepsy, intellectual disability/developmental delay, and gingival overgrowth; FTT, failure to thrive; KINSSHIP, horseshoe kidney, Nievergelt/Savarirayan type of mesomelic dysplasia, seizures, intellectual disability, pulmonary involvement; RXL, recessive X-linked.

PART 6: GENETIC DISORDERS

Table 66.2 Atrichias.

Disease name	MIM	Inheritance	Gene or genetic defect	Cutaneous features	Extracutaneous features
A Non-syndromic atrichias					
Alopecia universalis congenital	203655	AR	HR	Atrichia	None
Atrichia with papular lesions	209500	AR	HR	Atrichia Papular lesions	None
Ectodermal dysplasia 9, hair/nail type	614931	AR	HOXC13	Atrichia (some cases hypotrichosis) Koilonychia and micronychia	None
Lethal acantholytic epidermolysis bullosa	609638	AR	DSP	Generalised atrichia Generalised skin blistering Anonychia	None
B Syndromic atrichias					
AEC syndrome	106260	AD	TP63	Sparse, coarse, wiry hair	Hearing loss
EEC syndrome	604292	AD		Scalp erosions and red peeling skin	Ankyloblepharon, lacrimal duct
Rapp–Hodgkin syndrome	129400	AD		Palmoplantar keratoderma	atresia, blepharoconjunctivitis
ADULT syndrome	103285	AD		Dystrophic nails	Cleft lip/palate
					Abnormal dentition
					Syndactyly
					Cardiac defects
					Kidney defects
					Breast and mammary gland hypoplasia
Frontonasal dysplasia type 2	613451	AR	ALX4	Atrichia	Frontonasal dysplasia (large skull defect, coronal craniosynostosis, hypertelorism, severely depressed nasal bridge and ridge, bifid nasal tip) Cryptorchidism Agenesis of the corpus callosum and mental disability
Growth retardation, alopecia, pseudoanodontia, optic atrophy (GAPO) syndrome	230740	AR	ANTXR1	Scalp hair permanently lost in childhood	Facial dysmorphism with protruding ears and prominent lips Failure of tooth eruption Optic atrophy
Ichthyosis follicularis, atrichia, photophobia syndrome (allelic to keratosis follicularis spinulosa decalvans)	308205	RXL AD	MBTPS2 SREBF1	Atrichia or near-atrichia Dystrophic nails Erythroderma Ichthyosis Follicular hyperkeratosis Palmoplantar keratoderma	Photophobia, vascularising keratitis, BRESHECK syndrome
Keratitis–ichthyosis–deafness syndrome	148210	AD	GJB2	Atrichia/hypotrichosis Ichthyosis Oral leukoplakia Palmoplantar keratoderma Bacterial and fungal skin infections Squamous cell carcinoma	Keratitis Deafness
Mitochondrial complex III deficiency, nuclear type 10	618775	AR	UQCRF1	Atrichia	Fetal bradycardia, hypertrophic cardiomyopathy Delayed motor development Lactic acidosis Thrombocytopenia and normochromic anaemia
T-cell immunodeficiency, alopecia and nail dystrophy syndrome	601705	AR	FOXN1	Atrichia Dysplastic nails	Severe T-cell immunodeficiency
Vitamin D-dependent rickets, type 2A	277440	AR	VDR	Atrichia or near-atrichia Papular lesions	Growth retardation, rickets, dental abnormalities, delayed motor development, seizures

AD, autosomal dominant; ADULT, acro-dermato-ungual-lacrimal-tooth; AEC, ankyloblepharon-ectodermal defects-cleft lip/palate; AR, autosomal recessive; BRESHECK, brain anomalies, retardation, ectodermal dysplasia, skeletal malformations, Hirschsprung disease, ear/eye anomalies, cleft palate/cryptorchidism, and kidney dysplasia/hypoplasia; EEC, ectrodactyly, ectodermal dysplasia and cleft lip/palate; GAPO, wth retardation, alopecia, pseudoanodontia and optic atrophy; HR, hairless.

Table 66.3 Hypotrichoses.

Disease name	MIM	Inheritance	Gene or genetic defect	Cutaneous features	Extracutaneous features
A Non-syndromic hypotrichoses					
Autosomal dominant generalised basaloid follicular hamartoma syndrome	605827	AD	?	Hypotrichosis Milia Palmar pits Hypohidrosis Basaloid follicular hamartomata	None
Autosomal recessive localised hypotrichosis	–	AR	C3ORF52	Sparse hair over scalp, eyebrows, eyelashes	None
Autosomal recessive woolly hair 3 with hypotrichosis	616760	AR	KRT25	Scalp hypotrichosis Woolly hair	None
Ectodermal dysplasia with skin fragility	604536	AR	PKP1	Severe hypotrichosis Skin fragility Dystrophic nails Palmoplantar erosive keratoderma	None
Ectodermal dysplasia type 4, hair/nail type	602032	AR	KRT85	Localised to generalised hypotrichosis (with pili torti) Dysplastic nails	None
Generalised hereditary hypotrichosis simplex (hypotrichosis type 1)	605389	AD	APCDD1	Generalised hypotrichosis, progressing from childhood with sparing of eyebrows, eyelashes and facial hair	None
Hypotrichosis simplex of the scalp (hypotrichosis type 2)	146520	AD	CDSN	Scalp hypotrichosis, progressing from childhood	None
Hypotrichosis type 3	613981	AD	KRT74	Scalp hypotrichosis Woolly hair	None
Hypotrichosis type 9	614237	AR	Mapped to 10q11.23–q22.3	Hypotrichosis involving scalp, arms, and legs. Eyebrows and eyelashes are spared	None
Hypotrichosis type 10	614238	AR	Mapped to 7p22.3–p21.3	Generalised hypotrichosis Scalp papules	None
Hypotrichosis type 11	615059	AD	SNRPE	Generalised hypotrichosis with sparing of pubic hair	None
Hypotrichosis type 12	603636	AD	RPL21	Scalp hair loss, progressive, after 2–6 months of age, beard hair unaffected Body hair, axillary and pubic hair, eyebrows and eyelashes sparse or absent	None
Hypotrichosis type 13	608245	AD	KRT71	Woolly hair, scalp, eyebrows, eyelashes hair paucity Symptoms improve with time	
Hypotrichosis type 14	618275	AR	LSS	Sparse to absent lanugo-like scalp hair Sparse and brittle eyebrows, eyelashes, body hair, pubic and/or axillary hair	One patient with congenital cataract
Hypotrichosis and recurrent skin vesicles	613102	AR	DSC3	Generalised hypotrichosis Skin vesicles (?)	None
Keratoderma and woolly hair	–	AR	KANK2	Generalised hypotrichosis Woolly hair Striate palmoplantar keratoderma Leukonychia Pseudoainhum	None
Localised, AR hypotrichosis, type 1 (hypotrichosis type 6)	607903	AR	DSG4	Generalised hypotrichosis with sparing of secondary sexual hairs Monilethrix and other structural hair shaft abnormalities Follicular hyperkeratosis	None
Localised, AR hypotrichosis, type 2 (hypotrichosis type 7)	604379	AR	LIPH	Sparse scalp, eyebrows, eyelashes, up to generalised hypotrichosis; woolly hair in some patients (as well as other hair shaft abnormalities)	None
Localised, AR hypotrichosis, type 3 (hypotrichosis type 8)	278150	AR	LPAR6	Sparse and short scalp, eyebrows, eyelashes, up to generalised hypotrichosis; woolly hair in some patients (as well as other hair shaft abnormalities); fair hair in some patients; nail pitting or longitudinal ridging in some patients	None

(continued)

Table 66.3 (*continued*)

Disease name	MIM	Inheritance	Gene or genetic defect	Cutaneous features	Extracutaneous features
Marie Unna hereditary hypotrichosis (hypotrichosis type 4)	146550	AD	*U2HR*	Sparse to normal hair at birth; coarse, wiry, twisted hair in early childhood progressing to generalised hypotrichosis	None
Marie Unna hereditary hypotrichosis (hypotrichosis type 5)	612841	AD	*EPS8L3* (?)		None
Monilethrix	158000	AD	*KRT81* *KRT83* *KRT86*	Hypotrichosis (regional to generalised) due to hair fragility, starting during early childhood and typically improving over time; occipital area most severely involved Follicular hyperkeratosis Nail dystrophy	None
Rombo syndrome	180730	AD	?	Absent or dystrophic eyelashes and eyebrows Bluish discoloration of lips and hands Facial milia and telangiectasis Follicular atrophoderma Basal cell carcinomas	None
Skin fragility–woolly hair syndrome	607655	AR	*DSP*	Hypotrichosis Woolly hair Palmoplantar keratoderma Skin fragility and blistering Nail dystrophy	None
B Syndromic hypotrichoses					
Alopecia-mental retardation syndrome Type 1 Type 2	203650 618840	AR	*AHSG* *LSS* (note: in some families, *LSS* variants associated with non-syndromic hypotrichosis)	Hypotrichosis Ichthyosis (in some families)	Neurological abnormalities Autism spectrum Intellectual disability Psychomotor delay
Alopecia–neurological defects–endocrinopathy (ANE) syndrome	612079	AR	*RBM28*	Variable degrees of alopecia Flexural hyperpigmentation	Growth retardation Hypogonadism Addison disease Abnormal dentition
Argininosuccinic aciduria	207900	AR	*ASL*	Dry, sparse brittle hair with trichorrhexis nodosa	Failure to thrive Hepatic fibrosis and hepatomegaly Encephalopathy Poor feeding, vomiting Neurological defects Intellectual disability
AR ichthyosis with hypotrichosis	610765	AR	*ST14*	Generalised hypotrichosis with curly hair and long eyelashes Multiple hair shaft abnormalities Ichthyosis	Photophobia, corneal opacities, blepharitis Abnormal dentition
Bachmann–Bupp syndrome	619075	AD	*ODC1*	Hypotrichosis involving scalp, eyelashes and eyebrows	Macrocephaly and high forehead Hypertelorism Developmental delay and ADHD Short corpus callosum Pinched long nose Joint hypermobility
Bazex syndrome	301845	XLD	*ACTRT1*	Hypotrichosis with pili torti and trichorrhexis nodosa Facial hyperpigmentation and milia (which disappear in adulthood) Follicular atrophoderma Comedones Keratosis pilaris Localised hypohidrosis Basal cell carcinomas in second decade of life	

(*continued*)

Table 66.3 (continued)

Disease name	MIM	Inheritance	Gene or genetic defect	Cutaneous features	Extracutaneous features
Biotinidase deficiency	253260	AR	BTD	Alopecia Dermatitis Skin infections	Hepatosplenomegaly Vomiting, diarrhoea Hearing loss Vision loss Breathing problems Neurological defects
Björnstad syndrome	262000	AR	BCS1L	Hypotrichosis Coarse dry and fragile hair with pili torti	Nerve deafness Hypogonadism
Cardiofaciocutaneous syndrome	115150 615278 615279 615280	AD	BRAF KRAS MAP2K1 MAP2K2	Sparse, curly hair Absence of eyebrows and eyelashes Ichthyosis Haemangiomata Keratosis pilaris Lentigines Abnormal palmoplantar creases	Short stature Facial dysmorphism Eye defects Cardiac defects Osteopenia Neurological defects, including seizures and hypotonia Intellectual disability
Cartilage–hair hypoplasia	250250	AR	RMRP	Generalised hypotrichosis with fair sparse and fine hair	Skeletal dysplasia and short stature Malabsorption and Hirschprung disease Haematological anomalies Cellular immunodeficiency Increased risk of lymphoma and skin cancer
Cerebral arteriopathy, autosomal recessive, with subcortical infarcts and leukoencephalopathy (CARASIL) syndrome	600142	AR	HTRA1	Alopecia (sometimes preceding neurological defects)	Progressive encephalopathy (onset after puberty)
Chondrodysplasia punctate 2	302960	XLD	EBP	Patchy alopecia Coarse sparse hair Ichthyosis Follicular atrophoderma along Blaschko lines	Short stature Frontal bossing Hearing loss Cataracts, microphthalmia Skeletal dysplasia with epiphyseal stippling Impaired mental function
Cleft lip/palate–ectodermal dysplasia syndrome	225060	AR	PVRL1	Hypotrichosis Palmoplantar keratoderma Dystrophic nails	Facial dysmorphism Cleft lip/palate Hypodontia Syndactyly
Clouston syndrome	129500	AD	GJB6	Hypotrichosis with wiry, brittle and pale hair Palmoplantar keratoderma Dysplastic nails	Short stature Ophthalmological manifestations including cataracts, conjunctivitis, strabismus, photophobia
Costello syndrome	218040	AD	HRAS	Curly sparse hair Dystrophic nails Cutis laxa Periorifical papillomas Acanthosis nigricans	Short stature Facial dysmorphism with full cheeks, macrocephaly, thick lips and macroglossia Cardiac defects Lung defects Pyloric stenosis Kidney defects Delayed psychomotor development and neurological defects Malignancies
Cranioectodermal dysplasia type 1	218330	AR	IFT122	Fine sparse hair Thin short nails	Abnormal dentition Facial dysmorphism
Cranioectodermal dysplasia type 2	613610	AR	WDR35		Craniosynostosis Brachydactyly, short limbs
Cranioectodermal dysplasia type 3	614099	AR	IFT43		Bicuspid aortic valve Liver disease

(continued)

PART 6: GENETIC DISORDERS

Table 66.3 (*continued*)

Disease name	MIM	Inheritance	Gene or genetic defect	Cutaneous features	Extracutaneous features
Cranioectodermal dysplasia type 4	614378	AR	WDR19		Renal failure Osteoporosis Abnormal dentition
Dermatopathia pigmentosa reticularis	125595	AD	KRT14	Alopecia Reticulate hyperpigmentation Hypo-/hyperhidrosis Absent fingerprints Palmoplantar keratoderma Dystrophic nails	
Dilated cardiomyopathy with woolly hair and keratoderma	605676	AR	DSP	Hypotrichosis Woolly hair Palmoplantar keratoderma	Dilated left ventricular cardiomyopathy
Dilated cardiomyopathy with woolly hair, keratoderma and tooth agenesis	615821	AD	DSP	Hypotrichosis Woolly hair Palmoplantar keratoderma	Dilated cardiomyopathy Tooth agenesis/caries
Ectodermal dysplasia, ectrodactyly and macular dystrophy	225280	AR	CDH3	Generalised hypotrichosis Light-coloured hair	Progressive retinal macular degeneration Abnormal dentition Ectrodactyly, syndactyly
Ectodermal dysplasia 14, hair/tooth type with or without hypohidrosis	61810	AR	TSPEAR	Hypotrichosis of scalp and extremities (hypertrichosis of chest) Hypohidrosis	Hypodontia Conical teeth
Ectodermal dysplasia 15, hypohidrotic/hair type	618535	AR	CST6	Hypotrichosis involving scalp, eyelashes Dry skin with hypohidrosis	Blepharitis and photophobia
Ectodermal dysplasia-syndactyly syndrome 1	613573	AR	PVRL4	Generalised hypotrichosis with pili torti Dysplastic nails Palmoplantar keratoderma	Syndactyly Abnormal dentition
Ectodermal dysplasia-syndactyly syndrome 2	613576	AR	?	Generalised hypotrichosis Dysplastic nails Palmoplantar keratoderma Hyperhidrosis	Syndactyly Facial dysmorphism Abnormal dentition Cardiomegaly
Gomez-Lopez-Hernandez syndrome	601853	Sporadic	?	Parieto-occipital alopecia	Facial dysmorphism Short stature Neurological defects Corneal opacities
Hallerman–Streiff syndrome	234100	?	GJA1 (?)	Hypotrichosis Light hair Skin atrophy and telangiectases	Short stature Multiple skeletal abnormalities Facial dysmorphism with small pointed nose, thin lips, microstomia, frontal bossing, micrognathia Microphthalmia, cataracts, strabismus, coloboma Abnormal dentition Tracheomalacia Pulmonary hypertension and infections Neurological defects
Hephaestin-like 1 deficiency	261990	AR	HEPHL1 (single case)	Hypotrichosis with sparse eyebrows, absent lateral third of eyelashes, pili torti and trichorrhexis nodosa Hypoplastic nails	Elfin facies Cognitive delay Joint hypermobility Small teeth
Hutchinson–Gilford progeria syndrome	176670	AD	LMNA	Alopecia Absence of subcutaneous fat Wrinkled, atrophic and pigmented skin Scleroderma	Growth retardation Osteoporosis Premature ageing Premature cardiovascular disease Insulin resistance
Hypohidrotic ectodermal dysplasia types 1, 10A, 10B, 11A, 11B	305100 129490 224900 614940	XLR AD AR	EDA EDAR EDARADD	Generalised hypotrichosis Hypohidrosis Dysplastic nails Dry skin	Facial dysmorphism including pigmentation under the eyes, everted nose, prominent lips Conical teeth and hypodontia Heat stroke Hypoplastic mammary glands Hoarse voice

PART 6: GENETIC DISORDERS

Table 66.3 (*continued*)

Disease name	MIM	Inheritance	Gene or genetic defect	Cutaneous features	Extracutaneous features
Hypotrichosis with juvenile macular dystrophy	601553	AR	CDH3	Generalised hypotrichosis with pili torti Light-coloured hair	Progressive retinal macular degeneration
Hypotrichosis–lymphoedema–telangiectasia syndrome	607823	AD (?) AR	SOX18	Progressive hair loss since childhood involving scalp, eyebrows and eyelashes	Telangiectases (acral) Leg lymphoedema, congenital eyelid oedema, hydrocele, scrotal oedema
Macrocephaly, alopecia, cutis laxa, scoliosis (MACS) syndrome	613075	AR	RIN2	Alopecia Receding anterior hairline Cutis laxa	Short stature Coarse facies Abnormal dentition Scoliosis Joint hypermobility
Mandibulofacial dysostosis with alopecia	616367	AD	EDNRA	Hypotrichosis involving scalp, body hair, eyebrows and eyelashes	Facial dysmorphism Dental abnormalities
Menkes disease	309400	XLR	ATP7A	Steely, kinky sparse hair which can show pili torti, monilethrix and trichorrhexis nodosa Cutis laxa Hypopigmentation	Short stature Microcephaly Joint laxity Osteoporosis Neurodegenerative manifestations Variable vascular pathologies Chronic diarrhoea Urogenital anomalies Skeletal dysplasia (including occipital horns)
Naxos disease	601214	AR	JUP	Hypotrichosis Woolly hair Palmoplantar keratoderma	Arrhythmogenic right ventricular dysplasia Dilated cardiomegaly
Neonatal ichthyosis-sclerosing cholangitis (NISCH) syndrome	607626	AR	CLDN1	Hypotrichosis with loss of lateral eyebrows Sparse eyelashes Ichthyosis Jaundice	Sclerosing cholangitis Hepatomegaly Hypodontia
Neonatal inflammatory skin and bowel disease	614328	AR	ADAM17	Short and broken hair, disorganised eyebrows and eyelashes Perorificial erythema Pustular rash Dysplastic nails and paronychia	Chronic bloody diarrhoea, malabsorption Left heart ventricular dilatation High IgE
Netherton syndrome	256500	AR	SPINK5	Hypotrichosis with abnormal hair shaft structure (trichorrhexis invaginata) Congenital erythroderma Ichthyosis linearis circumflexa	Growth retardation Perinatal hypernatraemia Atopic diathesis Multiple food allergies Recurrent infections Gastroenteropathy High IgE levels
Nicolaides–Baraitser syndrome	601358	AD	SMARCA2	Hypotrichosis Low anterior hairline Wrinkled or eczematous skin	Short stature Skeletal dysplasia Facial dysmorphism Neuropsychiatric manifestations
Noonan syndrome-like disorder with loose anagen hair	607721	AD	SHOC2	Sparse light-coloured hair Hyperpigmentation Wrinkled skin	Developmental delay Macrocephaly Cardiac defects Hypotonia and intellectual disability Brain abnormalities
Oculodentodigital dysplasia	164200	AD	GJA1	Hypotrichosis Dry hair Palmoplantar keratoderma	Microphthalmia, cataracts, strabismus Abnormal dentition Cleft lip/palate Multiple skeletal abnormalities Hearing loss Lymphoedema Neurological defects

(*continued*)

Table 66.3 (continued)

Disease name	MIM	Inheritance	Gene or genetic defect	Cutaneous features	Extracutaneous features
Odonto-onychodermal dysplasia	257980	AR	WNT10A	Hypotrichosis Dry and thin hair Dystrophic nails Palmoplantar keratoderma Hyperhidrosis Decreased number of tongue papillae	Hypodontia
Olmsted syndrome Type 1 Type 2 Type 3	614594 619208 300918	AD, AR AD XLR	TRPV3 PERP MBTPS2	Hypotrichosis Woolly hair Palmoplantar keratoderma Ichthyosis Periorificial hyperkeratosis Pseudoainhum	Caries Leukokeratosis of buccal mucosa Corneal neo-vascularisation (MBTPS2)
Oro-facio-digital syndrome	311200	XLD	OFD1	Alopecia Sparse, coarse hair Facial milia	Short stature Microcephaly, frontal bossing, hypoplastic alar cartilage Hyperplastic oral frenulum, bifid/lobulated tongue, tongue hamartoma Cleft lip/palate Lip anomalies Abnormal dentition Liver, pancreas, ovarian, kidney cysts Clino-/syn-/brachy-/polydactyly Neuropsychiatric complications
Poikiloderma, hereditary fibrosing, with tendon contractures, myopathy, and pulmonary fibrosis	615704	AD	FAM111B	Hypotrichosis involving scalp, eyebrows and eyelashes Poikiloderma Hypohidrosis	Interstitial pulmonary fibrosis Contractures of limbs Delayed puberty
Rothmund–Thompson syndrome	268400	AR	RECQL4	Hypotrichosis involving scalp, face, eyebrows and eyelashes Poikiloderma mainly evident in sun-exposed areas Photosensitivity Hyperkeratotic lesions over soles and knees Nail dystrophy Non-melanoma skin cancers	Short stature Skeletal dysplasia Hypogonadism Cataracts Abnormal dentition Risk of osteogenic sarcoma
Schopf–Schulz–Passarge syndrome	224750	AR	WNT10A	Hypotrichosis Dry and thin hair Dystrophic nails Palmoplantar keratoderma Hyperhidrosis Decreased number of tongue papillae Eyelid hydrocystomata Non-melanoma skin cancer	Hypodontia Bird-like facies
Severe dermatitis, multiple allergies and metabolic wasting (SAM) syndrome	615508	AR	DSG1	Hypotrichosis Congenital erythroderma with acantholysis Palmoplantar keratoderma	Growth retardation Perinatal hypernatraemia Recurrent infections Oesophagitis Cardiac defects High IgE levels
Short stature, onychodysplasia, facial dysmorphism and hypotrichosis (SOFT) syndrome	614813	AR	POC1A	Generalised hypotrichosis Hypoplastic nails	Short long bones and other skeletal abnormalities resulting in short stature Macrocephaly Facial dysmorphism Oligospermia High-pitched voice
Trichohepatoenteric syndrome	222470 614602	AR	TTC37 SKIV2L	Hypotrichosis with trichorrhexis nodosa and woolly hair	Failure to thrive Prominent cheeks and forehead Congenital heart defects Cholestatic jaundice, hepatomegaly, cirrhosis Severe secretory diarrhoea Intellectual disability

(continued)

PART 6: GENETIC DISORDERS

Table 66.3 (*continued*)

Disease name	MIM	Inheritance	Gene or genetic defect	Cutaneous features	Extracutaneous features
Tricho-rhino-phalangeal syndrome types I, II, III	190350 150230 90351	AD	TRPS1	Hypotrichosis Dysplastic nails	Growth retardation Skeletal dysplasia including various developmental abnormalities of hand and feet Late-onset osteopenia and osteoarthritis Facial dysmorphism including large ears and pear-shaped nose Abnormal dentition Hypotonia
Trichothiodystrophy, non-photosensitive type	234050	AR	MPLKIP TARS1 GTF2E2 RNF113A	Hypotrichosis resulting from brittle sulphur-deficient hair	Short stature Intellectual disability Decreased fertility
Trichothiodystrophy, photosensitive type	601675	AR	ERCC2 ERCC3 GTF2H5	Hypotrichosis resulting from brittle sulphur-deficient hair Ichthyosis Photosensitivity Brittle nails Lack of adipose tissue	Short stature Progeroid facies Microcephaly Various ocular manifestations including cataracts and microcornea Joint contractures Hypogammaglobulinaemia Recurrent infections Hypogonadism Asthma Intellectual disability
Werner syndrome	277700	AR	RECQL2	Premature balding Poikiloderma Scleroderma-like changes Loss of adipose tissue Hyperpigmentation Calcinosis cutis Ulcers	Short stature Prematurely aged facies Cataracts Retinal degeneration Osteoporosis and avascular necrosis Premature cardiovascular disease Diabetes Hypogonadism Malignancies
Woodhouse–Sakathi syndrome	241080	AR	DCAF17	Scalp and eyebrows alopecia	Deafness Hypogonadism Diabetes Extrapyramidal abnormalities, intellectual disability and other neurological defects
Yunis–Yaron syndrome	216340	AR	FIG4	Hypotrichosis involving scalp, eyebrows and eyelashes Palmar crease Hypoplastic nails	Growth retardation Facial dysmorphism including dysplastic ears and protruding eyes Abnormal dentition Heart defects Pyloric stenosis Micropenis and hypospadias Severe neurological defects

AD, autosomal dominant; ADHD, attention deficit hyperactivity disorder; AR, autosomal recessive; XLD, X-linked dominant; XLR, X-linked recessive.

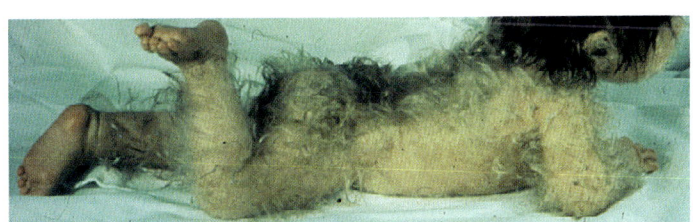

Figure 66.1 Generalised hypertrichosis. Courtesy of Professor Peter Itin.

Hypertrichosis universalis congenita, Ambras type

Children affected by this disorder present with generalised hypertrichosis which consists of large amounts of velus hair over the entire surface of the skin, with some predilection for the face, ears and shoulders. Hypertrichosis of the external ears is typical. Facial

PART 6: GENETIC DISORDERS

dysmorphism and skeletal abnormalities have also been reported [13]. The disorder has been found to be caused by chromosomal rearrangements over 8q23.1 leading to downregulation of the *TRPS1* gene [14], also known to be involved in the pathogenesis of tricho-rhino-phalangeal syndrome, another complex hair disorder (Chapter 65). Of interest, a similar defect was also found in a murine model of the disease, the 'Koala' mouse [14].

Generalised hypertrichosis terminalis

This disorder is inherited in an autosomal dominant fashion and is characterised by excess of terminal hair and a variable age of onset. Many patients demonstrate facial dysmorphism and often severe gingival hyperplasia [15]. In several cases, genomic changes on chromosome 17q24.2-q24.3 were found to segregate with the disease phenotype [16,17]. It has been suggested that these changes may impact on the function of SOX9, which is known to play a role in the regulation of hair growth. A mutation in the *ABCA5* gene, which maps to the same region, has been identified in a single case [18].

Cantu syndrome

Cantu syndrome is inherited in an autosomal dominant fashion and features congenital hypertrichosis with long curly eyelashes, macrosomia, facial dysmorphism, gingival hyperplasia, skeletal anomalies, cardiac defects and occasionally mild intellectual disability [19]. The disease was found to be caused by activating mutations in *ABCC9* encoding the sulfonylurea receptor 2 [20,21]. This is of interest as this molecule is part of an adenosine triphosphate (ATP)-sensitive potassium channel complex, targeted by minoxidil [22] which is used to treat male and female pattern baldness.

LOCALISED HYPERTRICHOSES

Congenital localised hypertrichosis has been reported as an isolated finding around the elbows (hypertrichosis cubiti) and the neck (posterior and anterior cervical hypertrichosis) [23,24]. Congenital localised hypertrichosis has been described in association with spinal (faun-tail naevus) or cranial dysraphism (hair collar sign) [25–28]. Localised hypertrichosis often accompanies pigmentation abnormalities as in congenital melanocytic naevi and Becker naevus. Localised hypertrichosis is also a classical feature of congenital porphyrias (Chapter 58).

The histiocytosis and lymphadenopathy syndrome (also known as H syndrome) is a complex disorder featuring a wide and variable constellation of cutaneous and systemic manifestations including skin hyperpigmentation, localised hypertrichosis, hepatosplenomegaly, heart anomalies, hearing loss, hypogonadism, short stature and hyperglycaemia/diabetes [29,30] (Figure 66.2). The disorder was found to be caused by mutations in *SLC29A3* encoding the human equilibrative nucleoside transporter (ENT3) [31,32]. Of note, the histiocytes present in dermal infiltrates in the

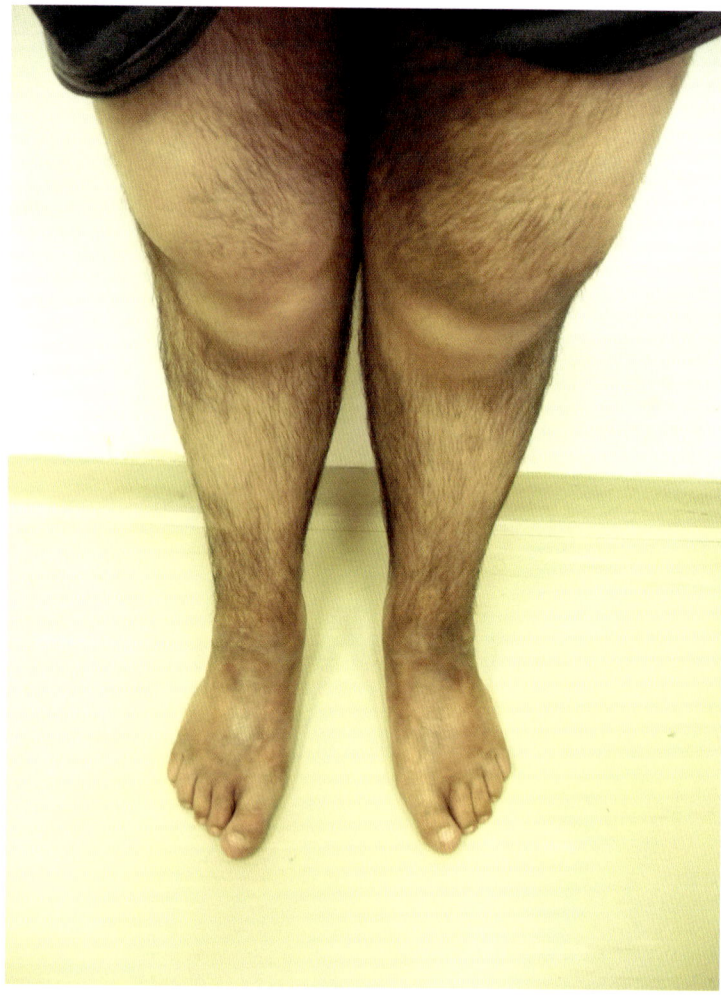

Figure 66.2 Hypertrichosis and hyperpigmented plaques localised to the lower limb in an adult patient with H syndrome. Courtesy of Professor Avraham Zlotogorski.

skin of the patients resemble those seen in Rosai–Dorfman disease [33]. ENT3 deficiency was shown to affect hematopoietic and mesenchymal stem cell fates [34].

DIFFERENTIAL DIAGNOSIS

The most important diagnosis to exclude in any form of hypertrichosis is hirsutism, which results from excessive growth of hair in a male pattern distribution and warrants thorough investigations in search for an endocrinological, drug or paraneoplastic cause (Chapter 148). The late onset of hypertrichosis should always raise the possibility of an underlying malignancy [35].

TREATMENT

Hair removal using depilation or laser techniques has been successfully employed [36]. Surgical debulking of the gums and total tooth extraction have been reported to result in improved oral function in generalised hypertrichosis terminalis [37]. Treatment of H syndrome with mycophenolate mofetil and tocilizumab has been reported [38,39].

ATRICHIAS

Atrichias refer to a group of very rare disorders characterised by total or near total absence of visible scalp and body hair.

Atrichia with papular lesions

Clinical features

Children affected with atrichia with papular lesions (APL) are usually born with normal hair that is shed during the first months of life, never to regrow thereafter. During the first to second decades of life, patients develop a diffuse papular rash that has been noted to be particularly prominent over the cheeks and scalp but can involve almost any part of the body [40–42] (Figure 66.3). Although APL has been described with mental disability, gastrointestinal polyposis and delay in bone age, these associations are considered spurious. On histology, APL is characterised by the conspicuous presence of dermal cysts, which reflect abortive development of different regions of the hair follicles (Figure 66.3c) [43].

Pathogenesis

APL is caused by mutations in the *HR* gene, encoding a transcription co-repressor factor called hairless [40,42,44]. Hairless has been shown to function as a histone H3K9 demethylase [45]. Hairless may regulate hair cycling through its effect on the WNT signalling pathway [46], through its effect on polyamine synthesis [47] or

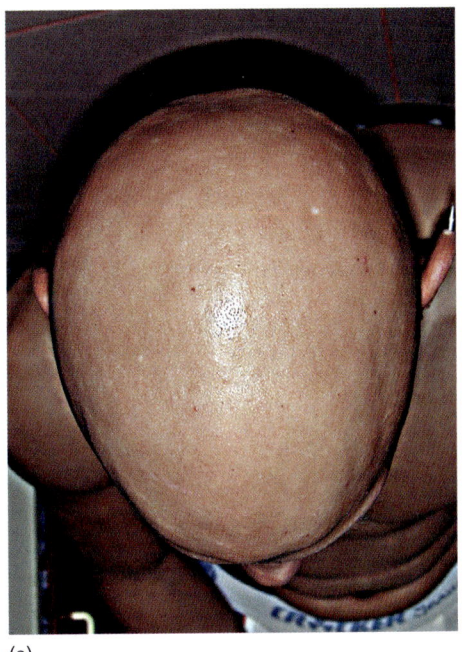
(a)

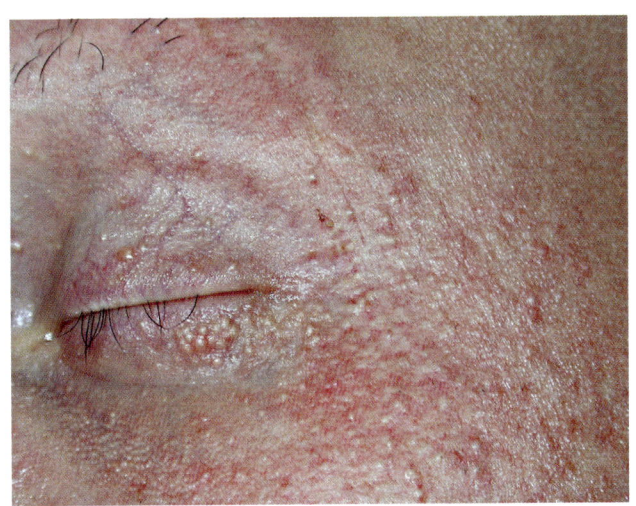
(b)

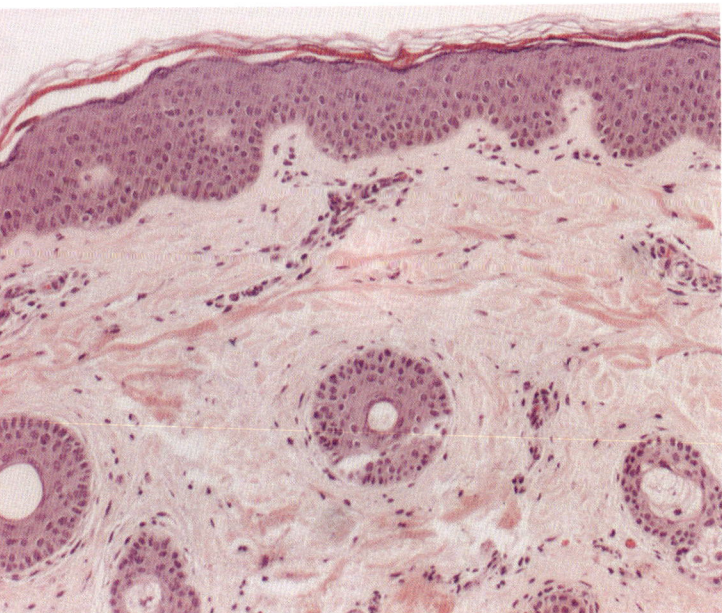
(c)

Figure 66.3 Total lack of hair (a) and follicular lesions (b) in atrichia with papular lesions. On histology, note the conspicuous presence of dermal cysts (c).

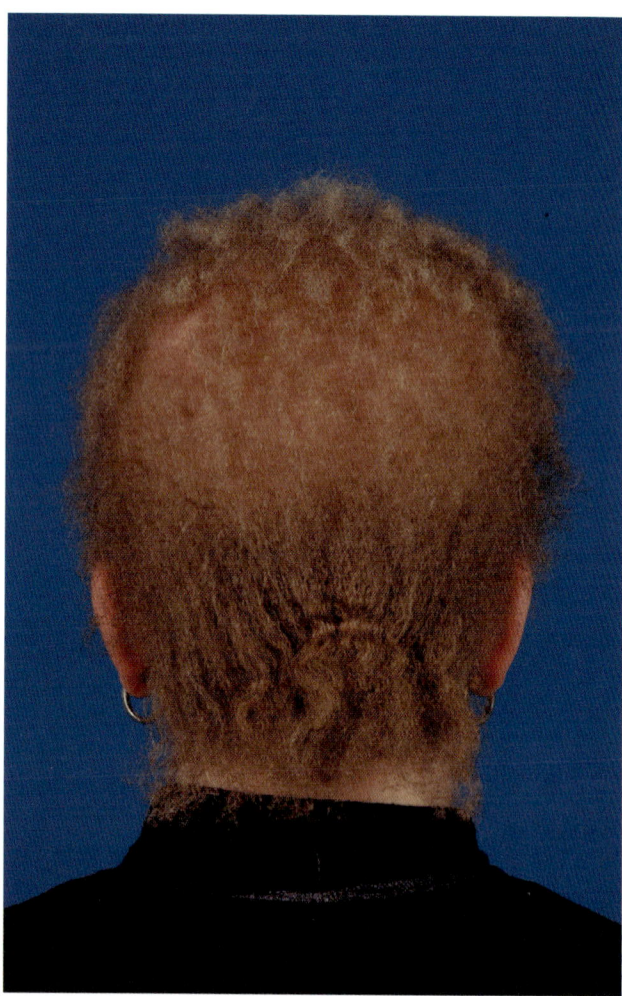

Figure 66.4 Wiry, coarse and sparse hair in Marie Unna hereditary hypotrichosis. Courtesy of Professor Maurice Van Steensel.

through additional targets [48]. Regardless of its exact mechanism of action, downregulation of hairless is associated with abnormal catagen and interferes with the normal hair cycle, leading to the abnormal development of hair follicles into epidermal cysts that manifest at the clinical level as papules [49]. Of note, overexpression of hairless due to heterozygous mutations in a short regulatory open reading frame located upstream to the *HR* gene also leads to abnormal hair development in patients affected with Marie Unna hereditary hypotrichosis [50], indicating that absence and increased expression of hairless are equally detrimental to hair growth and development. Marie Unna hereditary hypotrichosis (also known as hypotrichoses 4 and 5) is in contrast with APL inherited in an autosomal dominant fashion. Affected individuals display sparse to normal hair at birth, develop coarse, wiry and twisted hair in early childhood, followed by the development of generalised alopecia in adulthood [51] (Figure 66.4).

Differential diagnosis

Another inherited form of congenital atrichia, termed alopecia universalis congenita (MIM: 203655), is also caused by mutations in *HR* and is clinically identical to APL except for the absence of skin papules [40,42]. Vitamin D resistant rickets (VDRR; MIM: 277440) is inherited in an autosomal recessive fashion. It results from end organ unresponsiveness to 1,25-dihydroxycholecalciferol. Affected patients display normal serum 25-hydroxyvitamin D, high serum 1,25-$(OH)_2$-cholecalciferol and profound hypocalcaemia, leading to rickets and loss of teeth [52]. VDRR with hair loss (type IIa) must be differentiated from VDRR without hair loss (type IIb). VDRR type IIa patients are born with normal hair, which is shed during the first year of life and never significantly regrows thereafter (Figure 66.5).

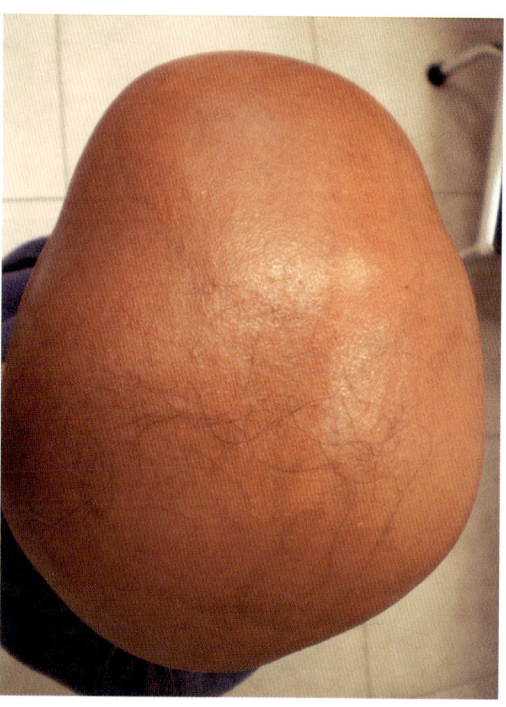

(a)

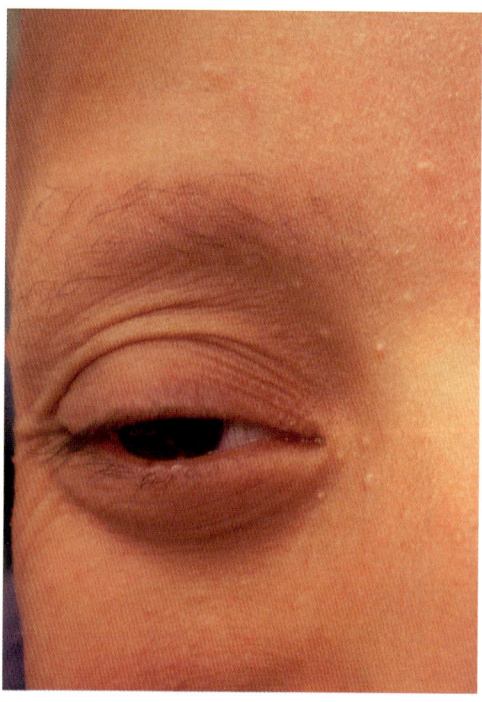

(b)

Figure 66.5 Near total absence of hair in a young patient with vitamin D resistant rickets type IIa (a); note the whitish papules over the central part of the face (b).

In contrast, bony changes can improve with age. Milia-like lesions similar to those observed in APL have also been described in VDRR [52]. VDRR is caused by mutations in the gene encoding the vitamin D_3 receptor (*VDR*). Most VDRR type IIa-causing mutations affect the N-terminal DNA-binding domain of the receptor, which harbours two zinc finger domains responsible for DNA binding and interactions with other proteins. In contrast, mutations in the vitamin D binding domain, situated at the C-terminus, do not cause alopecia [53]. Thus, vitamin D binding to the VDR is not necessary for normal hair development, which may explain why other forms of inherited rickets, with defective vitamin D binding, are not associated with alopecia [52,53]. These studies emphasised the importance of VDR binding to DNA and its interactions with other transcription factors during hair cycling. The fact that hairless functions under physiological conditions in association with the VDR explains the clinical similarities of the two phenotypes [48].

Bazex syndrome should also be included in the differential diagnosis of alopecia associated with a papular rash. This X-linked recessive disorder [54] manifests with hypotrichosis, milia, atrophoderma of the dorsa of the hands and feet, face and extensor surfaces of the elbows and knees, and hypohidrosis of the face [55,56]. Hair microscopy can reveal trichorrhexis nodosa and pili torti. Basal cell neoplasms often develop after the second decade of life [56]. Bazex syndrome (also known as Bazex–Dupre–Christol syndrome) was recently shown to result from a genetic variant affecting the expression of ARP-T1 which inhibits *GLI1* expression; thus, loss of ARP-T1 leads to activation of the Hedgehog pathway in individuals with the syndrome [57]. In addition, ARP-T1 regulates cilia formation [58]. Generalised basaloid follicular hamartoma syndrome is clinically similar although basal cell carcinomas do not develop [59].

Another disorder featuring total absence of hair is the *G*rowth retardation, *A*lopecia, *P*seudoanodontia, *O*ptic atrophy (GAPO) syndrome [60] (Figure 66.6). This autosomal recessive complex disorder is caused by mutations in the *ANTXR1* coding for the anthrax toxin receptor, which seems to play an important role in actin assembly [61].

Treatment

An accurate diagnosis is critical to prevent unnecessary treatment of APL with systemic steroids when misdiagnosed as alopecia universalis. Oral or intravenous calcium and active vitamin D metabolites may attenuate the bone disease of patients with VDRR but do not affect hair status [62].

Ichthyosis follicularis with atrichia and photophobia

Clinical features

This disorder manifests with congenital total or partial atrichia, severe and diffuse follicular hyperkeratosis, different degrees of scaling and vascularising keratitis leading to photophobia and blindness [63]. Ichthyosis follicularis with atrichia and photophobia (IFAP) is transmitted as a recessive X-linked trait or in an autosomal dominant fashion. Disease severity is highly variable. IFAP has been reported in association with a wide range of extracutaneous manifestations including the BRESHECK constellation of signs (*B*rain anomalies (including mental disability, corpus callosum dysgenesis, olivo-pontocerebellar atrophy), growth *R*etardation, *E*ctodermal dysplasia, *S*keletal deformities (scoliosis, rib and pelvic anomalies), *H*irschsprung disease, *E*ar (hearing loss)/*E*ye anomalies, *C*left palate/cryptorchidism and *K*idney dysplasia/hypoplasia) [64]. IFAP has been shown to overlap clinically with keratosis follicularis spinulosa decalvans (KFSD), which features scarring alopecia, typically prominent over the occiput and involving the eyelashes and eyebrows, facial erythema, follicular hyperkeratosis, keratoderma, blepharitis, conjunctivitis and keratitis [65].

Pathogenesis

IFAP, BRESHECK syndrome and KFSD as well as Olmsted syndrome (and possibly osteogenesis imperfecta, type XIX) have been found to result from mutations in the membrane-bound transcription factor protease, site 2 (*MBTPS2*) gene [64,66–69] which encodes a protein involved in endoplasmic reticulum stress response as well as in cholesterol homeostasis. MBTPS2 regulates the translocation of regulatory molecules and transcription activating factors to the nucleus [70]. As the *MBTPS2* gene is located on the X chromosome, female carriers are either phenotypically normal or show patchy alopetic linear lesions of atrophoderma or follicular ichthyosis along the lines of Blaschko, reflecting Lyonisation [71].

More recently, IFAP has been shown to result from dominant mutations in the *SREBF1* gene which encodes the sterol regulatory element (SRE) binding transcription factor 1 (SREBP1). SREBP1 regulates the biosynthesis of fatty acids and cholesterols [72]. Of note, hereditary mucoepithelial dysplasia (featuring non-scarring alopecia, xerosis and abnormal mucosal tissues) is also caused by

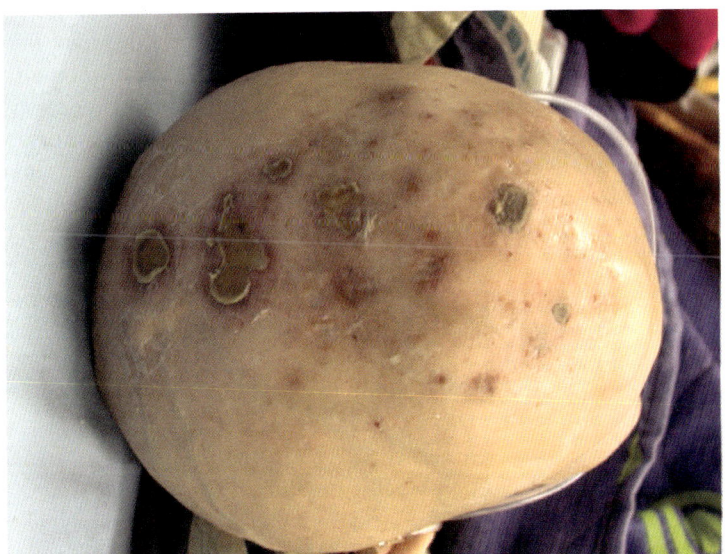

Figure 66.6 Alopecia totalis in a patient with growth retardation, alopecia, pseudoanodontia and optic atrophy (GAPO) syndrome. Courtesy of Professor David Enk.

mutations in *SREBF1* [73] and shares many clinical manifestations with IFAP [74].

Treatment

Treatment is mainly aimed at maintaining visual function [75] as well as preventing or correcting systemic complications of the syndrome. A variable response to acitretin has been reported in several patients with improvement in ichthyosiform changes and corneal erosions but no change in alopecia or photophobia [63,76–78].

HYPOTRICHOSES

Hypotrichoses represent a very heterogeneous and vast group of disorders characterised by a reduced density of hair follicles. Phenotypic variability is the rule and can be striking even amongst affected members of the same family, which often complicates the diagnosis. These disorders are traditionally classified based on their mode of inheritance and based on the presence of extracutaneous features [3]. Table 66.3 provides a full list of this group of diseases. The major forms of hypotrichoses are described in detail in the following subsections.

NON-SYNDROMIC AUTOSOMAL DOMINANT HYPOTRICHOSES

Autosomal dominant hypotrichosis comprises two major disorders known as generalised hereditary hypotrichosis simplex (also known as hypotrichosis type 1) and hypotrichosis simplex of the scalp (also known as hypotrichosis type 2).

Individuals with generalised hereditary hypotrichosis simplex typically show normal hair at birth, with progressive hair loss and thinning starting during early childhood and involving to a variable extent all parts of the body except for eyelashes, eyebrows and beard [79]. Hair pigmentation can be affected as well but hair shaft structure is normal. The disorder has been found to result from a recurrent mutation in the *APCDD1* gene [79], encoding a regulator of the WNT signalling pathway, which is known to play a critical role during hair follicle development [46,80,81]. Of note, the Wnt/β-catenin pathway requires the lymphoid enhancer-binding factor 1 (LEF1) to activate hair follicle ontogenesis and recently haploinsufficiency for LEF1 has been shown in two individuals to be associated with oligodontia, hypotrichosis and hypohidrosis [82].

Similar clinical findings are observed in hypotrichosis simplex of the scalp except for the fact they are limited to the scalp (Figure 66.7). The disease has been found to result in several families from mutations in the *CDSN* gene encoding corneodesmosin, a component of the corneodesmosomes [83]. Of note, genetic alterations in the same gene have been linked to the inflammatory subtype of peeling skin syndrome [84] and to psoriasis [85,86]. Each type of mutation seems to exert a different deleterious effect: dominant mutations associated with hypotrichosis result in the perifollicular accumulation of a toxic amyloidosis-like material [87]; recessive mutations causing peeling skin syndrome lead to absence of expression of

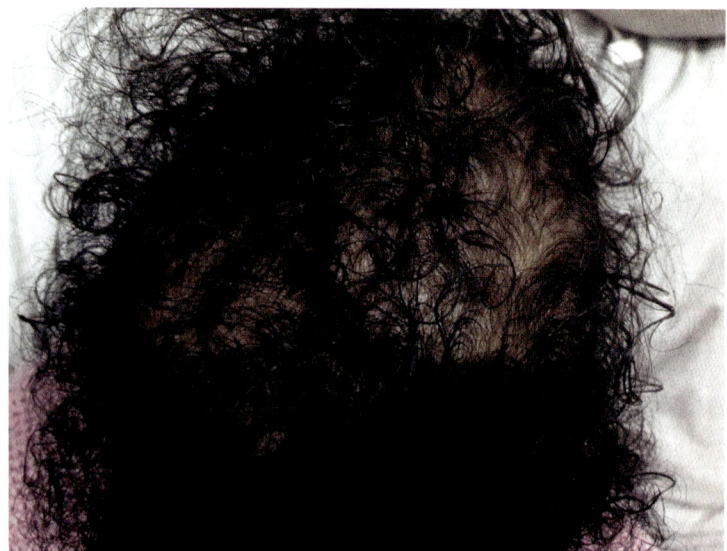

Figure 66.7 Autosomal dominant hypotrichosis of the scalp, caused by a mutation in *CDSN*.

corneodesmosin [84]; while a polymorphism in the *CDSN* gene associated with an increased risk for psoriasis seems to result in increased *CDSN* mRNA stability [85].

A recent open-labelled clinical trial suggested a beneficial effect of topical gentamycin in *CDSN*-associated hypotrichosis [88].

NON-SYNDROMIC AUTOSOMAL RECESSIVE HYPOTRICHOSES

Autosomal recessive localised hypotrichosis (alias hypotrichosis types 7 and 8) features varying degrees of hair paucity over most parts of the body, with occasionally decreased pigmentation [89,90] (Figure 66.8). The disorder overlaps with woolly hair [91], which refers to the growth of fine and tightly curled hair (unlike normal curly hair, woolly hair grows slowly to a shorter distance than normal hair and can be associated with several structural anomalies such as trichorrhexis nodosa) [92]. The hypotrichosis is progressive and can be limited to the scalp or involve the whole body surface including the eyebrows, eyelashes and facial hair [92]. Autosomal recessive localised hypotrichosis has been found to be caused by mutations in three genes: *LIPH* [93], *LPAR6* [94,95] and *C3ORF52* [96]. *LIPH* encodes lipase H, which promotes the synthesis of lysophosphatidic acid, the natural ligand of a G protein-coupled receptor encoded by *LPAR6* which is expressed in both the Henle and the Huxley layers of the inner root sheath of the hair follicle [97]. *C3ORF52* is co-expressed with lipase H in the inner root sheath of the hair follicle. *C3ORF52* serves as a cofactor to *LIPH* and is essential for LPA biosynthesis [98].

In a single centre, open-label, prospective interventional study, topical minoxidil 1% was found to benefit eight patients with *LIPH*-associated hypotrichosis [99]. Minoxidil 5% was also found to benefit a single case with hypotrichosis associated with *DSP* mutations [100].

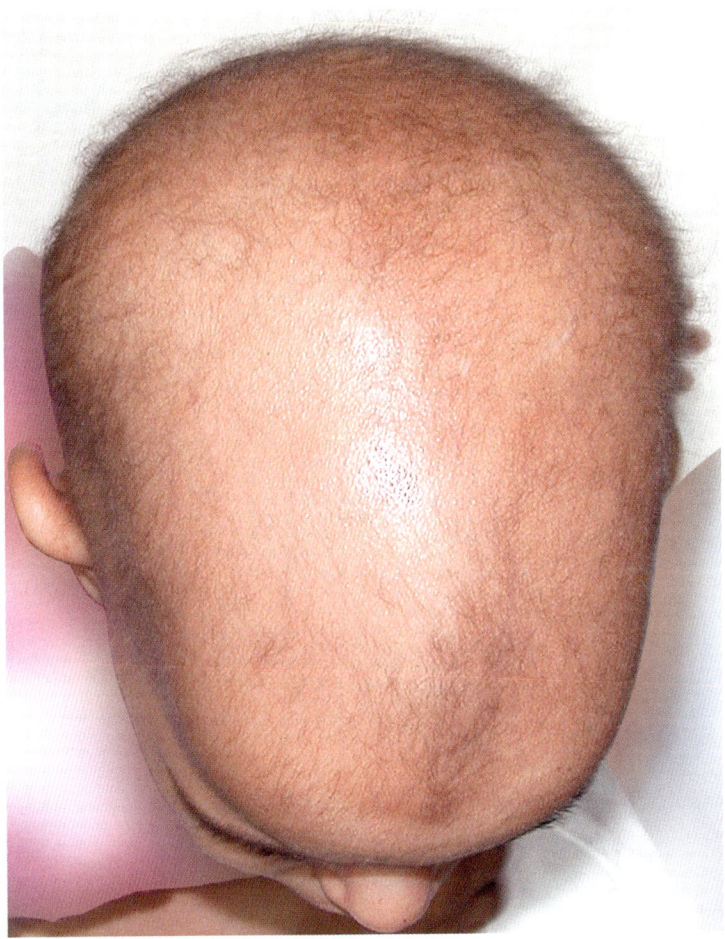

Figure 66.8 Sparse, short and light-coloured hair in a patient carrying a mutation in *LIPH*.

SYNDROMIC AUTOSOMAL DOMINANT HYPOTRICHOSES

Tricho-rhino-phalangeal syndrome

For a detailed description of the syndrome, see Chapter 65. Three subtypes of tricho-rhino-phalangeal syndrome (TRPS) have been described. TRPS I patients feature sparse scalp hair as well as thin and malformed nails associated with a typical bulbous nose, a long philtrum, abnormal dentition and large ears. Patients display short metacarpals and metatarsals, brachydactyly with cone-shaped epiphyses at the (middle) phalanges, scoliosis, lordosis, hip malformations, abnormal patellae, short stature and suffer from osteopenia and osteoarthritis in adulthood [101]. The disorder was found to be caused by mutations in the *TRPS1* gene which codes for a GATA-type zinc finger transcription factor regulating cartilage, kidneys and hair follicle formation [102]. TRPS III is associated with more severe skeletal manifestations than TRPS I but is also due to mutations in *TRPS1* [103].

TRPS II (Langer–Giedion syndrome) is characterised by the same features as TRPS I apart from the conspicuous presence of multiple exostoses and borderline intelligence in some patients [104]. Eyebrows are thickened medially and absent laterally (*signe du sourcil*)

in TRPS I and III but normal in TRPS II. TRPS II is a contiguous gene syndrome caused by deletion mutations affecting both *TRPS1* as well as *EXT1* encoding exostosin 1 [105].

Connexin disorders

A number of dominant syndromes caused by defective function of connexins are associated with various forms of alopecia [**106**]. Keratitis–ichthyosis–deafness syndrome can manifest with alopecia and dense follicular papules over the scalp (Figure 66.9) and results from mutations in the *GJB2* gene encoding connexin-26 [107]. Clouston syndrome is characterised by focal to total alopecia (Figure 66.10) associated with palmoplantar keratoderma and nail dystrophy and results from mutations in the *GJB6* gene encoding connexin-30 [108]. Mutations in the *GJA1* gene coding for connexin-43 cause oculodentodigital dysplasia (ODDD) syndrome which presents with fine and slow-growing sparse hair, palmoplantar keratoderma, facial dysmorphism, a wide range of eye anomalies, abnormal teeth, cleft lip or palate, hyperostosis and other skeletal problems and numerous neurological defects [109,110].

SYNDROMIC AUTOSOMAL RECESSIVE HYPOTRICHOSES

Hypotrichosis with juvenile macular dystrophy

In hypotrichosis with juvenile macular dystrophy (HJMD), short, light and sparse hair in early childhood is associated with the later development of progressive degeneration of the retinal macula leading to blindness during the second to third decades of life [111] (Figure 66.11). The disorder was found to result from mutations in the *CDH3* gene [112] encoding P-cadherin, a component of the adherens junction which was shown to be expressed in the retinal pigment epithelium [113] and to regulate hair growth and pigmentation [114,115]. HJMD has been shown to be allelic to *E*ctodermal dysplasia, *E*ctrodactyly and *M*acular dystrophy (EEM) syndrome, which is characterised by the same clinical features as HJMD in association with abnormal development of the teeth and limbs [116].

Autosomal recessive ichthyosis with hypotrichosis

Affected individuals are born with sparse and short hair and display generalised scaling (Figure 66.12) with ophthalmological manifestations including photophobia, corneal opacities and pinguecula [117]. Abnormal dentition has also been noticed. Structural defects are observed on hair microscopy [117]. The disorder was found to result from mutations in the *ST14* gene [117] that encodes matriptase, a serine protease that functions as a

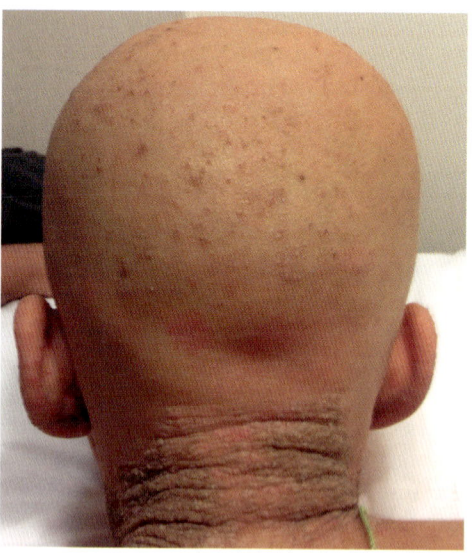

(a)

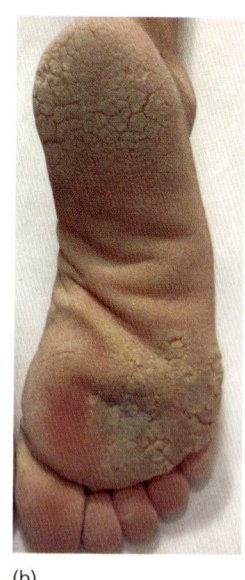

(b)

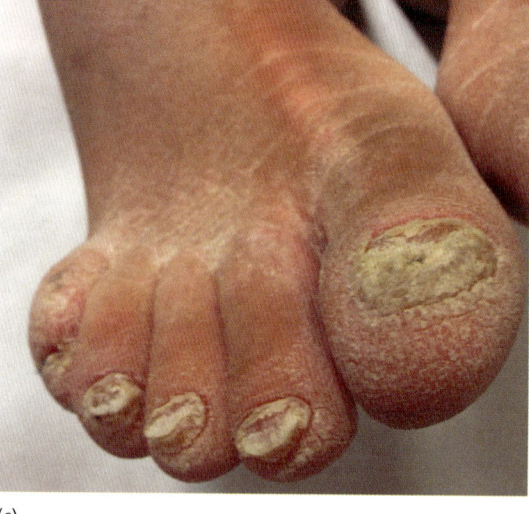

(c)

Figure 66.9 A patient with keratitis–ichthyosis–deafness syndrome demonstrates atrichia associated with follicular papules in the nape area (a), plantar keratoderma (b) and severe nail dystrophy (c).

membrane-bound cell surface protein or as a soluble extracellular protease following release of its ectodomain [118]. Matriptase has been shown to have a role in filaggrin processing and regulates epidermal proliferation and differentiation [118,119]. Mutations in the same gene have been found to cause a disorder called ichthyosis, follicular atrophoderma, hypotrichosis and hypohidrosis, which in many aspects resembles autosomal recessive ichthyosis with hypotrichosis [120].

HAIR SHAFT STRUCTURAL ABNORMALITIES

These disorders are easily identified when suspected since examination of a hair sample under a light microscope is very often sufficient to pose a diagnosis [121]. Rarely, scanning electron microscopy is

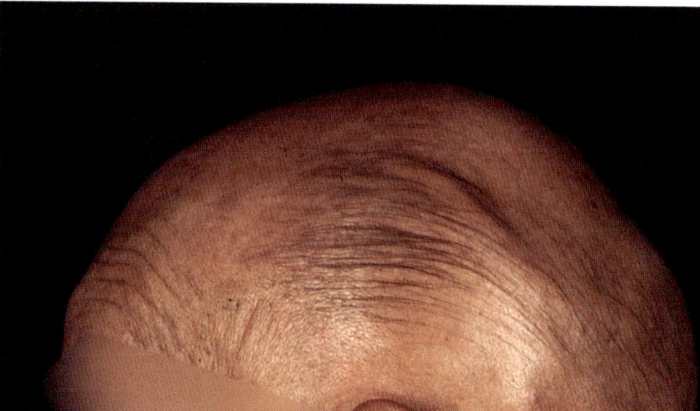

Figure 66.10 Diffuse hypotrichosis in an adult patient with Clouston syndrome. Courtesy of Professor Maurice Van Steensel.

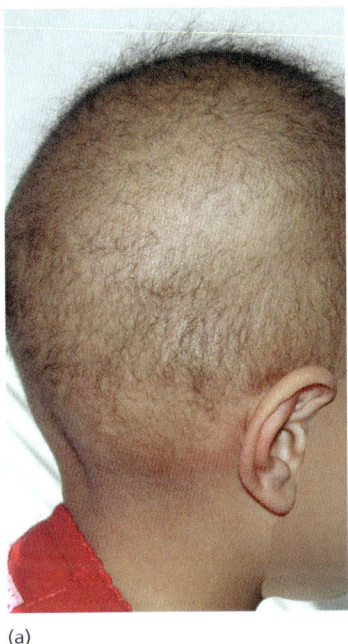

(a)

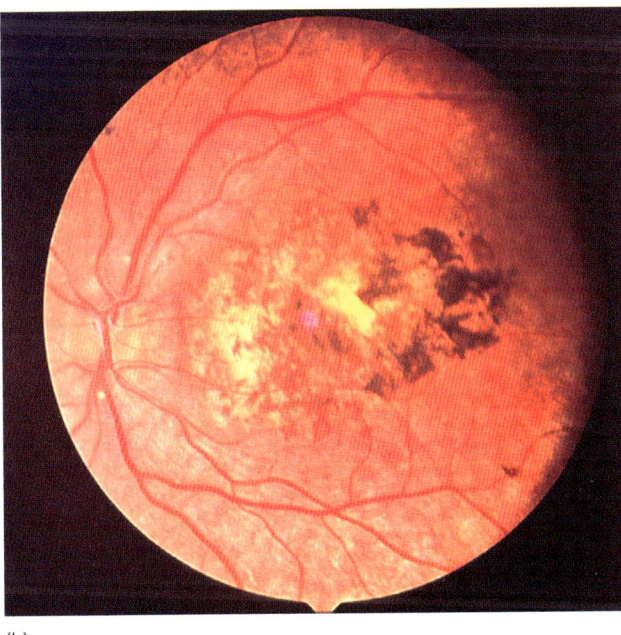

(b)

Figure 66.11 Sparse and short hair on the scalp of a young patient with hypotrichosis and juvenile macular dystrophy (a); fundus examination reveals severe degenerative pigmentary changes in the retinal macula (b).

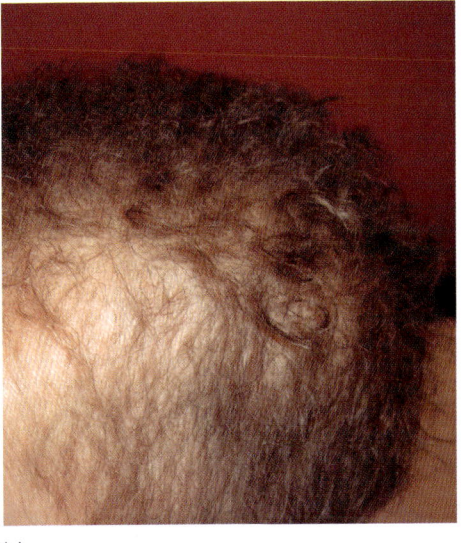

(a)

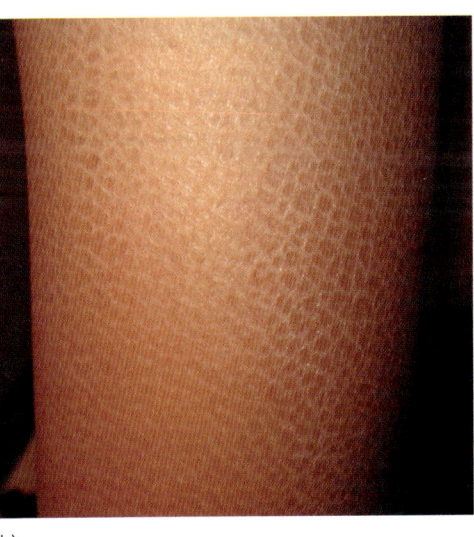

(b)

Figure 66.12 Hypotrichosis (a) and lamellar ichthyosis (b) in a patient with autosomal recessive ichthyosis with hypotrichosis.

Table 66.3). This group of hair disorders is reviewed in detail in Chapter 87.

needed to establish the diagnosis. More recently, dermoscopy has been recognised as a useful and cost-efficient adjunct technique for the rapid diagnosis of hair shaft abnormalities [122].

As a group, hair shaft disorders largely overlap at the clinical and molecular level with hypotrichoses because hair shaft anomalies often (but not always) result in hypotrichosis [92]. As with other genotrichoses, the first step in the diagnosis of hair shaft structural disorders is to determine whether the hair disease is isolated or is part of a more complex disorder. The following sections review those hair shaft disorders inherited as monogenic traits (see

Monilethrix

Clinical features
Beaded hair is the hallmark of monilethrix. Scalp hair is fragile at constricted sites leading to apparent hypotrichosis [91,121] (Figure 66.13). Gradual improvement with age is the rule, with hair looking sometimes normal by puberty or early adulthood. Improvement has also been noted during pregnancy and summertime. Body hair as well as eyelashes and eyebrows are less frequently involved. Intrafamilial phenotypic variability is common [123]. Associated features include follicular papules in the nape area as well as keratosis pilaris and nail dystrophy [91,121].

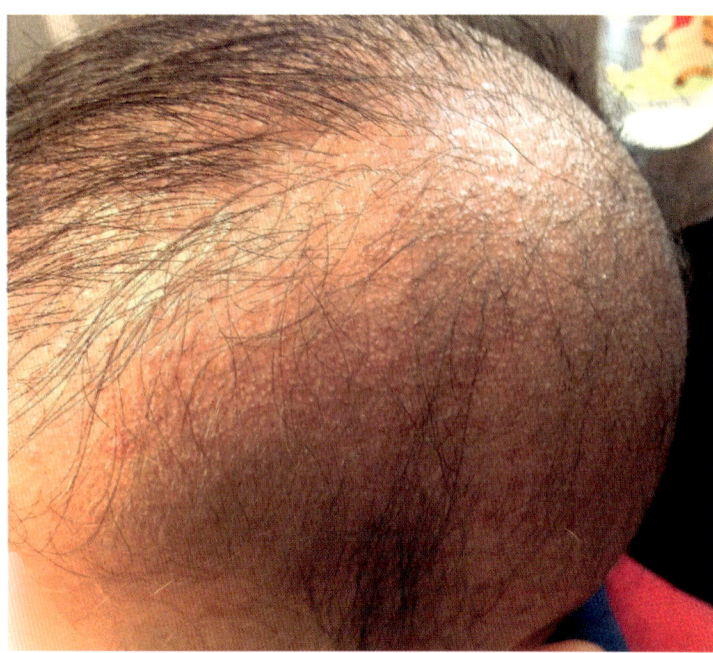

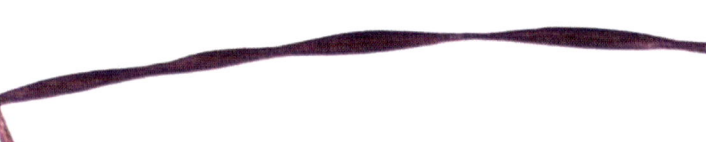

Figure 66.13 Short and sparse hair associated with follicular papules a patient with monilethrix; hair beading typical of monilethrix on microscopy.

Pathogenesis

Monilethrix is usually transmitted in an autosomal dominant fashion and is due to mutations in genes encoding several hair keratins (*KRT81*, *KRT83*, *KRT86*) [124–126]. Recessive inheritance of mutations in the *DSG4* gene encoding desmoglein 4 have been reported in localised autosomal recessive hypotrichosis which is characterised by monilethrix-like hairs, fragile scalp and body hairs that break easily, and are associated with hyperkeratotic follicular papules [127]. Monilethrix has been observed in syndromic forms of hypotrichosis such as Menkes disease [128].

Differential diagnosis

Monilethrix must be distinguished from pili torti in which hair shaft twisting can generate the false impression of beading [121]. Pseudo-monilethrix refers to a poorly defined form of hypotrichosis due to fragile and easily breakable hair shafts. On electron microscopy, irregular nodes represent the edges of depressions within the shafts; in other cases, the beaded appearance of the hair shafts reflects irregular twisting without flattening of the hair shafts as in pili torti; finally, pseudomonilethrix can result from breaks within the shafts. Although autosomal inheritance of pseudomonilethrix has been described, many authorities considered it as an artefactual finding due to trauma to the hair shafts [129].

Treatment

Monilethrix has been successfully treated in uncontrolled studies with minoxidil [130,131] and with oral retinoids [132–134].

Woolly hair

Clinical features

Woolly hair refers to generalised or localised occurrence of curly hair, which usually demonstrates slow growth and/or easy breakage, sometimes associated with hypopigmentation (Figure 66.14). The disorder can appear as an isolated dominant trait, and in this case can be allelic to autosomal recessive localised hypotrichosis [92], but has also been reported in the context of various cardiocutaneous disorders [135].

Patients with woolly hair may in some cases be affected with Noonan syndrome, especially in combination with ulerythema ophryogenes [136]. These patients tend to display a short stature, ptosis, borderline intelligence, a webbed neck and pulmonic stenosis.

Pathogenesis

Isolated autosomal recessive woolly hair has been shown to be allelic to autosomal recessive localised hypotrichosis (see Non-syndromic autosomal recessive hypotrichoses) caused by mutations in *LPAR6* and *LIPH* [91,95]. Autosomal recessive woolly hair has been shown to result from mutations in *KRT25*, encoding keratin 25 [137,138]. Autosomal dominant inheritance has also been described and linked to mutations in two hair keratin genes, *KRT71* and *KRT74* [139,140].

Woolly hair has been described in the context of complex syndromes. Naxos disease and Carvajal syndrome manifest with woolly hair, hypotrichosis, diffuse palmoplantar keratoderma and cardiac disease, and are caused by recessive mutations in *JUP* and *DSP*, respectively, which encode two desmosomal proteins, plakoglobin and desmoplakin [141,142]. In fact, pathogenic variants in different desmosomal proteins have been found to be associated with hypotrichosis and woolly hair [143].

Pili torti

Clinical features

Pili torti refers to hair showing 180 degree twists under the microscope [121] (Figure 66.15b). Patients with pili torti usually display breakable, short and sparse hair over the scalp (Figure 66.15a) and body. Isolated pili torti can be congenital but often becomes apparent in childhood only, with spontaneous improvement with time.

Pathogenesis

Pili torti can be inherited in an autosomal dominant fashion. The molecular cause for isolated pili torti remains elusive.

Differential diagnosis

Pili torti has been reported in the context of complex syndromes. Pili torti is typically found in Menkes disease (Chapter 61), an X-linked metabolic disorder usually fatal in early life [144]. Menkes disease is characterised by paucity of hair that is fine, wiry, fragile and silver or white. Phenotypic variability is the rule. Hair microscopy usually

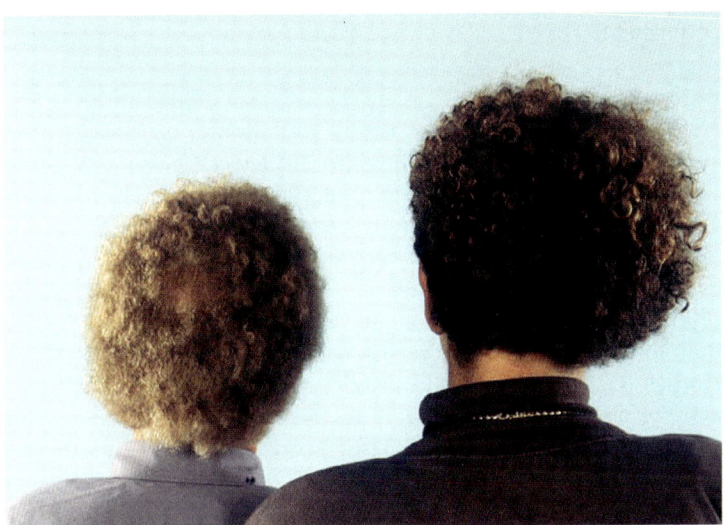

Figure 66.14 Woolly hair in a white woman and her son. Courtesy of Professor Rudolf Happle.

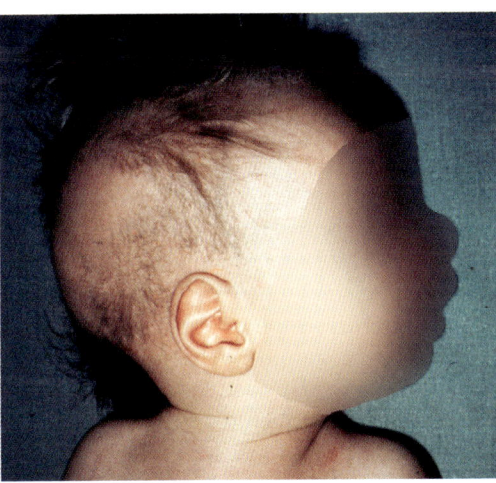

(a)

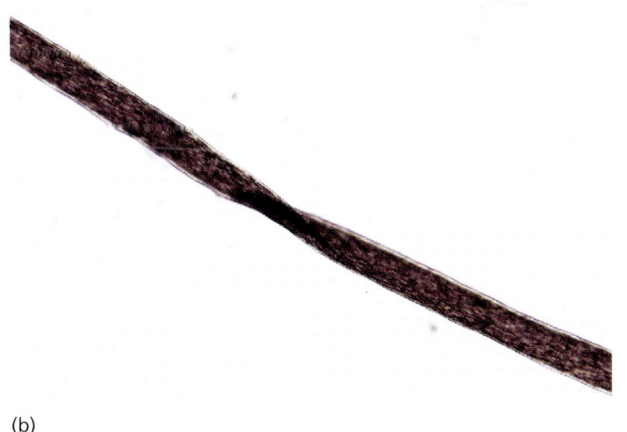

(b)

Figure 66.15 (a) Pale and sparse hair in a child with Menkes disease. Courtesy of Professor Rudolf Happle. (b) Hair twisting along its axis, typical of pili torti. Courtesy of Professor Reuven Bergman.

reveals pili torti as well as monilethrix and trichorrhexis nodosa. The skin can show a mottled discoloration and is often lax. The upper lip has an exaggerated 'cupid bow' configuration. Of interest, asymptomatic female carriers can display foci of pili torti and uneven skin pigmentation along the Blaschko lines. Systemic manifestations include early onset of neurological signs including hypotonia, seizures, psychomotor retardation as well as periodic hypothermia. Tortuous vessels in the central nervous system can be seen on magnetic resonance angiogram (MRA) and are characterised on histology by fragmentation of the internal elastic lamina. Osteoporosis, skeletal dysplasia and dental and ocular anomalies are also observed [145]. The disorder is caused by mutations in the *ATP7A* gene [146,147] which encodes a trans-Golgi membrane bound copper transporter. Accordingly, serum copper and ceruloplasmin levels are low. As a result, numerous copper-dependent enzyme activities are lost. Among the enzymes most prominently affected are tyrosinase, lysyl oxidase, mono-amine oxidase, cytochrome oxidase and ascorbate oxidase, which explain the pigment defects, lax skin, hair abnormalities, hypothermic episodes and skeletal changes typically found in patients, respectively. Occipital horn disease is allelic to Menkes disease and manifests with more severe skin changes, less prominent neurological manifestations and the presence of exostoses on the occiput (hence the name of the syndrome) and other bones [148].

Björnstad syndrome features a combination of pili torti and progressive sensorineural hearing loss [149]. The syndrome is caused by mutations in the *BCS1L* gene, which plays an important role in mitochondrial function [150]. Pili torti has also been seen in Netherton syndrome [151] (see later), hypotrichosis with juvenile macular dystrophy (see earlier) [112], Bazex syndrome [152], citrullinaemia [153], pachyonychia congenita [154], Clouston syndrome [155], hephaestin like-1 deficiency [156] and autosomal recessive ichthyosis with hypotrichosis [117] (see earlier).

In addition to the inherited conditions mentioned previously, pili torti has been described in association with systemic acquired diseases such as lupus erythematosus and other forms of cicatricial alopecia [157].

Trichorrhexis nodosa

Clinical features

Trichorrhexis nodosa is diagnosed under the microscope as irregularly spaced swellings along the hair shaft which appear to be the consequence of cuticle loss and exposure of cortical fibres. These areas are prone to fracture. Trichorrhexis nodosa has seldom been described as an isolated finding. It rather accompanies conditions manifesting with hair fragility, inherited and acquired alike [158–161].

Pathogenesis

No single gene has been associated with isolated trichorrhexis nodosa. Trichorrhexis nodosa has been described in the context of Netherton syndrome [151] (Chapter 63), Menkes syndrome [128] (Chapter 79) and trichothiodystrophy [162]. It is also typically found

PART 6: GENETIC DISORDERS

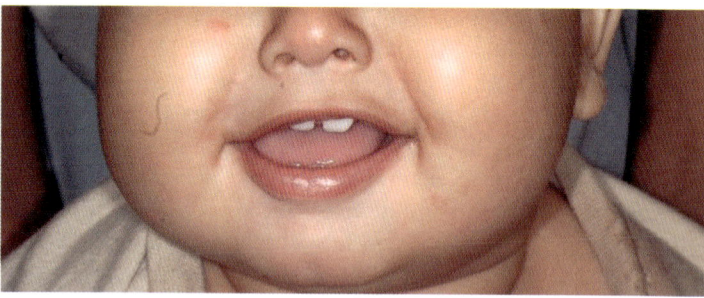

(a)

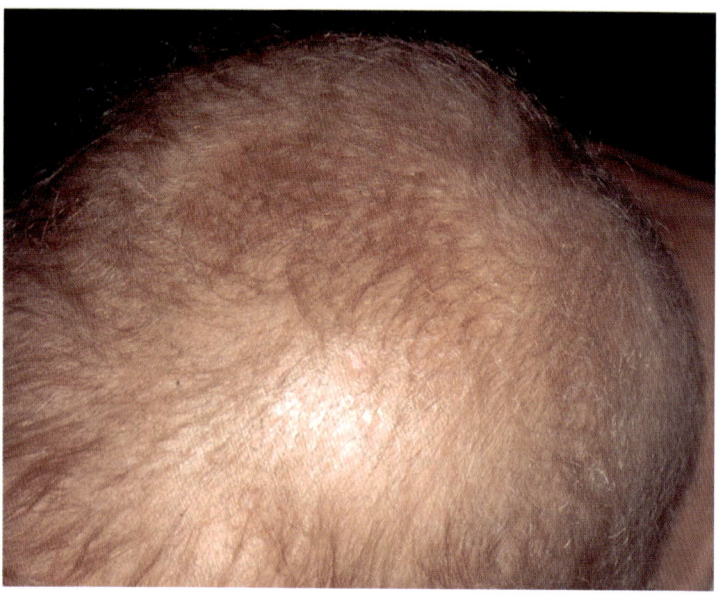

(b)

Figure 66.16 Typical cutaneous features of the trichohepatoenteric syndrome including puffy cheeks (a) and hypotrichosis (b).

in argininosuccinic aciduria [160] also featuring failure to thrive, liver disease and neurological manifestations and caused by mutations in *ASL* encoding argininosuccinate lyase [163]. Trichorrhexis nodosa has also been observed in association with hypotrichosis as part of the trichohepatoenteric (THE) syndrome, which features intractable diarrhoea and is caused by mutations in two regulatory genes, *TTC37* and *SKIV2L* [164,165] (Figure 66.16).

Trichorrhexis invaginata

Clinical features

Hair is sparse, short, very thin and shows under the microscope the typical ball and socket ('bamboo hair') appearance in which the distal part of the hair shaft is compressed against the dilated and cupped proximal shaft. Trichorrhexis invaginata is considered as a hallmark of Netherton syndrome [166] (Chapter 63) although it can be seen in other ichthyosiform disorders as well [167]. Trichorrhexis invaginata is often seen only after the first year of life. Examination

of the eyebrows is recommended to demonstrate the hair shaft abnormality [168].

Pathogenesis

Netherton syndrome is caused by mutations in *SPINK5*, which encodes a serine protease inhibitor called LEKTI [169]. LEKTI deficiency causes increased degradation of corneodesmosin and desmoglein 1 [170]; interestingly, corneodesmosin deficiency does not cause hair anomalies [84] and although defective desmoglein 1 has been linked to hypotrichosis in the context of severe dermatitis, multiple allergies and metabolic wasting (SAM syndrome) [171], hair microscopy did not reveal trichorrhexis invaginata. Mouse studies suggest that LEKTI physiologically inhibits kallikrein 14 activity; since kallikrein 14 degrades desmoglein 4 which is essential for hair shaft formation, LEKTI deficiency may lead to hair shaft abnormalities in Netherton syndrome due to kallikrein 14 increased activity [172].

Trichothiodystrophy

Clinical features

Trichothiodystrophy refers to a strikingly heterogeneous group of disorders, all sharing in common brittle and fragile hair, which demonstrates on polarised hair microscopy a typical 'tiger tail banding' pattern [162,173]. Various hair shaft defects such as pili torti and trichorrhexis nodosa have also been described. Hypotrichosis involves typically the scalp (Figure 66.17), eyebrows and eyelashes, but can also sometimes affect other areas. Nails demonstrate a wide range of dystrophic changes. Other clinical features include short stature, progeroid facies with loss of adipose tissue, microcephaly, various ocular manifestations including cataracts and microcornea, joint contractures and asthma [174]. The disorder has been reported in association with a number of clinical manifestations which demarcate distinct subsets including mental disability and dental caries reported in Sabinas syndrome (MIM: 211390), infertility, developmental delay found in hair–brain syndrome (MIM: 234050), ichthyosis featured in Tay syndrome (MIM: 242170), photosensitivity seen in *P*hotosensitivity *I*chthyosis, *B*rittle hair, *I*ntellectual impairment, *D*ecreased fertility and *S*hort stature (PIBIDS) syndrome (MIM: 278720) and immune defects (MIM: 258360) (Table 66.4).

Pathogenesis

The hair defect results from a decrease in high sulphur protein contents in the hair shaft, which are a major component of the hair cuticle. The disorder has been found to be caused by mutations in a number of genes. Mutations in *C7ORF11* (*MPLKIP*), encoding a protein whose function is poorly understood, cause non-photosensitive trichothiodystrophy [175]. Mutations in a number of genes encoding elements of the transcription factor complex, TTFIH [176], and involved in nucleotide excision repair cause photosensitive trichothiodystrophy including *ERCC3*, *ERCC2* and *GTF2H5* [177–179].

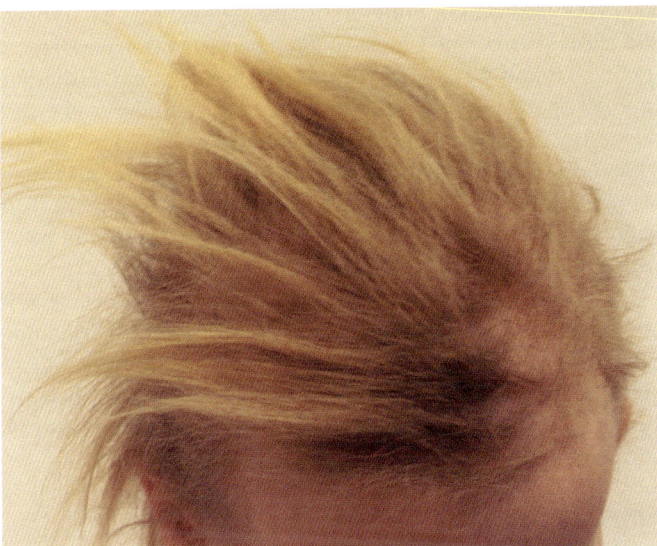

(a)

Table 66.4 Trichothiodystrophy variants.

Type	Clinical features	Syndrome eponym
A	Hair ± nails	–
B	Hair ± nails + intellectual disability	Sabinas
C	Hair ± nails + intellectual disability, folliculitis, retarded bone age + caries	Pollitt
D	(Brittle) hair ± nails + infertility, developmental delay, short stature	BIDS
E	Ichthyosis + BIDS + intellectual disability ± decreased gonadal function + cataracts + progeroid appearance + microcephaly ± ataxia ± basal ganglia calcifications	Tay/IBIDS
F	Photosensitivity and IBIDS	PIBIDS
G	Hair ± intellectual disability + immune defects	Itin
H	Trichothiodystrophy with severe intrauterine growth retardation, developmental delay, recurrent infections, cataracts, hepatic angioendotheliomas	–

PIBIDS, photosensitivity ichthyosis, brittle hair, intellectual impairment, decreased fertility and short stature.

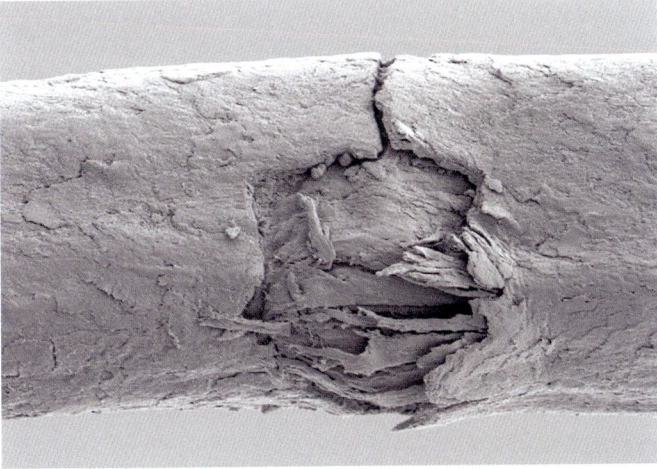

(b)

Pili triangulati et canaliculi

Clinical features

Isolated pili triangulati et canaliculi cause the uncombable hair syndrome [180]. This structural hair defect usually becomes apparent in early childhood as dry, coarse, frizzy and light hairs which stand straight up from the scalp and cannot be combed (Figure 66.18). Microscopic examination of pulled hair can be misleading as the triangular cross-sectional appearance (at the origin of the name of the hair shaft defect) and the typical longitudinal grooves, which confer to the hair its rigidity, are visible only on transverse section (or on scanning electron microscopy) [181].

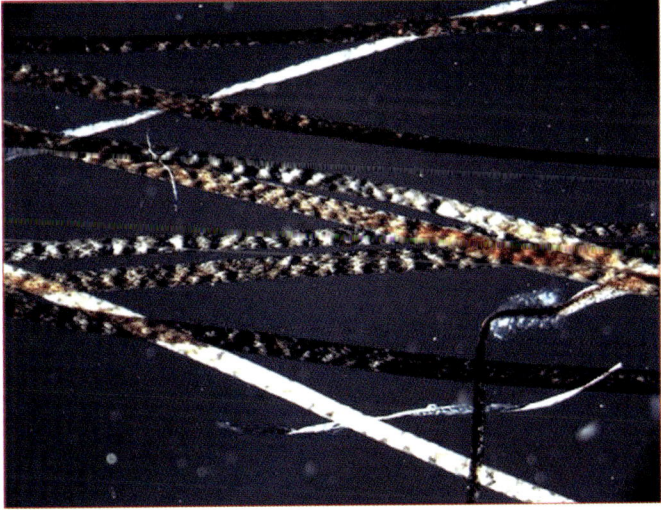

(c)

Figure 66.17 (a) Light-coloured and coarse hair in a patient with trichothiodystrophy. Courtesy of Professor Peter Itin. (b) Defective cuticle visualised by scanning electron microscopy. Courtesy of Professor Peter Itin. (c) Tiger tail banding under polarising light microscopy. Courtesy of Professor Reuven Bergman.

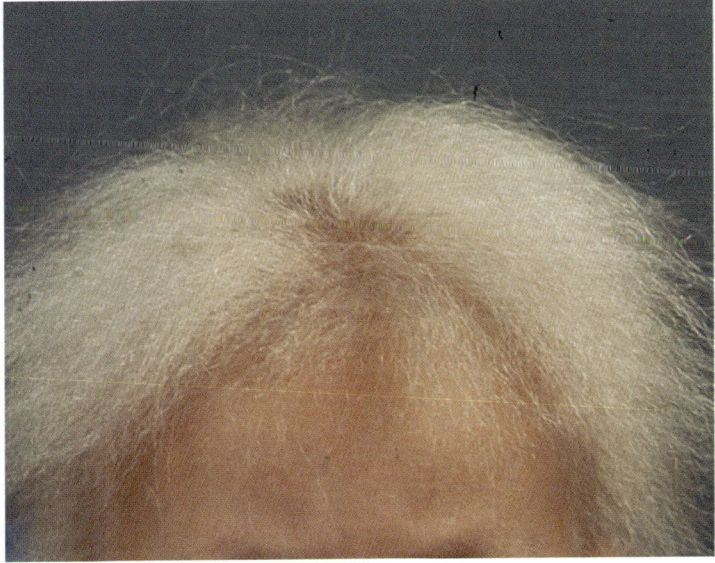

Figure 66.18 Uncombable hair syndrome. Courtesy of Professor Peter Itin.

PART 6: GENETIC DISORDERS

Pathogenesis

The uncombable hair syndrome can occur sporadically or be transmitted as an autosomal trait [182]. It has been shown to be caused by mutations in three genes: *PADI3* encoding peptidylarginine deiminase 3, *TGM3* encoding transglutaminase 3 and *TCHH* encoding trichohyalin [183]. The peptidylarginine deiminase 3 and transglutaminase 3 enzymes mediate post-translational modification of trichohyalin, which is a critical component of the hair shaft [183]. Of great interest, mutations in *PADI3* also explain the propensity of a large proportion of women of African origin to develop central centrifugal cicatricial alopecia [184] (Chapter 87).

Other inherited hair shaft defects

Pili annulati and pseudoannulati

Pili annulati reflects the presence of air-filled cavities within the hair shaft, which results in alternating dark and light bands under the microscope [185,186]. The disorder has been shown to be inherited as an autosomal dominant trait [187]. Pili pseudoannulati results from reflection of the light over flattened or twisted surfaces of the hair shaft and is considered as a normal variant.

Loose anagen syndrome

This disorder starts in early childhood and features hair which is easily pulled away from the scalp. The disease is thought to result from poor adhesion between the cuticle and the inner root sheath. Autosomal dominant inheritance has been suggested. Patients often seek medical advice because of slow-growing hair and ensuing patchy alopecia. Hair can be short, sparse, unruly and is often light coloured. Increased shedding is noted [188] (Figure 66.19). Improvement over time is the rule. A diagnosis of loose anagen hair syndrome is based on the presence of 70% or more loose anagen hairs on a standard trichogram [189].

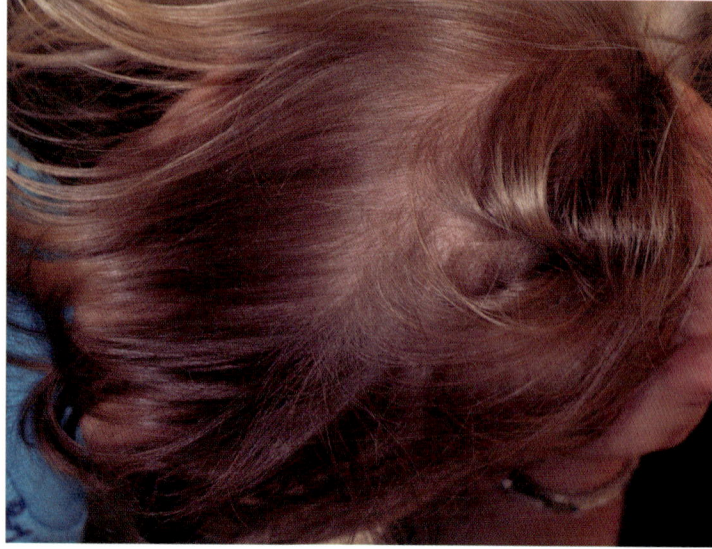

Figure 66.19 Loose anagen syndrome. Courtesy of Professor Peter Itin.

Because symptoms are often mild, the disease may be underdiagnosed. However, because loose anagen hair can often be seen in normal children and adults, the disorder may also be overdiagnosed. A report suggesting that a keratin defect may underlie the disease [190] has not been subsequently replicated. Loose anagen syndrome has been reported in association with pili triangulati and canaliculi as well as with a Noonan-like phenotype [191]. Treatment of loose anagen syndrome with topical or low-dose oral minoxidil has been reported to be beneficial [192].

Loose anagen syndrome should be distinguished from the short anagen syndrome [193] which is characterised by the inability to grow long hair because of an idiopathic short anagen phase. In contrast with loose anagen syndrome, it is not associated with hair unruliness, systemic diseases or skin disorders. Here too, some improvement is typical after puberty.

Kinky hair

Neonatal kinky hair is typical of the trichodento-osseous syndrome, caused by mutations in the *DLX3* gene [194,195]. The disorder is also associated with dysplastic nails, abnormal teeth and skeletal abnormalities including increased bone density and dolichocephaly due to premature fusion of the cranial sutures. Kinky hair is also found in Menkes disease, giant axonal neuropathy 1, Noonan syndrome and oculodentodigital dysplasia [196,197].

Spiky hair

Spiky hair is a hallmark of the athyroidal hypothyroidism with spiky hair and cleft palate (Bamforth–Lazarus) syndrome, which also features choanal atresia and bifid epiglottis [198]. The disorder is transmitted in an autosomal recessive fashion and is caused by mutations in the *FOXE1* gene [199], which is a downstream target of the Sonic hedgehog signalling pathway during hair follicle morphogenesis [200].

OVERALL APPROACH TO THE DIAGNOSIS OF GENOTRICHOSES

The most important step in the diagnosis of this group of disorders is to differentiate them from acquired diseases. Family history, neonatal or early onset, and associated clinical features can favour Mendelian inheritance although they cannot rule out an acquired form of hypertrichosis or alopecia. For example, the diagnosis of alopecia universalis congenita may require a skin biopsy because it is often difficult to distinguish this disorder from autoimmune alopecia areata.

Once it is clear that a patient is affected by an inherited form of hypertrichosis (see Table 66.1), atrichia (see Table 66.2) or hypotrichosis (see Table 66.3), it is important in order to make a diagnosis to establish (i) the mode of inheritance; (ii) the absence (see Tables 66.1A, 66.2A and 66.3A) or presence (see Tables 66.1B, 66.2B and 66.3B) of extracutaneous manifestations; and (iii) the absence or presence of microscopic structural hair shaft abnormalities [3]. Although evidence-based treatment options are mostly non-existent at this stage for most genotrichoses, a correct diagnosis may suggest the need for systemic work-up (see Tables 66.1B, 66.2B and 66.3B) and is essential to direct the subsequent molecular analysis appropriately, which in turn will set the stage for proper genetic counselling and prenatal diagnosis, when indicated.

Key references

The full list of references can be found in the online version at https://www.wiley.com/rooksdermatology10e

3 Betz RC, Cabral RM, Christiano AM *et al.* Unveiling the roots of monogenic geno-dermatoses: genotrichoses as a paradigm. *J Invest Dermatol* 2012;132:906–14.

6 Paus R, Cotsarelis G. The biology of hair follicles. *N Engl J Med* 1999;341:491–7.

46 Thompson CC, Sisk JM, Beaudoin GM 3rd. Hairless and Wnt signaling: allies in epithelial stem cell differentiation. *Cell Cycle* 2006;5:1913–17.

56 Parren LJ, Frank J. Hereditary tumour syndromes featuring basal cell carcinomas. *Br J Dermatol* 2011;165:30–4.

81 Myung PS, Takeo M, Ito M *et al.* Epithelial Wnt ligand secretion is required for adult hair follicle growth and regeneration. *J Invest Dermatol* 2013;133:31–41.

89 Sprecher E. Genetic hair and nail disorders. *Clin Dermatol* 2005;23:47–55.

92 Shimomura Y. Congenital hair loss disorders: rare, but not too rare. *J Dermatol* 2012;39:3–10.

106 Lai-Cheong JE, Arita K, McGrath JA. Genetic diseases of junctions. *J Invest Dermatol* 2007;127:2713–25.

170 Hovnanian A. Netherton syndrome: skin inflammation and allergy by loss of protease inhibition. *Cell Tissue Res* 2013;351:289–300.

174 Itin PH, Sarasin A, Pittelkow MR. Trichothiodystrophy: update on the sulfur-deficient brittle hair syndromes. *J Am Acad Dermatol* 2001;44:891–920;quiz 1–4.

CHAPTER 67

Genetic Defects of Nails and Nail Growth

Samantha Gordon and Amy S. Paller

Departments of Dermatology and Pediatrics, Northwestern University, Chicago, IL, USA

Introduction

Nail changes are a component of many genodermatoses, especially the ectodermal dysplasias. Included in this chapter are the more common hereditary nail disorders that are not described in detail elsewhere and have distinctive manifestations. A comprehensive list of additional non-syndromic and syndromic genodermatoses with nail abnormalities and their features is given in Table 67.1.

Pachyonychia congenita

Definition and nomenclature

Pachyonychia congenita (PC) is a group of disorders caused by dominant mutations in one of five genes encoding nail keratins. The clinical features seen in virtually all affected patients are toenail thickening and plantar keratoderma, often associated with plantar pain (Table 67.2). Despite the name of the disorder (pachy = large, onyx = nail), about 4% of PC patients lack nail involvement and plantar foot pain is the most problematic issue for most patients.

PC was originally classified into two subtypes based on clinical features, the Jadassohn–Lewandowsky type (PC type 1; MIM: 167200) and the Jackson–Lawler type (PC type 2; MIM: 167210). Based on genotype–phenotype analyses of more than 250 patients showing that correlations of clinical features with underlying genotype were not absolute, this old terminology has been abandoned [1]. The new classification is based on genotype, with defects in one of five different genes encoding keratins underlying the disorder (*KRT6A*, *KRT6B*, *KRT6C*, *KRT16* and *KRT17*). The new designations are PC-K6a, PC-K6b, PC-K6c, PC-K16 and PC-K17 [2].

Synonyms and inclusions
- Congenital pachyonychia
- Pachyonychia congenita syndrome
- Pachyonychia ichthyosiformis

Introduction

PC is a group of disorders marked by nail dystrophy, painful focal palmoplantar keratoderma, mucosal leukokeratosis, cysts, follicular keratoses and, less commonly, natal teeth. This group of disorders is typically autosomal dominant in inheritance, although biallelic (autosomal recessive) cases have been described. Features of PC are generally present by 3 years of age.

Epidemiology

Approximately 5000–10 000 affected individuals have been described globally, with a prevalence of 0.9 cases per million [2].

Pathophysiology

The keratins affected in individuals with PC (*KRT6A*, *KRT6B*, *KRT6C*, *KRT16* and *KRT17*) are expressed in the nail bed, palmoplantar epidermis, mucosae and follicular upper outer root sheath [2]. Because keratins provide structural integrity to epithelial structures, mutations in the genes encoding keratins cause cell fragility and compensatory hyperkeratosis [3]. The severity of nail changes may be mutation dependent. For example, individuals with PC-K16 and p.Leu132Pro mutations have dystrophy of all fingernails, whereas those with p.Asn125Ser or p.Arg127Cys mutations in the same gene generally have no fingernail changes [1].

Studies in *Krt16* null mice have shown early defects in terminal differentiation, with reduction in *Krt9* expression and increases in expression of compensatory differentiation markers [4], which in humans with a missense mutation in *KRT6/16* correlates with reduction of *KRT9* but increases in the mutant *KRT6/16*. *Krt16* null mice also show increased oxidative stress responses within palmoplantar lesions, with decreased antioxidant glutathione and glutathione synthesis genes, attenuated Keap1-Nrf2 signalling (regulate cellular antioxidant responses), and misregulation of Danger Associated Molecular Patterns (DAMPS) [4,5].

Clinical features

Although the nail dystrophy can cause embarrassment, the often exquisitely *painful plantar keratoderma* exerts the greatest functional

---

Rook's Textbook of Dermatology, Tenth Edition. Edited by Christopher Griffiths, Jonathan Barker, Tanya Bleiker, Walayat Hussain and Rosalind Simpson.
© 2024 John Wiley & Sons Ltd. Published 2024 by John Wiley & Sons Ltd.

Table 67.1 Key genetic syndromes with nail manifestations and known underlying genetic basis.

Name (alternative names)	MIM number/ primary ref.	Inheritance	Gene mutation	Nails	Phenotypic characteristics Other
Syndromic genodermatoses with nail anomalies					
Acro-dermato-ungual-lacrimal-tooth syndrome (adult syndrome) [1]	103285	AD	TP63	Finger and toenail dysplasia	Intensive freckling, hypodontia, frontal alopecia; lacrimal duct atresia; ectrodactyly, syndactyly; hypoplastic breasts and nipples
Adams–Oliver syndrome [2–4]	614814 100300 614219 615297	AD	RBPJ2 EOGT DOCK6 ARHGAP31	Nail aplasia	Cutis aplasia, syndactyly, microcephaly, short palpebral fissures, short distal phalanges, absent toes, asymmetric shortening of the hands, asymmetric reductions of the feet, intellectual deficits
Anaemia, dyserythropoietic congenital, type I [5]	224120	AR	CDAN1 (codanin 1)	Nail hypoplasia or anonychia	Brown pigmentation of skin; absence of distal phalanges, syndactyly (esp. of toes); neurological deficits; macrocytic anaemia with absolute or relative reticulocytopenia
Ankyloblepharon-ectodermal defects–cleft lip and palate (AEC) syndrome (which includes Rapp–Hodgkin syndrome) [6,7]	106260	AD	TP63	Severe dystrophy	Dry and smooth skin; palmoplantar hyperkeratosis with obliteration of dermatoglyphic patterns; occasional reticulate hyperpigmentation; supernumerary nipples, severe recurrent scalp pustulation and erosion; hypotrichosis, coarse, wiry hair; poorly formed and pointed teeth, severe hypodontia; ankyloblepharon filiforme adnatum with partial fusion of eyelids at birth; broad nasal bridge; hypoplastic maxilla; ear canal atresia; cleft lip/palate; lacrimal duct atresia; photophobia
Autoimmune polyendocrinopathy, candidiasis, ectodermal dystrophy (APECED) syndrome; autoimmune polyendocrinopathy syndrome, type I [8]	240300	AR	AIRE	Thickened and dystrophic	Chronic mucocutaneous candidiasis; primary adrenal insufficiency; autoimmune endocrinopathies (hypoparathyroidism, hypergonadotropic hypogonadism, insulin-dependent diabetes, autoimmune thyroid diseases and pituitary defects); autoimmune or immune-mediated gastrointestinal diseases (chronic atrophic gastritis, pernicious anaemia and malabsorption); chronic active hepatitis; autoimmune skin diseases (vitiligo and alopecia); squamous cell carcinoma of oral mucosa and oesophagus; keratoconjunctivitis; immunological defects (cellular and humoral); asplenia and cholelithiasis
Brachydactyly, type b1 [9,10]	113000	AD	ROR2 (receptor tyrosine kinase-like orphan receptor 2)	Nail hypoplasia/aplasia	Hypoplastic or absent distal phalanges of digits 2–5; fusion of middle and distal phalanges; broad or bifid thumb
Cleft lip/palate–ectodermal dysplasia syndrome (CLEPD1) (formerly known as Margarita Island ectodermal dysplasia and Zlotogora–Ogur syndrome) [11]	225060	AR	PVRL1	Dysplastic	Dry or eczematous skin; sparse, brittle and fine hair; teeth dysplasia; hypohidrosis, cleft lip/palate; malar hypoplasia; micrognathia; ear anomalies; syndactyly of fingers and/or toes; intellectual disability in some
Coffin–Siris syndrome (fifth digit syndrome) [12]	135900	AD, most commonly de novo	SMARCB1, SMARCA4, SMARCA2, ARID1A ARID1B	Absent to hypoplastic fifth fingernails and toenails; other nails occasionally hypoplastic or absent	Dermatoglyphic changes; simian crease; sparse scalp hair (esp. temporal regions); hirsutism/hypertrichosis, thick eyebrows, long eyelashes, coarse face with thick everted lips, broad nasal bridge and tip with anteverted nares, retardation of psychomotor and growth development; hypotonia; lax joints; clinodactyly of the fifth fingers; absence of terminal phalanges of fifth fingers and toes; aplasia or variable hypoplasia of middle and proximal phalanges of other fingers and toes; bilateral or unilateral dislocation of the radial heads; small or absent patellae; frequent respiratory infections; umbilical and inguinal hernias; cleft palate; feeding problems in infancy; six lumbar vertebrae; sternal anomalies; microcephaly; patent ductus arteriosus

Disorder	MIM	Inheritance	Gene	Nails	Clinical features
Cranio-ectodermal syndrome (Levin syndrome I; Sensenbrenner syndrome) [13, 14]	218330	AR	IFT122	Broad and short	Cutis laxa; thin, sparse, and slow-growing hair, rhizomelic shortness; dolichocephaly; sagittal craniosynostosis; hypertelorism; frontal bossing; shortening of upper and lower limbs; short and narrow thorax with protuberant abdomen; pectus excavatum, retinal dysfunction; progressive renal disease
Deafness, onychodystrophy, osteodystrophy, intellectual disability and seizures syndrome (DOOR syndrome) [15]	220500	AR	TBC1D24	Anonychia, hypoplastic or rudimentary nails; abnormal colour, structure, shape, or texture of nails	Dermatoglyphic abnormalities (arched pattern), enamel hypoplasia, irregular placement of teeth, congenital sensorineural deafness; apparently low-set ears; antimongoloid eye slant, slight ptosis, long philtrum, highly arched palate; myopia; nystagmus; optic atrophy; cataracts; seizures and intellectual disability; triphalangy of both thumbs and halluces; hypoplasia or aplasia of terminal phalanges of fingers and toes
Dyskeratosis congenita – see text [16, 17]	305000, 127550, 613990, 613989, 224230, 613276, 613937, 613938, 615190, 613589	XR, AD, AR	DKC1, TERC, TINF2, TERT, ACD, C16orf57, NOP10, NHP2, RTEL1, WRAP53, PARN, CTC1	Thin dystrophic nails, late-onset paronychia occasionally leading to anonychia; hypoplasia	**Skin:** reticular skin pigmentation, telangiectatic erythema; acrocyanosis; palmoplantar hyperkeratosis; hyperhidrosis; malignant leukoplakia on lips, mouth, anus, urethra and conjunctiva **Teeth:** poorly aligned, early carious degeneration **Hair:** hypotrichosis; absence of eyebrows and lashes
Ectodermal dysplasia with ectrodactyly and macular dystrophy (EEM syndrome) [18]	225280	AR	CDH3	Dysplastic	Hypotrichosis of scalp hair, eyebrows, and eyelashes, partial anodontia, ectrodactyly; syndactyly (hands > feet); macular dystrophy
Ellis–van Creveld syndrome (chondroectodermal dysplasia, mesoectodermal dysplasia) [19, 20] See Weyer acrofacial dysostosis later	225500	AR	EVC1, EVC2	Hypoplastic, dystrophic, friable (brittle, furrowed and underdeveloped)	Thin, brittle, and hypochromic; absent or scanty eyebrows and lashes, natal teeth; precocious exfoliation; hypodontia; occasional hypoplastic enamel, disproportionate dwarfism; bilateral postaxial polydactyly; brachydactyly, clinodactyly, small phalanges, syndactyly; cardiac anomalies; chest wall changes, pulmonary malformations, hypospadias, cryptorchidism, renal anomalies, haematologic abnormalities, CNS abnormalities, intellectual disability; strabismus, malar hypoplasia, dolichocephaly, prominent nose, low set ears
Epidermolysis bullosa group					
Epidermolysis bullosa dystrophica, autosomal recessive (RDEB) [21]	226600	AR	COL7A1 (collagen, type VII, alpha 1)	Anonychia, dystrophy	Severe scarring blisters, contractures of hands and feet, mitten deformities, abnormal teeth, milia, gastrointestinal strictures
Epidermolysis bullosa dystrophica, autosomal dominant (DDEB) [21]	131750	AD	COL7A1 (collagen, type VII, alpha 1)	Anonychia, dystrophy	Blisters, atrophic scarring, milia, oral blisters, rare oesophageal strictures
Epidermolysis bullosa dystrophica, nails only (DEB-na) [22]		AD, AR	COL7A1 (collagen, type VII, alpha 1)	Dystrophy, majority isolated toenail involvement	No skin fragility or trauma-induced blisters
Epidermolysis bullosa, junctional, generalised intermediate (formerly known as JEB non-Herlitz) [23]	226650	AR	COL17A1 (collagen XVII, alpha-1 polypeptide), LAMA3 (alpha-3 laminin), LAMB3 (beta-3 laminin), LAMC2 (gamma-2 laminin gene), ITGB4 (integrin, beta 4)	Nail dystrophy	Localised blisters that improve with age, dental enamel hypoplasia, scarring alopecia

(continued)

Table 67.1 (continued)

Name (alternative names)	MIM number/primary ref.	Inheritance	Gene mutation	Nails	Phenotypic characteristics — Other
Epidermolysis bullosa, junctional, generalised severe (formerly known as JEB-Herlitz) [23]	226700	AR	LAMA3 (alpha-3 laminin), LAMB3 (beta-3 laminin), LAMC2 (gamma-2 laminin gene), ITGB4 (integrin, beta 4)	Nail dystrophy, paronychial inflammation, granulation tissue of nail beds, nail loss	Blisters that heal without scarring, significant granulation tissue, mucosal involvement (weak hoarse cry), failure to thrive, neonatal sepsis, congenital malformations of urinary tract and bladder, tooth enamel pitting, scarring alopecia
Epidermolysis bullosa simplex, generalised severe (previously known as Dowling–Meara type) [23]	131760	AD	KRT5, KRT14 (keratin 5, keratin 14)	Nail dystrophy, nail shedding, hyperkeratotic nails	Widespread and severe blisters and/or multiple grouped small blisters (herpetiform appearance); progressive palmoplantar hyperkeratosis; oral blisters
Erythrokeratodermia variabilis et progressiva (EKVP) [24]	133200	AD	GJA1 (gap junction protein alpha 1), (connexin 43)	Prominent porcelain-white proximal nails without dystrophy during childhood; nails may be dystrophic in affected adults	**Skin:** symmetric hyperkeratotic hyperpigmented or erythematous plaques with accentuated skin markings and fine scale, some with corrugated scale. Plaques can be stationary, migratory, or transient. Palmoplantar keratoderma
Focal dermal hypoplasia syndrome (Goltz syndrome) [25]	305600	XD	PORCN	Micronychia, V-shaped nicking, longitudinal ridging with splitting, anonychia	**Skin and hair:** absent of skin from various parts at birth; linear hypo- or hyperpigmentation; telangiectasia; herniation of subcutaneous fat; multiple papillomas of mucous membranes and periorificial skin; lipomatous skin changes; follicular hyperkeratotic papules; angiofibromatous nodules around lips and anus; palmoplantar hyperkeratosis; thin wiry hair, patchy alopecia; hypohydrosis **Other:** occasional hearing loss; colobomas; microphthalmia; irregularity of pupils; clouding of cornea or vitreous; blue sclerae; malformed auricles; asymmetry and notching of the alae nasi; pointed chin; triangular face; hypertelorism; intellectual disability; short stature; syndactyly; polydactyly; hypoplasia of the external genitalia; umbilical and/or inguinal hernia; vertebral anomalies (scoliosis, spina bifida, etc.), highly arched palate
Growth retardation, alopecia, pseudoanodontia, optic atrophy (GAPO syndrome) [26]	230740	AR	ANTXR1	Hyperconvexity on fingers and toes (two patients)	**Skin:** dry, redundant; fragile with inadequate wound healing (small, depressed scars); depigmented areas; prominent scalp veins; alopecia; hypotrichosis **Face:** craniofacial dysostosis; wide anterior fontanelle, frontal bossing, micrognathia, protruding ears; protruding and thickened lips; depressed nasal bridge; pseudoanodontia **Other:** sensorineural hypoacusia; optic atrophy; glaucoma; keratoconus; nystagmus; growth retardation; hypoplasia of mammary glands; umbilical hernia
Haim–Munk syndrome [27]	245010	AR	CTSC (cathepsin C)	Onychogryphosis	Congenital palmoplantar keratosis, pes planus, periodontitis, arachnodactyly, acro-osteolysis
Hidrotic ectodermal dysplasia (Clouston syndrome/ECTD2) [28,29]	129500	AD	GJB6 (connexin-30)	Milky white and small in infancy, progressive nail plate thickening with age; hyperconvex nail plates; shortened nails (micronychia), onychorrhexis; triangular nail plates; pincer nails	Wiry, sparse and brittle hair; patchy alopecia; palmoplantar hyperkeratosis; recurrent conjunctivitis and blepharitis; spares teeth and eccrine glands

Disorder	OMIM	Inheritance	Gene	Nails	Clinical features
Hyperphosphatasia with intellectual disability syndrome 2 [30]	614749	AR	Phosphatidylinositol glycan anchor biosynthesis, class O (PIGO)	Nail hypoplasia, especially 2nd, 4th, and 5th digits; absent nails with broad halluces	Facial dysmorphism with wide-set eyes, long palpebral fissures, short nose with broad nasal bridge and tip, tented mouth; moderate to severely delayed psychomotor development; anal stenosis or anal atresia; persistently elevated serum alkaline phosphatase
Hypohidrotic ectodermal dysplasia–X-linked (ED1; Christ–Siemens–Touraine (CST) syndrome) [29,31,32]	305100	XR	EDA (ectodysplasin A)	Usually normal; sometimes dystrophic or absent at birth and/or fragile and brittle with incomplete development	Hypohidrosis, hypotrichosis (thin, lightly pigmented, slow-growing), hair fragility, hypodontia with peg-shape, smooth dry skin (absent eccrine pores), periorbital pigmentation; dry eyes; lack of dermal ridges; absent or supernumerary nipples and areolae, midface hypoplasia and depressed nasal bridge frontal bossing; raspy voice; recurrent pneumonia and asthma-like symptoms
Hypohidrotic ectodermal dysplasia 10A-autosomal dominant [29,31,32]	129490	AD	EDAR (ectodysplasin A receptor)	Usually normal; sometimes hypoplastic	Sparseness of the hair, patchy distribution of sweat dysfunction; few small or missing teeth; underdeveloped nipples
Hypohidrotic ectodermal dysplasia 10B-autosomal recessive [29,31,32]	224900	AR	EDAR (ectodysplasin A receptor)	Usually normal; sometimes hypoplastic	Hypohidrosis, hypotrichosis (thin, lightly pigmented, slow-growing), hair fragility, hypodontia, smooth dry skin, periorbital pigmentation; dry eyes; lack of dermal ridges; absent or supernumerary nipples and areolae, midface hypoplasia and depressed nasal bridge; raspy voice; recurrent pneumonia and asthma-like symptoms
Hypohidrotic ectodermal dysplasia with immunodeficiency [31]	300291	XR	IKBKG/NEMO	Usually normal; sometimes hypoplastic	Hypohidrosis, hypotrichosis, conical incisors; failure to thrive, recurrent infections; dysgammaglobulinaemia
IFAP (ichthyosis follicularis with atrichia and photophobia) syndrome with or without BRESHECK syndrome [33]	308205	XR	MBTPS2 (membrane-bound transcription factor peptidase, site 2)	Dystrophic nails, thick nails	IFAP: ichthyosis follicularis, atrichia and photophobia. BRESHECK: brain anomalies, intellectual disability, ectodermal dysplasia, skeletal deformities, Hirschsprung disease, ear/eye anomalies, cleft palate/cryptorchidism and kidney dysplasia/hypoplasia
Incontinentia pigmenti (familial male-lethal type IP, Bloch–Sulzberger syndrome) [34]	308300	XL	IKBKG (inhibitor of kappa light polypeptide gene enhancer in B cells, kinase gamma)	Dystrophic with ridging and pitting	Vesicular-bullous eruption in the neonatal period followed or accompanied by verrucous lesions, followed by swirling macular hyperpigmentation and linear hypopigmentation; alopecia and/or abnormal hair texture; delayed dentition, conical teeth, and hypodontia, occasional congenital hearing loss; ophthalmological alterations in about one fifth of the patients include blindness, strabismus, cataract, uveitis, retrolental fibroplasias, optic nerve atrophy, microphthalmia; occasional clubfoot, cleft palate, microcephaly; about one third of the cases present severe CNS anomalies: spastic tetraplegia, hemiplegia, diplegia; epilepsy; intellectual disability; occasional short stature
Keratitis, ichthyosis and deafness (KID) syndrome [33]	148210	AD	GJB2	Absent at birth; delayed development; leukonychia (most marked in the fingernails); destructive dystrophy	Ichthyosiform erythroderma with sebaceous dysfunction; furrowing around mouth and chin; erythematous hyperkeratotic plaques on elbows, knees, and the dorsa of hands and feet; marked thickening (leather-like consistency) of palms and soles; increased susceptibility to squamous cell carcinoma; progressive alopecia; congenital sensorineural deafness; keratitis with corneal neovascularisation
Laryngo-onycho-cutaneous syndrome (Shabbir syndrome) [35]	245660	AR	LAMA3 (laminin, alpha 3)	Dystrophic nails, loss of nails	Excessive granulation tissue in the skin and submucosal tissue (larynx, conjunctiva), hoarseness and laryngeal webs, skin ulcers, conjunctival injection and erosions
Limb–mammary syndrome [36]	603543	AD	TP63 (tumour protein p63)	Nail dysplasia	Hand and foot anomalies; hypoplasia/aplasia of the mammary glands and nipples; cleft palate +/–bifid uvula; lacrimal duct atresia

(continued)

5

Table 67.1 (continued)

Name (alternative names)	MIM number/ primary ref.	Inheritance	Gene mutation	Phenotypic characteristics	
				Nails	Other
Multiple self-healing palmoplantar carcinoma (formerly known as corneal intraepithelial dyskeratosis and ectodermal dysplasia) [37]	615225	AD	NLRP1 (family, pyrin domain containing 1)	Dystrophic nails with prominent thickening of nail beds	Recurrent keratoacanthomas on the palms and soles, palmoplantar hyperkeratosis, dyshidrosis, hyperkeratosis pilaris, keratopathy with neovascularisation, corneal opacification with dyskeratosis, maxillary decalcification with tooth loss
Nail-patella syndrome – see text [38,39]	161200		LMX1B (LIM homeobox transcription factor 1, beta)	Triangular lunulae, ulnar nail dystrophy, poorly formed lunulae, anonychia, dystrophic nails	Absent or hypoplastic patellae, elbow abnormalities, iliac horns, nephropathy, glaucoma, Lester sign (flower or clover leaf shape of pigmentation around the central portion of iris)
Odonto-onychodermal dysplasia [40]	257980	AR	WNT10A (wingless-type MMTV integration site family, member 10A)	Dystrophic nails	Palmoplantar keratoderma, hyperhidrosis, erythematous atrophic patches on face; anodontia or hypodontia with peg-shaped incisors, enamel hypoplasia, and widely shaped teeth; dry hair; sparse eyebrows; mild intellectual disability; smooth tongue with reduction in fungiform and filiform papillae
Pachyonychia congenita – see text [41,42]	167200 167210	AD	KRT6A KRT6B KRT6C KRT16 KRT17	Severe wedge-shaped thickening	Focal palmoplantar keratoderma; verrucous lesions on the knees, elbows, buttocks, ankles, and popliteal regions; follicular keratoses/keratosis pilaris, multiple pilosebaceous cysts (steatocystomas); oral leukokeratosis; hoarseness
Pallister–Hall syndrome [43,44]	146510	AD	GLI3	Nail hypoplasia	Hypothalamic hamartoblastoma, pituitary dysfunction, polydactyly, brachydactyly with brachytelephalangy, imperforate anus; bifid epiglottis; dysmorphic facies (small ears, small retroverted nose with flat nasal bridge, small tongue); microphallus; internal organ abnormalities (renal, cardiac, pulmonary); intrauterine growth retardation
Palmoplantar keratoderma, mutilating, with periorificial keratotic plaques (Olmsted syndrome) [45,46]	614594	AD	TRPV3 (Transient receptor potential cation channel, subfamily V, member 3)	Lusterless, ridged and rough nails; leukonychia; irregular curvatures; onycholysis; paronychia; subungual hyperkeratosis; anonychia	Painful and mutilating palmoplantar keratoderma with flexion deformities and autoamputation periorificial hyperkeratosis; alopecia; perifollicular keratosis; leukokeratosis; erythromelalgia
Papillon–Lefèvre syndrome [27]	245000	AR	CTSC	Occasional dystrophy (spoon-shaped and striated; onychogryphosis)	Palmoplantar hyperkeratosis, severe periodontitis; mild intellectual disability; calcification of the dura mater; hyperhidrosis; increased susceptibility to infections
Poikiloderma with neutropenia (Navajo poikiloderma) [47]	604173	AR	USB1 (U6 snRNA biogenesis 1), C16orf57	Pachyonychia	Eczematous rash in infancy followed by postinflammatory poikiloderma; palmoplantar hyperkeratosis; calcinosis cutis; non-healing skin ulcers; non-cyclical neutropenia with recurrent sinopulmonary infections and bronchiectasis; increased risk of myelodysplastic syndrome; short stature, midfacial retrusion; hypogonadotropic hypogonadism
Popliteal pterygium syndrome [48]	119500	AD	IRF6	Pyramidal skinfold overlying the nail of the hallux	Cleft palate/lip, cutaneous syndactyly of fingers and/or toes, popliteal pterygium (eponymous skin fold extending from ischial tuberosities to the heels), genital anomalies (bifid scrotum, cryptorchidism, small labia)
Popliteal pterygium syndrome, lethal type (Bartsocas-Papas syndrome) [49]	263650	AR	RIPK4 (receptor-interacting serine-threonine kinase 4)	Nail dysplasia	Popliteal pterygia, syndactyly of hands and feet, midface hypoplasia, ankyloblepharon, orofacial clefts, filiform bands between jaws, severe growth retardation, death in utero or infancy

Syndrome	OMIM	Gene	Inheritance	Nail features	Other features
Robinow syndrome, autosomal recessive [50]	268310	ROR2 (receptor tyrosine kinase-like orphan receptor 2)	AR	Nail hypoplasia or dystrophy	Short stature, rib and vertebral abnormalities, brachydactyly, hypoplastic genitalia, empty sella, gum hypertrophy, macrocephaly, face with hypertelorism, wide palpebral fissures, depressed nasal bridge with flared nostrils, micrognathia, cleft lip and/or palate
Rothmund–Thomson syndrome [51,52]	268400	RECQL4	AR	Dystrophy or pachyonychia	**Skin:** poikiloderma including hyperpigmentation and hypopigmentation, telangiectasias, and atrophy; palmoplantar hyperkeratosis; sensitivity to sunlight; initial rash is red, elevated with oedematous patches appearing symmetrically on the cheeks, hands, forearms and buttocks **Hair:** sparse, thin or absent hair on scalp, eyebrows and/or eyelashes **Teeth:** microdontia, rudimentary teeth, caries **Other:** bilateral cataracts, corneal and retinal atrophy, blue sclerae; small hands and feet; short terminal phalanges, syndactyly: absence of metacarpals, rudimentary ulna and radius; increased risk of osteosarcoma; short stature; saddle nose, frontal bossing; occasional intellectual disability; sensorineural deafness; pyloric stenosis and anal atresia
Scalp-ear-nipple syndrome [53] (Finlay-Marks syndrome)	181270	KCTD1	AD	Nail dysplasia	Aplasia cutis of scalp; breast abnormalities; anomalies of external ears; cutaneous syndactyly; dental anomalies; renal malformations
Schinzel–Giedion midface-retraction syndrome [54]	269150	SETBP1	AD	Hyperconvex nails with hypoplastic distal phalanges	**Face:** short, upturned nose; prominent forehead; midface hypoplasia; orbital hypertelorism; low-set ears **Other:** developmental delay; seizures; hydronephrosis; skeletal abnormalities (sclerotic skull base, wide occipital synchondrosis, increased cortical density or thickness, broad ribs, wormian bones); cardiac defects; malignant tumours (neuroepithelial)
Schopf–Schulz–Passarge syndrome (cystic eyelids–palmoplantar keratosis–hypodontia–hypotrichosis) [55]	224750	WNT10A (wingless-type MMTV integration site family, member 10A)	AR	Nail fragility, dystrophic nails	Cysts along the eyelid margin (apocrine hidrocystomas); palmoplantar keratosis; hypodontia; hypotrichosis; bilateral early senile cataract; arteriosclerotic fundi; myopia; cysts of eyelids developing late
Sclerosteosis 1 [56]	269500	SOST (sclerostin)	AR	Nail dysplasia	Syndactyly; progressive skeletal overgrowth, square jaw, frontal bossing; facial palsy; increased intracranial pressure
Sclerosteosis 2 [57]	614305	LRP4	AD, AR	Hypoplastic nails, nails separated into two parts	Facial asymmetry, thickening of the skull and long bones; variable syndactyly and brachyphalangy
SOFT syndrome (short stature, onychodysplasia, facial dysmorphism and hypotrichosis) [58]	614813	POC1 centriolar protein A (POC1A)	AR	Hypoplastic fingernails	Short and thick long bones, growth retardation, relative macrocephaly, long, triangular face with prominent nose and small ears, unusual high-pitched voice; postpubertal sparse and short hair; clinodactyly, brachydactyly, hypoplastic distal phalanges
T-cell immunodeficiency, congenital alopecia and nail dystrophy (TIDAND) [59]	601705	FOXN1 (forkhead box N1)	AR	Nail dystrophy: leukonychia, koilonychia, canaliform dystrophy, Beau's lines	Congenital alopecia, severe T-cell immunodeficiency and congenital thymic aplasia
Trichodento-osseous syndrome [60]	190320	DLX3	AD	Nail dystrophy, brittle nails	Curly hair, bone sclerosis, taurodontism ('bull teeth'), amelogenesis imperfecta, mandibular prognathism
Trichorhinophalangeal syndrome types I and III [61,62]	190350 190351	TRPS1	AD	Thin and dystrophic nails (feet > hands)	Pear-shaped nose; long and wide philtrum; thick and broad eyebrows; sparse, depigmented, and slow-growing hair; large, prominent ears; small breasts; short stature; brachydactyly; cone-shaped epiphyses at the phalanges; hip dysplasia/malformations Type III: severe brachydactyly and severe short stature

(continued)

Table 67.1 (continued)

Name (alternative names)	MIM number/primary ref.	Inheritance	Gene mutation	Phenotypic characteristics	
				Nails	Other
Trichorhinophalangeal syndrome type II (Langer–Giedion syndrome) [61]	150230	AD	Contiguous deletion of TRPS1, RAD21 and EXT1 genes	Occasional thin, short, with long longitudinal grooves; flattened, koilonychia-like and normal in colour; racket thumbnails	As above plus multiple osteochondromas; intellectual disability (mild to moderate)
Trichothiodystrophy, photosensitive [63]	601675	AR	ERCC2 (XPD), ERCC3(XPB), or GTF2H5 (TTDA)	Hypoplastic and brittle nails, dysplastic nails	Brittle sulphur-deficient hair (tiger-tail pattern under polarised light); ichthyosis; short stature; intellectual impairment; microcephaly; decreased fertility; osteoporosis; premature ageing; dental caries; proneness to infections
Ulnar-mammary syndrome [64]	181450	AD	TBX3	Duplication of the nail on the ventral 5th digit; absence of digits with radial shortening	Hypoplasia of mammary and apocrine glands, upper limb defects/posterior limb duplications or deficiencies, abnormal dentition, genital abnormalities, delayed puberty in males
Weaver syndrome [65]	277590	Sporadic, AD	EZH2 (enhancer of zeste homolog 2 (Drosophila))	Thin, deep set nails	Generalised overgrowth, advanced bone age, macrocephaly, ocular hypertelorism, deep horizontal chin groove, prominent wide philtrum, microganthia, intellectual disability
Weyers acrofacial dysostosis [66]	193530	AD	EVC2 *Allelic to Ellis-van Creveld syndrome (see previously)	Hypoplastic/dysplastic	Other: mild short stature; postaxial polydactyly; dental anomalies (hypodontia, irregular and small teeth, single central incisor)
Witkop syndrome (tooth and nail syndrome) [67]	189500	AD	MSX1	Koilonychia; longitudinal ridging; easily breakable; toenails more affected than fingernails; nail dysplasia improves with age (may be absent in adults)	Lip eversion, hypodontia, tooth malalignment
Yunis–Varon syndrome [68]	216340	AR	FIG4	Absent/hypoplastic nails, absent thumbs and halluces; hypoplasia or loss of phalanx of other digits	Skeletal abnormalities (wide fontanelles, aplasia or hypoplasia of clavicles, pelvic bone dysplasia); cleidocranial dysplasia, severe neurological involvement with neuronal loss; enlarged vacuoles are present in neurons, muscle, and cartilage; sparse and pale hair
Non-syndromic genodermatoses with nail anomalies					
Candidiasis, familial, 7 (familial chronic mucocutaneous candidiasis, autosomal dominant; immunodeficiency 31C) [69,70]	614162	AD	STAT1 (signal transducer and activator of transcription 1)	Candida onychomycosis causing dystrophy and paronychia	Candida infections of skin and mucous membranes. Variable features: recurrent bacterial, viral, fungal and mycoplasmal infections; disseminated dimorphic fungal infections; enteropathy with villous atrophy; autoimmune disorders; osteopenia; delayed puberty; intracranial aneurysms
Darier disease [71]	124200	AD	ATP2A2	V-shaped notching and alternating white and red longitudinal streaks	Greasy keratotic yellow to brown verrucous papules and plaques in a seborrhoeic distribution, palmoplantar punctuate keratoses, palmoplantar pits; flat-topped acral papules; acrokeratosis verruciformis of Hopf; intraoral cobblestoning of hard palate, buccal mucosa, tongue and gingiva; associated neuropsychiatric disorders
Ectodermal dysplasia 9, hair/nail type [72,73]	614931	AR	HOXC13 (homeobox C 13)	Short fragile nails or koilonychia; all 20 digits	Hypotrichosis starting after birth, ranging from mild hair loss to complete atrichia

Disorder	OMIM	Inheritance	Gene	Nail changes	Associated abnormalities
Ectodermal dysplasia 4, pure hair/nail type [74]	602032	AR	KRT85	Congenital onychodystrophy; micronychia; irregularly shaped and fragile distal ends of nails	Mild absence to complete loss of scalp hair; brittle and fragile hair; diffuse follicular papules on the scalp; absent facial and body hair
Ectodermal dysplasia/skin fragility syndrome (McGrath syndrome) [75]	604536	AR	PKP1 (plakophilin 1)	Thick and dystrophic nails	Skin fragility, alopecia/hypotrichosis, focal palmoplantar keratoderma, hypohidrosis, perioral fissuring/cheilitis, perianal and perineal erosions/fissuring, pruritus, failure to thrive
Hailey–Hailey disease (benign chronic pemphigus) [76]	169600	AD	ATP2C1	Longitudinal leukonychia of fingernails	Flexural erosions, blisters and warty papules
Kindler syndrome [77]	173650	AR	FERMT1 (Fermitin family homolog 1)	Nail dystrophy	Acral blistering in infancy and childhood, progressive poikiloderma, skin atrophy, photosensitivity and gingival fragility
Monilethrix [78]	158000	AD	KRT81, KRT83, KRT86	Koilonychia, brittle nails	Short and fragile hair (normal at birth), keratosis pilaris, occasional syndactyly, cataracts, dental abnormalities
Disorders with changes limited to the nails					
Anonychia congenita (nail disorder, non-syndromic congenital, 4) [79]	206800	AR	R-spondin 4 (RSPO4)	Congenital absence of the nails, involving fingernails and/or toenails	No other associated abnormalities
Hereditary koilonychia (nail disorder, non-syndromic congenital, 2) [80]	149300	AD	NK	Koilonychia/spoon nails – abnormally thin and concave from side to side with the edges turned up	No other confirmed associations
Leukonychia totalis and/or partialis (nail disorder, non-syndromic congenital, 3) [81]	151600	AD and AR	PLCD1	White discoloration of a portion or of the entire nail plate	No other confirmed associations
Partial onycholysis with scleronychia/hereditary distal onycholysis (nail disorder, non-syndromic congenital, 5) [82]	167800	AD	NK	Decreased rate of growth of the nail, scleronychia (thick and hard nails), and a straight or concave proximal edge of detachment	Palmoplantar hyperhidrosis, marked sensitivity of fingers to cold
Twenty nail dystrophy (nail disorder, non-syndromic congenital, 1) [83]	161050	AR	FZD6 (Frizzled family receptor 6)	Excessive longitudinal striations and superficial pits on the nails	No other confirmed associations

AD, autosomal dominant; AR, autosomal recessive; XR, X-linked recessive.

Table 67.2 Clinical features of pachyonychia congenita. From the International PC Research Registry.

Clinical feature	Overall %	PC-K6a %	PC-K6b %	PC-K6c %	PC-K16 %	PC-K17 %
Toenail dystrophy	96	98	97	62	97	95
Fingernail dystrophy	74	97	43	06	57	84
Plantar keratoderma	90	86	97	100	98	80
Plantar pain	94	95	100	91	96	84
Palmar keratoderma	63	67	48	35	71	51
Oral leukokeratoses	52	86	24	26	33	25
Natal teeth	14	05	0	09	01	76
Cysts	51	58	65	24	23	93
Follicular hyperkeratoses	36	48	39	0	10	63

Modified from https://www.pachyonychia.org/pc-data/ Last updated January 2021.

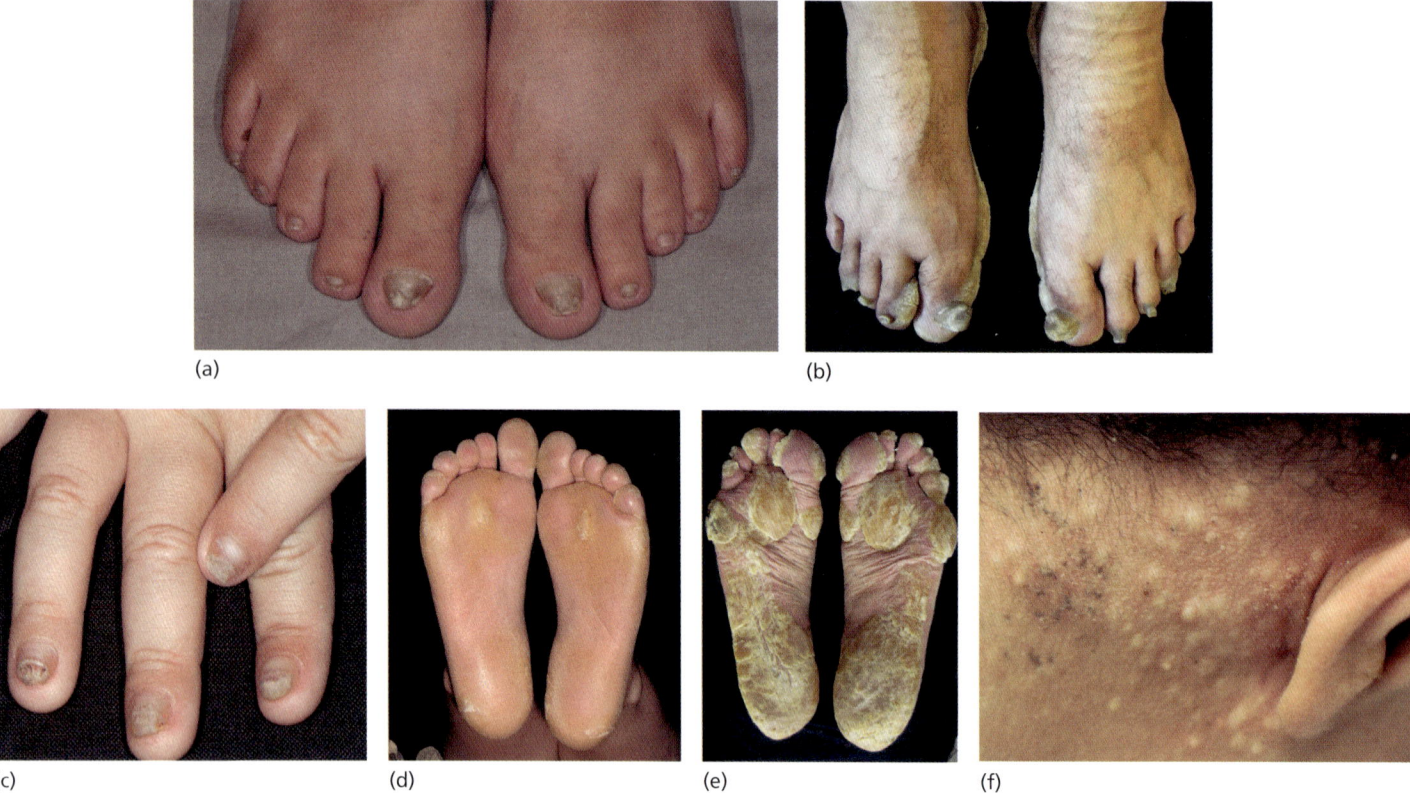

(a)

(b)

(c) (d) (e) (f)

Figure 67.1 Nail dystrophy and plantar keratoderma are the principal features of pachyonychia congenita. (a) Toenails are dystrophic in this patient with PC-K17 (mutation K17 N92S). (b) Severe nail dystrophy and obvious plantar keratoderma in PC-K16 (mutation K16 L132P). (c) Fingernail dystrophy in PC-K6a (mutation K6a N172del). (d) Mild plantar keratoderma in PC-K6a (mutation K6a N171K). (e) Severe plantar keratoderma in PC-K16 (mutation K16 N125D). Parts a–e courtesy of patients in the International Pachyonychia Congenita Research Registry (IPCRR) sponsored by the PC Project. (f) Multiple sebaceous cysts on the neck of a patient with PC.

limitation and effect on quality of life [3] (Figure 67.1d,e). The plantar keratoderma is present at birth in fewer than 10% of patients, but is usually present by 5 years of age in PC-K6a, -K16 and -K17 (the majority of patients), and occurs after 5 years of age in most individuals with milder forms, PC-K6b and -K6c [3]. Thickening tends to be focal and is most prominent at pressure points on the heel and ball of the foot; diffuse plantar involvement has occasionally been described. Secondary skin infection is common [3]. Transgrediens spread (to the dorsal surface of the foot) has also been noted, especially with PC complicated by infection, trauma from standing or shoes, or exposure to foot moisture [6]. Palmar keratoderma occurs in fewer than 60% of patients, most often in PC-K16, and can involve the fingertips [2,3].

Hoarseness and *oral leukokeratoses* typically present in the first year of life, particularly in babies with PC-K6a, leading to misdiagnosis of a variety of airway issues and thrush, respectively. Overall, 53% have oral leukokeratoses, with PC-K6a and PC-K17 having more severe or earlier onset of the oral leukokeratosis. The most commonly affected site is the tongue [3]. *Natal teeth* in PC are virtually always a sign of PC-K17 [2]. Other features are *pilosebaceous cysts* (Figure 67.1f), found in most patients with PC-K6a, -K6b and -K17, and *follicular hyperkeratoses*. Cysts and hyperkeratoses most often develop in school-aged children, but can occur in younger children [3]. *Hyperhidrosis* affects more than 50% of PC patients, particularly in adults.

The nail changes lead to considerable embarrassment, particularly in adolescents, resulting in various strategies to conceal the nails [3]. The keratoderma can impede function, including walking, playing, schoolwork, a variety of other tasks and social development, especially in school-age patients and adults.

Differential diagnosis

Nail trauma in children from shoe friction can lead to changes that resemble PC, but typically affects the fifth toenail without other nail involvement. The genetic disorder most often confused with PC is hidrotic ectodermal dysplasia (Clouston syndrome; MIM: 604418; see Chapter 65), which results from mutations in GJB6, encoding connexin 30. Patients typically show toenail and fingernail alterations at birth and keratoderma that can be indistinguishable from PC. However, the plantar keratoderma is typically not as painful as that seen in PC. Hearing loss, if present, and thin sparse hair during childhood (not a feature of PC unless biallelic keratin gene mutations) are distinguishing features of hidrotic ectodermal dysplasia. Mutations on both alleles of *FZD6*, which encodes frizzled 6, a Wnt-signalling pathway receptor in the nail matrix, similarly lead to hypertrophic nail dystrophy at birth [7,8]. The so-called 'recessive PC' was found to represent a different disorder, PLACK (Peeling skin, Leukonychia, Acral punctate keratoses, Cheilitis, Knuckle pads) syndrome, caused by defective function of calpastatin [9].

Investigations

Genotyping is currently performed at no cost on a research basis for patients registered with the International Pachyonychia Congenita Research Registry (IPCRR) (www.pachyonychia.org, last accessed February 2022).

Management

Mechanical treatment of the nails, such as filing, grinding and cutting, is most effective, particularly after soaking the nails [10]. While antibiotics and antifungal therapy are helpful in managing secondary paronychia, they do not improve the nail dystrophy. Surgical removal of nails can also be performed but results in regrowth unless complete ablation is performed [10]. Mechanical intervention can also ameliorate the keratoderma, but topical agents, such as retinoids, steroids, keratolytics and moisturisers, have had mixed results.

Pain control is critical for the many patients with chronic debilitating plantar pain, especially with weight bearing [11]. While blisters underlying the keratoderma have been shown, there is also evidence through sensory testing that the chronic pain has a neuropathic component, suggesting utility of neuropathic pain medications, such as tricyclic antidepressants, serotonin-norepinephrine reuptake inhibitors, and GABA receptor agonists [5,11]. Botulinum toxin injections using a standardised protocol of 500 U of abobotulinumtoxin A or 200 U of onabotulinumtoxin A, diluted in 5 mL sterile normal saline 0.9% (0.5–1 mL of toxin (50–100 U of abobotulinumtoxin A or 20–40 U of onabotulinumtoxin A) per injection site) have been demonstrated to greatly reduce pain, but only for a period of up to 3 months; nevertheless, subsequent treatments were associated with progressive improvement [12].

Oral retinoids can decrease plantar thickening in 50% of patients, but only decreased plantar pain in about one-third of cases, led to worsening or no improvement in nails in 87% of patients, and caused unacceptable side effects, especially at higher doses (more than 25 mg acitretin daily) [13]. Administration of systemic rapamycin, which suppresses activation of mTOR but also expression of keratin 6a, partially reversed the plantar thickening and pain in PC-K6a during a 12-week trial (without affecting the appearance of nails) but had unacceptable side effects [14]. Topical 1% sirolimus ointment resulted in decreased pain and reduced keratoderma thickness in two patients with twice daily use [15], and a double-blind, placebo-controlled trial is currently in progress (NCT02152007) [16]. Statins have also been shown to decrease expression of *KRT6A* in keratinocytes *in vivo* through inhibition of the cholesterol/mevalonate pathway [17]; however, only one case describing the clinical use of oral rosuvastatin for PC has been reported to date [18]. siRNA injections directed against a mutant KRT6A led to dramatic improvement in the plantar keratoderma at the localised site of injection in the proof-of-concept human trial, but could not be sustained because of pain [19,20]. Topical treatment with small natural molecule sulforaphane, which activates Nrf2 signalling (thought to contribute to the pathogenesis of palmoplantar keratoderma in PC – see pathophysiology earlier), prevents PPK-like lesions in *Krt16* null male mice, but has not been studied in humans [4].

Resources

Patient resources

Support group: International Pachyonychia Congenita Research Registry or IPCR (www.pachyonychia.org; last accessed February 2022).

Dyskeratosis congenita

Definition and nomenclature

Synonyms and inclusions
- Zinsser–Engman–Cole syndrome
- X-linked recessive dyskeratosis congenita (MIM: 305000)
- Autosomal dominant dyskeratosis congenita (MIM: 127550)
- Autosomal recessive dyskeratosis congenita (MIM: 224230)

Introduction and general description

Dyskeratosis congenita (DC) is a heterogeneous group of inherited disorders of telomere maintenance, characterised by nail dysplasia, oral leukoplakia, reticulated hyperpigmentation and a tendency towards bone marrow failure, pulmonary fibrosis, and malignancy [1].

Epidemiology

The prevalence of DC is estimated to be 1 in 1 000 000 individuals. Most patients are male, and X-linked recessive inheritance accounts for approximately half of the cases. Females with heterozygous *DCK1* mutations may show clinical findings if skewed X-inactivation

PART 6: GENETIC DISORDERS

Table 67.3 Underlying gene mutations in dyskeratosis congenita [2].

Inheritance pattern	MIM number	Gene location	Gene	Protein name	Protein function	Percentage of cases*
XLR	305000	Xq28	DKC1	Dyskerin	Component of telomerase complex that converts uridine residues of ribosomal RNA to pseudouridine	20–25
AD	613990	14q12	TINF2	TRF1-interacting nuclear factor 2	Shelterin complex component that protects telomere ends during DNA replication	12–20
AD	127550	3q26.2	TERC	Telomerase RNA component	Acts as a template for adding telomere repeats	5–10
AD or AR	613989	5p15.33	TERT	Telomerase	Catalytic component of telomerase, which synthesises telomere repeats	1–7
AD or AR			ACD	ACD Shelterin Complex Subunit and Telomerase Recruitment Factor	Telomerase recruitment to telomeres	<1
AD or AR	615190	20q13.33	RTEL1	Telomere replication	DNA helicase that is crucial for telomere maintenance, DNA repair and prevention of excess meiotic crossovers; interacts with TRF1	2–8
AR	613276	16q21	C16orf57	Mpn1 RNA exonuclease	Processes small nuclear RNAs post-transcriptionally	2
AR	224230	15q14	NOP10	Nuclear protein, Family A, member 3	Small nucleolar RNA-binding protein that is associated with NHP2 and dyskerin in telomerase complex; involved in uridine to pseudouridine conversion	<1
AR	613987	5q35.3	NHP2	Nuclear protein, Family A, member 2	Small nucleolar RNA-binding protein that is associated with NOP10 and dyskerin in telomerase complex; involved in uridine to pseudouridine conversion	<1
AR	613988	17p13.1	WRAP53	WD repeat-containing protein encoding RNA Antisense to p53; also called TCAB1: telomerase Cajal body protein 1	Important for telomerase trafficking	<1
AR			PARN	Poly(A)-Specific Ribonuclease	Removes oligo(A) tails to prevent degradation of mature or precursor miRNAs	<1
AR			CTC1	Conserved telomere maintenance component 1	Part of a complex that protects telomeres from degradation	1–3

*Not all cases have been associated with a particular genotype, so that the numbers do not add to 100%.
ACD encodes a protein formerly called Adrenocortical Dysplasia Protein Homology. AD, autosomal dominant; AR, autosomal recessive; XLR, X-linked recessive.

leads to significant expression of the mutant allele. Autosomal recessive and autosomal dominant inheritance patterns have also been reported (Table 67.3) [2,3]. Autosomal dominant forms exhibit genetic anticipation, with disease presenting earlier in life and increased penetrance in subsequent generations [4].

Pathophysiology

Dyskeratosis congenita is considered a 'telomeropathy', because most patients show severe shortening of telomeres. Mutations in one of 12 genes are found in approximately 70% of patients, and the protein products of these genes affect telomerase maintenance (Table 67.3) [2]. Telomeres provide a repetitive template (TTAGGG) for repair at the 3' ends of chromosomes that prevents the loss of genetically encoded information after replication. When too short, telomeres signal the arrest of cell proliferation and lead to senescence and apoptosis, which particularly impacts rapidly dividing cells. Telomerase catalyses DNA synthesis to maintain telomere length; the telomerase catalytic unit contains telomerase reverse transcriptase (TERT) and its template, telomerase RNA component (TERC) [5]. 'Shelterin' is a protein complex of six proteins that regulate telomere length by acting as a cap at the telomere (TERF1, TERF2, TINF2, TERF2IP, ACD and POT1); mutations in TINF2 cause at least 10% of cases of DC [5]. Other components of the telomerase complex that are mutated in DC are DKC1, encoding

dyskerin, a small nucleolar protein that binds to RNA, and the stabilisers NHP2, NOP10, and GAR1 [5]. The most common cause of DC is mutations in DKC1, but features of DC have been described from mutations affecting other telomerase complex components (Table 67.3).

Clinical features

The phenotype of DC varies widely, including among DC patients with mutations in the same gene. Dyskeratosis congenita should be considered in patients with at least two of the three features of the classic triad: abnormal nails, reticular skin pigmentation, and/or oral leukoplakia, or one feature of the triad plus two or more other recognised features (Table 67.4) [2,5]. The complete triad may be present in up to 37% of patients, whereas a complete absence of triad features can be seen in 10% of patients, the latter of which is more common in AD DC [3]. A higher number of triad features (two or three) is associated with a greater incidence of bone marrow failure and death as compared with those with no or one feature [3].

The thin *dystrophic nails* usually appear first, between the ages of 5 and 13 years (Figure 67.2a,b). Mildly affected nails show ridging and longitudinal grooving; severely affected nails are shortened and show pterygium formation or near complete loss. Cutaneous

Table 67.4 Clinical features of dyskeratosis congenita [3].

Major features (>75% of patients)
Nail dystrophy
Leukoplakia
Abnormal skin pigmentation
Bone marrow failure

Other recognised features (10–75% of patients)
Short stature
Sparse hair or premature greying
Hyperhidrosis
Epiphora
Blepharitis
Abnormal eyelashes
Developmental delay
Pulmonary disease
Oesophageal stricture
Tooth decay and loss
Squamous cell carcinoma
Intrauterine growth retardation
Liver disease, enteropathy
Hypogonadism, undescended testes, phimosis, urethral stenosis
Microcephaly
Osteoporosis, scoliosis, avascular necrosis of the hips or shoulders
Deafness

changes usually develop after the onset of nail changes, most commonly during late childhood to teenage years. A fine *reticulated dusky brown hyperpigmentation*, sometimes surrounding hypopigmented, atrophic, telangiectatic patches ('poikilodermatous'), on the face, neck, shoulders, upper back and thighs is characteristic (Figure 67.2b,c). Other cutaneous changes may include:
- Telangiectasia of the trunk.
- Redness and atrophy of the face with irregular macular hyperpigmentation.
- Acrocyanosis.
- Palmoplantar hyperkeratosis.
- Hyperhidrosis and bullae of the palms and soles.
- Wrinkled atrophic skin over the elbows, knees and penis.
- A diffuse atrophic, transparent and shiny appearance on the dorsal aspects of the hands and feet.
- Sparse and lustreless hair of the scalp, eyebrows, and eyelashes.

The most common mucous membrane change is *leukoplakia* (Figure 67.2d), which is associated with a 1000-fold increased risk of malignant transformation to oral squamous cell carcinoma (SCC) compared with oral leukoplakia in the general population. Oral cutaneous graft-versus-host disease, which is often seen after stem cell transplantation (see management later), is another risk factor for development of oral SCC [6]. Rarely, periodontitis and blisters and erosions of the oral and anal mucosae, oesophagus and urethra may develop. Inflammation of the tarsal conjunctivae may result in atresia of the lacrimal ducts, excessive lacrimation, chronic blepharitis, conjunctivitis and ectropion. The teeth tend to be defective and subject to early decay.

Overall, almost 90% of patients develop life-threatening *bone marrow failure*, characterised by severe aplastic anaemia with neutropenia, splenomegaly and a haemorrhagic diathesis. Cytopenia is often the first sign in DC [5]. Haematologic involvement tends to be more severe in patients X-linked recessive, autosomal recessive or

TINF2-associated DC [3]. Acute myeloid leukaemia and myelodysplastic syndrome have also been described at rates of 73 and 500 times that of the general population, respectively [4]. Pulmonary fibrosis and hepatic cirrhosis are other life-threatening complications [4]. Idiopathic pulmonary fibrosis, liver disease, aplastic anaemia, myelodysplasia and leukaemia as isolated features have each been described in patients with mutations in DC genes, especially single allele mutations in TERT and TERC.

Epithelial tumours often first develop by the mid-teens, frequently in areas of mucosa with leukoplakia. SCC of the tongue is most common, but other oral sites, oesophageal, anogenital and cutaneous SCC can also occur (Figure 67.2e) [2]. These carcinomas are not driven by human papillomavirus (HPV) infection and thus HPV vaccination is not predicted to decrease the risk.

A severe variant, Hoyeraal–Hreidarsson syndrome (HH), shows the major features of DC, but in addition cerebellar hypoplasia, microcephaly, developmental delay, intrauterine growth retardation, and sometimes severe immunodeficiency, enteropathy and/or aplastic anaemia. Most patients have mutations in *DKC1*, but mutations in *TERT* and *TINF2* or have been described [5]. Another severe variant of DC, Revesz syndrome (RS), has bilateral exudative retinopathy, growth retardation, bone marrow failure, and central nervous system calcifications, in addition to nail dystrophy, oral leukoplakia and sparse fine hair [5]. Mutations have been found in *TINF2* [5].

The average life expectancy of individuals with DC is 44 years, although the life expected is shorter in patients with HH (5 years) and RS (11 years) [5]. Patients usually die of bone marrow failure (~60–70%), pulmonary disease (~10–15%) or malignancy (~10%).

Pterygium nail changes of DC can be seen in patients with lichen planus and graft-versus-host disease. The poikilodermatous change is sometimes confused with Rothmund–Thomson syndrome (*RECQL4* mutations), epidermolysis bullosa simplex with mottled pigmentation (usually *KRT5* mutation), Naegeli–Franceschetti–Jadassohn syndrome/dermatopathia pigmentosa reticularis (*KRT14* mutation) or Clericuzio-type poikiloderma with neutropenia (another *C16orf57* mutation).

Investigations

Screening for DC is best performed by flow cytometry and fluorescence *in situ* hybridisation (flow-FISH) of leukocyte subsets to detect telomere shortening [3]. This should be complemented by genetic testing using a panel for bone marrow failure (BMF) disorders in order to establish a diagnosis [3]. Recommended disease surveillance includes annual complete blood counts, pulmonary functional tests, gynaecological exams and cancer screening (annually by dermatology and otolaryngology and twice annually by a dentist) [2].

Management

Treatment of bone marrow failure is recommended when the haemoglobin is persistently below 8 g/dL, platelets <30 000/mm³ and neutrophils <1000/mm³ [4]. Allogeneic stem cell transplantation is the only definitive therapy for the haematopoietic and immunologic defects in DC. Long-term survival after transplant has been poor, generally attributed to fatal pulmonary or vascular complications [4], but increases with reduced intensity conditioning regimens [3]. Androgens, such as oxymetholone or danazol, have

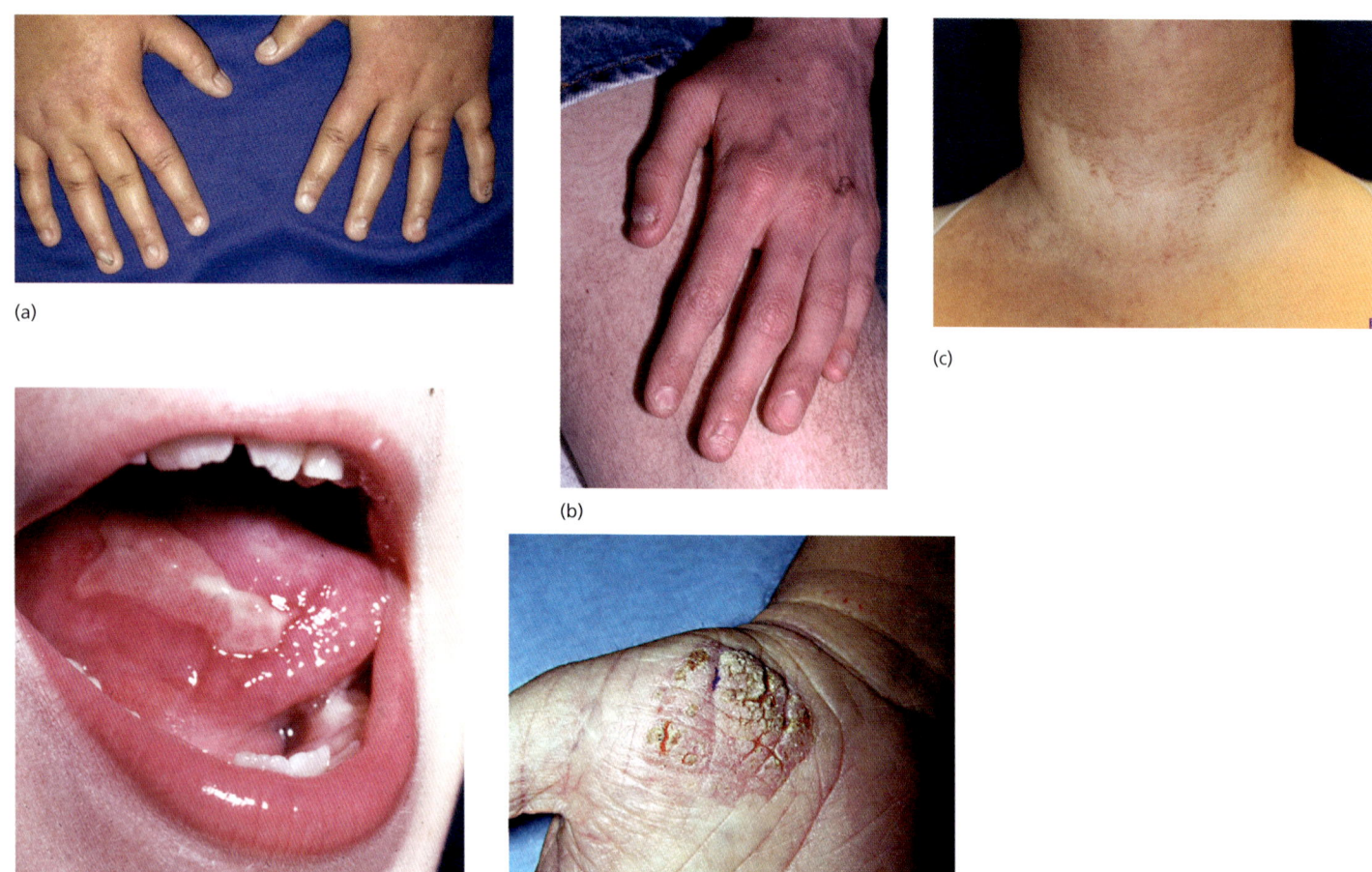

Figure 67.2 Nail dystrophy, poikiloderma and oral leukoplakia are the major mucocutaneous findings of dyskeratosis congenita. (a) Pterygium formation. (b) Nail dystrophy with poikiloderma (telangiectasia, atrophy and dyspigmentation) of the underlying thigh. (c) Poikiloderma on the neck of a young woman. (d) Leukoplakia on the tongue. (e) Squamous cell carcinoma on the hand; mucosa is a more typical location. (e) Courtesy of Dr E. Sprecher.

been reported to improve blood counts in 80% of treated patients [3]. Limiting side effects include virilisation in female patients and dyslipidemia, along with hepatic toxicity [3]. Management of patients otherwise consists of bougienage for oesophageal stenosis; fulguration, curettage and surgical excision of leukokeratosis of the buccal and anal mucosae; and lifelong regular supervision for early detection of mucosal or cutaneous carcinomas [4].

Resources

Patient resources

Support group: Team Telomere (https://teamtelomere.org, last accessed February 2022).

National Cancer Institute, Inherited Bone Marrow Failure Syndrome Study (IBMFS). https://marrowfailure.cancer.gov/disorders/telomere.html (last accessed February 2022).

Nail–patella syndrome

Definition and nomenclature

Nail–patella syndrome (NPS) is an inherited disorder of nail and bone dysplasia.

Synonyms and inclusions
- Hereditary onycho-osteodysplasia (HOOD)
- Fong disease
- Turner–Keiser syndrome

Introduction and general description

NPS is an autosomal dominant disorder classically characterised by nail changes, dystrophy of the knees and elbows, and the presence of iliac horns. Interfamilial and intrafamiliar variability is seen [1]. The diagnosis is often missed for several generations, although features tend to be present at birth. Males and females are affected equally.

Epidemiology

NPS has an estimated prevalence of 1 in 50 000 individuals, although the prevalence could be higher, given the many affected individuals with a mild phenotype [2]. *De novo* mutations occur in 12% of affected individuals (i.e. 88% have an affected parent) [2,3].

Pathophysiology

NPS results from mutations in *LMX1B* on chromosome 9q33.3, which encodes the LIM homeobox transcription factor 1-β. *LIMX1B* is induced by Wnt7a and is required for establishing dorsoventral polarity in the dorsal limb mesenchyme during development, as well as the development of the kidneys, anterior eyes and bones. For additional details on the anatomy and embryological development of the nails, the reader is referred to Chapter 93. Mutations in *LMX1B* can also lead to nail–patella-like renal disease, in which skeletal and nail findings are absent [4].

Clinical features

The nails may be absent (anonychia) or underdeveloped and discoloured, split, ridged or pitted, but *nail dysplasia with the characteristic triangular lunula*, instead of the normal crescent-shaped lunula, occurs in most affected individuals and may be the only feature (Figure 67.3). Changes are present at birth in 95% of individuals with NPS and are usually bilateral and symmetrical [3]. The fingernails are more likely to be affected than the toenails, and the thumbnails are usually the most severely affected with severity decreasing from the index toward the fifth fingers [1]. In addition, the ulnar side of the fingernail is more severely affected than the radial side [4]. Patients often show flexion of the distal interphalangeal joints but hyperextension of the proximal interphalangeal joints, leading to 'swan-necking' [2]. Creases overlying the distal interphalangeal joints tend to be absent [4].

Knees are involved in 74% of patients [2] and tend to have a flattened profile. Patellar involvement is often asymmetrical and commonly characterised by a *small irregularly shaped or absent patella* with recurrent dislocation or subluxation. Flexion contractures and early degenerative arthritis are common; as a result, patients often develop knee pain, locking, instability, and inability to straighten the knee. Elbow involvement, resulting in limited elbow extension,

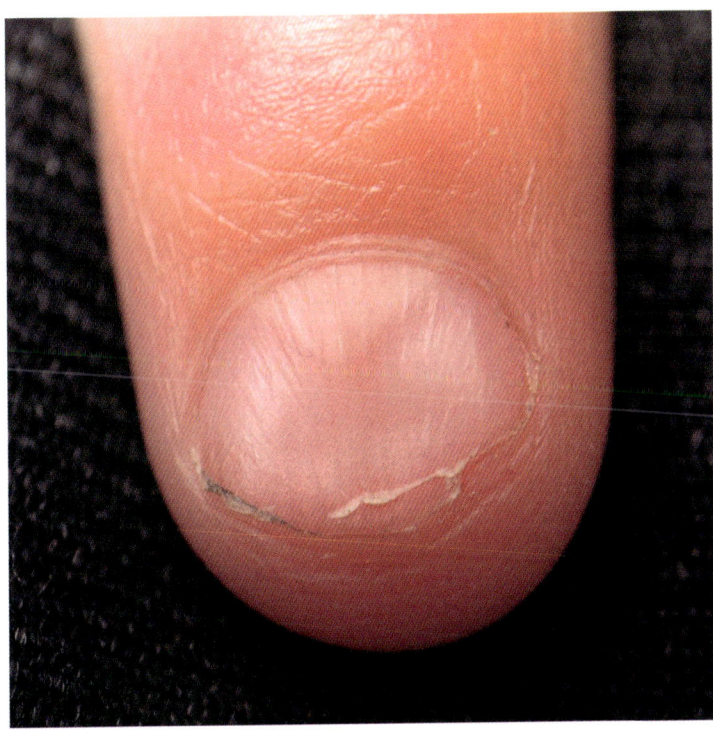

Figure 67.3 Nail dystrophy with triangular lunula of the nail–patella syndrome. Courtesy of Dr Mark Holzberg.

Table 67.5 Clinical features of nail–patella syndrome.

Features	% of patients
Nail changes, especially triangular lunula	96–98
Digital changes	90
Small or absent patella	74
Elbow deformity	70
Iliac horns	70–76
Renal dysfunction	30–50
End-stage renal disease	Rare to 15
Ocular hypertension, glaucoma	10–25

pronation, and supination, is often asymmetrical and occurs in 70% of individuals [4]. The characteristic *iliac horns* are bilateral conical bone projections that extend posteriorly and laterally from the centre of the pelvic iliac bones. They affect approximately 80% of affected individuals, are asymptomatic and are pathognomonic for the disorder [1]. Renal changes occur in 30–50% of affected individuals, initially as *proteinuria with or without haematuria and hypertension*. Up to 15% of patients show end-stage renal disease, which may occur rapidly or develop gradually [2]. Primary open-angle glaucoma and ocular hypertension occur overall in one-third of patients and at a younger age than in the general population [4]. Lester iris, hyperpigmentation of the central part of the iris, is seen in nearly 50% of patients [5]. Crumbling teeth and thin dental enamel have been described [2]. Patients have an increased risk of attention deficit hyperactivity disorder and major depressive disorder, possibly because of *LMX1B* expression in embryonic dopaminergic and serotonergic neurons [6]. Sensorineural hearing loss, peripheral neuropathy and epilepsy have also been described [4]. See Table 67.5.

Investigations

The diagnosis of NPS is based on clinical findings, supplemented by laboratory testing to show the radiographic changes and evidence of renal disease, if present. Radiographic evaluation is necessary to detect the iliac horns, although large horns may be palpable. X-rays are also helpful to confirm the bony changes of the elbows and knees. Characteristic modifications of the glomerular basement membrane can be observed by electron microscopy.

Management

No treatment intervention is needed for the nail abnormalities. Orthopaedic complications are treated by physiotherapy, splinting or bracing, analgesics and occasionally surgery. However, chronic administration of non-steroidal anti-inflammatory drugs (NSAIDs) should be avoided because of the risk of renal disease. Annual monitoring for hypertension, renal disease (urinalysis) and glaucoma is recommended. Hypertension should be controlled medically but renal transplantation is occasionally necessary. Dual-energy X-ray absorptiometry (DEXA) bone density scans are recommended, beginning in young adults.

Resources

Patient resources
Support groups: Nail Patella Syndrome Worldwide (www.npsw.org) (last accessed March 2021).

Hereditary anonychia

Definition and nomenclature

Hereditary anonychia is a rare autosomal recessive non-syndromic disorder characterised by isolated congenital anonychia or hypoplasia of the fingernails and/or toenails [1].

Synonyms and inclusions
- Congenital anonychia
- Onychodystrophy-anonychia

General description of hereditary anonychia

In hereditary anonychia, anonychia or hypoplasia of the fingernails and/or toenails is congenital and usually involves all of the nails. The disorder results from mutations in the *R-spondin 4 (RSPO4)* gene on chromosome 20p13 [2]. RSPO4 is a member of the R-spondin family of secreted proteins, which activates Wnt/β-catenin signalling and presumably Wnt7a, which is crucial for embryonic nail development. Other RSPO proteins are able to compensate for the absence of RSPO4 at all sites except the digital tip, which results in the observed isolation of clinical findings at the nail [3,4].

Key references

The full list of references can be found in the online version at https://www.wiley.com/rooksdermatology10e

Pachyonychia congenita
2 Samuelov L, Smith FJD, Hansen CD, Sprecher E. Revisiting pachyonychia congenita: a case-cohort study of 815 patients. *Br J Dermatol* 2020;182:738–46.

3 Shah S, Boen M, Kenner-Bell B, Schwartz M, Rademaker A, Paller AS. Pachyonychia congenita in pediatric patients: natural history, features, and impact. *JAMA Dermatol* 2014;150(2):146–53.
4 Zieman AG, Coulombe PA. Pathophysiology of pachyonychia congenita-associated palmoplantar keratoderma: new insights into skin epithelial homeostasis and avenues for treatment. *Br J Dermatol.* 2020;182:564–73.
5 Rittié L, Kaspar RL, Sprecher E, Smith FJD. Report of the 13th annual international pachyonychia congenita consortium symposium. *Br J Dermatol* 2017;176:1144–7.
12 Koren A, Sprecher E, Reider E, Artzi O. A treatment protocol for botulinum toxin injections in the treatment of pachyonychia congenita-associated keratoderma. *Br J Dermatol* 2020;182:671–7.

Dyskeratosis congenita
3 Ward SC, Savage SA, Giri N *et al.* Beyond the triad: Inheritance, mucocutaneous phenotype, and mortality in a cohort of patients with dyskeratosis congenita. *J Am Acad Dermatol* 2018;78:804–6.
4 Agarwal S. Evaluation and management of hematopoietic failure in dyskeratosis congenita. *Hematol Oncol Clin North Am* 2018;32:669–85.
5 Savage SA, Alter BP. Dyskeratosis congenita. *Hematol Oncol Clin North Am* 2009;23:215–31.

Nail–patella syndrome
1 Figueroa-Silva O, Vicente A, Agudo A *et al.* Nail–patella syndrome: report of 11 pediatric cases. *J Eur Acad Dermatol Venereol* 2016;30:1614–17.

Hereditary anonychia
1 Afsar FS, Karakuzu A. Total congenital anonychia. *Pediatr Dermatol* 2014;31:743–4.

CHAPTER 68

Genetic Disorders of Pigmentation

Fanny Morice-Picard and Alain Taïeb

Service de Dermatologie et Dermatologie Pédiatrique, Hôpital St André, Bordeaux, France

PART 6: GENETIC DISORDERS

Introduction and general description

Normal skin colour is determined by a number of variables, the most important of which is melanin. Differences in skin and hair colour are principally the result of differences in the melanin content of skin although other chromophores and skin thickness may also determine shade variation in the skin. Besides melanin, haemoglobin (in both the oxygenated and reduced state) and carotenoids also contribute significantly to skin colour (see Chapter 86).

Melanocytes are responsible for the synthesis of melanin, a complex quinone/indole-quinone-derived mixture of biopolymers. Melanocytes migrate from the neural crest into the epidermis during the first 2 months of gestation. They produce melanin within specialised vesicles known as melanosomes. Racial and ethnic differences in skin colour are related to variation in the number, size, composition and distribution of melanosomes to surrounding keratinocytes. *Constitutive* pigmentation refers to the amount of melanin pigmentation that is genetically determined in the absence of sun exposure and other influences. *Facultative* (inducible) pigmentation, or 'tan', results from sun exposure (or other exogenous influences including drugs). The regulation of human pigmentation is complex and intertwined with other factors affecting epidermal or dermal–epidermal homeostasis. It involves both systemic and local factors secreted in the dermal or epidermal compartment. This is reflected in physiological pigmentary changes, such as normal palmar hypopigmentation more striking in black skin, pigmentary lines enhanced during pregnancy and systemic disorders with hyperproduction of pigmentation stimulators, such as α-melanocyte-stimulating hormone (MSH) in Addison disease.

The major precursor of melanins is tyrosine. Tyrosinase catalyses the hydroxylation of tyrosine to DOPA (3,4-dihydroxyphenylalanine). Once completely formed within melanocytes, melanosomes are transported along dendrites towards adjacent keratinocytes. The next step involves the extrusion of the melanosomes and their transfer into neighbouring keratinocytes, by a mechanism which is still debated. After being transferred to keratinocytes, melanosomes are translocated to the apical pole of the keratinocyte where they protect the nucleus from UV mutagenic damage. Keratinocyte terminal differentiation is accompanied by concomitant degradation of melanosomes so that no melanosomes are normally visible in the very upper part of the epidermis (Chapter 86).

Hundreds of genes are known to modulate pigmentation type or pattern in the skin, hairs/coat and eyes in mammals during or after development by acting directly or indirectly on the pigment cell lineage. Among these, only a few have been also found to underlie inherited monogenic pigmentation disorders (Table 68.1). Of interest, some genes known to be important for normal variation in skin, eye or hair colour are in this list. These disorders can be classified into three major groups: (i) disorders of hypopigmentation, (ii) disorders of hyperpigmentation and (iii) disorders featuring combined hypo- and hyperpigmentation, known as the dyschromatoses. This classical clinical classification is, however, in part misleading, since an overlap of phenotypes exist between the last two groups, as illustrated in this chapter.

Rook's Textbook of Dermatology, Tenth Edition. Edited by Christopher Griffiths, Jonathan Barker, Tanya Bleiker, Walayat Hussain and Rosalind Simpson.
© 2024 John Wiley & Sons Ltd. Published 2024 by John Wiley & Sons Ltd.

Table 68.1 Major monogenic inherited pigmentation disorders.

Disease name	Inheritance	Genes	Clinical features
Hypopigmentation disorders			
Defects in melanocyte lineage migration			
Piebaldism	AD	KIT SNAI2	Well-demarcated ventral midline hypopigmentary macules, white forelock
Waardenburg syndrome			
WS1	AD	PAX3	White forelock, hypopigmented patches, dystopia canthorum, iris heterochromia, deafness, synophris and mild facial dysmorphism (broad nose root)
WS2	AD	MITF/SNAI2	Same as WS1, but no facial dysmorphism
WS3	AD	PAX3	Same as WS1 with musculoskeletal anomalies (syndactyly, carpal bone fusion)
WS4	AR	EDN3/EDNRB /SOX10	(Shah–Waardenburg syndrome) WS phenotype accompanied by Hirschsprung disease, neurological symptoms if caused by SOX10 mutation
Albinism: defects in melanin synthesis			
OCA1	AR	TYR	Variable degrees of hypopigmentation extending from a complete absence of pigmentation to normal pigmentation
OCA2	AR	OCA2	Prevalent in black people, blond to red brown hair with age, ephelides
OCA3	AR	TYRP1	Rufus albinism in black people
OCA4	AR	SLC45A2	Similar to OCA1, more common in Japan
OCA5	AR	Unknown	One family described in Pakistan
OCA6	AR	SLC24A5/NCKX5	One family described from China and five from Europe
OCA7	AR	C10orf11	Faroe albinism
OCA8	AR	DCT	Mild skin and hair hypopigmentation
OA1	XLR	GPR143	Isolated ocular albinism
Defects in lysosomal biogenesis and transport, including melanosomes			
Hermansky–Pudlak syndrome			
HPS1	AR	HPS1	
HPS2	AR	AP3B1	
HPS3	AR	HPS3	
HPS4	AR	HPS4	Decreased pigmentation in eyes, hair and skin, easy bruisability and bleeding tendency, lung interstitial fibrosis, granulomatous colitis
HPS5	AR	HPS5	
HPS6	AR	HPS6	
HPS7	AR	DTNBP1	
HPS8	AR	BLOC1S3	
HSP9	AR	BLOC1S6	
HPS10	AR	AP3D1	
HPS11	AR	BLOC1S5	
Chediak–Higashi syndrome	AR	CHS1/LYST	Partial albinism (blond hair, fair skin) accompanied by immunodeficiency (pyogenic infections, haemophagocytic syndrome) and cerebellar syndrome
Griscelli–Pruniéras syndrome			
GS1	AR	MYO5A	Silvery grey hair and fair skin, neurological defects
GS2	AR	RAB27A	Silvery grey hair and fair skin, immunological defects
GS3	AR	MLPH	Silvery grey hair and fair skin
Hyperpigmentation disorders			
Generalised/diffuse			
Familial progressive hyperpigmentation	AD	KITLG	Congenital sharply and irregular hyperpigmentary patches involving both the mucosae and the skin which increase in size and number with age. Hypopigmented patches also noted
Linear			
Incontinentia pigmenti	XLD	IKBKG	Pigmentation abnormalities consisting of whorls and streaks located over the trunk
Linear and whorled naevoid hypermelanosis	SO	Report of mosaicism for KITLG	Usually no extracutaneous features although rarely associated with cardiovascular, neurological and musculoskeletal abnormalities

Table 68.1 (continued)

Disease name	Inheritance	Genes	Clinical features
Punctate/reticulate			
Dyskeratosis congenita	DKC/XLR	*DKC1*	Reticulated pattern of hyperpigmentation, bone marrow dysplasia, haematological and epithelial malignancies
	DKC/AD1	*TERC*	
	DKC/AD2	*TERT*	
	DKC/AD3	*TINF2*	
	Incl. Revesz sy DKC/AD4		
	DKC/AD6	*RTEL1*	
	DKC/AR1	*ACD?*	
	DKC/AR2	*NOP10*	
	DKC/AR3	*NHP2*	
	DKC/AR4	*WRAP53*	
	DKC/AR5	*TERT*	
	DKC/AR6	*RTEL1*	
	DKC/AR6	*PARN*	
		ACD?	
Naegeli–Franceschetti–Jadassohn syndrome and dermatopathia pigmentosa reticularis	AD	*KRT14*	Complete absence of dermatoglyphics, reticulate pattern of skin hyperpigmentation, alopecia, palmoplantar keratoderma, abnormal sweating, dental anomalies and nail dystrophy
Dowling–Degos disease (including Galli–Galli disease)	AD	*KRT5*	Postpubertal reticulate hyperpigmentation of the flexures
		POFUT1	Comedo-like lesions on the neck and pitted perioral acneform scars and genital and perianal reticulated pigmented lesions have also been described
		POGLUT1	Generalised lesions in *POGLUT1* mutation
		PSENEN	Reticulated pigmentation associated with acne inversa
Reticulate acropigmentation of Kitamura	AD	*ADAM10*	Hyperpigmented atrophic macules on the hand dorsa and 'pits' on the palms and soles with abnormal dermatoglyphics
Peutz–Jeghers–Touraine syndrome	AD	*STK11*	Macules of the lips, buccal mucosa and digits, gastrointestinal hamartomatous polyps, may be associated with an increased risk of neoplasms
Dyschromatoses			
Dyschromatosis symmetrica hereditaria	AD	*ADAR1*	Small hyperpigmented and hypopigmented macules on the back of the hand and feet
Dyschromatosis universalis hereditaria	AD	*ABCB6*	Hypopigmented and hyperpigmented macules distributed over the entire surface of the skin

Adapted from Hershkovitz and Sprecher 2008 [103].
AD, autosomal dominant; AR, autosomal recessive; SO, sporadic; XLR, X-linked recessive.

HYPOPIGMENTATION DISORDERS

Piebaldism

Introduction and general description

Piebaldism is a rare autosomal dominant trait characterised by well-demarcated irregular hypopigmented macules [1]. The incidence of piebaldism is estimated at fewer than 1 in 20 000. Both sexes are affected equally and no population is spared.

Pathophysiology

The disease results from heterozygous mutations in *KIT*, encoding c-KIT, a membranal tyrosine kinase receptor responsible for triggering cell proliferation and migration [2]. Dominant mutations in *KIT* result in impaired migration of melanocytes to the skin, as reflected by the absence of melanocytes and melanin in

hypopigmented patches [2]. Piebaldism can also be caused by heterozygous mutation in the gene encoding the zinc finger transcription factor *SNAI2* [3].

Morphological studies have shown either an absence of melanocytes and melanosomes in the hypomelanotic areas or sometimes reduced numbers of abnormal large melanocytes. In the hypermelanotic islands situated in areas of hypomelanosis, melanocytes produce normal melanosomes but also abnormal spherical and granular melanosomes.

Clinical features

The most typical and common clinical feature of the disease is a white forelock, often associated with a V-shaped area of leukoderma on the mid-forehead. The hypopigmented lesions of piebaldism have a predilection for the anterior part of the body and the mid-portion of the limbs (Figure 68.1). Often, white patches occur on the upper chest, abdomen and limbs, bilaterally but not necessarily symmetrically. Occasionally, they are found on the face,

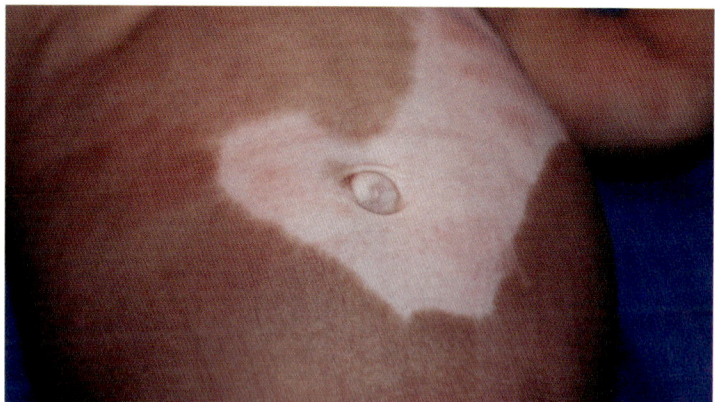

Figure 68.1 Typical trunk pattern of hypopigmentation in piebaldism.

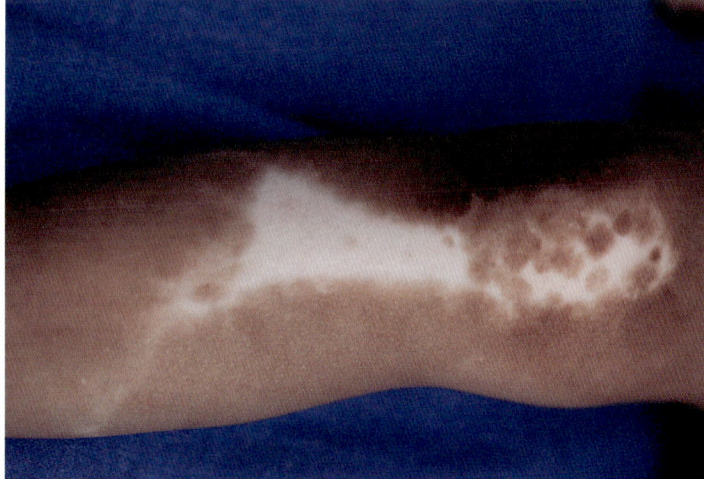

Figure 68.2 Partial repigmentation pattern on the leg in piebaldism.

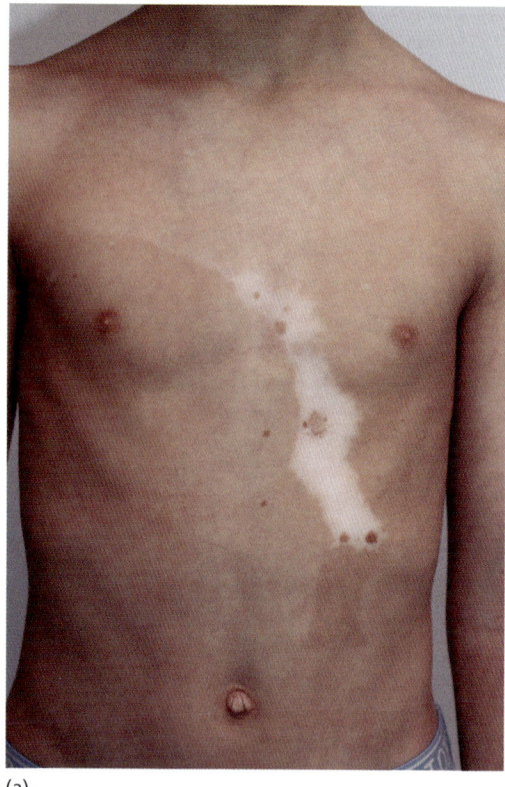

(a)

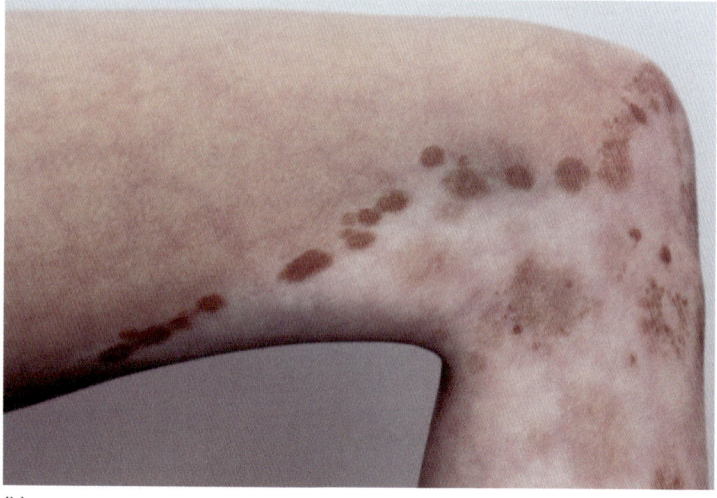

(b)

Figure 68.3 (a) Note the mosaic pattern on the trunk in piebaldism. (b) Detail of repigmentation pattern (leg).

particularly the chin. The hands and feet, as well as the back, remain normally pigmented. In addition, small spots of hyperpigmentation arise subsequently within the hypopigmented lesions or even on the background of normal skin (Figure 68.2).

The extent of the areas of depigmentation is variable. Rarely, the white forelock may be the only lesion. Piebaldism is usually not associated with extracutaneous manifestations; however, mental retardation or deafness have been reported in the context of a large deletion [4].

Although the skin lesions in piebaldism are quite typical, the occurrence of isolated poliosis or skin hypopigmentation can suggest a number of inflammatory disorders affecting pigmentation (e.g. vitiligo, alopecia areata, Vogt–Koyanagi syndrome, Alezzandrini syndrome, Woolf syndrome), as well as monogenic (e.g. tuberous sclerosis, Waardenburg syndrome (WS)) or somatic (naevus depigmentosus) disorders.

Piebaldism can be distinguished from vitiligo because of the neonatal presence of white patches. In cases of fair skin and poorly detectable lesions at birth, the medial distribution of lesions is quite different from that of vitiligo; hyperpigmented patches

which appear at the border or centre of hypopigmented patches are quite distinctive (Figure 68.3) and, overall, lesions remain stable in adults.

If the interpupillary distance is increased or the patient is deaf, the diagnosis of WS must be considered. The evolution of piebaldism is benign. Sun protection is recommended to protect the amelanotic areas from burning. Epidermal cell or skin grafting have been successfully tried in piebaldism [5]. In contrast, phototherapy is inefficacious, as are topical corticosteroids.

Waardenburg syndrome

Introduction and general description
Waardenburg syndrome is an autosomal dominant genetic disorder characterised by piebaldism and sensorineural deafness. A molecular classification is used (WS1–4) based on the mutant gene (Table 68.1). It is an autosomal dominant condition except for the recessive WS4 with an estimated incidence of 1 in 20 000–40 000.

Pathophysiology
All abnormalities seen in WS involve the neural crest lineage. Type 1 and type 3 result from loss-of-function mutations in the *PAX3* gene [5]. Mutations in *MITF* result accordingly in WS type 2 [6]. WS type 2 is characterised by genetic heterogeneity: it was shown to also result from mutations in *SNAI2* encoding a zinc finger transcription factor [7].

Type 4 disease is caused by mutations in at least three genes including *EDNRB*, encoding the endothelin-B receptor, *EDN3*, encoding the ligand of EDNRB, and *SOX10*, which, like *PAX3*, regulates the expression of *MITF*. Bi-allelic mutations in *EDNRB* and *EDN3* result in WS type 4 whereas heterozygous mutations in the same genes cause isolated Hirschsprung disease [8]. Loss of *SOX10* expression leads to abnormal expression of *RET*, which is known to cause Hirschsprung disease [9]. In addition, lack of *SOX10* expression is associated with abnormal myelination and neurological signs.

Clinical features
Waardenburg syndrome features congenital leukoderma reminiscent of piebald pattern in association with sensorineural deafness of varying severity. Areas of hypopigmentation may diminish in size or even disappear with time [10,11].

Clinical variants
Waardenburg syndrome type 1 is inherited in an autosomal dominant fashion and is characterised by a white forelock, alopecia, hypopigmented patches, dystopia canthorum (increased distance between the inner canthi without any change in the distance between the pupils) and heterochromia irides associated with deafness in one third to one half of cases. Patients may also display dysmorphic features including a broad nasal root and synophrys (medial hyperplasia of the eyebrows) and mild skeletal anomalies (Figure 68.4). WS type 2 (Klein–Waardenburg syndrome) is inherited as an autosomal dominant trait. Clinical signs are similar to those seen in WS type 1 except for absence of facial dysmorphism and dystopia canthorum, and a higher frequency of deafness and heterochromia. WS type 3, an autosomal dominant disorder, is rarer than the other types and presents the same clinical manifestations as type 1 in association with musculoskeletal anomalies. WS type 4 (Shah–Waardenburg syndrome) is inherited in an autosomal recessive fashion, features the white forelock and is accompanied by Hirschsprung disease [5].

Management
Management of the hearing loss associated with WS1 depends on its severity. The hearing loss in WS1 is typically non-progressive.

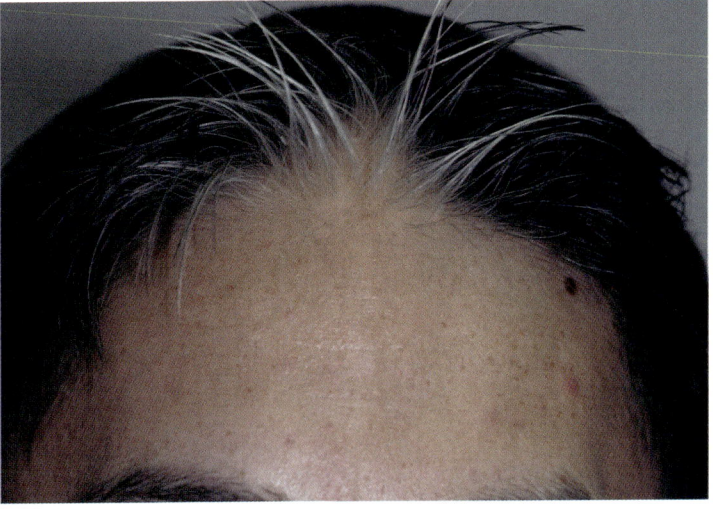

(a)

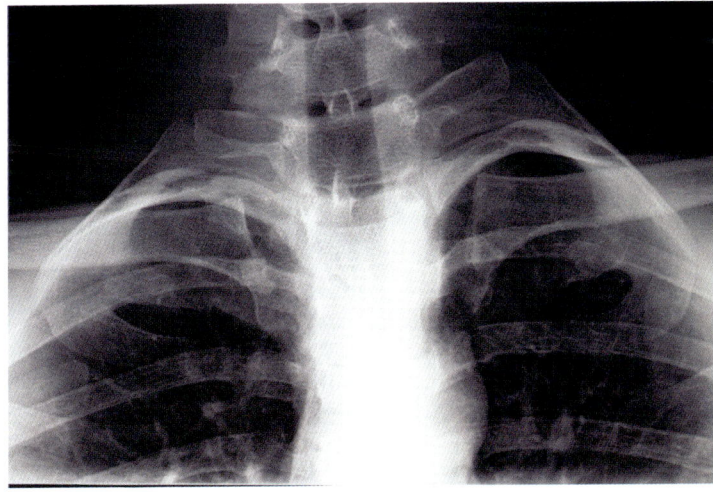

(b)

Figure 68.4 (a) Typical facial dysmorphic features and (b) supernumerary ribs in Waardenburg syndrome.

Oculocutaneous albinism

Introduction and general description
Oculocutaneous albinism (OCA) is a rare genetic disorder characterised by generalised depigmentation of the skin, hair and eye, and by ophthalmological anomalies caused by a deficiency in melanin biosynthesis [12].

A molecular classification is used (OCA1–7) derived from mutant genes (Table 68.1).

The appellation of the various OCA subtypes, initially centred on clinical findings, has moved towards a molecular classification based upon the identification of causative genes. OCA is a genetically heterogeneous disorder. Initially, four types of OCA were known and recently three additional forms of OCA have been reported. Altogether seven genes have been implicated in the pathogenesis of OCA: *TYR* in OCA1, *OCA2* in OCA2, *TYRP1* in OCA3, *SLC45A2* in OCA4, *SLC24A5* in OCA6, *LRMD5* in OCA7

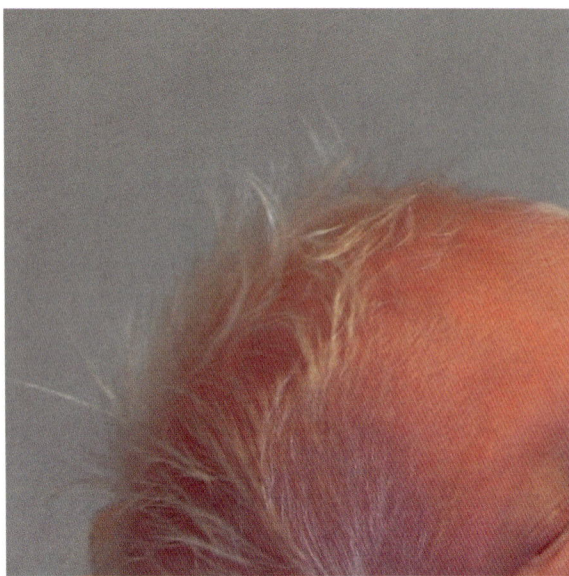

Figure 68.5 White hair in a patient with oculocutaneous albinism type 1A (OCA1) at birth.

and *DCT* in OCA8 [13–19]. OCA5 has been mapped to 4q24 but the gene still remains to be identified [20].

Epidemiology

Oculocutaneous albinism is the most frequent form of diffuse hypopigmentation worldwide with a prevalence estimated around 1/20 000.

The prevalence of the various OCA subtypes varies considerably from one continent to another, but OCA1 is the most frequent form worldwide. OCA2 is the most frequent form among African patients with a prevalence that reaches 1/1000 in some populations in Western Africa.

Pathophysiology and genetics

Oculocutaneous albinism is due to a deficiency of melanin biosynthesis whereas melanocytes are normally present and distributed. The reduction of the amount of melanin is responsible for an increased sensitivity to UV radiation and for a predisposition to skin cancers. The ophthalmological anomalies associated with albinism are not only a consequence of a lack of melanin but also of a lack of levodopa an early intermediate of the synthesis of melanin, which has been shown to be required for normal retinal and visual development [21].

Oculocutaneous albinism type 1 (OCA1) is caused by mutations in *TYR*, encoding tyrosinase, which is the essential and rate-limiting enzyme for melanin production [13]. Variable degrees of hypopigmentation extending from a complete absence of pigmentation to normal pigmentation are observed in OCA1 depending on the residual level of tyrosinase activity, which constitutes the key step in melanogenesis (Figure 68.5) [22].

Oculocutaneous albinism type 2 is caused by mutations in the *OCA2* gene, encoding the P protein, a transmembrane protein of importance for melanin biosynthesis and for processing and transport of other melanosomal proteins such as tyrosinase. It seems that OCA2 exerts at least some of its effects by maintaining an acidic pH in melanosomes [23].

Mutations in *TYRP1* are responsible for oculocutaneous albinism type 3. The protein encoded by this gene catalyses the oxidation of dihydroxyindole-2-carboxylic acid (DHICA) monomers into eumelanin and serves also to stabilise tyrosinase. It is not required for phaeomelanin production, explaining the accumulation of the latter in the skin and hair in OCA3 [4].

Oculocutaneous albinism type 4 is caused by mutations in *SLC45A2*, encoding the membrane-associated transporter protein (MATP), a membrane transporter in melanosomes [5].

Oculocutaneous albinism type 6 is caused by mutations in *SLC24A5*, coding for a membrane-associated transporter protein (NCKX5). This protein is involved in proper maturation of melanosomes [6].

Mutations in *LRMD5*, coding a protein involved in melanocyte differentiation and function, are associated with oculocutaneous albinism type 7 [7].

Oculocutaneous albinism type 8 is associated with dopachrome tautomerase variants in patients with oculocutaneous albinism [8].

Clinical features

The pigmentation of the skin, hair and eyes is in general reduced but its degree varies with the type of albinism. It is important to check pigmentary characteristics in siblings and parents to consider the diagnosis of albinism in its subtle variants (Figure 68.6).

All types of OCA and ocular albinism (OA) have similar ocular findings, including various degrees of congenital nystagmus, hypopigmentation of the iris leading to iris translucency, reduced pigmentation of the retinal pigment epithelium, foveal hypoplasia, reduced visual acuity usually in the range 20/60 to 20/400 and refractive errors, and sometimes a degree of colour vision impairment [13,14].

Photophobia may be prominent. Iris translucency is demonstrable by slit lamp examination. A characteristic finding is misrouting of the optic nerves, consisting of an excessive crossing of the fibres in the optic chiasma, which can result in strabismus and reduced stereoscopic vision [13]. The abnormal crossing of fibres can be demonstrated by monocular visual evoked potential [2].

Clinical variants

In the severe OCA1 form, there is a complete absence of pigmentation with white hair and pink skin (Figure 68.5). There is no tendency to tan. Naevi are achromic. The visual impairment is severe with nystagmus, photophobia and errors of refraction.

In other types initially described as tyrosinase positive, pigmentation is highly variable and influenced by the phototype of the patient. Hair colour may range from white to blond to light brown (Figures 68.6 and 68.7). Pigmentation can increase with age. Dark-brown freckles may develop with age in sun-exposed areas, particularly in African patients with OCA2 (Figure 68.8). Visual acuity may improve as patients get older and they may have less severe nystagmus.

Rufous albinism (OCA3) was originally described in African patients with *TYRP1* mutations, but recent molecular investigations indicate that it is not restricted to African populations [15,24].

Differential diagnosis

The presence of OA excludes a large number of diseases associated with pigment dilution. Diagnoses to be considered in the

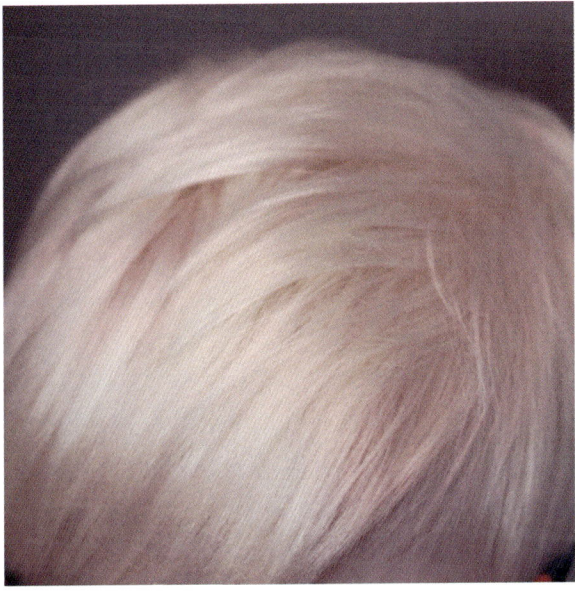

(a)

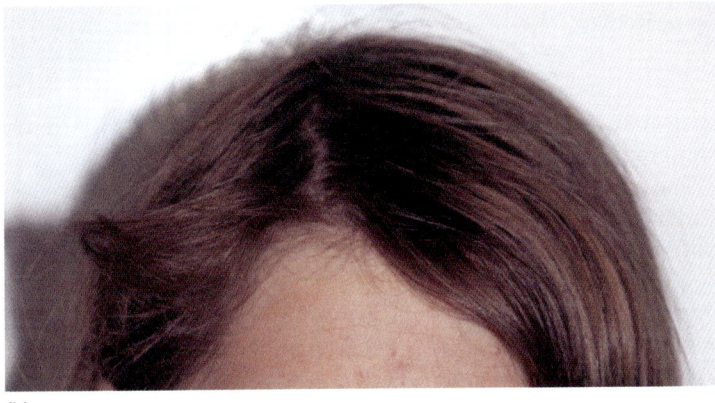

(b)

Figure 68.6 Variability of hair colour among patients with OCA1. Patient with OCA1 and white hair (a) contrasting with light brown hair in a patient with a mild form of OCA1 (b).

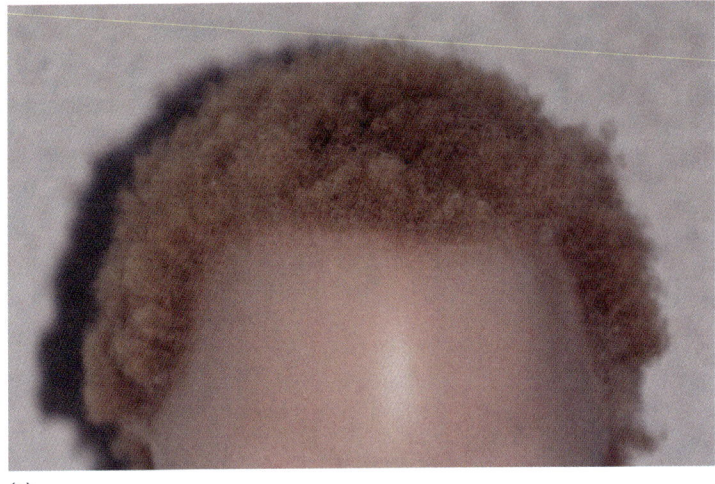

(a)

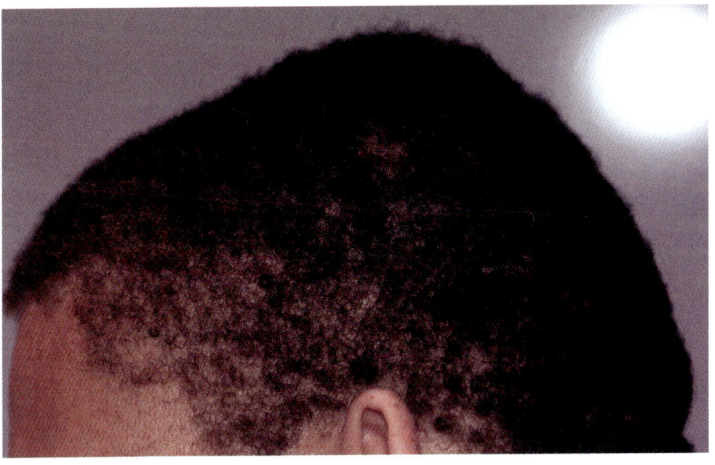

(b)

Figure 68.7 (a) Yellow blond hair in a child presenting with oculocutaneous albinism type 2 (OCA2). (b) Brown hair in an adult patient with OCA2.

case of ocular and cutaneous hypopigmentation include histidinaemia, homocystinuria, phenylketonuria, Hermansky–Pudlak and Chedlak–Higashi syndromes, as well as Cross and Tietz syndromes. Pure OCA has to be distinguished from syndromic forms of OCA, especially Hermansky–Pudlak syndrome, and a platelet secretion test is recommended in the initial assessment of an OCA patient without family history of albinism.

Complications and co-morbidities

The incidence of skin cancer is increased in patients with OCA, especially spinous cell carcinoma, which is a cause of mortality in Africans with OCA2. Melanoma is far less common, suggesting that melanin production is a key factor for melanoma risk in the context of UV exposure.

Disease course and prognosis

Lifespan in patients with OCA is normal and medical problems are generally not increased compared with those in the general population. Skin cancers may occur and regular skin checks should

be offered. Development and intelligence are normal. Persons with OCA have a normal fertility.

Investigations

The diagnosis of OCA is based on the association of ophthalmological manifestations with hypopigmentation of the skin and hair. Ophthalmological examination should include an examination with optical coherence tomography (OCT) of the retina showing characteristic foveal hypoplasia. Electrophysiological testing can demonstrate misrouting of the optic nerves, resulting in strabismus and impaired stereoscopic vision [25].

Due to the clinical overlap between the OCA subtypes, molecular diagnosis is necessary to establish a correct diagnosis, and subsequently provide patients and their families with prognostic information and genetic counselling.

Management

Sun protection is mandatory to avoid skin sunburns and skin cancers with a special emphasis in patients living in high UV risk environments. Early referral to an ophthalmologist is mandatory. Decreased visual acuity is usually managed with corrective lenses

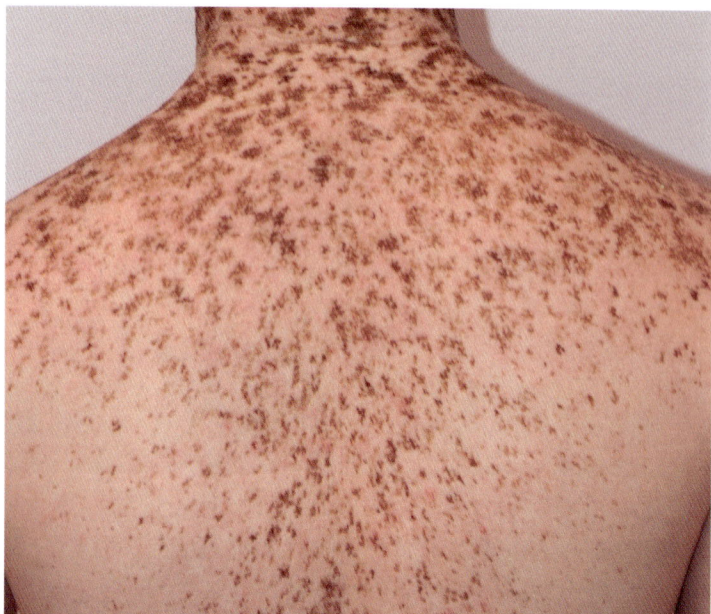

Figure 68.8 Dark-brown freckles may develop with age in sun-exposed areas particularly in African patients with OCA2.

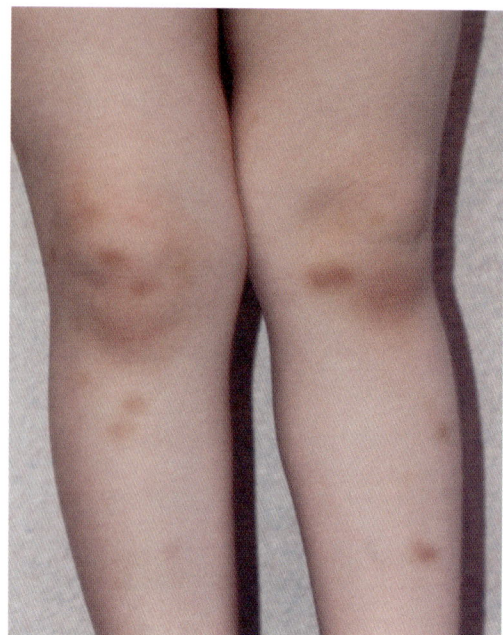

Figure 68.9 White skin with ecchymotic lesions in a young patient with Hermansky-Pudlak syndrome type 4.

while strabismus requires eye patching or surgical correction. Dark glasses are important to protect the eyes and prevent photophobia.

Hermansky–Pudlak syndrome

Introduction and general description
Hermansky–Pudlak syndrome is a rare type of OCA associated with a haemorrhagic diathesis [26,27]. Here too, a molecular classification has now been universally accepted recognising nine clinicogenetic subtypes of the disease (Table 68.1). The disorder is rare except in Puerto Rico.

Pathophysiology
The disease results from abnormal biogenesis of lysosome-related organelles with impaired melanosome maturation and absent dense bodies in thrombocytes [27]. Hermansky–Pudlak syndrome is associated with mutations in nine distinct genes: *HPS1* (type 1) and *HPS4* (type 4) encode components of the BLOC3 lysosomal complex, which is essential for the proper formation of lysosome-related organelles; *AP3B1* (type 2) encodes a subunit of the AP3 complex, which is responsible for mediating protein sorting to lysosomes; *HPS3* (type 3), *HSP5* (type 5) and *HSP6* (type 6) all encode components of BLOC2 and *DTNBP1* (type 7), *BLOC1S3* (type 8), *BLOC1S6* (type 9) and *BLOC1S5* (type 11) encode components of BLOC1 which are all required for proper melanosome maturation [28–33]. Mutation in AP3D1 encoding a subunit of the AP3 adaptor-like complex, involved in trafficking to lysosomes [34].

Clinical features and complications
All subtypes of the syndrome share common clinical manifestations including decreased pigmentation in the eyes, hair and skin, easy bruisability and bleeding tendency, interstitial pulmonary fibrosis and granulomatous colitis (Figure 68.9) [35].

The complications of Hermansky–Pudlak syndrome are secondary to bleeding problems, pulmonary fibrosis and colitis. Prognosis is guarded with a life expectancy of 30–50 years.

Investigations
Absence of dense bodies on whole mount electron microscopy of platelets constitutes a standard diagnostic test. Moreover, upon stimulation of platelets, the dense bodies, which contain adenosine diphosphate (ADP), adenosine triphosphate (ATP), serotonin, calcium and phosphate, release their contents to attract other platelets, which can be tested to screen for Hermansky–Pudlak syndrome [33]. For detection and evaluation of lung fibrosis, pulmonary function tests should be performed on a regular basis in adulthood and computed tomography (CT) scans when necessary. Molecular analysis of the Hermansky–Pudlak syndrome genes helps to confirm the diagnosis and to give appropriate genetic counselling.

Chédiak–Higashi syndrome

Introduction and general description
Chédiak–Higashi syndrome is a rare autosomal recessive disorder characterised by hypopigmentation of the skin and eye, immunodeficiency and possibly neurological symptoms [36].

Pathophysiology and genetics
The disease results from loss-of-function mutations in *CHS1* (*LYST*) encoding a protein known as lysosomal trafficking regulator. The melanocytes contain giant pigment granules which arise by autophagocytosis and defective fission of large melanosomes [37].

Clinical features

The skin is fair, the retinae are pale and the irides translucent. The diagnosis of Chédiak–Higashi syndrome is suspected in individuals with clinical criteria for OCA combined with a significant history of pyogenic infections. Neutropenia is noted. The most reliable diagnostic clinical criterion for Chédiak–Higashi syndrome is the finding of giant inclusions in polymorphonuclear neutrophils. Neurological manifestations (e.g. progressive intellectual decline, cranial nerve palsies, decreased deep tendon reflexes, tremor and abnormal gait, seizures) can appear any time from childhood to early adulthood.

Attenuated forms have been described with genotype–phenotype correlation. Loss-of-function mutations are associated with severe childhood-onset form [38,39]. The accelerated phase corresponding to a haemophagocytic lymphohistiocytosis, occurs in 85% of individuals at any age and can be fatal [40,41].

Of note, the tricho-hepato-enteric syndrome caused by mutations in the *TTC37* gene share diffuse hypopigmentation, platelet defects and immunodeficiency with Chédiak–Higashi syndrome. The presence of brittle hair, liver failure and diarrhoea distinguishes this rare condition (Chapter 66).

Investigations

Peroxidase-positive giant inclusions seen in leukocytes is a first line diagnostic test. Light microscopy of hairs shows pigment clumping.

Management

The only curative treatment available for Chédiak–Higashi syndrome is bone marrow transplantation. A case of complete remission after a combination therapy with rituximab and ciclosporin has been reported [42].

Griscelli–Pruniéras syndrome types I and II

Introduction and general description

Griscelli–Pruniéras syndrome is a rare autosomal recessive disorder that associates hypopigmentation, characterised by a silver-grey sheen of the hair and the presence of large clusters of pigment in the hair shaft, and the occurrence of either a primary neurological impairment or a severe immune disorder.

Pathophysiology and genetics

All genetic alterations associated with Griscelli–Pruniéras syndrome result in defective transport of melanosomes and consequently abnormal accumulation of melanosomes in melanocytes. Griscelli–Pruniéras syndrome type 1 results from mutations in *MYO5A*, encoding myosin 5a [43]. Type 2 disease results from mutations in the *RAB27A* gene whereas type 3 is caused by mutations in *MLPH* encoding melanophilin or by a specific genetic defect in MYO5A [44,45].

Clinical features

In 1978, Griscelli *et al.* described two patients with partial albinism of the hair and skin, frequent pyogenic infections and acute episodes of fever, hepatosplenomegaly, neutropenia and thrombocytopenia [46].

Dermatological findings included pigmentary abnormalities of the hair variably described as silvery grey, silvery, greyish-golden or dusty [47]. Neurological involvement is a prominent feature. Patients with Griscelli–Pruniéras syndrome type 1 have primary central nervous system dysfunction, type 2 patients commonly develop haemophagocytic lymphohistiocytosis and type 3 patients have only partial albinism. The differential diagnosis of the disease in the patient presenting with silvery hair includes primarily the Griscelli–Pruniéras, Chédiak–Higashi, and Elejalde syndromes. Elejalde syndrome is inherited in an autosomal recessive fashion and is characterised by pigment dilution, silvery grey hair and neurological defects [48]. Some authors suggest that the disease may in fact be identical to Griscelli–Pruniéras syndrome type 1 [48].

Patients with Griscelli–Pruniéras syndrome are predisposed to the occurrence of 'accelerated phases' similar to those encountered in Chédiak–Higashi syndrome. Griscelli–Pruniéras syndrome has been successfully treated with bone marrow transplantation.

Oculocerebral syndrome with hypopigmentation (Cross syndrome/Kramer syndrome)

The disorder was initially described in an inbred Amish family and is characterised by generalised hypopigmentation with white/silvery hair, severe mental retardation with spastic tetraplegia and athetosis [49]. Ocular anomalies include microphthalmos, a small opaque cornea and coarse nystagmus.

About 10 cases of Cross syndrome have been described in Amish and Gipsy families and in South Africa. It is an autosomal recessive disorder. The disorder maps to chromosome 3q27.1q29 but the defective gene remains to be identified [50].

Albinism–deafness syndrome (Ziprkowski–Margolis syndrome/Woolf syndrome)

Albinism–deafness syndrome is an X-linked disorder consisting of congenital deafness and partial albinism (without OA) [51,52]. The disease has been mapped to Xq26.3-q27.1 but the causative gene is unknown. [53]. Hypopigmentation has a piebald pattern, but more diffuse. Deafness is of the subtotal sensorineural nerve type.

Hypomelanosis of Ito

In 1952, Ito described the occurrence of a bilateral systematised depigmented naevus in a 22-year-old Japanese woman [54]. Hypomelanosis of Ito is a rare neuroectodermal disorder often associated with mental retardation and epilepsy [55,56]. Prevalence

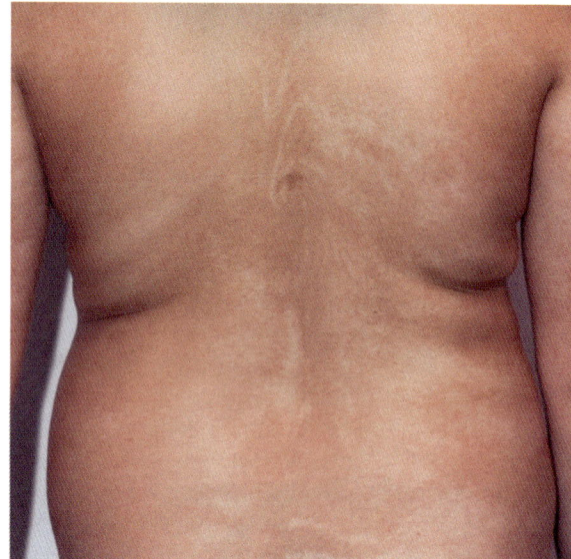

Figure 68.10 Hypomelanosis of Ito.

is unknown but incidence has been estimated between 1/10 000 and 1/8500. The phenotypic presentation is highly variable. The skin abnormalities are characterised by unusual unilateral or bilateral cutaneous macular hypopigmented whorls, streaks and patches, corresponding to the lines of Blaschko (Figure 68.10) [57]. Extracutaneous findings include neurological, ophthalmological and skeletal defects. The skin lesions have to be distinguished from other mosaic depigmented lesions and from focal dermal hypoplasia where the skin shows atrophic changes. Nearly all cases are sporadic suggesting a postzygotic mutation, which is assumed to be lethal when transmitted to offspring. Various chromosomal anomalies have been identified in some patients and the current consensus is that the phenotype of hyper- or hypopigmentation following Blaschko lines is the result of cutaneous mosaicism, either for a monogenic or a chromosomal disorder, rather than being a distinct disease [57–59]. Postzygotic activating mutations in *MTOR* and *RHOA* have been found in patients with complex phenotype including pigmentary mosaicism [60,61].

HYPERPIGMENTATION DISORDERS

Familial progressive hyperpigmentation/progressive hyperpigmentation and generalised lentiginosis without associated systemic symptoms/familial progressive hyper- and hypopigmentation

Familial progressive hyperpigmentation is a very rare autosomal dominant disorder. The disease is characterised by sharply and irregular hyperpigmented patches involving both the mucosae and the skin. These patches are present either at birth or in early infancy and increase in size and number with age.

Familial progressive hyperpigmentation-1 (FPH1) has been mapped to chromosome 19pter-p13.1 [62] whereas familial progressive hyperpigmentation-2 (FPH2; MIM: 145250) is caused by mutation in the *KITLG* gene (MIM: 184745) on chromosome 12q22 [63], which is also associated with the hyper–hypopigmented variant [64].

Incontinentia pigmenti

Definition
Incontinentia pigmenti (IP) is a rare X-linked dominant multisystemic ectodermal dysplasia that is usually lethal in males and presents classically in females with skin lesions, teeth abnormalities, alopecia, nail dystrophy, and ocular and neurological findings [65].

Epidemiology
Birth prevalence is 0.6–0.7/1 000 000. The female to male ratio is 20 : 1.

Pathophysiology and genetics
IP is caused by mutations of the *IKBKG* gene encoding the nuclear factor (NF)-κB essential modulator (NEMO), also known as the inhibitor of the NF-κB kinase subunit gamma (IKK-γ) [66]. NEMO (IKK-γ) is the regulatory subunit of the inhibitor of the I-κB kinase (IKK) complex, which activates NF-κB resulting in activation of genes involved in inflammation, immunity, cell survival and other pathways [67]. IP cells are highly sensitive to tumour necrosis factor-induced apoptosis that could explain the development of skin, retinal and neurological lesions in patients with IP. IP is an X-linked dominant disorder. A recurrent exon 4–10 deletion of the gene underlies 85% of cases. The mutation can be inherited from an affected mother or occur *de novo*. When the mother of an affected female carries the mutant *IKBKG*, the risk to siblings of inheriting the mutant *IKBKG* allele at conception is 50%; most male conceptuses with loss-of-function mutation of *IKBKG* are miscarried. Fertility is normal except for the miscarriage of affected males. Genetic prenatal diagnosis is available [68].

Clinical features
IP cutaneous findings typically present perinatally with a red vesicular rash (bullous stage I; Figure 68.11a) following Blaschko's lines. Stage I evolves within a few months to a verrucous stage II, occurring mainly on the limbs (Figure 68.11b). Stage III hyperpigmented streaks and whorls along Blaschko's lines begin within months and fade in adolescence (Figure 68.11c). Stage I rash can recur during febrile illness. Stage IV patients have pale, hairless, atrophic linear streaks or patches mostly on the lower extremities at adolescence. Extracutaneous abnormalities observed in IP include delayed dentition and missing or malformed cone-shaped teeth (Figure 68.12). Other manifestations include onychodystrophy, alopecia and a wide range of ophthalmological abnormalities with retinal neovascularisation (Figure 68.13). Central nervous system (CNS) abnormalities may comprise microcephaly, seizures and

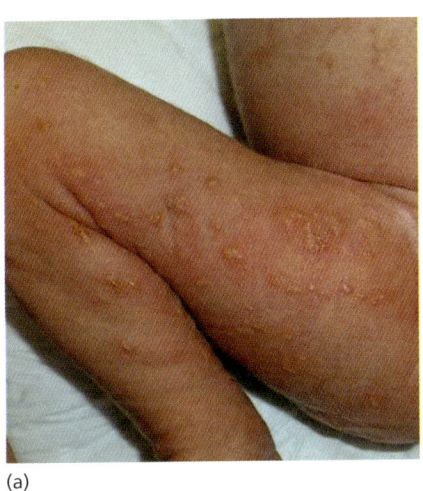
(a)

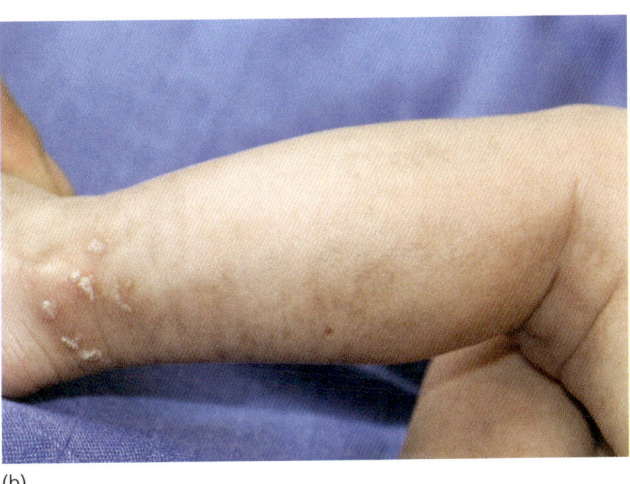
(b)

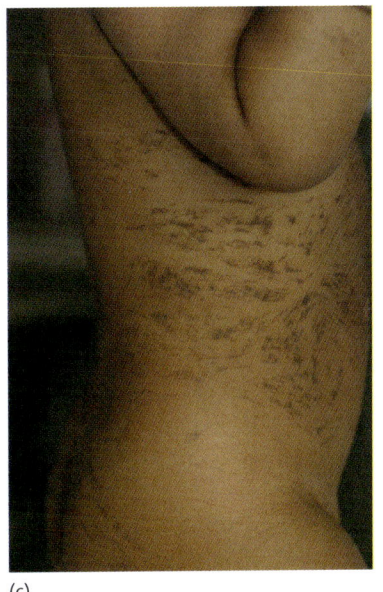
(c)

Figure 68.11 (a) Incontinentia pigmenti, vesiculobullous stage, frequently wrongly diagnosed as bullous impetigo. (b) Verrucous stage. (c) Pigmentary stage, with an obvious linear pattern following Blaschko's lines.

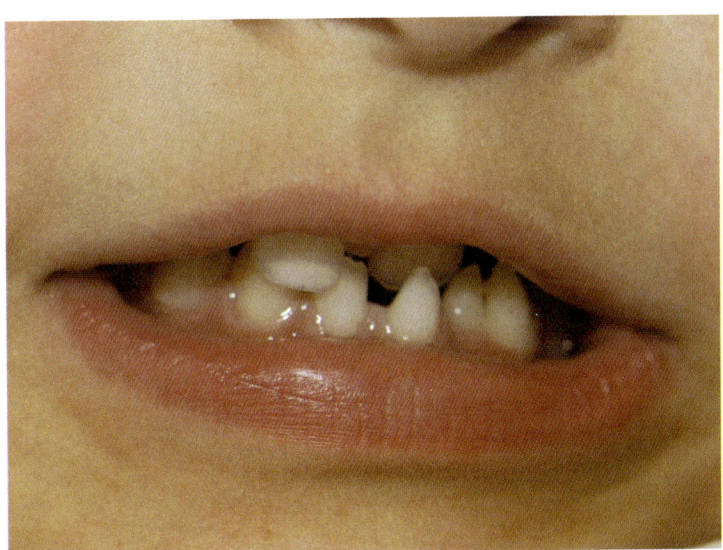

Figure 68.12 Dystrophic teeth in a child with incontinentia pigmenti.

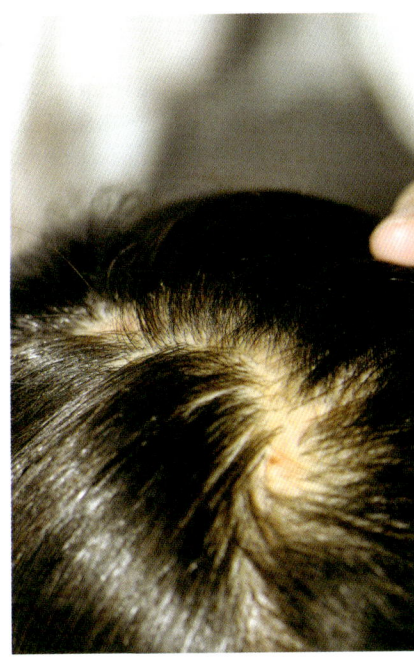

Figure 68.13 Cicatricial alopecia of incontinentia pigmenti.

neurocognitive and motor impairments. The majority (>60%) of patients are neurologically normal [69].

Differential diagnosis

Stage I lesions have to be distinguished from other bullous dermatoses (bullous impetigo, epidermolysis bullosa, herpes or varicella). Differential diagnosis of stage II includes warts or epidermal naevus syndrome. Any condition with 'linear and swirled' pigmentation overlaps with stage III. Stage IV resembles scarring, Ito's hypomelanosis or other hypopigmentary disorders with localised alopecia.

Complications and co-morbidities

Life expectancy is normal. Patients without neonatal CNS abnormalities typically have normal physical and cognitive development.

Management

No specific treatment is available for IP. Symptomatic treatment includes standard management of blisters. Ophthalmological follow-up is required for retinal neovascularisation monitoring and treatment (cryotherapy and laser photocoagulation) and treatment of retinal detachment if it occurs. Dental abnormalities should be managed by a paediatric orthodontist in combination with speech therapy and a paediatric nutrition programme. Patients should be referred to a paediatric neurologist for evaluation if microcephaly, seizures, spasticity or focal deficits are present. Brain magnetic resonance imaging is indicated in any child with functional neurological abnormalities or retinal neovascularisation.

PART 6: GENETIC DISORDERS

Linear and whorled naevoid hypermelanosis

Linear and whorled hypermelanosis (LWNH) is a benign skin condition characterised by the onset in infancy of hyperpigmented regions that follow the lines of Blaschko on the trunk and limbs. The soles, palms, face and mucous membranes are spared. In general, affected individuals have no accompanying extradermal features [70] although the condition has been rarely associated with cardiovascular, neurological and musculoskeletal abnormalities [2]. This phenotype is the reverse of hypomelanosis of Ito (Figure 68.10). Mosaic chromosomal abnormalities have been detected [71]. As stated above for hypomelanosis of Ito, the phenotype of either hyper- or hypopigmentation following Blaschko lines (Figures 68.10 and 68.11) is the result of cutaneous mosaicism, either for a monogenic or a chromosomal disorder, rather than being a distinct disease. *KITLG* mutations in a mosaic state have been associated in LWNH [**72**].

Dyskeratosis congenita

Dyskeratosis congenita (DKC) is a genetically heterogeneous disorder, showing autosomal recessive, autosomal dominant and X-linked inheritance (Table 68.1). DKC is a disease with a highly variable phenotype that is classically defined by reticulated skin pigmentation, nail dystrophy and leukoplakia of the oral mucosa often undergoing malignant transformation (Figure 68.14) [73]. The pigmentary change may be limited to the neck, upper chest and proximal parts of the limbs initially, but within affected areas the involvement is always diffuse. Overall, predisposition to malignancy is an important feature and bone marrow dysplasia, haematological and epithelial malignancies are frequent complications [74]. The disease is caused by mutations in multiple genes coding for proteins involved in telomere function and maintenance [**75**].

Differential diagnosis includes Fanconi anaemia, a clinically and genetically heterogeneous disorder that causes genomic instability. Fanconi anaemia is also sometimes associated with pigmentation anomalies including reticulated pigmentation and café-au-lait spots. The diagnosis is based mostly on haematological anomalies, especially pancytopenia and there is an increased risk of neoplasia [76].

Naegeli–Franceschetti–Jadassohn syndrome and dermatopathia pigmentosa reticularis

These two diseases are closely related autosomal dominant ectodermal dysplasia syndromes that are both caused by mutations specifically located at the start of the *KRT14* gene sequence [77]. These mutations result in haploinsufficiency for keratin 14 and

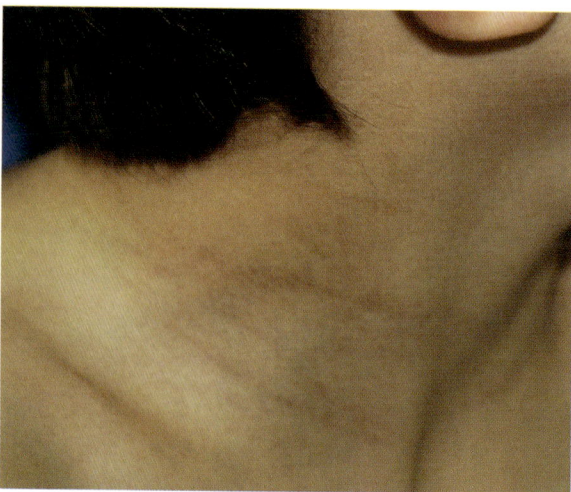

(a)

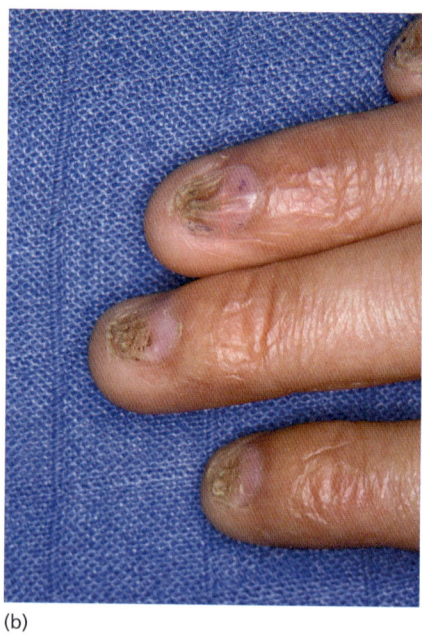

(b)

Figure 68.14 (a) Pigmentation of the neck associated with (b) dystrophic nails in a patient with dyskeratosis congenita.

are associated with increased susceptibility of keratinocytes to proapoptotic stimuli [78].

The cardinal features of Naegeli–Franceschetti–Jadassohn syndrome are reticular cutaneous pigmentation (Figure 68.15) starting in early life without a preceding inflammatory stage, discomfort provoked by heat with diminished sweat gland function, poor teeth and moderate hyperkeratosis of the palms and soles [79]. Males and females are equally affected. In dermatopathia pigmentosa reticularis, cutaneous findings include reticulate hyperpigmentation, non-cicatricial alopecia and onychodystrophy. These two diseases clinically share complete absence of dermatoglyphics, a reticulate pattern of skin hyperpigmentation mainly involving the trunk and face, palmoplantar keratoderma, abnormal sweating and other subtle developmental anomalies including plantar bullae in early childhood, dental anomalies and nail dystrophy.

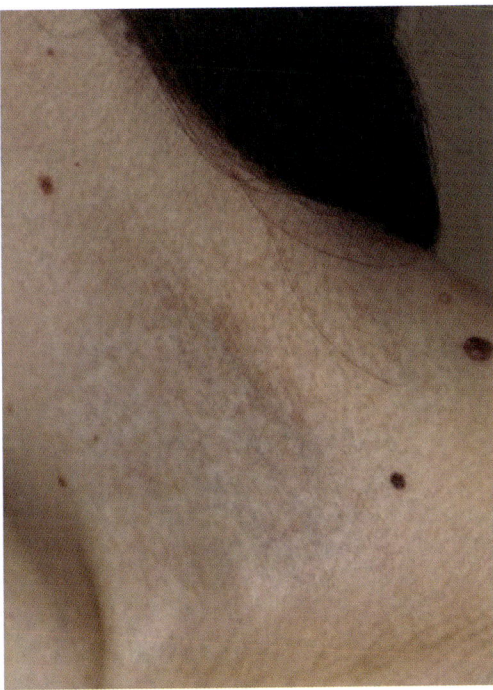

Figure 68.15 Naegeli–Franceschetti–Jadassohn syndrome: case of the original family. Courtesy of P. Itin.

Dowling–Degos disease

Dowling–Degos disease is an autosomal dominant form of reticulate pigmentary genodermatosis with variable penetrance that was first described by Dowling and Freudenthal [80]. The reticulate pigmentation usually has a flexural distribution. Comedo-like lesions on the neck and pitted perioral acneform scars and genital and perianal reticulated pigmented lesions have also been described (Figure 68.16) [81,82]. Onset is usually postpubertal and the reticulate hyperpigmentation is progressive and disfiguring. No abnormalities of the hair or nails have been reported. Generalised Dowling–Degos disease can also occur, with numerous hyperpigmented or red macules and papules on the neck, chest and abdomen [5]. Histopathology from pigmented lesions discloses characteristic thin branch-like patterns of epidermal downgrowth.

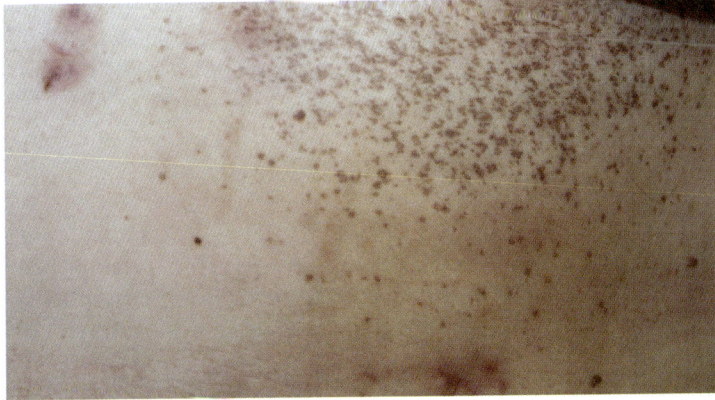

Figure 68.16 Dowling–Degos disease.

At least, four genes have been shown to be associated with Dowling–Degos disease. Flexural Dowling–Degos disease was found to be caused by loss of function mutations affecting the *KRT5* gene region encoding the initial part of keratin 5 [81]. Galli–Galli disease, which features acantholysis on histology in addition to clinical and histological signs of Dowling–Degos disease, was also shown to result from mutations in *KRT5* [83]. Generalised Dowling–Degos disease was found to be associated with mutations in *POFUT1*, which encodes protein O-fucosyltransferase 1 and in *POGLUT1*, which encodes protein O-glucosyltransferase 1 [84,85]. Knockdown of *POFUT1* was shown to reduce the expression of KRT5 in keratinocytes [84]. Mutations in PSENEN are responsible for a subtype of DDD associated with an increased susceptibility to acne inversa in the presence of particular risk factors [86]. POGLUT1, POFUT1 and PSENEN are regulators of Notch activity [87].

Reticulate acropigmentation of Kitamura

Reticulate acropigmentation of Kitamura (RAK) is a rare pigmentary disorder that has an autosomal dominant pattern of inheritance. Typical features include reticulate hyperpigmented atrophic macules on the dorsa of the hands (Figure 68.17) and 'pits' on the palms and soles in the first or second decade of life [88,89]. The macules gradually darken and tend to spread to the proximal regions of the extremities with progression of the eruptions that stops in middle age. Histopathologically, the pigmented lesions show pigmentation in the tip of rete ridges with thinning of the epidermis, elongation and thinning of the rete ridges, and slight hyperkeratosis without parakeratosis [90]. RAK was found to be caused by mutations in *ADAM10* [91].

Peutz–Jeghers–Touraine syndrome

Peutz–Jeghers–Touraine (PJT) syndrome is a rare but very distinctive lentiginosis syndrome with an autosomal dominant pattern of inheritance. Typical cutaneous features include lentigines of the lips of early onset (Figure 68.18). Associated melanocytic macules of buccal mucosa and digits are common.

Non-cutaneous features are dominated by hamartomatous polyps, which may occur in any part of the gastrointestinal tract but more consistently in the jejunum. They may lead to intussusception and bleeding. Malignant degeneration of the small intestinal polyps is rare [92]. Other polyps have been described in the kidney pelvis, ureter, bladder, bronchus and nose. Among non-gastrointestinal associated tumours in PJT syndrome, granulosa cell ovarian tumours are the most distinctive, but other malignant tumours (especially breast and pancreas) have been described [93].

Histologically, the oral mucosal lesions resemble lentigo simplex. In acral lesions there is an increased number of melanocytes with long dendrites filled with melanosomes, but few melanosomes in keratocytes, suggesting a pigment block [94]. Gastrointestinal hamartomas in PJT syndrome are distinct from those of other

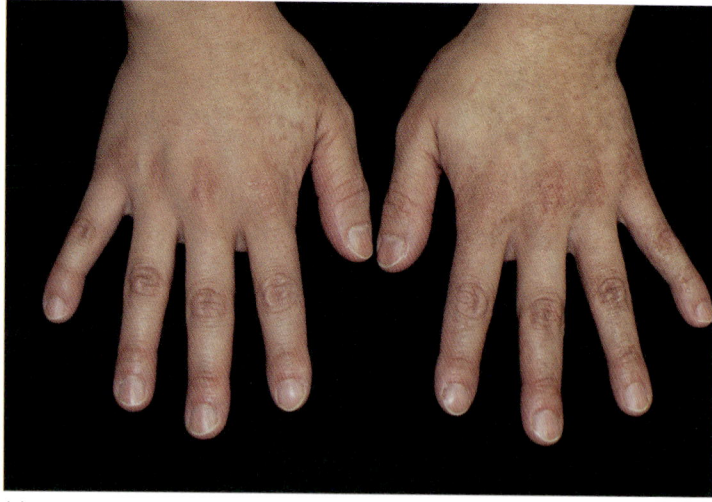

(a)

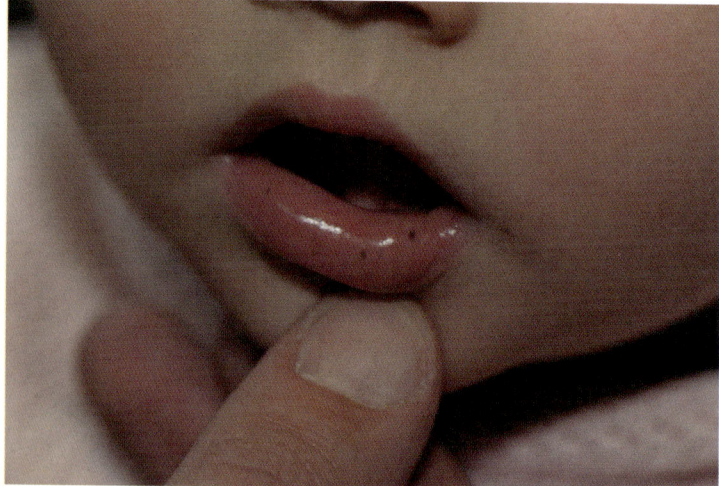

Figure 68.18 Peutz–Jeghers–Touraine syndrome. Lentigines on the lower lip of a 2-year-old girl.

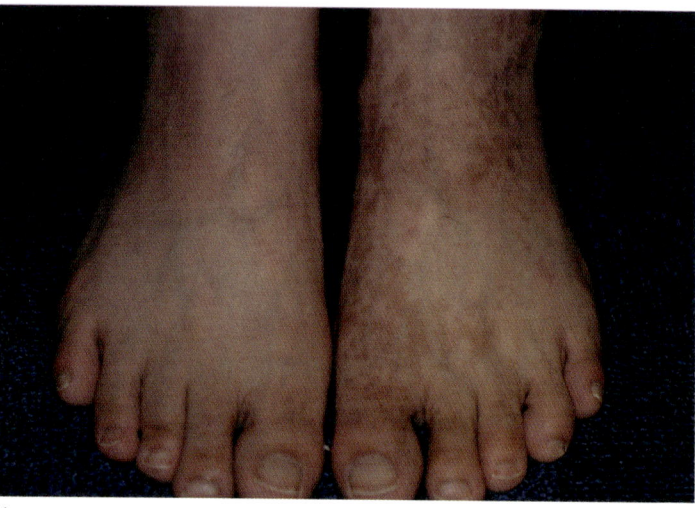

(b)

Figure 68.17 (a,b) Reticulate hyperpigmentation of Kitamura. Molecular diagnosis was confirmatory. Courtesy of Dr H. Ujiie and Professor H. Shimizu.

types and show an elongated, frond-like epithelium with cystic dilatation of glands overlying an arborising network of smooth muscle bundles [92]. The disorder is due to mutations in the serine/threonine kinase (*STK11*) gene [95]. Mutations in the part of the gene involved in ATP binding and catalysis are rarely associated with cancer, whereas mutations in the part of the gene involved in substrate recognition are more frequently associated with malignancies. Patients with PJT syndrome with breast cancers have predominantly truncating mutations [96].

DYSCHROMATOSES

Dyschromatosis symmetrica hereditaria

Dyschromatosis symmetrica hereditaria (DSH) – also called symmetrical dyschromatosis of the extremities and symmetrical or

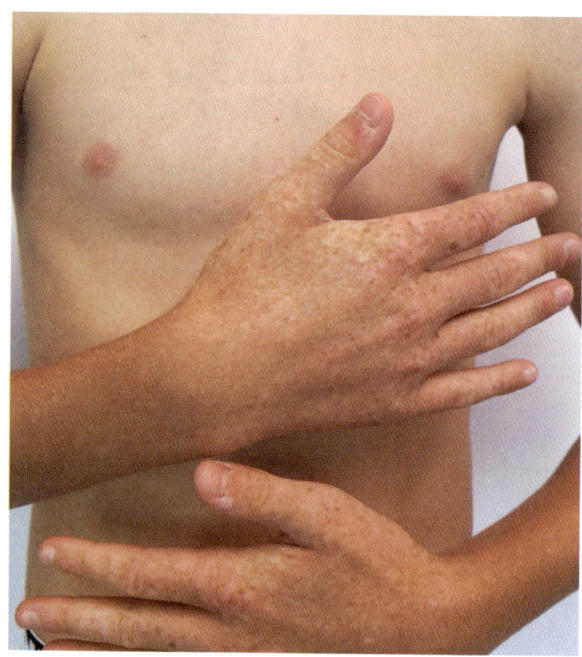

Figure 68.19 Dyschromatosis symmetrica hereditaria. Molecular diagnosis was confirmatory.

reticulate acropigmentation of Dohi [90] – is characterised by freckle-like pigmented macules on the face associated with small hyper- and hypopigmented macules affecting the back of the hands and feet (Figure 68.19). The condition usually begins in early childhood and has been predominantly reported in Japanese and Chinese individuals. The prevalence of DSH in the Japanese population is estimated to be 1.5 per 100 000 [97].

Dyschromatosis symmetrica hereditaria has a dominant pattern of inheritance and is caused by a heterozygous mutation in the *ADAR1* gene (adenosine deaminase acting on RNA1) located on chromosome 1q21 [97]. ADAR1 mediates a post-transcriptional modification of the messenger RNA known as RNA editing. Miyamura *et al.* postulated that impaired RNA editing during melanoblast migration causes their differentiation into either

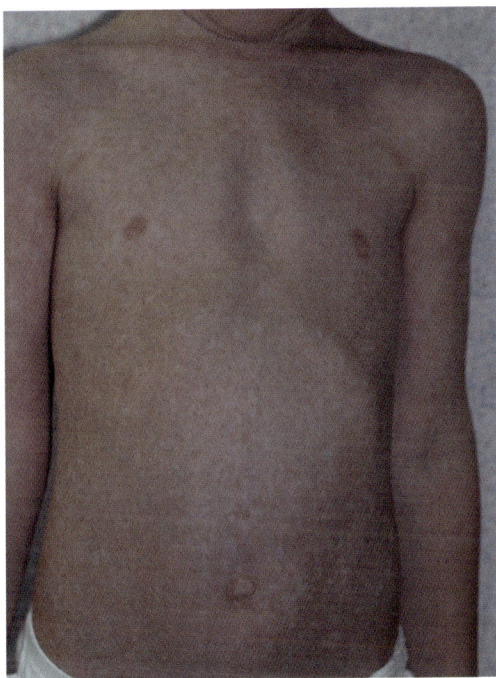

Figure 68.20 Dyschromatosis universalis hereditaria.

hyper- or hypoactive melanocytes and that the most affected melanocytes are those that migrate farthest, to the extremities, i.e. the hands and feet [98].

Dyschromatosis universalis hereditaria

Dyschromatosis universalis hereditaria (DUH) is a rare autosomal genodermatosis characterised by hyper- and hypopigmented macules distributed over the entire surface of the skin (Figure 68.20). The lesions usually appear in infancy or early childhood. Involvement of the palms or soles is unusual. Abnormalities of the hair and nails have also been reported. Also, DUH has been associated with neurological, ophthalmological and haematological complications [99].

There is now evidence for genetic heterogeneity in DUH. Heterozygous mutations in *SASH1* have associated with DUH1 [99,100], DUH2 maps to chromosome 12q21-q23a [99] and DUH3 is caused by mutation in the *ABCB6* gene on chromosome 2q35 [102].

Key references

The full list of references can be found in the online version at https://www.wiley.com/rooksdermatology10e

5 Tomita Y, Suzuki T. Genetics of pigmentary disorders. *Am J Med Genet C Semin Med Genet* 2004;131C:75–81.

6 Kubic JD, Young KP, Plummer RS, Ludvik AE, Lang D. Pigmentation PAX-ways: the role of Pax3 in melanogenesis, melanocyte stem cell maintenance, and disease. *Pigment Cell Melanoma Res* 2008;21:627–45.

25 Kruijt CC, de Wit GC, Bergen AA, Florijn RJ, Schalij-Delfos NE, van Genderen MM. The phenotypic spectrum of albinism. *Ophthalmology* 2018;125:1953–60.

27 Wei A-H, Li W. Hermansky–Pudlak syndrome: pigmentary and non-pigmentary defects and their pathogenesis. *Pigment Cell Melanoma Res* 2013;26:176–92.

57 Nehal KS, PeBenito R, Orlow SJ. Analysis of 54 cases of hypopigmentation and hyperpigmentation along the lines of Blaschko. *Arch Dermatol* 1996;132:1167–70.

67 Smahi A, Courtois G, Rabia SH *et al*. The NF-kappaB signalling pathway in human diseases: from incontinentia pigmenti to ectodermal dysplasias and immune-deficiency syndromes. *Hum Mol Genet* 2002;11:2371–5.

72 Sorlin A, Maruani A, Aubriot-Lorton M-H *et al*. Mosaicism for a KITLG mutation in linear and whorled nevoid hypermelanosis. *J Invest Dermatol* 2017;137: 1575–8.

75 Nelson ND, Bertuch AA. Dyskeratosis congenita as a disorder of telomere maintenance. *Mutat Res* 2012;730:43–51.

78 Lugassy J, Itin P, Ishida-Yamamoto A *et al*. Naegeli–Franceschetti–Jadassohn syndrome and dermatopathia pigmentosa reticularis: two allelic ectodermal dysplasias caused by dominant mutations in KRT14. *Am J Hum Genet* 2006;79:724–30.

99 Zhang J, Li M, Yao Z. Updated review of genetic reticulate pigmentary disorders. *Br J Dermatol* 2017;177:945–59.

CHAPTER 69

Genetic Blistering Diseases

John A. McGrath

St John's Institute of Dermatology, School of Basic and Medical Biosciences, Faculty of Life Sciences and Medicine, King's College London, London, UK

PART 6: GENETIC DISORDERS

Introduction

Inherited blistering skin disorders are uncommon but often have a dramatic impact on the patient and their family, as well as severe economic consequences for individuals and health services. These rare diseases have been the subject of intensive study in recent years, initially with a focus on trying to identify causative genes and mutations, but more recently considerable activity has centred on translational work, developing new clinical services such as multidisciplinary clinics and prenatal diagnosis, as well as generating disease models and research that lead to clinical trials and the possibility of disease-modifying interventions and improvement in symptoms. Inherited blistering skin disorders are clinically and genetically heterogeneous and classification tends to undergo periodic revisions as new discoveries are made and disease nomenclature is updated. The term epidermolysis bullosa (EB) is sometimes used to encompass the spectrum of inherited blistering skin diseases, although precisely which disorders should be included within the classification of EB continues to be debated and changed by international consensus, especially with the discovery of new candidate genes and disease entities in which inherited skin or mucosal fragility can be a major or minor clinical feature. Deciphering the molecular basis of EB (and related disorders) is fundamental to improving our understanding of inherited blistering skin diseases, although it is important to maintain a practical and clinically useful framework to assist

Rook's Textbook of Dermatology, Tenth Edition. Edited by Christopher Griffiths, Jonathan Barker, Tanya Bleiker, Walayat Hussain and Rosalind Simpson.
© 2024 John Wiley & Sons Ltd. Published 2024 by John Wiley & Sons Ltd.

dermatologists and other health care personnel in providing best care for patients [1].

Definition and classification

EB comprises a group of genetically determined skin fragility disorders characterised by blistering of the skin and mucosae following mild mechanical trauma. The alternative term therefore is *mechanobullous diseases*. The descriptive term *epidermolysis* is somewhat illogical because epidermal disruption is not the primary change in several categories of EB. Nevertheless, the name *epidermolysis bullosa*, as originally used by Koebner [1] in 1886, is now so well established in the literature that it remains the preferred term. Classification of EB, however, is difficult and not helped by the large variety of names and eponyms that have traditionally been used. Initial classification schemes were based largely on the mode of inheritance and clinical studies involving relatively few patients and families. While these early observations were clearly important in establishing EB as an entity, a major step forward was made by Pearson [2] in the 1960s who used transmission electron microscopy to show that the ultrastructural level of tissue cleavage (blister formation) in the skin is distinctive in the three major groups: EB simplex, junctional EB and dystrophic EB. In addition to defining specific levels of blistering in the different subtypes of EB, ultrastructural studies were also able to identify distinct morphological abnormalities such as keratin filament disruption in EB simplex, poorly formed hemidesmosomes in junctional EB, and rudimentary anchoring fibrils in dystrophic EB. During the 1980s, the immunohistochemical labelling of EB skin with basement membrane zone antibodies became a useful diagnostic addition, for example showing reduced immunostaining for proteins such as laminin 332 in some forms of junctional EB and type VII collagen in recessive dystrophic EB, respectively. Then in the 1990s, the discovery of candidate genes and pathogenic mutations, such as mutations in *KRT14* in EB simplex (keratin 14) and *COL7A1* in dystrophic EB (type VII collagen), heralded the era of molecular diagnostics. Subsequent advances in next generation sequencing have led to the identification of further skin fragility genes, including *EXPH5* (exophilin-5), *DST* (bullous pemphigoid antigen 230, the epithelial isoform of dystonin), *KLHL24* (Kelch-like family member 24) in EB simplex and *ITGA3* (α3 integrin subunit) in junctional EB. Originally viewed as a disorder of blistering at or close to the dermal–epidermal junction, the protean variants of EB now include both classic forms and other skin fragility disorders (Figure 69.1); the major classic subtypes of EB are listed in Table 69.1 and the related disorders are shown in Table 69.2.

This plethora of discoveries has had an impact on the diagnostic classification of EB and left dermatologists wondering whether to favour a classification based on phenotype, skin pathology or gene mutations – or a combination thereof. Mindful of that dilemma, over the last two decades an international consensus group has met on a number of occasions to review and revise the classification of EB. Their most recent guidelines were published in October 2020 [3]. There has been a trend to eliminate use of historical eponyms and instead to use straightforward terms that refer to the extent of disease and severity.

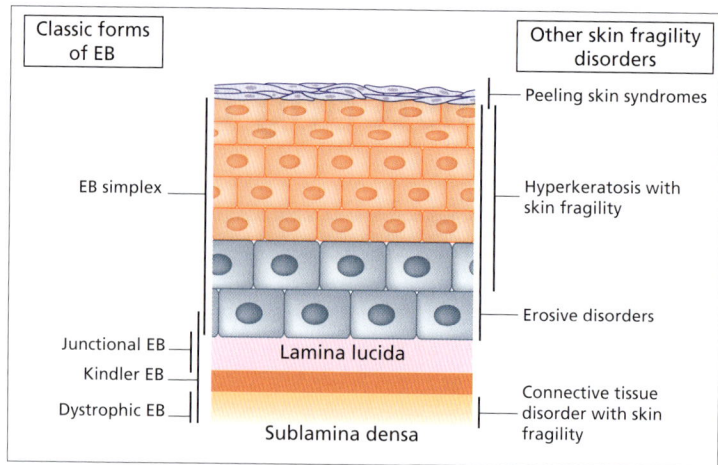

Figure 69.1 Epidermis and basement membrane illustrating the different levels where blisters occur in classic subtypes of epidermolysis bullosa (EB) as other types of skin fragility that are within the broader classification of EB.

Prevalence and incidence

The most accurate data available on the incidence and prevalence of EB are derived from the National EB Registry (USA) project, a longitudinal study of approximately 3300 patients in the USA [1]. The incidence and prevalence of EB are estimated to be 19.60 per million live births and 8.22 per million population, respectively. Similarly, the incidence and prevalence rates for EB simplex are 10.75 and 4.60; junctional EB 2.04 and 0.44; dominant dystrophic EB 2.86 and 0.99; and recessive dystrophic EB 2.04 and 0.92, respectively. In other parts of the world, where consanguinity rates are higher, the prevalence of EB may be three to four times higher for autosomal recessive forms of EB, with further differences in disease subtypes and epidemiology [2,3]. It should be remembered, however, that all reported rates probably underestimate the true prevalence and incidence of EB, especially the clinically milder forms, because of recruitment or selection bias.

Skin proteins and genes implicated in classic epidermolysis bullosa

Currently, 16 different genes have been shown to harbour mutations germane to the pathogenesis of classic forms of EB (Figure 69.2). These genes encode proteins involved in the structural adhesion of cell–matrix junctions as well as keratinocyte integrity. Understanding the function and tissue distribution of these proteins provides a useful platform for understanding the clinicopathological basis of the protean forms of EB. With increasing understanding of the molecular pathology of EB, it is feasible that future classifications of this group of disorders will be based on the nature of the gene/protein relevant to a particular case, and thus an overview of the relevant proteins is presented here before the clinical variants of EB are described.

Keratins 5 and 14: *KRT5, KRT14*

Keratins are the most abundant structural proteins in the cytoplasm of epithelial cells, forming a network of 10 nm diameter intermediate filaments [1]. The keratin filament network helps

Table 69.1 Classification of classic epidermolysis bullosa (EB).

Level of skin cleavage	EB type	Inheritance	Mutated gene(s)	Targeted protein(s)
Intraepidermal	EB simplex	Autosomal dominant	KRTS, KRT14	Keratin 5, keratin 14
			PLEC	Plectin
			KLHL24	Kelch-like member 24
		Autosomal recessive	KRTS, KRT14	Keratin 5, keratin 14
			DST	Bullous pemphigoid antigen 230 (BP230) (syn. BPAG1e, dystonin)
			EXPHS (syn. SLAC2B)	Exophilin-5 (syn. synaptotagmin-like protein homolog lacking C2 domains b, Slac2-b)
			PLEC	Plectin
			CD1S1 (syn. TSPAN24)	CD151 antigen (syn. tetraspanin 24)
Junctional	Junctional EB	Autosomal recessive	LAMA3, LAMB3, LAMBC2	Laminin 332
			COL17A1	Type XVII collagen
			ITGA6, ITGB4	Integrin α6β4
			ITGA3	Integrin α3 submit
Dermal	Dystrophic EB	Autosomal dominant	COL7A1	Type VII collagen
		Autosomal recessive	COL7A1	Type VII collagen
Mixed	Kindler EB	Autosomal recessive	FERMT1 (syn. KIND1)	Fermitin family homologue 1 (syn. kindlin-1)

Reproduced from Has *et al.* [3] with permission from Wiley.

Table 69.2 Other forms of inherited skin fragility disorders within the classification of EB.

Level of skin cleavage	Disorder name	Inheritance	Mutated gene(s)	Targeted protein(s)
Peeling skin disorders				
Intraepidermal	Peeling skin disorders	Autosomal recessive	TGMS	Transglutaminase 5
			CSTA	Cystatin A
			CTSB	Cathepsin B
			SERPINB8	Serpin family B member 8
			FLG2	Filaggrin 2
			CDSN	Corneodesmosin
			CAST	Calpastatin
			DSG1[a]	Desmoglein 1
			SPINKS	LEKTI
Erosive disorders				
Intraepidermal	Erosive skin fragility disorders	Autosomal recessive	DSP	Desmoplakin
			JUP	Plakoglobin
			PKP1	Plakophilin 1
			DSC3	Desmocollin 3
			DSG3	Desmoglein 3
Hyperkeratotic disorders with skin fragility				
Intraepidermal	Keratinopathic ichthyoses	Autosomal dominant	KRT1, KRT10, KRT2	Keratin 1, 10, 2
		Autosomal recessive	KRT10	Keratin 10
Intraepidermal	Pachyonychia congenita	Autosomal dominant	KRT6A, KRT6B, KRT6C, KRT16, KRT17	Keratin 6A, 6B, 6C, 16, 17
Connective tissue disorder with skin fragility				
Dermal	Syndromic connective tissue disorder with skin fragility	Autosomal recessive	PLOD3	Lysyl hydroxylase 3

[a] Also hyperkeratotic features.
Reproduced from Has *et al.* [3] with permission from Wiley.

maintain the shape of keratinocytes by providing both structural stability and flexibility. Many keratin isoforms exist, with keratin 5 and 14 representing the major keratins in basal keratinocytes. Autosomal dominant mutations in *KRT5* or *KRT14* result in disruption to keratin tonofilament assembly and function [2], and underlie the most common EB subtype, localised EB simplex, a condition affecting *c*.8000 people in the UK and close to 400 000 worldwide. EB simplex usually results in minor blistering that is typically worse in the summer months and that does not result in scarring. There are several other clinical variants of EB simplex that also result from *KRT5* or *KRT14* mutations; most of these are dominant but semidominant and autosomal recessive keratin mutations have been reported [3–5].

Kelch-like family member 24: *KLHL24*
KLHL24 is part of the family of more than 40 genes with a Kelch-like motif that forms part of a ubiquitin-ligase complex [1]. First reported in 2016, autosomal dominant mutations in *KLHL24* have been

PART 6: GENETIC DISORDERS

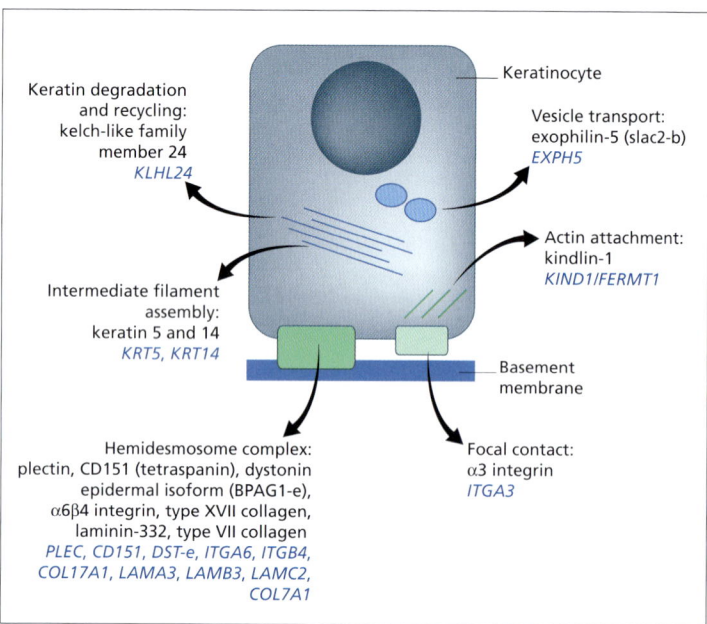

Figure 69.2 The collection of proteins involved in the pathogenesis of classic forms of epidermolysis bullosa. The genes encoding these proteins are indicated in blue text.

reported in >40 families worldwide [2,3]. All mutations detected thus far reside within the methionine initiation codon which leads to adoption of a downstream methionine to initiate transcription and consequently truncation of the protein by 28 amino acids. The truncated protein is more stable than wild-type protein and it promotes excessive ubiquitination and degradation of keratin 14. Intermediate filaments become irregular and fragmented leading to a variant of EB simplex with cleavage through the lower pole of basal keratinocytes. KLHL24 is ubiquitously expressed and in addition to skin fragility, individuals with *KLHL24* mutations have an increased risk of developing cardiomyopathy [4].

CD151 antigen/tetraspanin: *CD151*

CD151 is a cell surface protein which in skin is expressed on the basolateral surface of basal keratinocytes concentrated within the hemidesmosomes [1]. It contributes to cell adhesion, motility and intracellular vesicular transport of integrins. CD151 is also thought to be important for signal transduction and cytoskeleton formation due to its association with phosphatidylinositol-4-kinase. A previous report described two teenage siblings with hereditary nephritis, EB and β-thalassaemia minor [2]. Both showed multiple recurrent infected skin blisters of the lower limbs followed by atrophy, nail dystrophy, bilateral lacrimal duct stenosis, sensorineural deafness, proteinuria and anaemia. These siblings, and one other individual, were subsequently shown to be homozygous for a 1 bp insertion in *CD151*. Identification of a further individual with bi-allelic *CD151* mutations has led to inclusion of *CD151* as a listed gene for a classic form of autosomal recessive EB simplex, although skin fragility is only a minor part of the phenotype [3].

Exophilin-5: *EXPH5*

A consanguineous pedigree has been reported with minor trauma-induced skin scaling/crusting and intermittent skin blistering associated with mottled dyspigmentation [1]. Whole exome sequencing was used to identify a homozygous loss-of-function mutation in *EXPH5* which encodes exophilin-5, also known as Slac2-b. *EXPH5* is an effector protein of Rab GTPase Rab27B, which is thought to have an important role in intracellular vesicle trafficking along actin and tubulin networks, as well as in the transfer of vesicles to cell membranes [2]. Patients with this condition demonstrate a loss of exophilin-5 immunostaining, disrupted keratinocyte adhesion within the lower epidermis and increased numbers of perinuclear vesicles. This form of inherited skin fragility has been classified as an autosomal recessive form of classic EB simplex.

Plectin: *PLEC*

Plectin is an epidermal plakin protein, also found within the Z-lines of striated muscle [1]. Although present throughout much of the epidermis, in basal keratinocytes it plays a key role in linking the keratin filament network to hemidesmosomes at the plasma cell membrane. Autosomal recessive mutations in *PLEC* cause EB simplex associated with muscular dystrophy, which manifests as relatively minor skin blistering and progressive muscle weakness [2]. Autosomal recessive mutations in *PLEC* can also cause skin blistering with pyloric atresia, or, occasionally, both manifestations. Autosomal dominant mutations in plectin may also occur in other forms of EB simplex; these cases do not usually have extracutaneous features. Mutations in *PLEC* are a common but underrecognised cause of EB simplex, accounting for almost one-tenth of all cases [3].

Dystonin epidermal isoform (BP230): *DST*

Autosomal recessive mutations in the epidermal isoform of dystonin, also known as the 230 kDa bullous pemphigoid antigen (BP230), have been shown to result in a relatively mild form of inherited skin blistering [1]. Loss-of-function mutations on both alleles of the epidermal isoform of *DST* lead to a complete absence of the hemidesmosomal inner plaques – the sites at which keratin intermediate filaments anchor to the hemidesmosomes. It is therefore perhaps somewhat surprising that the clinical blistering is relatively trivial. In part, this can be accounted for by a compensatory upregulation in keratin 14 and plectin [2]. Pathogenic mutations are usually sited within the coiled-coil rod domain or within the intermediate filament binding domain. Although dystonin isoforms have a wide tissue distribution, neurological or cardiac involvement does not appear to be a clinical feature of the subtype classified as an autosomal recessive form of EB simplex.

α6β4 integrin: *ITGA6, ITGB4*

Integrins represent a family of cell adhesion receptors that have important roles in ligand binding and signalling; the α6β4 integrin is involved in hemidesmosome assembly and in epithelial–mesenchymal signalling [1]. Mutations in *ITGA6* or *ITGB4* (that encode the α6 and β4 integrin subunits, respectively) have been shown to result in autosomal recessive junctional EB associated with pyloric atresia [2]. The clinical severity of both the skin fragility and degree of gastric outflow obstruction in this condition can vary but surgical correction of the pylorus is usually required. More severe forms of the disease usually result from loss-of-function mutations on both alleles of *ITGA6* or *ITGB4*, although missense mutations in certain critical cysteine residues may also have devastating clinical consequences [2]. Other missense mutations can result in different forms of intermediate junctional EB.

α3 integrin subunit: *ITGA3*

The α3 integrin subunit is a component of focal contacts at the dermal–epidermal junction, where it may dimerise with β1 integrin and contribute to epithelial–mesenchymal signalling [1]. Autosomal recessive loss-of-function mutations have been reported in association with trauma-induced skin fragility [2], but affected individuals also displayed more striking clinical pathology with pulmonary inflammation and congenital nephrotic syndrome, reflecting the important role of α3 integrin in lung and kidney biology. The clinical disorder is sometimes referred to as interstitial lung disease, nephrotic syndrome and EB (ILNEB). Although initial reports indicated early demise because of lung/kidney disease, it is evident that *ITGA3* mutations may result in varying involvement of the key organs with different prognoses [3].

Kindlin-1: *KIND1/FERMT1*

Kindlin-1 is a component of different cell–matrix complexes at the dermal–epidermal junction – focal contacts, which are important in cell migration [1]. Kindlin-1, which is also known as fermitin family homologue-1, is associated with anchorage of the actin cytoskeleton to focal contacts and the formation of a signalling platform via β1 integrin. Autosomal recessive mutations in *KIND1/FERMT1* result in Kindler EB, a blistering genodermatosis that may resemble dystrophic EB in early life [2]. With increasing age, the blistering often diminishes and new features develop: photosensitivity and poikiloderma (a combination of hyperpigmentation, hypopigmentation, telangiectases and skin atrophy), which are most evident in sun-exposed areas. Individuals with Kindler EB may also have an increased risk of cutaneous malignancy (squamous cell carcinoma).

Type XVII collagen: *COL17A1*

Type XVII collagen, also known as the 180 kDa bullous pemphigoid antigen, is a transmembranous protein located within the hemidesmosome and lamina lucida [1]. It is the antigenic target in the autoimmune blistering disease bullous pemphigoid, but loss-of-function mutations on both alleles result in intermediate junctional EB (previously known as non-Herlitz or generalised atrophic benign EB) [2]. The finding that a complete loss of type XVII collagen results in a less severe blistering disease than complete loss of laminin 332 provides some physiological insight into the respective contributions of these two proteins in normal epidermal–dermal adhesion [2]. Some dominant missense mutations in type XVII collagen may result in defective dental enamel and occasionally skin fragility, but most pathogenic mutations in *COL17A1* are autosomal recessive.

Laminin-332: *LAMA3, LAMB3, LAMC2*

Laminin-332, previously known as laminin-5, is a heterotrimeric protein consisting of α3, β3 and γ2 laminin polypeptide chains located within the lamina lucida/lamina densa of the epidermal basement membrane [1]. Autosomal recessive mutations affecting both alleles of any of the three genes can give rise to severe, intermediate or more localised forms of junctional EB. Severe disease (previously known as Herlitz junctional EB) is the most devastating form of EB, often resulting in widespread mucocutaneous fragility and a poor prognosis, with most affected individuals not surviving beyond infancy [1]. Clinically less severe forms of junctional EB are usually associated with mutations that allow for some residual functional laminin-332 protein. Mutations in the *LAMA3A* isoform of the *LAMA3* gene are associated with a form of junctional EB known as laryngo-onycho-cutaneous syndrome, in which excessive granulation tissue can develop leading to laryngeal obstruction and blindness [2].

Type VII collagen: *COL7A1*

Type VII collagen is the major component of anchoring fibrils [1]. These adhesion complexes insert into the dermal side of the lamina densa and are traversed by dermal collagen fibres to provide adhesion between the epidermis and dermis. Mutations in *COL7A1* underlie both autosomal dominant and autosomal recessive forms of dystrophic EB. Typically, loss-of-function mutations on both alleles of *COL7A1* underlie the severe forms of recessive dystrophic EB, where affected individuals develop widespread trauma-induced blistering [2]. Poor wound healing results in chronic wounds, mutilating scar formation and an increased incidence of early, aggressive cutaneous malignancy. However, there is a spectrum of clinical severity in recessive dystrophic EB with some less disruptive mutations giving rise to milder phenotypes. Dominant dystrophic EB is usually clinically less severe than recessive disease and most cases result from heterozygous missense mutations within the type VII collagen triple helix.

Other proteins and genes linked to skin fragility

In addition to the above proteins and genes that are currently implicated in the classic forms of EB, a number of other genetic disorders associated with skin fragility have also been described. Whether these proteins/genes and clinical entities all should be included in the classification of EB is much debated and currently not resolved, but they all feature in the latest umbrella classification [1] and are therefore detailed in this chapter.

Transglutaminase 5: *TGM5*

Autosomal recessive mutations in *TGM5* have been shown to underlie acral peeling skin syndrome [1]. Transglutaminase 5 is one of eight different transglutaminase enzymes expressed in the skin and has a distinct role in the formation of the cornified cell envelope [2]. In acral peeling skin syndrome, the level of blister formation occurs above the granular layer, just below the stratum corneum. However, given the increased thickness of the stratum corneum in the palms and soles relative to other body sites, the clinical appearances often resemble the most common form of localised EB simplex and indeed may cause some clinical confusion [2]. Acral peeling skin associated with *TGM5* mutations may be more common than is currently appreciated since up to 1.5% of individuals in some populations, particularly in northern Europe, may be carriers of a common mutant ancestral allele.

Cystatin A: *CSTA*

Cystatin A (also known as stefin A) is a protease inhibitor which targets papain-like lysosomal cysteine proteases, such as cathepsins B, H and L [1]. Cystatin A mainly has an intracellular localisation but is also detectable in sweat and in the medium of cultured keratinocytes. Loss-of-function mutations in *CSTA* result in autosomal recessive exfoliative ichthyosis [2], although the phenotype is sometimes also referred to as acral peeling skin syndrome, other cases of which are caused by mutations in *TGM5*. Dysadhesion occurs within the basal and lower spinous layer; loss of the cystatin A protein leads to a cell–cell adhesion defect in keratinocytes that is prominent when cells are subject to mechanical stress.

Cathepsin B: *CTSB*

Abnormalities in the functioning of the *CTSB* gene encoding cathepsin B have been implicated in keratolytic winter erythema [1]. Initially disregarded as a candidate gene, the molecular pathology for this peeling skin condition was finally established as tandem duplications in a non-coding genomic region containing an active enhancer element for *CTSB*, resulting in upregulation of this gene in affected individuals. Cathepsin B is a cysteine protease involved in keratinocyte homeostasis that is found throughout the spinous layer and in intercellular spaces [2], but which shows enhanced expression in keratolytic winter erythema, particularly in the granular layer. Levels of the protease may be modified by environmental factors thereby accounting for the seasonal changes in phenotype.

Serpin B8: *SERPINB8*

SERPINS comprise a large and functionally diverse family of serine protease inhibitors. Loss-of-function mutations in *SERPINB8* result in an autosomal recessive form of exfoliative ichthyosis [1]. Functionally, loss of SERPINB8 leads to dysadhesion between keratinocytes, particularly when cells are subjected to mechanical stress. Serine protease cascades appear to be involved in various processes that are essential for epidermal differentiation, such as lipid barrier formation and assembly of the cornified envelope [2]. Clinically, the skin fragility manifests as superficial peeling on the hands and feet (palmoplantar and dorsal aspects) and may be aggravated by heat, humidity and friction.

Filaggrin 2: *FLG2*

Mutations in *FLG1* are known to be implicated in the pathobiology of ichthyosis vulgaris and atopic dermatitis, but mutations in a different filaggrin gene, *FLG2*, result in a skin fragility disorder referred to as autosomal recessive peeling skin syndrome type A [1] or generalised ichthyotic peeling skin syndrome [2]. Filaggrin 2 is expressed throughout the cornified cell layers and co-localises with corneodesmosin which plays a crucial role in maintaining cell–cell adhesion in this region of the epidermis. Lack of filaggrin 2 markedly decreases corneodesmosin expression, which may contribute to the peeling phenotype displayed by individuals with biallelic *FLG2* mutations. In this setting, keratinocyte dysadhesion is also aggravated by temperature elevation.

Corneodesmosin: *CDSN*

Corneodesmosin is an essential component of corneodesmosomes and must undergo degradation so that desquamation can occur.

Surprisingly, autosomal dominant mutations in *CDSN* have been shown to underlie hereditary hypotrichosis simplex rather than a skin barrier abnormality [1]. However, autosomal recessive mutations in *CDSN* have been described in patients with a form of generalised skin peeling disease [2]. Clinically, loss of corneodesmosin expression results in profound skin barrier disruption with marked inflammation and a predisposition to atopy and food allergy as well as symptoms of pruritus. The barrier disruption associated with corneodesmosin loss does not resemble trauma-induced fragility and the clinical syndrome does not show much overlap with other desmosomal blistering genodermatoses.

Calpastatin: *CAST*

Calpastatin is an endogenous specific inhibitor of calpain, a calcium-dependent cysteine protease. Loss-of-function mutations in the calpastain gene, *CAST*, are the genetic cause of an autosomal recessive condition characterised by generalised *P*eeling skin, *L*eukonychia, *A*cral punctate keratoses, *C*heilitis and *K*nuckle pads, which gives rise to the acronym PLACK syndrome [1]. In normal skin, calpastatin is localised throughout the epidermis and has a cytoplasmic localisation but is absent in PLACK syndrome skin. Calpastatin is a specific endogenous protease inhibitor of calpains (μ-calpain and m-calpain), cysteine proteases that are involved in keratinocyte growth, migration and cell cycle regulation [2].

Desmoglein-1: *DSG1*

Desmoglein-1 is a transmembranous desmosomal cadherin predominantly expressed in the superficial epidermis. It is the autoantigen targeted in the autoimmune blistering skin disease pemphigus foliaceus, and the target for bacterial toxins in staphylococcal scalded skin syndrome [1]. Autosomal dominant mutations in *DSG1* have been reported in striate palmo-plantar keratoderma, although semidominant inheritance may occur in some pedigrees [2]. This condition is not normally associated with skin blistering, although histological changes of impaired cell–cell adhesion are often present and clinical signs of skin fragility are seen in some cases. Biallelic mutations in *DSG1* have also been described in individuals with disruption of the skin barrier [3]. Notably, loss of cell adhesion within the epidermis led to severe dermatitis, multiple allergies and metabolic wasting. An upregulation of allergy-related cytokines, including interleukin-17, secondary to the loss of cell adhesion was also observed.

Serine protease inhibitor Kazal-type 5: *SPINK5*

One of the major proteases involved in stratrum corneum desquamation is kallikrein 5, the major inhibitor of which is lympho-epithelial Kazal-type inhibitor (LEKTI) encoded by the serine protease inhibitor Kazal-type 5 (*SPINK5*) [1]. Biallelic loss-of-function mutations in *SPINK5* have been shown to result in Netherton syndrome, a severe autosomal recessive form of ichthyosis with defective cornification, hypotrichosis with trichorrexis invaginata, and atopic manifestations such as atopic dermatitis and hay fever, along with high serum IgE levels and hypereosinophilia [2]. Increased proteolytic activity in the superficial epidermis caused by *SPINK5* mutations leads to diminution or loss of the granular and horny layers and a distinctive defect in skin barrier function.

Desmoplakin: *DSP*

Desmoplakin is the major intracellular structural component of the desmosomal plaque. Autosomal dominant mutations in *DSP* can give rise to striate palmo-plantar keratoderma, a disorder characterised by linear thickening (but no blisters) on trauma-prone sites on the palms or weight-bearing areas on the soles [1]. Other dominant mutations underlie cases of arrhythmogenic cardiomyopathy, often in the absence of any cutaneous abnormalities. Furthermore, autosomal recessive mutations in *DSP* can result in woolly hair and keratoderma with or without cardiomyopathy. Some recessive mutations in *DSP* can result in devastating mucocutaneous skin fragility, with pan-epidermal acantholysis [2]. Loss of desmoplakin expression in these cases leads to early death because of the profound skin loss and potential involvement of other organs, notably the heart.

Plakoglobin: *JUP*

Plakoglobin is an intracellular armadillo protein component of the desmosome which helps anchor the constituents of the desmosomal plaque to the keratin intermediate filaments [1]. Autosomal recessive mutations have been reported in individuals with Naxos disease – a combination of woolly hair, palmo-plantar keratoderma and cardiomyopathy; heterozygous carriers may also be prone to cardiac arrhythmias or heart failure [2]. Other autosomal dominant mutations may cause cardiomyopathy although skin fragility may be an unusual feature. In contrast, individuals with recessive mutations in JUP may have variable skin fragility, hair abnormalities and keratoderma with early or late onset cardiac abnormalties [3]. Some JUP mutations may result in pan-epidermal acantholysis resulting in widespread erosions, transcutaneous fluid loss, onycholysis, alopecia and early demise [4].

Plakophilin-1: *PKP1*

Inherited skin fragility has also been shown to result from autosomal recessive mutations in the desmosomal protein plakophilin-1 resulting in ectodermal dysplasia-skin fragility syndrome [1]. The skin fragility results from a loss of keratinocyte adhesion within the desmosomal inner plaque; the ectodermal dysplasia partly results from altered differentiation and proliferation in the epidermis but also from the fact that plakophilin-1 is present in the nuclei of cells that lack desmosomes. In those cells, the interactions of plakophilin 1 with other signalling molecules involved in epithelial development may be disrupted. Plakophilin-1 is essential for desmosome assembly and stabilisation, particularly in the spinous and granular epidermal layers [2], with pathogenic mutations leading to acantholysis in the spinous layer but with intact basal keratinocyte adhesion.

Desmocollin 3: *DSC3*

Desmocollin 3 is one of the transmembranous desmosomal cadherins that is expressed throughout the epidermis, particularly in the basal keratinocyte layer [1]. Interactions between DSC3 and other desmosomal proteins such as DSG1 and plakophilin-3 are crucial for keratinocyte cohesion and epidermal integrity. Autosomal recessive mutations in *DSC3* result in pan-epidermal acantholysis with clinical features of skin fragility and hypotrichosis [2,3], although the blistering is highly variable and may not be present in early life. Perifollicular hyperkeratosis and ghost follicles are noted on dermoscopy [3]. Mice lacking *Dsc3* show widespread trauma-induced skin fragility and telogen hair loss and thus resemble the key features of the human genodermatosis [1].

Desmoglein 3: *DSG3*

Desmoglein-3 is a demosomal cadherin that is found predominantly in the basal and spinous layers of the cutaneous epidermis, and which is expressed in stratified squamous non-cornified epithelia [1]. The only case thus far of genetic inactivation of *DSG3* was a Korean girl with congenital blistering and erosions of the oral and laryngeal mucosa [2]. A homozygous nonsense mutation in *DSG3* led to absent DSG3 expression in the skin and oral mucosa, although no clinical manifestations in the skin. Furthermore, the conjunctival and genital mucosa, nails and hair were also unremarkable [2]. The compensatory mechanisms underlying the lack of skin blistering remain to be characterised.

Keratins 1, 10 and 2: *KRT1, KRT10, KRT2*

The major epidermal keratins in the spinous layer of the epidermis (i.e. superficial to the basal keratinocytes) are keratins 1 and 10, mutations in which result in epidermolytic ichthyosis, sometimes also called keratinopathic ichthyosis [1]. Also expressed in the superficial spinous layer is keratin 2, mutations in which cause superficial epidermolytic ichthyosis [1]. Although these conditions cause microscopic evidence of keratinocyte cytolysis (hence the term epidermolytic), and there may be clinical overlap with some EB subtypes, particularly with EB simplex in neonates, the major pathological consequences are altered epidermal differentiation and proliferation leading to scaling (ichthyosis). For that reason, genodermatoses involving mutations in *KRT1*, *KRT10* and *KRT2* are classified as forms of ichthyosis rather than primary blistering genodermatoses [2].

Keratins 6A, 6B, 6C, 16 and 17: *KRT6A, KRT6B, KRT6C, KRT16, KRT17*

Within the family of epithelial keratins are the differentiation-specific keratins that include keratins 6A, 6B, 6C, 16 and 17, which are expressed in certain sites including skin, nails and oral mucosa [1]. Mutations in these keratins result in a group of autosomal dominant conditions called pachyonychia congenita [2]. Affected individuals have a painful and debilitating plantar keratoderma, variable hypertrophic nail dystrophy, oral leukokeratosis and epidermal cysts. Painful keratoderma can occur due to deep blisters forming under the callus.

Procollagen-lysine,2-oxoglutarate 5-dioxygenase 3: *PLOD3*

PLOD3 encodes lysyl hydroxylase 3 (LH3) which glycosylates hydroxylysine residues and, amongst other functions, contributes to the post-translational modification of type VII collagen, the major component of anchoring fibrils within the cutaneous basement membrane zone. Recessive mutations in *PLOD3* compromise type VII collagen function and lead to skin blistering resembling a form of dystrophic EB [1]. However, blistering is a minor part of the phenotype which involves widespread connective tissue and bony anomalies [2]. Mutations in *PLOD3* are therefore proposed to result in a syndromic form of dystrophic EB.

Clinical subtypes of classic forms of EB

The classic forms of EB are divided into four groups: EB simplex, junctional EB, dystrophic EB and Kindler EB.

EB simplex

The subtypes of EB simplex are subdivided into autosomal dominant and autosomal recessive variants, some of which are listed as syndromic disorders because of their extracutaneous manifestations (Table 69.3).

Autosomal dominant localised EB simplex

This is the most common type of EB. Inheritance is autosomal dominant. The soles and palms (Figures 69.3 and 69.4) are mainly affected, with the exception of the sides of the toes, and blistering may be painful [1]. Many patients have blisters only on the feet, and a minority (*c*.10%) will have blisters at other sites, such as the hands, waist or neck, especially in hot weather and after friction from clothing or other sources. In most individuals blistering starts in childhood, but onset may be delayed until early adult life, only manifesting after strenuous physical activity. The condition is typically worse in warm weather. Hyperhidrosis of the feet is common; this increases friction, which also exacerbates blistering. The blisters usually heal without clinically significant scarring or milia formation, although both may infrequently be seen. Discrete and sometimes punctate calluses are very common, especially in adults. Although troublesome

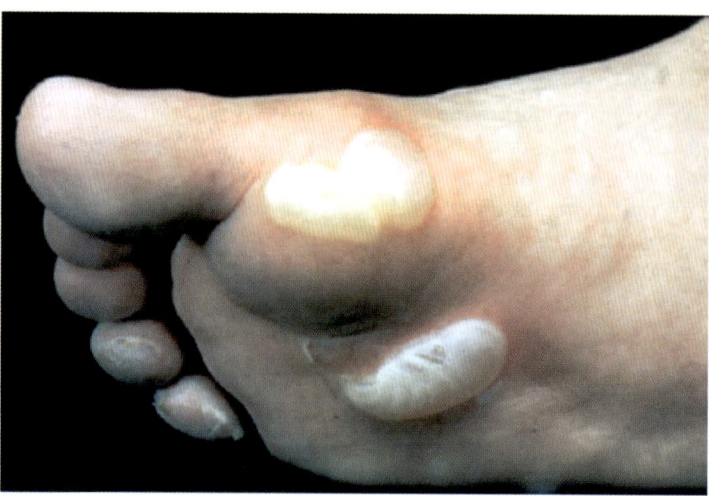

Figure 69.3 Blisters on the foot in a patient with localised epidermolysis bullosa simplex.

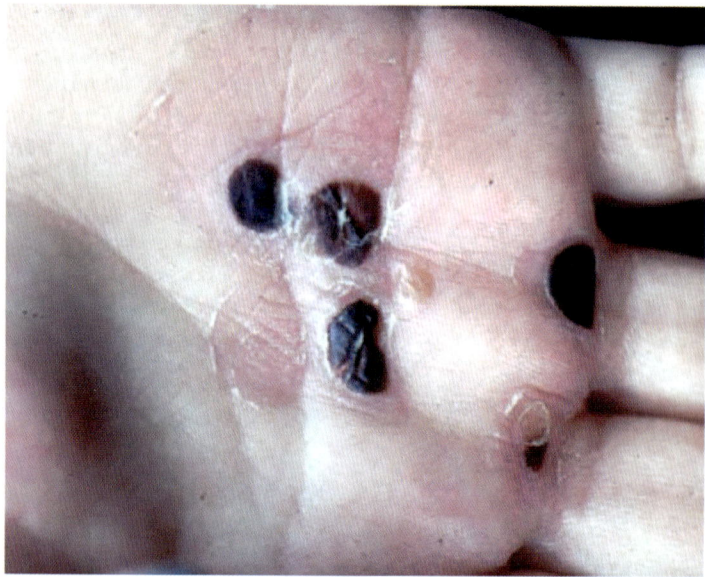

Figure 69.4 Blisters, some of which are haemorrhagic, and erosions on the palm in a patient with localised epidermolysis bullosa simplex.

Table 69.3 Epidermolysis bullosa simplex (EBS) clinical subtypes.

Most common EBS clinical subtypes	Targeted protein(s)
Autosomal dominant EBS	
Localised	Keratin 5, keratin 14
Intermediate	Keratin 5, keratin 14
Severe	Keratin 5, keratin 14
With mottled pigmentation	Keratin 5[a]
Migratory circinate erythema	Keratin 5
Intermediate	Plectin
Intermediate with cardiomyopathy	**Kelch-like member 24**
Autosomal recessive EBS	
Intermediate or severe	Keratin 14, keratin 5
Intermediate	Plectin
Localised or intermediate with BP230 deficiency	Bullous pemphigoid antigen 230 (BP230) (syn. BPAG1e)
Localised or intermediate with exophilin-5 deficiency	Exophilin-5 (syn. Slac2-b)
Intermediate with muscular dystrophy	**Plectin**
Severe with pyloric atresia	**Plectin**
Localised with nephropathy	**CD151 (CD151 antigen) (syn. tetraspanin 24)**

[a] Typical recurrent mutation in keratin 5, but cases with other keratin 5, keratin 14 or exophilin-5 mutations have been reported; **bold**, syndromic EBS subtypes. Reproduced from Has *et al.* [3] with permission from Wiley.

blistering or ulceration of the oral mucosa is rare, at least 25% of infants may develop occasional small intraoral lesions, especially palatal and worsened by trauma from narrow bore bottle feeding. The hair and teeth are normal; nail dystrophy is infrequent and is usually localised and mild when it does occur. Most cases result from point mutations in *KRT5* or *KRT14* (encoding keratin 5 and 14, respectively) that lead to amino acid substitutions [2].

Autosomal dominant intermediate EB simplex

This subtype of EB includes inherited blistering previously known as Koebner EB simplex and generalised intermediate EB simplex [1]. Most cases are autosomal dominant. Although usually mild, approximately 60% of patients have localised scarring and approximately 15% have milia. The development of hair, teeth and nails is normal. The nails rarely may be affected by acral blisters but are only temporarily shed. Blisters appear within the first year and may be present at birth. In infancy, they commonly appear on the occiput, back and legs, while in childhood the hands and feet are often affected, although the palms and soles are not preferentially involved, as in localised EB simplex. In common with other forms of EB simplex, blistering is worse in warm weather. Although blistering occurs throughout life, some patients are alleged to improve after puberty. In some authors' experience, this subtype of EB simplex is rare in comparison with the localised or severe forms of EB simplex. At times it may be difficult to readily distinguish this EB simplex subtype from patients with localised EB simplex who are experiencing a disease flare. Missense mutations in keratins 5 and 14 have been shown in most cases [2]. Some intermediate forms of EB simplex may also arise from mutations in plectin (*PLEC*); such cases may or may not have additional extracutaneous anomalies. Within this subtype of EB simplex is the condition previously referred to as the Ogna variant.

Severe EB simplex

A further common subtype of EB simplex is the severe variant, previously known as Dowling–Meara or generalised severe EB simplex. Inheritance is autosomal dominant although approximately 30% of cases are sporadic (new mutations). Blisters tend to occur in groups reminiscent of those seen in dermatitis herpetiformis, hence the earlier use of the term EB herpetiformis. In infancy, blistering may be severe and extensive with involvement of the mucous membranes, shedding of nails and formation of milia, the latter often occurring during the first week of life [1]. The differential diagnosis at this age may include both the junctional and recessive dystrophic forms of EB. After several months, blistering of the palms and soles becomes more frequent, as it does elsewhere. The distinctive feature of this condition is spontaneous herpetiform, annular or arcuate blistering on the trunk, limbs and neck (Figure 69.5). Healing of blisters may leave mild hyperpigmentation; localised atrophic scarring affects approximately 40% of patients. Irregular hyperkeratosis of the palms and soles, eventually developing into a confluent keratoderma, first appears in childhood. The general condition tends to improve with age. Most cases result from heterozygous missense mutations in *KRT5* or *KRT14* but unlike those in localised EB simplex, the amino acid substitutions involve key residues involved in keratin filament polymerisation [2].

Autosomal dominant EB simplex with mottled pigmentation

This autosomal dominant condition can be distinguished from other forms of EB simplex by the associated pigmentary changes, which are present at birth or appear during infancy [1]. There is a reticulate pattern of small, tan-coloured macular lesions, which may spread from acral sites to the trunk and which fade with age (Figure 69.6). They may cover the entire skin surface but preferentially involve the neck, upper trunk or extremities. Blistering may be localised or become more generalised. Punctate keratoses on the palms and soles sometimes progressing to keratoderma have been noted in some cases. Mild localised skin atrophy and nail dystrophy are also features of the condition. Previously thought to be rare, more cases have been reported in recent years. This increase has been facilitated by the discovery that most cases harbour the same heterozygous missense mutation in keratin 5 [2], although other mutations in keratin 14 or exophilin-5 have also been implicated.

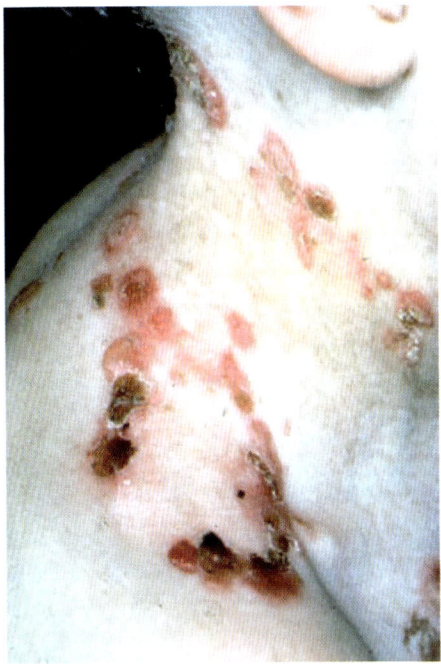

Figure 69.5 Grouped blisters on an erythematous base in severe epidermolysis bullosa simplex.

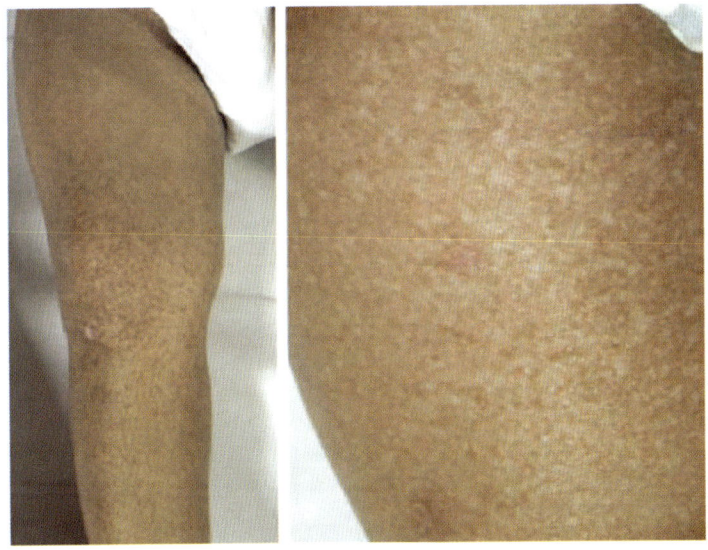

Figure 69.6 Epidermolysis bullosa simplex with mottled pigmentation on the lower limb in an 18-month-old child. Courtesy of Prof. J. E. Mellerio, St John's Institute of Dermatology, London, UK.

Autosomal dominant EB simplex with migratory circinate erythema

A small number of individuals and families have been reported with an autosomal dominant form of EB simplex characterised by migratory circinate redness and postinflammatory hyperpigmentation [1]. Present at birth, blistering may be generalised. Following signs of skin fragility, there are often centrifugally expanding circinate erythematous plaques which may also be itchy. Some cases have been misdiagnosed as tinea corporis. The underlying cause of this entity typically involves heterozygous frameshift mutations in *KRT5* (encoding keratin 5) leading to skin inflammation with a T-cell infiltrate [2].

Autosomal dominant intermediate EB simplex with cardiomyopathy

Following advances in next generation sequencing technology, a new form of autosomal dominant EB simplex was described in 2016 [1,2]. Affected individuals often have quite marked birth trauma, especially on the lower legs, with additional early blistering often involving the trunk and upper limbs. These lesions typically heal quickly with subtle atrophic scarring, but blistering persists throughout childhood. Nails defects and oral ulceration are common; transient milia may also occur (Figure 69.7). With increasing age, blistering severity tends to lessen. The molecular pathology involves mutations affecting the methionine initiation codon of Kelch-like family member 24 (KLHL24). The truncated protein results in abnormal autoubiquitination of keratin 14 and reduced levels of functional keratin 14. A key clinical point is that individuals with *KLHL24* mutations are prone to develop cardiac arrythmias and cardiomyopathy which may manifest in teenagers and adults [3].

Intermediate or severe autosomal recessive EB simplex

Although most mutations in *KRT5* or *KRT14* in EB simplex are autosomal dominant, pathogenic recessive mutations in both these genes have been reported that give rise to autosomal recessive forms of EB simplex. Clinically, cases may resemble intermediate EB simplex although the latter is typically autosomal dominant (Figure 69.8). Blisters are often scattered and there is usually minor palmo-plantar keratoderma and varying degrees of nail dystrophy, atrophic scarring, hyperpigmentation and oral and genital blistering [1]. Nevertheless, it is perhaps surprising that a complete absence of keratin 14 usually leads to a less severe phenotype than some heterozygous missense mutations, such as those that occur in severe EB simplex [2]. Heterozygous carriers of these nonsense mutations usually show no phenotypic abnormalities (although other heterozygous nonsense mutations in *KRT14* underlie Naegeli–Franceschetti–Jadassohn ectodermal dysplasia). Homozygous missense mutations or nonsense mutations have also

been reported in *KRT5* [3]. Most cases are phenotypically similar to *KRT14* knockouts although complete loss of *KRT5* in one individual was associated with neonatal lethality [3]. Autosomal recessive mutations in *PLEC* may also result in an intermediate form of EB simplex that is indistinguishable from other clinical intermediate subtypes. Genotype–phenotype correlation for *PLEC* mutations is complex and may relate to the multiple different isoforms of plectin expressed in various tissues [4].

Autosomal recessive EB simplex with BP230 deficiency

The 230 kDa bullous pemphigoid antigen (BP230) is a structural component of the hemidesmosomal inner plaque. An autosomal recessive form of EB simplex has been described in which nonsense mutations lead to a complete loss of BP230 protein expression in skin [1]. Blistering is lifelong and generalised but clinically is mild, with only a few predominantly acral blisters that can extend to several centimetres in size but which are non-inflammatory and which heal with no scarring and only mild postinflammatory pigmentary anomalies (Figure 69.9) [2]. Oral and genital mucosae are not affected. The gene encoding BP230 is an isoform of dystonin (*DST*) but the encoded protein is different from the *DST* transcripts expressed in brain and muscle and therefore no extracutaneous abnormalities have been noted in patients with inherited skin fragility. A variant of this form of EB simplex has been described with prurigo-like features [3].

Autosomal recessive localised or intermediate EB simplex with exophilin-5 deficiency

Autosomal recessive loss-of-function mutations in *EXPH5* (encoding exophilin-5, also known as Slac2-b) result in mild, scattered, trauma-induced skin fragility, although blistering can be generalised shortly after birth [1,2]. In later infancy, however, the clinical features mostly comprise crusted erosions on the limbs with few intact blisters. No mucosal abnormalities are noted. Exophilin-5 is involved in the intracellular transport of vesicles in keratinocytes and in focal adhesion dynamics. The loss of exophilin-5 leads to keratin filament disruption and intraepidermal skin fragility, as well as intercellular keratinocyte separation, particularly within the

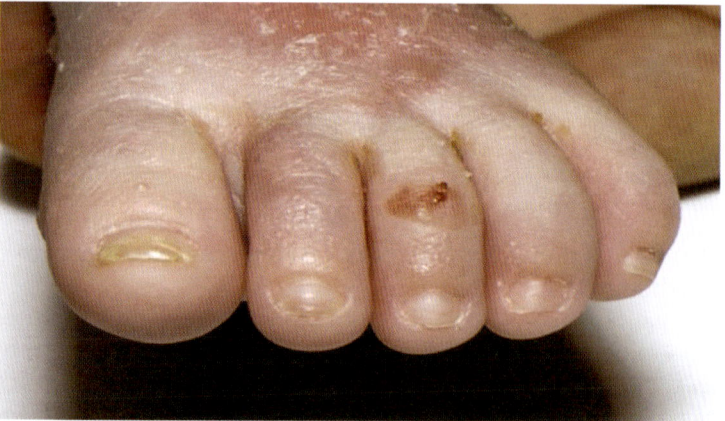

Figure 69.7 Epidermolysis bullosa simplex with cardiomyopathy due to a mutation in KLHL24. Acral blistering, mild atrophic scarring, scattered milia (transient) and minor nail dystrophy on the foot in an 8-month-old child.

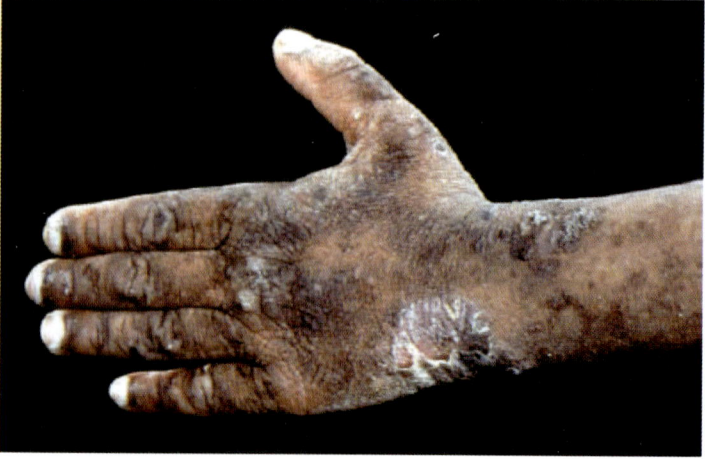

Figure 69.8 Acral blistering in a patient with autosomal recessive epidermolysis bullosa simplex with loss of keratin 14 expression in the skin.

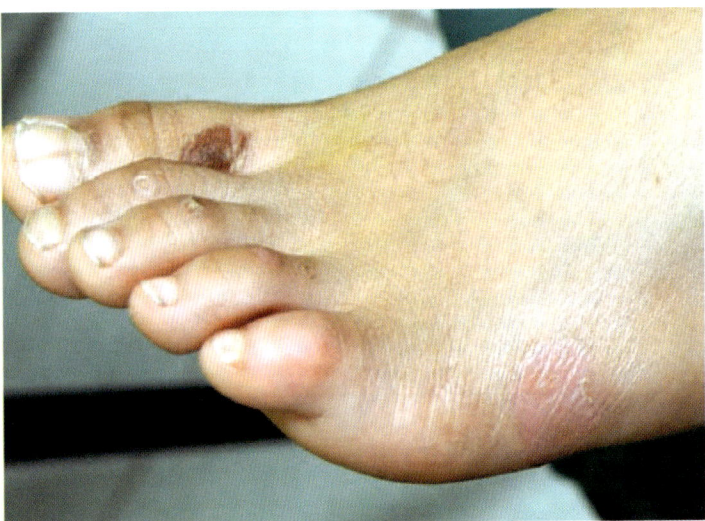

Figure 69.9 Localised blistering on the foot in a patient with autosomal recessive epidermolysis bullosa simplex due to autosomal recessive mutations in BP230. Courtesy of Dr A. Nanda, Kuwait.

lower epidermis. In some cases there may be pigmentary changes in the skin resembling autosomal dominant EB simplex with mottled pigmentation (see earlier) [3].

Autosomal recessive intermediate EB simplex with muscular dystrophy

Several families have been described in which skin fragility and blistering are associated with a neuromuscular disorder, chiefly muscular dystrophy, although myasthenia gravis and spinal muscular atrophy have also been described; cardiomyopathy can occur too [1]. The blisters, which affect the skin and oral mucosa, are present at birth or soon afterwards. Muscle weakness and wasting may be severe and evident in early childhood, or milder and only detectable later in life. The blistering may be widespread but can be limited to the hands and feet (Figure 69.10). There is associated atrophic scarring, milia, nail dystrophy and alopecia, which can mimic junctional or dystrophic EB. Supraglottic scarring and hoarseness that may necessitate tracheostomy are an important potential complication [2]. The disorder is autosomal recessive and results from mutations in *PLEC*, encoding plectin, a component of the hemidesmosomal inner plaque in the skin basement membrane but also found in the Z-lines of striated muscle. Nevertheless, there is a considerable range of phenotypes associated with *PLEC* mutations; *PLEC* has at least eight isoforms with varying expression patterns in different tissues and the sites of the underlying mutations have implications for cutaneous and extracutaneous manifestations.

Autosomal recessive severe EB simplex with pyloric atresia

Pyloric atresia may rarely occur in the setting of EB simplex – most cases are classified as a junctional form of EB [1]. Affected infants tend to have generalised skin disease. Although only a few cases have yet been reported, this entity appears to be as severe as junctional EB with pyloric atresia and clinically impossible to differentiate from it. There are widespread blisters and erosions that increase infection risk with early demise in the neonatal period. As such, this

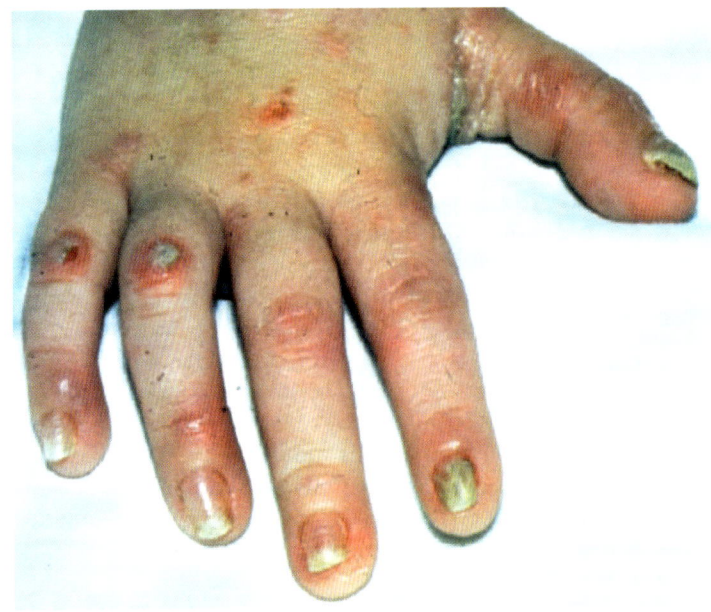

Figure 69.10 Acral blisters and nail dystrophy in a patient with epidermolysis bullosa simplex with muscular dystrophy due to autosomal recessive mutations in plectin.

is one of the forms of EB simplex that is associated with a generally poor prognosis. Inheritance is autosomal recessive and involves mutations in *PLEC* – usually outside exon 31, the exon in which most of the pathogenic mutations that associate with muscular dystrophy are located [2]. *PLEC* mutations are typically associated with a low level of cleavage within basal keratinocytes but focal detachment within the lamina lucida is also often evident, making the distinction between classification as EB simplex or junctional EB challenging.

Autosomal recessive localised EB simplex with nephropathy

A recent addition to the classification of classic forms of EB simplex is a disorder resulting from biallelic mutations in *CD151*, encoding the CD151 antigen which is also known as tetraspanin 24. Although autosomal recessive mutations in CD151 were first reported in 2008 in which skin blistering was documented [1], the predominant clinical pathology involved the kidneys and therefore the clinicopathological manifestations were not included in the list of recognised EB subtypes. However, a further case in 2018 led to a classification amendment [2]. In that report, the clinical features resembled Kindler EB with widespread blistering, especially on the shins, as well as poikiloderma, loss of teeth, early-onset alopecia and oseophageal stricture. As in the earlier cases, nephropathy with proteinuria was a major co-pathology.

Molecular pathology of classic EB simplex

To date, mutations in 7 different genes underlie the disease phenotypes denoted as classic forms of EB simplex. Mutations in *KRT5* (keratin 5), *KRT14* (keratin 14) or *PLEC* (plectin) may result in autosomal dominant or autosomal recessive forms of EB simplex. Mutations in *KLHL24* (Kelch-like family member 24) exclusively result in autosomal dominant EB simplex, whereas mutations in *DST* (dystonin epithelial isoform, 230-kDa bullous pemphigoid antigen), *EXPH5* (exophilin-5) or *CD151* (tetraspanin 24) all under-lie recessive forms of EB simplex. Occasionally digenic (*KRT5* and *KRT14*) inheritance can occur. Approximately two-thirds of all EB simplex cases have underlying mutations in *KRT5* or *KRT14*. With regard to genotype–phenotype correlation, mutations in the severe forms of classic autosomal dominant EB simplex are usually located within the helix initiation and termination motifs of the keratins, critical sites for stacking and assembling keratin monomers in the process of intermediate filament polymerisa-tion. Other milder intermediate or localised forms of EB simplex typically have mutations in less critical parts of the protein such as the linker or tail regions. Nevertheless, perhaps up to 25% of all cases of classic localised forms of EB simplex do not harbour mutations in *KRT5* or *KRT14*; the molecular basis of such cases is currently unknown. Heterozygous mutations in *PLEC* may result in autosomal dominant intermediate forms of EB simplex, whereas biallelic *PLEC* mutations are usually associated with autosomal recessive EB simplex associated with extracutaneous abnormalities: recessive mutations in exon 31 of *PLEC* are typically associated with muscular dystrophy whereas recessive mutations in other parts of the gene may feature pyloric atresia, although genotype–phenotype discrepancy for this paradigm may occur. Mutations in *KLHL24* result in widespread birth trauma but with clinical lessening of the blistering severity with age. In contrast to most other forms of EB simplex, some scarring may be present. The major concern for *KLHL24* gene pathology, however, is the associated risk of cardiac arrythmias and cardiomyopathy. *KLHL24* mutations affect autoubiquitination of keratin 14 leading to reducing functional keratin 14 protein. All reported mutations in *KLHL24* reside within the methionine initiation codon. Mutations in *EXPH5* result in accumulation of endosomal vesicles close to keratinocyte nuclei. Precisely how the loss of exophilin-5 disrupts keratinocyte integrity is not yet known. Recessive mutations in *KRT14* lead to generalised skin fragility, although the phenotypic features are often less severe than some of the dominant mutation within the helix initiation and termination motifs. Recessive mutations in *KRT5* have recently been added to the molecular pathology of autosomal recessive EB simplex; the clinical features may resemble recessive *KRT14* muta-tions but may also result in a more severe form of skin blistering. Recessive mutations in the epithelial isoform of *DST* compro-mise hemidesmosome integrity through lack of expression of the 230-kDa bullous pemphigoid antigen. Blisters are typically large and acral. Although *DST* has several different isoforms, including some expressed in brain and muscle, the pathogenic *DST* mutations in EB have skin-only manifestations. Mutations in *CD151* have been reported to result in a Kindler EB-like phenotype with widespread blisters, particularly on the shins, poikiloderma, nail dystrophy, loss of teeth, early-onset alopecia and oesophageal stricture. However, nephropathy with proteinuria occurs and may be the predominant abnormality in some cases.

Junctional EB

Junctional EB encompasses a collection of autosomal recessive forms of EB. Heterozygous carriers of junctional EB mutations do not usually have any clinical abnormalities although some may have dental enamel anomalies. The latest classification of junctional EB no longer uses the word 'generalised' because it is often not

Table 69.4 Junctional epidermolysis bullosa (JEB) clinical subtypes.

Most common JEB clinical subtypes	Targeted protein(s)
Severe	Laminin 332[a]
Intermediate	Laminin 332
Intermediate	Type XVII collagen
With pyloric atresia	**Integrin α6β4**
Localised	Laminin 332, type XVII collagen, integrin α6β4, integrin α3 subunit
Inversa	Laminin 332
Late onset	Type XVII collagen
LOC syndrome	Laminin α3A
With interstitial lung disease and nephrotic syndrome	**Integrin α3 subunit**

LOC, laryngo-onycho-cutaneous. [a] JEB severe is rarely caused by pathogenic variants affecting the type XVII collagen gene; **bold**, syndromic JEB subtypes.
Reproduced from Has *et al.* [3] with permission from Wiley.

an indication of overall severity; instead, the main subtypes are described as severe, intermediate and localised.

The full classification of classic junctional EB is shown in Table 69.4.

Severe junctional EB

This is the most devastating form of junctional EB, previously referred to as Herlitz or generalised severe junctional EB. Blistering and erosions are present at or soon after birth and rapidly become generalised [1]. The whole skin is extremely fragile and lifting or turning the baby may cause extensive blistering or peeling away of the epidermis (Figure 69.11). Eroded areas are often very slow to heal. Healing may result in atrophic scarring. Milia are not generally seen, although they may occur after secondary infection. Involvement of the oral and pharyngeal mucosa is frequent and may be severe; hoarseness and stridor may indicate laryngeal or supraglottic involvement, most notably potentially life-threatening stenosis or stricture. Many infants die early in infancy with over-whelming infection or from failure to thrive, but those surviving the first few months will often develop distinctive lesions char-acterised by non-healing, crusted erosions containing exuberant granulation tissue [2]. These typical lesions occur symmetrically around the nose and mouth but also in other sites, including the neck, trunk, buttocks and rarely within the upper respiratory tract. The combination of chronic infection and loss of protein and iron from the skin, in addition to poor feeding, contributes to impaired healing and refractory anaemia. The teeth show abnormal enamel formation, but normal dentine, and as a result are malformed, pitted and lost prematurely. Following blistering and erosions, the formation of exuberant granulation tissue on the nail folds and nail bed leads to shedding of the nails and bulbous changes of the fingertips (Figure 69.12). Blisters may occur on the cornea, resulting in pain, erosions and scarring. A variety of genito-urinary tract complications may occur including urethral meatal stenosis, urinary retention, hydronephrosis and bladder hypertrophy.

Intermediate junctional EB

This form of junctional EB was previously referred to as non-Herlitz disease and included entities such as generalised atrophic benign

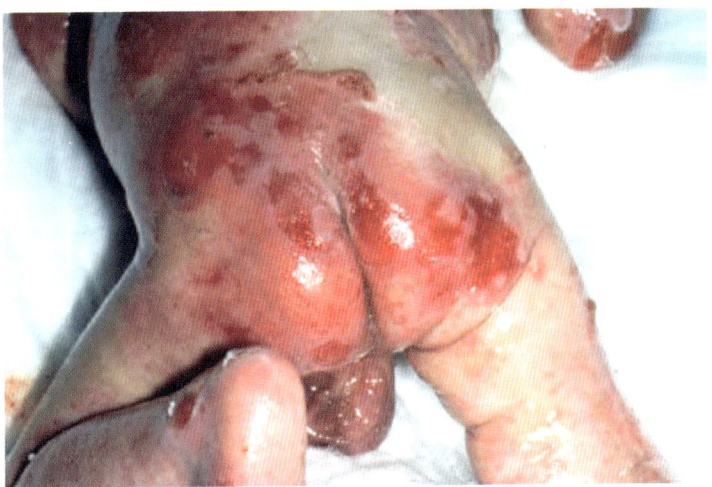

Figure 69.11 Extensive erosions over the buttocks in an infant with severe junctional epidermolysis bullosa.

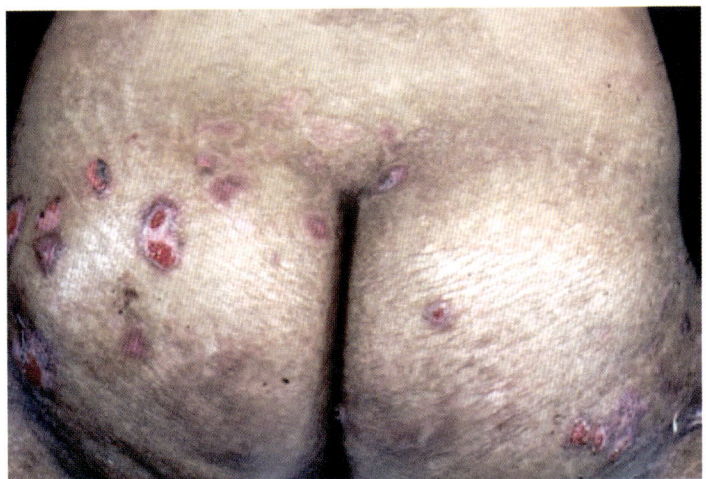

Figure 69.13 Erosions, scarring and atrophy on the buttocks in a patient with intermediate junctional epidermolysis bullosa.

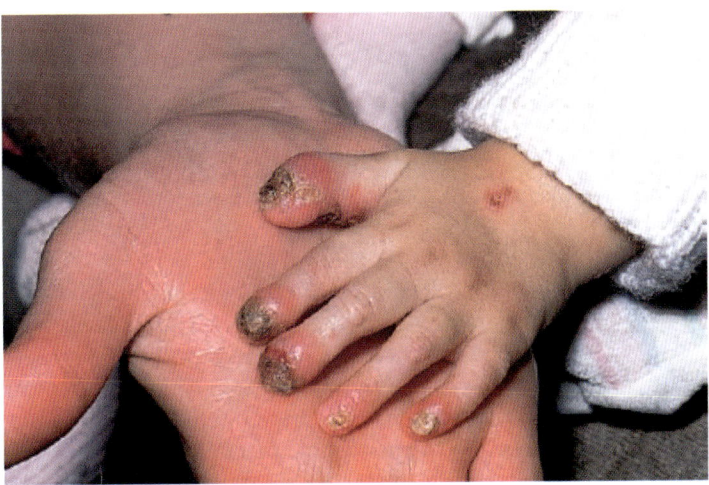

Figure 69.12 Nail changes with classical paronychia in severe junctional epidermolysis bullosa.

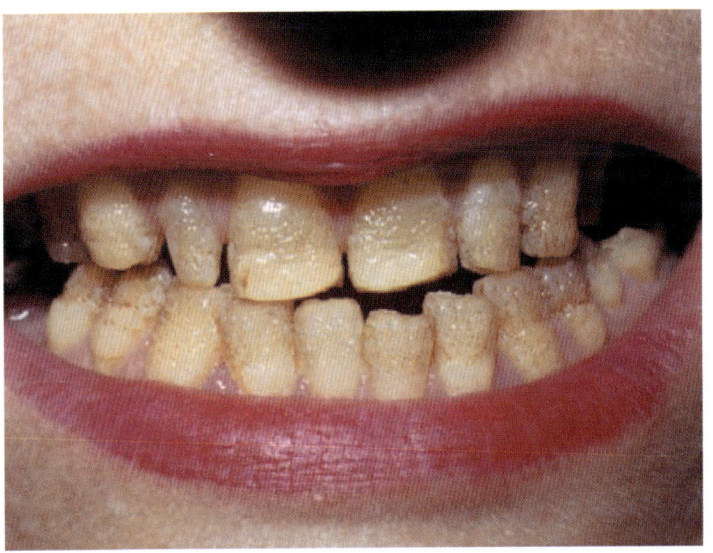

Figure 69.14 Pitting and discoloration of teeth in intermediate junctional epidermolysis bullosa.

EB. The early clinical course of this subtype of junctional EB may be similar to the severe variant with widespread skin fragility and blistering, but the patients usually survive to adulthood [1]. Although blistering persists, there is a gradual lessening in severity of the disease with age (Figure 69.13). Mucous membranes are involved, but less severely than in severe junctional EB. The teeth show severe enamel defects (Figure 69.14) and may fail to erupt normally. The nails are dystrophic or frequently missing (Figure 69.15), especially on the toes. Up to 5% of patients may develop a degree of pseudosyndactyly, clinically suggestive of dystrophic EB. Typically, the lesions in intermediate junctional EB heal with atrophic scarring, which can easily be mistaken for the scarring seen in dystrophic EB, especially on the lower legs or backs of the hands. Postinflammatory hypopigmentation or depigmentation may be present in areas of scarring. An important sign of this form of EB is poor hair development; the alopecia affects the scalp, eyebrows and eyelashes, and body hair is also sparse or absent (Figure 69.16).

Pigmented naevi, or acquired macular hyperpigmented lesions with irregular borders, are common, although these are not specific for this subtype of EB as they are also observed in EB simplex and dystrophic EB. Oesophageal stricture, laryngeal involvement, oral erosions, corneal ulcers and urethral stricture have all been reported. In this type of junctional EB, it is common to observe small patches of skin that do no blister and which, in pale-skinned individuals, may appear slightly darker than regions which blister [2]. This phenomenon is called revertant mosaicism or natural gene therapy; it represents a spontaneous correction of one copy of the mutant gene.

Junctional EB with pyloric atresia

This rare disorder is normally included as a subtype of junctional EB, although, not uncommonly, the true level of blistering has been found to be in the cytoplasm of basal keratinocytes, just above the plasma membrane, rather than within lamina lucida. Hence

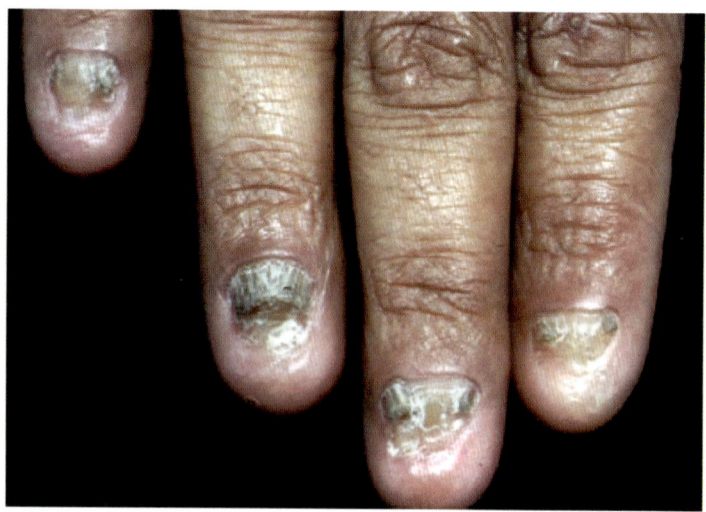

Figure 69.15 Nail dystrophy in intermediate junctional epidermolysis bullosa.

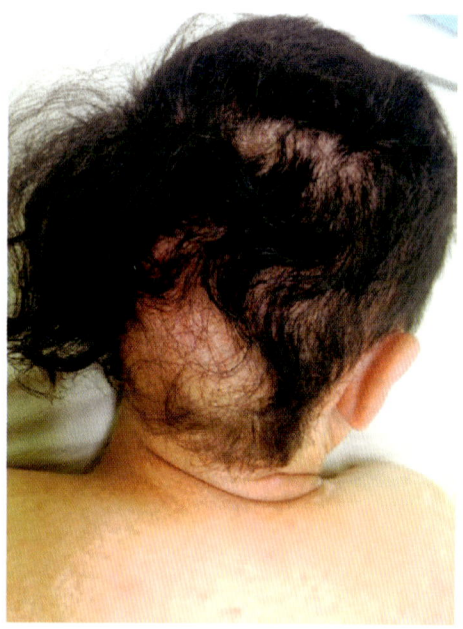

Figure 69.16 Scalp alopecia and hair thinning in intermediate junctional epidermolysis bullosa. Courtesy of Professor E. Sprecher, Tel Aviv, Israel.

there is an overlap with EB simplex both clinically and in the classification of EB. Blistering is usually present at birth, following a pregnancy complicated by polyhydramnios. The lesions are usually widespread and can result in atrophic scarring [1]. The teeth are hypoplastic, lacking normal enamel, and the nails are dystrophic. Early attempts at feeding result in vomiting. The majority of cases do not survive early infancy. In those children who survive, other features include haematuria, dysuria and recurrent urinary tract infections. Surgical correction of the congenital pyloric atresia improves prognosis although the nature of the underlying molecular pathology, which involves mutations in *ITGA6* (α6 integrin) and *ITGB4* (β4 integrin), determines the extent of the mucocutaneous fragility and whether the disease course will then resemble severe junctional EB or an intermediate variant [2].

Localised junctional EB

Localised forms of junctional EB occur: typical clinical manifestations include nail dystrophy, dental enamel changes and blistering involving the lower legs and feet only [1]. In some individuals, chronic, painful erosions associated with hyperkeratosis develop on the soles, although it is not clear why the lower legs should be a predilection site for blistering. In some cases, blistering starts in neonates, while in others there may be late-onset disease. Some cases may result from mutations in *COL17A1* (type XVII collagen) in which missense rather than nonsense or frameshift mutations usually (but not always) predominate, thus providing some genotype–phenotype correlation for localised or generalised disease [2].

Inversa junctional EB

In the neonatal period in the rare inversa subtype of junctional EB, the whole skin may be fragile with generalised blistering. Later, however, the lesions affect chiefly the groins, perineum and axillae, hence the description of 'inversa' [1]. Healing may result in small, atrophic, white streaks. Dysplastic teeth, erosions of the cornea and feet and nail dystrophy are all features. Why there should be a preference for flexural site involvement is not known; for those cases associated with mutations in *COL17A1* (type XVII collagen) it is possible that certain mutant proteins may be more unstable in warmer body regions, although genetic heterogeneity is likely [2]. Moreover, some historical reports may have combined cases of both junctional and dystrophic EB with inversa descriptions.

Late-onset junctional EB

This is a rare subtype of autosomal recessive junctional EB that may encompass several closely related entities. The clinical features overlap with intermediate junctional EB, except that the onset of symptoms is delayed – often not starting until childhood, typically between 5 and 8 years of age [1]. Initially, the trauma-induced blisters mainly occur on the hands and feet, although they may be preceded by nail dystrophy. Later, knees and elbows are involved. Progressive atrophic changes lead to early loss of fingerprint patterns and mild finger contractures. The tooth enamel may be defective and the tongue papillae may disappear. The oral mucosa is sometimes involved. Underlying mutations in *COL17A1* (type XVII collagen) provide support for this type of junctional EB being a specific clinicopathological entity [2], although genetic heterogeneity is also evident.

Laryngo-onycho-cutaneous syndrome

This subtype of junctional EB starts in infancy with chronic erosions affecting the face (mainly around the nose and mouth) although erosions are also seen on the limbs, trunk and genitalia. The nails are also involved with marked periungual and subungual inflammation and a universal feature is hoarseness. The teeth may be notched. There is prominent skin and mucosal granulation tissue that can lead to delayed wound healing, laryngeal obstruction and blindness. The disorder results from autosomal recessive mutations in a particular splice variant of one of the laminin-332 genes, *LAMA3A* (and not *LAMA3*) [1]. Originally thought to exist only in people of Punjabi descent, other mutations in *LAMA3A* have been reported in the laryngo-onycho-cutaneous syndrome [2]. Moreover, considerable overlap with some forms of intermediate junctional EB can occur in some cases.

Junctional EB with interstitial lung disease and nephrotic syndrome

This is a syndromic form of junctional EB in which there is congenital nephrotic syndrome, interstitial lung disease and skin fragility [1]. In most cases the renal and respiratory features predominate clinically, but considerable variability in the severity of organ involvement can occur. Blisters or erosions may or may not be present at birth. In early reports of this form of junctional EB, small blisters and erosions developed after trauma, healed slowly without scarring, but with residual redness. There was no mucosal involvement. The scalp hair, eyebrows and eyelashes were fine and sparse, and some nails were dystrophic. All cases died during infancy with recurrent lung infections and multiorgan failure consistent with the known distribution of the mutated α3 integrin in several tissues [1], but other cases have been associated with better prognoses [2].

Molecular pathology of classic junctional EB

The molecular basis to classic junctional EB may involve mutations in eight different genes: *LAMA3* (laminin α3), *LAMA3A* (laminin α3A), *LAMB3* (β3 laminin), *LAMC2* (γ2 laminin), *COL17A1* (type XVII collagen, also known as 180-kDa bullous pemphigoid antigen), *ITGA6* (α6 integrin subunit), *ITGB4* (β4 integrin subunit) and *ITGA3* (α3 integrin subunit). Severe junctional EB results from biallelic loss-of-function mutations in any of the *LAMA3*, *LAMB3* or *LAMC2* genes, which encode the α3, β3 and γ2 polypeptide chains of heterotrimeric laminin-332, respectively. Intermediate variants may also result from mutations in these three genes although the nature of the underlying mutations usually has less disruptive consequences, such that there is some residual protein, reduced in amount and with impaired function. However, a similar phenotype of intermediate severity can also result from loss-of-function mutations in *COL17A1* leading to a complete absence of type XVII collagen protein. Rarely, digenic inheritance may contribute: junctional EB can result from a combination of mutations in *COL17A1* and *LAMB3*. Localised forms of junctional EB, including some cases of the inversa subtype, may also result from a range of less disruptive mutations in *LAMA3*, *LAMB3*, *LAMC2*, *COL17A1* or occasionally *ITGA6* or *ITGB4*. Loss-of-function mutations in *ITGA6* or *ITGB4* (nonsense, frameshift or occasionally involving critical cysteine residue substitutions) underlie junctional EB with pyloric atresia. Autosomal recessive nonsense or splice site mutations in *ITGA3* (α3 integrin) are found in junctional EB with interstitial lung disease and nephrotic syndrome. *LAMA3A* mutations occur in laryngo-onycho-cutaneous syndrome, although compound heterozygosity for *LAMA3A/LAMA3* mutations can also occur with a phenotype that overlaps with intermediate junctional EB.

Dystrophic EB

Dystrophic EB can be autosomal recessive or autosomal dominant. Clinically, dystrophic EB is characterised by skin fragility, blistering, scarring, nail dystrophy and milia formation. Mucosal involvement is common, and erosions and scarring can affect the mouth, oesophagus, genitalia and anus. There may be clinical overlap between some cases of recessive and dominant dystrophic EB which, in

Table 69.5 Dystrophic epidermolysis bullosa (DEB) clinical subtypes.

DEB subtypes	Targeted protein
Autosomal dominant DEB (DDEB)	
Intermediate	Type VII collagen
Localised	
Pruriginosa	
Self-improving	
Autosomal recessive DEB (RDEB)	
Severe	Type VII collagen
Intermediate	
Inversa	
Localised	
Pruriginosa	
Self-improving	
Dominant and recessive (compound heterozygosity)	
DEB, severe	Type VII collagen

bold, most common subtypes.
Reproduced from Has *et al.* [3] with permission from Wiley.

the absence of molecular diagnosis, can make genetic counselling difficult, particularly in sporadic cases. All cases of dystrophic EB, irrespective of the genotype, result from mutations in a single gene, *COL7A1*, which encodes type VII collagen, the major component of anchoring fibril structures beneath the lamina densa. The most recent classification of dystrophic EB is presented in Table 69.5.

Intermediate dystrophic EB (autosomal dominant or autosomal recessive)

Blisters in intermediate forms of dominant or recessive dystrophic EB mainly occur following trauma to the skin overlying the bony prominences, such as the knees and ankles, and dorsa of the hands or feet (Figure 69.17) [1]. The most consistent findings are localised scarring with milia formation and dystrophic nails. Nail dystrophy is probably the most important diagnostic feature of the disease, especially in adults, because many patients have only limited scarring, which becomes less noticeable with age. The nail plates, particularly of the large toes, are often diminutive (Figure 69.18) or entirely absent, where the normal nail is replaced by atrophic scar tissue. Blistering in the mouth is usually mild and the teeth are generally normal. However, perianal lesions may cause considerable pain, especially in children. Terms such as Bart syndrome are obsolete as the original pedigree described was found to have *COL7A1* gene pathology typical of a number of families with various forms of dominant dystrophic EB [2]. Cutaneous features such as albopapuloid lesions, once thought to be pathognomonic for subtypes of dominant dystrophic EB, are now recognised to occur in several forms of dominant and even recessive dystrophic EB and are therefore not relevant to disease subtyping.

Localised dystrophic EB (autosomal dominant or autosomal recessive)

The nature of this subtype of dominant or recessive dystrophic EB is not precisely defined but embraces individuals with a more localised pattern of skin involvement, usually involving the hands and feet [1]. Oral or oesophageal involvement can occur despite the relative lack of involvement of much of the skin. Trauma-induced

PART 6: GENETIC DISORDERS

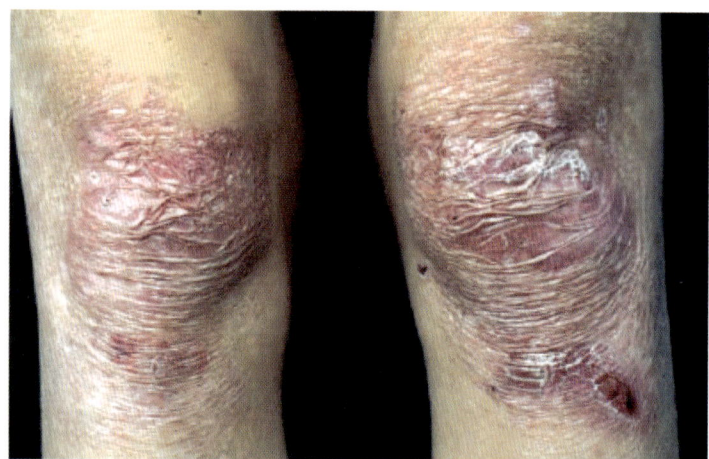

Figure 69.17 Scarring on the knees in a 14-year-old patient with intermediate recessive dystrophic epidermolysis bullosa.

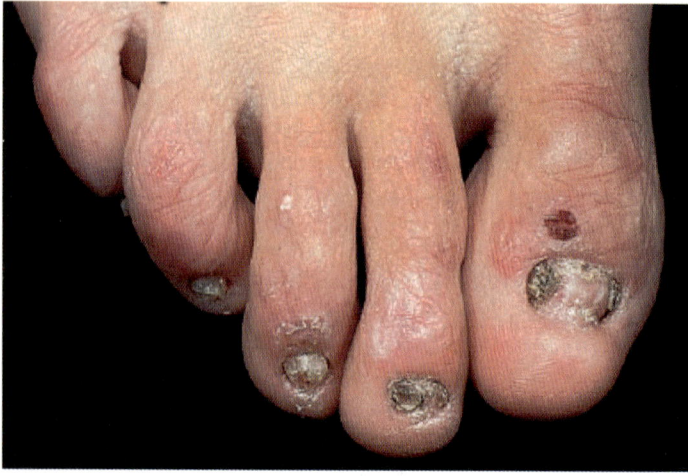

Figure 69.18 Nail changes and scarring of skin on the toes in dominant dystrophic epidermolysis bullosa.

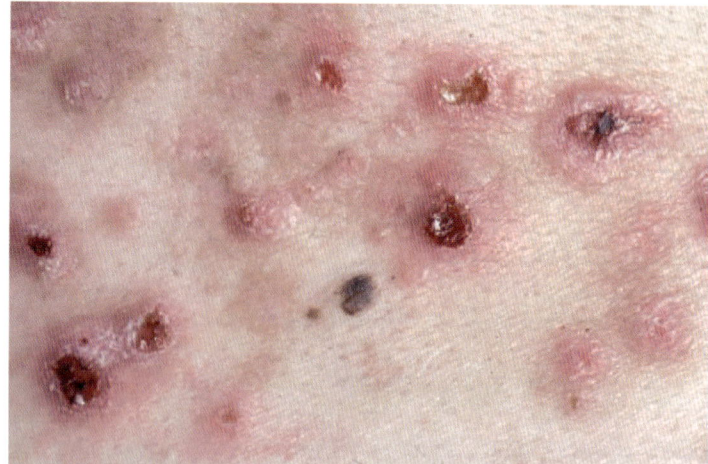

Figure 69.19 Inflammatory skin blistering in epidermolysis bullosa pruriginosa (dystrophic EB) resembling an acquired immunobullous disease.

blistering, scarring and milia are typically present in acral sites. In some cases, blistering may be mainly localised to the shins with just minor lesions elsewhere; these cases are often referred to as pretibial dystrophic EB. Other individuals may only have nail dystrophy with no evident skin fragility, with the condition previously known as nails only dystrophic EB [2].

Pruriginosa dystrophic EB (autosomal dominant or autosomal recessive)

This subtype of dystrophic EB overlaps with the pretibial variant, clinically and genetically. The main difference is the intense pruritus, the aetiology of which is uncertain. Studies have excluded concomitant atopy and a range of possible metabolic, biochemical and endocrine factors in disease pathogenesis [1]. Moreover, there is no specific genotype–phenotype correlation to implicate certain types of *COL7A1* mutation in dystrophic EB pruriginosa [2]. The clinical features can resemble hypertrophic lichen planus or nodular prurigo or autoimmune inflammatory blistering (Figure 69.19), or even dermatitis artefacta. Like the pretibial subtype, the initial onset

of symptoms and signs may be delayed for several decades, often leading to a genetic cause for the skin lesions being erroneously discounted. Although the shins are often involved, pruritic skin lesions can occur at any site.

Self-improving dystrophic EB (autosomal dominant or autosomal recessive)

One curious variant of dystrophic EB is when localised or generalised blistering in neonates starts to show signs of spontaneous clinical improvement over the first few weeks or months of life (Figure 69.20). The amelioration in phenotype is mirrored by improvement of the underlying skin pathology with increased type VII collagen at the dermal–epidermal junction. Initial skin biopsies reveal punctate intraepidermal labelling for type VII collagen and ultrastructural signs of dilated perinuclear vacuoles with a granular appearance (stellate bodies). Initially, it was thought that complete correction of the type VII collagen secretion and assembly into anchoring fibrils occurred, leading to the diagnostic label of 'transient bullous dermolysis of the newborn' [1]. Now, however, it is appreciated that most cases do not resolve completely and that there may be permanent stigmata of dominant or recessive dystrophic EB, albeit less severe than in early life [2]. This pattern of incomplete resolution led to the modified nosology 'bullous dermolysis of the newborn' but the preferred term now is self-improving dystrophic EB. Intraepidermal type VII collagen is not an exclusive finding in self-improving dystrophic EB as it can also occur in other subtypes of dystrophic EB depending on the nature of the underlying *COL7A1* mutation(s).

Severe recessive dystrophic EB

Bullae are present at birth or appear in early infancy and the skin is very fragile (Figure 69.21). The clinical presentation may include localised absence of skin especially affecting the lower legs. Blisters develop spontaneously or after the mildest trauma on any part of the skin and may be haemorrhagic [1]. Healing lesions leave atrophic scars, although thicker scars may occur particularly over the large joints, such as the knees. Milia formation is a nearly constant feature. Although the whole of the skin is fragile and at high risk of developing blisters, the main sites of predilection are those

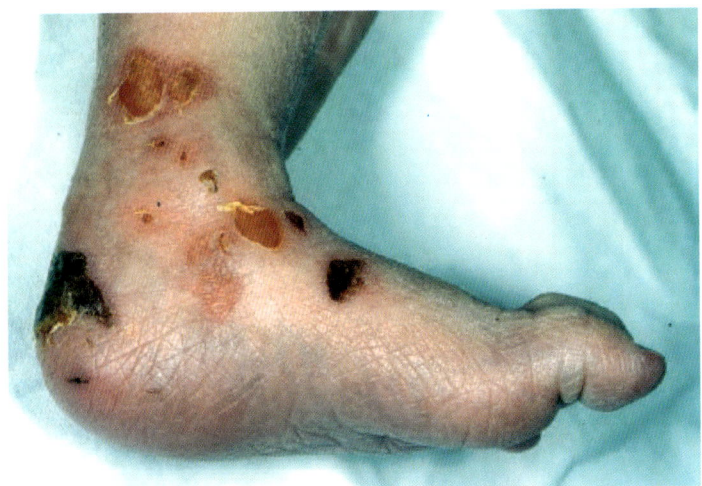

Figure 69.20 Acral blistering in (autosomal dominant) self-improving dystrophic EB in a 2-month-old male infant. By the age of 9 months the blistering had ceased and only a few small scars and some toenail dystrophy persisted (lifelong).

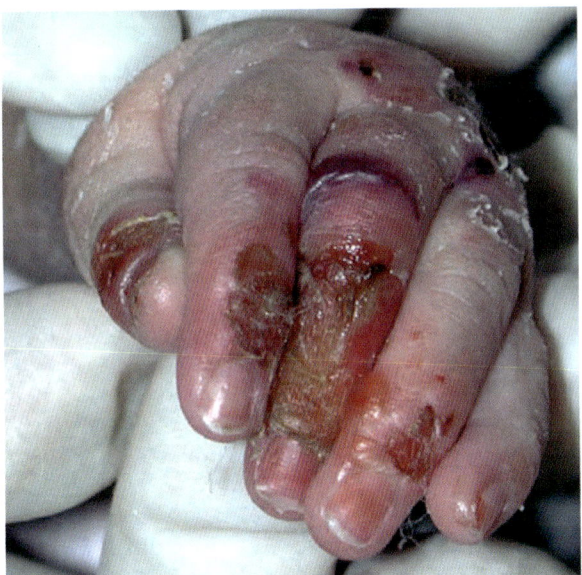

Figure 69.21 Blisters and erosions on the hand in a 4-week-old child with severe recessive dystrophic epidermolysis bullosa.

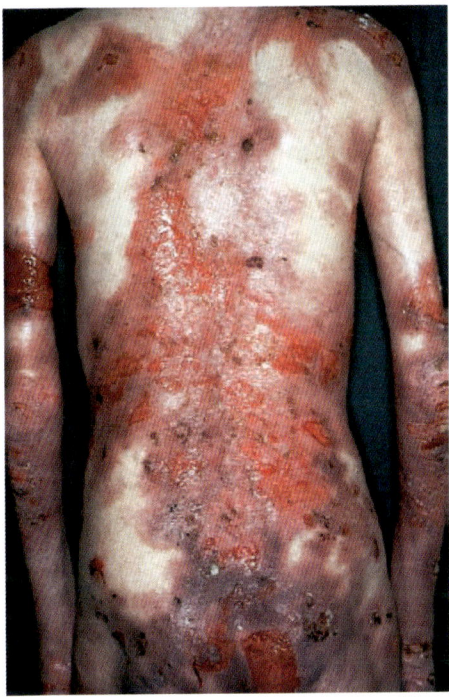

Figure 69.22 Extensive lesions on the back in severe recessive dystrophic epidermolysis bullosa.

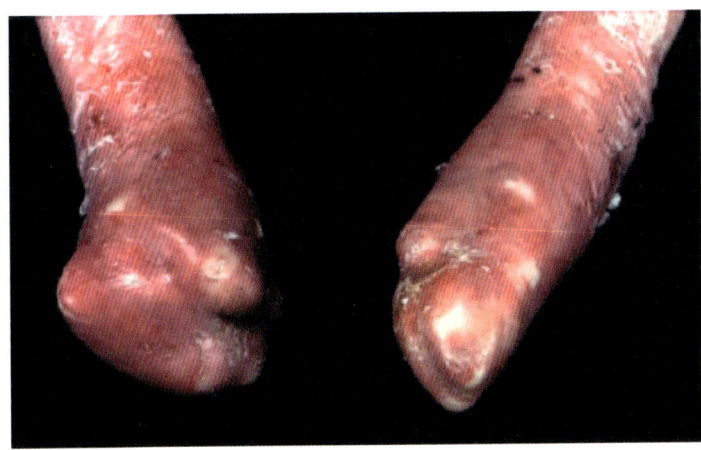

Figure 69.23 Mitten hand deformity in severe recessive dystrophic epidermolysis bullosa.

subjected to repeated friction and other forms of physical trauma. These include the knees, elbows, hands, feet, back of the neck, shoulders and over the spine (Figure 69.22). Chronic erosions and ulcers tend to become covered with a slough, often associated with heaped-up crusting and scaling, increasing the risk of secondary infection. Pruritus is frequent and constant rubbing and scratching may induce blisters. Considerable pain may be present and exacerbated with dressing changes. The scalp is often involved. Hair growth on the scalp and body is impaired and scarring alopecia may occur. During childhood, repeated blistering with progressive scarring leads to fusion ('pseudosyndactyly') of adjacent fingers and toes. Digits can undergo progressive contractures and gradually become encased in a cocoon-like covering of thin scar tissue, resembling a mitten (Figure 69.23). Disuse of the hands results in

bony resorption and muscle atrophy. Non-cutaneous epithelia are also at risk of developing blisters, erosions and scars.

Oral lesions may be severe, leading to marked ankyloglossia and microstomia [2]. The gums are fragile, and gentle tooth brushing may induce epithelial disruption with bleeding. The lingual papillae are lost, and the surface of the tongue becomes smooth, shiny and atrophic. Although there is limited evidence for a primary abnormality of dental enamel in dystrophic EB, the teeth are at a high risk of developing caries (Figure 69.24). Oesophageal involvement is a serious and invariable complication. It may occur very early in life, even in infancy, and by the age of 20–30 years will have affected most patients. Blistering in the oesophagus may cause acute pain and dysphagia, with difficulty in swallowing solids. With

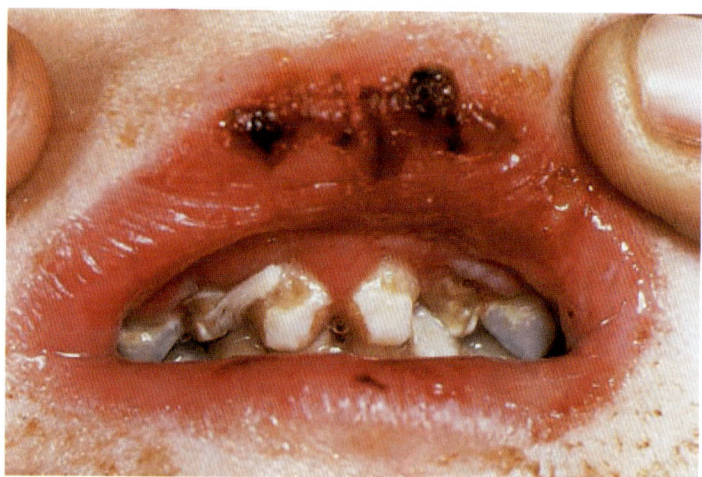

Figure 69.24 Dental caries and blistering on the lips in severe recessive dystrophic epidermolysis bullosa.

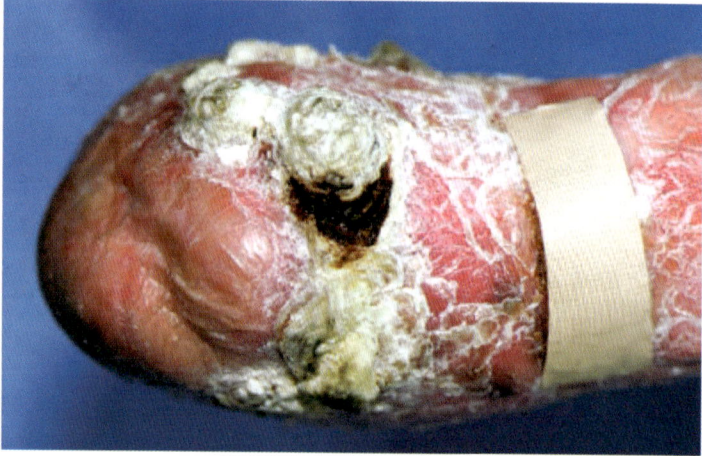

Figure 69.25 Squamous cell carcinoma on the scarred hand of a 35-year-old patient with severe recessive dystrophic epidermolysis bullosa.

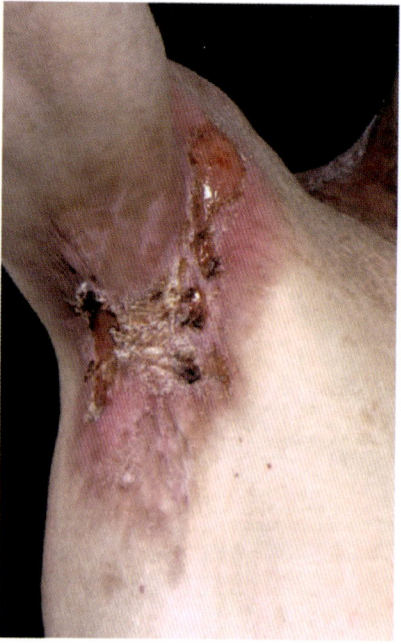

Figure 69.26 Scarring and erosions affecting the axilla and neck in inversa recessive dystrophic epidermolysis bullosa.

Inversa recessive dystrophic EB

In this variant of recessive dystrophic EB, the primary areas of blistering and scarring include the groins, axillae (Figure 69.26), neck and lumbar area, although in early life the distribution of the blistering may be generalised and not indicative of the subsequent pattern [1]. Traumatic corneal erosions and oesophageal lesions are common. Nail dystrophy, mucous membrane involvement and dental changes are similar to those in the other recessive variants. Patients are also at risk of developing squamous cell carcinoma. The reason for the predominance of flexural involvement is not clear, although the specific underlying mutations in *COL7A1* and their impact on type VII collagen thermal stability may be implicated in some cases [2].

Combined dominant and recessive dystrophic EB

Co-inheritance of a dominant *COL7A1* mutation and a recessive *COL7A1* mutation on separate alleles has been reported in a number of families [1,2], and the clinicopathological entity is now recognised as a distinct subtype of recessive dystrophic EB. In several instances, mothers with a localised or intermediate form of dominant dystrophic EB gave birth to a child with a more severe form of dystrophic EB. The explanation was that the father was an asymptomatic carrier of a recessive *COL7A1* mutation, and the child had inherited both the dominant maternal and recessive paternal *COL7A1* gene pathology. Clinically, most individuals with combined dominant and recessive dystrophic EB have clinical features towards the more severe end of the recessive dystrophic EB spectrum, i.e. they are phenotypically similar to individuals with two recessive *COL7A1* mutations resulting in severe recessive dystrophic EB.

Molecular pathology of dystrophic EB

All forms of dystrophic EB, dominant and recessive, result from mutations in *COL7A1* (type VII collagen). More than 1000 different

time, partial or complete obstruction may result from oesophageal stricture, caused by scarring and fibrosis, or from web formation. Perianal blistering, erosions and painful fissures are common in childhood. Later, anal stenosis from scarring may develop leading to constipation. The main ocular complications include symblepharon, corneal erosions and corneal opacity or scarring. Most patients with severe generalised recessive dystrophic EB are very thin and have a short stature. Some blood vitamin and trace metal levels are low and refractory anaemia is evident. Osteopenia and osteoporosis are not uncommon. Rarely, secondary amyloidosis can also develop in cases associated with persistent chronic inflammation and extensive scarring. A more common and clinically very important complication of this form of EB is the development of squamous cell carcinomas (Figure 69.25), even in individuals as young as 6 years of age. Most carcinomas are on the limbs, often in areas of chronic, non-healing ulceration. Multiple primary tumours with progressive loss of differentiation for each subsequent cancer is the usual course, and death typically occurs within 5 years of the first malignancy.

mutations have been reported with few recurrent mutations; most are specific to families or occasional regional founder effects. The spectrum of mutations predominantly includes nonsense, small insertions/deletions, missense and splice site mutations. In severe recessive subtypes there is usually a complete absence of type VII collagen resulting from nonsense or frameshift mutations on both *COL7A1* alleles. Intermediate variants usually express some type VII collagen, with at least one of the pathogenic *COL7A1* mutations having a less deleterious effect on protein structure and function. Most cases of dominant dystrophic EB result from heterozygous glycine substitutions within the type VII collagen triple helix, although a minority result from in-frame splice site mutations or small insertions/deletions that lead to in-frame exon skipping. There is no clear genotype–phenotype correlation for specific glycine substitutions which are present in most cases of dominant dystrophic EB as well as in some individuals with recessive dystrophic EB. Moreover, a minority of glycine substitutions can cause both dominant and recessive disease. What factors determine the genotypic implications of certain glycine substitutions remains to be determined. Apart from glycine substitutions, a small number of missense changes involving other amino acid residues can underlie both dominant and recessive dystrophic EB.

Kindler EB

Kindler EB, previously termed Kindler syndrome, is listed as a separate fourth category of the classic forms of EB. It is an autosomal recessive disorder. Initially it can resemble intermediate or localised forms of dystrophic EB, although skin biopsy typically shows a variable plane of cleavage and a fragmented or duplicated lamina densa in contrast to the specific planes of tissue separation that underlie EB simplex, junctional EB and dystrophic EB [1]. In most cases of Kindler EB, the initial skin blistering lessens during childhood and instead signs of a progressive poikiloderma develop (Figure 69.27). At this stage the differential diagnosis includes other congenital poikilodermatous disorders, including dyskeratosis congenita and Rothmund–Thomson syndrome. The poikilodermatous skin changes are particularly marked in individuals who live in sunny climates. Other somewhat variable clinical features include gingival inflammation, ectropion, corneal erosions, periodontal disease, scarring of the external urethral meatus and an increased risk of developing cutaneous squamous cell carcinoma, particularly on the hands [2]. Chronic colitis may also complicate some cases of Kindler syndrome. The hands can also show evidence of pseudosyndactyly, similar to some cases of dystrophic EB.

Molecular pathology of Kindler EB

Kindler EB arises due to loss-of-function mutations on both alleles of the *KIND1* gene that encodes kindlin-1, a protein involved in the attachment of actin microfilaments to focal contact junctions at the dermal–epidermal junction [1,2]. The gene/protein is also known as *FERMT1* or fermitin family homologue-1, and both terminologies are currently used. Thus far, the only other focal contact junction protein implicated in the pathophysiology of EB is α3 integrin (junctional EB with respiratory and renal involvement). Most pathogenic mutations in *KIND1/FERMT1* are nonsense, frameshift or splice site mutations; less commonly, missense mutations, large intragenic deletions and promoter region mutations can occur. Heterozygous carriers of mutations are asymptomatic with no mucocutaneous

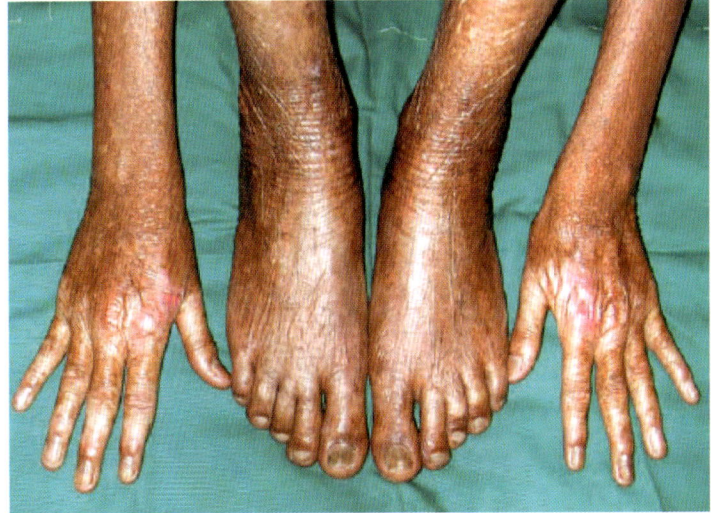

Figure 69.27 Poikiloderma in a 12-year-old Indian patient with Kindler epidermolysis bullosa.

abnormalities. Thus far there has been no evidence for genetic heterogeneity in Kindler EB, although the advent of next generation sequencing may lead to a widening of the spectrum of focal contact protein genodermatoses, some of which may feature in future classifications of EB, if skin fragility is a core clinical feature.

Other conditions included within the umbrella classification of skin fragility disorders

In addition to the four classic categories of EB (simplex, junctional, dystrophic, Kindler), the latest classification of skin fragility disorders also includes four categories of 'other disorders': these are divided into peeling skin disorders, erosive disorders, hyperkeratotic disorders with skin fragility, and a connective tissue disorder with skin fragility (Table 69.5). Some of these disorders were previously classified as forms of EB and are therefore discussed briefly here.

Peeling skin disorders

Within the peeling skin disorder subgroup is the entity of acral peeling skin syndrome, an autosomal recessive disorder caused by mutations in *TGM5* (transglutaminase 5) [1,2]. This condition was previously classified as a form of EB because of its clinical similarity to some classic forms of EB simplex resulting from mutations in *KRT5* and *KRT14* (Figure 69.28). In acral peeling skin syndrome, blisters typically occur on the feet although some of the blisters may be more evident on the sides or dorsal aspects of the toes. The level of blistering occurs above the granular layer but because of the thicker stratum corneum in acral skin, the clinical consequences may appear almost identical to blistering through the basal keratinocyte layer. The reason why acral peeling skin syndrome resulting from mutations in *TGM5* has been removed from within the classification of EB simplex relates to the very large number of other peeling skin disorders that have been characterised at a molecular level: mutations in at least nine genes have now been implicated in peeling

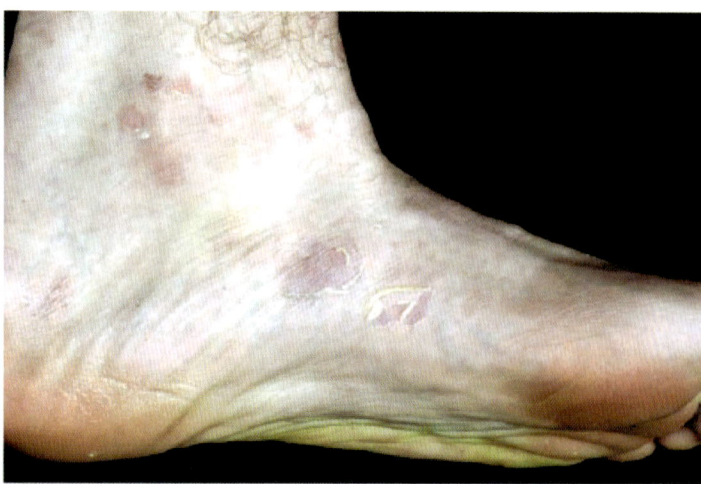

Figure 69.28 Autosomal recessive acral peeling skin syndrome resembling autosomal dominant localised epidermolysis bullosa simplex.

skin disorders (see Table 69.5), several of which are phenotypically distinct from what clinicians would diagnose as a form of EB.

Erosive disorders

The group of erosive skin fragility conditions comprises five autosomal recessive desmosomal disorders. Three of these were included in previous classifications of EB: mutations in *PKP1* (plakophilin 1) result in ectodermal dysplasia skin fragility syndrome (Figure 69.29) [1], whereas mutations in *DSP* (desmoplakin) and *JUP* (plakoglobin) result in more extensive skin fragility that can be associated with extracutaneous abnormalities. The two new desmosomal disorders involve mutations in *DSG3* (desmoglein-3) and *DSC3* (desmocollin-3). Clinically, mutations in genes encoding desmosomal proteins result in a spectrum of erosive skin and mucosal phenotypes that also may affect hair or heart [2]. Notably, mutations in *DSP* or *JUP* can result in cardiocutaneous syndromes, in which the cardiac manifestions can include cardiomyopathy, arrhythmias and sudden death.

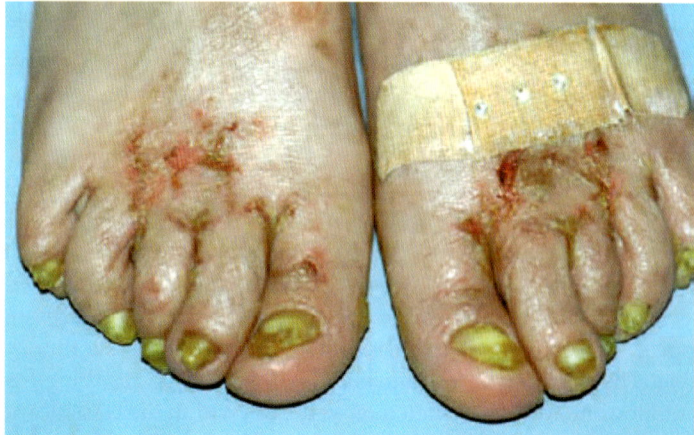

Figure 69.29 Erosions on the feet and nail dystrophy in ectodermal dysplasia-skin fragility syndrome.

Hyperkeratotic disorders with skin fragility

The category of other skin fragility disorders referred to as hyperkeratotic disorders with skin fragility comprises the various forms of keratinopathic ichthyoses and pachyonychia congenita, conditions that are more typically classified as inherited forms of ichthyosis, keratoderma or nail dystrophy. These disorders have a shared pathology in resulting from mutations in keratin genes; they also have skin histology features of epidermolysis although in most cases this does not manifest as clinical blistering. These disorders are discussed in more detail elsewhere (Chapter 63).

Connective tissue disorder with skin fragility

This category comprises a single entity with skin blistering only a minor part of the phenotype. Affected individuals have widespread connective tissue abnormalities and bony deformities [1,2]. However, the condition is referred to as a syndromic form of dystrophic EB because the causative gene pathology impacts directly on type VII collagen function. Notably, autosomal recessive mutations occur in *PLOD3*, which encodes LH3 (lysyl hydroxylase 3), an enzyme that has an important function in the post-translational modification of type VII collagen. Some of the blistering and scarring, although minor, have clinicopathological overlap with dystrophic EB.

Diagnosis of EB

Despite impressive advances in elucidating the molecular basis of the different forms of EB, optimal diagnosis of EB does not depend on next generation sequencing of EB gene panels. Rather, initial diagnosis still relies largely on careful clinical examination, enquiry into the family history and establishing the level of blister formation. Because the clinical features may be unhelpful or even misleading, especially in a neonate, the diagnosis will often rely on microscopic analysis of a skin biopsy. Traditionally, transmission electron microscopy and immunofluorescence microscopy using a panel of antibodies against the candidate proteins implicated in EB are the preferred methods. However, with increased access to molecular diagnostics, some cases of EB – such as clearly autosomal dominant EB simplex or dominant dystrophic EB – may merit DNA sequencing as a primary diagnostic method and thus avoid the need for a skin biopsy. For most recessive forms of EB, however, skin biopsy remains key to establishing a rapid diagnosis – although the diagnostic information that can be gained from the different microscopic techniques has evolved in recent years. Many recessive forms of EB are characteristically associated with a reduction or complete absence of one particular protein, and thus a skin biopsy submitted for skin immunolabelling alone often can be fully informative in establishing a diagnosis and in identifying a candidate gene for sequencing. Thus, the value of transmission electron microscopy as a diagnostic tool has diminished somewhat in recent years, although it remains a useful investigation in a significant minority of cases.

Skin biopsy

The main objectives of skin biopsy are first to establish the level of blistering or tissue separation and, second, to search for other

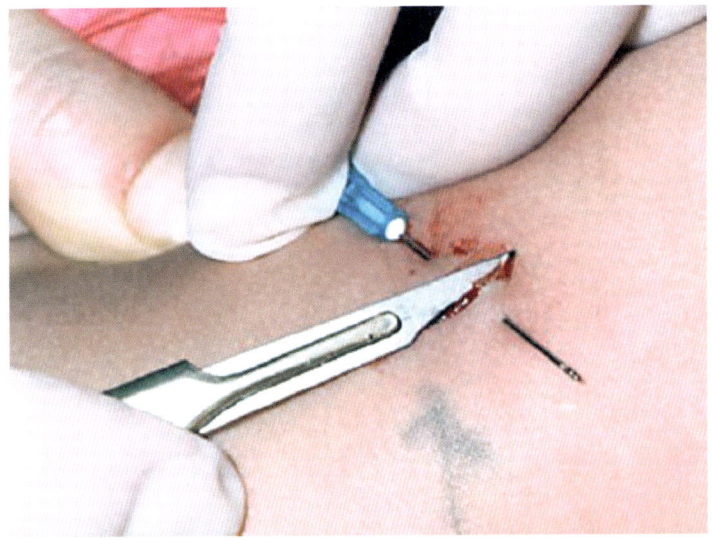

Figure 69.30 Shave biopsy technique suitable for the investigation of suspected epidermolysis bullosa.

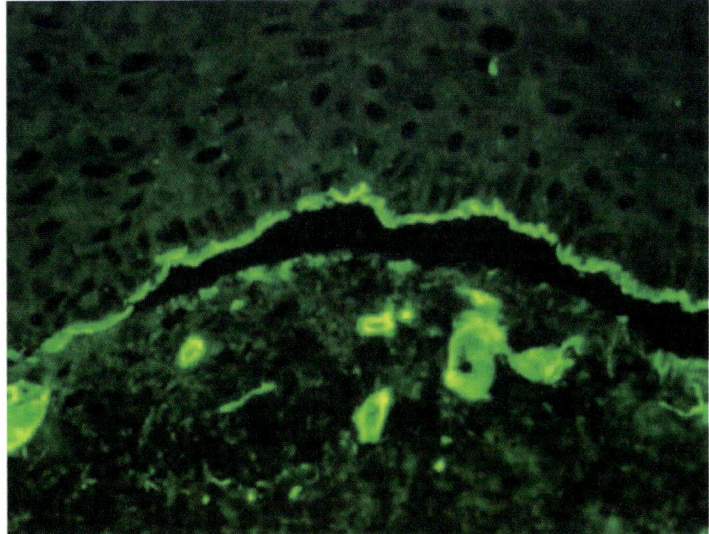

Figure 69.31 Antigen mapping of type IV collagen to a blister roof in a patient with dystrophic epidermolysis bullosa (sublamina densa blistering).

clues that may be indicative of the underlying disorder and therefore helpful in the diagnosis [1]. The importance of the correct biopsy technique cannot be overstressed. Most blisters that are clinically evident, and especially those with bloodstained contents, are often more than 12 h old and therefore too old for diagnostic purposes. Older blisters may cause severe diagnostic difficulty because false negative immunostaining caused by proteolytic antigen degradation can occur. Old blister sampling can also reveal re-epithelialisation under the blister roof and multiple cleavage planes. A sample of non-blistered skin that has been gently rubbed to produce a mild redness is preferable, because this will usually contain a cleavage plane with few if any secondary changes. Because the diagnostic signs are mostly seen in and around the dermal–epidermal junction, shave biopsy samples are preferable to thicker specimens (Figure 69.30). Care must be taken to ensure that a sufficient amount of dermis is present, to allow examination of the entire dermal–epidermal junction. The samples should be immediately immersed in suitable fixative for electron microscopy or in Michel's transport medium for immunofluorescence [2]. If facilities are available, the skin for immunofluorescence can be snap frozen.

Antigen mapping and antibody probes

The level of blister formation can be determined using indirect immunohistochemical staining. The aim is not to look for reduced expression of skin antigens, but to stain the dermal–epidermal junction or other junctional complexes using antibodies to proteins that are strongly expressed in both normal skin and skin from patients with different forms of EB [1]. For example, antitype IV collagen antibody will stain the lamina densa. If this antibody labels the roof of a blister then the level of separation must be beneath the lamina densa (Figure 69.31). Diagnostically, this indicates dystrophic EB since for EB simplex and junctional EB, type IV collagen immunostaining would map to the blister base. Most diagnostic laboratories perform the immunohistochemical studies on frozen skin sections, although antigen mapping studies (e.g. with antibodies to keratin 14 or type IV collagen) may be informative

on paraffin-emebdded sections. In addition to antibodies that are expressed in all skin, it is also possible to use antibodies against proteins that are mutated in the different forms of EB. This strategy has been particularly useful for diagnosing recessive forms of EB in which the underlying mutations tend to lead to reduced expression of the mutated protein, resulting in a reduction or sometimes complete absence of immunolabelling for the antibody probe targeting that particular protein [2]. For example, in recessive dystrophic EB, there are mutations in *COL7A1* encoding type VII collagen. Immunolabelling recessive dystrophic EB skin with an antibody against type VII collagen shows reduced labelling, or a complete absence of labelling, at the dermal–epidermal junction compared with control skin (Figure 69.32). This reveals the diagnosis because immunolabelling with other basement membrane antibody probes (e.g. to laminin-332 or α6β4 integrin) shows no differences from the control in dystrophic EB patients. Paraffin-emebdded sections are not suitable for labelling with antibodies to transmembranous proteins (e.g. integrins) and frozen skin is necessary.

Immunofluorescence microscopy, however, may not be sufficient to make the diagnosis in all cases of EB. For example, if there is no blister in an EB skin biopsy and there are no clear differences in immunolabelling of the skin compared with the control, despite using a panel of antibodies targeting all the candidate proteins in EB, it cannot be concluded that the skin is normal since some cases of autosomal dominant EB simplex and dominant dystrophic EB cannot be discounted. Additional diagnostic tests, such as transmission electron microscopy or DNA sequencing, may be necessary in such cases to reach a precise diagnosis.

Transmission electron microscopy

The main purpose of ultrastructural analysis of the skin in cases of EB is to demonstrate the level of tissue separation or blistering. Viewing skin sections by light microscopy alone is not usually sufficient to establish a precise diagnosis, although vacuolar changes may sometimes be seen in EB simplex, particularly if semi-thin

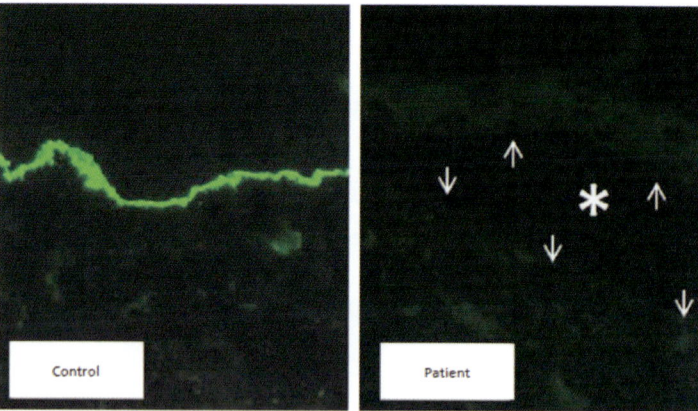

Figure 69.32 Immunolabelling for type VII collagen in normal skin showing bright linear staining at the dermal–epidermal junction. In contrast, in a patient with severe recessive dystrophic epidermolysis bullosa, there is a complete absence of type VII collagen immunoreactivity. Asterisk indicates blister; arrows depict roof and base of blister.

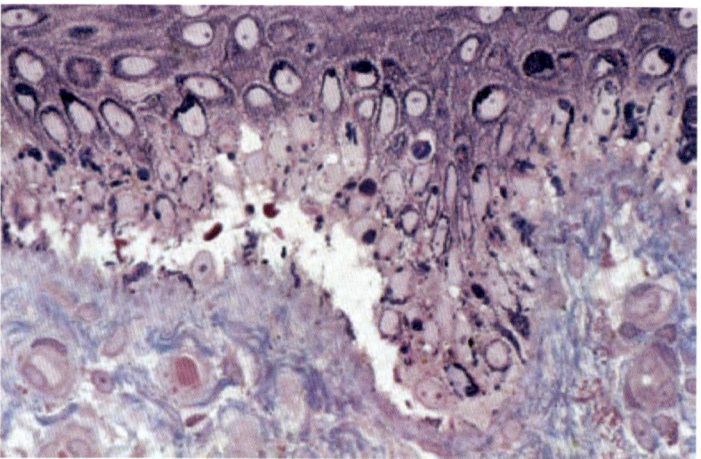

Figure 69.33 Intraepidermal cleavage revealed by light microscopy (semi-thin section) in severe epidermolysis bullosa simplex (Huber stain).

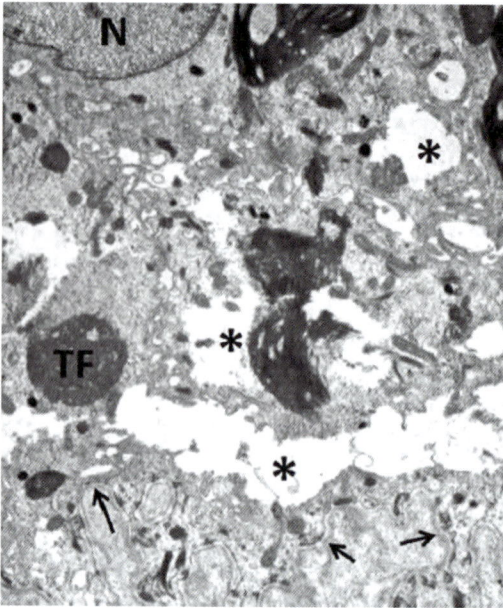

Figure 69.34 Electron microscopy of part of a basal keratinocyte in severe epidermolysis bullosa simplex showing tonofilament clumping (TF) and cytolysis (asterisks). N, nucleus; arrows indicate dermal–epidermal junction.

resin-embedded sections (0.5 μm thick) are viewed instead of conventional paraffin-embedded tissue (Figure 69.33). However, most levels of split need to be established by ultrastructural examination. In EB simplex the split is intraepidermal, in junctional EB it is through the lamina lucida, and in dystrophic EB it is beneath the lamina densa [1]. In Kindler EB, the cleavage plane may be variable and mixed (all of the above levels). Cleavage in EB simplex may feature cytolysis or acantholysis, depending on the underlying pathology in certain subtypes (Figure 69.34). Other ultrastructural features important for diagnosis are that keratin filaments in the basal keratinocytes tend to be disrupted or aggregated or, for other variants, desmosome cell junctions, granular layer or cytoplasmic vesicles may be abnormal. Hemidesmosomes are generally sparse and small in the more severe forms of junctional EB and anchoring fibrils are reduced in number, absent or structurally abnormal in dystrophic EB [2]. A clear distinction cannot be made between some dominant and localised recessive dystrophic forms, even with morphometrical analysis of the anchoring fibrils. Certain ultrastructural findings in particular subtypes of EB can be diagnostically

useful. For example, ball-like clumping of tonofilaments in basal keratinocytes is found in severe EB simplex; pallor and lack of tonofilaments in basal keratinocytes are associated with recessive knock-out mutations in keratin 14 or dominant mutations in KLHL24; grouped perinuclear vesicular endosomes typify EB simplex with exophilin-5 pathology; and intracellular stellate bodies can indicate self-improving dystrophic EB.

It is important to remember that preparing skin for electron microscopy requires attention to detail, which includes choice of optimal fixative, tissue processing and recognition of what represents genuine pathology or artefact. Overall, electron microscopy now provides a useful contribution to EB diagnostics in fewer than 10% of cases; the remainder can usually be diagnosed through a combination of immunofluorescence microscopy and DNA sequencing. Thus, it is now common practice to process the initial diagnostic skin biopsy and mount in resin but only continue to tissue sectioning and examining the skin if the other techniques fail to reveal a clear diagnosis.

Sanger sequencing

To date 16 different genes have been implicated in the molecular pathology of classic forms of EB, which increases to 40 genes if the other skin fragility disorders are included. Most of the pathogenic mutations are point mutations or involve small insertions or deletions. As such, mutation detection strategies have been established that are based on Sanger sequencing of DNA – directly sequencing polymerase chain reaction (PCR) products spanning the exons and flanking intronic sequences that cover all the coding regions and splice sites of all known EB genes (Figure 69.35) [1]. Thus, for the known EB genes, this equates to more than 400 PCR products. However, it is not usual practice to sequence all these PCR products for all patients. Usually, the genes to amplify and sequence are influenced (or determined) by a preceding combination of the clinical features and skin biopsy data implicating a candidate

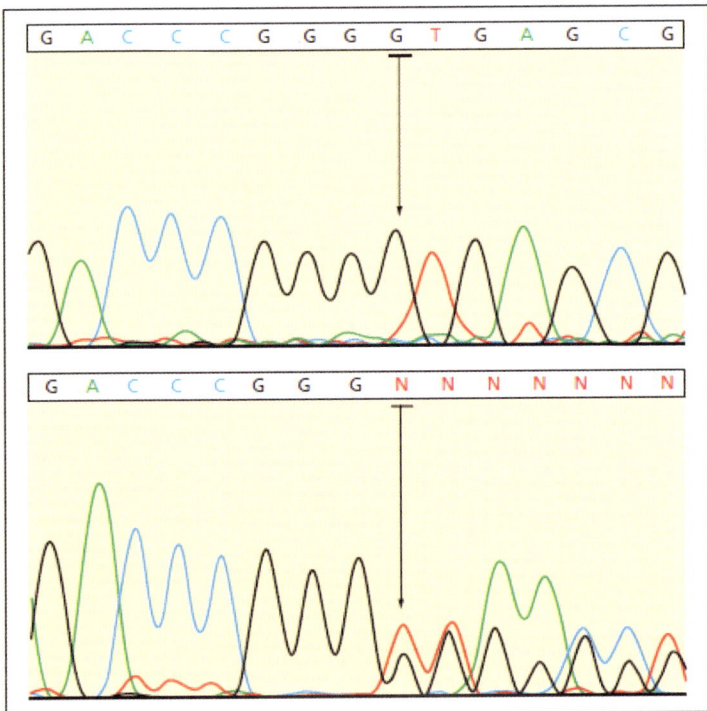

Figure 69.35 Sanger sequencing. The upper image shows a wild-type DNA sequence but in the lower image there is a 1 bp deletion (G nucleotide) that induces a frameshift, resulting in a downstream premature termination codon. This type of mutation can be found in several recessive forms of epidermolysis bullosa.

gene/protein. For example, if a patient's skin biopsy showed a reduction in type VII collagen, the Sanger sequencing would focus on the *COL7A1* gene and not the other genes [2]. For some subtypes of EB, including autosomal dominant EB simplex and dominant dystrophic EB, Sanger sequencing of the *KRT5* (keratin 5), *KRT14* (keratin 14) and *COL7A1* (type VII collagen) genes may be used as a first line diagnostic. Most diagnostic DNA sequencing in cases of EB is undertaken using DNA extracted from peripheral blood or saliva samples, although in cases of mosaic disease (including revertant mosaicism) it is usually also necessary to obtain DNA from affected and unaffected skin for sequencing and mechanistic studies.

Next generation sequencing
Recent advances in DNA technologies have led to the introduction of next generation sequencing (NGS) techniques that have had a major impact on DNA diagnostics for inherited disorders such as EB [1]. The aim of NGS is to sequence in one go all of the genome (whole genome sequencing) or all the exons and flanking introns of the 21 000 or so known genes (whole exome sequencing) and then apply a series of bioinformatic filters to identify disease-causing mutations. This approach has been highly informative in a research setting in identifying novel disease–gene associations (e.g. the identification of *EXPH5* mutations in autosomal recessive EB simplex) and is now used for diagnostic purposes [2]. The overall costs of using NGS for EB diagnostics are similar to the combination of skin biopsy and Sanger sequencing, but costs of NGS are expected to fall further in coming years. The major obstacle, however, is the time it takes to make a diagnosis. Establishing a rapid diagnosis is often

important to clinicians, especially for those involved in the management of neonates with suspected EB. Currently, a skin biopsy can be used to make the diagnosis of most forms of EB within 2–3 days. By contrast, NGS may take several weeks or months to complete. Even with preferential access to sequencing machines and with the sequencing focused on a limited panel of known EB genes, a minimum of 1 week (and often considerably longer) is needed to reach the diagnosis. Nevertheless, technology continues to evolve rapidly and the era of being able to sequence a 'genome in a day' is not too far away. NGS, if backed by adequate bioinformatic support, has the potential to become a preferred diagnostic modality for all inherited skin diseases, with the capacity to identify pathogenic mutations without detailed *a priori* clinical or skin biopsy data, and to provide a data file of other known and unknown potential genetic modifiers. As a technology, additional techniques have been added to the repertoire of NGS diagnostic tools, for example RNA sequencing for transcriptomics or whole genome sequencing with long-read sequencing.

Differential diagnosis

Differentiating EB from non-EB, or one form of EB from another, can be very difficult, especially in the neonatal period (Figure 69.36). At this stage, the following disorders may need to be included in the differential diagnosis of EB: bullous congenital ichthyosiform erythroderma; staphyloccocal scalded skin syndrome; bullous impetigo; incontinentia pigmenti; neonatal herpes simplex; autoimmune bullous disease, such as pemphigus or pemphigoid gestationis, acquired transplacentally; aplasia cutis; focal dermal hypoplasia; and Gunther disease. In infants, older children or adults, some autoimmune bullous diseases, such as bullous pemphigoid, mucous membrane pemphigoid or linear IgA disease, may show overlapping features with junctional EB or severe generalised EB simplex. EB acquisita may resemble dystrophic EB. Usually, the timing of the onset of blistering will allow inherited EB to be distinguished from the autoimmune immunobullous disorders. Pachyonychia congenita and epidermolytic ichthyosis may also be confused with EB in some children or adults. Peeling skin syndromes are heterogeneous and some may resemble EB. Finally, factitial skin damage, including child abuse, may also be a diagnostic consideration in some cases.

Other blistering genodermatoses

In addition to the classic forms of EB, and the entities listed as other skin fragility disorders in the most recent international consensus classification of EB [1], two other groups of disorders may have features of skin fragility: calcium pump disorders and certain metabolic or signalling disorders.

Calcium pump disorders
Darier disease is a severe dominant genetic skin disorder characterised by the loss of cell-to-cell adhesion and abnormal keratinisation. The defective gene, *ATP2A2*, encodes sarco/endoplasmic reticulum Ca^{2+}-ATPase isoform 2 (SERCA2), an intracellular

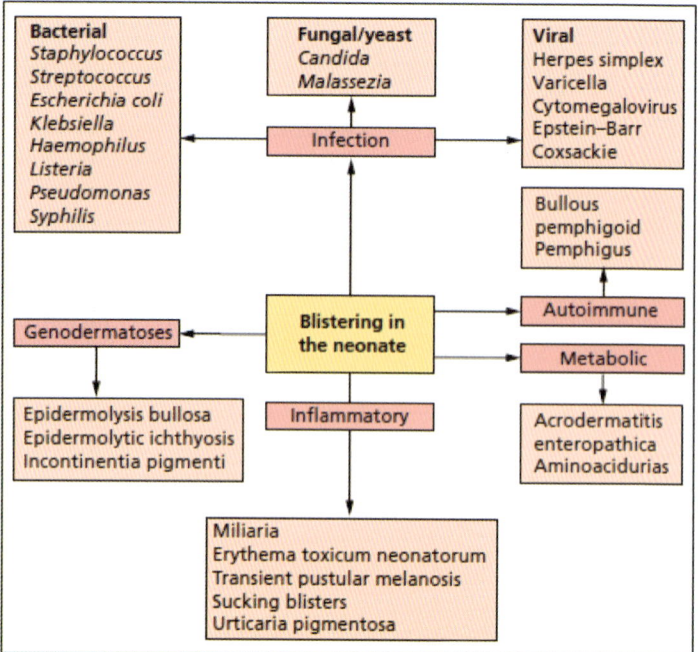

Figure 69.36 Differential diagnosis of skin blistering in a neonate.

Ca²⁺-ATPase pump. Mechanistically, desmosome and adherens junctions are immature and there is abnormal keratinocyte differentiation [1]. Acantholytic dyskeratosis is seen on light microscopy. Greasy papules and plaques arise on the seborrhoeic areas and in the flexures and almost all patients have nail abnormalities, with V-shaped nail plate notches and longitudinal violaceous/white band-like streaks. Hailey–Hailey disease (familial benign chronic pemphigus) is also autosomal dominantly inherited and manifests as uncomfortable erosions or vegetating lesions at sites of friction. It results from mutations in a different calcium pump gene, *ATP2C1* [2]. In Hailey–Hailey disease the skin is more fragile than in Darier disease. Flexural skin may become somewhat thickened and papillomatous, but patients do not develop the hyperkeratotic papules seen in Darier disease.

Metabolic and signalling disorders

Acrodermatitis is an inherited disorder of zinc deficiency. The clinical manifestations include eczematous, pink, scaly plaques that can become vesicular, bullous, pustular or desquamative skin lesions that mostly occur around the body orifices and on the extremities. Angular cheilitis, also known as perlèche, is a common early manifestation followed closely by paronychia. Subsequently, the features include alopecia and diarrhoea. The condition usually presents in infancy within days if an infant is bottle-fed and days to weeks after weaning in breast-fed infants. The disorder is caused by autosomal recessive mutations in a zinc transporter gene, *SLC39A4* [1], and responds to zinc supplementation. Incontinentia pigmenti is an X-linked dominant genodermatosis that is lethal *in utero* in males. It results from abnormalities affecting the transcription factor NF-κB with dysregulation of the immune and stress responses, inflammation, cell adhesion and protection against apoptosis [2]. An internal deletion within the *IKBKG* (previously known as *NEMO*, NF-κB essential modulator) gene accounts for 85% of incontinentia

pigmenti patients and results in absent NF-κB activation. Clinically there is an inflammatory and vescular eruption along Blaschko lines that later becomes hyperpigmented and warty in appearance.

Treatment of EB

At present there is no curative treatment for any form of EB, and the mainstay of clinical management is based on protection and avoidance of provoking factors and attention to patient symptoms such as itch and pain [1,2]. In the more severe forms of EB, it should be remembered that the whole skin and other stratified squamous epithelia, including the oral mucosa, are extremely fragile and vulnerable to blistering from the slightest friction or scrapes. In the milder forms, blistering may not always result from minor friction and may only follow sharp knocks to the skin. Major challenges include the treatment of the neonate with severe disease and the older child, adolescent or adult with the chronic disability that accompanies severe recessive dystrophic EB.

Management of neonates and infants

Because severe blistering and erosions may be associated with junctional, dystrophic or simplex forms of EB in the neonate, an early objective is to establish the diagnosis from an appropriate skin biopsy. This may be particularly relevant for a newborn with severe EB simplex, where the clinical appearance may be confused with generalised forms of junctional EB or even dystrophic EB, suggesting a much graver prognosis. A key to successful management of neonates with EB is expert nursing care [1]. Paediatric nurse specialists with experience of caring for babies and children with EB are often best placed to help with coordinating hospital or home treatment, initiating diagnostic tests and training parents. Ideally, babies with EB are nursed on thick foam pads, which are covered by a silk sheet. This allows the babies to be held, fed and nursed without subjecting them to undue trauma. The erosions are cleaned with sterile normal saline and covered in comfortable non-adherent dressings [2]. Some EB specialists may prefer to use a topical antiseptic such as stabilised hydrogen peroxide cream (e.g. Hioxyl®, Quinoderm, UK) or 1% chlorhexidine cream, rather than topical antibiotics, chiefly because of the risk of emergence of antibiotic-resistant bacteria. Another preference is to treat open wounds with 1% silver sulfadiazine cream (Flamazine®, Smith and Nephew, UK) or an ointment containing polymyxin B or bacitracin, although use of topical silver preparations should be limited because of the potential for systemic absorption. The topical antibiotic mupirocin is not recommended for regular use, especially in hospital practice, because of the emergence of mupirocin-resistant *Staphylococcus aureus*. However, its use for short periods (up to 7 days) in the home, for localised infected areas, is normally safe and effective. Among the newer dressings now favoured for use in children and older patients are Mepitel® and Mepilex® (Molynycke, Luton, UK). Mepitel is a porous, mildly adherent silicone-based material, which can be left in place for up to 7 days. Any exudate is usually able to pass through the holes in this dressing to be absorbed by a secondary gauze dressing, which can be changed more frequently. Mepilex has a foam backing that provides more protection where needed. Other dressings that have been found to be useful include Urgotul® (Urgo Medical, Loughborough, UK) and PolyMem® (Ferris Mfg. Corp., Fort Worth, TX, USA).

Management of EB simplex

Heat and humidity lower the threshold for blistering in patients with EB simplex, and measures to reduce both these factors are therefore important [1]. Patients with localised or more extensive forms of EB simplex should wear well-fitting, well-ventilated shoes, preferably with a soft inner lining. Cooling insoles such as CoolSorb® (Algeos Ltd, Liverpool, UK) can be helpful, especially in hot weather. Cotton socks are preferable to wool or synthetic fibres, and double-layer sports socks provide extra protection from friction and absorb sweat well. Heat-dissipating silver fibre socks, such as Carnation Silversocks® (Cuxson Gerrard and Co., Oldbury, UK) can be useful for many patients. Turning ordinary socks (and sometimes T-shirts) inside out can be helpful in reducing friction between the creases on clothes and the skin. Use of 20% aluminium chloride hexahydrate for the hyperhidrosis that can exacerbate blistering can be used for the treatment of localised EB simplex, although it does not help everyone. Botulinum toxin injections can also improve acral hyperhidrosis in some individuals. Dressings are not always needed in EB simplex – sometimes they can exacerbate the blistering. The use of non-sterile cornflour (cornstarch) can sometimes be preferable in reducing blisters and improving wound healing. The cornflour can be applied directly to the skin (including blistered sites) or sprinkled into socks or shoes. There are no proven systemic therapies to improve EB simplex, although in some people oral tetracycline may reduce the numbers of new blisters [2].

Management of severe junctional EB

Individuals with the more severe form of junctional EB usually have a poor prognosis and mostly do not survive for more than a few weeks or months. However, the prognosis is variable and in a small minority of cases there can be a lessening of clinical severity and survival for several years. Extreme care should be taken in handling affected children because of the profound muco-cutaneous fragility. Non-adhesive dressings should be used (see section on neonatal management). Assessment should also be made for extracutaneous abnormalities, that is, whether this is a subtype of junctional EB associated with muscular dystrophy, pyloric atresia, etc. Facial erosions and periungual inflammation are common. Many wounds display exuberant granulation tissue that can improve following the application of potent topical steroids for a few days. Skin grafting may also help, although the extent of the erosions and underlying tissue fragility, in combination with the poor prognosis, may influence what is clinically feasible [1]. Some children require tracheostomy because of vocal hoarseness and airways obstruction [2].

Management of severe recessive dystrophic EB

Patients with the more severe forms of recessive dystrophic EB will often survive into middle age and will therefore require continuing care throughout life. Ideally, they should be seen at 6-monthly intervals in a multidisciplinary clinic with expertise to help with the particular needs of these patients. Special precautions should be taken in the use of adhesive tapes, blood presssure cuffs, tourniquets and any other instruments or appliances that might lead to blister formation or shearing of the skin or mucous membranes. The following systems require particular attention.

Oral and dental care

Microstomia, intraoral fibrosis and tethering of the tongue (ankyloglossia) make access and examination of the teeth and mucosa difficult [1]. Treatment should start in early childhood, so the involvement of a paediatric dentist with specialist knowledge of the dental complications affecting children with EB is important [2]. Whenever necessary, reconstructive measures should be applied to permanent and primary teeth to maintain function; this includes treatment of caries and meticulous cleaning of tooth surfaces (paediatric electric toothbrushes are ideal). Crown placement and even tooth implants (in adults) have been used successfully in some patients. More frequent preventative measures include daily fluoride supplements and the use of a mouthwash containing sodium fluoride and aqueous chlorhexidine.

Gastrointestinal tract and nutrition

Dysphagia and pain on swallowing are common [1]. Oesophageal strictures may be demonstrated by X-ray examination (including barium swallow and cine radiography) (Figure 69.37) or by endoscopy. Oesophageal spasm, often accompanying an acute obstruction, can sometimes be relieved by the administration of calcium-channel blocking agents (e.g. sublingual nifedipine). The treatment of established strictures requires an endoscopically guided balloon dilatation, which will usually have to be repeated every few months. Most patients have gastro-oesophageal reflux, which should be treated with a proton pump inhibitor to prevent further damage to the lining of the oesophagus. Constipation is inevitable and often chronic. The cause is complex and associated, to some degree, with inadequate fibre in the diet. A high-fibre diet is therefore important, and patients who have difficulty in eating sufficient fibre may benefit from nutritional supplements such as Enrich® (Abbot Laboratories Ltd, Maidstone, UK). Osmotic and stimulant laxatives, as well as faecal softeners, may all have a role and be prescribed according to an individual patient's needs. Anal blistering and erosions contribute to the constipation and faecal retention, especially in children. Glycerol suppositories used in conjunction with a topical anaesthetic preparation may help. Trying to ensure adequate nutrition with a balanced diet is especially important to maintain growth in children. A deficiency of vitamins and trace elements (including zinc, iron and selenium) is frequent [2]. Comprehensive nutritional supplementation is only partly effective in maintaining adequate growth and in controlling anaemia and wound healing. Feeding through a gastrostomy allows appropriate nutrition in addition to the administration of supplements, which children may find difficult to take by mouth. Gastrostomy feeding can be delivered overnight in the home and is well tolerated.

Eyes

External abrasions should be dealt with urgently; they usually require topical treatment with an antibiotic and anaesthetic [1]. Eyepads may need to be worn for 2–3 days following corneal injury until pain diminishes. Scarring of the lids following blistering may result in inadequate lid closure and loss of normal protection to the eyes [2]. Plastic surgical reconstruction may be indicated. Artificial

PART 6: GENETIC DISORDERS

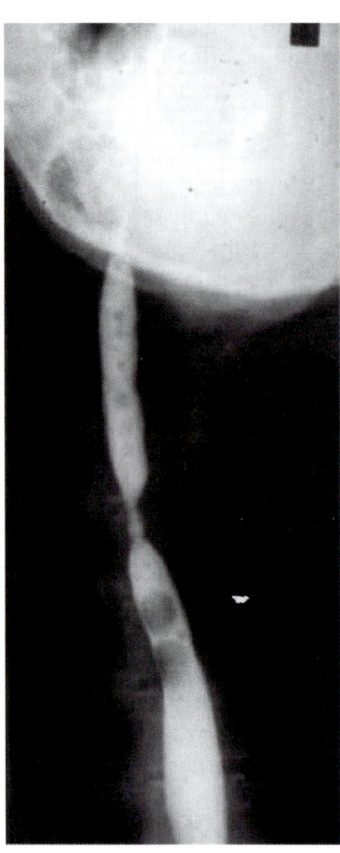

Figure 69.37 Barium swallow radiograph showing constriction in the upper oesophagus in recessive dystrophic epidermolysis bullosa. Courtesy of Professor R.A.J. Eady, St John's Institute of Dermatology, London, UK.

tears are a useful lubricant during the daytime, with lubricant ointments applied at night.

Musculoskeletal system

Although early exercises and physiotherapy may be helpful, the progress of finger and hand contractures with eventual mitten-type deformity is virtually inevitable [1]. Contractures and tight tethering by scar tissue may also affect elbows and knees. Surgical release of the contracted fingers is a highly specialised procedure and requires skin grafting, postoperative splinting and intensive physiotherapy and occupational therapy [2]. The benefit from surgery is only temporary, however, and most patients need further surgical treatment within a few years. The feet may be involved in a similar scarring process, but surgery is rarely undertaken because the foot deformities do not usually prevent patients from standing or walking.

Anaemia

All patients with the more severe forms of recessive dystrophic EB are anaemic, and the picture is that of anaemia of chronic disease [1]. Despite the administration of oral iron supplements, the iron stores are usually low as assessed by serum ferritin levels. In patients with widespread lesions and secondary infection, the serum ferritin may not accurately reflect the need for supplementary iron. Instead, the serum iron level may be a better indicator of the requirement for iron replacement in these patients. Parenteral iron is painful if given intramuscularly, especially where the muscles are thin and wasted, and intravenous administration is preferred [2]. Anaphylaxis is a potential risk of intravenous administration although the risk is low with preparations such as Ferinject® (ferric carboxymaltose; Vifor Pharma, Wigan, UK). Following intravenous iron, haemoglobin levels generally increase, and the patient's sense of well-being improves. Transfusion of packed red cells may be required in some patients, especially when the blood haemoglobin level falls below c.7.00 g/dL or when the patient becomes short of breath and more easily fatigued than usual.

Bony abnormalities

Virtually all patients have bony changes, mainly osteoporosis [1]. The cause is multifactorial and is related to poor nutrition, vitamin D deficiency, relative immobility in some patients and previous treatment with systemic glucocorticoids. This last point is especially relevant in older patients. Regular checking of bone density, especially of the hips and spine, usually by dual-energy X-ray absorptiometry (DEXA), is now part of routine management [2]. Treatment with calcium supplements, vitamin D and biphosphonates is usually indicated.

Genito-urinary tract abnormalities

Patients may infrequently develop a variety of genito-urinary and renal complications [1]. These may include stenosis of the external urethral meatus. Urological intervention is recommended whenever function is compromised although occasionally may result in more scar formation [2]. Dialysis has been successfully performed in occasional patients with end-stage renal disease.

Systemic treatments for recessive dystrophic EB

Long-term systemic corticosteroid treatment is not used now because of the high risk of complications, and phenytoin has not proved to be more effective than placebo [1]. Other systemic drugs that have been tried with mixed results in small numbers of patients include vitamin E, minocycline, ciclosporin and retinoic acid, although the number of randomised clinical trials in EB has been few [2]. Although, theoretically, the systemic use of a retinoid such as isotretinoin or acetretin might reduce the risk of squamous cell carcinomas in these patients, there is no evidence yet in support of this presumably lifelong treatment. In addition, increased mechanical fragility, blistering and/or itching may occur for doses approaching 0.5 mg/kg/day.

Cancer and recessive dystrophic EB

Squamous cell carcinomas (SCCs) are expected to occur in nearly every patient with severe recessive dystrophic EB, as well as in a minority of patients with intermediate and inversa variants [1]. Meticulous surveillance of the skin, particularly over bony prominences and in areas of greatest scarring and delayed wound healing, preferably with the aid of serial photography, should be performed regularly (at least every 6 months) from the age of 5 years, and any suspicious lesion should be immediately biopsied. Those lesions that fail to reveal cancer histologically, and yet remain atypical in appearance or healing pattern, such as a non-healing erosion, should be re-biopsied. This is because it is possible to miss an early

SCC, given the tendency of these tumours to be well-differentiated histologically and to show only focal areas of neoplastic change. Large SCCs (>5 cm in diameter) or those overlying difficult anatomical sites should be imaged with magnetic resonance imaging or computed tomography to assess tumour extent. Surgical excision is recommended, and careful serial follow-up examinations should be implemented, seeking possible local or regional recurrences. Amputation of an affected limb may eventually be required in some cases. Although still unproven, there may be a role for sentinel node biopsy in the management of these patients. There is no evidence to support use of Mohs micrographic surgery instead of conventional surgical excision. Regional metastases, for example those arising within the axillary vault, may benefit from at least partial surgical debulking, even if extensive, to reduce the size of non-healing, painful, malodorous or chronically infected lesions. Neither conventional chemotherapy nor radiotherapy has been shown to provide lasting benefit in the treatment of primary or secondary tumours, although epidermal growth factor receptor antagonists or immune checkpoint inhibitors may have some impact in lessening early-stage cancer progression. Radiotherapy, like surgery, may be used for reducing the tumour mass. Best practice guidelines for managing malignancy in EB have been published [2].

Pain management

Patients with EB frequently experience severe pain, which is unresponsive to conventional treatment with non-opiate-based or non-steroidal anti-inflammatory agents [1]. Unfortunately, systemic opiates are addictive and tend to exacerbate chronic constipation, making their long-term use highly undesirable. However, the use of topical opiates, including diamorphine, may be effective in the treatment of pain in EB patients, reducing the need for powerful systemic analgesia [2]. Its use is particularly beneficial when chronic pain is associated with chronic ulcers and erosions, accompanied in some patients by SCC. Amitriptyline is useful in pain management in both adults and children, and benzodiazipines such as midazolam can be helpful in reducing pain associated with changing dressings. Psychological support and cognitive–behavioural techniques may also be helpful in managing pain.

Skin grafting

Autologous split-thickness skin grafts have had short- to longer-term beneficial effects in the treatment of chronic ulcers or erosions in patients with some forms of recessive dystrophic EB or pretibial EB. Cultured autologous keratinocytes have also been used successfully in the treatment of junctional EB. Allogeneic keratinocyte grafting may be helpful in reducing wound pain although the cells do not survive more than a few days post-transplantation [1]. Skin bioequivalents (use of epidermal and dermal components in the skin grafts) have also been used in the treatment of EB simplex, junctional EB and dystrophic EB, with mixed results [2]. Concerns have been raised about the relative efficacy, especially in the long term, of treatment with bioequivalents, until more comprehensive data based on controlled trials become available (or alternative therapies are introduced). Some data from the National EB Registry suggest that such treatments are often either ineffective or any benefits may be relatively short lived.

Innovative therapies

Although there is currently no cure for EB, clinical testing of different forms of gene, cell, protein, small molecule and other forms of therapy is widely pursued. An update on the status of clinical trials in EB is available online: www.clinicaltrials.gov. At any given time, there are usually more than 100 active clinical trials assessing innovative therapies for EB. Selected examples of some of these treatments follow.

Recombinant protein therapy

One potentially attractive approach is recombinant protein therapy – if conditions such as recessive dystrophic EB lack type VII collagen protein in the skin, then why not simply make artificial type VII collagen and restore this to the defective skin? Topically applied recombinant protein therapy is unlikely to be successful because of the degree of infection and protease activity in EB wounds. Moreover, the extent of both cutaneous and mucosal and other organ involvement in EB makes systemic protein replacement a more attractive option. Following testing in small and large animal models of dystrophic EB [1,2], trials of intravenous type VII collagen protein therapy started in humans in February 2019. Although full data are yet to be published, thus far no safety concerns have been raised, either in the form of allergic reactions or autoantibodies to the type VII collagen as a neoantigen.

Gene therapy

Most recessive blistering genodermatoses are associated with loss-of-function mutations on both alleles. The result of these mutations is that no functional protein is being generated and therefore gene replacement strategies are being pursued. The most dramatic example of successful gene therapy for EB was reported in 2017 [1]. *Ex vivo* keratinocyte gene therapy using a *LAMB3* transgene was used to correct 80% of the skin of a boy with an intermediate form of junctional EB. This study also showed the importance of targeting keratinocyte holoclone stem cells for permanent correction; physical functional correction of the skin has been maintained for >5 years. For recessive dystrophic EB, attempts to replace *COL7A1* gene expression have been assessed in autologous keratinocyte sheets grafted on to wounds, as well as autologous fibroblasts injected into intact and wounded skin. For optimal gene replacement therapy in recessive dystrophic EB wounds, it may be advantageous to *COL7A1* correct both keratinocytes and fibroblasts and to graft composite skin equivalents. Delivering *COL7A1* gene therapy topically to wounds in a gel or cream base is also being assessed but no clinical trial results have yet been published. Gene editing approaches have not yet been tested in clinical trials in EB but technological advances in a technique called prime editing offer great promise for future clinical translation [2].

Cell therapy

Keratinocytes (autologous, allogeneic), fibroblasts (allogeneic), mesenchymal stromal cells (autologous, allogeneic, haploidentical – from bone marrow, umbilical cord, adipose tissue) and bone marrow transplantation have all been tested in patients with EB, particularly in severe forms of recessive dystrophic EB [1]. At present, no single approach provides universal benefit. Some approaches address the primary genetic abnormality underlying the EB, such as punch grafting of revertant mosaic skin or bone marrow transplantation. For these therapies, there may be restoration of the defective protein underlying the EB. Most other approaches, however, target inflammation in the skin, for example intravenous allogeneic mesenchymal stromal cells release various cytokines and chemokines that reduce redness, pain and itch and promote wound healing [2], albeit for just a few months. Inducible pluripotent stem cells currently present a means of generating model systems for studying EB and for therapeutic screening but have yet to feature in human clinical trials for any subtype of EB.

Small molecule therapy

Small molecules are chemicals of <900 Da that can pass across cell membranes and interact or interfere with target biomolecules. For EB, there are typically more than 30 active clinical trials of small molecule therapy ongoing at any time [1]. Of current interest is gentamicin (results in readthrough of nonsense mutation-associated RNA decay), which is being tested topically, intradermally and intravenously in individuals with dystrophic and junctional forms of EB in which the underlying gene pathology involves nonsense mutations [2]. Other studies are assessing topical betulin (betulin-enriched triterpene extract from birch bark to improve wound healing), topical diacerin (derived from rhubarb root to target interleukin-1β associated inflammation) in severe EB simplex, oral serlopitant (a neurokinin-1 receptor antagonist) to reduce itch severity, and epigallocatechin-3-gallate (inhibitor of matrix metalloproteinase 7) to reduce blister numbers in recessive dystrophic EB. Additional clinical testing is being undertaken for coenzyme Q10 (topically to improve wound healing); intradermal botulinum toxin for plantar pain and blistering in EB simplex; oral pregabalin (neurotransmitter modulation) to reduce pain and itch in recessive dystrophic EB; topical sirolimus (mTOR inhibitor) for EB simplex keratoderma; oral/intravenous rigosertib (a polo-like kinase-1 inhibitor) for SCC in recessive dystrophic EB; and topical ropivocaine (local anaesthetic) to reduce wound pain.

Key references

The full list of references can be found in the online version at https://www.wiley.com/rooksdermatology10e

Introduction

1 Bardhan A, Bruckner-Tuderman L, Chapple ILC et al. Epidermolysis bullosa. *Nat Rev Dis Primers* 2020;6:78.

Definition and classification

3 Has C, Bauer JW, Bodemer C et al. Consensus reclassification of inherited epidermolysis bullosa and other disorders with skin fragility. *Br J Dermatol* 2020;183:614–27.

Erosive disorders

2 Lee JYW, McGrath JA. Mutations in genes encoding desmosomal proteins: spectrum of cutaneous and extracutaneous abnormalities. *Br J Dermatol* 2021;184:596–605.

Diagnosis of EB

Skin biopsy

1 Has C, Nyström A, Saeidian AH, Bruckner-Tuderman L, Uitto J. Epidermolysis bullosa: molecular pathology of connective tissue components in the cutaneous basement membrane zone. *Matrix Biol* 2018;71:313–29.

2 Takeichi T, Liu L, Fong K et al. Whole-exome sequencing improves mutation detection in a diagnostic epidermolysis bullosa laboratory. *Br J Dermatol* 2015;172:94–100.

Cancer and recessive dystrophic EB

2 Mellerio JE, Robertson SJ, Bernardis C et al. Management of cutaneous squamous cell carcinoma in patients with epidermolysis bullosa: best clinical practice guidelines. *Br J Dermatol* 2016;174:56–67.

Gene therapy

1 Hirsch T, Rothoeft T, Teig N et al. Regeneration of the entire human epidermis using transgenic stem cells. *Nature* 2017;551:327–32.

Cell therapy

1 Rashidghamat E, McGrath JA. Novel and emerging therapies in the treatment of recessive dystrophic epidermolysis bullosa. *Intractable Rare Dis Res* 2017;6:6–20.

Small molecule therapy

1 Wally V, Reisenberger M, Kitzmüller S et al. Small molecule drug development for rare genodermatoses – evaluation of the current status in epidermolysis bullosa. *Orphanet J Rare Dis* 2020;15:292.

2 Woodley DT, Cogan J, Hou Y et al. Gentamicin induces functional type VII collagen in recessive dystrophic epidermolysis bullosa patients. *J Clin Invest* 2017;127:3028–38.

CHAPTER 70

Genetic Disorders of Collagen, Elastin and Dermal Matrix

Nigel Burrows

Department of Dermatology, Addenbrooke's Hospital, Cambridge University Hospitals NHS Foundation Trust, Cambridge, UK

PART 6: GENETIC DISORDERS

INHERITED DISORDERS OF COLLAGEN

Ehlers–Danlos syndrome

Definition and nomenclature

The Ehlers–Danlos syndromes (EDS) are a heterogeneous group of inherited disorders of connective tissue that variably impair the structure and function of the skin, joints, internal organs, eyes and blood vessels. They are characterised by joint hypermobility, skin hyperextensibililty and tissue fragility.

Synonyms and inclusions
• Cutis hyperelastica

Introduction and general description

The original classification divided EDS into 11 clinical types and, in 1986, the International Nosology of Heritable Disorders of Connective Tissue redefined EDS into subtypes I–VIII and X [1]. Progress in molecular biology led to the Villefranche classification in 1997 [2]. Further subtypes have been described, with molecular characterisation, resulting in the 2017 International Classification which recognises 13 subtypes [3]. Since then, another distinct subtype has been identified [4].

Epidemiology

Incidence and prevalence

Data for the prevalence of EDS is incomplete. All types of EDS combined are estimated to occur in 1 per 5000–10 000 [5]. Hypermobility type (hEDS) is the most common (1/10 000–15 000), although its true incidence is unknown. hEDS combined with hypermobility spectrum disorder, using data from Wales, UK suggests a prevalence of 194.2 per 100 000 [6]; classical EDS (cEDS) is 1/20 000–40 000 and vascular type is 1/50 000–250 000 [7,8]. The other subtypes are much rarer, with only a small number of patients reported for each.

Age

Whilst features may be present at birth most patients present later in childhood as the diagnosis can be difficult to make, particularly in classical and hypermobile types, until the child starts to walk.

Sex

There is no sex predilection although more females present with hypermobility type.

Ethnicity

There is no racial variation.

Associated diseases

Type III collagen production by fibroblasts is decreased in some patients with ruptured cerebral aneurysm, even though they have no other stigmata of EDS [9]. The collagen deficiency in these patients does not appear to arise from COL3A1 mutations, but may relate to abnormal post-translational modification or altered collagen metabolism [10].

Hypermobile EDS and hypermobility spectrum disorder patients are increasingly reported to exhibit extra-articular manifestations involving postural orthostatic intolerance, gastrointestinal symptoms and features of mast cell activation syndrome (MCAS) [11].

Pathophysiology

Defects directly affecting fibrillar collagens and in intracellular trafficking, secretion and assembly of extracellular matrix (ECM) molecules, including proteoglycans and tenascin-X, are causal in different types of EDS [3].

Pathology

Skin histology is variable and often within normal limits. Typically, there is a loose, disordered dermal collagen network. Elastic fibres are usually increased and orientated irregularly. The 'pseudotumours' seen in cEDS consist of fat and mucoid material in fibrous capsules; they may be calcified. Bone mineralisation is decreased, and the collagen fibres are irregular. Adventitial defects of the small arteries and inadequate support from the surrounding connective tissue account for the vascular vulnerability in vascular EDS (vEDS) [12,13]. Often, in vEDS, the skin is reduced to 25% of normal thickness, with small collagen fibre bundles. Fibril diameter is markedly variable in some patients [13]. In many patients, the fibroblasts contain prominent rough endoplasmic reticulum containing abnormal type III procollagen [14,15]. Although bruising can be explained on the basis of skin and blood vessel fragility, a few patients also exhibit both ultrastructural and functional platelet defects [16,17]. Clotting factor deficiencies have been only rarely reported.

Electron microscopy of dermal collagen may show irregularities of fibril shape and size. Although reliable subclassification of the more common subtypes is not possible, it can help contribute to the diagnosis [18,19]. Cauliflower-like fibrils mainly occur in cEDS, and variable small diameter fibrils in vEDS. Tenascin-X-deficient patients have uniform collagen fibrils which are less densely packed and not as well aligned [16]. In musculo-contractural EDS, the collagen fibrils are less densely packed although their size and shape are not altered [20]. In contrast, arthrochalasia-type EDS is characterised by angular fibrils in cross-section, and dermatosparaxis by grossly distorted hieroglyphic fibrils.

Genetics

Spontaneous mutations occur in 30–50% of the autosomal dominant subtypes. The less common types are autosomal recessive. The previously described X-linked variant has been removed from the classification.

The different molecular abnormalities corresponding to the varying subtypes are listed in Table 70.1 [20,29,**30**,31–50].

Clinical features

Presentation

A diagnosis of EDS should be considered in anyone with the cardinal manifestations of skin hyperextensibility, skin fragility, easy bruising and joint laxity. Further features will depend on the EDS subtype. However, great phenotypic overlap occurs often making it difficult to rely on clinical features alone. Skin fragility, for example, may not be apparent until the child is at walking age [51].

Clinical variants

Classical Ehlers–Danlos syndrome (cEDS). The skin is soft, velvety and hyperextensible (Figure 70.1) but retains its normal recoil. The skin on the palms and soles may be hyperlinear and loose. The skin is not usually otherwise lax until later in life, when redundant folds occur on the eyelids (blepharochalasis), face and limbs. Secondary cutis laxa has been described on the lower back of a patient with mild cEDS [52]. Striae often do not develop during pregnancy. Trivial lacerations form gaping wounds that heal very slowly to leave broad, atrophic 'cigarette paper' scars (Figures 70.2 and 70.3). Sutures may tear out repeatedly. Blue-grey, spongy tumours (molluscoid pseudotumours), due to accumulation of connective tissue, may form on the skin, especially in scars or over pressure points. Smaller, firm, subcutaneous nodules (spheroids), which show calcification on X-ray, develop on the shins and forearms in up to a third of patients.

Easy bruising may be the presenting symptom, and pigmentation due to haemosiderin deposition is often found on areas of repeated trauma.

The facies may be distinctive, with widely spaced eyes, a wide nasal bridge and epicanthic folds. Gorlin sign, the ability to touch the nose with the tip of the tongue, is more common in those with EDS. The sclerae are sometimes blue.

There is marked joint hypermobility, which can impair walking, especially during pregnancy. Subluxation of the large joints may occur [53]. Muscle tone is often poor, and hernias develop. Pedal piezogenic papules are seen more frequently. Diaphragmatic eventration and gastric torsion have been reported [54]. Symptomatic bladder diverticula may develop [55]. Varicose veins may develop in early life. Prematurity due to ruptured fetal membranes is common.

As physical and mental developments are normal, life expectancy is not reduced, hence large family pedigrees are not unusual.

Hypermobile Ehlers–Danlos syndrome (hEDS). The 2017 classification of EDS has redefined hEDS and distinguishes it from other hypermobility disorders, referred to as hypermobility spectrum disorders [3,56]. Currently no molecular cause has been identified. The Beighton score (Table 70.2) is the most common, quick method for assessing global joint hypermobility and a score of 5 or more out of 9 under the age of 50 years old is considered diagnostic for joint hypermobility [3,57]. Ultimately, molecular analysis will determine whether these two groups are genetically heterogeneous. Haploinsufficiency of tenascin-X results in reduced dermal collagen and may account for 5–10% of hEDS, although this has been found only in females [58].

The skin is only minimally affected by scarring and hyperextensibility, whereas joint mobility is markedly increased, and dislocation

Table 70.1 Clinical and molecular subtypes of the Ehlers–Danlos syndrome (EDS).

EDS subtype	Mode of inheritance	Major diagnostic clinical criteria [3]	Minor diagnostic clinical criteria [3]	Gene-specific minor criteria	Ultrastructural findings	Molecular defect (references in square brackets)
Classical (cEDS)	AD	1 Hyperextensible skin and atrophic scars 2 GJH	1 Easy bruising 2 Soft, doughy skin 3 Skin fragility 4 Molluscoid pseudotumours 5 Subcutaneous spheroids 6 Hernia 7 Epicanthal folds 8 Complications of joint hypermobility 9 First-degree relative who meets clinical criteria		'Cauliflower' fibrils	COL5A1 and COL5A2 mutations identified in up to 90% [21]; majority are COL5A1 null type with remainder structural mutations [22] Rare: COL1A1 (α1(I)) p.Arg312Cys associated with increased vascular fragility [23]
Classical-like (clEDS)	AR	1 Skin hyperextensibility, velvety texture and absence of atrophic scarring 2 GJH 3 Easy bruising	1 Foot deformities: broad/plump forefoot, brachydactyly with excessive skin, pes planus, hallux valgus, piezogenic papules 2 Oedema of legs 3 Mild proximal and distal muscle weakness 4 Axonal polyneuropathy 5 Atrophy of muscles in hands and feet 6 Acrogeric hands, mallet finger(s), clinodactyly, brachydactyly 7 Vaginal/uterus/rectal prolapse		Normal fibrils but reduced density	TNXB mutations that lead to nonsense-mediated mRNA decay, or biallelic deletion of TNXB resulting in complete lack of tenascin-X [24,25]
Classical-like type 2 (provisional) (clEDS2)[a]	AR	1 Hyperextensible skin with atrophic scarring 2 GJH 3 Foot deformities 4 Early-onset osteopenia			Moderate variation in fibril size and scattered composite collagen fibrils ('collagen flowers')	Biallelic mutations in AEPBI that encodes aortic carboxypeptidase-like protein (ACLP), which has a role in ECM remodelling following injury [4]
Cardiac-valvular	AR	1 Severe progressive cardiac/valvular problems (aortic valve, mitral valve) 2 Skin hyperextensibility, atrophic scars, thin skin, easy bruising 3 GJH or restricted to small joints	1 Inguinal hernia 2 Pectus deformity 3 Joint dislocations 4 Foot deformities: pes planus, pes planovalgus, hallux valgus		Variable fibre diameter but within normal range	Lack of the proα2-chain of type I collagen due to biallelic COL1A2 mutations, which leads to nonsense-mediated mRNA decay [26]
Hypermobile (hEDS)	AD	1 Hypermobile joints 2 Features of more generalised disorder of connective tissue 3 Exclusion of other heritable and acquired connective tissue disorders			As above, but less pronounced	Unknown

(continued)

4

Table **70.1** (*continued*)

EDS subtype	Mode of inheritance	Major diagnostic clinical criteria [3]	Minor diagnostic clinical criteria [3]	Gene-specific minor criteria	Ultrastructural findings	Molecular defect (references in square brackets)
Vascular (vEDS)	AD	1 Family history of confirmed vEDS 2 Arterial rupture at a young age 3 Spontaneous sigmoid colon perforation in the absence of bowel disease 4 Third trimester uterine rupture and/or severe peripartum perineum tears 5 Spontaneous carotid–cavernous sinus fistula	1 Severe bruising 2 Thin translucent skin 3 Characteristic facial appearance 4 Spontaneous pneumothorax 5 Acrogeria 6 Talipes equinovarus 7 Congenital hip dislocation 8 Small joint hypermobility 9 Tendon and muscle rupture 10 Keratoconus 11 Gingival recession/fragility 12 Early-onset varicose veins		Small variable fibrils	COL3A1 mutations. Mainly point mutations resulting in glycine substitution but exon skipping and deletions also occur [27–29,**30**] Null mutations may have a better prognosis [31]
Kyphoscoliotic (kEDS)	AR	1 Congenital muscle hypotonia 2 Congenital or early-onset kyphoscoliosis 3 GJH	1 Skin hyperextensibility 2 Easy bruising 3 Arterial rupture/aneurysm 4 Osteopenia/ osteoporosis 5 Blue sclerae 6 Hernia (umbilical or inguinal) 7 Pectus deformity 8 Marfanoid habitus 9 Talipes equinovarus 10 Myopia/hypermetropia	PLOD1: 1 Skin fragility and bruising 2 Scleral and ocular fragility/rupture 3 Microcornea 4 Facial dysmorphology FKBP14: 1 Congenital (sensorineural, conductive or mixed) hearing loss 2 Follicular hyperkeratosis 3 Muscle atrophy 4 Bladder diverticula	Small collagen bundles; fibrils normal or similar to classical type Normal collagen fibrils in skin, enlarged fibroblast endoplasmic cisterns, disorganised myofibrils (in muscle)	Lysyl hydroxylase (PLOD1) mutations. Most common is an intragenic duplication caused by a Alu-Alu recombination between introns 9 and 16 that leads to reduced lysyl hydroxylase activity [32] Biallelic mutations in FKBP14, encoding FKBP22, a member of the F506-binding family of peptidyl-prolyl cis/trans isomerases, resulting in collagen folding less efficiently [33,34] Deoxypyridinoline/pyridinoline cross-links in urine normal
Arthrochalasia (aEDS)	AD	1 Congenital bilateral hip dislocation 2 Severe GJH 3 Skin hyperextensibility	1 Muscle hypotonia 2 Kyphoscoliosis 3 Radiologically mild osteopenia 4 Atrophic scars 5 Easy bruising		Angular fibrils	A and B: COL1A1 and COL1A2 mutations, respectively, result in loss of exon 6 (procollagen N-proteinase/ADAMTS2 cleavage site), which reduces cross-link formation in collagen 1 [35–40]

Type	Inheritance	Clinical features		Ultrastructure	Molecular basis
Dermatosparaxis (dEDS)	AR	1 Extreme skin fragility with congenital or postnatal skin tears 2 Characteristic craniofacial features 3 Redundant skin 4 Increased palmar wrinkling 5 Severe bruising 6 Umbilical hernia 7 Postnatal growth retardation 8 Short limbs, hands and feet 9 Perinatal complications due to connective tissue fragility	1 Soft, doughy skin texture 2 Skin hyperextensibility 3 Atrophic scars 4 GJH 5 Visceral fragility 6 Delayed motor development 7 Osteopenia 8 Hirsutism 9 Tooth abnormalities 10 Myopia, astigmatism 11 Strabismus	Hieroglyphic fibrils (but may be almost indistinguishable from those observed in aEDS)	Procollagen N-proteinase (ADAMTS2) mutations result in inability to cleave N-propeptide of type I and II procollagens [41]
Periodontal	AD	1 Severe and intractable early-onset periodontitis 2 Lack of attached gingiva 3 Pretibial plaques 4 Family history of an affected first-degree relative	1 Easy bruising 2 Distal joint hypermobility 3 Skin hyperextensibility and atrophic scars 4 Increased infections 5 Hernias 6 Marfanoid facial features 7 Acrogeria 8 Prominent vasculature	Small fibrils in some patients	Heterozygous gain-of-function mutations in C1R or C1S, encoding subunits C1r and C1s of the first component of the classical complement pathway [42]
Spondylodysplastic (spEDS)	AR	1 Short stature (progressive in childhood) 2 Muscle hypotonia (ranging from severe congenital to mild late onset) 3 Bowing of limbs	1 Hyperextensible, soft, translucent skin 2 Pes planus 3 Delayed motor development 4 Osteopenia 5 Delayed cognitive development B4GALT7: 1 Radioulnar synostosis 2 Bilateral elbow contractures or limited elbow movement 3 GJH 4 Single transverse palmar crease 5 Characteristic cranio-facial features 6 Characteristic radiographic findings 7 Severe hypermetropia 8 Clouded cornea B3GALT6: 1 Kyphoscoliosis 2 GJH or restricted to distal joints, with joint dislocations 3 Joint contractures 4 Peculiar fingers (slender, tapered, arachnodactyly, spatulate, with broad distal phalanges) 5 Talipes equinovarus 6 Characteristic cranio-facial features 7 Tooth anomalies	Collagen fibrils appear normal	Biallelic mutations in B4GALT7 resulting in reduced galactotransferase I activity and therefore glycosaminoglycans production [43] Biallelic mutations in B3GALT6 resulting in reduced galactotransferase II activity and therefore glycosaminoglycans production [44]

(continued)

Table 70.1 (continued)

EDS subtype	Mode of inheritance	Major diagnostic clinical criteria [3]	Minor diagnostic clinical criteria [3]	Gene-specific minor criteria	Ultrastructural findings	Molecular defect (references in square brackets)
				SLC39A13: 1 Protuberant eyes with bluish sclerae 2 Hands with finely wrinkled palms 3 Atrophy of the thenar muscles, and tapering fingers 4 Hypermobility of distal joints 5 Characteristic radiological findings		SLC39A13 mutations resulting in reduced activity of transmembrane zinc transporter [45] Biallelic mutations in SLC39A13, encoding the ZIP13 protein, impairs regulation of the influx of zinc into the cytosol
Musculocontractural (mcEDS)	AR	1 Congenital multiple contractures, characteristically adduction-flexion contractures and/or talipes equinovarus (clubfoot) 2 Characteristic cranio-facial features 3 Skin hyperextensibility 4 Easy bruisability, skin fragility with atrophic scars, increased palmar wrinkling	1 Recurrent/chronic dislocations 2 Pectus deformities 3 Scoliosis/kyphoscoliosis 4 Peculiar fingers (tapering, slender, cylindrical) 5 Progressive talipes deformities (valgus, planus, cavum) 6 Large subcutaneous haematomas 7 Chronic constipation 8 Colonic diverticulae 9 Pneumothorax/ pneumohemothorax 10 Nephrolithiasis/cystolithiasis 11 Hydronephrosis 12 Cryptorchidism in males 13 Strabismus 14 Refractive errors (myopia, astigmatism) 15 Glaucoma/elevated intraocular pressure		Small collagen bundles with variable diameter collagen fibrils. Dilated endoplasmic reticulum in fibroblasts	Biallelic mutations in CHST14, encoding D4ST1 (dermatan 4-O-sulfotransferase 1) or dermatan sulfate epimerase (DSE), both enzymes involved in the biosynthesis of the GAG dermatan sulfate [20,46–48]
Brittle cornea syndrome	AR	1 Thin cornea, with or without rupture 2 Early-onset progressive keratoconus 3 Early-onset progressive keratoglobus 4 Blue sclerae	1 Enucleation or corneal scarring due to previous rupture 2 Progressive loss of corneal stromal depth, especially in central cornea 3 High myopia, with normal or moderately increased axial length 4 Retinal detachment		Not reported	Biallelic mutations in either ZNF469, a zinc finger protein which may act as a transcriptional regulator in the synthesis or assembly of collagen fibrils, or PRDM5, encoding a DNA binding transcription factor of the PR/SET protein family, that appears to regulate ECM development [49]

Type	Inheritance	Major criteria	Minor criteria	Other features	Genetic basis
		5 Deafness, often with mixed conductive and sensorineural components, progressive, higher frequencies often more severely affected ('sloping' pure tone audiogram) 6 Hypercompliant tympanic membranes 7 Developmental dysplasia of the hip 8 Hypotonia in infancy, usually mild if present 9 Scoliosis 10 Arachnodactyly 11 Hypermobility of distal joints 12 Pes planus, hallux valgus 13 Mild contractures of fingers (especially fifth) 14 Soft, velvety skin, translucent skin	1 Soft, doughy skin 2 Atrophic scarring 3 Motor developmental delay 4 Myopathy on muscle biopsy	Increased collagen fibril diameter and increased interfibrillar spacing [50]	
Myopathic (mEDS)	AD or AR	1 Congenital muscle hypotonia and/or muscle atrophy that improves with age 2 Proximal joint contractures (knee, hip, elbow) 3 Hypermobility of distal joints			Heterozygous or biallelic mutations in COL12A1, encoding type XII collagen which binds to fibrillar collagens and tenascin-X

a Described after the Villefranche classification.

AD, autosomal dominant; AR, autosomal recessive; ECM, extracellular matrix; GJH, generalised joint hypermobility.

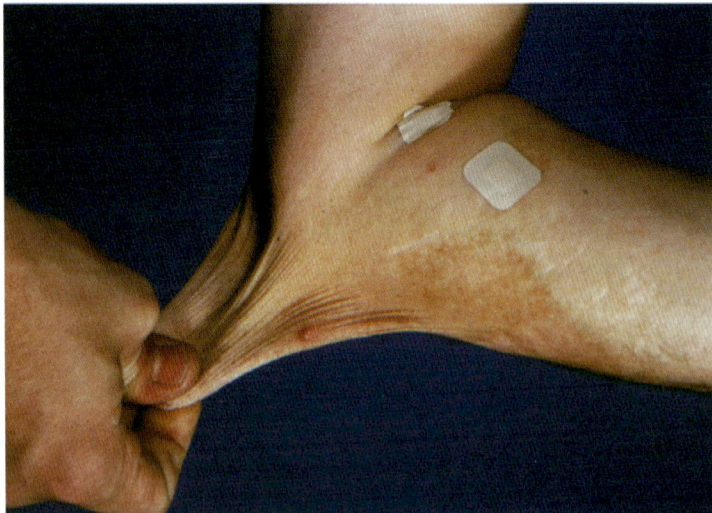

Figure 70.1 Cutaneous hyperextensibililty in classical Ehlers–Danlos syndrome.

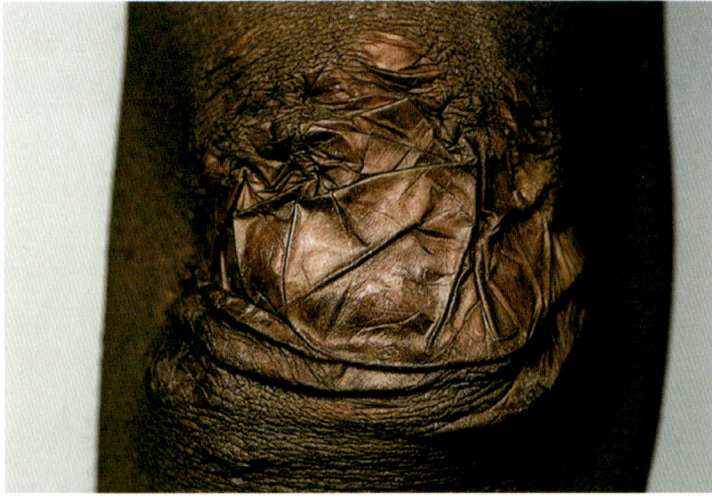

Figure 70.2 Atrophic scarring of the elbow in classical Ehlers–Danlos syndrome.

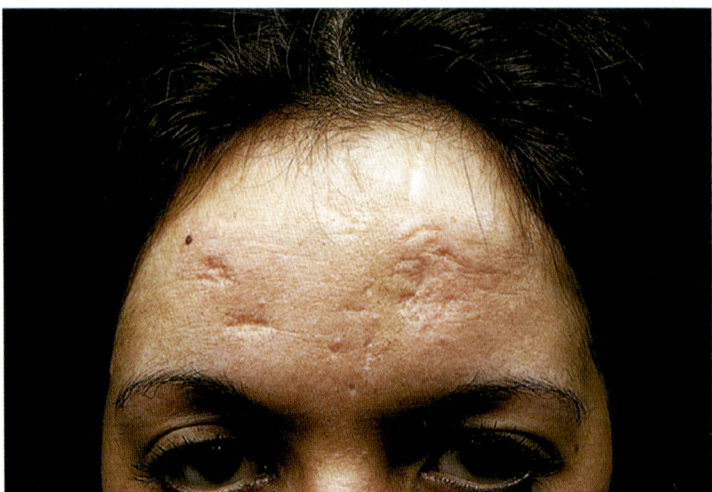

Figure 70.3 Scarring of the forehead in classical Ehlers–Danlos syndrome.

Table 70.2 The Beighton score.

Movement	Score
Dorsiflex L and R fifth finger >90°	2
Apposition L and R thumb to forearm	2
Hyperextend L and R elbow >10°	2
Hyperextend L and R knee >10°	2
Palms to floor	1
Total	9

Adapted from Beighton PH *et al.* 1973 [57].

and joint pains are common [3]. Extra-articular manifestations of dysautonomia are significantly more common in joint hypermobility patients [59]. Although the mechanisms remain unclear there is increasing evidence suggesting a link to mast cell activation disorder [11]. The symptoms include tachycardia, hypotension, gastrointestinal dysmotility and disturbed bladder function and sweating regulation [60,61]. Failure to respond adequately to local anaesthetic is reported more commonly in this subgroup [62,63].

Vascular Ehlers–Danlos syndrome (vEDS). This severe form is inherited as an autosomal dominant trait. Tissues rich in type III collagen, notably arterial media, bowel and uterus are mainly affected.

Clubfoot and/or congenital dislocation of the hips may be present at birth. Other features include prematurity (due to rupture of friable placental membranes), easy bruising, which may lead to the mistaken accusation of child abuse [64], inguinal hernia and pneumothorax [65]. Many individuals have an acrogeric appearance consisting of prematurely aged, thin, translucent and fragile skin (Figure 70.4), a hollow-eyed appearance, thin peaked nose and thin lips. Elastosis perforans serpiginosa is seen more commonly in vEDS [66]. Unlike other forms of EDS, the skin is not hyperextensible, and joint hypermobility is chiefly restricted to the small joints of the hands and feet. Surface veins are usually readily visible. There is a tendency to form keloid scars.

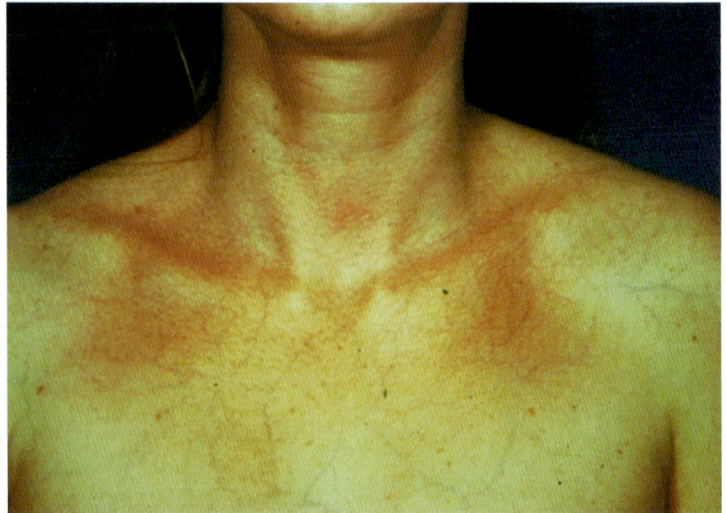

Figure 70.4 Cutaneous atrophy in vascular Ehlers–Danlos syndrome.

The major complications arise following spontaneous rupture of large arteries, the colon and gravid uterus. The largest case series to date of vEDS patients showed a median survival of 48 years, with 25% of index cases having their first significant complication by 20 years [30]. Most deaths follow arterial dissection or rupture, mainly of the thoracic and abdominal vessels. In the same series, complications of pregnancy led to death in the peripartum period in 12 of 81 women who had a total of 183 pregnancies [30]. Seven died following vessel rupture and five following uterine rupture.

Kyphoscoliotic Ehlers–Danlos syndrome (kEDS). This autosomal recessive condition was the first true disorder of collagen structure to be described [32,67,68]. The biochemical abnormality is a deficiency of lysyl hydroxylase, now known as procollagen-lysine 2-oxoglutarate 5-dioxygenase, which is encoded by the *PLOD1* gene. Deficiency of this enzyme leads to reduced hydroxylation of lysyl residues in types I and III collagen in skin; hydroxylysine-containing cross-links are not formed [69] and lysine-derived cross-links are not as stable as those from hydroxylysine [70]. The detection of abnormal pyridinoline cross-links in urine can be used as a diagnostic aid [71].

Clinical features include soft, velvety, hyperextensible skin and joint hypermobility and (sub)luxations. Kyphoscoliosis is congenital or early onset. Eye manifestations include microcornea, glaucoma, keratoconus and ocular fragility. Some patients have a Marfanoid habitus. Bleeding may occur from major wounds, and there may be delayed motor development [72].

A second type of autosomal recessive kEDS with additional features of congenital hearing impairment, muscle atrophy and bladder diverticulae is caused by mutations in *FKBP14* resulting in impaired collagen folding [32,33]. Urinary pyridinoline cross-links levels are normal.

Musculocontractural Ehlers–Danlos syndrome (mcEDS). This form of EDS was originally reported under the terms adducted thumb–clubfoot syndrome, Kosho type and D4ST1-deficient EDS [20,44–46]. Features in addition to EDS include a distinctive cranio-facial appearance and congenital multiple contractures, typically adduction/flexion contractures and talipes equinovarus [73].

Spondylodysplastic Ehlers–Danlos syndrome (SpEDS). Three conditions caused by *B4GALT7*, *B3GALT6* and *SLC39A13* mutations with overlapping phenotype are now grouped in this subtype [73]. In addition to hyperextensible skin which is soft, doughy, thin and translucent, patients commonly exhibit short stature, muscle hypotonia (ranging from severe congenital to mild later-onset) and bowing of the limbs [74]. Other features more specific to the molecular subtype occur (see Table 70.1) [75].

Arthrochalasia Ehlers–Danlos syndrome (aEDS). This rare autosomal dominant condition, like osteogenesis imperfecta, results from mutations causing defects in type I collagen. Phenotypic overlap therefore occurs. The most important clinical features for the diagnosis of aEDS are hypermobility and recurrent joint dislocations, typically bilateral congenital hip dislocation. The cutaneous features are milder than in most other EDS types. There is significant skin redundancy, resulting in one of the key features of arthrochalasia type, namely a criss-cross pattern on the palms and soles [40,73].

Cardiac-Valvular Ehlers–Danlos syndrome (cvEDS). This is due to recessive mutations in *COL1A2* and manifests with EDS features in association with severe, progressive aortic and mitral valve diseases [24,73].

Dermatosparaxis Ehlers–Danlos syndrome (dEDS). This very rare autosomal recessive form is characterised by premature rupture of the membranes, extreme skin fragility and laxity and bruising (Figure 70.5) [41,76–79]. Facial appearance is characterised by blue sclera, puffy eyelids, epicanthic folds, downslanting palpebral fissures, micrognathia with gingival hyperplasia and dental anomalies [80]. Other features include umbilical hernia, variable joint laxity that becomes more prominent with age, delayed closure of the fontanelles, short stature and brachydactyly. Serious complications include spontaneous rupture of the bladder or diaphragm.

Two cases with congenital skull fractures and skin lacerations after birth have been reported [81,82].

Periodontal Ehlers–Danlos syndrome (pEDS). The features are similar to cEDS but often with only moderate small joint hypermobility and milder skin manifestations. The distinguishing clinical features are premature periodontal recession (Figure 70.6), resulting in loss of teeth by the third decade, and heavily pigmented pretibial plaques (Figure 70.7) [42,83,84]. pEDS arises due to mutations in the classical complement pathway, resulting in activation of the local complement cascade in the periodontal region, with possible other effects on ECM proteins at sites of complement 1 expression [42,85].

Classic-like Ehlers–Danlos syndrome (clEDS). Tenascin-X deficiency causes a clinically distinct, autosomal recessive form of EDS [24,25]. Patients have hyperextensible skin, bruising and joint laxity, but no

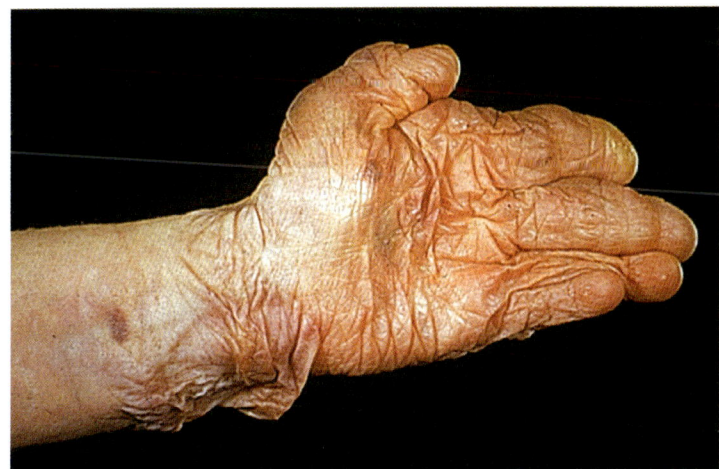

Figure 70.5 Extreme cutaneous fragility and laxity in dermatosparaxis Ehlers–Danlos syndome.

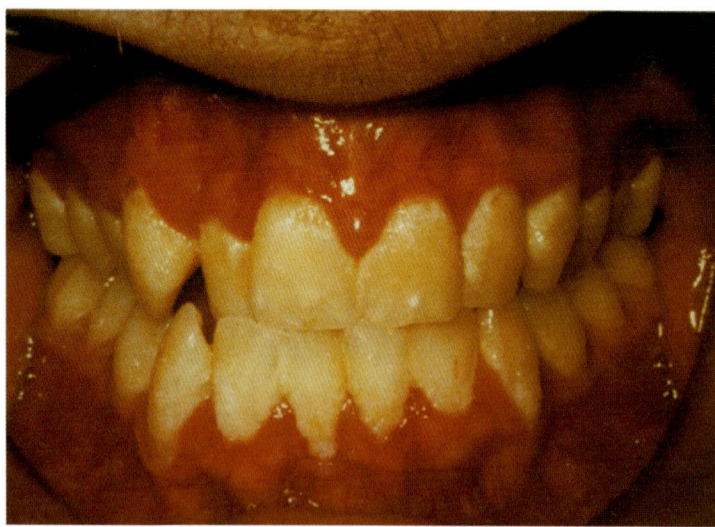

Figure 70.6 Premature periodontal recession in periodontal Ehlers–Danlos syndrome.

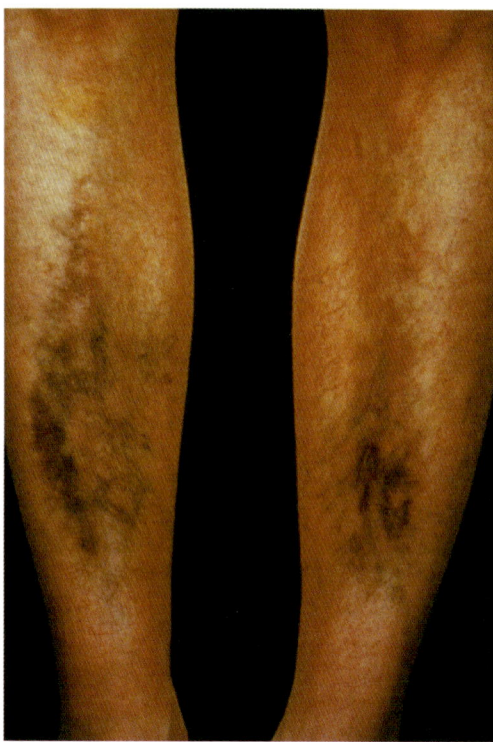

Figure 70.7 Pigmented pretibial plaques in periodontal Ehlers–Danlos syndrome.

scarring [86,87]. Generalised muscle weakness and distal contractures are also features [86]. Tenascin-X encodes a large ECM protein that appears to be an essential regulator of collagen deposition by dermal fibroblasts and interacts with many other ECM components in the organisation of the ECM [88,89].

The diagnosis is confirmed by the absence of tenascin-X in serum and mutation analysis of the *TNX-B* gene.

Classic-like (type 2) Ehlers–Danlos syndome (clEDS2). This subtype was described after the 2017 classification and has provisionally been referred to as type 2 clEDS. Pronounced cEDS

skin changes occur in addition to generalised joint hypermobility, foot deformities and early-onset osteopenia. Autosomal recessive mutations in *AEBP1*, which encodes the aortic carboxypeptidase-like protein, alter the association with fibrillar collagens [4].

Brittle cornea syndome (BCS). Brittle cornea syndrome is a rare autosomal condition due to mutations in *ZNF469* or *PRDM5* genes encoding zinc finger proteins. It shows significant phenotypic overlap with kEDS [90,91]. Thin brittle cornea and ocular fragility, blue sclera and keratoconus are prominent features but it can be associated with skin fragility, joint hypermobility and kyphoscoliosis [3].

Myopathic Ehlers–Danlos syndrome (mEDS). This autosomal recessive phenotype shows features of EDS and a myopathy, combined with proximal joint contractures and distal hypermobility. It occurs due to abnormalities of type XII fibril-associated collagen with interrupted triple helices (FACIT) collagen [3,50].

Differential diagnosis

Ehlers–Danlos syndrome should be distinguished from cutis laxa (Chapter 77), in which the skin hangs in flaccid, redundant folds. In EDS, redundant skin folds may develop in late adult life, but they are usually limited to the elbows and around the eyes. Hyperextensible soft skin is seen as a minor feature of many other genetic conditions including Williams syndrome, Down syndrome, arterial tortuosity syndrome and Costello syndrome. These syndromes can be easily differentiated by their other major features.

Vascular EDS overlaps clinically with an autosomal dominant aneurysmal disorder, Loeys–Dietz syndrome (LDS). LDS type I patients overlap clinically with Marfan syndrome and hEDS, whereas type II patients have a phenotype similar to vEDS [92]. LDS occurs due to mutations in the transforming growth factor β (TGF-β) receptor genes *TGFBR* and less commonly *SMAD* genes.

Marfan syndrome should be considered if the presenting vascular complication is an aortic aneurysm or dissection.

Complications and co-morbidities

Complications vary according to the underlying molecular mechanisms and phenotype of the different EDS subtypes.

Disease course and prognosis

The prognosis depends on the subtype of EDS. Life expectancy is reduced in those who have vascular or bowel fragility.

Investigations

Molecular characterisation should be sought whenever possible. A baseline echocardiogram will enable assessment for valvular prolapse. Views of the aortic arch should also be obtained to look for aortic dilatation. This is, however, much less common in the classical and hypermobility types. Adults with vEDS are at risk for arterial aneurysm and rupture, and non-invasive visualisation of the arterial tree from head to iliac arteries may be indicated [93].

Analysis of the urine for an increased deoxypyridinoline: pyridinoline ratio may be used as a screening test for *PLOD1*-related kEDS.

In patients with significantly reduced physical activity, a dual-energy X-ray absorptiometry (DEXA) scan should be considered to assess for low bone density.

Management

Attempts should be made to delineate the clinical and, if possible, the molecular abnormalities in a patient with EDS in view of the widely differing prognosis between different types. A multidisciplinary approach is required with involvement of appropriate specialists. Patients should receive genetic counselling.

First line

Joints. Patients should avoid excessive activities that produce additional stress on their hypermobile joints. Physiotherapy is aimed at increasing tone and strength around joints, neuromuscular coordination and joint proprioception.

Skin. Advice should be given about simple precautionary measures to lessen the chances of accidental trauma, scarring or bruising. It is advisable for children to avoid contact sports. Excessive sun exposure to minimise skin damage should be started early. High-dose (1–4 g/day) ascorbic acid (vitamin C) therapy may reduce bruising and can also improve wound healing in patients with kEDS [94,95].

Wounds should be closed without tension, preferably in two layers. Deep stitches should be applied generously. Cutaneous stitches should be left in place twice as long as usual, and additional fixation of adjacent skin with adhesive tape can help prevent stretching of the scar.

Pregnancy. There is a greater prevalence of obstetric and gynaecological symptoms reported by women with EDS than in the general population [96]. Pregnancy represents a special issue in patients with certain types of EDS. Maternal risks include cervical insufficiency, uterine prolapse, uterine tear, poor wound healing during the postpartum period and excessive bleeding both during and after delivery [97].

Infant risks include premature rupture of membranes with secondary premature delivery and all the inherent complications.

Patients with vEDS should be advised to avoid pregnancy as maternal mortality is high. The largest series found 12 maternal deaths in 81 women due to uterine and arterial rupture [**30**]. It is unclear whether elective caesarean section reduces these risks. Patients should be managed in specialist obstetric units with multidisciplinary input.

Vascular EDS-specific precautions. Patients should avoid trauma, including physical contact sports, and avoid activities that raise intracranial pressure by the Valsalva effect. Bleeding should be managed conservatively if at all possible.

Celiprolol, a long-acting β_1-antagonist with partial β_2-agonist properties, has been shown in a randomised trial to reduce the incidence of arterial dissection or rupture [98]. Patients should be advised to carry medical alert identifiers in case of an acute complication.

Resources

Patient resources
Ehlers–Danlos Support UK: https://www.ehlers-danlos.org/.
The Ehlers–Danlos Society, the International Consortium on EDS and HSD: https://www.ehlers-danlos.com/international-consortium/
(Both last accessed February 2022.)

Prolidase deficiency

Definition

Deficiency of prolidase is a rare inborn error of collagen metabolism, associated with chronic skin ulceration, intellectual disability, splenomegaly and recurrent respiratory infections [1,2].

Introduction and general description

Prolidase (peptidase D) is involved in the latter stages of degradation of endogenous and dietary proteins and is particularly important in collagen catabolism. Deficiency of prolidase is a rare, clinically heterogeneous, multisystem disorder.

Epidemiology

Incidence and prevalence

This is a rare disorder occurring in approximately 1/1–2 million births. Approximately 100 cases have been reported.

Age

Features typically first appear in infancy to young adult life.

Sex

There is equal sex incidence.

Ethnicity

It is more common in certain areas in northern Israel [3].

Associated diseases

Approximately 10% of cases have been reported to also have features of systemic lupus erythematosus. It is therefore possible that prolidase deficiency is a risk factor for the development of systemic lupus erythematosus due to loss of immune tolerance to lupus-associated autoantigens [4,5].

Pathophysiology

Collagen is degraded to iminodipeptides, which are then broken down into amino acids that can be recycled to form collagen. Prolidase cleaves dipeptides with proline or hydroxyproline at the C-terminus end. Decreased prolidase activity therefore leads to impaired collagen synthesis and wound healing [6]. It is not well understood how prolidase deficiency causes the other different clinical features.

Pathology

Light and electron microscopy of cultured fibroblasts from affected patients suggest necrosis-like cell death with abnormal morphology and increased cytosolic vacuolisation, and abnormal plasma membranes and mitochondria [7].

PART 6: GENETIC DISORDERS

Genetics

The deficiency is inherited as an autosomal recessive trait [2,8]. Mutations in the prolidase gene *PEPD* result in loss of prolidase activity [**7**]. Heterozygotes have no clinical features [9].

Clinical features

History

The severity of symptoms varies greatly among affected individuals; however, the most characteristic feature is recalcitrant skin ulcers.

Presentation

Most patients have intellectual and developmental impairment and abnormal facies, which includes prominent eyes with hypertelorism, a high forehead, saddle nose and micrognathia. Skin changes occur in about 85% of cases. The skin may feel spongy, with pitting and scarring, especially on the legs (Figure 70.8). The skin is fragile and leg ulcers are common. Occasionally, there may be photosensitivity, telangiectasia, purpura, premature greying and lymphoedema [10].

Splenomegaly, recurrent skin, ear or chest infections and obesity or a protuberant abdomen occur in about 30% of cases. Families have been described with associated chronic lung disease, resembling cystic fibrosis [11].

Differential diagnosis

The presence of splenomegaly, photosensitive rash and autoantibodies can mimic systemic lupus erythematosus [12].

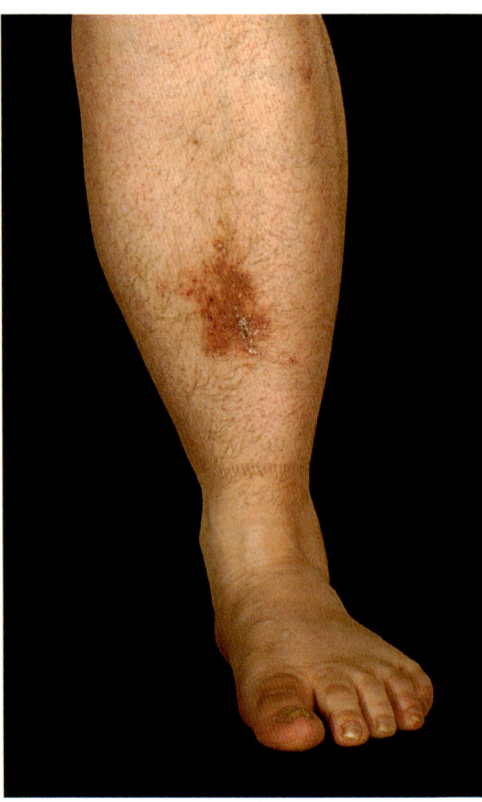

Figure 70.8 Pitted skin in prolidase deficiency. Courtesy of Addenbrooke's Hospital, Cambridge, UK.

Complications and co-morbidities

Recurrent infections and skin ulceration are the most troublesome complications.

Disease course and prognosis

Prolidase deficiency is a chronic disorder with quite variable prognosis.

Investigations

Large amounts of imidodipeptides are excreted in the urine [13,14], and the proline : hydroxyproline ratio in collagen is increased. Reduced or absent prolidase activity can be detected in the red and white blood cells or cultured fibroblasts. Other abnormal laboratory findings include mild anaemia, thrombocytopenia and hypergammaglobulinaemia.

Management

Treatment is limited to improving the skin ulcers.

First line

Topical 5% proline and 5% glycine combined in an ointment base have been shown to be more effective in healing the ulcers than topical 5% proline in ointment alone [**15**]. Oral proline administration produces no clinical improvement.

Second line

A combination of topical and systemic growth hormone healed recalcitrant leg ulcers in one patient [16] and dapsone in another [17]. Enzyme replacement by transfusion of prolidase-containing red cells [18], pulsed corticosteroids [19] and apheresis exchange [20] and low-molecular-weight anticoagulants [21] have all improved skin ulceration. Various combination therapies have also been used [22].

Resources

Patient resources

Genetic and Rare Diseases Information Center: https://rarediseases.info.nih.gov/diseases/7473/prolidase-deficiency (last accessed February 2022).

Osteogenesis imperfecta

Definition and nomenclature

This is a heterogeneous group of heritable disorders characterised by osteoporosis with fractures, due predominantly to type I collagen abnormalities.

Synonyms and inclusions
• Brittle bone disease

Introduction and general description

In 1979 Sillence classified osteogenesis imperfecta (OI) into types I–IV [1], with these four accounting for 85% of all subtypes that have been identified. The classification has been expanded due to new molecular findings [2,3].

Epidemiology

Incidence and prevalence

This condition affects approximately 1 in 10 000–20 000 [3].

Age

The age of onset depends on the severity of the disease. The severest forms are lethal perinatally, with the mildest forms not being diagnosed until adulthood.

Sex

There is no sex bias.

Ethnicity

There is no racial bias.

Associated diseases

An overlap may be seen with some forms of EDS due to collagen I abnormalities [4].

Pathophysiology

Pathology

Clinical features arise due to defects in collagen synthesis, assembly and processing as well as bone mineralisation and osteoblast differentiation. The bones are markedly collagen deficient, and often have a distorted architecture [5]. The dermis is thin, with a relative increase of argyrophilic and elastic fibres, and a deficiency of adult collagen [6].

Genetics

Osteogenesis imperfecta is usually inherited in an autosomal dominant fashion, with a high frequency (c.25–30%) of *de novo* mutations; autosomal recessive forms are much less common. Mutations in *COL1A1* and *COL1A2* genes cause the autosomal dominant subtypes and account for approximately 85% of all cases [3].

Clinical features [1,3,7]

Presentation

In addition to fractures, patients may also have blue sclerae (Figure 70.9), deafness, skeletal deformity, abnormal dentine formation (dentinogenesis imperfecta), mild joint hypermobility, hernias, mitral valve prolapse, microvascular fragility leading to bruising and thin fragile skin [1].

Clinical variants

The most common types are types I–IV relating to collagen I abnormalities, with rarer types V–XVIII showing molecular heterogeneity.

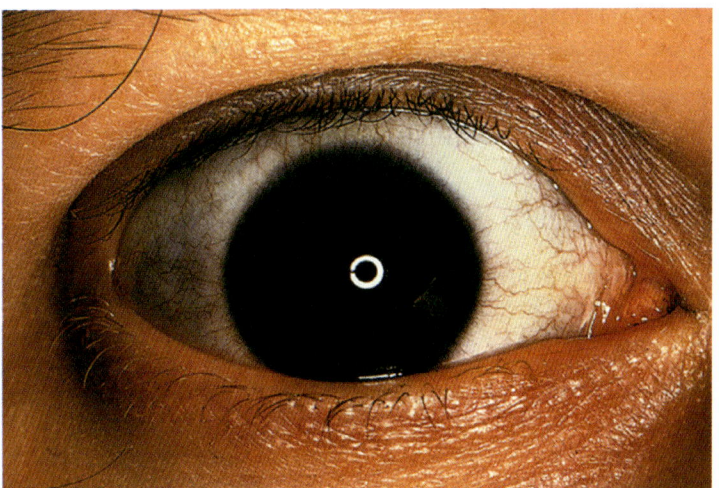

Figure 70.9 Blue sclera in osteogenesis imperfecta.

Type IA: classical form. This is the commonest form. It is inherited as an autosomal dominant trait, although sporadic cases also occur [8]. Fractures are common in childhood. The sclerae are blue or grey, and easy bruising and early-onset deafness are common, but skeletal deformity is absent or mild. Joint laxity is common. The incidence of mitral valve prolapse is increased, and the aortic valves are thin and occasionally incompetent [9,10]. A few patients (type IB) have dentinogenesis imperfecta, but this is more common in the type IV group. Most patients have increased skin collagen, with an increased ratio of type I : type III collagens [11]. Other patients have an abnormal α_2-chain, which is unduly susceptible to proteolysis by pepsin [12].

Type II: lethal perinatal form. There are multiple fractures *in utero* and infants rarely survive for more than a few days after birth [3]. Avulsion of the limbs may occur during delivery due to a generalised connective tissue fragility. Radiography shows beaded ribs, crumpled femora and little skull calcification. This form has been subdivided on the basis of rib and limb bone abnormalities [13]. Inheritance is usually autosomal dominant. Multiple recurrence due to gonadal mosaicism can mimic autosomal recessive inheritance [14].

Type III: progressively deforming form. This is the most severe form of OI compatible with survival beyond infancy [3]. The long bones are thin and occasionally cystic. As the child grows older, progressive scoliosis and bowing of the long bones cause crippling deformities. The sclerae are blue in childhood but become normal in the adult.

Type IV: mild form with normal sclerae. This condition is similar to type I in clinical features and inheritance, but the sclerae are not blue, dentinogenesis imperfecta is frequent and deafness is rare [1,3].

Differential diagnosis

Patients with short extremities and a large skull may be confused with having achondroplasia, but bone fragility and thin skin do not occur in achondroplasia. The multiplicity of fractures seen in OI commonly raises the issue of possible child abuse.

Classification of severity

The different subtypes of OI reflect not only molecular but also phenotypic variability.

Complications and co-morbidities

These will vary according to the subtype.

Disease course and prognosis

The prognosis varies depending on the severity of symptoms. Respiratory failure followed by accidental trauma are the commonest causes of premature death. However, despite complications of OI, most children and adults lead productive and successful lives.

Investigations

Prenatal diagnosis of the more severe forms is possible using ultrasonography from week 16 [15]. The preferred examination for the initial investigation of OI is plain radiography. Some radiographic features are specific to certain subtypes [16].

Management

A multidisciplinary approach, including medical, orthopaedic, physiotherapy and rehabilitation input, is required with the aim of preventing fractures and disability, and improving function and quality of life [17].

Bisphosphonates have become standard care for patients although they are not associated with a significant reduction in long bone fracture in children [18]. It is also unclear how long therapy should be maintained [19]. Ongoing prevention of vitamin D and calcium deficiency is important.

Denosumab, an anti-RANK (receptor activator of nuclear factor κB) ligand antibody that inhibits osteoclastic activity, and teriparatide, a human parathyroid analogue, have shown preliminary effectiveness [3]. Somatic cell therapy using allogeneic bone marrow and mesenchymal stromal cell transplantation have been used [20,21].

Resources

Further information

National Center for Biotechnology Information, OMIM: http://www.ncbi.nlm.nih.gov/omim.

National Organization for Rare Disorders: http://rarediseases.org/.

Steiner RD, Basel D. *COL1A1/2* osteogenesis imperfecta. *GeneReviews® [Internet]* 2005;PMID 20301472. https://pubmed.ncbi.nlm.nih.gov/20301472/.

Patient resources

Brittle Bone Society: http://www.brittlebone.org.

(All last accessed February 2022.)

INHERITED DISORDERS OF ELASTIC FIBRES

ELASTINOPATHIES

Inherited generalised cutis laxa

Definition and nomenclature

Cutis laxa is characterised clinically by lax pendulous skin that only slowly recoils when pulled [1]. Histologically, there is loss and fragmentation of elastic tissue in the dermis. It is a heterogeneous condition and may be inherited or acquired. The inherited forms include autosomal dominant and recessive types and an X-linked type.

Synonyms and inclusions
- Generalised elastolysis
- Generalised elastorrhexis
- Generalised dermatochalasis

Introduction and general description

Generalised cutis laxa is rare. The clinical presentation and the mode of inheritance show considerable heterogeneity. Cutis laxa variably affects connective tissue in the skin as well as other parts of the body, including the heart, blood vessels, joints, intestines and lungs.

Epidemiology

Incidence and prevalence

No reliable data have been published but the prevalence at birth is estimated at around 1/1000 000. Autosomal recessive types (ARCL1 and ARCL2) are the most common [2].

Age

Presentation is at birth or early infancy although the autosomal dominant type has a later and milder onset.

Sex

Both sexes are affected equally in the autosomal dominant and recessive forms. X-linked cutis laxa affects males only.

Ethnicity

There is no racial variation.

Associated diseases

It is important to differentiate cutis laxa from other inherited disorders of connective tissue although it may also accompany disorders such as pseudoxanthoma elasticum and EDS [3].

Pathophysiology

Cutis laxa is caused by disruption to normal elastic tissue function. Three main groups of proteins have so far been identified as being responsible for the abnormal elastic fibre morphology:

- Proteins that are directly incorporated into elastic fibres, including fibulin-4, fibulin-5 and latent TGF-β-binding protein.
- Proteins involved with synthesis, modification and secretion of elastic fibres.
- Proteins involved in mitochondrial function [4].

Pathology

The skin is of normal thickness, but the elastic fibres are sparse, short, fragmented and clumped, particularly in the upper dermis, and they show granular degeneration [5]. Similar changes in elastic fibres may occur in the lungs and aorta.

Various ultrastructural changes have been described, depending on the subtype. These include separation of the elastin microfibrils from the amorphous matrix, the presence of a 'wood-grain' pattern and aggregation, fragmentation and clumping of the elastic fibres [5–7].

Genetics

There is genetic and phenotypic heterogeneity (Table 70.3). Approximately 30% of patients with autosomal dominant cutis laxa have *de novo* mutations with no family history [8].

Clinical features
Clinical variants

Various clinical types have been described (Table 70.3) [8–11,**12**].

Autosomal dominant cutis laxa. The skin changes may develop at any age (Figure 70.10a) but tend to be less pronounced, compared with the recessive forms, in those who present later (Figure 70.10b). A minority of patients (25%) show skin redundancy only in the facial, neck, inguinal and/or axillary regions, whereas it is more widespread in the remainder [**13**]. The skin is soft and variably hyperextensible. Facial dysmorphism is mild but a beaked nose is common. Inguinal hernias are also common. Although autosomal dominant cutis laxa is considered to be a milder form of the disease, systemic involvement can range from mild to severe, including bronchiectasis and emphysema, hernias, mitral and tricuspid valvular prolapse, pulmonary stenosis, aortic and arterial dilatation and tortuosity, gastrointestinal and uro-genital diverticuli [8,**12**,14]. In the largest series reported to date, 35% had lung and 57% had aortic involvement [**13**].

Autosomal recessive cutis laxa. Several autosomal recessive forms of cutis laxa (ARCL) are known, and categorised into types 1 (ARCL1A, -B and -C), 2 (ARCL2A and -B) and 3 (ARCL3A and B/de Barsy syndrome) [2,8,**12**,15]. Infant and childhood mortality is high. The typical facies comprises downward slanting palpebral fissures, a broad flat nose, sagging cheeks and large ears (Figure 70.11). There are prominent skin folds around the knees, abdomen and thighs. Herniae, diverticula, arterial tortuosity and aneurysms, severe pulmonary emphysema and cor pulmonale and developmental delay are variable but important complications. Death due to respiratory complications is common in the first few years of life. The various ARCL1 subtypes are characterised by prominent vascular and visceral involvement, while the different ARCL2 subtypes feature prominent neurological manifestations and brain structural abnormalities. Of note, the de Barsy syndrome which is distinguished by developmental delay and corneal clouding due to degeneration of the tunica elastica of the cornea [16–18], is caused by mutations in genes also involved in ARCL2 [19], suggesting that this subtype of cutis laxa does not need to be separately classified. Finally, beyond the current classification of ARCL, new forms of this condition continue to emerge but seem to share with classical types of ARCL similar manifestations, as in LTBP1-associated cutis laxa featuring facial dysmorphism, heart defects and prominent skeletal abnormalities [20].

X-linked recessive form (occipital horn syndrome). Affected males in occipital horn syndrome, previously known as EDS type IX, have a defect in the distribution of intracellular copper to copper-dependent enzymes [21]. Lysyl oxidase is a major copper-dependent enzyme, and its activity is markedly decreased in some patients [22], resulting in defective collagen and elastin cross-links. Occipital horn syndrome is considered a less severe form of Menkes syndrome, and both conditions are caused by mutations in the *ATP7A* gene [23,24]. Clinical manifestations include the development of bladder diverticula during childhood, inguinal herniae, mild laxity of the skin and skeletal defects such as short humeri and clavicles. Bony occipital horns appear during adolescence [22]. Other features include mild chronic diarrhoea and orthostatic hypotension.

Differential diagnosis

Although there are many similarities between the wrinkly skin syndrome and cutis laxa type 2 (both are caused by mutations in *ATP6V0A2*), the skin changes in the former are limited mainly to the abdomen, hands and feet. Facial dysmorphism is less pronounced in wrinkly skin syndrome and large fontanelles have not been described [25].

Acquired cutis laxa (Chapter 94) may rarely develop at any age but often follows an inflammatory process or an associated disorder.

In EDS the skin is hyperextensible but not lax, and it recoils quickly. In pseudoxanthoma elasticum the skin may be lax, but it is yellowish and the face is usually spared. It is distinguished histologically by the presence of calcification. There may be circumscribed folds of lax skin in neurofibromatosis, and loose folded skin may also occur in leprechaunism, Patterson syndrome and trisomy 18, but these conditions are distinguished by their associated features.

Excessive skin wrinkling of the forehead has been reported in Apert syndrome [26], although this and the other craniosynostosis syndromes are easily distinguished by their cranio-facial dysmorphism and recognised associations (Table 70.4).

Disease course and prognosis

The prognosis depends on the subtype of cutis laxa but in general autosomal dominant types tend to have a better prognosis.

Investigations

A skin biopsy can be helpful. An echocardiogram, chest X-ray and lung function testing should be performed. Neurological examination and imaging are mandatory in ARCL2. If acquired cutis laxa is suspected, a primary cause should be sought. Molecular testing is possible for congenital and inherited cutis laxa.

Table 70.3 Cutis laxa and related synromes [12].

Type	Molecular defect	Major clinical features	MIM	Additional references
Autosomal dominant (ADCL1 and 2)	ELN, FBLN5[a]	Symptoms less severe than autosomal recessive types	ADCL1 (ELN)123700	[30–32]
		Onset usually childhood/early adult	ADCL2 (FBLN5) 614434	[33]
Autosomal recessive type 1A	FBLN5	Cutis laxa, gastrointestinal diverticula, herniae, uterine prolapse, aortic dilatations	219100	[34]
		Cutis laxa, pulmonary emphysema, gastrointestinal and bladder diverticula, arterial tortuosity and aneurysms, pulmonary artery stenosis, hernia, bone fragility		
Autosomal recessive type 1B	FBLN4/EFEMP2	As for type 1A with additional propensity to supravalvular aortic stenosis	614437	[35]
Autosomal recessive type 1C/URDS	LTBP4	Cutis laxa, microretrognathia, flat mid face, receding forehead, wide fontanelle, minimal cardiovascular complications limited to pulmonary artery stenosis and patent foramen ovale, severe genito-urinary and gastrointestinal involvement	613177	[36]
Autosomal recessive type 2A	Loss-of-function mutations ATP6V0A2	Cutis laxa, growth and developmental delay, skeletal abnormalities, large fontanelle with delayed closure, oxycephaly, herniae, hip dislocations, abnormal glycosylation of proteins	219200	[37]
Autosomal recessive type 2B	PYCR1	Cutis laxa, growth and developmental delay, joint laxity, microcephaly, triangular face, large ears, premature aged appearance, osteoporosis, normal glycosylation of proteins	612940	[38,39]
Autosomal recessive type 3A and 3B (de Barsey syndrome)	ALDH18A1 and PYCR1	Cutis laxa, progeroid appearance, corneal opacities, intellectual disability, pseudoathetoid movements	ARCLIIIA (ALDH18A1) 219150	[40,41]
			ARCL3B (PYCR1) 614438	[42]
X-linked (occipital horn syndrome)	ATP7A (allelic with Menkes syndrome)	Bladder diverticula, inguinal hernias, slight skin laxity and hyperextensibility, joint laxity, coarse hair, skeletal abnormalities, including persistent open anterior fontanelle and occipital exostoses	304150	[22,23,43]
Other syndromes with cutis laxa				
Gerodermia osteodysplastica	GORAB/SCYL1BP	Dwarfism with premature aged appearance, lax skin, osteoporosis, Wormian bones, mandibular prognathism, malar hypoplasia	231070	[44,45]
MACS	RIN2	Macrocephaly, alopecia, cutis laxa	613075	[46]
SCARF syndrome	Unknown X-linked recessive	SCARF acronym: *skeletal abnormalities, cutis laxa/craniostenosis, ambiguous genitalia, retardation, facial abnormalities*	312830	[47]
Arterial tortuosity syndrome	SLC2A10	Long face, sagging cheeks, downslanting and short palpebral fissures, large ears, beaked nose, malar hypoplasia, micrognathia, hernia, cutis laxa, arterial tortuosity and aneurysms of large and medium vessels; lungs not affected	208050	[48]
Costello syndrome	HRAS	Phenotypic overlap with cardio-facio-cutaneous syndrome Characteristic coarse facies, short stature, cutis laxa particularly hands and feet, severe feeding difficulty and failure to thrive, cardiac anomalies, facial warts Often presents in childhood	218040	[49,50]
Transaldolase deficiency	TALDO1	Cutis laxa, growth retardation, dysmorphic features, congenital heart disease, hepatosplenomegaly, abnormal platelet aggregation	606003	[51]
Lenz–Majewski syndrome	PTDSS1	Intrauterine growth retardation, postnatal short stature, disproportionately large head, distinct cranio-facial and dental anomalies, distal limb anomalies, particularly brachydactyly and symphalangism. Progressive bone sclerosis evident on X-ray. Moderate to severe intellectual disability. Cutis laxa in infancy, thin skin with prominent veins especially on the scalp. Cutis marmorata	151050	[52,53]
COG7-related disorder	COG7	Hypotonia, hepatosplenomegaly, growth retardation, microcephaly, variable skeletal anomalies, developmental delay, loose wrinkled skin	608779	[54]

Adapted from Beyens *et al.* 2021 [12].

[a] Only one family reported.

COG, component of oligomeric Golgi complex; MACS, macrocephaly–alopecia–cutis laxa–scoliosis; URDS, Urban–Rifkin–Davis syndrome.

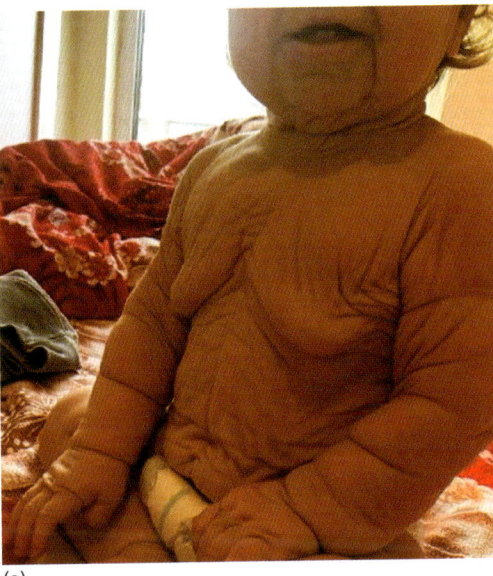

(a)

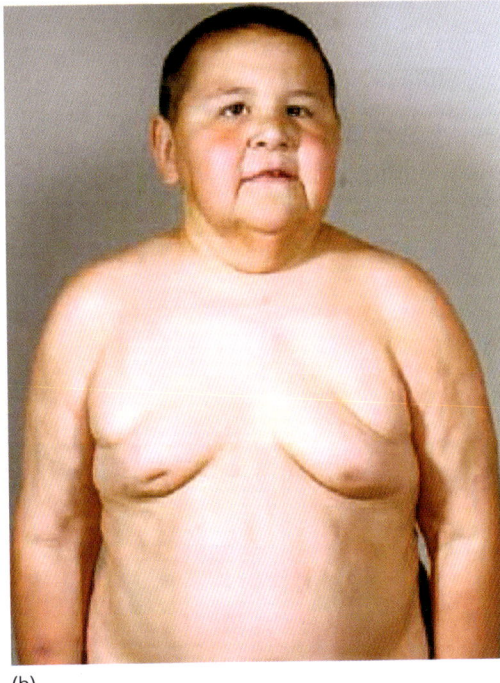

(b)

Figure 70.10 (a) A 1-year-old female with autosomal dominant cutis laxa due to a heterozygous *ELN* mutation. (b) Autosomal dominant cutis laxa in a 13-year-old male. (a) Courtesy of Dr Gabriela Petrof, consultant dermatologist at Great Ormond Street Hospital for Children, London, UK. (b) Reproduced from Berk *et al.* 2012 [8] with kind permission of Elsevier.

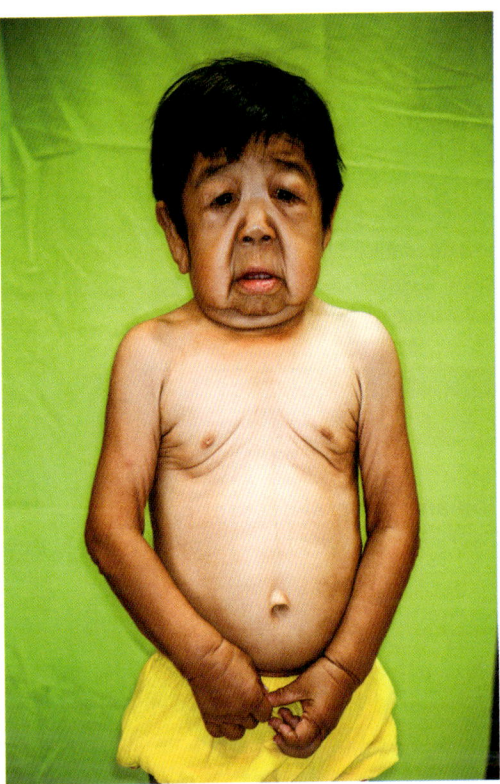

Figure 70.11 Autosomal recessive type 1A cutis laxa due to *FBLN5* mutation in a 4-year-old girl. Generalised loose skin affects the trunk and limbs and is most evident on the face, with a 'droopy' appearance giving the impression of downward slanting eyes. Reproduced with permission of Dr Nik Kantaputra, Chiang Mai University, Chiang Mai, Thailand.

Table 70.4 The main craniosynostosis syndromes.

Syndrome	Other features in addition to craniosynostosis	Chromosomal localisation	Gene
Apert	Mid-face malformations, syndactyly of hands and feet, acne	10q26	FGFR2
Crouzon	Proptosis, acanthosis nigricans (AN)	10q26	FGFR2
		4p16.3	FGFR3 (with AN)
Pfeiffer	Broad halluces and thumbs	8p11.2-11.1/ 10q26	FGFR1/FGFR2
Saethre–Chotzen	Ptosis, facial asymmetry, low hairline	7p21	TWIST1
Beare–Stevenson	Cutis gyrata	10q26	FGFR2

FGFR, fibroblast growth factor receptor gene; *TWIST1*, encoding a basic helix–loop–helix transcription factor.

Management

Treatment is limited and is directed towards alleviating complications. Surgical removal of lax skin can be undertaken as patients generally heal well although the benefits are not long term [13,27]. Botulinum toxin has been used successfully as a less invasive modality to improve facial defects in one case [28]. Although parenteral copper-histidine treatment has been of benefit to patients with Menkes disease, it appears to have less effect on the connective tissue abnormalities [29].

Resources

Patient resources

Contact.org: https://contact.org.uk/help-for-families/information-advice-services/. There is no support group for cutis laxa in the UK but this may be a useful resource for carers and patients.

Cutis Laxa Internationale: https://www.cutislaxa.org/.

(Both last accessed February 2022.)

PART 6: GENETIC DISORDERS

Williams–Beuren syndrome

Definition and nomenclature

The Williams–Beuren syndrome (WBS) is a multisystem disorder characterised by premature laxity of the skin, congenital heart disease (notably supravalvular aortic stenosis), metabolic abnormalities, dysmorphic facial features and developmental problems [1,2]. It is caused by deletion of the WBS chromosome region (chromosome 7), containing multiple genes [3].

Synonyms and inclusions
- Williams syndrome

Introduction and general description

Williams–Beuren syndrome is a rare genetic developmental disorder.

Epidemiology
Incidence and prevalence

Approximately 1/10 000 persons are affected [4].

Age

It can start in early adulthood.

Sex

There is equal sex incidence.

Ethnicity

No racial bias has been reported.

Pathophysiology

It is not understood which factors in the contiguous gene defect causes the phenotype but it is likely to be related to reduced expression of certain genes. Although WBS is not strictly an elastinopathy, this region includes the *ELN* gene [5,6] and WBS shares many clinical features associated with elastin deficiency.

Genetics

The syndrome is caused by a hemizygous deletion of 1.5–1.8 Mb on chromosome 7q11.23, which contains at least 28 genes [3]. The deletion arises on either the maternally or the paternally inherited chromosome 7 and is sporadic in virtually all cases [7]. Familial cases are autosomal dominant.

Environmental factors

An 'epidemic' of the Williams syndrome was reported in the UK following the administration of excessive doses of vitamin D to prevent rickets in pregnant women [8]. Vitamin D is known to downregulate elastin gene expression [9].

Clinical features
Presentation

The syndrome is characterised by premature laxity of the skin and congenital heart disease, notably supravalvular aortic stenosis.

Pulmonary artery stenosis is present at birth [10]. Metabolic abnormalities occur and dysmorphic facial features include a flat nasal bridge, short upturned nose and baggy connective tissue around the eyes [1]. Newborns have 'elfin-like' faces. As patients get older, their features become noticeable and coarser with full cheeks, prominent lips and dental malocclusion (Figure 70.12) [7,11]. Premature greying of the hair can start in young adulthood. Inguinal (and other) hernias may be present. A recent study demonstrated also an increased incidence of wrinkles (92%) and abnormal scarring (33%) as well as abnormal biomechanical properties of the skin [12].

Delayed motor and perceptual development are sometimes masked by above-average language skills allied to a 'cocktail party' personality [13].

Differential diagnosis

Identical cardiovascular abnormalities are seen in familial supravalvular aortic stenosis, due to elastin gene (*ELN*) mutations, but the other features of WBS are lacking [14,15].

Complications and co-morbidities

Endocrine abnormalities occur and include variable hypercalcaemia, sometimes with associated symptoms [16], impaired glucose tolerance [17] and subclinical thyroid disease [18]. Hypertension occurs in approximately 50% of patients [19]. Cardiovascular complications are the major cause of death [20].

Disease course and prognosis

Cardiovascular-associated mortality is 25–100 times that among controls [20].

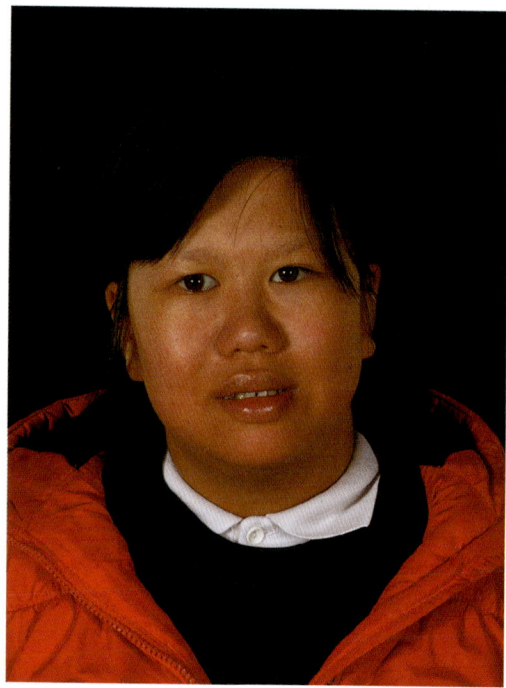

Figure 70.12 Child with Williams–Beuren syndrome exhibiting later facial features of full cheeks and lips, periorbital puffiness and epicanthic folds. Copyright of the Addenbrooke's NHS Trust, Cambridge, UK.

Investigations

Echocardiography will detect most stenoses. Regular monitoring of calcium levels and investigation of other endocrine associations should be performed.

Management

Therapy is directed to specific complications. Surgery is the preferred choice for arterial stenoses [7].

Resources

Further information

National Organization for Rare Disorders: http://rarediseases.org/.

Patient resources

Williams Syndrome Foundation: https://williams-syndrome.org.uk/. (Both last accessed February 2022.)

Michelin tyre baby syndrome

Definition and nomenclature

This syndrome is characterised by the folding of skin, which leads to symmetrical and circumferential ringed creases, primarily of the limbs. Affected individuals also exhibit intellectual disability, cleft palate and dysmorphic features.

Synonyms and inclusions
- Congenital symmetric circumferential skin creases
- Kunze–Riehm syndrome

Introduction and general description

The physical features resemble the mascot of the tyre manufacturer, Michelin, hence the name of the syndrome. The phenotype refers to most probably a very heterogeneous group of disorders manifesting with circumferential skin folds [1]. It can occur either in isolation or in association with additional anomalies, in particular facial dysmorphism, intellectual disability and cardiac and genital abnormalities [1,2]. It can be sporadic or inherited as an autosomal dominant or recessive trait [3,4].

Epidemiology
Incidence and prevalence

There are approximately 30 cases reported in the literature [5].

Age

It is present at birth

Sex

There is an equal sex incidence.

Ethnicity

No racial bias has been reported.

Pathophysiology

Mutations in *TUBB* or in *MAPRE2* that affect microtubule assembly or function underlie this genetic condition [2]. Tubulins constitute the structural units of microtubules, which are essential for a number of cellular processes including intracellular trafficking, chromosome separation and cell migration.

Pathology

Some cases are associated with underlying smooth muscle hamartomas [6] or adipose tissue hyperplasia [7]. Scarring instead of increased adipocytes has also been reported. Abnormal elastic fibres have been observed and in some cases the histology is normal [8].

Genetics

There is heterozygosity for a missense mutation in the *TUBB* gene and homozygous and heterozygous mutations in the *MAPRE2* gene [2].

Clinical features
Presentation

Multiple, symmetrical, circular skin creases are present at birth, on the forearms, lower legs and often the neck. Associated abnormalities vary and may include facial dysmorphism, growth retardation, upslanting palpebral fissures, hypertelorism, cleft palate, genital anomalies, mild developmental delay and ureterocele [5].

Differential diagnosis

It should be distinguished from other disorders with redundant skin folds such as leprechaunism and cutis laxa. Diagnostic criteria to help better delineate the syndrome have recently been proposed with the suggestion to rename the condition as circumferential skin folds syndrome [8].

Constriction ring syndrome due to intrauterine amniotic bands affects distal extremities like the fingers and toes.

Disease course and prognosis

The creases can disappear later in life [9].

Investigations

A skin biopsy may help identify the variable underlying changes that may be present.

Management

No specific therapy is required. Follow-up to monitor development and the possible associations is recommended [10].

Resources

Further information

National Center for Biotechnology Information, OMIM: http://www.ncbi.nlm.nih.gov/omim (last accessed February 2022).

FIBRILLINOPATHY

Marfan syndrome

Definition
The full syndrome is characterised by aortic dilatation, ectopia lentis and skeletal abnormalities. Individuals are disproportionately tall and thin with abnormally long extremities [1].

Introduction and general description
Marfan syndrome (MFS) is an autosomal dominant disorder of connective tissue with variable clinical manifestations, mainly affecting the cardiovascular, skeletal and ocular systems.

Epidemiology
Incidence and prevalence
Marfan syndrome affects 1/5000–10 000 individuals [1].

Age
Symptoms can appear at any age and vary greatly between individuals even within the same family.

Sex
There is no sex bias.

Ethnicity
There is no racial variation.

Associated diseases
Several patients have been reported with concomitant EDS and MFS [2]. A specific Marfanoid phenotype with congenital lipodystrophy and a neonatal progeroid appearance has been identified with truncating mutations in the penultimate exon 64 of *FBN1* as the cause [3,4]. A Marfanoid habitus has also been reported in association with distal pigmentation, neuroma of the eyelids and tongue, medullary carcinoma of the thyroid and phaeochromocytoma as part of the multiple endocrine neoplasia type 2B (MEN2B) syndrome [5], which has been found to be caused by a specific mutation in *RET*.

Pathophysiology
True cases of MFS are due to abnormalities in fibrillin 1 which is one component of the elastin-associated microfibrils. It is especially important in the ciliary zonule of the eye (the suspensory ligament of the lens). Changes in growth factor signalling are also critical in MFS. As well as its structural role, fibrillin-1 also binds TGF-β, and abnormal fibrillin leads to detrimental, increased TGF-β signalling [6].

Pathology
Patients with MFS lack fibrillin in their skin and on culture of their dermal fibroblasts [7,8], with accumulation of mucinous material in the media of the aorta [9]. Mild to severe degenerative changes in elastic tissue are also seen in the lungs [10].

Genetics
Mutations in the *FBN1* gene, which is located on chromosome 15q21.1 and encodes fibrillin-1, cause the majority if not all cases of MFS [11,12]. Up to 30% of cases are new mutations [13] and a strong paternal-age effect occurs. The mean age of fathers of individuals who appear to harbour 'new' mutations is from 5 to 10 years greater than average [14].

Mutations in the genes for the TGF-β receptors (*TGFBR1* and *TGFBR2*) have been identified in a number of disorders with phenotypic overlap with classical MFS [15].

Clinical features
History
The diagnostic criteria for MFS were revised in 2010 with aortic root aneurysm and ectopia lentis now considered cardinal manifestations [**16**].

Presentation
The full syndrome comprises skeletal, ocular and cardiovascular defects. The patient is often, but not invariably, exceptionally tall, and the skeletal proportions are abnormal. The limbs are long, the excess being greatest distally, giving rise to arachnodactyly. Simple screening tests include the thumb sign (positive if the thumb when completely opposed in the clenched hand projects beyond the ulnar border), the wrist sign (positive if the thumb and little finger overlap when wrapped around the opposite wrist) and the ratio of the lower segment (pubic ramus to floor) to the upper segment (height minus lower segment); but this latter ratio varies with age and sex.

The skull is dolichocephalic, the paranasal sinuses are large and the palate high and arched [17]. Other skeletal changes include hyperextensible joints, kyphoscoliosis, pectus excavatum and flat foot. Muscles may be underdeveloped and hypotonic, and subcutaneous fat is sparse.

The common ocular abnormalities [18,19] include ectopia lentis (usually upward), a trembling iris (iridodonesis), myopia and retinal detachment; less frequent are blue sclerae and heterochromia of the iris.

Aneurysmal dilatation of the ascending aorta is the most important abnormality of the cardiovascular system. Aortic dilatation may begin in childhood. Aortic and mitral incompetence are common, with mitral valve prolapse occurring in 80% of cases [20].

Striae atrophicae were observed in 7% of children and 35% of adults [21]. Other features include papyraceous scars and skin hyperextensibility [21]. The MASS syndrome (MIM: 604308), standing for mitral valve prolapse, myopia, borderline and non-progressive aortic enlargement, and non-specific skin and skeletal features, has been used to describe a subset of MFS patients with prominent cutaneous manifestations [22].

Other abnormalities include nerve deafness, which occurs in 6%; pulmonary malformations, which are often reported at autopsy; and renal abnormalities, which manifest as proteinuria and microhaematuria [23,24].

Clinical variants
There is significant phenotypic variability of true MFS as well as considerable overlap with closely related syndromes. Neonatal

MFS is at the most severe end of the spectrum, often with death in the first year of life due to congestive heart failure as a consequence of significant atrioventricular valve dysfunction. This phenotype arises due to mutations in two specific regions of the *FBN1* gene [25].

Differential diagnosis

Homocystinuria (due to cystathionine β-synthetase) should be considered in Marfanoid patients with myopia or downward ectopia lentis. Urine screening is unreliable; blood levels of methionine and homocysteine should be measured. Prompt diagnosis and treatment of homocystinuria, for example, with pyridoxine supplements reduces the risk of coronary artery or cerebrovascular thrombosis [26].

Significant phenotypic overlap occurs with LDS, caused by mutations in the TGF-β receptor genes *TGFBR1* and *TGFBR2* [12,27].

MFS also shares some clinical features with the other fibrillinopathies, and in particular: dominant ectopia lentis, Shprintzen–Goldberg syndrome (craniosynostosis, cardiac features, delayed neurodevelopment and Marfanoid features), Weill–Marchesani syndrome (ectopia lentis, short stature, brachycephaly and joint stiffness), as well as Beals syndrome (congenital contractural arachnodactyly). Overlap is also seen with some forms of EDS (see earlier in this chapter), familial thoracic aortic aneurysms and arterial tortuosity syndrome [16,28].

Disease course and prognosis

Aortic dissection is the most common cause of mortality; 50% of patients <40 years old who remain undiagnosed die from aortic dissection, with an increased risk during adolescence [29]. However, with the introduction of β-blocking agents, angiotensin II receptor 1 blockers and improvements in vascular and cardiac surgery, the prognosis has improved greatly and treated patients can have near-normal life expectancy [30,31].

Investigations

Regular surveillance is recommended with careful imaging and monitoring of aortic root width and of the function of the aortic and mitral valves.

Management

Identification of presymptomatic patients is critical to reduce the frequency of catastrophic aortic events [29]. The two most important risk factors for aortic dissection are maximal dimension and family history of dissection.

Beta-blocker therapy has been used for many years. More recently, treatment with angiotensin-converting enzyme inhibitors has been advocated due to their inhibitory effect on circulating TGF-β. The addition of angiotensin receptor blockers to β-blocker therapy slows the progression of aortic route dilatation further [31].

A number of criteria exist to determine the need for aortic root surgical intervention in adults including those with aortic root diameter >50 mm (this is indexed for body surface area) [28].

The majority of *FBN1* mutations are unique to one affected individual or family, but despite this, and the presence of sporadic cases, prenatal and preimplantation diagnosis is feasible [32].

Resources

Further information

National Center for Biotechnology Information, OMIM: http://www.ncbi.nlm.nih.gov/omim.
National Organization for Rare Disorders: http://rarediseases.org/.

Patient resources

Marfan Trust: https://www.marfantrust.org/
(All last accessed February 2022.)

INFANTILE STIFF SKIN SYNDROMES

Hyaline fibromatosis syndrome

Definition and nomenclature

Hyaline fibromatosis is one of several rare syndromes causing hard, stiff skin and joint contractures in early life.

> **Synonyms and inclusions**
> - Systemic hyalinosis
> - Hyaline fibromatosis incorporates both infantile systemic hyalinosis (ISH) and juvenile hyaline fibromatosis (JHF)

Introduction and general description

Both JHF and ISH are rare allelic autosomal recessive disorders of the connective tissue with overlapping clinical features comprising progressive joint contractures, skin papules and nodules and chronic pain [1–3].

Epidemiology

Incidence and prevalence

These are very rare disorders, with JHF being reported more frequently than ISH [4].

Age

Presentation is in infancy or childhood.

Sex

There is no sex predilection.

Ethnicity

No racial variation has been reported.

Pathophysiology

Anthrax toxin receptor 2 (*ANTXR2* or *CMG2*) encodes a transmembrane protein that plays a role in basement membrane matrix assembly and endothelial cell morphogenesis. Defects in this protein leads to extravasation of plasma (hyaline material) [4].

Pathology [4,5–7]

The dermis is thickened with deposition of hyaline eosinophilic material which appears fibrogranular on electron microscopy. The hyaline material may also be present in other tissues including bowel, muscle and bone. The dermal collagen is decreased and the collagen fibrils are fewer and thinner than in normal skin. An absence of pro-α2 chains and type III collagen has been demonstrated in affected skin.

Genetics

Hyaline fibromatosis is caused by homozygous or compound heterozygous mutation in the gene encoding the anthrax toxin receptor 2 gene also known as capillary morphogenesis protein 2 (*ANTXR2/CMG2*) [1–3,**4**].

Clinical features

Presentation

Infantile systemic hyalinosis is the more extreme variant characterised by the skin becoming diffusely thickened and hard in the first few weeks of life, with limited joint mobility. Papules or nodules may be present at birth or develop in early childhood, particularly on the face, neck or perianal region. In the milder phenotypic spectrum of JHF, onset may be delayed until 3 months to 4 years [8]. Other variable features include gingival hypertrophy, hyperpigmentation, painful swollen joints with contractures, hypotonia, osteopenia, diarrhoea with hypoproteinaemia, severe infections and growth failure.

Differential diagnosis

Winchester syndrome, stiff skin syndrome, lipoid proteinosis (Urbach–Wiethe disease), congenital generalised multiple fibromatosis (MIM: 228550) and mucopolysaccharidosis type II (Hunter syndrome) should be considered in the differential diagnosis. Similarly, infants with Farber disease (MIM: 228000) can present with a clinical picture very similar to ISH. Here, the yellowish colour of the nodules and the presence of granulomas on histology allows the diagnosis of Farber disease to be made; this is caused by decreased acid ceramidase activity.

Classification of severity

Denadai *et al.* [**4**] have proposed a grading system of 1–4 for the severity of clinical manifestations.

Disease course and prognosis

The prognosis is poorer with ISH, with survival beyond the age of 2 years being unlikely mostly due to recurrent respiratory infections and severe diarrhoea [9]. Most patients with JHF survive until the fourth decade [10].

Investigations

Molecular testing can be performed, if appropriate.

Management

Treatment of these diseases is limited to symptomatic relief. Joint contractures and small skin nodules may respond to intralesional steroid injections in the early stages and may also respond to systemic steroids and physiotherapy [11].

The tumours do not respond to radiotherapy and they may recur after excision [12].

Stiff skin syndrome

Definition

Stiff skin syndrome is one of several rare syndromes causing hard stiff skin and joint contractures in early life.

Epidemiology

Incidence and prevalence

Approximately 40 cases have been reported in the literature [1].

Age

Features present in infancy or early childhood.

Sex

There is no sex bias.

Ethnicity

Of the 43 cases published five have been from Brazil [2].

Pathophysiology

Mutations in the integrin-binding domain of fibrillin 1 leads to altered cell-matrix interactions, impaired elastogenesis and increased TGF-β signalling in the dermis. Similar observations are found in systemic sclerosis [1].

Pathology

A deep sclerosis is found with a lattice-like array of thickened, horizontally orientated collagen bundles in the absence of inflammation [3].

Genetics

This is an autosomal dominant disorder due to mutations in the *FBN1* gene region encoding the integrin-binding domain of fibrillin 1 [1]. Segmental stiff skin syndrome has been associated with IL17C mutation in one case [4].

Clinical features

Presentation

Patients have diffuse, firm, thick skin, leading to reduced joint mobility and causing flexion contractures [5]. More variable features include hypertrichosis, short stature, lipodystrophy, muscle weakness, cutaneous nodules over distal interphalangeal joints and diffuse entrapment neuropathy [1]. Internal organs are not involved [**6**]. Localised (segmental) involvement accounts for about a third of cases and is less severe, with older onset [7].

Differential diagnosis

Mucopolysaccharidoses need to be excluded. Scleroderma and neonatal scleredema can be distinguished on skin histology. Infantile hyalinosis, restrictive dermopathy and Hutchinson–Gilford progeria all present with tight skin but can be excluded by molecular analyses [**6**].

There are overlapping features with congenital fascial dystrophy (CFD) (MIM: 28020), although this appears to be a distinct, probable autosomal recessive disorder [8]. CFD is characterised by mild hirsutism, limitation of joint mobility affecting the gait and localised areas of stony-hard skin, most pronounced on the buttocks and legs, which are otherwise normal in appearance [9]. Thickening of the thoracic fascia may cause hypoventilation due to thoracic underdevelopment. Stiff skin syndrome and CFD also show some similarities to the tight-skin mouse [10,11] although the gene defect for CFD is not known.

Disease course and prognosis
There is slow progression of skin involvement.

Investigations
Whilst skin histology can be helpful, it is not pathognomonic. Other laboratory tests are usually normal.

Management
There is no specific treatment but physiotherapy is important to help with reduced mobility. Mycophenolate mofetil, losartan and more recently secukinumab have all been used with variable degree of success for segmental stiff skin syndrome [7].

Resources

Further information
National Center for Biotechnology Information, OMIM: http://www.ncbi.nlm.nih .gov/omim (last accessed February 2022).

Winchester syndrome

Definition and nomenclature
This is one of several rare syndromes causing thickened stiff skin, osteolysis, joint contractures, as well as other features, in early life [1].

Synonyms and inclusions
- Hereditary contractures with sclerodermatoid changes of the skin
- Stiff skin syndrome [2]

Introduction and general description
Winchester syndrome is included in the heterogeneous group of inherited osteolyses, or 'vanishing bone' syndromes. Bone and joints abnormalities are the main features seen.

Epidemiology
Incidence and prevalence
The condition is very rare and the true prevalence is not known.

Age
Onset is in infancy.

Sex
More female cases have been reported although it is an autosomal recessive disorder.

Ethnicity
There is no known racial variation.

Pathophysiology
Mutations in matrix metalloproteinase 14 (*MMP14/MT1MMP*) decrease the membrane location of the metalloproteinase resulting in impairment of MMP2 activation [3]. It is known in mouse fibroblasts that this leads to a reduced ability to degrade type I collagen [4].

Pathology
Defective collagen remodelling is central to the underlying pathology [5]. The changes in the dermis are variable and may relate to the stage of evolution of the disease [6]. In a young patient, fibroblastic proliferation was present in the deep dermis, whilst an older patient exhibited only swirling masses of abnormal collagen with a paucity of fibroblasts throughout the entire depth of the dermis. In both patients a lymphocytic perivascular infiltrate was present. On electron microscopy, mitochondrial abnormalities are present in dermal fibroblasts and include swelling, degeneration and vacuolisation.

Genetics
Winchester syndrome is an autosomal recessive condition due to mutations in *MMP14*, encoding for a matrix metalloproteinase.

Previously, Torg syndrome, multicentric osteolysis, nodulosis and arthropathy (MONA) and Winchester syndrome were considered allelic [7], but with the identification of causal mutations in the *MMP14* gene exclusive to Winchester syndrome, this is no longer the case [3].

Clinical features
Presentation
This is a disease of infancy characterised by joint contractures, gingival hypertrophy, dwarfism, osteolysis, particularly of the hands and feet, osteoporosis, arthralgia, corneal opacities and hypertrichosis [1,8,9]. Diffusely thickened, leathery skin with areas of hyperpigmentation as well as widespread symmetrical restrictive banding of the skin have been reported [10]. Abnormal electrocardiogram changes suggesting myocardial damage can also occur [1].

Differential diagnosis
Patients share clinical similarities to MONA (MIM: 259600) caused by heterozygous or homozygous mutations in *MMP2*, but subcutaneous nodules are characteristically absent. Frank–ter Haar syndrome is a rare disorder characterised by cranio-facial malformations, skeletal and cardiac abnormalities and dermal fibrosis [5].

The skin changes resemble those of scleroedema of Buschke but are distinguished by their early onset. The condition must also be distinguished from sclerema neonatorum, but this is a disorder of subcutaneous fat rather than the skin. There is also some clinical overlap with the mucopolysaccharidoses.

Complications and co-morbidities
Progressive osteolysis can lead to loss of function of large and small joints.

Disease course and prognosis
The prognosis is relatively good, and many patients survive into adult life.

Investigations
The osteolytic changes will be detectable by plain radiographs.

Management
No specific therapies are reported and treatment is aimed at symptomatic relief.

Resources

Further information
National Organization for Rare Disorders: http://rarediseases.org/.

Patient resources
MPS Society: www.mpssociety.org.uk.
(Both last accessed February 2022.)

PART 6: GENETIC DISORDERS

Restrictive dermopathy

Definition and nomenclature
Restrictive dermopathy is a very rare autosomal recessive and lethal laminopathy that presents at birth with a taut, shiny skin restricting movement of the joints.

Synonyms and inclusions
• Lethal tight skin contracture syndrome

Epidemiology
Incidence and prevalence
Restrictive dermopathy is very rare with approximately only 60 cases published [1].

Age
The skin changes are present at birth.

Sex
There is no sex bias.

Pathophysiology
Mutations in *ZMPSTE24* and *LMNA* lead to accumulation of prelamin A with detrimental effect on nuclear function [2,3].

Pathology
The epidermis shows hyperkeratosis and parakeratosis, and the keratohyaline granules are abnormal. The dermal–epidermal junction is flat, with a thin dermis and a thick layer of subcutaneous fat. The eccrine and pilosebaceous glands are underdeveloped. The collagen bundles appear stretched, and orientated in parallel lines, as they are in a tendon [4,5].

Genetics
Restrictive dermopathy is autosomal recessive and caused in most cases by homozygous or compound heterozygous mutation in the *ZMPSTE24* gene or less commonly by heterozygous mutations in the *LMNA* gene [1].

Clinical features
Presentation [6–9]
It is characterised by intrauterine growth retardation and premature birth due to ruptured fetal membranes. At birth, the skin is tight, red and shiny with flexural erosions. The typical facies comprise a small, fixed, round, open mouth, micrognathia, small nose with choanal atresia/stenosis, low-set ears and widely spaced cranial sutures. Half of the children have neonatal teeth. Skeletal changes include enlarged fontanelles, clavicular dysplasia and reduced bone density. The joints are all fixed in flexion, and there is gross restriction of the respiratory movements. Respiratory insufficiency and secondary infections cause death within a few weeks from birth.

Differential diagnosis
Hutchinson–Gilford progeria syndrome (also caused by *LMNA* mutations) shares some clinical features including hypoplastic clavicles, bone density reduction, sparse eyebrows and eyelashes, micrognathia and joint contractures. Neu–Laxova syndrome very much resembles restrictive dermopathy except for the presence of brain structural abnormalities. Collodion membrane may confer to the skin an appearance that can be confused with the skin of patients with restrictive dermopathy. Sclerema neonatorum should also be considered in the differential diagnosis of restrictive dermopathy.

Disease course and prognosis
Death usually occurs within the first week of life due to respiratory failure [10].

Investigations
Radiological investigations for skeletal changes, skin biopsy and molecular analysis can be undertaken.

Management
No specific therapies are available.

Resources

Further information
National Center for Biotechnology Information, OMIM: http://www.ncbi.nlm.nih.gov/omim (last accessed February 2022).

PREMATURE AGEING SYNDROMES

Progeria

Definition and nomenclature
This is a very rare disorder characterised by retarded physical development, abnormal facies, skeletal abnormalities and the onset in early childhood of scleroderma-like changes. Although progressive senile degeneration occurs, many of the more common features of ageing, such as cataracts, presbycusis and presbyopia, are not seen.

Introduction and general description
Progeria is derived from the Greek word *geras*, meaning old age. Although death usually occurs in the second decade as a result of severe generalised atherosclerosis, Hutchinson–Gilford progeria syndrome is considered a segmental ageing syndrome as some of the other typical features of ageing, such as cataracts, presbycusis, presbyopia, increased incidence of cancer and dementia do not occur.

Epidemiology
Incidence and prevalence
Hutchinson–Gilford progeria syndrome is ultra-rare but is the commonest of the progeria syndromes, with a prevalence of approximately 1 in 20 million newborns worldwide [1].

Age
Clinical features may not be obvious at birth. The mean age at diagnosis reported in the literature cases is 2.6–2.9 years [2]. Rarely, some patients present with cutaneous manifestations in the third decade of life [3].

Sex
There is a slight male predilection; the male to female ratio is 1.5 : 1.2 [2].

Ethnicity
Approximately 150 cases have been reported with a significant majority in people with white skin. It is possible that this racial disparity is due to publication bias.

Pathophysiology
Lamin A is an intermediate filament protein which acts as an intranuclear scaffold as well having cellular functions affecting DNA repair, regulation of gene expression and telomere stability. Mutations in *LMNA* produce an abnormal lamin A protein precursor, progerin, which retains a farnesyl group, that is usually removed. This results in genomic instability, decreased cell proliferation and premature cell senescence and death [4–6].

Pathology
The major changes are in the skin, bone and cardiovascular tissues [7]. The skin shows atrophy of epidermis and dermis. There may be progressive hyalinisation of dermal collagen and loss of subcutaneous fat. Scanning electron microscopy of hairs from one patient showed unusual longitudinal depressions with minor cuticular defects [8].

The cardiovascular system shows extensive atherosclerosis and there may be extensive myocardial fibrosis, with extensive lipofuscin ('age pigment') deposition characteristic of elderly adults [9,10].

The bones show a variety of changes including osteolysis, osteoporosis, necrosis, dislocations and poorly healing fractures [11,12].

Genetics
It occurs due to *de novo* heterozygous mutations of the lamin A gene (*LMNA*) which encodes for a major constituent of the inner membrane lamina [13,14]. Prelamin A is blocked at a critical step mediated by the zinc metalloproteinase ZMPSTE24. A small group of atypical patients have LMNA mutations with normal processing linked to later onset disease [3].

Clinical features
Presentation (Table 70.5) [15,16]
The commonest presenting feature is failure to thrive, with reduced subcutaneous fat on the face and limbs [2,17]. The facial appearance is reminiscent of a fledgling bird. By the second year of disease, the skin has become thin, taut and shiny in some areas but lax and finely wrinkled in others. Mid-facial cyanosis is often seen. After several years, progressive mottled hyperpigmentation develops, most marked on exposed sites, but there is no photosensitivity. Thickened sclerotic areas may be present on the lower trunk or thighs, and in one case multiple keloids developed on the hands and arms [8]. The nails are usually small, thin and dystrophic. The nipples may be hypoplastic.

The dentition is abnormal and delayed, and there may be skeletal abnormalities such as dystrophic clavicles and coxa valga, with joint contractures and a 'horse-riding' stance. Progressive bone resorption may lead to frequent fractures [12]. Sexual maturation is absent but intelligence is normal.

Angina and strokes are common. Insulin resistance can often be detected although overt diabetes is rare.

Differential diagnosis
Other progeroid syndromes that share some similarities include mandibuloacral dysplasia [18], Mulvihill–Smith syndrome [19] and neonatal pseudohydrocephalic progeroid syndrome of Wiedemann–Rautenstrauch [20–22] (see later in this chapter).

Stunting of growth from early childhood is associated with senile changes in the skin but normal scalp hair in gerodermia osteodysplastica (see Table 70.3) [23]. Gerodermia osteodysplastica, wrinkly skin syndrome and autosomal recessive cutis laxa type 2 show some phenotypic overlap [24–26].

A progeroid appearance with distinct facial features is seen in neonates with MFS which is associated with congenital lipodystrophy, premature birth and an accelerated linear growth and is due to truncating mutations in the penultimate exon 64 of *FBN1* [27].

Table 70.5 Clinical features of the classical premature ageing syndromes.

	Pangeria (Werner syndrome)	Progeria (Hutchinson–Gilford syndrome)	Acrogeria (Gottron syndrome)
Stature	Small stature; cessation of growth at 12 years	Small stature	Usually normal but some have low birth weight and short stature
Facies	Beaked nose; skin of ears atrophic and tightly bound down giving bird-like facies	Bird-like facies with protruding ears, beaked nose, thin lips with centrofacial cyanosis, prominent eyes, frontal and parietal bossing with pseudohydrocephaly, mid-face hypoplasia with micrognathia and large anterior fontanelle; prominent frontal tuberosities and scalp veins	Micrognathia; atrophy of skin on tip of nose
Skin	Dry atrophic skin; mottled hyperpigmentation and telangiectasia particularly over limbs, face and neck	Dry, thin and wrinkled with progressive mottled pigmentation; may present with scleroderma-like changes on limbs; eccrine sweating is decreased	Atrophic transparent skin with telangiectasia and mottled hyperpigmentation on extremities; easy bruising and prominent veins
Scalp hair	Premature greying at 20 years; loss of hair at 20–25 years	Hair lost in first 2 years of life	Normal
Eyes	Bilateral juvenile cataracts (20–30 years); keratopathy; glaucoma	Prominent eyes; otherwise normal	Normal
Nails	Normal	Thin and brittle	Dystrophic or thickened
Limbs	More generally affected than trunk; sclerodactyly; restricted movement of joints; lower limb ulcers; hyperkeratosis over bony prominences; generalised loss of subcutaneous fat	Prominent joints; coxa valga; generalised subcutaneous fat loss; poorly developed muscular system; no acrosclerosis or Raynaud phenomenon	Atrophy of skin most marked on extremities; no leg ulcers; hands and feet may be small

Cockayne syndrome (Chapter 76) may cause confusion, but progeria is distinguished by the loss of hair, the lack of photosensitivity and ocular changes, and the absence of disproportionately large extremities.

In metageria, sexual maturation and skeletal growth are normal [28].

The firm skin of sclerema neonatorum may be confused with this syndrome, but these infants lack the other skeletal features.

Disease course and prognosis
Death occurs at an average age of 13 years with 80% from myocardial infarction or stroke [29]. The prognosis for the rarer, atypical, later onset presentation is better, with death expected in middle age due to cardiovascular disease [3].

Investigations
Molecular confirmation of the diagnosis is important. Monitoring for cardiovascular and cerebrovascular disease is required.

Management
First line
Infants and children may experience feeding difficulties and failure to thrive and require advice regarding nutrition. Measures to reduce the risk of atherosclerotic disease are important. Early input from physiotherapy and occupational therapy should be arranged to help reduce the complications of arthritis.

Second line
A clinical trial in children of a farnesyl transferase inhibitor, lonafarnib, improved weight gain, vascular stiffness, bone structure and audiological status [30]. Neurological sequelae were also reduced [31]. The results from ongoing trials of lonafarnib combined with everolimus are waited [1].

Resources

Further information
National Center for Biotechnology Information, OMIM: http://www.ncbi.nlm.nih .gov/omim.
National Organization for Rare Disorders: http://rarediseases.org/.

Patient resources
Progeria Research Foundation (USA), patient support group: www.progeriaresearch .org.
(All last accessed February 2022.)

Werner syndrome

Definition and nomenclature
Werner syndrome is an inherited premature ageing disorder in which the ageing process is accelerated, starting after puberty. Cutaneous changes include atrophy, loss of cutaneous fat, wrinkling, canities (greying of the hair), hair loss, nail dystrophy, defective pigmentation, poikiloderma, sclerosis and ulceration.

Synonyms and inclusions
- Pangeria
- Adult premature ageing syndrome

Introduction and general description
More than 150 diseases manifest one or more features of apparent premature ageing, but there are discrepancies between this process and true ageing. Werner syndrome is characterised by multisystem involvement and an increased risk of malignancy [1,2]. It is caused by mutations in the *RECQL2* gene [3].

Epidemiology
Incidence and prevalence
Werner syndrome is estimated to affect 1/200 000 individuals in the USA [4]. It is more common in Japan, affecting 1/20 000–40 000 people [5].

Age
Development is usually not until the second or third decade.

Sex
There is no sex bias.

Ethnicity
Relatively higher incidence has been reported in Japan (approximately 75% of all cases) and northern Sardinia with founder mutations in these countries [6,7].

Pathophysiology
RECQL2 (previously denoted WRN) is a member of the RecQ family of DNA helicases and appears to play a critical role in the rescue of impaired replication forks (sites on DNA that unwind thus allowing synthesis). Lack of this helicase results in genome instability which may lead to cancer [8].

Pathology
Many tissues show premature ageing, but the changes are not uniform. Microsplanchnia and generalised atherosclerosis are usually present. The epidermis is atrophic and some appendages are sparse. The dermis is thickened, with replacement of subcutaneous fat by hyalinised collagen, increased glycosaminoglycans, abnormal elastic fibres, disorganised nerves and vessel changes, which resemble those seen in diabetes. These abnormalities are more marked in the acral skin than on the trunk [9].

Genetics
Werner syndrome is transmitted as an autosomal recessive trait and is observed more commonly with parental consanguinity. More than 70 disease-causing mutations have been described in *RECQL2*. The majority are stop codon mutations, splice mutations or small indels producing truncations of the protein and/or nonsense-mediated decay of mutant mRNA [10].

Clinical features
Presentation (Table 70.5) [2]
Greying at the temples is usually the earliest sign and develops between the ages of 14 and 18 years but may rarely be present as early as 8 years. The first significant changes are usually noticed between 18 and 30 years but may begin earlier. A delay in diagnosis of up to 15 years is common [11].

Cutaneous findings include, in addition to hair thinning and greying, loss of subcutaneous tissue and scleroderma-like changes with associated telangiectases, calcinosis and ulcerations. Patchy pigmentary changes are also typical.

A high pitched or hoarse voice from thinning of the vocal cords and fixation of the epiglottis is characteristic. Intelligence is usually normal. Most patients are of small stature. Hypogonadism and premature menopause are characteristic, with sparse or absent pubic and axillary hair. Some patients yet achieve normal stature and successful pregnancies.

Diffuse early atherosclerosis results in ischaemic and valvular heart disease and is a major cause of premature death among patients. Diabetes occurs in at least 30%. The diabetes is characterised by peripheral insulin resistance [12,13]. Cataracts develop between the ages of 20 and 35 years in most cases. Other ocular defects may occur [14]. Osteoporosis and arthritis can be the source of severe morbidity.

Differential diagnosis
This includes progeria, Rothmund–Thomson syndrome (Chapter 75), systemic sclerosis (Chapter 54) and Huriez syndrome (Chapter 63).

Scleroderma can also be misdiagnosed in patients with early Werner syndrome.

The differentiation from some of the other ageing syndromes is indicated in Table 70.5.

Complications and co-morbidities
A recent study of neoplasias in 189 Werner syndrome patients [15] has identified that the most frequent tumours are thyroid carcinomas (16.1%) and, along with malignant melanoma, meningioma, soft-tissue sarcoma, haematological and bone neoplasms account for two-thirds of all the malignancies reported.

Disease course and prognosis
Death usually occurs in the fourth to sixth decade, due to myocardial infarction or malignancy [16].

Investigations
Mutations in *WRN* are identified in approximately 90% of individuals with Werner syndrome [17].

Investigations should be directed to assess the known complications especially diabetes, arteriosclerosis and hypogonadism. There may be calcification of the arteries, ligaments, tendons and subcutaneous tissues, with osteoporosis of the extremities, especially the legs. Osteosclerosis of the distal phalanges of the fingers and/or toes can also be detected on radiographs [18].

Management
Only symptomatic measures are available. The management of recurrent painful ulceration of the feet and legs is difficult, and amputation may be needed. Cataract surgery should be undertaken with special caution, for it is often complicated by severe degenerative changes of the cornea [14].

Resources

Further information
National Center for Biotechnology Information, OMIM: http://www.ncbi.nlm.nih.gov/omim.
National Organization for Rare Disorders: http://rarediseases.org/.

Patient resources
National Organization for Rare Disorders: http://rarediseases.org/.
(All last accessed February 2022.)

Acrogeria

Definition and nomenclature

This disorder, first described by Gottron in 1941 [1], is characterised by cutaneous atrophy and loss of subcutaneous fat, particularly over the distal extremities, but with no tendency to atherosclerosis, diabetes or decreased life expectancy. The term 'acrogeria' refers to premature ageing of the extremities.

> **Synonyms and inclusions**
> • Metageria
> • Acrometageria
> • Gottron syndrome

Introduction and general description

It remains unclear whether Gottron syndrome is a distinct or heterogeneous group of disorders.

Epidemiology

Incidence and prevalence

It is extremely rare with only about 40 cases described.

Age

It begins at birth or soon afterwards.

Sex

Most patients have been female [2,3].

Pathophysiology

Pathology

The subcutaneous fat is absent in the most severely affected regions. The dermis is atrophic, with sparse thin collagen bundles, but there is abundant elastin, which appears clumped due to the deficiency of collagen [3,4].

Clinical features

Presentation (Table 70.5)

The changes develop at or soon after birth. The skin becomes dry, thin, transparent and wrinkled, especially over the hands and feet, although the trunk and face may be affected to a lesser extent. The face appears 'pinched', with a hollow-cheeked 'owl-eyed' appearance, a beaked nose and thin lips. The lack of subcutaneous fat accentuates the appearance of premature senility.

Clinical variants

It is likely that acrogeria includes several subtypes. Firstly, with type III collagen deficiency as occurs in vEDS [5,6]. The ultrastructural changes in fibroblasts resemble those seen in vEDS [7]. Secondly, acrogeria affecting the acral skin but with normal type III collagen [4,8]. *LMNA* mutations have been identified in this type and more recently *ZMPSTE24* mutations have been implicated [9,10]. Thirdly, cases are occasionally described which do not fit easily into any of the previously recognised categories and have been termed metageria and acrometageria [11,12]. It is not entirely clear, however, whether these are separate entities.

Differential diagnosis

The lack of other system involvement helps to distinguish the condition from progeria and pangeria.

Phenotypic overlap is seen with the LDS due to mutations in *TGFBR1* and -2 [13]. It is possible that some of the earlier cases reported with normal collagen III could be LDS.

Disease course and prognosis

General health and life expectancy are normal.

Investigations

Vascular EDS and LDS should be excluded by molecular analysis.

Management

There is no specific treatment.

Resources

Further information

National Organization for Rare Disorders: http://rarediseases.org/ (last accessed February 2022).

Familial mandibuloacral dysplasia

Definition and nomenclature

This is a rare, genetically and phenotypically heterogeneous, autosomal recessive disorder characterised by variable progeroid features, skeletal abnormalities including hypoplasia of the mandible and clavicles, and acro-osteolysis, cutaneous atrophy and lipodystrophy [1,2].

> **Synonyms and inclusions**
> • Craniomandibular dermatodysostosis

Epidemiology

Incidence and prevalence

The incidence is less than 1/1 000 000.

Age

Affected individuals have a normal appearance at birth, then progressively develop lipodystrophy and dysmorphic cranio-facial and skeletal features.

Sex

There is an equal sex incidence.

Ethanicity

There is no reported racial variation.

Pathophysiology

The underlying fault in mandibuloacral dysplasia is alteration of lamin A through mutations in either the *LMNA* or *ZMPSTE24* genes [3,4]. Lamin A is an intermediate filament protein which acts as an intranuclear scaffold as well as having cellular functions affecting DNA repair, regulation of gene expression and telomere stability. Cellular senescence probably occurs via a variety of these molecular processes [5].

Genetics

Both types of mandibuloacral dysplasia are autosomal recessive, with mutations in two genes: *LMNA*, which encodes lamin A/C and is associated with mandibuloacral dysplasia type A, and *ZMPSTE24*, which is associated with mandibuloacral dysplasia type B and codes for an endoprotease involved in lamin A maturation [3,4]. Some patients with mandibuloacral dysplasia do not have mutations in either the *LMNA* or *ZMPSTE24* genes, suggesting the existence of other loci for this disorder.

Clinical features

Presentation

The main features are mandibular hypoplasia, delayed cranial suture closure, dysplastic clavicles, club-shaped terminal phalanges associated with acro-osteolysis and atrophy of the skin over the hands and feet (Figure 70.13) [1,2]. Other characteristics may include short stature, multiple Wormian bones, prominent eyes and a sharp nose [6,7]. Some patients show progeroid features such as bird-like facies, high-pitched voice and ectodermal defects, such as skin atrophy, mottled pigmentation, alopecia and nail dysplasia [8,9].

Clinical variants

Two types of body fat distribution patterns, both of which are associated with insulin resistance, diabetes and hyperlipidaemia, may be evident: partial lipodystrophy of the extremities (type A) and generalised loss of subcutaneous fat (type B) [10].

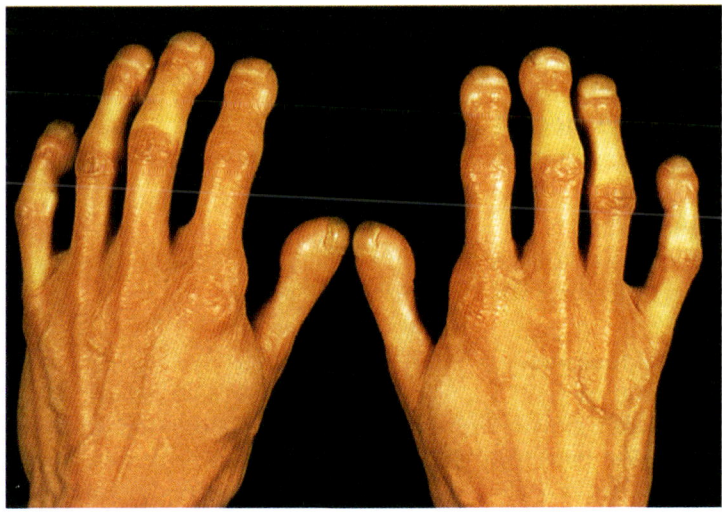

Figure 70.13 Familial mandibuloacral dysplasia, showing the short club-shaped terminal phalanges, the so-called 'tree-frog' appearance. Courtesy of Dr A. M. Zina, Turin University, Turin.

Mandibuloacral dysplasia patients with *LMNA* mutations usually have normal development during the first 4 years of life, whereas patients with *ZMPSTE24* mutations have a more severe phenotype [11]. A form of mandibuloacral dysplasia associated with hearing loss and lipodystrophy occurs due to heterozygous POLD1 mutations [12].

Differential diagnosis

The cutaneous changes resemble a mild form of progeria and some cases have been mistakenly diagnosed in the past as acrogeria or Werner syndrome. Néstor–Guillermo progeria (MIM: 614008) is a newly described progeria syndrome characterised by severe osteolysis, osteoporosis, generalised lipoatrophy and a relatively long survival [13,14]. Normal development occurs until the age of around 2 years and may therefore be confused with mandibuloacral dysplasia. It is caused by mutations in the *BANF1* gene, the product of which is implicated in nuclear envelope assembly and interacts with lamin A [15].

Complications and co-morbidities

Due to the association of the development of metabolic disorders, the risk of cardiovascular disease is likely to be increased.

Disease course and prognosis

The severity of the clinical features increases with time although the true prognosis is unclear.

Investigations

Molecular analysis and appropriate investigations targeted at possible metabolic associations should be undertaken.

Management

There is no specific therapy but treatment is aimed at reducing any metabolic complications.

Resources

Further information

National Center for Biotechnology Information, OMIM: http://www.ncbi.nlm.nih.gov/omim.
National Organization for Rare Disorders: http://rarediseases.org/.

Patient resources

National Organization for Rare Disorders: http://rarediseases.org/.
(All last accessed February 2022.)

Mulvihill–Smith syndrome

Definition and nomenclature

This is a rare progeroid syndrome with multisystem involvement.

Synonyms and inclusions
• Premature ageing with short stature and pigmented naevi

PART 6: GENETIC DISORDERS

Epidemiology
Incidence and prevalence
Only 11 cases have been described in the literature [1].

Age
Symptoms become apparent in childhood.

Sex
Although both sexes should be affected equally, more male cases have been reported.

Ethnicity
No variation has been noted.

Pathophysiology
The cause is unknown.

Pathology
In one patient investigated, the skin fibroblasts were slow to grow in culture and they were morphologically different from normal controls in terms of their size, with a large number of inclusions and absence of primary cilia [2].

Genetics
The underlying genetic cause is not yet known. Reported cases support probable autosomal recessive inheritance.

Clinical features
Presentation
This rare progeroid syndrome is characterised by low birth weight, short stature and moderate intellectual disability, associated with multiple pigmented naevi and distinctive bird-like facies with microcephaly [2,3]. There is a small chin with a broad forehead, and the lack of facial subcutaneous fat gives an appearance of premature ageing. Other features include sensorineural hearing loss, hypospadias, a high-pitched voice, irregular dentition, fine hair, cataracts, hepatomegaly and low immunoglobulin G with immunodeficiency.

Differential diagnosis
Cockayne syndrome patients exhibit similar facial features, short stature and intellectual disability. Patients with multiple lentigines syndrome (formerly called LEOPARD syndrome) also have retarded growth and the lentigines may be confused.

Complications and co-morbidities
Four cases have developed cancers in their twenties involving the stomach, tongue, pancreas and skin (melanoma) [4–6].

Disease course and prognosis
The clinical features tend to become more noticeable with increasing age. Adult manifestations include the development of tumours, a sleep disorder with severe insomnia (agrypnia excitata) and cognitive decline [4].

Investigations
No specific investigations are available but diagnosis will depend on the identification of characteristic and associated findings.

Management
Treatment is targeted to specific symptoms.

Resources

Further information
National Center for Biotechnology Information, OMIM: http://www.ncbi.nlm.nih.gov/omim.
National Organization for Rare Disorders: http://rarediseases.org/.
(Both last accessed February 2022.)

Neonatal progeroid syndrome

Definition and nomenclature
This is a rare autosomal recessive disorder with features including intrauterine growth retardation, failure to thrive, short stature, decreased subcutaneous fat, a progeroid appearance with macrocephaly, variable mental impairment and death in childhood [1].

Synonyms and inclusions
- Wiedemann–Rautenstrauch syndrome
- Neonatal pseudohydrocephalic progeroid syndrome

Epidemiology
Incidence and prevalence
It is very rare with only less than 40 cases reported [2].

Age
It may present pre- and postnatally with growth retardation.

Sex
There is no sex bias.

Ethnicity
There is no ethnic variation.

Pathophysiology
An increased chromosomal breakage is observed in some cases.

Genetics
Biallelic loss-of-function variants of *POLR3A*, which encodes for the largest subunit of RNA polymerase III, are causal [2,3].

Clinical features
Presentation [1–7]
Intrauterine growth is observed. The facial features include frontal and lateral bossing of the skull with small facial bones, a small beak-shaped nose, low-set ears, small mouth with dysodontia and ectropion. The scalp hair and eyebrows are long and sparse, the extremities are thin and the hands are large with long fingers and atrophic nails. The subcutaneous fat is decreased, the skin is thin

and wrinkled and the veins are prominent. It is characterised by mild to moderate mental and physical retardation.

Differential diagnosis

Wiedemann–Rautenstrauch syndrome should be differentiated from other syndromes that exhibit a progeroid phenotype at birth, for example Petty–Laxova–Wiedemann syndrome [7] and Hallerman–Strieff syndrome [8]. The true progeria syndromes usually do not show the characteristics of premature ageing until some time after birth. A rare variant of MFS is reminiscent of some of the major features of Wiedemann–Rautenstrauch syndrome [9].

Disease course and prognosis

It is usually lethal by the first year of life often due to respiratory tract infections. Only a few individuals have lived to their twenties [10].

Management

There is no specific therapy.

DISORDERS OF ECTOPIC CALCIFICATION AND ABNORMAL MINERALISATION

Pseudoxanthoma elasticum

Definition and nomenclature

Pseudoxanthoma elasticum (PXE) is an autosomal recessive multisystem disorder characterised by generalised fragmentation and progressive calcification of elastic tissue predominantly in the dermis, blood vessels and Bruch membrane of the eye.

Synonyms and inclusions
- Systematised elastorrhexis
- Gronblad–Strandberg syndrome

Introduction and general description

Pseudoxanthoma elasticum is an inherited multisystem disorder with considerable morbidity and occasional mortality. Abnormal mineralisation of peripheral tissues occurs due to reduced plasma levels of inorganic pyrophosphate inhibitor (PPi), an inhibitor of ectopic mineralisation. A number of potential therapies are currently undergoing trials [1].

Epidemiology
Incidence and prevalence

The precise prevalence is unknown but it is thought to occur in about 1/50 000 [2].

Age

The first manifestation of PXE is commonly skin changes which are usually noticed around the teenage years but can appear earlier in childhood [3].

Sex

Although PXE is autosomal recessive, slightly more women present with the disease than men (<2: 1). This may in part reflect self-selection bias as it appears that women are more likely to have skin involvement [3].

Ethnicity

No racial predilection has been observed.

Associated diseases

Pseudoxanthoma elasticum-like cutaneous changes are seen in several other inherited disorders including PXE-like disorder with multiple coagulation factor deficiency caused by mutations in *GGCX* [4]; and generalised arterial calcification of infancy type 1 (CAGI1), a disorder that is characterised by extensive vascular calcification and a poor prognosis, which is due to mutations in *ENPP1* [4]. CAGI1 can also be caused by mutations in *ABCC6*, which is normally associated with classical PXE [4]. Arterial calcification due to CD73 deficiency also results in reduced plasma levels of PPi and manifests with juxta-articular joint-capsule and arterial calcification in adults [5].

Skin changes of PXE and/or angioid streaks are occasionally seen in patients with osteitis deformans (Paget disease), sickle cell anaemia and familial tumoural calcinosis. PXE has also been reported in association with osteoectasia, which is characterised by dwarfism, bizarre radiographic changes and elevated serum alkaline phosphatase levels [6].

Pathophysiology

Pseudoxanthoma elasticum is caused by mutations in the *ABCC6* gene [7–9]. This is a member of the adenosine triphosphate binding cassette (ABC) family and acts as a transmembrane transporter. It facilitates transport of adenosine triphosphate (ATP) out of hepatocytes where it is converted to adenosine monophosphate (AMP) and PPi [10–12].

Pathology

In the fully developed skin lesions, the elastic fibres in the mid-dermis are clumped, degenerate, fragmented and swollen, and the abnormal fibres stain positively for calcium. Similar changes occur in the connective tissue of the media and intima of the blood vessels, the Bruch membrane of the eye, and in the endocardium and pericardium. The heart may occasionally be enlarged, with extensive calcification [13], and rarely pulmonary calcification has been reported [14]. Calcification may occur in other viscera including the placenta, liver, kidneys, testes, spleen and mammary tissue [15–17].

In patients with angioid streaks but no obvious skin abnormalities, a biopsy of scar tissue, regardless of site, may provide diagnostic pathology [18]. A biopsy of normal-looking flexural skin, in those with angioid streaks, may also show pathognomonic changes but the yield is lower [19,20].

Genetics

Causative mutations occur in the *ABCC6* gene located on chromosome 16p13.1. Approximately 40% of mutations are accounted for by two recurrent mutations p.R1141X and g.del23-29 [21]. Familial inheritance is autosomal recessive. Several large studies have failed to identify any convincing signs of PXE in heterozygotes [22]. There is no genotype–phenotype correlation [21].

In keeping with the clinical overlap with generalised arterial calcification of infancy, occasional reports of *ABCC6* mutations leading to a predominance of this phenotype and *ENPP1* leading to a PXE phenotype have been described [4,23,24].

Clinical features
History
The complete syndrome consists of asymptomatic flexural skin lesions, visual disturbances and cardiovascular manifestations due to calcification. The features are late onset and slowly progressive.

Presentation
An updated diagnostic classification has been proposed [25]. This is summarised in Box 70.1.

Box 70.1 Revised diagnostic criteria for pseudoxanthoma elasticum (PXE)

Major diagnostic criteria
1 **Skin**
  a. Yellowish papules and/or plaques on the lateral side of the neck and/or flexural areas of the body; *or*
  b. Increase of morphologically altered elastin with fragmentation, clumping and calcification of elastic fibres in a skin biopsy taken from clinically affected skin
2 **Eye**
  a. Peau d'orange of the retina; *or*
  b. One or more angioid streaks, each at least as long as one disc diameter. When in doubt, fluorescein or indocyanine green angiography of the fundus is needed for confirmation
3 **Genetics**
  a. A pathogenic mutation of both alleles of the *ABCC6* gene; *or*
  b. A first-degree relative (parent, sibling, child) who meets independently the diagnostic criteria for definitive PXE

Minor diagnostic criteria
1 **Eye**
  a. One angioid streak shorter than one disc diameter; *or*
  b. One or more 'comets' in the retina; *or*
  c. One or more 'wing signs' in the retina
2 **Genetics**
  a. A pathogenic mutation of one allele of the *ABCC6* gene

Requirements for the diagnosis of PXE
1 **Definitive diagnosis**
  a. The presence of two (or more) major criteria not belonging to the same category (skin, eye, genetic)
2 **Probable diagnosis**
  a. The presence of two major eye or two major skin criteria; *or*
  b. The presence of one major criterion and one or more minor criteria not belonging to the same category as the major criterion
3 **Possible diagnosis**
  a. The presence of a single major criterion; *or*
  b. The presence of one or more minor criteria

Reproduced from Plomp *et al.* 2010 [25] with permission from Wiley.

Skin changes. The characteristic skin lesions consist of small (1–3 mm), yellowish papules in a linear or reticular pattern, which tend to coalesce into confluent plaques. The skin is soft, lax and slightly wrinkled, and may hang in folds, especially in elderly people. There may be a slightly pebbly surface, which has been variously described as a 'cobblestone', 'Moroccan leather' or 'chicken skin' appearance (Figure 70.14). The sites of predilection are the sides of the neck, below the clavicles, the axillae (Figure 70.15),

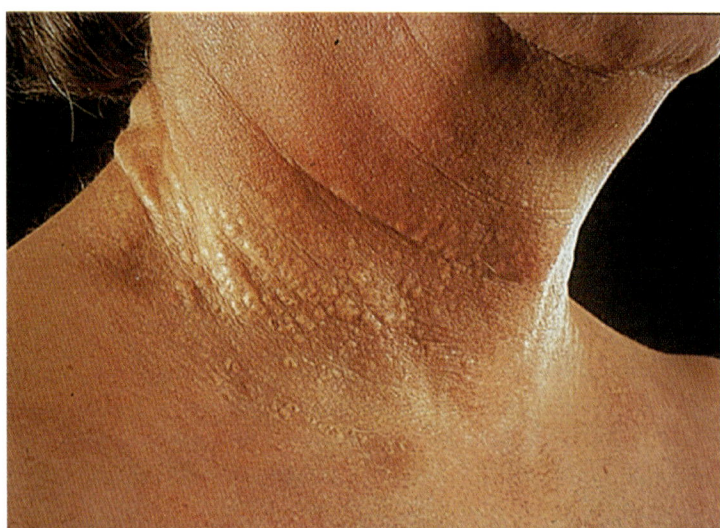

Figure 70.14 Pseudoxanthoma elasticum, showing the typical 'chicken skin' appearance involving the neck.

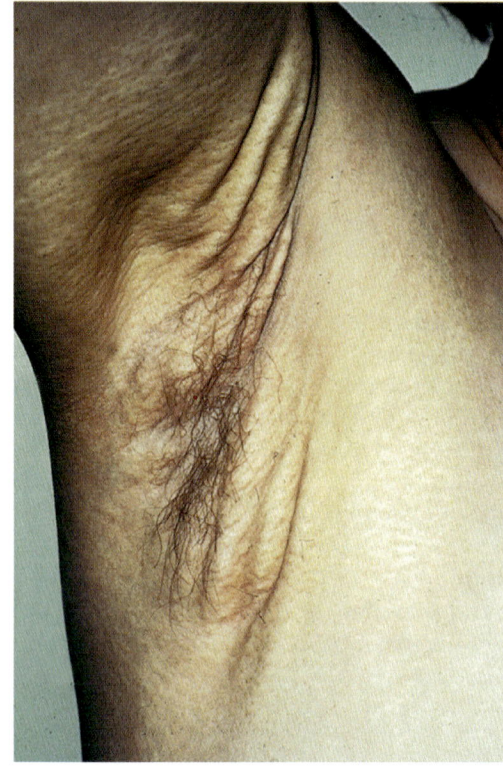

Figure 70.15 Pseudoxanthoma elasticum of the axilla, showing the characteristic yellow discoloration of the skin and the loose folds. The changes in this condition are often much more subtle than in this patient.

abdomen, groins, perineum and thighs. Although usually limited, the eruption may occasionally involve most of the body. It rarely develops in early childhood, and usually does so in teenage years, but it may also first appear in old age. Similar changes may occur in the soft palate, inside the lips and in the mucous membranes of the stomach, rectum and vagina. In the mouth, the lesions may mimic sebaceous glands (Fordyce spots). Reticulate pigmentation on the abdomen may occur [26]. Numerous comedonal lesions have been reported [27]. Rarely, chronic granulomatous nodules have developed in the skin lesions [28].

Occasionally, there may be spontaneous perforating lesions, with transepidermal elimination of the fragmented elastic fibres (sometimes assuming the typical appearance of elastosis serpiginosa perforans).

The presence of an exaggerated mental (chin) crease has recently been shown to be a sensitive and highly specific finding in patients under the age of 30 years with PXE [29].

Cardiovascular changes. Arterial involvement does not usually clinically manifest until adult life. Involvement in early childhood raises the possibility of overlap with generalised arterial calcification of infancy [30]. The vascular involvement may be generalised or may involve predominantly the larger arteries, the mesenteric and visceral arteries or those of the extremities [31]. Calcification of the internal elastic lamina of the arteries leads to vascular occlusion. There may be intermittent claudication with diminished peripheral pulses, and accelerated atherosclerosis, often with hypertension [32,33]. Lower extremity with periarticular calcification is more in keeping with the rare arterial calcification disease due to CD73 deficiency [5].

Aneurysms are infrequent [34]. Rarely death may result from cerebral haemorrhage, coronary occlusion or massive haemorrhage into the gut [35]. Intermittent claudication and angina have occurred in early childhood [36] but more commonly occurs in (up to 50%) adults [35]. More recent studies report less frequent cardiac complications although cardiomyopathy has been reported [37–39].

Nephrolithiases and strokes may be more common than initially reported [40]. In fact, *ABCC6* variants were found to confer a significant risk for ischaemic stroke [41].

Ocular changes. The ocular changes are variable. A 'peau d'orange' fundus, which corresponds to yellowish lesions of the retinal pigment epithelium can be present in childhood as the earliest ophthalmic sign, but it tends to become less distinct with age (Figure 70.16). Angioid streaks of the retina are seen as slate grey, poorly defined streaks radiating from an incomplete greyish ring surrounding the nerve head (Figure 70.17) [42,43]. They are usually symmetrical and have only rarely been described before 15 years of age as they usually first appear between the ages of 20 and 40 years [36]. Comet-tail lesions are small round white bodies and are considered pathognomonic for PXE [44,45]. They appear earlier than the other ocular changes.

Other associated ocular findings include small raised pearly white *drusen*, or punched-out atrophic areas in focal areas of dehiscence of the Bruch membrane [46]. There may also be speckled yellowish mottling (leopard spotting) and this may antedate the angioid streaks [47]. About 50% of patients also have a random

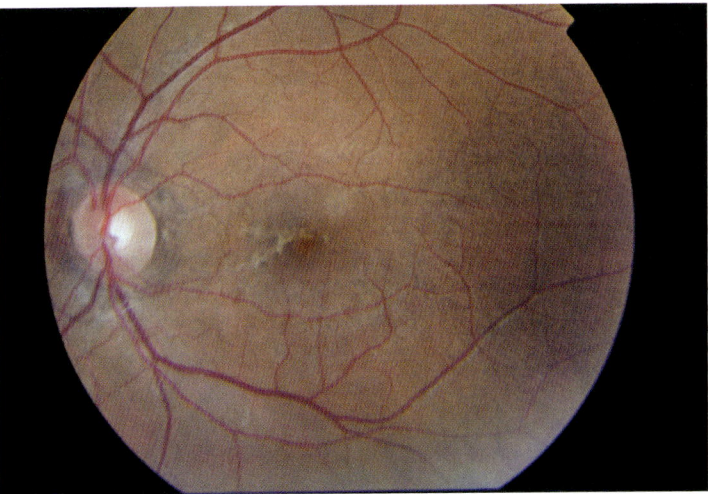

Figure 70.16 Left fundus showing angioid streaks at the macula which have caused deterioration of the central vision. A mottled appearance 'peau d'orange' can be seen in the peripheral retina. Courtesy of Miss Louise Allen, Cambridge University Hospitals NHS Foundation Trust, Cambridge, UK.

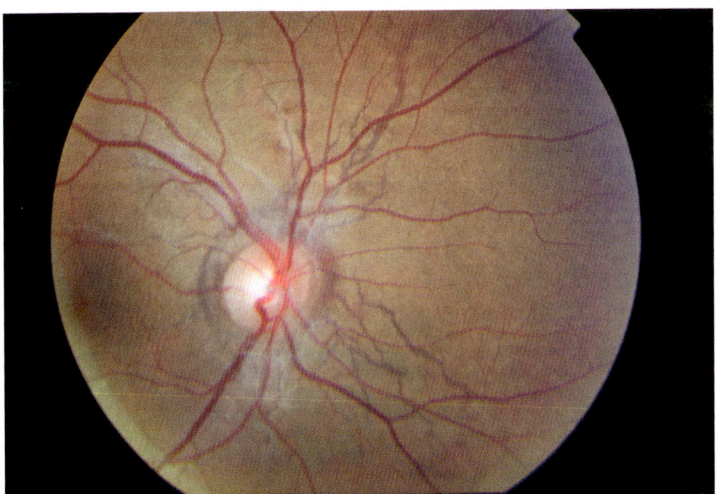

Figure 70.17 Right fundus showing angioid streaks radiating from the optic nerve in pseudoxanthoma elasticum. Courtesy of Miss Louise Allen, Cambridge University Hospitals NHS Foundation Trust, Cambridge, UK.

scattering of small round pigment dots throughout the macula and optic nerve [48].

By the age of 50 years, the majority of patients have some visual impairment (usually not more than 6/60) which occurs due to macular atrophy, choroidal rupture or choroidal neovascularisation, with or without choroidal haemorrhage from angioid streaks [49]; retinal dysfunction in PXE may also contribute to visual loss [50].

Gastrointestinal changes. The most common problem is upper gastrointestinal bleeding, particularly the stomach. Approximately 10% develop bleeding complications [51]. The exact cause is unknown but may reflect fragility of calcified submucosal vessels which are unable to constrict.

Obstetric risk. Initial reports suggested that there is an increased risk of miscarriage in the first trimester, possibly related to failure of placental development [52,53] but a larger study of 795 pregnancies in 306 women showed no increased fetal loss or adverse reproductive outcomes. Furthermore, the incidence of gastric bleeding and retinal complications, at <1%, is lower than previously thought [**54**]. Twelve per cent of pregnancies were associated with worsening of skin manifestations [55].

Clinical variants

In most cases, the serum calcium and phosphate levels are normal, but in a few patients the phosphate levels are increased, with mild hypercalcaemia and abnormalities of vitamin D metabolism [56,57]. The biochemical changes resemble those of tumoural calcinosis [58], although the clinical changes are those of PXE. This seems to be a distinctive rare type of PXE which may be associated with renal failure in other members of the family. Some of these patients also have systemic sclerosis [59].

Other patients have been reported with multiple calcified cutaneous nodules, with angioid streaks and hyperphosphataemia, but without pseudoxanthoma [59].

The development of both clinical and histopathological PXE-like changes, involving the skin, eyes and vasculature, occurs with sickle cell disease and β-thalassaemia [60]. The abnormalities are most probably acquired and related to the consequences of the primary disease. The clinical features are of later onset and milder than in inherited PXE.

A group of patients with PXE-like phenotype with cutis laxa and deficiency of vitamin K-dependent clotting factors has been identified. This occurs due to mutations in the *GGCX* gene which encodes vitamin K-dependent γ-glutamyl carboxylase, which is important in the activation of several coagulation factors and a systemic inhibitor of calcification, matrix gla protein (MGP) [61,62]. Further overlap can occur with typical skin and histological features of PXE and pathogenic (compound heterozygote) mutations in both *GGCX* and *ABCC6* [62].

Differential diagnosis

The disseminated form of dermatofibrosis lenticularis (Buschke–Ollendorff) can be clinically similar, and juvenile elastoma, which is a feature of this condition, shows thickened elastic fibres on histology.

Papular elastorrhexis is an uncommon acquired disorder of elastic fibres that presents as multiple, whitish or skin-coloured, non-follicular papules, with symmetrical distribution on the trunk and upper extremities and may be confused with PXE [63].

If laxity of the involved skin is extreme, other forms of cutis laxa must be excluded. The diagnosis can be difficult in the presence of marked solar elastosis and/or macular degeneration.

There are a number of *acquired* syndromes that have PXE-like features (Chapter 94).

Complications and co-morbidities

Some degree of visual impairment is common in older adults. Up to 10% will experience gastrointestinal bleeding and peripheral and cardiac complications may occur. Skin changes may progress to localised cutis laxa.

Disease course and prognosis

Pseudoxanthoma elasticum causes considerable morbidity and only occasional mortality [**3**,64].

Investigations

Calcium and phosphate levels should be checked. The histological changes of PXE are often distinctive and a skin biopsy from the side of the neck can be helpful (elastic fibres in the mid-dermis are clumped, degenerate, fragmented and swollen, and the abnormal fibres stain positively for calcium). Soft-tissue or vascular calcification may be detectable radiologically [17].

Although the true incidence of cardiac anomalies is unclear, it is advisable to perform at least a baseline echocardiogram with further investigations according to symptoms. Vitamin K clotting factors should be assayed if a *GGCX* gene deficiency is suspected.

The definitive diagnosis is made by molecular analysis of the *ABCC6* gene.

Management

No specific treatment for PXE exists. The most important aspect of management is to ensure that complications are prevented or dealt with quickly by the appropriate specialist. Annual ophthalmology and cardiovascular assessments are often recommended. Patients and their families should also receive genetic counselling.

Dietary. It has been suggested that individuals with a history of high intake of dairy products (rich in calcium and phosphate) during adolescence developed more severe disease later in life [65]. However, when studied in mouse models of PXE dietary calcium did not affect mineralisation and to date there is no strong evidence linking dietary calcium intake with severity of PXE [**1**]. Dietary intervention in humans has been with oral phosphate binders but this did not result in either a reduction in calcification levels or clinical improvement [66]. Recent studies in PXE knock-out mice have shown that supplementation with magnesium carbonate completely abolishes the abnormal mineralisation [67,68] A 2-year study of magnesium supplementation in PXE patients shows promising trends in the reduction of skin elastic fibres [69].

Ocular. Ophthalmologists will recommend that the patient learns to use an Amsler grid in the early detection of visual loss. Patients should avoid any activity that might cause a sudden increase in blood pressure or contact injury to the eyes. Laser photocoagulation may be helpful in preventing further retinal haemorrhage but recurrence is common [50]. Intravitreal antivascular endothelial growth factor (anti-VEGF) therapy is beneficial for the treatment of choroidal neovascularisations secondary to angioid streaks, especially in the early stages of the disease [70]. Surgical intervention may be required for gastrointestinal bleeding and severe peripheral vascular disease.

Cardiovascular. Cardiovascular risks should be minimized with control of blood pressure, weight and serum lipids, avoidance of smoking and advice about regular exercise.

Gastrointestinal. Aspirin and non-steroidal anti-inflammatory medications should be avoided whenever possible to reduce the risk of gastrointestinal bleeding.

Surgical. The cosmetic appearance of the skin lesions, particularly secondary cutis laxa, can be improved by plastic surgery. However, in one report two out of nine patients developed complications with calcium extruding from the wound which delayed wound healing and resulted in a poorer cosmetic outcome [71].

Resources

Patient resources

PiXiE (UK support group): www.pxe.org.uk.
PXE International (US support group): www.pxe.org.
(Both last accessed February 2022.)

Fibrodysplasia ossificans progressiva

Definition

Fibrodysplasia ossificans progressiva is a severe and disabling disorder of ectopic ossification involving the skeletal muscle, fascia, tendons and ligaments.

Epidemiology

Incidence and prevalence

The incidence is 1 in 2 million [1].

Age

Ossification is not present at birth but affected individuals have abnormalities of the great toe, namely shortening, deviation and monophalangic great toe.

Sex

There is no sex bias [2].

Ethnicity

There is no racial variation [2].

Pathophysiology

Genetics

Sporadic (95%) or autosomal dominant gain-of-function mutations in the *ACVR1* gene encode a type I bone morphogenetic protein (BMP) transmembrane receptor [3,4].

Environmental factors

Minor trauma or viral illnesses can trigger acute inflammatory myositis leading to progressive ossification, which is further aggravated by surgical intervention [5].

Clinical features

Presentation

Malformed big toes are present at birth but other limb skeletal malformations may be present. The average age of onset of ossification is 5 years with progressive involvement of muscles, ligaments, tendons and fascia, such that by 15 years of age more than 95% have functional restriction of limb movement [6]. The sternocleidomastoid and masseter muscles as well as those of the dorsal trunk and proximal limb are particularly affected. Bony exostoses may also develop.

Differential diagnosis

In progressive osseous heteroplasia, bone formation can occur in skeletal muscle tendon and ligaments but additionally, and initially, there is dermal involvement [7].

Disease course and prognosis

Most patients are confined to a wheelchair by the third decade of life and require lifelong care. The median lifespan is around 40 years due to thoracic restriction and accompanying pneumonia or right-sided heart failure [8].

Management

High-dose steroids can be used for acute inflammatory flares. There is currently no cure but several approaches in animal models look promising [9].

Primary hypertrophic osteoarthropathy

Definition and nomenclature

Primary hypertrophic osteoarthropathy (PHO) is a group of inherited disorders with shared clinical features involving the bones and skin.

Synonyms and inclusions

- Pachydermoperiostosis
- Touraine–Solente–Gole syndrome

Epidemiology

Incidence and prevalence

This is a rare condition.

Age

It presents in infancy in type 1 and puberty in type 2.

Sex

It is more commonly seen in males possibly due to higher levels of prostaglandins.

Pathophysiology

Predisposing factors

Primary PHO has a genetic basis whereas secondary PHO is associated with underlying malignancies and cardiopulmonary and less commonly inflammatory bowel disease [1].

Genetics

Homozygous mutations in the *HPGD* (15-hydroxyprostaglandin dehydrogenase) gene, which is the main enzyme in prostaglandin degradation, cause autosomal recessive type 1 [2]. It is also responsible for the allelic variant of craniosteoarthropathy. Autosomal recessive type 2 is caused by homozygous or compound heterozygous mutation in the *SLCO2A1* gene, involved in cellular prostaglandin transport [3]. Autosomal dominant PHO is also caused by heterozygous mutation in the *SLCO2A1* gene.

PART 6: GENETIC DISORDERS

Clinical features
Presentation
Primary hypertrophic osteoarthropathy is characterised by digital clubbing osteoarthropathy and acro-osteolysis (more common in type 1), variable features of pachydermia, with furrowing of the face and scalp and delayed closure of the fontanelles. Oily skin, hyperhidrosis, flushing and palmoplantar hyperkeratosis are all described. Severe cutis verticis gyrate and myelofibrosis are seen in type 2 [4,5].

Investigations
Diagnosis is based on imaging to look for bone abnormalities such as diaphyseal periostosis and acro-osteolysis.

Management [6]
Non-steroidal anti-inflammatory drugs provide symptomatic relief. In addition, corticosteroids or colchicine have been tried. Clinical improvement of the dermatological symptoms is achieved by retinoids.

MISCELLANEOUS DERMAL DISORDERS

Adermatoglyphia

Congenital absence of epidermal ridges, known as adermatoglyphia, is a rare autosomal dominant condition. It was coined the 'immigration delay disease' because affected individuals report significant difficulties entering countries which require fingerprint recording [1]. To date, only a few families with isolated congenital absence of fingerprints have been described [1,2]. Associated features may include abnormal palmoplantar sweating, skin blisters, congenital facial milia, nail clubbing, calluses and fissures associated with heat or trauma [3–5]. Adermatoglyphia with congenital acral bullae, congenital milia, hypohidrosis, palmoplantar keratoderma and nail dystrophy is known as Basan syndrome [6].

Adermatoglyphia and Basan syndrome are caused by mutations affecting a skin-specific isoform of *SMARCAD1* [7–9], a member of the SNF subfamily of the helicase protein superfamily [10]. Of note, Huriez syndrome featuring adermatoglyphia, palmoplantar hypohidrosis and keratoderma, nail anomalies and scleroatrophy of hands and feet associated with squamous cell carcinoma, was also found to be associated with mutations in *SMARCAD1* [11]. Surprisingly, all causative mutations in the three disorders disrupt the same conserved splice site, resulting in haploinsufficiency for the skin-specific isoform of *SMARCAD1* [8,10]. Although mostly expressed in skin fibroblasts [8], the skin-specific SMARCAD1 isoform was recently found to regulate the expression of numerous genes involved in epidermal differentiation [9].

Of note, adermatoglyphia is also a feature of several complex ectodermal dysplasias [8,12]. In addition, acquired adermatoglyphia has been reported in chronic dermatitis [10].

Lipoid proteinosis

Definition and nomenclature
Lipoid proteinosis is a rare autosomal recessive disorder, characterised by infiltration of hyaline material into the skin, oral cavity, larynx and internal organs [1]. The exact nature of the hyaline material is still uncertain.

Synonyms and inclusions
- Urbach–Wiethe disease
- Hyalinosis cutis et mucosae
- Lipoglycoproteinosis

Epidemiology
Age
This presents in early infancy with hoarseness.

Sex
There is no sex bias.

Ethnicity
Lipoid proteinosis is common in the Namaqualand region of South Africa, where cases can be traced back to a German immigrant [2].

Pathophysiology
Pathology
The epidermis shows acanthosis and irregular acanthosis. The dermis is thickened and the upper dermis contains large deposits of extracellular hyaline material that stains strongly with periodic acid–Schiff (PAS). There is also thickening of the (PAS-positive) basement membranes at the dermal–epidermal junction and around the blood vessels and sweat glands. Immunofluorescence labelling for type IV collagen confirms the basement membrane thickening [1]. Ultrastructurally, there are multiple concentric rings of basement membrane around the blood vessels and irregular reduplication of the lamina densa at the dermal–epidermal junction. The hyaline deposits are featureless. Histochemical diagnosis is now possible using an antibody to extracellular matrix protein 1 (ECM1) [3].

Genetics
The disorder is caused by homozygous or compound heterozygous mutation in *ECM1* [4]. ECM1 binds to various proteins (perlecan, fibulins and MMP9) but its function is unknown [1]. Interestingly, antibodies to ECM1 are present in 75% of patients with lichen sclerosus [5].

Clinical features
Presentation
Lipoid proteinosis usually presents in infancy with hoarseness, which can progress to complete aphonia. The vocal cords are thickened, with nodules here and on the epiglottis. Occasionally, stridor necessitates a tracheostomy [6]. The lips, pharynx, soft palate, uvula and tonsils develop yellow-white submucous infiltrates. The tongue is enlarged and firm with infiltrates on its

undersurface. The frenulum becomes short and thick, restricting tongue movement, such that it cannot be protruded. There may be recurrent inflammation of the salivary glands [2].

The first skin lesions are often blistering in early childhood, which become eroded and crusted after minor trauma [2]. Acneform, pock-like scars appear on the face and elsewhere, either following trauma or spontaneously. Infiltration of the skin can cause waxy papules, hyperkeratosis or warty plaques, which may become darker with time. These lesions may affect the palms or backs of the hands, forehead or elbows, where they can be prominent and resemble xanthomas. Characteristic 'beaded' papules are present along the margins of the eyelids but they may be subtle (moniliform blepharosis) (Figure 70.18). There may be loss of eyelashes or patchy alopecia due to scalp involvement [7]. Some patients complain of itching or increased sensitivity to sunlight [2]. Visceral involvement has also been reported [8]. Problems progress until early adult life but subsequently stabilise.

Differential diagnosis
Erythropoietic protoporphyria causes waxy papules and depressed scars but the scars are confined to sun-exposed skin. Rarely, hyaline deposition in facial skin caused by erythropoietic protoporphyria may mimic lipoid proteinosis [9]. Xanthomatosis and amyloidosis are also excluded by the histological appearances. In adults, other differential diagnoses include lichen myxoedematosus and myxoedema with hoarseness.

Complications and co-morbidities
Epilepsy and psychiatric problems occur in a number of patients and may be associated with intracranial calcification (e.g. in the temporal lobes or amygdala) [10].

Investigations
Histological and ultrastructural analysis of affected skin will show the features outlined earlier. The identification of pathogenic mutations in *ECM1* provides a definitive diagnosis.

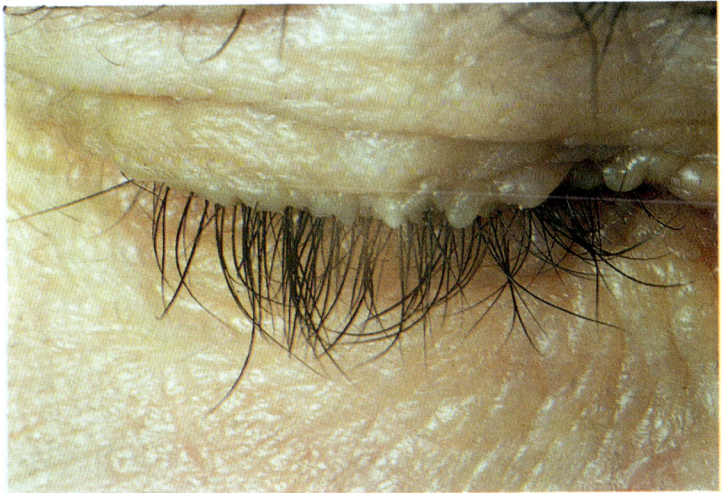

Figure 70.18 Lipoid proteinosis. Typical 'beaded' papules present along the margins of the upper eyelids. Courtesy of Dr R. C. D. Staughton, Chelsea and Westminster Hospital, London, UK.

Management
Microlaryngoscopy and dissection of the vocal cords can be successful. Dermabrasion [11], chemical skin peeling, blepharoplasty and carbon dioxide laser therapy [12] may be helpful. Oral dimethyl sulfoxide was reported to help one patient [13] but not others [14]. Beneficial effects of etretinate [15], acitretin [16] and of penicillamine [17] have also been reported.

Pterygium syndromes

Definition and nomenclature
The pterygium syndromes are characterised by skin webbing around the joints with a tendency to restricted movement and variable oro-facial features, most commonly cleft lip and/or palate. Some forms are lethal.

> **Synonyms and inclusions**
> • Multiple pterygium syndromes
> • Politeal pterygium syndromes

Epidemiology
Incidence and prevalence
These are rare disorders.

Age
The features present at birth.

Pathophysiology
Genetics
- Popliteal pterygium syndrome 1: autosomal dominant mutations in *IRF6*.
- Popliteal pterygium syndrome 2, lethal type: autosomal recessive mutations in *RIPK4*.
- Multiple pterygium syndrome, Escobar type: autosomal recessive mutations in *CHRNG*.
- Multiple pterygium syndrome, Escobar type with myopathy: autosomal recessive mutations in *TPM2*.
- Multiple pterygium syndrome, lethal type: autosomal recessive mutations *CHRNA1*, *CHRND* or *CHRNG*.

Clinical features
Presentation
Multiple pterygium syndromes present at birth with webbing (pterygium) typically involving the neck, antecubital and popliteal fossae. Muscle weakness leads to joint contractures (arthrogryposis).

Escobar type is the milder of the two types, whereas the lethal form is associated with hypoplastic organ development and is typically fatal in the second or third trimester of pregnancy or shortly after birth [1]. The associated complications of hydrops fetalis or cystic hygroma of the neck can be picked up on antenatal screening. Escobar type with associated myopathy occurs due to mutation in one of the genes encoding tropomyosin [2,3]. Skeletal and external genitalia malformations may also be present.

In type I popliteal pterygium syndrome, webbing of the neck and arms does not occur. Most have congenital cleft lip and/or palate with a similar oro-facial phenotype to van der Woude syndrome (MIM: 119300) to which it is allelic [4]. Some patients with the lethal variety of popliteal pterygium syndrome (syn: Bartsocas–Papas syndrome) have widespread pterygium. Death is usually in infancy, although survival into early adulthood has been reported [5,6].

Key references

The full list of references can be found in the online version at https://www.wiley.com/rooksdermatology10e

Ehlers–Danlos syndrome

3 Malfait F, Francomano C, Byers P et al. The 2017 international classification of the Ehlers–Danlos syndromes Am J Med Genet C Semin Med Genet 2017;175C:8–26.
30 Pepin M, Schwarze U, Superti-Furga A, Byers PH. Clinical and genetic features of Ehlers–Danlos syndrome type IV, the vascular type. N Engl J Med 2000;342:673–80.
56 Castori M, Tinkle B, Levy H et al. A framework for the classification of joint hypermobility and related conditions. Am J Med Genet C Semin Med Genet 2017;175C:148–57.
73 Brady AF, Demirdas S, Fournel-Gigleux S et al. The Ehlers–Danlos syndromes, rare types. Am J Med Genet C Semin Med Genet 2017;175C:70–115.

Prolidase deficiency

7 Forlina A, Luupi A, Vaghi P et al. Mutation analysis of five new patients affected by prolidase deficiency; the lack of enzyme activity causes necrosis-like cell death in cultured fibroblasts. Hum Genet 2002;111:3114–22.
15 Jemec GB, Moe AT. Topical treatment of skin ulcers in prolidase deficiency. Pediatr Dermatol 1996;13:58–60.

Osteogenesis imperfecta

1 Sillence DO, Senn A, Danks DM et al. Genetic heterogeneity in osteogenesis imperfecta. J Med Genet 1979;16:101–16.
3 Marini JC, Dang Do AN. Osteogenesis imperfecta. In: Feingold KR, Anawalt B, Boyce A, eds. Endotext [Internet]. South Dartmouth, MA: MDText.com, Inc.; 2000.
19 Glorieux FH. Experience with bisphosphonates in osteogenesis imperfecta. Pediatrics 2007;119:S163–5.

Inherited generalised cutis laxa

2 Morava E, Guillard M, Lefeber DJ, Wevers RA. Autosomal recessive cutis laxa syndrome revisited. Eur J Hum Genet 2009;17:1099–110.
4 Urban Z, Davis EC. Cutis laxa: Intersection of elastic fiber biogenesis, TGFβ signaling, the secretory pathway and metabolism. Matrix Biol 2014;33C:16–22.
12 Beyens A, Boel A, Symoens S, Callewaert B. Cutis laxa: a comprehensive overview of clinical characteristics and pathophysiology. Clin Genet 2021;99:53–66.
13 Hadj-Rabia S, Callewaer BL, Bourrat E et al. Twenty patients including 7 probands with autosomal dominant cutis laxa confirm clinical and molecular homogeneity Orphanet J Rare Dis 2013;8:36.

Williams–Beuren syndrome

7 Pober BR. Williams–Beuren syndrome. N Engl J Med 2010;362:239–52.

Michelin tyre baby syndrome

2 Isrie M, Breuss M, Tain G et al. Mutations in either TUBB or MAPRE2 cause circumferential skin creases Kunze type. Am J Hum Genet 2015;97:790–800.

Marfan syndrome

16 Loeys BL, Dietz HC, Braverman AC et al. The revised Ghent nosology for the Marfan syndrome. J Med Genet 2010;47;476–85.
28 Meester JAAN, Verstraeten A, Schepers D et al. Differences in manifestations of Marfan syndrome, Ehlers-Danlos syndrome, and Loeys-Dietz syndrome. Ann Cardiothorac Surg 2017;6:582–94.

Hyaline fibromatosis syndrome

4 Denadai R, Raposo-Amaral CE, Bertola D et al. Identification of 2 novel ANTXR2 mutations in patients with hyaline fibromatosis syndrome and proposal of a modified grading system. Am J Med Genet A 2012;158A:732–42.

Stiff skin syndrome

6 Liu T, McCalmont TH, Frieden IJ et al. The stiff skin syndrome: case series, differential diagnosis of the stiff skin phenotype, and review of the literature. Arch Dermatol 2008;144:1351–9.

Winchester syndrome

5 De Vos IJHM, Wong ASW, Coull BJ, van Steensel MAM. Multicentric osteolytic syndromes represent a phenotypic spectrum defined by defective collagen remodelling. Am J Med Genet 2019;179A:1652–64.

Progeria

1 Gordon LB, Tuminelli K, Andrés V et al. The progeria research foundation 10th international scientific workshop; researching possibilities, ExTENding lives – webinar version scientific summary. Aging (Albany NY) 2021;13:9143–51.

Pseudoxanthoma elasticum

1 Luo H, Li Q, Cao Y, Uitto J. Therapeutics development for pseudoxanthoma elasticum and related ectopic mineralization disorders: update 2020. J Clin Med 2021;10:114.
3 Neldner KH. Pseudoxanthoma elasticum. Clin Dermatol 1988;6:1–159.
4 Nitschke Y, Baujat G, Botschen U et al. Generalized arterial calcification of infancy and pseudoxanthoma elasticum can be caused by mutations in either ENPP1 or ABCC6. Am J Hum Genet 2012;90:25–39.
25 Plomp AS, Toonstra J, Bergen AAB et al. Proposal for updating the pseudoxanthoma elasticum classification system and a review of the clinical findings. Am J Med Genet A 2010;152A:1049–58.
36 Naouri M, Boisseau C, Bonicel P et al. Manifestations of pseudoxanthoma elasticum in childhood. Br J Dermatol 2009;161;635–9.
54 Bercovitch L, Leroux T, Terry S, Weinstock MA. Pregnancy and obstetrical outcomes in pseudoxanthoma elasticum. Br J Dermatol 2004;151:1011–18.

CHAPTER 71

Disorders Affecting Cutaneous Vasculature

Anne Dompmartin[1], Nicole Revencu[2], Laurence M. Boon[2] and Miikka Vikkula[2,3]

[1]Consultation of Vascular Anomalies, Université de Caen Basse Normandie, Caen; Department of Dermatology, CHU Caen, Caen, France
[2]Center for Vascular Anomalies, Cliniques Universitaires Saint-Luc, Université catholique de Louvain (a VASCERN VASCA European Reference Centre), Brussels, Belgium
[3]Human Molecular Genetics, de Duve Institute, Université catholique de Louvain, Brussels, Belgium

PART 6: GENETIC DISORDERS

Introduction

The localised structural abnormalities that develop during vasculogenesis, angiogenesis and/or lymphangiogenesis lead to vascular anomalies. On the basis of clinical and biological criteria, they are divided into vascular tumours and vascular malformations [1]. This classification has been adopted by the International Society for the Study of Vascular Anomalies (ISSVA) and is detailed enough to cover all reported entities [2]. The identification of disease-causing genes associated with precise clinical delineation of the phenotypes has become the foundation for better management of these diseases [3]. For several of the familial forms, a paradominant inheritance has been established, with a combination of a germinal mutation and a local somatic second hit, whereas somatic/mosaic genetic defects cause the more common sporadic vascular malformations [4,5]. Links between phenotypes and genotypes have been unravelled for several vascular malformations.

These genetic mutations associated with inherited and sporadically occurring vascular anomalies lead to hyperactivity of two major signalling pathways: the RAS/mitogen-activated protein kinase (MAPK)/extracellular signal-regulated kinase (ERK) pathway and the phosphatidylinositol 3-kinase (PI3K)/protein kinase B (AKT)/mammalian target of rapamycin (mTOR) pathway (Figure 71.1). They are important regulators of cellular growth, proliferation, migration and apoptosis, and often implicated in cancers. The fact that similar mutations are observed in vascular anomalies may be explained by the occurrence of second-hits and somatic mutations in vascular endothelial cells and in the context of a stable genome, whereas in cancers other cell types are affected, and commonly an accumulation of somatic mutations occur. These discoveries paved the way for the development of a theranostic approach for vascular anomalies, testing targeted molecular inhibitors already used as anticancer drugs [6]. In contrast, various primary lymphoedemas are associated with mostly loss-of-function mutations in a central vascular endothelial growth factor C (VEGFC)/vascular endothelial growth factor receptor 3 (VEGFR3) signalling pathway. However, emerging data suggest that the complicated lymphatic anomalies (CLAs), with dysfunction of the central conducting lymphatic channels, often associated with primary lymphoedema, are due to similar somatic/mosaic mutations as seen in localised vascular malformations.

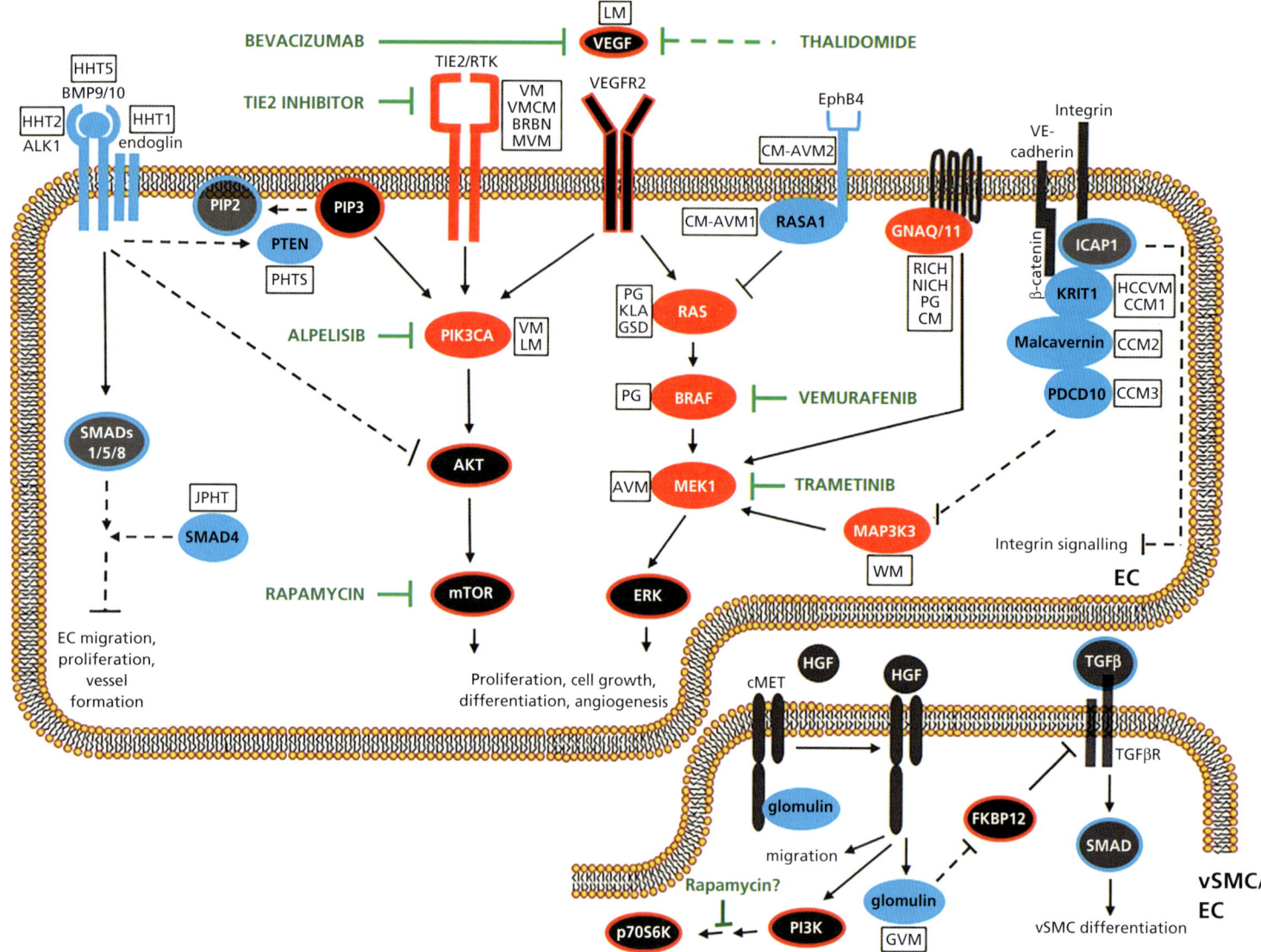

Figure 71.1 Proteins mutated in vascular anomalies with some inhibitors to be studied for therapeutic intervention. PI3K (phosphoinositide 3-kinase)/AKT (protein kinase B)/mTOR (mammalian target of rapamycin) signalling and RAS (rat sarcoma)/RAF (rapidly accelerated fibrosarcoma)/MEK (mitogen-activated protein kinase kinase)/ERK (extracellular signal-regulated kinases) signalling in vascular anomalies. Red: gain-of-function; blue: loss-of-function; black, circled with red: enhanced signalling; grey, circled with blue: decreased signalling. ALK, activin receptor-like kinase; AVM, arteriovenous malformation; BMP, bone morphogenetic protein; BRAF, B-raf proto-oncogene; BRBN, blue rubber bleb naevus syndrome; CCM, cerebral cavernous malformation; CLOVES, congenital lipomatous overgrowth, vascular malformations, epidermal naevi and scoliosis; CM, capillary malformation; CM-AVM, capillary malformation–arteriovenous malformation; EC, endothelial cell; EphB4, ephrin B4; FKBP12, FK506 binding protein 12; GNAQ, G protein subunit alpha Q; GSD, Gorham–Stout disease; GVM, glomuvenous malformation; HCCVM, hyperkeratotic cutaneous capillary–venous malformations; HHT, hereditary haemorrhagic telangiectasia; ICAP, integrin cytoplasmic-associated protein; JPHT, juvenile polyposis/HHT syndrome; KLA, kaposiform lymphangiomatosis; KRIT, Krev interaction trapped; KTS, Klippel–Trenaunay–Weber syndrome; LM, lymphatic malformation; MAP3K3, mitogen-activated protein kinase kinase kinase 3; MCAP, megalencephaly–capillary malformation syndrome; MVM, multifocal venous malformation; NICH, non-involuting congenital haemangioma; PDCD, programmed cell death 10; PG, pyogenic granuloma; PHTS, PTEN hamartoma tumour syndrome; PIK3CA, phosphatidylinositol-4,5-bisphosphate 3-kinase catalytic subunit alpha; PIP2, phosphatidylinositol-4,5-bisphosphate; PIP3, phosphatidylinositol-3,4,5-trisphosphate; PROS, PIK3CA-related overgrowth spectrum; PTEN, phosphatase and tensin homologue; RASA, RAS p21 protein activator; RICH, rapidly involuting congenital haemangioma; RTK, receptor tyrosine kinase; SMAD, mothers against decapentaplegic homologue; SMC, smooth muscle cell; TGF, transforming growth factor; VEGF, vascular endothelial growth factor; VEGFR, vascular endothelial growth factor receptor; VM, venous malformation; VMCM, inherited cutaneomucosal venous malformation; vSMC, vascular smooth muscle cells; VVM, verrucous venous malformations. Reproduced from Queisser A *et al.* [3] with permission of Wolters Kluwer Health, Inc.

CAPILLARY DISORDERS

Capillary malformation

Synonyms and inclusions
- Port-wine stain

Classification links
- ICD-10: Q82.5
- ICD-11: L90.0
- Snomed CT: 234118009
- MIM: 163000, 600998
- Orphanet: ORPHA211247

Introduction and general description
A capillary malformation (CM) is a sporadic, homogeneous, pink, red or purple macule present at birth. It is usually located on the skin, sometimes on the mucosa (Figure 71.2).

Epidemiology
It is the most common vascular malformation. It is present at birth in approximately three of 1000 newborns [7] and has equal sex distribution.

Pathophysiology
A CM is characterised by the dilatation of normal numbers of capillaries of the papillary and upper reticular dermis combined with areas of increased numbers of normal-looking capillaries. Endothelial cells are flat. Immunohistochemistry shows normal

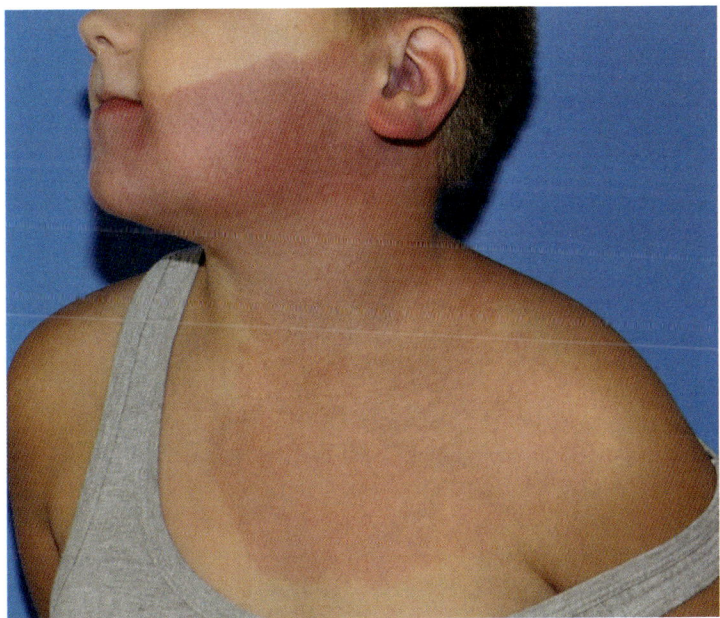

Figure 71.2 A 10-year-old boy with extensive capillary malformation involving V3, the neck and thorax.

factor VII, fibronectin and basement membrane proteins, but S100 staining shows abnormal innervation [4]. A recurrent somatic activating change (c.548G→A; p.Arg183Gln) has been found in the *GNAQ* gene in several patients with CMs [5]. Other somatic mutations leading to a substitution of Q209 by another amino acid in GNAQ have been identified in blue naevi, naevus of Ota and uveal melanoma [6]. This may explain the co-occurrence of vascular and pigmentary changes in phakomatosis pigmentovascularis. The homologous protein GNA11 is mutated in some CMs, especially at position p.Arg183Cys [8].

Clinical features
Capillary malformations are pink, red or purple flat lesions of variable size and with geographic borders (Figure 71.2). They are usually located on the head and neck, but can also be seen on the trunk or limbs. A CM grows proportionately with the child and persists throughout life. The lesion darkens and often thickens with age, and the underlying tissues (skin, fat, muscle and bone) can be hypertrophic. It is generally an isolated, sporadic and solitary malformation. Multiple lesions can be observed in more complex disorders.

Investigations
Most CMs do not require any investigation. However, associated signs and symptoms, large size and multifocality evoke a possible 'syndromic' form. For example, on the upper face, the larger the lesion, the higher the risk for Sturge–Weber syndrome. Segmental lower extremity CMs need scaniometry at around 8 years of age to evaluate growth discrepancy and management.

Management
Capillary malformations are asymptomatic, but can generate important psychosocial distress. Pulsed-dye laser is the first line treatment [9]. It reduces coloration in 75% of patients without modifying skin texture. Laser treatment consists of several consecutive sessions. Due to pain, general anaesthesia is often used for children. Surgery is done to correct tissue hyperplasia associated with CM, commonly seen on the lip.

Sturge–Weber syndrome

Classification links
- ICD-10: Q85.8
- ICD-11: LD23
- Snomed CT:19886006
- MIM: 185300, 600998
- Orphanet: ORPHA3205

Introduction and general description
Sturge–Weber syndrome (SWS) is a severe neurocutaneous sporadic disorder characterised by a CM located on the territory of the first branch of the trigeminal nerve. It is associated with a leptomeningeal and/or retinal capillary–venous malformation on the same side (Figure 71.3).

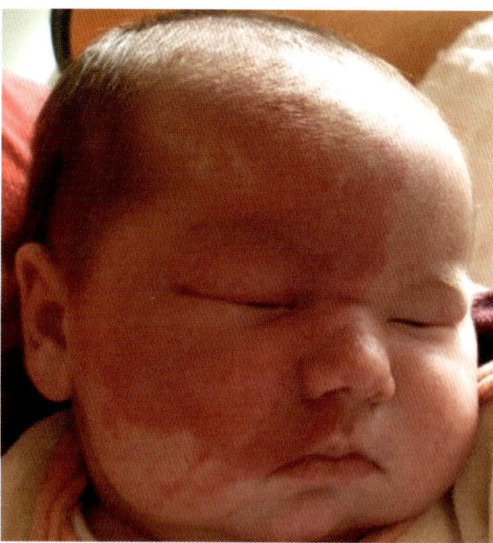

Figure 71.3 Sturge–Weber syndrome showing an 8-month-old boy with capillary malformation involving the left V1, V2 and V3 and right V3.

Epidemiology

The estimated incidence is one in 50 000. Males and females are equally affected.

Pathophysiology

As for the common CM, a somatic activating change (c.548G→A; p.Arg183Gln) has been identified in the *GNAQ* gene in several patients with SWS [10]. The fact that the same mutation can cause either SWS or CM most probably reflects different embryonic stages (earlier in SWS than in CM) at which the somatic change occurs.

Clinical features

Sturge–Weber syndrome is characterised by a CM located on the forehead and the upper eyelid (V1) associated with an ipsilateral leptomeningeal capillary–venous anomaly and/or ocular involvement [11]. The CM can be bilateral and/or more extensive, covering the territory of the maxillary (V2) and mandibular (V3) branches of the trigeminal nerve, and sometimes the trunk and the limbs (Figure 71.3). About 75% of children with intracranial vascular anomaly develop seizures, most often before the age of 2 years, with a risk of contralateral neurological deficit and learning difficulties. Gyral calcifications can be observed. The major ocular complication is glaucoma, occurring in more than 50% of patients.

Investigations

Frontopalpebral CMs necessitate brain magnetic resonance imaging (MRI), and an ophthalmological evaluation of the fundus of the eye as well as regular assessment of intraocular pressure. An abnormal MRI warrants a neurological evaluation.

Management

Pulsed-dye laser can be used to treat the CM. Management of epilepsy and glaucoma is an emergency. It is still questioned if prophylactic anticonvulsant treatment is recommended or not. In patients with intractable seizures, surgery (lobectomy) can be required. Regular ophthalmological follow-up is needed throughout life, with reduced intervals during infancy. Targeted therapies are being developed to various vascular anomalies [3,6]. For SWS,

there is special interest in the mTOR inhibitor rapamycin, which seemed to improve cognitive function in a small series [12].

Capillary malformation with dilated veins

Synonyms and inclusions
- CVM

Classification links
- ICD-10: Q27.8
- Snomed CT: 2341 33001
- Orphanet: ORPHA458837

Introduction and general description

Capillary malformation with dilated veins (CMDV) is a sporadic, usually homogeneous light pink, macule present at birth located on the upper or lower limb, and associated with prominent veins and minor growth disturbance in length or girth [13,14]. Using the term CM with dilated veins avoids confusion, as the entity CVM refers to a combined capillary–venous malformation in the ISSVA classification.

Epidemiology

Prevalence is unknown, with 32 patients reported [13,14].

Pathophysiology

The aetiology is unknown.

Clinical features

Capillary malformation with dilated veins is commonly characterised by a faint pink-red homogeneous CM, the majority of which have indistinct borders. Ectatic veins are seen on the affected area of the limb. Most patients can exhibit minor hyper- or hypotrophy of the affected extremity. Patients have no consumptive coagulopathy, but almost half of them complain of pain and less frequently of swelling.

Investigations

Doppler ultrasound shows dilatation of the superficial venous system, and sometimes ectasia of the deep venous system and veins in the muscles. D-dimers are not elevated, in contrast to venous and capillary–venous malformations, in which they can be raised.

Management

Pulse-dye laser, which is used to lighten the CM, seems to be more efficient on the proximal part of the limb. Sclerotherapy or endovascular laser can be proposed to treat the ectatic veins.

Angioma serpiginosum

Synonyms and inclusions
- Progressive patchy capillary malformation

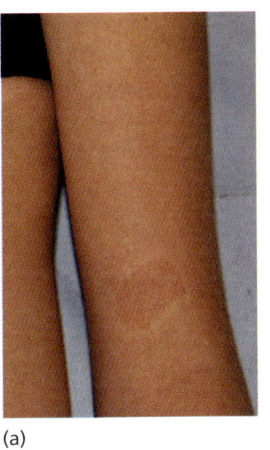 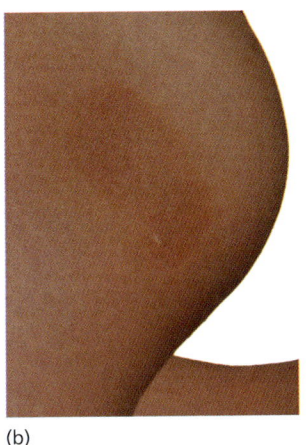 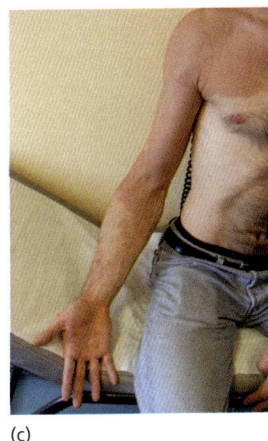 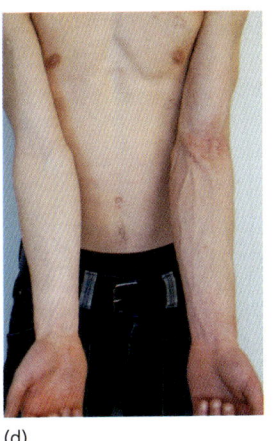 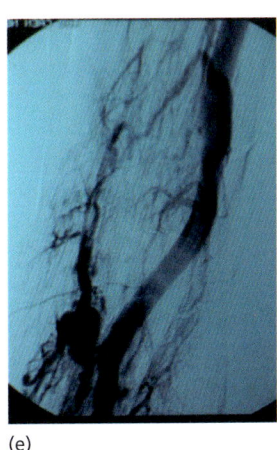

(a)   (b)   (c)   (d)   (e)

Figure 71.4 Capillary malformation–arteriovenous malformation spectrum. (a, b) A 14-year-old girl with multiple capillary malformations. (a) Note the white halo on the arm lesion. (b) The lesion on the buttock showed hypervascularity on Doppler ultrasound. (c–e) Parkes Weber syndrome in two patients with a *RASA1* mutation. Note the red blush on the thorax and arm (c), which is warm on palpation, and dilated veins (d) secondary to arteriovenous fistulae and confirmed by arteriography (e).

Classification links
- Snomed CT: 49465005
- MIM: 106050
- Orphanet: ORPHA95429

Introduction and general description
Angioma serpiginosum or progressive patchy CM is a rare congenital skin disorder characterised by non-purpuric, red, punctate lesions on a reddish background. The lesions follow the Blaschko lines.

Epidemiology
Females are more often affected than males with a sex ratio of 9 : 1 [15]. It is a rare disease with a prevalence less than 1 : 1 000 000.

Pathophysiology
Histologically, angioma serpiginosum appears as capillary ectasias in the superficial papillary dermis. The disorder seems to be genetically heterogeneous with X-linked dominant and autosomal dominant inheritance. One family was linked to Xp11.3-Xq12, and subsequently a deletion of the *PORCN* gene was identified [16,17]; these investigators suggested that angioma serpiginosum could be a mild allelic variant of focal dermal hypoplasia or Goltz–Gorlin syndrome (MIM: 305600) (Chapter 65).

Capillary malformation–arteriovenous malformation

Synonyms and inclusions
- Parkes Weber syndrome

Classification links
- ICD-10: Q82.5, Q87.8
- ICD-11: LD2F.1Y
- Snomed CT: 703533007
- MIM: 608354, 618196, 139150
- Orphanet: ORPHA137667

Introduction and general description
Capillary malformation–arteriovenous malformation (CM-AVM) is an autosomal dominant disorder characterised by multifocal CMs and an increased risk for fast-flow vascular malformations (Figure 71.4) [9]. The disorder has been reported in well over 100 families [18,19].

Epidemiology
The incidence is estimated to be around 1 in 50 000, but the disorder is likely underdiagnosed [18,19]. There is no sex difference, the penetrance is high (>95%) and there is an important intrafamilial clinical variability.

Pathophysiology
Capillary malformation–arteriovenous malformation is caused by heterozygous loss-of-function mutations in the *RASA1* or *EPHB4* genes (CM-AVM1 and CM-AVM2, respectively) [19–23]. A germline mutation is identified in about two-thirds of patients [18,19,24]. Intragenic deletions and mosaicism may underlie additional patients [25,26]. Somatic second-hits explain the intrafamilial clinical variability and the multifocality of lesions at least in CM-AVM1 [18]. *RASA1* encodes p120RASGAP, a negative regulator of RAS (name derived from rat sarcoma virus), and it can be downregulated by miR-132 [23]. p120RASGAP is involved in EPHB4→p120RASGAP→RAS→MAPK→ERK signalling [27].

Clinical features
There are two different types of CM-AVM: CM-AVM1 and -2. In both types all affected individuals have cutaneous CMs (Figure 71.4a, b). These are distinct from common CMs and represent the clue for diagnosis. Typically, they are multifocal, but a few patients have a single lesion. They are of variable size, with haphazard distribution. In contrast to common CMs, additional lesions can appear with time, until young adulthood. The CMs are pink, red or brownish, homogeneous or telangiectatic, and about half of them have a characteristic white halo around the lesion. Some patients have areas of multiple punctate telangiectasias surrounded by white halos, especially on extremities. These bier spots are more frequent

in CM-AVM2. The concurrence of CM with multiple telangiectasia, especially on the lips, perioral region and thorax, is an important clinical difference between CM-AVM1 and -2. Epistaxis can occur especially in CM-AVM2, but it is not a major symptom as in hereditary haemorrhagic telangiectasia (HHT).

In about one-third of patients with CM-AVM1, and 18% of patients with CM-AVM2, fast-flow vascular malformations are observed: arteriovenous malformation (AVM), arteriovenous fistula (AVF) or Parkes Weber syndrome (capillary blush on an upper or lower extremity, bony and soft tissue hypertrophy, and multiple arteriolo-venular microfistulae) (Figure 71.4c–e). The AVMs and AVFs are located either within the central nervous system (intracranial or intraspinal) or outside the central nervous system (above all in the extremities, face and neck).

The CMs of CM-AVM1 and -2 are asymptomatic. The intra-central nervous system AVMs/AVFs are usually symptomatic early in life: perinatally or during childhood [10,14]. Associated symptoms are cardiac failure, hydrocephaly, epilepsy, developmental delay, para- or tetraplegia and neurogenic bladder. The AVMs/AVFs located on the face, neck and extremities tend to worsen with time, and cause pain, local destruction and bleeding and cardiac failure. Often the skin, subcutis, muscles and bones are affected. The major problem associated with Parkes Weber syndrome is leg length discrepancy causing scoliosis. Cardiac overload or failure can occur.

In rare cases, CM-AVM1 has been associated with primary lymphoedema, non-immune hydrops fetalis, pleural effusions, chylothorax or chylous ascites [18,24,28–30]. Interestingly, EPHB4 cases of non-immune hydrops fetalis have also been reported [31]. These patients do not have CM-AVM, and the mutations seem to act differently.

Investigations

The small CMs do not require any investigation, unless they are warm on palpation. Such findings should be evaluated by Doppler ultrasound for the presence of fast-flow lesions. The AVMs/AVFs are followed by Doppler ultrasound and/or MRI and arteriography [32]. Leg length discrepancy in patients with Parkes Weber syndrome is followed radiographically. Screening for cerebral and spinal fast-flow lesions by MRI in asymptomatic patients can be proposed. *RASA1* and *EPHB4* testing is required in patients with suggestive clinical features.

Management

The CMs of CM-AVM respond only partially or not at all to pulsed-dye laser treatment. Patients with AVM or AVF should be followed by a multidisciplinary team specialised in vascular anomalies. The risks and benefits of treating or not are based on symptoms, patient age, lesion size and location, angio-architecture and expected evolution. The treatment of patients with Parkes Weber syndrome is as conservative as possible (e.g. elastic stocking) and the leg length discrepancy is monitored until the end of puberty. Epiphysiodesis may be necessary; however, this procedure should be avoided whenever possible as it may aggravate the fast-flow lesion [33]. CM-AVM patients may also benefit in the future from the development of targeted therapies [3,6]. As at least

the RAS-MAPK signalling pathway seems to be activated, there is interest in studying inhibitors of this pathway for efficacy.

Genetic consultation is needed to assess family history and to provide counselling. It is also needed for risk assessment, and to inform on the possibilities of IVF, prenatal testing and the importance of close follow-up during pregnancy.

Cutis marmorata telangiectatica congenita

Synonyms and inclusions
- Livedo reticularis
- Naevus vascularis reticularis

Classification links
- ICD-11: LC52
- Snomed CT: 254778000
- MIM: 219255
- Orphanet: ORPHA1556

Introduction and general description
Cutis marmorata telangiectatica congenita (CMTC) is a rare capillary malformation characterised by persistent, reticulated, atrophic, purplish skin [34].

Pathophysiology
The aetiology of CMTC is unknown.

Clinical features
Cutis marmorata telangiectatica congenita is a rare, sporadic CM characterised by a reticulated, marbled, dark purple skin patch which blanches with pressure, but its aspect does not change in regard to modification in temperature [34]. The atrophic purplish reticulated bands involve telangiectasias and venous ectasias. They are depressed and fragile and can ulcerate. The lesions occur mostly in a regional pattern and less often in a generalised distribution. During the first year of life and throughout childhood the purple network fades and becomes less depressed.

Associated anomalies, such as body asymmetry, glaucoma and neurological delay, have been noted in more than half of the reported patients. This prevalence can be disputed because the term CMTC has often been used to describe various mimicking marble-like vascular birthmarks.

Investigations
Cutis marmorata telangiectatica congenita does not usually require any investigation, unless incited by clinical multidisciplinary examination. In generalised or facial CMTC, ophthalmological examination for glaucoma is indicated [34].

Management
Ulcerations can be treated with wound dressings, and laser photocoagulation may be useful to treat residual vascular lesions.

Microcephaly–capillary malformation syndrome

Classification links
• ICD-10: Q82.5, Q87.8
• ICD-11: LD2F.1Y
• MIM: 614261, 606247
• Orphanet: ORPHA294016

Introduction and general description
Microcephaly–capillary malformation (MIC-CAP) syndrome is an autosomal recessive congenital disorder. It is characterised by severe congenital microcephaly, early-onset refractory epilepsy, profound developmental delay, spastic quadriparesis and multiple small cutaneous CMs. The CMs are present at birth, spread over the body and vary from 2 to 20 mm in diameter [35,36].

Epidemiology
Prevalence is unknown, but MIC-CAP is a very rare disease. Fewer than 20 patients have been reported.

Pathophysiology
The MIC-CAP syndrome is caused by homozygous or compound heterozygous recessive mutations in the *STAMBP* gene. This gene encodes a deubiquitinating isopeptidase that plays a role in PI3K/AKT/mTOR and RAS/MAPK signalling [37]. These pathways seem to be dysregulated in MIC-CAP.

Investigations
Investigation includes neuroimaging studies, an electroencephalogram in case of seizures and visual and hearing assessment. Genetic testing can confirm the clinical diagnosis.

Management
Management is symptomatic and mainly includes follow-up of neurological and cognitive development, physiotherapy and speech therapy and anticonvulsant medications. It might be possible to develop novel targeted therapies for MIC-CAP using molecules inhibiting the PI3K/AKT/mTOR and RAS/MAPK signalling pathways. Genetic consultation is needed to assess family history and counselling.

Capillary malformation with overgrowth

Classification links
• Snomed CT: 234118009
• MIM: 163000
• Orphanet: ORPHA458830

Introduction and general description
Capillary malformation with overgrowth (CMO) is characterised by a purple or dark red CM of an extremity associated with soft tissue and bony hypertrophy.

Pathophysiology
It was associated in three patients with a somatic p.Arg183Cys *GNA11* mutation [38].

Clinical features
Capillary malformation with overgrowth is characterised by a purple or dark red homogeneous capillary malformation, which is mostly well delineated with distinct borders. It is limited to a regional pattern usually on an upper or lower limb. It is associated with length and/or girth overgrowth which can appear with time. It is associated with pain on the affected extremity without coagulopathy, or other vascular or neurological anomalies.

Investigations
Doppler ultrasound, MRI and neurological investigations may be useful for differential diagnosis, for instance of CMDV and capillaro-lymphatico-venous malformation (CLVM) with hypertrophy.

Management
The CM can be managed the same way as a common CM. Pain is difficult to manage with classic analgesic drugs.

PI3K-RELATED OVERGROWTH SYNDROMES

Capillary malformations are seen in several disorders with overgrowth, including Parkes Weber syndrome and CMO (see earlier in this chapter). Moreover, PI3K-related overgrowth syndromes (PROS) is a term used for various overgrowth syndromes related to a somatic *PIK3CA* mutation. Recently, next generation sequencing (NGS) enabled the discovery of *PIK3R1* somatic mutations within 17 patients with vascular malformation associated with overgrowth. PIK3R1 regulates the PI3K/AKT pathway [39]. In the following, the entities with clearly recognisable PROS phenotypes are described separately: diffuse CM with overgrowth (DCMO), macrocephaly–CM (M-CM), Klippel–Trenaunay–Weber syndrome (KTS) and CLOVES syndrome (congenital lipomatous overgrowth, vascular malformations, epidermal naevi and scolosis). Clinical phenotypes in individuals with *PIK3R1* variants are similar to those attributed to somatic mosaic hotspot variants in *PIK3CA*. Therefore, the term PROS could be extended to include overgrowth syndromes related to PIK3R1, and thus understood as PI3K-related overgrowth syndrome.

Disseminated capillary malformation with overgrowth

Introduction and general description

Diffuse capillary malformation with overgrowth belongs to the spectrum of the vascular anomaly–overgrowth syndrome. It is characterised by an extensive reticular vascular staining with proportionate overgrowth which is different from other disorders with CM and hypertrophy.

Pathophysiology

It was associated in two patients with a somatic non-hotspot variant in the *PIK3CA* gene [40].

Clinical features

Diffuse capillary malformation with overgrowth is characterised by a sporadic extensive reticulate CM which can be associated with focal areas of homogeneous stains mostly located on acral sites, that is, the head and neck, hands and feet. CM is present at birth and lightens over the first months of life. It is associated with soft-tissue and/or bony proportionate overgrowth. Associated digital anomalies can be seen in 30% of patients: syndactyly, sandal gap or macrodactyly. Children with DCMO have a normal developmental growth [41].

Investigations

It does not require any investigation and is a more benign common condition than other overgrowth syndromes.

Management

Capillary stain of DCMO lightens with time and does not require laser treatment. Overgrowth is often mild and proportionate, and does not need treatment.

Macrocephaly–capillary malformation syndrome

Introduction and general description

Macrocephaly–capillary malformation (M-CM) syndrome was initially described as macrocephaly–cutis marmorata telangiectatica congenita [42,43]. The disorder is characterised by macrocephaly (megalencephaly) and capillary malformation, plus a variable combination of other features: overgrowth, brain and body asymmetry, syndactyly, polydactyly, developmental delay and joint hyperlaxity [44,45]. Cortical brain malformations, especially polymicrogyria, are frequent [46]. The CM in M-CM has a patchy reticular pattern with no cutaneous atrophy. As this is different from CMTC, the name macrocephaly–capillary malformation was proposed in 2007 [47]. Subsequently, as macrocephaly is secondary to a large brain and perisylvian polymicrogyria, the name of megalencephaly–capillary malformation–polymicrogyria syndrome was proposed in 2012 [48].

Epidemiology

This is a rare disorder with a prevalence below one in 1 000 000, which is probably underestimated.

Pathophysiology

The M-CM syndrome is associated with somatic, activating, commonly non-hotspot *PIK3CA* mutations [49].

Investigations

Investigations include neuroimaging studies and neurocognitive evaluation. Genetic testing can be used to help the clinical diagnosis.

Management

The management of patients with M-CM is symptomatic and mainly includes the follow-up of neurological and cognitive development, and management of growth asymmetry because of their possible progressive development. Targeted therapy with the mTOR inhibitor rapamycin, AKT inhibitor miransertib or the PI3K-specific inhibitor alpelisib via clinical trials may allow the development of a targeted molecular therapy [3,6].

Klippel–Trenaunay–Weber syndrome

Introduction and general description

Klippel–Trenaunay–Weber syndrome (KTS) is characterised by capillaro-lymphatico-venous malformation with overgrowth most commonly affecting one lower extremity (Figure 71.5). Important differential diagnoses are Parkes Weber syndrome, CMO and DCMO.

Epidemiology

This is a rare sporadic disorder. Prevalence estimates vary around one in 50 000–100 000.

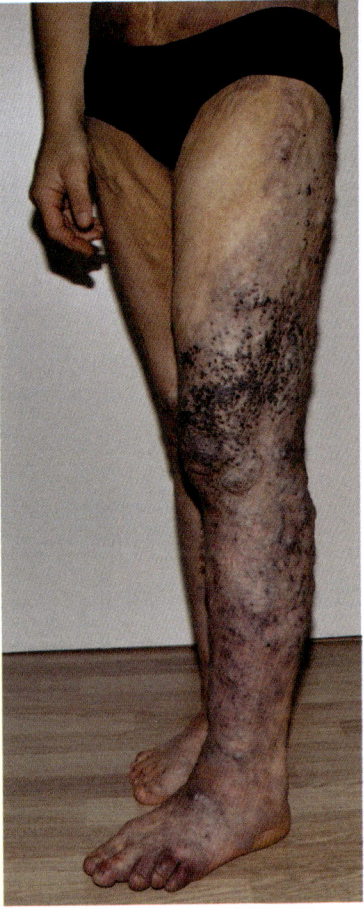
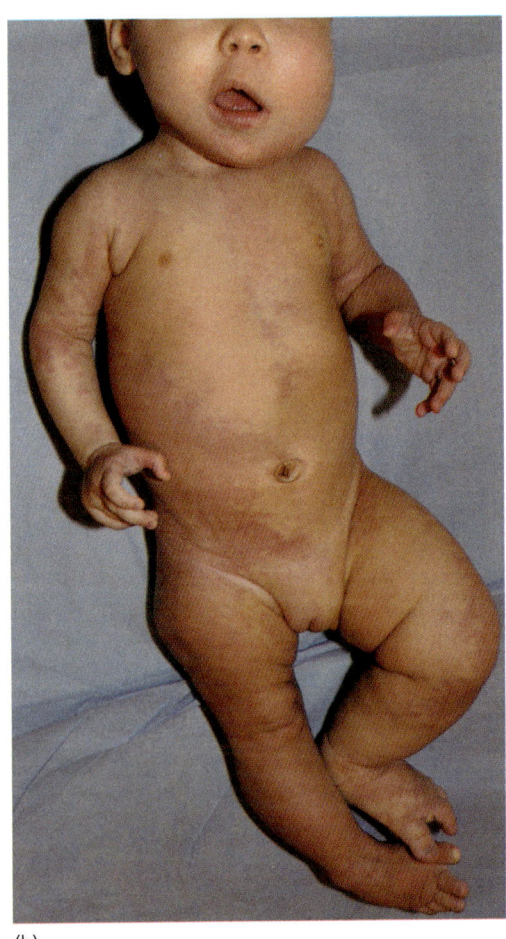

Figure 71.5 Capillary malformation in overgrowth syndromes. (a) Klippel–Trenaunay–Weber syndrome with a capillaro-lymphatico-venous malformation on the left lower extremity with overgrowth. (b) An 8-month-old girl with CLOVES syndrome showing extensive capillary malformation, hemifacial and left lower extremity hypertrophy and a sandal gap.

(a)   (b)

Pathophysiology

Happle proposed that KTS is caused by a postzygotic mutation that is lethal in a non-mosaic state [50]. Somatic, activating mutations are found in *PIK3CA* in patients with KTS [49,**51**]. They are mostly hotspot mutations, as in isolated vascular malformations with a *PIK3CA* mutation (see the sections 'Venous malformation' and 'Lymphatic malformation' later in this chapter) [52].

Clinical features

Klippel–Trenaunay–Weber syndrome is sporadic and congenital, characterised by asymmetrical overgrowth in girth and length of an extremity with a vascular lesion consisting of combined capillary, lymphatic and venous malformation (Figure 71.5) [53,54]. There is often persistence of the embryonic vein of the lateral thigh (vein of Servelle) and anomalies of the deep venous system (stenosis, hypoplasia, aplasia). KTS is often associated with localised intravascular coagulopathy (see 'Venous malformation' later in this chapter). There is a high risk for thromboembolism and subsequent pulmonary arterial hypertension [53].

Investigations

The vascular malformations are investigated as their sporadic, isolated counterparts. A skeletal survey, especially for scoliosis, is indicated. Patients with PROS and especially those with KTS need Doppler ultrasound to perform an extensive analysis of their deep and superficial venous and arterial system of the affected extremity and the trunk. D-dimer and fibrinogen measurements assess the severity of localised intravascular coagulopathy. MRI is useful before surgery. Genetic testing for mosaic mutations can disclose the underlying cause.

Management

Management of patients with KTS is multidisciplinary and includes management of overgrowth (debulking and epiphysiodesis with or without amputation), treatment of scoliosis and treatment of vascular malformations (sclerotherapy, embolisation and surgery). Low-molecular-weight heparin (LMWH) is indicated before any intervention to avoid pulmonary embolism, especially when coagulopathy is severe (D-dimer level >1000 ng/mL and low fibrinogen). It is also used long term as a prophylactic treatment for those with documented pulmonary embolism [55,56]. KTS can be treated with sirolimus when refractory to conventional treatments. A recent trial demonstrated that the patients experienced improvement in mobility, bleeding and oozing, and an improvement in their general quality of life. Sirolimus also decreased coagulation abnormalities and long-term treatment with LMWH may be interrupted for some patients [57,58]. Genetic counselling is needed. Clinical trials are ongoing (see EudraCT (https://eudract.ema.europa.eu/) and ClinicalTrials.gov; both last accessed April 2022) to establish how to improve outcomes and reduce adverse effects [59–62].

CLOVES syndrome

Synonyms and inclusions
- Congenital lipomatous overgrowth, vascular malformations, epidermal naevi and scoliosis syndrome

Classification links
- ICD-10: Q87.2
- ICD-11: LD26.60
- Snomed CT: 719475006
- MIM: 612918
- Orphanet: ORPHA140944

Introduction and general description

CLOVES is characterised by lipomatous overgrowth associated with vascular malformations in different parts of the body (Figure 71.5b). Epidermal naevi and scoliosis are also regularly present. Scoliosis is progressive. Careful clinical examination and genetic testing are needed to differentiate Proteus syndrome and CLOVES.

Epidemiology

CLOVES is a rare sporadic disorder. Prevalence estimates vary around 1 in 50 000–100 000. True prevalence may be higher due to difficulties in diagnosis.

Pathophysiology

Somatic, activating mutations are found in *PIK3CA* in patients with CLOVES [51]. They are mostly non-hotspot mutations, as seen in M-CM, and thus may help diagnostic work-up [52].

Clinical features

CLOVES is characterised by asymmetrically overgrown feet and extensive, usually truncal, arteriovenous, venous, capillary, lymphatic or combined vascular malformations (Figure 71.5) [63]. It was described in patients earlier diagnosed with Proteus syndrome, although several specific criteria were lacking and the natural history was different [63,64]. Mainly, patients with CLOVES syndrome have enlarged, but not distorted, bony structures and no cerebriform connective tissue thickening [65].

Investigations

The vascular malformations are investigated as their sporadic, isolated counterparts. A skeletal survey, especially for scoliosis, is indicated. Patients need Doppler ultrasound to characterise soft-tissue masses. D-dimer and fibrinogen measurements assess the severity of localised intravascular coagulopathy. MRI is useful before surgery. Genetic testing for mosaic mutations can disclose the underlying cause.

Management

CLOVES is a complex multiorgan disease that is mainly treated by supporting care based on extensive and multiple surgical procedures. Sirolimus and the PIK3CA inhibitor alpelisib (BYL719) have been used successfully to improve the outcome for some PROS patients, with only a few side effects during a short-term follow-up [59,60]. Two children with severe PROS were treated with miransertib (ARQ092), a highly selective pan-AKT inhibitor [61]. Treatment response and tolerability confirmed the potential utility of this inhibitor in selected patients [62]. Clinical trials are ongoing (see EudraCT (https://eudract.ema.europa.eu/) and ClinicalTrials.gov; both last accessed April 2022) to establish how to improve outcomes and reduce adverse effects.

Proteus syndrome

Classification links
- ICD-10: Q87.2
- ICD-11: LD26.60
- Snomed CT: 23150001
- MIM: 176920
- Orphanet: ORPHA744, 2969

Epidemiology

Prevalence is below one in 1 000 000.

Pathophysiology

The KTS, CLOVES and Proteus syndromes are all sporadic. Happle proposed that KTS and Proteus syndrome are caused by a postzygotic mutation that is lethal in a non-mosaic state [50]. Somatic, activating mutations are found in *AKT1* in patients with the Proteus syndrome [66].

Clinical features

The Proteus syndrome is characterised by an asymmetrical, progressive, disproportionate, severely deforming, overgrowth of body parts with bony hypertrophy, dysregulated adipose tissue, epidermal naevi, vascular malformations and increased tumour risk [67]. Typically, some overgrowth can be observed at birth, but it is greatly accelerated postnatally. A very distinctive feature and a clue for diagnosis is the cerebriform connective tissue thickening mainly located in the soles and palms. Vascular malformations have been described: capillary, venous or lymphatic malformations. They resemble those observed in patients with KTS and CLOVES syndrome. Other anomalies, including intellectual disability, cerebral malformations and ocular and renal anomalies have been reported [67,68]. Proteus syndrome is overdiagnosed, and it seems that at least half of the patients have another diagnosis [68].

Investigations

The vascular malformations are investigated as their sporadic, isolated counterparts. Doppler ultrasound is indicated to diagnose soft-tissue masses in Proteus syndrome. MRI is useful before surgery. Genetic testing for mosaic mutations can disclose the underlying cause.

Management

Management of patients with Proteus syndrome is multidisciplinary and includes the management of overgrowth (debulking and epiphysiodesis with or without amputation), treatment of scoliosis and treatment of vascular malformations (sclerotherapy, embolisation and surgery). Genetic counselling is needed. Six patients (children and adults) with a somatic *AKT1* c.49G>A (Glu17Lys) variant were treated with miransertib, a selective pan-AKT inhibitor, with a dose of 5 mg/m^2/day [62]. A decrease in the cerebriform connective tissue naevus and a reduction of pain were observed. The dose was well tolerated. Treatment response and tolerability confirmed the potential utility of this inhibitor in selected patients.

ARTERIOVENOUS DISORDERS

Arteriovenous malformation

Synonyms and inclusions
- AV malformation (AVM)
- Arteriovenous anomalies

Classification links
- ICD-10: Q27.3
- ICD-11: 585997617
- Snomed CT: 24551003
- Orphanet: ORPHA211266

Introduction and general description
Arteriovenous malformations are congenital, destructive, fast-flow vascular malformations that tend to worsen with time. They can occur in any body part (Figure 71.6).

Epidemiology
Males and females are equally affected. The incidence is not known. The AVM can be isolated or part of a disorder, such as CM-AVM, HHT or phosphatase and tensin homologue (PTEN) hamartoma tumour syndrome (PHTS). Intracranial AVM can be asymptomatic. Based on autopsy and imaging studies, brain AVM prevalence varies from 0.01–0.5% [69] to 4.3% [70]. Extracranial AVMs are less frequent.

Pathophysiology
Arteriovenous malformations consist of distorted arteries, and veins with thickened muscle walls due to arteriovenous shunting and fibrosis [71]. In AVM, the normal capillary bed is replaced by a nidus, via which blood shunts from feeding arteries into draining veins. An arteriovenous fistula consists of a direct communication between an artery and a vein. They are less frequent than AVMs, and usually post-traumatic. It is usually sporadic, but an underlying predisposing genetic defect exists when it is part of CM-AVM, HHT or PHTS.

Somatic activating mutations have been identified in series of sporadic intracerebral and peripheral AVMs in the RAS/MAK pathway proteins KRAS, BRAF and MAP2K1 [72,73].

Clinical features
Arteriovenous malformations are localised, affecting the brain, skin, muscles, bone or viscera. Parkes Weber syndrome consists

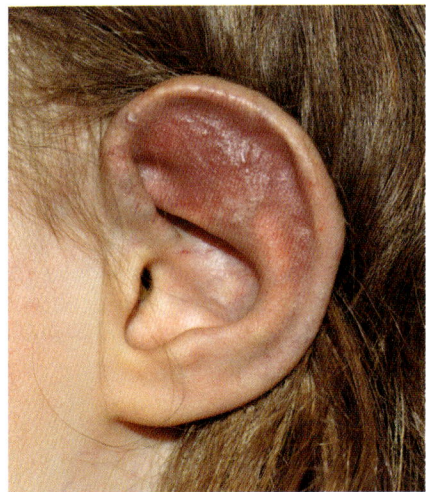

(a)

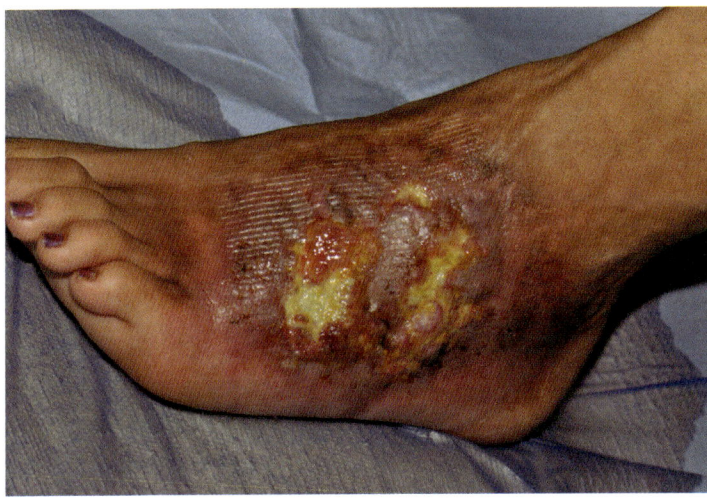

(b)

Figure 71.6 Arteriovenous malformation (AVM) spectrum. (a) A 4-year-old girl with stage 2 AVM of the left ear. (b) Extensive ulcerated stage 3 AVM of the left foot.

of multiple microfistulae (see the section on CM-AVM earlier in this chapter). AVMs expand slowly, but can worsen rapidly at puberty, during pregnancy, after trauma and, particularly, after incomplete treatment. At birth or in infancy, an AVM involving the skin can appear as a capillary blush, which can be misdiagnosed as a CM (Figure 71.6a). The presence of increased warmth, thrill or bruit suggests a fast-flow component. Evolution is variable and unpredictable, but many worsen with time and can become life-threatening. Clinical manifestations depend on size, rheology and localisation of the lesion, and the age of the patient. In neonates, large cerebral AVMs usually present with congestive cardiac failure. Symptoms in childhood and adulthood vary: hydrocephaly, headache, epilepsy, haemorrhage and focal neurological deficit in intracranial lesions; cyanosis, clubbing, polycythaemia and right-to-left shunt with cerebral abscess and embolic stroke in pulmonary lesions; cardiac failure, portal hypertension and biliary disease in hepatic lesions; and heaviness, pain, pulsatile mass, thrill, trophic changes (deformation, ulceration, destruction) and bleeding in cutaneous, subcutaneous and muscular lesions.

Investigations

Radiological investigations are mandatory to confirm the clinical diagnosis, to delineate the lesion and to evaluate the therapeutic options: Doppler ultrasound shows high-velocity arterial and pulsatile venous flow with low resistance. It differentiates AVMs from vascular tumours (haemangiomas) and other (vascular) malformations [74]. T_2-weighted MRI shows dilated veins and arteries within normal or hypertrophied tissue. It defines the extent of AVMs and, for intracranial lesions, differentiates them from other (vascular) malformations. Arteriography is done as a pre-treatment examination to identify the feeding arteries and to localise the nidus.

Management

The therapeutic approach depends on the lesion type, location and symptoms. Evaluation should be made by a multidisciplinary team, including a dermatologist, internist or paediatrician, surgeon and interventional radiologist. It varies from conservative follow-up to aggressive treatment consisting of embolisation and/or surgical resection. Conservative treatment includes antihypertensive medications, pain killers, elastic stockings and wound management. Antiangiogenic molecules are being tested [75,76]. The effects of invasive treatment can be devastating, especially if not performed properly (e.g. proximal ligation should not be used), and thus should be performed only in reference centres by trained physicians. Treatment should be as complete as possible to avoid recruitment of new feeding arteries and aggravation of the malformation. Otherwise, AVMs can aggravate suggesting that interventions can stimulate lesions. Therefore, a medical antiangiogenic approach may help management. Thalidomide, a potent antiangiogenic drug can reduce bleeding, pain, ulceration and vascularity of some AVMs with a low-dose regimen [76]. Recently, trametinib, a MEK (mitogen-activated extracellular signal-regulated kinase) inhibitor, was used to control large progressive AVMs in two case studies harbouring a *MAP2K1* or *KRAS* mutation [77,78]. Tolerance and efficacy were good after 6 months of treatment with a significant decrease in the volume of the malformation and arterial inflow. A theragnostic approach is also used in the ongoing clinical trametinib trial TRAMAV (EudraCT 2019-003573-26) to manage complex AVMs.

Capillary malformation–arteriovenous malformation

See the previous section on CM-AVM earlier in this chapter.

Hereditary haemorrhagic telangiectasia

Synonyms and inclusions
• Rendu–Osler–Weber syndrome

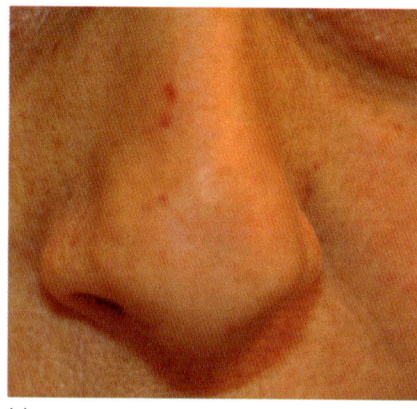

(a)

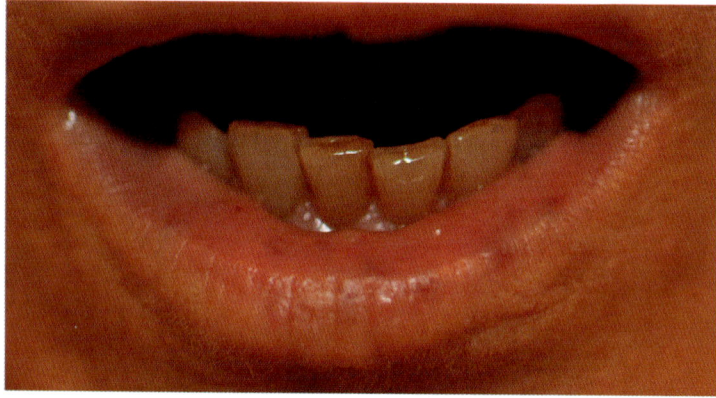

(b)

Figure 71.7 A 62-year-old female with multiple (a) cutaneous and (b) mucosal telangiectasias associated with recurrent epistaxis typical of hereditary haemorrhagic telangiectasia.

Classification links
• ICD-10: 178.0
• ICD-11: 714406192
• Snomed CT: 21877004
• MIM: 187300, 600376, 601101, 601284,600993, 615506, 131195
• Orphanet: ORPHA774

Introduction and general description

Hereditary haemorrhagic telangiectasia is an autosomal dominant disorder characterised by mucocutaneous and gastrointestinal telangiectasias, associated with AVMs/AVFs in the lungs, liver or brain (Figure 71.7).

Epidemiology

Its incidence is about 1 : 5000 to 1 : 8000. Males and females are equally affected.

Pathophysiology

Ultrastructurally, the telangiectasias of HHT are micro-AVFs [79]. Histological analysis of a cerebral and a pulmonary AVM in two HHT1 patients showed vessel dilatation, and variable thickness and disorganisation of the smooth muscle cell layer [80]. It has been proposed that the telangiectasias and AVMs represent a continuum spectrum [81].

At least six genes are involved: four identified (*ENG*, *ACVRL1*, *SMAD4*, *GDF2*) and two localised (*HHT3* on chromosome 5q31.3-q32 and *HHT4* on chromosome 7p14) [82–88]. More than 80% of HHT patients have mutations in *ENG*, *ACVRL1* or *SMAD4* (61%, 37% and 2%, respectively) [88]. These three genes, as well as *GDF2*, encode components of the TGF-β signalling pathway: Endoglin, ALK1, SMAD4 and BMP9, respectively. Causative mutations probably exert a loss-of-function effect. The TGF-β signalling pathway plays an important role in the development and homeostasis of many organs, including the vascular system.

Clinical features
The diagnosis of HHT is based on the Curaçao criteria, which include epistaxis, telangiectasias, visceral fast-flow lesions and family history. The diagnosis is considered 'definite' if three or more criteria are present, 'possible' when two criteria are present and 'unlikely' when only one criterion is present. Patients with mutations in *ENG* or *ACVRL1* are clinically similar. However, patients with *ACVRL1* mutations are characterised by later onset, lower penetrance, less frequent cerebral and pulmonary AVMs, more frequent liver involvement and a risk of developing pulmonary arterial hypertension. Patients with mutations in *SMAD4* have HHT combined with juvenile polyposis. The HHT phenotype in these patients is similar to those caused by mutations in *ENG* or *ACVRL1* [84].

Investigations
Contrast echocardiography is indicated [**89**]. Cerebral MRI, thoracic computed tomography (CT) scan and hepatic Doppler ultrasound can be performed to screen for asymptomatic AVMs in children and young adults, as they are at higher risk for haemorrhage than the general population [90]. Symptomatic AVMs necessitate radiological investigations similar to those for the sporadic forms of AVMs. Genetic consultation is needed to assess family history and to perform genetic testing. Blood haemoglobin and haematocrit should be measured annually. Genetic testing can confirm the clinical diagnosis.

Management
International guidelines have been proposed for the diagnosis and management of patients with HHT [91]. Treatment is symptomatic and multidisciplinary: regular follow-up of oximetry and blood count for anaemia or polycythaemia; iron supplementation and transfusion for anaemia; and nasal humidification, lubricants and haemostatic products for nasal bleeding. Laser can be used for cutaneous, nasal or gastrointestinal telangiectasias. The treatment of fast-flow lesions is similar to that described for sporadic AVMs. Antiangiogenic molecules, such as thalidomide and bevacizumab (antivascular endothelial growth factor A (anti-VEGF-A)), tyrosine kinase inhibitors and PI3K inhibitors are currently under investigation [75,92,93]. Genetic consultation is needed to assess family history and counselling.

PTEN hamartoma tumour syndrome

Synonyms and inclusions
- Bannayan–Riley–Ruvalcaba syndrome (BRRS) and Cowden syndrome (CS)

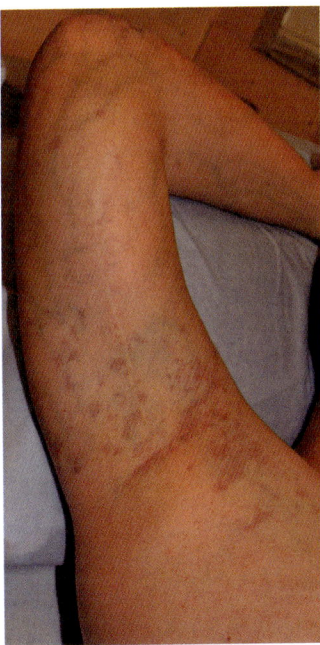

Figure 71.8 A 14-year-old boy with an inherited *PTEN* mutation showing patchy capillary malformations with underlying venous anomalies, and hypertrophy of the right upper extremity. The patient also has typical penile freckles.

Classification links
- Snomed CT: 722859001
- MIM: 158350; 601728; 608309
- Orphanet: ORPHA306498

Introduction and general description
PTEN hamartoma tumour syndrome is an autosomal dominant disorder that regroups patients with Bannayan–Riley–Ruvalcaba syndrome (BRRS) and Cowden syndrome. These patients often have macrocephaly, facial trichilemmomas, papillomatous papules, acral keratoses, benign thyroid disease, lipomatous masses, increased risk of developing cancer, and vascular anomalies (Figure 71.8). These signs have sex-specific differences in prevalence [94].

Epidemiology
The prevalence is estimated at 1 : 200 000 [95], but the disorder is probably underdiagnosed [96].

Pathophysiology
Heterozygous *PTEN* mutations are identified in approximately 60% of BRRS and 81% of Cowden syndrome patients. *PTEN* codes for a dual specificity phosphatase, which antagonises PI3K and MAPK signalling [97,98]. Most *PTEN* mutations cause premature termination codons, suggesting a loss-of-function effect and haploinsufficiency [98,99].

Clinical features
Most vascular anomalies (86%) in PHTS patients are fast-flowing [**100**]. The extracranial ones are in general intramuscular or subcutaneous, and associated with ectopic fat, disrupted architecture and severe and progressive enlargement of affected muscles. In addition to swelling, patients can have pain and a cutaneous capillary stain

(Figure 71.8) [100]. BRRS is characterised by macrocephaly, variable degrees of developmental delay, hamartomatous intestinal polyposis, lipomas and pigmented macules of the glans penis [101,102]. Cowden syndrome is characterised by macrocephaly, multiple hamartomas with an increased risk for benign and malignant tumours (especially thyroid, breast and endometrial cancer), and mucocutaneous lesions (trichilemmomas, acral keratosis, papillomatous lesions) (Chapter 78). Both are part of the phenotypic spectrum of PHTS [94].

Investigations

Radiological investigations of PHTS vascular lesions include Doppler ultrasound, T_2-weighted MRI and magnetic resonance angiography (MRA) [100]. Cancer surveillance should be done according to guidelines [103]. *PTEN* genetic testing is required in patients with suggestive clinical features.

Management

Management of patients with *PTEN* mutations includes surveillance for cognitive development in children and for benign and malignant tumours in adults. The papillomatous papules are treated when symptomatic with topical agents, curettage, cryosurgery, laser or surgery. Treatment of PHTS fast-flow or slow-flow vascular malformations is similar to that for sporadic forms. Rapamycin seems effective in clinical trials [104]. Genetic counselling is needed. This complex vascular malformation may be improved with sirolimus treatment and studies are ongoing to confirm these clinical results [58]. Genetic consultation is needed to assess family history and counselling.

VENOUS DISORDERS

Venous malformation

Synonyms and inclusions
- Venous angioma
- Cavernoma
- Cavernous angioma
- Multifocal sporadic VM

Classification links
- ICD-10: Q27.10, Q27.4
- ICD-11: L90.2
- Snomed CT: 234124003, 703198009, 724842007
- MIM: 6001195, 600221
- Orphanet: ORPHA211252

Introduction and general description

Venous malformations (VMs) are congenital, sporadic, vascular lesions characterised by localised light-to-dark blue lumps consisting of malformed veins (Figure 71.9). They can affect any tissue or organ. They can be emptied by compression or in the upright position [80].

Epidemiology

Venous malformations have an incidence estimated at around 1 : 10 000 [105]. Males and females are equally affected. They are the most frequent vascular malformations referred to specialised centres [106,107]. They are sporadic, and most are unifocal (99%).

Associated diseases

D-dimer levels are elevated in 42% of patients, reflecting increased fibrinolysis. This localised intravascular coagulopathy (LIC) is associated with size, deepness and presence of palpable phleboliths. Most multifocal sporadic VMs have LIC [106,108,109]. In 25% of patients with LIC, D-dimers are very high (over twice the normal range); 40% have concomitant low fibrinogen levels. The latter are at high risk of disseminated intravascular coagulopathy with severe bleeding during interventional or surgical procedures. Within vascular anomalies, LIC has 96% specificity for venous malformations [106].

Pathophysiology

Histologically, VMs are characterised by enlarged, convoluted, venous channels lined by a single flattened layer of endothelial cells surrounded by irregularly distributed smooth muscle cells [110,**111**]. Somatic mutations in *TEK* encoding the endothelial cell tyrosine kinase receptor TIE2 are present in about 50% of VMs [**112**,113]. The most common one, p.L914F, accounts for 75% of all mutations. It has not been observed as an inherited mutation suggesting it may be lethal when germline [113]. It causes strong hyperphosphorylation of TIE2. Some sporadic patients, especially those with multifocal lesions, have two different *TEK* mutations on the same *TEK* allele [**112**,114]. Both mutations singly cause increased TIE2 phosphorylation, which is stronger for *cis*-mutated alleles. The hyperphosphorylated TIE2 activates the PI3K→AKT→FOXO1 signalling pathway leading to decreased platelet-derived growth factor β (PDGF-β) production. This may explain the scarcity of vascular smooth muscle cells in VMs [115]. Another 20% of patients with a VM have a somatic activating PIK3CA hotspot mutation [116].

Clinical features

Venous malformations are mainly solitary; <1% are multifocal. They vary from small blebs to large, bluish lesions (Figure 71.9). Palpation is not painful, unless thrombosis occurs. There is no thrill or bruit, and the malformation is not warmer than non-lesional areas. VMs can affect the skin, mucosa, muscles, joints, nerves, bones and internal organs, such as the brain or the gastrointestinal or urinary tract. Depending on their size and location, and the hormonal status and physical activity of the patient, VMs can be painful, cause bleeding and/or functional impairment, and even be life-threatening. Intrabuccal VMs are often associated with sleep apnoea. Migraine is a common feature in VMs located in the temporal muscle. On the extremities, VMs can cause muscle weakness.

Clinical variants

A few patients have multifocal sporadic VMs. Their lesions are cutaneous and subcutaneous, and rarely involve deeper structures. They are commonly smaller in diameter (<5 cm²), more superficial and less compressible. Additional VMs can develop with time [110,117].

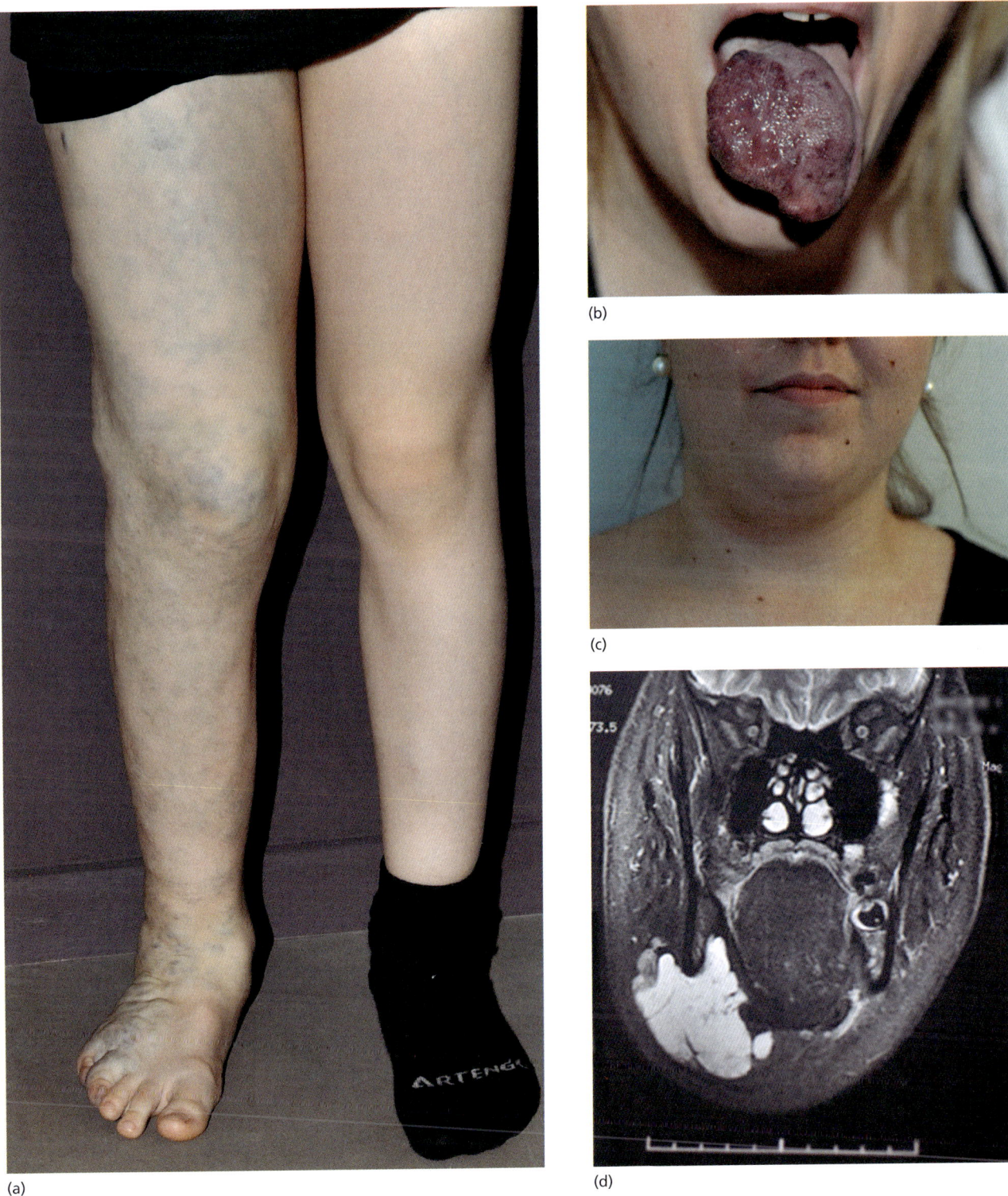

(a)

(b)

(c)

(d)

Figure 71.9 Venous malformation (VM) spectrum. (a) Extensive VM of the right lower extremity invading the skin, muscles and knee joint. (b) VM of the tongue causing sleep apnoea. (c, d) Deep VM of the right cheek causing swelling (c), and seen on T_2-weighted MRI as a bright mass (d).

Differential diagnosis

Various pathologies may present with similar lesions, including inherited mucocutaneous venous malformation, blue rubber bleb naevus syndrome, glomuvenous malformation, hyperkeratotic cutaneous capillaro-venous malformation, lymphatic malformation with intracystic bleeding, subcutaneous haemangioma, iatrogenic venous stenosis and blue naevus. Differentiation is based on clinical history, and medical and Doppler ultrasound examination. Histopathological examination is sometimes necessary. Genetic testing may be helpful.

Complications and co-morbidities

Pulmonary thromboembolism with or without pulmonary arterial hypertension has been reported in some patients with extensive VM of the extremities with LIC. Radiologically, they all had large draining veins [118,119].

Disease course and prognosis

Venous malformations grow proportionately with the individual. They never regress spontaneously. Initially, asymptomatic lesions often become painful at puberty. Aesthetic and functional impairment worsen with time because of expansion or bleeding. Depending on location, they can be life-threatening.

Investigations

Doppler ultrasound is the best examination to confirm the vascular nature of the lesion (slow flow) and to identify the anatomy of the draining vessels. MRI with spin-echo T_1- and T_2-weighted and fat-saturation sequences depict the anatomical relationship between the vascular lesion and adjacent structures [110]. These two radiological examinations are mandatory for pre-therapeutic assessment of VMs and to evaluate efficacy of treatment. A blood test is needed to identify associated coagulation abnormalities.

Management

A tailored compression garment is used for symptomatic and extensive VMs of the extremities to reduce pain and thrombosis [110,120]. Aspirin may help children with painful VMs and elevated D-dimer levels. LMWH (100 anti-Xa/kg/day) is used to relieve pain associated with elevated D-dimer levels and to prevent bleeding during a surgical procedure [108,109]. Sclerotherapy followed by surgical resection (whenever possible) is the treatment of choice. Pulsed-dye and/or yttrium-aluminium-garnet (YAG) laser can be efficient for small superficial lesions. Well-localised VMs can be surgically resected. Extensive VMs should undergo several sessions of sclerotherapy by an experienced interventional radiologist, sometimes followed by (partial) surgical resection. Sclerosing agents include detergents (sodium tetradecyl sulphate, polidocanol, sodium morrhuate), microfoam, bleomycin, absolute ethanol and radio-opaque ethylcellulose-ethanol [121,122]. With the understanding of the underlying aetiopathogenic mechanisms, targeted molecular therapies are becoming possible. Rapamycin is promising in clinical trials with adequate monitoring [4,57,58,123,124].

Cutaneo-mucosal venous malformation

Synonyms and inclusions
- Venous malformations, multiple cutaneous and mucosal
- Mucocutaneous venous malformation

Classification links
- ICD-10: Q27.8
- Snomed CT: 6993011008
- MIM: 600195, 600221
- Orphanet: ORPHA2451

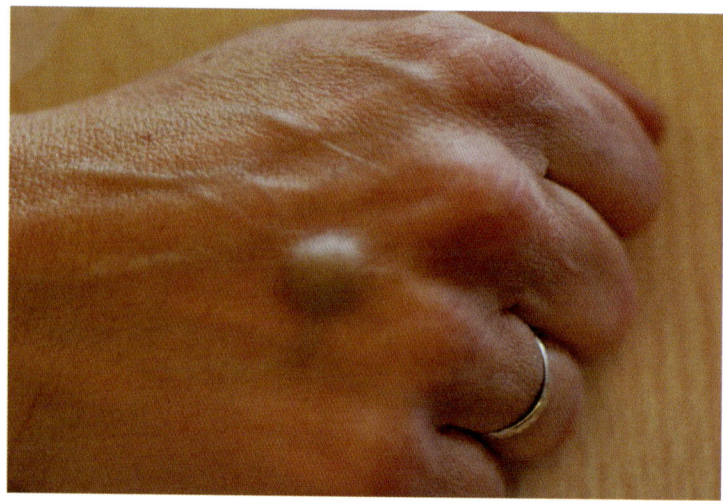

(a)

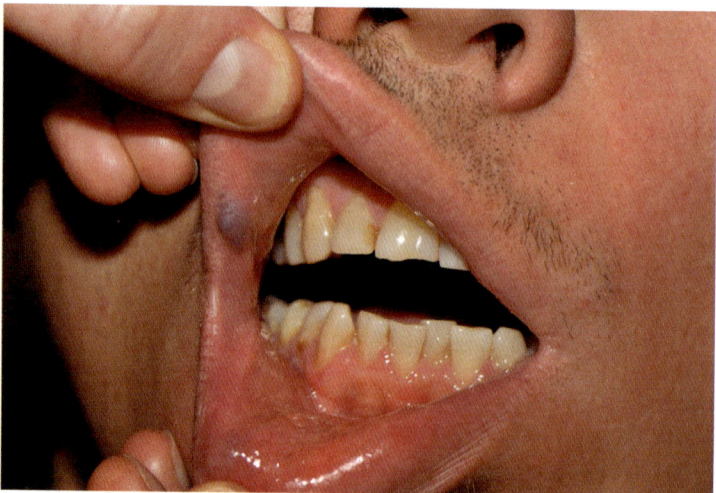

(b)

Figure 71.10 Mucocutaneous venous malformation spectrum showing (a) a small subcutaneous venous malformation on the right hand, and (b) lip mucosa. These patients have additional lesions elsewhere.

Introduction and general description

Cutaneo-mucosal VM (VMCM), more commonly known as mucocutaneous VM, is an inherited, autosomal dominant, venous anomaly characterised by multifocal, small, bluish lesions (Figure 71.10). They mainly involve the skin and oral mucosa, but can rarely affect the muscles, gastrointestinal tract, lungs and brain [**111**,125–127].

Epidemiology

The VMCMs account for <1% of venous malformations [128]. Prevalence is unknown. Males and females are equally affected.

Pathophysiology

Like sporadic venous malformations, VMCM is caused by activating *TEK* mutations [**111**,126,128]. However, the mutations differ in nature. VMCM mutations are inherited in an autosomal dominant fashion and are found in a heterozygous state in all cells of the patient, whereas VM mutations are somatic and are therefore exclusively present in VM tissues. Moreover, the most common

VMCM mutation is p.R849W, which causes mild activation of TIE2, whereas the most common somatic mutation is p.L914F, which causes strong TIE2 activation. The multifocal localised lesions in VMCM probably result from somatic second-hits on the normal allele. The single reported second-hit was shown to result in loss of function, presumably abolishing the protective effect of the wild-type allele [112].

Clinical features
Mucocutaneous VM lesions are commonly multifocal and small in diameter (<5 cm^2) [117]. Most have only a few inconspicuous, tiny, blue spots (<5 mm^2), whereas others have additional egg-size symptomatic lesions [110]. There is great intra- and interfamilial variability in the number, size and location of lesions, confirming that the germline mutation is not sufficient to explain the disease. Additional VMs can develop with time [110]. Some are associated with LIC [126].

Investigations and management
See the section on VMs earlier in this chapter. Genetic analysis can give a definite diagnosis. Genetic counselling is needed to assess family history and counselling.

Blue rubber bleb naevus syndrome

Synonyms and inclusions
- Bean syndrome

Classification links
- ICD-10: Q27.8
- ICD-11: LA90.2Y
- Snomed CT: 254784002
- MIM: 112200
- Orphanet: ORPHA1059

Introduction and general description
Blue rubber bleb naevus (BRBN) syndrome is a rare, sporadic, congenital, slow flow vascular anomaly. It is characterised by numerous, widely distributed, cutaneous and internal VMs. Pathognomic are small, rubbery, dark bluish, palmoplantar lesions and gastrointestinal VMs (Figure 71.11) [129,130].

Epidemiology
Prevalence is unknown, and there is no sex preponderance.

Associated diseases
Like venous malformation, BRBN syndrome is associated with LIC [106].

Pathophysiology
Like VM and VMCM, BRBN syndrome is caused by activating *TEK* mutations [114]. However, these are somatic double mutations in *cis* on the same allele. They cause strong receptor activation. Distinct lesions even at distance have the same *cis* mutations [114,131].

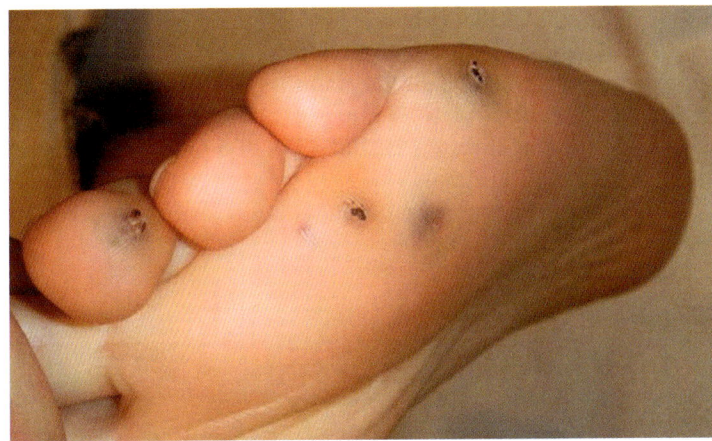

(a)

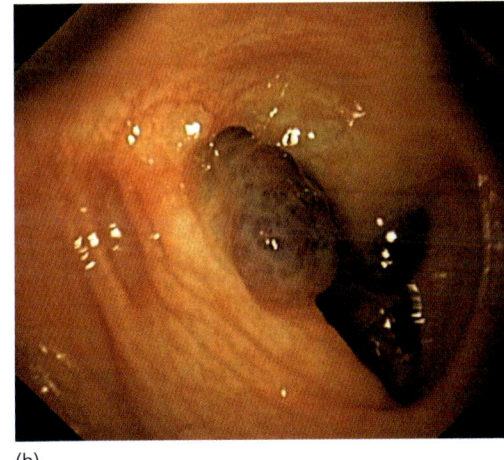

(b)

Figure 71.11 Blue rubber bleb naevus spectrum. (a) Typical multifocal hyperkeratotic lesions on the sole. (b) Gastrointestinal venous malformations seen on gastroscopy.

Clinical features
Most patients are born with a large VM. Additional small (<1–2 cm) cutaneous lesions are usually present at birth, and increase in size and number with age, often around puberty [132]. They are dark bluish to purple in colour, often hyperkeratotic, and of rubbery consistency. They are especially frequent on the palms and soles (Figure 71.11a). Gastrointestinal VMs are most commonly located in the small intestine, but may be found anywhere on the mucosae from the mouth to anus (Figure 71.11b). They can cause gastrointestinal haemorrhage with chronic iron deficiency and severe anaemia, intussusception, volvulus and infarction [133]. VMs can also involve the brain, kidneys, lungs and other organs. There is great variability in the number, size and location of lesions between affected individuals [114]. Life expectancy should not be reduced if bleeding is managed.

Investigations and management
See the sections on VM and VMCM earlier in this chapter. Endoscopy, colonoscopy, wireless capsule endoscopy or MRI are needed to document gastrointestinal lesions [110,134].

Chronic anaemia due to gastrointestinal bleeding necessitates iron supplementation and even blood transfusions. Aggressive

PART 6: GENETIC DISORDERS

surgical excision of all gastrointestinal lesions should be performed in patients who require blood transfusions or who have frequent intermittent abdominal pain due to intussusception [133]. Targeted molecular therapies, such as rapamycin, may become an option after validation in clinical trials [57,135]. In a prospective phase II monocentric trial, sirolimus was efficient in 19 patients with extensive LM, VM and complex malformations refractory to conventional treatments, and was well tolerated [57,58].

Glomuvenous malformation

Synonyms and inclusions
- Glomangioma
- Glomangiomatosis
- Hereditary multiple glomangiomas
- Venous malformation with glomus cells
- Glomus tumour

Classification links
- ICD-10: Q27.8
- ICD-11: LA90.2Y
- Snomed CT: 715644000
- MIM: 138000, 60179
- Orphanet: ORPHA83454

Introduction and general description

Glomuvenous malformation (GVM) is an inherited, autosomal dominant, venous anomaly characterised by multifocal bluish purple lesions mainly located on the extremities (Figure 71.12) [117].

Epidemiology

Glomuvenous malformation accounts for about 5% of venous anomalies [117]. Prevalence is unknown and there is no sex preponderance. More than 80% of GVMs are inherited as an autosomal dominant trait. For the rest, family history is not necessarily available [136,**137,138**,139]. GVMs have an age-dependent penetrance, which reaches its maximum of 93% by 20 years of age [117,**137**].

Associated diseases

In contrast to VM, VMCM and BRBN syndrome, GVM is not associated with coagulation abnormalities [106].

Pathophysiology

Histologically, GVMs are characterised by the presence of ill-differentiated mural smooth muscle cells, called 'glomus' cells, surrounding enlarged and convoluted venous channels [**137,140**]. GVM is caused by loss-of-function dominant mutations in the *GLMN* gene, encoding glomulin [**137,138,141**]. In addition to the inherited mutation, a somatic second-hit is needed for GVM to develop [**137**,139]. The most common second-hit is acquired uniparental isodisomy, which leads to cellular homozygosity for the inherited mutation [139]. This leads to complete loss of function of

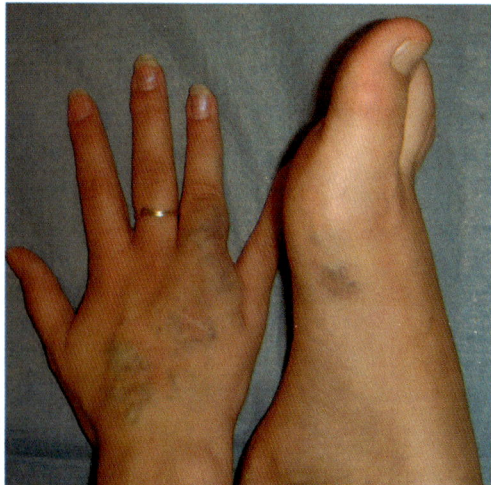

(a)

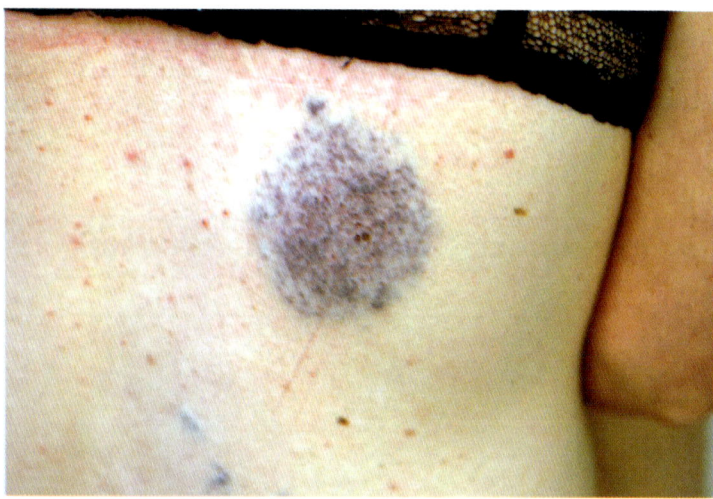

(b)

Figure 71.12 Glomuvenous malformation (GVM) spectrum. (a) A 20-year-old woman with cutaneous/subcutaneous cobblestone lesions on the right foot and right hand. (b) A plaque-like GVM on the back.

glomulin. It is still unclear how glomulin dysfunction leads to the disease phenotype.

Clinical features

Glomuvenous malformations are congenital, and never regress spontaneously. Additional small lesions can develop until young adulthood. There is great variability in the number, size and location of lesions between affected individuals. Some have a few inconspicuous, tiny, blue spots (often grouped), whereas others have extensive lesions [117]. GVMs are usually small in diameter (<5 cm^2), pink to purple, raised, with a cobblestone appearance, and slightly hyperkeratotic, especially when located on the extremities (Figure 71.12) [117]. They are cutaneous and subcutaneous, and rarely involve the mucosa, deep muscles, joints or bones. They are not compressible, but painful on palpation. Plaque-like GVM is a rare variant characterised by a solitary large lesion that can mimic a capillary–venous malformation, especially at birth [117,142]. When thoracic, plaque-like GVM may be associated with pleural effusion [143].

Investigations

Normal D-dimer and fibrinogen levels help in differentiating GVM from VM, VMCM and BRBN. Doppler ultrasound is the best examination to confirm the slow-flow nature of the malformation, and the higher cellularity and weaker compressibility compared with VM. MRI with spin-echo T_1- and T_2-weighted and fat-saturation sequences depict the extension into underlying tissues [110]. These radiological examinations are mandatory for pre-therapeutic evaluation. Histological and/or genetic analysis can give a definite diagnosis.

Management

Tailored compression garments are contraindicated in GVM as they increase pain [110,120]. The treatment of choice is surgical resection. A skin graft is often needed. Sclerotherapy can be used, but it is often less effective and has a higher risk for ulceration than with VMs. Pulsed-dye and/or YAG lasers may be efficient for small lesions. Genetic counselling is needed to assess family history and counselling.

Cerebral cavernous malformation-associated cutaneous lesions

Synonyms and inclusions
- HCCVM
- Angiokeratoma associated with CCM
- Nodular venous malformation associated with CCM

Classification links
- ICD-10: Q28.3
- ICD-11: 8B22.41
- Snomed CT: 254788004
- MIM: 116860, 604214, 607929, 609118
- Orphanet: ORPHA221061

Introduction and general description

Cerebral cavernous malformations (CCMs) are well localised vascular lesions of the central nervous system. They are histologically characterised by dilated capillary-like channels and/or large caverns. The endothelial cells have defective tight junctions.

Epidemiology

The prevalence is estimated to be 1 : 200 to 1 : 1000. Sporadic and familial forms exist; usually one cerebral vascular lesion is observed in sporadic cases and multifocal lesions in familial cases. The familial forms comprise around 10–20% of white patients and up to 50% of Hispanic American patients of Mexican descent. There is no sex difference and the intrafamilial clinical variability is important.

Pathophysiology

The familial form has an autosomal dominant inheritance and has been associated with loss-of-function mutations in three genes: *CCM1* (*KRIT1*), *CCM2* and *CCM3* (*PDCD10*), and a fourth locus was suggested on 3q26.3-27.2. Molecular genetic screening reveals heterozygous mutations in about 95% of patients with multifocal CCMs and positive family history, but only in about half of patients with multifocal CCMs and unaffected parents [144,145]. It has been shown that a somatic second-hit on the normal allele explains the multifocality of the lesions [146]. Using laser capture microdissection, the mutations were shown to occur in a subset of endothelial cells, but not in non-endothelial cells, and this was consistent with the immunohistochemistry studies [147].

Clinical features

Cerebral cavernous malformations are localised in the central nervous system. Associated cutaneous vascular lesions are found in approximately 9% of patients, mainly with *KRIT1* mutations. They consist of CMs (34%), VMs (21%) or, more specifically, hyperkeratotic cutaneous capillaro-venous malformations (39%) [**148**]. About 60% of mutation carriers are symptomatic; associated symptoms are mainly seizures and cerebral haemorrhages, but also headaches and focal neurological deficit, irrespective of the gene involved. Radiological penetrance is much higher, but not complete, even with very sensitive gradient-echo MRI. This is important for genetic counselling. Even if symptoms can be observed at any age, most often the onset is around 30 years in familial CCM. Importantly, new lesions appear with age and the size of the lesions tends to increase. Symptoms do not seem to correlate with the number of lesions, but with their location. The most severe outcome is associated with those in the brainstem and basal ganglia [149].

Investigations

Gradient-echo MRI is generally used to diagnose CCM in symptomatic patients. Some clinicians recommend brain MRI for surveillance of asymptomatic patients, but this is controversial as asymptomatic lesions are usually not treated. Genetic testing of *CCM1–3* allows the molecular subtype to be distinguished, and to evaluate the risk for transmission, when no family history exists.

Management

Current clinical guidelines for symptomatic patients recommend medical treatment for seizures and surgical removal in cases of haemorrhage, focal neurological deficit or intractable epilepsy. Anticoagulant treatment should be avoided. Genetic counselling is needed to assess family history and counselling.

Verrucous venous malformation

Synonyms and inclusions
- Verrucous hemangioma

Classification links
- ICD-10: Q27.8
- ICD-11: LA90.2Y
- Orphanet: ORPHA464318

PART 6: GENETIC DISORDERS

Introduction and general description

A verrucous venous malformation (VVM) is a non-hereditary vascular anomaly that occurs on an extremity in 91% of cases. It is a raised purple hyperkeratotic papule or nodule that can extend in the subcutis. The diagnosis is clinical.

Epidemiology

The incidence is currently unknown. Similar lesions are seen in some patients with *KRIT1*-related familial cerebral cavernous malformations.

Pathophysiology

Somatic activating mutations have been identified in the *MAP3K3* gene [150].

Clinical features

Verrucous venous malformations are single or multiple lesions that occur mainly on the extremities during infancy. Initially the lesions are dark blue or purple and non-keratotic and, in time, they become increasingly hyperkeratotic and do not regress. Histologically the affected tissue contains clusters of venule-like channels that immunostain positively for *GLUT1* and negative for D2-40 [151].

Investigations

They are cutaneous lesions that do not require any investigations. A differential diagnosis between VVMs and hyperkeratotic cutaneous capillary VMs is important (see the section on CCMs earlier in this chapter). The latter are observed in the context of inherited CCMs.

Management

Verrucous venous malformations require a wide surgical excision as they often involve the subcutis or the fascia, and the lateral extent is larger than the verrucous lesion. Recurrence follows if lesions are incompletely resected [150,151].

Maffucci syndrome

Synonyms and inclusions
- Multiple enchondromatosis, Maffucci type

Classification links
- ICD-10: Q87.4
- ICD-11: LD2F.1Y
- Snomed CT: 46041001
- MIM: 614569
- Orphanet: ORPHA163634

Introduction and general description

First described in 1881, Maffucci syndrome is characterised by multiple enchondromas associated with superficial and deep, slow-flow, venous-like malformations, containing areas with spindle cells (Figure 71.13) [152]. These lesions are called spindle cell haemangiomas. The signs and symptoms progress with time, causing grotesque deformities especially on the hands and feet. The risk for malignancy increases with age.

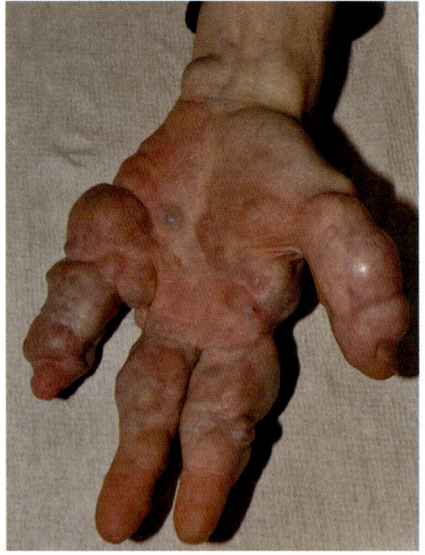

(a)

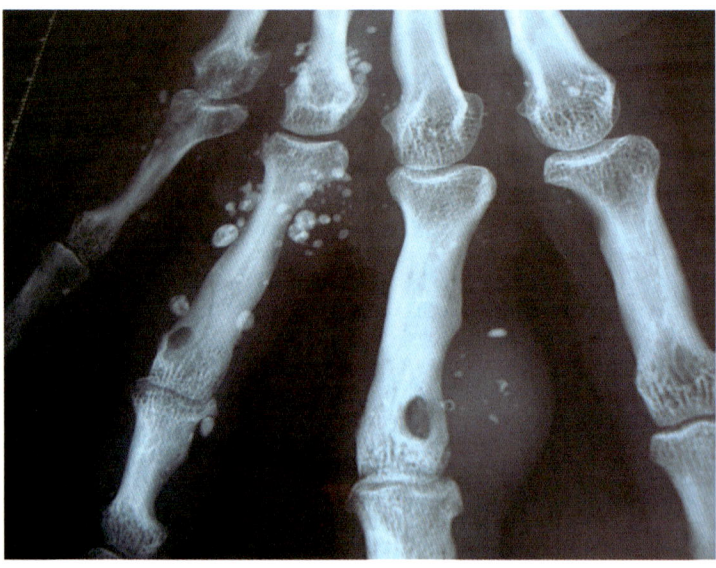

(b)

Figure 71.13 Maffucci syndrome in a 15-year-old girl with multiple enchondromas and spindle cell haemangiomas on the left hand. (a) The fourth finger has been amputated. (b) Enchondromas and phleboliths on plain radiograph.

Epidemiology

The prevalence is unknown. It is a rare disease with less than 200 cases reported. The disease appears early in life, around the age of 4–5 years, with 25% being congenital, as a mesodermal dysplasia [71]. There is no sex preponderance.

Pathophysiology

Spindle cell haemangiomas are composed of thin-walled, venous-like channels separated by spindled fibroblastic cells. Maffucci syndrome is a sporadic, non-inherited disease and germline karyotypes are usually normal. A mutation in *PTHR1* encoding the parathyroid hormone receptor 1 has been identified in the clinically similar Ollier disease but not in the Maffucci syndrome [153]. Likewise, mutations in *PTPN11* encoding the protein-tyrosine phosphatase non-receptor type 11, which are found in enchondroma patients, were not detectable in Maffucci patients [154]. In contrast, somatic mutations in *IDH1* and *IDH2* encoding isocitrate dehydrogenase 1 and 2, respectively, have been identified in enchondromas and spindle cell haemangiomas of Maffucci patients [155,156]. Seventy-seven per cent of subjects carried *IDH1* (98%) or *IDH2* (2%) mutations in their lesions; the most frequent was a p.R132C substitution in *IDH1*. *IDH1* mutations are associated with genomic hypermethylation and transcriptional downregulation of several genes. Additional genes implicated in the pathogenesis of the syndrome may reside on 2p22.3, 2q24.3 and 14q11.2, which are frequently altered in enchondromas and spindle cell haemangiomas [157].

Clinical features

The Maffucci syndrome belongs to the spectrum of enchondromatoses [158–160]. Enchondromas are hamartomatous proliferations of chondrocytes leading to an abnormal endochondral ossification of the diaphysis or metaphysis of the bones. They can appear anywhere. When bilateral, they are asymmetrical [157].

Spindle cell haemangiomas are subcutaneous, firm, bluish nodules, which usually appear around puberty on the fingers and toes (Figure 71.13) [160,161]. Patients with Maffucci syndrome have a significant risk for the appearance of skeletal and non-skeletal malignant lesions [162]. Their exact prevalence is unknown, but incidence increases with age. Enchondromas may degenerate into chondrosarcomas, and differentiation may be difficult. The appearance of pain and/or increase in volume are clues. Most chondrosarcomas are of low histological grade (1 or 2) and they are successfully treated with surgical resection [163]. Other mesodermal neoplasms associated with Maffucci syndrome include fibrosarcoma, glioma, astrocytoma, ovarian tumours, haemangiosarcoma and leukaemia [164]. A third of the tumours are non-mesodermal, such as adenocarcinoma. Therefore, special emphasis on careful and prolonged clinical follow-up and imaging studies is indicated.

Investigations

On conventional radiographs, enchondromas are radiolucent. Multiple, oval-shaped osteolytic lesions with well-defined margins in the metaphysis and/or diaphysis of the long tubular and flat bones are often seen [164–166]. Phleboliths can be observed [109]. D-dimer levels are normal in contrast to venous malformations. Histological analysis confirms the clinical diagnosis.

Management

When there is functional impairment, surgical excision of spindle cell haemangiomas and enchondromas is necessary. Malignant lesions are surgically treated as early as possible.

LYMPHATIC DISORDERS

Lymphatic anomalies comprise lymphatic malformations (LMs) and various types of lymphoedema. LMs are focal lesions; they can occur isolated or be part of a syndrome. Lymphoedema is an accumulation of lymphatic fluid in the connective tissue. Lymphoedema is divided into primary and secondary forms. The latter is caused by extrinsic factors such as infection or surgery. Primary lymphoedema can be inherited. Depending on the age of onset, primary lymphoedema can be divided into: type I, congenital lymphoedema, present at birth; type II, praecox (Meige disease), appearing after puberty; and lymphoedema tarda, appearing after the age of 35 years. More than a dozen forms with the underlying gene identified are currently known and these explain about 40% of familial cases and 10% of sporadic cases [167,168].

Lymphatic malformation

Synonyms and inclusions
- Cavernous lymphangioma
- Cystic hygroma
- Cystic lymphangioma
- Lymphangioma
- Lymphangioma circumscriptum
- Lymphangiomatosis
- Macrocystic lymphatic malformation
- Microcystic lymphatic malformation

Classification links
- ICD-10: D18.1
- Snomed CT: 234095009, 400016000
- MIM: 616843, 617300, 618773, 153100, 613480, 611944, 153200, 136352
- Orphanet: ORPHA2415

Introduction and general description

Lymphatic malformations are focal lesions composed of dilated lymphatic channels disconnected from the lymphatic system. LMs can be macrocystic, microcystic or combined (Figure 71.14). LMs occur sporadically.

Epidemiology

Lymphatic malformation is a rare disease. The exact prevalence is unknown. There is no sex preponderance.

Pathophysiology

Macrocystic LMs are composed of a single or multiple lymphatic cysts surrounded by a thick fibrous membrane. Microcystic LMs are characterised by dilated lymphatic channels with variable thickness of the walls. Blood can be seen in the spaces after intracystic bleeding or in a combined lymphatico-venous malformation. Endothelial cells express specific lymphatic markers, such as podoplanin, D2-40 and VEGFR-3 [169].

No familial case of LM has been reported. It is an isolated, sporadic disease. LMs can be seen in combined vascular malformations (e.g. lymphatico-venous malformation, capillaro-lymphatic malformation, capillaro-lymphatico-venous malformation) or as a component of a syndrome, such as Klippel–Trenaunay–Weber syndrome (capillary–lymphatico-venous malformation with overgrowth) [63,71,170,171] and CLOVES syndrome. Isolated and combined LMs are caused by somatic-activating usually hotspot mutations in *PIK3CA*, which encodes the PI3K catalytic alpha subunit. Syndromic forms of LMs, with the exception of Klippel–Trenaunay–Weber syndrome, are more commonly caused

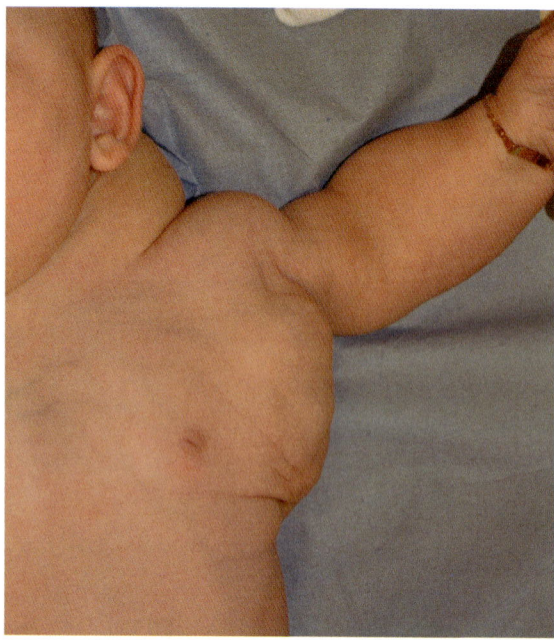

(a)

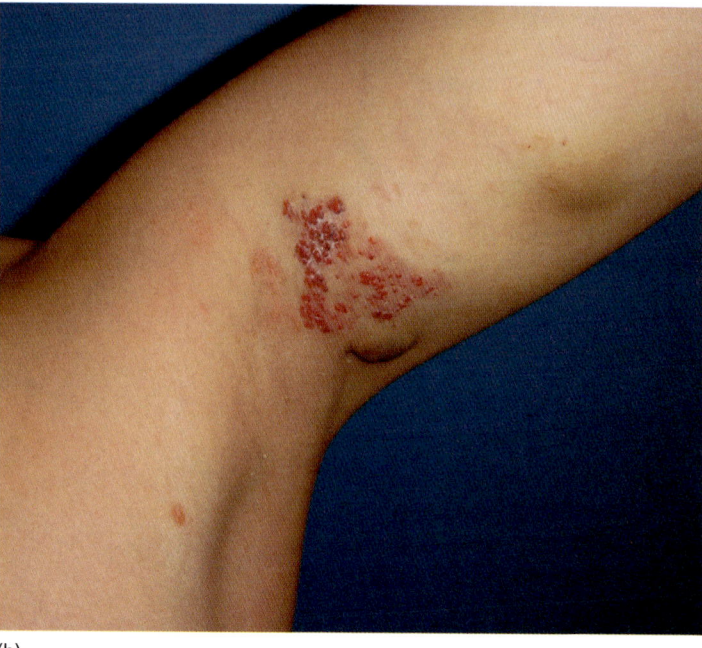

(b)

Figure 71.14 Lymphatic malformation (LM) spectrum. (a) A 10-month-old girl with extensive macrocystic/microcystic LMs of the neck, thorax and axilla. (b) Microcystic dermal and subcutaneous LM of the left arm with intracystic bleeding.

by non-hotspot *PIK3CA* mutations [28,52,172] (see the PIK3CA section earlier in this chapter). In addition, somatic mutations in the *PIK3R1* gene have recently been reported in patients with combined lymphatic malformations [39].

Clinical features

Macrocystic LMs can be diagnosed *in utero* as early as the first trimester of pregnancy [173]. They are often located on the neck, chest wall and axilla. They manifest as multilobulated, well-defined lesions that are translucent, soft, but only slightly compressible on palpation. Microcystic LMs are mostly located on the head and neck. They are ill-defined vesicular plaques, which often invade adjacent structures. The skin can be normal in colour, but becomes blue or purple when intracystic bleeding occurs (Figure 71.14). Capillaro-lymphatic malformation or angiokeratoma circumscriptum is a hyperkeratotic plaque often located on the extremity.

An LM often causes asymmetry with bone overgrowth, especially on the face. It can suddenly become painful and enlarge due to intralesional bleeding or infection. Recurrent erysipelas or cellulitis are major complications that need to be treated rapidly as they can evolve into septicaemia. Visceral LMs can cause protein-losing enteropathy and hypoalbuminaemia.

Investigations

Doppler ultrasound is the best examination to confirm the cystic nature of this slow-flow vascular malformation. In contrast to VM, the cysts cannot be completely emptied by compression and often contain echogenic debris. Microcystic LMs appear as ill-defined, echogenic, subcutaneous fat. MRI imaging with spin-echo T_1- and T_2-weighted and fat-saturation sequences depicts the anatomical relation between the vascular lesion and adjacent structures. Differential diagnosis with VM is difficult unless there are fluid–fluid levels associated with rim, septal or no contrast enhancement [110,174–177]. The two radiological examinations are mandatory for pre-therapeutic assessment of LMs and to evaluate efficacy of treatment. As extensive LMs are often combined with venous lesions, D-dimer and fibrinogen measurement is helpful to evaluate associated coagulation abnormalities.

Management

Bacterial infection should be managed with systemic antibiotics and pain medications. Sometimes, a subsequent involution of a macrocystic lesion may occur. Complete surgical excision can be proposed depending on the anatomical site and extension of the lesion. Recurrence is frequent for microcystic LMs since it is difficult to differentiate the abnormal tissue from adjacent structures. Macrocystic LMs are treated by fluid aspiration followed by percutaneous intralesional injection of a sclerosing agent by an interventional radiologist. Several sclerosing agents are available: OK-432 (extract from a killed strain of group A *Streptococcus pyogenes*) [178], doxycycline, bleomycin [179,180] and ethanol [180]. Multi-injection sclerotherapy, especially using bleomycin, is efficient for microcystic LMs. Sclerosis can be followed by fever, redness of the skin and oedema. Microcystic dermal LMs can be treated by laser by experienced physicians [181]. The unravelling of the underlying aetiopathogenic mechanisms allows the design of targeted molecular therapies. Systemic and topical rapamycin is promising in clinical trials [58,104,182–184]. Sildenafil was also reported, but its effect has not been confirmed [185].

Complicated/complex lymphatic anomalies

Synonyms and inclusions
- Generalised lymphatic anomaly (GLA)
- Gorham–Stout disease (GSD) (cystic angiomatosis of bone, diffuse)
- Kaposiform lymphangiomatosis (KLA)
- Central conducting lymphatic anomaly (CCLA)

Classification links
- ICD-10: Q28.8
- ICD-11: LA90.1Y
- Snomed CT: 703298001
- MIM: 123880 (Gorham–Stout disease), 617300 (central conduction lymphatic anomaly)
- Orphanet: ORPHA141209

Introduction and general description

Complicated lymphatic anomalies (CLAs) are a group of rare sporadic disorders, comprising generalised lymphatic anomaly (GLA), Gorham–Stout disease (GSD), kaposiform lymphangiomatosis (KLA) and central conducting lymphatic anomaly (CCLA). These are severe disorders, associated with high morbidity and mortality. The differential diagnosis and management are challenging.

Epidemiology

Complicated lymphatic anomalies are rare, and the exact prevalence is unknown. There is no sex preponderance.

Pathophysiology

Somatic mutations have recently been identified in a limited number of patients with CLA: *PIK3CA* in GLA [186], *KRAS* in GSD [187,188] *NRAS* and *CBL* in KLA [189,190] and *ARAF* in CCLA [184,186,189,191–193]. In addition, heterozygous germline kinase-dead *EPHB4* mutations have been identified in a family with CCLA [194].

Clinical features

Gorham–Stout disease or 'vanishing bone disease' is characterised by progressive destruction and resorption of bones, which are replaced by lymphatic vessels and capillaries [195,196]. It can also involve viscera and soft tissues. Depending on the location, it manifests as bone pain, spontaneous fractures, deformity, neurological deficit, pleural or pericardial effusion, ascites and cerebrospinal fluid rhinorrhoea. It is lethal in 16% of cases.

Generalised lymphatic anomaly is more widespread than GSD, affecting multiple organs and tissues (bones, lungs, mediastinum, liver, spleen, soft tissues). In contrast to GSD, the bone lesions are not associated with cortical bone resorption. Symptoms depend on the location (pleural effusion, ascites, skin involvement). Respiratory insufficiency is the major cause of morbidity and mortality.

Kaposiform lymphangiomatosis is a subtype of GLA, histologically characterised by foci of spindle-shaped, lymphatic endothelial cells (PROX1 and D2-40 positive). It is often associated with severe, life-threating coagulopathy (hypofibrinogenaemia and thrombocytopenia).

Central conducting lymphatic anomaly is characterised by dilatation and dysfunction of large lymphatic vessels, mainly leading to ascites or pleural effusion or protein-losing enteropathy. It can be associated with peripheral lymphoedema, and it can be part of GSD, GLA and KLA.

Investigations

Complicated lymphatic anomalies have overlapping features. Differential diagnosis is challenging and it might require X-rays,

MRI, CT, lymphangiography, histology (PROX1 and D2-40), coagulation studies and analysis of the fluid of pleural effusion or ascites. X-ray reveals progressive osteolysis and cortical destruction in GSD.

Genetic testing for mosaic mutations in the tissues of patients with CLA and for germline *EPHB4* in patients with CCLA can disclose the underlying cause. Genetic testing on cell-free DNA (plasma, pleural effusion, ascites) are in development.

Management

The management of patients with CLA is multidisciplinary and depends on the location and type of the lesions. Current treatments include embolisation, surgery and bisphosphonates with limited efficacy. Some clinical trials and off-label case reports have shown promising results with the mTOR inhibitor rapamycin in patients with CLA, mainly GLA [58,197,198]. The MEK inhibitor trametinib has been successfully used in some patients with CLA and a mutation in the RAS/MAPK pathway [191,193].

Schimmelpenning–Feuerstein–Mims syndrome

Synonyms and inclusions
- Schimmelpenning syndrome
- Linear sebaceous naevus syndrome
- Jadassohn naevus phakomatosis
- Epidermal naevus syndrome

Classification links
- MIM: 163200
- Orphanet: ORPHA2612

Introduction and general description

Schimmelpenning–Feuerstein–Mims (SFM) syndrome is characterised by cognitive developmental delay and naevus sebaceus (usually on the face, neck and scalp), and is associated with central nervous system, ocular, skeletal and cardiovascular anomalies. Vascular anomalies are present in more than 10% of patients [199].

Epidemiology

The SFM syndrome is rare and its exact prevalence is unknown. There is no sex preponderance.

Pathophysiology

The syndrome is due to postzygotic activating mutations in genes encoding HRAS (Harvey murine sarcoma virus oncogene) and KRAS (Kirsten rat sarcoma viral oncogene) [200]. Mutations in these genes are also found in naevus sebaceous (5% in *KRAS*, 91% in *HRAS*). The SFM syndrome belongs to the RASopathies.

Clinical features

The vascular anomalies in SFM syndrome can be arterial (aortic coarctation, aneurysm and/or stenosis of the renal and carotid arteries), capillary, lymphatic (LM, chylothorax, lymphoedema) or venous.

Investigations

Genetic analysis can help in diagnosis.

Management

The associated vascular anomalies are managed similarly to the isolated counterparts. Future targeted therapies could target the RAS signalling pathway.

PRIMARY LYMPHOEDEMAS

The primary lymphoedemas are a large group of clinically and genetically heterogeneous disorders. Only entities with primary lymphoedema as a principal feature are presented here. For a more detailed review, see Brouillard *et al*. [201].

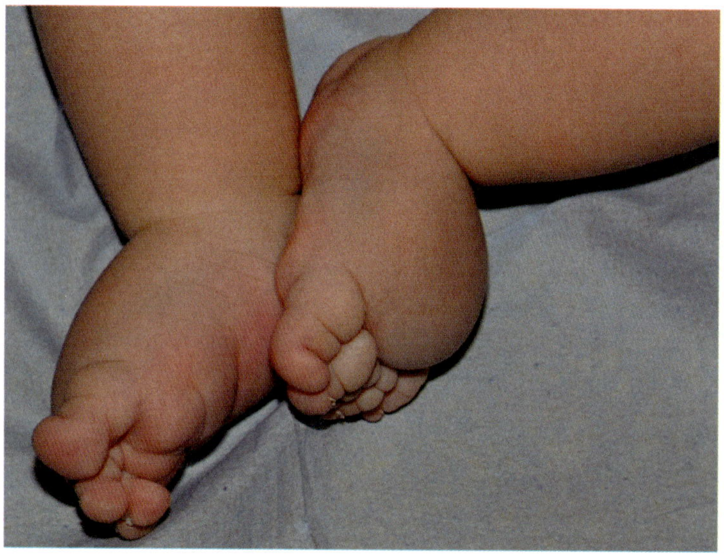

Figure 71.15 A 20-month-old boy with bilateral lymphoedema of the feet and calves.

Hereditary lymphoedema type IA

Synonyms and inclusions
- Nonne–Milroy disease

Classification links
- Snomed CT: 30213001, 399889006, 400040008
- MIM: 153100
- Orphanet: ORPHA79452

Introduction and general description

Lymphoedema, hereditary, type IA (LMPH1A) is an autosomal, dominantly inherited, congenital lymphoedema. It consists of an accumulation of lymphatic fluid in the connective tissue (Figure 71.15).

Epidemiology

The prevalence is unknown, but this is probably the most frequent form of primary lymphoedema [167]. Males and females seem to be equally affected. There is large intrafamilial variability and the penetrance is around 85–90%.

Pathophysiology

Hereditary lymphoedema type IA is caused by loss-of-function dominant mutations in *FLT4* affecting the intracellular tyrosine kinase domains of VEGFR-3 [202,203]. A homozygous recessive mutation was identified in one family [204]. Mutations in *FLT4* are identified in approximately 70% of patients.

Clinical features

Hereditary lymphoedema type IA is characterised by lower limb bilateral lymphoedema, localised below the knees, and usually present at birth (Figure 71.15). Occasionally, lymphoedema is observed prenatally. A few families with pleural effusion, chylous ascites or hydrops have been reported [204–206]. Other associated features include hydrocele, prominent veins, up-slanting toenails and papillomatosis [207]. Lymphoedema can improve spontaneously, even prenatally [208]. Patients with mutations in *VEGFC* (LMPH1D) have similar signs and symptoms.

Investigations

Genetic investigations are useful tools for primary lymphoedema and give a definite diagnosis when a mutation is identified. In selected patients, invasive and non-invasive imaging techniques can be required to diagnose the type of lymphatic pathology and guide the interventions when possible/necessary. Lymphoscintigraphy is preferred to lymphography in the investigation of lymphoedema. Nevertheless, even if there are differences in the uptake of the radioactive tracer patterns, they are usually not discriminative. However, in LMPH1A, a lack of uptake of the tracer is seen, suggesting lymphatic aplasia/hypoplasia or peripheral malfunction, whereas in lymphoedema–distichiasis (see next section), lymphatic hyperplasia is present [207,209]. Additional techniques exist and are used in specialised centres, such as non-contrast-enhanced or dynamic contrast-enhanced magnetic resonance lymphangiography and CT [201].

Other forms of hereditary primary lymphoedema

Apart from LMPH1A, other forms of autosomal dominant or recessive primary lymphoedemas have been described.

1 Hereditary lymphoedema type IB (MIM: 611944) is mapped to chromosome 6q16.2-q22.1. It is an autosomal dominant disorder characterised by lower leg lymphoedema starting in childhood, and improving in adulthood.
2 Hereditary lymphoedema type IC (MIM: 613480) is an autosomal dominant disorder caused by heterozygous mutations in *GJC2* encoding Cx47 [210,211]. The penetrance is incomplete.

The onset of lymphoedema is in childhood or adolescence, and later in males than in females [210]. All four extremities can be affected. Other associated features are ptosis, cellulitis and venous insufficiency; recurrent skin infections are common.

3 Hereditary lymphoedema type ID (MIM: 615907), also known as Nonne–Milroy-like lymphoedema, is an autosomal dominant disorder characterised by a neonatal or very early onset lymphoedema of the lower legs, associated with dysplastic toenails, leg papillomatosis and hyperkeratosis. Exome sequencing led to the identification of heterozygous mutations in *VEGFC* [212,213]. This gene encodes one of the ligands of VEGFR-3.

4 Hereditary lymphoedema type II (MIM: 153200; ORPHA: 90186), also known as Meige lymphoedema or lymphoedema praecox, features late onset (puberty) of lymphoedema predominantly involving the lower extremities, but also the face and upper limbs.

5 Hereditary lymphoedema type III (MIM: 616843) is an autosomal recessive disorder caused by biallelic homozygous or compound heterozygous mutations in the *PIEZO1* gene. The disorder is characterised by generalised lymphatic dysplasia with systemic involvement: pleural and pericardial effusion, ascites and intestinal and/or pulmonary lymphangiectasia. The onset is prenatally, with a high incidence of non-immune hydrops fetalis, or during childhood [214].

6 Primary lymphoedema caused by *ANGPT2* mutation (MIM: 619369) is an autosomal dominant disorder characterised by congenital lymphoedema in the lower extremities. The upper extremities can also be involved. Hydrocele is frequent in boys. The lymphoedema can improve spontaneously. The penetrance is incomplete [215].

Management

Lymphoedema patients are followed in specialised clinics [**201**]. The management is symptomatic. Elastic garments and manual lymphatic drainage are the gold standard approaches. Cellulitis and recurrent cellulitis are treated with appropriate antibiotics and prophylactic antibiotics, respectively. Lymphatico-venous micro-anastomosis has been beneficial in some patients [216]. Suction-assisted lipectomy in combination with postoperative elastic compression can be helpful [217]. Understanding the molecular mechanisms at the origin of the different subtypes of primary lymphoedema is an important step in developing targeted therapies in the future. Genetic counselling is needed.

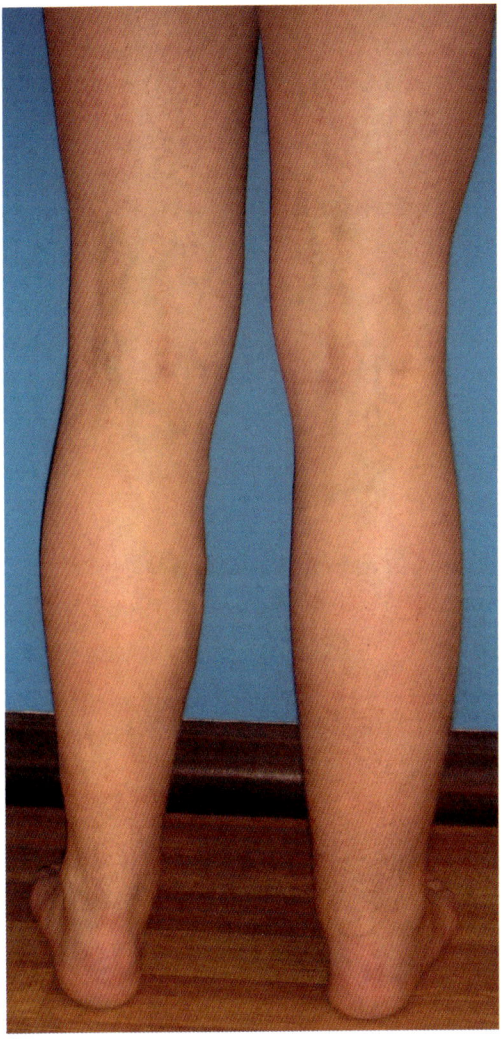

(a)

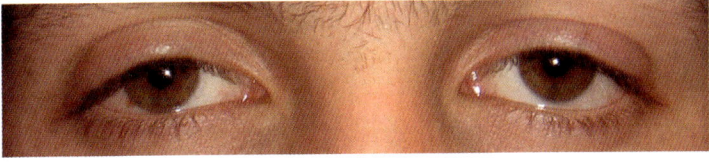

(b)

Figure 71.16 A patient with *FOXC2* mutation and (a) bilateral lymphoedema of the lower extremities (right leg more affected) and (b) bilateral ptosis.

Lymphoedema–distichiasis syndrome

Classification links
- MIM: 153400
- Orphanet: ORPHA33001

Introduction and general description

Autosomal dominant lymphoedema–distichiasis syndrome is characterised by late-onset lower limb lymphoedema associated with double rows of eyelashes from the meibomian glands (distichiasis) (Figure 71.16). Lymphoedema–distichiasis syndrome seems to be allelic with several inherited forms of lymphoedema including hereditary lymphoedema type II, lymphoedema and ptosis and the yellow nail syndrome [218].

Epidemiology

The prevalence is unknown and there is important intrafamilial variability. After LMPH1A, lymphoedema–distichiasis is the primary lymphoedema with the most frequently identified genetic cause. Males seem to develop symptoms earlier than females [209].

Pathophysiology

Lymphoedema–distichiasis and yellow nail syndrome are caused by loss-of-function mutations in *FOXC2* encoding the forkhead box C2 transcription factor [218,219]. FOXC2 acts downstream of the VEGFC/VEGFR-3 complex. *FOXC2* is regulated by GATA2, and it regulates the expression of connexin CX47/GJC2 and KIF11 [**168**]. FOXC2 is important for valve development in the collecting lymphatics [220].

Clinical features

Usually lymphoedema develops around puberty, but early presentation as hydrops fetalis is possible [208]. The distichiasis has a high penetrance and is a clue to diagnosis. When symptomatic, distichiasis can cause corneal irritation, infection and photophobia. Other associated features are varicose veins, cardiac malformations, cleft palate, ptosis and yellow nails [209,218].

Investigations and management

See the section on LMPH1A earlier in this chapter.

Hypotrichosis–lymphoedema–telangiectasia syndrome

Synonyms and inclusions
- Hypotrichosis–lymphoedema–telangiectasia–renal defect syndrome

Classification links
- MIM: 607823
- Orphanet: ORPHA69735

Introduction and general description

This syndrome is an autosomal dominant or recessive disorder with onset in childhood or puberty.

Epidemiology

It is very rare with only a few families reported [221–223].

Pathophysiology

Hypotrichosis–lymphoedema–telangiectasia syndrome is caused by recessive or dominant mutations in *SOX18* encoding a transcription factor [221]. A particular stop codon mutation (p.C240*) in *SOX18* causes severe glomerulonephritis, leading to end-stage renal disease necessitating renal transplantation [222]. SOX18 regulates PROX1 expression and thus is a major regulator of lymphangiogenesis [**168**].

Clinical features

The disorder is characterised by lymphoedema in the lower extremities, which develops during childhood or at puberty, sparse hair, absent eyelashes and eyebrows, and telangiectasias in the palms, soles, scalp and scrotum [221]. Renal malfunction is associated with a specific mutation [222]. Hydrops fetalis can occur [221].

Investigations and management

See the section on LMPH1A earlier in this chapter. Patients with the dominant premature stop codon mutation should be specifically monitored for renal function.

Hennekam lymphangiectasia–lymphoedema syndrome

Synonyms and inclusions
- Lymphoedema–lymphangiectasia–mental retardation syndrome
- Lymphoedema–intestinal lymphangiectasia–intellectual disability syndrome

Classification links
- MIM: 235510, 616006, 618154
- Orphanet: not listed

Introduction and general description

This syndrome is an autosomal recessive, generalised, lymphatic dysplasia characterised by intestinal lymphangiectasias associated with severe and progressive lymphoedema of the limbs, genitalia and face. Intellectual deficit can be observed [224].

Epidemiology

The prevalence is unknown.

Pathophysiology

Hennekam lymphangiectasia–lymphoedema syndrome is caused by homozygous or compound heterozygous mutations in *CCBE1* (encoding collagen and calcium-binding EGF domain 1) [225] or *FAT4* (encoding homologue of *Drosophila* FAT tumor suppressor 4) [226] or *ADAMTS3* (ADAM metallopeptidase with thrombospondin type 1 motif 3) [105]. Compound heterozygous *CCBE1* mutations have also been identified in patients with generalised lymphatic dysplasia, without other features of the Hennekam lymphangiectasia–lymphoedema syndrome [227]. CCBE1 regulates lymphangiogenesis via ADAMTS3 and VEGFC activation [228].

Clinical features

Hennekam lymphangiectasia–lymphoedema syndrome is characterised by generalised lymphatic dysplasia, distinct facial features (flat face, low nasal bridge, hypertelorism, epicanthal folds, small mouth) and dental and ear anomalies. This may mimic Down syndrome. Syndactyly, camptodactyly, craniosynostosis, hypothyroidism and ectopic kidney may be present. Hydrops fetalis can occur [229].

Investigations and management

See the section on LMPH1A earlier in this chapter. Protein-losing enteropathy secondary to intestinal lymphangiectasias is treated with careful nutritional management, including fat restriction, medium-chain triglyceride supplementation or parenteral nutrition [230]. Octreotide administration may be helpful [231]. Surgical ligation of leaky channels, if visible, can be tried [232].

Microcephaly with or without chorioretinopathy, lymphoedema and mental retardation

Synonyms and inclusions
- Microcephaly, lymphoedema and chorioretinal dysplasia syndrome
- Microcephaly and chorioretinopathy with or without mental retardation

Classification links
- MIM: 152950
- Orphanet: ORPHA2526

Introduction and general description

Microcephaly with or without chorioretinopathy, lymphoedema and mental retardation (MCLMR) is an autosomal dominant disorder with incomplete penetrance and intrafamilial variable expressivity. Lymphoedema is inconstant.

Epidemiology

The prevalence is unknown.

Pathophysiology

This syndrome is caused by heterozygous mutations in *KIF11* encoding kinesin family member 11 [172,233]. *KIF11* expression is regulated by FOXC2. KIF11 is involved in microtubule activity. The pathophysiological mechanisms underlying the phenotypic expression of *KIF11* mutations are unknown.

Clinical features

When lymphoedema is present it is usually congenital and confined to the lower limbs with or without dilated veins. Microcephaly is congenital and present in over 90% of patients and varies from mild to severe; there is also cognitive delay, present in two-thirds of patients [172,233]. The most frequent eye finding is chorioretinopathy, present in two-thirds of patients. Distinct facial features can be present: prominent ears, up-slanting palpebral fissures, broad nose with a rounded tip, long philtrum, thin upper lip and prominent chin [172].

Investigations and management

See the section on LMPH1A earlier in this chapter

Choanal atresia and lymphoedema

Classification links
- MIM: 613611
- Orphanet: ORPHA99141

Introduction and general description

Choanal atresia and lymphoedema is a very rare autosomal recessive disorder characterised by onset in childhood [234].

Epidemiology

One family has been reported.

Pathophysiology

In a large consanguineous pedigree with lymphoedema and choanal atresia, autozygosity mapping and analysis of potential candidate genes led to the identification of a 2 kb genomic deletion. This deletion includes exon 7 of the *PTPN14* gene encoding the protein tyrosine phosphatase non-receptor-type 14 (PTPN14) [234]. PTPN14 interacts with VEGFR3, and probably regulates the activity of the receptor complex.

Clinical features

Choanal atresia and lymphoedema is a very rare autosomal recessive disorder characterised by choanal atresia and lower limb lymphoedema sometimes associated with pericardial effusion and pectus excavatum [234].

Investigations and management

See the section on LMPH1A earlier in this chapter.

Primary lymphoedema with myelodysplasia

Synonyms and inclusions
- Emberger syndrome

Classification links
- MIM: 614038
- Orphanet: ORPHA3226

Introduction and general description

This is an autosomal dominant disorder.

Epidemiology

Primary lymphoedema with myelodysplasia is a very rare syndrome with only a few families reported.

Pathophysiology

It is caused by loss-of-function heterozygous mutations in the transcription factor gene *GATA2* [211,235]. GATA2 is highly expressed in lymphatic valves and regulates FOXC2 expression.

Clinical features

It is characterised by lymphoedema in the lower extremities and genitalia, occurring during childhood. The patients are at risk of congenital deafness, immune dysfunction, cellulitis, myelodysplasia and acute myeloid leukaemia [183].

Investigations and management

See the section on LMPH1A earlier in this chapter. Periodic follow-up is needed for early detection of myelodysplasia.

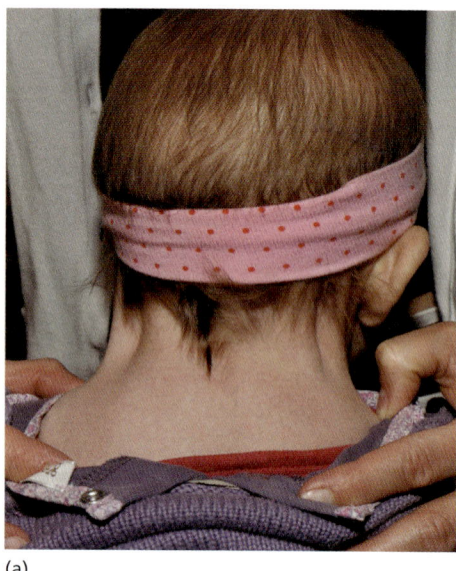
(a)

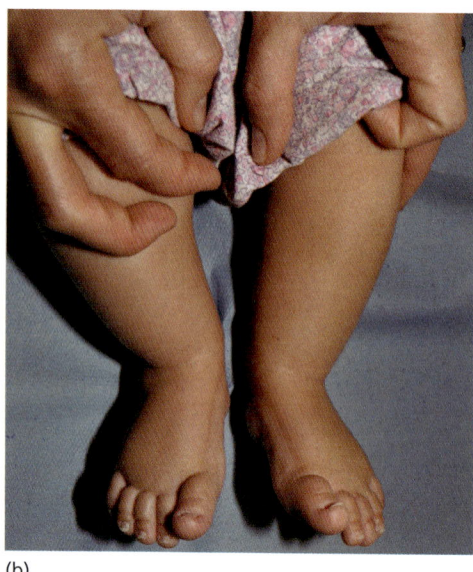
(b)

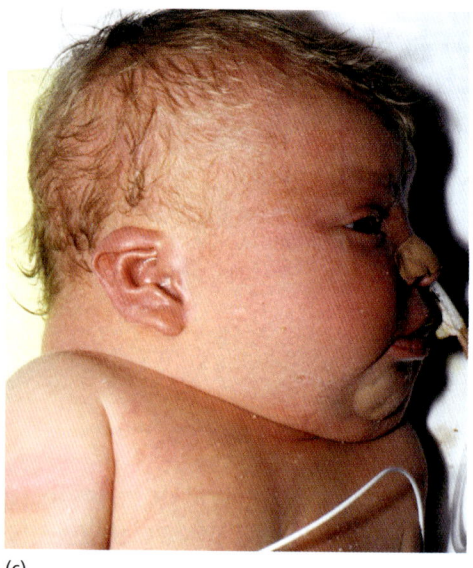
(c)

Figure 71.17 Other syndromes with lymphoedema. (a, b) A 7-month-old girl with Turner syndrome showing nuchal webs (a) and right foot lymphoedema (b). (c) A newborn with Noonan syndrome and cervico-facial oedema.

Other syndromes with lymphoedema

Lymphoedema can be observed in many syndromes. It can be localised or generalised, prenatal and/or postnatal, and with high variability even among patients with the same syndrome. Often there are other, more specific, features that orientate toward the diagnosis, as in Turner syndrome (Figure 71.17a, b), Noonan syndrome (Figure 71.17c), Costello syndrome and cardio-facio-cutaneous syndrome.

Conclusions

There are numerous disorders that affect the cutaneous vasculature. The adoption of the biological classification for vascular anomalies has helped differentiate various entities. This has enabled genetic studies on their aetiopathogenesis, and led to the identification of several genes that are mutated in the inherited forms. Moreover, somatic changes have been identified as the cause for isolated, non-hereditary vascular malformations. The surge of next generation sequencing (exomes or targeted) has further empowered these genetic analyses, and make an efficient and relatively fast panel approach possible for diagnostic testing.

Many of the disorders have an intrinsic vascular endothelial dysfunction due to a genetic mutation. Most of these are now known, and the signalling pathways in which they are involved, although we still lack understanding of the detailed molecular mechanisms that lead from the causative mutations to the disease. Yet this basic knowledge has allowed us to start to generate animal models and to test molecular therapies using drugs that have been developed for other disorders, but which target the pathways also implicated in vascular anomalies. The receptor tyrosine kinases seem to be central, along with their downstream signalling pathways, including PI3K/AKT and RAS/ERK. Several molecules that are able to modulate the activity of these pathways exist, and thus there is hope for the not-too-distant development of novel therapies.

Key references

The full list of references can be found in the online version at https://www.wiley.com/rooksdermatology10e

18 Revencu N, Boon LM, Mendola A *et al*. RASA1 mutations and associated phenotypes in 68 families with capillary malformation-arteriovenous malformation. *Hum Mutat* 2013;34:1632–41.
51 Kurek KC, Luks VL, Ayturk UM *et al*. Somatic mosaic activating mutations in PIK3CA cause CLOVES syndrome. *Am J Hum Genet* 2012;90:1108–15.
89 Shovlin CL. Hereditary haemorrhagic telangiectasia: pathophysiology, diagnosis and treatment. *Blood Rev* 2010;24:203–19.
100 Tan WH, Baris HN, Burrows PE *et al*. The spectrum of vascular anomalies in patients with PTEN mutations: implications for diagnosis and management. *J Med Genet* 2007;44:594–602.
111 Vikkula M, Boon LM, Carraway KL *et al*. Vascular dysmorphogenesis caused by an activating mutation in the receptor tyrosine kinase TIE2. *Cell* 1996;87:1181–90.
112 Limaye N, Wouters V, Uebelhoer M *et al*. Somatic mutations in angiopoietin receptor gene TEK cause solitary and multiple sporadic venous malformations. *Nat Genet* 2009;41:118–24.
137 Brouillard P, Boon LM, Mulliken JB *et al*. Mutations in a novel factor, glomulin, are responsible for glomuvenous malformations ("glomangiomas"). *Am J Hum Genet* 2002;70:866–74.
138 Brouillard P, Ghassibe M, Penington A *et al*. Four common glomulin mutations cause two thirds of glomuvenous malformations ("familial glomangiomas"): evidence for a founder effect. *J Med Genet* 2005;42:e13.
140 Boon LM, Brouillard P, Irrthum A *et al*. A gene for inherited cutaneous venous anomalies ("glomangiomas") localizes to chromosome 1p21-22. *Am J Hum Genet* 1999;65:125–33.
141 Brouillard P, Boon LM, Revencu N *et al*. Genotypes and phenotypes of 162 families with a glomulin mutation. *Mol Syndromol* 2013;4:157–64.
148 Sirvente J, Enjolras O, Wassef M *et al*. Frequency and phenotypes of cutaneous vascular malformations in a consecutive series of 417 patients with familial cerebral cavernous malformations. *J Eur Acad Dermatol Venereol* 2009;23:1066–72.
168 Brouillard P, Boon LB, Vikkula M. Genetics of lymphatic anomalies. *J Clin Invest* 2014;124:898–904.
201 Brouillard P, Witte MH, Erickson RP *et al*. Primary lymphoedema. *Nat Rev Dis Primers* 2021;7:77.

CHAPTER 72

Genetic Disorders of Adipose Tissue

George W. M. Millington

Dermatology Department, Norfolk and Norwich University Hospital, Norwich, UK

PART 6: GENETIC DISORDERS

Introduction

Subcutaneous fat consists of white (WAT), brown (BAT) and beige adipose tissue, as well as capillaries, which facilitate its metabolic functions [1]. In adults, it comprises almost entirely WAT, where its functions include insulation, energy storage and secretion of regulatory peptides called adipokines [1–4]. Adipokine secretion varies according to adipose tissue type, distribution and energy status, with diverse paracrine and endocrine effects on metabolic and immune functions [1–4]. Adipose tissue disorders are therefore associated with cardiometabolic, inflammatory and malignant diseases [1–5].

BAT also secretes adipokines, but its main functions include fatty acid metabolism and thermogenesis [1]. BAT is most detectable in the neonate, but adults also have small distinct BAT deposits in their upper body subcutaneous fat, which are thought to be metabolically important [1]. Beige adipose tissue describes adipocytes that possess functional similarities to BAT, but are dispersed amongst WAT [1,6]. Beige adipocytes are derived from white adipocyte progenitors, and an increased ratio of beige adipose tissue to WAT contributes to a favourable metabolic profile [6].

Disorders of adipose tissue can be divided principally into disorders of distribution of fat, the lipodystrophies [7], lipoedema [8] and adipose hyperplasia [9]; disorders of excess generalised accumulation of fat, in other words obesity [10], and tumours [11]; and finally inflammation, such as panniculitis [12,13]. There is increasing evidence of a hereditary component in the pathogenesis of all of these conditions [7–13].

CONGENITAL (FAMILIAL) LIPODYSTROPHIES

Lipodystrophies are characterised by selective loss of adipose tissue at various anatomical sites [1,2]. The reduced adipocyte storage capacity causes excess triglycerides to accumulate within the blood, liver and muscles [1,2]. The resultant metabolic complications of lipodystrophy include dyslipidaemia, hepatic steatosis and insulin resistance [1–3]. Serum leptin levels decrease in association with lipodystrophies, which causes hyperphagia, and may exacerbate the metabolic complications [1]. Additionally, the cosmetic appearance of lipodystrophy frequently causes psychological distress [4]. Management strategies include lifestyle modification, antidiabetic medication and metreleptin, a recombinant human leptin analogue [1,5–7].

Lipodystrophies are classified according to their pattern of fat loss, which may vary from localised involvement to near complete absence of adipose tissue [1,2], as well as their aetiopathogenesis. Acquired lipodystrophies are discussed in Chapter 98. Inherited lipodystrophies include the congenital generalised lipodystrophies (CGLs) and familial partial lipodystrophies (FPLs), as well as a number of additional syndromes where lipodystrophy is a variable feature within a complex phenotype. Some patients with inherited lipodystrophies do not have any of these defined mutations or exact clinical phenotypes, and their pathogenesis remains uncertain [8,9].

CONGENITAL GENERALISED LIPODYSTROPHIES

The CGLs (Beradinelli–Seip syndrome) are a group of rare autosomal recessive conditions that first present in neonates [1,2]. The phenotype is characterised by a virtual absence of subcutaneous and visceral adipose tissue, distinctive muscular appearance and prominent veins (Figure 72.1) [1,8]. Mechanical adipose tissue of the palms, soles, orbits, scalp and joints is usually spared, but it is deficient in CGL2 [8]. This severe lack of metabolically active adipose tissue results in childhood-onset metabolic complications, including hypertriglyceridaemia, hepatic steatosis, palpable hepatosplenomegaly and acanthosis nigricans [2,8]. Type 2 diabetes develops during adolescence or early adulthood [1,8]. Focal

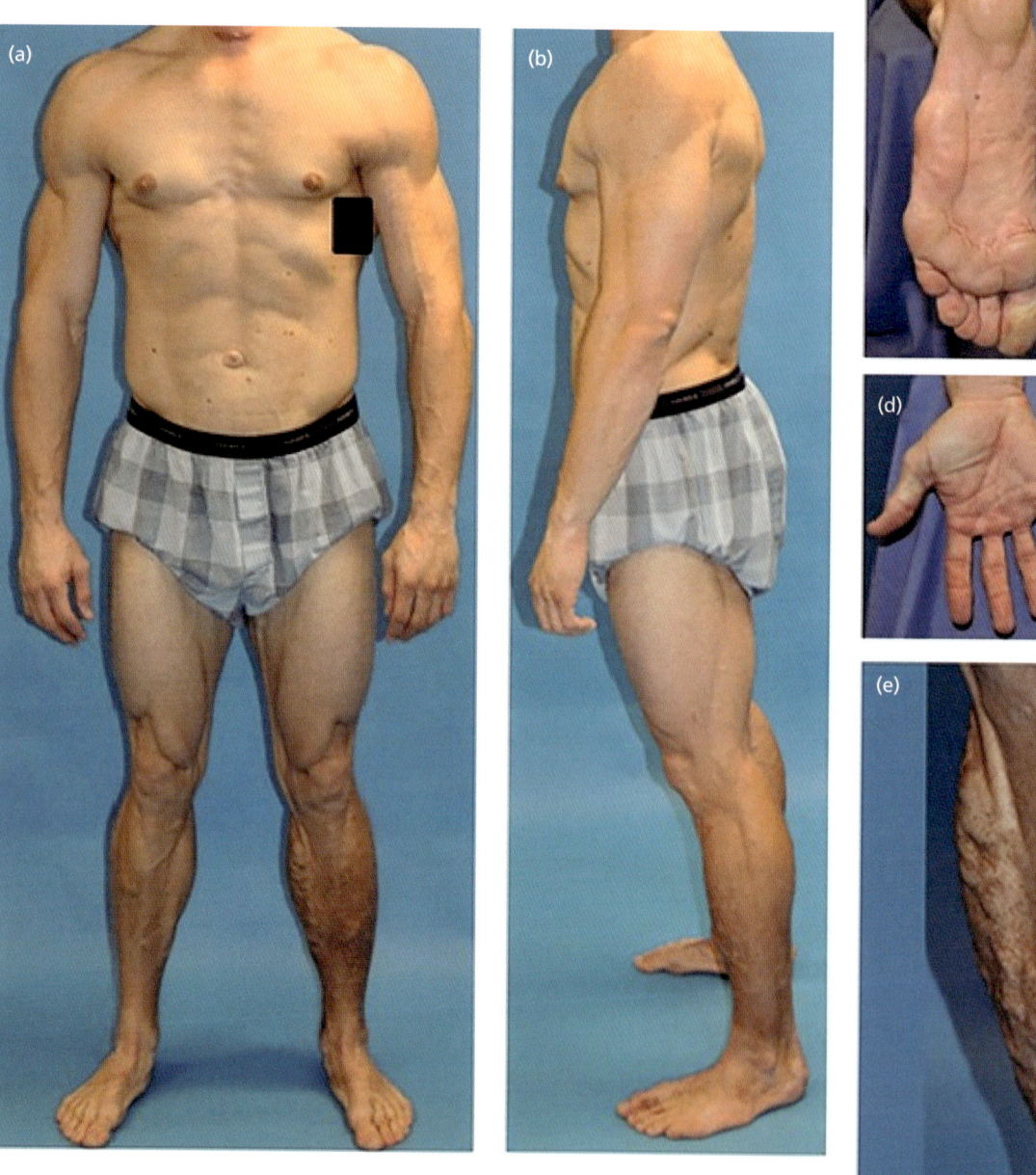
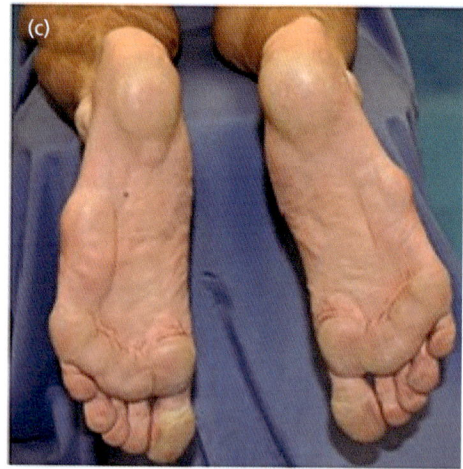
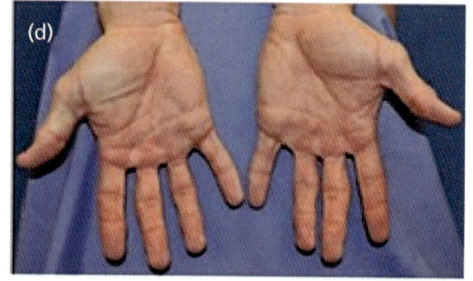
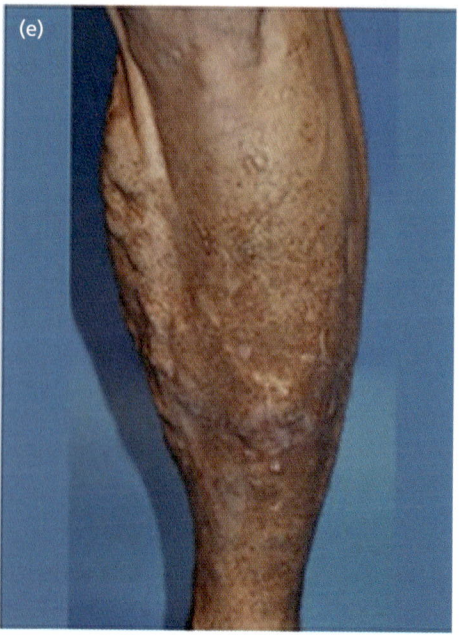

Figure 72.1 A patient with a heterozygous missense *LMNA* mutation affecting lamin C showing (a, b) generalised loss of subcutaneous fat and muscular prominence, including involvement of the soles (c) and palms (d) with prominent veins on the lower leg (e). Reproduced from Patni *et al.* 2017 [13] with permission of John Wiley & Sons.

Table 72.1 Congenital generalised lipodystrophies.

Syndrome	Mode of inheritance	Gene	Gene function	Clinical summary	MIM
CGL1	AR	AGPAT2	Encodes an enzyme which catalyses triglyceride and phospholipid synthesis within adipocytes	Generalised lipodystrophy, metabolic complications, focal lytic lesions in long bones, pseudoacromegalic features	608594
CGL2	AR	BSCL2	Encodes seipin with a function in lipid droplet formation within preadipocytes, neurons and testes	Generalised lipodystrophy, including loss of palmoplantar fat, metabolic complications, intellectual disability, hypertrophic cardiomyopathy, teratozoospermia	269700
CGL3	AR	CAV1	Encodes caveolin-1, the main structural component of caveolae, which are plasma membrane invaginations involved in signal transduction and lipid trafficking	Generalised lipodystrophy, metabolic complications, vitamin D resistance, hypocalcaemia, short stature	612526
CGL4	AR	CAVIN1	Encodes caveolae-associated protein 1 involved in the biogenesis of caveolae in adipocytes and muscle cells	Generalised lipodystrophy, metabolic complications, congenital myopathy, cervical spine instability, cardiac arrhythmias, pyloric stenosis	613327

AR, autosomal recessive.

lytic lesions in the long bones represent defective bone marrow fat production, and cause an increased risk of pathological fractures [8]. Affected adolescents may develop pseudoacromegalic features with enlargement of the mandible, hands and feet [1,2,8]. Women with CGL may develop hirsutism, clitoromegaly, polycystic ovarian syndrome and infertility [1,8]. Men with CGL usually have normal fertility but spermatogenesis may be impaired [8]. The genetic basis and pathophysiology of these disorders are provided in Table 72.1. For example in CGL2, the abnormal gene is seipin [9].

FAMILIAL PARTIAL LIPODYSTROPHIES

The FPLs mostly demonstrate autosomal dominant inheritance (Table 72.2), and present in childhood or early adulthood with unevenly distributed adipose tissue [1,2]. In contrast to CGL, body fat distribution is normal during infancy and early childhood [10,11]. FPLs are characterised by the gradual loss of adipose tissue, usually from the limbs [10,11,12]. The face, neck and trunk are variably affected, and FPLs can be associated with paradoxical accumulation of fat at these sites [10,11,12], which may cause confusion with Cushing syndrome [1,2]. FPL is thought to be underrecognised in males due to physiological sex differences in body fat distribution and muscularity [1,2]. As for CGLs, metabolic complications include hypertriglyceridaemia, hepatic steatosis, insulin resistance and type 2 diabetes [9]. Acanthosis nigricans tends to be milder than in CGL [9]. Females with FPL are reported to be at higher risk of metabolic complications and atherosclerotic cardiovascular disease than men [2]. Details regarding the genetic basis and pathophysiology of these disorders can be found in Table 72.2.

OTHER INHERITED LIPODYSTROPHIES

Lipodystrophy is a recognised feature within the phenotype of a number of other syndromes, which are outlined in Table 72.3.

These other inherited lipodystrophy syndromes demonstrate varied inheritance and fat distribution, may not necessarily be associated with the metabolic complications of CGL and FPL, and display additional multisystemic features [1]. The premature ageing disorders (Chapter 77) account for a significant proportion of these other inherited lipodystrophies [13–27].

HEREDITARY OBESITY

Obesity is a serious public health concern [1]. Adipose hyperplasia and hypertrophy cause dysregulated adipokine production, which contributes to cardiovascular disease, metabolic disease, musculoskeletal disorders, certain cancers, Alzheimer disease and dermatological conditions [1,2,3]. Altered gut and skin microbiomes may also contribute to obesity-associated disease, with increased skin-resident *Corynebacterium* shown to promote cutaneous inflammation [4,5].

Primary obesity results from complex gene–environment interactions [6]. There is growing acknowledgement of genetic influence in the development of obesity, especially where the onset is in childhood [3,6–8]. In the majority of cases, this represents polygenic susceptibility, but obesity can also result from single-gene disorders, which may present with obesity alone [3,7,8]. However, more often than not, they display other clinical features. Some of these syndromes have a clear dermatological phenotype [3,7,8].

MONOGENIC OBESITY WITHOUT CUTANEOUS FEATURES

Certain rare monogenic human obesity syndromes exist that do not have primary cutaneous features (Table 72.4) [3,7,8]. However, affected individuals are likely to develop the secondary consequences of obesity, including skin problems (Box 72.1) [1,2].

Table 72.2 Familial partial lipodystrophies.

Syndrome	Mode of inheritance	Gene	Gene function	Clinical summary	MIM
FPL1 (Kobberling type)	AD	Unknown	Unknown	Lipoatrophy: limbs, buttocks Lipohypertrophy: trunk, face, neck Metabolic complications	608600
FPL2 (Dunnigan type)	AD	LMNA	Encodes lamin A/C, which are intermediate filament proteins that provide structural integrity to the nuclear envelope; mutations cause adipocyte apoptosis	Lipoatrophy: limbs, trunk Lipohypertrophy: face, neck, labia majora Metabolic complications There may be associated features of other laminopathies including cardiomyopathy, skeletal myopathy and neuropathies	151660
FPL3	AD	PPARG	Encodes perixisome proliferator-activated receptor-gamma, which is a transcription factor that facilitates adipocyte differentiation	Lipoatrophy (milder than FPL2): limbs, buttocks Trunk, face and neck are unaffected or demonstrate mild fat reduction Metabolic complications	604367
FPL4	AD	PLIN1	Encodes perilipin, which is a phosphoprotein that assembles lipid droplets for storage	Lipoatrophy: lower limbs, buttocks, sometimes trunk Face and neck unaffected Metabolic complications Muscular hypertrophy Small adipocytes, adipose fibrosis	613877
FPL5	AR	CIDEC	Encodes cell death-inducing DNA fragmentation factor-like effector C; mutations cause adipocyte apoptosis	Lipoatrophy: lower limbs, buttocks Face, neck and trunk unaffected Metabolic complications Multiple small lipid droplets within adipocytes	615238
FPL6	AR	LIPE	Encodes lipase E, which is a hormone-sensitive enzyme that mediates lipolysis of triglycerides to free fatty acids	Lipoatrophy: lower limbs Lipohypertrophy: back, triceps, axillae, neck Metabolic complications Proximal myopathy Hypopigmented cutaneous lesions	615980
FPLD7	AD	CAV1	Encodes caveolin-1, the main structural component of caveolae, which are plasma membrane invaginations involved in signal transduction and lipid trafficking	Lipodystrophy: all sites except buttocks, palms, soles Absence of hypertriglyceridaemia and insulin resistance Thin skin with prominent vessels, sparse hair, triangular face, mandibular hypoplasia, thin nose, cataracts, ataxia, neuropathy	606721

AD, autosomal dominant; AR, autosomal recessive.

Box 72.1 Secondary skin complications of primary obesity

- Striae
- Poor wound healing
- Cutaneous infection
- Lymphovascular disorders and ulceration
- Hyperandrogenism and hirsutism
- Psoriasis
- Atopic eczema
- Keratosis pilaris
- Irritant contact dermatitis
- Skin cancer
- Hidradenitis suppurativa
- Scleredema
- Livedo reticularis
- Pilonidal sinus
- Skin changes associated with diabetes

MONOGENIC OBESITY WITH CUTANEOUS FEATURES

Rare monogenic obesity syndromes with primary cutaneous features are summarised in Table 72.5 [3]. Deficiency in the pro-opiomelanocortin (POMC) pathway and Prader–Willi syndrome (PWS) are discussed here as specific examples.

Pro-opiomelanocortin and prohormone convertase deficiency

The gene POMC, which encodes pro-opiomelanocortin, and PCSK1, which encodes prohormone convertase 1 (PC1), are involved in

Table 72.3 Other inherited lipodystrophies.

Syndrome	Mode of inheritance	Gene	Gene function	Clinical summary	MIM
MAD type A	AR	LMNA	Encodes lamin A/C which are intermediate filament proteins that provide structural integrity to the nuclear envelope	Bone abnormalities: mandibular and clavicular hypoplasia, thin beaked nose, acro-osteolysis, dental crowding, delayed dentition, late closure of cranial sutures, joint stiffness. Skin abnormalities: atrophy, prominent vessels, mottled hyperpigmentation, alopecia. Partial lipodystrophy similar to FPL2 and metabolic complications	248370
MAD type B	AR	ZMPSTE24	Encodes a zinc metalloproteinase involved in processing and maturation of lamin A	Bone and skin abnormalities as for MAD type A. Generalised lipodystrophy and metabolic complications. Focal segmental glomerulosclerosis	608612
MDPL syndrome	AD	POLD1	Encodes polymerase delta 1, which provides the catalytic and proofreading functions of DNA polymerase delta	Mandibular hypoplasia, sensorineural deafness, progeroid features, partial lipodystrophy, insulin resistance, dyslipidaemia	615381
Hutchinson–Gilford progeria syndrome	AD	LMNA	Mutations alter splicing and delete the cleavage site required to convert prelamin A to mature lamin A. Accumulated abnormal prelamin A (progerin) disrupts nuclear integrity	Short stature, low body weight, lipodystrophy (partial or generalised), alopecia, scleroderma-like skin, midface hypoplasia, micrognathia, joint contractures, osteolysis, insulin resistance, atherosclerosis, cardiovascular disease	176670
Atypical progeroid syndrome	AD	LMNA	As above	Progeroid features, but late onset. Variable lipodystrophy	–
Wiedemann–Rautenstrauch syndrome	AR	POLR3A	Encodes a subunit of RNA polymerase III	Progeroid features, variable lipodystrophy, short stature, hypotonia	264090
Werner syndrome	AR	RECQL2	Encodes a member of the RECQ family of DNA helicases involved in telomere maintenance	Progeroid features, partial lipodystrophy, premature bilateral cataracts, osteoporosis, diabetes mellitus, atherosclerosis, neoplasms	277700
Ruijs–Aalfs syndrome	AR	SPRTN	Encodes a molecular regulator for DNA repair	Progeroid features, generalised lipodystrophy, early-onset hepatocellular carcinoma	616086
Keppen–Lubinsky syndrome	AD	KCNJ6	Encodes an ATP-sensitive K+ channel linking cellular metabolism to electrical excitability of the plasma membrane	Intellectual disability, hypertonia, hyperreflexia, generalised lipodystrophy, microcephaly, large prominent eyes, aged facial appearance	614098
SHORT syndrome	AD	PIK3R1	Encodes the regulatory subunit of phosphaditylinositol 3-kinase influencing PI3K/AKT/mTOR signalling	Triangular face, prominent forehead, hypoplastic nasal alae, ocular depression, progeroid features, short stature, lipodystrophy (partial or generalised), insulin resistance but no hypertriglyceridaemia, thin skin, prominent vessels, delayed dentition, iris hypoplasia, hyperextensibility, inguinal hernia, hearing loss, cardiac malformation	269880
Pentinnen syndrome	AD	PDGFRB	Encodes the tyrosine kinase receptor platelet-derived growth factor beta	Epidermal and dermal atrophy, lipoatrophy, hypertrophic scars, thin hair, underdeveloped malae, acro-osteolysis	601812
Kosaki overgrowth syndrome	AD	PDGFRB	As above	Thin hyperelastic fragile skin, lipodystrophy (partial or generalised), hypertelorism, prominent supraorbital ridges, broad nasal bridge, downslanting palpebral fissures, tall stature, scoliosis, iris hypoplasia, myofibroma, arachnoid cysts, fusiform coronary and cerebral aneurysms	616592

AD, autosomal dominant; AR, autosomal recessive; ATP, adenosine triphosphate; MAD, mandibuloacral disease; MDPL, mandibular hypoplasia, deafness, progeroid features and lipodystrophy; PI2K, phosphatidylinositol 3-kinase; SHORT, short stature, hyperextensibility of joints and/or inguinal herna, ocular depression, rieger anomaly and teething delay.

PART 6: GENETIC DISORDERS

Table 72.4 Monogenic obesity syndromes without cutaneous features.

Syndrome	Mode of inheritance	Gene(s) or chromosome	Other clinical features	MIM
Leptin receptor deficiency	AR	LEPR	Hypogonadism, hyperleptinaemia, susceptibility to infection	614963
Melanocortin-4 receptor deficiency	AD>AR	MC4R	Accelerated growth, tall stature	618406
TrkB deficiency	AD	NTRK2	Developmental delay, hyperactivity, memory problems, reduced pain sensation, hypotonia, epilepsy, craniosynostosis	613886
SIM1 deficiency	AD	SIM1 1p22.1 6q16.2 transl	Developmental delay, intellectual disability, round face with small nose and depressed nasal bridge, hypogonadism	–
MYT1L deficiency	AD	MYT1L 2p25.3 delet	Developmental delay, autism, epilepsy	–
Bardet–Biedel syndrome	AR	ARL6, BBS1, BBS2, BBS4, BBS5, BBS7, BBS10, BBS12, CEP19, MKKS, MKS1, PTHB1, TTC8	Developmental delay, polydactyly, retinal dystrophy, renal anomalies, hypogonadism, high arched palate, dental crowding	209900; 600151; 604896; 615981-90
Carpenter syndrome	AR	RAB23 MEGF8	Craniosynostosis, polysyndactyly, cardiac defects, undescended or underdeveloped testes	201000 614976
Börjeson–Forssman–Lehmann syndrome	XLR	PHF6	Developmental delay, epilepsy, hypogonadism, facial swelling, narrow palpebral fissures, large ears	301900
MOMO syndrome	?AD	?LINC00237	Macrosomia, macrocephaly, retinal coloboma, nystagmus, downslanting palpebral fissures, intellectual disability, delayed bone maturation	–
Cohen syndrome	AR	VPS13B	Developmental delay, microcephaly, downslanting palpebral fissures, maxillary hypoplasia, micrognathia, myopia, retinopathy, neutropenia	216550
MORM syndrome	AR	INPP5E	Intellectual disability, early-onset non-progressive retinal dystrophy, micropenis	610156

AD, autosomal dominant; AR, autosomal recessive; MOMO, macrosomia, obesity, macrocephaly and ocular abnormalities; MORM, mental retardation, truncal obesity, retinal dystrophy and micropenis; XLR, X-linked recessive.

the same biochemical pathway [9,10]. POMC undergoes sequential enzymatic processing (involving PC1), in a tissue-specific manner, to yield multiple biologically active peptides, including melanocyte-stimulating hormones (MSHs), corticotrophin (ACTH) and β-endorphin (Figure 72.2) [9,10]. Severe obesity, fair skin and red hair are features of autosomal recessive mutations in the POMC and PCSK1 genes.

In the fed state, adipocyte-derived leptin levels are increased, which act via the leptin receptors (LEPRs) to stimulate POMC expression within hypothalamic neurons. MSHs bind to the melanocortin 4 receptor (MC4R) to induce satiety [10]. LEPR, POMC, PCSK1 and MC4R mutations cause defective MC4R signalling, severe hyperphagia and early-onset obesity. MC4R agonists are a potential treatment for obesity caused by LEPR or POMC deficiency [11].

α-MSH and ACTH bind to melanocortin 1 receptor (MC1R) and stimulate eumelanin synthesis [9]. MC1R mutations are associated with fair skin and red hair, but not necessarily obesity [9]. In contrast, biallelic POMC mutations are associated with both the obesity and cutaneous phenotypes, but red hair may be absent or late onset in non-white children (Figure 72.3) [9,12,13]. Alterations in signalling in the POMC pathway may also be associated with psychiatric problems [6].

Prader–Willi syndrome

Imprinting is the process by which genetic alleles responsible for a phenotype are inherited from one parent only. It is an epigenetic phenomenon resulting from altered DNA methylation, histone modification or the effect of non-coding microRNAs [14,15]. PWS and Albright hereditary osteodystrophy (Figure 72.4) demonstrate autosomal dominant inheritance and feature imprinting [14].

PWS results from loss of paternally expressed genes at the 15q11-q13 imprinted locus [14]. This is usually associated with a large deletion of the imprinted region, but less frequently results from maternal uniparental disomy [16]. The SNORD116 cluster is thought to represent the PWS critical region, given that microdeletions of this region result in a PWS phenotype [17]. SNORD116 encodes non-coding RNAs, for which the function has not been clearly established [16]. Human and mouse models of PWS demonstrate reduced nescient helix loop helix 2 (NHLH2) and PC1 neuronal expression [18]. NHLH2 transcriptionally regulates PCSK1, and the characteristic neuroendocrine features of PWS are thought to be caused by PC1 deficiency [18].

Table 72.5 Monogenic obesity syndromes with cutaneous features.

Syndrome	Mode of inheritance	Gene(s) or chromosome	Cutaneous features	Other clinical features	MIM
POMC deficiency	AR	POMC	Red hair, fair (type 1) skin	Tall stature, hypoadrenalism	609734
PC1 deficiency	AR	PCSK1	Red hair, fair (type 1) skin	Elevated proinsulin, postprandial hypoglycaemia, hypogonadism, malabsorption	600955
Prader–Willi syndrome	Imprinted	15q11-q13, SNORD116	Generalised hypopigmentation, acanthosis nigricans	Developmental delay, hypotonia, short stature, small hands and feet, hypogonadotrophic hypogonadism, decreased pain sensitivity	176270
McCune–Albright syndrome[a]	Mosaic disorder	GNAS	Atypical café-au-lait patches, linear epidermal naevi, pigmentation of the nape of the neck	Polyostotic fibrous dysplasia, thyrotoxicosis[b], precocious puberty, Cushing syndrome[b], acromegaly[b]	174800
Albright hereditary osteodystrophy	Imprinted	GNAS	Subcutaneous ossification, dimpling over the metacarpophalangeal joints, dermal hypoplasia (Figure 72.4)	Short stature, skeletal defects and brachydactyly, round facies, multiple hormone resistance (including PTH)	103580
Carney complex[a]	AD	PRKAR1A	Lentigines, oral and mucosal pigmentation, blue naevi, schwannomas, café-au-lait macules, cutaneous and mucosal myxomas, skin tags, lipomas, pilonidal sinus	Cardiac myxoma, cardiomyopathy, precocious puberty, Cushing syndrome[b], gigantism[b], acromegaly[b], thyroid nodules and carcinoma, pituitary adenoma, osteochondromyxoma, breast ductal adenoma	160980
Fragile X syndrome	XLD	Xq27.3 >200 CGG repeats in FMR1	Regional hyperpigmentation	Developmental delay, hyperactivity, autism, prominent mandible, large ears, elongated face, hypermobility, macro-orchidism, muscle hypotonia, rapid growth but adult short stature, mitral valve prolapse	300624
MOMES syndrome	AR	4q35.1 del, 5p14.3 dup	Atopic eczema	Developmental delay, ocular abnormalities, macrocephaly, maxillary hypoplasia, prognathism	606772
Ulnar–mammary syndrome	AD	TBX3	Hypohidrosis, mammary hypoplasia, absent axillary hair, nail duplication	Ulnar ray defects, hypogonadism, delayed growth, cardiac conduction abnormalities, dental anomalies, genital anomalies	181450
Microcephalic osteodysplastic primordial dwarfism type II	AR	PCNT	Generalised hyperpigmentation, freckling, regional hypopigmentation, café-au-lait macules, xerosis, hypotrichosis, sacral dimples, cutis marmorata	Delayed growth, microcephaly, prominent nose and ears, bony dysplasia, scoliosis, hypoplastic dentition, developmental delay, cerebrovascular malformations	210720
Coffin–Lowry syndrome	XLD	RPS6KA3	Lax skin	Developmental delay, growth retardation, delayed puberty, kyphoscoliosis, cervical ribs, pectus carinatum/excavatum, prominent forehead, hypertelorism, downslanting palpebral fissures, prominent and low-set ears, enlarged lips, deafness, seizures, 'drop' attacks, cardiac anomalies	303600
Diploid/triploid mosaicism	Chromosomal defect	Diploid/triploid mosaicism	Transverse palmar crease, irregular skin pigmentation	Developmental delay, growth retardation, asymmetrical growth, prominent forehead, micrognathia, low-set ears, hypotonia, clinodactyly, syndactyly, narrow small hands, precocious puberty, micropenis, cryptorchidism	–
Prolidase deficiency	AR	PEPD	Leg ulcers, papular, erythematous and necrotic lesions, telangiectasias, pruritus, impetigo-like and eczema-like lesions, photosensitivity, hirsutism	Developmental delay, recurrent respiratory infections, hypertelorism, exophthalmos, micrognathia, saddle nose, splenomegaly	170100
Rubinstein–Taybi syndrome	AD	CREBBP, EP300	Keloids	Short stature, broad thumbs and halluces, facial dysmorphism, microcephaly, intellectual disability Ocular, cardiac, renal and dental problems	180849
Alström syndrome	AR	ALMS1	Acanthosis nigricans	Retinal dystrophy, deafness, dilated cardiomyopathy, insulin resistance, pulmonary, hepatic, urological and renal dysfunction	203800
Leptin deficiency	AR	LEP	Hair loss?	Hypogonadism, frequent infections, hypoleptinaemia	614962

[a] Only obese if Cushing syndrome is present.
[b] Secondary skin changes.
AD, autosomal dominant; AR, autosomal recessive; MOMES, mental retardation, obesity, mandibular prognathism with eye and skin anomalies; PC1, prohormone convertase 1; POMC, pro-opiomelanocortin, PTH, parathyroid hormone; XLR, X-linked recessive.

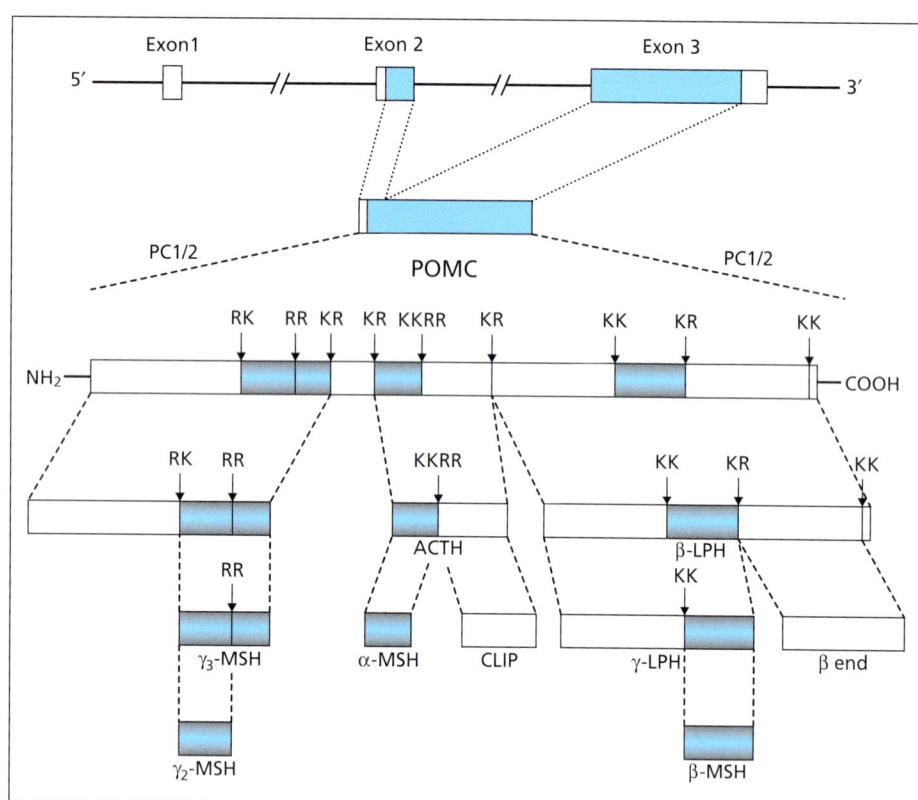

Figure 72.2 Gene structure and post-translational processing of pro-opiomelanocortin (POMC). POMC in mammals consists of three exons, of which exons 2 and 3 are translated. Prohormone convertases 1 and 2 (PC1/2) break the parent POMC peptide into successively smaller peptides by cleavage at paired dibasic amino acid residues consisting lysine (K) and/or arginine (R). ACTH, corticotrophin; β end, β-endorphin; MSH, melanocyte-stimulating hormone. Reproduced from Millington 2006 [9] with permission of John Wiley & Sons.

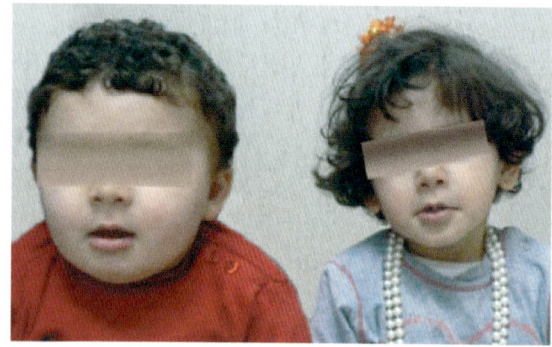

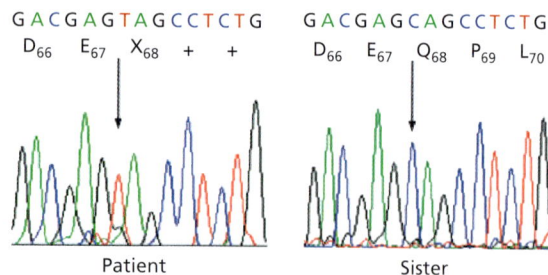

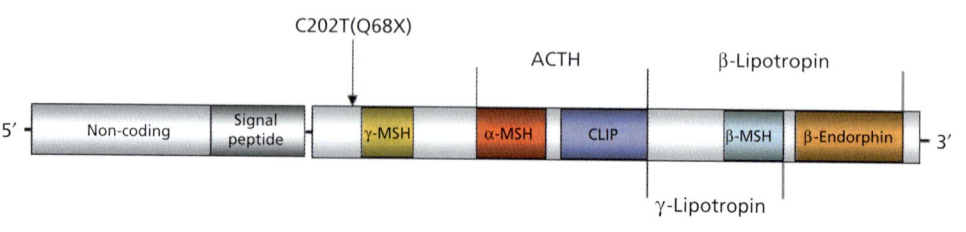

Figure 72.3 A pro-opiomelanocortin (POMC) deficient patient and his unaffected sister showing a lack of red hair. The arrows show a C202T mutation leading to a premature stop within the protein just upstream of the γ-melanocyte-stimulating hormone peptide. Reproduced from Cirillo et al. 2012 [12] with permission of John Wiley & Sons.

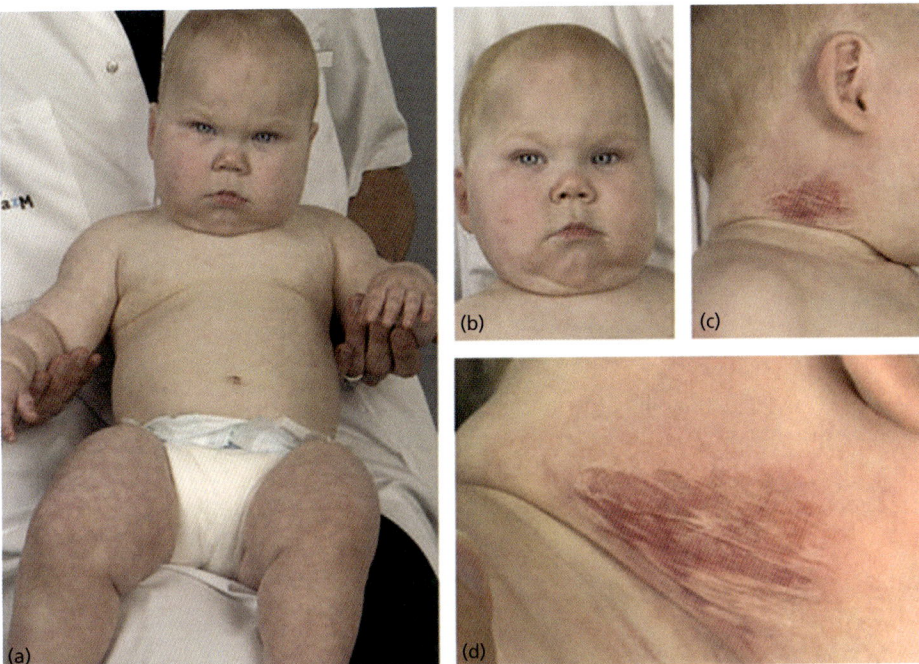

Figure 72.4 Clinical features of Albright hereditary osteodystrophy: (a) obesity; (b) round facies; (c) hypoplastic skin lesion; and (d) detailed view of a skin lesion. Reproduced from Klaasens *et al.* 2009 [26] with permission of John Wiley & Sons.

The 15q11-q13 region also contains the *OCA2* gene; homozygous or compound heterozygous *OCA2* mutations are implicated in oculocutaneous albinism type 2 [16]. Hypopigmentation in PWS is caused by single copy deletion of *OCA2*, and thus occurs in individuals with a large deletion but not uniparental disomy [16].

Other monogeneic obesity syndromes

These are described in Table 72.5 and other sources [19–25].

GENETIC ASSOCIATIONS WITH LIPOMA

Lipoma, benign tumours of adipocytes, are discussed in detail in Chapter 136. Table 72.6 summarises genetic associations with lipoma [1,2,3–7].

PIK3CA-RELATED OVERGROWTH SPECTRUM

Somatic activating *PIK3CA* mutations drive abnormal activation of the phosphatidylinositol 3-kinase (PI3K)/AKT signalling pathway, which causes cellular proliferation through the mTOR1 pathway [1]. The resultant disorders are collectively termed the PIK3CA-related overgrowth spectrum (PROS) due to their common genetic basis plus evidence of tissue overgrowth. Clinical features include adipose tissue, musculoskeletal or nerve overgrowth, vascular malformations and epidermal naevi [1]. CLOVES (congenital lipomatous overgrowth, vascular malformations, epidermal naevi and skeletal/spinal) syndrome [2], fibroadipose hyperplasia and hemihyperplasia–multiple lipomatosis syndrome and facial infiltrating lipomatosis present with overgrowth of adipose tissue, and thus are described in more detail in this chapter.

CLOVES syndrome

Lipomatous masses predominantly involve the thorax, and may be anatomically associated with capillary, arteriovenous or lymphatic malformations (Figure 72.5) [2]. Lipomatous hyperplasia is present at birth and demonstrates age-related progression. Complications include scoliosis, and occasionally lipomatous infiltration into the paraspinal or intraspinal spaces causing nerve root or spinal cord compression [2,3]. Other features include large wrinkled hands and feet, macrodactyly and linear epidermal naevi [2].

Fibroadipose hyperplasia and hemihyperplasia–multiple lipomatosis syndrome

These disorders display phenotypic overlap; clinical features include segmental overgrowth of adipose, fibrous, skeletal and muscular tissue (Figure 72.6) [4,5]. The lower extremities, distal more so than proximal, are most commonly involved. However, anatomical involvement, severity and progression demonstrate interindividual variability.

Table 72.6 Hereditary lipomatoses.

Syndrome	Mode of inheritance	Gene(s) or chromosome	Gene function	Clinical summary	MIM
Adiposis dolorosa (Dercum disease)	Usually sporadic, autosomal dominant in some families	Unknown	Unknown	Painful adipose tissue and/or lipomas; late onset; female : male ratio of 5 : 1 Obesity, easy bruising, sleep disturbances, impaired memory, depression, anxiety, rapid heartbeat, shortness of breath, diabetes, bloating, constipation, fatigue, weakness, joint pains	103200
Multiple symmetrical lipomatosis (Madelung disease)	Unknown, maternally inherited in some families	Mitochrondrial mutations (m.A8344G, m.T8357C) identified in some families	Unknown	Unencapsulated lipomas in the neck area ('collar of fat'); excess alcohol intake accelerates its progression. Associated with sensory, motor and autonomic neuropathies	151800
Mutliple lipomatosis (familial multiple lipomatosis)	AD	Chromosomal rearrangements (12q13 or12q14)	Unknown	Encapsulated non-painful lipomas; late onset; no other syndromic features	151900
Multiple endocrine neoplasia type 1	AD	MEN1 (MENIN)	Tumour suppressor	Parathyroid, gastrointestinal endocrine and pituitary tumours; lipomas; facial angiofibromata and collagenomata; CALMs; meningioma, ependymoma	131100
Frontonasal dysplasia type 1	AR	ALX3	Homeodomain-containing protein	Frontonasal dysostosis; hypertelorism; anterior cranium bifidum occultum; cutaneous and intracranial lipomas	136760
PTEN hamartoma tumour syndrome (Cowden syndrome; Bannayan–Riley–Ruvalcaba syndrome) (Chapter 71)	AD	PTEN	Cell-cycle, tumour suppressor	Benign and malignant tumours of the thyroid, breast and endometrium; lipomas; macrocephaly; trichilemmomas; acral keratosis; papillomatous lesions; developmental delay; pigmented macules of the glans penis	158350
Neurofibromatosis type 1 (Chapter 80)	AD	NF1	Negative regulator of RAS-MAPK pathway	CALMs; axillary freckling; neurofibromata; Lisch nodules; lipomas; macrocephaly; optic gliomas; predisposed to solid cancers and CNS tumours	162200
Legius syndrome (Chapter 80)	AD	SPRED1	Negative regulator of RAS-MAPK pathway	CALMs; axillary freckling; macrocephaly; lipomas; predisposition to solid cancers (note no neurofibromata)	611431
Nasopalpebral lipoma–coloboma syndrome	AD	Unknown	Unknown	Upper eyelid and nasopalpebral lipomas; eyelid colobomas; telecanthus; maxillary hypoplasia	167730
Familial adenomatous polyposis 1 (Gardner syndrome) (Chapter 80)	AD	APC	Tumour suppressor	Multiple gastrointestinal adenomatous polyps; abnormal dentition; osteomas; epidermoid cysts; lipomas; hyperpigmentation; keloids; colorectal and other cancers	175100
Proteus syndrome (Chapters 73 and 103)	Mosaic disorder	AKT1	Oncogene, protein kinase	Asymmetrical overgrowth (usually limb); intradermal, linear verrucous, epidermal and connective tissue naevi; shagreen patches, haemangiomata; lipomas; vascular lesions	176920
Aicardi syndrome	XLD	Unknown	Unknown	Infantile spasms; chorioretinal lacunae; agenesis of the corpus callosum; may have cavernous haemangioma, angiosarcoma, lipomas	304050
Lipomyelomeningocele	Unknown	Unknown	Unknown	Cutaneous and intraspinal lipomas (linked anatomically)	609537
Encephalocraniocutaneous lipomatosis	Mosaic disorder	FGFR1	Receptor tyrosine kinase	Ocular choristomas; naevus psiloliparus; cutaneous lipomas; skin tags; scalp cutis aplasia; non-scarring alopecia; blaschkoid pigmentary change; intracranial/intraspinal lipomas, arachnoid cysts, enlarged ventricles, leptomeningeal angiomatosis, gliomas; bone cysts; coarctation of the aorta	613001
Overgrowth and lipomata	One sporadic case	Pericentric inversion of chromosome 12 – deletion of HMGA2	Adipogenesis, osteogenesis, control of growth	Somatic overgrowth; advanced endochondral bone and dental ages with epiphyseal dysplasia; multiple lipomas; thrombocytopenia; arthritis; brachydactyly; cerebellar tumour; facial dysmorphic features	–

AD, autosomal dominant; AR, autosomal recessive; CALMs, café-au-lait macules: CNS, central nervous system; RAS-MAPK, RAS-mitogen-activated protein kinase; XLR, X-linked recessive.

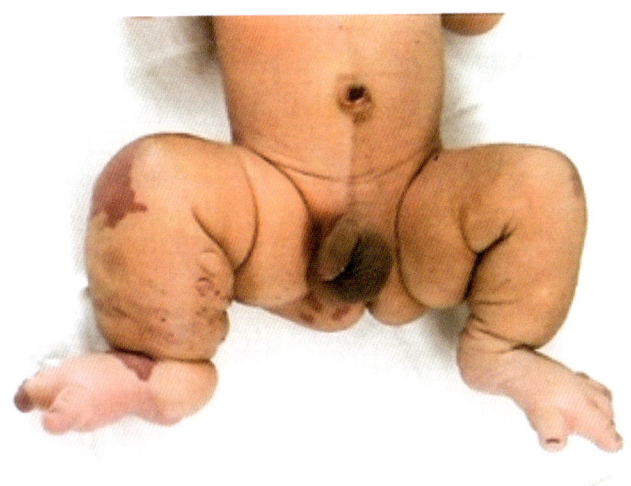

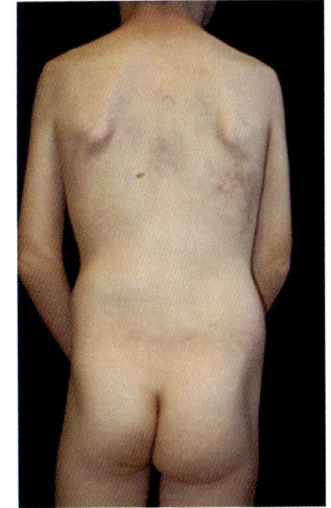

Figure 72.5 A patient with CLOVES syndrome showing congenital lipomatous overgrowth of the right leg with vascular malformation and epidermal naevus. Reproduced from Harit *et al.* 2010 [8] with permission of John Wiley & Sons.

Figure 72.6 A patient with hemihyperplasia-multiple lipomatosis syndrome demonstrating subtle hyperplasia of the right buttock and thigh, mixed capillary/venous malformation on the upper back and lipomas on the lower back and right hip. Reproduced from Craiglow *et al.* 2014 [9] with permission of John Wiley & Sons.

Facial infiltrating lipomatosis

Affected individuals develop unilateral facial hypertrophy caused by skeletal and adipose tissue overgrowth [6,7]. Additional features include mucosal neuromas, hemimacroglossia, advanced dentition and macrodontia [7].

HEREDITARY PANNICULITIS

Panniculitis, inflammation of adipose tissue, is discussed in detail in Chapter 97. Table 72.7 summarises the genetic associations with panniculitis [1,2–8].

Table 72.7 Hereditary panniculitis.

Syndrome	Mode of inheritance	Gene(s)	Gene function	Clinical summary	MIM
Proteasome-associated autoinflammatory syndrome 1 (CANDLE syndrome, Nakajo–Nishimura syndrome) (Chapter 45)	AR	PSMB8	Encodes a catalytic subunit of the immunoproteasome, which influences the antigenic repertoire presented on major histocompatibility complex (MHC) class I molecules	Annular erythematous plaques (Figure 72.7), violaceous eyelids, panniculitis-induced lipoatrophy affecting the face and extremities, elevated temperature, inflammatory markers, microcytic anaemia, failure to thrive, joint contractures, muscular atrophy	256040
Autoimmune lymphoproliferative syndrome (Canale–Smith syndrome)	AD	FASLG, FAS	Encodes FAS cell surface death receptor, and causes apoptosis in cells of haematological and immunological lineage	Lymphadenopathy, hepatosplenomegaly, anaemia, thrombocytopenia, urticaria, vasculitis, panniculitis, increased risk of malignant lymphoma	601859
Alpha1-antitrypsin deficiency	AR	SERPINA1	Encodes alpha1-antitrypsin, a serum protease inhibitor that inhibits tissue elastase	Emphysema, liver disease, panniculitis (Figure 72.8), glomerulonephritis, arthritis, vasculitis, uveitis	613490
Autoinflammation, panniculitis and dermatosis syndrome	AR	OTULIN	Encodes a deubiquitinating enzyme that cleaves linear polyubiquitin chains and inhibits NF-κB signalling	Neonatal onset of episodic fever, elevated inflammatory markers, diarrhoea, erythematous subcutaneous nodules (neutrophilic panniculitis), swollen painful joints, lipodystrophy	617099
Subacute panniculitis-like T-cell lymphoma	AR	HAVCR2	Encodes T-cell immunoglobulin mucin 3, which is an immune checkpoint inhibitor	Multiple subcutaneous nodules, haemophagotic lymphohistiocytosis, increased risk of autoimmune disorders, e.g. systemic lupus erythematosus	618398

AD, autosomal dominant; AR, autosomal recessive; CANDLE, chronic atypical neutrophilic dermatosis with lipodystrophy and elevated temperature; NF-κB, nuclear factor κB.

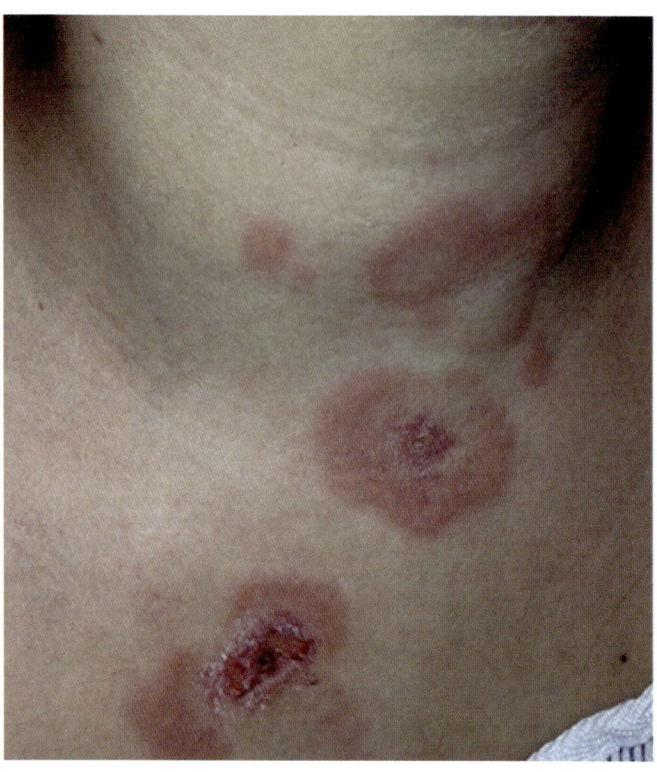

Figure 72.7 A patient with chronic atypical neutrophilic dermatosis with lipodystrophy and elevated temperature (CANDLE) syndrome demonstrating the violaceous annular and figurate plaques. Reproduced from Patel *et al.* 2021 [**1**] with permission of John Wiley & Sons.

FAMILIAL LIPOEDEMA

Lipoedema is the persistent accumulation of fat, which disproportionately affects the lower limbs (Figure 72.9) (Chapter 98). Lipoedema may occur as part of a syndrome (Table 72.8) [1,2,**3**,4–6]. Familial clustering is reported in non-syndromic lipoedema [1], but its molecular basis has not been identified.

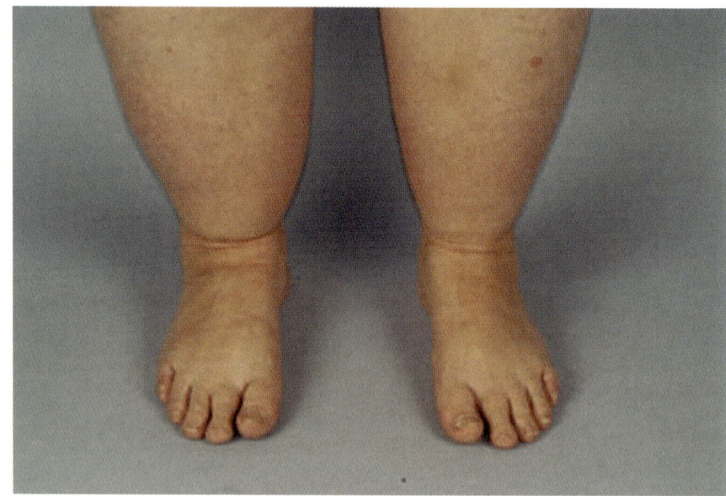

Figure 72.9 Lipoedema. Reproduced from Langendoen *et al.* 2009 [2] with permission of John Wiley & Sons.

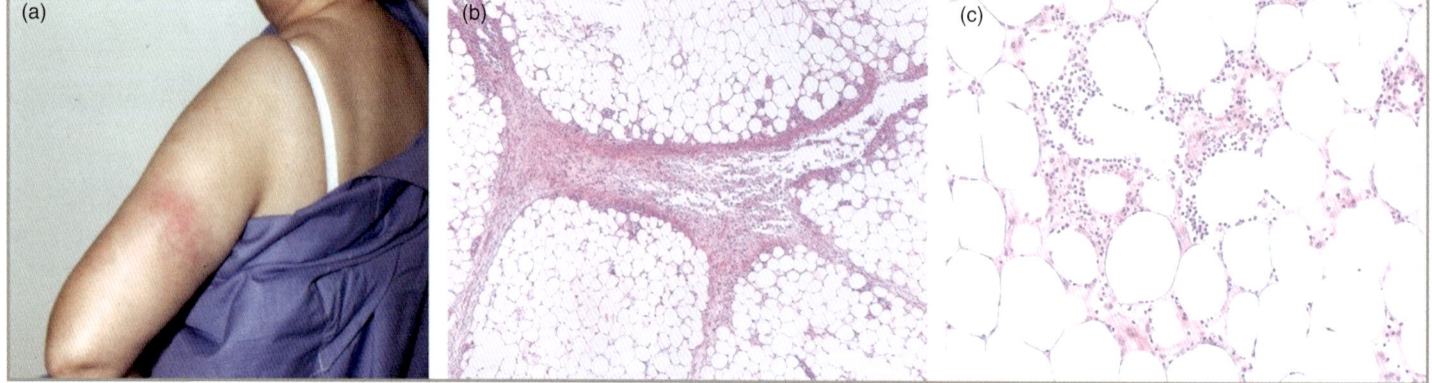

Figure 72.8 Hereditary panniculitis caused by homozygous ZZ α_1-antitrypsin deficiency. Reproduced from Blanco *et al.* 2015 [2] with permission of John Wiley & Sons.

Table 72.8 Familial lipoedema.

Syndrome	Mode of inheritance	Gene(s)	Clinical summary	MIM
Short stature/lipoedema	AD	*POU1F1*	Short stature, lipoedema of the lower limbs, growth hormone deficiency, secondary hypothyroidism, hypoprolactinaemia	–
Sotos syndrome 1	AD	*NSD1*	Overgrowth, macrocephaly, acromegalic features, developmental delay, lipoedema of the lower limbs	117550
Williams–Beuren syndrome (Chapter 70)	AD	*7q11.23 del.*	Flat nasal bridge and anteverted nares, prominent lips, intellectual disability, lax skin, increased wrinkles, abnormal scarring, lipoedema of the lower limbs, congenital heart disease, impaired glucose tolerance	194050

AD, autosomal dominant.

Key references

The full list of references can be found in the online version at https://www.wiley.com/rooksdermatology10e

Congenital (familial) lipodystrophies

8 Patni N, Garg A. Congenital generalized lipodystrophies – new insights into metabolic dysfunction. *Nat Rev Endocrinol* 2015;11:522–34.

10 Bagias C, Xiarchou A, Bargiota A *et al.* Familial partial lipodystrophy (FLPD): recent insights. *Diabetes Metab Syndr Obes* 2020;13:1531–44.

Hereditary obesity

1 Cotter C, Walsh S. Cutaneous sequelae of a national health crisis: obesity and the skin. *Skin Health Dis* 2020;1:e7.

3 Millington GWM. Obesity, genetics and the skin. *Clin Exp Dermatol* 2013;38:50–6.

4 Brandwein M, Katz I, Katz A *et al.* Beyond the gut: skin microbiome compositional changes are associated with BMI. *Hum Microb J* 2020;13:100063.

Genetic associations with lipoma

2 López-Gallardo E, Cammarata-Scalisi F, Emperador S *et al.* Mitochondrial DNA pathogenic mutations in multiple symmetric lipomatosis. *Clin Genet* 2020;97:731–5.

PIK3CA-related overgrowth spectrum

2 Martinez-Lopez A, Blasco-Morente G, Perez-Lopez I *et al.* CLOVES syndrome: review of a PIK3CA-related overgrowth spectrum (PROS). *Clin Genet* 2016;91:14–21.

Hereditary panniculitis

1 Patel PN, Hunt R, Pettigrew ZJ *et al.* Successful treatment of chronic atypical neutrophilic dermatosis with lipodystrophy and elevated temperature (CANDLE) syndrome with tofacitinib. *Pediatr Dermatol* 2021;38:528–9.

Familial lipoedema

3 Bano G, Mansour S, Brice G *et al.* Pit-1 mutation and lipoedema in a family. *Exp Clin Endocrinol Diabetes* 2010;118:377–80.

CHAPTER 73

Congenital Naevi and Selected Naevoid Conditions

Veronica A. Kinsler[1] and Neil J. Sebire[2]

[1] Paediatric Dermatology, Great Ormond St Hospital for Children NHS Foundation Trust and UCL GOS Institute of Child Health; Mosaicism and Precision Medicine Laboratory, The Francis Crick Institute, London, UK
[2] Paediatric Pathology, Great Ormond Street Hospital for Children NHS Foundation Trust and UCL GOS Institute of Child Health, London, UK

PART 6: GENETIC DISORDERS

CONGENITAL NAEVI

Introduction

The understanding of congenital naevi has changed substantially over the last decade, with the discovery of the genetic basis of many lesions. With this new understanding has come the opportunity to reclassify the well-recognised phenotypes into simpler and potentially more clinically relevant groups. This classification comes with the caveat that research in this field is still revealing findings at a startling rate, and it will likely need to accommodate further changes in the future.

Principles underlying naevus phenotypes

1 Congenital naevi are ultimately caused by a postzygotic mutation in a cell that resides in or will eventually reside in the skin.
2 Only some parts of the skin are affected, with other areas or the rest of the skin appearing entirely normal, at least macroscopically. This is the dermatological phenotypic correlate of genotypic mosaicism, defined as the presence of two or more genetically distinct populations of cells within an individual derived from a single zygote, at the time of birth, and leading to a disease phenotype [1].
3 The phenotype will largely be dictated by the normal function of the gene during development, and the specific mutation that

occurs. In congenital naevi there is often exquisite specificity of genotype–phenotype association, down to codon and even base pair level.
4 The extent and/or number of lesions is an important (although not absolute) guide to the possibility of non-dermatological associations. More than one distinct naevus in the same individual suggests a single somatic event affecting a precursor cell before full commitment to one area of the skin, which could therefore potentially have led to non-dermatological features as well; however this is a guideline only.
5 The cell type affected by the mutation is, of course, central to the clinical phenotype, both in appearance and distribution. However, the exact cell type affected is not yet known with certainty for some congenital naevi.
6 It is becoming apparent that the dermatological phenotype of mosaic lesions is not necessarily the same as that associated with exactly the same mutation in a germline form. This phenomenon is yet to be explained but is likely to relate to the interactions of mutant and non-mutant cells during development.

Classification
Clinical phenotypic classification
1 Congenital epidermal naevi.
2 Congenital pigment cell naevi.
3 Congenital connective tissue naevi.

Rook's Textbook of Dermatology, Tenth Edition. Edited by Christopher Griffiths, Jonathan Barker, Tanya Bleiker, Walayat Hussain and Rosalind Simpson.
© 2024 John Wiley & Sons Ltd. Published 2024 by John Wiley & Sons Ltd.

These can each be divided into:
- Cutaneous involvement only – single or multiple lesions.
- Syndromic – associated with non-cutaneous features.

Histological classification

Within congenital epidermal naevi (CEN) there are classifications based on the predominant (although usually not only) cell type seen on histology:
- Keratinocytic naevi.
- Sebaceous naevi.
- Follicular naevi.
- Eccrine/apocrine naevi.

Further histological subclassifications of these groups of epidermal naevi can also be made (Box 73.1).

Within congenital pigment cell naevi there are subclassifications based on the histology of the lesions:
- Melanocytic naevi.
- Blue naevi.
- Spitz naevi.
- Naevus spilus.

Within congenital connective tissue naevi there are subclassifications based on the predominant cell type seen on histological examination:
- Collagen naevi.
- Elastic tissue naevi.
- Mucinous naevi.
- Fat naevi.

Although there are other lesions with the epithet 'naevus', this list is proposed to cover those that can occur congenitally, and attempts to group together a wide variety of rarely described histological subtypes. Note that CEN have sometimes been divided into 'organoid' and 'non-organoid' types, which is simply a differentiation between those where the predominant histological cell type is adnexal (organoid – i.e. sebaceous glands, sweat glands or hair follicles) and those where it is keratinocytic (non-organoid).

Box 73.1 List of terms applied to congenital naevi and 'naevus-like' lesions

Epidermal naevi
- Keratinocytic/hyperkeratotic/verrucous epidermal naevus
- Epidermolytic hyperkeratotic/verrucous epidermal naevus
- Inflammatory linear verrucous epidermal naevus (ILVEN)
- Papular epidermal naevus with 'skyline' basal cell layer (PENS)
- Rounded and velvety epidermal naevus (RAVEN)/naevus-like acanthosis nigricans
- Naevus sebaceous
- Linear syringocystadenoma papilliferum
- Comedo naevus/acne naevus
- Hair follicle naevus/follicular naevus
- Linear basaloid follicular hamartoma
- Hairy malformation of the palms and soles
- Naevus trichilemmocysticus
- Apocrine naevus
- Eccrine naevus
- Porokeratotic eccrine ostial and dermal duct naevus (PAON)
- Porokeratotic adnexal and ostial duct naevus (PAON)

Pigment cell naevi
- Congenital melanocytic naevus
- Congenital blue naevus
- Congenital naevus spilus
- Congenital Spitz naevus
- Mongolian blue spot (dermal melanocytosis)

Connective tissue naevi
- Eruptive collagenoma
- Shagreen patch
- Isolated collagenomas
- Elastic naevus
- Juvenile elastoma
- Naevus anelasticus
- Proteoglycan naevus
- Mucinous naevus
- Mixed connective tissue naevus

Muscle 'naevi'
- Congenital smooth muscle hamartoma
- Becker naevus and segmental odonto-maxillary dysplasia
- Diffuse smooth muscle hamartoma
- Congenital leiomyoma
- Striated muscle naevus

Fat 'naevi'
- Naevus lipomatosus cutaneous superficialis
- Congenital lipoma
- Congenital lipomatosis
- Naevus psiloliparus

'Naevus-like' entities
- Angora hair naevus (naevus, but difficult to classify thus far)
- Linear atrophodermas, including of Moulin, and linear presentations of atrophoderma of Pierini and Pasini
- Linear scleroderma/morphoea
- Lichen striatus
- Incontinentia pigmenti, CHILD syndrome naevus and other X-linked conditions with a linear pattern
- Linear Darier disease and other linear presentations of generally non-linear skin disorders

Details of some entities are covered in other chapters.

Genetic classification

For congenital naevi there are also subclassifications based on the causative genetic mutation, where known, for example mutations in: fibroblast growth factor receptors (*FGFR1*, *FGFR2*, *FGFR3*), RAS family members (*NRAS*, *HRAS*, *KRAS*), other signalling pathway genes (*AKT1*, *PIK3CA*, *BRAF*), keratins (*KRT10*, *KRT1*), connexins (*GJB2*, *GJA1*) and others such as *ACTB*, *CARD14* and *NEK9*.

A clinical diagnosis may therefore be initially of a CEN syndrome, which with histological and genetic investigation becomes *AKT1*-mutated keratinocytic CEN syndrome. Where this systematic classification leads to a clear diagnosis of a well-defined syndrome (such as Proteus syndrome in this case), then the eponymous name can be used if preferred. This systematic classification allows for the description of new syndromes, and of the approximation of previously distinct diagnoses such as Schimmelpenning syndrome and phakomatosis pigmentokeratotica.

Inheritance of naevus mutations

Mosaic mutations cannot by definition be inherited. Dominant mosaic mutations, however, can be passed on to future generations as a germline heterozygous disease, meaning that the genetic abnormality will not then be in mosaic form but affecting the whole body. This can happen if the mosaic mutations fulfil two criteria: firstly that they affect the gametes of the individual, which can generally not be tested, and secondly that the mutations are compatible with life in the germline. As new mosaic genotypes are being discovered this is becoming an increasingly complex area, and it is important to consider when managing individuals with mosaic cutaneous disease. It has sometimes been suggested that the percentage of skin affected by the CEN may be an indication of the percentage of gametes affected; however there is no published evidence to support this hypothesis. A summary of the recent knowledge of which conditions can definitely or theoretically be passed on to offspring is included in tabulated form in a recent consensus publication [1].

Table 73.1 Genetic basis of epidermal naevi.

Epidermal naevus subtype	Gene mutated
Keratinocytic, non-inflammatory	FGFR3 (in isolated naevi and as part of the FGFR3 epidermal naevus syndrome) [5,6], PIK3CA (in isolated naevi and as part of the CLOVES syndrome) [7,8], HRAS, KRAS and BRAF (in isolated naevi and as part of unique epidermal naevus syndromes) [9–12], AKT1 (so far as part of the Proteus syndrome) [4], KRT1 [13] and KRT10 [14]
Keratinocytic, inflammatory (ILVEN)	GJA1 (single case) [15] and CARD14 (two cases) [16], arguably ABCA12 [17] (single case, classified clinically as mosaic ichthyosis)
Sebaceous	HRAS or KRAS (both in individual naevi and as part of phakomatosis pigmentokeratotica/Schimmelpenning syndrome) [18], or in a papillomatous subtype by FGFR2 [19]
Follicular/acne/comedo	Linear lesions mutated in FGFR2 [20], and more recently NEK9 [21]
Porokeratotic eccrine	GJB2 [22]

Congenital epidermal naevi

Definition and nomenclature

Congenital epidermal naevi are benign naevi of epidermal components present at birth, or appearing in the first few years of life, in a characteristic developmental pattern.

Introduction and general description

Congenital epidermal naevi is a descriptive term for congenital hamartomas of epidermal structures. This encompasses a wide range of clinical and histological phenotypes, and can occur as isolated cutaneous lesions or associated with extracutaneous features as part of diverse syndromes. The clinical diagnosis of CEN is not usually difficult, but a thorough history and physical examination of the patient is required to look for associated features, and in many cases histopathology is required to make a more accurate diagnosis. In addition, follow-up of a newborn or young child is recommended for all but small single lesions, as the full phenotype may not be apparent for several years. Rarely CEN in an embryonic distribution appear later in life [2,3].

CEN syndromes are the association of CEN with extracutaneous features, with a predilection for neurological, ophthalmological, skeletal and endocrinological abnormalities. A very wide range of extracutaneous associations has been reported in the literature, with significant overlap between historically distinct diagnoses, but with many cases appearing to be unique. The elucidation of the underlying genetic basis of increasing numbers of the CEN syndromes has not only proven that certain phenotypes are truly distinct diagnoses (for example in the case of Proteus syndrome), but that others are in fact a spectrum of manifestations of the same disorder (e.g. Schimmelpenning–Feuerstein–Mims syndrome and phakomatosis pigmentokeratotica).

Epidemiology

Sufficiently large-scale studies are lacking for all but the commonest CEN, namely isolated sebaceous naevi, which have a prevalence of 1–3 in 1000. This figure is therefore a minimum birth prevalence for all CEN grouped together. Data are also lacking for whether there are differences between the sexes and ethnic groups.

The birth prevalence of CEN syndromes is also unknown; however, they are extremely rare, with Proteus syndrome for example quoted by experts as occurring in less than 1 in 1 million [4].

By definition, CEN are usually present at birth, although some lesions appear in the first few years of life with a characteristically embryonic distribution.

Pathophysiology

Most CEN are caused by single postzygotic mutations in an epidermal precursor cell, leading to epidermal mosaicism, with or without mosaicism in other organs. As a result the same mutation is found in all affected tissues in an individual with a CEN syndrome. The current state of genetic knowledge is shown in Table 73.1.

Individual phenotypes in CEN so far are to some extent linked to genotype, with codon-specific mutation hotspots predominating in the majority of cases. So far the same mutations have been found in isolated CEN as in the corresponding CEN syndrome.

Rarely, CEN are a feature of germline conditions, for example CHILD (congenital hemidysplasia with ichthyosiform erythroderma and limb defects) syndrome and Cowden syndrome. This cutaneous CEN phenotype can only be due to further genetic mechanisms, or we would expect the entire skin to be affected. In CHILD syndrome this mechanism is X-inactivation, revealing the effects of the mutation in areas where the mutant NSDHL allele is not inactivated. In Cowden syndrome this mechanism is a second genetic hit to PTEN [23].

Pathology

Epidermal naevi are localised hamartomatous processes of the epidermis that may show varying histopathological changes, most of which include varying degrees of hyperkeratosis, acanthosis and papillomatosis. The lesions are most easily identified when compared with the surrounding normal skin – that is, in a biopsy

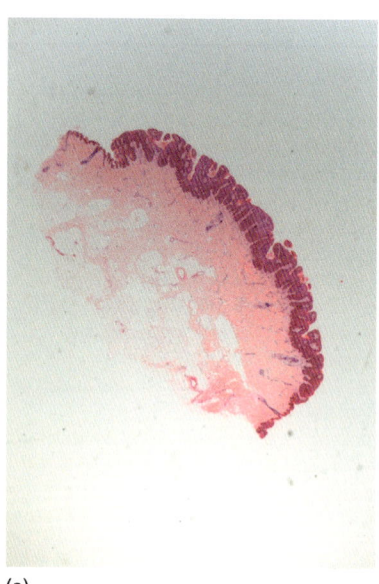

(a)

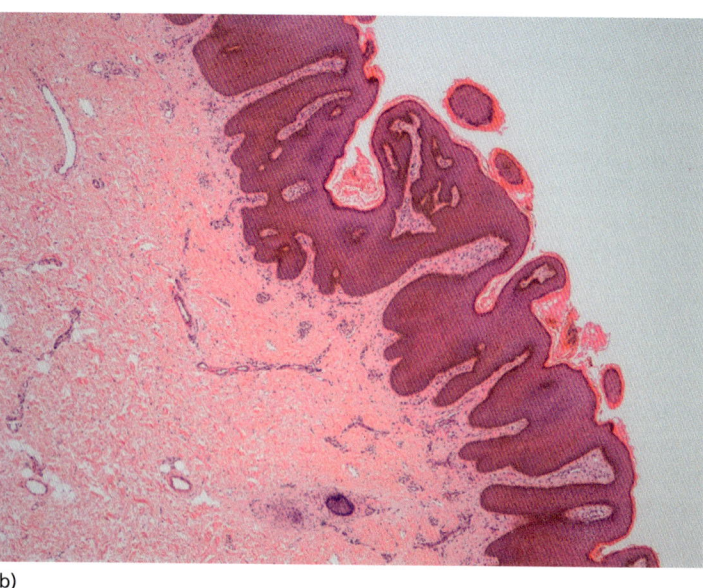

(b)

Figure 73.1 Photomicrographs of an epidermal naevus demonstrating an area of thickened epidermis with papillomatosis and mild hyperkeratosis. Original magnifications (a) ×20 and (b) ×40 (H&E). Courtesy of Professor N. J. Sebire.

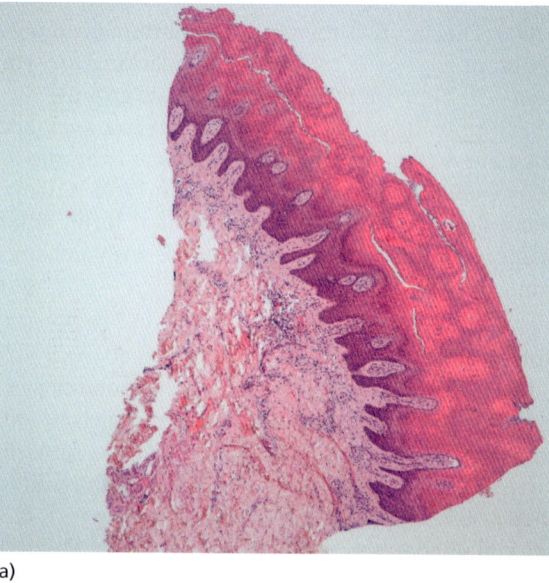

(a)

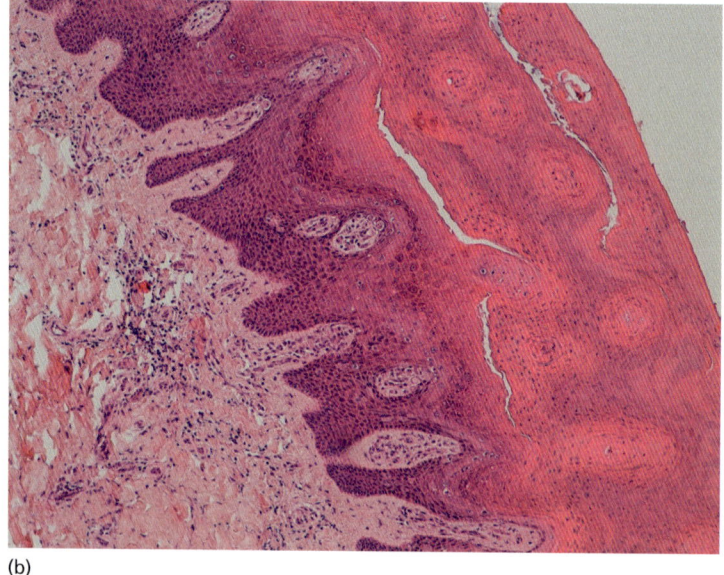

(b)

Figure 73.2 Photomicrograph of inflammatory linear verrucous epidermal naevus demonstrating marked epidermal thickening with hyperkeratosis and an associated inflammatory reaction. Original magnifications (a) ×40 and (b) ×100 (H&E). Courtesy of Professor N. J. Sebire.

spanning the edge of the lesion. The lesions are classified histologically based on the predominant epidermal component (sebaceous, keratinocytic, follicular, eccrine/apocrine) and whether or not there is an associated significant inflammatory component (Figure 73.1). In inflammatory linear verrucous epidermal naevus (ILVEN) there is usually a marked inflammatory component, including a psoriasiform appearance with epidermal hyperplasia and a dense associated superficial dermal inflammatory infiltrate (Figure 73.2).

Importantly, the histopathological features may vary with the patient's age, such that, for example in sebaceous naevi in younger individuals, the epidermis often remains flat but in the dermis there are characteristic immature rudimentary hair follicles associated with only small sebaceous glands. Following puberty, the lesion becomes more prominent with a particular increase in the size of the sebaceous glands (Figure 73.3).

An important aspect of histopathological examination of keratinocytic naevi is the presence or absence of epidermolysis, as when present this distinguishes epidermolytic naevi.

Clinical features

Congenital epidermal naevi are by definition present at birth or become apparent in the first years of life. The phenotype can develop in extent over the first years, and often become more pronounced with age, particularly with increasing hyperkeratosis in keratinocytic naevi.

Single small CEN lesions can be either round or linear, but larger or multiple lesions are always Blaschkolinear in distribution. The only exception to this thus far are the recently described naevi of the PENS (papular epidermal naevus with 'skyline' basal cell layer) syndrome which are multiple but round/ovoid. This suggests to

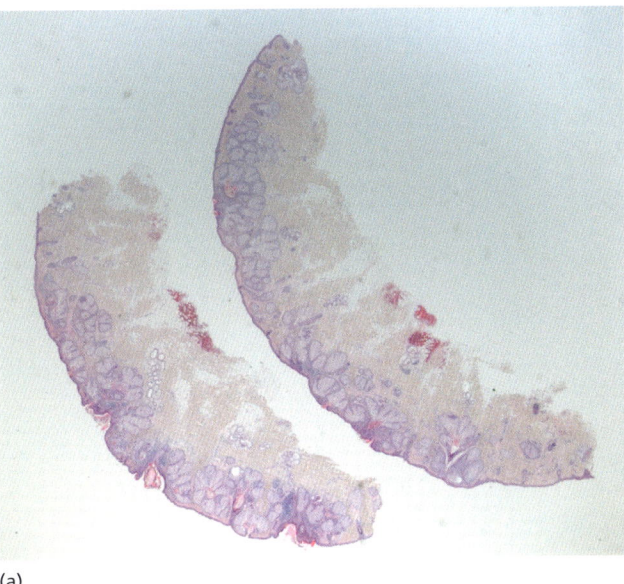

(a)

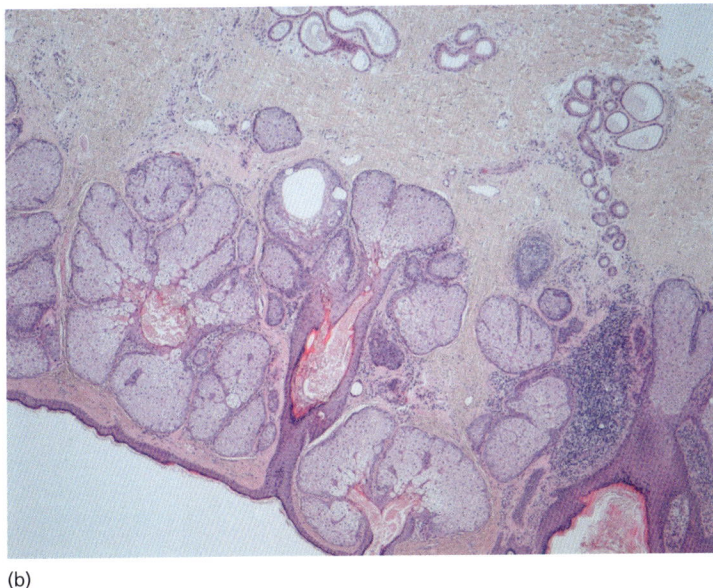

(b)

Figure 73.3 Photomicrographs of a typical sebaceous naevus demonstrating a lesion composed of prominent sebaceous glands within the dermis. Original magnifications (a) ×20 and (b) ×40 (H&E). Courtesy of Professor N. J. Sebire.

the authors of this chapter that this may turn out to either be a *de novo* germline mutation, or that the cell type affected is not an epidermal precursor, or that a second-hit is required to produce the cutaneous phenotype. Epidermal naevi are by their nature very superficial and are therefore raised, and can have the appearance of being 'stuck on' to the surface of the skin rather than intrinsic to it. Their surface characteristics depend on the cell type that predominates.

Keratinocytic naevi vary from pale brown and nearly macular with a soft velvety feel, to brown or red, verrucous or hyperkeratotic, and can have a prominent inflammatory component. ILVEN commonly appears in the first few years of life rather than at birth, and spreads gradually until stabilising in a classic Blaschkolinear distribution. It is characterised clinically by inflamed and hyperkeratotic skin that can be pruritic. It is usually confined to a single limb, but can be more extensive (Figure 73.4). Clinically and histologically, there can be a significant overlap between ILVEN and psoriasis [24,25].

Sebaceous naevi have a greasy feel and appearance, are often yellowish or pink (Figure 73.5a), but can sometimes be deeply pigmented (Figure 73.5b). Follicular naevi (naevus comedonicus or acne naevus) are very characteristic in appearance and skin coloured with a high density of multiple, comedo-like lesions. Congenital eccrine or apocrine naevi are particularly rare, but are recognisable by localised hyperhidrosis, with porokeratotic variants of eccrine naevi exhibiting the classic signs of porokeratosis (Figure 73.6). Although syringocystadenoma papilliferum is thought to be a hamartoma of eccrine/apocrine glands, it most commonly arises in clinical practice from a sebaceous naevus.

Clinical variants

There are several clearly delineated CEN syndromes. Note that other patterns of signs in association with CEN have been described, but are either extremely rare or unique cases.

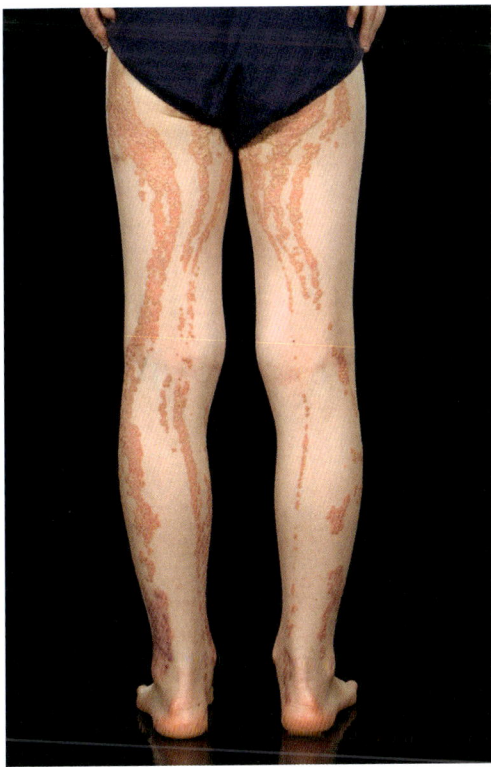

Figure 73.4 Extensive inflammatory linear verrucous epidermal naevus on the lower limbs in a Blaschkolinear distribution.

***HRAS/KRAS* mosaicism.** Schimmelpenning–Feuerstein–Mims syndrome [26,27] and phakomatosis pigmentokeratotica [28] were originally described as separate phenotypes, but since the discovery of the same underlying mutations [18,29] can be viewed as a spectrum of the same mosaic RASopathy. Clinical features are sebaceous epidermal naevi (Figure 73.5b) with or without the following: areas of keratinocytic epidermal naevus, naevus spilus

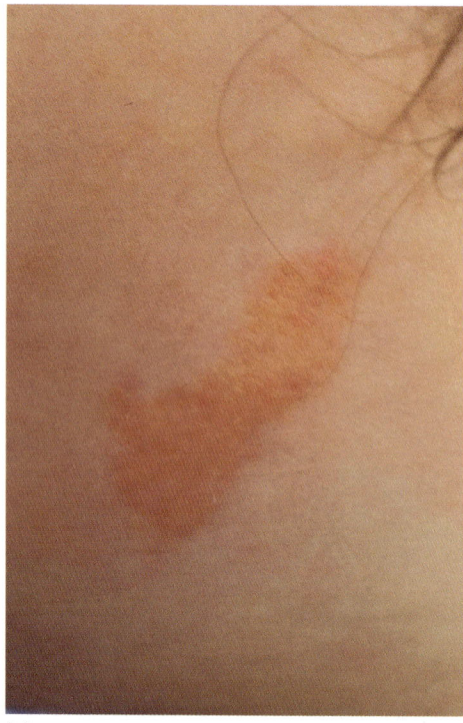

(a)

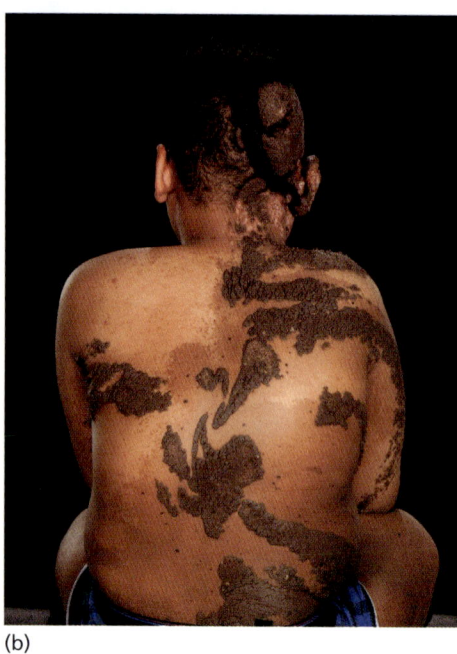

(b)

Figure 73.5 (a) Single sebaceous naevus on the cheek, with a yellowish hue and characteristic greasy texture. (b) Multiple pigmented sebaceous epidermal naevi on the trunk and scalp in a Blaschkolinear distribution, accompanied by large areas of café-au-lait macular pigmentation with superimposed melanocytic lesions.

(synonym: speckled lentiginous naevus) or areas of café-au-lait macular pigmentation, neurological abnormalities, developmental skeletal abnormalities and hypophosphataemia leading to rickets. Many other less common associations have been described with *HRAS* mosaicism. Woolly hair naevus with epidermal naevi has recently also been identified as part of this spectrum of HRAS mosaicism [30].

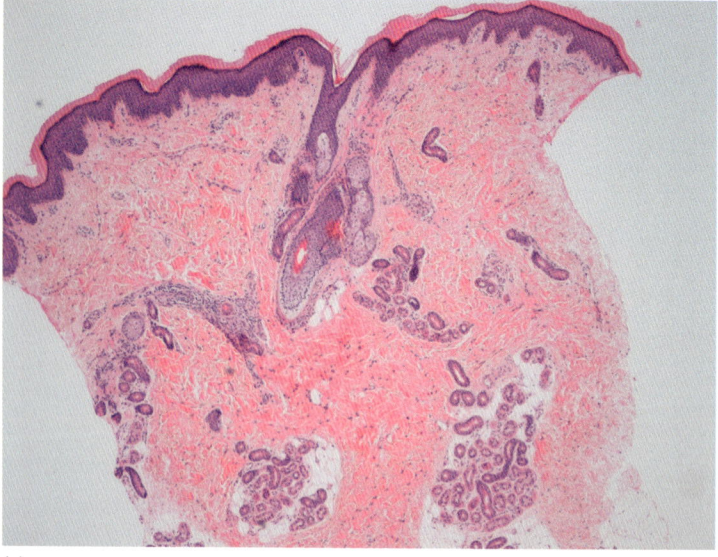

(a)

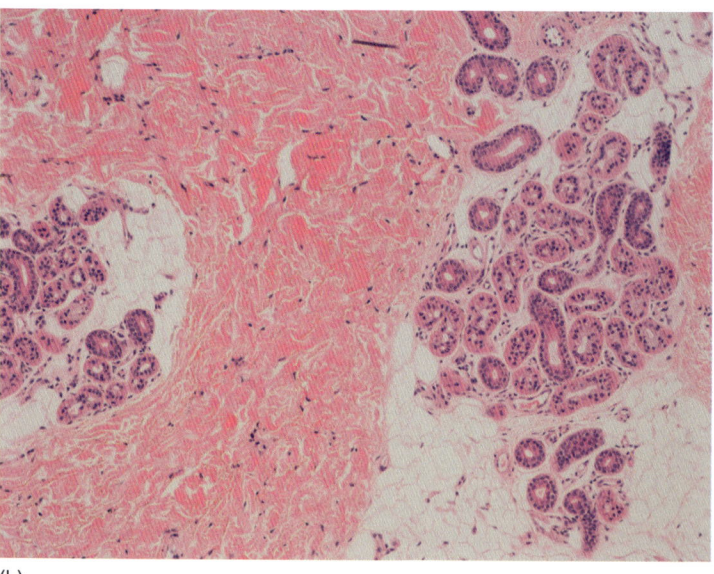

(b)

Figure 73.6 Photomicrographs of an eccrine naevus demonstrating prominent eccrine glands within the dermis. Original magnifications (a) ×40 and (b) ×100 (H&E). Courtesy of Professor N. J. Sebire.

Proteus syndrome. Proteus syndrome is a mosaic disorder of growth. Diagnostic criteria are well established [31], and cutaneous lesions include keratinocytic epidermal naevi, connective tissue naevi, lipomas, vascular naevi and patchy lipohypoplasia or dermal hypoplasia. The number of skin lesions correlates to some degree with the severity of the phenotype in an affected individual [32], and can progress over time [33]. Proteus syndrome as defined by the diagnostic criteria is caused by somatic mosaicism for mutations in *AKT1* [4].

CLOVES syndrome. This acronym is the description of associated congenital lipomatous overgrowth, vascular malformation, epidermal naevi (keratinocytic type) and skeletal abnormalities [34]. This overgrowth syndrome can also be associated with neurological abnormalities [35]. Despite sharing many similar clinical features

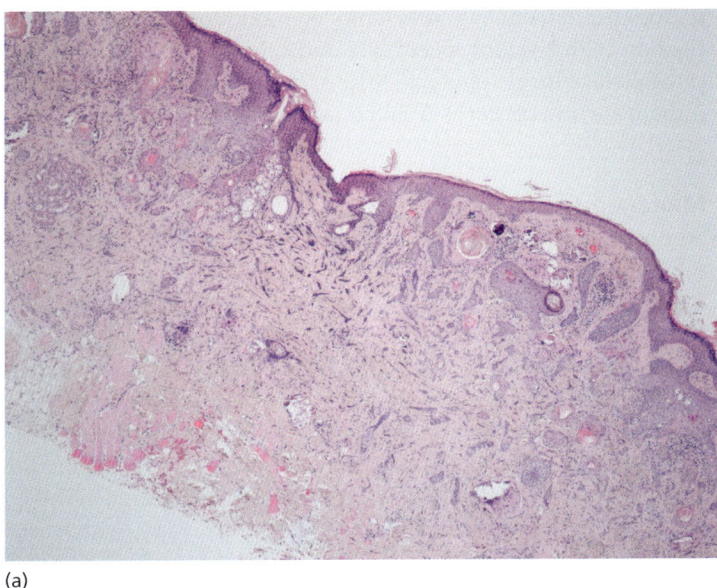

(a)

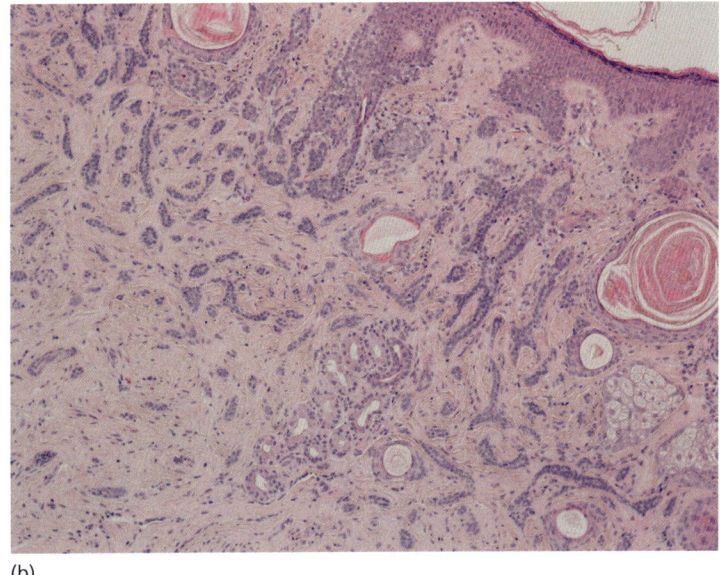

(b)

Figure 73.7 Photomicrographs of a desmoplastic trichoepithelioma arising in a sebaceous naevus demonstrating epithelial strands infiltrating the dermis surrounded by a desmoplastic, collagenous stroma. Original magnifications (a) ×40 and (b) ×100 (H&E). Courtesy of Professor N. J. Sebire.

it can be distinguished both clinically and genotypically from Proteus syndrome [30]. It is caused by somatic mosaicism for *PIK3CA* mutations [8].

***FGFR3* epidermal naevus syndrome.** The association of a *FGFR3*-variant keratinocytic epidermal naevus with a neurological phenotype has been rarely described with *FGFR3* mutation mosaicism [6,36]. Unusually, the mutation was detectable in blood leukocyte DNA [6,37].

PENS syndrome. This newly delineated familial or sporadic syndrome is characterised by multiple, round/ovoid, papular, white/yellowish, keratotic lesions of 0.1–1.5 cm diameter. They are present at birth or develop shortly after, and have a characteristic histological appearance of a 'skyline' basal cell layer [38,39]. Many of the cases described have had mild neurodevelopmental delay and/or epilepsy [38]. The genetic basis is currently unknown.

Curry–Jones syndrome/Happle–Tinschert syndrome. These two rare syndromes are now thought to be on the same spectrum. Curry–Jones syndrome was described in 1995 as the association of asymmetrical face, craniosynostosis, corpus callosum agenesis and Blaschkolinear skin atrophy and hypopigmentation [40]. Happle–Tinschert syndrome was described in 2008 as the association of segmental basaloid follicular hamartomas with similar extracutaneous abnormalities in the dental, skeletal and neurological systems [41,42]. The genetic basis of Curry–Jones syndrome was recently demonstrated to be mosaic mutations in gene *SMO* [43], and was later confirmed in a case of Happle–Tinschert syndrome [44].

Follicular naevus/naevus comedonicus syndrome. Naevus comedonicus has been described in association with cataracts, skeletal abnormalities and neurological abnormalities [45–47].

Complications and co-morbidities

Some CEN have an increased risk of superimposed benign tumour development, and in some there is a risk of malignant transformation. Due to the rarity of the individual phenotypes these risks are not well quantified. For isolated sebaceous naevi the evidence suggests that benign tumours with a risk of malignant transformation occur at a rate of approximately 1% (syringocystadenoma papilliferum being the commonest), whereas basal cell carcinoma occurs in less than 1% [48] and squamous cell carcinoma is rarer although well documented (Figures 73.7 and 73.8). Single, small CEN therefore do not require routine resection for medical reasons; however, in practice, as epidermal naevi are rare and can also pose a cosmetic problem, these lesions are often resected. In the authors' experience of *HRAS* mosaicism with extensive sebaceous naevi, multiple syringadenoma papilliferum are common from puberty onwards and can pose a serious management problem. Melanoma has been described in Becker naevus [49,50].

Hypophosphataemic rickets and osteomalacia is a serious and specific complication of RAS gene mosaicism, seen most commonly with *HRAS* mosaicism, but also very rarely with congenital melanocytic naevus syndrome (*NRAS* mosaicism) [50]. Recently the molecular basis of this has been described with the finding of RAS mutated cells within the bone of affected individuals [51]. This provides an explanation for the known association with elevated serum bone-derived FGF23 levels [52], previously suggested to emanate from the skin lesions. This condition requires phosphate replacement, and specialist endocrinology management.

Neurological abnormalities associated with CEN are many and varied, and are usually congenital structural malformations of the brain [6,53–55]. They have not so far been described with keratinocytic CEN due to *KRT10* or *KRT1* mutations. Central nervous system (CNS) lesions where they do occur tend to manifest as neurodevelopmental delay and/or seizures, both of which can be severe. High-risk cutaneous phenotypes for neurological involvement have not been firmly established, however one study

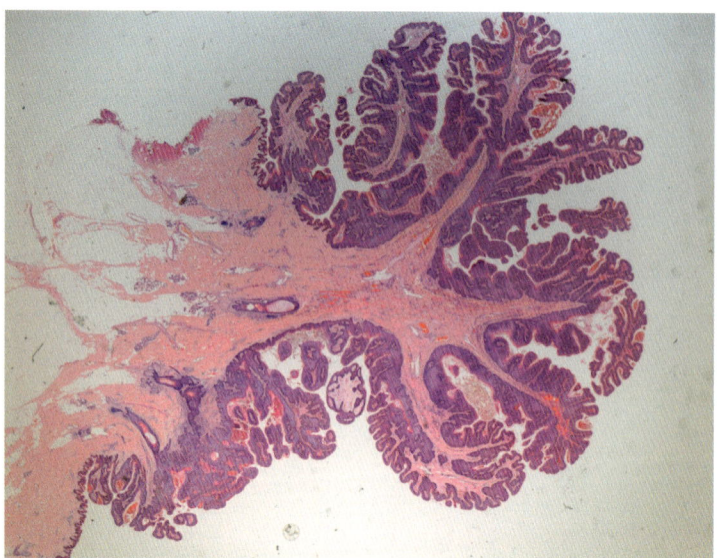

Figure 73.8 Photomicrograph of a syringocystadenoma arising in a sebaceous naevus showing a prominent papillary architecture. Original magnification ×20 (H&E). Courtesy of Professor N. J. Sebire.

encompassing various types of CEN suggested an increase when naevi were located on the head [56]. It is the authors' practice to perform magnetic resonance imaging (MRI) of the brain for any individual with neurological symptomatology at any time.

Disease course and prognosis

All CEN are permanent if not surgically removed. The prognosis for patients with CEN without extracutaneous involvement is excellent, although the prognosis for patients with CEN syndrome remains guarded with respect to neurological, ophthalmological, skeletal and other organ system abnormalities.

Investigations

History, examination and relevant investigations for non-cutaneous associations are essential to distinguish isolated from syndromic CEN. Small single non-Blaschkolinear CEN do not require biopsy for diagnosis and do not need further investigation if the child is well. For Blaschkolinear CEN a biopsy of the epidermal naevus is required to make an exact diagnosis, particularly for keratinocytic CEN of any size, to look for epidermolysis. There is no evidence that the size of the naevus is related to the chance of gonadal mosaicism in this condition. Should the biopsy reveal epidermolytic CEN, referral should be made to a clinical geneticist for counselling at an appropriate age as there is a possibility of transmitting the trait as a germline heterozygous dominant mutation if there is gonosomal mosaicism. Similarly CEN that have an inherited dimension (e.g. CHILD syndrome, Cowden syndrome) should trigger a referral to clinical genetics.

Investigation for extracutaneous abnormalities is not yet standardised in the literature as these conditions are rare, and presentations are often unique. In the absence of systematic studies, current investigation varies with the type of naevus, and should be dictated by the clinical presentation and the known associations of that particular CEN (e.g. dental, ophthalmological, neurological, orthopaedic or metabolic assessment). The association of multiple keratinocytic or sebaceous epidermal naevi with

hypophosphataemia is sufficiently common to merit routine investigation with baseline electrolyte and calcium/phosphate/alkaline phosphatase measurements. MRI of the CNS should be performed if there are any concerns from neurological assessment.

Management

Appropriate treatment options vary with the type of naevus, and whether the patient has associated abnormalities. Large-scale studies of therapy are lacking, but this is an area likely to expand in the future given recent genetic advances. Surgical excision can be suitable for small, single, epidermal naevi, but for more extensive lesions this is now rare. Keratinocytic and sebaceous naevi are candidates for ablative laser therapy to reduce thickness and/or hyperkeratosis of the lesion, and smaller verrucous lesions have been treated successfully with cryotherapy in a large series [57]. ILVEN have been treated with CO_2 laser therapy with variable response [58], and case reports describe treatment with therapies for psoriasis such as topical calcipotriol, etanercept and oral retinoids.

Congenital melanocytic naevi

Definition, nomenclature and classification

Congenital melanocytic naevi (CMN) are benign, pigmented, melanocytic naevi present at birth (Chapter 131).

Synonyms and inclusions
- Multiple CMN
- CMN syndrome
- Naevocellular naevus
- Naevus spilus-type CMN
- *NRAS* mosaicism
- Mosaic RASopathy
- Giant or giant hairy naevus – these should be avoided as the terms hairy and giant are understandably not generally acceptable to patients
- Neurocutaneous melanosis – this should be avoided in favour of CMN syndrome as many of the neurological associations are not melanotic, and the term NCM in the literature also included all cases of CNS melanoma

Classification links
- ICD-11: 887489797
- MIM: 137550
- Orphanet: ORPHA626

Epidemiology

Incidence and prevalence

It is not possible to estimate the true incidence of CMN as it is a congenital condition and affected fetuses could be miscarried. The prevalence at birth of small, single CMN is found consistently over time to be 1–2% of new births [59–61]. The prevalence of multiple CMN or of CMN syndrome as defined here is not known. The prevalence of CMN of greater than 20 cm projected adult size has only been systematically established in one study, at one in 20 000 new births [62].

Age

Congenital melanocytic naevi should be by definition present at birth. However, a small minority of lesions are either invisible or barely visible at birth, and then become clinically apparent as otherwise typical CMN in the first year of life – these are termed 'tardive'. These 'darken' as they fully appear over a period of years. There can occasionally be a tardive element to a normal CMN, where a subtle café-au-lait colouring adjacent to the main CMN becomes darker after birth. This can give the appearance of the CMN growing out of proportion to the child, which is not the usual clinical behaviour of CMN.

Sex

Most studies of patients with CMN show a slight preponderance of females to males of 1.2 : 1 [63–65], although a large prospective neonatal study showed no difference between the sexes [62].

Ethnicity

Congenital melanocytic naevi are seen in all ethnic groups. Overall incidence rates are consistent in the different worldwide studies so far. However, subgroup analysis of the largest study suggested a small but significant increase in children of black African descent [62], and in the absence of large studies in African and Asian populations we cannot yet conclude that there is no variability between ethnic groups.

Associated diseases

There has been controversy over whether CMN and neurofibromatosis type 1 can coexist, stemming from confusion due to the well-documented neuroid change that can be seen in CMN [66]. As a result, the current literature is not an easily interpretable source of data on this point. However, in the authors' experience, a single CMN can occasionally be the presenting feature of neurofibromatosis type 1, and very rarely a full-blown phenotype of multiple CMN can coexist with neurofibromatosis type 1 as defined by diagnostic criteria. A full physical examination is therefore always advised.

Pathophysiology

Predisposing factors

Germline predisposing factors were proposed to exist when a family history of some size of CMN was reported in second-degree relatives in approximately 25–30% of cases in a UK cohort [64]. Subsequently, homozygosity and compound heterozygosity for germline variants in the *melanocortin-1-receptor* (*MC1R*) gene were found to be more common in individuals with CMN, and certain variants were associated with a more severe cutaneous phenotype [67]. This increase in *MC1R* germline variants in CMN patients was confirmed in a second cohort, but no phenotype modification was identified in that cohort [68]. Predisposing germline duplications of Xp22.33 including gene *PPP2R3B* have also recently been described as predisposing to CMN as well as sporadic melanoma [69]. The mechanism for these genetic predispositions to both CMN and melanoma are not yet understood, but could involve either a predisposition to somatic mutation, or a promotion of the clinical phenotype should the somatic mutation occur.

Pathology

Melanocytic naevi of congenital type are almost always compound naevi with junctional, and predominant dermal, components, composed of bland melanocytes that characteristically extend around adnexal structures and often into the underlying muscle and fat. There is no cytological atypia. Melanocyte phenotypes often vary with depth such that they show a less differentiated and more spindled to ovoid appearance in the deep dermis (Figure 73.9).

Microscopic or macroscopic nodules may arise within CMN that almost always represent proliferative or hamartomatous nodules rather than melanoma (Figure 73.10). Melanoma may rarely occur within a CMN; when it does it is characterised by a poorly circumscribed, infiltrating proliferation of cells often with focal necrosis and demonstrating marked cytological atypia and mitotic activity (Figure 73.11).

It is not yet known exactly which cell type is affected by the somatic mutation as naevus cells exhibit many of the characteristics of undifferentiated and multipotent cells. Proposed candidate cell types have included mature melanocytes, immature melanocytes, melanocyte or dermal stem cells and neural crest stem cells [70–75], with recent evidence supporting some type of stem cell of origin.

Genetics

Congenital melanocytic naevi are caused by a somatic mutation *in utero*. A possible mechanism for single versus multiple skin lesions hinges on the timing of the mutation, with CMN syndrome occurring earlier in development. Germline background genotype may also play an important role in their development.

Single CMN were initially described to carry multiple different oncogenic mutations, including *BRAF* [76–82], *NRAS* [76,77,83–86], *MC1R* [76,87], *TP53* [76] and *GNAQ* [85]. At this stage the cause of CMN was still considered unknown, as causality of common driver mutations is difficult if not impossible to prove when sampling a single lesion. A study of multiple CMN and CMN syndrome then sampled multiple cutaneous and/or neurological lesions and established that there was conservation of specific mutations in multiple lesions from any individual [88]. This proved clonality, and that therefore the mutation detected was the phenotype-causing mutation. In this study *NRAS* was therefore identified as the cause of CMN in the majority of patients [88], and confirmed recently to be the commonest cause of all sizes of CMN, responsible for approximately 70% of cases [89]. *BRAF* was first demonstrated in more than one lesion in a single patient [90], and recently confirmed as a recurrent cause of CMN in 7% of a larger cohort [89].

The CMN-causing mutations in *NRAS* are codon-specific, with p.Q61K being the most common amino acid change, and p.Q61R being less frequent [88]. Codon 61 is within the active site of the NRAS GTPase, and these mutations lead to constitutive activation of the protein. Subsequently, a remarkable phenotype–genotype correlation has been shown for p.Q61H and p.G13R mutations that were shown to be associated with naevus spilus-type CMN (see 'Clinical variants' later in this section) [91], but have never been described in classic CMN.

ALK gene fusions have been described in two patients with multiple CMN [92,93], in one case demonstrated in more than one lesion [92], and therefore this may be a recurrent cause of CMN.

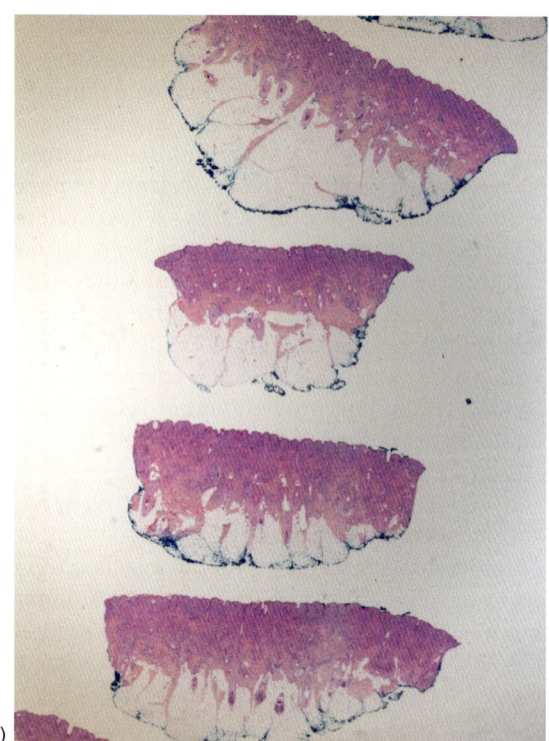

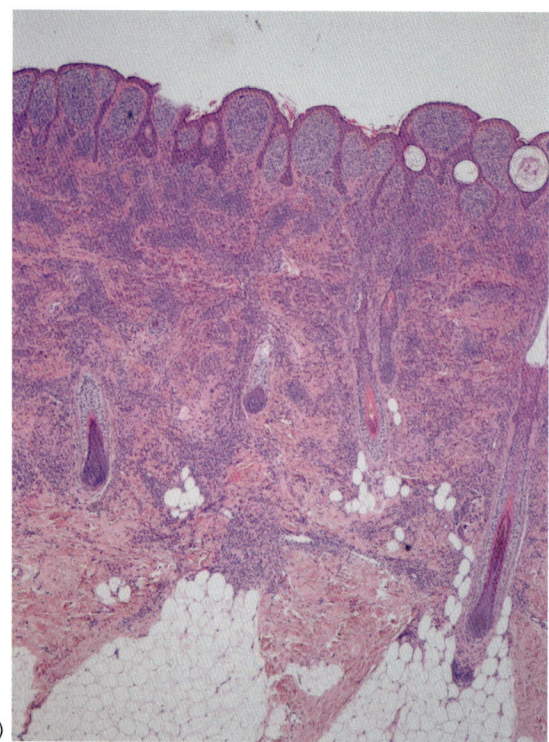

(a)   (b)

Figure 73.9 Photomicrographs of a typical congenital melanocytic naevus demonstrating a predominantly dermal lesion composed of bland naevus cells that extend around adnexal structures with no cytological atypia. Original magnifications (a) ×20 and (b) ×40 (H&E). Courtesy of Professor N. J. Sebire.

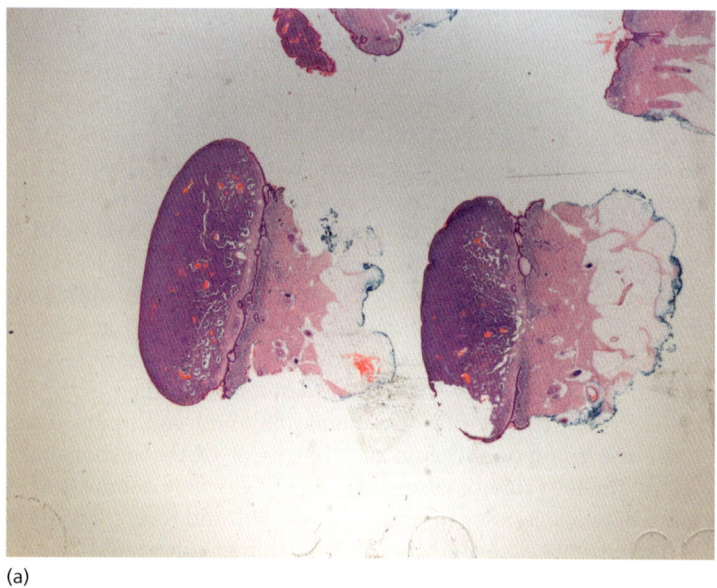

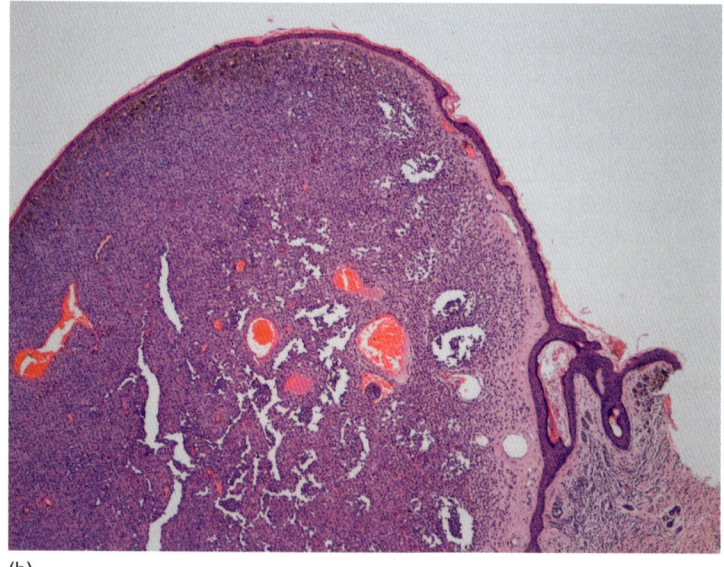

(a)   (b)

Figure 73.10 Photomicrographs demonstrating a proliferative nodule arising in a congenital melanocytic naevus composed of sheets of bland naevus cells forming a distinct nodule but with no cytological atypia. Original magnifications (a) ×20 and (b) ×40 (H&E). Courtesy of Professor N. J. Sebire.

A single patient with a *SOX5-RAF1* fusion in more than one lesion has also been described [92], potentially implicating one or both of these genes as a cause.

A study of genotype versus phenotype and clinical outcomes has found that the genotype of CMN is not currently indicated in clinical practice unless the patient develops melanoma, as it will not alter the management of non-malignant CMN [89]. It is important,

however, to genotype if the patient develops melanoma as it will guide targeted therapies [94].

Environmental factors

Environmental factors have not been shown to play a significant role in the development of CMN. A retrospective questionnaire cohort study examined the question of potential environmental

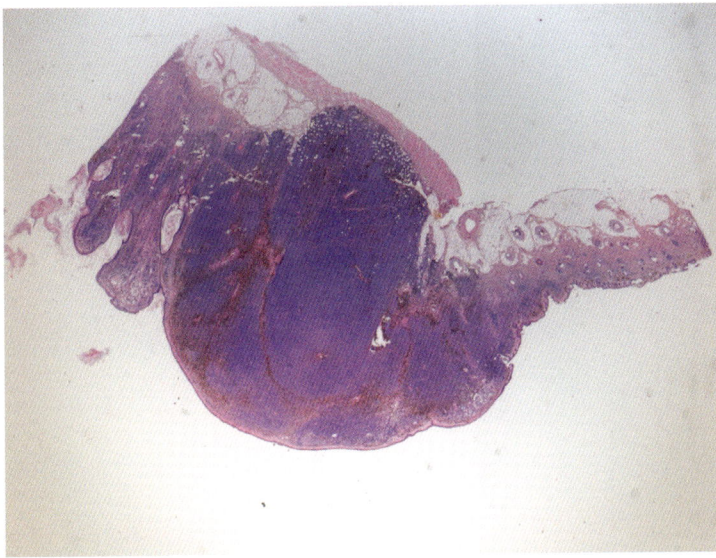

Figure 73.11 Photomicrograph of a melanoma developing within a congenital melanocytic naevus demonstrating a proliferative subpopulation, which infiltrates widely and distorts the surrounding architecture, associated with cytological atypia. Original magnification ×20 (H&E). Courtesy of Professor N. J. Sebire.

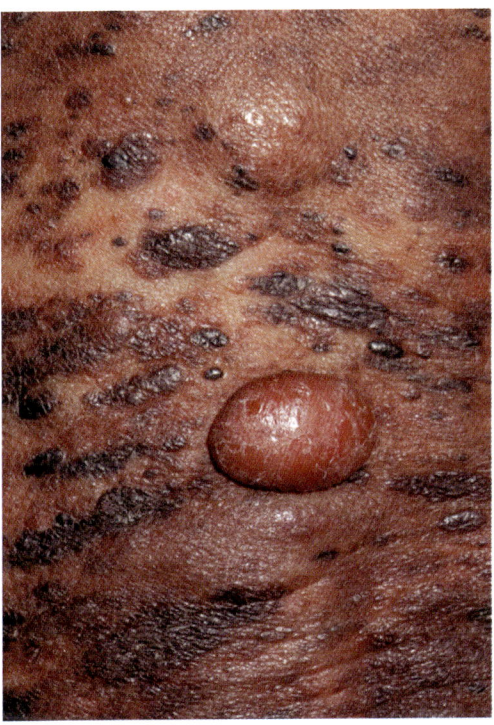

Figure 73.12 Benign proliferative nodule in a large congenital melanocytic naevus, present from birth and stable in behaviour.

factors in the pathogenesis of CMN, suggesting that smoking during pregnancy could be associated with a small excess risk, but excluding sunbed use, medications, radiographs, alcohol ingestion, maternal infections and anaesthetics. Mothers of children born with CMN were, however, more likely to have suffered a threatened miscarriage, severe nausea/vomiting or raised blood pressure than a control group [64]. These features could be either cause or effect of the mutation, or due to a common independent factor.

Clinical features
History and presentation
Congenital melanocytic naevi are most commonly brown or black, but can also appear purplish or red, particularly at birth. They are frequently heterogeneous in colour and/or texture. Apart from the very smallest lesions they are usually palpable, with increased surface markings. Lesions are darkest at birth, and usually lighten to some degree over the first few years of life, occasionally dramatically [95,96].

For non-scalp CMN, overlying hair is often not apparent at birth and may develop in the first year. Scalp CMN often have thick luxuriant or wiry hair at birth, which grows at a significantly greater rate than the surrounding scalp hair. The colour of the hair usually approximates to the scalp colour over time, but may remain of a different texture. Occasionally, CMN even on the scalp are not hair-bearing. CMN on the scalp can produce white hairs after some years, and patchy hair loss within the CMN is not uncommon.

CMN can be single or multiple. Smaller CMN in association with a larger one have traditionally been termed 'satellite' lesions, however multiple CMN is a more accurate term [97]. This is because the term satellites probably stems from its use in melanoma where it means local seeding/metastasis from a central lesion, which has not been shown to be the case in CMN.

A CMN can contain at birth or develop benign proliferative areas or well-defined nodules (Figure 73.12) [98,99]. These can cause clinical and histological difficulties in differentiation from melanoma

[66], and specialist opinions should be obtained in this situation. The management of a new lump is detailed later in this section. The authors recognise two commonly arising benign proliferative lesions, although many variants exist. These two can be termed proliferative nodules and diffuse neuroid proliferations:

- Proliferative nodules are often present at birth, are well circumscribed, symmetrical, round or oval, soft to firm and of any uniform colour. They are usually half to a few centimetres in diameter. These nodules can usually be resected relatively easily if required.
- Diffuse neuroid proliferations are usually not present at birth, but can develop at any point during childhood, and often continue to grow slowly over time. They can become more active around puberty. They have less well-defined edges, can be a few centimetres to very large, are firm, and often become pendulous when larger. In the authors' experience they are often difficult to resect, as they tend to recur, often quickly. Histopathologically, they show poorly circumscribed areas showing neuroid-type differentiation of CMN cells.

BRAF-variant CMN appear to be associated with a higher chance of a multinodular phenotype. This was first described as a phenotypic feature in a single case [90], and the association demonstrated in a larger cohort [89]. It is, however, possible to have a multinodular phenotype with other genotypes, and it is possible to have no nodules with a *BRAF*-variant CMN [89].

Clinical variants
Naevus spilus-type CMN is defined by a café-au-lait macular background, onto which are superimposed multiple CMN of different sizes and colours [100,101]. Importantly, however, the café-au-lait macular background may not be evident at birth, and the diagnosis

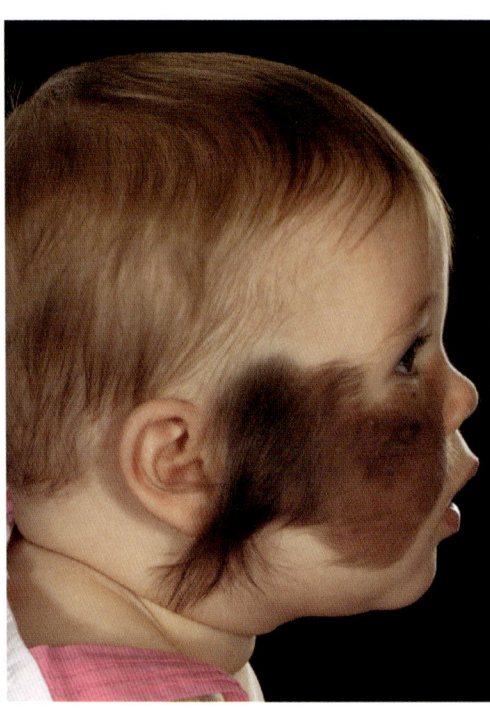

(a)

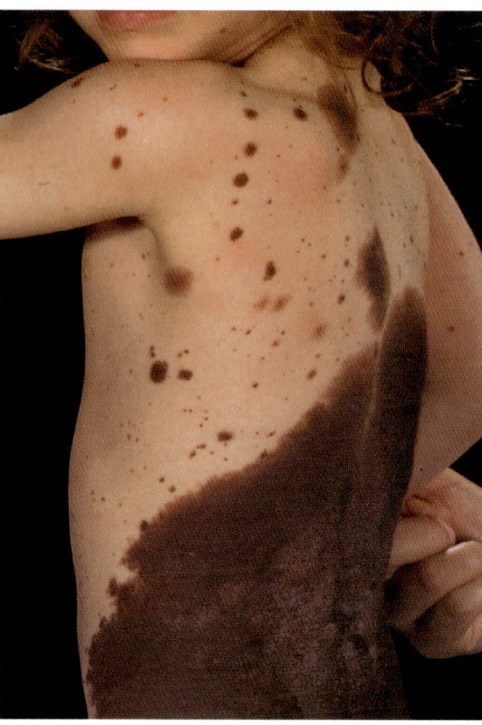

(b)

Figure 73.13 Congenital melanocytic naevi (CMN). (a) Single CMN on the face showing marked hypertrichosis. (b) Multiple CMN of different sizes on the trunk.

should therefore be suspected where CMN are agminated. The background generally appears in the first few years. These naevus spilus CMN can occur on the body as single or multiple lesions. Where multiple, the smaller 'satellite' lesions are often not present at birth, and when they do appear are often indistinguishable from café-au-lait macules as they only present initially with the café-au-lait macular background [91]. Naevus spilus-type CMN has a subtly different genetic basis (see 'Genetics' earlier in this section).

CMN have recently been described in association with low-flow vascular malformations in the same area as the CMN [90,**102**]. This appears to be a rare finding.

Differential diagnosis

Congenital melanocytic naevi can sometimes be difficult to distinguish from congenital blue naevi, but the latter are usually blue/black rather than brown/black. If in doubt a biopsy will help differentiate.

Classification of severity

The most clinically useful phenotypic measure in terms of clinical outcomes remains the distinction between a single lesion and more than one lesion (Figure 73.13). It is therefore extremely important that the patient is examined thoroughly, to look for a second or subsequent small CMN, which may be relatively pale at birth.

If the patient has more than one CMN there is some degree of association between the severity of the cutaneous phenotype and the risk of neurological and malignant complications. The clinical cutaneous feature that has been shown to have the best statistical correlation with neurological outcomes is the projected adult size (PAS) [64,103]. The total number of naevi is also associated with the neurological outcome, however as the PAS of the largest lesion

and the total number of lesions are themselves closely connected, these are confounders in statistical models, and PAS is consistently more reliable. A complete classification of phenotype in an individual with CMN should also include the presence of neurological lesions on MRI, clinical neurological abnormalities, characteristic facial features and the presence of malignancy. Some clinicians also include other details of cutaneous phenotype such as rugosity and colour [104], however these have not been shown so far to be connected to outcome measures.

Assessment of PAS can be done in various ways, *none of which is accurate*. There is a method that involves a multiplication factor applied to a measured diameter, which takes into account the differential rate of growth of the head and body in children. However, these authors do not find this method useful as the largest lesion frequently affects more than one body part (e.g. extending from the head onto the torso). Therefore, until better measures exist, we suggest that the patient is examined fully and the largest lesion identified; the outline is drawn onto a standard adult body map, and the projected adult size of the largest non-circumferential diameter is then estimated.

Complications and co-morbidities

Neurological abnormalities. Single CMN have not so far been described in association with neurological abnormalities on MRI, independent of the size and site of the CMN. For multiple CMN, however, neurological abnormalities are the commonest co-morbidity [103]. The term neurocutaneous melanosis was initially proposed to describe the association of cutaneous and melanotic CNS lesions [105–107]. However, this term is no longer appropriate due to many subsequent reports of non-melanocytic, structural and tumoral lesions in these patients [103,108–110], and the term CMN syndrome has therefore been proposed to encompass anyone with CMN and non-cutaneous features [111].

The description of a characteristic signal for melanin on MRI and the first reports of neurological findings in individuals with CMN [105,106,112–114] opened the door to studying the neurological features. All previous reports had been necessarily biased by postmortem findings only. Since those initial studies, larger cohorts have been studied prospectively, and a new classification has been recently proposed based on long-term follow-up of affected individuals [115]. Most importantly, the long-held tenant that anyone with 'symptomatic' neurological lesions (i.e. seizures or neurodevelopmental delay) is always at high risk of death is incorrect. This confusion has arisen from the complicating feature of melanoma arising within the CNS (see the section on melanoma).

CNS abnormalities can be classified into two clinically relevant groups based on MRI findings: intraparenchymal melanosis alone, and 'other' (everything else). Intraparenchymal melanosis alone is the commonest finding in association with multiple CMN (approximately 20% of cases with more than one CMN in a large prospective study), and very importantly is not in itself associated with an increased risk of death. In approximately 50% of cases the lesions are asymptomatic, but in the other 50% they can be associated with neurodevelopmental delay, attention deficit hyperactivity disorder and autistic spectrum disorder, or seizures. As the commonest site for intraparenchymal melanosis is the amygdala [96,103,105,112], seizures are most commonly temporal lobe epilepsy. These lesions do not need to be either biopsied or resected if they show characteristic MRI changes, and MRI scans do not need to be repeated routinely if the patient is well. Very occasionally, seizures are refractory to medical therapy, and epilepsy surgery has been successfully employed in suitable cases [116–118]. Infants with intraparenchymal melanosis only can therefore be given a normal prognosis but should have neurodevelopmental follow-up in the first few years of life, and referral to a paediatric neurologist in the event of clinical abnormalities.

All other findings on MRI should be viewed with more caution. These are much rarer and there are many unique reports of associations. These lesions require re-scanning at regular intervals until behavioural stability has been determined. In particular, leptomeningeal involvement has to be viewed with a high level of suspicion and monitored carefully as rapid diffuse growth of melanocytic cells can occur, behaving clinically as a malignant process. Hydrocephalus has so far always required shunting in patients with CMN, even when there is no apparent obstructive cause. This is presumed to be due to leptomeningeal disease below the level of MRI resolution, which then usually becomes radiologically apparent within weeks. It can be the presenting feature of a new malignant process, either within the leptomeninges or sometimes separately from an intraparenchymal melanoma, but can rarely also be stable over years. Dandy–Walker malformation and other posterior fossa malformations are also well described. A variety of non-melanoma brain tumours have been described in individual cases and should be treated in the usual way, with the caveat that they should be genotyped for *NRAS* codon 61 mutations [88], as this could alter oncological management.

Importantly, individuals with CMN can have abnormal neurodevelopment and occasionally seizures in the absence of any detectable lesion on MRI [119]. The recent discovery of intraparenchymal lesions and subtle cortical dysplasia on histology that were below the resolution of MRI is the most likely explanation for this [116]. Again, these neurological symptoms do not equate to an increased risk of death, and they should be managed as for any other child.

Melanoma. Melanoma occurs more commonly in individuals with CMN. The risk in adulthood has not been systematically studied. The risk in childhood is polarised and associated with the severity of the congenital neurocutaneous phenotype. For small single cutaneous lesions the risk is very low, estimated at less than 0.1% [120].

It is now fairly well established that the risk of melanoma in childhood in all sizes of CMN is 0.1–2% [64,121–124]. However, this risk is variable, being very low for small single lesions [120], with a range extending up to as high as 10–14% in individuals with naevi of >60 cm PAS [64]. The median age for developing melanoma was estimated at approximately 7 years in a retrospective literature review [121], however in a prospective cohort study the median age was approximately 2 years [**94**]. The relative risk in childhood is therefore very high compared with the normal population where melanoma is virtually unknown in this age group. Management of a new cutaneous lump and new neurological presentation is detailed later.

Importantly, primary melanoma does not only arise within affected skin, but within the CNS in at least 50% of cases [64,121]. So far there have been no reliable reports of melanoma arising in the CNS of an individual with a normal screening MRI scan taken in the first 6 months of life. However, given the presence of lesions below the resolution of MRI it cannot be ruled out as a possibility, and any child with CMN presenting with an acute change in CNS symptoms or signs should have an urgent MRI with contrast enhancement. Melanoma has also rarely been reported arising in other organ systems.

Other tumours. There are rare reports of other malignancies arising within CMN, most notably rhabdomyosarcoma [125–128].

Characteristic facial features. Children with CMN have been found to have characteristic facial features using strictly defined dysmorphology criteria, and in statistical comparison with a large cohort of normal schoolchildren [111]. At least three characteristic facial features were seen in 74% of the CMN cohort studied. The characteristic features are wide or prominent forehead, hypertelorism, eyebrow variants, periorbital fullness, small/short nose, narrow nasal ridge, broad nasal tip, broad or round face, full cheeks, prominent premaxilla, prominent/long philtrum and everted lower lip. These features are likely to be due to involvement by the mosaic mutation of the precursors of facial bone and/or cartilage and/or dermis, all of which are derived from the neural crest in humans. RAS pathway genes are known to alter facial development, as is seen in germline RASopathies, with widening of the face a described feature of *NRAS* mutations in animal models and humans [129,130]. Furthermore, characteristic facial features are well described in other mosaic conditions such as Pallister–Killian syndrome [131], *PIK3CA* mosaicism [132] and Cornelia de Lange syndrome [133].

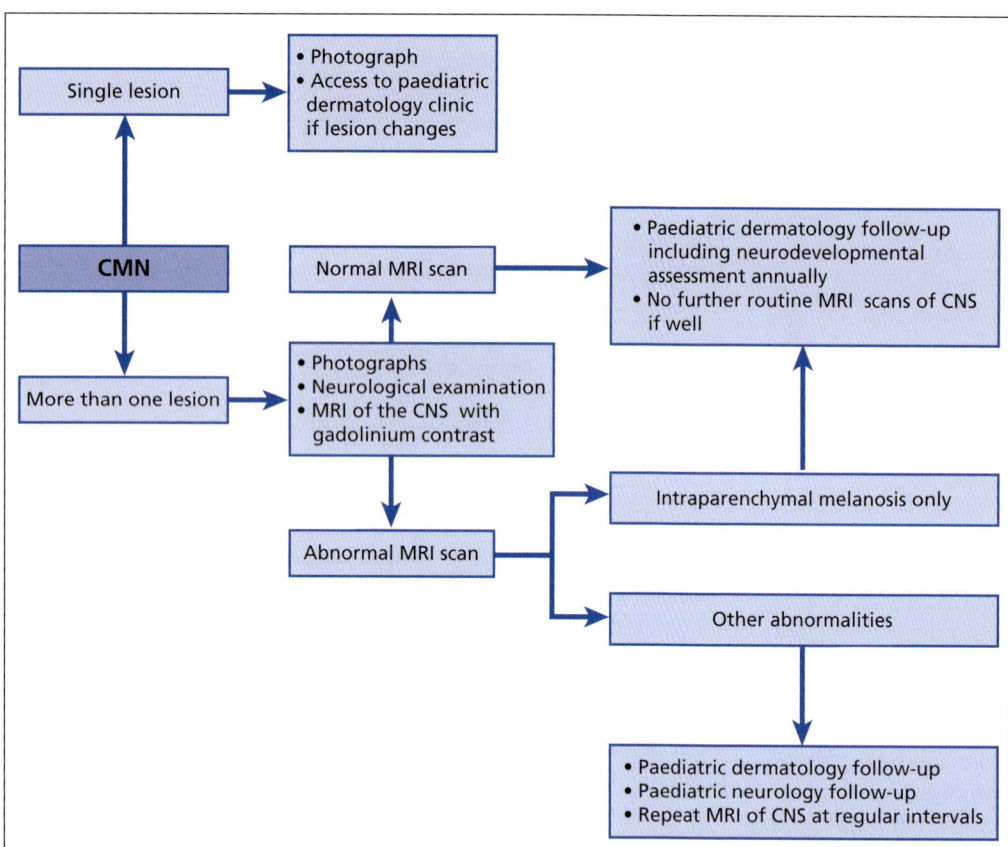

Figure 73.14 Clinical management algorithm for neurological investigation and follow-up of patients with congenital melanocytic naevi (CMN). CNS, central nervous system; MRI, magnetic resonance imaging.

Investigations

The diagnosis of CMN is usually a clinical one. Neurological investigations and monitoring for cutaneous or extracutaneous melanoma should be undertaken as in Figure 73.14.

Management

All children with CMN should have a clinical neurological history and examination after birth (Figure 73.14). Any child with clinical abnormalities should have an MRI of the CNS. In the absence of abnormal clinical neurology, children with a single CMN (independent of size or site) do not require routine MRI of the CNS. Children with multiple (i.e. two or more) CMN at birth (independent of size or site) should have a routine MRI of the brain and whole spine with contrast injection, preferably within the first 6 months of life [134]. In large paediatric centres this can usually be done without the need for a general anaesthetic. If the MRI is either normal or shows classic intraparenchymal melanosis only, no further imaging needs to be undertaken during childhood if the patient remains clinically neurologically normal (which should be assessed at each visit). If, however, the MRI reveals other intracranial pathology, the child should have an urgent referral to paediatric neurology and/or neurosurgery depending on the appearances. Further imaging in these cases is highly likely to be required.

Acute presentation at any age with neurological symptoms such as those of raised intracranial pressure or seizures should trigger urgent MRI of the whole CNS with contrast. Hydrocephalus in these cases is always in our experience caused by leptomeningeal disease, but this is not always visible on MRI at the time of the initial presentation of raised intracranial pressure. Raised intracranial pressure in the presence of normal MRI should therefore be treated as if due to an obstructive problem at the level of the leptomeninges (usually by ventriculo-peritoneal shunting), and a repeat scan undertaken within a few weeks to look for progression. If none is seen it is sensible to continue to repeat scans at 3-monthly intervals until it is certain that its appearance is stable. Leptomeningeal disease presenting acutely with hydrocephalus is most often a malignantly behaving process, which should be considered to be diffuse leptomeningeal melanoma, although very rarely it can stabilise and persist with issues pertaining to spinal cord compression only. There is no proven benefit in sampling of the cerebrospinal fluid as this usually contains melanin-containing cells, and the histology of these cells is very difficult to interpret. Currently, the best way of assessing for malignancy in the leptomeninges is to look for radiological progression until stable or clearly progressive. If clearly progressive, a biopsy of the leptomeningeal tissue is indicated to assess for melanoma. Copy number measurement of DNA from leptomeningeal tissue demonstrates abnormalities in leptomeningeal melanoma but not in benign leptomeningeal proliferation, mirroring the situation in the skin [135,136]. This has therefore been found to be a clinically very useful investigation in distinguishing between a benign proliferation and melanoma in the CNS. Occasionally, a diffuse leptomeningeal melanoma is accompanied by a spatially distinct intracerebral melanoma. This is difficult to comprehend as it suggests two primaries, but is an observable phenomenon and both lesions need to be considered for treatment. In the authors' experience it is most commonly the leptomeningeal disease that is the cause of death, due to rapidly progressive spinal cord progression. For potential treatment options see later.

Acute presentation with a new lump in the CMN, if clinically diagnosed as a benign proliferative nodule, should be photographed with a scale and a thorough search should be made for lymphadenopathy. If none is present, a clinical review should be undertaken within 4 weeks. If local lymphadenopathy is present, the nodule should be removed immediately. If at review in 4 weeks the nodule is continuing to change, biopsy is indicated, with histology, NRAS and BRAF mutation analysis, and array comparative genomic hybridisation (CGH) where available [88,137]. Array CGH has been well documented to be clinically useful at distinguishing benign bland CMN from proliferative nodules, and from melanoma, and is frequently helpful in cases of difficult histology [88,137]. If the nodule is clinically unchanged after 4 weeks, continue to observe unless there is another indication for removal (such as catching on clothing).

It is important to stress again that cutaneous melanoma is frequently overdiagnosed in patients with CMN, and expert clinical and histopathological opinions should always be sought. Where melanoma is definitely confirmed, the outlook in patients with multiple CMN is extremely poor, and death usually occurs within 6–12 months from diagnosis [94]. Standard management used for adult melanoma (where no CMN is present) is not sufficiently aggressive in most cases. The patient should be referred to a specialist centre with paediatric oncology experience and a melanoma multidisciplinary team. Work-up to look for metastases includes a full-body positron emission tomography scan, a chest X-ray, abdominal ultrasound and an MRI of the CNS if this has not already been undertaken. Bloods should include a lactate dehydrogenase level. Treatment of cutaneous melanoma will usually include surgery. MEK (mitogen-activated extracellular signal-regulated kinase) inhibition has been demonstrated to improve symptoms in a small cohort of patients with NRAS-variant CMN-associated melanoma of the CNS [138], and further unpublished data in similar patients suggest that survival is prolonged. BRAF inhibitors would be contraindicated in NRAS-variant CMN, however if the CMN was BRAF-variant these would be an appropriate therapy.

Importantly, there are no current data to suggest that surgical removal of multiple CMN reduces the risk of malignancy in an affected individual. In addition, surgical removal of all affected tissue is not possible in those cases with highest risk, as some of this tissue will be within the CNS, and the skin is usually extensively affected. Lastly, more cases of CMN melanoma arise within the CNS than in the skin in childhood, and surgical removal of skin lesions does not remove this risk.

Where there are no immediate medical problems to consider, however, cosmetic management of CMN is important to discuss with the family and patient. There are many different opinions on how best to deal with CMN from a cosmetic viewpoint, and to a large degree the decision on what to do is dependent on the individual. Hair can be removed most easily by shaving, which may not have to be done very often to improve the appearance significantly. Hair removal creams and waxing are usually too harsh to use on CMN in children, causing irritation or skin removal. Superficial removal techniques such as dermabrasion or curettage or laser therapy have been shown not to improve the final colour

of CMN. In a large study of colour change in CMN over time it was demonstrated that the degree of spontaneous lightening is related to the underlying pigmentary phenotype of the individual. In other words, children with lighter skin get more lightening of the CMN, and this is genetically determined. In addition, no correlation was found between the colour of the CMN at birth and its final colour, indicating that pigmentary phenotype of the CMN at birth is as unreliable a predictor as hair and eye colour at birth, all of which are likely affected by maternal factors [139]. While superficial removal techniques lighten the CMN initially this is solely a function of removal of the top layer of pigmented cells, which are replaced (rapidly in some cases) with new pigmented cells. The apparent improvement in final colour comes about due to comparison of photographs from birth, with photographs after superficial removal. This has been demonstrated in cases where part of the CMN was lasered and part was not, with both areas ending up at exactly the same digitally measured colour [139]. In addition, superficial removal can leave areas of scarring. Superficial removal techniques should not therefore be used for the cosmetic treatment of CMN.

Serial excision of single lesions or cosmetically prominent lesions (e.g. on the face) can produce good results although inevitably will leave a scar. Some centres favour large-scale removal using balloon skin expansion techniques, and cosmetic results can be good, albeit again with the caveat of scarring and the impact of multiple operations and the associated pain. In each individual case the pros and cons of surgery should be discussed with the families.

Resources

Patient resources
Caring Matters Now: www.caringmattersnow.co.uk.
Nevus Outreach: www.nevus.org.
Contact (for families with disabled children): http://www.cafamily.org.uk.
(All last accessed February 2022.)

Congenital Spitz naevus, congenital blue naevus and congenital naevus spilus

Congenital Spitz naevi are rare with no reliable estimates of prevalence at birth. As in later life, they can mimic melanoma [140], and the diagnosis is therefore often made after excisional biopsy as the histological features are characteristic of acquired Spitz naevi [141] (Chapter 131). Spitzoid change is also described within congenital melanocytic naevi [141]. The incidence of malignant transformation in congenital lesions is not known. Agminated or eruptive Spitz naevi can rarely present at birth [142].

Congenital blue naevi are rare and can be of either the common, cellular or epithelioid blue naevus types. Congenital common blue naevi exhibit the same clinical and histological features (Figure 73.15) as their acquired counterpart, in which somatic mutations have been described in GNAQ [143]. Where the clinical appearance is typical, resection is not required for medical reasons. Congenital cellular blue naevi on the other hand are frequently significantly larger than their acquired counterparts, and occur most frequently on the scalp. This variant has been described in association with various underlying scalp and neurological defects [144,145], and with malignant transformation [146]. Multiple congenital blue naevi at birth have very rarely been described (Figure 73.16) [147,148] and can rarely be familial [149].

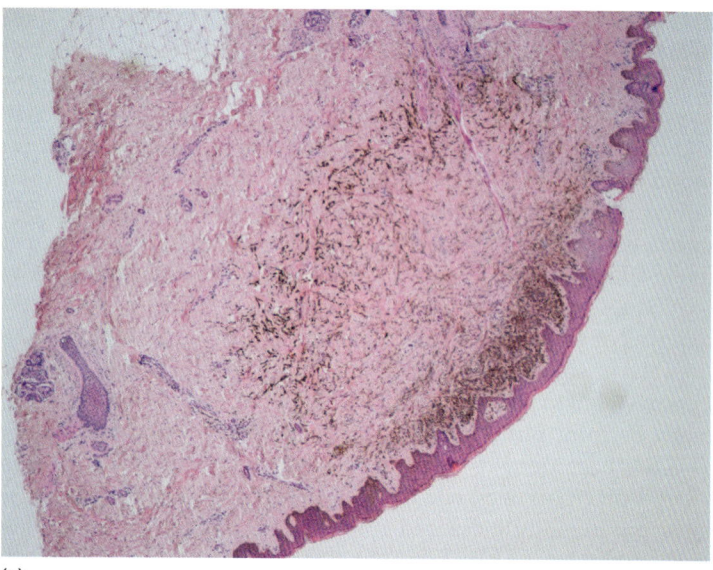

(a)

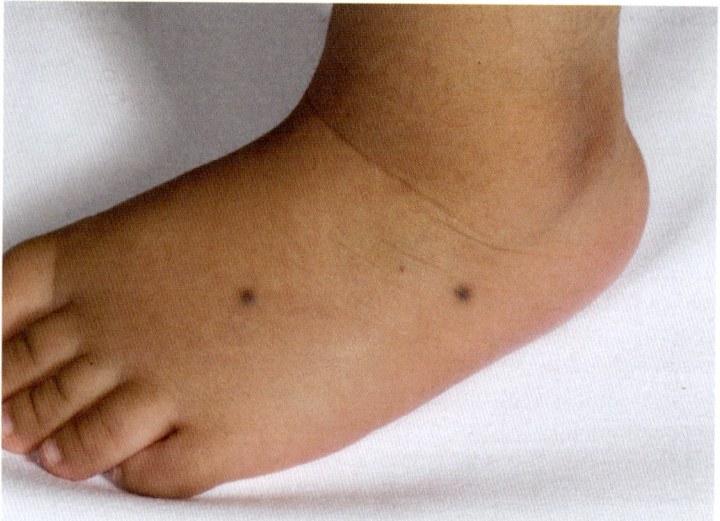

Figure 73.16 Two congenital blue naevi on the foot of a child with multiple similar lesions from birth, and developing over the first year of life.

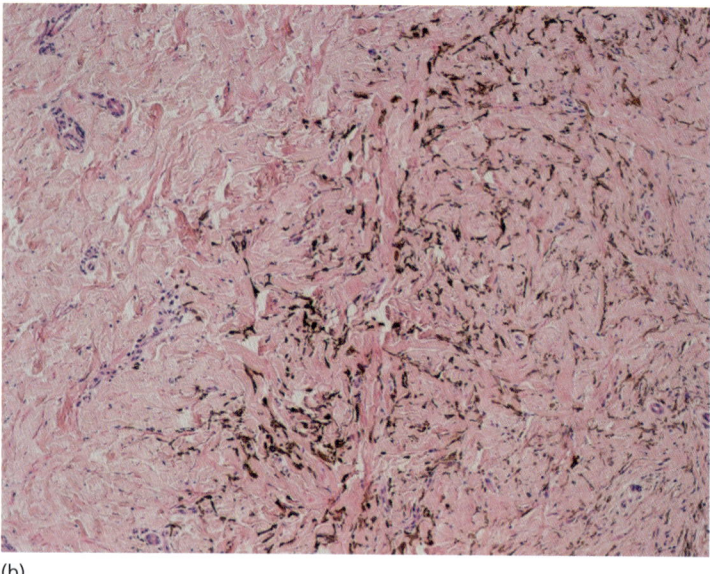

(b)

Figure 73.15 Photomicrographs of a blue naevus demonstrating spindle-shaped pigmented naevus cells extending into the deep dermis. Original magnifications (a) ×40 and (b) ×100 (H&E). Courtesy of Professor N. J. Sebire.

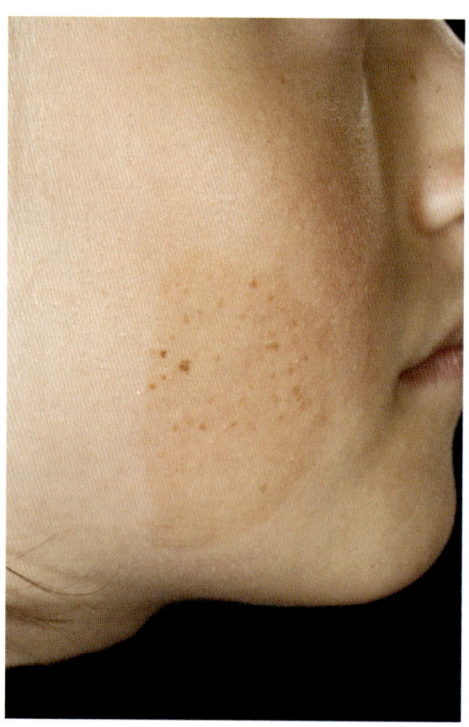

Figure 73.17 Single naevus spilus on the face showing a café-au-lait macule background with superimposed darker areas.

Congenital naevus spilus (or speckled lentiginous naevi) are pigmented lesions with a café-au-lait macule background and super-imposed, more darkly pigmented areas (or speckles) (Figure 73.17). The background may not be apparent at birth, and the superimposed speckles may increase in number over time. Some lesions are entirely macular, and some have papular and less uniformly distributed speckles [150]. Histologically, naevus spilus is lentigo simplex with superimposed benign junctional or compound melanocytic naevi [151]. Naevus spilus are more often single but the size varies from about a centimetre in diameter to covering a whole limb in a segmental or zosteriform distribution. Larger lesions can form part of phakomatosis pigmentokeratotica [152], or the speckled lentiginous naevus syndrome with hyperhidrosis, dysaesthesia, underlying muscular defects and neurological abnormalities [153,154]. Some smaller and larger lesions have been found to be due to somatic-activating mutations in *HRAS* [29,155], at least partly explaining the predilection for these lesions to develop superimposed Spitz naevi [156,157], previously described to harbour *HRAS* mutations [158]. More recently, congenital naevus spilus either alone or in the context of phakomatosis pigmento-vascularis type III or spilorosea type have been found to be due to variants in gene *PTPN11* [159]. These patients are at risk of *PTPN11*-driven melanoma arising in the naevus spilus.

Congenital connective tissue naevus and fat naevus

Definition and nomenclature

Congenital connective tissue naevi are benign cutaneous hamartomas of connective tissue components present at birth.

Synonyms and inclusions
- Collagen naevus
- Elastic tissue naevus
- Juvenile elastoma
- Naevus anelasticans
- Naevus mucinosus
- Mixed connective tissue naevus
- Congenital lipoma
- Naevus psiloliparus

Introduction and general description

Congenital connective tissue naevi are a clinically heterogeneous group of hamartomas, named by the predominant cell type on histology, and therefore usually requiring biopsy for diagnosis.

Epidemiology

Congenital connective tissue naevi as a group are rare at birth but exact prevalences have not been established. No sex predilection is known. No differences between ethnic groups have been described.

Pathophysiology

Histologically, connective tissue naevi are hamartomatous lesions of the dermis usually with a mixed histological composition [160] but in which a predominant component is present, giving the lesion its name, or by the absence of a component as in naevus anelasticus. Lesions are poorly circumscribed and non-encapsulated and show thickening of the dermis with replacement of the normal dermis or subcutis with lesional tissue. This lesional tissue is often composed of irregularly arranged collagen fibres with or without variable amounts of abnormal elastic tissue (Figure 73.18). Comparison with normal skin, in addition to special stains to highlight particular components, are helpful in making the diagnosis.

Clinical features

By definition, these lesions are present at birth, although the average age for presentation of any connective tissue naevus is 2 years [160]. They can be single or multiple, and can be associated with extracutaneous features. Some can continue to grow or develop adjacent new lesions, particularly plantar collagenomas in Proteus syndrome [161] and elastomas in Buschke–Ollendorf syndrome.

Isolated, congenital collagenomas are soft to firm, skin-coloured, brownish or yellowish nodules or plaques (Figure 73.19). This is in contrast to eruptive collagenomas, an acquired disease of multiple lesions appearing after puberty. Familial cutaneous collagenomas again present later in life, and are usually multiple, often larger lesions. Collagenomas associated with Proteus syndrome occur characteristically on the soles of the feet in the first few years of life, and are cerebriform in appearance. Similar lesions can be seen in other overgrowth syndromes due to *PIK3CA* mosaicism [8,34].

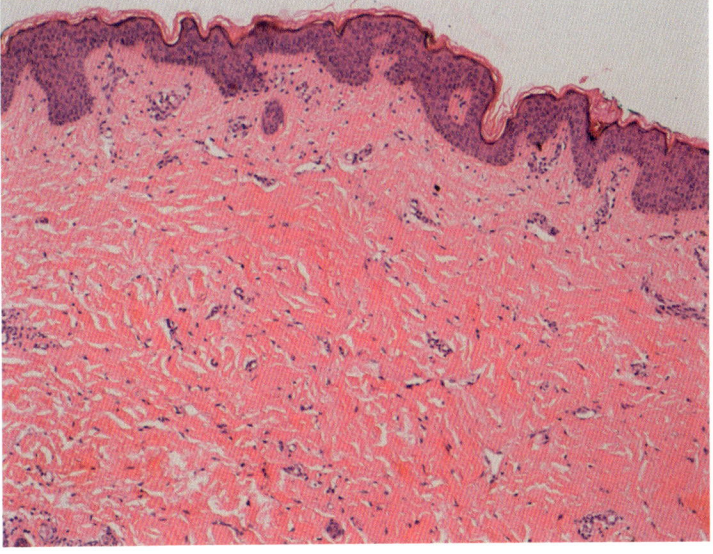

(a)

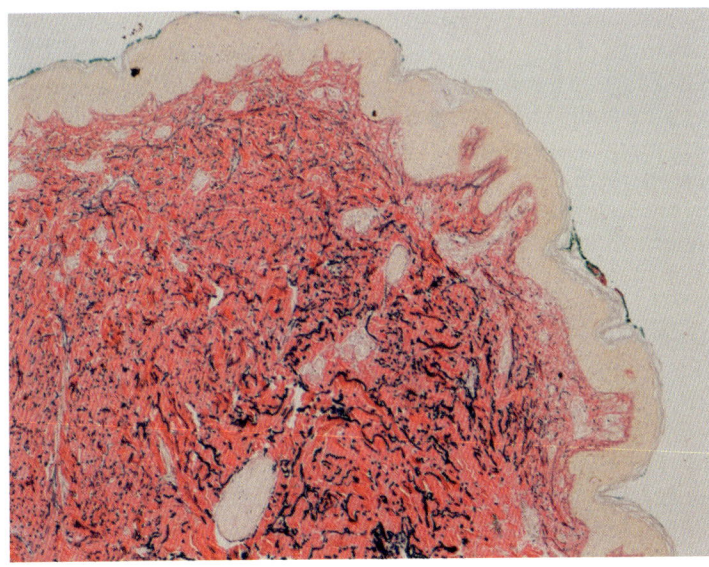

(b)

Figure 73.18 Photomicrographs of a connective tissue naevus demonstrating a poorly circumscribed dermal lesion composed of abnormal bundles of collagen and admixed elastic fibres within the dermis. Original magnifications ×100 (a, H&E; b, elastic van Gieson stain). Courtesy of Professor N. J. Sebire.

Congenital elastomas are firm, skin-coloured or creamy/yellowish papules or nodules, with a diameter ranging from millimetres to a centimetre, that often coalesce to form plaques or clusters. Single lesions can present at any site; however in Buschke–Ollendorf syndrome they classically present in groups or plaques on the lower abdominal wall, trunk, arms and buttocks. Naevus anelasticus is not described congenitally but does start in the first two decades. This is a histopathological diagnosis due to the absence or fragmentation of elastic fibres within a papule or plaque, and controversy exists regarding the diagnostic overlap between this and eruptive collagenomas or papular elastorrhexis [162–164].

Congenital lipomas present as localised, skin-coloured, soft proliferations with indistinct edges. The 'Michelin tyre' baby phenotype

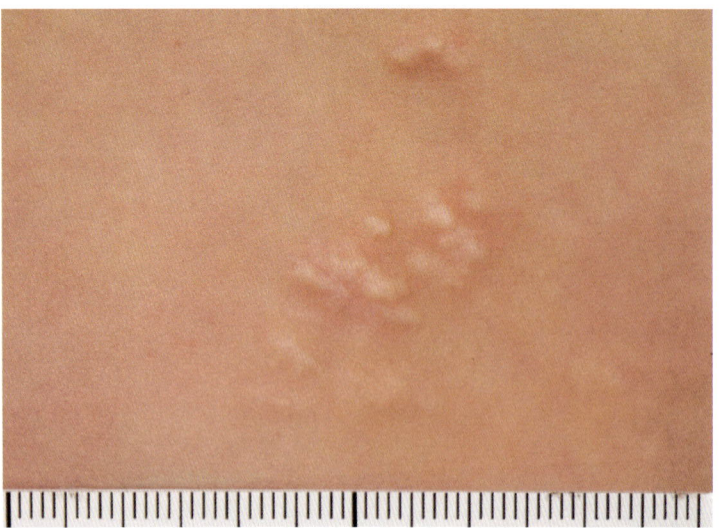

Figure 73.19 Collagenoma-type connective tissue naevus on the lower abdomen.

has been associated with both fat naevus and diffuse smooth muscle hamartoma [165,166]. In this phenotype the infant has generalised thickening of the skin with pronounced folds. Naevus psiloliparus is a rare entity characterised by aberrant hair follicle development and prominent dermal fat deposition [167], which presents as a smooth, skin-coloured or yellowish, flat or slightly raised lesion on the scalp. These naevi can be single lesions without associated abnormalities [168], or can be found in encephalo-cranio-cutaneous lipomatosis.

Associations, syndromes and genetics

The genetic basis of isolated congenital connective tissue naevi remains to be fully delineated, although in one case *LEMD3* has also been implicated in the pathogenesis of isolated familial collagenomas [169]. The genetic basis of single, non-syndromic, non-familial connective tissue naevi is not yet known.

Elastomas (and occasionally collagenomas) can be the presenting feature of Buschke–Ollendorf syndrome, an autosomal dominant disorder caused by germline loss-of-function mutations in *LEMD3* [170]. Suspected cases should have limited plain radiographs to look for the characteristic findings of osteopoikilosis and melorheostosis.

Plantar collagenomas are seen in both Proteus syndrome (*Akt1* mosaicism [4]; see the section on CEN earlier in this chapter) and *PIK3CA*-related overgrowth syndromes [132], differentiated clinically in this naevus by the characteristic cerebriform appearance in the former condition.

Naevus mucinosis has been described in association with the lysosomal storage disease Hunter syndrome, an X-linked recessive condition due to germline mutations in the *IDS* gene. As this condition is progressive and the full phenotype evolves over time, suspected cases should be referred urgently for specialist investigation of storage disorders.

Fibrous connective tissue naevi are a frequent feature of tuberous sclerosis, an autosomal dominant hamartoma syndrome caused by mutations in one of two genes (*TSC1* and *TSC2*). However, these lesions would not usually be present congenitally, and as such are not usually an isolated presenting feature of the disease.

The principal importance of congenital lipomas in paediatric dermatology lies in the association of lumbo-sacral lesions and underlying spinal defects [171], which should be sought using appropriate imaging techniques. Congenital lipomas and naevus psiloliparus can also form part of the neurocutaneous disorder encephalo-cranio-cutaneous lipomatosis, and the highly phenotypically similar oculo-ectodermal syndrome. Ophthalmological and neurological investigations are required if these are suspected. The genetic basis of these conditions has recently been demonstrated to be mosaic mutations in either *KRAS* [172] or *FGFR1* [173] genes.

Investigations

Histopathological examination of a full-thickness skin biopsy is often useful for accurate diagnosis of connective tissue naevi, with adjacent normal skin being helpful for comparison of subtle dermal changes.

Management

Family history, examination and follow-up for any associated non-cutaneous or syndromic features are important. In the absence of these, single lesions can be followed up or resected non-urgently.

OTHER DEVELOPMENTAL ABNORMALITIES AFFECTING THE SKIN

Becker naevus and segmental odonto-maxillary dysplasia

Becker naevus (or Becker melanosis) is a relatively common hyperpigmented, generally non-linear lesion with an incidence of around 0.25% [1], and is commoner in males than females. It is only rarely congenital, with the majority of lesions appearing in the first two decades, classically at puberty. It is frequently but not always hypertrichotic and is commonest on the upper trunk. Becker naevus is in the authors' opinion currently unclassifiable within the above classification, as it shows features of lentiginous melanocytic hyperplasia, epidermal hyperplasia and smooth muscle hyperplasia. Becker naevus is not uncommonly associated with extracutaneous abnormalities [2], and is then termed Becker naevus syndrome [3], which can involve underlying structures, namely aplasia or hypoplasia of the underlying breast tissue, or the pectoralis major muscle (or sometimes shoulder muscles) or lipoatrophy. Other extracutaneous associations described are ipsilateral limb growth disturbance, supernumerary nipples [4] and scoliosis. Very rarely Becker naevus has been described in a linear form [5]. The genetic basis of Becker naevus in 60% of cases tested has been shown to be mosaicism for *ACTB* variants, also found as the cause of a single case of Becker naevus syndrome, and thought to arise within smooth muscle cells of the hair follicles [6]. The biology of this disease mechanism is not yet understood, but has been proposed to be via activation of Hedgehog pathway signalling [6].

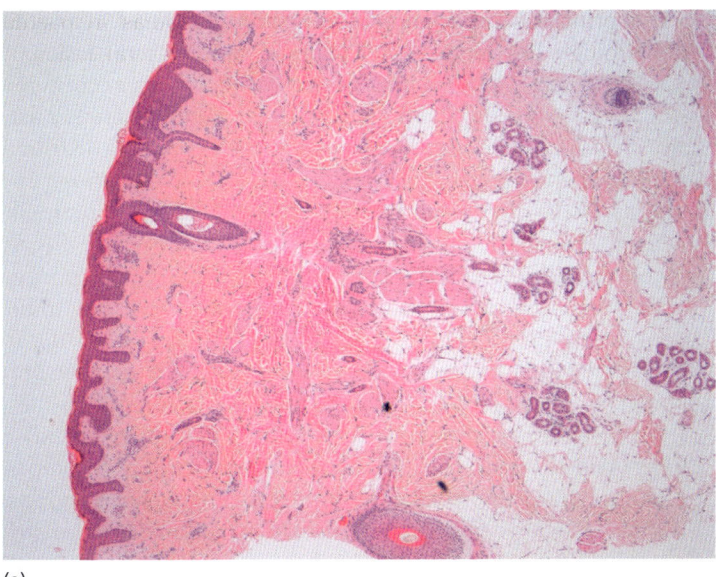
(a)

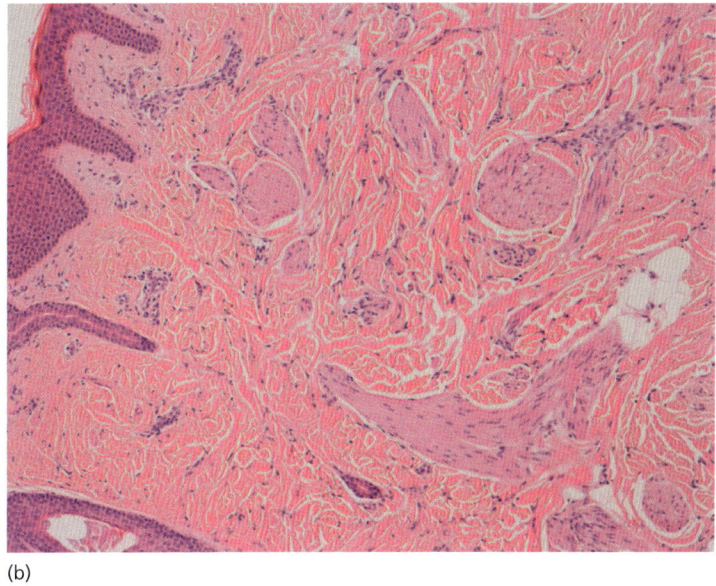
(b)

Figure 73.20 Photomicrographs of a smooth muscle hamartoma demonstrating a poorly circumscribed dermal lesion composed of abnormal bundles of smooth muscle within the dermis. Original magnifications (a) ×40 and (b) ×100 (H&E). Courtesy of Professor N. J. Sebire.

Mosaic *ACTB* variants have also been described as the cause of segmental odonto-maxillary dysplasia, a maxillary and dental condition which presents to dermatologists with pigmentary and/or hypertrichotic changes on the face, and which can be considered to be a cranial variant of Becker naevus syndrome [7].

Congenital muscle hamartomas

Smooth muscle hamartomas are benign collections of mature smooth muscle fibres within the dermis [8,9]. They have an estimated prevalence at birth of 0.04–0.2% [9,10]. Clinically they are soft, skin-coloured or slightly pink-brown lesions with indistinct edges, with overlying hair that may not be present at birth. Characteristically they demonstrate induration or worm-like fasciculation when the lesion is rubbed (pseudo-Darier sign), with raising of overlying hairs. The lesions are usually up to a few centimetres in diameter and solitary, most commonly in the lumbo-sacral region [9]. Once established they are static in behaviour, and as malignant transformation is not a reported feature, resection is not medically required. There are rare case reports of diffuse smooth muscle hamartomas leading to the Michelin tyre baby phenotype [11,12] and rare familial cases of multiple smooth muscle hamartomas [13,14].

These lesions demonstrate a characteristic histopathological appearance in which a poorly circumscribed, non-encapsulated lesion within the dermis demonstrates numerous well-defined bundles of smooth muscle which are characteristically orientated in varying directions (Figure 73.20).

The genetic basis of smooth muscle hamartomas has recently been established to be somatic *ACTB* mutations in approximately 70% of cases [15]. The spectrum of *ACTB* mosaicism therefore extends from a single smooth muscle hamartoma, through a classic Becker naevus, to syndromic forms involving musculoskeletal and neurological abnormalities.

Striated muscle hamartoma is an uncommon congenital lesion, usually arising on the head or neck, with a particular propensity for the chin. Clinically it is usually soft and often polypoid, and histologically it shows benign striated muscle fibres within the dermis and/or subcutis, with or without hamartomatous collections of other cutaneous components [16]. These lesions can be isolated or associated with extracutaneous abnormalities [17].

Heterotrimeric G-protein mosaic disorders

Heterotrimeric guanosine nucleotide-binding protein (G-protein) mosaic disorders are a new grouping of previously distinct disorders that have recently been identified to have a common genetic basis, namely mosaicism for G-protein subunit mutations. Heterotrimeric G-proteins are key molecular switches that assemble from alpha, beta and gamma subunits to transduce signals from G-protein-coupled receptors on the cell surface to intracellular signalling pathways. These are distinct from monomeric G-proteins, which belong to the RAS family of GTPases, and are homologous to the α-subunits of the heterotrimeric complexes.

There are currently three known conditions in this group, namely McCune–Albright syndrome, Sturge–Weber syndrome and phakomatosis pigmentovascularis. The clinical presentation in these conditions is highly variable from case to case due to variation in the percentage of mosaicism, and the particular tissues affected by the mutations.

McCune–Albright syndrome

The classic triad that is McCune–Albright syndrome is the association of café-au-lait macules, polyostotic fibrous dysplasia and autonomously hyperfunctioning endocrinopathies [18]. The clinical diagnosis can be made in the presence of two of these three features, and the genetic diagnosis can be made in the presence of one of these three with a detected mutation [19].

The café-au-lait pigmentation in this condition has to be differentiated from the innumerable other causes of café-au-lait macules. Typically (but not universally) the café-au-lait macules in McCune–Albright syndrome are large, are present at birth or appear early in the first decade, are in a 'segmental' type distribution respecting the midline, and have irregular edges likened to the coast of Maine. Oral pigmentation can arise later in childhood or early adulthood [20]. Bony involvement can present with pathological fracture, visible deformity and bone or joint pain. The commonest endocrinological abnormality is gonadotrophin-independent precocious puberty, which has earlier onset in girls than in affected boys [21]. A wide range of other endocrinopathies has been described, including growth hormone excess, hyperthyroidism, Cushing syndrome and hyperparathyroidism [22]. Investigation of endocrinological abnormalities should be undertaken by a paediatric endocrinologist, and treatment instigated as appropriate.

If the condition is suspected from dermatological findings alone, then plain radiographs of the skull, mandible, pelvis and long bones should be performed to look for polyostotic fibrous dysplasia. If fibrous dysplasia is suspected or confirmed, further investigation should be guided by recent expert guidelines, as there is a small but significant risk of osteosarcoma in McCune–Albright syndrome [23].

McCune–Albright syndrome is caused by mosaicism for activating mutations in the gene *GNAS* [24], which encodes one of the family of G-protein α-subunits, resulting in ligand-independent activation of G-protein-coupled receptor signalling pathways. Traditionally, genetic diagnosis has been maximised using DNA extracted directly from affected tissue other than skin, and rather than leukocyte DNA [19]. Skin biopsy has not been considered the best investigation due to low sensitivity, probably due to the very small percentage of mutated cells in a pigmented macular lesion. However, the mutation is present in a substantial percentage of blood samples from affected patients, particularly in those with more widespread disease [19], so blood is worth testing in the absence of easy access to other affected tissues. Furthermore, next generation sequencing has greatly improved the sensitivity of mutation detection, now down to below 1% mosaicism [25].

Sturge–Weber syndrome

The first description of what came to be known as Sturge–Weber syndrome was of the association of extensive facial and truncal port-wine stains (capillary malformations), contralateral focal seizures thought to be due to an ipsilateral abnormality on the surface of the brain (later confirmed in other cases) and ipsilateral intraocular vascular malformations presenting with glaucoma [26]. The definition of what constitutes a diagnosis of Sturge–Weber syndrome has altered many times subsequently, now encompassing cases without skin features [27] and with contralateral as well as ipsilateral brain or eye abnormalities [28,29]. The variably present clinical complications of these vascular malformations include seizures, neurodevelopmental delay, headache, stroke-like episodes, behavioural problems, hemiparesis, glaucoma, postnatal asymmetrical overgrowth (e.g. of the face or limbs) and growth hormone deficiency [30–32].

As port-wine stains are common, but Sturge–Weber syndrome is relatively rare (unconfirmed estimates of incidence are 1 : 20 000 to 1 : 50 000), many attempts have been made to predict oculo-cerebral associations from the phenotype of the port-wine stains. Historically it was surmised that the facial lesions followed the distribution of the branches of the trigeminal nerves, and that those in the ophthalmic division or on both sides of the face were more likely to be associated with Sturge–Weber syndrome [33,34]. Recently, however, a new classification of the distribution of facial port-wine stains in this condition has been proposed, which has found a strong association between lesions affecting any part of the forehead (defined as any part of the forehead with the lower border defined by a line joining the outer canthus of the eye to the top of the ipsilateral ear helix and including the upper eyelid) and Sturge–Weber syndrome [35]. This forehead region encompasses parts of all three divisions of the trigeminal nerve, confirming that all three divisions can be involved [36,37], and that the distribution of facial port-wine stains in this condition does not seem to follow a neurological pattern but that of the embryonic vasculature brought from the neural crest [35]. Guidelines have been proposed that urgent ophthalmological investigation of infants with facial port-wine stains should be targeted to those with lesions involving any part of the forehead (as defined above), as well as MRI of the CNS [35]. Glaucoma can be present from birth, and ophthalmology referral should therefore be made urgently to reduce potential morbidity. The timing of MRI of the CNS is controversial, as early scans can miss disease that becomes apparent later [30]. However, there is now some supportive evidence for the prophylactic use of oral therapy in infants with cerebral involvement to reduce the venous stasis-induced cerebral atrophy and calcification [38,39], and ongoing debate regarding prophylactic anticonvulsants in the presence of radiological abnormalities [30]. Recent suggested guidelines from a dermatological viewpoint suggest scanning within the first 3 months of life in the high-risk group only (with neurological referral where there are positive findings), and repeat scanning at a later stage if there is clinical suspicion but the first scan was clear [35].

Sturge–Weber syndrome is caused in approximately 90% of cases by codon-specific mosaic-activating mutations in the gene *GNAQ* [**40**], with the same mutation responsible for a similar proportion of isolated, non-syndromic port-wine stains in the one cohort tested so far. Recently a case of *GNA11*-mutant Sturge–Weber syndrome has been reported [41].

Phakomatosis pigmentovascularis

Phakomatosis pigmentovascularis (PPV) is a descriptive term currently applied to a group of phenotypes that are unified by the coexistence of different pigmentary and vascular cutaneous lesions. In practice the term was originally used to describe one particular phenotype [42], and as that phenotype is so much more common than all the others it has been argued that it alone should be termed PPV [43]. This particular phenotype is the combination of a capillary malformation (port-wine stain/naevus flammeus) and dermal melanocytosis (Mongolian blue spots) (Figure 73.21). In the largest study thus far of PPV, this phenotype had a prevalence of 0.006% in a large Mexican hospital paediatric population, and was the only type encountered in a 5-year period [43]. However, there is not only

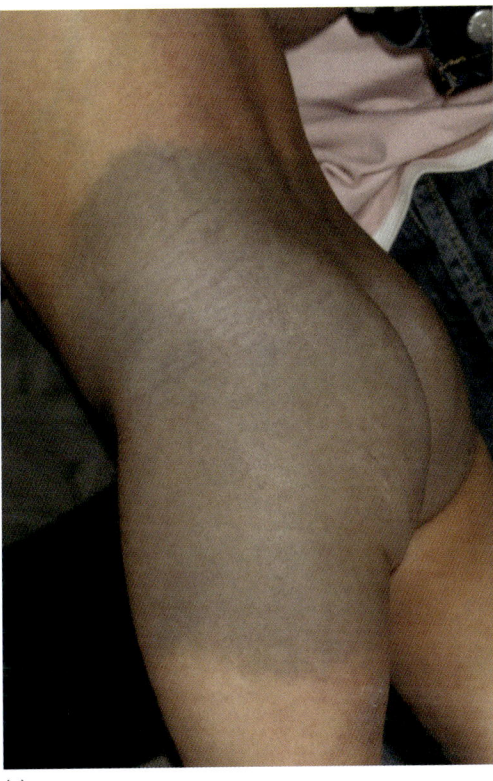

(a)

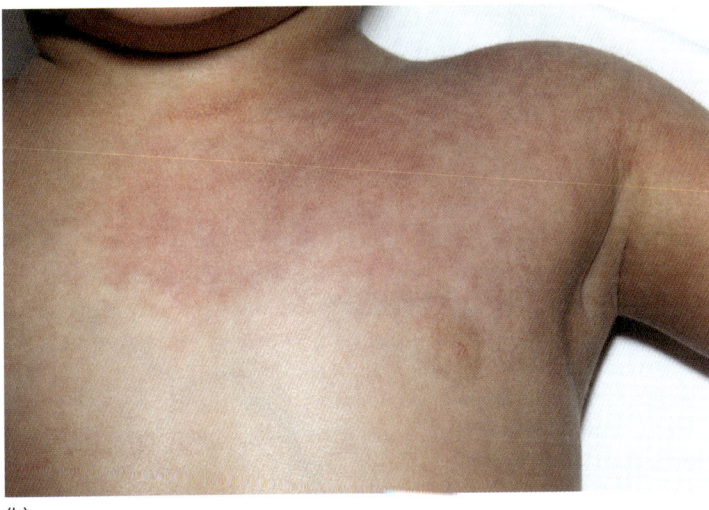

(b)

Figure 73.21 Phakomatosis pigmentovascularis type II (or cesioflammea type), showing the characteristic combination of (a) a capillary malformation (port-wine stain) and (b) dermal melanocytosis (Mongolian blue spot).

clear phenotypic evidence of other subtypes, but now genotypic evidence as well. In addition not all phenotypes described in the literature are classifiable, and recent genetic advances will help with recognition of the spectrum of this disease. There may be significant differences in the incidence of PPV between ethnic groups, as most cases described thus far have been in non-white individuals, however there are still too few series described to draw definite conclusions in this regard

Two phenotypic subclassifications have previously been proposed, which can be roughly equated as shown in Table 73.2.

As this condition is rare, the following associations and management suggestions are based on the existing literature, the phenotypic and genotypic promixity of this disease to the better studied Sturge–Weber syndrome, and err on the side of caution until larger series of patients can be studied. The known associations of PPV are:

- Naevus anaemicus (described in all types).
- Scleral or intraocular melanocytosis. Importantly, this may not be evident without dilatation and slit lamp examination, therefore an ophthalmology review should be arranged for all patients with this diagnosis [46].
- Glaucoma, for which an urgent referral to ophthalmology should be made as soon as the diagnosis is suspected, and regular follow-up given. This appears to be more related to the episcleral vascular malformations than the pigmentary abnormality [47], and examination of the literature suggests that those at risk of glaucoma may be primarily those with cutaneous vascular lesions around the eye.
- Intracerebral vascular malformations, for which we would suggest MRI of the brain should be performed within the first few months of life. Radiologically, these lesions are often indistinguishable from those seen in Sturge–Weber syndrome, which has led to the misunderstanding that the two diagnoses coexist, and has now been explained by the genetic proximity in pathogenesis. Clinically, these lesions can be accompanied by macrocephaly, developmental delay and/or seizures. Potentially prophylactic medication can be given to try to reduce the effects of venous stasis and underlying cortical atrophy (see 'Sturge–Weber syndrome' earlier in this chapter).
- Overgrowth, either as full hemihypertrophy, or as localised asymmetry of the face or limbs, which has led to concurrent diagnoses of phakomatosis pigmentovascularis and Klippel–Trenaunay–Weber syndrome.
- Melanoma of the choroid and conjunctiva and melanocytoma of the optic disc are all described [46,48,49]. Regular ophthalmological screening should be undertaken to screen for this complication, and the patient should be made aware to report any ocular symptoms promptly. This predisposition is explained by the genetic basis of the cases described thus far.

A recent cohort study of individuals with PPV types which included dermal melanocytosis (types I, II, IV and V, or cesiomarmorata and cesioflammea) has described additional phenotypic features – namely café au-lait macules, macrocephaly and hypertension associated with renal artery anomalies [41]. Recommendations were to measure head circumference and blood pressure at follow-up visits. A second cohort study of patients with known GNAQ/GNA11 mosaicism also described macrocephaly and hypertension associated with renal artery anomalies [50].

The genetic basis of PPV has been established in recent years. Clinically distinguishable phenotypes are caused, therefore, in at least a percentage of cases by mosaicism for activating mutations in the same gene GNA11, a close paralogue of the gene causing Sturge–Weber syndrome, GNAQ, and a known melanoma gene [51]. There is conservation of the same mutation in one individual in both pigmentary and vascular lesions, but no mutation generally detectable in the blood. This further refutes the now-retracted hypothesis of twin spotting as the mechanism in this and similar

Table 73.2 Two historical phenotypic subclassifications of phakomatosis pigmentovascularis.

Pigmentary lesions	Vascular lesions	Classification 1 [44]	Classification 2 [45]
Linear epidermal naevus	Capillary malformation (port-wine stain/naevus flammeus)	Type I	Does not exist in this classification
Dermal melanocytosis (Mongolian blue spot)	Capillary malformation (port-wine stain/naevus flammeus)	Type II	Cesioflammea type
Naevus spilus	Capillary malformation (port-wine stain/naevus flammeus in classification 1, pale pink telangiectatic naevus in classification 2)	Type III	Spilorosea type
Dermal melanocytosis (Mongolian blue spot) and naevus spilus	Capillary malformation (port-wine stain/naevus flammeus)	Type IV	Extremely rare, unclassifiable in this classification
Naevus spilus	Capillary malformation (cutis marmorata telangiectatica congenita)	Type V	Cesiomarmorata type

mosaic disorders where two types of lesion coexist [52]. Rather, the pathogenetic mechanism is likely to be a single mutation affecting a precursor cell which gives rise to both the pigmentary and vascular lesions during development. The cell type affected is yet to be confirmed, although in Sturge–Weber syndrome it is thought to be endothelial [53].

Extensive or atypical dermal melanocytosis

Extensive or atypical dermal melanocytosis has to be differentiated from the self-resolving congenital dermal melanocytosis previously known as Mongolian blue spots. In general these lesions are in unusual sites outside the lumbo-sacral area, may be more deeply pigmented, better defined at the edges, multiple and more likely to persist. A small percentage of patients with this clinical presentation are mosaic for *GNAQ* mutations [54], the same as are found in Sturge–Weber syndrome and the dermal–melanocytosis-associated types of PPV. Key associated abnormalities are ocular melanocytosis and other ocular abnormalities, and cutaneous and ocular melanoma.

Naevus-like entities

Angora hair naevus

The angora hair naevus [55] is an extremely rare hypertrichotic naevus with increased pigmentation in the basal layer, where the hypertrichosis has a hypopigmented and fine nature. It has been described in linear and non-linear forms. Angora hair naevus has been associated with extracutaneous abnormalities. The genetic basis remains unknown.

Linear atrophoderma of Moulin

This entity describes an acquired hyperpigmented atrophy of subcutaneous tissue rather than a naevus, but in a Blaschkolinear distribution [56]. It generally appears in the first two decades of life, and usually stabilises after its initial development, although very slow progression has been described [57]. Most commonly lesions are truncal and unilateral [56,58]. No familial cases have been described thus far, and the genetic basis is still unknown although hypotheses have been suggested [59].

Lichen striatus

See Chapter 37.

Linear morphoea/scleroderma

See Chapter 37.

Linear manifestations of X-linked skin disease

This group of 'naevus-like' lesions are identifiable by being hereditary in their Blaschkolinear forms, a pattern of inheritance that cannot be seen in mosaic disorders. The classic example is incontinentia pigmenti. The overarching molecular basis for the cutaneous phenotype is random X-inactivation, producing a functional or expression-level mosaicism, rather than mosaicism at the DNA level.

CHILD syndrome (congenital hemidysplasia with ichthyosiform erythroderma and limb defects) (MIM: 308050) is a rare and in its classic form a striking condition affecting either the right or left of the body, with a sharp midline cut-off [60]. The underlying genetic defect is known to be germline loss-of-function mutations in *NSDHL* [61], which encodes an enzyme involved in cholesterol metabolism, with X-inactivation postulated to be responsible for the hemidysplasia phenotype (although the exact mechanism of this is not clear). The inheritance is X-linked dominant, and the condition is almost universally lethal in males. Importantly for diagnosis, bilateral cutaneous involvement has rarely been described [62], and limb defects are not always seen. CHILD syndrome lesions have previously been notoriously difficult to treat, with variable success with CO_2 laser and topical calcipotriol. Recently, however, novel topical therapy has been highly successful in two children with CHILD syndrome, based on the role of the affected gene in cholesterol metabolism [63]. Treatment of extensive epidermolytic, hyperkeratotic, epidermal naevi is often with systemic retinoids, and topical vitamin D analogues have also been used with success [64,65].

Other conditions in this group are dealt with in other chapters in detail.

Linear manifestations of generalised skin disease

These can rarely occur either as single linear lesions, or as a linear component of generalised disease. Examples of the first presentation are linear Darier disease caused by mutations in *ATP2A2* [66] or linear porokeratosis caused by *PMVK* and *MVK* [67], the latter successfully treated recently with a topical cholesterol and statin mix [68]. The molecular mechanism of the second presentation was hypothesised to be due to loss of heterozygosity of the normal allele in the linear area [69], and an example of this is linear Hailey–Hailey disease [70].

Blaschkolinear areas of conditions where the genetic basis is not fully understood such as atopic dermatitis, psoriasis, juvenile xanthogranuloma, granuloma annulare, lichen planus and pemphigus vulgaris, are rarely described as a concomitant, antecedent or only manifestation of more typical disease [71]. For inflammatory conditions this is sometimes termed 'Blaschkitis' and should be considered as a differential diagnosis in Blashko linear lesions. They are not as a rule congenital. Although hypotheses concerning pathogenesis have been evinced, there are thus far no data explaining this phenomenon.

Key references

The full list of references can be found in the online version at https://www.wiley.com/rooksdermatology10e

Congenital naevi

1 Kinsler VA, Boccara O, Fraitag S, Torrelo A, Vabres P, Diociaiuti A. Mosaic abnormalities of the skin – review and guidelines from the European Reference Network for rare skin diseases (ERN-Skin). *Br J Dermatol* 2020;182:552–63.

4 Lindhurst MJ, Sapp JC, Teer JK *et al*. A mosaic activating mutation in AKT1 associated with the Proteus syndrome. *N Engl J Med* 2011;365:611–19.

18 Groesser L, Herschberger E, Ruetten A *et al*. Postzygotic HRAS and KRAS mutations cause nevus sebaceous and Schimmelpenning syndrome. *Nat Genet* 2012;44:783–7.

89 Polubothu S, McGuire N, Al-Olabi L *et al*. Does the gene matter? Genotype–phenotype and genotype–outcome associations in congenital melanocytic naevi. *Br J Dermatol* 2020;182:434–43.

94 Kinsler VA, O'Hare P, Bulstrode N *et al*. Melanoma in congenital melanocytic naevi. *Br J Dermatol* 2017;176:1131–43.

102 Al-Olabi L, Polubothu S, Dowsett K *et al*. Mosaic RAS/MAPK variants cause sporadic vascular malformations which respond to targeted therapy. *J Clin Invest* 2018;128:1496–508.

Other developmental abnormalities affecting the skin

6 Cai ED, Sun BK, Chiang A *et al*. Postzygotic mutations in beta-actin are associated with Becker's nevus and Becker's nevus syndrome. *J Invest Dermatol* 2017;137:1795–8.

7 Polubothu S, Abdin D, Barysch M *et al*. Dermatological signs lead to discovery of mosaic ACTB variants in segmental odontomaxillary dysplasia. *Br J Dermatol* 2020;183:1128–30.

40 Shirley MD, Tang H, Gallione CJ *et al*. Sturge–Weber syndrome and port-wine stains caused by somatic mutation in GNAQ. *New Engl J Med* 2013;368:1971–9.

63 Paller AS, van Steensel MA, Rodriguez-Martin M *et al*. Pathogenesis-based therapy reverses cutaneous abnormalities in an inherited disorder of distal cholesterol metabolism. *J Invest Dermatol* 2011;131:2242–8.

CHAPTER 74

Chromosomal Disorders

Neil Rajan[1], Alan D. Irvine[2] and Jemima E. Mellerio[3]

[1] Translational and Clinical Research Institute, Newcastle University, Newcastle upon Tyne, UK
[2] Trinity College, Dublin, Ireland
[3] St John's Institute of Dermatology, Guy's and St Thomas' NHS Foundation Trust, London, UK

Introduction

Chromosomal disorders may be due to abnormalities of chromosome number or structure and may involve autosomes or sex chromosomes. Somatic cells are *diploid*, with a complement of 46 chromosomes, whereas gametes (ova and sperm) are *haploid*, with only 23 chromosomes following reduction division in meiosis. Abnormalities of chromosome number that involve the gain or loss of one or more chromosomes are known as aneuploidies. Structural chromosome rearrangements result from chromosome breakage with subsequent reunion in a different configuration. They may be balanced or unbalanced, depending on whether or not gain (or loss) of genetic material occurs. DECIPHER is a catalogue of genetic causes of developmental disorders that is an excellent resource for chromosomal disorders, and reports genetic changes and associated phenotypes [1].

Approximately 7.5% of all conceptions have a chromosomal disorder, but most of these are spontaneously aborted, so the birth frequency is 0.6%. Among early spontaneous abortions, the frequency of chromosomal disorders is 60%, whereas in late spontaneous abortions and stillbirths the frequency is 5%. Chromosomal abnormalities generally cause multiple congenital malformations. Children with more than one physical abnormality, particularly if developmentally delayed, should undergo chromosomal analysis as part of their investigation. Chromosomal disorders are incurable but can be reliably detected by prenatal diagnostic techniques [2].

Recent advances for detecting chromosomal aneuploidies leverage the ability of sensitive DNA sequencing technologies to detect fetal (cell free) DNA circulating in the maternal circulation. These assays, termed 'non-invasive prenatal assays (NIPT)' have been shown to exceed sensitivity of combined screening approaches in the context of some conditions like Down syndrome. These approaches are combined with additional testing as discussed below. Invasive diagnostic testing approaches such as chorionic villus sampling or amniocentesis allow access to tissue or amniocytes that can be tested for fetal chromosomal abnormalities. DNA from such tissues are now typically subject to chromosomal microarray analysis [3], which involve assays such as SNP arrays, which can detect abnormalities of chromosome number (aneuploidy) and structure (deletions/duplications/inversions).

A growing number of inherited skin conditions have been found to be associated with submicroscopic genomic aberrations such as copy-number variations (CNVs) [4] including cornification, hair and connective tissue disorders [5–7]. They do not fit the strict definition of chromosomal disorders and are discussed throughout the chapters of the present section.

AUTOSOMAL CHROMOSOME DEFECTS

Down syndrome (trisomy 21)

Down syndrome is the most common autosomal abnormality, with a frequency of about 1/700 live births [1].

Aetiology

There are three genetic scenarios that give rise to the phenotype of Down syndrome [2]. Most cases (95%) result from germline trisomy of chromosome 21, in which the extra chromosome is derived by non-disjunction at meiosis, usually from the mother; the incidence of this type rises with maternal age. Some patients also have translocation Down syndrome, where an extra part of chromosome 21 is present, and is attached to another chromosome, such that the

Rook's Textbook of Dermatology, Tenth Edition. Edited by Christopher Griffiths, Jonathan Barker, Tanya Bleiker, Walayat Hussain and Rosalind Simpson.
© 2024 John Wiley & Sons Ltd. Published 2024 by John Wiley & Sons Ltd.

PART 6: GENETIC DISORDERS

affected child has the normal number of 46 chromosomes. Finally, some patients have mosaic Down syndrome, and only some of the cells in their body demonstrate trisomy 21; these patients tend to have less marked physical signs and higher intelligence [3].

Pathology

The effects of having an increased gene dosage of chromosome 21 are widespread. Congenital heart defects are common and the brain is small with flat convolutions. Renal tract anomalies are less common but recognised. Immunological defects are frequent. Autoimmune disease is common in Down syndrome, T-cell function is impaired and the atopic state is often seen [4]. There is an increased risk of developing acute leukaemia, estimated at 150× higher than expected, usually under the age of 5 years. Recent studies suggest that increased expression of microRNAs from chromosome 21 play a role in the development of leukaemia [5].

Clinical features [6]

The facial appearance often allows for a clinical diagnosis. Head size is small, the facial profile is flat, the nose short and the ears small. The eyes are usually conspicuously almond shaped, with slanting palpebral fissures. The eyelids are thickened and the eyelashes short and sparse. Epicanthic folds are frequent in early childhood but tend to become less noticeable with age. The iris tends to be hypoplastic and may show light areas in its outer third (Brushfield's spots). The limbs are short and the joint ligaments lax. The fingers are also short and cone shaped and are sometimes webbed. The little finger is often curved. The presence of these features varies in affected individuals.

Intellectual disability is a common feature. Congenital heart malformations, especially endocardial cushion defects, are present in 40%, and duodenal atresia may occur. Other complications include cataracts (2%), epilepsy (10%), hypothyroidism (3%), leukaemia (1%), atlantoaxial instability (2–3%) and recurrent respiratory infections. Puberty is often delayed and incomplete, with adult height at about 150 cm. Presenile dementia is common after 40 years of age.

Dermatological conditions in Down syndrome are common and patients may benefit from dermatologist review as part of their care [7,8]. The skin is normal at birth and in early childhood is soft and velvety [7]. Between the ages of 5 and 10 years it becomes increasingly dry and less elastic, and by the age of 15 over 70% show generalised xerosis of mild to moderate degree with evidence of accelerated skin ageing [9]. Patchy lichenification is present in some 30% under 10 years and more than 80% over 20 years of age. The patches resemble lichen simplex and most commonly occur on the upper arm, wrists, the fronts of the thighs, the back of the ankle and the back of the neck, and are probably correctly regarded as manifestations of atopic eczema, the incidence of which some authorities have considered to be low. The lichenified patches of skin show no distinctive pattern on histology, with hyperkeratosis, acanthosis and a dermal inflammatory infiltrate.

A chronic follicular papular eruption of the presternal and interscapular regions is frequently present, consistent with *Malassezia* folliculitis. In a clinical trial, oral itraconazole produced a significant clinical improvement accompanied by a decrease in the skin *Malassezia* count, but relapse occurred when therapy was discontinued and was accompanied by recurrence of *Malassezia* yeasts [10].

Hidradenitis suppuritiva and generalised folliculitis are recognised in patients with Down syndrome [11].

The hair may be normal but is often fine and may be hypopigmented. The prevalence of alopecia areata is high and it tends to be extensive and persistent [6,12]. The teeth are hypoplastic and late to erupt. Fissuring and thickening of the lips are frequent and increase in prevalence and severity with age. The tongue is fissured in almost all cases. Elastosis perforans serpiginosa and syringomas, especially in adult females with Down syndrome [13–15], occur more often than in normal subjects.

Skin infections, angular cheilitis, chronic blepharitis and a purulent nasal discharge are common. There is a high prevalence of onychomycosis [6,16]. The cheeks are often red. The peripheral circulation is poor, acrocyanosis is frequent and livedo reticularis is often conspicuous throughout the year, on the thighs, buttocks and trunk.

There is no evidence that the prevalence of other dermatoses is significantly different in individuals with Down syndrome compared with individuals with intellectual disability from other causes. Acral lentiginous melanoma has been described in association with Down syndrome [17]. Psoriasis runs its normal course, although an unusual hyperkeratotic form has been described. There is some evidence that seborrhoeic dermatitis is commoner [11,18] and also premature greying.

Trisomy 18 (Edwards syndrome) [1–3]

This is the second most common multiple malformation syndrome. It occurs in about 1/3000 live births; 95% of affected fetuses abort spontaneously. Parental non-disjunction at either the first or second meiotic division results in the extra copy of chromosome 18. Rarely, a parental translocation is responsible. Occasionally, mosaicism is seen with a milder phenotype and can give rise to pigmentary skin changes, as seen in hypomelanosis of Ito [4,5]. The syndrome comprises severe intellectual disability, a characteristic skull shape with a small chin and prominent occiput, low-set malformed ears, clenched hands with overlapping index and fifth fingers, single palmar crease, 'rocker-bottom' feet and a short sternum. Malformations of the heart, kidneys and other organs are frequent. Cutaneous features include aplasia cutis, cutis laxa of the neck, hypertrichosis of the forehead and back, and capillary haemangiomas. Fingerprints show a distinctive low-arch dermal ridge pattern. Death within a month occurs in 30%. Only 10% survive beyond the first year and these infants show profound developmental delay.

Trisomy 13 [1–4]

The incidence of trisomy 13 is 1/5000 live births. Non-disjunction at either the first or second meiotic division in either parent may cause trisomy 13. In about 20% of cases, one parent is a translocation carrier. In about 5% of patients, mosaicism is present, which may be associated with prolonged survival [5]. The characteristic features of the syndrome are intellectual disability, sloping forehead reflecting underlying holoprosencephaly (a developmental defect of the forebrain), eye defects including microphthalmia or anophthalmia, cleft palate and cleft lip, low-set ears, rocker-bottom feet, cardiac defects and a variety of other visceral abnormalities. Survival for more than 6 months is unusual. Cutaneous features include vascular anomalies, especially of the forehead, hyperconvex nails and localised defects of the scalp. Cutis laxa of the neck has also been reported. The palm print shows a distal palmar axial triradius.

Other autosomal abnormality syndromes

Although the syndromes to which these autosomal abnormalities give rise include distinctive craniofacial malformations, they do not exhibit constant or frequent dermatological features, apart from abnormal dermatoglyphics. Other chromosomal disorders are reviewed elsewhere [1,2].

Chromosome 4, short-arm deletion syndrome [3]
These children have microcephaly, intellectual disability, hypospadias and multiple malformations, such as cleft lip and/or palate, low-set ears and pre-auricular pits. There are scalp defects in some cases.

Chromosome 5, short-arm deletion syndrome (cri du chat syndrome) [4–6]
This is a clinically heterogeneous syndrome. The patients have severe intellectual delay and microcephaly with a cat-like cry. In some cases, a pre-auricular skin tag accompanies low-set malformed ears. There may be premature greying of the hair.

Chromosome 18, long-arm deletion syndrome [7]
Hypoplasia of the mid-face gives these children deep-set eyes. The antihelix is very prominent and there are multiple skeletal and ocular abnormalities. Eczema has been reported to occur in 25% of cases.

SEX CHROMOSOME DEFECTS

Turner syndrome

Turner syndrome [1,2] occurs when one of the two copies of the X chromosome is missing or structurally defective. Turner syndrome is thought to account for 10% of all spontaneous miscarriages in the first trimester [3].

Aetiology [2]
The frequency of Turner syndrome is 1/2500 female births [4]. In 80% of cases, there are 45 chromosomes, with the presence of one copy of the X chromosome, designated 45,X. The incidence of 45,X was reported to be increased in the offspring of teenage mothers [5], but in a study from Denmark there was no significant relation between the mother's age and the risk of Turner syndrome [6].

The remaining cases are mosaic, or in some cases have a partial deletion of one X chromosome [7,8]. Mosaicism of various types has been reported (45,X/46,XX or 45,X/47,XXX) [9]. Such individuals may not differ significantly in their phenotype from the common 45,X genotype but they may be less severely affected [10].

Pathology
In place of the normal gonads, ovarian streaks are present that are composed of stroma-like cells and quiescent germinal epithelium without follicular activity or germ cells. However, both follicles and germ cells have occasionally been present. Lymphangiographic studies have shown hypoplasia of cutaneous and subcutaneous lymphatics [11].

A lack of feedback inhibition by hormones from the defective ovaries produces elevated levels of follicle-stimulating hormone (FSH) and luteinising hormone (LH) in the serum by 5 days of age [12].

Clinical features [10,13,14,15]
Growth failure is a consistent finding at birth in infants with Turner syndrome, which begins in early gestation and is well established by mid-pregnancy [16]. The diagnosis may be suggested in the newborn by redundant neck skin and peripheral oedema. However, the diagnosis is usually made later as a result of investigation for short stature and primary amenorrhoea.

The characteristic clinical features of Turner syndrome include: small stature; a broad shield-shaped chest with widely spaced nipples; a wide carrying angle of the arms; a webbed neck (pterygium colli); low, misshapen ears; high, arched palate; short fourth, and sometimes fifth, metacarpals and metatarsals; hypoplastic nails; and a tendency to keloidal scar formation. Skeletal abnormalities are a common feature, but are also very variable. Among the most frequent are cubitus valgus, kyphoscoliosis and epiphyseal defects and pathological fractures. Cardiovascular abnormalities are present in some 25% of cases, especially coarctation of the aorta. Ocular defects, squints or ptosis, are also a feature of some cases. Intelligence is usually normal. Progress has been made in identifying foundational deficits in attention and executive function that could explain visuospatial and arithmetical impairments [17].

Dermatological features in Turner syndrome are numerous but variable [18]. Apart from a low posterior hairline and cutis laxa, especially on the neck and buttocks, individuals with Turner syndrome have increased numbers of melanocytic naevi and an increased risk for melanoma [19] as well as other skin and non-cutaneous neoplasias (although cancer relative risk in Turner is still a matter of debate) [20]. Halo nevi are particularly frequent in Turner syndrome [21]. Lymphangiectatic oedema of the hands and feet may be present at birth and clear in the first 2 years. Alopecia areata and psoriasis have been reported in association with Turner syndrome, which may relate to the fact that Turner syndrome patients are prone to develop autoimmune diseases, mainly autoimmune thyroiditis and inflammatory bowel syndrome [22].

Endocrinological investigations reveal an increased output of pituitary gonadotrophins accompanied by low oestrogen levels. Thus, there is usually primary amenorrhoea with failure to develop full secondary sexual characteristics [23]. Some patients menstruate and, exceptionally, may be fertile. Adrenal androgens are present, and pubic and axillary hair may be present in the absence of other manifestations of normal pubertal development. A few examples are known [24] in which otherwise typical Turner syndrome (XO chromosome complement) is accompanied by some degree of genital virilisation and hirsutism.

Diagnosis

Diagnosis may be made prenatally by amniocentesis if suspected based on ultrasound findings [5]. Diagnosis can also be made in infancy or childhood, but if they are inconspicuous or absent, the diagnosis may be unsuspected until puberty. Increased urinary excretion of FSH supports the diagnosis, which can be confirmed by testing peripheral blood leukocyte DNA or buccal smears for karyotyping.

Treatment

Oestrogen replacement will allow the development of secondary sexual characteristics but does not seem to influence stature or infertility. Treatment with human growth hormone may improve the ultimate adult height. Melanocytic naevi may grow more rapidly during growth hormone therapy [25]. Therefore, individuals with Turner syndrome, especially those on growth hormone therapy, should have periodic skin examinations and be advised on the regular use of sunscreens. For a comprehensive recent review of clinical care please see [**26**].

Klinefelter syndrome [1,2]

Aetiology

The frequency of Klinefelter syndrome is 1/600 male births [2]. Klinefelter patients have 47 chromosomes with an XXY sex chromosome complement [3]. The differentiation of the developing gonad proceeds along male lines but the testis fails to develop fully and many seminiferous tubules are replaced by fibrous tissue. Leydig cells are present in normal or increased numbers.

Clinical features [1,2,4,**5**,6]

There are no clinical manifestations before puberty, which occurs at the normal age. The testes are small and fail to produce adult levels of testosterone, which leads to poorly developed secondary sexual characteristics and infertility. Hair growth on the trunk, limbs and face tends to be reduced. Psychiatric disorders are common but intellectual disability is not. Klinefelter syndrome patients typically are taller than average, mainly attributed to abnormally long legs, and an arm span exceeding height by 2 cm [7]. Some patients may be obese and develop gynaecomastia. Associated features include osteoporosis [8] and taurodontism (vertical enlargement of the molar pulp chamber) [9]. Various minor dermatoglyphic changes have been recorded [10].

An association between systemic lupus erythematosus (SLE) and Klinefelter syndrome has been postulated [11], and this is interesting in view of the fact that SLE is more frequent in women than men and that oestrogens may provoke SLE in some patients [12]. In a case report of SLE in a hypogonadal male with Klinefelter syndrome treated with testosterone in doses sufficient to normalise the serum

level of this hormone to the adult male range, haematological and serological abnormalities, including elevated levels of anti-DNA antibodies and depressed complement levels, returned to normal within 9 months of increasing the testosterone dose [13]. Men commonly have SLE that is more severe than that found among women, but patients with Klinefelter syndrome seem to have SLE of the same degree of severity as women [14]. A study of 213 men with SLE demonstrated that five had Klinefelter syndrome, two of whom had not been previously diagnosed [15].

Patients with Klinefelter syndrome have an increased risk of developing leg ulcers, especially in combination with hyperpigmentation or atrophie blanche [16–18]. Some authors have attributed the cause of leg ulceration to venous insufficiency, others have implicated increased activity of plasminogen activator inhibitor 1 [19].

The presence of an extra X chromosome in Kleinfelter syndrome allows for the birth of male children with X-linked dominant genodermatoses such as Conradi–Hünermann–Happle syndrome [20] or incontinentia pigmenti [21].

Diagnosis

The association of gynaecomastia with small testes and otherwise apparently normal genitalia should suggest the diagnosis, which is supported by finding an increased urinary excretion of gonadotrophin. The diagnosis is confirmed by chromosome studies.

Treatment

Testosterone replacement therapy will improve secondary sexual characteristics, but infertility is the rule, except in mosaic patients [22].

Other abnormalities of the sex chromosomes

There are several other syndromes affecting the sex chromosomes. However, they are very rare and the cutaneous features are not so prominent.

XXYY syndrome

Individuals with XXYY syndrome [1] show many of the main features of Klinefelter syndrome, including sparse body hair. Additional features reported are multiple cutaneous angiomas, acrocyanosis and early peripheral vascular disease.

XYY syndrome

Patients with XYY syndrome [2] are phenotypic males, often tall and with, perhaps, an increased incidence of severe acne (see Chapter 88). They may have intellectual disability and have a reputation for aggressive behaviour [3], not accepted by all authorities. There is no evidence of increased secretion of FSH or LH [4].

XXXXY syndrome

Patients with XXXXY syndrome [5] are of low birth weight, are slow to grow physically and are intellectually impaired. There are multiple skeletal defects, of which limited elbow pronation is the most characteristic. The ears are large, low set and malformed.

There is hypogenitalism. No consistent dermatological defects are reported, but some patients have hypotrichosis.

Fragile X syndrome

Fragile X syndrome [6–8] is associated with a folate-sensitive fragile site in band Xq27.3 due to a triplet DNA repeat that is expanded and unstable. Subjects have intellectual disability and mild dysmorphic features, with mild connective tissue abnormality that leads to fine skin, hyperextensible joints and flat feet. Males are more commonly affected than females. The disorder is common, with about 1/2000 children affected.

CHROMOSOMAL MOSAICISM

Chromosomal mosaicism is the coexistence within an individual of two or more distinct cell lines that are genetically identical except for the chromosomal difference (total number/ploidy, deletions, duplications, other chromosomal abnormalities) between them. Chromosomal mosaicism results from a post-zygotic event typically caused by an error in mitosis in a cell during embryogenesis that contributes to multiple cells in the developing embryo [1]. This can result in uneven development and growth of abnormal mosaic cells in the tissues that they contribute to throughout the body. The degree of mosaicism (the proportion or percentage of cells that are chromosomally normal as compared with chromosomally abnormal) very roughly correlates to phenotype severity. Low-level mosaicism is more likely to result in a less abnormal phenotype.

Mosaicism often involves the skin and this commonly is expressed as patchy pigmentary, vascular, atrophic or hyperkeratotic changes along the lines of Blaschko. Any child with patchy pigmentary abnormalities, especially if asymmetrical or following the lines of Blaschko, should be considered to possibly have chromosomal mosaicism. An awareness of this possibility is important for dermatologists as they will often make or suggest the diagnosis. The possibility of chromosomal mosaicism should be entertained in any child or adult with patchy Blaschkoid pigmentation occurring in association with syndromic developmental anomalies.

It is relatively straightforward to confirm mosaicism in the skin if the fibroblast lineage is affected. Fibroblasts collected via skin biopsy can be cultured and chromosome analysis can take place using either traditional karyotyping or comparative genomic hybridisation (CGH) arrays. If keratinocytes are affected in the absence of fibroblast involvement, keratinocytes will need to be isolated and cultured separately [1]. Recent work has highlighted the important role that array CGH plays in the detection of mosaicism [2]. Low-level mosaicism for several chromosomal abnormalities has been detected on array CGH in individuals in whom the routine karyotype was normal. A recent study of 73 patients with pigmentary mosaicism highlighted that 23 had chromosomal alterations [3].

Key references

The full list of references can be found in the online version at https://www.wiley.com/rooksdermatology10e

Down syndrome (trisomy 21)

7 Ryan C, Vellody K, Belazarian L et al. Dermatologic conditions in Down syndrome. *Pediatr Dermatol* 2021;38(Suppl 2):49–57.

8 Wentworth AB, Hand JL, Davis DM et al. Skin concerns in patients with trisomy 21 (Down syndrome): a Mayo Clinic 22-year retrospective review. *Pediatr Dermatol* 2021;38(Suppl 2):73–8.

11 Ercis M, Balci S, Atakan N. Dermatological manifestations of 71 Down syndrome children admitted to a clinical genetics unit. *Clin Genet* 1996;50:317–20.

18 Bilgili SG, Akdeniz N, Karadag AS, Akbayram S, Calka O, Ozkol HU. Mucocutaneous disorders in children with Down syndrome: case-controlled study. *Genet Couns* 2011;22:385–92.

Turner syndrome

15 Chacko E, Graber E, Regelmann MO, Wallach E, Costin G, Rapaport R. Update on Turner and Noonan syndromes. *Endocrinol Metab Clin North Am* 2012;41:713–34.

18 Lowenstein EJ, Kim KH, Glick SA. Turner's syndrome in dermatology. *J Am Acad Dermatol* 2004;50:767–76.

20 Larizza D, Albanesi M, De Silvestri A et al. Neoplasia in Turner syndrome. The importance of clinical and screening practices during follow-up. *Eur J Med Genet* 2016;59:269–73.

26 Gravholt CH, Andersen NH, Conway GS et al. Clinical practice guidelines for the care of girls and women with Turner syndrome: proceedings from the 2016 Cincinnati International Turner Syndrome Meeting. *Eur J Endocrinol* 2017;177: G1–G70.

Klinefelter syndrome

5 Becker KL, Hoffman DL, Albert A et al. Klinefelter's syndrome. Clinical and laboratory findings in 50 patients. *Arch Intern Med* 1966;118:314–21.

Chromosomal mosaicism

1 Kinsler VA, Boccara O, Fraitag S et al. Mosaic abnormalities of the skin: review and guidelines from the European Reference Network for rare skin diseases. *Br J Dermatol* 2020;182:552–63.

PART 6: GENETIC DISORDERS

CHAPTER 75

Poikiloderma Syndromes

Alan D. Irvine[1] and Jemima E. Mellerio[2]

[1] Children's Health Ireland at Crumlin; St James's Hospital, Dublin; and Trinity College, Dublin, Ireland
[2] St John's Institute of Dermatology, Guy's and St Thomas' NHS Foundation Trust, London, UK

Introduction

Poikiloderma is defined as the constellation of skin atrophy, hypo- and hyperpigmentation and telangiectasia. It is a finding in a number of genodermatoses that have variable and potentially serious and life-limiting extracutaneous features. Delineation of the clinical phenotype in these disorders helps to direct subsequent molecular genetic testing to refine the diagnosis and inform the likely associated features and prognosis. Table 75.1 summarises some of the more common or significant mucocutaneous and extracutaneous features of the major poikiloderma syndromes.

Dyskeratosis congenita

Definition and nomenclature

Dyskeratosis congenita (DKC) is a group of rare, inherited disorders characterised by a mucocutaneous triad of reticulate pigmentation and atrophy of the skin, nail dystrophy and leukoplakia, as well as bone marrow failure and a predisposition to malignancy. It is clinically and genetically heterogeneous, arising from mutations in genes involved in maintaining telomere length during cell division [1,2,3].

Synonyms and inclusions
- Zinsser–Cole–Engman syndrome
- Hoyeraal–Heidarsson syndrome
- Revesz syndrome

Pathophysiology
Pathology
The cutaneous changes are not pathognomonic and are unimpressive. The epidermis is flattened; the dermis is vascular and contains pigment-laden macrophages and a variable lymphocytic infiltrate. The connective tissue is usually normal.

Genetics
All forms of DKC arise from mutations in genes involved in telomere maintainance or protection. Telomeres are structures composed of tandem nucleotide repeats and a protein complex at the ends of chromosomes that are required to maintain chromosomal integrity. In humans, they are usually 10–15 kb long. With every cell division, telomeres are shortened by the loss of nucleotide repeats. If this shortening becomes critical, cells may undergo senescence with apoptosis, genetic instability or reduced potential for proliferation [2,4]. In DKC, the telomeres are greatly shortened (under the first percentile), a phenomenon also observed in inherited and acquired haematological diseases such as some cases of inherited bone marrow failure, aplastic anaemia and myelodysplasia [1,2,4].

Normally, a series of cellular mechanisms exist by which telomere length is maintained. Telomerase extends telomeres following cell division by replacing nucleotide repeats on the 5′ end of the telomeric DNA [5]. It comprises a reverse transcriptase activity, TERT, and an RNA template for the nucelotide repeats, TERC. Assembly and stability of the telomerase complex rely on H/ACA small nucleolar ribonucleoprotein (snoRNP) complexes which include dyskerin, NOP10 and NHP2 [6]. The ends of the telomeres are protected from degradation from exonucleases and the cell's DNA repair mechanisms by a protein complex called shelterin, which includes TIN2 along with five other proteins [7]. To date, 11 different genes involved in telomere maintainance have been implicated in different forms of DKC [1,5,8], which are summarised in Table 75.2. However, only approximately 70% of individuals fulfilling the clinical criteria for DKC harbour mutations in one of these genes, suggesting that further genes remain to be identified.

X-linked recessive DKC is the most common form [9] although autosomal inheritance, both dominant [10] and recessive [11], is

PART 6: GENETIC DISORDERS

Table 75.1 Major clinical features of poikiloderma syndromes.

Disease	Poikiloderma	Other mucocutaneous features	Extracutaneous features	Prognosis
Dyskeratosis congenita	Mainly neck, trunk and thighs from late childhood	Nail dystrophy and leukoplakia from childhood	Bone marrow failure Mucocutaneous carcinoma Pulmonary or hepatic fibrosis Growth delay Microcephaly Retinopathy (RS) Cerebellar hypoplasia (HHS and RS)	Very variable Death at 30–50 years of age from bone marrow failure or carcinoma
Rothmund–Thomson syndrome	Early-onset redness and telangiectasia on face and exposed sites then replaced by poikiloderma over the face, limbs and buttocks	Variable photosensitivity Keratoses from adolescence BCC or SCC development Sparse hair	Juvenile cataracts (RTS1) Osteosarcoma (RTS2) Small stature Myelodysplasia, lymphoma and leukaemia Craniosynostosis (BGS)	Normal life expectancy if no malignancy
Poikiloderma with neutropenia	Redness or eczematous changes in first 6 months replaced by poikiloderma on limbs spreading centripetally	Variable photosensitivity Pachyonychia Palmoplantar hyperkeratosis	Variable neutropenia Respiratory infections Increased risk of myelodysplasia and leukaemia Variable short stature and dysmorphism	Depends on associated pulmonary or haematological disease
Hereditary fibrosing poikiloderma with tendon contractures, myopathy and pulmonary fibrosis	Early-onset photosensitivity, eczematous changes and poikiloderma on sun-exposed sites	Scleroderma Reduced sweating Alopecia	Limb contractures in first decade Progressive myopathy from childhood Variable development of pulmonary fibrosis Pancreatic insufficiency	Reduced life expectancy due to pulmonary fibrosis and myopathy
Acrokeratotic poikiloderma of Weary	Generalised poikiloderma accentuated in flexures, sparing the face	Palmoplantar hyperkeratosis Linear hyperkeratosis Clubbing	Tissue calcinosis Variable cardiac abnormalities	Not known
Kindler syndrome (see also Chapter 69)	Progressive poikiloderma from childhood, especially in exposed sites	Variable photosensitivity Skin fragility in childhood improving with age Atrophic scarring and wrinkled skin Partial syndactyly Periodontitis Ectropion Meatal, anal or oesophageal stenosis Increased risk of mucocutaneous SCC	Occasional colitis	Usually normal
Bloom syndrome (see also Chapter 77)	From infancy, redness and telangiectasia of the face, hands and forearms	Variable photosensitivity Variable loss of subcutaneous fat Early adulthood skin malignancies common	Pre- and postnatal growth restriction Immunodeficiency Increased risk of various malignancies from second and third decades Type 2 diabetes	Death in early to mid adulthood due to malignancy

BCC, basal cell carcinoma; BGS, Baller–Gerold syndrome; HHS, Hoyeraal–Hreidarsson syndrome; RS, Revesz syndrome; RTS1, Rothmund–Thomson syndrome type 1; RTS2, Rothmund–Thomson syndrome type 2; SCC, squamous cell carcinoma.

Table 75.2 Causative genes and modes of inheritance in dyskeratosis congenita (DKC).

Gene	Protein	Chromosomal location	Function	Inheritance	MIM number	Frequency of all cases of DKC [1]
DKC	Dyskerin	Xq28	Component of H/ACA snoRNPs and telomerase	XLR	300126	20–25%
TINF2	TIN2	14q12	Component of shelterin	AD	613990	12–20%
TERC	TERC	3q26	RNA component of telomerase	AD	127550	5%
RTEL1	RTEL1	20q13	DNA helicase in telomere maintainance and DNA repair	AD AR	615190	2–8%
TERT	TERT	5p15	Telomerase reverse transcriptase	AD AR	613989	1–7%
CTC1	CTC1	17p13.1	Component of CST complex	AR	612199	1–3%
NOLA3	NOP10	15q14	Component of H/ACA snoRNPs	AR	224230	<1%
NOLA2	NHP2	5q33	Component of H/ACA snoRNPs	AR	613987	<1%
WRAP53	TCAB1	17p13	Control of telomerase trafficking	AR	613988	<1%
ACD	TPP1	16q22.1	Component of shelterin	AD AR	616553	<1%
PARN	PARN	16p13.12	Exonuclease required for 3'-end maturation of TERC	AR	616353	<1%

AD, autosomal dominant; AR, autosomal recessive; snoRNP, small nucleolar ribonucleoprotein; XLR, X-linked recessive.

observed in other pedigrees. The clinical severity, somatic and haematological abnormalities, age at onset and age of death vary greatly in different individuals with DKC.

The first mutations in patients with X-linked DKC were identified in *DKC1*, the gene encoding dyskerin, an H/ACA snoRNP component involved in the modification of ribosomal RNA, and a component of the telomerase complex [9]. One or both of these mechanisms may be affected by *DKC1* mutations in X-linked DKC [12]. Female carriers of X-linked DKC show skewed X inactivation suggesting that wild-type haematopoietic cells have a growth and survival advantage over cells carrying *DKC1* mutations [13]. Mutations in *TERC* and *TERT* encoding telomerase components have been identified in families with autosomal dominant DKC [14]. In addition, there is evidence of anticipation in families with *TERC* and *TERT* mutations, which has been attributed to progressive telomere shortening in successive generations [15]. *TERC* and *TERT* mutations have also been demonstrated in families with adult-onset aplastic anaemia and shortened telomeres but no other features of DKC [15–17]. Autosomal recessive *TERT* mutations have also been identified in a few kindreds with a severe DKC phenotype [18]. Mutations in *TINF2* (which encodes TIN2, a component of shelterin) have been delineated in other families with autosomal dominant DKC [10,14]. Autosomal recessive DKC may also result from mutations in genes encoding two other components of telomerase and snoRNP complexes, *NOLA2* and *NOLA3*, as well as in *WRAP53* which encodes the TCBA1 protein thought to be involved in telomerase trafficking [11,19,20]. A severe DKC phenotype has also been associated with autosomal recessive mutations in the *RTEL1* gene, which is implicated in DNA replication at the ends of telomeres [8]; heterozygous carriers may exhibit a milder phenotype [21]. Autosomal recessive pathogenic variants in the *CTC1* gene, which encodes a component of a telomere stabilising complex, are usually associated with cerebro-retinal microangiopathy with calcification and cysts (Coats plus syndrome) but have also been identified in individuals with the classic triad of DKC [22]. Mutations in *ACD* encoding a component of shelterin have been described in families with autosomal dominant [23] and autosomal recessive [24] DKC. A further rare form of autosomal recessive DKC results from mutations in the *PARN* gene, encoding an exonuclease required for TERC function [25–27]. New genes associated with DKC keep appearing. Recently, pathogenic variants in NMP1 encoding nucleophosmin, an essential regulator of rRNA methylation, were identified in patients with DKC [28].

Clinical features [1,29,30]

Because of the relatively late onset of the characteristic features of this syndrome, their relationship may be overlooked for some years and diagnosis delayed. The median age of diagnosis of DKC is 15 years (range 0–75 years). The essential mucocutaneous features of the syndrome are reticulate pigmentation and atrophy of the skin, nail dystrophy and mucosal leukoplakia. The nail changes are usually the first to appear. Between the ages of 5 and 13 years, the nails become dystrophic and are shed: they may be reduced to horny plugs or be completely destroyed. There may be recurrent episodes of suppurative paronychia.

The pigmentary changes may appear simultaneously or 2–3 years after nail changes and reach their full development in 3–5 years.

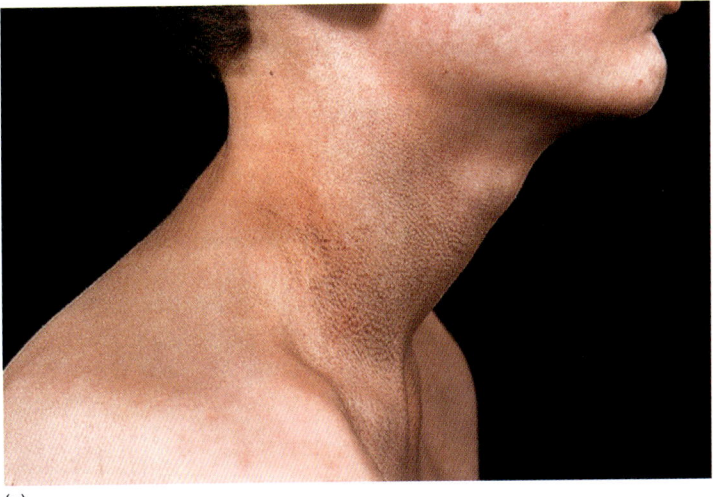

(a)

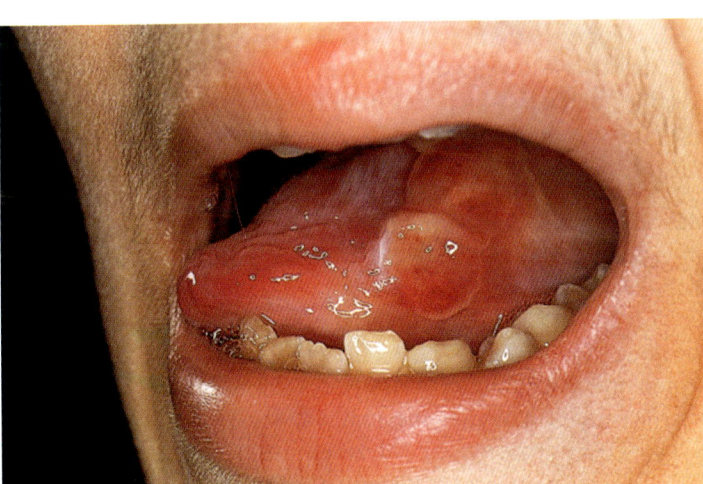

(b)

Figure 75.1 Dyskeratosis congenita. (a) Reticulate pigmentation on the neck. (b) The development of leukoplakia.

Fine, reticulate, grey-brown pigmentation is most conspicuous on the neck (Figure 75.1a) and thighs, but involves the greater part of the trunk. The skin is atrophic, and telangiectasia may be sufficiently prominent to give a poikilodermatous appearance. The skin of the face is red and atrophic, with irregular macular pigmentation, while that of the dorsa of the hands and feet is diffusely atrophic, transparent and shiny. The palms and soles may be thickened and hyperhidrotic, and may form bullae with trauma. Premature canities and cicatricial alopecia have occasionally been noted [31]. The teeth tend to be defective and irregularly implanted, and periodontal disease and early caries are usual.

The onset of mucous membrane lesions may coincide with, or follow, the nail and skin changes. Small blisters and erosions of the lingual and buccal mucous membranes are succeeded by irregular patches of leukoplakia (Figure 75.1b). Similar changes on the tarsal conjunctiva may obliterate the lacrimal puncta, resulting in excessive lacrimation and soreness and scarring of the lids. Ano-rectal, oesophageal or urethral leukoplakia may produce stenosis. Similar changes may occur throughout the gastrointestinal tract and on the uro-genital mucous membranes. Pulmonary and hepatic fibrosis have also been described [10]. Growth and psychomotor development may be delayed, and immunodeficiency and osteoporosis can occur.

Hoyeraal–Hreidarsson and Revesz syndromes are more severe forms of DKC, usually presenting in early childhood and characterised by intrauterine growth retardation, profound developmental delay and early-onset bone marrow failure [**1,30**]. Additionally, cerebellar hypoplasia is a feature of Hoyeraal–Hreidarsson syndrome which results from *DKC1*, *TERT*, *TINF2*, *RTEL1*, *NHP2*, *WRAP53*, *ACD* or *PARN* gene mutations [32–35]. Revesz syndrome is characterised by bilateral exudative retinopathy and intracranial calcifications [31]; it is caused by pathogenic variants in *TINF2* [35–37].

Co-morbidities

Haematological abnormalities. The incidence of bone marrow failure in DKC is high: in one series, it arose in 93% of patients, with pancytopenia as the cause of death in 71% [29]. The timing of onset is variable but the risk increases from 10 years of age. Myelodysplasia and acute myeloid leukaemia have been reported in other patients.

Malignancy. In addition to an increased incidence of haematological malignancy in DKC, the risk of squamous cell carcinoma (SCC) of the head and neck (particularly in areas of tongue leukoplakia), the skin and ano-genital region is increased [38]. A review of the literature and prospective data collection in a group of DKC patients demonstrated a cumulative risk of developing cancer of 40–50% by age 50 years and a median survival of 42 years [38]. Other neoplasms reported include pancreatic carcinoma and Hodgkin disease.

Associated allelic disorders. Improved understanding of the molecular pathology of genes important in telomere maintainance has led to the identification of mutations in *TERT*, *TERC* and *ACD* in patients without a full DKC phenotype, but with aplastic anaemia and bone marrow failure with, or without, pulmonary and hepatic fibrosis [16,17,23]. In addition, heterozygous mutations in *TERT*, *TERT*, *PARN* and *RTEL1* have been identified in individuals with autosomal dominant idiopathic pulmonary fibrosis [26,39–41]. Variants of *TERC* and *TERT* associated with telomere shortening have also been identified with greater frequency in patients with chronic liver disease who have progressed on to cirrhosis [42,43].

Prognosis

The prognosis is usually poor as a result of the blood dyscrasia or carcinoma, although the age at which these complications occurs is generally very variable. Individuals with *TINF2* or *DKC1* mutations, or those with autosomal recessive *RTEL*, *PARN* or *ACD* mutations, tend to have more severe and early-onset disease, including Hoyeraal–Hreidarsson and Revesz syndromes [23–26,44,45]. In contrast, autosomal dominant *RTEL* and *ACD* variants tend to result in milder phenotypes with better outcomes. In some patients, only mucocutaneous features are present and life expectancy is into late adulthood [46].

Investigations and diagnosis

It is important to enquire about a personal and family history of the following: bone marrow failure, head and neck, ano-genital or other cancers below the age of 50 years, and pulmonary or hepatic fibrosis. As mentioned earlier, the clinical features of DKC may be variable and present at different time points. An examination of other family members may also be helpful. A blood count and film should be undertaken with a bone marrow biopsy if abnormal. Pulmonary function tests and liver ultrasonography may also be indicated in view of possible fibrosis. Bone density assessment may reveal osteoporosis. A telomere length assay will demonstrate telomere shortening which is characteristic of this condition. Molecular analysis should reveal the underlying mutation(s) in around 70% of patients and can be undertaken as single gene sequencing, as a multigene panel or a next generation sequencing approach. Carrier testing of relatives should be considered due to the variable penetrance and variability in timing of presentation; this should detect relatives at risk of developing bone marrow failure or other complications of the disease. A molecular diagnosis may also enable DNA-based first trimester prenatal or preimplantation genetic testing for affected families.

Management

Management of individuals with DKC should be provided by a multidisciplinary team comprising all relevant medical specialties. The aplastic anaemia associated with DKC is not responsive to immunosuppressive treatment but can be treated with the anabolic steroids danazol, nandrolone or oxymethalone [47]. Bone marrow failure or leukaemia associated with DKC should be treated with haematopoietic cell transplantation ideally if a matched, related donor is available, and can be considered if there is an unrelated donor [48]. Caution should be taken to use reduced conditioning to minimise the risks of problems due to underlying hepatic or pulmonary disease.

Retinoids have been reported to cause regression of lesions in leukoplakia [49] and so may reduce the incidence of malignancy.

Rothmund–Thomson syndrome

Definition and nomenclature

Rothmund–Thomson syndrome (RTS) is a rare, autosomal recessive disorder characterised by early-onset poikiloderma, skeletal abnormalities, short stature, premature ageing, sparse hair, dental problems and an increased susceptibility to malignancy [**1**].

Synonyms and inclusions
- Poikiloderma congenitale
- Baller–Gerold syndrome
- RAPADILINO syndrome

Pathophysiology
Pathology [2]
In childhood, the histological changes are flattening and atrophy of the epidermis, with oedema of the dermal–epidermal junction.

There may be some vasodilatation and perivascular lymphocytic infiltration in the dermis. In adults, exposed skin shows a combination of fragmentation of elastic tissue in the dermis with patchy Bowenoid dyskeratosis of the epidermis.

Genetics

Around 60% of affected individuals with RTS have compound heterozygous or homozygous mutations in the DNA helicase gene, *RECQL4*, on chromosome 8q24.3 [3]. The RECQL4 protein is essential for the initiation of DNA replication and is necessary for efficient removal of ultraviolet (UV)-induced DNA damage [4]. Reduced DNA repair capacity and increased sensitivity to UVC have been reported in individual patients with RTS [5,6]. Recently, a second gene, *ANAPC1*, on chromosome 2q13, has been implicated in around 10% of cases of RTS [7]. It encodes APC1, a component of anaphase-promoting complex/cyclosome, which plays a role in cell cycling as well as senescence, DNA replication and repair, cell differentiation and metabolism [8]. Failure to identify causative mutations in around 30% of cases with clinical features suggestive of RTS suggests that an additional gene or genes remain to be elucidated [1].

Patients can be classified depending on the underlying molecular pathology. Patients with RTS type I have poikiloderma and may have juvenile cataracts, but do not have an increased incidence of malignancy; this cohort have been shown to harbour *ANAPC1* mutations. In contrast, in RTS type II, *RECQL4* mutations are found, and patients have typical poikiloderma and an increased risk of osteosarcoma [9]. Identification of *RECQL4* mutations in patients with a clinical diagnosis of RTS, therefore, may have implications for the need for ongoing surveillance for malignancy. Trisomy 8 mosaicism has also been described in some patients [10].

Mutations in *RECQL4* have also been identified in two other disorders with a clinical overlap with RTS. Firstly, Baller–Gerold syndrome (BGS), which is characterised by craniosynostosis and radial defects, in which poikiloderma may be a feature. It has been proposed that the clinical and genetic similarities between RTS and BGS may indicate that these are a single entity [11], although BGS patients without poikiloderma do not harbour *RECQL4* mutations and therefore probably represent a separate entity [3]. Secondly, RAPADILINO syndrome, which encompasses growth retardation, bony abnormalities (particularly radial defects) and an increased risk of certain malignancies but no poikiloderma [12]. Genotype–phenotype correlation has been shown for a number of families with these disorders and *RECQL4* mutations [9].

Clinical features [1,3,13,14]
Presentation

The skin appears normal at birth. The earliest lesions usually develop between the third and sixth months, but sometimes as late as the second year. Plaques of red skin and oedema, or more transitory diffuse redness, are succeeded by varying combinations of atrophy, telangiectasia, pigmentation and depigmentation (Figure 75.2). The pigmentation, dull brown in colour, irregularly macular or reticulate, develops later than the atrophy and telangiectasia on which it is superimposed (Figure 75.3), although it may extend much beyond these areas, especially on the neck and trunk where it may be the only change. On the face and hands, telangiectasia predominates.

The cheeks are first and most severely affected, but the forehead, chin and ears are also usually involved. The hands, forearms and lower legs are next affected, and the buttocks and thighs are frequently involved. Light sensitivity is a feature of many cases, and exposure to sunlight may extend the distribution of the eruption on the upper trunk; however, it is not limited to light-exposed skin, and the poikiloderma may develop without any preceding redness. Light sensitivity may be so severe that a bullous response is elicited, and although this tends to diminish after early childhood, it may persist into adult life [15].

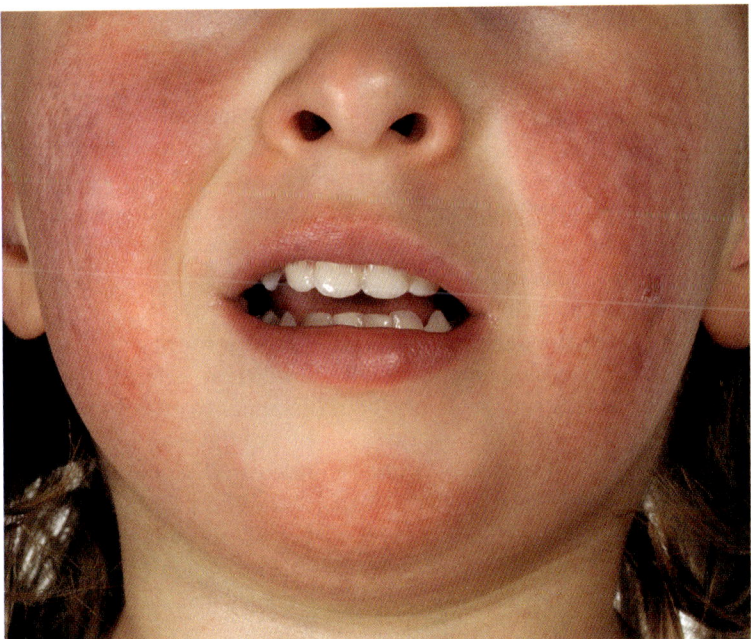 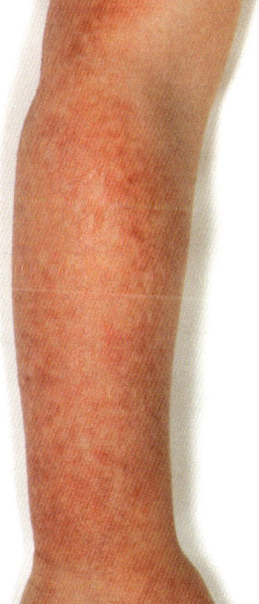

Figure 75.2 Rothmund–Thomson syndrome. (a) Facial telangiectasia, redness and early poikiloderma in a young child. (b) Telangiectasia, redness and poikiloderma on the arm of a young child showing sparing in the elbow flexure. Courtesy of Dr H. Fassihi, St John's Institute of Dermatology, London, UK.   (a)   (b)

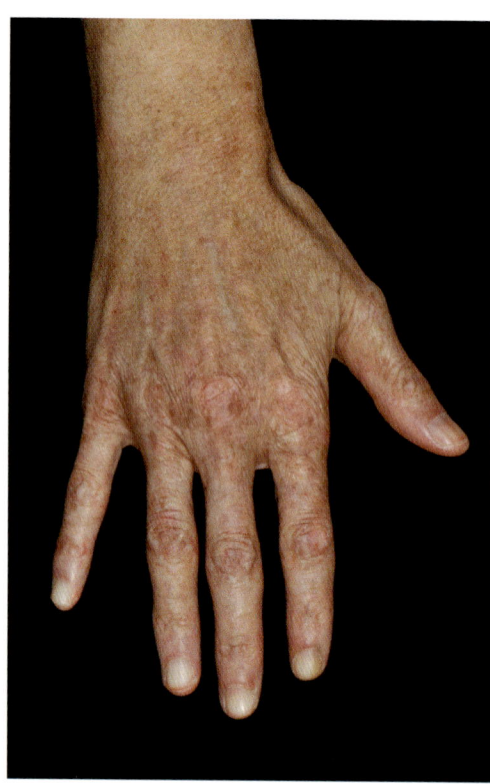

Figure 75.3 Poikiloderma of the dorsa of the hand in an adult woman with Rothmund–Thomson syndrome.

Once fully developed in early life, the skin lesions tend to remain unchanged, but in many cases keratoses develop on exposed skin from adolescence onwards, and large warty keratoses of the hands, wrists, feet, ankles and elsewhere may occur [16]. Skin cancer arises in around 5% of individuals; squamous or basal cell carcinoma may develop in the keratoses or in the surrounding atrophic skin [17], and malignant melanoma has also been reported [18].

Scalp hair, eyebrows, eyelashes and pubic and axillary hair are often sparse or absent. Nails are normal or small and dystrophic. Teeth may be normal, but microdontia, hypodontia or anodontia, delayed dental eruption and early caries have been reported.

Bilateral cataracts, usually developing between the fourth and seventh years, occur in around 10–40% of reported cases, and are particularly associated with *ANAPC1* mutations [7,13].

Skeletal abnormalities include radial ray defects, which may present as thumb hypoplasia with an abnormal radial head, or complete absence of the radius. Ulnar defects, patellar hypoplasia or aplasia, abnormal trabeculation and osteopenia may also arise [19,20]. There is a recognised risk of osteosarcoma, notably in patients with *RECQL4* mutations, especially in the bones of the lower leg, which can present in childhood [9,13,14]. In a series of 41 patients with RTS, Wang *et al.* identified osteosarcoma in 32% (higher than previous estimates) and radial defects in 20% [13].

Most patients are of proportionate small stature, with slender delicate limbs, small hands and feet and short fingers. The skull may be small and the features bird-like, sometimes with a saddle nose. Hypogonadism of variable degree is frequent and the incidence of

hyperparathyroidism appears also to be increased [21]. The association of RTS and Addison disease has also been reported [22].

Other associations reported include myelodysplastic syndrome [23], lymphoma, leukaemia [24], malignant eccrine poroma [25], malignant fibrous histiocytoma [26], gastrointestinal adenocarcinoma [27,28] and annular pancreas with duodenal stenosis [29]. Individuals with RTS are usually of normal intelligence.

Differential diagnosis
The essential features in differential diagnosis are the age of onset and the distribution of the poikiloderma, which is most intense on light-exposed skin but not necessarily confined to it.

In Werner syndrome, the skin changes are essentially scleroder-matous, and both skin and ocular lesions develop later than in RTS. In DKC, reticulate pigmentation develops between the ages of 5 and 13 years, and is most marked on the neck, trunk and thighs. Atrophy and telangiectasia may appear later. The nail changes are constant and severe. In progeria, the child is often small but otherwise normal during the first year; thereafter development is delayed. Scalp hair, eyebrows and eyelashes are lost and the skin assumes an increasingly senile appearance. In Cockayne syndrome, light sensitivity is a conspicuous feature after the first year, but there is no poikiloderma. Xeroderma pigmentosum should not cause confusion: in mild forms, only freckle-like macules are present, whereas in mild forms of RTS, telangiectasia is the conspicuous feature. In Kindler syndrome, skin fragility is present in the early years ahead of the development of poikiloderma, and photosensitivity is variable. Characteristic fine, atrophic scarring and limited webbing of the digits occurs from adolescence onwards, and gingival involvement may lead to marked periodontal disease and dental loss. Telangiectasia, often irregular, linear and present at birth, is a feature of focal dermal hypoplasia. In Bloom syndrome, redness, and not poikiloderma, is the essential change.

Prognosis
Life expectancy depends on the development of an associated malignancy; otherwise, it appears to be normal.

Investigation
Genetic testing can be undertaken by single gene sequencing, via a gene panel or through next generation sequencing methods [1]. Identification of causative mutations in *ANAPC1* or *RECQL4* enables DNA-based prenatal or preimplantation genetic testing in at-risk pregnancies.

Management
Protection against sunlight is important. Careful supervision is essential to ensure the detection of malignancy. Baseline radiography of the long bones by the age of 5 years has been recommended since underlying skeletal dysplasias can make X-ray interpretation difficult if there is a later suspicion of osteosarcoma [13]. It is not known whether patients with RTS have increased sensitivity to chemotherapy and radiotherapy. Improvement of cutaneous changes has been described with retinoids [30]. Telangiectasia, especially on the face, can be improved significantly by treatment with a vascular pulsed dye laser [31].

Poikiloderma with neutropenia, Clericuzio type

Definition
The dermatological manifestations of this autosomal recessive genodermatosis include a red rash evolving into poikiloderma, and paronychia [1,2–4]. It is associated with neutropenia, respiratory infections and susceptibility to myelodysplasia and leukaemia.

Pathophysiology
Homozygous or compound heterozygous mutations in the *USB1* (*C16ORF57*) gene have been identified in individuals with poikiloderma with neutropenia [5,6–10]. This gene encodes the USB1 protein, an exonuclease involved in the regulation of RNA splicing [11]. Although the precise mechanisms by which mutations give rise to the clinical phenotype are not yet fully understood, USB1 is known to interact with RECQL4 through SMAD-mediated signalling [5,12].

Clinical features
Skin manifestations usually start in the first 6 months of life with red, eczematous or ichthyosiform changes on the limbs, subsequently spreading more centrally and being replaced by poikiloderma [2–4,5]. Photosensitivity is variable. The nails show an early onset of pachyonychia and there may be an associated palmoplantar keratoderma. Early-onset cutaneous SCC has been reported [9,10]. In contrast to RTS, alopecia is not a feature, and unlike DKC, leukoplakia is not seen.

The presence of neutropenia is variable and may be cyclical [2,3], and myelodysplasia or acute myeloid leukaemia may occur [5,7]. Recurrent airway infections with chronic cough and reactive airway changes are common, and otitis media has also been described [3]. Affected individuals may have short stature and facial dysmorphism [8].

Hereditary fibrosing poikiloderma with tendon contractures, myopathy and pulmonary fibrosis

Definition and nomenclature
This relatively newly described entity is a rare autosomal dominant condition characterised by early-onset poikiloderma associated with myopathy, joint contractures, pulmonary fibrosis and pancreatic insufficiency caused by mutations in the *FAM111B* gene.

Synonyms and inclusions
- POIKTMP

Pathophysiology
Hereditary fibrosing poikiloderma with tendon contractures, myopathy and pulmonary fibrosis (HFP) has been described in a number of families from various ethnic backgrounds. Heterozygous missense mutations in the *FAM111B* gene have been shown to be causative [1]. The function of the gene product is currently unknown, but it is expressed in numerous tissues including skin and skeletal muscle [1]. Histopathology of the skin shows the loss of adnexal structures due to fibrosis and elastic degeneration and globules in the papillary dermis [2].

Clinical features [1,2–6]
Cutaneous features of HFP include early-onset photosensitivity with pain and redness of sun-exposed skin starting in the first 6 months of life. Poikiloderma also occurs early in predominantly sun-exposed sites which may also have an eczematous or psoriasiform appearance. Transient bullae of exposed skin may arise. Later, there may be more sclerodermatous or lymphoedematous skin changes and reduced sweating, which can lead to overheating. There is marked alopecia of the scalp, eyelashes, eyebrows and body hair, but the nails and teeth are normal. In the first decade, progressive tendon contractures of the lower and, in some cases, upper limbs develop. Myopathy also starts in the early years with atrophy with fatty infiltration of the skeletal muscle. Some affected individuals develop progressive pulmonary fibrosis from the second decade leading to breathlessness and diminished pulmonary function, which may be fatal in adulthood. Pancreatic insufficiency may occur, and pancreatic carcinoma has also been described. Hepatomegaly and transaminitis are also recognised in some individuals.

Acrokeratotic poikiloderma of Weary

Definition and nomenclature
This syndrome, probably determined by an autosomal dominant gene, appears to be a distinct entity that has been described in a handful of families [1,2,3]. It is characterised by generalised poikiloderma with accentuation in the flexures and sparing of the face, scalp and ears, sclerosis of the palms and soles, linear hyperkeratosis and sclerosis of the flexures, and finger clubbing. Tissue calcinosis, Raynaud phenomenon and cardiac abnormalities have also been described [1,3].

Synonyms and inclusions
- Hereditary sclerosing poikiloderma

Key references

The full list of references can be found in the online version at https://www.wiley.com/rooksdermatology10e

Dyskeratosis congenita
1 Savage SA. Dyskeratosis congenita. 2009 (updated 2019). In: Adam MP, Ardinger HH, Pagon RA *et al.*, eds. *GeneReviews® [Internet]*. Seattle, WA: University of Washington, 1993–2022.
2 Mason PJ, Bessler M. The genetics of dyskeratosis congenita. *Cancer Genet* 2011;204:635–45.

30 Vulliamy TJ, Marrone A, Knight SW *et al*. Mutations in dyskeratosis congenita: their impact on telomere length and the diversity of clinical presentation. *Blood* 2006;107:2680–5.

Rothmund–Thomson syndrome

1 Wang LL, Plon SE. Rothmund–Thomson syndrome. 1999 (updated 2020). In: Adam MP, Ardinger HH, Pagon RA *et al*., eds. *GeneReviews® [Internet]*. Seattle, WA: University of Washington, 1993–2022.

9 Siitonen HA, Sotkasiira J, Biervliet M *et al*. The mutation spectrum in RECQL4 diseases. *Eur J Hum Genet* 2009;17:151–8.

13 Wang LL, Levy ML, Lewis RA *et al*. Clinical manifestations in a cohort of 41 Rothmund–Thomson syndrome patients. *Am J Med Genet* 2001;102:11–17.

Poikiloderma with neutropenia, Clericuzio type

1 Clericuzio C, Hoyme HE, Aase JM. Immune deficient poikiloderma: a new genodermatosis. *Am J Hum Genet* 1991;49(Suppl.):131.

5 Volpi L, Roversi G, Colombo EA *et al*. Targeted next-generation sequencing appoints C16orf57 as Clericuzio-type poikiloderma with neutropenia gene. *Am J Hum Genet* 2010;86:72–6.

Hereditary fibrosing poikiloderma with tendon contractures, myopathy and pulmonary fibrosis

1 Mercier S, Kury S, Shabodien G *et al*. Mutations in FAM111B cause hereditary fibrosing poikiloderma with tendon contracture, myopathy, and pulmonary fibrosis. *Am J Hum Genet* 2013;93:1100–7.

Acrokeratotic poikiloderma of Weary

1 Weary PE, Hsu YT, Richardson DR *et al*. Hereditary sclerosing poikiloderma: report of two families with an unusual and distinctive genodermatosis. *Arch Dermatol* 1969;100:413–22.

CHAPTER 76

DNA Repair Disorders with Cutaneous Features

Hiva Fassihi

St John's Institute of Dermatology, Guy's and St Thomas' NHS Foundation Trust, London, UK

Introduction

The human genome is made up of about 3 billion DNA base pairs containing an estimated 30 000 protein-encoding genes. This DNA is continually being damaged by a variety of endogenous sources (such as reactive oxygen species) and exogenous sources (such as ultraviolet and ionising radiation).

Cells have evolved a number of complex and effective systems, including nucleotide excision repair, double-strand break repair and mismatch repair, to recognise and repair this damage in actively transcribed genes. Successful repair of damaged DNA is also dependent on the unzipping of the DNA double helix by enzymes of the helicase group.

Defects in these DNA repair pathways result in a number of disorders, many with skin involvement, commonly photosensitivity, cancer and premature ageing (Table 76.1).

Xeroderma pigmentosum

Definition

Xeroderma pigmentosum (XP) is a rare autosomal recessive disorder of DNA repair. It is characterised by progressive pigmentary changes at exposed sites, an increased risk of ultraviolet radiation (UVR)-induced skin and mucous membrane cancers, severe photosensitivity in about 50%, and neurodegeneration in approximately 30% of affected cases. It is divided into eight complementation groups: XP-A to XP-G and XP-V (XP variant), corresponding to the affected DNA repair gene. There is wide variability in clinical features both between and within XP complementation groups [1].

Introduction and general description

XP is a rare disorder of DNA repair, which presents clinically with progressive pigmentary abnormalities, and an increased incidence of UVR-induced skin and mucous membrane cancers at sun-exposed sites. About half of affected individuals also show an exaggerated and prolonged sunburn response on minimal exposure. In a minority of cases, there is progressive neurological degeneration [2].

The initial report of this disorder was made by Hebra and Kaposi in 1874 [3] and the term xeroderma pigmentosum, meaning pigmented dry skin, was introduced in 1882 [4]. The first neurological problems were reported in 1883 by Neisser [5], and in 1932 De Sanctis and Cacchione reported three brothers with XP, with severe progressive neurological degeneration and associated dwarfism and gonadal hypoplasia; they called this De Sanctis–Cacchione syndrome [6]. This term is no longer in general use as it is now appreciated that XP can be associated with neurological problems of widely varying severity, and that De Sanctis–Cacchione syndrome is at the extreme end of a continuous spectrum.

DNA repair abnormalities in XP were reported by Cleaver in 1968. He discovered deficient excision repair in cultured skin fibroblasts from these patients [7]. UVR-induced DNA photoproducts were identified by Setlow and Setlow [8] and XP cells were found to be defective in the excision repair of these photoproducts *in vivo* [9]. The excision repair-proficient form of XP was first described in 1971 [10], named 'variant' by Cleaver in 1972 [11]. These 'variant' cultured fibroblasts were able to repair UVR-induced damage but were found to be defective in another DNA repair pathway, post-replication repair [12]. This subtype is now known as XP variant (XP-V).

Cell fusion studies by De Weerd-Kastelein in 1972 demonstrated molecular heterogeneity in XP [13]. The fusion of fibroblasts from different XP patients to form heterokaryons was found to correct the defect in DNA repair. This suggested that patients had different defects in nucleotide excision repair, and one defect could be corrected by the fusion of cells from a patient with a different defect because of the availability of the protein that the other was lacking. This led to the characterisation of XP into different complementation groups (XP-A through to XP-G).

Rook's Textbook of Dermatology, Tenth Edition. Edited by Christopher Griffiths, Jonathan Barker, Tanya Bleiker, Walayat Hussain and Rosalind Simpson.
© 2024 John Wiley & Sons Ltd. Published 2024 by John Wiley & Sons Ltd.

Table 76.1 DNA repair disorders with cutaneous features.

Disorder	DNA repair defect
Xeroderma pigmentosum	Nucleotide excision repair
Cockayne syndrome	Nucleotide excision repair
Cerebro-oculo-facio-skeletal syndrome	Nucleotide excision repair
UV-sensitive syndrome	Nucleotide excision repair
Trichothiodystrophy	Nucleotide excision repair
Rothmund–Thomson syndrome	Recombination Q helicase
Bloom syndrome	Recombination Q helicase
Werner syndrome	Recombination Q helicase
Ataxia telangiectasia	Double-strand break repair
Fanconi anaemia	Interstrand cross-link repair
Muir–Torre syndrome	Mismatch repair

Epidemiology

Incidence and prevalence

Estimates from the 1970s suggested an incidence of XP in the USA of one in 250 000 [14] and in Japan of one in 80 000 [15]. A more recent survey in Western Europe suggests an incidence of approximately 2.3 per million live births [16]. The incidence of XP in Japan is significantly higher than in western countries, with the majority of XP patients in Japan belonging to the XP-A complementation group (90% of patients are homozygous for the *XPA* founder mutation, carried by 1% of the Japanese population [17]).

The prevalence is higher in North Africa and the Middle East, especially in communities in which consanguinity is common. Amid Indian and Middle Eastern areas, the incidence is quoted at

one per 10 000–30 000 [18–21]. In 2010, Soufir *et al.* reported that 85% of XP families in the Maghreb region (Algeria, Tunisia and Morocco) carried a founder mutation in the *XPC* gene [22]. More recently, it has been reported that one in 5000 individuals of the black Mahori population in the Comoro Islands have XP-C. This is linked to another founder mutation [23].

Sex

XP affects males and females equally.

Ethnicity

It has been reported to occur in all ethnic groups worldwide.

Pathophysiology

XP is an autosomal recessive disorder and results from mutations in any one of eight genes. The products of seven of these genes (*XPA* through to *XPG*) are involved in the recognition and repair of UVR-induced photoproducts in DNA (cyclobutane pyrimidine dimers (CPDs) and pyrimidine (6-4) pyrimidone photoproducts (6-4PPs)) by the process of nucleotide excision repair (NER) [24].

NER is made up of two pathways (Figure 76.1): global genome nucleotide excision repair (GG-NER) in which damage to DNA not undergoing transcription is repaired, and transcription-coupled nucleotide excision repair (TC-NER) in which damage in transcribed regions of DNA is rapidly repaired [25,26]. In GG-NER, the photoproducts are recognised by the proteins XPC and XPE. In TC-NER, these bulky lesions block the progress of RNA

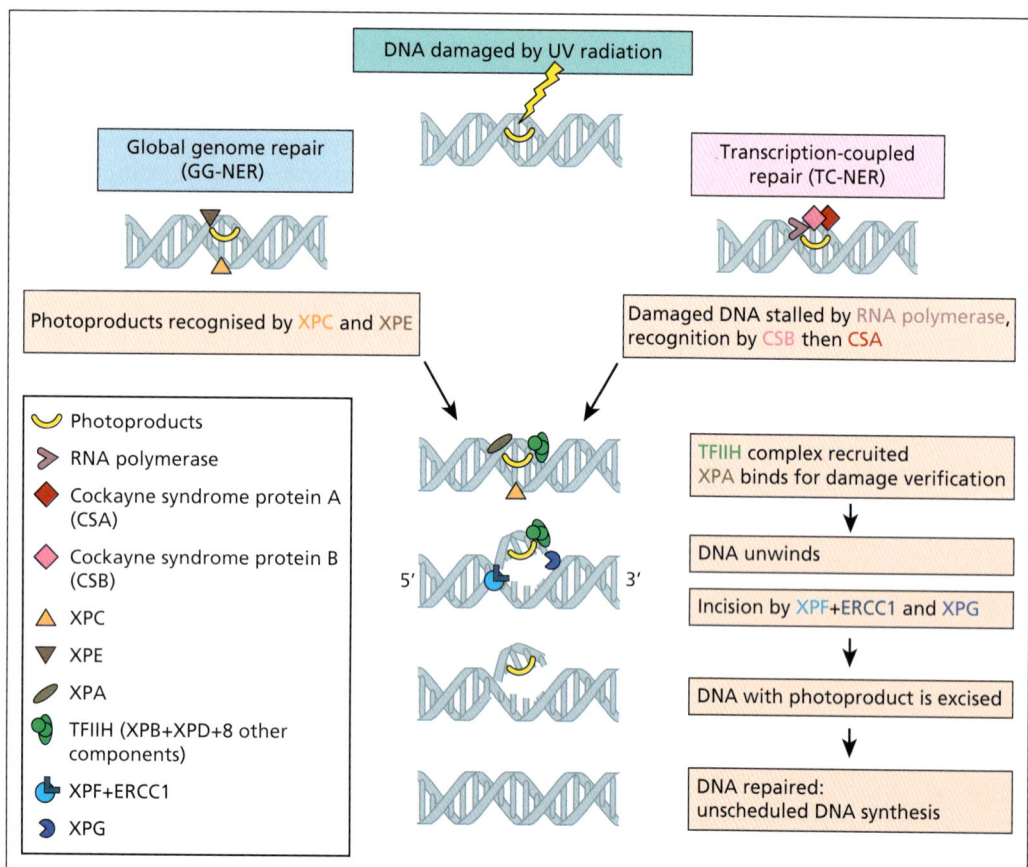

Figure 76.1 In global genome nucleotide excision repair (GG-NER), XPE (with its partner protein DDB1) binds to the photoproduct and recruits another protein, XPC, which recognises and binds to the strand opposite the photoproduct. In transcription-coupled NER (TC-NER), RNA polymerase II stalls at the site of the photoproduct. This then leads to the recruitment of CSA and CSB protein (defective in Cockayne syndrome and not xeroderma pigmentosum). The two pathways then converge. TFIIH (a complex containing 10 peptides including the helicases XPB and XPD) then opens up the DNA and subsequently XPA binds to verify the correct positioning of all the proteins. The heterodimeric nucleases ERCC1/XPF and XPG then cleave the damaged DNA strand at the 5' to 3' ends, on either side of the photoproduct. The gap is filled in by using the undamaged DNA strand as template. This process is referred to as unscheduled DNA synthesis. Adapted from Sethi *et al.* 2013 [26].

Table 76.2 The genes, chromosomal locations, protein functions and the main clinical features in different XP complementation groups.

XP complementation group	Gene	Chromosomal location	Protein function	Defective pathway	Clinical features
XP-A	*XPA*	9q22.23	Damage verification	NER	Severe subtype Common in Japan Exaggerated sunburn Variable neurological abnormalities dependent on genetic mutations
XP-B	*ERCC3* (*XPB*)	2q14.3	Helicase Part of TFIIH	NER	Extremely rare subtype Exaggerated sunburn Mild neurological abnormalities (Mutations in *XPB* can also result in XP/CS and TTD)
XP-C	*XPC*	3p25.1	Damage recognition	NER (GG-NER)	Most common subtype No abnormal sunburn reaction Severely atypical and dense lentigines at exposed sites Severe ocular surface disease No neurological abnormalities
XP-D	*ERCC2* (*XPD*)	19q13.32	Helicase Part of TFIIH	NER	Severe exaggerated sunburn Variable neurological abnormalities dependent on genetic mutations (Mutations in *XPD* can also result in XP/CS and TTD)
XP-E	*DDB2* (*XPE*)	11p11.2	Damage recognition	NER (GG-NER)	Rare subtype No abnormal sunburn reaction Large number of skin cancers from thirties onwards No neurological abnormalities
XP-F	*ERCC4* (*XPF*)	16p13.12	Nuclease	NER	Mildly exaggerated sunburn Skin signs tend to be mild Variable neurological abnormalities dependent on genetic mutations (Mutations in *XPF* can also result in XP/CS)
XP-G	*ERCC5* (*XPG*)	13q33.1	Nuclease	NER	Rare subtype Exaggerated sunburn Variable neurological abnormalities dependent on genetic mutations (Mutations in *XPG* can also result in XP/CS)
XP-V	*POLH* (*XPV*)	6p21.1	Polymerase	TLS	No abnormal sunburn reaction Diagnosed in thirties/forties after multiple skin cancers No ocular disease No neurological abnormalities

Adapted from Lehmann *et al*. 2011 [**27**].

GG-NER: global genome nucleotide excision repair subpathway; NER, nucleotide excision repair; TLS, translesion synthesis; TTD: trichothiodystrophy; XP/CS: xeroderma pigmentosum/Cockayne syndrome complex.

polymerase II in a process involving two proteins not involved in XP, CSA and CSB (Cockayne syndrome proteins A and B). Following this initial damage recognition, the pathways converge. XPB and XPD are part of a protein complex, TFIIH, which opens up the structure of the DNA around the site of the photoproduct. XPA protein verifies that the proteins are in the correct position and then the endonucleases XPG and XPF cut the DNA on either side of the damage, so that the damaged section, in a fragment of about 30 nucleotides, can be removed. The gap is filled in by *de novo* DNA synthesis and the new stretch of DNA is finally joined up to the pre-existing strand. This is referred to as unscheduled DNA synthesis (UDS).

Mutation(s) in any of the seven genes encoding for these proteins (XPA to XPG) result in abnormal NER and the different XP complementation groups (XP-A to XP-G, respectively) (Table 76.2) [**27**]. More specifically, mutations in the *XPA*, *ERCC3* (*XPB*), *ERCC2* (*XPD*), *ERCC4* (*XPF*) and *ERCC5* (*XPG*) genes result in defects in both GG-NER and TC-NER. However, mutations in the *XPC*

and *DDB2* (*XPE*) genes only affect GG-NER and therefore some preservation of NER via the TC-NER pathway.

Defects in the eighth XP gene do not affect NER. About 20% of patients with XP, the so-called XP variant (XP-V), have problems replicating DNA containing UVR-induced damage [28]. They have defects in the *POLII* (or *XPV*) gene, which encodes for DNA polymerase η, one of the specialised enzymes required for replication beyond the damaged sites (translesion synthesis) [12,29].

Clinical features
History and presentation
Patients with XP are a clinically heterogeneous group with a wide variability in clinical features both between and within XP complementation groups (Table 76.2). The clinical manifestations, severity of disease and age of onset are in part dependent on the cumulative UVR exposure, the complementation group and the precise nature of the pathogenic mutation(s).

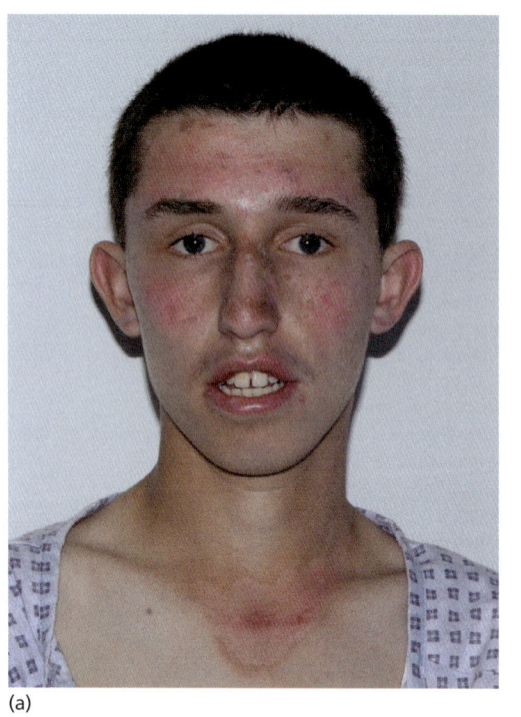
(a)

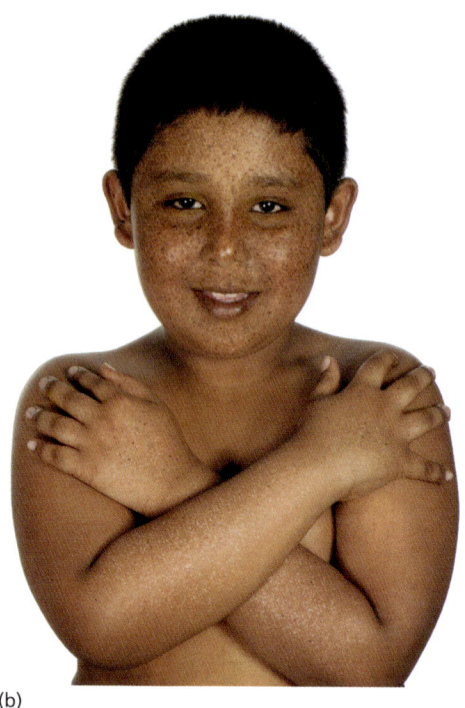
(b)

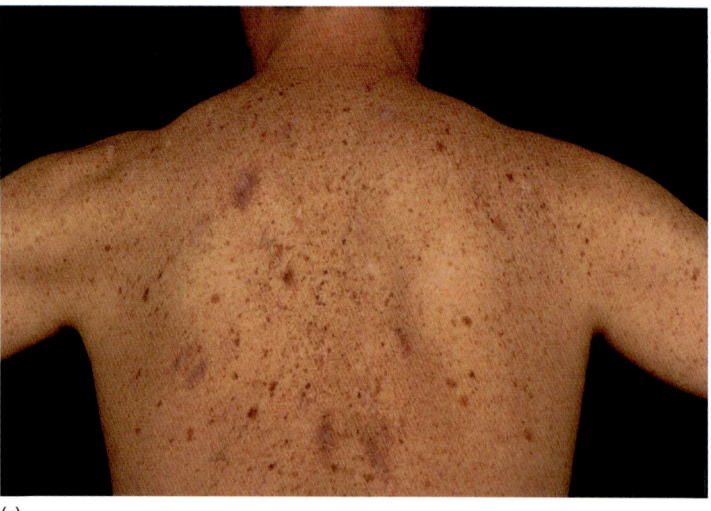
(c)

Figure 76.2 Xeroderma pigmentosum. (a) Severe and exaggerated sunburn on minimal sun exposure. (b) Lentigines and hypopigmented macules (seen on the forearms) at sun-exposed sites. (c) Pigmentary change and multiple surgical scars at sites of previous skin cancers.

Exaggerated sunburn and pigmentary changes. The skin is normal at birth. The changes in XP are the result of exposure to UVR, therefore the severity of these changes is totally dependent on the amount of sun exposure and the degree of UVR protection. Delayed diagnosis and poor sun protection will exacerbate the cutaneous features, resulting in significant pigmentary changes, multiple skin cancers and a worse prognosis.

Acute and severe sunburn on minimal sun exposure (Figure 76.2a), taking weeks to resolve, was once considered a cardinal presenting feature of XP. However, it is now known that only 50% of XP patients suffer from severe and prolonged sunburn reactions [30]. The remaining 50% have sunburn reactions that are normal for skin type, and these patients present with lentigines and hypopigmented macules at sun-exposed sites, initially on the face and dorsal aspect of the hands and, later, on other exposed parts (Figure 76.2b). The lentigines are fixed and progress over time to become more dense and irregular.

Patients in complementation groups XP-A, XP-B, XP-D, XP-F and XP-G suffer from severe sunburn reactions, whereas those in groups XP-C, XP-E and XP-V have normal sunburn reactions for skin type [30]. XPA, XPB, XPD, XPF and XPG proteins are all required for the common stem of NER, whereas XPC and XPE proteins are only required for GG-NER. In XP-C and XP-E, the TC-NER pathway remains active, and so does the ability to selectively remove photoproducts from the transcribed strand of active genes with kinetics similar to those observed in normal cells [31]. XP-V patients with mutations affecting DNA polymerase η, also have normal functioning TC-NER (and GG-NER). It is therefore hypothesised that normal sunburn reactions in approximately half of the XP patients relate to the preservation of TC-NER [32] and this is supported by *XPC* knock-out mice model studies [33,34].

Skin cancer. Absorption of UVR by DNA results in the formation of photoproducts (CPDs and 6-4PPs) that are recognised and repaired by NER. If left unrepaired, they can result in the classic 'UVB signature' mutations found in skin cancers [35,36]. The molecular defects in XP cells result in abnormal recognition and repair of UVR-induced DNA damage, and a subsequent significantly increased induction of 'UVB signature' mutations in the sun-exposed skin of affected individuals. This increased mutation frequency is likely to account for the pigmentary changes and the skin cancers in XP patients [37]. Indeed, examination of mutations in the *p53* gene in tumours from XP patients revealed mutations characteristic of UVR exposure in the majority of tumours [38].

XP patients who have severe and exaggerated sunburn reactions generally have a lower frequency of skin cancer than those patients with sunburn reactions that are normal for skin type. This may be due to severe sunburn reactions prompting earlier diagnosis and an earlier age of initiating more rigorous photoprotection, therefore resulting in less cumulative UVR exposure [30].

Other malignancies. DNA damage caused by carcinogens in cigarette smoke (chemical compounds such as benzopyrene) is repaired by NER in normal cells [39] and therefore patients with XP are potentially at higher risk of smoking-induced lung cancers.

XP patients also have an approximately 50-fold increase in cancers of the brain, including medulloblastoma, glioblastoma, spinal cord astrocytomas [40] and schwannoma. These malignancies are not UVR related and the precise relationship to DNA damage is unknown. High-dose X-ray irradiation can be used for the treatment of some of these brain tumours as the pathways involved in the repair of DNA damage by X-rays are normal in patients with XP [40,41].

Ocular manifestations. UVR exposure resulting in DNA damage of the eyelids and periocular skin can result in the development of cicatricial skin changes as well as skin cancers that require excision [42]. The ocular surface (conjunctiva and cornea) can develop UVR-related damage including dry eye, conjunctival injection and inflammation, as well as the development of premature pinguecula and pterygia. Prolonged corneal exposure can result in corneal scarring and visual impairment. Ocular surface cancers, mainly squamous cell carcinomas, have also been reported in patients with significant UVR exposure and poor ocular photoprotection [43]. Patients with XP-related neurodegeneration may also develop neuro-ophthalmological features, including sluggish pupils, nystagmus and strabismus. Photophobia is also common and often the earliest presenting ophthalmic symptom in XP.

Neurodegeneration. Approximately 30% of XP patients will develop neurodegeneration. The age at onset and rate of progression of the neurological abnormalities is variable between and within different complementation groups. Patients with XP-A, XP-B, XP-D, XP-F and XP-G have an increased susceptibility [1,30,32,44]. XP-C, XP-E and XP-V patients have not been reported to develop clinically detectable neurodegeneration.

The pathogenesis of the neurological abnormalities is poorly understood. It is not related to UVR exposure. Current theories suggest that oxidative DNA damage is generated during normal metabolism in the central nervous system, and that some of this damage, such as the generation of 8,5-cyclopurine-2-deoxynucleosides, is repaired by NER [45]. In the absence of functional repair, the lesions persist and result in neuronal cell death.

Neurological manifestations of XP typically present before the age of 2 years. Parents notice mild cognitive impairment first, usually when the child is starting school. Cerebellar signs manifest usually between 4 and 16 years of age, commonly dysarthria and difficulties with balance. Ataxia and areflexia follow. Nerve conduction studies show evidence of axonal sensory and motor neuropathy although this is not usually seen before the second decade of life. Patients develop progressive microcephaly. Magnetic resonance imaging demonstrates atrophy of the cortex of the brain with concomitant dilatation of the ventricles, and a secondary thickening of the skull bones. Most XP patients with neurological abnormalities will also develop sensorineural deafness. Patients eventually become wheelchair- and then bed-bound, a few years before death [46]. The presence of neurological abnormalities is associated with a worse prognosis.

Clinical variants
Xeroderma pigmentosum variant (XP-V). Approximately 20% of XP patients have XP-V. This subtype is caused by mutations in the *POLH* (*XPV*) gene encoding DNA polymerase η, one of the specialised enzymes required for replication past UVR-damaged sites [12,28]. The NER pathway is normal. XP-V is often diagnosed after the age of 30, once the patient has developed multiple skin cancers. No neurological manifestations are observed.

Xeroderma pigmentosum/Cockayne syndrome complex (XP/CS). This is a very rare autosomal recessive disorder characterised by cutaneous features of XP together with systemic and neurological features of CS such as short stature, microcephaly, cachexia, abnormal development, photosensitivity, premature ageing, retinal degeneration, sensorineural deafness and progressive neurological dysfunction (see the section on Cockayne syndrome). In contrast to the neurological abnormalities in XP, which are predominantly secondary to neuronal degeneration, in the XP/CS complex dysmyelination typical of CS is observed. Mutations in *ERCC3* (*XPB*), *ERCC2* (*XPD*), *ERCC4* (*XPF*) and *ERCC5* (*XPG*) genes have been reported in the XP/CS complex.

Xeroderma pigmentosum/trichothiodystrophy (XP/TTD) syndrome. The XP/TTD syndrome, with mutations reported in the *ERCC3* (*XPB*) and *ERCC2* (*XPD*) genes, is characterised by phenotypic features of TTD such as sulphur-deficient hair with 'tiger-tail' banding of hair shafts, developmental delay/intellectual impairment, short stature and ichthyosis (see the section on trichothiodystrophy), with clinical and cellular findings of XP.

Differential diagnosis
Differential diagnoses include trichothiodystrophy, Cockayne syndrome, cerebro-oculo-facio-skeletal syndrome, UV-sensitive syndrome, erythropoietic protoporphyria and Rothmund–Thomson syndrome.

PART 6: GENETIC DISORDERS

Classification of severity

Disease severity scores for sunburn, ocular disease and neurodegeneration have been designed for patients with XP [1]. Those for ocular and neurological disease, together with number of skin cancers as well as photoprotection scores, are a good way of documenting the progression of disease over time.

Complications and co-morbidities

The main complications of XP are related to the high risk of mucocutaneous cancers at sun-exposed sites and the possibility of neurodegeneration in some complementation groups.

Disease course and prognosis

There is no cure for XP. The overall median age of death is reported as 32 years [44], with skin cancer and neurodegeneration the main causes of death. Sun avoidance and regular follow-up to assess and treat any skin cancers increases life expectancy. For those without neurological disease, who practise meticulous UVR protection, the prognosis is good. However, the neurological abnormalities are progressive and the median age at death in these patients (29 years) is significantly younger than in XP patients without neurological degeneration (37 years) [44].

Investigations

In most cases, a clinical diagnosis can be made on the presence of extreme and exaggerated sunburn reactions in those individuals who show this feature, or on the appearance and progressive development of lentigines on the face and other exposed sites from an early age.

The diagnosis can be confirmed definitively by cellular tests for defective DNA repair. The most commonly used test is the measurement of unscheduled DNA synthesis in cultured skin fibroblasts. After UVR-induced DNA damage has been removed by NER, a patch of newly synthesised DNA replaces the damaged section. Synthesis of this new DNA is therefore referred to as unscheduled DNA synthesis (UDS) (Figure 76.1). Skin fibroblast cultures are established from a 4 mm punch biopsy taken from an unexposed area of the skin. Fibroblasts are UV irradiated in a Petri dish, and UDS can be measured as incorporation of nucleotides into DNA of the irradiated cells either by autoradiography [47] or liquid scintillation counting [48], or more recently using a fluorescence assay [49]. A reduced level of UDS confirms the diagnosis of XP.

XP-V patients do not show this defect in UDS, as NER is unaffected. Furthermore XP-V cells are not hypersensitive to killing by UVR. However, it has been found empirically that caffeine specifically sensitises XP-V cells to killing by UVR [50]. To diagnose XP-V cells, cultures are exposed to UVR, incubated in caffeine for a few days and their viability compared with that of normal cells. Specific sensitivity to UVR in the presence of caffeine together with normal UDS confirms the diagnosis of XP-V [51].

Subsequently, analysis of DNA, extracted from a blood sample, can identify the defective gene (confirming the complementation group) and the causative mutation(s) in patients. This can give further insight into genotype–phenotype correlations and enable genetic counselling and prenatal testing if requested.

Management

The mainstay of management is the avoidance of UVR exposure from sunlight through the application of high-factor sunscreen, UVR-protective clothing, hats, gloves and sunglasses, and UVR-blocking window films (at home and in cars). Fluorescent light sources emit UVR and should be avoided or covered in UVR filter film. Vitamin D deficiency is common and supplements should be prescribed. Smoking is prohibited.

Management requires a multidisciplinary approach. Regular skin and eye review and appropriate and early management of any cancers is essential. Early identification of skin cancer is critical but can be challenging due to the presence of numerous pigmentary lesions. Dermoscopy and reflectance confocal microscopy are important tools in this context [52]. Mohs micrographic surgery should be considered for facial skin cancers. This has been used in children as young as eight [53]. Topical 5-fluorouracil and imiquimod may be useful for early or premalignant lesions. Retinoids may have a role in the prevention of skin cancer [54]. Photodynamic therapy should not be used as the irradiation involved is likely to result in further skin damage and carcinogenesis [55].

Patients should be given appropriate genetic counselling. Psychosocial issues including social isolation from peers at school and at home, limited career prospects and the impact of meticulous sun protection on the quality of life need to be addressed.

In vitro and *ex vivo* experiments have established that correction of the underlying genetic defect in different forms of XP is possible. Animal studies using viral vectors have also established that gene therapy approaches for patients with this disease may become possible [56].

Resources

Further information

UK National Xeroderma Pigmentosum Service: www.guysandstthomas.nhs.uk/xp

Patient resources

Enfants de la lune: http://www.enfantsdelalune.org
Xeroderma Pigmentosum Society: http://www.xps.org/
XP Family Support Group: http://www.xpfamilysupport.org
XP Freu(n)de: http://www.xerodermapigmentosum.de
XP Support Group: http://xpsupportgroup.org.uk/
Teddington Trust: https://www.teddingtontrust.com
(All last accessed April 2022.)

Cockayne syndrome

Definition

Cockayne syndrome (CS) is a rare autosomal recessive disorder of DNA repair. It is characterised by short stature, photosensitivity, a distinctive facial appearance, ocular defects, premature ageing and progressive neurological dysfunction associated with extensive demyelination.

Introduction and general description

CS is a rare disorder of DNA repair first described by Cockayne in 1936 [1]. The disease is defined by progressive postnatal growth failure, short stature, microcephaly, cachexia, abnormal development, photosensitivity, premature ageing, retinal degeneration and sensorineural deafness [2]. Patients have a characteristic facial appearance with enophthalmia. CS is divided into three clinical types (types I, II and III) based on severity of disease.

Epidemiology

The annual incidence of CS is about one in 200 000 in European countries.

Age

Photosensitivity is present from birth and the abnormal growth and development becomes evident within the first few years of life.

Sex

It affects males and females equally.

Ethnicity

CS has been reported to occur in many ethnic groups worldwide.

Pathophysiology

CS is an autosomal recessive disorder and results from mutations in one of two genes, *ERCC8* (*CSA*) and *ERCC6* (*CSB*). The products of these genes are involved in NER (Figure 76.1) [3].

The skin fibroblasts of patients with CS are abnormally sensitive to UVR [4–6]. Unlike cells from patients with XP, the GG-NER process occurs normally in CS cells. However, CS cells are defective in the important transcription-coupled subpathway of NER (Figure 76.1). Following DNA damage, it is of prime importance for the cell to remove damage from actively transcribed regions of DNA. This preferential repair is referred to as transcription-coupled NER (TC-NER), and it is this repair that is specifically defective in CS cells [7].

Two complementation groups have been identified [8], CS-A (accounting for approximately 20% of CS patients) and CS-B (Table 76.3). CS-A is caused by mutation in the *ERCC8* gene and CS-B is caused by mutation in the *ERCC6* gene [9,10]. These genes encode proteins involved in TC-NER [10]. Among patients with CS, approximately 80% have mutations in the *ERCC6* gene [11,12]. So far, no correlation has been found between the three clinical subtypes (I, II, III) of CS and the genes involved.

CS can rarely be found in combination with XP. Mutations in the *XPB*, *XPD*, *XPF* and *XPG* genes have been implicated in XP/CS complex.

Clinical features

History and presentation

CS is characterised by cutaneous photosensitivity, progressive postnatal growth failure, short stature, microcephaly, characteristic bird-like facies (Figure 76.3) (prognathism, enophthalmia, a prominent thin nose, large ears and loss of subcutaneous fat), disproportionately large hands and feet, cachexia, premature ageing and dental caries. The skin is dry and thin, and the hair is often sparse and is sometimes prematurely grey [2,13,14]. In contrast to XP, patients with CS have no increased incidence of skin cancer [2].

Neurological features comprise extensive demyelination of the peripheral and central nervous system, microcephaly, progressive

Table 76.3 Genes, protein products and main clinical features in different Cockayne syndrome (CS) complementation groups and associated diseases.

Disorder	Gene	Defective pathway	Clinical features
CS-A	*ERCC8* (*CSA*)	TC-NER	Rare subtype (20% of cases). Milder phenotype
CS-B	*ERCC6* (*CSB*)	TC-NER	Common subtype (80% of cases). More severe phenotype
COFS1	*ERCC6* (*CSB*)	TC-NER	Extreme prenatal form of CS
COFS2	*ERCC2* (*XPD*)	NER	
COFS3	*ERCC5* (*XPG*)	NER	
COFS4	*ERCC1*	NER Stabilizing and enhancing XPF activity	
UVSS1	*ERCC6* (*CSB*)	TC-NER	Photosensitivity
UVSS2	*ERCC8* (*CSA*)	TC-NER	No increase in risk of skin cancers
UVSS3	*UVSSA*	Stabilization of TC-NER machinery Ubiquitination of stalled RNA polymerase	No evidence of neurological disease

COFS, cerebro-oculo-facio-skeletal; NER, nucleotide excision repair; TC-NER, transcription-coupled nucleotide excision repair; UVSS, UV-sensitive syndrome.

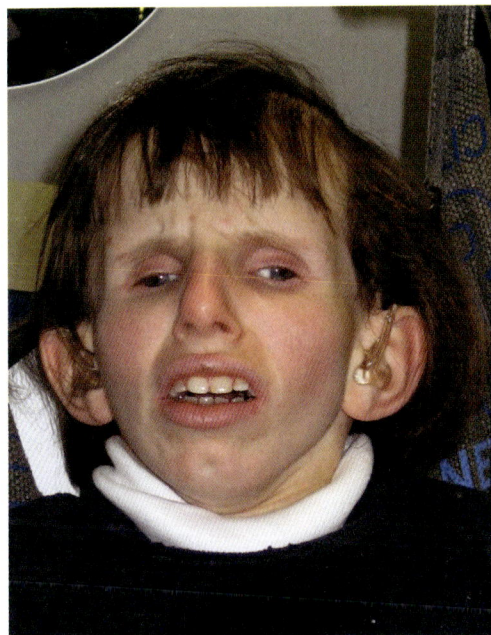

Figure 76.3 Cockayne syndrome demonstrating the characteristic bird-like facies with prominent enophthalmia.

cognitive decline, choreoathetosis, hydrocephalus and spasticity. There is progressive sensorineural deafness and skeletal abnormalities with flexion deformity. Ophthalmological problems include retinal degeneration, cataracts and optic atrophy leading to loss of vision [15].

Failure to thrive and growth difficulties are among the most consistent features of CS, leaving affected individuals vulnerable to numerous medical complications, including adverse effects of undernutrition, abrupt overhydration and overfeeding. Therefore, disease specific growth charts have been designed to improve the nutritional management of children with CS [16].

The age of onset and severity of disease are variable. In classic CS type I, the first symptoms usually appear during the first year of life. Type II refers to early-onset cases with more severe symptoms and type III are late-onset cases with milder symptoms. In general, CS-A is milder in clinical course than CS-B, but within each type, no clear genotype–phenotype correlation has been established [11,17–19].

Clinical variants

Cerebro-oculo-facio-skeletal syndrome. Cerebro-oculo-facioskeletal (COFS) syndrome is a very rare autosomal recessive disorder of DNA repair and constitutes the prenatal extreme form of CS [20,21]. Clinically it is characterised by congenital microcephaly, congenital cataract and/or microphthalmia, arthrogryposis, severe developmental delay, growth delay and facial dysmorphism (prominent metopic suture, micrognathism). The axial hypotonia contrasts with the peripheral hypertonia and is associated with feeding difficulties. Peripheral neuropathy, sensorineural hearing loss and pigmentary retinopathy can be observed. In COFS syndrome, photosensitivity is an inconstant feature [22]. Prenatal diagnosis can be suspected by the presence of cataracts, arthrogryposis and microcephaly, and is subsequently confirmed by examination of DNA repair in the chorionic villi or amniotic cells, or by checking for the familial mutation(s) if known.

In COFS, mutations have been identified in the *ERCC6*, *ERCC2* (*XPD*), *ERCC5* (*XPG*) and *ERCC1* genes (Table 76.3), designated as COFS1, COFS2, COFS3 and COFS4 syndromes respectively [23–26]. All these genes encode for proteins involved in NER (Figure 76.1).

COFS syndrome is a severe disease with death in the first years of life, usually from respiratory tract infections [21].

UV-sensitive syndrome. UV-sensitive syndrome (UVSS) is an autosomal recessive disorder of DNA repair characterised by sensitivity to UVR but without any increased risk of skin cancers or any evidence of neurological disease [27]. Despite this mild clinical phenotype, the cellular and biochemical responses of UVSS and CS cells to UVR are indistinguishable, and result from defective TC-NER of photoproducts in actively transcribed genes [28]. Mutations in the CS genes, *ERCC6* and *ERCC8*, have been reported in UVSS cases, designated UVSS1 and UVSS2 respectively [29,30]. More recently mutations in the *UVSSA* gene have been found in cases designated UVSS3 (Table 76.3). The *UVSSA* gene encodes for a protein that interacts with the TC-NER machinery and stabilises the CSB complex, and also facilitates ubiquitination of RNA polymerase stalled at DNA damage sites [31]. The mild phenotype and lack of neurological disease in these patients is not fully understood but may be associated with normal repair of oxidative damage in these patients [29].

Differential diagnosis

Differential diagnoses include progeria, XP, COFS syndrome, UVSS, Rothmund–Thomson syndrome, Werner syndrome, Bloom syndrome and Hartnup disease.

Classification of severity

A disease severity score for CS has been designed based on five items (head circumference, growth failure, sensory neural signs, motor autonomy, and communication skills). This will allow monitoring of patients under long-term follow-up and facilitate evaluation of future therapeutic interventions [32].

Disease course and prognosis

Patient with CS type I commonly die before the end of the second decade as a result of progressive neurological degeneration. Patients with type II have a worse prognosis, whereas patients with type III often survive into adulthood. There is no cure for CS. Survival beyond the second decade is unusual and the mean age at death in reported cases is 12.5 years.

Investigations

A clinical diagnosis can be made based on the presence of short stature, photosensitivity, distinctive facial appearance, ocular defects and premature ageing. Early cerebral imagery is not very specific, but it can reveal cerebral and cerebellar atrophy. Diffuse myelinisation anomalies and calcifications of the basal ganglia can appear secondarily.

The clinical diagnosis can be confirmed definitively by cellular tests for defective DNA repair, specifically TC-NER. A skin biopsy should be taken for fibroblast culture as in patients with XP. CS cells are specifically deficient in TC-NER, which results in a prolonged inhibition of RNA synthesis following UVR. The test for CS therefore involves ultraviolet irradiation of cells, followed by measurement of RNA synthesis 24 h later. In normal cells, RNA synthesis will have recovered to untreated levels, whereas in CS cells it remains depressed [8].

Subsequently, analysis of DNA extracted from the blood can identify the defective gene and the causative mutation(s) in patients. This can enable genetic counselling and prenatal testing if requested.

Management

Management is purely supportive and requires a multidisciplinary approach with input from clinical genetics, ophthalmology, neurology, dermatology, audiology (for hearing aids) and physiotherapy. Psychosocial issues for the patient and their family need to be addressed.

Patients avoid UVR exposure because of their increased photosensitivity, and therefore vitamin D deficiency is common and supplements should be given. There is no increased risk of skin cancers.

The use of metronidazole in patients with CS is considered an absolute contraindication because of the significant risk of severe hepatoxicity [33].

Patients should be given appropriate genetic counselling. Prenatal diagnosis is possible by amniocentesis or from chorionic villus samples [34,35], using the RNA synthesis recovery test or by looking for causative familial mutation(s), if known.

Resources

Patient resources

Amy and Friends: https://www.amyandfriends.org (last accessed April 2022)

Trichothiodystrophy

Definition

Trichothiodystrophy (TTD) is a rare autosomal recessive disorder of DNA repair. It is a multisystem disorder characterised by short, brittle, sulphur-deficient hair with a pattern of alternating light and dark 'tiger-tail' bands under polarised light microscopy, along with photosensitivity, ichthyosis, developmental delay and short stature.

Introduction and general description

Trichothiodystrophy is a rare disorder of DNA repair that is characterised by sulphur-deficient hair with alternating dark and light banding on polarised light microscopy [1–4]. Other clinical features include photosensitivity in about half of the affected individuals, ichthyosis, developmental delay, short stature, haematological abnormalities, skeletal abnormalities and maternal pregnancy complications [5].

The term trichothiodystrophy was first introduced by Price *et al.* in 1979 and soon after they reported two patients with sulphur-deficient, brittle hair and a variety of other features [6]. Since then, many variants of TTD based on the different clinical associations have been proposed, including BIDS syndrome (TTD type D or Amish brittle hair syndrome), IBIDS syndrome (TTD type E or Tay syndrome), PIBIDS syndrome (TTD type F), Sabinas syndrome (TTD type B), SIBIDS syndrome, ONMRS (Itin syndrome) and Pollitt syndrome (TTD type C) [7–10]. However, a recent comprehensive review of 112 TTD patients reported in the literature demonstrated that many patients did not fit into these designated subtypes and that these acronyms were poor descriptors of TTD patients' clinical manifestations [5]. These acronyms should therefore no longer be used, and TTD is now divided in photosensitive and non-photosensitive subtypes.

Epidemiology
Incidence and prevalence

The incidence of TTD is estimated as one per million live births.

Sex

It affects males and females equally.

Ethnicity

It has been reported to occur in many ethnic groups worldwide although it is more common in populations where consanguinity is frequent.

Pathophysiology

Trichothiodystrophy is an autosomal recessive disorder. Photosensitive TTD results from mutations in the DNA repair genes *ERCC2* (*XPD*) [11], *ERCC3* (*XPB*) [12] or *GTF2H5* [13,14]. Most patients carry mutations in the *ERCC2* (*XPD*) gene. These three genes encode the XPD, XPB and p8/TTDA subunits, respectively, of the TFIIH complex in the NER pathway (Figure 76.1) [15]. Mutations in these subunits can affect both DNA repair and transcription. Mutations in a gene of unknown function, *MPLKIP* (*TTDN1*), have been found in a few cases of non-photosensitive TTD [16,17].

Although mutations in *ERCC2* (*XPD*) and *ERCC3* (*XPB*) genes are also found in XP, a disorder of DNA repair associated with a 10 000-fold increased risk of skin cancer, TTD patients have not been reported to have an increased risk of cancer. This is thought to be because the mutations in these genes in patients with XP predominantly affect DNA repair, while mutations in the same genes in patients with TTD predominantly affect transcription [5,18]. Therefore, the clinical features in XP are related to an abnormal repair of UVR-induced DNA damage in the skin, whereas TTD is primarily a disorder of development, related to transcriptional abnormalities. This would explain the multisystem involvement in TTD, particularly the fetal developmental abnormalities and the haematological features.

Clinical features
History and presentation

Trichothiodystrophy is characterised by short, brittle, sulphur-deficient hair with a pattern of alternating light and dark bands under polarised light microscopy (Figure 76.4a,b) [4]. About 50% have photosensitivity with severe and exaggerated sunburn reactions. However, unlike patients with XP, there is no increased risk of skin cancer. Other cutaneous features include ichthyosis (Figure 76.4c), dry skin and collodion membrane at birth. The nails may be brittle and demonstrate onychodystrophy. Pregnancy complications including intrauterine growth retardation, pre-eclampsia and eclampsia, low birth weight (<2500 g) and premature birth (before 37 weeks' gestation) occur in about 30% of cases [19,20]. Other common features are developmental delay/intellectual impairment (85% of cases), short stature (73%) and facial dysmorphism with microcephaly, large ears and micrognathia. Neuroimaging shows dysmyelination and cerebral atrophy. Ocular abnormalities occur in about 50% of cases and include congenital cataracts, nystagmus and strabismus [21]. Patients gradually develop joint abnormalities with contractures and dislocations. Skeletal abnormalities include axial osteosclerosis and distal osteopaenia. Many patients are anaemic and neutropaenic and show haematological features of β-thalassaemia trait [22]. Severe and recurrent infections, especially respiratory, occur in the first year of life.

The spectrum of clinical features varies from mild disease with only hair involvement to severe disease with profound developmental defects and recurrent infections [5,23]. The abnormalities at birth and during pregnancy suggest that the pathophysiology of TTD involves a developmental abnormality affecting pregnancy as well as transcriptional abnormalities after birth.

Clinical variants
Xeroderma pigmentosum/trichothiodystrophy (XP/TTD) syndrome.

XP/TTD syndrome with mutations reported in the *ERCC2* (*XPD*) and *ERCC3* (*XPB*) genes is characterised by phenotypic features of TTD with clinical and cellular findings of XP.

Differential diagnosis

Differential diagnoses include CS, XP and congenital alopecias, especially Menkes disease and Netherton syndrome.

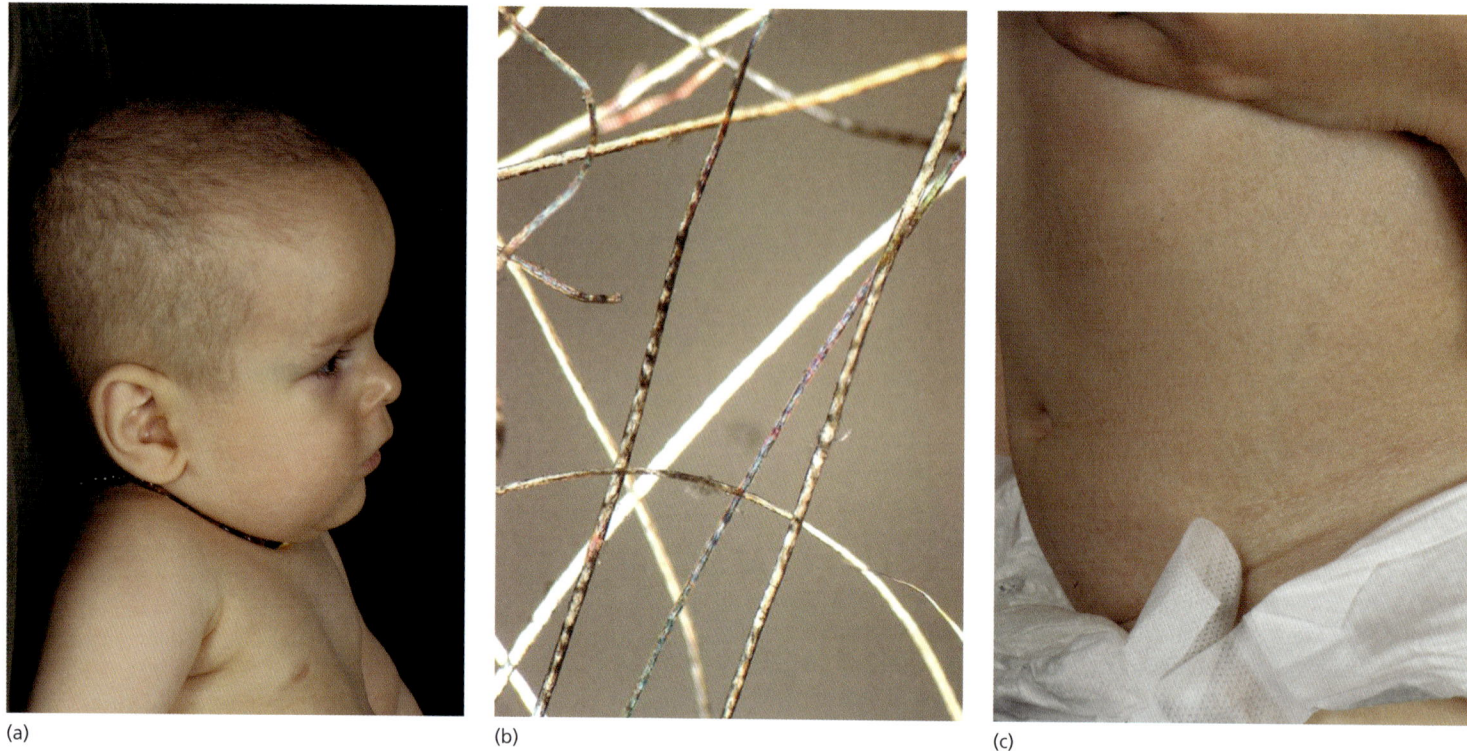

(a)   (b)   (c)

Figure 76.4 Trichothiodystrophy. (a) Short, brittle, sulphur-deficient hair. (b) The pattern of alternating light and dark 'tiger-tail' bands under polarised light microscopy. (c) Ichthyosis on the trunk.

Complications and co-morbidities

The main complications of TTD are related to the high risk of developing severe and potentially fatal infections.

Disease course and prognosis

There is no cure for TTD. There is significant morbidity and mortality in the neonatal and childhood years. The overall median age of death is reported as 3 years [5], with pneumonia and other infections (especially sepsis) being the main causes of death.

Investigations

A clinical diagnosis can be made on the presence of 'tiger-tail' bands of hair shafts under polarised light microscopy as well as the other clinical features.

The diagnosis can be confirmed definitively by cellular tests for defective DNA repair. Although the clinical features of TTD and XP are quite different, TTD cells, like XP cells, are defective in NER and this defect can be measured using UDS (see the section on XP investigation earlier in this chapter). A reduced level of UDS confirms the diagnosis of TTD.

Subsequent analysis of DNA extracted from the blood can identify the defective gene and the causative mutation(s) in patients. This can give further insight into genotype–phenotype correlations and enable genetic counselling and prenatal testing if requested.

Management

Management requires a multidisciplinary approach with input from obstetrics, paediatrics, genetics, ophthalmology, neurology, orthopaedics, infectious diseases and radiology. There is no cure. Any infections should be aggressively treated as mortality from

infections is significant (20-fold higher compared with the US population) [5]. Sun protection advice, in those patients who are photosensitive, should be given.

Patients and their families should be given appropriate genetic counselling and prenatal diagnosis offered if required.

Patient resources

Amy and Friends: https://www.amyandfriends.org (last accessed April 2022)

OTHER DISORDERS

Ataxia telangiectasia (Louis-Bar syndrome)

Ataxia telangiectasia (AT) is a rare autosomal recessive disorder of DNA repair. It was first reported by Denise Louis-Bar in 1941, but it was Boder and Sedgwick who introduced the term ataxia telangiectasia in 1958 [1]. It is a multisystem disorder characterised by ataxia and mucocutaneous telangiectasia. Telangiectasia initially appears in the conjunctiva and is most prominent in the facial areas. Additional cutaneous features include premature hair greying, café-au-lait spot and pigmentary changes, including poikiloderma. Progressive cerebellar degeneration is the first clinical manifestation in AT, starting at about 1 year of age. Immunodeficiency with increased susceptibility to infections, hypogonadism, sensitivity to ionising radiation, insulin resistance and a predisposition to cancer are cardinal features in AT [2,**3**].

AT is a chromosome instability disorder with inactivating mutations in the *ATM* gene. The ATM protein kinase plays a key role in the control of double-strand break DNA repair [4,5]. It is also involved in cell cycle regulation and telomere length maintenance. Management is symptomatic and involves a multidisciplinary approach with input from physiotherapy, speech therapy, neurology and early treatment of infections. As the cells of AT patients are sensitive to ionising radiation, X-rays and radiotherapy should be used with caution. The prognosis is poor because of severe respiratory infections, progressive neurodegeneration and an increased risk of cancer.

Fanconi anaemia

Fanconi anaemia is an autosomal recessive disorder of DNA repair. It was first described in 1972 by the Swiss paediatrician, Guido Fanconi. It is clinically heterogeneous and characterised by congenital developmental defects, early-onset bone marrow failure and a high predisposition to cancer. There is cellular hypersensitivity to DNA interstrand cross-link agents such as mitomycin C [**1**]. Two-thirds of patients are born with congenital malformations of the kidneys, heart and skeleton (absent or abnormal thumbs and radii). Other features include a typical facial appearance with small head, eyes and mouth, hearing loss, hypogonadism and reduced fertility. Cutaneous abnormalities include reticulate or patchy hyper- or hypopigmentation and café-au-lait spots [2]. Bone marrow failure usually presents in the first decade of life. Fanconi anaemia is associated with the occurrence of an unusual number of viral warts due to a decrease in cell-mediated immunity. Subsequently, patients develop tumours such as lymphomas, oesophageal carcinomas, basal cell and squamous cell carcinomas of the head and neck [3], liver and brain tumours, and acute myeloid leukaemia. Patients with Fanconi anaemia may develop Sweet syndrome either just before or shortly after the diagnosis of acute myeloid leukaemia [4].

So far mutations in at least 15 *FANC* genes, representing 15 Fanconi anaemia complementation groups, have been identified [**5**]. These gene products make up the 'FA pathway' involved in DNA repair, interstrand cross-link repair and maintenance of genome stability [6]. Diagnosis is based on the evaluation of chromosomal breakage induced by alkylating agents such as mitomycin C. Bone marrow failure and cancers result in a poor prognosis and the life expectancy of patients is reduced to an average of 20 years [5]. Management involves supportive care with transfusions as necessary. Haematopoietic stem cell transplant is curative for the haematological features, but this increases the risk of solid tumours, which must be monitored.

Muir–Torre syndrome

Muir–Torre syndrome is a rare autosomal dominant disorder of DNA repair. It was independently reported by Muir in 1967 and Torre in 1968 [1,2]. There is a lot of clinical variation but it is characterised by the occurrence of sebaceous gland neoplasms and/or keratoacanthomas associated with one or more visceral malignancies, in particular gastrointestinal or genito-urinary [3–5]. Although the malignancies are often multiple, they behave less aggressively and are often low grade. Muir–Torre syndrome occurs as a result of a mutation in one of the DNA mismatch repair genes (*MSH-2*, *MLH-1* and *MSH-6*). The management involves a multidisciplinary approach with genetic counselling, regular skin reviews and appropriate cancer screening [**6**].

Key references

The full list of references can be found in the online version at https://www.wiley.com/rooksdermatology10e

Xeroderma pigmentosum

1 Fassihi H, Sethi M, Fawcett H *et al*. Deep phenotyping of 89 xeroderma pigmentosum patients reveals unexpected heterogeneity dependent on the precise molecular defect. *Proc Natl Acad Sci USA* 2016;113:E1236–45.

2 Kraemer KH, Lee MM, Scotto J. Xeroderma pigmentosum. Cutaneous, ocular, and neurologic abnormalities in 830 published cases. *Arch Dermatol* 1987;123:241–50.

7 Cleaver JE. Defective repair replication of DNA in xeroderma pigmentosum. *Nature* 1968;218:652–6.

25 Cleaver JE, Lam ET, Revet I. Disorders of nucleotide excision repair: the genetic and molecular basis of heterogeneity. *Nat Rev Genet* 2009;10:756–68.

27 Lehmann AR, McGibbon D, Stefanini M. Xeroderma pigmentosum. *Orphanet J Rare Dis* 2011;6:70.

30 Sethi M, Lehmann AR, Fawcett H *et al*. Patients with xeroderma pigmentosum complementation groups C, E and V do not have abnormal sunburn reactions. *Br J Dermatol* 2013;169:1279–87.

32 Totonchy MB, Tamura D, Pantell MS *et al*. Auditory analysis of xeroderma pigmentosum 1971–2012: hearing function, sun sensitivity and DNA repair predict neurological degeneration. *Brain* 2013;136:194–208.

42 Lim R, Sethi M, Morley AMS. Ophthalmic manifestations of xeroderma pigmentosum: a perspective from the United Kingdom. *Ophthalmology* 2017;124:1652–61.

44 Bradford PT, Goldstein AM, Tamura D *et al*. Cancer and neurologic degeneration in xeroderma pigmentosum: long term follow-up characterises the role of DNA repair. *J Med Genet* 2010;48:168–76.

46 Anttinen A, Koulu L, Nikoskelainen E *et al*. Neurological symptoms and natural course of xeroderma pigmentosum. *Brain* 2008;131:1979–89.

Cockayne syndrome

2 Nance MA, Berry SA. Cockayne syndrome: review of 140 cases. *Am J Med Genet* 1992;42:68–84.

3 Cleaver JE, Lam ET, Revet I. Disorders of nucleotide excision repair: the genetic and molecular basis of heterogeneity. *Nat Rev Genet* 2009;10:756–68.

11 Calmels N, Botta E, Jia N *et al*. Functional and clinical relevance of novel mutations in a large cohort of patients with Cockayne syndrome. *J Med Genet* 2018;55:329–43.

13 Laugel V. Cockayne Syndrome. 2000 Dec 28 [updated 2019 Aug 29]. In: Adam MP, Ardinger HH, Pagon RA *et al*., eds. *GeneReviews*® [Internet]. Seattle: University of Washington, Seattle; 1993–2021.

14 Frouin E, Laugel V, Durand M *et al*. Dermatologic findings in 16 patients with Cockayne syndrome and cerebro-oculo-facial-skeletal syndrome. *JAMA Dermatol* 2013;149:1414–18.

16 Baer S, Tuzin N, Kang PB *et al*. Growth charts in Cockayne syndrome type 1 and type 2. *Eur J Med Genet* 2021;64:104105.

17 Lehmann AR, Thompson AF, Harcourt SA *et al*. Cockayne's syndrome: correlation of clinical features with cellular sensitivity of RNA synthesis to UV-irradiation. *J Med Genet* 1993;30:679–82.

32 Spitz MA, Severac F, Obringer C *et al*. Diagnostic and severity scores for Cockayne syndrome. *Orphanet J Rare Dis* 2021;16:63.

33 Wilson BT, Strong A, O'Kelly S, Munkley J, Stark Z. Metronidazole toxicity in Cockayne syndrome: a case series. *Pediatrics* 2015;136:e706–8.

Trichothiodystrophy

4 Liang C, Morris A, Schlucker S et al. Structural and molecular hair abnormalities in trichothiodystrophy. *J Invest Dermatol* 2006;126:2210–16.

5 Faghri S, Tamura D, Kraemer KH et al. Trichothiodystrophy: a systematic review of 112 published cases characterises a wide spectrum of clinical manifestations. *J Med Genet* 2008;45:609–21.

15 Hashimoto S, Egly JM. Trichothiodystrophy view from the molecular basis of DNA repair/transcription factor TFIIH. *Hum Mol Genet* 2009;18:R224–30.

17 Stefanini M, Botta E, Lanzafame M et al. Trichothiodystrophy: from basic mechanisms to clinical implications. *DNA Repair (Amst)* 2010;9:2–10.

23 Kraemer KH, Patronas NJ, Schiffmann R et al. Xeroderma pigmentosum, trichothiodystrophy and Cockayne syndrome: a complex genotype–phenotype relationship. *Neuroscience* 2007;145:1388–96.

Ataxia telangiectasia (Louis-Bar syndrome)

3 Knoch J, Kamenisch Y, Kubisch C, Berneburg M. Rare hereditary diseases with defects in DNA-repair. *Eur J Dermatol* 2012;22:443–55.

Fanconi anaemia

1 Deakyne JS, Mazin AV. Fanconi anemia: at the crossroads of DNA repair. *Biochemistry* 2011;76:36–48.

5 Joenje H, Patel KJ. The emerging genetic and molecular basis of Fanconi anaemia. *Nat Rev Genet* 2001;2:446–57.

Muir–Torre syndrome

5 Abbas O, Mahalingam M. Cutaneous sebaceous neoplasms as markers of Muir–Torre syndrome: a diagnostic algorithm. *J Cutan Pathol* 2009;36:613–19.

6 John AM, Schwartz RA. Muir-Torre syndrome (MTS): an update and approach to diagnosis and management. *J Am Acad Dermatol* 2016;74:558–66.

CHAPTER 77

Syndromes with Premature Ageing

Alan D. Irvine[1] and Jemima E. Mellerio[2]

[1]Children's Health Ireland at Crumlin; St James's Hospital, Dublin; and Trinity College, Dublin, Ireland
[2]St John's Institute of Dermatology, Guy's and St Thomas' NHS Foundation Trust, London, UK

Introduction

Progeroid syndromes comprise a heterogeneous group of conditions with variable cutaneous features that lead to a prematurely aged appearance, including poikiloderma, photosensitivity, pigmentation, sclerodermatous changes, alteration of the subcutaneous fat, or skin laxity and wrinkling. Broadly, these diseases can be grouped according to the underlying pathology. For example, conditions with impaired DNA repair mechanisms including Bloom and Werner syndromes, and xeroderma pigmentosum, may be associated with skin photosensitivity, pigmentation and telangiectasia as well as an increased incidence of skin and other malignancies. Aberrant lamin A processing leading to an accumulation of prelamin A in the nucleus is another mechanism leading to a progeroid appearance, for example in Hutchinson–Gilford progeria syndrome (HGPS) and forms of mandibulo-acral dysplasia. In contrast, defects in genes involved in the formation of elastic fibres in the skin and other tissues lead to forms of cutis laxa. Importantly, many progeroid syndromes are associated with severe extracutaneous disease, notably early systemic ageing, malignancy, developmental and neurological impairment and premature death. Often, the cutaneous features of these rare disorders occur early and are key to helping identify the underlying disorder, with important implications for genetic counselling, management and prognosis. Table 77.1 summarises the major syndromes of premature ageing, some of which are discussed in other chapters.

Werner syndrome

Definition

Clinically, the syndrome is characterised by premature ageing with sclerodermatous skin changes, subcutaneous calcification, short stature, prematurely aged facies, premature arteriosclerosis, diabetes and a predisposition to malignancy [1].

Pathophysiology

Werner syndrome is a rare, autosomal recessive disorder caused by mutations in gene *RECQL2* (*WRN*) on 8p12-p11.2, encoding a DNA helicase [1,2–6]. Aberrant repair of double-stranded DNA damage in the absence of WRN helicase activity leads to an accumulation of DNA damage, telomere shortening, genetic instability and a reduction in cellular replicative lifespan [7,8]. It is possible that WRN is an intrinsic inhibitor of progerin, an abnormal splicing product of lamin A, which may explain the phenotypic overlap between Werner syndrome and HGPS [9]. Clinically normal heterozygous carriers of *WRN* mutations have also been shown to have increased genetic instability compared with normal controls [10]. Tissues of mesenchymal origin are preferentially affected compared with tissues of neural origin, reflected phenotypically by absent neurological involvement such as Alzheimer or Parkinson diseases [11]. Werner syndrome occurs worldwide but there appears to be a higher frequency in Japan where the incidence is estimated at approximately three per million [12].

Clinical features [1,12–14]

A subset of patients have 'atypical' Werner syndrome, characterised by more severe clinical features. Some of these individuals have heterozygous mutations of the *LMNA* gene encoding lamin A/C [15], and therefore this should probably be more correctly considered a milder, later-onset variant of HGPS [14]. In other cases, however, mutations have not been identified in either *RECQL2* or *LMNA*, indicating an alternative genetic aetiology [14].

Management

Complications of Werner syndrome such as cardiovascular disease, diabetes and cataract are treated conventionally as and when they arise. Recent *in vitro* research suggests that the abnormal cellular phenotype in Werner syndrome might be amenable to treatment with mitogen-activated protein (MAP) kinase inhibitors [16] or the mTOR inhibitor rapamycin [17]. Reprogramming Werner

Rook's Textbook of Dermatology, Tenth Edition. Edited by Christopher Griffiths, Jonathan Barker, Tanya Bleiker, Walayat Hussain and Rosalind Simpson.
© 2024 John Wiley & Sons Ltd. Published 2024 by John Wiley & Sons Ltd.

PART 6: GENETIC DISORDERS

Table 77.1 Progeroid disorders.

Disease	MIM	Inheritance	Gene	Cutaneous features	Photo-sensitivity	Neuro-logical	Immuno-deficiency	Growth restriction	Non-cutaneous malignancy	Death
Werner syndrome	277700	AR	RECQL2	Scleroderma	–	–	–	From puberty	+ (10%)	In fifties (malignancy and cardiovascular)
Bloom syndrome	210900	AR	RECQL3	Poikiloderma, facial telangiectasia	+	–	+	Pre- and postnatal	+ (15%), mean age 32 years	Early death from malignancy
XP-A[a]	278700	AR	XPA	Freckles, telangiectasia, skin cancer	+	+	–	–	–	For all XP types, it depends on complementation subgroup and occurrence of skin malignancy and/or neurological involvement
XP-B[a]	610651	AR	ERCC3	Freckles, telangiectasia, skin cancer	+	+	–	+	–	
XP-C[a]	278720	AR	XPC	Freckles, telangiectasia, skin cancer	–	–	–	–	–	
XP-D[a]	278730	AR	ERCC2	Poikiloderma, telangiectasia, skin cancer	+	+	–	–	–	
XP-E[a]	278740	AR	DDB2	Freckles, poikiloderma, skin Cancer	–	–	–	–	–	
XP-F[a]	278760	AR	ERCC4	Freckles, skin cancer	+	+/–	–	+/–	–	
XP-G[a]	278780	AR	ERCC5	Mild freckling	+	+/–	–	–	–	
XP-V[a]	278750	AR	POLH	Freckles, poikiloderma, skin cancer	–	–	–	–	–	
Cockayne syndrome type A[a]	216400	AR	ERCC8	Progeria, pigmentation, atrophy, brittle hair and nails, reduced subcutaneous fat	+	+	–	Pre- and postnatal	–	Usually death in childhood or adolescence
Cockayne syndrome type B[a]	133540	AR	ERCC6	Progeria, pigmentation, atrophy, brittle hair and nails, reduced subcutaneous fat	+	+	–	Pre- and postnatal	–	Death in childhood
Trichothiodystrophy[a]	601675	AD	ERCC3 GTF2H5 ERCC2	Thin dry hair, ichthyosiform erythroderma, brittle hair and nails, reduced subcutaneous fat	+/–	+	+	Postnatal	–	Variable
Classic HGPS	176670	AD	LMNA	Scleroderma, premature ageing, alopecia	–	–	–	Progressive from first year	–	Death in teens from cardiovascular disease, mean 13 years
Atypical HGPS and other progeroid laminopathies	176670	AD AR	LMNA LMNA	Variable scleroderma, premature ageing, sparse hair	–	–	–	May be marked	–	Variable
MADA	248370	AR	LMNA	Scleroderma, pigmentation, alopecia	–	–	–	Postnatal	–	–
MADB	608612	AR	ZMPSTE24	Atrophy, pigmentation, sparse hair	–	–	–	–	–	–
MDPL	615381	AD	POLD	Scleroderma, aged appearance, reduced subcutaneous fat	–	–	–	–	–	–
MDPS	619127	AR	MTX2	Poikiloderma, atrophic skin, nail dystrophy, palmoplantar keratoderma, sparse hair, reduced subcutaneous fat	–	–	–	Postnatal	–	Variable
Neonatal progeria syndrome (Wiedemann–Rautenstrauch syndrome)	264090	AR	POLR3A	Sparse hair, aged appearance, reduced subcutaneous fat	–	+	–	IUGR	–	Death in childhood
Hallermann–Streiff syndrome	234100	Sporadic	–	Skin atrophy, telangiectasia, hypotrichosis	–	+/–	–	Short stature	–	–
Restrictive dermopathy	275210 275210	AD AR	LMNA ZMPSTE24	Tight, sclerotic skin, erosions and fissures, thin and translucent	– –	– –	– –	IUGR IUGR	– –	Often premature or stillborn. Death in first to second week of life

AR, autosomal recessive; AD, autosomal dominant; HGPS, Hutchinson–Gilford progeria syndrome; IUGR, intrauterine growth retardation; MADA, mandibulo-acral dysplasia with type A lipodystrophy; MADB, mandibulo-acral dysplasia with type B lipodystrophy; MDPL, mandibular hypoplasia, deafness, progeroid appearance and generalised lipodystrophy; MDPS, mandibulo-acral dysplasia progeroid syndrome; XP, xeroderma pigmentosum.

[a] See also Chapter 76.

syndrome cells into induced pluripotent stem cells can restore telomere function *in vitro* and may have therapeutic potential [18,19]. In another approach, readthrough drugs such as aminoglycoside antibiotics and ataluren can lead to full length protein and restored *WRN* function from nonsense mutations and may be applicable for future clinical use [20].

Bloom syndrome

Definition

This syndrome is characterised by photosensitivity, telangiectatic facial redness, proportionate pre- and postnatal growth deficiency, distinctive facies, abnormal immune responses and a predisposition to malignancy [1,2,3].

Pathophysiology

Bloom syndrome is a rare, autosomal recessive disorder. The gene for Bloom syndrome (*RECQL3*) lies on chromosome 15q26.1 and encodes a DNA helicase, RecQ protein-like-3 [4]. This helicase forms a complex with topoisomerase III alpha (TopIIIα), and RecQ-mediated genome instability 1 and 2 (RMI1 and RMI2, respectively) to resolve abnormal structures that can arise during DNA replication and may additionally be involved in transcriptional regulation [5]. Without normal DNA replication there is chromosomal instability that results in the observed predisposition to malignancy. Cultured lymphocytes and fibroblasts from patients with Bloom syndrome show a high incidence of chromosomal aberrations, and cells with abnormally high rates of sister chromatid exchange (SCE) are uniquely characteristic of this condition [6].

Bloom syndrome occurs with greater frequency in Ashkenazi Jews, accounting for approximately one-third of all cases. A common ancestral mutation has been identified in most of these patients, with an estimated carrier frequency of 1%. Other founder mutations have also been identified in patients from other geographical regions [7,8].

Recently, mutations in the genes encoding RMI2 [9] and TopIIIα [10] have been identified in individuals with a Bloom-like syndrome, also associated with increased rates of SCE.

Clinical features [1,3,11–13]

Cutaneous features

Telangiectatic redness of the face develops during infancy or early childhood as red macules or plaques, which may simulate lupus erythematosus. They are most numerous on the 'butterfly' area of the nose and cheeks, but may involve the margins of the eyelids, the forehead, the ears, and sometimes the dorsa of the hands and forearms. There may be slight scaling. Sun exposure usually exacerbates these changes and may also provoke bullae, bleeding and crusting of the lips.

Extracutaneous features

Patients with Bloom syndrome have a characteristic appearance. There is moderate and proportionate growth deficiency both *in utero* and postnatally (Figure 77.1). Patients have a narrow, slender, delicate facies with a relatively prominent nose and small jaw. The

limbs tend to be long with large hands and feet, and there may be reduced subcutaneous fat.

Other associated abnormalities include café-au-lait patches, clinodactyly, syndactyly, congenital heart disease, annular pancreas and a high-pitched voice, possibly due to the cranio-facial anatomy and high-arched palate. Many associated developmental defects have been reported. T- and B-cell immunodeficiencies may occur, and IgA and IgM levels may be reduced, predisposing to pneumonia, bronchiectasis and chronic lung disease. Gastro-oesophageal reflux is common and may lead to aspiration, contributing to the risk of chronic lung disease.

Testicular atrophy is common and males are infertile. Although the tubular elements of the testes function poorly, the androgen-secreting portions are spared, thus permitting normal puberty [13]. Fertility in female patients appears reduced, although full-term pregnancies have been reported [14]. Bloom syndrome patients have an increased incidence of type II diabetes [15]. Neurological development is normal.

The mortality from neoplastic disease, particularly acute leukaemia, during the second or third decade is significantly increased [1,3,4,6,12]; there is an estimated 150–300 times increased risk of malignancy relative to normal. Cancers of the types and sites seen in the general population arise frequently and unusually early, as do rare cancers of early childhood [12]. They are predominantly internal such as those of the upper and lower gastrointestinal tract, genito-urinary cancers and haematological malignancies, but cutaneous malignancies are also more common with approximately 15% of patients in the Bloom Syndrome Registry having had skin cancer, with a mean age of 32 years [1,11]. There is no increased frequency of malignancies in most heterozygous carriers of *RECQL3* mutations [16].

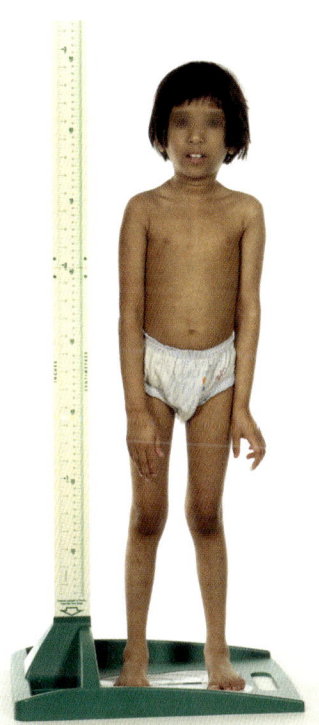

Figure 77.1 Child with Bloom syndrome showing short stature and characteristic facies. Courtesy of Dr H. Fassihi, St John's Institute of Dermatology, London, UK.

Management

Early diagnosis of Bloom syndrome is important for awareness of possible malignancies and for photoprotection. Chromosomal analysis may demonstrate increased numbers of SCEs and abnormal chromosomal configurations. Genetic testing of *RECQL3* will confirm the diagnosis. In the Ashkenazi Jewish population, where women have a 1 in 200 risk of having an affected child, targeted screening of the recurrent founder mutation may be indicated.

Patients should minimise sun exposure and use a high-factor sunscreen. Regular screening for diabetes and malignancies (e.g. skin surveillance, colonoscopy and faecal occult blood testing in adults) may be indicated. Symptoms suggestive of possible malignancy should prompt appropriate investigations. However, ionising radiation from cancer surveillance or treatment and alkylating agents may predispose to further DNA damage and carcinogenesis and should therefore be minimised where possible [17]. Aside from this, standard cancer treatments are recommended, as are treatments of associated diseases such as diabetes.

Prenatal testing for Bloom syndrome has been successfully undertaken by SCE analysis in chorionic villus cell cultures [18] as well as from *RECQL3* screening from chorionic villi or amniotic cells. Preimplantation genetic diagnosis has also been carried out [1].

Progeroid laminopathies and related conditions

Lamins comprise a type of intermediate filament which are important structural proteins of the nuclear lamina beneath the inner nuclear membrane; they have a role in maintaining the size and shape of the nuclear membrane. The *LMNA* gene encodes prelamin A, which undergoes post-translational modification to lamin A. Autosomal dominant or recessive *LMNA* mutations result in a number of different syndromes, termed laminopathies, with variable phenotypic features depending on the site and nature of the mutations, but which essentially cause accumulation of prelamin A in the nucleus [1,2]. While some disorders are characterised by progeroid features, others involve cardiomyopathy, muscular dystrophy, peripheral neuropathy or lipodystrophy (Table 77.1) [2]. Mutations in a zinc metalloproteinase gene, *ZMPSTE24*, which is involved in post-translational lamin A processing, give rise to clinically similar conditions, also from accumulation of unmodified prelamin A within nuclei.

Hutchinson–Gilford progeria syndrome

Definition

Growth retardation with premature and accelerated ageing from early childhood are the cardinal features of HGPS [1]. Affected individuals usually die in childhood or teenage years due to cardiovascular disease.

Pathophysiology

HGPS is an autosomal dominant condition with a birth prevalence estimated at 1 in 4 million [2]. Almost all cases arise from *de novo* mutations in the gene encoding lamin A/C, *LMNA*, on chromosome 1q22 [3,4]. A single recurrent mutation, c.1824C>T, causes the classic form of HGPS, accounting for around 90% of cases [3–5]; this mutation causes abnormal gene splicing and the deletion of 50 amino acids leading to an abnormal prelamin A protein termed progerin. This deletion interferes with the normal post-translational modification of prelamin A leading to persistent farnesylation of progerin, which accumulates at the inner nuclear membrane causing increased cellular damage with age. Other dominant *LMNA* mutations have been identified in cases of non-classic HGPS which may be more or less severe, dependent on the molecular consequences of the mutation [5–8].

Fibroblasts from patients with classic HGPS show changes in nuclear morphology on light and electron microscopy, including nuclear envelope lobulation, nuclear lamina thickening, clustering of nuclear pores and loss of peripheral heterochromatin [9]. These changes are due to increased accumulation of progerin with cellular age and result in the progressive premature ageing seen in HGPS.

Histopathologically, during the early sclerodermatous phase in the skin, thickening of the dermis with hypertrophic collagen bundles but a normal epidermis have been described [10], although changes may be non-specific [11]. Later in life the epidermis may be thinned, the dermis replaced by fibrotic hyaline material, with a reduction of sweat glands and subcutaneous tissue [12].

Clinical features [1,2,13]

Intrauterine growth is usually normal but may be reduced; by the first year of life, however, failure to thrive is the norm and this growth retardation persists and worsens thereafter. Over the first few years of life, individuals develop typical facies with a small receding mandible, and the nose develops a pointed tip and narrow bridge. The head appears large for the face and scalp veins are prominent, made more noticeable due to partial or total alopecia which may also affect the eyebrows and eyelashes. The eyes tend to be prominent, the lips are thin and may have surrounding cyanosis, and earlobes may be absent. Sclerodermatous changes of the skin also manifest early, particularly on the trunk and limbs, with reduced subcutaneous fat and joint contractures. Nails are frequently dystrophic. The clavicles may be short, leading to sloping shoulders and a pear-shaped chest. Bony changes include osteolysis of the distal phalanges and delayed closure of the anterior fontanelle. Primary dentition is often late to erupt and may not be lost, leading to overcrowding. There may also be partial failure of eruption of secondary teeth.

Later in childhood, features of accelerated ageing become more wide ranging, including a pigmented, aged appearance to the skin, conductive hearing loss, osteoarthritis, atherosclerosis leading to ischaemic heart disease and cerebrovascular disease, Raynaud phenomenon and insulin resistance, although not usually diabetes. Growth delay means that individuals do not reach completion of secondary sexual characteristics and do not, therefore, have children. Of note, motor and intellectual development are normal and there is no immunodeficiency or predisposition to malignancy.

In classic HGPS the usual survival is around 6–20 years with a mean of 13 years [2]; death usually results from myocardial infarction, heart failure or stroke.

Diagnosis

Diagnosis is usually suspected clinically from a combination of profound growth failure, typical physical appearances and consequences of premature ageing. If suspected, targeted sequencing of known *LMNA* mutations can be undertaken, followed, if negative, by full sequencing of the gene [1]. Other genes such as *ZMPSTE24* may be implicated in other progeroid syndromes and may warrant testing if *LMNA* screening is negative. Alternatively, multigene panel testing of known progeroid syndrome genes can be undertaken as a primary screening approach [1].

Management

Management should focus on monitoring disease progress, preventative care where possible, and treatment of complications as and when they arise [1,2]. Patients should have 6–12-monthly growth, cardiovascular, neurological, musculoskeletal, dental, ear and eye assessments. Lipids, electrocardiogram, echocardiogram, carotid duplex scanning, hip X-rays and bone densitometry scans should form part of annual care. Low-dose aspirin may be recommended in view of the increased risk of cardiovascular disease, and sun avoidance to limit cutaneous signs of increased ageing. Lipid levels are usually normal but may require statin treatment if elevated.

Recent research has highlighted some potential therapeutic agents to reverse the underlying molecular defect in HGPS, specifically by reducing the farnesylation of progerin which results in its nuclear accumulation [14]. Following successful clinical trials in HGPS, the farnesyl transferase inhibitor lonafarnib has been approved for clinical use in the USA [15] and is currently in clinical trials in combination with the mTOR inhibitor everolimus (ClinicalTrials.gov NCT025790440). A number of other drug therapies including JAK inhibitors [16,17], tocilizumab [18] and progerinin [19] have been the focus of recent preclinical studies, as have a variety of genome editing approaches [20–22] (for review see [23]).

Mandibulo-acral dysplasia with type A and type B lipodystrophy

Definition

Mandibulo-acral dysplasia with type A (MADA) and type B (MADB) lipodystrophy are autosomal recessive conditions with growth delay, skeletal abnormalities, lipodystrophy and pigmentary skin changes [1,2,3].

Pathophysiology

MADA lipodystrophy is caused by homozygous or compound heterozygous *LMNA* mutations [1,2–5], whereas MADB results from compound heterozygous mutations in the zinc metalloproteinase STE24 gene, *ZMPSTE24*, which is involved in post-translational modification of prelamin A [1,3,5,6].

Clinical features [1,2–7]

Affected individuals have postnatal growth retardation and develop progressive osteolysis of the clavicles and distal phalanges. Cranio-facial changes include mandibular hypoplasia, leading to dental crowding, and delayed closure of the fontanelles and cranial sutures, with a progeroid appearance in some. In general, MADB tends to be more severe and presents earlier in the first year or two of life with skeletal manifestations and skin atrophy compared with individuals with MADA. In MADA, lipodystrophy results in the loss of acral fatty tissue with an increase in subcutaneous fat in the trunk in some individuals, whereas in type B the lipodystrophy also tends to be more generalised. Impaired insulin resistance and diabetes may occur. Cutaneous changes include patchy pigmentation, atrophy, sclerodermatous changes with stiff joints, sclerotic, calcified acral skin and alopecia.

Cutis laxa: autosomal dominant and autosomal recessive

Definition

Cutis laxa is a group of conditions in which skin lacks elasticity leading to a loose, wrinkly and prematurely aged appearance. In addition, these heterogeneous disorders are variably associated with connective tissue problems as a result of loss, disorganisation or fragmentation of elastic tissues in other organs, notably the lungs, cardiovascular system, joints and gastrointestinal and genito-urinary systems. Some forms are associated with developmental delay and neuromuscular compromise. Cutis laxa is very rare, with an estimated incidence of 1 in 4 million [1].

Pathophysiology

The formation of elastic fibres is a stepwise process and involves interplay between a number of different proteins. Microfibrils consisting of fibulin, fibrillin and various glycoproteins act as a scaffold for soluble tropoelastin monomers, which are then cross-linked by lysyl oxidase into an insoluble elastin core [2]. The resulting elastic fibres are responsible for the resilience of organs such as the skin, blood vessels, intestine, bladder and joints. Defects in some of the proteins involved in elastic fibre formation, such as fibulins and elastin, cause different cutis laxa phenotypes. Histological and ultrastructural changes depend on the underlying defect.

Clinical features

Table 77.2 summarises the different forms of cutis laxa, the main ones being autosomal dominant cutis laxa (ADCL) and autosomal recessive cutis laxa (ARCL).

Autosomal dominant cutis laxa

Autosomal dominant mutations of the elastin gene, *ELN*, cause lax skin and a prematurely aged appearance with onset between childhood and early adulthood, as well as gastrointestinal diverticula and inguinal hernias (ADCL type 1) [3,4]. Less common manifestations include emphysema, aortic aneurysm and aortic or mitral valve prolapse. Elastic fibres in the skin are sparse and fragmented with a paucity of amorphous elastin on electron microscopy [5].

PART 6: GENETIC DISORDERS

Table 77.2 Cutis laxa subtypes, causative genes and predominant phenotypes.

Disease	MIM	Gene	Chromosome	Cutis laxa	Emphysema	Cardiovascular involvement	Intellectual impairment	GI/GU diverticula	Skeletal manifestations
Autosomal dominant									
ADCL1	123700	ELN	7q11.23	+	+	+	–	–	–
ADCL2	614434	FBLN5	14q32.12	+	+	+	–	–	–
ADCL3 (progeroid)	616603	ALDH18A1	10q24.1	++	–	++	++	+	+++
Autosomal recessive									
ARCL1A	219100	FBLN5	14q32.12	+++	+++	+	–	+	–
ARCL1B	614437	EFEMP2 (FBLN4)	11q13.1	++	++	+++	–	–	–
ARCL1C	613177	LTBP4	19q13.2	++	+++	+	–	+++	+
ARCL2A	219200	ATP6V0A2	12q24.31	++	–	+	++	–	+
ARCL2B	612940	PYCR1	17q25.3	++	–	–	++	–	++
ARCL2C	617402	ATP6V1E1	22q11.21	++	+	++	–	++	++
ARCL2D	617405	ATP6V1A	3q13.31	++	–	+	++	–	++
ARCL3A	219150	ALDH18A1	10q24.1	+	–	+	+++	–	++
ARCL3B	614438	PYCR1	17q25.3	+	–	+	+++	–	++
X-linked									
XLCL (OHS)	304150	ATP7A	Xq21.1	+	–	+	+	+	+++
Associated disorders									
MACS	613075	RIN2	20p11.23	++	–	–	–	–	++
GO	231070	SCYL1BP1	1q24.2	++	–	–	–	–	+++
ATS	208050	SLC2A10	20q13.12	++	–	+++	–	–	+

ADCL, autosomal dominant cutis laxa; ARCL, autosomal recessive cutis laxa; ATS, arterial tortuosity syndrome; GI/GU, gastrointestinal/genito-urinary; GO, geroderma osteodysplasticum; MACS, macrocephaly, alopecia, cutis laxa, scoliosis syndrome; OHS, occipital horn syndrome; XLCL, X-linked cutis laxa.

Type 2 ADCL with a similar phenotype has been reported due to a heterozygous mutation of the fibulin 5 gene, *FBLN5* [6]. A progeroid form of ADCL (type 3) results from heterozygous mutations in the *ALDH18A1* gene, associated with lax skin, an aged appearance, intellectual disability and growth delay [7].

Autosomal recessive cutis laxa

A number of different genes have been implicated in recessive forms of cutis laxa, including those encoding fibulins 5 and 4, *FBLN5* and *EFEMP2* (*FBLN4*), respectively [1]. Other causative genes have less well characterised functions but encode proteins involved in amino acid metabolism, regulation of transforming growth factor β1 (TGF-β1) activity, or transport and/or modification of components of the extracellular matrix [1].

ARCL type 1 comprises severe forms with life-threatening complications and death occurring between infancy and young adulthood usually from cardiorespiratory compromise [1]. Three main types are recognised depending on the underlying gene pathology (Table 77.2): in general, ARCL type 1A (*FBLN5* mutations) is associated with more severe and early respiratory complications [8,9]; type 1B (*EFEMP2* mutations) has greater vascular fragility and tortuosity [10,11]; and type 1C (*LTBP4* mutations) results in problems with diverticula of the gut or bladder [9,12]. In all types, skin changes are generalised but may be particularly prominent over the axillae, neck and groins, and give the face a droopy, aged appearance. Atelectasis and emphysema usually present in early childhood and vascular anomalies, notably supravalvular aortic stenosis, pulmonary artery stenosis or aortic aneurysm, occur commonly. There may be multiple diverticula of the gastrointestinal and genito-urinary tracts and, less commonly, inguinal hernias, joint laxity, hip dislocation and delayed closure of the fontanelles. Facial dysmorphism and postnatal growth delay may be seen but intellectual development is normal. Histology shows normal or reduced elastic fibres with mild fragmentation in the dermis [12]; ultrastructurally there is a reduction in elastic fibres and accumulation of elastin globules [13]. Arterial tortuosity syndrome has similarities to ARCL type 1B with a variable phenotype of extensible or lax skin, prominent cardiovascular features with arterial tortuosity and a propensity to arterial aneurysms and other systemic manifestations [14]. This recessive form of cutis laxa is caused by bilallelic mutations in a glucose transporter gene, *SLC2A10* [15].

Type 2 ARCL comprises a number of different forms of cutis laxa with variable severity but overlap in phenotypic features. It results from mutations in genes encoding proteins involved in the function of mitochondria, endosomes and Golgi apparatus. Most cases result from mutations in the *ATP6V0A2* ATPase gene (ARCL type 2A) [16,17], and less often from mutations in *PYCR1* (ARCL type 2B), *ATP6V1E1* (ARCL type 2C) and *ATP6V1A* (ARCL type 2D) [18,19]. Cutaneous phenotypes vary between wrinkly skin and more pronounced cutis laxa with excess folds of skin over the face, large flexures and dorsa of the hands and feet, which may improve over time. Unlike type 1 ARCL, there is often pronounced developmental delay, seizures and neurological impairment, with most individuals showing cerebral and cerebellar malformations. Other features include delayed growth, congenital hip dislocation, joint laxity, inguinal hernias, osteoporosis, high myopia and facial dysmorphism. De Barsy syndrome is a form of type 3 ARCL in which there is generalised cutis laxa giving a progeroid appearance, pre- and postnatal growth delay, clouding of the corneas or cataracts, and severe developmental delay in the majority [20–23]. There may also be agenesis of the corpus callosum, joint laxity, hypotonia, tortuosity of blood vessels and facial dysmorphism. Causative mutations have been identified in *ALDH38A1* [21,22],

PYCR1 [23] or *P14K2A* [24]. Macrocephaly, alopecia, cutis laxa and scoliosis (MACS) syndrome is another variant of ARCL with coarse facial sagging and developmental delay. It results from mutations in *RIN2* which encodes a Rab5 effector protein of endosomal vesicles [25]. At the milder end of the phenotypic spectrum, geroderma osteodysplasticum is characterised by progeroid skin wrinkling mainly on the hands, feet and abdomen presenting in infancy or early childhood [26]. There is osteoporosis and bony fractures, and there may be hernias or hip dislocation. Intellectual development is normal. The causative gene, *SCYL1BP1*, encodes a protein involved in Golgi trafficking and structure [26]. Types 2 and 3 ARCL show variable histopathological and ultrastructural abnormalities; cases due to impaired vesicle trafficking tend to demonstrate sparse elastic fibres with disintegrated cores [**1**,17,19], whereas defects of cellular metabolism show thin elastic fibres with an increased microfibrillar mantle [**1**,27].

X-linked cutis laxa (XLCL), also termed occipital horn syndrome because of characteristic calcifications over the occipital bone at the sites of muscle insertion, also features lax skin, inguinal hernias, joint laxity, tortuous blood vessels and, in some, intellectual impairment [28–30]. It is caused by mutations in the copper-transporting ATPase gene, *ATP7A*. Mutations in the same gene can also cause Menke disease; in contrast to XLCL, these patients have severe neurological degeneration, growth retardation and death in early childhood, with milder skin laxity and sparse, kinky hair [29,30].

Management [1]

Investigation of an individual with cutis laxa should aim to identify possible systemic complications. Hip dislocation should be checked for clinically and with ultrasonography if indicated. Clinical examination should also look for inguinal herniation and any abnormalities of the cardiovascular system. An echocardiogram, chest computed tomography scan, magnetic resonance (MR) imaging, MR angiogram and pulmonary function tests may be indicated. Similarly, a renal ultrasound, voiding cystourethrogram and barium enema may demonstrate diverticular disease. A full ophthalmological examination may be needed, particularly if ARCL type 3 is suspected, and neurological evaluation, electroencephalograph and brain MR scan if indicated.

Routine management is indicated for complications such as refractive errors, emphysema, hip dislocation, inguinal hernias and seizures. A β-blocker or angiotensin-converting enzyme inhibitor may be indicated if dilatation of the aortic root is identified and surgical management of aneurysms and other cardiovascular anomalies may be warranted. Avoidance of sunbathing and smoking should be recommended. Although botulinum toxin injections and plastic surgery for facial involvement by cutis laxa have been advocated, longer term, redundant skin folds tend to recur [31,32].

Key references

The full list of references can be found in the online version at https://www.wiley.com/rooksdermatology10e

Werner syndrome

1 Oshima J, Martin GM, Hisama FM. Werner syndrome. In: Adam MP, Ardinger HH, Pagon RA *et al.*, eds. *GeneReviews [Internet]*. Seattle, WA: University of Washington, 2002–2016.

Bloom syndrome

1 Flanagan M, Cunniff CM. Bloom syndrome. In: Adam MP, Ardinger HH, Pagon RA *et al.*, eds. *GeneReviews [Internet]*. Seattle, WA: University of Washington, 2006–2016.

8 German J, Sanz MM, Ciocci S *et al.* Syndrome-causing mutations of the BLM gene in persons in the Bloom's Syndrome Registry. *Hum Mutat* 2007;28:743–53.

Progeroid laminopathies and related conditions

2 Bertrand AT, Chikhaoui K, Ben Yaou R, le Bonne G. Clinical and genetic heterogeneity in laminopathies. *Biochem Soc Trans* 2011;39:1687–92.

Hutchinson–Gilford progeria syndrome

1 Gordon LB, Brown WT, Collins FS. Hutchinson–Gilford progeria syndrome. In: Adam MP, Ardinger HH, Pagon RA *et al.*, eds. *GeneReviews [Internet]* . Seattle, WA: University of Washington, 2003–2019.

2 Hennekam RCM. Hutchinson–Gilford progeria syndrome: review of the phenotype. *Am J Med Genet A* 2006;140A:2603–24.

Mandibulo-acral dysplasia with type A and type B lipodystrophy

1 Cenni V, D'Apice MR, Rivieri F *et al.* Mandibuloacral dysplasia: a premature ageing disease with aspects of physiological ageing. *Ageing Res Rev* 2018;42:1–13.

Cutis laxa: autosomal dominant and autosomal recessive

1 Beyens A, Boel A, Symoens S, Callewaert B. Cutis laxa: a comprehensive overview of clinical characteristics and pathophysiology. *Clin Genet* 2021;99: 53–66.

PART 6: GENETIC DISORDERS

CHAPTER 78

Inherited Skin Tumour Syndromes

Neil Rajan[1], Jemima E. Mellerio[2] and Alan D. Irvine[3]

[1] Translational and Clinical Research Institute, Newcastle University and Newcastle Hospitals NHS Foundation Trust, Newcastle upon Tyne, UK
[2] St John's Institute of Dermatology, Guy's and St Thomas' NHS Foundation Trust, London, UK
[3] Children's Health Ireland at Crumlin, Dublin; St James's Hospital, Dublin; Trinity College, Dublin, Ireland

Introduction

This chapter covers three exemplar inherited skin tumour syndromes: neurofibromatosis type 1 (NF1), the tuberous sclerosis complex and familial adenomatous polyposis, as well as providing an overview of inherited tumour syndromes with cutaneous manifestations. NF1, tuberous sclerosis complex and familial adenomatous polyposis have diverse clinical and genetic features and require disease-specific knowledge for diagnosis, along with targeted interventions and cancer surveillance plans. All three share in common the clinical presentation of multiple benign skin tumours, which are often pathognomonic for these genetic conditions, and a significant risk of cutaneous and non-cutaneous neoplasia.

NEUROFIBROMATOSES

The neurofibromatoses comprise several distinct genetic disorders that lead to the formation of tumours surrounding the nerves and many other pathological features. There are three main forms: NF1, NF2 and schwannomatosis. The spectrum of these disorders has been reviewed elsewhere [1–5]. The most common type, NF1, is characterised by multiple café-au-lait macules and the occurrence of neurofibromas along the peripheral nerves. NF2 is characterised by vestibular schwannomas (acoustic neuromas), which are usually bilateral, as well as meningiomas. Cutaneous schwannomas may be seen and present as dermal plaques or nodules [6,7]. The third form, schwannomatosis, causes tumours to develop on the cranial, spinal and peripheral nerves resulting in chronic pain, altered sensation and muscle weakness, and has been linked to germline pathogenic variants in *SMARCB1* and *LZTR1* [8]. Schwannomatosis does not have cutaneous manifestations.

Neurofibromatosis type 1

Classification links
- MIM: 162200

Introduction and general description

Neurofibromatosis type 1 is an inherited neuroectodermal abnormality, characterised by the presence of six or more café-au-lait spots, axillary freckles (Figure 78.1), cutaneous neurofibromas (Figure 78.2), plexiform neurofibromas and Lisch nodules (pigmented iris hamartomas) (Figure 78.3) [1,9,10]. Box 78.1 lists the diagnostic criteria [11].

Pathophysiology
Genetics

The mode of inheritance is autosomal dominant, with almost 100% penetrance by the age of 5 years [10,12]. Sporadic cases account for up to 50% of all cases and may be explained by both parental gonadal mosaicism and a high gene mutation rate (*de novo* mutations). The prevalence of NF1 has been estimated at about 1 in 2500–3300 births [1,9,10]. Mosaic forms with incomplete features are frequent [13–15].

The *NF1* gene is located on chromosome 17 [16,17], and encodes a protein named neurofibromin [18,**19,20**]. The gene spans 335 kb and has at least 59 exons, producing four major alternatively spliced transcripts. Neurofibromin has been shown to be expressed in both keratinocytes and melanocytes in normal adult human skin [21]. Neurofibromin is a Ras guanosine triphosphatase (GTPase) activating protein (RasGap) and negatively regulates the Ras-mitogen activated protein kinase (MAPK) pathway, an important pathway in neuroectodermal cells such as neuronal cells and melanocytes.

Rook's Textbook of Dermatology, Tenth Edition. Edited by Christopher Griffiths, Jonathan Barker, Tanya Bleiker, Walayat Hussain and Rosalind Simpson.
© 2024 John Wiley & Sons Ltd. Published 2024 by John Wiley & Sons Ltd.

PART 6: GENETIC DISORDERS

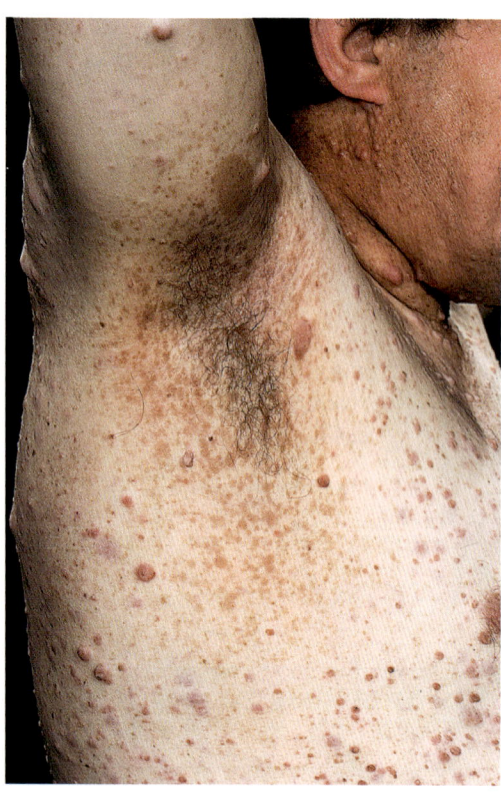

Figure 78.1 Neurofibromatosis: axillary freckling and multiple neurofibromas. Courtesy of Professor J. Harper, Great Ormond Street Hospital, London, UK.

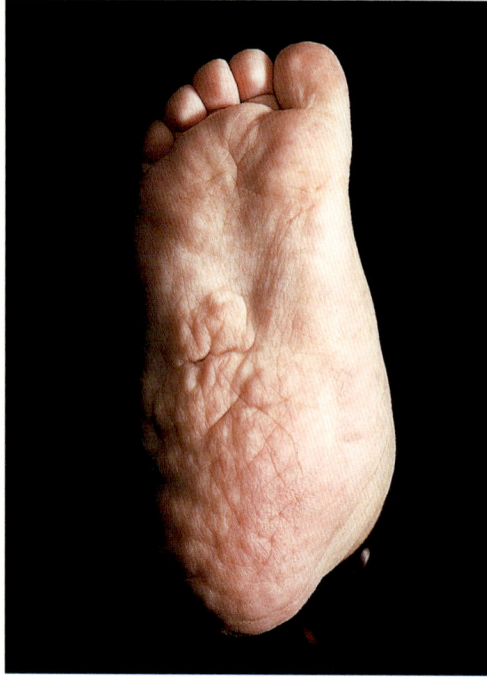

Figure 78.2 Neurofibromatosis: extensive plexiform neurofibroma of the foot. Courtesy of Professor J. Harper, Great Ormond Street Hospital, London, UK.

NF is now considered a 'RASopathy' – one of several conditions where pathogenic variants in genes result in the deregulation of Ras signalling which is a key step towards the development of the phenotype (see 'RASopathies' later in this chapter).

The majority of *NF1* germline pathogenic variants alter the reading frame or insert a premature stop codon, resulting in loss of

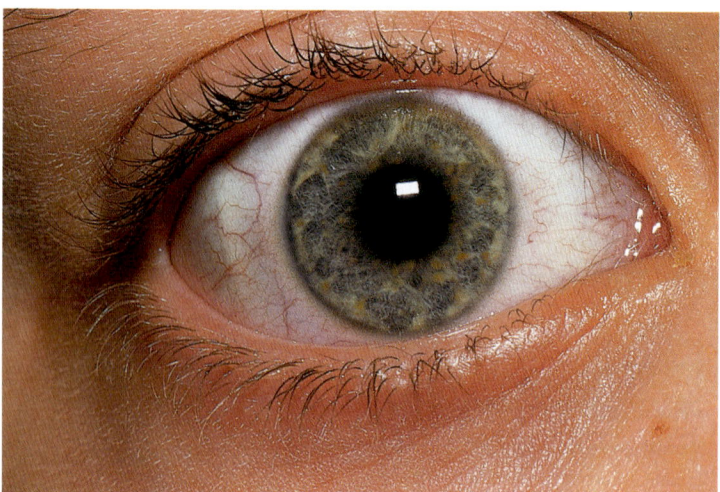

Figure 78.3 Neurofibromatosis: Lisch nodules (pigmented iris hamartomas). Courtesy of Professor J. Harper, Great Ormond Street Hospital, London, UK.

function. No mutational hotspot has been recognised, and individuals and families have private pathogenic variants. Contiguous gene deletions that include neurofibromin and adjacent genes lead to a more severe NF phenotype, often with associated developmental delay.

Box 78.1 Revised diagnostic criteria for neurofibromatosis type 1 (NF1)

A: The diagnostic criteria for NF1 are met in an individual who does not have a parent diagnosed with NF1 if two or more of the following are present:
- Six or more café-au-lait macules over 5 mm in greatest diameter in prepubertal individuals and over 15 mm in greatest diameter in postpubertal individuals[a]
- Freckling in the axillary or inguinal region[a]
- Two or more neurofibromas of any type *OR* one plexiform neurofibroma
- Optic pathway glioma
- Two or more iris Lisch nodules identified by slit-lamp examination or two or more choroidal abnormalities (CAs), defined as bright, patchy nodules imaged by optical coherence tomography (OCT)/near-infrared reflectance (NIR) imaging
- A distinctive osseous lesion such as sphenoid dysplasia,[b] anterolateral bowing of the tibia or pseudarthrosis of a long bone
- A heterozygous pathogenic *NF1* variant with a variant allele fraction of 50% in apparently normal tissue such as white blood cells

B: A child of a parent who meets the diagnostic criteria specified in A merits a diagnosis of NF1 if one or more of the criteria in A are present

[a] If only café-au-lait macules and freckling are present, the diagnosis is most likely NF1 but exceptionally the person might have another diagnosis such as Legius syndrome. At least one of the two pigmentary findings (café-au-lait macules or freckling) should be bilateral.
[b] Sphenoid wing dysplasia is not a separate criterion in the case of an ipsilateral orbital plexiform neurofibroma.

Reproduced from Legius *et al.* [11] with permission of Springer Nature / CC BY 4.0.

NF1 is a tumour suppressor gene, with patients carrying heterozygous germline pathogenic variants, and homozygous pathogenic variants demonstrated in cutaneous neurofibromas, in keeping with the classic Knudson 'two-hit' hypothesis of tumourigenesis. The requirement of somatic mutations in the remaining normal parental copy of *NF1* [22] partly explains the delayed age of onset of neurofibromas associated with NF1 and the variability of expression [23]. Conversely, second hits in the *NF1* gene *in utero* before development is complete are thought to explain the formation of plexiform neurofibromas [24].

Clinical features [2,9,10]

The National Institutes of Health Consensus Development Conference Statement on diagnostic criteria for NF1, developed in 1988, is widely employed in clinical practice [25] and was revised in 2019 [11]. This requires two or more of the criteria listed in Box 78.1 to be fulfilled.

Café-au-lait macules (CALMs). These are sharply defined, light brown patches that vary in size from 0.5 to 50 cm, although the majority are 10 cm or less in size. CALMs are the first feature of the disease to appear in all children [1,10]. In a population study of NF1, parents of all affected children reported the appearance of CALMs by the age of 4 years, and within the first year of life in 82%. CALMs increase in size and number during the first decade.

Cutaneous neurofibromas. These are soft tumours, sessile and dome shaped, and sometimes pedunculated. Cutaneous neurofibromas are derived from peripheral nerves and their supporting structures, including neurilemmal cells. These lesions are most numerous on the trunk and limbs; hundreds may be present, ranging from a few millimetres to several centimetres in diameter. Blue-red macules and pseudoatrophic macules also occur [26] and are often variants of neurofibromas. Pruritus may be a symptom of NF1. The presence of large numbers of mast cells in the skin in this condition, and the response of itch to antihistamines, suggest that histamine mediates pruritus in NF1 [27]. Long-term treatment with ketotifen, a mast cell-blocking agent, has not however resulted in resolution of cutaneous neurofibromas, and its utility as a preventative treatment for cutaneous neurofibromas remains unclear in the absence of suitably controlled interventional studies.

Plexiform neurofibromas. These are diffuse, elongated fibromas that run along the course of a nerve, frequently involving the trigeminal or upper cervical nerves and usually present within the first 2 years of life. They may also arise in peripheral nerves and within the spinal cord. Plexiform neurofibromas have a distinctive 'bag of worms' feeling on palpation. They may involve underlying sensory and motor nerves as well the viscera and blood vessels.

Freckling. Freckling occurs frequently in the axillae, where it is virtually pathognomonic (Crowe sign) [28]. It is present in about 70% of affected subjects and appears a little later than the café-au-lait spots, the youngest case in one series being 3 years old [1]. It may also occur in other intertriginous areas, especially the groin.

Lisch nodules. Lisch nodules (pigmented iris hamartomas) appear as dome-shaped lesions found superficially around the iris on slit-lamp examination. They occur in over 90% of patients and increase in incidence with age [1]. They do not occur in mosaic NF1 or NF2 [2].

Oral lesions. Oral lesions are present in up to 37% of cases, as papillomatous neurofibromas of the palate, buccal mucous membrane, tongue and lips [29].

Skeletal abnormalities. These are well described in NF1. Kyphoscoliosis occurs in 2% of cases. Sphenoid wing dysplasia is a characteristic abnormality. Pseudarthrosis involving the tibia or radius occurs in 1% but may be asymptomatic [2]. Short stature and macrocephaly [30] are also uncommon features of the condition. A generalised bone metabolic defect due to loss of function of neurofibromin has been identified [31], explaining the increased risk for osteopenia and osteoporosis in NF1 [32]. Early identification of NF1 patients with osteoporosis may permit more timely and aggressive treatments to prevent the likely substantial morbidity associated with increased fracture risk later in life.

Additional extracutaneous features. The severity of cutaneous involvement gives no reliable indication of the extent of the disease in other organs. Between 25% and 30% of children may exhibit learning difficulties [1,33] and physical development may be impaired. Speech impediments, hypertelorism and headaches are also common [2,34]. Endocrine disturbances of many types may be associated [35]: precocious puberty, acromegaly [36], Addison disease, hyperparathyroidism, gynaecomastia and phaeochromocytoma. Renovascular hypertension may occur in children [37]. Involvement of the lower urinary tract [38] may give rise to urinary symptoms. Constipation occurs due to dysfunction of the colonic musculature. Gastrointestinal stromal tumours may also cause recurrent haemorrhage or obstruction. There is a high prevalence of cardiovascular abnormalities [39,40] and NF1 can be complicated by pulmonary hypertension [41].

Neurological disease secondary to NF1-related tumours. The most common solitary intracranial tumour is an optic nerve glioma; astrocytomas and schwannomas also occur. Some reports suggest that these tumours may be sex dependent and more symptomatic in female patients [42,43]. Intracranial tumours may cause epilepsy, although seizures may occur in the absence of any demonstrable focal lesion.

Malignant tumours in NF1. Sarcomatous change within a neurofibroma occurs in 1.5–15% of cases, more often in deeper lesions than in cutaneous lesions [1,44]. This is rare before the age of 40 years but has occurred in early childhood. Growth is often slow and metastasis late, but local recurrence is frequent. In contrast, malignant peripheral nerve sheath tumours (MPNSTs) are highly aggressive sarcomas [45]. Enlargement or pain of cutaneous neurofibromas should suggest the possibility of malignant change, although rapid enlargement may also occur secondary to intralesional haemorrhage.

Other malignant diseases associated with NF1 include Wilms tumour and rhabdomyosarcoma. Children with NF1 and juvenile xanthogranulomas (JXGs) have been reported to develop juvenile myelomonocytic leukaemia (JMML) [46–48]. JXGs are seen in 5–10% of children under 2 years of age with NF1, and a recent case–control designed study [49] suggested that the risk of JMML in NF1 patients with JXG may have been previously overestimated. The presentation of multiple CALMs and acute lymphoblastic leukaemia or lymphoma should raise the alternate diagnosis of constitutional mismatch repair deficiency (CMMRD) [50,51].

Disease course and prognosis [2,52]

The course of the condition varies considerably in individual patients and the majority will have a benign course without developing major complications. In fact, a diagnosis of NF1 is frequently made after childhood.

Characteristically, café-au-lait spots are present at birth or, more commonly, develop in early childhood and increase in number throughout life. Cutaneous neurofibromas appear during childhood and increase rapidly in number at puberty, suggesting a possible hormonal influence. However, lesions may be present at birth and become progressively more extensive [53]. It is difficult to prognosticate based on the extent of cutaneous symptoms. Extensive involvement of the urinary or gastrointestinal tract or the central nervous system carries a poor prognosis.

Pregnancy in some cases appears to induce rapid progression of existing lesions and the development of new cutaneous neurofibromas [54], however a recent small controlled study of 26 pregnant NF1 patients suggests that this is not generally the case [55]. Long-term follow-up information on cohorts of NF1 patients has shown a reduced life expectancy related to the development of malignancy and other complications, such as hypertension due to renal artery stenosis or phaeochromocytoma [56,57].

Investigations

Diagnosis of germline NF1 is established based on clinical criteria. Cutaneous neurofibromas are clinically and histologically distinctive. CALMs, usually the earliest manifestation of NF1 in children, may be seen as isolated lesions in 10–20% of normal individuals. If only one or two are present, they have little diagnostic significance in the absence of other diagnostic criteria. Other clinical conditions (Table 78.1) may also be important to consider when multiple early-onset CALMs are seen.

Molecular genetic testing is now a relatively inexpensive test and is more widely used in clinical practice when the diagnosis is uncertain, but the majority of cases are diagnosed on the basis of characteristic clinical features [58]. Identification of the *NF1* gene means that prenatal/presymptomatic diagnosis for this disease is now possible, as is preimplantation genetic diagnosis [59].

Management

A detailed clinical assessment of the proband is essential and examination of all other members of the family may identify other affected individuals. It is recommended that individuals with NF1 have an annual clinical review, which includes the measurement of blood pressure, head circumference measurements, assessment of potential scoliosis, presence of painful lumps consistent with MPNSTs and eye examination. The Manchester checklist is widely used in the UK as a guide to patient management (Figure 78.4). Further investigations will depend upon the detection of specific associated features. Magnetic resonance imaging (MRI) should be performed in children who have macrocephaly or who demonstrate focal neurological signs or symptoms. In the UK, MRI screening is only suggested if there are neurological or ophthalmological anomalies, whereas practice in the USA is to screen all infants routinely with cranial MRI scanning. Patients with NF1 may require monitoring by a number of different specialists, with one physician acting as the coordinator. Ideally this is delivered in a multidisciplinary clinic, now established in several centres [60,61].

The management of symptomatic or growing cutaneous neurofibromas is usually surgical [62,63]. Ablative laser surgery is a treatment modality that can be employed for smaller cutaneous neurofibromas, but hypertrophic and atrophic scars can result, and a preliminary test treatment is recommended [62,64]. Surgery is also indicated when an increase in size and pain suggests possible malignant change. In 2020, the Ras-MAPK pathway inhibitor selumetinib (which targets the MEK (mitogen-activated extracellular signal-regulated kinase) protein in this pathway) was licenced by the US Food and Drug Administration (FDA) for the treatment of paediatric patients 2 years of age and older with NF1 who have symptomatic, inoperable plexiform neurofibromas [65,**66**]. New therapeutic strategies are being investigated in clinical trials [67].

Genetic counselling is important. Informing families about the varied complications of NF1 is a difficult counselling task, and there is a fine balance between providing adequate information and causing unnecessary alarm. It should be made clear to affected NF1 patients that 50% of their children are likely to be affected and the disease may be severe. First-degree relatives who have no stigmata of the disease are unlikely to carry the gene, and cascade genetic testing can be done to reassure if needed.

Table 78.1 Selected conditions apart from neurofibromatosis that feature café-au-lait macules as part of their clinical phenotype.

Condition	Gene
Legius syndrome	*SPRED1*
Constitutional mismatch repair deficiency (CMMRD)	*MLH1, MSH2, MSH6, PMS2*
Cowden syndrome	*PTEN*
Noonan syndrome with multiple lentigines	*PTPN11*
McCune–Albright syndrome	*GNAS*
Naevoid basal cell carcinoma syndrome	*PTCH1*

Adapted from Ponti *et al.* [77].

Mosaic neurofibromatosis 1

Mosaic NF1 can present as café-au-lait spots, cutaneous neurofibromas and sometimes visceral neurofibromas, limited typically to one side or a region of the body (Box 78.2) [68–71]. The condition represents somatic mosaicism involving the *NF1* gene, where only some cells in an affected patient carry a heterozygous pathogenic variant in *NF1*. A systematic review of mosaic NF1 patients suggests that

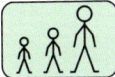

Neurofibromatosis type 1
Review guidelines

Annual Review Recommended

At time of diagnosis, or possible diagnosis, ALL patients should be seen in a genetics department.
Those with significant complications will be followed up as appropriate through the nationally-funded Complex NF1 Service.
Annual review should be undertaken by a community/district paediatrician and GP throughout childhood, and by a GP in adulthood. Patients, paediatricians and GPs have telephone access to the NF Service in Genetic Medicine for NF-related concerns.

Age	Genetics appointment	NF1 reviews carried out by	Vision checks
<6 and 50% risk	In first year and then at 2 and 5*¹	Care coordinated by genetics	Symptom check at NF1 review
<8 affected	Confirmation of diagnosis and assessment. Genetic counselling for family	GP and Community/ District Paediatrician. Liaison with NF service for complex cases	At least annual with paediatric ophthalmologist
8–15 affected	On request		Annual with optician/orthoptist
16–18 affected	Appointment for counselling re: adult complications and genetics	Care coordinated by GP	Symptom check at NF1 review
>16 affected *²	On request		

*¹ If no café-au-lait spots by 5 years, NF1 can be excluded in the majority of NF1 families.
Mutation testing can be considered to confirm or exclude the diagnosis and clarify the need for follow-up.

*² Women aged 40–50 should be referred for annual mammography as per 'moderate risk' NICE guidelines.

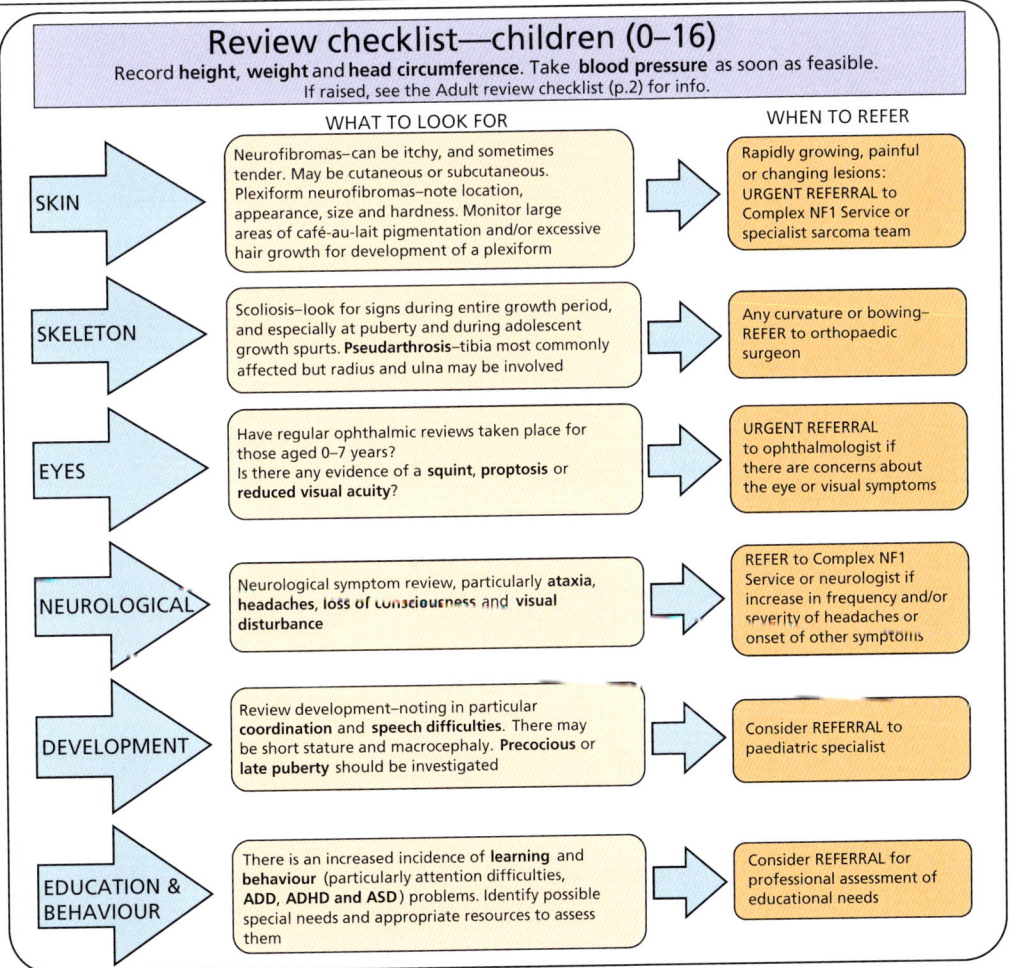

Review checklist—children (0–16)
Record **height**, **weight** and **head circumference**. Take **blood pressure** as soon as feasible.
If raised, see the Adult review checklist (p.2) for info.

WHAT TO LOOK FOR — **WHEN TO REFER**

SKIN — Neurofibromas–can be itchy, and sometimes tender. May be cutaneous or subcutaneous. Plexiform neurofibromas–note location, appearance, size and hardness. Monitor large areas of café-au-lait pigmentation and/or excessive hair growth for development of a plexiform — Rapidly growing, painful or changing lesions: URGENT REFERRAL to Complex NF1 Service or specialist sarcoma team

SKELETON — Scoliosis–look for signs during entire growth period, and especially at puberty and during adolescent growth spurts. **Pseudarthrosis**–tibia most commonly affected but radius and ulna may be involved — Any curvature or bowing– REFER to orthopaedic surgeon

EYES — Have regular ophthalmic reviews taken place for those aged 0–7 years? Is there any evidence of a **squint**, **proptosis** or **reduced visual acuity**? — URGENT REFERRAL to ophthalmologist if there are concerns about the eye or visual symptoms

NEUROLOGICAL — Neurological symptom review, particularly **ataxia**, **headaches**, loss of consciousness and **visual disturbance** — REFER to Complex NF1 Service or neurologist if increase in frequency and/or severity of headaches or onset of other symptoms

DEVELOPMENT — Review development–noting in particular **coordination** and **speech difficulties**. There may be short stature and macrocephaly. **Precocious** or **late puberty** should be investigated — Consider REFERRAL to paediatric specialist

EDUCATION & BEHAVIOUR — There is an increased incidence of **learning** and **behaviour** (particularly attention difficulties, **ADD, ADHD and ASD**) problems. Identify possible special needs and appropriate resources to assess them — Consider REFERRAL for professional assessment of educational needs

Figure 78.4 Manchester checklist for screening for neurofibromatosis. ADD, attention deficit disorder; ADHD, attention deficit hyperactivity disorder; ASD, autism spectrum disorder; GP, general practitioner; NF, neurofibromatois. Courtesy of Dr Judith Eeloo and Professor Gareth Evans. *Continued overleaf.*

PART 6: GENETIC DISORDERS

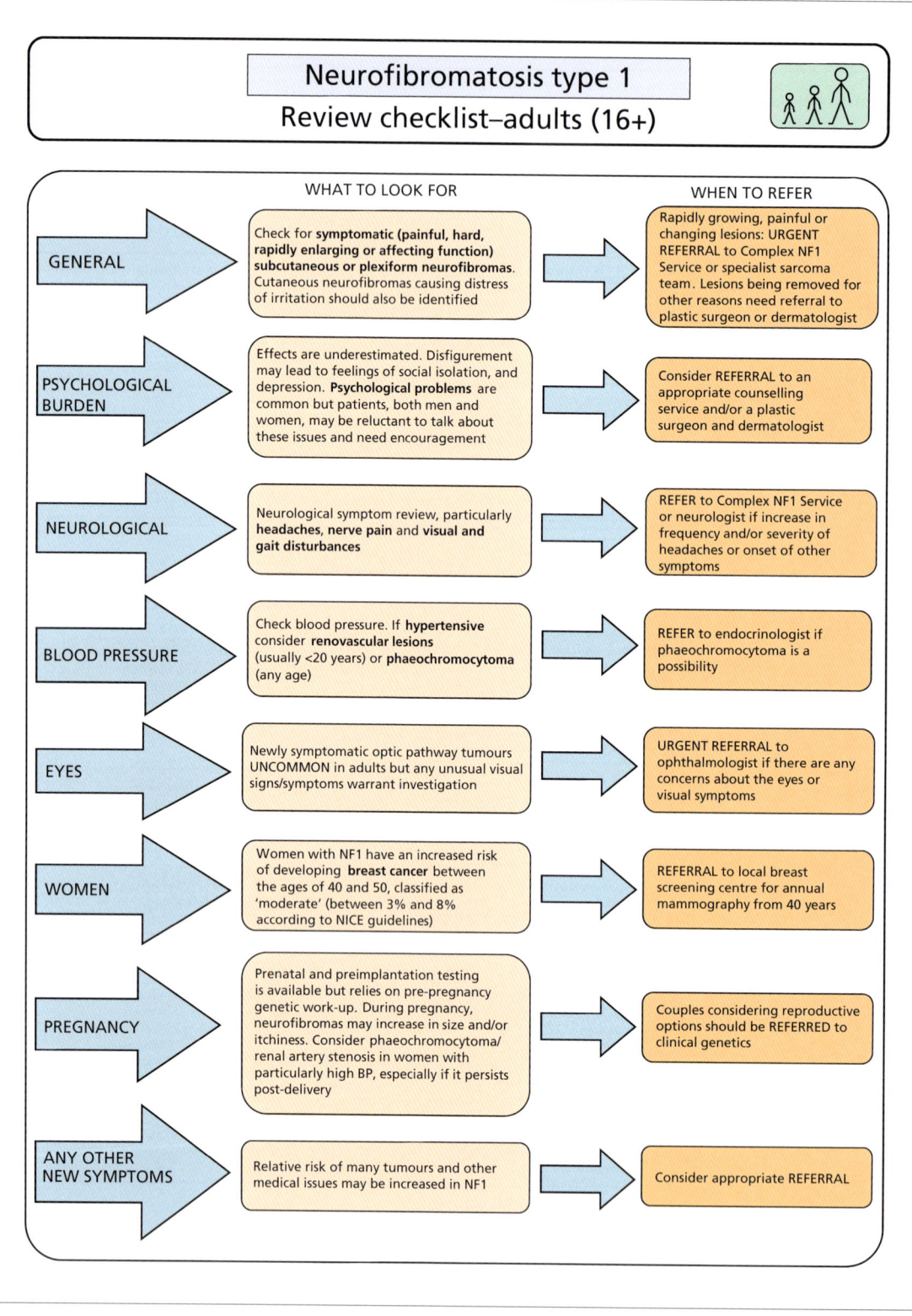

Neurofibromatosis type 1
Review checklist–adults (16+)

WHAT TO LOOK FOR | WHEN TO REFER

GENERAL
Check for **symptomatic (painful, hard, rapidly enlarging or affecting function) subcutaneous or plexiform neurofibromas.** Cutaneous neurofibromas causing distress of irritation should also be identified
Rapidly growing, painful or changing lesions: URGENT REFERRAL to Complex NF1 Service or specialist sarcoma team. Lesions being removed for other reasons need referral to plastic surgeon or dermatologist

PSYCHOLOGICAL BURDEN
Effects are underestimated. Disfigurement may lead to feelings of social isolation, and depression. **Psychological problems** are common but patients, both men and women, may be reluctant to talk about these issues and need encouragement
Consider REFERRAL to an appropriate counselling service and/or a plastic surgeon and dermatologist

NEUROLOGICAL
Neurological symptom review, particularly **headaches, nerve pain** and **visual and gait disturbances**
REFER to Complex NF1 Service or neurologist if increase in frequency and/or severity of headaches or onset of other symptoms

BLOOD PRESSURE
Check blood pressure. If **hypertensive** consider **renovascular lesions** (usually <20 years) or **phaeochromocytoma** (any age)
REFER to endocrinologist if phaeochromocytoma is a possibility

EYES
Newly symptomatic optic pathway tumours UNCOMMON in adults but any unusual visual signs/symptoms warrant investigation
URGENT REFERRAL to ophthalmologist if there are any concerns about the eyes or visual symptoms

WOMEN
Women with NF1 have an increased risk of developing **breast cancer** between the ages of 40 and 50, classified as 'moderate' (between 3% and 8% according to NICE guidelines)
REFERRAL to local breast screening centre for annual mammography from 40 years

PREGNANCY
Prenatal and preimplantation testing is available but relies on pre-pregnancy genetic work-up. During pregnancy, neurofibromas may increase in size and/or itchiness. Consider phaeochromocytoma/renal artery stenosis in women with particularly high BP, especially if it persists post-delivery
Couples considering reproductive options should be REFERRED to clinical genetics

ANY OTHER NEW SYMPTOMS
Relative risk of many tumours and other medical issues may be increased in NF1
Consider appropriate REFERRAL

Figure 78.4 (*Continued*)

transmission to the next generation of germline NF1 is reported in between 2.5% and 6.4% of patients affected with mosaic NF [72].

Box 78.2 Revised diagnostic criteria for mosaic neurofibromatosis type 1 (NF1)

Diagnostic criteria for mosaic NF1 [11] are met in an individual if any of the following are present:
- A pathogenic heterozygous NF1 variant with a variant allele fraction of significantly less than 50% in apparently normal tissue such as white blood cells *AND* one other NF1 diagnostic criterion (except a parent fulfilling diagnostic criteria for NF1)
- An identical pathogenic heterozygous NF1 variant in two anatomically independent affected tissues (in the absence of a pathogenic NF1 variant in unaffected tissue)[a]
- A clearly segmental distribution of café-au-lait macules or cutaneous neurofibromas *AND*
  - Another NF1 diagnostic criterion (except a parent fulfilling diagnostic criteria for NF1)[b]
      OR
  - Child fulfilling diagnostic criteria for NF1
- Only one NF1 diagnostic criterion from the following list: freckling in the axillary and inguinal region, optic pathway glioma, two or more Lisch nodules or two or more choroidal abnormalities, distinctive osseous lesion typical for NF1, two or more neurofibromas or one plexiform neurofibroma *AND* a child fulfilling the criteria for NF1

[a] Neurofibroma and overlying hyperpigmented skin count for one tissue only; different tissues originating from the same primary affected lesion count for one tissue only.
[b] If only café-au-lait macules and freckling are present, the diagnosis is most likely mosaic NF1 but rarely might be mosaic Legius syndrome or constitutional mismatch repair deficiency (CMMRD) syndrome.

RASopathies

Neurofibromatosis type 1 is recognised to be part of a family of related conditions that arise due to deregulated Ras-MAPK signalling, termed RASopathies. These autosomal dominant disorders are caused by pathogenic variants affecting genes that encode proteins that regulate components of the Ras-MAPK signalling pathway [73] (Figure 78.5). These disorders include capillary malformation–arteriovenous malformation syndrome, cardio-facio-cutaneous syndrome, Costello syndrome, Legius syndrome, NF1, Noonan syndrome (NS) and NS with multiple lentigines (previously termed LEOPARD syndrome).

Because these various disorders affect the same signalling pathway, they share many phenotypic features, including cardinal cutaneous manifestations such as skin tumours, and pigmentary and hair abnormalities [74]. Table 78.2 summarises their major clinical features. Additional genes that are recognised as associated with RASopathies include *RIT1*, *SOS2*, *RASA2* and *RRAS*, which have been detected in patients with the NS phenotype [75]. The regrouping of these various disorders under one clinical entity

has been driven by the recognition of the possibility of designing therapeutic interventions targeting the Ras-MAPK pathway as a general approach to their treatment [74,76].

OTHER INHERITED SKIN TUMOUR SYNDROMES

Tuberous sclerosis complex

Classification links
- MIM: 191100 (TSC1), 613254 (TSC2)

Introduction and general description
Tuberous sclerosis complex (TSC) represents a genetic disorder of hamartoma formation in many organs, particularly the skin, brain, eye, kidney and heart [1,2]. The term 'complex' emphasises the multisystem involvement and highly variable expression of the disease. Characteristic skin lesions include angiofibromas, connective tissue naevi, periungual fibromas and 'ash-leaf' white macules. These features are typically seen in association with epilepsy and intellectual impairment.

Studies have shown the incidence to be 1 in 10 000 in the Oxford region [1] and one in 27 000 in the west of Scotland [3]. Osborne *et al.* [4] have estimated that the birth incidence may be in the region of 1 in 5800, which makes TSC, along with NF1, one of the more common single-gene disorders.

TSC is an autosomal dominant condition, showing great variability of expression of phenotypes, even within a single family. It is now recognised that about half the TSC families are linked to pathogenic variants in *TSC1* and the other half to *TSC2* [5,6]. A minority of families do not carry coding pathogenic variants in either gene. The *TSC1* gene encodes a protein named hamartin and the *TSC2* gene encodes tuberin. Both genes are tumour suppressor genes, with evidence of loss of heterozygosity for the *TSC1* and *TSC2* gene regions in various hamartomas from TSC patients [7–9]. No obvious phenotypic differences have been found between families linked to *TSC1* and *TSC2* [10]. Analysis of deletions of the *TSC2* locus has identified one specific correlation, namely severe polycystic kidney disease, caused by a contiguous gene deletion involving both *TSC2* and the polycystic kidney disease gene *PKD1* [11].

Clinical features
The characteristic features of the syndrome are skin lesions, intellectual impairment and epilepsy, but these show a very wide variation in age of onset and severity [12–16]. Onset before the age of 5 years with cutaneous changes or with epilepsy is typical, although the disease may remain undiagnosed until adolescence or adult life. Diagnostic criteria (Box 78.3) have been agreed by the Tuberous Sclerosis Alliance [17,18,19]. A definitive clinical diagnosis of TSC requires two major features.

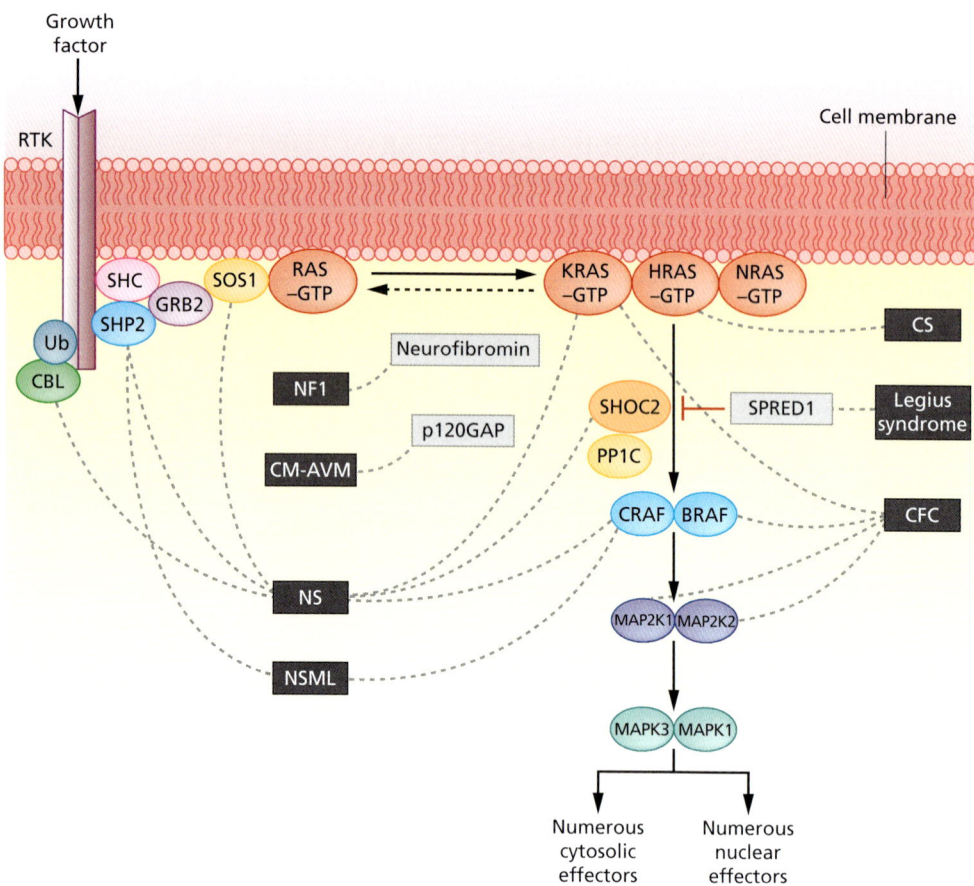

Figure 78.5 The Ras–mitogen-activated protein kinase (MAPK) signal transduction pathway. The MAPK signalling pathway of protein kinases is critically involved in cellular proliferation, differentiation, motility, apoptosis and senescence. The RASopathies are medical genetic syndromes caused by pathogenic variants in genes that encode components or regulators of the Ras-MAPK pathway (indicated by dashed lines). These disorders include neurofibromatosis type 1 (NF1), Noonan syndrome (NS), Noonan syndrome with multiple lentigines (NSML), capillary malformation–arteriovenous malformation syndrome (CM-AVM), Costello syndrome (CS), cardio-facio-cutaneous syndrome (CFC) and Legius syndrome. RKT, receptor tyrosine kinase; Ub, ubiquitin. Reproduced from Rauen 2013 [74] with permission of Annual Reviews.

Skin lesions. Skin lesions are found in 60–70% of cases; four types are pathognomonic:

1 *Angiofibromas.* Angiofibromas (Figure 78.6) may rarely be present at birth or develop in infancy, but usually appear between the ages of 3 and 10 years, and sometimes later. They often become more extensive at puberty and then remain unchanged. Firm, discrete, red-brown, telangiectatic papules, 1–10 mm in diameter, extend from the naso-labial furrows to the cheeks and chin, and are occasionally found in the ears.

2 *Periungual fibromas.* Periungual fibromas (Koenen tumours) appear at or after puberty as smooth, firm, flesh-coloured protuberances emerging from the nail folds. They are usually 5–10 mm in length but may be very large. This can be the only clinically evident abnormality.

3 *Connective tissue naevi.* Connective tissue naevi (also termed shagreen patches) present as irregularly thickened, slightly elevated, soft, skin-coloured plaques, usually in the lumbo-sacral region.

4 *White ovoid or ash-leaf-shaped macules.* These are 1–3 cm in length, most easily detectable by examination under Wood light, and are frequently present on the trunk or limbs [20]. They are a valuable physical sign as they may be found at birth or in early infancy, some years before other signs of the disease develop, and may suggest the correct diagnosis of TSC in infants with convulsions. However, it is important to appreciate that hypopigmented macules are seen in 2–3 per 1000 of apparently normal newborn babies and therefore their presence alone is not indicative of TSC [21].

Other cutaneous manifestations include:
- Firm fibromatous plaques, especially on the forehead [12] and scalp (Figure 78.7).
- Soft pedunculated fibromas around the neck and axillae.
- Eyelash poliosis [22].
- Fibromatous tumours, which are occasionally present on the gums and palate.
- Small pits, which commonly occur in the tooth enamel in adult patients and have been used as an early diagnostic sign in children with TSC [23].

Mosaic forms of TSC. These are reported where only one component of the syndrome is clinically evident [24,25], although postmortem findings in such cases often show the involvement of other organs. Unilateral, multiple, facial angiofibromas have been reported in two patients with a mosaic form of TSC [26].

Neurological features. Learning difficulties are present in 60–70% of cases and may be progressive, but if intellectual development has been normal throughout childhood subsequent deterioration is uncommon [27]. Some patients have presented with behavioural disorders, with normal intelligence. In particular, self-injury behaviour is quite common, occurring in up to 10% of patients [28].

Table 78.2 Genetic syndromes of the Ras-MAPK pathway.

Syndrome	Ras-MAPK pathway gene	Protein	Protein function	Clinical phenotype
Neurofibromatosis type 1	NF1	Neurofibromin	RasGAP	Café-au-lait macules; intertriginous freckling; neurofibromas and plexiform neurofibromas; iris Lisch nodules; osseous dysplasia; optic pathway glioma; normal neurocognitive function or mild impairment; predisposition to other cancers
Noonan syndrome	PTPN11	SHP2	Phosphatase	Cranio-facial dysmorphic features, including a broad forehead, hypertelorism, down-slanting palpebral fissures, ptosis, a high-arched palate and low-set, posteriorly rotated ears; congenital heart defects; short stature; undescended testicles; ophthalmological abnormalities; bleeding disorders; normal neurocognitive function or mild impairment; predisposition to cancer
	SOS1	SOS1	RasGEF	
	RAF1	CRAF	Kinase	
	KRAS	KRAS	GTPase	
	NRAS	NRAS	GTPase	
	SHOC2	SHOC2	Scaffolding	
	CBL	CBL	E3 ubiquitin ligase	
Noonan syndrome with multiple lentigines	PTPN11	SHP2	Phosphatase kinase	Same as Noonan syndrome, but with possible development of multiple skin lentigines as individuals age; unclear predisposition to cancer
	RAF1	RAF1/CRAF		
Capillary malformation–arteriovenous malformation	RASA1	p120-RasGAP	RasGAP	Multifocal capillary malformations, which may be associated with arteriovenous malformations and fistulae; unclear predisposition to cancer
Costello syndrome	HRAS	HRAS	GTPase	Cranio-facial features similar to those of Noonan syndrome but potentially more coarse; congenital heart defects; failure to thrive; short stature; ophthalmological abnormalities; multiple skin manifestations, including papilloma; normal neurocognitive function or mild impairment; hypotonia; predisposition to cancer
Cardio-facio-cutaneous syndrome	BRAF	BRAF	Kinase	Cranio-facial features similar to those of Noonan syndrome; congenital heart defects; failure to thrive; short stature; ophthalmological abnormalities; multiple skin manifestations, including progressive formation of naevi; normal neurocognitive function or mild impairment; hypotonia; unclear predisposition to cancer
	MAP2K1	MEK1	Kinase	
	MAP2K2	MEK2	Kinase	
	KRAS	KRAS	GTPase	
Legius syndrome	SPRED1	SPRED1	SPROUTY-related, EVH1 domain-containing protein 1	Café-au-lait macules; intertriginous freckling; macrocephaly; normal neurocognitive function or mild impairment; no apparent predisposition to cancer

Adapted from Rauen 2013 [74] with permission of Annual Reviews.
GTPase, guanosine triphosphatase; RasGAP, Ras GTPase activating protein; RasGEF, Ras-guanine nucleotide exchange factors.

Psychotic symptoms, including schizophrenia, sometimes develop, but may not be higher than in the general population [27].

Epilepsy is seen in 84% of patients [29]. It usually begins in infancy or early childhood, thus often preceding the skin lesions by many years. Less frequently, the onset of epilepsy is delayed until puberty or adult life. The attacks may be focal and often become progressively more frequent and severe, but there may be long remissions. Treatment can be quite challenging and in some cases requires surgery. Intracranial malignant change occurs in a few patients.

Ocular signs. These occur in 50% of cases but may be hard to detect [30,31]. Retinal phacomas are seen as white streaks along the vessels or as small, rounded tumours near the disc. Pigmentary and other retinal abnormalities can occur. Symptoms are rare but there may be scotomas or amaurosis. Hypopigmented spots in the iris also occur and these may be analogous to the ash-leaf macule in the skin [32].

Cardiac rhabdomyomas. Cardiac rhabdomyomas, detected by echocardiography, occur in over 50% of infants [33–35]. These tumours may result in early death; however, recent evidence suggests that in the majority these tumours regress in early infancy and again in adolescence [35]. Prenatal detection of these tumours is now possible by fetal echocardiography [36,37] and is often the initial clue to the diagnosis.

Renal involvement. This includes angiomyolipoma [38], a benign tumour of the renal parenchyma and, less commonly, renal cysts [39,40].

Pulmonary involvement. Pulmonary involvement is uncommon [41]. Lymphangio-leiomyomatosis (LAM) is almost exclusively seen in females [42] and tends to become clinically manifest in the second decade as increasing dyspnoea and recurrent spontaneous pneumothorax [43]. Male patients may develop multifocal micronodular pulmonary hyperplasia (MPPH) [44].

Gastrointestinal tumours. These are usually hamartomatous colonic polyps.

Endocrine disorders. Endocrine disorders frequently reported are pituitary–adrenal dysfunction, thyroid disorders and premature puberty.

Disease course and prognosis

Mortality is significantly increased in patients with TSC, with one study estimating a fivefold higher mortality than that in an age- and gender-matched population [45]. One review of disease burden estimated a mortality of between 4.8% and 8.3% associated with TSC, during a follow-up period of 8–17.4 years [46]. Death is usually due

Box 78.3 Diagnostic criteria for the tuberous sclerosis complex

Major features

- Hypomelanotic macules (≥3, at least 5 mm diameter)
- Angiofibromas (≥3) or fibrous cephalic plaque
- Ungual fibromas (≥2)
- Shagreen patch
- Multiple retinal hamartomas
- Cortical dysplasias[a]
- Subependymal nodules
- Subependymal giant cell astrocytoma (SEGA)
- Cardiac rhabdomyoma
- Lymphangioleiomyomatosis (LAM)[b]
- Angiomyolipomas (≥2)[b]

Minor features

- 'Confetti' skin lesions
- Dental enamel pits (>3)
- Intraoral fibromas (≥2)
- Retinal achromic patch
- Multiple renal cysts
- Non-renal hamartomas

Definite diagnosis: two major features or one major feature with two or more minor features

Possible diagnosis: either one major feature or two or more minor features

[a] Includes tubers and cerebral white matter radial migration lines.
[b] A combination of the two major clinical features (LAM and angiomyolipomas) without other features does not meet criteria for a definite diagnosis.

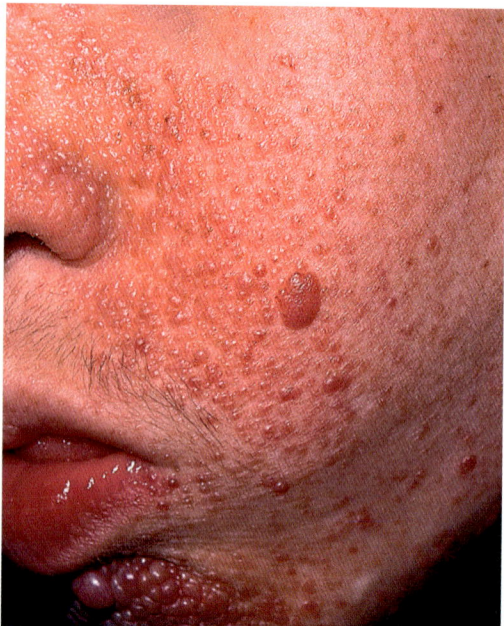

Figure 78.6 Tuberous sclerosis: angiofibromas. Courtesy of Professor J. Harper, Great Ormond Street Hospital, London, UK.

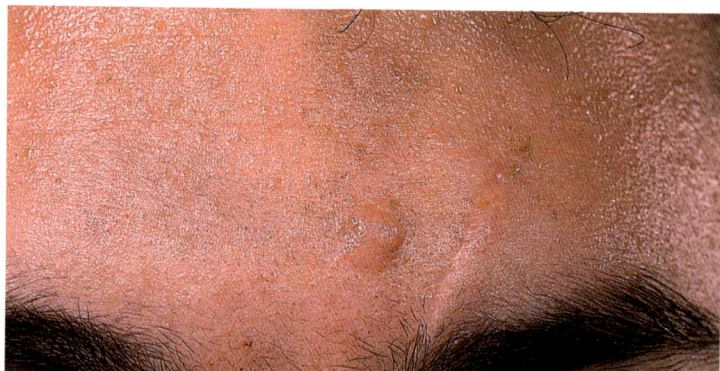

Figure 78.7 Tuberous sclerosis: fibromatous nodule on the forehead. Courtesy of Professor J. Harper, Great Ormond Street Hospital, London, UK.

to sudden unexplained death in epilepsy (SUDEP), kidney-related complications or complications relating to infection [46].

Investigations

The telangiectasia and lack of comedones and pustules distinguish angiofibromas from acne vulgaris, and biopsy may be useful if there is diagnostic uncertainty to distinguish this from other genetic conditions that present with facial papules (e.g. CYLD cutaneous syndrome, Birt–Hogg–Dubé syndrome). White ash-leaf-shaped macules may be evident under Wood light examination. MRI of the brain, computed tomography (CT) of the kidneys and ophthalmological examination should be requested.

Genetic testing of *TSC1* and *TSC2* is positive in 85% of cases and is routinely performed in new patients. Approximately 60–70% of TSC cases are thought to be the result of *de novo* mutations. Genetic testing of parents is available when a *TSC* pathogenic variant has been identified in an affected child to determine if either parent carries the variant, as this may influence genetic counselling. Any child of a person diagnosed as having TSC has a 50% chance of inheriting the disease. Family screening and genetic counselling should be carried out by referral to a clinical genetics service.

Management

Patients with TSC are increasingly managed by dedicated TSC multidisciplinary teams that involve renal physicians, neurologists, geneticists and dermatologists [47]. From a cutaneous perspective,

the cosmetic appearance may be improved by treating angiofibromas with topical mammalian target of rapamycin (mTOR) inhibitors in patients who are not receiving systemic mTOR inhibitors such as everolimus [48]. The more papular/nodular lesions may be treated surgically or using ablative lasers [49]. The surveillance and management recommendations specific for organ-related complications of TSC have been reviewed and summarised in a UK guideline [47]. It is important to recognise that systemic everolimus is now licensed and may be useful in the therapy of many of the visceral tumours and neurological complications, including epilepsy, in TSC.

Familial adenomatous polyposis

Classification links
- MIM: 175100

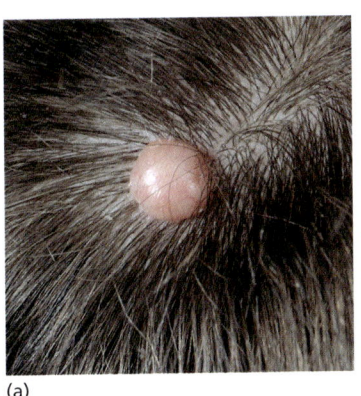 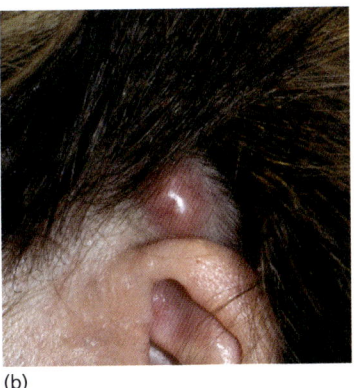

(a)   (b)

Figure 78.8 (a) Sclerosing collagenoma seen in a patient with Cowden syndrome and (b) cutaneous cylindroma in a patient with CYLD cutaneous syndrome demonstrating similar clinical features and showing the importance of histological diagnosis.

Introduction and general description

Familial adenomatous polyposis (FAP) is dominantly inherited. It is one of the *APC*-associated polyposis conditions [**50**], a group of disorders with familial polyposis as a central feature. Disorders in this spectrum include (i) FAP; (ii) attenuated FAP, which has a lower colonic polyp burden and lower cancer risk; and (iii) gastric adenocarcinoma and proximal polyposis of the stomach (GAPPS) [51]. All are caused by pathogenic variants in the *APC* gene and these variant syndromic combinations can be seen as an example of variable expressivity [52,**53**,54]. Eponymous terms such as Gardner and Turcot syndrome are considered historical terms.

Patients with FAP have the complex phenotype comprising multiple epidermoid cysts, fibrous tissue tumours, osteomas and polyposis of the colon. Congenital hypertrophy of the retinal pigment epithelium (CHRPE) is a frequent finding in FAP and is a valuable clue to the presence of the gene defect in persons who have not yet developed other manifestations [55,56].

Clinical features [53,54,57–60]

Cutaneous epidermoid cysts. These may be numerous and are usually irregularly distributed on the face, scalp and extremities, and are less frequent on the trunk. They may first appear between the ages of 4 and 10 years, but often considerably later, and are ultimately present in almost all cases. Pilomatrixomas have been reported. Fibromas or desmoid tumours affect 10–30% of patients with FAP. They are usually poorly localised tumours in incisional scars of the abdomen but may occur at other sites. Lipomas in the subcutaneous tissues, and in other organs, have frequently been noted.

Gastrointestinal polyposis of the colon or rectum. This usually arises during the second decade but may occur in early childhood. It is present in about 50% of patients by the age of 20 years. Malignant change develops some 15–20 years later in over 40% of reported cases. Gastric fundus polyps and small bowel polyps may also occur, with an increased risk of duodenal carcinoma reported. Patients with FAP are also at increased risk of hepatoblastoma.

Skeletal osteomas. These develop mainly in the maxilla, mandible and sphenoid bones, but also in other bones of the skull and, less frequently, in the long bones. They are usually small, multiple and present in some 50% of cases. The age of onset is often not accurately known, but they may be present at puberty.

Extracutaneous tumours. Extracutaneous tumours such as fibrosarcomas have also been associated with the syndrome. Fibromatous growths of the mesentery may be discovered at operation, and severe peritoneal scarring may follow surgery. Leiomyomas of the stomach or ileum, or retroperitoneal tissue, are sometimes present. Patients with APC pathogenic variants are at increased risk of benign thyroid disease and thyroid cancer, particularly the cribriform-morular variant of papillary thyroid cancer. Adrenal tumours are reported to occur [61]. FAP patients are at increased risk of central nervous system tumours, usually medulloblastoma.

Investigations

A diagnosis of FAP is considered in a patient with typically >100 colorectal adenomatous polyps. Genetic testing of the *APC* gene is usually offered as part of a gene panel as there are several polyposis genes. Skin biopsy may helpfully distinguish epidermoid cysts from trichilemmal cysts (*PLCD1*) and sebaceous cysts (*KRT17*) if the initial presentation is to dermatology and there is uncertainty.

Management

The mainstay of management of FAP is surveillance for somatic cancers, ideally under the direction of a cancer geneticist with specific knowledge in this area [**62**,63]. Surveillance investigations include colonoscopy, which may need to start from the age of 10–12 years, and ultrasound imaging for thyroid cancer and hepatoblastoma. Colectomy is usually recommended after adenomas emerge. Cascade genetic testing is helpful and will identify other affected members who may also benefit from cancer surveillance.

INHERITED TUMOUR SYNDROMES INVOLVING THE SKIN

The identification of a tumour predisposition syndrome can be challenging and relies on good phenotyping and a family history. Frequently, skin biopsy and a dermatopathology review are helpful aids. Identification of a pathogenic variant by genetic testing of the affected proband is a helpful diagnostic tool, and allows for cascade testing of related members of the family. As demonstrated with the exemplar syndromes earlier, diagnosis may lead to screening tests and, in some disorders, consideration for cancer chemoprevention (e.g. mismatch repair deficiencies such as Lynch syndrome), pre-emptive surgery to reduce cancer risk and consideration for emerging clinical trials. Tables 78.3, 78.4 and 78.5 give an overview of inherited tumour predisposition syndromes to aid recognition of these genetic disorders.

PART 6: GENETIC DISORDERS

Table 78.3 Skin syndromes linked with skin and other cancers. Recessive conditions are coloured blue.

Syndrome	Gene	MIM number	Skin phenotype	Extracutaneous features	Reference
Loss of function of a tumour suppressor gene					
Familial melanoma	*CDKN2A*[a]	606719	Dysplastic naevi Melanoma	Pancreatic cancer CNS tumours	[1]
Naevoid basal cell carcinoma syndrome	*PTCH1* *SUFU*	109400	Basal cell carcinoma Basal cell naevi Palmar pits	Odontogenic keratocysts Ovarian fibromas Mesenteric cysts Medulloblastoma	[2,3]
CYLD cutaneous syndrome (syn. Brooke–Spiegler) (Figure 78.8b)	*CYLD*	132700 605041 601606	Cylindromas Spiradenomas Hybrid cylindroma and spiradenoma Trichoepithelioma Milia	Salivary gland membranous basal cell adenoma Pulmonary metastases	[4]
Bazex–Christol–Dupré	*ACTRT1*	301845	Hypotrichosis Hair shaft abnormalities Milia Follicular atrophoderma Basal cell carcinoma Trichoepithelioma		[5]
Happle–Tinschert, Curry–Jones	*SMO*	601707	Basaloid follicular hamartomas Basal cell carcinoma	Polysyndactyly Unicoronal craniosyntosis Microphthalmia Intestinal malrotation	[6,7]
Increased susceptibility to DNA damage					
Dyskeratosis congenita	*TERC* Multiple genes, dominant and recessive forms: *ACD, CTC1, DKC1, NHP2, NOP10, PARN, RTEL1, TERC, TERT, TINF2, WRAP53*	602322	Skin hyperpigmentation, dysplastic nails, premature greying of the hair and increased risk of skin cancer associated with abnormal telomere maintenance	Bone marrow failure Pulmonary and hepatic fibrosis	[8]
Xeroderma pigmentosum	*XPA-G* *XPV* *POLH*	Multiple	Premature ageing Poikiloderma Wrinkling Early-onset BCC, SCC and melanoma	Ocular disease Neurological disease	[9]
Rothmund–Thomson 1	*ANAPC1*	618625	Poikiloderma Sparse hair Abnormal nails Bilateral juvenile cataracts Short stature	Skeletal abnormalities	[10]
Rothmund–Thomson 2, RAPADILINO, Baller–Gerold	*RECQL4*	268400 266280	Poikiloderma Sparse hair Abnormal nails Short stature	Osteosarcoma	[11,12]
Werner	*RECQL2* *LMNA*	604611	Premature ageing Melanoma	Short stature Bilateral cataracts Hypogonadism Thyroid cancer Meningiomas Sarcomas Leukaemia	[13,14]

Table 78.3 (*continued*)

Syndrome	Gene	MIM number	Skin phenotype	Extracutaneous features	Reference
Bloom	*RECQL3*	210900	Poikiloderma Photosensitivity	Short stature Immune deficiency Leukaemia Lymphoma Gastrointestinal tumours	[15,16]
Ataxia telangiectasia	*ATM*	208900	Telangiectasia	Ataxia Leukaemia Lymphoma	[17]
Reduced UV protection					
Oculocutaneous albinism	*TYR* *OCA2* *TYRP1* *SLC45A2* *SLC24A5* *C10orf11*	Multiple	Reduced UV protection associated with reduced or absent melanin production and increased risk of skin cancer	Reduced visual acuity Nystagmus	[18]
Hermansky–Pudlak	*HPS1, 3, 4, 5, 6* *AP3B1* *BLOC1S3* *BLOC1S6* *DTNBP1*	203300	Reduced skin pigmentation Squamous cell carcinoma	Prolonged bleeding Pulmonary fibrosis Granulomatous colitis Immunodeficiency	[19]
Diverse mechanisms mediating increased skin cancer risk					
Carney complex	*PRKAR1A*	160980 605244	Lentigines Myxoid neurofibromas	Atrial myxomas Primary pigmented nodular adrenocortical disease (PPNAD) Thyroid, testicular and ovarian tumours	[20]
Rombo, Nicolau–Balus, MALTA	*MYH9*	180730	Syringoma Microcystic adnexal carcinoma Atrophoderma vermiculata Milia		[21]
Ferguson–Smith	*TGFBR1*	132800	Multiple 'self-healing' squamous epitheliomas		[22]
Huriez	*SMARCAD1*	181600	Scleroatrophy of the distal fingers Palmoplantar keratoderma Nail hypoplasia Poikiloderma Early-onset SCC		[23]
Tylosis with oesophageal cancer	*RHBDF2*	148500	Palmoplantar hyperkeratosis	Oesophageal cancer	[24]
Clouston	*GJB6*	129500	Syringofibroadenoma Palmoplantar keratoderma Hypotrichosis Nail dystrophy	Some patients with *GJB2* mutations may have deafness in addition to the skin phenotype	[25,26]
Myotonic dystrophy	*DMPK*	160900	Pilomatrixomas	Myotonic dystrophy	[27]
Familial pilomatrixoma	*PLCD1*	132600	Pilomatrixomas		[28]
Schöpf–Schultz–Passarge	*WNT10a*	224750	Eyelid apocrine hirocystomas Hypotrichosis Basal cell carcinoma Palmoplantar keratoderma (eccrine syringofibroadenoma)	Hypodontia	[29]

(Continued)

Table 78.3 (*continued*)

Syndrome	Gene	MIM number	Skin phenotype	Extracutaneous features	Reference
Cartilage–hair hypoplasia	*RMRP*	250250	Hypotrichosis BCC	Skeletal dysplasia Immunodeficiency	[30]
Epidermodysplasia verruciformis	*EVER1* *EVER2* *CIB1*	226400	HPV susceptibility in the absence of lymphopenia Multiple warts SCC		[31]
Recessive dystrophic epidermolysis bullosa	*COL7A1*	226600	Recurrent blistering and scarring from birth associated with an increased risk of cutaneous SCC		[32]
Netherton	*SPINK5*	605010	Ichthyosis Bamboo hair Isolated reports of BCC and SCC		[33,34]

[a] Other genes are reported.

BCC, basal cell carcinoma; CNS, central nervous system; HPV, human papillomavirus; MALTA, MYH9-associated elastin aggregation; RAPADILINO, radial ray defect, patellar aplasia and palate abnormalities, diarrhoea and dislocated joints, limb abnormalities and little size, slender nose and normal intelligence; SCC, squamous cell carcinoma; UV, ultraviolet.

Table 78.4 Syndromes linked with gastrointestinal cancer.

Syndrome	Gene	MIM number	Skin phenotype	Extracutaneous features	Reference
Muir–Torre, Lynch	*MSH2* *MSH6* *PMS2* *MLH1*	158320	Sebaceous adenoma Sebaceous carcinoma Squamous cell carcinoma	Colorectal cancer Endometrial cancer Urothelial malignancies CNS tumours	[35]
Peutz–Jehghers	*STK11*		Perioral lentigines	Small bowel polyps Gastrointestinal cancer	[36]
Cowden (Figure 78.8a)	*PTEN*	158350	Trichilemmomas Oral papillomas Acral keratoses Mucocutaneous neuromas Sclerosing collagenoma Lipomas Fibromas Milia Macular pigmentation of the glans penis	Breast cancer Endometrial cancer Colon cancer Renal cell carcinoma Thyroid cancer (follicular)	[37]
Hereditary haemorrhagic telangiectasia	*SMAD4*	175050	Labial papular vascular lesions	Colorectal cancer	[38]

CNS, central nervous system.

Table 78.5 Syndromes linked with renal cancer.

Syndrome	Gene	MIM number	Skin phenotype	Extracutaneous features	Reference
Birt–Hogg–Dubé (Figure 78.9)	*FLCN*	315150	Fibrofolliculoma Trichodiscoma Skin tags (acrochordons)	Pulmonary cysts and associated risk of pneumothorax Renal cysts Renal cell carcinoma Rhabdomyoma	[39]
Hereditary leiomyomatosis and renal cell cancer (Figure 78.10)	*FH*	605839	Pilar leiomyomas	Uterine leiomyomas Leiomyosarcoma Renal cell carcinoma (type 2 papillary subtype)	[40]

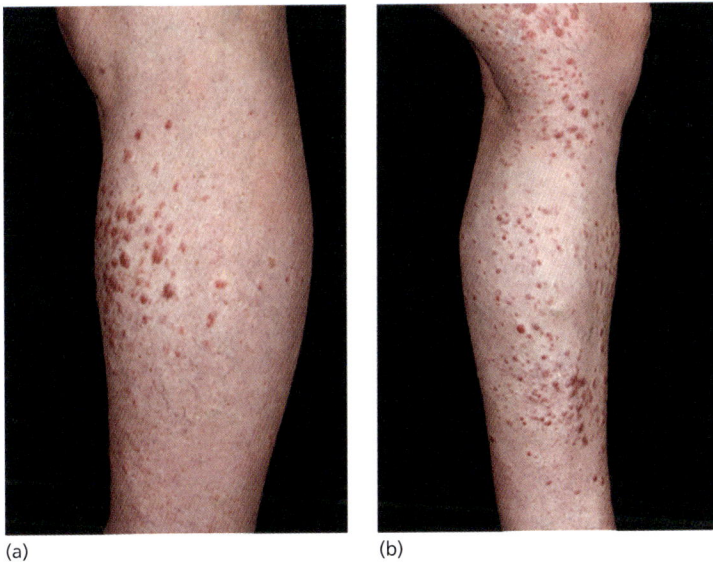

(a)   (b)

Figure 78.9 (a, b) Hereditary leiomyomatosis and renal cell cancer showing clustered pilar leiomyomas. Reproduced from Brown *et al.* [41] with permission of Royal College of Physicians.

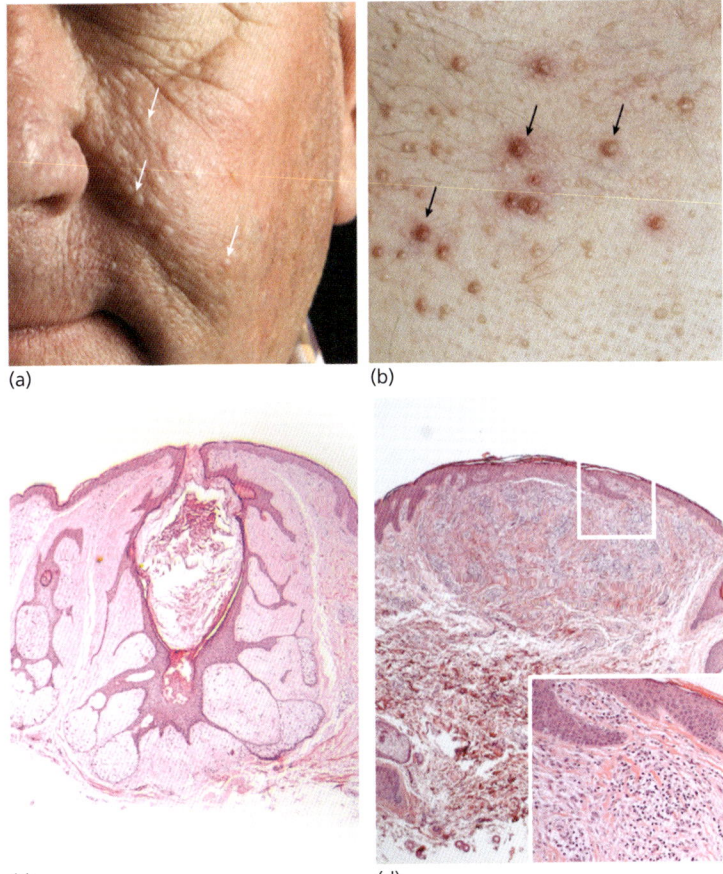

(a)   (b)

(c)   (d)

Figure 78.10 Birt–Hogg–Dubé syndrome. (a, b) Fibrofolliculomas. (c) Histology of a fibrofolliculoma. (d) Histology of a trichodiscoma. Reproduced from Brown *et al.* [41] with permission of Royal College of Physicians.

Conclusions

The syndromes outlined in this chapter highlight how a range of genes are important in the normal function of multiple tissues, and how the skin can be an indicator of an underlying genetic disease. A personal and family history, a full skin examination and in some cases a biopsy are important steps in determining the underlying genetic diagnosis and the selection of relevant genetic tests. These may be important in confirming the diagnosis, genetic counselling and family planning, as well as the selection of therapeutic approaches, and are often performed in the context of a multidisciplinary team.

Key references

The full list of references can be found in the online version at https://www.wiley.com/rooksdermatology10e

Neurofibromatoses

6 Evans DG. Neurofibromatosis type 2 (NF2): a clinical and molecular review. *Orphanet J Rare Dis* 2009;4:16.

11 Legius E, Messiaen L, Wolkenstein P *et al.* Revised diagnostic criteria for neurofibromatosis type 1 and Legius syndrome: an international consensus recommendation. *Genet Med* 2021;23:1506–13.

19 Viskochil D, Buchberg AM, Xu G *et al.* Deletions or translocation interrupt a cloned gene at the neurofibromatosis type 1 locus. *Cell* 1990;62:187–92.

20 Wallace MR, Marchuk DA, Anderson LB *et al.* Type 1 neurofibromatosis gene: identification of a large transcript disrupted in three NF1 patients. *Science* 1990;249:181–6.

66 Gross AM, Dombi E, Widemann BC. Current status of MEK inhibitors in the treatment of plexiform neurofibromas. *Childs Nerv Syst* 2020;36:2443–52.

72 García-Romero MT, Parkin P, Lara-Corrales I. Mosaic neurofibromatosis type 1: a systematic review. *Pediatr Dermatol* 2016;33:9–17.

75 Tidyman WE, Rauen KA. Expansion of the RASopathies. *Curr Genet Med Rep* 2016;4:57–64.

Other inherited skin tumour syndromes

3 Sampson JR, Scahill SJ, Stephenson JBP *et al.* Genetic aspects of tuberous sclerosis in the west of Scotland. *J Med Genet* 1989;26:28–31.

19 Northrup H, Krueger DA, International Tuberous Sclerosis Complex Consensus Group. Tuberous sclerosis complex diagnostic criteria update: recommendations of the 2012 International Tuberous Sclerosis Complex Consensus Conference. *Pediatr Neurol* 2013;49:243–54.

24 Happle R, Torrelo A. Superimposed mosaicism in tuberous sclerosis complex: a key to understanding all of the manifold manifestations? *J Eur Acad Dermatol Venereol* 2020;34:2511–17

25 Tyburczy ME, Dies KA, Glass J *et al.* Mosaic and intronic mutations in TSC1/TSC2 explain the majority of TSC patients with no mutation identified by conventional testing. *PLOS Genet* 2015;11:e1005637.

27 De Vries PJ, Wilde L, de Vries MC, Moavero R, Pearson DA, Curatolo P. A clinical update on tuberous sclerosis complex-associated neuropsychiatric disorders (TAND). *Am J Med Genet C Semin Med Genet* 2018;178:309–20.

48 Kingswood JC, Belousova E, Benedik MP *et al.* TuberOus SClerosis registry to increase disease Awareness (TOSCA) post-authorisation safety study of everolimus in patients with tuberous sclerosis complex. *Front Neurol* 2021;12:630378.

50 Jasperson KW, Patel SG, Ahnen DJ. APC-associated polyposis conditions. In: Adam MP, Ardinger HH, Pagon RA *et al.*, eds. *GeneReviews® [Internet]*. Seattle, WA: University of Washington, 1993–2022.

53 Juhn E, Khachemoune A. Gardner syndrome: skin manifestations, differential diagnosis and management. *Am J Clin Dermatol* 2010;11:117–22.

62 Aihara H, Kumar N, Thompson CC. Diagnosis, surveillance, and treatment strategies for familial adenomatous polyposis: rationale and update. *Eur J Gastroenterol Hepatol* 2014;26:255–62.

CHAPTER 79

Inherited Metabolic Diseases

Andrew A.M. Morris

Manchester Centre for Genomic Medicine, Manchester University Hospitals NHS Foundation Trust, Manchester, UK

PART 6: GENETIC DISORDERS

Introduction

Inherited metabolic diseases or 'inborn errors of metabolism' are caused by deficiencies of enzymes or transport proteins. They are extremely diverse and often multisystem diseases. They are classified according to the organelle or pathway involved. Groups of inherited metabolic diseases with dermatological features are listed in Table 79.1, which indicates whether the disorder is described here or elsewhere.

LYSOSOMAL STORAGE DISORDERS

Lysosomes contain more than 50 acid hydrolases for the degradation of macromolecules, which accumulate if a hydrolase is deficient. The clinical features vary depending on the precise disorder and the severity of the deficiency. The characteristic dermatological findings are angiokeratomas (as in Fabry disease) and thickened skin and hypertrichosis, which lead to a 'coarse' facial appearance when combined with abnormalities of the facial skeleton (as in the mucopolysaccharidoses).

Mucopolysaccharidoses

MPSs are caused by impaired degradation of long sugar chains called glycosaminoglycans (or mucopolysaccharides), which are found in connective tissue, bound to core proteins to form proteoglycans. The clinical features are summarised in Table 79.2 and

include a 'coarse' facial appearance, hepatosplenomegaly, bone dysplasia and developmental regression.

Incidence
The total incidence of MPS is approximately 1 in 25 000.

Genetics
All mucopolysaccharidoses show autosomal recessive inheritance except for MPS II, which is X-linked recessive.

Clinical features
Patients usually present in early childhood with developmental delay. Ear, nose and throat infections, upper airway obstruction and deafness are common. Valvular heart disease is often the cause of death.

Dysmorphism. The coarse facial appearance is seldom noticeable at birth and becomes more apparent with time (Figure 79.1). Hypoplasia of the mid facial bones leads to a flat nasal bridge. The skin and lips are thickened and the tongue is enlarged. Mouth breathing is common due to adenoidal hypertrophy. Many patients have generalised hypertrichosis and some have synophrys. Corneal clouding is seen in MPS I, VI and VII. The hands appear podgy with short, broad digits. The facial dysmorphism is absent in MPS IV and subtle in MPS III.

Other dermatological features. Ivory white papules or nodules are often seen on the back of patients with severe MPS II and may occur in MPS I. Individual nodules range from 1 to 10 mm in size and they may coalesce to form ridges or a reticular pattern [1]. Typically,

Table 79.1 Inherited metabolic diseases with dermatological features.

Group of disorders	Examples	Dermatological features	Where considered
Lysosomal disorders	Mucopolysaccharidoses	Coarse features, hirsute	This chapter
	Fabry disease	Angiokeratomas	This chapter
Mitochondrial disorders	MERRF syndrome	Lipomatosis	This chapter
	Ethylmalonic encephalopathy	Acrocyanosis	This chapter
Congenital defects of glycosylation	Phosphomannomutase 2 deficiency	Fat pads, inverted nipples	This chapter
	Other defects	Cutis laxa, ichthyosis	This chapter and Chapter 94
Amino acid disorders	Phenylketonuria	Hypopigmentation	This chapter
	Tyrosinaemia type 2	Hyperkeratoses	This chapter and Chapter 63
	Various	Oculocutaneous albinism	Chapter 68
	Prolidase deficiency	Ulcers, scarring	This chapter and Chapter 72
	Argininosuccinic aciduria	Trichorrhexis nodosa	This chapter and Chapter 66
	Serine, proline and glutamine synthesis disorders	Ichthyosis, cutis laxa, erythroderma	This chapter
Carbohydrate disorders	Glycogen storage diseases	Xanthomas	Chapter 60
Lipid disorders	Hyperlipidaemias	Xanthomas	Chapter 60
	Cerebrotendinous xanthomatosis	Xanthomas	Chapter 60
	Smith–Lemli–Opitz syndrome	Photosensitivity	This chapter
	Complex lipid disorders	Ichthyosis	Chapter 63
	Berardinelli-Seip syndrome, etc.	Lipodystrophy	Chapter 72
Haem disorders	Porphyrias	Photosensitive rashes	Chapter 58
Vitamin disorders	Biotin disorders	Alopecia, rash	This chapter and Chapter 66
Mineral disorders	Acrodermatitis enteropathica	Alopecia, periorificial rash	This chapter and Chapter 63
	Menkes disease	Pili torti, cutis laxa	This chapter and Chapter 94
	Wilson disease	Xerosis, blue lunulae	This chapter
	Haemochromatosis	Hyperpigmentation	Chapter 86
	Familial tumoral calcinosis	Calcinosis	This chapter

Table 79.2 Classification of the mucopolysaccharidoses.

Number	MIM	Eponym	Clinical features	Enzyme deficiency	Glycosaminoglycans excreted
MPS I	252800	Hurler or Scheie[a]	Dysmorphism, corneal clouding, DM, heart disease, HSM, ±PI	α-L-Iduronidase	DS, HS
MPS II	309900	Hunter	Dysmorphism, DM, HSM, heart disease, ±PI	Iduronate sulphatase	DS, HS
MPS III	252900	Sanfilippo	PI, regression, hyperactivity, mild somatic features	4 possible enzymes	HS
MPS IVA	253000	Morquio A	DM, joint laxity, corneal clouding, normal intelligence	Galactose 6-sulphatase	Keratan sulphate
MPS IVB	253010	Morquio B	Milder DM, slow neurodegeneration	β-Galactosidase	Keratan sulphate
MPS VI	253200	Maroteaux–Lamy	Dysmorphism, DM, corneal clouding, normal intelligence	N-Acetyl-galactosamine 4-sulphatase	DS
MPS VII	253220	Sly	Hydrops fetalis, dysmorphism, DM, HSM, PI	β-Glucuronidase	DS, HS
MPS IX	601492	Natowicz	Soft periarticular masses, arthritis	Hyaluronidase	Hyaluronan

[a] Scheie syndrome refers to mild MPS I with normal intelligence and potentially normal lifespan.
DM, dysostosis multiplex; DS, dermatan sulphate; HS, heparan sulphate; HSM, hepatosplenomegaly; PI, psychomotor impairment.

they are found laterally, between the angles of the scapulae and posterior axillary lines (Figure 79.2). Papules may also be found on the upper arms and outer thighs. They appear at 1–4 years but may clear in older patients. Mongolian blue spots are common in MPS I and II and may be found on the upper back, the anterior trunk or the limbs, in addition to the sacro-coccygeal region. The spots fade more slowly than normal: in Japanese patients they persist until the teenage years [2].

Developmental regression. This is the dominant feature in MPS III. After a period of hyperactivity, behaviour problems and sleep disturbance, patients gradually deteriorate into a vegetative state. Learning difficulties are also present in severe cases of MPS I, II and VII. Other neurological problems may include seizures, hydrocephalus, spinal cord compression and carpal tunnel syndrome.

Bone dysplasia (dysostosis multiplex). This is a particular problem in patients with MPS IV. These patients have very short stature and joint laxity leading to arthritis of the hip and knee and a risk of atlanto-axial dislocation. In the other MPSs, the joints are stiff and short stature is associated with kyphosis.

Differential diagnosis

Mucopolysaccharidosis-like problems (including coarse facial features) occur in other lysosomal disorders, such as glycoproteinoses, mucolipidoses and a few sphingolipidoses (the severe forms of galactosialidosis and G_{M1} gangliosidosis). Patients presenting with an MPS-like phenotype at birth are likely to have mucolipidosis type II or G_{M1} gangliosidosis. The differential diagnoses can be identified by analysis of urinary oligosaccharides, combined with lysosomal enzyme assays in plasma and leukocytes.

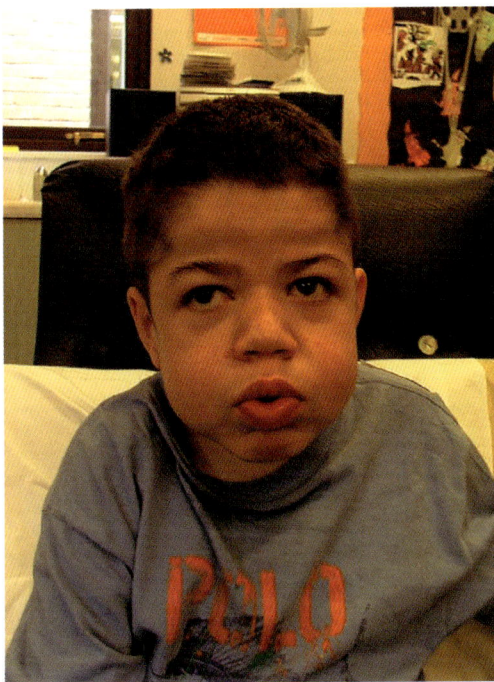

Figure 79.1 Facial features of an 8-year-old boy with MPS II.

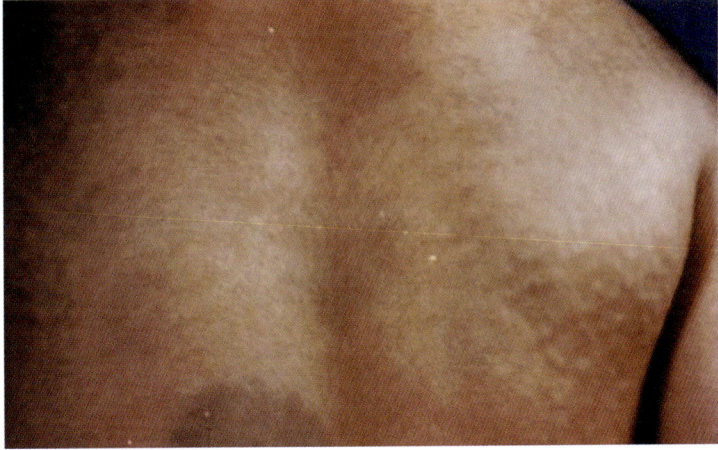

Figure 79.2 'Pebbling' of the skin and large Mongolian blue spot on the back of a boy with MPS II. Reproduced from Wraith 2006 [78] with permission of Springer Nature.

Investigations
The initial investigation is analysis of urine glycosaminoglycans. Diagnoses are confirmed by enzyme assays on leukocytes or by mutation analysis.

Histology
Malpighian cells in the epidermis are distended with pale cytoplasm. The papules in MPS II show pooling of metachromatic material between the collagen bundles of the lower reticular dermis. Fibroblasts and Schwann cells show cytoplasmic metachromasia when stained with toluidine blue; ultrastructurally, they contain membrane-bound cytoplasmic vacuoles [3].

Management
Symptomatic treatment may include ear, nose and throat care, and orthopaedic and neurosurgery involvement. Medication can be

useful for sleep and behaviour problems, especially in MPS III. Haematopoietic stem cell transplantation (HSCT) is an established treatment for Hurler and Maroteaux–Lamy syndromes, using bone marrow or umbilical cord blood [4]. Transplantation in infancy leads to an improvement in most systems and can preserve normal developmental progress in Hurler syndrome but the skeletal problems progress and ophthalmological problems persist. Moreover, HSCT has significant morbidity and mortality. Enzyme replacement therapy (ERT) is now available for MPS I, II, IV, VI and VII. Its major limitation is the inability of the enzyme to cross the blood–brain barrier. Bone and heart valve disease are also resistant to ERT but starting treatment early improves outcomes [5].

Glycoproteinoses

Introduction and general description
Most secreted and cell surface proteins are glycosylated. The oligosaccharide components of glycoproteins are degraded by lysosomal hydrolases, deficiency of which leads to the storage of oligosaccharides and/or glycopeptides. All the glycoproteinoses show autosomal recessive inheritance and are very rare. Their features are summarised in Table 79.3. Many have a coarse facial appearance or angiokeratomas.

Clinical features

Fucosidosis. (MIM: 230000) presents in early childhood with developmental delay, followed by neurological deterioration. Other clinical features include a slightly coarse facial appearance, short stature, hypohydrosis and hepatosplenomegaly. Angiokeratomas appear in mid to late childhood and are present in 85% of patients aged over 20 years [6]. The angiokeratomas usually have the same appearance and distribution as in Fabry disease but may be confined to the limbs (Figure 79.3). Similar lesions may occur on the lips, gums or tongue.

Alpha-mannosidosis. Alpha-mannosidosis (MIM: 248500) is associated with coarse facial features, learning difficulties, deafness, corneal clouding, cataracts, dysostosis multiplex, hepatosplenomegaly and frequent infections.

Beta-mannosidosis. Beta-mannosidosis (MIM: 248510) presents with learning difficulties, deafness and frequent infections; the face is not coarse but angiokeratomas are occasionally present.

Sialidosis. There are two main types of sialidosis (MIM: 256550). Mildly affected patients (type I) present as adolescents or adults with myoclonus, visual impairment and a macular 'cherry red spot' on fundoscopy. Severely affected patients (type II) present in early childhood with coarse facies, developmental delay, dysostosis multiplex and hepatosplenomegaly.

Aspartylglucosaminuria. Aspartylglucosaminuria (MIM: 208400) is extremely rare except in Finland. Patients have developmental

Table 79.3 Glycoproteinoses, sphingolipidoses and mucolipidoses with cutaneous features.

Name	Enzyme deficiency	Cutaneous features	Other clinical features
Glycoproteinoses			
Fucosidosis	α-L-Fucosidase	Coarse (mild), angiokeratomas	PI
α-Mannosidosis	α-Mannosidase	Coarse	PI, deafness, DM, HSM, frequent infections
β-Mannosidosis	β-Mannosidase	Angiokeratomas	PI, deafness, frequent infections
Sialidosis type II	Neuraminidase	Coarse	PI, DM, HSM
Aspartylglucosaminuria	Aspartylglucosaminidase	Coarse, angiofibromas, angiokeratomas	PI, regression, seizures
Kanzaki	α-*N*-Acetylgalactosaminidase	Angiokeratomas, coarse (mild)	PI
Sphingolipidoses			
Fabry	α-Galactosidase A	Angiokeratomas, hypohydrosis	Acroparaesthesia, renal failure, heart disease, strokes
G_{M1} gangliosidosis (early-onset form)	β-Galactosidase	Coarse, angiokeratomas, telangiectasia	Hydrops, HSM, DM, PI, regression, spasticity, CRS
Galactosialidosis (early-onset form)	PPCA	Coarse, telangiectasia	Hydrops, HSM, heart disease, DM, PI, CRS
Galactosialidosis (later-onset form)	PPCA	Angiokeratomas, coarse (mild)	Myoclonus, ataxia, PI, CRS
Gaucher types I and III	β-Glucosidase	Pigmentation, telangiectasia	Bone pain, DM, HSM ± regression (type III)
Gaucher type II	β-Glucosidase	Collodion baby	HSM, squint, stridor, dysphagia, spasticity
Niemann–Pick A	Sphingomyelinase	Papules, pigmentation	HSM, lymphadenopathy, PI, regression, spasticity, CRS
Niemann–Pick B	Sphingomyelinase	Papules, pigmentation	HSM, lung disease
Farber	Ceramidase	Nodules	Hoarse voice, arthritis, PI, regression, CRS
Mucolipidoses and other disorders			
Mucolipidosis type II	Multiple	Coarse	Gum hypertrophy, DM, PI, cardiomyopathy
Mucolipidosis type III	Multiple	Coarse (mild)	Arthritis, DM, PI
Multiple sulphatase deficiency	Multiple	Coarse ± ichthyosis	PI, regression, HSM, DM
Infantile sialic acid storage disease	Sialic acid transporter	Coarse, hypopigmentation	PI, HSM, DM, hydrops/ascites

CRS, cherry red spot; DM, dysostosis multiplex; HSM, hepatosplenomegaly; PPCA protective protein/cathepsin A; PI, psychomotor impairment.

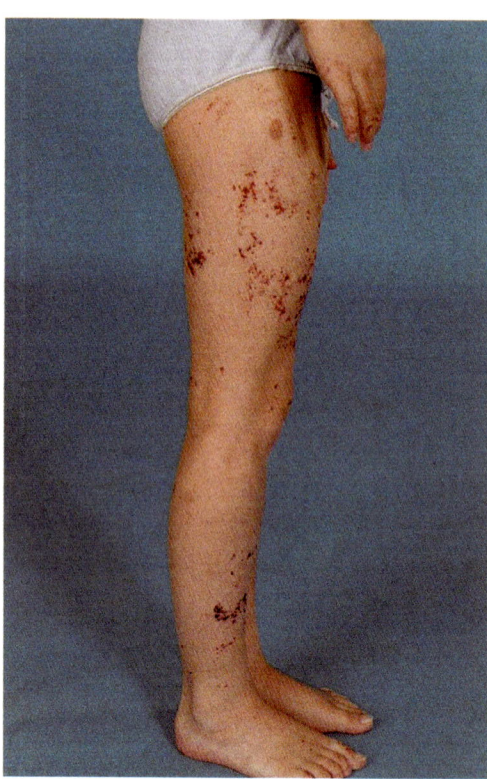

Figure 79.3 Angiokeratoma corporis diffusum on a 7-year-old girl with fucosidosis.

Alpha-*N*-acetyl-galactosaminidase deficiency. Alpha-*N*-acetyl-galactosaminidase deficiency (MIM: 104170) is an extremely rare cause of angiokeratomas in adults, sometimes with lymphoedema and polyneuropathy (Kanzaki disease). The angiokeratomas may have a similar distribution to Fabry disease or may be more widespread [8]. The enzyme deficiency has been reported in infants with neurodegeneration (Schindler disease) but it may not have been responsible.

Investigations

These diagnoses are generally established by enzyme assays, usually on leukocytes but, for sialidosis, neuraminidase can only be assayed in cultured cells. Many laboratories offer a set of lysosomal enzyme assays on leukocytes for screening patients with relevant features. Electron microscopy of the skin often shows cytoplasmic vacuoles, particularly in endothelial cells, fibroblasts, Schwann cells and the myoepithelial cells of sweat glands [8,9].

Management

For most of these disorders, only symptomatic treatment is available. ERT is being developed for α-mannosidosis and bone marrow transplantation may improve the neurological outcome in fucosidosis.

delay in childhood and regress after puberty, eventually becoming severely disabled. There is gradual coarsening of the facial features, with sagging skin, thick lips, a broad low nasal bridge and coarse hair. Facial angiofibromas, gingival overgrowth and buccal oedema are common in adults [7]. Angiokeratomas are less common.

Mucolipidoses types II and III

Introduction and general description

These are autosomal recessive disorders, in which multiple lysosomal enzymes fail to enter their organelle. Mucolipidosis II (MIM: 252500) refers to the severe end of the spectrum: patients often present at birth with coarse facial features. They also have gum hypertrophy, severe neurological involvement, dysostosis multiplex and cardiomyopathy. In mucolipidosis III (MIM: 252600), the main problem is arthritis (due to skeletal dysplasia); there may also be mild learning difficulties (Table 79.3).

Investigations
The diagnosis is established by demonstrating raised levels of the mis-targeted lysosomal enzymes in plasma. Skin histology reveals membrane-bound vacuoles and cytoplasmic bodies in fibroblasts and other mesenchymal cells.

Management
Only symptomatic treatment is available.

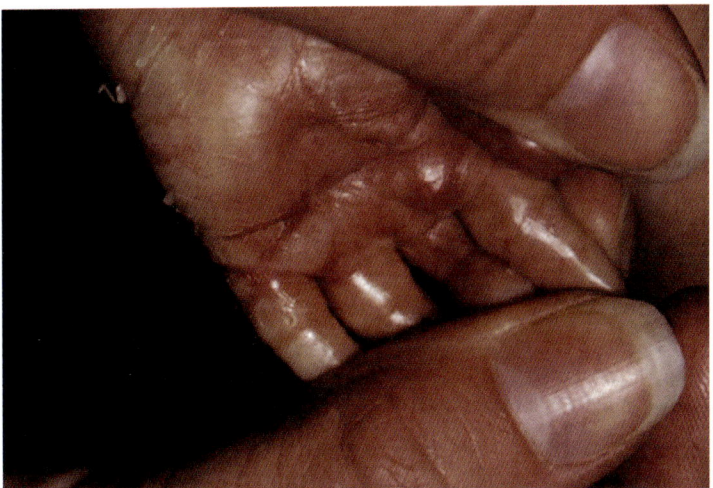

Figure 79.4 The hand of a 'collodion baby' with Gaucher disease type II.

Sphingolipidoses

Introduction and general description
Sphingolipids are amphiphilic molecules found in cell membranes. They are degraded by lysosomal hydrolases and deficiencies of these enzymes (or their protector proteins) cause the sphingolipidoses. Some sphingolipidoses (e.g. Tay–Sachs disease) only affect the nervous system. Other sphingolipidoses may be associated with coarse facial features, angiokeratomas or other dermatological abnormalities and are included in Table 79.3. Fabry disease is described separately, later.

Genetics
All the sphingolipidoses are autosomal recessive disorders, except Fabry disease, which is X-linked.

Clinical features

G_{M1} **gangliosidosis.** G_{M1} gangliosidosis (MIM: 230500) is very rare and has a wide clinical spectrum. Severe cases present as neonates with hydrops fetalis or hypotonia, hepatosplenomegaly and facial dysmorphism (including macroglossia, gum hypertrophy and a depressed nasal bridge). Neurodegeneration is the main feature in other cases. The mildest cases present in late childhood with dysarthria, dystonia and skeletal dysplasia (affecting the spine and hip). Angiokeratomas are prominent in a few patients with infantile G_{M1} gangliosidosis, affecting the trunk, thighs and upper arms [10]. Telangiectasia and extensive Mongolian blue spots have also been reported in infantile cases.

Galactosialidosis. Galactosialidosis (MIM: 256540) is extremely rare. Deficiency of protective protein/cathepsin A leads to a combined deficiency of neuraminidase and β-galactosidase. Neonatal-onset patients resemble those with G_{M1} gangliosidosis and often have telangiectasia. Later-onset cases have mild facial coarsening and neurodegeneration; angiokeratomas are commoner in these patients [11].

Gaucher disease. Gaucher disease (MIM: 606463) is the most prevalent lysosomal disorder (1 in 50 000). It is classified clinically into three types [12]. Type I (non-neuronopathic) is much the commonest: children and adults present with hepatosplenomegaly, thrombocytopenia, bone pain or pathological fractures. Type II (acute neuronopathic) patients present by 6 months of age with neurological problems, poor weight gain and hepatosplenomegaly; most die by 2 years. Type III (subacute neuronopathic) patients present as young children with hepatosplenomegaly, followed by an eye movement disorder and other neurological problems.

Cutaneous features are common in type I but not troublesome and include diffuse yellow-brown pigmentation, easy tanning, brown macules and telangiectasia [13]. Thrombocytopenia may lead to petechiae or ecchymoses. A few type II patients have congenital ichthyosis leading to the collodion baby phenotype (Figure 79.4). The baby is encased in thick, tight, shiny skin that cracks and desquamates to leave erythroderma [14]. There is ectropia of the eyes. The skin may return to normal if the baby survives for more than a month.

Niemann–Pick disease. Niemann–Pick disease (MIM: 257200) due to sphingomyelinase deficiency is classified into type A (neuronopathic) and type B (non-neuronopathic); type C is an *unrelated* disorder of intracellular lipid trafficking and is not considered here. Type A usually causes diarrhoea and vomiting, poor weight gain, hepatosplenomegaly and neurological problems in early infancy; these patients die by 3 years of age. Less severely affected type A patients have juvenile- or adult-onset neurological disease. Type B patients present as children or adults with splenomegaly or hepatosplenomegaly; complications include interstitial lung disease, poor growth, hyperlipidaemia and thrombocytopenia.

The skin may be involved in types A or B, with patches of waxy induration and brownish yellow pigmentation. Papular, papulonodular or suppurative lesions may be found on the face or trunk, occasionally becoming confluent [15,16]. Histology shows foamy macrophages. Mongolian blue spots occur in children.

Farber disease. Farber disease (MIM: 228000) is extremely rare. Patients usually present in early infancy with a hoarse cry, painful swollen joints and subcutaneous nodules. The most commonly affected joints are those of the hand and wrist, elbows, knees and ankles. The subcutaneous nodules may be associated with red papules and are generally close to affected joints and over pressure points, such as the occiput and lower spine. Histology reveals granulomas containing large, foamy histiocytes; electron microscopy shows that these have cytoplasmic vacuoles containing curvilinear inclusions (Farber bodies) [17]. Most patients have psychomotor impairment, poor weight gain and die in early childhood from respiratory infections.

Investigations

These diagnoses are usually established by enzyme assays on leukocytes.

Histology

'Foam cells' are found in the bone marrow and, to a lesser extent, in the skin. Niemann–Pick cells are typical examples – large, usually mononucleate histiocytes, whose cytoplasm is filled with lipid droplets that take up Sudan stains. Ultrastructurally, the cytoplasm of Niemann–Pick cells contains granular lipid inclusions that may appear lamellar [15]. Gaucher cells differ markedly from the foam cells seen in other lipidoses. They are large cells with pale-staining cytoplasm that has a delicate, striated, 'wrinkled tissue paper' appearance. Ultrastructurally, Gaucher cells have vesicles that contain twisted tubular structures [18].

Management

ERT is available for Fabry disease and Gaucher disease types 1 and 3 but it is expensive and requires slow intravenous infusion at least every 2 weeks [12]. It is recommended for symptomatic patients with Gaucher disease type 1; ERT also alleviates the systemic complications in Gaucher disease type 3 but HSCT should be considered if there is neurological deterioration. ERT will soon be licensed for Niemann–Pick disease type B; in clinical trials, it led to improvements in all the features, including growth.

Miglustat and Eliglustat are oral drugs that decrease the accumulation of glucocerebroside by reducing the synthesis of glycosphingolipids (substrate reduction therapy) [12]. They are used mainly in Gaucher disease type 1 patients who cannot tolerate ERT. Miglustat is also used in Niemann–Pick disease type C; diarrhoea and weight loss are common side effects. Only symptomatic treatment is available for the other sphingolipidoses.

Fabry disease

Synonyms and inclusions
• Anderson–Fabry disease

Introduction and genetics

Fabry disease causes angiokeratomas, pain in the extremities, renal failure, and cardiac and cerebrovascular disease [**19**]. Inheritance is X-linked recessive but many heterozygous females develop symptoms; onset is later than in men. About 1000 variants have been identified in *GLA*, the gene for α-galactosidase A; none is highly prevalent and establishing pathogenicity can be difficult. Some cause milder disease (e.g. the p.Asn215Ser 'cardiac' variant [20]).

Incidence

The incidence is at least 1 in 40 000–60 000 males.

Pathophysiology

α-Galactosidase A deficiency prevents the degradation of glycosphingolipids with terminal galactose residues, predominantly globotriaosylceramide (Gb3). Gb3 accumulation in vascular endothelial, perithelial and smooth muscle cells leads to aneurysmal dilatation of blood vessels, ischaemia and infarction. Glycosphingolipids also accumulate in the renal glomeruli and tubules, cardiac muscle, autonomic ganglion cells and corneal epithelium.

Clinical features

The first symptoms are usually episodes of severe burning pain in the palms and soles (acroparesthesiae). These occur in 70–85% of male patients, usually starting between 5 and 15 years of age, although diagnosis is often delayed [21]. Acroparesthesiae occur in 50–70% of female patients, with a mean age of onset of 15 years [22]. Painful crises are often triggered by fever or exertion and may last hours or days. Pain may diminish spontaneously in older men.

Angiokeratoma corporis diffusum occurs in 65–70% of male patients and 35–40% of female patients [21,22]. In males, angiokeratomas often start to appear shortly before puberty (mean age of onset 19 years) whereas in females they usually appear later (mean 28 years). The initial lesion is a dark red or black telangiectatic macule or papule, up to 4 mm across, that does not blanch with pressure; there is usually mild hyperkeratosis over larger lesions. Angiokeratomas are clustered and may be numerous or sparse. In men, the commonest sites are around the umbilicus (Figure 79.5) and in the bathing trunk area: inner thighs, lower back, buttocks, penis and scrotum. Lesions may also be found on the upper arms, around the border of the lips, around the nail folds and on the palms and soles – these are usually macular angiomas with minimal hyperkeratosis. In women, lesions are most frequent on the trunk and proximal limbs; genital lesions are rare. Telangiectases are present in 23% of male patients and 9% of female patients, usually on the lips, buccal mucosa, ears or conjunctiva [23].

Anhidrosis or hypohidrosis occurs in 53% of male patients and 28% of female patients, usually starting in the third decade [23]. It probably results from autonomic neuropathy and is associated with heat and exercise intolerance. Hyperhidrosis occurs in 10% of patients, predominantly females, often starting in adolescence. Later, vasomotor disturbances may cause flushing, cyanosis or blanching of the hands. Lymphoedema is common and may be due to lymphatic microangiopathy.

Clinical variants

Men with the 'cardiac variant' usually present after the age of 40 years with cardiomyopathy and proteinuria.

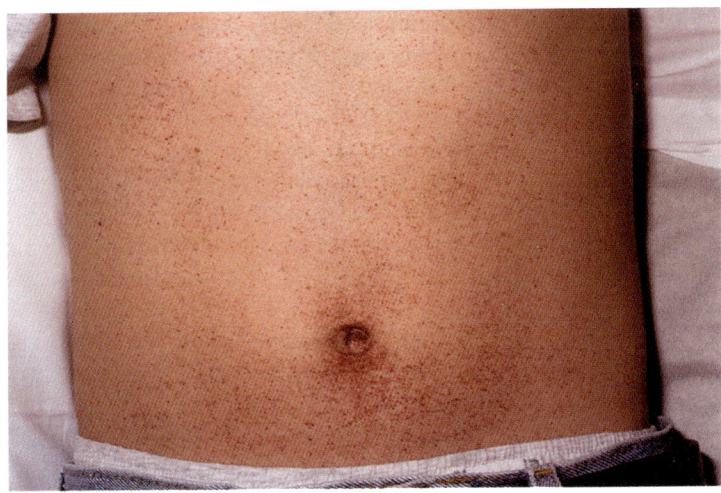

Figure 79.5 Angiokeratoma corporis diffusum around the umbilicus in a man with Fabry disease.

Differential diagnosis

Angiokeratoma corporis diffusum occurs in several other lysosomal disorders, although Fabry disease is much the commonest cause (Table 79.4). There have been a few reports of patients with angiokeratoma corporis diffusum in whom no enzyme deficiency was identified. The differential diagnosis also includes purpura, angioma serpiginosum and localised types of angiokeratoma (Chapter 101).

Complications and co-morbidities

Almost all men with Fabry disease develop cardiac problems, such as left ventricular dilatation and hypertrophy, mitral valve regurgitation, arrhythmias and ischaemic heart disease. Most men have proteinuria, hypertension and slowly deteriorating renal function. Without treatment, end-stage renal failure is usually reached at 40–50 years of age [21]. Cerebrovascular disease leads to early strokes or transient ischaemic attacks. Heterozygous women may also develop heart and cerebrovascular disease: in a survey of 248 women, 26% had left ventricular hypertrophy and 7% had suffered a stroke at a mean age of 50 years [24]. Vertigo, dizziness and hearing loss are common. Other complications include abdominal pain and diarrhoea, achalasia of the oesophagus and arthritis in the fingers.

Prognosis

Without treatment, the median survival is 60 years in males with classic disease and 75 years in females.

Investigations

The diagnosis of Fabry disease can be established by skin histology or slit lamp examination of the cornea. In males, the diagnosis should be confirmed by demonstrating α-galactosidase A deficiency in plasma, leukocytes or cultured skin fibroblasts. In women, the diagnosis is confirmed by molecular analysis because enzyme activity is often normal.

Slit lamp examination of the eye

Most adult patients (male and female) have an asymptomatic corneal dystrophy. Initial haziness progresses to characteristic whorled streaks radiating to the periphery (cornea verticillata). Identical appearances can result from long-term treatment with chloroquine or amiodarone. Other findings include lens opacities and tortuosity of the conjunctival and retinal vessels.

Histology

Light microscopy of the angiokeratomas shows dilated vessels in the upper dermis beneath a thinned epidermis, with or without hyperkeratosis (Figure 79.6). The diagnostic feature is the presence of vacuolated cells in the media and intima of small blood vessels. The accumulating glycosphingolipids are birefringent and, in frozen sections, they appear as 'Maltese crosses' in polarised light. Electron microscopy shows cytoplasmic inclusion bodies in the endothelial cells of blood vessels (Figure 79.7), smooth muscle and dermal macrophages. The inclusions are present in clinically unaffected skin; they are electron dense and lamellar, with a periodicity of 4–6 nm [25]. In contrast, other lysosomal disorders associated with angiokeratomas have electron-lucent vacuoles containing scanty fibrillary or granular material.

Management

The acroparesthesiae may respond to carbamazepine, gabapentin, venaflexine or phenytoin or they may require opiates. Angiokeratomas can be removed by laser therapy for cosmetic or other reasons but this is seldom requested. Cardiac complications should be managed conventionally. Aspirin may reduce the risk of stroke and angiotensin-converting enzyme inhibitors should be started if there is proteinuria. Renal failure is treated with dialysis or transplantation: glycolipids do not reaccumulate in the graft.

ERT reduces neurogenic pain and left ventricular hypertrophy and attenuates renal deterioration, particularly in patients with normal baseline renal function [26]. ERT is usually started following diagnosis in symptomatic males; in females, it is started if there is cardiac, neurological or renal disease, troublesome gastrointestinal

Table 79.4 Lysosomal diseases associated with angiokeratomas.

Name/eponym	Gene	Age of onset of angiokeratomas	Ultrastructure of lysosomal storage in mesenchymal cells
Fabry	GLA	>10 years (males), adulthood (females)	Dense concentric lamellar inclusions
Fucosidosis	FUCA1	Mid to late childhood	Vacuoles with granular material
Kanzaki	NAGA	Adulthood	Vacuoles with fibrillary material
Galactosialidosis	CTSA	Adulthood	Vacuoles with granular material
G$_{M1}$ gangliosidosis	GLB1	Infancy	Vacuoles with fibrillogranular material
Aspartylglycosaminuria	AGA	Late childhood or adulthood	Vacuoles with fibrillogranular material
β-Mannosidosis	MANBA	Late childhood or adulthood	Vacuoles with granular material

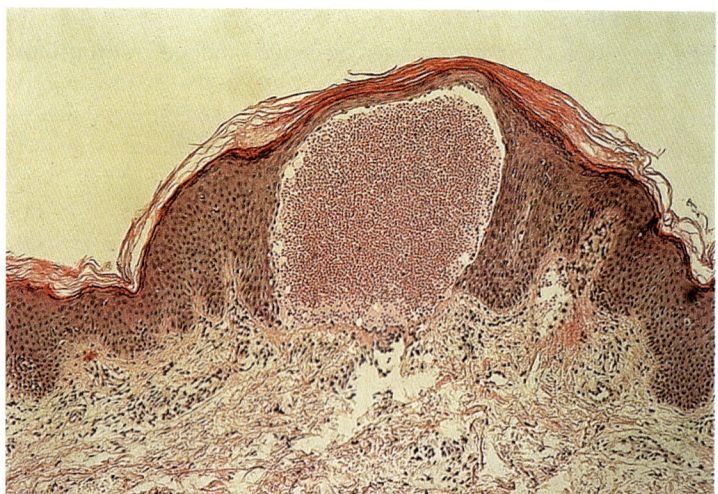

Figure 79.6 Angiokeratoma corporis diffusum showing dilated blood-filled vessels in the papillary dermis.

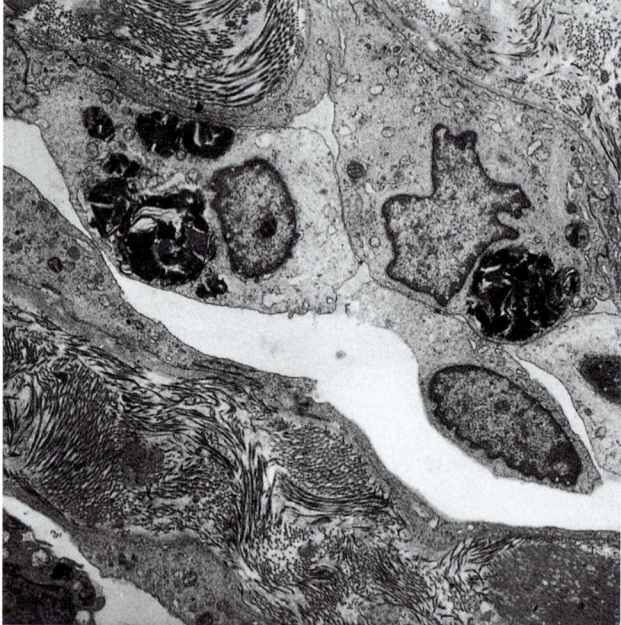

Figure 79.7 Electron-dense cytoplasmic inclusion bodies within endothelial cells in Fabry disease. Courtesy of Dr P.H. McKee, King's College, London, UK.

symptoms or pain that cannot be controlled by other means. ERT is costly and requires intravenous infusion every 2 weeks. Migalastat now provides an oral alternative in patients aged over 16 years with specific 'amenable' mutations [27,28]. It acts as a chaperone, stabilising these mutant forms of the enzyme and facilitating transport to the lysosome.

MITOCHONDRIAL RESPIRATORY CHAIN DISORDERS

The mitochondrial respiratory chain is responsible for the production of adenosine triphosphate using energy released during the oxidation of cellular fuels. Due to the ubiquitous need for energy,

mitochondrial disorders can affect any tissue; neuromuscular problems are commonest but, as the disease progresses, it often involves an increasing number of apparently unrelated organs. Multisystem presentations are particularly common in childhood but mitochondrial disorders can present at any age.

Mitochondrial disorders have unusually varied patterns of inheritance. Though most mitochondrial proteins are encoded by nuclear genes, mitochondria also have their own genome (mtDNA), which is inherited exclusively from the mother and there are hundreds of copies in each cell. MtDNA mutations can be homoplasmic, when they affect all the mtDNA copies, or heteroplasmic, when they only affect a proportion of the copies. For heteroplasmic mutations, the level of mutant mtDNA can vary within a maternal pedigree and clinical problems only occur when the level exceeds a threshold. Symptoms are generally more severe if the level of mutant mtDNA is very high than if it is just above the threshold.

Dermatological features of mitochondrial disorders

Multiple symmetrical lipomatosis

Lipomas are seen in adults with certain mtDNA mutations. Typically, there are multiple lipomas symmetrically distributed over the back of the neck and shoulders; they often recur following removal [**29**]. They are most frequently associated with the m.8344A>G and m.8363G>A mutations, both of which affect the gene for mitochondrial tRNA^{Lys} [**30**]. Patients with these mutations at a high level of heteroplasmy often have neurological problems. The classic combination of *m*yoclonus *e*pilepsy and myopathy with *r*agged *r*ed *f*ibres is given the acronym MERRF syndrome (MIM: 545000); other patients may have deafness, ataxia or a childhood neurodegenerative disorder called Leigh syndrome. Lipomas can occur in patients with neurological problems and in subjects with a lower level of the mutation who are otherwise asymptomatic. Within a single patient, the level of the mutation varies from one tissue to another and it is higher in the lipomas than in other tissues (such as unaffected adipose tissue). Cells within the lipomas are derived from brown fat [**29**] and have altered expression of genes involved in regulating adipogenesis [**30**].

Palmoplantar keratoderma

Non-epidermolytic palmoplantar keratoderma has been reported in a number of families with the m.7445A>G mtDNA mutation [31]. All affected individuals have also had sensorineural hearing loss. There is diffuse or circumscribed epidermal thickening particularly over pressure points, such as the metatarsal heads, without intraepidermal blistering. Hyperkeratosis appears from mid-childhood onwards, the soles of the feet being affected earlier and more frequently than the palms. Skin biopsy shows orthokeratotic and parakeratotic hyperkeratosis with some acanthosis. Interestingly, although the m.7445A>G mutation has always been homoplasmic, only 60% of individuals had deafness and fewer than 40% had keratoderma: other genetic or environmental factors must affect expression of the disorder. Palmoplantar keratoderma with deafness can also result from mutations in *GJB2*, which encodes a gap junction protein; these cases show autosomal dominant inheritance.

Acrocyanosis

Orthostatic acrocyanosis is a characteristic finding in patients with ethylmalonic encephalopathy (MIM: 602473) [32]. Patients have intermittent red or purple discoloration of the feet (± hands) without trophic changes. They may also have a recurrent petechial rash and bruising (with normal platelets and clotting studies). Other problems include chronic diarrhoea, poor growth, developmental delay and regression, seizures and episodes of coma. Most patients present in infancy and die in early childhood, although some follow a less severe course. Ethylmalonic encephalopathy is an autosomal recessive disorder caused by mutations in *ETHE1*, a mitochondrial sulphur dioxygenase. Deficiency of this enzyme leads to the accumulation of hydrogen sulphide, which is vasoactive and damages small blood vessels, accounting for the acrocyanosis and petechiae [33]. Hydrogen sulphide also inhibits cytochrome oxidase (leading to mitochondrial dysfunction) and short-chain fatty acid oxidation (leading to ethylmalonic aciduria). Treatment with *N*-acetylcysteine and metronidazole can be helpful [34]. *N*-acetylcysteine is a precursor of glutathione, which can detoxify hydrogen sulphide, and metronidazole reduces the formation of hydrogen sulphide in the gut.

Other dermatological features

Several other dermatological abnormalities are associated with mitochondrial disorders but they are non-specific and overshadowed by other symptoms. Hypertrichosis occurs in several disorders, including Leigh syndrome due to *SURF1* mutations [35], infantile lactic acidosis due to *SUCLG1* mutations and MELAS syndrome (*m*itochondrial myopathy, *e*ncephalopathy, *l*actic *a*cidosis and *s*troke-like episodes) due to the m.3243A>G mtDNA mutation. Redness, ichthyosis, pruritus, reticular hyperpigmentation and poikiloderma have also been reported in m.3243A>G patients [36].

CONGENITAL DISORDERS OF GLYCOSYLATION

This is a heterogeneous group of rare disorders with impaired glycosylation of proteins or lipids. Most are multisystem disorders affecting the brain and various other organs, such as muscle, heart and the eyes. The skin is often involved, problems including ichthyosis and cutis laxa [37] (Table 79.5).

Incidence

At least 130 congenital disorders of glycosylation (CDGs) have been described and more are identified each year. Much the commonest is phosphomannomutase 2 deficiency, with an incidence of 1 in 40 000 in Sweden. Other CDGs are extremely rare.

Pathophysiology

Many proteins, including most secreted and cell surface proteins, require glycosylation to function properly. Oligosaccharides are attached to the side chain of asparagine (N-linked) or serine/threonine residues (O-linked). Some lipids also require glycosylation (e.g. glycosylphosphatidylinositol, GPI, which anchors many proteins to the cell membrane). Phosphomannomutase 2 catalyses the isomerisation of mannose 6-phosphate to mannose 1-phosphate, which is needed to synthesise the oligosaccharides for N-linked glycoproteins. Other disorders affect other steps in the complicated glycosylation pathways.

Genetics

The name for each disorder is now based on its gene. Phosphomannomutase 2 deficiency (previously called CDG type 1a) is caused by mutations in the *PMM2* gene and is called PMM2-CDG. More than 115 *PMM2* mutations have been identified, of which p.R141H is the commonest. PMM2-CDG and most other CDGs are inherited as autosomal recessive traits. The exceptions mentioned here are POFUT1-CDG and POGLUT1-CDG (autosomal dominant) and ATP6AP1-CDG (X-linked).

Clinical features

PMM2-CDG (MIM: 212065) usually presents in the newborn period with hypotonia, internal strabismus and dysmorphic features [38]. Some patients have subcutaneous fat pads, usually located over the iliac crests in the superolateral portions of the buttocks, with lipodystrophy of the rest of the buttocks (Figure 79.8). They may also occur in the suprapubic area, lateral thighs or upper arms. The fat pads are most prominent in infancy and usually disappear later in childhood. The skin may have loose folds or feel thick and there may be peau d'orange; later, lipoatrophy can lead to streaks over the legs. The nipples are often inverted. Dysmorphic features may include large dysplastic ears and skeletal abnormalities, such as long fingers and toes. Most patients have severe psychomotor impairment and are unable to walk. Feeding problems, poor growth, hepatomegaly and hypogonadism are also common. Approximately 20% of patients die in the first few years but subsequently the mortality is low. There is a wide range of severity: patients at the mild end of the spectrum have no dysmorphic or dermatological features and only mild learning difficulties.

The main dermatological features in other CDGs are ichthyosis, cutis laxa, Ehlers–Danlos syndrome and abnormal pigmentation (including Dowling–Degos disease). CDGs can also cause Adams–Oliver syndrome and hyperphosphataemic familial tumoral calcinosis (see end of this chapter). There is a range of severity for each CDG and many patients only exhibit some of the features. Thus, most patients with PIGA-CDG, PIGO-CDG, COG5-CDG, MAN1B1-CDG and ATP6A1-CDG have no dermatological abnormalities.

Investigations

Serum transferrin isoelectric focusing is a useful screening test that detects many CDGs, including PMM2-CDG. Transferrin is an N-linked glycoprotein and the attached oligosaccharides give it a negative charge; in defects of N-glycosylation, some oligosaccharides are abnormal or missing, causing transferrin to migrate

Table 79.5 Congenital defects of glycosylation with dermatological features.

Gene	Glycosylation pathway affected	Dermatological features	Other features
Fat pads, inverted nipple			
PMM2	N-glycosylation	Fat pads, inverted nipples, peau d'orange	PI, strabismus, dysmorphism
ALG8	N-glycosylation	Fat pads, inverted nipples, cutis laxa	Dysmorphism, cataracts, neurological problems
Ichthyosis			
DOLK	N-glycosylation & GPI anchor	Ichthyosis ± alopecia, neonatal collodion bands	Cardiomyopathy
SRD5A3	N-glycosylation & GPI anchor	Ichthyosis or palmoplantar keratoderma	PI, eye signs
PIGL	GPI anchor	Erythematous rash at birth then ichthyosis (esp. flexures)	Congenital heart disease, PI, seizures
PIGA	GPI anchor	Ichthyosis, linear plaque-like scales, eczema	Profound PI, seizures
PIGO	GPI anchor	Palmoplantar keratoderma	PI, seizures
MPDU1	GPI anchor	Ichthyosis	Severe PI
COG5	N- & O-glycosylation	Hyperkeratosis, hypohidrosis	PI
COG6	N- & O-glycosylation	Hyperkeratosis, hypohidrosis	PI, liver disease
Cutis laxa			
ATP6VOA2	N- & O-glycosylation	Cutis laxa, improves with age	Microcephaly, joint laxity, strabismus
COG7	N- & O-glycosylation	Cutis laxa	PI
MAN1B1	N-glycosylation	Cutis laxa	PI, obesity
Ehlers–Danlos syndrome			
B4GALT7, B3GALT6	O-glycosylation	Hyperextensible, thin, fragile, doughy skin	Spondylodysplasia, joint laxity, mild PI
B3GAT3	O-glycosylation	Hyperextensible, thin, fragile, doughy skin	Spondylodysplasia, joint laxity, cardiovascular disease
Abnormal pigmentation			
POFUT1, POGLUT1	O-glycosylation	Hypopigmented macules and reticular hyperpigmentation (Dowling–Degos disease)	None
ST3GAL5	N- and O-glycosylation and glycolipids	Hyper- and hypopigmented macules, ichthyosis	Severe PI, epilepsy
ATP6AP1	N- and O-glycosylation	Alopecia, increased skin pigmentation	Immunodeficiency, deafness
Hyperphosphataemic familial tumoral calcinosis			
GALNT3	O-glycosylation	Tumoral calcinosis	Hyperostosis
Adams–Oliver syndrome			
EOGT	O-glycosylation	Aplasia cutis congenita of scalp	Terminal limb malformations

PI, psychomotor impairment.

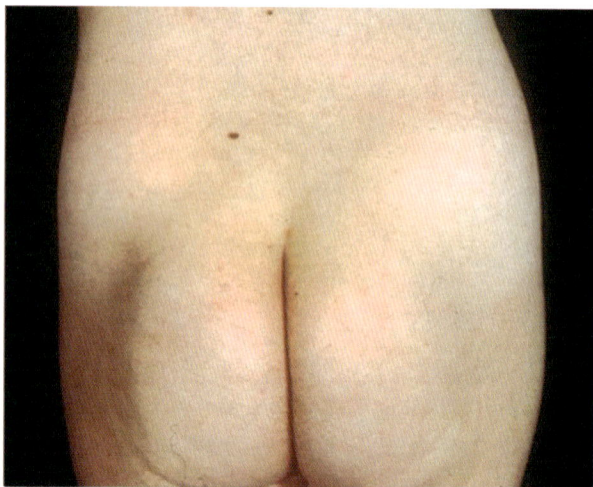

Figure 79.8 Fat pads over the iliac crests in a child with phosphomannomutase 2 deficiency. Courtesy of Professor P.T. Clayton, Institute of Child Health, London, UK.

abnormally on isoelectric focusing. PMM2 deficiency can be confirmed by measuring its activity in leukocytes. Unfortunately, transferrin isoelectric focusing is normal in many CDGs (such as defects of O-glycosylation); these are usually diagnosed by exome sequencing or a gene panel.

Management
Unfortunately, only symptomatic treatment is available for the CDGs mentioned here.

DISORDERS OF AMINO ACID METABOLISM AND TRANSPORT

In these disorders, neurological and other problems are caused by the deficiency or accumulation of an amino acid or a related chemical. Amino acid disorders are often treated with a special diet. Those with dermatological features are listed in Table 79.6.

Phenylketonuria

Introduction, genetics and incidence
Phenylketonuria (PKU, MIM: 261600) is an autosomal recessive disorder caused by mutations in the *PAH* gene. Deficiency of phenylalanine hydroxylase leads to high blood phenylalanine concentrations. Without treatment, it causes severe neurodevelopmental problems. The incidence is about 1 in 12 000.

Table 79.6 Disorders of amino acid metabolism with dermatological features.

Disorder	Dermatological features	Other features
Phenylketonuria (PKU)	Hypopigmentation of skin and hair, eczema	Cognitive problems, seizures
Tyrosinaemia type 2	Painful palmoplantar hyperkeratoses	Corneal ulcers, cognitive problems
Alkaptonuria	Pigmentation of pinna, sclera, skin and mucosa	Arthritis
Prolidase deficiency	Ulcers, eczema, purpura, scarring, predisposition to SLE	Cognitive problems, facial dysmorphism, splenomegaly
Argininosuccinic aciduria	Trichorrhexis nodosa	Cognitive problems, hyperammonaemia
Hartnup disease	Photosensitive dermatitis	Cerebellar ataxia
Serine synthesis defects	Ichthyosis	Cognitive problems
Proline synthesis defects	Cutis laxa	Cognitive problems
Glutamine synthetase deficiency	Erythroderma and blistering	Epilepsy
Classical homocystinuria	Pale skin and hair, ulcers, livedo reticularis on legs	Cognitive problems, dislocated lenses, Marfanoid habitus, thromboembolism
Lysinuric protein intolerance	Predisposition to SLE	Poor weight gain and growth, osteopenia, hepatosplenomegaly, hyperammonaemia
Methylmalonic, propionic, isovaleric acidaemias	Periorificial dermatitis, alopecia if excessive protein restriction	Acute ketoacidosis, vomiting, cognitive problems

SLE, systemic lupus erythematosus.

Clinical features

In most developed countries, PKU is detected by newborn screening. *Without screening*, patients present during infancy or early childhood, with psychomotor impairment and behaviour problems sometimes followed by seizures. Untreated patients have an increased incidence of eczema (20–40%) [39]. They also have reduced pigmentation of the hair, skin and iris [39]. Hair tends to be blonde in children who might otherwise have brown hair and it is brown in children expected to have black hair. White children often have blue irides. The altered pigmentation is caused by the impaired synthesis of melanin and improves with tyrosine supplements, indicating that it is at least partly due to tyrosine deficiency, although the high phenylalanine concentrations may also inhibit tyrosinase.

Investigations

PKU is usually diagnosed following newborn screening. Plasma amino acid analysis should be undertaken if PKU is suspected in unscreened patients.

Management

PKU is treated with a diet that is extremely low in natural protein and a supplement containing all the amino acids except phenylalanine. Dietary phenylalanine restriction can control the blood level because phenylalanine is not synthesised in the body. The diet also corrects the tyrosine deficiency, so treated patients have normal pigmentation. Pharmacological doses of the enzyme's cofactor (tetrahydrobiopterin) reduce blood phenylalanine concentrations in some patients with relatively mild PKU [40] but they usually still require some dietary restriction.

Target phenylalanine concentrations are less strict in older children and adults because the damage caused by high phenylalanine levels diminishes with age. Indeed, many adults revert to a normal diet without major problems. Strict dietary treatment is essential during pregnancy to avoid adverse effects on the fetus. Adults who stop dietary treatment may have a slightly increased risk of eczema [41] but low tyrosine concentrations and hypopigmentation are not seen.

Tyrosinaemia type 2

Synonyms and inclusions
- Richner–Hanhart syndrome

Introduction, genetics and incidence

Tyrosinaemia type 2 (MIM: 276600) is a very rare autosomal recessive disorder caused by mutations in the *TAT* gene. This encodes tyrosine aminotransferase, which catalyses the first step in tyrosine degradation. The eye, skin and brain can be affected but some patients are probably asymptomatic.

Pathophysiology

The ophthalmological problems are thought to result from tyrosine crystals precipitating in corneal epithelial cells, disrupting lysosomes and leading to inflammation [42]. In contrast, skin biopsies show no tyrosine crystals and minimal inflammation. There is hyperkeratosis, acanthosis and parakeratosis with homogeneous refractile eosinophilic inclusions in the stratum corneum and upper Malpighian layer. Electron microscopy shows keratinocytes with increased tonofibrils and microtubules [42].

Clinical features

Corneal ulcers occur in approximately 75% of patients, palmoplantar hyperkeratoses in 80% and learning difficulties in 60%. Manifestations may vary within a single pedigree.

Patients usually present with photophobia and eye pain in infancy. The eye is red with lacrimation; slit lamp examination shows dendritic corneal erosions that resemble herpetic ulcers. Without treatment, scarring can cause visual loss.

Painful hyperkeratotic plaques usually appear on the digits, palms and soles after the first year [43]. They are commonest at pressure points, such as the fingertips. The lesions may start as blisters and may ulcerate (Figure 79.9). There may be hyperhidrosis of the palms and soles and leukokeratosis of the tongue.

PART 6: GENETIC DISORDERS

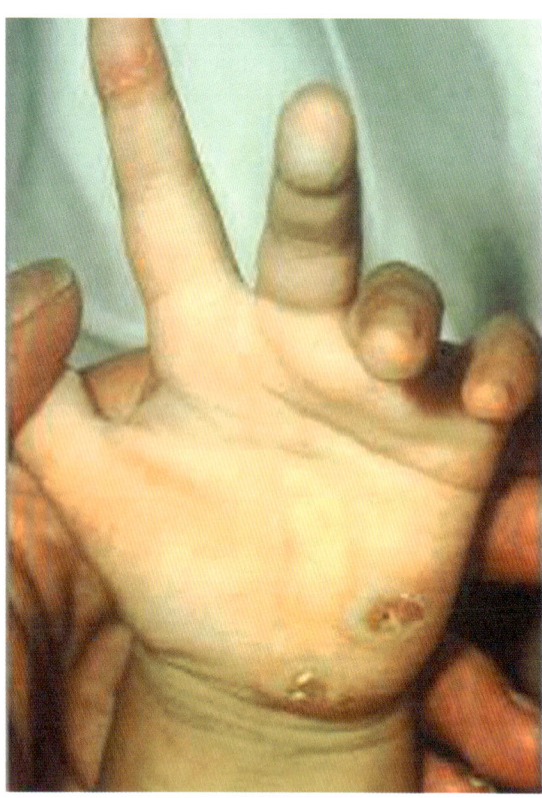

Figure 79.9 Hyperkeratotic lesion in tyrosinaemia type 2. Reproduced from Sarafoglou *et al.* 2009 [79] with permission of McGraw Hill Education.

Some patients have cognitive impairment, behaviour problems, seizures or poor coordination.

Investigations
Plasma amino acid analysis shows marked increased tyrosine concentrations, often above 1200 µmol/L. The diagnosis is confirmed by mutation analysis.

Differential diagnosis
Tyrosine concentrations are usually less raised in tyrosinaemia types 1 and 3 and skin lesions have not been reported. The main problems are liver disease in type 1 and learning difficulties in type 3.

Management
Tyrosinaemia type 2 is treated with a low protein diet; if severe protein restriction is needed, patients are given an amino acid supplement free of tyrosine and phenylalanine. Most centres aim to keep plasma tyrosine concentrations below 500 µmol/L.

Alkaptonuria

Introduction, genetics and incidence
Alkaptonuria (MIM: 203500) is an autosomal recessive disorder caused by *HGD* mutations. It is very rare (1 in 250 000 to 1 000 000). It causes adult-onset backache and arthritis.

Pathophysiology
Homogentisate dioxygenase catalyses the third step in tyrosine degradation. Its deficiency leads to accumulation of homogentisic acid. Derivatives of this are polymerised to form a dark pigment, which is deposited in connective tissue. It is uncertain why this causes arthritis but the pigment may act as a chemical irritant.

Clinical features
Most patients present with low back pain between 25 and 40 years of age [44]. This progresses to kyphosis and, often, ankylosis. Arthritis in the hip or knee may require joint replacement. Children are asymptomatic but their urine darkens after a few hours, particularly if alkalinised: cloth nappies and contaminated sheets may turn black when washed. Ochronosis (melanin-like black pigmentation) occurs from 30 years onwards. The cartilage of the ears develops grey or blue-black discoloration and feels inflexible [44]. There may also be brown deposits in the sclera, brown nails or dusky discoloration of the skin, especially over the cheeks, forehead and genital region; cerumen is sometimes black.

Investigations
The diagnosis is established by finding homogentisic acid on urine organic acid analysis.

Management
Nitisinone inhibits the first step in tyrosine breakdown and, even at low doses, it reduces plasma and urine homogentisic acid by >95%. A 4-year controlled trial in adults showed slowing of disease progression [45].

Prolidase deficiency

Introduction, genetics and incidence
Prolidase deficiency (MIM: 170100) is a very rare autosomal recessive disorder due to mutations in the *PEPD* gene. It is characterised primarily by skin lesions, especially ulcers.

Clinical features
Patients have presented at any age from birth to 22 years and some may remain asymptomatic throughout life. Recurrent ulcers are the commonest problem, mostly on the lower legs (Figure 79.10) [46]. The skin is fragile and the ulcers sometimes follow an injury. The ulcers are resistant to treatment and there may be secondary infection. Other skin problems include dermatitis (with crusting), fine scarring or pitting (Figure 79.11), telangiectasia, purpura or bruising. There may be lymphoedema or a doughy consistency to the skin. Many patients have psychomotor impairment and some have a shallow nasal bridge and hypertelorism [47]. There may be recurrent infections or chronic lung disease resembling cystic fibrosis. Other features include splenomegaly, anaemia, thrombocytopenia or hypergammaglobulinaemia; there is an increased risk of systemic lupus erythematosus [47].

Pathophysiology and investigations

Prolidase is needed to degrade dipeptides with an N-terminal proline or hydroxyproline. Why these 'imidodipeptides' cause the clinical problems is unknown. They are revealed by plasma or urine amino acid analysis. The diagnosis is confirmed by mutation analysis.

Management

No specific treatment is known to help, although there have been anecdotal reports of success with ointments containing glycine and proline or systemic ascorbic acid or manganese (the co-factor of prolidase). Skin grafts have been unsuccessful. Infections should be treated aggressively.

Argininosuccinic aciduria

Introduction, genetics and incidence

This autosomal recessive disorder is caused by argininosuccinate lyase deficiency (MIM: 207900), with mutations in the *ASL* gene. The incidence is approximately 1 in 70 000.

Clinical features

Most patients present with lethargy or coma due to acute hyperammonaemia. This occurs 12–72 h after birth or triggered by infection later in childhood. Patients with residual enzyme activity often present at a few years of age, with learning difficulties and thinning of the hair, which is dry and brittle (Figure 79.12). Examination with a microscope reveals nodular swellings on the hair shafts and frayed cortical fibres, consistent with trichorrhexis nodosa [48].

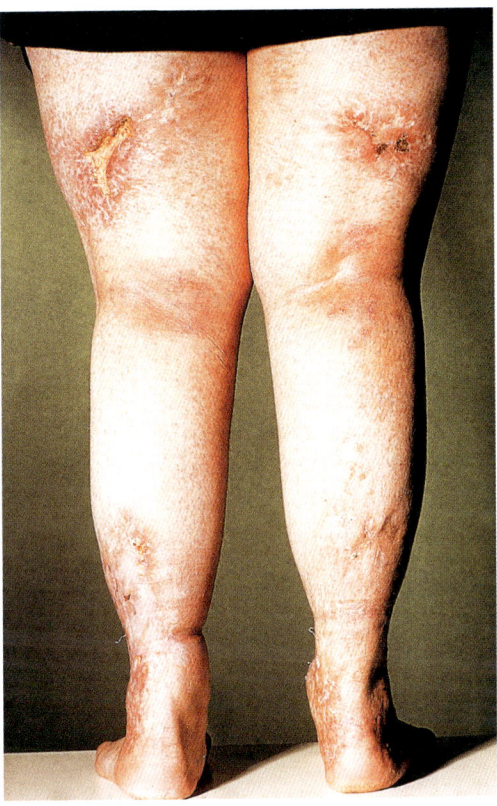

Figure 79.10 Multiple ulcers with an unusual distribution in prolidase deficiency.

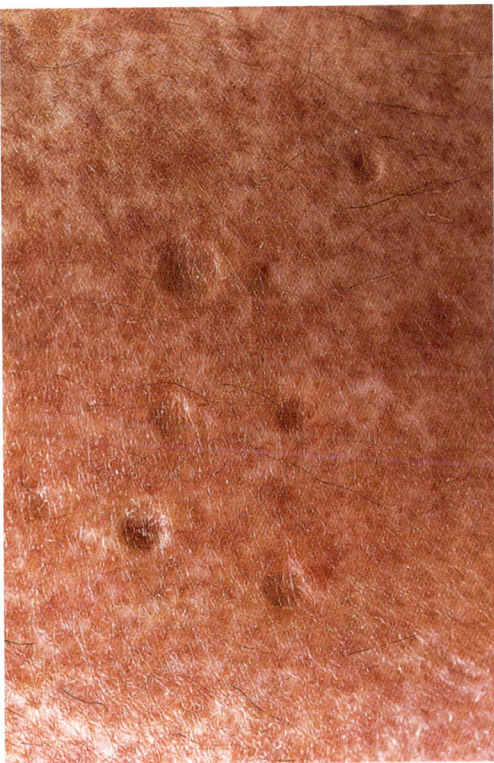

Figure 79.11 Pitted skin in prolidase deficiency. Courtesy of Dr D.A. Burns, Leicester Royal Infirmary, Leicester, UK.

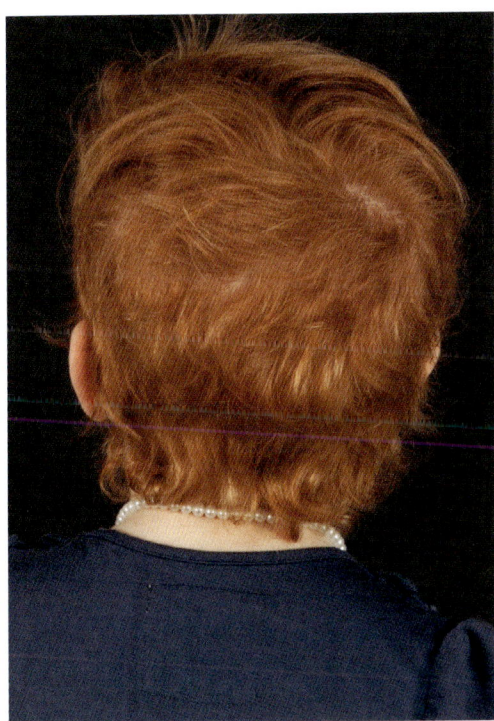

Figure 79.12 Trichorrhexis nodosa in a 4-year-old with argininosuccinic aciduria. Courtesy of Manchester University Hospitals NHS Foundation Trust, Manchester, UK.

PART 6: GENETIC DISORDERS

Pathophysiology

The defect interrupts the urea cycle, explaining the episodes of hyperammonaemia. The trichorrhexis nodosa may be related to chronic arginine deficiency. Argininosuccinate lyase stabilises nitric oxide synthase and some long-term complications may be due to nitric oxide deficiency [49].

Investigations

Argininosuccinic acid is best detected by urine amino acid analysis, although it is also present in plasma.

Management

Treatment involves dietary protein restriction and drugs (sodium benzoate and/or sodium phenylbutyrate). L-Arginine is also given to correct the deficiency of this amino acid and to facilitate the elimination of ammonia. These measures prevent hyperammonaemia and lead to resolution of the trichorrhexis nodosa.

Prognosis

Despite treatment, most patients have learning difficulties and those with severe defects develop neurological problems, epilepsy and chronic liver disease.

Hartnup disease

Introduction, genetics and incidence

Hartnup disease (MIM: 234500) can cause a pellagra-like rash and neurological problems. It is an autosomal recessive disorder caused by mutations in *SLC6A19*, which encodes the neutral amino acid transporter in renal tubular and intestinal epithelial cells. The incidence on newborn screening is 1 in 14 000–45 000 but most patients remain asymptomatic.

Pathophysiology

Nicotinamide is essential for many reactions and can be formed from dietary niacin or from tryptophan. In patients with Hartnup disease, impaired intestinal absorption of tryptophan (a neutral amino acid) leads to a reduced synthesis of nicotinamide. The absence of symptoms in some patients may reflect their dietary niacin intake or the absorption of tryptophan in oligopeptides [50].

Clinical features

Patients usually present with a rash between 3 and 9 years of age. Well-demarcated, dry, scaly patches occur on sun-exposed skin, such as the face, backs of the hands and exposed parts of the arms. Exposure to sunlight causes redness, sometimes with blistering, and may be followed by desquamation and depigmentation [51]. Cerebellar ataxia is the commonest neurological problem and starts after the rash. There may also be nystagmus, tremor, weakness or psychiatric symptoms.

Investigations

There are increased neutral amino acids in the urine with low or low–normal concentrations in the plasma.

Management

The rash and neurological problems generally resolve with oral nicotinamide (50–300 mg/day). A high protein diet is also recommended.

Prognosis

Symptoms tend to improve with age, even without treatment.

Serine, proline and glutamine synthesis defects

Introduction and incidence

Disorders of serine, proline and glutamine synthesis cause a combination of neurological and skin disorders [52]. They are all extremely rare.

Genetics

Impaired serine synthesis is caused by autosomal recessive mutations in *PHGDH*, *PSAT1* or *PSPH*. Proline synthesis disorders are caused by autosomal recessive mutations in *ALDH18A1* or *PYCR1* or dominant mutations in *ALDH18A1* (often *de novo*). Glutamine synthetase deficiency is an autosomal recessive disorder caused by *GLUL* mutations.

Pathophysiology

Deficiency of the amino acid impairs protein synthesis. Proline and hydroxyproline comprise 17% of the amino acids in collagen, explaining why proline deficiency causes cutis laxa.

Clinical features

Serine synthesis defects. Severely affected patients die perinatally with Neu-Laxova syndrome (ichthyosis, fetal growth retardation, microcephaly and dysmorphism). Less severely affected patients have cognitive impairment and seizures but no ichthyosis.

Proline synthesis disorders. Most patients present in infancy with cutis laxa, joint laxity, progeroid features, cognitive impairment and sometimes seizures. Other patients present as adults with spastic paraplegia and normal skin.

Glutamine synthetase deficiency. This presents with epileptic encephalopathy in early infancy. Most patients develop a generalised red rash with intraepidermal blistering and die in infancy or childhood.

Investigations

Plasma and CSF concentrations of the relevant amino acid are usually low but they can be normal in proline synthesis disorders, particularly *PYCR1* defects, which can only be diagnosed by DNA sequencing.

Management

Treatment with serine ameliorates the neurological problems in non-lethal serine synthesis defects, particularly if started very early.

Prognosis

Outcomes are poor for patients presenting in infancy, except for promptly treated serine deficiency.

DISORDERS OF LIPID METABOLISM

Many hyperlipidaemias cause *xanthomas* (Chapter 60) and several rare disorders of lipid synthesis or metabolism cause *ichthyosis* (Chapter 63) or *lipodystrophy* (Chapter 72). *Mevalonate kinase deficiency* and *Majeed syndrome* are defects of lipid synthesis that cause inflammatory disorders involving the skin (Chapter 45).

Smith–Lemli–Opitz syndrome

This autosomal recessive disorder is caused by 7-dehydrocholesterol reductase deficiency (MIM: 270400). It is much the commonest disorder of cholesterol synthesis, with an incidence of 1 in 15 000–60 000. There is a wide range of severity: most patients have facial dysmorphism, syndactyly of the second and third toes, undescended testes, failure to thrive, microcephaly, intellectual disability and autism. The main dermatological problem is photosensitivity, which may be severe [53]. Other features may include hypopigmented hair, hyperhidrosis of the palms, eczema, cutis marmorata and acrocyanosis [54]. The diagnosis is made by demonstrating elevated plasma 7-dehydrocholesterol levels. Treatment with cholesterol does not alter the cognitive outcome but it is said to improve the photosensitivity [55].

VITAMIN AND MINERAL DISORDERS

Disorders of biotin metabolism

Introduction, genetics and incidence

Biotin, a water-soluble vitamin, is the co-factor for four carboxylase reactions involved in amino acid degradation, gluconeogenesis and fatty acid synthesis. Holocarboxylase synthetase is needed to bind biotin to the apoenzymes. Biotinidase is needed for the recycling of biotin and the use of dietary protein-bound biotin. Deficiency of either biotinidase or holocarboxylase synthetase leads to multiple carboxylase deficiency. They are both autosomal recessive disorders. The incidence of severe biotinidase deficiency is about 1 in 100 000; partial deficiency has a similar frequency but its clinical significance is debatable. Holocarboxylase synthetase deficiency is rarer.

Clinical features

Holocarboxylase synthetase deficiency (MIM: 253270) usually presents in the first days of life with vomiting, lethargy, lactic acidosis, ketoacidosis and hyperammonaemia; without treatment, this leads to coma and death. Patients with some residual enzyme activity may present later in childhood with similar symptoms or with developmental impairment, hair loss or rashes. The rash is usually widespread, red and scaly, particularly affecting the napkin area. It may resemble ichthyosis or seborrhoeic dermatitis [56].

Biotinidase deficiency (MIM: 253260) usually presents between 2 and 6 months of age, although symptoms may occur earlier and a few patients present later in childhood [57, 58]. The initial features are usually hypotonia and seizures (generalised tonic clonic or myoclonic). Patients also have psychomotor retardation, hearing loss and visual impairment due to optic atrophy. Dermatological problems are common but may be delayed [**58**]. Most patients develop a patchy red or exudative rash, particularly around the mouth. The rash may be widespread and there may be skin infections, conjunctivitis, blepharitis or onychoschizia. Hair is sparse and some patients have complete alopecia, including loss of eyelashes and eyebrows.

Investigations

Patients with holocarboxylase synthetase deficiency excrete characteristic organic acids, including lactate, 3-hydroxyisovalerate, 3-hydroxypropionate, methylcitrate and 3-methylcrotonylglycine. The diagnosis is confirmed by mutation analysis.

Biotinidase deficiency is diagnosed by measuring biotinidase activity in plasma; the organic acids may be normal. Some countries undertake newborn screening for biotinidase deficiency.

Management

In biotinidase deficiency, the seizures and dermatological problems respond promptly to treatment with biotin (5–10 mg/day). Unfortunately, cognitive and hearing problems persist unless treatment is started early.

Most patients with holocarboxylase synthetase deficiency respond to biotin at 10–20 mg/day but some require higher doses. A few patients only show a partial response and have learning difficulties despite early treatment.

Acrodermatitis enteropathica

Introduction, genetics and incidence

Acrodermatitis enteropathica (MIM: 201100) is an autosomal recessive disorder affecting the intestinal absorption of zinc. The resulting zinc deficiency leads to dermatitis, alopecia and diarrhoea. It is caused by mutations in *SLC39A4*, the gene for ZIP4, which is the main intestinal zinc transporter. Acrodermatitis enteropathica is very rare (1 in 500 000).

Pathophysiology

Zinc is a co-factor for many enzymes. The skin, intestine and immune system are most severely affected by zinc deficiency because of their rapid cell turnover.

PART 6: GENETIC DISORDERS

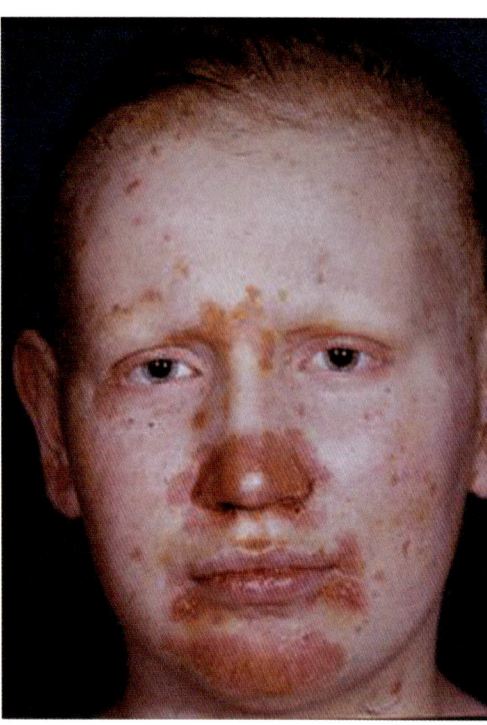

Figure 79.13 Acrodermatitis enteropathica with eczematous skin lesions and sparse hair.

Clinical features

Patients present with apathy or irritability and a rash around the mouth and anus and on the hands and feet [59]. Symptoms start after weaning in breastfed babies and at 4–10 weeks of age in formula-fed babies. Redness progresses to vesicles, bullae, pustules, desquamation and crusting (Figure 79.13). There is alopecia and frequently blepharitis, conjunctivitis and photophobia. Infections are common, including secondary infections of the skin, for example with *Candida albicans*. Wound healing is poor and many patients have diarrhoea and growth faltering. The condition can be fatal but some patients survive into adulthood without treatment.

Differential diagnosis

Similar problems occur in zinc deficiency due to other causes, such as gastrointestinal disorders. Biotinidase deficiency and protein malnutrition lead to a similar rash.

Investigations

The serum zinc concentration is usually low but can be normal [59]. Patients respond within a week to a trial of zinc therapy [60] and relapse after stopping treatment. *SLC39A4* sequencing confirms the diagnosis.

Management

During childhood 150–400 mg/day of zinc sulphate is given orally; a lower dose may suffice after puberty but 400–500 mg/day is needed during pregnancy. If zinc sulphate causes gastric problems, other zinc salts or encapsulated preparations have been recommended but they are not widely available. Monitoring for copper deficiency should be undertaken.

Menkes disease and occipital horn syndrome

Introduction, genetics and incidence

Menkes disease (MIM: 209400) is an X-linked recessive disorder due to mutations in *ATP7A*. Copper deficiency leads to neurodegeneration, 'kinky hair' and connective tissue abnormalities. Occipital horn syndrome (MIM: 304150) is an allelic variant with connective tissue abnormalities but no neurodegeneration. Both diseases are very rare (approximately 1 in 250 000).

Pathophysiology

The ATP7A protein exports copper from the intestinal mucosa into the portal circulation. Copper is essential for many enzymes, including lysyloxidase (which is involved in collagen cross-linking) and tyrosinase (which is necessary for melanin synthesis). Copper is also involved in mitochondrial function and neurotransmitter synthesis, explaining the neurological features of Menkes disease.

Clinical features

Boys with Menkes disease typically present at 2–3 months with hypotonia and seizures. Developmental regression and spasticity appear later in the first year. The hair is usually normal for the first few weeks but soon becomes sparse and brittle. In typical cases, there is scanty colourless or blond hair over the vertex with stubble elsewhere (Figure 79.14); in milder cases, the hair may be pigmented with occipital baldness due to trauma. Microscopic examination reveals pili torti and occasionally trichorrhexis nodosa [61]. Patients acquire a characteristic facial appearance with sagging cheeks and frontal bossing. The skin is loose, especially on the back of the neck. Diarrhoea, osteoporosis and subdural haemorrhages are common. Untreated patients generally die by 3 years of age.

Clinical variants

Occipital horn syndrome is a mild variant with demineralisation and exostoses, especially over the occiput, giving rise to the name [62]. The skin and joints are lax and the disorder was previously called X-linked cutis laxa. Patients often have diarrhoea or urine infections due to bladder diverticulae. There may be mild learning difficulties but other neurological problems and pili torti are rare.

Investigations

Low serum copper and caeruloplasmin concentrations are only diagnostic after 3 months of age; low levels can be found in normal babies below this age. The diagnosis is confirmed by mutation analysis.

Management

Daily subcutaneous injections of copper histidine can improve the outcome, but only if started within a month of birth [63]. Even with early treatment, patients with severe mutations have psychomotor impairment. Copper histidine injections do not correct the connective tissue abnormalities.

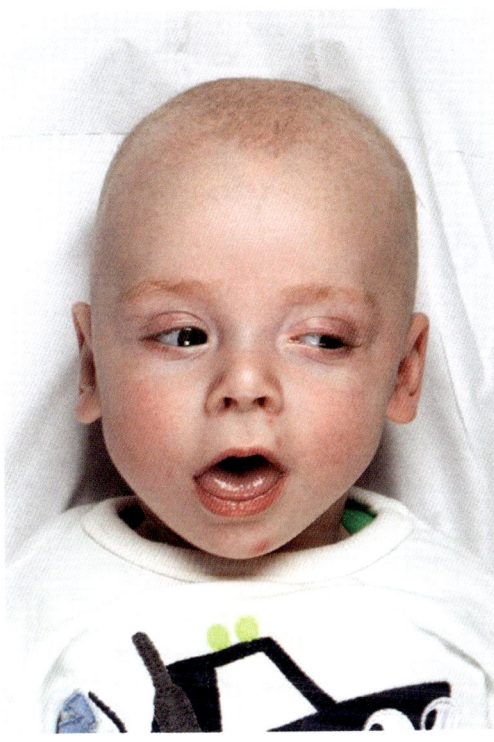

Figure 79.14 Infant with Menkes disease. Courtesy of Dr A. Chakrapani, Birmingham Children's Hospital, Birmingham, UK

MEDNIK syndrome

This extremely rare autosomal recessive disorder is caused by mutations in *AP1S1* or *AP1B1* [64,65]. These defects impair the intracellular trafficking of ATP7A, leading to low serum copper and caeruloplasmin concentrations. Patients present as neonates with erythrokeratoderma and diarrhoea or constipation. The acronym stands for Mental retardation, Enteropathy, Deafness, peripheral Neuropathy, Ichthyosis and Keratoderma; neuropathy does not occur with *AP1B1* mutations. Improvement with zinc acetate has been reported [64].

Wilson disease

Introduction, genetics and incidence

Wilson disease (MIM: 277900) is an autosomal recessive disorder caused by *ATP7B* mutations. The incidence is 1 in 30 000 to 100 000. Impaired copper excretion in bile leads to its accumulation in the liver, brain and other tissues; the dermatological features are mild.

Clinical features

Patients typically develop liver disease at 8–20 years of age or neurological symptoms (dysarthria, tremor, dystonia and drooling) at 12–30 years. Other problems may include behavioural changes, renal tubulopathy or haemolytic anaemia. A brown Kayser–Fleischer ring may be seen at the limbus of the cornea, particularly in patients with neurological symptoms.

Blue lunulae of the nails are the most specific dermatological feature and are present in 10% of adults at diagnosis. Commoner dermatological findings include xerosis, cheilitis and grey-brown hyperpigmentation, especially on the extensor surfaces of the legs [66]. There may also be pruritus or spider naevi due to liver disease, or drug-induced rashes.

Investigations

Serum copper and caeruloplasmin concentrations are generally low, with raised 24-hour urine copper excretion and raised liver copper. No test is entirely reliable and *ATP7B* sequencing is often undertaken [67].

Management

Copper excretion is promoted using chelators (penicillamine, trientine or tetrathiomolybdate) or zinc, which increases the faecal excretion of copper bound to metallothionein [68]. Penicillamine is recommended for patients with liver disease; a few require liver transplantation. Zinc is often used for presymptomatic patients and those with neurological symptoms as it has fewer side effects. Unfortunately, neurological problems seldom resolve completely and treatment may cause an initial deterioration.

Familial tumoral calcinosis

Introduction, genetics and pathophysiology

Hyperphosphataemic and normophosphataemic familial tumoral calcinosis (HFTC and NFTC) are extremely rare autosomal recessive disorders that cause ectopic calcification in the skin [**69**]. HFTC can result from mutations in three genes: *FGF23* encodes a phosphaturic hormone, *GALNT3* encodes a glycosyltransferase that modifies FGF23 and *KL* encodes Klotho, a co-receptor for FGF23 [70–72]. *GALNT3* defects are congenital defects of O-glycosylation (see earlier).

NFTC is caused by mutations in *SAMD9* [73]. *SAMD9* regulates EGR-1, a transcription factor involved in the regulation of tissue calcification, inflammation and cell migration [74]. *SAMD9* may also be a tumour suppressor gene as *SAMD9* deletions are associated with haematological cancers [75].

Clinical features

HFTC presents with calcified masses deep in the dermis and subcutaneous tissues, mainly over the large joints. These cause pain and can affect joint mobility. Dental problems are common, particularly affecting the roots. Some patients have recurrent episodes of pain in the tibia and other long bones, with redness and warmth of the overlying skin ('hyperostosis') [76].

NFTC presents with a vasculitis-like rash at a young age, followed years later by the appearance of calcified masses in cutaneous and subcutaneous tissues (Figure 79.15) [73]. The calcified lesions are smaller and more superficially located than in HFTC, and tend to perforate the skin, leading to painful ulcers and secondary infections. Gingivitis and conjunctivitis are common.

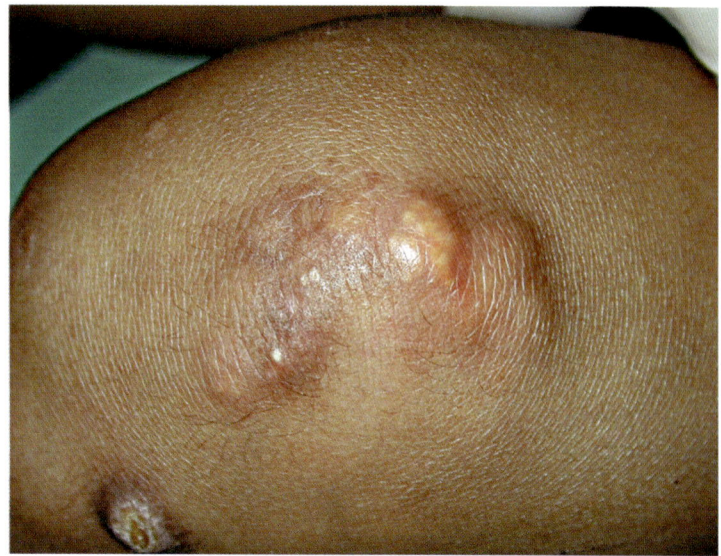

Figure 79.15 Calcinosis over knee of a child with normophosphataemic familial tumoral calcinosis.

Differential diagnosis

Cutaneous calcinosis may complicate Albright hereditary osteodystrophy, Rothmund–Thomson syndrome, hereditary sclerosing poikiloderma and pseudoxanthoma elasticum. It can also occur with acquired hyperphosphataemia or hypercalcaemia (as in chronic renal failure) or following tissue damage (due to autoimmune diseases, atherosclerosis or cancer) (Chapter 59).

Management

Surgical removal of calcified masses may be needed if there is significant functional impairment or an unacceptable cosmetic appearance. Treatment with phosphate binders seldom helps patients with HFTC but acetazolamide may be beneficial [77].

Key references

The full list of references can be found in the online version at https://www.wiley.com/rooksdermatology10e

19 Germain DP. Fabry disease. *Orphanet J Rare Dis* 2010;5:30.
29 Plummer C, Spring PJ, Marotta R *et al*. Multiple symmetrical lipomatosis – a mitochondrial disorder of brown fat. *Mitochondrion* 2013;13:269–76.
33 Tiranti V, Viscomi C, Hildebrandt T *et al*. Loss of ETHE1, a mitochondrial dioxygenase, causes fatal sulfide toxicity in ethylmalonic encephalopathy. *Nat Med* 2009;15:200–5.
37 Rymen D, Jaeken J. Skin manifestations in CDG. *J Inherit Metab Dis* 2014 37:699–708.
43 Rabinowitz LG, Williams LR, Anderson CE, Mazur A, Kaplan P. Painful keratoderma and photophobia: hallmarks of tyrosinemia type II. *J Pediatr* 1995;126:266–9.
47 Ferreira C, Wang H. Prolidase deficiency. In: Adam MP, Ardinger HH, Pagon RA iet al., eds, GeneReviews [Internet]. Seattle, WA: University of Washington, 2015.
58 Wolf B, Heard GS, Weissbecker KA, McVoy JR, Grier RE, Leshner RT. Biotinidase deficiency: initial clinical features and rapid diagnosis. *Ann Neurol* 1985;18:614–17.
59 Van Wouwe JP. Clinical and laboratory diagnosis of acrodermatitis enteropathica. *Eur J Pediatr* 1989;149:2–8.
61 Kaler SG. Diagnosis and therapy of Menkes syndrome, a genetic form of copper deficiency. *Am J Clin Nutr*. 1998;67(Suppl):1029S–34S.
69 Sprecher E. Familial tumoral calcinosis: from characterization of a rare phenotype to the pathogenesis of ectopic calcification. *J Invest Dermatol* 2010;130:652–60.

CHAPTER 80

Inherited Immunodeficiency

Tim Niehues[1] *and Andrew R. Gennery*[2]

[1] Centre for Child Health and Adolescence, HELIOS Klinikum, Krefeld; Academic Hospital, RWTH, Aachen; Immunodeficiency and Rheumatology Centre, Krefeld, Germany
[2] Translational and Clinical Research Institute, Newcastle University, and Paediatric Haematopoietic Stem Cell Transplant Unit, Great North Children's Hospital, Newcastle upon Tyne, UK

PART 6: GENETIC DISORDERS

Introduction

Definition

Inborn errors of immunity (IEI) have been traditionally defined as a group of inherited disorders resulting from defects in the immune system that lead to an increased susceptibility to infection, manifest by recurrent, persistent or opportunistic infectious episodes. With a greater understanding of the immune system and normal immunological responses, it has become clear that defects in immune responses can also present with the following:

- Susceptibility to single ubiquitous pathogens.
- Autoimmune disease.
- Autoinflammation.
- Failure of the inflammatory response.
- Failure of lymphocyte apoptosis following infection.
- Neoplasia.

IEI are differentiated from secondary immunodeficiencies, which result from HIV infection, use of immunosuppressive drugs (e.g. biologics, chemotherapy agents, radiotherapy, ciclosporin, etc.), nutritional deficiencies, splenectomy, uraemia, protein-losing states such as enteropathy or nephrotic syndrome, hepatic failure or cirrhosis, metabolic disorders (e.g. diabetes), atopic eczema and autoimmune diseases (e.g. systemic lupus erythematosus (SLE)) and extremes of age. IEI represent 'experiments of nature' and the clinical phenotype can help demonstrate the function of a particular molecule in the human immune system.

Given the complexity of disease, and wide variety of presentations, along with the specialised knowledge required to direct appropriate therapy, IEI patients are best cared for by physicians with a high level of specialisation and knowledge about the immune system, who are committed to an interdisciplinary approach.

Epidemiology

While each of the more than 450 genetic defects associated with IEI is extremely rare, IEI as a group are seen with increased frequency and have an estimated prevalence in Europe of 4.1/100 000 individuals [1].

Diagnosis

Clinical features suggesting inborn errors of immunity

Physiological susceptibility to infection is age dependent. While between 0 and 4 years of age, individuals experience almost five infections per year; this frequency decreases with increasing age from approximately three infections per year in the age group 5–19 years and two infections per year between 20 and 39 years of age and 1.5 infections above the age of 40 years. Some IEI do not manifest before adulthood. The most common IEI in adults is common variable immunodeficiency (CVID), with a twin peak incidence at 20–40 years of age and between 50 and 60 years of age.

The physician needs to differentiate between physiological or pathological susceptibility to infection. In adults, it has been defined that more than three infections per year which require treatment (including antibiotics), and each of which lasts more than 4 weeks, are defined as pathological susceptibility to infection. Other clues for pathological susceptibility to infection are unusual pathogens (e.g. pneumocystis), long duration of infection, unusual localisations (organ abscesses), unusually severe infection with common pathogens or recurring infections with the same infectious agent. Other manifestations of IEI include signs of immune dysregulation often referred to under the acronym of GARFIELD:

- **G**ranuloma.
- **A**utoimmune disease.
- **R**ecurring **F**ever and chronic **I**nflammation.
- Unusual **E**czema.
- **L**ymphoproliferation.
- Chronic, inflammatory bowel **D**isease.

The 10 Warning Signs of the Jeffrey Modell Foundation were proposed by an expert panel but were never validated prospectively. In a retrospective analysis in Great Britain, 430 children with IEI were tested for the predictive value of these warning signs. Only four signs had a positive predictive value (positive family history, more than 2 months of antibiotic treatment, failure to thrive, deeply seated abscesses). Thus, while they are used frequently in clinical practice, immunodeficiency should be considered even if the presentation does not fulfil these warning signs:

- Four or more new ear infections within 1 year (children), two or more new ear infections within 1 year (adults).
- Two or more serious sinus infections within 1 year (in the absence of allergy, adults).
- Two or more months of antibiotics with little effect (children).
- Two or more pneumonias within 1 year (children), one pneumonia for more than 1 year (adults).
- Failure of an infant to gain weight or grow normally.
- Recurring deep skin or organ abscesses.
- Persistent oro-pharyngeal *Candida* or fungal infection on the skin.
- Need for intravenous antibiotics to clear infections.
- Two or more deep-seated infections, including septicaemia.
- Family history of IEI.

Other warning signs include recurrent bacterial or fungal infections, recurrent viral infections (e.g. herpes, warts, condylomata), in association with chronic diarrhoea with weight loss, one pneumonia per year for more than 1 year, lymphoreticular malignancy (e.g. lymphoma in diseases of increased chromosomal breakage, intestinal lymphoma in CVID), syndromal aspects (e.g. DiGeorge syndrome, autosomal dominant hyper-IgE syndrome), albinism (e.g. Chediak–Higashi syndrome) and a history suggestive of X-linked inheritance, or parental consanguinity. The type of microorganism involved, especially if atypical, should direct further investigation. In immunodeficient patients, cutaneous infections are either caused by microorganisms not usually pathogenic in normal individuals or follow a more severe course due to infection with a common microorganism as compared with those with normal immunity. Allergic/atopic manifestations are common in IEI and may be unusually severe. Autoimmune and malignant diseases, though not common, have an increased incidence. Photosensitivity rashes may be a particular feature in some disorders, for example in immunodeficiencies associated with DNA repair disorders.

In some conditions, e.g. immunoglobulin A (IgA) deficiency, there may be a family history of collagen vascular or other immunopathological disease. Older relatives who are carriers of an inherited immunodeficiency or who are affected by milder variants of primary immune defects may have autoimmune manifestations

(e.g. mouth ulcers and SLE variant in chronic granulomatous disease (CGD)) or have a history of malignant disease (lymphoma in X-linked lymphoproliferative disease (XLP) or Wiskott–Aldrich syndrome (WAS)).

Infectious disease-related manifestations of inborn errors of immunity

Furuncular lesions or abscesses can be an overlooked manifestation of an IEI. They are most characteristically seen in neutrophil disorders such as CGD, Chediak–Higashi syndrome, leukocyte adhesion deficiency and neutrophil-specific granule deficiency but also in STAT3-loss-of-function (autosomal dominant hyper-IgE syndrome) and antibody deficiencies such as X-linked agammaglobulinaemia (XLA) or in complement disorders. In these disorders it is, however, usual for infections of the skin to be accompanied by infection at other sites.

Cutaneous and mucosal ulceration are features of several immunodeficiency states and are the hallmark of leukocyte adhesion deficiency. Although infection is believed to be the likely cause of skin ulceration, it can be difficult to identify the microorganisms responsible and the accumulation of neutrophils in small blood vessels to the point where blockage and tissue necrosis occur probably plays an important part in their genesis. Such ulcers are a characteristic feature of disorders featuring neutropenia, including congenital neutropenia, cyclical neutropenia and the Chediak–Higashi syndrome. Gradually extending cutaneous ulcers due to herpes simplex virus (HSV) are suggestive of T-lymphocyte defects but have also been reported in XLA.

Unusually severe or extensive infections with HSV or varicella-zoster virus, including the haemorrhagic vesicles seen in haemorrhagic chickenpox, are characteristic of T-lymphocyte defects. Bullous impetigo with clear blisters may be a presentation of neutropenia. A vesicular presentation of the hyper-IgE syndrome in infancy has been described.

Ordinary viral warts are virtually never indicative of immunodeficiency. However, exceptionally rapid growth of warts, exceptionally large size or unusually extensive infections are suggestive of underlying defects of immunity [2]. Severe extensive persistent molluscum contagiosum is seen in similar disorders such as WAS, CD40 ligand deficiency and DOCK8 deficiency.

Refractory mucosal and cutaneous *Candida* infections are a characteristic presenting sign of several immunodeficiency disorders, particularly severe combined immunodeficiency (SCID) and severe T-lymphocyte defects. Surprisingly, systemic *Candida* infections are rather rare in these conditions. Persistent mucosal and cutaneous *Candida* infection, which responds poorly to systemic treatment, suggests chronic mucocutaneous candidiasis. Invasive fungal infection is a hallmark of neutrophil deficiency [3].

Non-infectious non-specific manifestations of inborn errors of immunity

Eczema is a characteristic cutaneous feature of some IEI such as WAS, and has been recorded as occurring, more frequently than one would expect, in various other disorders, including selective IgA deficiency, selective IgM deficiency, ataxia telangiectasia and combined immunodeficiencies. It is also typically seen with more complex immune dysfunction as in Comèl–Netherton and related syndromes (Chapter 63) as well as in disorders associated with abnormal CARD-BCL-10-MALT1 signalling [4].

Morbilliform eruptions are sometimes caused by viral infections, as in other children, but in SCID they are quite frequently manifestations of acute graft-versus-host reactions, due either to maternofetal engraftment or to engraftment of viable lymphocytes from a third party after the transfusion of non-irradiated blood products after birth. A rash may be seen after vaccination with live vaccines such as measles, mumps and rubella or varicella, in patients with severe T-lymphocyte immunodeficiency who develop disease.

Petechiae, due to thrombocytopenia, are a highly characteristic feature of WAS and may also occur in Fanconi anaemia, dyskeratosis congenita, Schwachman–Diamond syndrome and the Chediak–Higashi syndrome.

Vasculitic lesions may rarely be seen as an autoimmune manifestation and have been documented in XLP, autoimmune lymphoproliferative syndrome (ALPS) and immunodysregulation polyendocrinopathy enteropathy X-linked (IPEX) syndrome, as well as CVID.

Ichthyosis can be seen in nuclear factor κB essential modulator mutation (NEMO) deficiency and Comèl–Netherton syndrome.

A combination of erythroderma of early onset with failure to thrive in early infancy is highly suggestive of immunodeficiency and often results from dysregulated activated T lymphocytes invading the skin. In some cases these are maternally derived and represent true graft-versus-host disease while in other cases aberrant clones of the infant's own T lymphocytes cause a similar reaction which results in the condition known as Omenn syndrome, a 'leaky' form of SCID.

Patients with primary immunodeficiencies can display indurated erythematous papules and plaques with central scaling, scarring, atrophy or ulceration, which demonstrated caseating granulomas histologically. The conditions in which these have been reported include common variable immunodeficiency, XLA, ataxia telangiectasia, CGD, recombinase activating gene (RAG) deficiency and RNA component of mitochondrial RNA processing endoribonuclease (RMRP) deficiency [5]. In combined immunodeficiencies, these lesions have been associated with vaccine-derived rubella virus.

As well as classic systemic and discoid lupus erythematosus, a syndrome resembling SLE from the cutaneous point of view, but having only very mild non-cutaneous manifestations, and either absent or very low-titre plasma antinuclear antibodies, has been described in patients with a variety of complement deficiencies, most commonly C2 deficiency but also C3, C4, C1q and C1 esterase inhibitor deficiency. In such patients, this syndrome can occasionally have its onset as early as the first year of life, and, because many of these patients are susceptible to certain infections, such as meningococcal meningitis, the association of a disorder resembling lupus erythematosus and recurrent infections of appropriate type is highly suggestive of a hereditary complement deficiency.

There is an increased incidence of SLE in patients with IgA deficiency, and skin lesions closely resembling discoid lupus erythematosus have occurred in female carriers of the gene for X-linked CGD.

Hypo- or hyperpigmented lesions are characteristic of a few inborn errors of immunity, particularly those with an underlying DNA repair disorder, such as Bloom syndrome or Nijmegen breakage syndrome. Hypopigmentation of the skin or hair is also characteristic of Chediak–Higashi and Griscelli syndromes.

Diagnostic laboratory tests

Genetic diagnosis is best directed in the context of clinical and laboratory immunological findings. Although whole exome sequencing is becoming cheaper and more easily accessible, in the absence of clinical and laboratory immunological information, interpretation of the data can be difficult. Simple immunological investigations are useful before more specialised investigations are performed: IgG, IgA, IgM and IgE, blood count and a differential leukocyte count are of paramount importance in screening for immunodeficiency (e.g. neutropenia, lymphocytopenia, monocytopenia or eosinophilia may give important clues). In paediatrics, these values must be compared with age-related normal values. A titre of specific antibodies after vaccination indicates that there is sufficient B- and T-lymphocyte interaction as well as antibody production. Only rarely is there an indication to determine IgG subclasses; this is reserved for cases that show normal IgG but a classic picture of humoral immunodeficiency. Flow cytometric analysis of lymphocyte subpopulations is an important tool for the clinical immunologist, performed in a specialised laboratory that is experienced in the interpretation of results obtained from patients with IEI.

Functional tests of the immune system include tests for complement function (e.g. CH50, AP50), lymphocyte proliferation cell cycle (e.g. ataxia telangiectasia), cytotoxicity (immunodeficiencies with immune dysregulation), apoptosis (e.g. ALPS) and simulation of peripheral blood mononuclear cells with cytokines as well as calcium mobilisation assays. Genetic analyses and data can only be interpreted in the context of clinical and immunological findings, as finding a mutation does not necessarily imply that it is causing the disease.

Management

While a few IEI do not require specific treatment (e.g. selective IgA deficiency), others necessitate highly intensive treatment (e.g. haematopoietic stem cell transplantation or gene therapy for SCID, CGD and other IEI). In many IEI, regular immunoglobulin substitution has changed the prognosis significantly, e.g. in CVID and agammaglobulinaemia. Once a sufficient IgG trough level is established, most infectious complications significantly diminish. Supportive treatment is key in some IEI (e.g. CGD: antibacterial and antifungal prophylaxis). Autoimmune or autoinflammatory complications may require immunosuppressive or immunomodulatory treatment (e.g. steroids in granulomatous organ disease, anti-CD20 therapy in Epstein–Barr virus complications), or treatment with small molecule inhibitors (JAK inhibitors) or anticytokine therapies.

Inborn errors of immunity with skin manifestations

IEI are classified on a regular basis by an expert committee of the International Union of Immunological Societies (IUIS) [1]. IEI are classified as follows:

- I: Combined immunodeficiencies.

- II: Combined immunodeficiencies with associated or syndromic features.
- III: Predominantly antibody deficiencies.
- IV: Diseases of immune dysregulation.
- V: Congenital defects of phagocyte number and function.
- VI: Defects in intrinsic and innate immunity.
- VII: Autoinflammatory disorders.
- VIII: Complement deficiencies.
- IX: Bone marrow failure.

The skin is a critical mechanical barrier, and a vital component of the innate immune system and the site where many innate and adaptive immune responses to infection are seen. It is not surprising therefore that skin infections and other dermatological manifestations are common features of IEI. It is estimated that almost 50% of children who present with IEI have skin manifestations. In this chapter, we will not cover all of the more than 450 genetically defined IEI but will focus on IEI with prominent skin manifestations as well as manifestations affecting the hair, nails and sweat glands (Table 80.1).

Table 80.1 Inborn errors of immunity with prominent skin manifestations as well as manifestations affecting the hair, nails and sweat glands (see text for definitions of abbreviations).

Disease	MIM	Gene	Major immune defect	Major skin manifestations
Severe combined immune deficiencies				
X-linked	300400	*IL2RG*	SCID	Bacterial, viral, fungal skin infection, BCG nodules
JAK3-deficient	600173	*JAK3*	SCID	Bacterial, viral, fungal skin infection, BCG nodules
IL7Ra-deficient	146661	*IL7Ra*	SCID	Bacterial, viral, fungal skin infection, BCG nodules
ADA-deficient	608958	*ADA*	SCID	Bacterial, viral, fungal skin infection, BCG nodules Dermatofibrosarcoma protuberans
Artemis-deficient	602450	*DCLRE1C*	SCID	Bacterial, viral, fungal skin infection, BCG nodules
RAG1-deficient	601457	*RAG1*	SCID/CID	Bacterial, viral, fungal skin infection, BCG nodules, occasionally granuloma
RAG2-deficient	179616	*RAG2*	SCID/CID	Bacterial, viral, fungal skin infection, BCG nodules Occasionally granuloma
ORAI-1	610277	*ORAI1*	SCID	Ectodermal dysplasia
STIM-1	605921	*STIM1*	SCID	Ectodermal dysplasia
FOXN1	601705	*FOXN1*	SCID	Congenital alopecia, nail dystrophy
DiGeorge syndrome	188400	*TBX1*	SCID/CID/Omenn	Omenn features, autoimmune vitiligo
CHARGE syndrome	214800	*CHD7*	SCID/CID/Omenn	Omenn features, autoimmune vitiligo
Omenn syndrome	603554	Commonly *RAG1/2*, but other SCID genes described	SCID/CID	Erythroderma, alopecia, lymphadenopathy
Combined immune deficiencies				
Wiskott–Aldrich syndrome	301000	*WAS*	CID	Eczema, petechiae, bruising, severe molluscum contagiosum and varicella-zoster infection
DOCK8 deficiency	243700	*DOCK8*	CID	Atopic eczema, extensive, disfiguring, concurrently occurring cutaneous herpes simplex virus, human papillomavirus, molluscum contagiosum and varicella-zoster virus infections
X-linked hyper-IgM syndrome	308230	*CD40LG*	CID	Oral ulceration. Severe cutaneous *Pseudomonas aeruginosa* infections
CD40 deficiency	606843	*CD40*	CID	Oral ulceration. Severe cutaneous *Pseudomonas aeruginosa* infections
MHC class I deficiency	604571	*TAP1, TAP2, TAPBP*	CID	Necrotising granulomatous skin lesions, located on the extremities and midface
X-linked lymphoproliferative syndrome	300490	*SH2D1A*	CID	Vasculitis, polyarteritis nodosa
X-linked inhibitor of apoptosis	300079	*BIRC4*	CID	Fistulating skin abscesses
Comèl–Netherton syndrome	256500	*SPINK5*	CID	Trichorrhexis invaginata, ichthyosiform erythroderma and atopic eczema
Cartilage hair hypoplasia	250250	*RMRP*	CID/SCID	Sparse, thin hair, alopecia, short-limbed dwarfism, skin carcinoma, rarely cutaneous granulomas
DNA repair defects				
Ataxia telangiectasia	607585	*ATM*	CID	Telangiectasia, café-au-lait spots, granulomas (some patients)
Nijmegen breakage syndrome	602667	*NBS1*	CID	Microcephaly, photosensitivity, psoriatic-like lesions and hypo- or hyperpigmented lesions
LIG4 syndrome	606593	*LIG4*	CID/SCID	Photosensitivity, psoriatic-like lesions and hypo- or hyperpigmented lesions

(continued)

Table 80.1 (continued)

Disease	MIM	Gene	Major immune defect	Major skin manifestations
SCID with microcephaly, growth retardation and sensitivity to ionising radiation	611291	NHEJ1	CID/SCID	Photosensitivity, psoriatic-like lesions and hypo- or hyperpigmented lesions
Bloom syndrome	604610	BLM	CID	Photosensitivity, malar rash
Immunodeficiency, centromeric instability, facial anomalies (ICF) syndrome	242860	DNMT3B, ZBTB24	CID	Extensive cutaneous warts and fungal infections
Dyskeratosis congenita	305000, 127550, 613989, 604319, 606471, 613987, 604173, 613988, 612199, 615190	DKC1, TERC, TERT, TINF2, NOP10, NHP2, C16orf57, TCAB1, CTC1, RETL1	CID	Leukoplakia, oral ulceration and reticulated hyperpigmentation, palmar hyperkeratosis, perioral reticular hyperpigmentation, nail dystrophy
Fanconi anaemia	227650, 300514, 227615, 605724, 227646, 600901, 603467, 614082, 609053, 609054, 614083, 614087, 610832, 613390, 613951, 615272	FANCA, FANCB, FANCC, BRCA2, FANCD2, FANCE, FANCF, FANCG, FANCI, BRIP1, FANCL, FANCM, PALB2, RAD51C, SLX4, ERCC4	CID	Cutaneous macular brownish hyperpigmentation, resembling freckles in sun-exposed areas or more diffusely. Guttate macular hypopigmentation. Hypopigmentation and café-au-lait spots
Antibody deficiencies				
X-linked agammaglobulinaemia	300755	BTK	Antibody deficiency	Skin sepsis, Stevens–Johnson syndrome, vitiligo, alopecia areata
Autosomal recessive agammaglobulinaemia	601495, 613500, 613501, 613502, 613506, 612692, 615214	IGHM, IGLL, CD79A, BLNK, LRCC8, CD79B, PIK3R1	Antibody deficiency	Skin sepsis
PIK3CD	602839	PIK3CD	Antibody deficiency	Skin, salivary gland, lacrimal gland, dental abscess, orbital cellulitis
Common variable immunodeficiency	607594, 240500, 613493, 613494, 613495, 613496, 614699, 614700, 615577, 615767	ICOS, TNFRSF13B, CD19, TNFRSF13C, MS4A1, CD81, CR2, LRBA, NFKB2, IL21	CID, autoimmunity	Vitiligo, eczema, vasculitis, petechiae, skin infections, sarcoid-like skin granulomas, dermatomyositis, SLE
Immune dysregulation				
Chediak–Higashi syndrome	214500	LYST	Immune deficiency with albinism	Oculocutaneous albinism, partial albinism
Griscelli syndrome type 2	607624	RAB27A	Immune deficiency with albinism	Pigmentary dilution of skin, silvery-grey hair, cytophagic histiocytic panniculitis
Hermansky–Pudlak syndrome type 2	608233	AP3B1	Immune deficiency with albinism	Oculocutaneous albinism with neutropenia
Immunodysregulation, polyendocrinopathy, enteropathy, X-linked (IPEX) syndrome	304790	FOXP3		Neonatal exanthema or eczema often with early-onset insulin-dependent diabetes, autoimmune enteropathy
Autoimmune lymphoproliferative syndrome	601859, 603909, 607271	FASLG, TNFRSF6, CASP10, CASP8		Rarely linear IgA disease, vasculitis and urticarial – more usually lymphadenopathy
Phagocytic defects				
Chronic granulomatous disease	306400, 233700, 233690, 233710, 613960	CYBB, NCF1, CYBA, NCF2, NCF4	Functional phagocytic defect	Neonatal pustulosis, non-specific, impetiginised periorificial rash, impetiginised or ecthymatous broken skin followed by nodular lesions forming necrotic ulcers. Translucent papular lesions around the nose, eyes, lips and cheeks. Subcutaneous nodules at immunisation sites, which ulcerate. Poor healing of surgical wounds. Perianal abscesses, chronic suppurative paronychia, scalp folliculitis, ulcerative stomatitis

(continued)

PART 6: GENETIC DISORDERS

PART 6: GENETIC DISORDERS

Table 80.1 (*continued*)

Disease	MIM	Gene	Major immune defect	Major skin manifestations
Congenital neutropenia	202700, 610738, 612541, 615285, 616022, 232220, 600871, 245000, 604173, 300299	*ELANE, HAX1, G6PC3, VPS45A, JAGN1, GFI1, GSD1b, CTSC, WAS*	Neutrophil differentiation defect	Omphalitis, skin abscesses, oral ulceration, gingivitis and early loss of permanent teeth
Neutrophil adhesion defects	116920, 266265, 612840	*ITGB2, SLC35C1, KIND3*	Neutrophil migration defect	Delayed umbilical cord separation, omphalitis, rapidly progressive erosive perianal ulcers, gingivitis, ulcerative stomatitis, periodontitis, inflammatory lesions affecting the skin and resembling pyoderma gangrenosum
Defects in innate immunity				
NF-κB pathway-related immunodeficiencies	300291, 164008	*IKBKG, IKBKA*		Sparse scalp hair, conical teeth, absent sweat glands
Toll-like receptor pathway defects	607676, 612260	*IRAK4, MYD88*		Skin sepsis
Warts, hypogammaglobulinaemia, infections, myelokathexis (WHIM) syndrome	193670	*CXCR4*		Severe, generalised verrucosis, involving all cutaneous and mucosal tissues, associated with hypogammaglobulinaemia and neutropenia
Epidermodysplasia verruciformis	226400	*TMC6 TMC8 CIB1*		Similar to WHIM syndrome with increased susceptibility to human papillomavirus infections manifesting as widespread flat warts and pityriasis versicolor-like lesions. Verrucous skin carcinomas, neutropenia and hypogammaglobulinaemia are not features
Autosomal dominant hyper-IgE syndrome	147060	*STAT3*		Chronic dermatitis and repeated lung and skin infections, a non-specific, excoriated, papular and pustular eruption in infancy, over scalp, scalp margins, buttocks and proximal flexures, furunculosis and staphylococcal lung infections. Oral candidiasis and *Candida* nail infections are common
Chronic mucocutaneous candidiasis	240300, 212050, 607644, 613108, 613953, 613956, 614162	*AIRE, CARD9, CANDN1, CLEC7A, IL17RA, IL17F,* gain-of-function *STAT1*		Ectodermal dystrophy with onychomycosis, superficial chronic mucocutaneous candidiasis affecting particularly oro-pharyngeal mucosa and the perineal region
Autoinflammatory diseases				See Table 80.2
Complement diseases				
C1q	613652	*C1QA, C1QB, C1QC*		Systemic lupus erythematosus, recurrent skin lesions
C1r	216950	*C1R*		Lupus-like symptoms
C1s	613783	*C1S*		Systemic lupus erythematosus
C2	217000	*C2*		Henoch–Schönlein purpura, systemic lupus erythematosus, polyarteritis, polymyositis, vasculitis
C3	613779	*C3*		Recurrent bacterial infections, particularly with encapsulated bacteria, systemic lupus erythematosus
C4	614380 614379	*C4A C4B*		Systemic lupus erythematosus, Henoch–Schönlein purpura Bacterial meningitis
C5	609536	*C5*		Systemic lupus erythematosus, neisserial infection
C6	612446	*C6*		Meningococcal infection
C7	610102	*C7*		Recurrent meningococcal infection, pyoderma gangrenosum
C8	613790 120690	*C8A C8B*		Recurrent neisserial infection
C9	613825	*C9*		Systemic meningococcal infection
C1 esterase inhibitor	106100	*C1NH*		Episodic local subcutaneous oedema, rarely systemic lupus erythematosus
Factor H	609814	*HF1*		Recurrent bacterial infection, atypical haemolytic uraemic syndrome
Factor I	610984	*CFI*		Recurrent bacterial infection, atypical haemolytic uraemic syndrome, rarely systemic lupus erythematosus

Combined immunodeficiencies
Severe combined immunodeficiency

SCID comprises over 20 genetic subtypes in all of which T-lymphocyte activity is compromised by either a lack of development or function of mature T lymphocytes. Moreover, B-lymphocyte activity and antibody production are severely impaired. Classic clinical manifestations are recurrent severe infections, chronic diarrhoea and associated failure to thrive. Unless haematopoietic stem cell transplantation (or, in selected diseases, gene therapy or thymic transplantation) is performed, children die within the first months of life. The skin manifestations of SCID may be one of the clues to clinical diagnosis.

Skin manifestations are multiple in SCID

Due to the decreased barrier function of the skin and the lack of adaptive immunity in SCID patients, skin infections can be very severe and ulcerating. A common finding in patients for whom the diagnosis is delayed is deep skin ulceration in the diaper area infected by Gram-negative bacteria or fungi (Figure 80.1). With the introduction in many countries of the live attenuated rotavirus infection, prolonged diarrhoea with subsequent localised skin inflammation has become more common.

Chronic oro-perineal candidiasis

Due to the T-lymphocyte deficiency, sometimes associated with natural killer (NK) cell deficiency, persistent cutaneous *Candida* infection may be found, particularly affecting the oropharynx or perineal region.

Erythroderma

A morbilliform rash with fever, evolving into a red exfoliating protein-losing rash, which becomes a confluent erythema, may be due to graft-versus-host disease. While conventionally this is a complication of posthaematopoietic stem cell transplantation, in patients who have severe T-lymphocyte immunodeficiency, non-host T-lymphocytes can cause severe, often fatal

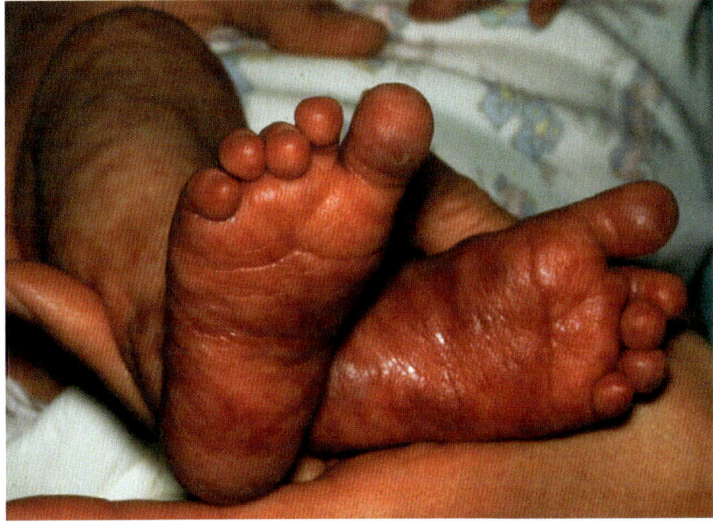

Figure 80.2 Maternofetal graft-versus-host disease in an infant with JAK3-deficient severe combined immunodeficiency.

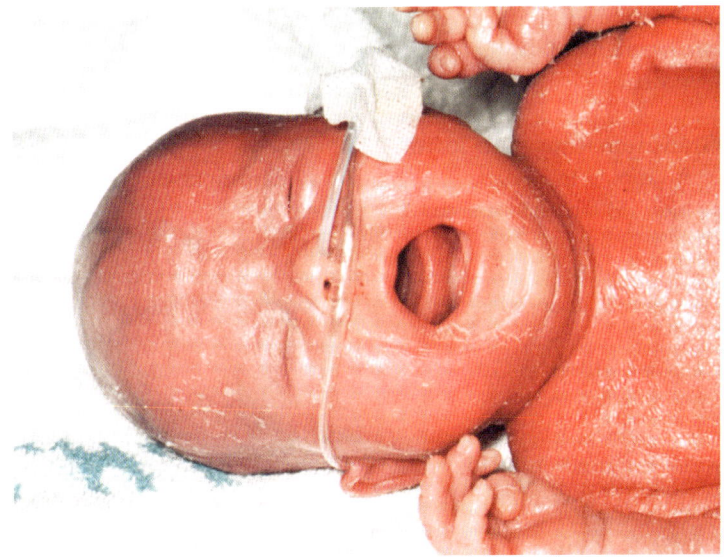

Figure 80.3 Omenn syndrome, with characteristic erythroderma and alopecia.

graft-versus-host disease. This is most commonly found following engraftment of transplacental maternal T lymphocytes (Figure 80.2), but transfusion of non-irradiated blood products may also transfer immune-competent HLA-reactive T lymphocytes. Histological examination will confirm the diagnosis, and genetic fingerprinting of circulating lymphocytes may help determine the origin of the cells.

Omenn syndrome is characterised by a generalised thickened erythematous rash, often with scaling and erythroderma [6]. The initial appearances may be papular, becoming confluent, and the skin often becomes thickened with a 'leathery' consistency. Hair, including the eyebrows, is often lost as the rash evolves (Figure 80.3). The rash may be present at birth or evolve over the first few weeks of life. There is also lymphadenopathy, particularly of the axillary and inguinal nodes, as well as increased serum IgE levels with a marked eosinophilia and combined immunodeficiency. Children usually present in early infancy but may present later in the first

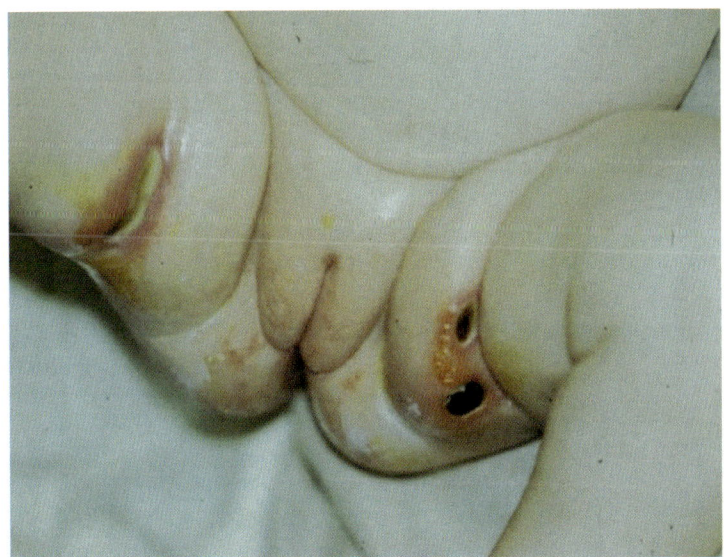

Figure 80.1 Ulcerated perineal region in an infant with severe combined immunodeficiency.

year of life and suffer from diarrhoea, failure to thrive and persistent infection as seen in other forms of SCID. There are abnormally high numbers of activated oligoclonal poorly functional T lymphocytes, which have a restricted Vβ repertoire, and there are high levels of circulating inflammatory cytokines. Peripheral B-lymphocyte numbers are low or absent, as are levels of immunoglobulin classes other than IgE. The clinical picture may resemble SCID with maternofetal engraftment. Histology of the skin shows a dense dermal perivascular lymphohistiocytic infiltrate, comprising activated T lymphocytes, with numerous eosinophils. S100-positive Langerhans cells are usually absent and there is no epidermotropism. Lymph node architecture is disordered, being replaced by a massive infiltrate of S100-positive interdigitating reticulum cells with absence of germinal centres, absent B lymphocytes and paucity of T lymphocytes. Activated oligoclonal lymphocytes in skin seemingly provoke Langerhans cells to migrate to lymph nodes, liver and spleen where lymphoid tissue architecture is severely disrupted. Molecular genetic studies to identify the origin of the T lymphocytes in the blood (maternal or autologous) will differentiate between Omenn syndrome and graft-versus-host reaction. Calcineurin inhibitors and interferon γ may ameliorate the clinical symptoms, but haematopoietic stem cell transplantation is the only curative treatment.

Granulomatous skin lesions

Granulomas may occur in the skin and present in a livedo-like fashion [5]. These skin granulomas have been observed in different IEI, including atypical SCID, where residual function of autologous T and B lymphocytes is retained. Histopathologically, these granulomas are epithelioid and non-caseating (Figure 80.4).

Bacille Calmette–Guérin infection

In certain geographical areas, infants with SCID may receive the live attenuated bacille Calmette–Guérin (BCG) vaccine in the first week of life, before the immunological diagnosis is considered. Surprisingly, in many the infection is latent, but a few present

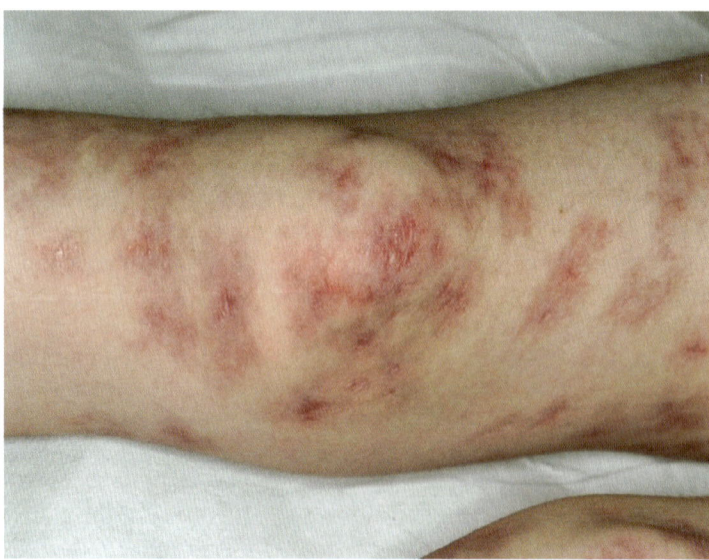

Figure 80.4 Inflammatory granulomatous skin lesions in a child with atypical severe combined immunodeficiency.

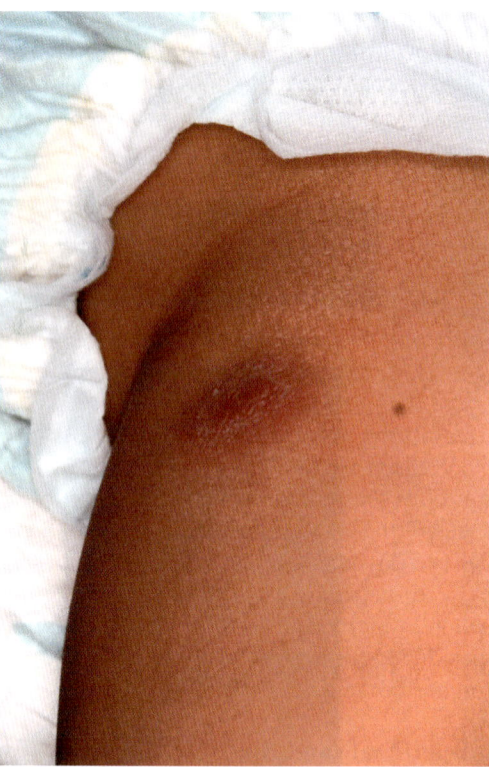

Figure 80.5 Cutaneous lesion in a child with severe combined immunodeficiency who had been immunised with the live bacille Calmette–Guérin (BCG) vaccine. On biopsy, acid-fast bacilli were seen, and BCG strain mycobacteria were subsequently isolated.

with disseminated BCG, which can affect many organs and may manifest on the skin as discrete nodules, which upon biopsy will be found to contain acid-fast bacilli (Figure 80.5). Many of these lesions become inflamed following transplantation, as effective T-lymphocyte immunity is established, and may progress to form draining abscesses, particularly over lymph nodes, often associated with fever.

Some particular SCID genotypes are associated with specific skin manifestations in addition to the ones already described:

- Adenosine deaminase (ADA) deficiency: these patients suffer from a rare malignant skin tumour, dermatofibrosarcoma protuberans, which is not prevented by curative treatment, and may occur after successful haematopoietic transplantation or gene therapy. In addition, skeletal abnormalities (cupping deformities of the ends of the ribs, as well as abnormalities of the transverse vertebral processes and the scapulae) are reported in up to 50% of cases of ADA deficiency.
- Calcium-channel deficiencies (*ORAI-1, STIM-1*): some patients have ectodermal dysplasia and myopathy.
- Winged helix deficiency (nude phenotype – *FOXN1*): this form of SCID is associated with congenital alopecia and nail dystrophy.
- Complete DiGeorge syndrome and CHARGE syndrome: DiGeorge syndrome is a relatively common (1/4000) syndrome, classically with cardiac anomalies, hypoplastic thymus and hypocalcemia as well as typical facial dysmorphic features. CHARGE syndrome is a related disorder, with cardiac and oesophageal anomalies. In both cases, the complete form of the syndrome results in thymic aplasia and absence of T lymphocytes. Skin manifestations consist of an eczematous dermatitis

with lymphadenopathy, similar to Omenn syndrome. In the partial forms of the disease, with some but a diminished number of T lymphocytes, autoimmune phenomena may include vitiligo.

Other combined immunodeficiencies
Wiskott–Aldrich syndrome

Immunodeficiency, thrombocytopenia, eczema and an increased risk of autoimmune disorders and malignancy characterise this X-linked recessive condition. The gene responsible for coding for the Wiskott–Aldrich syndrome protein (WASP) is only found in bone marrow derived cells and is essential for actin cytoskeleton polymerisation and consequently the correct assembly of cell surface receptors as well as cell movement. Patients who do express WASP, albeit in defective form, have a milder phenotype, known as X-linked thrombocytopenia, which is characterised by thrombocytopenia and bleeding tendency, but without eczema or immunodeficiency. Missense mutations in exons 1–3 lead to normal protein, whereas most other mutations result in the absence of WASP. Patients who do not express WASP at all usually exhibit the classic triad of thrombocytopenia, recurrent infections and eczema (Figure 80.6) but these vary in severity and in some patients the eczema is surprisingly mild. In general, it is indistinguishable from atopic eczema apart from the characteristic presence of purpura and bleeding from excoriation in many patients. The condition usually presents in early childhood with bruising, petechiae and bleeding; thrombocytopenia and bleeding episodes may require platelet transfusions. Herpesviruses, including herpes simplex and varicella-zoster virus, are poorly handled and may cause severe and recurrent disease. Impetigo, cellulitis and skin abscesses are surprisingly common, molluscum contagiosum and viral warts

may be very extensive and together with excessive bruising help to clinically distinguish WAS from uncomplicated eczema. Indeed, very extensive molluscum contagiosum is quite characteristic of WAS. Infection exacerbates the bleeding tendency and early death may result from bleeding. With increasing age, infectious complications replace bleeding as the major cause of death. Autoimmunity, particularly autoimmune haemolytic anaemia and vasculitis, and malignancy, particularly of the lymphoreticular system, become more common with increasing age and in many cases are related to abnormal persistence of Epstein–Barr viral infection. Thrombocytopenia with an abnormally small mean platelet volume (<5 fL) is pathognomonic. The severity of immunodeficiency is variable but progresses with age and affects cellular and humoral responses. Acute bleeding episodes may be controlled by platelet transfusions (irradiated to prevent graft-versus-host disease). Splenectomy and systemic steroids should be avoided if possible as they will increase the risk of infection and death. Topical steroids are required for the eczema. Intravenous immunoglobulin, with or without prophylactic antibiotics, reduces bacterial sinopulmonary infections and in high dose may help treat autoimmune phenomena. With only these supportive measures, the prognosis remains poor. Immunological and haematological reconstitution can be achieved by haematopoietic stem cell transplantation (HSCT) and despite a higher risk of Epstein–Barr virus driven lymphoproliferative disorders, results are good with a 5-year overall survival of 90% in transplants performed since 2000 [7].

DOCK8 deficiency

Mutations in dedicator of cytokinesis 8 (*DOCK8*) cause an autosomal recessive combined immunodeficiency with hyper-IgE. Cutaneous features include atopic eczema. The most significant feature of DOCK8 deficiency is susceptibility to extensive, disfiguring, concurrently occurring cutaneous viral infections, particularly HSV, human papillomavirus, molluscum contagiosum and varicella-zoster virus [8] (Figure 80.7). There are also *Staphylococcus aureus* skin abscesses and soft-tissue infections. Other invasive infections are described including recurrent sinopulmonary infection and meningitis from a wide spectrum of Gram-positive and Gram-negative bacteria, and intracellular fungi, such as *Histoplasma capsulatum*. Mucocutaneous candidiasis and recurrent gastrointestinal tract infections are common. Patients can also suffer from severe and extensive food allergies. Increased serum IgE levels and eosinophilia are found. Patients with DOCK8 deficiency are at high risk of developing malignancies, particularly lymphomas and squamous carcinomas. HSCT is curative.

CD40 ligand and CD40 deficiencies

Skin manifestations are related to the coexisting neutropenia and include oral ulceration. Severe cutaneous infections, particularly due to *Pseudomonas aeruginosa*, may occur.

OX40 deficiency

The T-lymphocyte co-stimulatory receptor OX40, one of the tumour necrosis factor superfamily proteins, enhances T-lymphocyte receptor-induced responses. It is expressed on many activated T lymphocytes, including CD8+ T-lymphocytes, and CD4+ T lymphocyte subtypes: T_H1, T_H2 and T_H17 and CD4+ Foxp3+ Tregs.

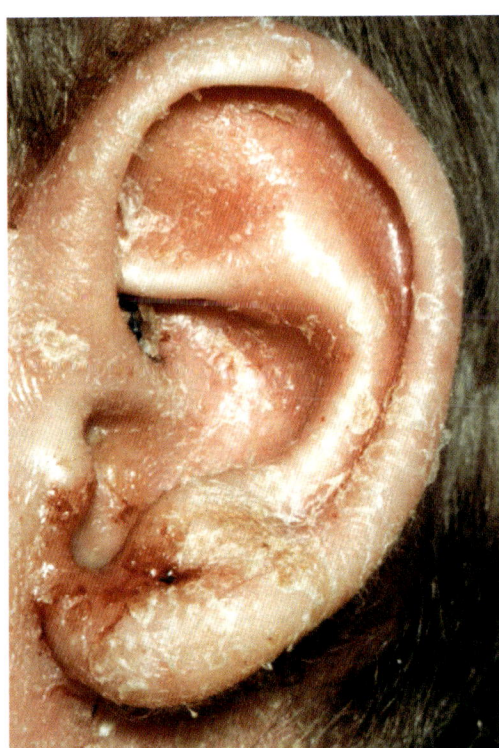

Figure 80.6 Severe eczema in a child with Wiskott–Aldrich syndrome.

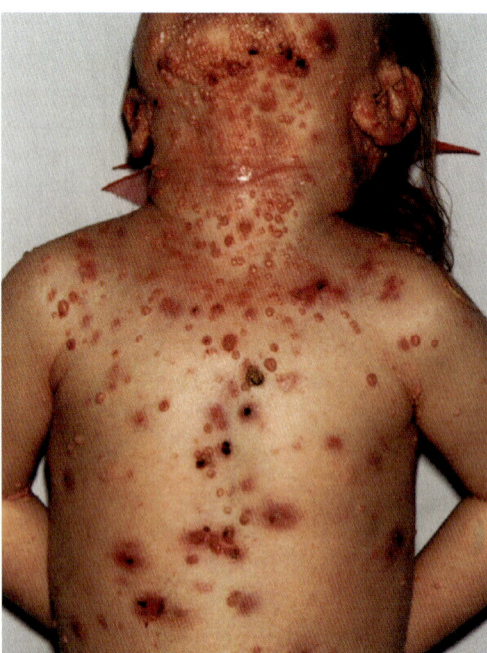

Figure 80.7 Severe molluscum contagiosum in a child with DOCK8 deficiency.

Loss-of-function mutations in *OX40*, described in only one patient to date, caused HHV8-associated Kaposi sarcoma. Given the high level of OX40 expressed in Kaposi sarcoma, OX40 deficiency may be selectively susceptible to this complication of HHV8 infection.

Major histocompatibility complex class I deficiency

Clinically, this disease has a milder phenotype than major histocompatibility complex (MHC) II deficiency with symptoms often not beginning until late childhood and is caused by deficiencies in the transporter associated with antigen processing (TAP) 1 or 2, or TAP-binding proteins. Recurrent respiratory tract infections leading to bronchiectasis and sinus problems are common. Gastrointestinal disease is rare. The most striking clinical manifestation is necrotising granulomatous skin lesions, which are located on the extremities (Figure 80.8) and also in the midface. The lesion begins with a small pustule or subcutaneous module, which slowly expands and ulcerates. The lesions are slow to heal, and usually leave hyperpigmented scars. Midface lesions can be particularly mutilating and resemble midline granuloma. Diagnosis is confirmed by showing absent HLA class I expression in peripheral blood. Treatment is directed towards prevention/limitation of lung disease with judicious use of antibiotics (directed by sputum cultures), and physiotherapy and bronchodilators as required. Prophylactic continuous antibiotics are of unproven benefit but may be helpful.

X-linked lymphoproliferative diseases

An X-linked immunodeficiency associated with fulminant fatal Epstein–Barr virus-driven infectious mononucleosis was first recognised in the Duncan kindred, a large midwestern American family in which six boys were affected, and after whom the disease was originally named (Duncan disease). There are three common clinical presentations: fulminant infectious mononucleosis (58%), dysgammaglobulinaemia, often evolving to CVID (31%), and

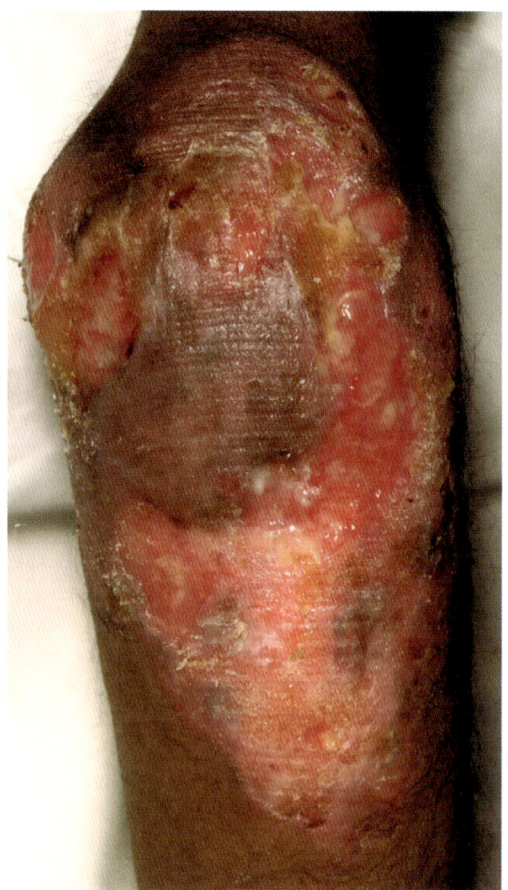

Figure 80.8 Sterile necrotising granulomatous lesion on the knee of a patient with TAP1 deficiency.

Epstein–Barr virus-driven B lymphoma, usually extranodal, and affecting the gastrointestinal tract or central nervous system (20%). Less commonly, patients present with vasculitis, aplastic anaemia, haemophagocytic lymphohistiocytosis, pulmonary lymphomatoid granulomatosis or vasculitis. Few cases of XLP-associated vasculitis have been published (Figure 80.9). Polyarteritis nodosa-like vasculitis has been reported. Vasculitic changes in small and medium-sized muscular arteries have also been reported. A clinical picture of polyarteritis nodosa in a boy with marked lymphadenopathy, erythrophagocytosis or recent infection should raise suspicion of this disease.

The prognosis is poor with a high risk of death during initial Epstein–Barr virus infection and no recorded survivors after 40 years of age. Most patients are well until infected with Epstein–Barr virus, although other viruses may act as triggers. Confirmation of the diagnosis involves demonstrating Epstein–Barr virus genome in blood by polymerase chain reaction, together with immune defects outlined earlier and an abnormal response to the Epstein–Barr virus with absent antibody response to Epstein–Barr nuclear antigen (EBNA). Haemophagocytic lymphohistiocytic (HLH) episodes are treated as per the HLH 2004 protocol, a combination of dexamethasone, etoposide and intrathecal methotrexate if there is evidence of central nervous system disease, and immunosuppression with ciclosporin; intravenous immunoglobulin is beneficial particularly when hypogammaglobulinaemia is present.

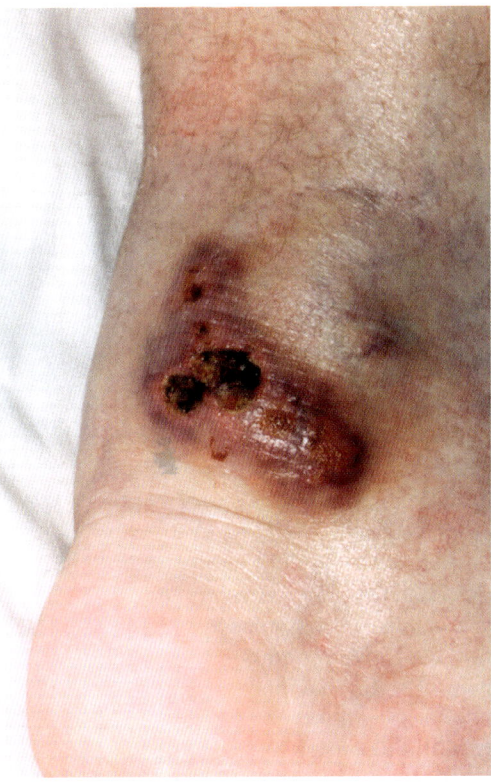

Figure 80.9 Vasculitis in a boy with X-linked lymphoproliferative disease.

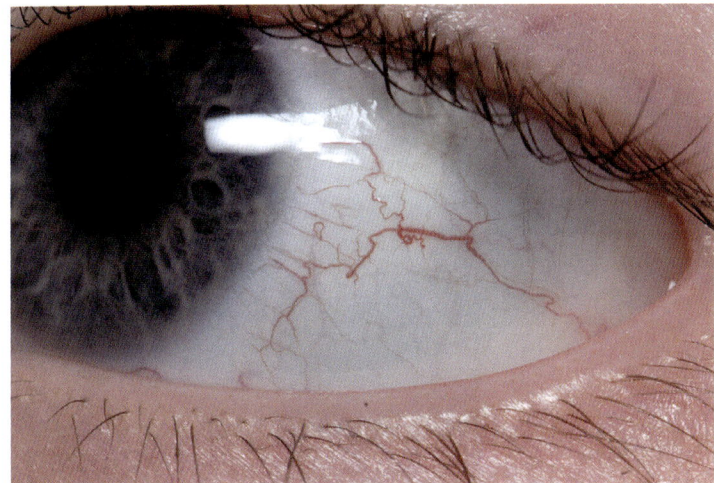

Figure 80.10 Bulbar telangiectasia in a patient with ataxia telangiectasia.

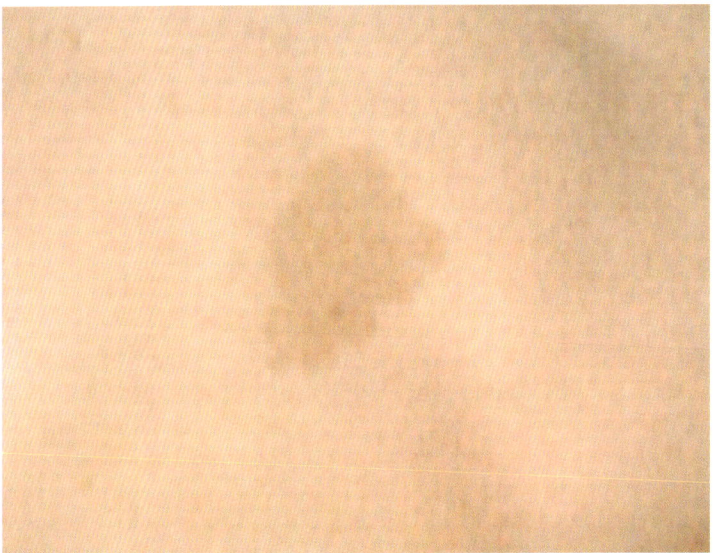

Figure 80.11 Hyperpigmented area on the back of a patient with Bloom syndrome.

X-linked lymphoproliferative disease II, known as XIAP due to X-linked inhibitor of apoptosis protein defects, is due to mutations in *BIRC4*. Patients also present with HLH, but other symptoms include inflammatory bowel disease, isolated splenomegaly and fistulating skin abscesses. HSCT is the only curative treatment for either genetic defect.

Combined immunodeficiencies with associated or syndromic features

DNA repair defects (Chapter 76)

These include ataxia telangiectasia, Nijmegen breakage syndrome, ligase 4 (LIG4) syndrome and SCID with microcephaly, growth retardation and sensitivity to ionising radiation (Cernunnos–XLF deficiency), Bloom syndrome, and immunodeficiency, centromeric instability–facial anomalies (ICF) syndrome. Patients with ataxia telangiectasia usually present with gait abnormalities before the development of characteristic telangiectasias, which usually appear first on the bulbar conjunctivae (Figure 80.10) but later elsewhere, particularly on the nose, ears and in the antecubital and popliteal fossae. The other DNA repair disorders are associated with facial dysmorphism and often with small stature. Microcephaly is typically a feature. Skin manifestations include photosensitivity, psoriatic-like lesions and hypo- or hyperpigmented lesions (Figure 80.11). Patients are at increased risk of developing lymphoreticular malignancy. Extensive warts or spreading cutaneous fungal infection are features of ICF syndrome (Figure 80.12).

Comèl–Netherton syndrome (Chapter 63)

Patients with Comèl–Netherton syndrome, due to mutations in *SPINK5* encoding the serine protease inhibitor LEKTI, present with a triad of generalised infantile ichthyosiform erythroderma and atopic diathesis, diarrhoea and failure to thrive, which may be associated with a variable immunodeficiency including mild lymphopenia and polysaccharide antibody deficiency. The clinical features may resemble those seen in Omenn syndrome or SCID with maternofetal engraftment, erythroderma and ichthyosis characterised by abnormal cornification, dryness and fish-like scaling of the skin. Hair shaft abnormalities (trichorrhexis invaginata or bamboo hair) are diagnostic but may not be seen until several months of age. Distinguishing these entities is important as the other conditions are treated by haematopoietic stem cell transplantation, whereas Comèl–Netherton syndrome is generally treated with conservative measures. Squamous cell carcinoma has been described in Comèl–Netherton syndrome.

Cartilage hair hypoplasia

This is an autosomal recessive T-lymphocyte deficiency, usually associated with short-limbed dwarfism and alopecia. Characteristically, the hair of the scalp, eyebrows and eyelashes is sparse

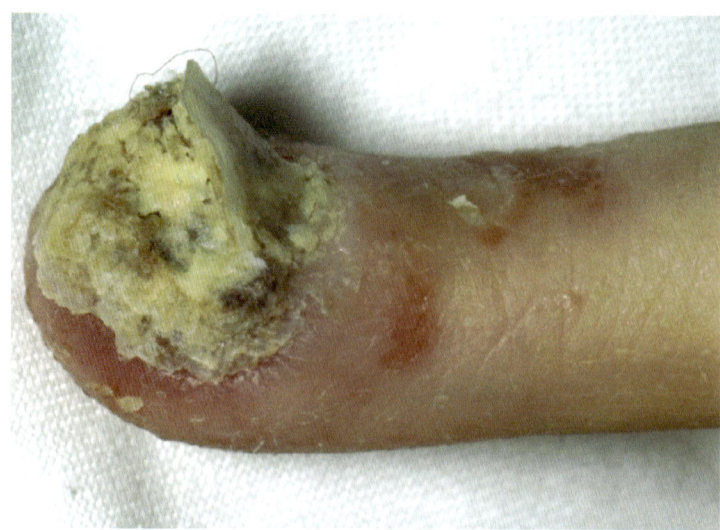

Figure 80.12 Extensive digital fungal infection in immunodeficiency, centromeric instability, facial dysmorphism syndrome.

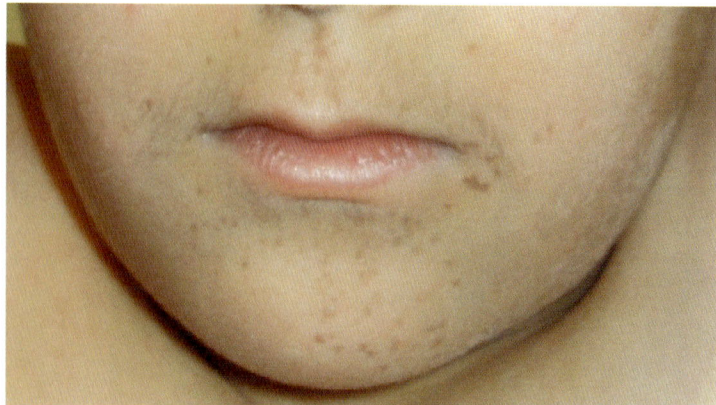

Figure 80.13 Characteristic perioral reticular hyperpigmentation in dyskeratosis congenita.

and upon hair microscopy there are characteristic findings of a lack of a central pigmented core. Cartilage hair hypoplasia, the best described of the immuno-osteochondrodysplasias, inherited in an autosomal recessive manner, is associated with mutations in *RMRP*, which encodes endoribonuclease RNase MRP. Severe short-limbed short stature (−11.8 SD to 2.1 SD) with X-ray appearances of metaphyseal and spondyloepiphyseal dysplasia are characteristic, although not always present, and most patients have sparse light hair. Severe anaemia and Hirschsprung disease are less common but well-recognised associations, as are malignancies, notably lymphoma and skin carcinoma. Cutaneous granulomatous lesions are also described. The immunodeficiency is surprisingly variable; most patients have T-lymphopenia, and impaired *in vitro* mitogen proliferative responses, but although half suffer from recurrent infections, a SCID-like presentation is well recognised. Patients are excessively vulnerable to viral infections, particularly varicella-zoster virus, Epstein–Barr virus and other human herpesvirus infections, and the risk of infective death is 300 times greater than normal. This condition should be considered in any child with severe chickenpox or herpes simplex infections who is short and has fine sparse hair. Severely affected patients should be assessed for HSCT, which has been successful in correcting the immunodeficiency.

Dyskeratosis congenita (Chapters 67 and 75)

Dyskeratosis congenita (DC) presents with recurrent infections, digestive tract involvement and pancytopenia. Cutaneous manifestations include leukoplakia, oral ulceration and reticulated hyperpigmentation, primarily in the regions of the neck, upper thorax and upper extremities. Some patients present with palmar hyperkeratosis and a characteristic perioral reticular hyperpigmentation (Figure 80.13). Nail dystrophy is typical and begins with longitudinal striations, increasing brittleness, deformation, onychoclasis and nail loss. Other cutaneous features include palmar and plantar hyperhidrosis, blistering, acrocyanosis and alopecia with sparse scalp hair and eyelashes. Mutations have been described in dyskerin (*DKC1*), *NOLA2*, *NOLA3*, *TERC*, *TERT*

as well as in *TINF2*, *ACD*, *RTEL1* and *WRAP53*, which code for proteins essential for telomere maintenance. A particularly severe variant of DC, Hoyeraal–Hreidarsson syndrome, is characterised by microcephaly, cerebellar hypoplasia, aplastic anaemia and growth retardation as well as a progressive combined immunodeficiency, with hypogammaglobulinaemia and lymphopenia.

Fanconi anaemia (Chapter 76)

Fanconi anaemia is a chromosomal instability disorder characterised by developmental defects, progressive bone marrow failure and cancer susceptibility. Children with Fanconi anaemia are generally small and elfin-like with a history of low birth weight. The major clinical manifestation of Fanconi syndrome is progressive bone marrow failure during childhood and adolescence. Easy bruising is a common presenting symptom, most often apparent between the ages of 4 and 10 years. In addition to thrombocytopenia, anaemia and leukopenia are frequent, and the bone marrow is aplastic.

The principal skeletal abnormality is absence or hypoplasia of at least one of the thumbs; hypoplasia or absence of the radius is also common. Structural renal abnormalities, endocrinopathies, genital hypoplasia, microcephaly and microphthalmia are other common features.

Cutaneous hyperpigmentation is characteristic. Macular brownish pigmentation is typical, either resembling freckles and occurring mainly in sun-exposed areas, or more diffusely in which case the abdomen, genital area and flexures appear to be predominantly affected. Guttate macular hypopigmentation is often also present in affected areas. Hypopigmentation and café-au-lait spots are reported. Persistent and exceptionally severe viral wart infection can occur.

There is a high risk of leukaemia and other malignancies in these children, probably due to the structural instability of chromosomes observed in Fanconi anaemia, which leads to a high frequency of chromosomal breaks and rearrangements.

Over 20 genes associated with Fanconi anaemia have been described to date. The Fanconi proteins are important for the repair of DNA cross-linking damage and some interact with other DNA repair pathways. The outlook for untreated patients with Fanconi anaemia is poor, with death usually occurring within a few years of the first signs of marrow failure. Initially, bone marrow function can be stimulated with corticosteroids and with the androgenic steroid oxymethalone. HSCT has been used successfully to treat patients, but care must be taken to avoid the use of alkylating agents in pretransplant conditioning. Patients are at increased risk of secondary malignancy post-transplantation.

Antibody deficiencies
X-linked agammaglobulinaemia (Bruton disease)
First described by Bruton in 1952, this X-linked defect prevents B-lymphocyte development beyond the pre-B-lymphocyte stage. It is caused by mutations in a gene that encodes a cytoplasmic enzyme, Bruton tyrosine kinase (*BTK*). Classically, affected boys demonstrate absence or severe depletion of all serum immunoglobulin classes, and antibody responses to vaccines are absent. There are normal numbers of T lymphocytes, but no B lymphocytes in peripheral blood, although pre-B lymphocytes (containing cytoplasmic μ chains) are found in bone marrow. Lymph nodes show absent follicles and germinal centres, and plasma cells cannot be demonstrated at any site. The diagnosis can be rapidly confirmed by demonstrating the absence of the BTK protein in cell lysates. Since the molecular basis has been defined, milder phenotypes have been recognised where some antibody function is present. Typically, recurrent pyogenic infections commence in the latter half of the first year of life, once maternal IgG levels have declined. The diagnosis is often made surprisingly late; in one series, the average age at diagnosis was 3.5 years and 2 years even when there was a positive family history. Sinopulmonary infections are most common, but gastroenteritis, arthritis, meningitis and osteomyelitis may be presenting features. Boils or impetigo, usually associated with neutropenia, are the most common dermatological features, frequently due to *Staphylococcus aureus* or *Pseudomonas* (Figure 80.14), although other organisms are also described. Chronic ulcerative cutaneous HSV infection has been reported. Stevens–Johnson syndrome, vitiligo and total alopecia areata have also been described. Immunoglobulin replacement therapy is the mainstay of treatment. Chronic lung damage and sinus disease may progress on treatment and for this reason vigorous and early antibiotic therapy should be used for respiratory tract infections.

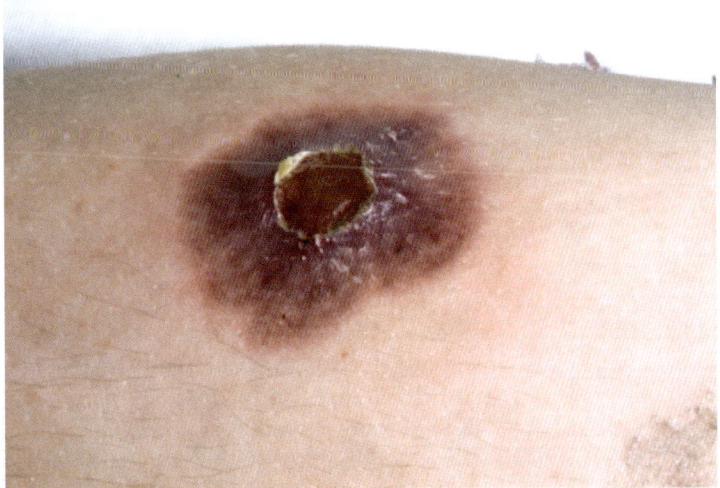

Figure 80.14 Cellulitis due to *Pseudomonas* infection in a patient with X-linked agammaglobulinaemia.

Autosomal recessive forms of agammaglobulinaemia
When hypogammaglobulinaemia is present in a female or a child with consanguineous parents, autosomal recessive genetic defects affecting B-lymphocyte differentiation should be considered. Mutations have been described so far in genes coding for μ heavy chain, Igα and Igβ (part of the signal transduction complex of the B-lymphocyte antigen receptor), λ5 light chain and BLNK (B-lymphocyte linker protein) molecules required for early B-lymphocyte development from pro-B lymphocyte to pre-B lymphocyte stage. Unlike XLA, pre-B lymphocytes are therefore not detectable in marrow samples. In all cases, the defect is B-lymphocyte specific. Skin sepsis is described as a feature, but less commonly than in XLA.

PI3Kδ deficiency
PI3Kδ deficiency, a common antibody deficiency due to dominant gain-of-function mutations in the gene encoding phosphoinositide 3 kinase δ, predominantly presents with recurrent sinopulmonary infections. Cutaneous signs are seen in the skin, salivary glands and lacrimal glands, or in dental abscess formation, as well as orbital cellulitis.

Common variable immunodeficiency
CVID is defined by low total concentrations of IgG as well as low IgA and/or IgM. Patients demonstrate recurrent infections, chronic lung disease including bronchiectases, gastrointestinal inflammatory diseases and other manifestations. Cutaneous manifestations include vitiligo, eczema, vasculitis and petechiae (as a result of autoimmune dysregulation and cytopenia) and skin infections. Autoinflammation manifests as sarcoid-like granulomas of the skin. Dermatomyositis and SLE also have an increased incidence in these kindreds.

Diseases with immune dysregulation
IEI with hypopigmentation are due to the lack of formation or trafficking of cytotoxic granules. Chediak–Higashi, Griscelli type 2 and Hermansky–Pudlak syndromes are examples of these diseases. In Chediak–Higashi and Hermansky–Pudlak syndromes, there is partial albinism. Chediak–Higashi syndrome is characterised by oculocutaneous albinism, recurrent infections and neuropathy. Photophobia and nystagmus are regular features, due to ocular pigment dilution. Severe gingivitis and oral mucosal ulceration are well described. Deficient cutaneous pigmentation may be obvious, but in some cases is more subtle (Figure 80.15), and only apparent if nipples and genitalia are carefully examined. Under light microscopy, characteristic giant lysosomal granules are seen in the cytoplasm of all cells containing these organelles and are easily detected on a peripheral blood film. Chediak–Higashi hair shafts show small aggregates of clumped pigmentation. The genetic defect is in *LYST*, which encodes a protein required for sorting endosomal resident proteins into late multivesicular endosomes by a mechanism involving microtubules. Patients usually, but not invariably, enter an accelerated lymphocyte and macrophage activation syndrome (similar to that seen in XLP), which if untreated is usually fatal. There is widespread tissue infiltration with activated lymphocytes and macrophages resulting in rapid enlargement of

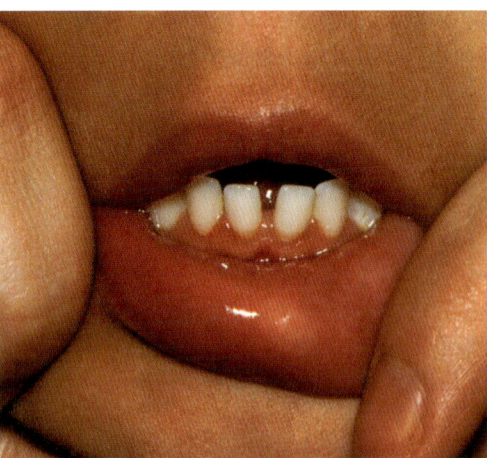

Figure 80.15 Partial albinism in Chediak–Higashi syndrome.

the liver, spleen and lymph nodes, together with jaundice, hepatic failure, respiratory distress, pancytopenia and bleeding. Death usually occurs in the first decade without HSCT, but survival into the second and third decades has been recorded. Progressive neurological deterioration is common in patients who survive early childhood and is not prevented by HSCT.

Hermansky–Pudlak syndrome is a disorder characterised by oculocutaneous albinism. Nine subtypes exist, but only type 2, caused by mutations in *AP3B1*, is also associated with congenital neutropenia. Other associations include platelet dysfunction and, occasionally, interstitial lung disease, pulmonary fibrosis and inflammatory colitis.

In Griscelli syndrome, there is a peculiar pigmentary dilution of the skin and hair. Microscopy demonstrates an uneven distribution of large pigment granules in the hair shafts. Three genes have been identified as causing the disease. Defects in *MYO5A*, which encodes myosin VA, and *MLPH,* encoding melanophilin, present with hypomelanosis, but no neurological or immunological defect. Patients with mutations in *RAB27A* present with similar features of hypopigmentation, characterised by typical silvery-grey hair, which persists even after haematopoietic stem cell transplantation (Figure 80.16), but also with recurrent pyogenic infections. In patients presenting with haemophagocytic lymphohistiocytosis, cytophagic histiocytic panniculitis has been rarely described.

Immunodysregulation polyendocrinopathy enteropathy X-linked syndrome

IPEX syndrome is a disease in which there is X-linked immune dysregulation due to mutations in *FOXP3*, encoding a transcription factor needed for the development of regulatory T lymphocytes. These children usually present in the neonatal or early infancy period with an impressive exanthema or eczema. There is often early-onset insulin-dependent diabetes, autoimmune enteropathy, thyroiditis and autoimmune cytopenias. Bruising may be apparent secondary to autoimmune thrombocytopenia. Defects with similar autoimmune manifestations, and particularly enteropathy, include deficiencies of CD25, IL-10, IL-10 receptor subunits, in which folliculitis may be a feature, and the gain-of-function mutations in *STAT3*.

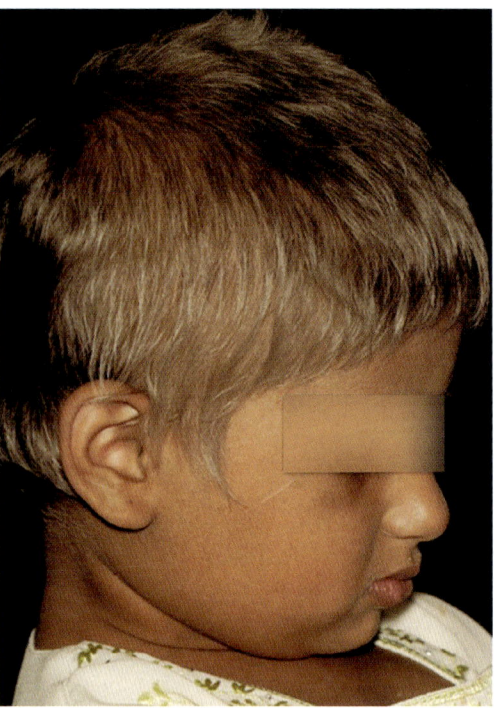

Figure 80.16 Patient with Griscelli syndrome demonstrating a silver sheen to the hair that has persisted post haematopoietic stem cell transplantation.

Autoimmune lymphoproliferative syndrome

Apoptosis, or programmed cell death, is important for regulating immune responses once an infection has been countered. Defects in apoptosis lead to autoimmune and lymphoproliferative features that characterise ALPS. There are a number of pathways through which apoptosis can be induced; one of the most important is initiated through a cell surface molecule Fas (CD95). Ligation of CD95 initiates a cascade of intracellular reactions culminating in apoptosis induced by proteolytic enzymes including caspases. Mutations in molecules in this cascade result in genetically distinct but clinically similar forms of ALPS. Fas is expressed as a trimeric surface protein. Heterozygotes with a Fas mutation in one allele often develop the full clinical syndrome because one abnormal protein chain is sufficient to impair the trimer's function significantly, a so-called dominant-negative effect. Most of the cases are due to heterozygous mutations, although a few homozygous cases have also been reported.

Many patients present in early childhood, but adult presentation and asymptomatic cases may occur. Patients usually remain well until the disease is triggered, often by human herpesvirus infection. Haematological autoimmunity is most common, but any system can be involved. Childhood linear IgA disease has been described (Figure 80.17). Other dermatological manifestations include vasculitis and urticaria. Lymphoproliferation leads to significant asymmetrical anterior cervical lymphadenopathy, with splenomegaly in nearly all cases and hepatomegaly in some. Malignant lymphoid disease (both Hodgkin and non-Hodgkin) is reported with increased frequency, although the histological picture of proliferation may be benign; clonality studies distinguish the two. Affected individuals usually have high lymphocyte counts and normal or high immunoglobulin levels. Autoantibodies are

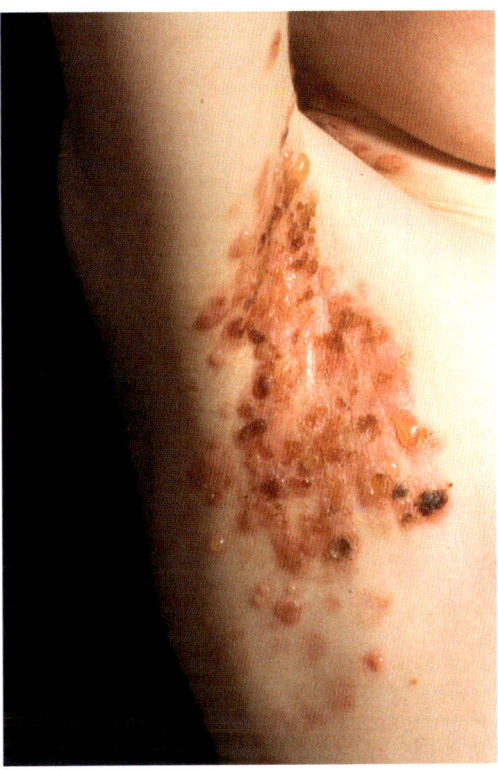

Figure 80.17 Childhood linear IgA disease in FAS-deficient autoimmune lymphoproliferative syndrome.

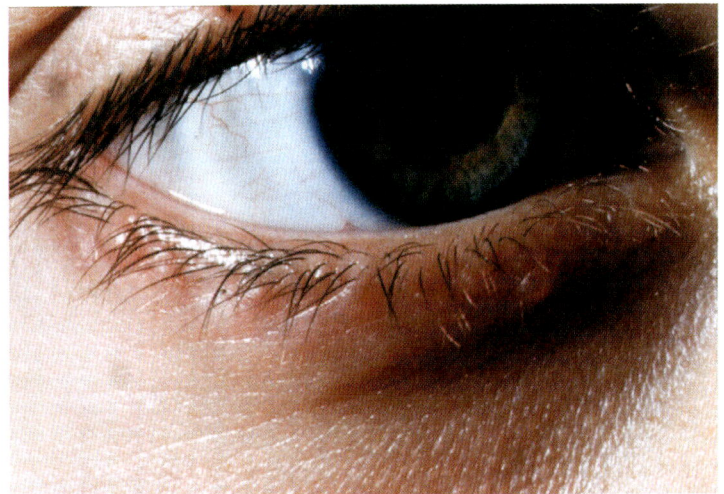

Figure 80.18 Translucent papular lesions around the eyelids of a patient with chronic granulomatous disease.

usually present. The occurrence of circulating CD3+ T lymphocytes expressing the αβ receptor but not expressing CD4 or CD8 (so-called double-negative T lymphocytes), and usually constituting between 5 and 20% of the total CD3 cell count, is helpful in making a diagnosis of FAS deficiency, but raised vitamin B$_{12}$ and soluble FAS ligand are more predictive. Autoimmunity usually responds to corticosteroids, high-dose intravenous immunoglobulin and dapsone in the case of ALPS-associated juvenile bullous dermatosis. Splenectomy should be avoided if possible because severe infective complications may follow.

Congenital defects of phagocyte function, differentiation and adhesion
Functional neutrophil defects
The prototype of functional phagocyte deficiency is CGD, a result of an inherited defect in one of the six components of the phagocyte nicotinamide adenine dinucleotide phosphate (NADPH) oxidase enzyme complex, which generates reactive oxygen species. The disease has numerous clinical manifestations, but the hallmark is acute, and potentially fatal, bacterial or fungal infection. Patients suffer from organ abscesses with staphylococci or fungi in the spleen, liver and lung, as well as lymph node abscesses. The earliest manifestations are often seen in the skin. Neonatal pustulosis is commonly the first sign of the disease. Subsequently, a rather non-specific, impetiginised periorificial rash is highly characteristic, most commonly seen around the nostrils, ears, mouth and eyes, and has sometimes been described as 'eczematous' or 'seborrhoeic'.

Any area where the skin has been broken, by abrasion for example, tends to become impetiginised or ecthymatous. Nodular lesions may follow, and these frequently break down to form necrotic

ulcers. Firm translucent papular lesions around the nose, eyes (Figure 80.18), lips and on the cheeks may mimic lupus vulgaris or sarcoidosis. Subcutaneous nodules may develop at immunisation sites, and these also tend in time to ulcerate. Poor healing of surgical wounds, and of the discharging nodular skin lesions, is characteristic. Perianal abscesses are a regular feature. Other frequent findings include chronic suppurative paronychia, folliculitis of the scalp and ulcerative stomatitis. Acute febrile neutrophilic dermatosis (Sweet syndrome) has been rarely described, as has chronic bullous disease of childhood. The importance of non-infectious inflammatory complications is increasingly recognised. These include inflammatory bowel disease, which clinically and histologically can be indistinguishable from Crohn disease, restrictive lung defects, acute genitourinary obstruction and cutaneous granulomata, particularly at vaccination sites. Female carriers not infrequently develop erythematous macular, papular and urticarial skin lesions following light exposure, and discoid lupus erythematosus or Jessner lymphocytic infiltrate (Figure 80.19).

Of note, the disease can manifest for the first time in older individuals so that a high degree of clinical suspicion must be maintained when encountering a clinical picture consistent with CGD regardless of the patient's age [9].

Defects of neutrophil differentiation
There are more than 20 subtypes of congenital neutropenia that have been described. Neutropenia may present as poorly healing, deep ulcerations of the skin and unusual abscesses. Patients with neutropenia present usually in infancy when omphalitis, skin and liver abscesses are most common. Moreover, there may be oral ulceration, gingivitis and early loss of permanent teeth. In Papillon–Lefèvre syndrome, there are mutations in *CTSC* encoding cathepsin C. Patients have aggressive periodontitis, leading to dental loss and palmoplantar hyperkeratosis.

Defects of neutrophil adhesion
In these disorders, adhesion molecules including CD18, FUCT1 (GDP-fucose transporter) or other integrins are affected. Patients present with poor wound healing despite marked leukocytosis in

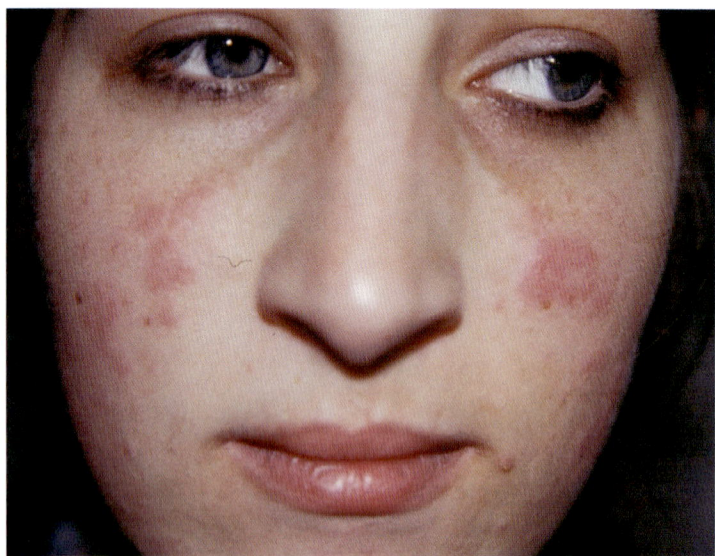

Figure 80.19 Malar erythematous photosensitive macular skin lesions in an X-linked carrier of chronic granulomatous disease.

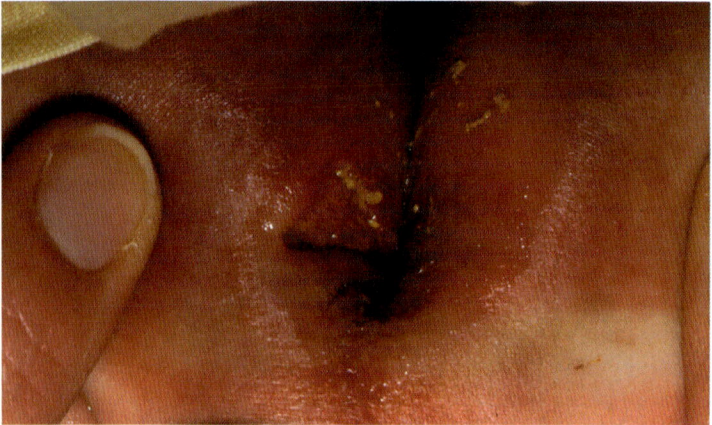

Figure 80.20 Erosive perianal ulcers in an infant with severe leukocyte adhesion deficiency type I.

their blood. The clinical picture is almost entirely explained by the way in which leukocytes are attracted to areas of infection and inflammation. Leukocytes normally attach to vessel walls at sites of inflammation but cannot pass out into the tissues. This leads to blockage of small vessels and rapidly expanding necrotic lesions without pus. Individuals with the most severe phenotype (<1% expression) present in the first weeks of life with delayed umbilical cord separation (the cord fails to shrink down and may not separate until 3–4 weeks of age) and omphalitis, together with rapidly progressive erosive perianal ulcers (Figure 80.20). Gingivitis, ulcerative stomatitis and periodontitis are common and severe, leading to loss of teeth. Inflammatory lesions, particularly affecting the skin and resembling pyoderma gangrenosum, can occur in the partial forms of the deficiency and may respond to steroid treatment.

Defects in innate immunity

NF-κB pathway-related primary immunodeficiencies

The NF-κB pathway is critical in the transduction of extracellular signalling from inflammatory cytokines and Toll-like receptor ligands to the cell nucleus, in order to induce transcription of target genes involved in immunity, inflammation, cell survival and apoptosis regulation. The IκB kinase (IKK) complex, a key protein complex in this signalling pathway, is composed of two kinases (IKK-α and IKK-β) and the non-catalytic regulatory protein NEMO. Mutations in genes encoding these molecules can lead to immunodeficiency associated with ectodermal dysplasia.

Incontinentia pigmenti is a rare X-linked dominant condition characterised by developmental abnormalities in the skin, hair, teeth and central nervous system. Carrier mothers demonstrate well-recognised cutaneous features of Blashko linear skin lesions occurring in four successive sometimes overlapping stages: (i) redness, vesicles, pustules; (ii) verrucous hyperkeratotic lesions; (iii) hyperpigmented whorls and streaks following lines of Blaschko; and (iv) pallor and scarring. In other respects, affected females are healthy. Previously, affected males were all reported to die before birth, but it is now recognised that hypofunctional mutations in *IKBKG* encoding NEMO lead to X-linked anhidrotic ectodermal dysplasia (EDA) and immunodeficiency which is characterised by sparse scalp hair, conical teeth and absent sweat glands. Some patients experience recurrent sinopulmonary infection, often with encapsulated organisms, and have poor antibody responses to polysaccharide antigens or frank hypogammaglobulinaemia. Affected infants share many of the cutaneous features of EDA, although they appear less severe than in children with 'classic' EDA without immunodeficiency, and the majority of patients have normal or sparse scalp hair. From early childhood, affected boys suffer from unusually severe life-threatening and recurrent bacterial infections of the lower respiratory tract, skin and soft tissues, bones, gastrointestinal tract, including meningitis and septicaemia. Causative pathogens are most often Gram-positive bacteria (*Streptococcus pneumoniae*, *Staphylococcus aureus*), followed by Gram-negative bacteria (*Pseudomonas* species, *Haemophilus influenzae*) and *Mycobacteria*. *Pneumocystis jiroveci* infection has also been described. Other related features include osteopetrosis and lymphoedema (osteopetrosis lymphodema ectodermal dysplasia immunodeficiency).

Autosomal dominant gain-of-function mutations in *IKBKA* encoding IκBα cause a similar clinical picture of immunodeficiency associated with ectodermal dysplasia, clinically indistinguishable from patients with hypomorphic mutations in *NEMO*.

MyD88 and IRAK-4 molecules are activated through toll-like receptors and signal through the nucleus via the NF-κB pathway. Patients with defects in these molecules experience severe pyogenic infection, most commonly meningitis or other deep-seated infections, but skin sepsis is reported.

WHIM syndrome

Gain-of-function mutations for the chemokine receptor CXCR4 cause Warts, Hypogammaglobulinemia, Infections, Myelocathexis (WHIM) syndrome, which results in a particular susceptibility to warts secondary to human papillomavirus infection, associated with neutropenia and hypogammaglobulinaemia. The generalised verrucosis may be severe and widespread, and involve all cutaneous and mucosal tissues. A similar clinical picture is apparent in epidermodysplasia verruciformis, with increased susceptibility to human papillomavirus infections manifesting as widespread flat warts and pityriasis versicolor-like lesions, and verrucous skin carcinomas. However, neutropenia and hypogammaglobulinaemia are not features of this disease. *EVER1* and *EVER2* genes are mutated in 75% of epidermodysplasia verruciformis cases.

Hyper-IgE syndrome due to STAT3 loss of function mutations

Hyper-IgE syndrome (previously Job syndrome), due to heterozygous autosomal dominant negative loss of function mutations in the gene coding for STAT3, is of special relevance to the dermatologist as the initial presentation may be cutaneous [10]. It is a complex disorder characterised by extreme elevation of the serum IgE level (usually in the range 2000–40 000 U/L), chronic dermatitis and repeated lung and skin infections. In the literature, these patients are frequently described as having eczema, although this is different from typical atopic eczema. Affected children develop a non-specific, excoriated, papular and pustular eruption in infancy, particularly over the scalp, scalp margins, buttocks and proximal flexures, such as the axillae, groins and neck. The rash may appear in the first few days of life, at which stage it may be vesicular, but crusting becomes a prominent feature. Typical eczematous features of lichenification or scales are absent or mild in hyper-IgE syndrome.

There is commonly a history of furunculosis and staphylococcal lung infections, abscesses and empyema. Many patients develop staphylococcal pneumatoceles, which strongly suggest the diagnosis. Although skin and lung infections predominate, infections of the ears, sinuses, joints and viscera are common. Lymphadenopathy may be complicated by the development of lymph node abscesses. *Staphylococcus aureus* is the predominant pathogen but infection is also seen with *Haemophilus influenzae*, pneumococci, group A streptococci and with *Candida*. Oral candidiasis and *Candida* nail infections are common. Pneumatoceles may provide the focus for the development of aspergillomas.

Non-immunological features that are variably present include abnormal, coarse often asymmetrical facies with a wide nasal bridge and large head; hypodense bones leading to frequent fractures; joint laxity; a high incidence of scoliosis; delayed resorption of primary dentition with consequent delayed eruption of secondary teeth; and cerebral aneurysms.

Peripheral blood eosinophilia may be marked (up to 50–60%). Serum IgE levels are consistently very high (more than 10 times the upper limit of normal), although they may be normal in infancy.

The mainstay of treatment is long-term antistaphylococcal antibiotic prophylaxis usually with flucloxacillin. Attention to skin hygiene is important, with judicial use of topical antimicrobials. *Candida* infections should be treated typically or, when refractory, with oral ketoconazole or fluconazole. Persistent pneumatoceles should be excised.

Chronic mucocutaneous candidiasis

Chronic mucocutaneous candidiasis is a heterogenous group of syndromes with non-invasive *Candida* infections that affect the skin, nails and mucous membranes. In many forms of the disease, there is a lack of T-lymphocyte helper 17 (Th17) cells or cell function [11]. Defects include gain-of-function *STAT1* mutations and mutations in *CARD9*, *STAT3*, *IL17RA*, *IL17F*, *IL22*, and *IL12RB* and

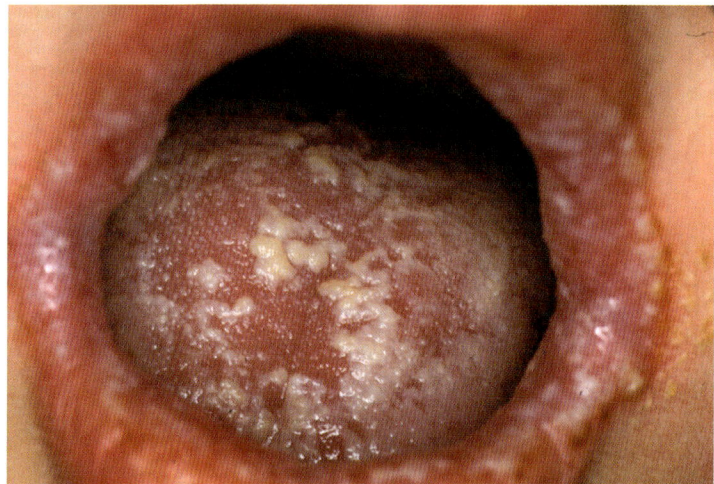

Figure 80.21 Oro-pharyngeal mucocutaneous *Candida* infection in a patient with a gain-of-function *STAT1* mutation.

CLEC7A encoding important mediators of Th17 cell development or function.

Autoimmune polyendocrine syndrome type 1, also known as autoimmune polyendocrinopathy candidiasis ectodermal dystrophy (APECED) syndrome, is caused by mutations in *AutoImmune REgulator* (*AIRE*) encoding a transcription factor required to establish central thymic self-tolerance. These patients suffer from many forms of autoimmunity, particularly involving parathyroid, adrenal and other endocrine organs. The cutaneous hallmark of this syndrome is ectodermal dystrophy with onychomycosis and superficial chronic mucocutaneous candidiasis, affecting particularly oro-pharyngeal mucosa and the perineal region (Figure 80.21). The defect is due to autoantibodies, which impair the development or function of Th17 cells, which are important in mucosal immunity and defects of which are associated with susceptibility to candidiasis.

Autoinflammatory disorders

Autoinflammatory diseases are clinical conditions characterised by episodes of apparently unprovoked inflammation, and due to dysregulation of the innate immune system, rather than autoreactive T lymphocytes or autoantibodies, differentiating them from classic autoimmune disease. Defects in several pathways can lead to autoinflammatory disease. The most frequently affected pathway is mediated by inflammasomes, and defects in intracellular innate immune system receptors (e.g. NOD-like receptor), downstream effector proteins as well as the inflammasome are described. The two other well-described pathogenic mechanisms causing autoinflammatory disorders are those related to activation of the NF-kB transcription factor and to type I interferons. Tightly controlled signalling is required to regulate gene transcription for immune cell activation, proliferation, differentiation, survival and signalling. NF-kB is a critical regulator involved in these processes. Activation occurs through signalling via cytokines and Toll-like receptors (the canonical pathway), or TNF-receptor family proteins (the non-canonical pathway), both of which are controlled by the ubiquitin system. Type I interferons are required to counter against virus and intracellular pathogens, and are activated through

PART 6: GENETIC DISORDERS

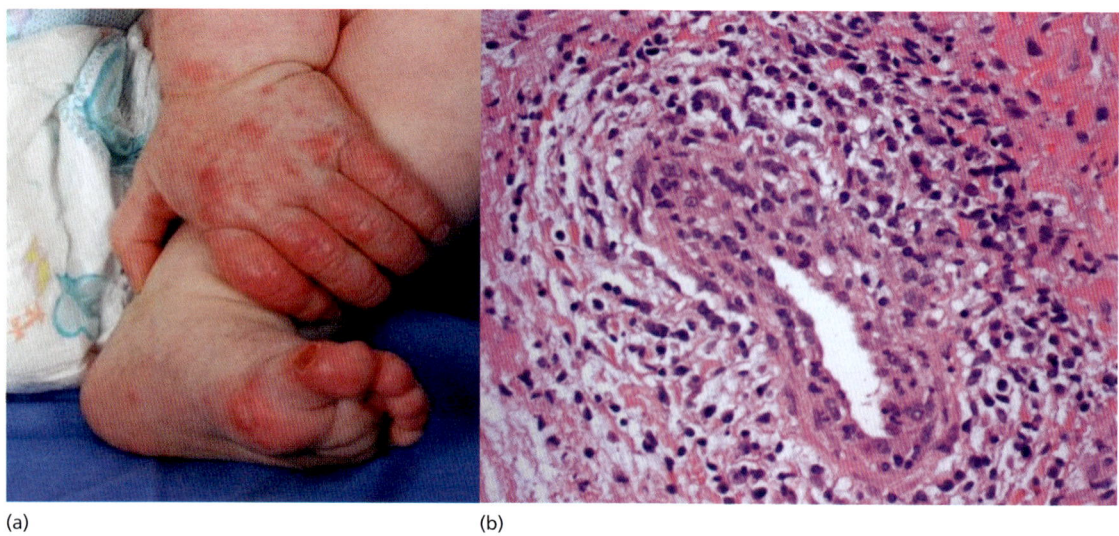

Figure 80.22 SLE-like vasculopathy (a) secondary to vasculitis (b) in an infant with STING-associated vasculopathy, infantile onset due to a mutation in *TMEM173*.

Toll-like receptors that detect endosomic viral nucleic acids and through cytosolic DNA and RNA sensors.

Clinical features are extremely variable and non-specific, and symptoms are often shared by different autoinflammatory conditions. Commonly described symptoms include recurrent fever, musculoskeletal symptoms, abdominal and thoracic serositis, headache, ophthalmic inflammation, and mucosal and skin lesions (Figure 80.22).

Cutaneous symptoms are common in monogenic autoinflammatory diseases and are often the initial presentation in some of them. Maculopapular rashes and urticaria are the most predominant symptoms, but recognition of skin disease as part of an autoinflammatory disorder may be difficult because of the range of skin disorders associated with these conditions. Severity of symptoms is variable between and within conditions, and not indicative of a particular disease. More than one manifestation may be present. Cutaneous manifestations of monogenic autoinflammatory disease can be classified as follows (Table 80.2):

- Urticarial rashes.
- Maculopapular rashes or inflammatory plaques.
- Vasculitis or vasculopathy.
- Panniculitis or subcutaneous nodules.
- Aphthous lesions.
- Pustular, pyogenic or neutrophilic dermatosis-like rashes.
- Bullous lesions.
- Hyperkeratotic lesions.
- Hyperpigmented lesions.

Treatment is largely symptomatic. Non-steroidal anti-inflammatory drugs and glucocorticoids may be used in an acute attack. For specific diseases, anticytokine directed therapy, e.g. anti-IL1 receptor, anti-IL6 or anti-TNF, can be useful. For selected diseases (ADA2 deficiency), hematopoietic stem cell transplantation has been used successfully.

Complement diseases

Deficiencies of isolated complement components are rare, deficiency of C2 being the most frequent, and with the exception of properdin and C1 esterase inhibitor deficiency, which are X-linked, are generally transmitted in an autosomal recessive manner. However, heterozygosity results in approximately half normal levels of the protein, which can sometimes be clinically important. A number of clinical patterns can occur depending upon which factor is deficient [12].

Complement defects predisposing to recurrent pyogenic infection

Recurrent pyogenic infections are a major feature of complement deficiencies. Encapsulated organisms such as streptococci and *Haemophilus influenzae* are the main problem because opsonisation of antibody and complement to bacteria is critical for microbial elimination. C3 deficiency is the most severe, thus meningococcal meningitis and pneumococcal pneumonia have been major problems. The clinical picture is similar to that of hypogammaglobulinaemia. Deficiency of the classic pathway components C1q and C2 and of factor D in the alternative pathway also predisposes to infection. Deficiencies of the alternative pathway control proteins, factors H or I, lead to uncontrolled consumption of C3, resulting in increased susceptibility to pyogenic infections including meningococcal disease, as well as atypical haemolytic uraemic syndrome. Defects in properdin also lead to neisserial disease. Defects in the terminal complement cascade (C5–C9) lead to recurrent meningococcal meningitis and disseminated gonococcal infections, the principal clinical consequence of deficiencies of all these complement components. Cutaneous infections are generally not a problem in these patients.

Complement defects predisposing to autoimmunity

A variety of clinical manifestations have been described in patients with C1q deficiency, including cutaneous vasculitis, SLE, membranous glomerulonephritis and problems with infections, particularly meningitis and septicaemia, but also including stomatitis, pyoderma and persistent candidiasis of the mouth and nails.

SLE or a disorder clinically suggestive of SLE, but lacking confirmatory serological findings, and/or membranous glomerulonephritis have similarly been reported in patients with deficiencies of either C1r or C1s. The majority of patients reported with C4 deficiency have been children or adolescents. Their principal clinical

Table 80.2 Main cutaneous manifestations of autoinflammatory diseases.

Major skin manifestations	Associated diseases	MIM	Gene
Urticarial rashes	Cryopyrin-associated periodic syndromes (CAPS)	191900	NLRP3
		120100	
	NLRP12-associated autoinflammatory disease (NLRP12-AD)	611762	NLRP12
	PLCγ2-associated antibody deficiency and immune dysregulation (PLAID)	614878	PLCγ2
	NLRC4-associated autoinflammatory diseases (NRLC4-AD)	616050	NLRC4
		616115	
Maculopapular rashes or	Familial Mediterranean fever (FMF)	249100	MEFV
inflammatory plaques	TNF receptor-associated periodic syndrome (TRAPS)	134610	TNFRSF1A
	Hyper-IgD syndrome/mevalonate kinase deficiency (HIDS/MKD)	142680	MVK
	Otulipenia/OTULIN-related autoinflammatory syndrome (ORAS)	260920	OTULIN
	HOIL-1 deficiency	615712	RBCK1
		610924	
Vasculitis or vasculopathy	Deficiency of adenosine deaminase 2 (DADA2)	607575	ADA2
	STING-associated vasculopathy with onset in infancy (SAVI)	612374	TMEM173
			TREX1
	Aicardi-Goutières syndrome (AGS) 1–7	606609	RNASEH2B
		610326	RNASEH2C
		610330	RNASEH2A
		606034	SAMHD1
		606754	ADAR1
		146920	IFIH1
		615846	ACP5
	Spondyloenchondrodysplasia with immune dysregulation (SPENCDI)	171640	
Panniculitis or subcutaneous nodules	Blau syndrome/early-onset sarcoidosis	186580	NOD2
	Chronic atypical neutrophilic dermatitis with lipodystrophy and elevated temperature (CANDLE)	256040	PSMB8
		609702	PSMG2
Aphthous lesions	Haploinsufficiency of A20 (HA20)	616744	TNFAIP3
	Autoinflammatory periodic fever, immunodeficiency and thrombocytopenia (PFIT)	604734	WDR1
	C/EBP+-associated autoinflammation and immune impairment of neutrophils (CAIN)	189965	CEBPE
	NFKB1-associated Behçet-like autoinflammatory disease	164011	NFKB1
			IL10
			IL10RA
	Monogenic forms of inflammatory bowel disease (IL-10 signalling defects)	124092	IL10RB
		146933	RIPK1
		123889	
	RIPK1 haploinsufficiency	618852	
Pustular, pyogenic or neutrophilic	Pyogenic sterile arthritis, pyoderma gangrenosum and acne (PAPA)	604416	PSTPIP1
dermatosis-like rashes	Deficiency of IL-1 receptor antagonist (DIRA)	612852	IL1RN
	Deficiency of IL-36 receptor antagonist (DITRA)	614204	IL36RN
	CARD-14 mediated psoriasis (CAMPS)	602723	CARD14
	Chronic recurrent multifocal osteomyelitis and congenital dyserythropoietic anaemia (Majeed syndrome)	609628	LPIN2
	ADAM17 deficiency	614328	ADAM17
	AP1S3 and autoinflammatory psoriasis	615781	AP1S3
Bullous lesions	Autoinflammation and PLCγ2-associated antibody deficiency and immune dysregulation (APLAID)	614468	PLCγ2 (missense mutations S707Y and L848P)
Hyperkeratotic lesions	NLRP-1 associated disease (NAIAD)	617388	NLRP1
Hyperpigmented lesions	H syndrome	602782	SLC29A3

abnormalities have comprised SLE, or an SLE-like syndrome, Henoch–Schönlein purpura or Sjögren syndrome.

C2 deficiency is the most common complement deficiency, shown to be associated with a variety of diseases, but deficient individuals are often entirely healthy. Disorders occurring in C2-deficient patients have included SLE, discoid lupus erythematosus, membranous glomerulonephritis, Henoch–Schönlein purpura, rheumatoid arthritis, dermatomyositis, Crohn disease and idiopathic thrombocytopenic purpura.

Transient maculopapular rashes have been reported to occur in association with infections in patients with C3 deficiency; histologically, these have shown the features of leukocytoclastic vasculitis. Other manifestations such as SLE and membranous glomerulonephritis have also been reported. While recurrent infection is the most common manifestation of defects in the terminal complement cascade (C5–C9), SLE, discoid lupus erythematosus, Sjögren syndrome, rheumatoid arthritis and ankylosing spondylitis have also been associated with these deficiencies.

Defects in the regulation of complement activation

Several proteins have regulatory effects on the complement system, and deficiencies in these components can lead to disease. The best known of these is C1 esterase inhibitor, deficiency of which results in hereditary angio-oedema (Chapter 43). Clinically, this manifests as angio-oedema, typically affecting the bowel mucosa, face or extremities, and, most seriously, laryngeal oedema, which may be life threatening.

Deficiency of factor 1, previously termed C3b inactivator, leads to unchecked cleavage of C3, and therefore to clinical manifestations closely resembling those seen in C3-deficient individuals. In this condition, plasma infusions may provoke anaphylaxis, because the contained C3 is so rapidly cleaved to form the anaphylotoxin C3a.

Key references

The full list of references can be found in the online version at https://www.wiley.com/rooksdermatology10e

1 Tangye SG, Al-Herz W, Bousfiha A, *et al*. Human inborn errors of immunity: 2019 Update on the Classification from the International Union of Immunological Societies Expert Committee. *J Clin Immunol* 2020;40:24–64.

2 Leiding JW, Holland SM. Warts and all: human papillomavirus in primary immunodeficiencies. *J Allergy Clin Immunol* 2012;130:1030–48.

3 Lanternier F, Cypowyj S, Picard C et al. Primary immunodeficiencies underlying fungal infections. *Curr Opin Pediatr* 2013;25:736–47.

4 Ruland J, Hartjes L. CARD-BCL-10-MALT1 signalling in protective and pathological immunity. *Nat Rev Immunol* 2019;19:118–34.

5 Rose CD, Neven B, Wouters C. Granulomatous inflammation: the overlap of immune deficiency and inflammation. *Best Pract Res Clin Rheumatol* 2014;28:191–212.

6 Marrella V, Maina V, Villa A. Omenn syndrome does not live by V(D)J recombination alone. *Curr Opin Allergy Clin Immunol* 2011;11:525–31.

7 Buchbinder D, Nugent DJ, Fillipovich AH. Wiskott-Aldrich syndrome: diagnosis, current management, and emerging treatments. *Appl Clin Genet* 2014;7:55–66.

8 Chu EY, Freeman AF, Jing H et al. Cutaneous manifestations of DOCK8 deficiency syndrome. *Arch Dermatol* 2012;148:79–84.

9 Schapiro BL, Newburger PE, Klempner MS, Dinauer MC. Chronic granulomatous disease presenting in a 69-year-old man. *N Engl J Med* 1991;325:1786–90.

10 Yong PF, Freeman AF, Engelhardt KR, Holland S, Puck JM, Grimbacher B. An update on the hyper-IgE syndromes. *Arthritis Res Ther* 2012;14:228.

11 Puel A, Cypowyj S, Maródi L, Abel L, Picard C, Casanova JL. Inborn errors of human IL-17 immunity underlie chronic mucocutaneous candidiasis. *Curr Opin Allergy Clin Immunol* 2012;12:616–22.

12 Lipsker D, Hauptmann G. Cutaneous manifestations of complement deficiencies. *Lupus* 2010;19:1096–106.

Psychological, Sensory and Neurological Disorders and the Skin

CHAPTER 81

Pruritus, Prurigo and Lichen Simplex

Sonja Ständer[1] and Gil Yosipovitch[2]

[1]Department of Dermatology, University Hospital Münster, Münster, Germany
[2]Dr Phillip Frost Department of Dermatology and Cutaneous Surgery, Miller School of Medicine, University of Miami, Miami, FL, USA

Pruritus

Definition and nomenclature

Chronic pruritus (CP) is defined as 'an unpleasant sensation leading to the desire to scratch' [1], lasting for at least 6 weeks and is a symptom of dermatological, systemic, neurological or psychiatric diseases [2]. Clinically, it may occur on diseased skin (international classification term: pruritus on inflamed skin; example: atopic eczema) or non-diseased, non-lesional skin (classification term: pruritus on non-inflamed skin; replaces the previous designation pruritus sine materia). Cutaneous signs secondary to scratching occur frequently (e.g. excoriations, erosions, ulcers, crusting, lichenification and dyspigmentation) and, if chronic, may form certain typical clinical pictures such as lichen simplex or prurigo nodularis (PN) (classification term: pruritus along with chronic scratch lesions). Several specific terms have been created to refer to unique clinical presentations of CP such as aquagenic pruritus (CP after contact with water), premonitory pruritus (CP occurring in advance of a disease) or paraneoplastic pruritus (CP in the context of a malignant disease).

Synonyms and inclusions
• Itch

Introduction and general description

During the past decades, pruritus research has improved our understanding of the neurobiology of this symptom [3], and led to the development of new itch classifications, questionnaires and guidelines [2,4]. CP may be generalised or localised. CP is a symptom occurring in a large variety of underlying diseases (Table 81.1), among which the most frequent are atopic eczema, chronic urticaria, psoriasis vulgaris, xerosis, chronic kidney disease (CKD) with or without dialysis, hepatobiliary or cholestatic liver disorders and haematological diseases [5]. A significant proportion of CP is unexplained. The heterogeneity of the underlying diseases results in a diversity of clinical presentation, itch characteristics (such as intensity, quality and course), dermatological, laboratory and radiological findings and therapy response. Most patients with CP have in common a high symptom burden, substantially impaired quality of life (QoL) including difficulties in everyday activities and social life, sleep disturbance and psychosomatic reactions such as reactive depression [6]. For example, in atopic eczema, the Dermatology Life Quality Index (DLQI) correlates with pruritus, xerosis and disturbed sleep [7]. In psoriasis, pruritus is among the factors significantly associated with severe impact on QoL (DLQI ≥10) [8]. In systemic sclerosis, pruritus severity is independently associated with severe sleep disturbance [9]. Polycythaemia vera-associated aquagenic pruritus leads to reduced overall health status and higher fatigue levels [10]. Patients with CKD-associated CP have poor sleep quality, physician-diagnosed depression and a 17% higher mortality risk [11]. Interestingly, female patients experience a higher negative impact on QoL than men, irrespective of the origin of CP [12].

Epidemiology

Incidence and prevalence

The incidence of CP in the general population is 7% as suggested by a German study with 1190 participants [13]. This is similar to a point prevalence in a previous study in an urban population (Oslo: 18 747 participants) in which 8.4% of all adults experienced pruritus [14]. The prevalence of CP in the general population (4500 participants) ranged from 13.5% (point prevalence) to 25.5% (lifetime prevalence) [15]. These data were confirmed by a study of a working age population (11 730 participants) which reported a point prevalence of 16.8% [16]. With increasing age, the prevalence of CP increased [16]: in the age group of 16–30 years, the prevalence was 12.3% while it increased to 20.3% in the oldest age group (61–70 years). Retrospective studies in Copenhagen, London and France found that pruritus occurred in 2.5%, 8.2% and 42% of dermatological patients, respectively [17–19].

PART 7: PSYCHOLOGICAL, SENSORY & NEUROLOGICAL

Table 81.1 Examples of diseases that can induce chronic pruritus (CP) [4,273–277].

Category of disease	Examples	Patients with this disease affected by CP (%)
Dermatological diseases	Atopic eczema	100
	Chronic urticaria (all forms)	100
	Bullous pemphigoid	100
	Erythroderma	97
	Post-burn scars	87
	Psoriasis	67–84
	Systemic sclerosis	42.6
	Pruritic papular eruption in HIV	11–46
	Elderly skin	20-46
Systemic diseases		
Metabolic and endocrine diseases	Hepatobiliary diseases with or without cholestasis including	80–100
	Primary biliary cholangitis	25–70
	Chronic kidney disease	10–77
	Anorexia	58
	Diabetes mellitus	2.7–49
	Hyperthyroidism	4–7.5
Infective diseases	HIV and AIDS	13
	Hepatitis C virus infection	15
	Varicella	17 (during shingles) 4.5 (CP after healing)
Haematological diseases and neoplasms	Myelofibrosis	69
	Hodgkin lymphoma	30
	Polycythaemia vera	28–42.2
	Non-Hodgkin lymphoma	10
	Iron deficiency (anaemia)	7.4–13.6
	Essential thrombocytosis	7.1–9.1
	Leukaemia	5
	Solid tumours	3
Drug-induced pruritus	All targeted cancer therapies	17.4 (14–47)
	Imatinib	10.2
	Infliximab	8
	Rituximab	20
Neurological diseases	Brachioradial pruritus	100
	Notalgia paraesthetica	100
	Postherpetic neuralgia	58
Psychiatric or psychosomatic diseases	Depression	17.5
	Fibromyalgia	60
	Stress and anxiety	56–72

AIDS, acquired immune deficiency syndrome; HIV, human immunodeficiency virus.

Age

There is no age limit for the development of CP. CP may even occur in newborns (e.g. atopic eczema, genetic disorders such as ichthyosis). The frequency increases with age [16].

Sex

Chronic pruritus occurs almost equally in women and men (women: 54.8%; men: 45.2%) [12]. Men are significantly older (mean 3 years) at the onset of CP, and have a larger number of co-morbidities (e.g. cardiovascular and uro-genital diseases) and co-medications. Women have more neuropathic and psychosomatic diseases and report more often that emotional and psychosomatic factors have a negative influence on CP. Prurigo nodularis occurs more commonly in women than men; women also complain of higher itch intensity and more severe impact on QoL than men.

Ethnicity

It is currently assumed that the prevalence of CP varies across different ethnic populations [20]. It is discussed that pruritus is more highly prevalent in individuals with darker skin types. Interestingly, a European study showed that healthy male immigrants from East Asia, the Middle East and North Africa had significantly more frequent acute pruritus (pruritus during the past week at the interview) than Norwegians and immigrants from western countries [21]. The difference between acute and chronic pruritus in skin type still has to be resolved. However, it was shown that after capsaicin application, African Americans had a lower rate of hypersensitivity towards pain than East Asians, Hispanics and people with white skin, suggesting a different sensitivity towards sensory symptoms [22]. US studies investigating itch severity in an itch centre, as well as in US veterans and eczema patients, demonstrated that African Americans have more severe pruritus compared with white people [23–25]. Together, these studies suggest neurobiological differences between ethnic groups and may indicate a different ethnic prevalence of CP.

Associated diseases

Chronic pruritus may evolve in association with dermatological, systemic, neurological and psychiatric diseases. In many cases, more than one disease is responsible for the evolution of CP; in others, no disease is found. There are different studies analysing the composition of the underlying diseases in CP patients. For example, the presence of an underlying systemic disease varied between 13% and 50% of CP patients in studies performed in small numbers of patients (34–132 CP patients) [26–30]. Based on an analysis of 3700 CP patients, the following underlying diseases were identified: dermatological disease 31.6%; systemic disease 8.6%; neurological disease 10.2% (e.g. stroke, multiple sclerosis); psychiatric disease 1.5%; multiple aetiologies 41.3%; and unknown origin 6.8% [31]. As long as interdisciplinary, national or international registries are unavailable, all such analyses are likely to be confounded by patient selection bias. A rare but important associated disease is malignancy. Analyses of large cohorts ($n = 8744$ and $n = 12\,813$) of patients with CP on non-lesional (i.e. normal-looking) skin identified haematological diseases and bile duct malignancies to be associated with occurrence of CP, particularly within the first year after onset [32,**33**].

Pathophysiology
Cutaneous induction of itch

Cutaneous sensory C and Aδ nerve fibres are involved in the pathophysiology of cutaneous itch. For decades, itch was considered as a weak pain signal transmitted by pain nerve fibres and mainly associated with histamine. In 1997, unmyelinated, mechano-insensitive C fibres specialised for the transmission of histamine-induced itch, but not pain, were identified [**34**]. It has been shown that nociceptors equipped with the thermoreceptor transient receptor potential cation channel subfamily V member 1 (TRPV1) are capable of transmitting histamine-induced itch via intracellular phospholipase Cβ3 (PLCβ3) [35,36].

Most CP types (except urticaria and several drug-related forms of itch) are now attributed to non-histaminergic pathways. In 2007, nociceptors of the mechano-sensitive C and Aδ nerve fibre class were demonstrated to be involved in the transmission of non-histaminergic itch [35,37]. The non-histaminergic pruritoceptors also require the ion channels of the transient receptor potential (TRP) channel family, TRPA1 and TRPV1, for itch signalling [38,**39**]. Studies have demonstrated that the proteinase cowhage (*Mucuna pruriens*) can activate mechano-sensitive, non-histaminergic C fibres and Aδ fibres thereby inducing itch. C fibres and Aδ fibres may transmit two distinct qualities of itch, a slow burning component and a faster pricking component, respectively [40]. This may explain the differing sensations described by patients which accompany itch. The most frequently reported qualities associated with itch are burning and stinging, but prickling, warmth and cold sensations are also described. Besides physiological transmission of itch, and independent of the involved nerve fibre class, spontaneous activity of C fibres was revealed in the symptomatic skin area in CP patients [41]. In addition, in various diseases, the cutaneous neuroanatomy is diseased and contributes to symptom induction and maintenance. Atopic eczema, PN and psoriasis are characterised by decreased epidermal nerve fibre number and increased substance P (SP) positive dermal nerve fibres [42–44].

Central transmission of itch

Peripheral afferent nerve fibres transmit the itch signal to the spinal cord, where the afferents enter the dorsal horn (superficial laminae I–II) and form a synapse with the secondary neuron [40]. Here, subsets of itch-specific spinal neurons are characterised by the expression of gastrin-releasing peptide receptor (GRPR) and natriuretic polypeptide B (nppB) [40,45,46]. Interestingly, gastrin-releasing peptide (GRP) seems also to have a role in the peripheral fibres (Table 81.2). Intradermal injection of GRP induced scratching through mast cell degranulation in an animal model [40,47]. It is currently assumed that spinal circuits of ascending neurons and interneurons form gates that control itch transmission, for example by counter-stimuli such as scratching. Dynorphin release by spinal neurons activates κ receptors on afferent neurons and interneurons resulting in a decrease of neuronal spinal activity. It was further shown that spinal interneurons expressing the atonal-related transcription factor Bhlhb5 inhibit the itch pathways within the dorsal horn. Furthermore, it was shown that they are most probably under the control of pain neurons [45,48]. This knowledge led to identification of novel pharmaceutical targets for antipruritic therapies.

The secondary itch neuron crosses over to the contralateral spino-thalamic tract and ascends to multiple brain areas such as prefrontal areas, supplementary motor areas (SMA), premotor cortex, anterior insular cortex, anterior midcingulate cortex, primary (S1) and secondary (S2) somatosensory cortices, thalamus, basal ganglia and cerebellum, all of which are involved in sensation, evaluative processes, emotion, reward and memory [40,**49**]. Current functional magnetic resonance imaging (MRI) studies suggest that there is no specific itch matrix in the brain but a broad overlapping of itch activation maps with pain areas [45]. In functional MRI studies, activation of brain areas such as the thalamus, primary and secondary somatosensory cortices, prefrontal cortex, anterior

Table 81.2 Examples of important mediators and receptors for itch.

Mediator	Receptor involved in itch	Clinically relevant mechanism or disease
Acetylcholine	Muscarinic acetylcholine receptor	Atopic eczema
Cutaneous and spinal neurotransmitters		
GRP	GRP receptor	Mast cell degranulation
Th2 and cytokines		
IL-31	IL-31RA/OSMR	Atopic eczema, familial primary cutaneous amyloidosis, prurigo nodularis, bullous pemphigoid, atopic eczema
IL-4, IL-13	IL-4R	
Periostin	Integrin receptor αVβ3	Atopic eczema, prurigo nodularis, stasis dermatitis, bullous pemphigoid
Histamine	H_1, H_4 receptor	Urticaria, insect bite reactions, cutaneous mastocytosis
Neuropeptide		
Endothelin 1	Endothelin A receptor	Release of nitric oxide, vasodilatation
Neurotrophin		
NGF	TrkA	Atopic eczema, psoriasis
Opioid peptides		
Endorphins	μ opioid receptor	Cholestatic pruritus
Dynorphin	κ opioid receptor	Uraemic pruritus
Proteases and Mrgpr agonists		
Tryptase, mucunain	PAR-2, PAR-4	Atopic eczema, cutaneous mastocytosis
Cathepsin S	PAR-2, PAR-4, MrgprC11	
Chloroquine	MrgprA3, TRPA1	Chloroquine-induced pruritus
Bilirubin	MrgprX4	Hepatic pruritus
Autotaxin	LPA	Hepatic pruritus
Tachykinins		
Substance P	Neurokinin 1 receptor	Atopic eczema, prurigo nodularis, psoriasis

Adapted from Akiyama and Carstens 2013 [40]. with permission of Elsevier.
GRP, gastrin-releasing peptide; IL, interleukin; LPA, lysophosphatidic acid; Mrgpr, Mas-related G-protein-coupled receptor; NGF, nerve growth factor; OSMR, oncostatin M receptor; PAR, proteinase activated receptor; Th2, T-helper 2; TrkA, tropomyosin-related kinase A; TRPA1, transient receptor potential ankyrin 1.

cingulate cortex, insular cortex, premotor and motor cortices and medial parietal cortex have been shown [45].

Scratching

Scratching is a reflex functioning at a spinal level, although modified greatly by higher centres. Scratching may also be habitual or triggered by boredom or emotional factors [50]. Scratching relieves itching for several minutes after cessation. Since the sensation of itching is reinforced by facilitating circuits in the relay synapses of the spinal cord, the prolonged scratch-induced relief could be due to temporary suppression of these circuits. Stimulation of fast-conducting myelinated afferents inhibits these circuits via pre- and postsynaptic mechanisms. These afferents could be activated by transepidermal electrical nerve stimulation (used therapeutically to allay itching) [51], by vibration, or more simply by scratching.

Alternatively, scratching could simply damage sensory nerve endings, repair occupying several minutes.

Why some itches evoke scratching and excoriation (as in scabies), whereas others prompt rubbing (as in lichen planus and urticaria), is unknown [52]. Scratching has been ingeniously utilised as an indirect objective method of quantifying itch and as such has been used in the evaluation of the treatment of itching [53].

Peripheral and central neuronal sensitisation

Several clinical observations favour the concept that peripheral and central neuronal sensitisation underlies the establishment of CP [**39**]. Sensitisation is defined as the increased responses of primary sensory neurons to itch and pain mediators. For example, measurable ongoing spontaneous neuronal activity, alloknesis (non-pruritogenic stimuli such as light touch in an area of CP elicit a sensation of itch) and hyperknesis (enhanced itch sensation elicited by a normal itch stimulus) are clinical pointers for sensitisation processes. In the skin, dysplasia of sensory neurons and a reduced threshold of neuroreceptors result in neuronal sensitisation mediated by several mediators such as bradykinin or nerve growth factor (NGF) [54]. Similarly, central neuronal sensitisation is based on spontaneous activity of superficial dorsal horn neurons, the enhancement of mechanically evoked responses and their increased response to mediators [**33**,40]. In the human brain, areas such as the parabrachial nucleus, periaqueductal gray, prefrontal cortex, anterior cingulate cortex and amygdala exhibit changes compatible with increases in excitability corresponding to central sensitisation of itch. More research in humans is required to delineate the brain mechanisms of central sensitisation.

Mediators of itching in skin diseases

Itch is the dominant symptom of inflammatory skin diseases, and in these dermatoses mediators of itch are assumed to play a central role. The concept of mediators in inflammatory skin diseases was pioneered by Lewis who proposed the involvement of 'H substances' [55]. Data on the identification and characterisation of mediators of itch in the skin has been obtained from several sources. Responses of skin of human volunteers to intradermal injection of the putative mediator depends on the measurement of subjective perception of itching, usually utilising a numerical rating scale (NRS) or visual analogue scale (VAS) or similar. Intradermal injection into mouse skin enables the frequency, duration and intensity of scratching to be measured. Mediators can also be directly identified and measured in tissue fluid from diseased skin by skin perfusion or microdialysis technology. Table 81.2 lists the mediators currently deemed to be important, and others that are potentially relevant.

Histamine and histamine receptors. Histamine is the archetypal mediator of inflammation and of acute itch. It causes itching if injected into the upper dermis but pain if it is injected more deeply into the dermis. However, repeated injection causes tachyphylaxis [56]. Histamine binds to G-protein-coupled receptors (GPCR). Four subclasses of histamine receptors have been identified and cloned. H_1 receptors are traditionally responsible for histamine-induced itching. The H_1-receptor-mediated itch involves the opening of TRPV1 receptors on histamine-sensitive C neurons via PLCβ3

[57]. In recent years, the spotlight has shifted to histamine H_4 receptors which appear to cause pruritus by direct action on a variety of immune and inflammatory cells, including mast cells and T helper 2 (Th2) lymphocytes in atopic eczema [58,59]. H_2 receptors seem not to be involved in histamine-evoked pruritus [60]. The main source of histamine in inflamed skin is the dermal mast cell, supplemented by infiltrating basophil leukocytes. In urticaria and in insect bite reactions these cells release histamine (and other mediators) via an energy-dependent signal transduction cascade triggered by a specific antigen (or in chronic urticaria by an autoantibody) cross-linking the high-affinity immunoglobulin E (IgE) receptor FcεR1. Elevated tissue fluid levels of histamine in lesional skin of chronic urticaria have been demonstrated [61]. The recognition that histamine is a mediator of itch in urticaria and can be abated by H_1 antihistamines, has led to these drugs being used indiscriminately for the treatment of pruritus in other conditions where there is little or no evidence that histamine is involved.

Acetylcholine. Acetylcholine, a neurotransmitter in the autonomic nervous system, acts on both muscarinic and nicotinic receptors. Intradermal injection of acetylcholine causes pain in healthy subjects, but evokes itch in atopic individuals [62]. Since tissue levels of acetylcholine are reported to be elevated in atopic eczema patients [63], it is possible that this mediator plays a role in the pruritus of atopic eczema. Botulinum toxin type A is known to inhibit the release of acetylcholine and was shown to suppress histamine-induced pruritus experimentally [64] and in notalgia paraesthetica [65].

Tachykinins. Substance P is an 11 amino acid neuropeptide that preferentially binds to the neurokinin 1 receptor (NK1R) which is widely expressed in the central nervous system, dorsal horn of the spinal cord and skin cells including keratinocytes and mast cells. SP is synthesised in the cell bodies of C fibres and released from these neurons along with depolarisation. In the skin, SP induces a neurogenic inflammation with redness, wealing and itching, at least in part due to degranulation of dermal mast cells [66,67]. Afferent neuron terminals enjoy close proximity to dermal mast cells consistent with presumed cross-talk between these structures [68]. NK1R expressed by mast cells are involved; for example, SP mediates release of the cytokine tumour necrosis factor α (TNF-α) by these cells, which in turn leads to afferent nociceptive neuronal sensitisation [69]. Further indirect evidence derives from reports of the beneficial effects of NK1R antagonists. Aprepitant, a selective NK1R antagonist, has been shown to be effective in case series suppressing pruritus in Sézary syndrome, dermatological pruritus including PN and in drug-induced pruritus by targeted cancer therapies [70–73]. However, phase II (aprepitant) and phase III (serlopitant) studies failed to show clinical meaningful itch reductions in PN and in chronic itch of unknown origin.

Opioid peptides. Opioid peptides are classified into three groups: endorphins, enkephalins and dynorphins; and their receptors are also classified into three types: μ (mu), δ (delta) and κ (kappa). The pruritic action of morphine and other opioids involves the μ opioid receptor and is antagonised by naloxone or naltrexone. However, ligation of the κ opioid receptor evokes an antipruritic effect. Opioids can cause pruritus by central mechanisms, due to imbalance between μ and κ opioid receptor activation [74]. The skin expresses μ and κ opioid receptors. Significant tissue levels of opioid peptides are found in human skin in cholestasis, a condition in which plasma levels of opioid peptides are elevated; cholestatic pruritus is ameliorated by the μ opioid receptor antagonist naloxone [75–77]. Nalfurafine, a κ opioid receptor agonist, also reduces end-stage CKD itch significantly and was licensed in Japan for this indication in 2009 [78]. Currently, other κ agonists difelikefalin and nalbuphine are being tested in CKD pruritus and PN; difelikefalin has shown significant antipruritic effects in a phase III trial and was recently approved for this indication [**79**].

Proteases, Mas-related G-protein-coupled receptor agonists and endothelin 1.

Peptide products from protease activity in the skin cause itching, an observation first reported by Shelley and Arthur [80]. They used spicules of cowhage which contains mucunain, a cysteine protease, which is more pruritic than histamine when injected into human skin. Its receptors proved to be proteinase-activated receptors (PAR) 2 and 4 which activate afferent mechano-sensitive C fibres (nociceptors). The naturally occurring counterpart of mucunain in human skin is mast cell-derived tryptase, which causes release of the pruritic tachykinin SP from afferent nociceptor C neurons. PAR-2 is overexpressed in the skin of patients with atopic eczema [81] and tryptase levels have been demonstrated to be increased in the lesional skin of patients with atopic eczema using a skin microdialysis technique [81]. It is likely that this receptor plays a central role in atopic pruritus.

Interestingly, a recent study reported that the chemical compound SLIGRL-NH2, a histamine-independent pruritogen, elicited scratching via Mas-related G-protein-coupled receptor 2 (MrgprC11) rather than PAR-2 [82]. The Mrgpr family consists of over 20 members (in mice) while only single analogues have been described in humans. MrgprAs, MrgprB4–5, MrgprC11 and MrgprD are involved in histamine-independent itch in mice [40]; human sensory neurons express MrgprX1 and MrgprX4. For example, chloroquine induces itch through MrgprA3, a receptor which is expressed in the skin and in addition defines a specific subpopulation of dorsal root ganglion neurons mediating itch [83]. It is also tempting to speculate that the itch of patients with the hereditary disorder Netherton syndrome, which is caused by a mutation in the *SPINK* (*Serine Peptidase Inhibitor Kazal*) gene leading to lack of a multidomain serine protease inhibitor, LEKT1 (lymphoepithelial Kazal-type related inhibitor), is due to consequential increased protease activity. The proteinase cathepsin E is an endogenous itch inducer via the production of endothelin 1 in the epidermis [84]. Endothelin 1 is produced by mast cells, endothelial cells and keratinocytes in the skin and is a pruritogen that can elicit scratching upon cutaneous injection [40]. Skin mast cells express MrgprX2; their activation triggers degranulation, proinflammatory mediator release, and itch induction in sensory neurons. MrgprX2 plays a role in chronic spontaneous urticaria, atopic dermatitis and psoriatic itch [85,**86**].

Neurotrophins.

Neurotrophins are neuropeptides that regulate growth and function of neurons, and those believed to be important in CP include NGF and neurotrophin 4. NGF is expressed by keratinocytes and mast cells and binds to the receptor tyrosine kinase receptor A (TrkA); it causes sprouting of nerve fibres and upregulates SP [87–89]. Involved skin in atopic eczema has been shown to express elevated levels of NGF in keratinocytes and increased TrkA in the epidermis and upper dermis [90].

Cytokines: interleukins 2, 4, 13 and 31.

There is increasing recognition of a functional interaction between the nervous system and the immune system. Neuropeptides such as SP can evoke transcription of cytokines and adhesion molecules [91]. Interleukin 2 (IL-2), a cytokine secreted by activated T lymphocytes, is one such candidate. Human recombinant IL-2 injected intradermally causes intense pruritus in atopic and non-atopic volunteers [92]. Both the presence of activated T lymphocytes in atopic eczema skin, and the antipruritic effect of ciclosporin, a suppressor of IL-2 secretion [93], indicates a role for this cytokine as a mediator of pruritus in atopic eczema.

The type 2 cytokines, IL-4 and its homologue IL-13, have an important role in itch and are closely related in their functions. Their receptors are on sensory neurons; when activated, they signal through the Janus kinase (JAK) pathway as well as both TRPA1 and TRPV1, causing itch [94,**95**]. More importantly, the IL-4 receptor α is involved in chronic pruritus as its activation may sensitise sensory neurons to multiple other pruritogens. In acute inflammation such as atopic dermatitis, IL-4 and IL-13 are released by Th2 T cells, mast cells and basophils. Both interleukins act on keratinocytes, fibroblasts, eosinophils, monocytes and B cells, and thereby enhance skin inflammation. For example, they impact the epidermal barrier via binding to keratinocytes to enhance the epidermal expression of the C-X-C motif chemokine ligand (CXCL) 9, 10 and 11, and thymic stromal lymphopoietin [96].

More recently, evidence has emerged that IL-31 functions as a mediator of pruritus in atopic eczema. IL-31 is a Th2 cytokine of the skin-homing cutaneous lymphocyte antigen (CLA) subtype found in increased quantities in the skin and serum of patients with atopic eczema [97,98]. Its heterodimeric receptor composed of IL-31 receptor A (IL-31RA) and oncostatin M receptor (OSMR) is located on keratinocytes and monocytes, and animal experiments utilising a mouse model of atopic eczema indicate its ability to induce itching and scratching in skin [99]. Subsequently, an antibody reactive with IL-31 receptor has been shown to ameliorate scratching in the same animal model [100]. It is interesting that IL-31 receptors have been demonstrated on dorsal root ganglia of afferent nociceptor neurons and can act on neurons at multiple loci [101]. IL-31 and its receptor have been highly associated with itch in numerous pruritic diseases beyond atopic eczema including PN, lichen amyloidosis, cutaneous T-cell lymphoma, stasis dermatitis, CKD-associated pruritus and dermatomyositis [102–109]. Periostin, an extracellular matrix and matricellular protein, binds to several types of integrins that transduce its signals. Recent studies have demonstrated a significant role of periostin in itch sensation via a direct integrin-mediated stimulation of nerve fibres and interaction with immune and non-immune cells inducing a Th2 response.

It appears to contribute to itch in various pruritic diseases including atopic eczema, PN, pemphigoid, stasis dermatitis and scabies [110,111].

Clinical features

History

History taking is an important step in the diagnostic work-up of CP patients [4]. It aims to narrow the spectrum of underlying diseases, which may be difficult to detect, especially in cases where CP precedes the evolution of the disease (premonitory pruritus). In order to obtain a comprehensive patient history, standardised questionnaires are recommended [112]. The most important points are summarised in Box 81.1. Intensive and long-lasting pruritus can lead to considerable psychological impairment. The attending clinician should not underestimate the negative psychological effects that pruritus can have on a patient. It is important that this issue is specifically addressed by when taking the history. In CP patients, there may be features of an adjustment disorder combined with a retreat from social and professional environments which may result in reactive depression [113]. A screen for distress is desirable as is a screen for other physical or psychological symptoms. Useful assessment tools include the Patient Health Questionnaires PHQ-15, PHQ-2 and PHQ-9 and the Hospital Anxiety and Depression Scale (HADS). Psychosomatic care may be indicated. Alternatively, the cause of CP might be primarily a disorder of a psychiatric nature. If this is suspected, the patient should be examined by a psychiatrist or initially seen in a psychodermatology clinic.

> ### Box 81.1 Important details in history taking in chronic pruritus (CP) patients
>
> **Pruritus-specific history**
> - Time point of start of CP and total duration
> - Localisation (start, spreading)
> - Quality: e.g. burning itch (classically seen in dermatitis herpetiformis or lupus erythematosus), pricking itch, tingling itch, itch resembling insects crawling on/under skin (formication), presence of pain
> - Intensity: average/worst intensity on the visual analogue scale (VAS) or numerical rating scale (NRS) in the past 24 h
> - Course: variations during the day (scabies typically worse at night), situational, continuous CP/attacks, spontaneous improvement/deterioration
> - Triggering factors, ameliorating factors, role of emotions pre-scratching
> - Behavioural response to itch: scratch, rub, role of habit – conscious vs subconscious scratching
> - Temporal association with previous illnesses, surgeries, medication intake, other events
> - Occupational/social exposure to possible causes, e.g. fibreglass, birds, dogs, cats, rats, farm animals
> - Travel history – consider rare infestations, e.g. onchocerciasis, gnathostomiasis, giardiasis
> - Other family members itching suggests scabies
> - Previous therapies: successful/unsuccessful
> - Self-treatment/over-bathing
> - Patient's own theory about the cause of CP
> - Psychogenic stress factors
> - Impairments in quality of life, burden, sleep disturbances

> **General history**
> - Previous illnesses including dermatoses
> - Drug intake (prescribed, over the counter, recreational), infusions, blood transfusions
> - Previous surgeries (stress reaction/medication-induced pruritus or nerve compression)
> - Allergies: type I/type IV allergies
> - Atopic predisposition
> - Clinical signs for malignancy (weight loss, fever, night sweats)
> - Pregnancy
> - Systematic enquiry/review of clinical systems
>
> Adapted from Ständer *et al*. 2012 [278].

Presentation

Chronic pruritus may initially occur on non-diseased skin (classification term: pruritus on non-inflamed skin; replaces the previous designation pruritus sine materia) or along with a dermatosis (pruritus on inflamed skin) (Figures 81.1 and 81.2). CP induces scratching that may change the initial clinical picture. Accordingly, patients may present with excoriations, erosions, papules, nodules, lichenification, scars and hyper- and hypopigmentation resulting from scratching (Figure 81.3). If these are predominant (classification term: pruritus along with chronic scratch lesions), they may conceal an initial dermatosis. Thus, it is important to distinguish a primary dermatosis from secondary scratch lesions and ask patients about the methods they use to relieve pruritus in order to interpret the clinical findings properly [4]. Certain recurrent clinical pictures have been summarised under specific names such as lichen simplex or PN. These also define clinical entities despite being initial reaction

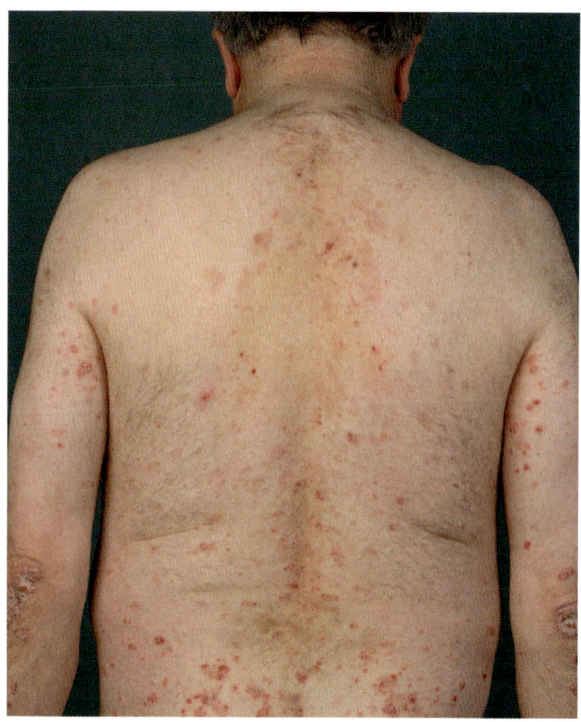

Figure 81.1 Patient with chronic pruritus on inflamed skin (psoriasis).

in great detail and current studies aim to show the antipruritic effect of new targeted therapies in these entities.

Pruritus of atopic eczema. The itch of atopic eczema is aggravated by scratch damage, which causes enhanced inflammation (itch–scratch cycle; see also Chapter 41). Itching is usually worse at night, and is aggravated by contact with wool, sweating and the ingestion of spicy foods and alcohol. The itch of atopic eczema is multifactorial, and is due to dryness (almost invariable in atopic eczema sufferers), inflammation and neural sensitisation in the peripheral and central nervous system. In this context, alloknesis (itchy skin) forms a major component of the itch suffered by the atopic eczema patient, explaining, for example, the paroxysms of itching experienced by patients in response to scratching, sweating, sudden changes of temperature, humidity, undressing or dressing, etc. Pruritus in atopic eczema involves skin barrier and keratinocyte signalling and immunological and neural mechanisms. Several studies have reported an enhanced and abnormally prolonged response to the application of pruritic pharmacological stimuli in unaffected skin in atopic patients. Studies of the itching response of atopic eczema patients to histamine iontophoresis suggest a decreased response of afferent cutaneous fibres to high doses, but an increased sensitivity to low concentrations; possibly because of increased permeability of clinically normal-looking skin of these atopic patients [116]. It is important to distinguish itching associated with inflammatory changes or chronic lichenification from that simply due to excessive drying of the skin in patients with atopic eczema. Emollients, which should always be recommended, and which in many cases may be all that is required, will be inadequate alone where inflammatory changes are responsible for the itching. Lowering skin pH and adding soothing topical emollients with oatmeal extracts and anaesthetics such as pramoxine and polidocanol further reduce the itch [116]. Molecular biological studies and dermal microdialysis studies have demonstrated the involvement of mediators other than histamine in lesional skin of atopic eczema patients such as IL-4, -13 and -31 and thymic stromal lymphopoietin [38,117]. Reviews of the effectiveness of H_1 antihistamines concluded that they are of little value in relieving pruritus [**118**]. However, most patients with itchy atopic eczema receive antihistamines, mainly of the sedative type, and find them of some value, presumably due to their central sedative effect. On the basis of a comparison of itching in atopic eczema patients receiving successively astemizole (low sedation antihistamine), trimeprazine (sedative antihistamine) and nitrazepam (non-antihistamine sedative), concluded that sedation was a required component of the successful systemic treatment of itching in atopics, and that, moreover, itching in atopic eczema involved a central component [119]. However, numbers of patients were small and subsequent studies have yielded conflicting results.

Systemic antibiotics might also modulate pruritus. Changes in skin microbiome in atopic eczema can cause dysbiosis and lead to robust colonisation of *Staphylococcus aureus* [120]. *Staphylococcus aureus* behaves as a superantigen leading to T-cell activation, and also activates nerves via serine proteases and dermal mast cells via Toll-like receptors and promotes the production of the pruritogen IL-31 [121].

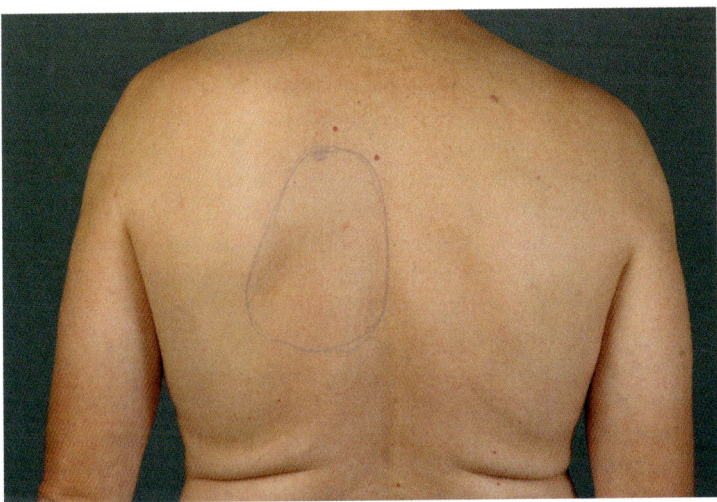

Figure 81.2 Patient with chronic pruritus on non-inflamed skin (notalgia paraesthetica; lesional area marked).

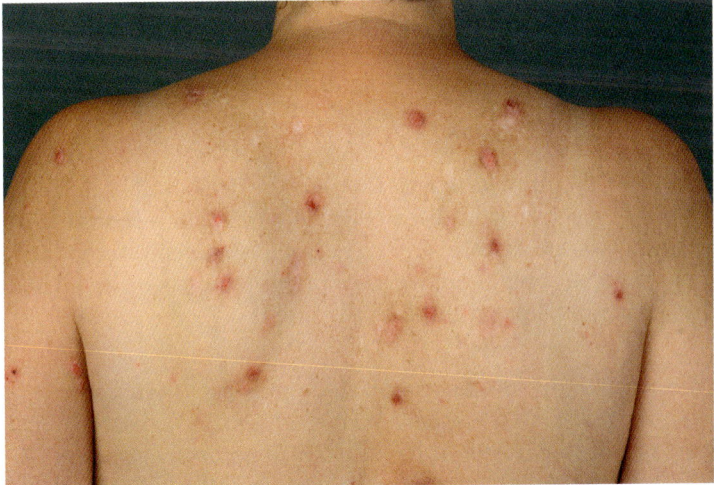

Figure 81.3 Patient with chronic pruritus and chronic scratch lesions (prurigo nodularis).

patterns resulting from chronic scratching. A common finding in all cases of generalised pruritus with the presence of scratch-related lesions is the so-called butterfly sign which describes the distribution of spared skin between the shoulder blades which cannot be reached. This part of the back is known as the acnestis.

Clinical variants

Pruritus in inflamed skin (dermatoses). The majority of dermatoses may induce pruritus, although itch occurs with interindividual variation. While all patients with atopic eczema, urticaria and bullous pemphigoid report itch, other diseases such as pityriasis rubra pilaris or lichen planus show itch only in a subset of patients. Intense widespread pruritus is also a major feature of Sézary syndrome and occurs in cutaneous mastocytosis if the skin is rubbed to provoke a weal (Darier sign). In mycosis fungoides, pruritus may be the presenting symptom without skin signs ('invisible mycosis fungoides'), but mainly occurs in late-stage mycosis fungoides and its follicular variant [114]. Subclinical urticaria is reported in the form of invisible dermographism [115]. Itch in atopic eczema (atopic itch) and psoriasis vulgaris (psoriatic itch) have been investigated

Topical corticosteroids are frequently effective in suppressing itching in the atopic eczema patient. Corticosteroids are not inherently antipruritic, but suppress the inflammatory component of the dermatosis thereby alleviating the itching indirectly. They are especially effective in highly pruritic children with atopic eczema treated with the 'wet wrap' technique [122]. The introduction of topical calcineurin inhibitors, tacrolimus and pimecrolimus, provides an effective measure for amelioration of pruritus of atopic eczema [123,124]. These agents owe their action to the downregulation of activated T cells [125].

Topical non-steroidal phosphodiesterase 4 inhibitors such as crisabarole have shown rapid antipruritic effect in atopic eczema [126,127]. Systemic immunosuppressive medications including systemic ciclosporin, methotrexate and azathioprine are highly effective in relieving the itching (and other signs and symptoms) of chronic atopic eczema in selected patients [84,103], due to their pan T-cell inhibition; however their safety profile limits their prolonged use [128].

In recent years a significant advancement in the treatment of atopic eczema has been achieved with the launch of dupilumab, a targeted biological inhibiting IL-4Rα. This drug has a significant antipruritic effect that shows meaningful improvement after the first dose [129]. Numerous drugs are currently being tested in clinical trials for atopic eczema and the majority have a very potent antipruritic effect including drugs targeting JAK/Stats signalling such as baricitinib, abrocitinib and upadacitinib, and IL-13 and IL-31 receptor antagonists such as tralokinumab and nemolizumab [130,131] (Chapter 41).

Other modalities that have shown an antipruritic effect are broad-band and narrow-band ultraviolet B (UVB), the latter being deemed superior and safer [132]. If this is not effective, the oral µ-opioid receptor antagonist naltrexone can be considered for itch control [133].

Pruritus of psoriasis vulgaris. Generalised pruritus is a feature of psoriasis in 80–89% of patients [134–136] (Chapter 35). The National Psoriasis Foundation collected the data of more than 5600 psoriasis patients from 2003 to 2011; pruritus was the most common symptom (93%) reported [137]. Pruritus may involve all areas of the body. The presence and intensity of itching did not depend on the age and gender of patients, type of psoriasis, duration of disease or last outbreak of psoriasis [135]. In approximately 80% of patients, pruritus appears on a daily basis and although usually confined to the psoriatic lesions and of moderate intensity [138,139], the pruritus significantly affects QoL [108] and induces feelings of stigmatisation and depressive symptoms [139]. In a web-based questionnaire study comparing atopic eczema and psoriasis, psoriasis respondents reported higher embarrassment associated with itch [139]. Important daily factors that were found to exacerbate the itch were ambient heat (81%), skin dryness (80%), sweating (65%) and stress (55%) [134]. To assess psoriasis symptoms including pruritus, an eight-item psoriasis symptom inventory (PSI) was developed and validated that assessed the severity of itch, redness, scaling, burning, cracking, stinging, flaking and pain [140].

It is very likely that inflammation, inflammatory T cells and neutrophils and their mediators such as IL-17 contribute to pruritus in psoriasis [86]. IL-31 mRNA expression was initially reported to not be involved in psoriasis itch [98,141], however recent studies have demonstrated it has a role and correlates with itch intensity [86]. Neuropeptides released by nerve fibres seem to contribute to the induction of itch in psoriasis [44]. A significant correlation was observed between the intensity of pruritus and protein gene product 9.5 immunoreactive intraepidermal nerve fibres (IENF), NGF immunoreactive keratinocytes (which showed a strong positivity throughout the entire epidermis) and expression of the high-affinity receptors for NGF TrkA in the epidermis. An increase in neuropeptide SP-containing nerve fibres in perivascular areas and decreased expression of neutral endopeptidase (enzyme degrading SP) in the epidermal basal layer and in the endothelium of blood vessels was described. An increase in the expression of TrkA next to basal keratinocytes and also in dermal nerves, as well as increased mast cell numbers showing degranulation in the papillary dermis, has been reported [44].

Interestingly, one study found that pruritus of psoriasis was found to be unresponsive to most available antipruritics, including phototherapy [134]. However, patients report a decline of itch accompanying effective clearance of psoriasis plaques. Novel therapies such as apremilast, a specific inhibitor of phosphodiesterase 4, and biologicals (inhibitors of IL-17 and -23) have demonstrated reduction of psoriatic itch [142].

Itching in systemic disease. This section deals with itch in skin devoid of primary skin disease, and occurring in response to systemic or internal disease, any signs in the skin being secondary to scratching or rubbing. An overview of this topic can be found in the European guideline on chronic pruritus [4].

Chronic kidney disease-associated pruritus (nephrogenic or uraemic pruritus). Persistent itching is a major cause of impairment of QoL in patients with CKD [143]. It occurs in around 10–77% of patients [144] but is rarely a feature in children or in patients with acute renal failure [145]; the reasons for this are unknown. It is more common in patients receiving haemodialysis than in those on continuous ambulatory peritoneal dialysis (CAPD) [146]. The clinical features have been comprehensively described [143]. Although the skin of some patients may appear dry, frequently it is essentially normal in appearance. The pruritus of CKD may be persistent, extensive and refractory to therapy, but in other patients it may be transitory and localised [143,145]. Secondary skin changes due to scratching and rubbing are very common. These include pigmentation and PN, often secondarily infected. Histologically, the clinically normal skin may show attenuation of sweat and sebaceous glands and an increased number of mast cells [147]. However, no correlation between mast cell population densities and pruritus has been established.

The pathophysiology of CKD pruritus is unclear but is likely multifactorial [148] and includes an imbalance of overexpression of µ opioid receptors and downregulation of κ opioid receptors, and upregulation of Th1 cytokines. Recent studies have demonstrated elevated levels of IL-31, 'the itchy cytokine' [111,149]. An abnormal sprouting of neuron-specific enolase-positive unmyelinated nerve fibres has also been reported in the skin of patients with CKD pruritus [150]. Other suggested factors in the pathogenesis include raised serum parathyroid hormone levels due to secondary hyperparathyroidism [151]; of note, parathyroid hormone increases the number of tissue mast cells [152]. However, although parathyroidectomy has relieved pruritus in some patients [153], no convincing correlation between parathormone levels and pruritus has been demonstrated in CKD [151]. The pruritus of CKD has been proposed to be related to aluminium overload during haemodialysis [154], treatable by the administration of desferrioxamine mesylate, but this has not been confirmed. Pharmacological mediators have been proposed to be responsible for CKD pruritus. Histamine is an improbable candidate, since treatment with antihistamines is ineffective. The DOPPS (Dialysis Outcomes and Practice Pattern Study), which included 29 000 patients, detected the following risk factors for the development of CKD pruritus: male sex, pre-existing diseases of lung, heart or liver (e.g. hepatitis C) and elevated serum calcium/phosphorus level but not uraemia. These findings question the term uraemic pruritus, which is now avoided and has been replaced by CKD pruritus [2].

Treatment of CKD pruritus is challenging. Urea-based topical humectants may help [155]. The topical calcineurin inhibitor tacrolimus 0.1% proved ineffective in a double-blind randomised placebo-controlled study in haemodialysis-related pruritus [156]. Opioid peptides have also recently been implicated in haemodialysis-related pruritus, elevated plasma met-enkephalin levels having been reported in haemodialysis patients [157], although a correlation has yet to be established [158]. Recent studies suggest that pruritus of renal failure responds to κ opioid agonist and this led to the approval of nalfurafine and difelikefalin for CKD pruritus [159,160]. The pathophysiology of CKD pruritus and its management has been reviewed recently [161].

Important general therapeutic measures include emollients for xerosis and treatment of scratch lesions [162]. The κ opioid receptor agonists seem to be a promising treatment. Nalfurafine is approved only in Japan but recent phase III clincial trials using difelikefalin have shown significant antipruritic effect in CKD which is approved now in the US and Europe [163].

Dialysis itself has little beneficial effect on CKD pruritus, although its frequency and severity has lessened since the advent of dialysis membranes with better bio-compatibility [164]. The only curative and reliably effective treatment for renal pruritus is renal transplantation. Parathyroidectomy may be followed by remission of pruritus in patients with secondary hyperparathyroidism [153]. Phototherapy with UVB is frequently effective and may act systemically as well as locally; its value is supported by a recent meta-analysis [165]. Ultraviolet therapy (combined UVA and UVB) depletes the skin of vitamin A and this has been proposed as a mode of action [166]. Only UVB phototherapy and activated charcoal have an established track record for this indication [167,168].

Other treatments have been advocated, including heparin, mexiletine, ion-exchange resin and intravenous lignocaine, but are of uncertain effectiveness and usually impractical to use. Opioid antagonists such as naltrexone have some efficacy but controlled studies are missing and this treatment remains to be independently confirmed [169]. Antihistamines and topical steroids are generally unhelpful in CKD pruritus, but emollients may provide relief in those with dry skin.

Since itching may be restricted to certain areas, topical capsaicin 0.025% has been reported to be effective in localised CKD pruritus [170]. In the longer term, only a greater availability of renal transplantation is likely to bring sustained relief to these greatly distressed patients.

Hepatobiliary diseases and cholestasis (cholestatic pruritus). Pruritus may be generalised or localised, for example to the hands and feet, and can be an early symptom of hepatobiliary disease. It is associated with rubbing rather than scratching, therefore secondary excoriation and infection are less common than in renal pruritus. It is a frequent and distressing symptom of hepatobiliary diseases; recent studies suggest that autotoxin and the bile acid receptor TGR5 are involved in the pathogenesis [171,172]. Hepatic pruritus is associated with cholestasis; about 70% of patients with cholestasis report pruritus. The most common are intrahepatic cholestasis of pregnancy (ICP), primary biliary cirrhosis (PBC), primary sclerosing cholangitis and hereditary paediatric cholestatic disorders [173]. Hepatitis C is also a cause of intense cholestatic pruritus, occurring in 15% of infected patients [174].

Cholestatic pruritus was speculated to be associated with elevated plasma levels of bile salts [175], but evidence of a direct correlation has been lacking except in ICP. Measurements of skin tissue levels of bile salts and their relationship to serum levels, and to intensity of itching, gave inconclusive results and the bile salt levels did not differ from values in control subjects [176]. Bile salts applied to blister bases in human skin, although causing pruritus, do so at minimal effective concentrations far exceeding those achieved in cholestatic jaundice [177]. A lack of demonstrable quantitative relationships has not, however, discouraged a number of investigators from exploring methods for lowering serum and skin bile salt levels in the management of itching due to cholestasis. For example, plasma perfusion through charcoal-coated glass beads was associated with a marked improvement in cholestatic pruritus, although a relationship between clinical response and fall in bile salt level was not demonstrated. Recent experimental evidence has implicated the lysophospholipase, autotaxin (ATX), and its product, lysophosphatidic acid (LPA), as potential mediators of cholestatic pruritus [171]. Serum ATX levels were demonstrated to be specific for cholestatic pruritus [171]. The treatment of patients with cholestasis with the bile salt sequestrant, colesevelam, but not placebo, effectively reduced total serum bile salts, but only marginally altered pruritus intensity and ATX activity. Rifampicin [178,179] significantly reduced itch intensity and ATX activity in patients with pruritus not responding to bile salt sequestrants [171] Similar results have been achieved clinically with ion-exchange resins, including cholestyramine [180–182]. These reports raise the possibility that other observed clinical improvements may be a consequence of removal of ATX following such procedures as extracorporeal albumin dialysis [183] and phototherapy [181]. Rifampicin is effective, but has to be administered with caution as it is associated with hepatotoxicity [184]. Ursodeoxycholic acid has proved disappointing in a recent meta-analysis [185]. Effective treatments of hepatobiliary pruritus have been reviewed [186].

Recent studies have demonstrated that bilirubin can elicit an itch sensation in humans by directly stimulating peripheral nerve fibres through mouse Mas-related G-protein-coupled receptor MrgprX4 receptors [187,188].

Earlier work highlighted the importance of dysregulation of central opioid peptides in patients with cholestatic pruritus [189]. Plasma levels of opioid peptides are elevated in human [189] and rat [190] cholestasis. Furthermore, plasma from patients suffering from pruritus of cholestasis induces facial scratching, reversed by naloxone, when injected into the medullary dorsal horn of the monkey [76]. Most importantly, carefully controlled trials established the effectiveness of parenteral and oral opioid antagonists in the treatment of cholestatic pruritus [191,192]. Thus, the conclusion that opioid antagonists are of value for treatment of the pruritus of cholestasis is based upon evidence of increased opioidergic tone in chronic cholestasis patients, and the impressive response to naloxone or naltrexone (specific opioid μ receptor antagonists). This response can be associated with opioid withdrawal symptoms [193]. Apart from biliary disease, cholestatic pruritus may also occur in pregnancy [194] and premenstrually [195]. However, the role of opioid peptides in these contexts has yet to be established.

Polycythaemia vera. Pruritus is a common symptom in polycythaemia vera (PV) patients (Chapter 149). As many as 50% of untreated patients with PV who have a mutation in JAK2V617 develop a severe, prickly and distressing discomfort within minutes of water contact, lasting 15–60 min [196]. As it frequently occurs after the patient emerges from bathing, it is often referred to as 'bath itch' or aquagenic pruritus. No visible changes are present in the skin, and the symptom may be associated with elevated serum and urinary histamine levels [196]. Platelet aggregation has been suggested as a possible mechanism and source of pruritogenic factors, including histamine [197]. Water-induced itching may precede development of PV by several years [198]. Bathing by regional sponging may mitigate the itch. Successful treatment of the underlying PV may not relieve the itching and although correction of venesection-induced iron deficiency may give relief, it may be at the expense of exacerbating the PV. Antihistamines are effective in around 30% based on the fact that the JAK2V617 mutation results in increased activation of mast cells. Psoralen and UVA (PUVA) photochemotherapy with 8-methoxypsoralen and UVA, has been successful in some patients [199]. Success has been claimed for narrow-band UVB phototherapy [200]. One report cites the use of long-term treatment with interferon-α2b for severe pruritus of PV [201], and another advocates the use of serotonin reuptake inhibitors such as paroxetine or the pain modulator pregabalin [202,203]. Some patients may respond to aspirin [197]. Inhibitors of JAK2 may reduce PV itch [204].

Thyrotoxicosis. Intractable itching associated with a warm moist skin is a recognised accompaniment of thyrotoxicosis and may be the presenting symptom [205] (Chapter 150). The cause is uncertain. Cutaneous vasodilatation, a regular feature of the disease, leads to increased skin surface temperature, which lowers the itch threshold [206].

Diabetes (diabetogenic pruritus). Contrary to past assumptions [207,208], generalised pruritus is a manifestation of diabetic [209,210] (Chapter 62). In a large-scale survey of 2656 diabetic out-patients and 499 non-diabetic subjects, 26.3% of the diabetic subjects and 14.6% of the non-diabetic participants (P <0.001) presented with CP. The prevalence of specifically located truncal pruritus in diabetic subjects was significantly higher than that in age-matched non-diabetic subjects (11.3 versus 2.9%, P = 0.0001). Further analysis revealed that abnormal sensation and Achilles tendon areflexia were independent risk factors suggesting that diabetic pruritus is significantly associated with the symptoms and signs of diabetic polyneuropathy [210]. Another recent study demonstrated positive associations between postprandial blood glucose and generalised diabetic pruritus [211]. In this study, 27.5% of 385 patients with type 2 diabetes suffered from itching. Scalp itch without rash was highly associated with diabetes in old age, suggesting a neuropathic cause [212].

Malignancy (paraneoplastic pruritus). The problem of pruritus as a manifestation of malignant diseases has been the subject of multiple publications [32,213,214] (Chapter 148). Large cohort studies showed that haematological malignancies and hepatobiliary neoplasms are associated with pruritus. However, it is well known that pruritus may precede the development of solid tumours or haematoproliferative diseases – so-called premonitory pruritus. For example, Hodgkin disease (5 years premonitory pruritus documented) and PV (13 years premonitory pruritus documented) are typical candidates for premonitory pruritus [196,215]. Other candidates for the development of paraneoplastic pruritus are Sézary syndrome, myelodysplastic syndrome and myelofibrosis; very rarely it occurs in non-Hodgkin lymphoma (including in children), multiple myeloma, chronic lymphocytic leukaemia and chronic myelomonocytic leukaemia [216]. In Hodgkin disease, about 30% of patients present with pruritus as a symptom; in one study this was associated with shorter life expectancy than if no itch was present [217]; however, this finding was not confirmed in recent studies [218,219].

Rarely, neoplasms may present as localised paraneoplastic pruritus; for example, unilateral facial pruritus is an early symptom of brainstem glioma; pruritus of the nose may be a presenting symptom of a cerebral tumour; and abdominal itching has been reported to be associated with an astrocytoma in neurofibromatosis [218,219]. Other solid tumours such as liver, breast, lung, gastric, laryngeal, prostate and cervical carcinoma are anecdotally reported to lead to localised or generalised pruritus [218,219].

Paraneoplastic itch can be relieved with selective serotonin reuptake inhibitors (e.g. paroxetine), combined κ opioid receptor agonists/μ opioid receptor antagonists, and pain modulators such as pregabalin, gabapentin as well as thalidomide in haematological malignancies, and short-course oral corticosteroids [220].

Drug-induced pruritus. Drug-induced pruritus without rash development is frequent; it is estimated that pruritus accounts for approximately 5% of all adverse skin reactions after drug intake [**221**] (Chapter 117). In general, drug-induced pruritus is divided into two groups: (i) the drug and its pathomechanism of CP induction are known, and there is a clear temporal relationship between intake of drug and onset of pruritus; and (ii) the role of the drug in causing pruritus is frequently unclear due to long latency between the start of drug intake and onset of itching, and, once identified, there is often no hypothesis on the pathomechanism involved. Typical examples for the first group of drugs are morphine, chloroquine and hydroxyethyl starch [222], the latter of which has been used widely as a plasma substitute, especially in Europe. It is also used to improve the function of the microcirculation. Generalised pruritus has been reported as a well-recognised complication, occurring in 15–42% of patients [223]. It results from deposits of hydroxyethyl starch in cutaneous peripheral nerves, and may be associated with severe, long-lasting, mechanically inducible itching [222,224]. It is poorly responsive to antihistamines, but may respond to topical capsaicin or systemic gabapentin or naltrexone [225,226].

The second group comprises a large number of substances such as angiotensin-converting enzyme inhibitors (e.g. captopril, enalapril), calcium channel blockers (e.g. amlodipine), β-blockers (e.g. atenolol, metoprolol), antidiabetics (e.g. glimepiride, metformin), diuretics (e.g. hydrochlorothiazide), hormones, statins and allopurinol [**221**].

Recently, pruritus has been reported as a common side effect of a number of molecularly targeted and immunotherapeutic antineoplastic agents, including inhibitors of epidermal growth factor, tyrosine kinase, BRAF (B-rapidly accelerated fibrosarcoma protein), MEK (mitogen-activated extracellular signal-regulated kinase), PD1 (programmed cell death receptor 1), PD-L1 (programmed cell death ligand 1) and CTLA-4 (cytotoxic T-lymphocyte-associated protein 4) [227–230].

Many other drugs are anecdotally reported to induce CP. The frequency of drug-induced pruritus following the use of particular medications, as well as the pathomechanisms involved, await further investigation [**221**].

Pruritus in pregnancy. Pruritus occurs in about 20% of pregnant women (Chapter 113). In the majority of these, itching is linked to pre-existing dermatoses such as psoriasis and atopic eczema. Atopic eruption of pregnancy (AEP) encompasses previous terms describing questionable entities such as prurigo of pregnancy and pruritic folliculitis of pregnancy [231,232]; it occurs in early pregnancy without fetal risk. Polymorphic eruption of pregnancy (PEP; previously known as pruritic urticated papules of pregnancy (PUPP)) occurs in about 21.6% of itchy pregnant women, and also does not risk fetal health. Pemphigoid gestationis is rare (4.2% of itchy pregnant women), and may lead to small-for-date babies. In ICP, generalised pruritus starts without skin lesions. Secondary scratch lesions and prurigo may be present. Typically, bile acids are elevated and jaundice may occur (after the onset of itching). Splicing mutations in the multidrug resistance P-glycoprotein 3 (*MDR3*) gene have been found to be related to ICP and may be associated with stillbirths and cholelithiasis [233].

No treatment for itching is absolutely safe in pregnancy, but it is a reasonable assumption that persistent intense pruritus is itself prejudicial to a healthy pregnancy. Loratadine has been used in over 5000 pregnancies with no increased risk for the fetus and can be taken in all trimesters. First generation antihistamines such as chlorpheniramine, hydroxyzine and dexchlorpheniramine are also not contraindicated in pregnancy and are considered safe although not licensed in pregnancy (Chapter 113). Topical corticosteroids may be applied if necessary; in late pregnancy UV therapy is possible.

Pruritus of senescence (previously known as senile pruritus). Persistent and widespread itching, often associated with extensive excoriation, is experienced by at least 50% of people in the seventh decade of life or beyond [234]. Because of the gradually increasing proportion of elderly persons in the population, it is also a burgeoning problem. In women, itching may be a manifestation of the postmenopausal syndrome. Pruritus of elderly people may be a symptom of subtle skin disease such as scabies, especially in the institutionalised, a manifestation of an underlying systemic disorder (including stroke disease, dementia, Parkinson disease, renal, hepatic or malignant disease), a skin manifestation of an adverse drug reaction or symptomatic of depression and loneliness or a combination of several of these factors (pruritus of multiple aetiologies). However, in many instances, itching is a result of excessive dryness of the skin (xerosis). There is evidence of reduced production of sebum production in association with ageing, and its composition also alters [235]; however, this is not thought to be a major factor in xerosis of the elderly. Senescence is frequently associated with failure of the skin to retain water and is often worse in the winter. The resulting dryness and fine cracking of the skin is associated with troublesome itching, which in most instances responds to emollients. Water-induced itching in elderly people [236] is a variant of senescent pruritus, being particularly common in those who are institutionalised and exposed to an overheated dry environment, resulting in skin desiccation, and both this and the common spontaneous variety respond to emollients. Analysis of senescent stratum corneum has shown greatly reduced water content [237]. Dystrophic changes in afferent nerve terminals may be involved in pruritic senescent skin and may have a pathogenetic role [238,239]. Immunosenescence is another cause of pruritus as there is a Th2 cytokine skew in the elderly associated with an eczematous itchy rash [240,241]. Pruritic skin diseases such bullous pemphigoid, stasis dermatitis, PN and cutaneous T cell lymphoma are more common in the elderly [2].

It is usually most expedient to prescribe several different emollients and encourage the patient to experiment with these, since it is not possible to predict individual responses with confidence. White soft paraffin ointment is cheap, occlusive and has been shown to accelerate recovery of barrier function in damaged skin. The use of a topical humectant such as 10% urea lotion can be effective [242]. The patient can be encouraged to apply emollients at least twice daily and more often if required and is practical. Also, if possible, ambient temperature and humidity should be modified. A trial of an appropriate psychopharmaceutical therapy such as mirtazapine at night is useful in patients in whom there is a significant element of depression and sleep disturbance. Corticosteroids, antihistamines and cooling lotions are not indicated in itching due to xerosis. In conditions where there is inflammation and eczema the use of methotrexate and dupilumab seem to be safer than immunosuppressants such as ciclosporin and systemic corticosteroids [243,244].

Neurological diseases (neuropathic pruritus). Chronic pruritus may occur in the context of a peripheral or central nervous system related nerve fibre injury or damage. Such damage causing overlapping symptoms of pruritus and pain, so-called 'pruralgia', spans a wide range of perceptions – feelings of stinging and burning, wet sensation, electric shock or pins and needles – and various symptoms of pain (e.g. mechanical dynamic allodynia) [245]. Accordingly, neuropathic pruritus cannot be clearly differentiated from neuropathic pain [246], while analysis of pruritic patients clearly demonstrates that neuropathic itch and neuropathic pain may occur in association [247]. Neuropathic CP may arise out of a local nerve fibre compression (e.g. brachioradial pruritus, notalgia paraesthetica) or nerve fibre degeneration (e.g. small fibre neuropathy) affecting different neuronal structures in the peripheral or central nervous system [245]. Pruritus due to nerve fibre compression is usually located in the corresponding dermatome while nerve fibre degeneration leads to localised or generalised pruritus. Accordingly, there are significant differences in the pathogenesis as well as in the clinical picture of neuropathic CP. The therapy of neuropathic pruritus is also challenging as the commonly used oral antipruritic drugs such as antihistaminergics, doxepin, chlorpromazine, diphenylhydantoin, and topical and intralesional corticosteroids do not lead to amelioration of symptoms [245]. Gabapentinoids are effective and indicated for neuropathy.

Notalgia paraesthetica. This is a fairly common cause of localised persistent pruritus. Characteristically, patients complain of persistent burning pruritus localised to the mid-scapular area, but possibly extending from there to a more widespread distribution, including the scalp. Apart from mild lichenification and pigmentation with or without macular amyloidosis (a consequence of rubbing; the amyloid results from the release of necrotic material from keratinocytes), there is usually little to see. Recent reports stress the importance of nerve root entrapment and sensory neuropathy of the primary dorsal rami of the spinal nerves from T2 to T6 [248–251]. It is more common in females than males [252–254]. Capsaicin cream or a patch can be effective in some patients [255–257]. Other localised neuropathic itch types are cheiralgia paraesthetica (radial nerve), meralgia paraesthetica (lateral femoral cutaneous nerve) and gonyalgia paraesthetica (infrapatellar branch of the saphenous nerve).

Brachioradial pruritus. Brachioradial pruritus (BRP) is located in the region of the elbow and adjacent lower and upper arm, in the C5/C6 dermatome, and the shoulder and neck may also be involved [245]. Sunlight may make it worse and it may be improved by cold applications ('ice pack sign'). More females than males are affected, mostly at an age over 60 years. Compressions of the spinal cord or nerve root of the cervical spine (cervical radiculopathy) by disc herniations, osteophytes, cervical rib or even cervical ependymomas are most probably responsible for the development of BRP [258]. Thus, MRI of the cervical spine is strongly recommended in addition to a comprehensive patient history and a neurological and orthopaedic examination [245]. Topical local anaesthetics or cooling compounds can ameliorate BRP. The most effective drug reported is the anticonvulsant gabapentin or pregabalin (dosage depending on age and co-morbidities) [4]. Other treatments used in anecdotal reports include topical capsaicin, ketamine–lidocaine, amitryptiline, oral carbamazepine and botulinium toxin injections [259,260].

Localised pruritus can further occur with or without dermatoses and is frequently found in the genito-anal area (e.g. pruritus ani

(Chapter 111), pruritus vulvae (Chapter 110) and trichodynia (Chapters 82 and 105)).

Psychiatric and psychosomatic diseases (psychogenic pruritus). Itching, either localised or generalised, can be a manifestation of psychiatric or psychosomatic diseases (Chapter 84). There are no satisfactory 'rule in, rule out' diagnostic paradigms; therefore, in practice, the conclusion that local or generalised itch is psychogenic in origin is arrived at by a process of exclusion of cutaneous or systemic causes [261]. In many chronic itch patients regardless of the underlying cause there are components of psychiatric co-morbidities such as stress, depression and anxiety. Diagnostic criteria have been proposed for functional itch disorder [262].

It is also self-evident that patients experiencing severe persistent pruritus become secondarily depressed, and that this may itself lower the threshold for pruritus, thus completing a 'vicious circle' of itch, depression and more itch [115,263–266]. Studies in psychiatric in-patients found a high prevalence of chronic itch, up to 32% [267]. Fibromyalgia is a complex condition, characterised by widespread somatic or physical symptoms such as pain, and often has a significant component of chronic itch and psychological manifestations [268].

Widespread psychogenic pruritus may result in extensive and disfiguring excoriations and scarring to the extent of self-mutilation. It is important to ask about the patient's concerns as to causation. Delusions of infestation of the skin is a rare psychiatric entity and is normally readily recognisable because of the patient's description of the itch (e.g. formication) and often the patient's presentation of particulate material considered by the sufferer to represent the supposed insects or their products, known as 'the specimen sign' [269]. Psychiatric advice should be sought, ideally in a joint dermatology/psychiatry clinic, and an appropriate psychopharmaceutical therapy tried (e.g. risperidone). Treatment options for these patients are covered in detail in Chapter 84 and have been extensively reviewed [270].

Classification of severity and measurement of pruritus

A uniform and generally valid method for documenting pruritus is currently being developed [271]. Itch is a subjective symptom and shows not only interindividual differences, but also intraindividual variations resulting from depression, anxiety or stress. In practice, the severity of pruritus can be determined, for instance, with a visual analogue scale (VAS). The VAS is a 100 mm long line marked with end points 0 (no pruritus) and 100 (the worst imaginable itch). The patient is asked to place a mark on this line, and the value represented by this can be determined by simply measuring its location in the line. The numerical rating scale (NRS) is a similar method of pruritus measurement by which patients can assess pruritus intensity by assigning a number between 0 (no pruritus) to 10 (the worst imaginable itch). The verbal rating scale (VRS) is used for assessing itch intensity in CP. The severity of pruritus is coded with graduated adjectives (from 0 = no pruritus to 4 = very severe pruritus) [271]. The three intensity scales VAS, NRS and VRS were shown to have a high degree of reliability and correlation. In a test–retest reliability analysis, a high degree of interclass correlation coefficients were found, confirming a good reproducibility of these instruments [271,272]. The severity of the intensity scale VAS is:

- 0 points: no pruritus.
- >0 points but <30 points: mild pruritus.
- ≥30 points but <70 points: moderate pruritus.
- ≥70 points but <90 points: severe pruritus.
- ≥90 points: very severe pruritus.

A diagnostic serum biomarker for confirmation of the presence of CP is not available. In dealing with CP running a severe course or of unclear origin, patients can be advised to keep a diary with daily entries of their pruritus experience. This can facilitate mapping and interpretation of symptoms by the treating physician.

Investigations

Dermatological examination of patients with CP includes a thorough inspection of the entire skin including the scalp, hair, nails, ano-genital region and mucous membranes [4]. Distribution of primary and secondary skin lesions as well as skin signs of systemic disease should be recorded. A general physical examination should include palpation of lymph node basins.

It is recommended that a diagnostic algorithm comprising laboratory and radiological investigations, compiled by the interdisciplinary European Guideline Expert Panel [4], be followed (Table 81.3). These investigations must be supplemented with symptom-specific diagnostic steps. A balance is needed between investigations based on clinical need versus an exhaustive 'rule out' approach.

Chronic pruritus can be prodromal, manifesting before the appearance of the initial symptoms of a malignant underlying disease such as Hodgkin lymphoma (so-called premonitory pruritus). Therefore, in CP of unclear origin, depending on the general health status of the patient, an annual physical examination may identify a possible underlying cause [4]. The patient can be encouraged to self-examine and to re-present if they develop any new symptoms.

Management

As detailed earlier, CP may be caused by a broad variety of underlying diseases and may have a heterogeneous clinical phenotype. Therefore, there are no general therapeutic recommendations but a few principles for the management of CP. First, it is important to gather data on the age, pre-existing diseases, medications and quality and intensity of pruritus; based on this information, a therapy regimen tailored to the individual patient can be planned. Most importantly, elderly patients, pregnant women and children require special attention [4]. General pruritus-relieving measures should be instituted in every patient with CP (Box 81.2). Prior to therapy beyond these general measures, the patient should undergo careful diagnostic evaluation and any underlying disease should be treated [4]. If pruritus persists, a step-by-step symptomatic treatment is recommended (Box 81.3). Specific pharmacological interventions must take into consideration the type of itch and should be performed according to the guideline for CP [4].

Table 81.3 Laboratory and radiological diagnostics in chronic pruritus.

First-step screening	Further investigations
Non-specific inflammatory markers including plasma viscosity, ESR, C-reactive protein (CRP)	Immunoelectrophoresis
	Hepatitis B and C antibodies
	Antimitochondrial antibodies
Differential blood cell count	HIV antibodies
Blood urea nitrogen, creatinine	ANA
Alkaline phosphatase, γ-GT, AST, ALT, bilirubin	PTH, calcium
	Erythrocyte fluorescence (erythropoietic protoporphyria screen)
TSH	
Glucose	PSA
Ferritin	Tryptase
Lactate dehydrogenase (LDH)	Bile acid when intrahepatic cholestasis of pregnancy is suspected
Age > 40 years: stool occult blood	
Ano-genital pruritus: stool test for parasites	Swab for *Candida* (mucocutaneous pruritus)
Urine dipstick for microscopic haematuria	Further imaging studies and bone marrow investigation depending on symptoms and previous findings, e.g. MRI thoracic and cervical spine in neuropathic pruritus
Chest X-ray	
Ultrasound abdomen	
Biopsy with routine histology and DIF (mastocytosis, pemphigoid, etc.)	Skin biopsy in cases of hydroxyethyl starch (electron microscopy)

Adapted from Weisshaar et al. 2019 [4].

ALT, alanine aminotransferase; ANA, antinuclear antibodies; AST, aspartate aminotransferase; DIF, direct immunofluorescence; ESR, erythrocyte sedimentation rate; γ-GT, gamma-glutamyl transferase; HIV, human immunodeficiency virus; MRI, magnetic resonance imaging; PSA, prostate-specific antigen; PTH, parathyroid hormone; TSH, thyroid-stimulating hormone.

Box 81.2 General measures for treating chronic pruritus

Avoidance of:
- Dry skin
- Factors that worsen dry skin (e.g. heat, frequent washing and bathing)
- Contact with irritant substances (e.g. poison ivy, poison oak, stinging nettle)
- Hot and spicy food, large amounts of hot drinks and alcohol
- Stress

Application of:
- Non-alkaline soaps, synthetic detergents, moisturising shower or bath oils
- Luke-warm bath water, bathing time not exceeding 20 min ± colloidal oatmeal
- Short, luke-warm showers
- Soft clothing permeable to air (e.g. cotton)
- Skin moisturisation on a daily basis especially after showering and bathing
- Topicals with symptomatic relief, especially for pruritus at night: creams/lotions/sprays containing antipruritics (e.g. 5–10% urea, 0.5–5% menthol in aqueous cream, tannin), calamine oily lotion, crotamiton cream, doxepin cream
- Topical emollients containg urea, ceramide, nicotinamide, lactic acid, glycerol, lauromacrogols, soya oil
- Wet, cooling wraps (e.g. with moisturiser, black tea)
- 20% zinc oxide ointment-impregnated rayon stockings (especially helpful for limbs if many chronic scratch lesions)
- Habit reversal training

Box 81.3 Guideline to recommended symptomatic therapy in chronic pruritus

Step 1
- General therapeutic measures (Box 81.2)
- Basic therapy with moisturisers
- Initial symptomatic therapy: systemic non-sedative H_1 antihistaminics, topical corticosteroids

Step 2
- If origin of chronic pruritus is known: symptomatic causative adapted therapy

Step 3
In pruritus of unknown origin or therapy-refractory cases to the second step:
- Symptomatic topical and/or systemic therapy, e.g. pramoxine, capsaicin, calcineurin inhibitors, topical polidocanol, ketamine–lidocaine and amitryptiline, systemic naltrexone, gabapentin, pregabalin, butorphanol, UV phototherapy, immunosuppressants (ciclosporin, methotrexate)

Concomitant treatment in every step
- Diagnostics and treatment of underlying disease
- General therapeutic measures
- In sleep disorders: sedative H_1 antihistaminics, tricyclical antidepressants or neuroleptics
- Psychosomatic care, habit reversal therapy for scratch behaviour
- In erosive scratch lesions: disinfecting measures, topical corticosteroids

Adapted from Weisshaar *et al.* 2019 [4].

Resources

Further information

International Forum for the Study of Itch (IFSI): http://www.itchforum.net/content. Butler DF. Pruritus and systemic disease. *Medscape*, last updated 2021. https://emedicine.medscape.com/article/1098029-overview.
(Both last accessed February 2022.)

Patient resources

Yosipovitch G, Kwatra SG. *Living with Itch: a Patient's Guide*. Baltimore: Johns Hopkins Press, 2013.

Prurigo nodularis

Definition and nomenclature

Prurigo nodularis (PN) is characterised by the presence of numerous symmetrically distributed hyperkeratotic or eroded pruriginous nodules, the presence of chronic pruritus and a history or signs of repeated scratching. The terminology around the term 'prurigo' was confusing and has been solidified by a consensus group [1]. The umbrella term chronic prurigo unites several subtypes including prurigo nodularis; PN is also referred to as chronic nodular prurigo. Nodules in PN are intensely itchy and thus a vicious itch–scratch cycle may evolve resulting in long-lasting and highly therapy-refractory PN. As in CP, PN may accompany numerous diseases and has a highly negative impact on patient QoL.

Synonyms and inclusions
- Chronic nodular prurigo
- Chronic prurigo
- Hyde disease

Introduction and general description

In 1901, the Chicago dermatologist James N. Hyde wrote in the sixth edition of his and F. H. Montgomery's dermatology textbook [2] that the term prurigo 'led to considerable confusion in the nomenclature of cutaneous disease'. This statement still holds true as the term is used for describing urticarial dermatoses (e.g. prurigo pigmentosa, actinic prurigo) as well as to describe scratch-associated, non-urticarial, inflammatory dermatoses (e.g. PN). There is continuing debate about conditions such as prurigo simplex acuta or prurigo simplex subacuta and their nature remains to be properly investigated. However, this chapter deals with the consequences of CP and chronic scratching leading to severe and therapy refractory skin lesions of PN.

Hyde used the term PN for the first time in 1909 [3]. In 1879, William Augustus Hardaway (1850–1923) described PN as 'multiple tumours of the skin accompanied by itching' in his 1880 paper in the *Archives of Dermatology* [4]. Hyde had noted PN in his own patients in 1879 and 1880, which he described in his textbook as early as 1883 [5]. The concept of *prurigo* was already established at this time, and several clinical variants were described such as prurigo Hutchinson (1879), prurigo Hebra, prurigo Hebra–Kaposi, prurigo Besnier (1892) and prurigo Jacquet (1894). In 1909, Hyde gave the name *prurigo nodularis* to the prurigo variant with rough hyperkeratinised nodes which were chronically refractory to therapy [3].

This definition is still valid today; PN can be defined as a highly pruritic condition with numerous, symmetrically distributed, hyperkeratotic or eroded nodules [3,6–8]. It evolves in patients with CP and is a consequence of chronic scratching. Thus, it may occur in a broad variety of diseases that induce pruritus.

Epidemiology

Incidence and prevalence

There are no epidemiological studies available. However, retrospective database analyses estimated the incidence at 100 per 100 000 population in Germany, and a prevalence of 36 to 72 per 100 000 population in the USA [9,10].

Age

Prurigo nodularis affects patients across all ages, including children [11], but is more common in older patients [12]. In one study analysing 108 patients [6], the age ranged from 12 to 96 years. The average age was 61.54 ± 16.70 (median: 61.9) [13]. In a European cohort of over 500 patients, the median age was 64 years.

Sex

Prurigo nodularis is more common in women [14]. In an analysis of 1037 patients with CP, women were significantly more frequently affected by PN than men (F: 22%; M: 13.9%).

Ethnicity

There are no data on ethnic differences of PN but in African Americans with atopic eczema PN seems to be more common than in other groups [15].

Pathophysiology
Predisposing factors
Prurigo nodularis is a reaction pattern occurring in CP. Accordingly, all factors which might induce CP may also lead in a subset of patients to PN. According to an analysis of over 100 PN patients, atopy is one key predisposing factor [6]. Nearly half (46.3%) of these patients had either an atopy or atopic eczema as an important cause for PN. Patients might have a variety of co-morbidities, however, their relevance as aetiological factors is uncertain [16].

Pathology
The development of CP may underlie a variety of diseases and mechanisms. Once established, in a subset of patients, CP causes severe and uncontrollable scratching, which leads to mechanical trauma of the skin. At first, there are excoriations and crust formation; prolonged scratching induces papules and nodules surrounded by areas of hyperpigmentation, which are characteristic for PN. It is not known which factors, besides predisposition for atopic eczema, contribute to the development of PN.

Prurigo nodularis involves collagen fibres, epidermal keratinocytes, mast cells, Merkel cells, dendritic cells, eosinophils, T cells, macrophages, endothelial cells and, possibly most importantly, the epidermal and dermal nerve fibres [17,18]. In a morphological study of 136 patients with PN, the nodules had the following histological characteristics: thick compact orthohyperkeratosis, the hairy palm sign (folliculosebaceous units in non-volar skin in conjunction with a thick and compact cornified layer, like that of volar skin), irregular epidermal hyperplasia or pseudoepitheliomatous hyperplasia, focal parakeratosis, hypergranulosis, fibrosis of the papillary dermis with vertically arranged collagen fibres, increased number of fibroblasts and capillaries, and a superficial, perivascular and/or interstitial inflammatory infiltrate of lymphocytes, macrophages and, to a lesser extent, eosinophils and neutrophils [17]. In sum, there is no strictly uniform histology but a constellation of different histological features [17]. There is an increased number of mast cells within the PN lesions and these show distinctive features including a dendritic appearance (normally round or elongated) with an enlarged cell body [19]. The volume of cytoplasm is increased but contains fewer granules suggesting the release of mast cell products into the surrounding tissue [19]. Such products may include histamine, tryptase and prostaglandins [7] which are all mediators of itch [20]. Other studies investigating smaller numbers of patients described a thickening of myelinated dermal nerves with neuroma formation (Pautrier neuroma) [21] and an occasional increase in the number of subepidermal and dermal nerve fibres (neuronal hyperplasia) with degeneration and fragmentation of axons and Schwann cells in PN [22,23]. These initial observations were followed up by a number of studies that aimed at defining in greater detail the immuno-neuro-anatomical structural changes in PN nodules by using specific staining techniques for neuropeptides (SP, calcitonin gene-related peptide), NGF and corresponding receptors (TrkA, p75NGF) (Table 81.4). As sensory, unmyelinated epidermal nerve fibres are suggested to play a major role in pruritus induction [16,21], the exact distribution of IENF in PN was investigated according to a guideline of the European Federation of Neurological Societies [18]. Interestingly, no hyperplasia was detected, in contrast to dermal nerves, but there was a significant decrease of sensory C fibres in the nodules and also in the non-lesional skin of PN patients.

Table 81.4 Morphological studies investigating nerve fibres in prurigo nodularis (PN).

Year, author[a]	No. of biopsies	Findings
1934, Pautrier	1	Hyperplasia of NF (Pautrier neuroma), SC proliferation
1985, Rowland Payne et al.	46	No Pautrier neuroma
		2/42: neural hyperplasia
1989, Vaalasti et al.	8	Increased numbers of papillary SP- and CGRP-positive NF bundles
1989, Lindley and Payne	26	5/26: neural hyperplasia (prominent dermal nerve bundles)
		Dermal NF density enhanced
1992, Harris et al.	25	24/25: increased numbers and thickened papillary NF
1992, Abadia Molina et al.	7	Increased numbers of epidermal and dermal PGP 9.5-, SP- and CGRP-positive NF
		1/7: Pautrier neuroma
1996, Liang et al.	6	Increased numbers of PGP 9.5 , NGF- and CGRP-positive NF in the papillary dermis (quantitative analysis)
		Epidermis: no NGF-positive NF, PGP 9.5-positive NF decreased, many branches, more elongated
1998, Liang et al.	8	Increased numbers of NGF-positive papillary NF
		Nerves: more branches, more tortuous
1998, Johansson et al.	6	Increased numbers of S100-positive papillary NF
1999, Liang et al.	8	Hyperplasia of p75 NGF-positive papillary NF
		Enlarged axons
2000, Johansson et al.	6	Increased numbers of PGP 9.5-positive NF in areas with increased eosinophils
2002, Johansson et al.	5	Dermis: huge number of NGF-positive cells, TrkA- and p75-positive hyperplastic NF
		Epidermis: weak NGF, p75 and TrkA
2011, Schuhknecht et al.	53	Significantly decreased intraepidermal NF density in nodules and non-lesional skin regardless of patient age, origin of PN, intensity or quality of pruritus
2016, Bobko et al. [31]	30	Intraepidermal NF density was increasing in sequence-lesional, inter-lesional, non-lesional and healed skin with significant differences between stages

Adapted from Schuhknecht et al. 2011 [18].
[a] All references in this table, except Bobko et al. 2016 [31], can be found in Schuhknecht et al. 2011 [18].
CGRP, calcitonin gene-related peptide; NF, nerve fibre(s); NGF, nerve growth factor; PGP 9.5, protein gene product 9.5; SC, Schwann cell; SP, substance P; TrkA, tyrosine kinase A.

The epidermal hyperplasia was independent of clinical parameters and suggests involvement of epidermal nerves in the pathophysiology of PN [18,24]. The degeneration of epidermal nerves might be related to scratching as no other signs of neuropathy could be detected [25]. In contrast, hyperplasia of SP-positive nerve fibres was found in the dermis. This might be of particular importance in the pathophysiology of PN, especially in light of the fact that aprepitant, an SP antagonist (= NK1 antagonist) led to relief of pruritus in PN in one trial [26].

Recently, Th2 cytokines including IL-31 and its receptor IL-31R and oncostatin in the dermis as well as IL-4, IL-13 and periostin (a matricellular protein involved in itch) were highly correlated to the itch of PN [27,28]. The important role of Th2 cytokines in PN is further exemplified by the significant effect of drugs such as dupilumab and nemolizumab in the reduction and improvement of itch in PN [29,30].

Clinical features

History

Patients may suffer from PN for years. According to one study, the average duration of PN before the patient presented to a specialist was 6.5 years [6]. Obtaining an accurate medical history from these patients is challenging as frequently they cannot remember exactly how their PN had started. As patients are unable to distinguish between primary and secondary skin lesions, they are also not able to say if a dermatosis was the initial cause of developing CP and the PN was subsequent, or if PN developed on skin with a normal appearance. As patients may have hundreds of lesions, they cannot describe the dynamics of developing lesions; some may be able to identify the initial lesions, however it is hard for them to comment on subsequent evolution and resolution. Therefore, the history taking should focus on the identification of the underlying origin of CP. Affected individuals can be very distressed with a large impact on their daily health-related QoL [32]. Secondary depression and suicide are reported [33].

Presentation

The typical lesion of PN is a skin-coloured or inflamed nodule with a hyperpigmented border. The lesion may have a hyperkeratotic or eroded surface. The nodules may be round or flat and large (plaques). In some patients, the PN lesion starts as a papule and then develops into a nodule. The term PN seems to restrict cases to where there is a clinical presentation of nodules, but patients may also have papular or plaque-type lesions (Figures 81.4, 81.5 and 81.6) [34].

Prurigo nodularis is usually disseminated bilaterally and symmetrically but preferentially on the dorsal areas of the extremities and trunk, back and buttocks. Usually the palms, soles and face are spared. In many patients, the central back (acnestis) is spared as this is an area that patients cannot reach easily with their hands to scratch. This area of sparing is known as the 'butterfly sign' [35]. PN may be confined to a specific area if pruritus is localised such as in BRP.

Clinical variants

The clinical variants concern only the underlying diseases. These may be as numerous as in CP itself. Accordingly, the underlying diseases in PN patients may be dermatological, systemic, neurological

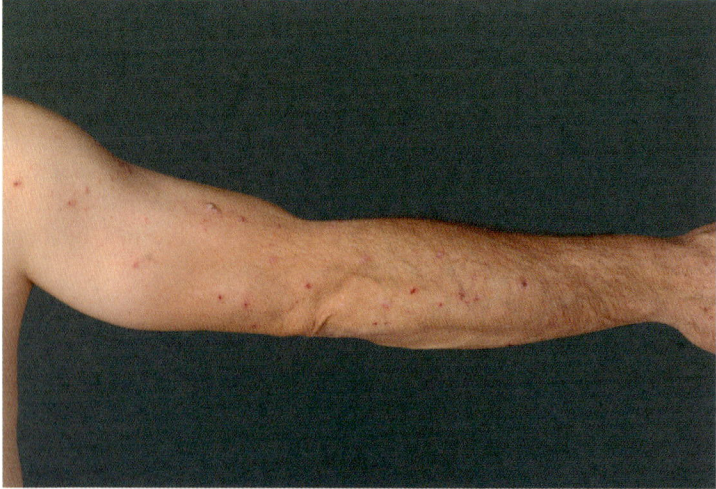

Figure 81.4 A 46-year-old patient with papular prurigo and an atopic predisposition.

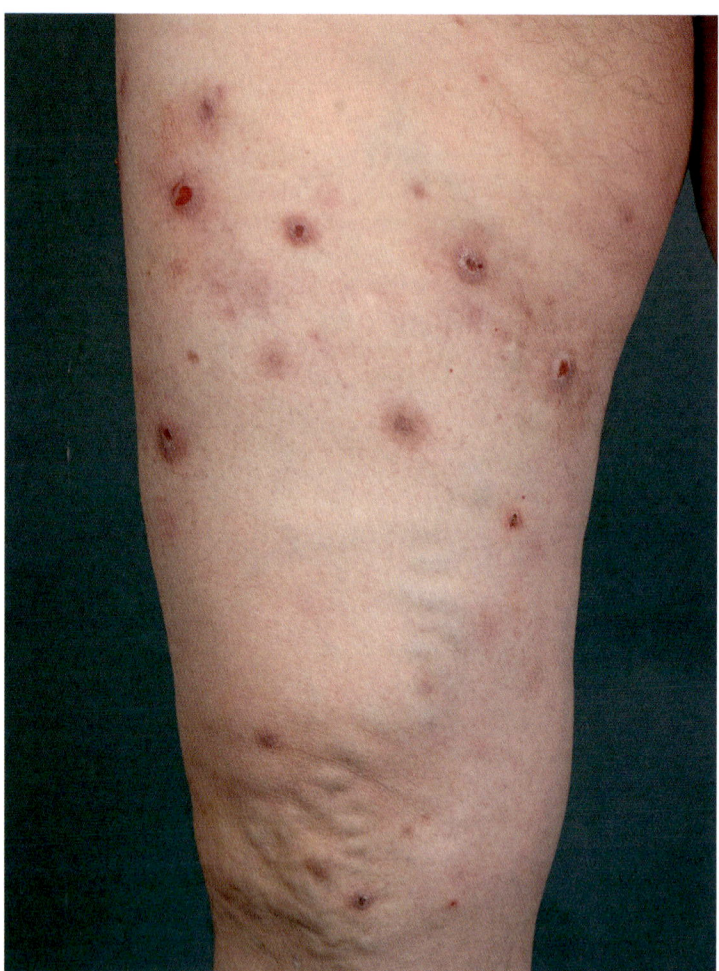

Figure 81.5 A 64-year-old patient with nodular prurigo of multiple aetiologies.

or psychiatric diseases or the PN may have multiple aetiologies. Table 81.5 summarises diseases underlying PN.

Patients suffer from high pruritus intensities (usually above 7 on the NRS (0–10 scale)) and a high symptom burden due to impact on the QoL and sleep loss [12,36]. There is no difference in itch intensity in PN with different underlying disease categories [6]. Further

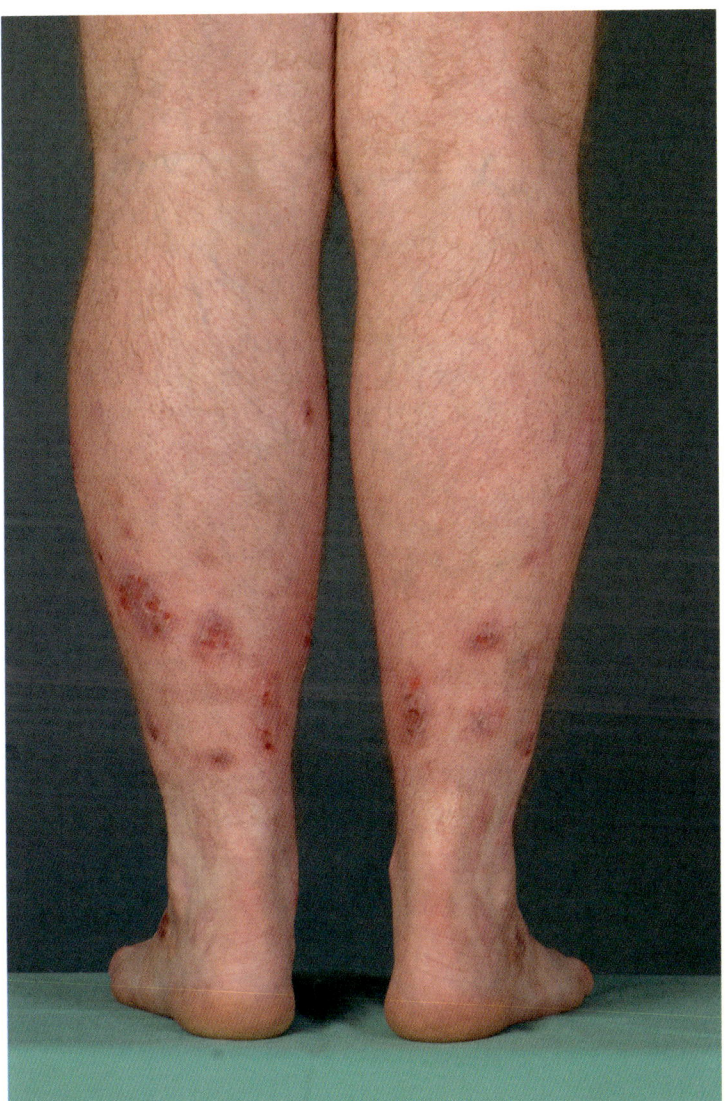

Figure 81.6 A 39-year-old patient with plaque prurigo in chronic venous insufficiency.

Table 81.5 Reported comorbidities in prurigo nodularis (PN).

Category of disease	Diagnosis
Dermatological diseases	Atopic eczema, atopic predisposition
	Nummular eczema
	Keratoacanthoma
	Psoriasis
	Grover disease
	Lichen planus
	Epidermolysis bullosa acquisita
	Dermatitis herpetiformis
	Bullous pemphigoid
	Cutaneous mycobacterial infection in PN nodules (different species, e.g. *Mycobacterium avium*)
	Mycosis fungoides
	Venous stasis
Systemic diseases	Chronic renal failure (may result in specific phenotype of umbilicated prurigo; previously termed reactive perforating dermatosis [39])
	Diabetes mellitus
	Hyperbilirubinaemia
	Sorbitol intolerance, lactose intolerance
	Gluten enteropathy
	Zinc deficiency, cobalamin deficiency
	Sarcoidosis
	Gastric *Helicobacter pylori* infection
	HIV infection
	Pulmonary tuberculosis
	Intestinal *Strongyloides stercoralis* infection
	Chronic HCV/HBV hepatitis
	Tonsillitis
	Iron deficiency, anaemia
	Hodgkin disease
	Angioimmunoblastic T-cell lymphoma
	HTLV1-positive adult T-cell leukaemia/lymphoma
	Neoplasms (bladder, breast, oesophagus, kidney, lung, rectum, stomach, uterus)
	Drug intake
Neuropathic diseases	Brachioradial pruritus
	Herpes zoster
	Neuropathy in alcoholics, hypothyroidism; multifocal motor neuropathy and conduction blocks in non-Hodgkin B-cell lymphoma
	Prolapsed intervertebral disc, lumbar disc herniation at L5–S1
Psychogenic diseases	Delusional infestation
	Emotional stress and psychological disorders
	Psychological disorder: depression, anxiety and other

Adapted from Iking *et al.* 2013 [**6**] and Schuhknecht *et al.* 2011 [**18**].
HBV/HCV, hepatitis B virus/hepatitis C virus; HTLV1, human T-cell leukaemia virus 1.

qualities of itch are reported by PN patients such as burning (59.3% of all patients), stinging (47.2%), tingling (35%), heat (21.3%) and cold (2.7%); there was no statistically significant difference in the distribution of these qualities among the different underlying disease groups of PN [**6**].

Disease course and prognosis

Prurigo nodularis is usually highly refractory to therapy and may last for years or even decades with slow progression [**37**]. However, it may resolve completely under treatment. One complication that can hinder healing is automatic habitual scratching behaviour that patients might have developed; in this case, they continue to scratch unknowingly even in the absence of itch sensations.

Investigations

The aim of dermatological examination is to identify any underlying dermatoses that may be masked by the presence of PN. For example, PN may be associated with bullous pemphigoid (also called pemphigoid nodularis) [**38**]. Hyperplastic lichen planus may look very similar to PN. For this reason, a skin biopsy is essential in PN of

unclear origin. To be thorough, a direct immunofluorescence test should also be performed especially if a patient had reported blisters and/or if redness or blisters were found on physical examination (Table 81.6).

The laboratory and radiological investigations are similar to those in the diagnostic work-up of CP. Despite thorough investigation, in about 13% of PN patients, an underlying disease or dermatosis is not found [**6**]. In another series, a large variety of co-morbidities was documented [**6**], some of which might be part of the pathogenesis of itch induction. Thus, some studies recommend performing a comprehensive diagnostic work-up including investigation of possible underlying diseases of PN (Table 81.6) [**40–43**]. However,

Table 81.6 Recommendations for diagnostic work-up in prurigo nodularis (PN) based on reported comorbidities [**6**,**37**,43].

Investigation level	Investigations
Skin	*Clinical examination*: search for signs of atopic eczema, bullous pemphigoid, lymphoma or other skin diseases *Skin biopsy*: H&E staining (routine histology) Direct immunofluorescence to rule out autoimmune diseases (bullous pemphigoid, epidermolysis bullosa acquisita) Polymerase chain reaction for mycobacteria if granulomatous inflammatory infiltrate is found on histological investigation *Allergy testing* to rule out type I or IV allergies
Laboratory – basic (associations reported)	Erythrocyte sedimentation rate Complete blood count (with differential) Ferritin, lactate dehydrogenase Kidney retention parameters: creatinine (with estimated GFR), urea Liver enzymes: AST, ALT, alkaline phosphate, γ-GT, bilirubin HBV/HCV serology Thyroid function test (TSH) Fasting glucose or HbA1c
Laboratory – advanced	Total IgE HIV Indirect and direct immunofluorescence, ELISA BP-180/-230
Functional and radiological	Chest X-ray (rule out sarcoidosis, neoplasm, lymphoma) Ultrasound abdomen (rule out liver or kidney disease in case of pathological lab values) Ultrasound lymph nodes (rule out lymphoma; especially if patient reports weight loss, fever or night-time sweating) Magnetic resonance tomography of cervical spinal column if patient has localised PN (e.g. on lower arms) PN on the lower leg: phlebological investigation if chronic venous insufficiency is suspected
Psychosomatics/ psychiatry	Assess for anxiety, depression, obsessive–compulsive disorders

ALT, alanine aminotransferase; AST, aspartate aminotransferase; ELISA, enzyme-linked immunosorbent assay; GFR, glomerular filtration rate; γ-GT, gamma-glutamyl transferase; HBV/HCV, hepatitis B virus/hepatitis C virus; H&E, haematoxylin and eosin; HIV, human immunodeficiency virus; IgE, immunoglobulin E; TSH, thyroid-stimulating hormone.

realistic principles of clinical practice apply and individualised work-up has to balance a rigid 'rule-out' approach with a 'clinical need' approach [44].

Management
The general principles of PN management are the same as in CP (Figure 81.7; see earlier section on pruritus). Recently, the first international guideline on PN was published [37] and management is discussed and compared with self-inflicted skin lesions in a comprehensive European position paper [44]. In brief, therapy must be multimodal, including therapy of the underlying disease, the use of topical emollients (especially in dry skin, atopic predisposition) and topical substances for short-term relief of itch (e.g. menthol), specific systemic antipruritic therapy and, if necessary, psychosomatic counselling. Novel systemic therapies are being tested in randomised controlled trials specifically for the treatment of PN; gabapentin, pregabalin, naltrexone, ciclosporin, methotrexate, dupilumab and nemolizumab have proved to be efficacious, as reported in case

series and trials of PN patients [37,45,46]. Several reports have focused on the effectiveness of thalidomide in PN [41]; however, this drug is not broadly recommended due to the risk of irreversible neuropathy. As PN patients may have subclinical neuropathy [**18**], this may be worsened by thalidomide. In randomised controlled trials, betamethasone valerate 0.1% tape, calcipotriol ointment, pimecrolimus cream, bath PUVA and bath PUVA + targeted UVB 308 nm excimer light have been demonstrated to be effective in the treatment of nodules [37]. Topical capsaicin was also reported to ameliorate the symptoms of PN; however, a randomised controlled trial has yet to be carried out [47]. Other topical measures of a more invasive nature such as cryosurgery and intralesional steroids or excimer laser have also been used to treat the nodular lesions of PN [48,49].

Resources

Further information
International Forum for the Study of Itch (IFSI): http://www.itchforum.net/content.

Patient resources
Prurigo Nodularis League: http://www.pruritussymposium.de/prurigonodularisleague.html.
(Both last accessed February 2022.)

Lichen simplex chronicus

Definition and nomenclature
Lichen simplex is a circumscribed, pruritus-associated dermatosis characterised by a small number of heavily lichenified plaques or, commonly, a single lesion.

Synonyms and inclusions
• Neurodermatitis circumscripta

Introduction and general description
Lichen simplex chronicus (LSC) is a highly pruritic, circumscribed plaque, the gross and microscopic features of which are due to incessant harmful scratching and rubbing.

Epidemiology
Age
The peak incidence is between 30 and 50 years of age, but it is seen at any age from adolescence onwards.

Sex
Women are more affected than men.

Pathophysiology
Lichen simplex chronicus is an entity and a reaction pattern to scratching similar to PN. It is most likely that the scratching behaviour of the patient influences the development of either nodules (PN) via scratching with the tip of fingers, or plaques

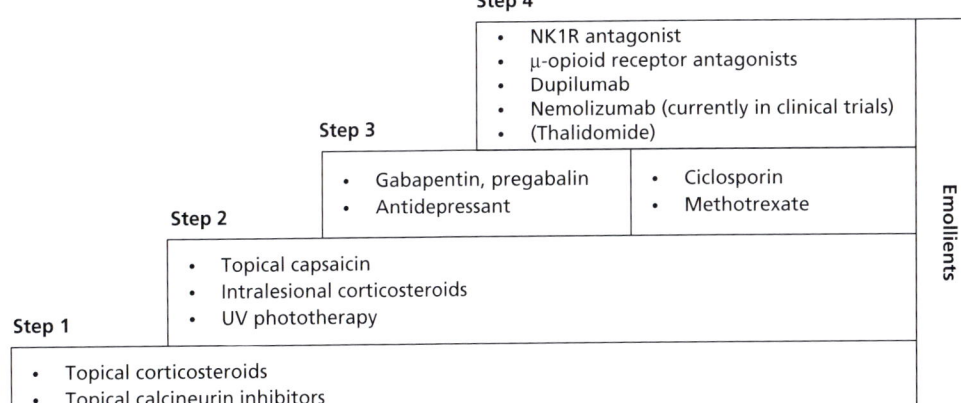

Figure 81.7 Treatment ladder of prurigo nodularis reflecting efficacy of therapy and time course [37]. In every step, emollients should be used. Following an interdisciplinary approach is recommended: treatment of the underlying disease and, in cases of suspected psychological factors, cooperation with specialists or other health professionals. Individualised therapy is recommended; the order in the box is not mandatory, therapies can be combined or steps can be skipped if necessary. In step 3, select depending on the need for therapy for a neuropathic or inflammatory component. NK1R, neurokinin 1 receptor; UV, ultraviolet.

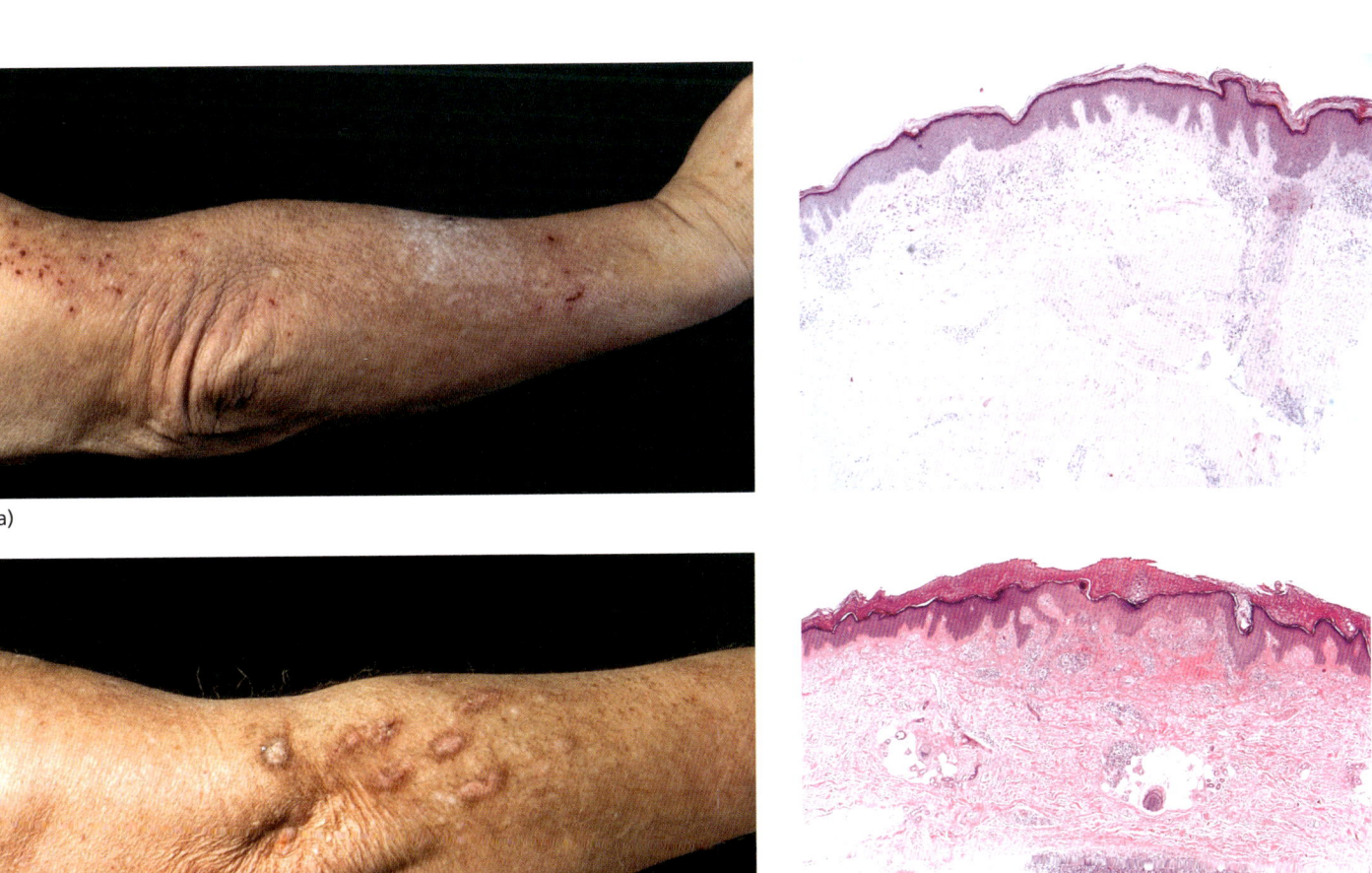

(a)

(b)

Figure 81.8 The arms of two patients with (a) lichen simplex and (b) prurigo nodularis. These diseases share 40% overlapping histological features. Courtesy of Dr Eduardo Calonje.

(LSC) via rubbing the skin (Figure 81.8). As in PN, the underlying diseases in LSC are numerous; patients often have an atopic background. Psychological factors such as anxiety, depression, or obsessive–compulsive disorder, may play a key role in inducing and maintaining LSC [1].

The population density of nerve fibres is often decreased in lesional skin and mast cell numbers may be increased. It has been proposed that these changes are central to the pathogenesis of lichen simplex, and there is evidence of increased immunoreactive NGF (see earlier) in affected skin [2]. There is also upregulated expression of neuropeptides in lesional skin, including tachykinins [3]. However, these changes may be reactive rather than primary.

Pathology

There is epidermal hyperplasia and hyperkeratosis and rete ridges are lengthened. Spongiosis is sometimes present, and small areas of parakeratosis are occasionally seen. The dermis contains a chronic inflammatory cell infiltrate. In very chronic lesions there may be fibrosis.

Clinical features

Characteristically, the history is of repeated bouts of intense itching and scratching, interspersed with itch-free intervals. During the early stages, the skin is reddened and slightly oedematous. With time the redness subsides and the affected skin becomes pigmented, thickened and slightly scaly. Accentuation of normal skin markings is characteristic (lichenification). There is clinical overlap of morphology with plaque prurigo.

Almost any area may be affected, but the commonest sites are those that are convenient to reach, namely the nape and sides of the neck, lower legs (Figure 81.9) and ankles, scalp, upper thighs, vulva, pubis or scrotum and extensor forearms. Interestingly, these sites are considered the most pleasurable for itch and LSC has the highest pleasurability of scratching an itch amongst all chronic itch conditions [4,5].

Disease course and prognosis

Lichen simplex chronicus usually resolves with appropriate treatment, but relapse at the same site is not uncommon.

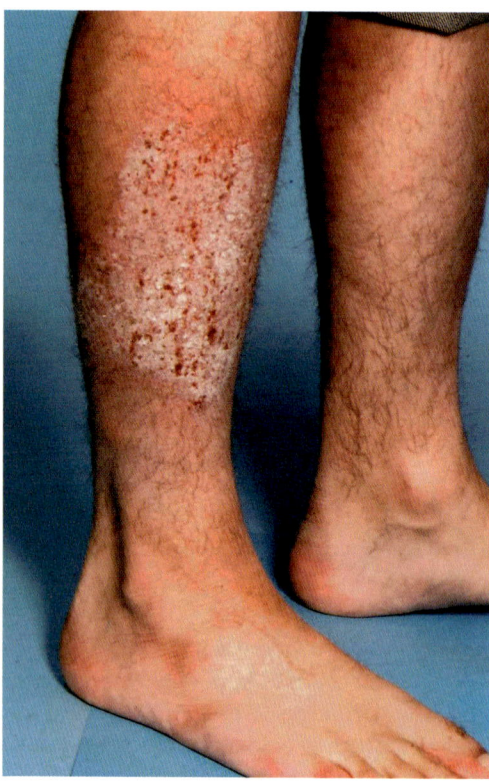

Figure 81.9 The right lower leg of a patient with lichen simplex chronicus.

Investigations

The morphological diagnosis of lichenification is not difficult, and the localised nature of LSC is usually easily recognised. However, hypertrophic lichen planus, lichen amyloidosis and psoriasis should be excluded.

Management

The nature of lichen simplex and the need to break the scratching habit must be explained. Habit reversal techniques can be employed and are easy to implement [6]. General principles are analogous to the treatment of pruritus and prurigo. Treatment is aimed at breaking the itch–scratch cycle and the suppression of pruritus, usually by topical corticosteroids or calcineurin inhibitors, topical capsaicin, doxepin or aspirin, systemic antihistamines, gabapentinoids or antidepressants, as well as transcutaneous electrical nerve stimulation, focused ultrasound or UV therapy (narrowband UVB) [7,8]. The application of an occlusive dressing or an occlusive bandage will intensify the effect of topical steroids and physically protect the affected area. For very thickened LSC, the use of topical keratolytic agents like salicylic acid can increase the efficacy of topical therapy. Self-adhesive, steroid-impregnated tape is often beneficial. Intralesional corticosteroids are also used in some cases.

Key references

The full list of references can be found in the online version at https://www.wiley.com/rooksdermatology10e

Pruritus

2 Ständer S, Weisshaar E, Mettang T *et al*. Clinical classification of itch: a position paper of the International Forum for the Study of Itch. *Acta Derm Venereol* 2007;87:291–4.

3 Ikoma A, Steinhoff M, Ständer S *et al*. The neurobiology of itch. *Nat Rev Neurosci* 2006;7:535–47.

4 Weisshaar E, Szepietowski JC, Dalgard FJ *et al*. European S2k Guideline on Chronic Pruritus. *Acta Derm Venereol* 2019;99:469–506.

5 Ständer S. Atopic dermatitis. *N Engl J Med*. 2021; 384:1136–43.

11 Pisoni RL, Wikström B, Elder SJ *et al*. Pruritus in haemodialysis patients: International results from the Dialysis Outcomes and Practice Patterns Study (DOPPS). *Nephrol Dial Transplant* 2006;21:3495–505.

33 Fett N, Haynes K, Propert KJ *et al*. Five-year malignancy incidence in patients with chronic pruritus: a population-based cohort study aimed at limiting unnecessary screening practices. *J Am Acad Dermatol* 2014;70:651–8.

34 Schmelz M, Schmidt R, Bickel A *et al*. Specific C-receptors for itch in human skin. *J Neurosci* 1997;17:8003–8.

39 Yosipovitch G, Rosen JD, Hashimoto T. Itch: from mechanism to (novel) therapeutic approaches. *J Allergy Clin Immunol* 2018;142:1375–90.

43 Tan Y, Ng WJ, Lee SZX *et al*. 3-Dimensional optical clearing and imaging of pruritic atopic dermatitis and psoriasis skin reveals downregulation of epidermal innervation. *J Invest Dermatol* 2019;139:1201–4.

44 Pogatzki-Zahn EM, Pereira MP, Cremer A *et al*. Peripheral sensitization and loss of descending inhibition is a hallmark of chronic pruritus. *J Invest Dermatol* 2020;140:203–11.

49 Yosipovitch G, Bernhard JD. Clinical practice. Chronic pruritus. *N Engl J Med* 2013;368:1625–34.

79 Fishbane S, Jamal A, Munera C, Wen W, Menzaghi F; KALM-1 Trial Investigators. A phase 3 trial of difelikefalin in hemodialysis patients with pruritus. *N Engl J Med*. 2020;382:222–32.

86 Nattkemper LA, Tey HL, Valdes-Rodriguez R *et al*. The genetics of chronic itch: gene expression in the skin of patients with atopic dermatitis and psoriasis with severe itch. *J Invest Dermatol* 2018;138:1311–17.

95 Oetjen LK, Mack MR, Feng J *et al.* Sensory neurons co-opt classical immune signaling pathways to mediate chronic itch. *Cell* 2017;171:217–28.

118 Apfelbacher CJ, van Zuuren EJ, Fedorowicz Z *et al.* Oral H1 antihistamines as monotherapy for eczema. *Cochrane Database Syst Rev.* 2013;2013:CD007770.

171 Kremer AE, van Dijk R, Leckie P *et al.* Serum autotaxin is increased in pruritus of cholestasis, but not of other origin, and responds to therapeutic interventions. *Hepatology* 2012;56:1391–400.

221 Reich A, Ständer S, Szepietowski JC. Drug-induced pruritus: a review. *Acta Derm Venereol* 2009;89:236–44.

231 Ambros-Rudolph CM, Müllegger RR, Vaughan-Jones SA *et al.* The specific dermatoses of pregnancy revisited and reclassified: results of a retrospective two-center study on 505 pregnant patients. *J Am Acad Dermatol* 2006; 54:395–404.

Prurigo nodularis

1 Pereira MP, Steinke S, Zeidler C *et al.* EADV Task Force Pruritus group members. European Academy of Dermatology and Venereology European Prurigo Project: expert consensus on the definition, classification and terminology of chronic prurigo. *J Eur Acad Dermatol Venereol* 2018;32:1059–65.

3 Hyde JN, Montgomery FH. *A Practical Treatise on Disease of the Skin for the Use of Students and Practitioners*, 8th edn. Philadelphia: Lea Brothers, 1909:174–5.

6 Iking A, Grundmann S, Chatzigeorgakidis E *et al.* Prurigo as a symptom of atopic and non-atopic diseases: aetiological survey in a consecutive cohort of 108 patients. *J Eur Acad Dermatol Venereol* 2013;27:550–7.

8 Metz M, Ständer S. Chronic pruritus – pathogenesis, clinical aspects and treatment. *J Eur Acad Dermatol Venereol* 2010;24:1249–60.

14 Ständer S, Stumpf A, Osada N *et al.* Gender differences in chronic pruritus: women present different morbidity, more scratch lesions and higher burden. *Br J Dermatol* 2013;168:1273–80.

18 Schuhknecht B, Marziniak M, Wissel A *et al.* Reduced intraepidermal nerve fibre density in lesional and nonlesional prurigo nodularis skin as a potential sign of subclinical cutaneous neuropathy. *Br J Dermatol* 2011;165:85–91.

22 Lindley RP, Payne CM. Neural hyperplasia is not a diagnostic prerequisite in nodular prurigo. A controlled morphometric microscopic study of 26 biopsy specimens. *J Cutan Pathol* 1989;16:14.

24 Boulais N, Misery L. The epidermis: a sensory organ. *Eur J Dermatol* 2008;18:119–27.

34 Schedel F, Schürmann C, Augustin M *et al.* Prurigo nodularis: introduction of a redefined classification and Prurigo Activity Score (PAS). *Acta Derm Venereol* 2013;93:610.

35 Kimura T, Miyazawa H. The 'butterfly' sign in patients with atopic dermatitis: evidence for the role of scratching in the development of skin manifestations. *J Am Acad Dermatol* 1989;21:579–80.

37 Ständer S, Pereira M, Berger T *et al.* IFSI-guideline on chronic prurigo including prurigo nodularis. *Itch* 2020;5:e42.

Lichen simplex chronicus

7 Juarez MC, Kwatra SG. A systematic review of evidence based treatments for lichen simplex chronicus. *J Dermatolog Treat* 2021;32:684–92.

8 Dereli T, Karaca N, Inanir I *et al.* Gabapentin for the treatment of recalcitrant chronic prurigo nodularis. *Eur J Dermatol* 2008;18:85–6.

CHAPTER 82

Mucocutaneous Pain Syndromes

Jon Goulding[1] and Anthony Bewley[2]

[1]Department of Dermatology, Solihull Hospital, University Hospitals Birmingham NHS Foundation Trust, Birmingham, UK
[2]Department of Dermatology, Barts Health NHS Trust, London; and Queen Mary University London, London, UK

Introduction

The mucocutaneous pain syndromes (MCPs) typically involve the head, neck, genitalia and mouth. Genital dysaesthetic syndromes (vulvodynia, vestibulodynia, penoscrotodynia) are particularly common and are discussed in this chapter, as well as in specific chapters on dermatoses of the genitalia (Chapters 109 and 110). For many MCPs no organic cause can be identified, and so they are considered idiopathic, unexplained or functional (with the exception of postherpetic neuralgia and the trigeminal trophic syndrome). Their aetiology is thought to be related in part to the complex physiological interactions between the central and peripheral nervous systems, accompanied by a variable but usually significant psychological component. It is essential that potential organic causes for MCPs are excluded before a firm diagnosis is established. Pain is often chronic and unresponsive to conventional first line analgesics. Co-existing morbidities are common including chronic fatigue, fibromyalgia, irritable bowel syndrome and chronic pain at other sites. The sensory symptoms often interfere with aspects of daily life. The management of patients with these diseases is often complex, and there is a growing consensus that these patients are best managed in specialist, multidisciplinary clinics. A thorough assessment of psychological distress and possible psychiatric co-morbidity is considered essential.

The dysaesthetic syndromes comprise a heterogeneous group of disorders in which there are abnormal, often unpleasant, sensations of the skin, e.g. burning, prickling, tingling or stabbing, generally in a specific anatomical site or region. A demonstrable cause for the abnormal skin sensations is usually absent. There may be little or nothing to see by way of cutaneous clinical signs, or there may be evidence of secondary excoriation, rubbing or skin traumatisation.

The disorders may be divided into those with no demonstrable neurological cause and those with a postulated or demonstrable neurological cause (Table 82.1).

Table 82.1 The dysaesthetic syndromes.

With (usually) demonstrable neurological deficit	Without demonstrable neurological deficit
Sensory mononeuropathies	Scalp dysaesthesia (trichodynia or allodynia)
Notalgia paraesthetica	Vulvodynia
Meralgia paraesthetica	Penodynia/scrotodynia
Postherpetic neuralgia	Atypical trigeminal trophic syndrome
Trigeminal trophic syndrome	Trigeminal neuropathic pain syndrome
Erythromelalgia	Burning mouth syndrome

Burning mouth syndrome

Definition and nomenclature

Burning mouth syndrome (BMS) describes the sensation of continuous burning intraoral discomfort, often accompanied by taste changes, for which no dental or systemic cause can be found and in which there are no gross clinical signs.

Synonyms and inclusions

- Glossodynia
- Stomatodynia
- Oropyrosis
- Scalded mouth syndrome
- Glossopyrosis
- Glossalgia

Introduction and general description

BMS is a disorder particularly encountered in perimenopausal women. In general, there are no abnormal clinical signs and, as a consequence, it is poorly understood and challenging to manage

PART 7: PSYCHOLOGICAL, SENSORY & NEUROLOGICAL

by health care professionals. BMS is characterised by a burning sensation with or without overt pain or discomfort localised to the oral mucosa without evident lesions. The diagnosis is therefore established by excluding secondary causes of burning oral discomfort and can present a diagnostic challenge [1].

Epidemiology
Incidence and prevalence
It is very difficult to establish the incidence and prevalence of this condition as there are so many varied definitions and since it is a diagnosis of exclusion. It is estimated that the prevalence is about 1%.

Age
There is a peak age of 50–60 years. It is relatively common in the elderly.

Sex
The female to male ratio is approximately 20 : 1.

Ethnicity
BMS presents clinically in all ethnicities.

Associated diseases
Patients often have a history of mental health co-morbidities, most commonly anxiety and depression [2]. The exclusion of organic oral disease is important.

Pathophysiology
BMS has previously been considered to reflect a form of neuropathic pain, and a variety of hypotheses have been postulated. It is known that some individuals have increased numbers of taste buds (so-called 'supertasters'). It has been proposed that for patients with BMS, neuropathic changes inside the taste neuronal connections induce the burning sensation by removing the inhibitory control on somatic small-fibre afferents [3]. BMS may be related to damage to the chorda tympani during the removal of wisdom teeth. Also, according to some authors, there is evidence of neuropathic changes in the mucosa and/or in the central nervous system [4]. Nonetheless, the possibility of somatoform illness has been raised by other authors, not least given the increased propensity for such patients to complain of multiple unexplained symptoms at other bodily sites [5]. In the latest International Classification of Orofacial Pain, the Orofacial and Head Pain Special Interest Group categorised BMS under idiopathic orofacial pain and defined it as pain/dysaesthesia recurring every day for more than 2 hours, for 3 months and beyond, with no evident causation on clinical examination and/or following investigations [6].

Genetics
The genetics of BMS are currently unknown.

Clinical features
History
Patients present with a history of several months to several years of increasing oral burning, pain or discomfort. The symptoms may be intermittent but are more often continuous. The intraoral area most frequently affected is the tongue, but BMS may involve the lips and occasionally the whole of the oral mucosa and does not usually follow the distribution of any one nerve. The symptoms do not radiate beyond the mouth. Patients will also describe altered taste sensations (dysgeusia) and even changes in salivation (most frequently dryness or xerostomia). Many describe a metallic or bitter taste. The burning pain may be triggered or exacerbated by certain (usually spicy or acidic) foods. However, in most patients, food or drink alleviates the pain, at least temporarily. Some patients have a habit of thrusting their tongue against the lower anterior teeth in an attempt to alleviate symptoms.

Examination
The oral mucosa looks normal on examination and there is usually no objective evidence of xerostomia. Some patients may have a (normal) fissured tongue or geographic tongue.

Differential diagnosis
The differential diagnosis is that of organic intraoral disease which leads to intraoral pain (Table 82.2).

Classification of severity
There is no classification system for BMS severity. Symptoms vary in intensity throughout the day, typically being worse towards the end of the day. Although some describe relatively mild pain, many describe it as the most severe pain imaginable. Attempts have been made to standardise the outcome (including patient reported) measures used, as well as the classification of BMS [7].

Table 82.2 Differential diagnoses for BMS and their appropriate investigation.

Differential diagnosis	Investigation
Allergic contact stomatitis	Usually from one of the components of the 'dental series' chemicals in patch tests (see Chapter 127), e.g. eugenol in mouth wash, and cinnamal in denture fixative cream
Medication side effects (e.g. fluoxetine, sertraline, clonazepam, venlafaxine, enalapril, captopril, lisinopril, candesartan, eprosartan, omeprazole, topiramate, clindamycin or HRT)	Exclusion and rechallenge
Dental (prostheses and procedures)	Examination
Microbiological: *Candida*, herpes	Clinical/microbiology testing
Primary dermatological disease (e.g. lichen planus, immunobullous disease, aphthosis, lingua plicata)	Usually clinically apparent, occasionally skin or mucosal biopsy
Parafunctional habits: bruxism, cheek biting	History or observation
Connective tissue disease: Sjögren syndrome, rheumatoid arthritis	Examination, appropriate immunology blood screen
Endocrinopathy: diabetes, thyroid disease	Glucose, TFT
Gastro-oesophageal reflux	History, dental examination
Nutritional deficiency	Where clinically suspected: iron, folate, B_{12} and zinc levels

HRT, hormone replacement therapy; TFT, thyroid function tests.

Complications and co-morbidities

BMS is commonly associated with affective disorders such as anxiety and depression. Sleep disturbance is common. Alexithymia is reported to be an association. Some patients have been known to attempt suicide. Most indicate that the disease severely affects their quality of life.

Disease course and prognosis

The prognosis is very variable. Spontaneous remission rates of 20% after 7 years or 3% after 5 years have been reported [8]. However, the vast majority of patients' disease can be improved with individualised multidisciplinary management in specialist centres.

Investigations

These are only undertaken to exclude other causes of BMS, if there are features in the history or on examination that suggest these may be possible (Table 82.2).

Management

BMS is a difficult condition to manage and there have been a wide variety of treatments proposed (Figure 82.1). Some therapies have been evaluated in open label studies. Randomised controlled clinical trials are of varying quality [7,9,10]. There have been attempts at a Cochrane review [9] and a meta-analysis of RCTs [7].

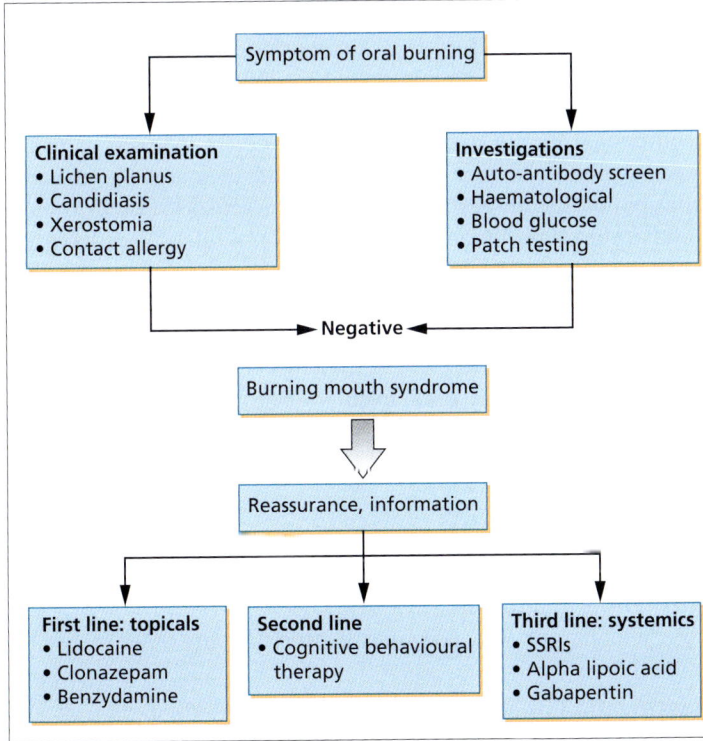

Figure 82.1 Burning mouth syndrome management. SSRI, selective serotonin reuptake inhibitors.

Treatment ladder

First line

- Detailed explanation with written information. Reassurance and highlighting that the physical symptoms experienced are real
- Sialogogue and oral lubricant
- Clonazepam 1 mg sucked slowly, without swallowing, has been shown to be effective in a very short randomised controlled trial [11]
- Lidocaine gel topically
- Benzydamine mouth wash
- Oral care gel

Second line

- Cognitive behavioural therapy (CBT), either alone or in combination with other treatments, may be very effective [12]

Third line

- Alpha-lipoic acid, which has been extensively trialled, with variable results [13,14]
- Oral gabapentin [13]
- Selective serotonin reuptake inhibitors (SSRIs) such as paroxetine,and serotonin-noradrenaline reuptake inhibitors (SNRIs) such as duloxetine have been used, often at relatively high doses, with some benefit
- Amitriptyline in very low doses (e.g. 5–10 mg OD)
- St John's wort has been used with limited benefit
- Low dose antipsychotics (e.g. aripiprazole)
- Herbal treatments (e.g. hypericum)
- Topical capsaicin
- Melatonin
- Cannabinoids
- Physical interventions
  - Sphenopalatine ganglion block in specialist anaesthetic centres
  - Mandibular nerve block
  - Laser treatment [15]
  - Acupuncture

Resources

Further information

The British and Irish Society for Oral Medicine: https://bisom.org.uk/wp-content/uploads/2020/08/BMS-PIL.pdf

Orofacial pain: http://www.orofacialpain.org.uk/

British Association of Oral and Maxillo-facial Surgeons: www.baoms.org.uk

(All last accessed April 2022)

PART 7: PSYCHOLOGICAL, SENSORY & NEUROLOGICAL

Postherpetic neuralgia

Definition

Pain from an acute herpes zoster reactivation (Chapter 25) results from viral damage and increased sensitisation of affected segmental sensory neurons during the first 30 days of onset, and is known as acute herpetic neuralgia (AHN). Postherpetic neuralgia (PHN) is defined as pain persisting for over one month after the healing of the rash and is one of the commonest neurological complications of herpes zoster. PHN is a neuropathic pain that develops in the distribution of one or more branches of the nerve affected. If the seventh cranial nerve is involved the acute phase is termed Ramsay Hunt syndrome.

Introduction and general description

PHN presents with a persistent burning, stabbing or itching pain with sharp exacerbations and associated sensory changes in a unilateral dermatomal distribution. If there is involvement of the seventh cranial nerve, the pain will be felt in the ear and tongue. If involving the trigeminal nerve, the ensuing facial and/or eye pain can be severe. PHN of the trigeminal nerve is probably the most common cause of trigeminal neuralgia and the trigeminal trophic syndrome (see later).

Epidemiology

Incidence and prevalence

The risk of developing PHN following acute herpes zoster virus reactivation may be as high as 20% [1]. The incidence in UK primary care has been estimated at 40 per 100 000 person years of observation [2].

Age

It is more common in people aged over 50 years.

Sex

The male to female ratio is equal.

Ethnicity

All ethnicities are affected.

Associated diseases

- PHN often results in low mood, poor sleep and social isolation. The psychosocial co-morbidities (e.g. anxiety and/or depression) and the effect on quality of life may be considerable, leading some to consider or attempt suicide
- Trigeminal neuralgia
- Trigeminal trophic syndrome
- Cervical trophic syndrome

Pathophysiology

Predisposing factors

Herpes zoster is more likely to affect immunocompromised individuals and elderly patients. Patients with severe or disseminated rash, involvement of the trigeminal nerve's ophthalmic division, allodynia, poor mood and viraemia during acute herpes zoster are at higher risk of PHN.

Pathology

PHN may be caused by neurological lesions at all levels of the nervous system (peripheral, central, autonomic). Why some patients develop PHN is not completely understood. *In vitro* studies suggest that the virus itself may cause normally silent neurons to produce spontaneous action potentials. Skin from a majority of PHN patients demonstrates loss of function and degeneration of small-fibre afferents in the affected dermatome. Ectopic impulses may occur at the site of dorsal root ganglion damage and these impulses can be evoked by mechanical or thermal stimuli (tactile allodynia). There is also some evidence that nociceptors in PHN patients have enhanced adrenergic sensitivity [3].

Causative organism

It results from prior infection with the herpes zoster virus. The virus lies dormant in the dorsal root ganglion after infection. When reactivated, patients present with shingles.

Clinical features

History

A history of shingles is usually, but not always, recalled. PHN most often commences in the 3 months after the acute infection, but may rarely eventuate many months to years later.

Presentation

Patients may report a variety of painful sensations with different components, including spontaneous and continuous deep aching and throbbing pain, burning, lancinating pain or paroxysms of burning pain, sometimes provoked by non-noxious stimuli, such as contact with clothing or changes in temperature [3]. The pain is accompanied by autonomic instability and its intensity is exacerbated by physical and emotional stress and alleviated by relaxation. Some patients with PHN have profound sensory loss in the area of maximum pain (anaesthesia dolorosa), while others have pronounced allodynia with minimal sensory loss. Some patients describe areas of sensory loss surrounded by a 'transition zone' within which a noxious stimulus can elicit a particularly unpleasant pain that radiates widely. These patients may go to extraordinary lengths to protect the area from innocuous stimuli, while firm compression of the skin may actually produce pain relief.

Clinical variants

The acute phase may not present with characteristic blisters.

Differential diagnosis

Trigeminal neuropathic pain may be due to many other causes.

Classification of severity

There may be mild to very severe pain.

Complications and co-morbidities

These include depression, isolation, poor sleep and a significant impact on the activities of daily living [4]. Screening for depression and/or anxiety should certainly be conducted, using validated indices, for those with severe or intractable pain.

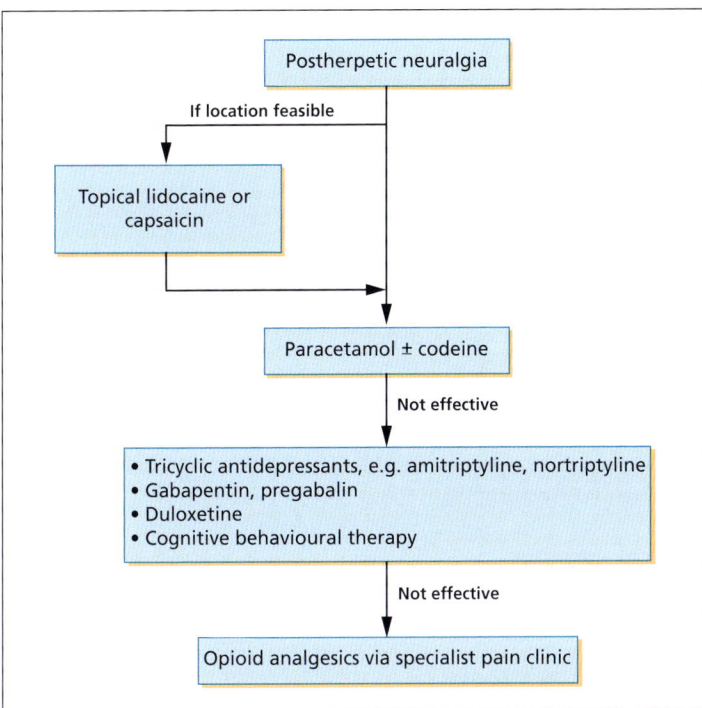

Figure 82.2 Managing neuropathic pain.

Disease course and prognosis

A long-term study over 8 years showed that there is a gradual improvement over time but that sensory changes take longer to recover, reflected in persistently abnormal skin innervation [4].

Investigations

Qualitative sensory testing will show areas of sensory change, which may be useful to monitor in the evaluation of progress.

Management

With the realisation that several pain mechanisms may be operating in any one individual, it is unrealistic to expect any one drug to completely alleviate the pain in all neuropathic pain disorders, or to significantly reduce the pain in all patients suffering from the same neuropathic condition. There are several national and international guidelines on managing neuropathic pain that include PHN [5,6,7], as well as specific reviews [8,9,10]. Figure 82.2 summarises the pharmacological options.

First line

In some guidelines it is suggested that topical lidocaine in the form of a 5% lidocaine patch should be used if the site is accessible. It is also available as a gel, which is cheaper. In patients with trigeminal PHN it is most useful to use topical lidocaine at night when it can reduce waking due to the tactile stimulus of facial skin on bedclothes. The patches can be worn for 12–18 h and should be used daily for 3–4 weeks in the first instance. There is a literature for the use of topical capsaicin, doxepin, gabapentin and ketamine. The former are reasonably readily available, the latter two are less so.

Systemic first line medication for mild to moderate PHN should comprise paracetamol, with or without codeine (assuming no contraindication) [11].

Second line

If pain remains uncontrolled, other medications to consider include the tricyclic antidepressants (e.g. amitriptyline, nortriptyline), the calcium channel $\alpha 2$-δ ligands (gabapentin, pregabalin), and the serotonin-noradrenaline reuptake inhibitor, duloxetine.

Non-pharmacological treatment including CBT should be considered, particularly for those with severe pain [12,13].

Third line

Opioid analgesics and tramadol may be used cautiously for short periods, but only if patients are monitored – ideally within a specialist pain clinic.

Prevention

Systemic corticosteroids given during acute herpes zoster reactivation are ineffective in preventing PHN and cannot therefore be recommended [14]. In older adults with localised herpes zoster, oral aciclovir reduces acute pain and healing times if treatment is initiated within 72 h of the onset of the eruption. A reduction in ocular complications, particularly keratitis and anterior uveitis, occurs with aciclovir treatment of herpes zoster ophthalmicus.

A systematic review of four placebo-controlled trials of oral aciclovir showed only marginal evidence for pain reduction after herpes zoster. Famciclovir and valaciclovir significantly reduced the duration but not the incidence of PHN in one placebo-controlled trial for each agent [15]. Famciclovir or valaciclovir may provide more prompt relief of zoster-associated pain than aciclovir in acute herpes zoster in older adults (over 50 years of age).

Vaccines have been developed that decrease the incidence both of herpes zoster reactivation and PHN. In a placebo-controlled primary prevention study of the vaccine, men and women aged 60 and over had a significant reduction in the burden of illness due to both clinical herpes zoster and PHN [16].

Resources

Further information

Clinical Knowledge Summaries: cks.nice.org.uk/topics/post-herpetic-neuralgia/
Patient.info: https://patient.info/skin-conditions/shingles-herpes-zoster-leaflet/
    postherpetic-neuralgia
(All last accessed April 2022)

Trigeminal neuropathic pain syndrome

Definition and nomenclature

Neuropathic pain is defined by the International Association for the Study of Pain (IASP) as 'pain arising as a direct consequence of a lesion or disease affecting the somatosensory system'. If the pain is in the distribution of the trigeminal nerve it can be termed a trigeminal neuropathic pain. In the updated International Classification of Headache Disorders, painful cranial neuropathies include trigeminal neuralgia, postherpetic neuralgia, post-traumatic trigeminal neuropathy and pain related to central causes such as multiple sclerosis, space-occupying lesions and following a stroke [1].

Synonyms and inclusions
- Painful post-traumatic trigeminal neuropathy
- Atypical odontalgia
- Persistent dento-alveolar pain disorder
- Phantom tooth pain [2]
- Trigeminal neuralgia

Introduction and general description

Although a range of conditions may cause neuropathic pain in the trigeminal region, only those causing intraoral pain will be discussed, acknowledging that such patients are unlikely to present to a dermatologist. PHN of the oro-facial region has the same clinical picture as elsewhere in the body and is managed in the same way. Trigeminal neuralgia, although often presenting in the mouth, also has extraoral features and is not discussed here.

Epidemiology

Incidence and prevalence

An accurate estimate of incidence and prevalence is not possible due to varying disease definitions and a lack of appropriate studies. The condition can occur in 3–6% of teeth that have been root-filled [3]. Pain can also occur after the removal of teeth, especially wisdom teeth when the inferior alveolar nerve or lingual nerve has been injured. Trigeminal neuropathic pain syndrome can also be triggered by the placement of implants or injection of local anaesthetic [4]. It may occur following healing of mucosal lesions, such as lichen planus. The term painful post-traumatic trigeminal neuropathy is used for pain outside the oral cavity.

Sex

From limited data, it is considered to be more common in females.

Associated diseases

It is often co-morbid with temporomandibular joint disorders and psychological factors [5].

Pathophysiology

Predisposing factors

It is more likely to occur after prolonged preoperative pain, and if there is a history of a painful procedure [3]. Multiple sclerosis is a reported association.

Pathology

Although often termed an idiopathic pain disorder, both psychological and neuropathic elements should be considered. Studies have shown that intraoral somatosensory abnormalities are present [6] and blink reflexes are altered [7]. There may also be central changes as not all patients get pain relief with the use of a local anaesthetic [8]. Psychosocial factors have also been implicated in case–control studies.

Clinical features

History

Most patients will link the start of their symptoms to some dental procedure ranging from root canal treatment, extraction, minor surgical procedure or trauma. Patients often find it hard to describe their symptoms.

Presentation

The pain is continuous, at least 8 h daily for over 15 days per month and of 3 months' duration. It is described as a dull, aching, throbbing pain that can occasionally be sharp and even burning. It is localised to an anatomical area around a tooth. There are often features of depression, anxiety and somatisation. Marked allodynia in the area is typical, as well as hyperaesthesia or hypoaesthesia/anaesthesia. One case series described patients with evidence of swelling and flushing [9].

Clinical variants

The location can vary. Trigeminal neuropathic pain can be unilateral or bilateral.

Differential diagnosis

This can include dental causes, such as a cracked tooth.

Classification of severity

It can vary in severity from moderate to severe.

Disease course and prognosis

From limited data, it is reported that up to a third of patients improve and 10% become pain-free over a 7-year period [10].

Investigations

Intraoral X-rays have often been performed prior to referral to a specialist centre. More sophisticated cone beam computerised tomography can help to identify other causes such as fractured teeth, inadequate root fillings or damage to local nerves.

Management

There are no randomised controlled trials, and treatments are based on expert opinions and extrapolated from those used in neuropathic pain. Antiepileptics and antidepressants may be helpful, and many patients will also turn to a wide range of non-pharmacological treatments such as acupuncture, TENS (transcutaneous electrical nerve stimulation) and relaxation techniques [10].

Treatment ladder

First line
- Reassurance and written information
- Avoidance of further invasive treatments which could cause more damage to the tissues
- Maintenance of good oral hygiene to prevent further dental problems is important
- Simple analgesia such as paracetamol and non-steroidal anti-inflammatory drugs

Second line
- Carbamazepine, amitriptyline, SSRIs, gabapentin and pregabalin may be considered

Third line
- Employing a multidisciplinary approach, such as using CBT in combination with other treatments, has been shown to be effective in a range of chronic facial pain conditions
- Botulinum toxin injections
- Lamotrigine

Trigeminal trophic syndrome

Definition
Trigeminal trophic syndrome (TTS) is an uncommon disorder in which chronic pain, burning and stinging sensations in the distribution of the trigeminal nerve are associated with an irresistible desire to pick at the involved skin. The skin itself may be relatively anaesthetic so that the patient does not realise the damage that he or she is doing. Alternatively, the involved skin may be dysaesthetic (i.e. patients experience an intractable itch, tickling or other sensations) from which temporary relief may be obtained by manipulating the skin. TTS (as opposed to atypical trigeminal trophic syndrome (ATTS), see later) is unilateral and an underlying cause can almost always be found (Table 82.3).

Epidemiology
Trigeminal trophic syndrome is rare but occurs in all ethnicities, usually in middle-aged individuals. It is reportedly more common in men (2 male : 1 female).

Pathophysiology
Neurotrophic changes in the trigeminal area may follow the destruction of fibres conveying pain and temperature sensation [1]. The commonest cause of TTS is either postherpetic (both herpes simplex and varicella-zoster) or post-stroke. Other causes of this disorder include central sensory neuronal damage, postencephalitic parkinsonism, syringobulbia, posterior fossa tumour or occlusion of the posterior inferior cerebellar artery [2], leprous neuritis and brainstem infarcts [3], or damage to the trigeminal nerve by attempts to relieve intractable trigeminal neuralgia (by maxillofacial surgery or alcohol injections into the Gasserian ganglion). TTS is usually a disease of adults, although a case has been described in a 14-month-old child secondary to herpes simplex trigeminal neuritis [4].

There are almost always demonstrable defects in the trigeminal nerve pathways (peripheral or central) which lead to this condition (e.g. from MRI scans or neurophysiological tests).

Clinical features
The patient complains of paraesthesiae or a sensation of itching, pain or burning discomfort in an area innervated by the trigeminal nerve. This is then picked, rubbed or scratched, and the resultant erosions increase in size and may extend to completely destroy the nasal cartilage (Figure 82.3). The appearance can mimic a primary skin cancer therefore taking a complete history is vital [1]. Patients freely admit to traumatising the area in an attempt to relieve the uncomfortable sensations. The pattern of ulceration may be sufficiently bizarre to suggest dermatitis artefacta. Ulcers may spread towards the cheek and the upper lip; subsequent scar formation in the area of the alar can lead to lip elevation, resulting in a disfiguring sneer [2]. Characteristically, the alar rim is involved and the tip of the nose spared. Sites less frequently involved include the forehead, scalp and cheeks. Neurological examination may reveal decreased perception of light touch and pain over the area, and sometimes an absent corneal reflex on the same side [2]. Ulcers may be complicated by secondary infection. Orbital cellulitis and corneal ulceration are recognised serious complications.

Investigations
Consider (if clinically indicated and not available from the history):
- MRI scan.
- Neurophysiological (i.e. nerve conduction) studies.
- Tests for mononeuropathy if clinically indicated (e.g. glucose, thyroid function, syphilis serology, B12, etc.).

Table 82.3 Differential features of trigeminal trophic syndrome (TTS), atypical trigeminal trophic syndrome (ATTS), dermatitis artefacta (DA) and skin picking disorder (SPS).

	Patient owns that they are manipulating their skin	Dysaesthesia	Unilateral	Compulsion to pick at the skin which leads to temporary resolution of the sensation	Other parts of the body involved	Neurological investigations usually show a cause
TTS	✓	✓	✓	✓	No	✓
ATTS	✓	✓	±	✓	No	± Neurophysiological studies usually abnormal
Dermatitis artefacta	No	No	±	±	±	No
Skin picking disorder	✓ Sometimes reluctantly	No	No	±	Usually unless a 'picker's nodule'	No

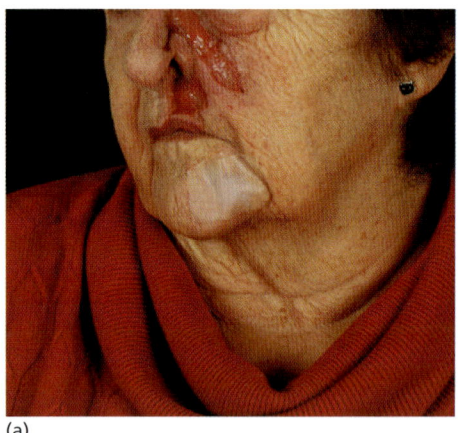
(a)

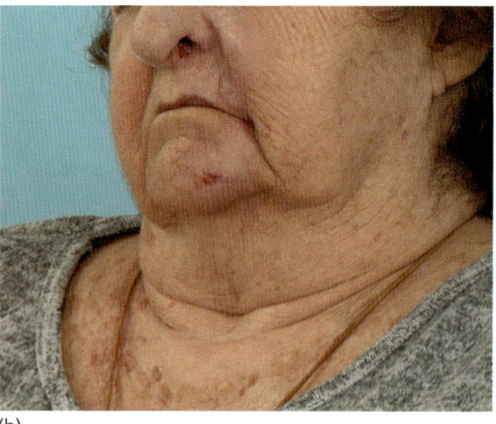
(b)

Figure 82.3 Trigeminal trophic syndrome (TTS) before (a) and after (b) treatment with pregabalin. Note the nasal alar ulcerations commonly seen with TTS.

Management

Treatment is aimed at trying to find a medication or approach that will relieve the patient's unpleasant sensations while promoting healing of the cutaneous changes.

Treatment ladder

First line

- Appropriate treatment of the skin with emollients and dressings (and if necessary antibiotics, etc.)
- Simultaneously treat the dysaesthesia with one of the following:
  - gabapentin, pregabalin (titrate the dose to that which controls the TTS)
  - amitriptyline in lower doses (e.g. 10– 30 mg at night)
    These agents should be tried according to side-effect profile and patient acceptability
- Attempts to limit self-inflicted skin trauma via the wearing of gloves can be helpful, but nonetheless the ulceration commonly persists, particularly in the elderly or in confused patients who compulsively pick at the skin
- Protection using appropriate dressings (e.g. occlusion with an aquaplast thermoplastic dressing sutured over the affected area and left in place for 1–2 weeks) has been shown to promote ulcer healing [5]

Second line

- Habit reversal CBT may be helpful
- Duloxetine and carbamazepine [6] have been tried with limited success
- Selective serotonin reuptake inhibitors (e.g. fluoxetine or citalopram)

Third line

- Surgical approaches in the past have included cervical sympathectomy [7], transcutaneous electrical stimulation [8] and grafting or the use of innervated transposition flaps [9]. These treatments will fail if the area continues to be traumatised
- Topiramate

Atypical trigeminal trophic syndrome

Definition

ATTS is newly described and different from TTS in that the distribution is unusual (often involving the neck or two areas of the trigeminal nerve supply) [10]. It appears to be distinct from skin picking disorders (Chapter 84) in that it only involves the trigeminal area of the face and the patient (similar to TTS) describes a sensation of tickling, itch or burning which is temporarily relieved by manipulating the skin in the involved area (Table 82.3).

Epidemiology

Atypical trigeminal trophic syndrome is rare but occurs in all ethnicities, usually in middle-aged individuals, and in men and women.

Clinical features

Atypical trigeminal trophic syndrome presents similarly to TTS except the ulceration may be bilateral and in atypical sites (Figure 82.4) [10]. Patients will volunteer that they traumatise the involved skin and by doing so they obtain relief of their symptoms. The condition may be mistaken for dermatitis artefacta.

Investigations

Trigeminal nerve abnormalities are frequently identified on neurophysiological testing, while MRI scans tend to show no demonstrable disease [10].

Management

Management of the condition is similar to that of TTS.

Cervical trophic syndrome

Definition

Cervical trophic syndrome (CTS) is similar to TTS in that the patient experiences intractable itch/pain/burning/irritation of the skin supplied by a specific nerve or branch of a nerve following iatrogenic

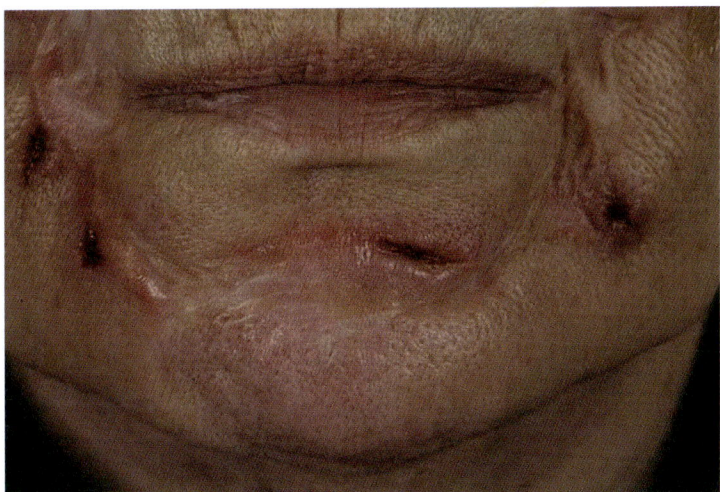

Figure 82.4 Patient with atypical trigeminal trophic syndrome.

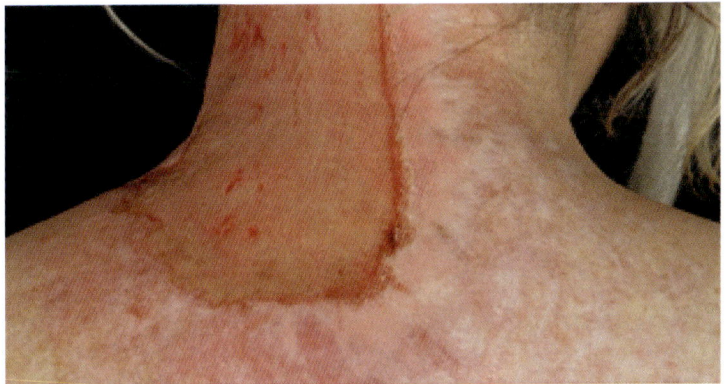

Figure 82.5 Patient with cervical trophic syndrome.

or other trauma. Patients pick, scratch or manipulate the involved skin in an attempt to relieve the sensations they are experiencing. The relief is usually temporary, and the patient will continue to interfere with the affected area even after a well-demarcated ulcer has developed. In CTS the implicated nerve is usually either the C2 or C3 nerve root.

Epidemlology
There are sporadic case reports of cervical trophic syndrome and it is rare [11].

Clinical features
Cervical trophic syndrome usually presents with a well-demarcated ulcer in the distribution of a cervical nerve (Figure 82.5). The patient will indicate that they experience burning/pain/irritation of the affected skin, and temporary relief of the sensation in response to manipulating the area. The involved area of skin will not usually cross the midline and will correspond to a recognised dermatomal distribution.

Aetiology
In case reports, CTS is thought to arise as a result of nerve dysaesthesia (usually postherpetic) or damage (e.g. from any potential mononeuropathic cause or postsurgical).

Management
Management of the condition is similar to that of TTS.

Midface toddler excoriation syndrome (MiTES)

MiTES is a recently described condition probably linked to *PRDM12* gene mutation. Patients usually present from infancy with excoriations, ulcers, dyspigmentation, lichenfication and erosions over the midface, with a predilection for the nasal bridge. Bi-allelic mutations in the *PRDM12* gene cause hereditary sensory and autonomic neuropathy type VIII (HSAN 8), a congenital pain insensitivity disorder, manifesting as ulceration of the digits, lips, tongue, as well as facial scratching. Since, MiTES is a genetically heterogeneous entity, genes other than *PRDM12* can also be involved. MiTES resembles HSAN 8 clinically and aetiologically but lacks ulceration of the acral parts. MiTES and genetic sensory neuronal causes of repeated skin excoriation (e.g. Lesch–Nyhan and hereditary sensory neuropathies) are rare but important to recognise clinically [12].

Vulvodynia

Definition and nomenclature
Vulvodynia is the term given to chronic vulvar discomfort, most commonly manifest as painful dysaesthetic skin sensations, with no visible clinical abnormalities, and in the absence of an alternative identifiable disorder.

> **Synonyms and inclusions**
> * Vulvodynia
> * Vestibulodynia (site-specific rather than a true synonym)

Introduction and general description
Vulvodynia (see also Chapter 110) may involve the female genital skin generally or be site-specific; it may be subdivided into vestibulodynia and other -dynias according to the area affected and the clinical presentation [1,2]. Some patients describe provocation factors such as sexual and non-sexual touch. Vulvodynia is considered to be an idiopathic, usually chronic disorder, unresponsive to simple analgesia, and almost invariably associated with significant psychosocial co-morbidities [3,4]. It commonly leads to significant functional impairment.

Epidemiology
Incidence and prevalence
Genital pain is said to occur in approximately 8% of women (range 3–14%) [5].

Age
It usually affects younger adults in their thirties to forties, but can affect any (usually) adult age.

PART 7: PSYCHOLOGICAL, SENSORY & NEUROLOGICAL

Ethnicity
It affects all ethnicities.

Associated diseases
There is a very common association with anxiety, depression and sexual dysfunction [3,4,6]. Vulvodynia may occur as part of a more generalised pelvic pain syndrome; urinary symptoms, painful bladder syndrome and interstitial cystitis may co-exist. Other chronic pain conditions such as irritable bowel syndrome, fibromyalgia and chronic fatigue syndrome are also more common in patients with vulvodynia [7].

Pathophysiology
The pathophysiology is unknown, though many potential factors have been implicated, including genetic, endocrine, trauma-related and pelvic floor muscular abnormalities. Previous theories have invoked dysfunction of the peripheral and/or central sensory nerve pathways which innervate the genital areas or are responsible for consciousness of genital sensation [8,9]. Vulvodynia has also been postulated to reflect a functional somatic symptom disorder [10]. It is a moot point as to whether the chronic pain of vulvodynia leads to the widely observed psychosocial and sexual dysfunction, or whether vulvodynia arises as a consequence of premorbid psychological abnormalities.

Clinical features
History
Patients often describe severe, chronic (usually months or longer) sensations of burning, stinging or stabbing pain or rawness affecting either the whole genital skin or a very specific genital site. The pain may be provoked (e.g. by sexual contact) or it may be present more or less continuously. A comprehensive screen for other potentially functional symptoms is desirable. Direct, albeit sensitive questioning on the possible impact on sexual function is needed as patients may be too ashamed or embarrassed to volunteer this information.

Presentation
There is usually very little, if anything, to see by way of physical signs. Patients may have subtle localised or more generalised redness affecting the skin or mucosa, but this is almost always well within the normal range and should not be overinterpreted. Often the initial misdiagnosis by a general practitioner is vulvovaginal candidiasis. Point tenderness (with cotton wool tips) is common. The diagnosis is one of exclusion, although the history and examination usually allows a firm diagnosis to be made clinically.

Differential diagnosis
The differential diagnosis includes the full range of genital dermatoses, which can usually be excluded clinically. Some patients have genital pain syndromes as a part of a more generalised chronic pain syndrome. Postherpetic neuralgia and pudendal neuropathy should be considered, as should vulvo-vaginal atrophy in postmenopausal women.

Complications and co-morbidities
Psychosexual (e.g. vaginismus, loss of libido) and psychosocial (e.g. anxiety, depression, hypervigilance, catastrophising) cognitions and co-morbidities are extremely common [6,11], with a resultant deleterious impact on quality of life and functional status.

Disease course and prognosis
Untreated disease may be recalcitrant. However, treatment is usually successful, although it may take some time to achieve remission or symptom amelioration. Clinicians and patients may have to search via trial and error for the treatment that best suits the individual, with both parties keeping an open mind, and seeking to employ a genuinely holistic approach.

Management
All patients should be offered referral to a patient advocacy organisation where available and given opportunities to learn as much as they wish to about their condition. A multidisciplinary approach to treatment is recommended [12], ideally involving dermatology, gynaecology, psychology, psychiatry, physiotherapy and pain specialists. Implementing a wider biopsychosocial conceptualisation of vulvodynia in the assessment and management process is strongly encouraged, and likely to improve patient outcomes [11]. All patients must be screened for co-morbid anxiety and depression using validated questionnaires and offered treatment accordingly.

Treatment ladder

First line
- Reassurance, validating symptoms, basic psychoeducation
- Topical lidocaine gel or ointment
- Amitriptyline (low-dose, e.g. 10 mg at night and build up slowly – 50 mg usual maximum tolerated dose)
- Other tricyclics (e.g. doxepin)
- Cognitive behavioural therapy (CBT), acceptance and commitment therapy (ACT) or other psychological talking therapies tailored to the individual's psychological formulation (especially if there are psychosexual or psychosocial co-morbidities)
- Mindfulness-based relaxation
- Pelvic floor physiotherapy

Second line
- SSRIs (e.g. sertraline, citalopram)
- Gabapentin and pregabalin (start low and titrate up according to response and tolerance)
- CBT or other psychological talking therapies if not already in place

Third line
- Nerve blocks
- Botulinum toxin
- Vestibulectomy

Resources

Further information

International Society for the Study of Vulvovaginal Disease: https://www.issvd.org/
Vulval Pain Society: http://www.vulvalpainsociety.org/vps/
(All last accessed April 2022)

Penoscrotodynia

Definition and nomenclature

Penoscrotodynia (PSD) describes persistent, unpleasant dysaesthetic skin sensations affecting the penis and/or scrotum, in the absence of any other identifiable cause.

Synonyms and inclusions

- Dysaesthetic penoscrotodynia
- Penodynia and scrotodynia (site-specific terms)
- Penile dysaesthetic syndrome
- Penile pain syndrome
- Angry or burning red scrotum syndrome

Introduction and general description

PSD (Chapter 109) may occur as a highly localised phenomenon or affecting the entirety of the genital skin. It tends to run a chronic course, is poorly responsive to neuropathic pain agents and is invariably associated with psychosocial comorbidities [1]. Men with PSD often struggle to receive an accurate diagnosis and timely, satisfactory treatment, on account of limited awareness of its existence and a sparse research literature.

Epidemiology

Incidence and prevalence

There are no reliable epidemiological data on PSD. It is, however, encountered frequently in specialist male genital dermatology clinics.

Age

PSD may affect adults of any age, although more commonly those in the 20–40 year age bracket.

Ethnicity

PSD affects all ethnicities.

Associated diseases

Akin to vulvodynia, there is a very common association with anxiety and depression [1]. Sexual dysfunction (e.g. dyspareunia, erectile and ejaculatory disturbance) is common. It may also present as part of a more generalised pelvic pain syndrome: so-called chronic prostatitis/chronic pelvic pain syndrome [2].

Pathophysiology

Historically, PSD has been assumed to reflect some kind of neuropathic pain disorder, despite a lack of supportive evidence. More recently, a functional somatic symptom disorder has been considered more likely, given the invariable presence of psychopathology and a reliable response to psychodermatological treatment, where this is accepted [1].

Clinical features

History

Patients describe severe, usually chronic, sensations of burning, stinging or stabbing pain, or extreme hypersensitivity. This may affect a very specific genital site (commonly the dorsal glans penis and coronal rim, or the scrotum), or lead to global genital discomfort which extends to involve adjacent skin in the groins, upper inner thighs, perineum and perianal region. The pain tends to be present more or less continuously, though patients are often completely distractible if busy with another activity. There may be a history of a stressful or traumatic antecedent trigger event, which is worth gently enquiring about. Themes such as guilt and remorse may be uncovered, not infrequently related to sexual misadventure [3,4]. Patients frequently become hypervigilant, ruminating excessively and checking their skin regularly through the day or taking multiple illustrative digital photographs.

Presentation

The clinical examination is always within normal limits. Patients are often focused on minute, fleeting areas of redness on the glans or distressed by the naturally dusky appearance of the scrotum and how this may vary according to ambient temperature. It helps to provide reassurance about other anatomical oddities such as angiokeratomata of Fordyce or Fordyce spots, which may have drawn the eye.

Differential diagnosis

PSD is a diagnosis of exclusion, which may usually be achieved with a careful history and clinical examination. Consider pudendal neuralgia, testicular pathology and sexually transmitted infections, which may occasionally merit limited, judicious investigation.

Complications and co-morbidities

There is almost always a very significant impact on quality of life, with patients typically resorting to extensive internet research in an attempt to find a cure, as well as becoming increasingly socially and sexually avoidant or isolated, which then compounds the severity of symptoms.

Disease course and prognosis

Treatment is usually successful, although this is dependent on establishing trust and rapport, arriving at a mutually acceptable psychological formulation, and assuming the patient has sufficient insight and willingness to engage in the suggested management plan.

Management

All patients must be screened for co-morbid anxiety and depression using validated questionnaires, and offered treatment accordingly [1,3]. Underlying affective disorders are not always obvious in this patient group, but by taking the time to sensitively and empathically enquire and treat, mutually satisfying outcomes may be achieved. It is important to provide sufficient time at the outset to allow a thorough patient-centred assessment, and regular follow-up thereafter to monitor progress. Most patients can be helped satisfactorily by the dermatologist working in conjunction with the local general practitioner, although a multidisciplinary psychodermatological approach is recommended in more challenging cases (involving dermatology, psychology, psychiatry and sometimes urology). Reiterating basic psychoeducation and healthy lifestyle advice (e.g. sleep hygiene, regular exercise, avoidance of internet searching) helps patients move away from an otherwise all-encompassing focus on their symptoms.

Treatment options
- Reassurance, validating symptoms, basic psychoeducation
- SSRIs (e.g. low-dose sertraline, citalopram)
- Psychological talking therapies tailored to the individual's psychological formulation

Chronic scalp pain and dysaesthesia

Definition and nomenclature
Scalp pain, dysaesthesia and tenderness without any obvious scalp disease is another mucocutaneous pain syndrome. It follows the pattern of other disorders in this group, in that patients complain of (usually) severe, chronic pain or discomfort affecting the scalp and/or hair, which may or may not be provoked by contact (e.g. combing the hair) and for which no underlying cause can be found.

> **Synonyms and inclusions**
> - Trichodynia
> - Scalp allodynia
> - Scalp dysaesthesia syndrome

Epidemiology
Incidence and prevalence
It is rare but probably under-reported; it is certainly encountered more commonly in specialist hair and psychodermatology clinics.

Pathophysiology
This is as for other cutaneous pain syndromes. Some authors indicate that the thalamus may be acting dysfunctionally and that this may lead to scalp allodynia amongst other cutaneous pain syndromes [1,2]. Psychological co-morbidities are exceedingly common.

Clinical features
Differential diagnosis
The differential diagnosis includes all scalp dermatoses. In the absence of scalp disease, the diagnosis of trichodynia can be made clinically with an appropriate history. Disproportionate pain with normal touch or pressure (allodynia) is very suggestive of the diagnosis.

Management

> **Treatment ladder**
>
> **First line**
> - Education and reassurance
> - Use gentle shampoos; avoid over-zealous styling and dyeing
> - Tricyclics (e.g. low-dose amitriptyline)
> - CBT or other talking therapies
>
> **Second line**
> - SSRIs (e.g. sertraline, citalopram)
> - Pregabalin and gabapentin
>
> **Third line**
> - Acupuncture [3]

Erythromelalgia

Definition and nomenclature
Erythromelalgia is defined by an intense burning sensation of the extremities (usually the feet) together with persistent redness and increased skin temperature (see also Chapter 101). It is subdivided into primary and secondary categories.

> **Synonyms and inclusions**
> - Weir-Mitchell disease
> - Acromelalgia
> - Red neuralgia
> - Erythermalgia

Epidemiology
Incidence and prevalence
The incidence of erythromelalgia is reported as 1.3 per 100 000 persons per year in one US county [1], though this is probably an underestimate.

Age
Patients with primary erythromelalgia tend to present in childhood, while those with secondary causes present on average aged 50–60 years.

Sex
Erythromelalgia is more common in females.

Pathophysiology
Primary erythromelalgia is now known to be caused by an autosomal dominant mutation in the *SCN9A* gene [2]. This gene codes for voltage-gated sodium channels, which are expressed in small nociceptive neurons, thought to play a crucial role in pain perception [3].

Secondary erythromelalgia has been linked with a vast array of disparate conditions including peripheral neuropathies, connective tissue disease, MS, chronic vibration and pregnancy. When associated with haematological disorders (e.g. leukaemia, thrombocytosis and polycythaemia vera) the pathogenesis is thought to be related to platelet activation and thrombotic occlusion [4].

Clinical features
The diagnosis of erythromelalgia is established clinically. Feet are most commonly affected, but cases involving legs, hands, ears, neck and face have also been described [5]. Symptoms may be intermittent but more usually there is a persistent background dysaesthesia with flares often at night.

Provoking and exacerbating factors include heat and exercise; relief often comes with cooling the extremities. Between attacks, the extremities may feel normal or may be mildly cool, cyanotic or uncomfortable [5]. Patients will often lie in bed with their feet facing an open window or lying on cooling ice packs (both of which probably exacerbate the disease). Once again, the impact on quality of life and mood may be profound and disabling. Patients will try anything to obtain relief of their disabling symptoms including use of topical aerosol anaesthetic skin refrigerants such as ethyl chloride. The severe chronic pain can lead to suicide.

Differential diagnosis
The differential diagnoses include peripheral neuropathy, connective tissue diseases, Raynaud phenomenon, acrocyanosis and peripheral vascular disease among others [5].

Investigations
Clinical diagnostic criteria have been proposed to encompass the typical symptoms and signs [6]. Genetic testing for *SCN9A* mutations is available for possible primary cases. Wide-ranging investigation may be required to pinpoint secondary causes, particularly to confirm or exclude cases of myeloproliferative disease [4].

Management
Treating the pain of erythromelalgia is difficult and usually achieved through trials of medication with the patient, unless there is a treatable secondary cause. For mild disease, first line topical treatment may be sufficient (e.g. lidocaine patches, doxepin cream or capsaicin cream). For moderate disease, topicals should be combined with oral systemic therapy such as gabapentin, pregabalin, SSRIs, amitriptyline or nortriptyline [7]. Aspirin usually relieves the symptoms associated with haematological disease [8]. Third line agents include intravenous lidocaine, sodium nitroprusside or prostaglandins (e.g. intravenous prostacyclin infusion). For patients unresponsive to medical therapy, invasive procedures such as sympathetic blockade, sympathectomy or dorsal cord stimulation may be considered [7]. More recently, agents directed specifically against the mutated sodium channels in primary erythromelalgia have been trialled successfully, including mexiletine [9] and ranolazine [10].

All patients should be educated to minimise provoking factors, such as warmth, dependent positioning, exercise and alcohol. Behaviours that may exacerbate the condition (such as using ice packs) should be discouraged. Some patients feel helpless and wretched and may consider suicide, so assessment and management of psychosocial co-morbidities and associated risk is important.

CBT and other talking therapies may be very helpful for some patients [7].

Resources

Further information
The Erythromelalgia Association: https://erythromelalgia.org
National Organization for Rare Disorders (NORD): rarediseases.org
(All last accessed April 2022)

Key references

The full list of references can be found in the online version at https://www.wiley.com/rooksdermatology10e

Burning mouth syndrome
7 Farag AM, Kuten-Shorrer M, Natto Z et al. WWOM VII: effectiveness of systemic pharmacotherapeutic interventions in the management of BMS: a systematic review and meta-analysis. *Oral Dis* 2021 Mar 12. doi: 10.1111/odi.13817. Online ahead of print.
9 McMillan R, Forssell H, Buchanan JA, Glenny AM, Weldon JC, Zakrzewska JM. Interventions for treating burning mouth syndrome. *Cochrane Database Syst Rev* 2016; Issue 11: CD002779. doi.org/10.1002/14651858.CD002779.pub3

Postherpetic neuralgia
6 Finnerup NB, Attal N, Haroutounian S et al. Pharmacotherapy for neuropathic pain in adults: a systematic review and meta-analysis. *Lancet Neurol* 2015;14:162–73.
9 Hempenstall K, Nurmikko TJ, Johnson RW, A'Hern RP, Rice AS. Analgesic therapy in postherpetic neuralgia: a quantitative systematic review. *PLOS Med* 2005;2:e164.
10 Schutzer-Weissmann J, Farquhar-Smith P. Post-herpetic neuralgia – a review of current management and future directions. *Expert Opin Pharmacother* 2017;18:1739–50.

Trigeminal neuropathic pain syndrome
1 The International Classification of Headache Disorders, 3rd edn (beta version). *Cephalalgia* 2013;33:629–808.
4 Renton T, Yilmaz Z. Profiling of patients presenting with posttraumatic neuropathy of the trigeminal nerve. *J Orofac Pain* 2011;25:333–44.

Trigeminal trophic syndrome/Atypical trigeminal trophic syndrome/MiTES
2 Ahmed A, Kentley J. Trigeminal trophic syndrome. In: Bewley AP, Lepping P, Taylor RE, eds. *Psychodermatology in Clinical Practice*. London: Springer Nature, 2021.
10 Gkini M-A, Ahmed A, Aguilar-Duran S et al. Atypical variant of trigeminal trophic syndrome successfully treated with pregabalin: a case report series. *Clin Exp Dermatol* 2019;44:225–8.
12 Moss C, Srinivas SM, Sarveswaran N et al. Midface toddler excoriation syndrome (MiTES) can be caused by autosomal recessive biallelic mutations in a gene for congenital insensitivity to pain, PRDM12. *Br J Dermatol* 2018;179:113–40.

Vulvodynia
2 Bornstein J, Goldstein AT, Stockdale CK et al. 2015 ISSVD, ISSWSH and IPPS Consensus Terminology and Classification of Persistent Vulvar Pain and Vulvodynia. *Obstet Gynecol* 2016;127:745–51.
11 Chisari C, Monajemi MB, Scott W, Moss-Morris R, McCracken LM. Psychosocial factors associated with pain and sexual function in women with vulvodynia: a systematic review. *Eur J Pain* 2021;25:39–50.

12 Mandal D, Nunns D, Byrne J *et al*. Guidelines for the management of vulvodynia. *Br J Dermatol* 2010;162:1180–5.

Penoscrotodynia

1 Anyasodor MC, Taylor RE, Bewley A, Goulding JMR. Dysaesthetic penoscrotodynia may be a somatoform disorder: results from a two-centre retrospective case series. *Clin Exp Dermatol* 2016;41:474–9.

3 Goulding JMR. Dysaesthetic disorders. In: Bewley AP, Lepping P, Taylor RE, eds. *Psychodermatology in Clinical Practice*. London: Springer Nature, 2021.

Erythromelalgia

4 Mann N, King T, Murphy R. Review of primary and secondary erythromelalgia. *Clin Exp Dermatol* 2019;44:477–82.

5 Davis MD, O'Fallon WM, Rogers RS, 3rd, *et al*. Natural history of erythromelalgia: presentation and outcome in 168 patients. *Arch Dermatol* 2000;136:330–6.

7 Durosaro O, Davis MD, Hooten WM *et al*. Intervention for erythromelalgia, a chronic pain syndrome: comprehensive pain rehabilitation center, Mayo Clinic. *Arch Dermatol* 2008;144:1578–83.

CHAPTER 83

Neurological Conditions Affecting the Skin

Andrew G. Affleck

Department of Dermatology, Ninewells Hospital & Medical School, NHS Tayside, Dundee, UK

Introduction and overview of genetic neurocutaneous disorders

The relationship between the nervous system and the skin is complex. Embryologically, both arise from the ectoderm and therefore a close relationship in health and disease is not surprising. Physiologically, stimulation of the skin by the nervous system is seen in responses such as sweating, flushing, pallor and goose bumps. Many inflammatory dermatoses including eczema, psoriasis and urticaria are exacerbated by stress via the central nervous system (CNS) and autonomic nervous system (ANS) culminating in neuropeptides; the term 'psychoneurogenic' emphasises this interaction. A broad definition of neurocutaneous disease would include all diseases, congenital and acquired, that exhibit both cutaneous and neurological features. Another definition would be genetic disorders with cutaneous and neurological features – this encompasses many diseases and syndromes with varying genetic inheritance patterns including autosomal dominant, autosomal recessive, x-linked male-lethal, x-linked non-lethal, lethal surviving by mosaicism and disorders caused by chromosomal aberrations. This genetic group of neurocutaneous disorders was first recognised by Van der Hoeve, an ophthalmologist from the Netherlands, who introduced the terms phakoma/phakomata (Greek – lentil, spot, lens-shaped) to define similar retinal lesions recorded in tuberous sclerosis (1920) and in neurofibromatosis (1923). He later applied this concept to similar lesions in other organs (e.g. brain, heart and kidneys) and to other disorders (i.e. von Hippel–Lindau disease and Sturge–Weber syndrome) (1933), and coined the term phakomatoses. At the same time, the American neurologist Paul Ivan Yakovlev and psychiatrist Riley H. Guthrie (1931) established the key role of the nervous system and cutaneous manifestations in these conditions and proposed to name them neurocutaneous syndromes (or ectodermoses, to explain the pathogenesis). The Belgian pathologist Ludo van Bogaert came to similar conclusions (1935) and suggested the term neuro-ectodermal dysplasias. 'Genodermatoses' and 'neurocristopathies' are alternative terms still used to define these conditions. However, in recent times, the most acclaimed terms are 'phacomatoses' and 'neurocutaneous disorders', which are used interchangeably. Neurocutaneous disorders are a heterogeneous group of conditions affecting the skin: with congenital pigmentary/vascular abnormalities and/or tumours, the CNS and peripheral nervous system (PNS); with congenital abnormalities and/or tumours and the eye; with variable abnormalities. Manifestations may involve many other organs or systems including the heart, vessels, lungs, kidneys and bones. Pathogenically, they are explained by interplay between intra- and extraneuronal signalling pathways encompassing receptor-to-protein and protein-to-protein cascades involving multiple pathways, which also shed light on phenotypic variability and overlap. Each disorder is described in detail and assigned a number in the Mendelian Inheritance in Man (MIM) clinical database. Ruggieri *et al.* [1] have attempted to classify neurocutaneous disorders in childhood into six groups according to predominant clinical features and genetics (Box 83.1).

Rook's Textbook of Dermatology, Tenth Edition. Edited by Christopher Griffiths, Jonathan Barker, Tanya Bleiker, Walayat Hussain and Rosalind Simpson.
© 2024 John Wiley & Sons Ltd. Published 2024 by John Wiley & Sons Ltd.

PART 7: PSYCHOLOGICAL, SENSORY & NEUROLOGICAL

Box 83.1 Subgroups of childhood neurocutaneous disorders

1 Predisposing to development of tumours (e.g. the neurofibromatoses and allelic/similar disorders and schwannomatosis; tuberous sclerosis complex; Gorlin–Goltz and Lhermitte-Duclos–Cowden syndromes)
2 With vascular malformations (e.g. Sturge–Weber and Klippel–Trenaunay syndromes; megalencephaly/microcephaly–capillary malformation syndromes; CLOVES, Wyburn–Mason and mixed vascular naevus syndromes; blue rubber bleb nevus syndrome; hereditary haemorrhagic telangiectasia)
3 With vascular tumours (von Hippel–Lindau disease; PHACE(S))
4 With pigmentary/connective tissue mosaicism (incontinentia pigmenti; pigmentary/Ito mosaicism; mTOR-related megalencephaly/focal cortical dysplasia/pigmentary mosaicism; RHOA-related ectodermal dysplasia; neurocutaneous melanocytosis; epidermal/papular spilus/Becker nevi syndromes; PENS and LEOPARD syndromes; encephalocraniocutaneous lipomatosis; lipoid proteinosis)
5 With dermal dysplasia (cerebello-trigeminal dermal dysplasia)
6 With twin spotting (paired patches of mutant tissue that differ genetically from each other and from the normal background tissue) or similar phenomena (phacomatosis pigmentovascularis and pigmentokeratotica; cutis tricolour)

CLOVES, *c*ongenital *l*ipomatous *o*vergrowth, *v*ascular malformations, *e*pidermal nevis, *s*pinal/skeletal anomalies, scoliosis; LEOPARD, *l*entigines, *e*lectrocardiographic conduction defects, *o*cular hypertelorism, *p*ulmonary stenosis, *a*bnormalities of the genitals, *r*etarded growth, *d*eafness or hearing loss; mTor, mammalian target of rapamycin; PENS, *p*apular *e*pidermal *n*aevus with 'skyline' basal cell layer; PHACE(S), *p*osterior fossa brain malformations, *h*aemangiomas, *a*rterial anomalies, *c*ardiac anomalies and coarctation of the aorta, *e*ye abnormalities and endocrine abnormalities, (S) *s*ternal cleft, supraumbilical raphe, or both.

When faced with a newborn, a child or sometimes an adult with a range of cutaneous and neurological anomalies, a dermatologist can work with colleagues including paediatricians, neurologists and geneticists to determine if the clinical features are suggestive of a known syndrome and whether genetic testing is indicated. Some neurocutaneous disorders remain unclassifiable according to formal genetics. Dedicated formal paediatric neurocutaneous multidisciplinary team (MDT) clinics have a valuable role [2]. Early recognition can be critical to surveillance for treatable complications and genetic counselling. Although many of the complications of genetic neurocutaneous diseases can only be treated symptomatically, advances in understanding of their pathogenesis are opening new approaches to molecularly targeted therapeutics, which promise to alter the natural history of the conditions in the future. For more information, see chapters in Volume 2, Part 6 – Genetic Disorders Involving the Skin. Detailed reference textbooks are also available [3,4].

In this chapter, only primary neurological disease with cutaneous manifestations will be discussed; such neurocutaneous disorders may be divided broadly into those associated with sensory abnormalities, and those associated with autonomic abnormalities, although there is overlap between the two groups. Cutaneous manifestations may occur where the pathology is predominantly located either in the CNS or in the PNS. Dermatologists will see patients with a known neurological disease presenting to them with cutaneous symptoms, or the underlying neurological disease may not be known. Therefore, knowledge of the cutaneous manifestations of neurological diseases is needed and an understanding of the skin's sensory and autonomic innervation is essential to appreciate the clinical manifestations of neurocutaneous disorders.

Cutaneous innervation

The skin is the largest sensory organ and is innervated by a dense three-dimensional network of highly specialised afferent sensory and efferent autonomic nerve branches. The sensory system contains receptors for touch, temperature, pain, itch and various other physical and chemical stimuli [1,2,3]. Information regarding these perceived sensations is transmitted to the CNS. Touch sensations are conveyed by distinct combinations of mechanosensory end organs and the low-threshold mechanoreceptors (LTMRs) that innervate them [3]. The autonomic system comprises post-ganglionic cholinergic parasympathetic nerves, and adrenergic and cholinergic sympathetic nerves. It plays a crucial role in maintaining cutaneous homeostasis by regulating vasomotor function, pilomotor activity and eccrine gland secretion. As many as 1000 such afferent neurons may innervate $1\,cm^2$ of skin. The afferent sensory neurons are unipolar, and each branches off with a single axon travelling towards the skin. The autonomic nerves innervate the skin in a different pattern. Post-ganglionic fibres originate in the sympathetic chain and are co-distributed with the sensory neurons until they arborise into plexuses around sweat glands, blood vessels and arrector pili muscles [1,2]. Skin nerves may contain myelinated and/or unmyelinated fibres: subgroups of sensory neurons are myelinated A fibres, whereas unmyelinated C fibres contain sensory and autonomic fibres. The sensory myelinated fibres can be further subdivided based on diameter into rapidly conducting Aα nerves that transmit tactile sensitivity, and slowly conducting Aδ nerves that transmit temperature, noxious sensation and itch [2,4,5]. In the upper dermis, small myelinated nerves lose their nerve sheaths and, together with the unmyelinated nerves, end in either free nerve endings, or in association with receptors, such as Merkel cells or nerve-ending organs [2,4].

Sensory innervation follows well-defined dermatomes, with some overlap if they are adjacent. Sensory nerves not only function as an afferent system to conduct stimuli back from the skin to the CNS, but also act in an efferent neurosecretory fashion, releasing neuropeptides with important visceromotor, inflammatory and trophic effects on the skin. Unmyelinated type C fibres terminate as either free nerve receptor endings, or in association with receptors such as the Pacinian or Meissner's corpuscles. Pacinian corpuscles, each innervated by a single myelinated sensory axon, are most densely located on the palms and soles, where they act as mechanoreceptors. Meissner corpuscles also occur in greatest density on the palms and soles; being innervated by one or more sensory nerve endings, they also act as mechanoreceptors, and in addition transmit touch sensation. Merkel cells, which occur at low density generally, with an increased density around hair follicles and at the palms, nail beds and lips, form synaptic-like contacts with sensory afferent terminals. The full function of Merkel cells is not yet fully understood, but recent molecular analysis has revealed that they express dozens of presynaptic molecules that are essential for synaptic vesicle release in neurons [6]. Merkel cells produce and contain a wide range of neuropeptides, which may be important in the local regulation of inflammation [2].

Afferent sensory nerves, either unmyelinated C fibres or myelinated Aδ fibres, derive from the dorsal root ganglion and are capable of the release of a variety of neuropeptides in response to noxious stimuli [2,4,5]. Sensory impulses are conducted in the peripheral and central axon of the spinal ganglion cell in the dorsal root ganglion, and pass via the lateral spino-thalamic tract and the lemniscus spinalis to the thalamus [5]. From the thalamus, the information reaches consciousness via the thalamic radiation to the postcentral gyrus of the parietal lobe.

C and Aδ fibres not only conduct nociceptive information to the dorsal root ganglion, but also have an important efferent function, in that they stimulate target tissues by releasing a range of neuropeptides in response to noxious stimuli, such as chemical, electrical, thermal and mechanical injury, or UV radiation. C fibres can also be stimulated by psychological stress, which activates the hypothalamopituitary–adrenal axis, and sensory nerves in the brain and skin [7,8]. More than 20 neuropeptides have been identified and characterised to a greater or lesser extent in the skin of various species [9,**10**]. Neuropeptides with an important neurotransmitter function contained in primary sensory neurons include three tachykinins: substance P (SP), neurokinin A (NKA) and calcitonin gene-related peptide (CGRP) [11]. These neuropeptides most frequently coexist in the same subpopulation of primary sensory neurons, the Aδ and C fibres, and are involved in the nerve transmission of impulses initiated by noxious stimuli. They usually occur in free nerve endings in the upper dermis (Figure 83.1) and epidermis throughout the body, but are at greatest density on the palms and soles, where some end in a plexus around Meissner corpuscles (Figure 83.2) [11].

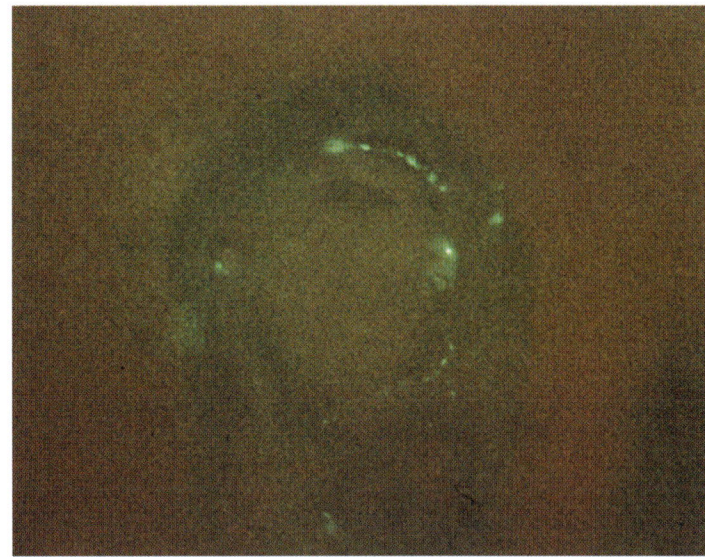

Figure 83.2 Substance P fibres ending in Meissner corpuscles of skin.

Capsaicin, a vanilloid alkaloid found in red pepper fruit [12], functions in nociception by binding to a specific receptor called the vanilloid receptor, the name referring to a homovanillyl group found in the ligands of the receptor. Vanilloid receptors have been found on the unmyelinated C and thinly myelinated Aδ fibre types, which transmit painful stimuli. When capsaicin stimulates the transient receptor potential vanilloid receptor 1 (TRPV1) – one of the vanilloid receptors particularly implicated in neurogenic inflammation [12] – this causes Ca^{2+} ion influx which is rapidly followed by receptor desensitisation. If calcium overload is sufficient, this can lead to cell death [12,13]. TRPV1 links with TRPA1 (transient receptor potential ankyrin 1) channels on the surface of keratinocytes, and their interlinked function has recently been associated with pain and neurogenic inflammation [14]. It has been suggested that neurogenic inflammation is involved in the pathogenesis of the common chronic cutaneous vascular disorders such as rosacea and a subtype known as neurogenic rosacea is now recognised [15]. Due to their involvement in the pathophysiology of rosacea, TRPV1 and TRPA1 may act as therapeutic targets for its inflammatory symptoms [16]. TRPV1 and TRPA1 are also expressed on a multitude of non-neuronal sites, which has led to a plethora of research into their possible function [14].

Release of neuropeptides often leads to neurogenic inflammation. The key components of neurogenic inflammation are precapillary vasodilation, plasma protein extravasation and leukocyte infiltration, which follow antidromic stimulation of peripheral nerves. Neuropeptides can regulate both acute and chronic inflammation by influencing vascular motility and cellular trafficking. After release, neuropeptides are metabolised by membrane-bound endopeptidases that occur on target structures such as blood vessels and eccrine sweat glands in skin [17]. Neutral endopeptidase (NEP) and angiotensin-converting enzyme (ACE) seem to play an important role in terminating the action of neuropeptide agonists [9].

A key receptor on sensory nerves that is involved in neurogenic inflammation is the proteinase-activated receptor 2 (PAR-2). PAR-2, bound to G protein, occurs on keratinocytes (especially in the stratum granulosum), endothelial cells, hair follicles and in

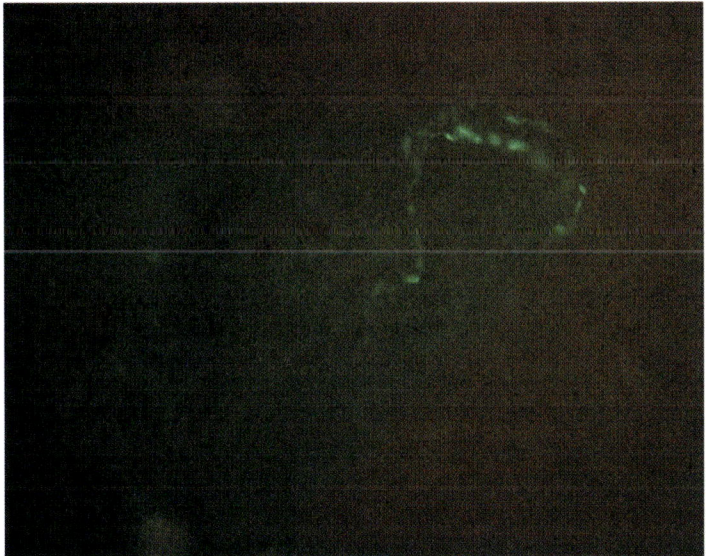

Figure 83.1 Substance P immunoreactive nerve endings in the epidermis of human skin.

the myoepithelial cells of the sweat glands [12]. Tryptase released from degranulated mast cells cleaves PAR-2 in the sensory nerve endings. This leads to its activation and stimulates the release of CGRP and neurokinins SP and NKA from sensory nerve endings. CGRP interacts with CGRP-1 receptors to induce arteriolar dilatation and hyperaemia, while SP interacts with NKA-1 receptors on the endothelial cells of postcapillary venules to induce plasma extravasation. The overall result is tissue oedema. SP may also stimulate degranulation of mast cells, leading to the release of tryptase, which produces positive feedback. Tryptase degrades CGRP and reduces its effects (CGRP inhibits SP degradation by NEP and enhances SP release). Other mediators from mast cells and other inflammatory cells stimulate the release of vasoactive peptides from sensory nerves [9,12].

Close interaction between the different neuromediators, target cells and neuropeptide-degrading enzymes is critical for the control of cutaneous neurogenic inflammation [9,**10**].

Autonomic nervous system

The ANS innervates the skin through postganglionic fibres originating in sympathetic ganglia, and terminating in autonomic plexuses that supply sweat glands, blood vessels and arrector pili muscles [1]. Histochemically, there are two main groups of postganglionic nerve fibres in the skin. First, adrenergic fibres synthesise and store catecholamines and norepinephrine (noradrenaline). The second major group consists of the cholinergic fibres containing acetylcholine. Co-localising with acetylcholine are 'secretory' neuropeptides, such as vasoactive intestinal peptide (VIP) and peptide histidine methionine (PHM). Nerves containing these should be regarded, at least physiologically, as parasympathetic. The secretory portions of the eccrine sweat glands, myoepithelial cells and nearby blood vessels are innervated by a basket-weave pattern of nerves, containing predominantly acetylcholine but also significant numbers of fibres containing 'secretory neuropeptides' including VIP (Figure 83.3), PHM (Figure 83.4), neuropeptide Y (NPY), CGRP, galanin, atrial natriuretic peptide (ANP) and norepinephrine.

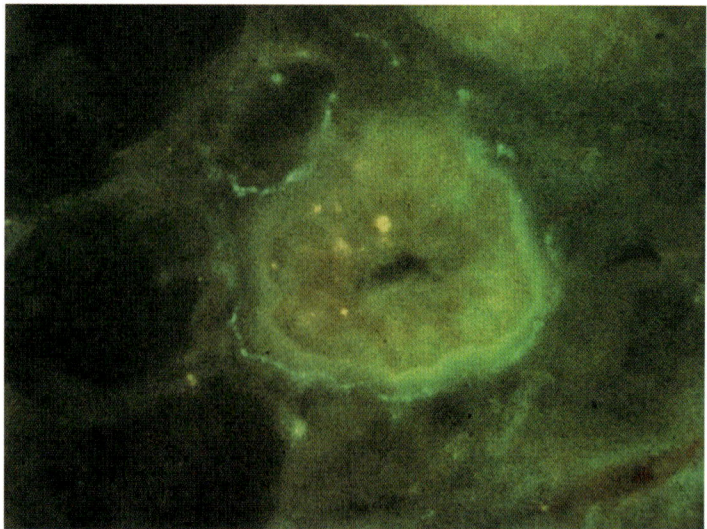

Figure 83.4 Peptide histidine methionine immunoreactive fibres surround eccrine sweat glands.

Secretory neuropeptides, mainly VIP and ANP, together with norepinephrine, are not as effective as acetylcholine at sweat production, and probably synergistically amplify acetylcholine-induced adenosine 3′,5′-cyclic monophosphate (cAMP) accumulation, which is the most important secondary messenger in sweat production. ANP may be responsible, at least in part, for the regulation of sodium and other electrolytes released in sweat [11]. NPY has been identified in the periarteriolar nerve fibres of the deep and superficial vascular plexus, and in eccrine sweat glands; and is likely to play a role in the regulation of skin blood flow and eccrine sweating [11]. Pituitary adenylate cyclase-activating polypeptide (PACAP) also plays a significant role in modulating cutaneous inflammation. It belongs to the VIP family and is capable of binding identical receptors to VIP in the same tissue but with different affinities. PACAP and VIP both participate in myelin maturation and synthesis [18]. PACAP leads to mast cell degranulation and dilatation of small blood vessels [19]. PACAP may have a pro-inflammatory effect on endothelial cells during acute inflammation, yet it exerts anti-inflammatory effects under chronic inflammatory conditions [9].

Blood vessels in the skin are innervated by adrenergic fibres, which are vasoconstrictors, while acetylcholine and neuropeptides, such as VIP and PHM, act as vasodilators and increase vascular permeability [11,20]. Thus, by increasing the release of acetylcholine and secretory neuropeptides, the body has a mechanism of increasing blood flow to the skin and increasing sweating, both of which act to reduce body temperature. If body temperature falls, this is detected in the preoptic region of the hypothalamus, which activates the sympathetic nervous system, which in turn reduces skin blood flow and sweating. Conversely, if warmer blood is detected in the hypothalamus, inhibition of sympathetic response allows skin sweating and blood flow to increase, thereby reducing core temperature [21,22].

Adrenergic fibres mediate strong vasoconstriction and arrector pili muscle activity, thus diverting blood from the skin, and pulling hairs into the upright position, in the classical 'fight or flight' reaction [1].

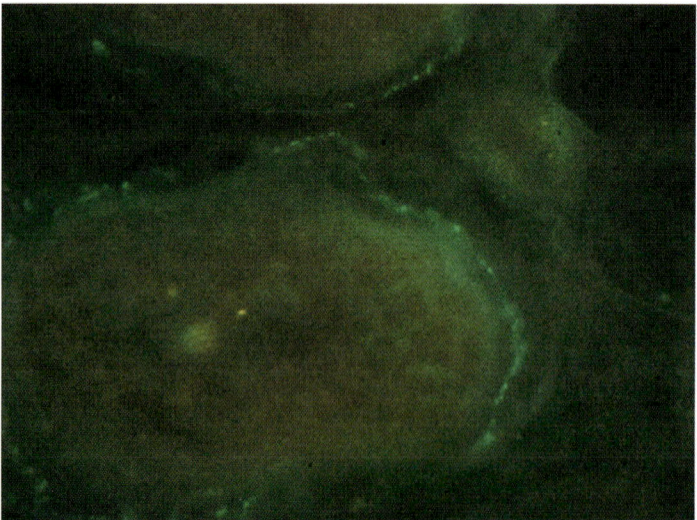

Figure 83.3 Vasoactive intestinal peptide immunoreactive fibres surround secretory cells of eccrine sweat glands.

The digital nerves in patients with Raynaud phenomenon and with systemic sclerosis are deficient in CGRP fibres [23]; intravenous infusions of CGRP increase digital blood flow in such patients. A similar depletion of CGRP fibres has been described in digital nerves of patients with vibration white finger, and this may be responsible for both the vasoconstriction and the sensory abnormalities characteristic of this condition [24].

Neurophysiological testing for skin innervation
Sympathetic skin response
Sympathetic skin response (SSR) is a safe, simple and non-invasive electrophysiological test used to evaluate sudomotor function in a variety of clinical settings [25–27]. It can be used to assess autonomic function in patients with suspected sympathetic nerve dysfunction. The SSR is a polysynaptic reflex associated with the activation of sweat glands. It is usually performed by electrical stimulation of the median, ulnar, peroneal or sural nerves, and measuring the change in galvanic resistance on glabrous skin brought about by sweating using a conventional electromyograph apparatus. The afferent component may be activated by non-specific sensory stimuli or repeated electrical stimulation; the efferent component depends on the functioning of the sympathetic cholinergic fibres from the sympathetic chain to the sweat glands. In autonomic failure the SSR cannot be elicited.

Cold-induced vasodilation
Hand cooling is a cold pressor test in which an extremity is placed in cold water, leading to a rapid decrease in skin temperature, accompanied by initial strong vasoconstriction aimed at limiting heat transfer to the environment [28–32]. After a few minutes, skin temperature starts increasing because of cold-induced vasodilation. The precise mechanism of this reflex is unknown, but it is thought to be mediated through an increase in sympathetic stimulation, although factors independent of the sympathetic nervous system may also play a role. Exposure of the human body to cold stress elicits generalised cutaneous vasoconstriction. This is a response mediated by a sympathetic control process, triggered partly by stimulation of cutaneous cold receptors and partly by cold blood returning to the general circulation and stimulating the temperature-regulating centre in the hypothalamus. The tone of cutaneous vessels is controlled mainly by vasoconstrictor skin sympathetic nerve activity. A reduction in this response has been reported in diabetic and neuropathic patients, and in the immature and elderly, probably resulting from reduced sympathetic nerve vasoconstriction in the skin [31,32].

Triple response of Lewis
Lewis described the capacity of the cutaneous microcirculation to vasodilate in response to direct stimulation with a firm mechanical stroke or with a dermographometer (the axon reflex) [32–34]. The amount of vasodilation can be measured by a Doppler flow meter. The axon reflex, known as 'antidromic vasodilation', does not occur in chronically denervated skin, or in skin in which neuropeptides have been depleted by capsaicin. The antidromic vasodilation and plasma extravasation, which occur in the skin following stimulation of the dorsal nerve roots or peripheral sensory nerves, can be mimicked by intra-arterial infusion of SP.

Histamine is known to be a principal mediator of the triple response of Lewis, and to act via H_1 and H_2 receptors to produce vasodilation and increased vascular permeability. However, it is known that SP, NKA and CGRP from primary sensory fibres are also mediators in the skin flares of the triple response of Lewis [35,36]. There is a bi-directional link between histamine and neuropeptides in neurogenic inflammation: neuropeptides induce the release of histamine from adjacent mast cells; and in turn, histamine evokes the release of SP and CGRP [37].

Skin biopsy as an aid to diagnosis of neurological disease and neuropathies
Skin biopsies can be useful to aid the diagnosis of various neurological conditions, although for diagnoses other than small fibre neuropathy it is becoming less important with advances in genetic testing using blood samples [1].

A discussion with the local histopathology department prior to the biopsy is important as only a limited number of departments provide this service. For example, in the UK, the national neuropathology referral centre is at King's College Hospital, London [2]. A 3 mm punch biopsy is recommended. The sample needs to be immediately immersed in periodate-lysine-paraformaldehyde fixative, which can be obtained in advance from the specialised laboratory. The sample should not remain in the fixative for more than 24 hours; immediate transport to the laboratory is important.

For the investigation of peripheral neuropathies, small-calibre sensory nerves, including somatic unmyelinated intraepidermal nerve fibres, dermal myelinated nerve fibres and autonomic nerve fibres, can be quantified and histologically assessed. To investigate a length-dependent process, a proximal biopsy 20 cm below the iliac spine on the leg can be compared to a distal biopsy 10 cm above the lateral malleolus [3].

The most used markers for nerve fibres are antibodies against PGP 95, which is a pan-axonal marker widely distributed throughout the PNS, but many other markers to specific components such as for example cytoskeleton or myelin are in use (Table 83.1).

Neuropathic pruritus and dysaesthesia
Dysaesthesia is defined as altered sensations in the skin without a primary skin disease. The abnormal sensory disturbance may be generalised but is usually localised and may be caused by organic neurological disease/injury originating in the CNS or PNS. Symptoms include itch, paraesthesia, burning, tingling, stinging, tickling, cold sensation and formication/crawling sensation. Itch may be provoked by stimuli that are not usually pruriceptive, i.e. do not ordinarily evoke itch, e.g. light touch; this is known as alloknesis. Increased itch can be perceived in response to a normal itch-evoking stimulus, hyperknesis. These two findings arise as part of itch sensitisation and are considered analogous to the pain-associated phenomena allodynia and hyperalgesia. A basic neurological history and examination are desirable specifically to assess for any red flags, e.g. objective signs of focal hypoaesthesia or anaesthesia, or motor signs and symptoms and sudden onset/rapid progression that would prompt referral to neurology. Imaging in individual cases may be requested. A combination of multilevel degenerative disc disease of the spine with associated spinal nerve root impingement, and/or nerve root traction, has been reported

Table 83.1 Antibodies and their targeted structures in skin biopsies [4].

Antibody	Target	Immunoreactive structures
Anti-PGP 9.5	Protein gene product 9.5	Axons
Anti-MBP	Myelin basic protein	Compact myelin
Anti-Col IV	Collagen type IV	Basal membrane, blood vessels
Anti-Nav[a]	Voltage-gated sodium channels	Node of Ranvier
Anti-Caspr	Contactin-associated protein	Paranodes
Anti-VIP	Vasoactive intestinal peptide	Autonomic cholinergic and adrenergic fibres (i.e. innervating sweat glands, hair follicles, AVAs, Merkel complexes)
Anti-DβH	Dopamine β-hydroxylase	Autonomic noradrenergic fibres (i.e. innervating arrector pili, AVAs)
Anti-sub P	Substance P	Peptidergic C fibres associated with Meissner corpuscles, NGF-dependent axons
Anti-CGRP	Calcitonin gene-related peptide	
Anti-S100	S100 protein	Schwann cells, myelinating or non-myelinating; Meissner corpuscle capsule
Anti-GAP43	Growth-associated protein 43	Primarily C fibres that are constantly remodelling
Anti-NF	Neurofilaments	Larger-diameter fibres (e.g. Aδ and Aβ)
Anti-TH	Tyrosine hydroxylase	Sympathetic C fibres innervating blood vessels and pilomotor muscles
Anti-p75	Low-affinity nerve growth factor receptor	Schwann cells

AVA, arteriovenous anastomoses; NGF, nerve growth factor.
[a] Pan sodium channel antibody stains all subtypes (e.g. 1.2 and 1.6–1.8 are found in peripheral nerves)

to possibly cause generalised symmetrical neuropathic pruritus (Box 83.2). The authors suggest the term 'multilevel symmetric neuropathic pruritus' for this subset of patients [2].

Box 83.2 Causes of neuropathic pruritus and dysaesthesia [1,2–7]

Peripheral nervous system
• Small fibre neuropathy
• Peripheral neuropathy
• Burning feet syndrome
• Erythromelalgia
• Radiculopathies
• Nerve entrapment syndromes
• Postherpetic neuralgia
• Trigeminal trophic syndrome
• Complex regional pain syndrome

Central nervous system
• Stroke disease
• Cortical atrophy
• Intracerebral haemorrhage
• Subarachnoid haemorrhage
• Dementia
• Parkinson disease
• Huntington disease
• Brain tumour
• Brain abscess
• Multiple sclerosis
• Neuromyelitis optica
• Motor neuron disease
• Spinal cord disease, e.g., syringomyelia, transverse myelitis, Brown–Sequard syndrome
• Degenerative spinal disc disease
• Meningitis
• Encephalitis
• HIV encephalopathy
• Prion disease
• Neurosyphilis

• Traumatic brain/spinal injury
• Post-traumatic epilepsy
• Normal pressure hydrocephalus
• Paraneoplastic (circulating neuropeptides)
• Iatrogenic, e.g. secondary to surgery

Nerve entrapment syndromes

When cutaneous sensory nerves are compressed, symptoms are produced which may lead to presentation to a dermatologist. There are several such cutaneous nerve entrapment syndromes.

Brachioradial pruritus

Brachioradial pruritus was first described in 1968 by Waiaman who termed it 'solar pruritus of the elbows' [1]. Patients present with itching and dysaesthesia (tingling, burning or stabbing sensations) localised to the proximal dorsolateral forearm without a primary skin change, which has been termed brachioradial pruritus. It can be intermittent, uni- or bilateral and may extend to the upper arm, shoulder, neck or upper trunk. Application of ice often eases symptoms ('ice-pack sign') [2].

The pathogenesis of brachioradial pruritus is not well understood. Current theories suggest cervical nerve root impingement at the levels of C5 to C8 as predisposing and solar radiation as an exacerbating factor [3].

Although most patients had primarily degenerative spinal joint abnormalities, neurological abnormalities were only found in a minority of these [3,4]. Therefore, it remains debatable if spinal imaging is of value [5]. Affected patients are often females of lighter skin types with significant cumulative UV exposure. Brachioradial pruritus frequently worsens during the summer. The subset of histamine sensitive C-fibres responsible for pruritus transmission is reduced and damaged by UV exposure causing alloknesis in affected patients, a pruritic response to a stimulus which would not normally cause pruritus [6]. There is evidence that excessive UV radiation causes damage to cutaneous nerve fibres similar to the histological changes seen after serial phototherapy and analagous to psoralen ultraviolet light A (PUVA) pain.

In rare cases of brachioradial pruritus associated with spinal tumours, additional sensory-motor symptoms are usually present [7].

Oral antihistamines rarely reduce the pruritus [8]. Treatment should start with UV protection. Topical application of capsaicin, corticosteroids, anaesthetics and antihistamines may help. Systemic treatment as for neuropathic pain with tricyclic antidepressants, antiepileptics and gabapentin can be tried but results are often disappointing with low efficacy and troublesome side effects. If a cervical spinal pathology is suspected then appropriate imaging is indicated, e.g. X-ray and magnetic resonance imaging (MRI). If imaging suggests cervical nerve impingement then the first line treatment should be cervical spine massage and exercises carried out by a physiotherapist or chiropractor.

Notalgia paraesthetica

Localised unilateral pruritus on the mid upper back medial of the scapular border is called notalgia paraesthetica (Greek 'notos' for back and 'algia' for pain). It is thought to arise from nerve entrapment of the posterior rami of the spinal nerves originating from T2 to T6 and mainly affects older women [9]. Rubbing and scratching may result in secondary skin changes such as lichenification, postinflammatory hyperpigmentation or amyloid deposition.

Physiotherapy and exercises can be tried initially [10]. Other treatment is as for brachio-radial pruritus, with gabapentin being most successful [11]. A small case series describes sustained improvement with narrow-band UVB and a 308 nm excimer lamp, applying a higher fluence to a more localised area [12,13]. The light might reduce the number of nerve fibres at the targeted area resulting in reduced pruritus.

Meralgia paraesthetica

Meralgia paraesthetica (Greek 'meros' for thigh and 'algia' for pain) is a relatively common [14] condition caused by compression of the lateral femoral cutaneous nerve [15]. This passes from the lumbar plexus through the abdominal cavity, under the inguinal ligament, where it is at risk of entrapment. Entrapment causes pain, numbness and altered sensation confined to the anterolateral thigh.

Risk factors include [16]:
- Obesity, large abdominal apron [17,18]
- Pregnancy [19,20]
- Diabetes
- Older age
- Ascites causing intra-abdominal pressure
- Tight belts or waistbands or other external pressure [15,21]
- Long-distance walking, cycling or circuit training, possibly related to local ischaemia during repetitive muscle stretching [22,23]
- Groin trauma
- Avulsion fracture of anterior superior iliac spine
- Local or regional surgery, e.g. after caesarean section, hysterectomy or laparoscopic inguinal hernia repair [24].

Examination may find:
- Loss of light touch and/or pinprick sensation in a small area on the upper lateral thigh.
- Pain or dysaesthesia on tapping the lateral aspect of the inguinal ligament (Tinel's sign).
- The pelvic compression test by relaxing pressure on the lateral cutaneous nerve may temporarily mitigate symptoms and can be used as a pointer towards the diagnosis.
- Negative straight leg test.

Imaging can be performed to exclude lumbar nerve root compression, e.g. if distribution is dermatomal.

Meralgia paraesthetica is usually self-limiting, but may recur. Reduction of pressure over the groin area should be advised as well as weight loss in obese patients [25]. Manual therapy and exercise have been reported to help during pregnancy. Treatment options included topical capsaicin or lignocaine, oral tricyclics, gabapentin and injection with lignocaine, with or without corticosteroids, around the nerve where it passes under the inguinal ligament [26,27].

Pulsed radiofrequency nerve ablation or surgical neurectomy of the lateral femoral cutaneous nerve may give permanent pain relief, but results in permanent loss of sensation [28–30].

Ilioinguinal, iliohypogastric, genitofemoral or pudendal neuropathic pain/neuralgia and dysaesthesia

Vulval, scrotal or penile dysaesthesia and pain may be due to ilioinguinal, iliohypogastric, genitofemoral or pudendal neuralgia. This may be due to idiopathic entrapment or secondary to physical trauma, e.g. injury, surgery, pregnancy and obesity. Symptoms include a sensation of burning, heat, irritation, discomfort, pain or increased sensitivity to touch/allodynia [31–33] and pain, dysaesthesia, hair loss and trophic changes in the distribution of the respective nerve – superior to the mons pubis, the anterior surface of the scrotum and root of the penis in males or labia majora and mons pubis in females, as well as lower abdomen and thighs, inguinal, pubic and gluteal regions, and the abdominal muscles.

Symptoms are aggravated by stretching of the respective nerve, coughing/sneezing and the Valsalva manoeuvre. Examination may reveal trigger points, which cause lancinating pain when touched. Painful pressure points suggest the diagnosis:
- Iliohypogastric nerve – tenderness above the midpoint of the inguinal ligament.
- Ilioinguinal nerve – tenderness 2.5 cm medial and inferior to the anterior superior iliac spine.
- Pudendal nerve – depending on entrapment site, tenderness medial to the ischium, the greater sciatic notch, the piriformis or the obturator internus muscle. Intrapelvic entrapment results in vaginal or rectal pressure points.
- Genitofemoral neuralgia – lumbar extension provokes pain; patients may adopt a bent-over posture to alleviate it.

The diagnosis can be confirmed if a regional nerve block results in resolution of the symptoms and in such cases, neurectomy can be considered. More than 90% of patients had resolution of pain after neurectomy of the involved nerve [31]. Postoperative side effects were persistent numbness below the resected nerve.

Pudendal neuralgia

The pudendal nerve is formed from branches of the sacral nerves S2–S4 and can become entrapped at several points during its course through the pelvis and obturator internus muscle resulting in ulvodynia, penoscrotodynia, dyspareunia with pain, numbness and erectile dysfunction and urinary symptoms [34]. It can be caused by pelvic surgery, pelvic tumours, pelvic radiation, trauma to buttocks or back, after childbirth, chronic constipation, excessive cycling and prolonged sitting [35].

The diagnosis is made clinically. Imaging with a pelvic and lumbosacral X-ray ± MRI pelvis can be done to exclude an underlying cause if suspected. Routine electroneuromyographic studies are not recommended [36]. Diagnostic criteria have been been proposed (Nantes criteria) [37] but need further validation:

1 Pain in the area innervated by the pudendal nerve (e.g. ipsilateral clitoris/penis, distal urethra, labia/scrotum, perineum and anus).
2 Pain increased by sitting.
3 Patient is not awakened by pain.
4 No sensory loss on clinical examination (sensory deficits are suggestive of a sacral nerve root lesion).
5 Resolution of pain with pudendal nerve block.

The differential diagnosis is idiopathic/functional scrotodynia and vulvodynia (Chapters 109 and 110).

Pudendal neuralgia may also cause male impotence, persistent arousal, sphincter dysfunction (associated with a defective reflex on defecation, faecal incontinence or urinary hesitancy) and a foreign-body sensation in the anus, rectum, urethra or vagina.

Ultrasound examination can sometimes reveal nerve entrapment. An MRI of the lumbosacral spine can exclude lumbar radiculopathies. Response to an ultrasound-, fluoroscopy- or CT-guided nerve block can confirm the diagnosis. The benefit of electrophysiological examination is questionable as sensory deficit is usually not captured.

Lifestyle modification to avoid painful stimuli is most important. The mainstay of management is physical therapy including pelvic floor exercises, stretches and lumbosacral physiotherapy. Pelvic floor physical therapy works by releasing spasms and lengthening muscles. Medication used includes analgesics, muscle relaxants, antidepressants and anticonvulsants such as gabapentin and pregabalin. Treatment options include nerve blocks, non-steroidal anti-inflammatories (NSAIDs), cryotherapy and neurectomy. In other conditions with neuropathic pain, medications including tricyclic antidepressants and venlafaxine may give some relief [38].

An area encircling the respective nerves can be infiltrated with local anaesthetic or steroid (nerve block) either 'blind', i.e. unguided, or with the aid of ultrasonography, fluoroscopy or CT. Surgical decompression is considered the best treatment for nerve entrapment and can in some cases can be done laparoscopically [39,40]. Other surgical options include neurectomy and dorsal root gangliotomy.

Neuromodulation with minimally invasive transforaminal sacral neurostimulation and pulsed radiofrequency are new, promising treatments [41,42].

Peripheral neuropathy

Peripheral polyneuropathy is common, affecting 8% of the population over 55. It may be sensory, motor or mixed [1]. The majority of patients have a typical distal 'glove and stocking' symmetrical sensory loss with depressed or absent tendon reflexes and associated acquired toxic or metabolic medical conditions such as diabetes, monoclonal gammopathy and chronic renal failure [2]. In contrast, patchy involvement of peripheral nerves known as mononeuritis multiplex is seen with conditions like polyarteritis nodosa and sarcoidosis.

The predominant fibre type affected is large myelinated nerve fibres, and in general pain is not a prominent symptom. Large fibres involved may include joint position and vibration sense, promoting alteration of gait due to sensory ataxia. Significant weakness is less typical and will prompt urgent neurology referral for further investigation.

Symptoms and signs reflect the underlying neuropathology and nerves involved. Referral to neurology is recommended when onset is acute, and there is asymmetry, non-length-dependent weakness and/or sensory loss, diffuse areflexia, pure or predominant motor symptoms, pure or predominant autonomic symptoms, and mononeuropathy multiplex. Typical clinical features are listed in Box 83.3 [3].

Box 83.3 Clinical features in sensory and motor polyneuropathy [1]

Early symptoms
- Distal numbness and paraesthesia/tingling
- Distal neuropathic pain
- Gait imbalance
- Toe weakness

Later symptoms
- Progression of numbness and tingling to proximal body parts
- Prominent neuropathic pain
- Tripping easily
- Worsening of gait
  - Frequent falls

Early signs
- Distal sensory loss to cold, pinprick and/or vibration
  - Reduced or lost ankle reflex
  - Romberg sign
- Impaired tandem walking
- Toe extensor weakness

Later signs
- Distal loss of cold, pinprick, vibration and joint position sense
- Areflexia at ankles and knees
  - Foot drop
- Inability to toe-and-heel walk

Many different aetiologies have been identified. Box 83.4 lists some common causes of distal symmetrical polyneuropathy. A stepwise approach to the evaluation and work-up of peripheral neuropathy is needed. Pattern recognition of various neuropathies can help to build a differential diagnosis based on the presentation. Such patterns include acute versus chronic, primary demyelinating versus axonal, hereditary versus acquired, asymmetrical versus symmetrical, presence of facial palsies, sensory or motor predominant, and presence of prominent autonomic symptoms [4]. Early categorisation of the type of neuropathy can help focus the work-up. Nerve conduction studies and electromyography are the primary diagnostic tools in the evaluation of patients with large fibre polyneuropathy. The finding of a primary demyelinating polyneuropathy narrows the differential diagnosis of polyneuropathy significantly and increases the chances of finding a treatable cause. Laboratory work-up includes a complete blood count, comprehensive metabolic panel, thyroid stimulating hormone, vitamin B_{12}, HbA1c, methylmalonic acid, serum protein electrophoresis, and potentially cerebrospinal fluid, genetic studies and immunological markers. Skin biopsy may be used to assess intraepidermal nerve fibre density if small fibre neuropathy is suspected, and nerve biopsy may be useful in select cases. A fat pad biopsy can be done in individual patients to look for amyloidosis. In recent years, MRI and neuromuscular ultrasound have also shown promise in the evaluation of peripheral neuropathy. Identification of the aetiology of neuropathy is crucial and often time-sensitive, as an increasing number of causes are now reversible or treatable.

Box 83.4 Common causes of distal symmetrical polyneuropathy

- Autoimmune/inflammatory – connective tissue disease, vasculitis, inflammatory bowel disease, sarcoidosis, primary systemic amyloidosis, primary biliary cholangitis, critical illness
- Neoplastic – paraneoplastic neuropathy, myeloma, Waldenstrom macroglobulinaemia, monoclonal gammopathy of uncertain significance (MGUS), lymphoma
- Endocrine/metabolic – diabetes, thyroid disease, chronic renal failure, liver disease, porphyria
- Infectious – HIV, HTLV-1, leprosy, diphtheria, mumps, Guillain-Barré syndrome, Lyme disease
- Inherited/genetic – Charcot–Marie–Tooth (CMT) disease, familial amyloidosis, Refsum disease, hereditary sensory and autonomic neuropathy (HSAN), Fabry disease, Roussy–Levy syndrome, metachromatic leukodystrophy
- Nutritional – deficiency of vitamins B_1, B_6, B_{12} and E, vitamin B_6 toxicity, copper deficiency, postgastric bypass, malabsorption syndrome including coeliac disease
- Toxic – alcohol, heavy metals, organic solvents
- Medications – chemotherapy, amiodarone, chloroquine, colchicine, dapsone, disulfiram, ethambutol, hydralazine, isoniazid, leflunomide, metronidazole, nitrofurantoin, nucleoside reverse transcriptase inhibitors, phenytoin
- Trauma – pressure neuropathy, ischaemia, pressure from tumours, electric shock

---

Small fibre neuropathy (SFN) is common and can be associated with many medical conditions (Box 83.5) [5]. Most patients with SFN suffer from painful paraesthesia which can negatively impact their quality of life. Patients with length-dependent small fibre

neuropathy promoting pain in the peripheries will usually have some large fibre involvement detectable on examination.

Box 83.5 Conditions associated with small fibre neuropathy

Hereditary
- Amyloidosis
- Hereditary sensory neuropathy I (HSAN I)
  - IA: *SPTLC1* gene
  - IC: *SPTLC2* gene
- Insensitivity to pain
  - Congenital insensitivity to pain sensation
    - Without anhidrosis
    - With reduced hidrosis: *PRDM12* gene
  - Congenital sensory neuropathy with anhidrosis (HSAN4)
  - Hereditary sensory neuropathy with loss of pain perception (HSAN5)
  - Congenital absence of pain perception (HSAN7)
- Hereditary ataxia with thermoanalgesia and loss of fungiform papillae
- An-α-lipoproteinaemia (Tangier)
- α-Galactosidase (Fabry's)
- Pain syndromes
  - *SCN9A* (Na$_v$1.7) gene mutations: erythromelalgia
  - *SCN10A* gene
  - *SCN11A* gene
- Hereditary sensory neuropathy and spastic paraparesis (Cavanagh variant)
- Sensory neuropathy, and deafness-dystonia and ichthyosis: *FITM2* gene
- Congenital indifference to pain
- Navajo neuropathy with arthropathy
- Cold-induced sweating
- Sensory and autonomic neuropathy with chronic diarrhoea: *PRNP* gene

Metabolic
- Diabetes mellitus: not pre-diabetes
- Hypertriglyceridaemia

Toxic
- Kepone; ciguatera

Infection
- Leprosy

Immune
- FGFR3 antibodies
- TS-HDS antibodies
- M-proteins

Idiopathic: often painful
- Burning mouth
- Fibromyalgia
- Fatigue syndromes

CNS disorders that may have loss of small skin axons
- Parkinson disease
- α-Synucleinopathies: rapid eye movement (REM) sleep behaviour disorder (RBD)
- Amyotrophic lateral sclerosis

Skin biopsy with intraepidermal nerve fibre density evaluation is the gold standard diagnostic test. Autonomic function testing is useful when autonomic symptoms are present. Screening for associated conditions should be done in every patient, even when a known underlying associated condition is present. Aetiology-specific treatment, lifestyle modification and pain control are the key elements of management in SFN.

Burning feet and restless leg syndromes

Definition and nomenclature

Burning feet syndrome (BFS) is characterised by a burning and aching sensation of the feet (hyperaesthesia), accompanied by vasomotor changes causing excessive sweating.

BFS often arises in association with restless leg syndrome (RLS) which is characterised by an uncomfortable twitching sensation in the leg muscles when sitting or lying down, which is only relieved by moving the legs.

Synonyms and inclusions

- Grierson–Gopalan syndrome
- Willis–Ekbom disease (RLS)

Introduction and general description

RLS is a common sleep and movement disorder. It is characterised by leg paraesthesia accompanied by an irresistible, uncomfortable urge, occurring at rest, to move the legs. Movement of the legs or getting up to walk gives relief. Symptoms tend to be worse at night. RLS may be primary (idiopathic) or secondary to pregnancy or a variety of systemic disorders, especially iron deficiency and chronic renal insufficiency. Genetic predisposition with a family history is common. RLS significantly impacts patients' quality of life and remains a therapeutic area sorely in need of innovation and new, biologically informed therapies.

BFS is a poorly recognised and underdiagnosed condition consisting of a burning sensation of the feet which is accentuated by heat or cold [1]. Associated autonomic features include dry skin, eyes and mouth, and vasomotor symptoms with peripheral coldness, burning or flushing, hypertension and impotence [1].

Epidemiology
Incidence and prevalence
One population study estimated 7.2% to have had RLS symptoms at least weekly during the preceding year; 2.7% reported moderately or severely distressing RLS symptoms at least twice-weekly [2].

Age
The conditions appear on average between the ages of 30 and 40 years.

Sex
F > M.

Predisposing factors
- Diabetes
- Chronic kidney disease (uraemia)
- Haemodialysis
- Pregnancy
- Vitamin deficiency (B_{12} and occasionally B_6)
- Iron deficiency
- Alcohol abuse
- Hypothyroidism
- Lyme disease
- HIV/AIDS
- Amyloid polyneuropathy
- Medication side effects, including chemotherapy, vitamin B_6 overdose, HIV medicines, isoniazid, amiodarone, metformin and others
- Heavy metal poisoning (lead, mercury, arsenic)
- Vasculitis
- Sarcoidosis
- Guillain–Barré syndrome
- Arterial disease
- Hypertension

Pathophysiology
RLS is a clinically pleomorphic syndrome, probably reflecting multiple genetic and acquired factors. It may represent a subclinical sensory neuropathy [3]. The pathogenesis of RLS remains unclear but is likely to involve CNS dopaminergic dysfunction, as well as other, undefined contributing mechanisms. Dopamine imbalance is implicated due to the presence of dyskinetic movements and response to levodopa. Basal ganglia studies using positron emission tomography (PET) scanning have shown decreased binding of dopamine to its receptor, and involvement of the endogenous opioid system has recently been implicated [1]. Up to 30% of patients have iron deficiency [4]. RLS is common in haemodialysis patients [4] and associations have been noted with pregnancy, fibromyalgia, rheumatoid arthritis and multiple sclerosis [1].

Loss of small fibre sensory nerves has been found both in type II diabetics [1] and idiopathic cases. Tests on the autonomic system have shown predominantly cholinergic defects, unlike with other autonomic neuropathies. There is a close correlation between quantitative abnormalities in the sudomotor axon reflex test and the loss of small nerve fibres in the skin.

Genetics
There is a link between RLS and chromosome 12q [5]. A familial form of BFS has been described [6] and there are BFS families with autosomal dominant inheritance [7].

Clinical features
Presentation
The main clinical features of BFS are a burning sensation on the feet, accentuated by heat or cold. Associated autonomic features often accompany foot dysaesthesia, including dry skin, dry eyes and mouth, vasomotor symptoms with peripheral coldness, burning or flushing, hypertension and impotence [1].

RLS is characterised by paraesthesiae of the legs associated with an irresistible urge, occurring at rest, to move the legs. Movement of the legs provides relief [1]. Symptoms are worse at night – with both circadian rhythms and recumbency playing a role [1] – and often lead to disruption of normal life and chronic sleep deprivation. Children may struggle at school and display symptoms of attention deficit hyperactivity disorder (ADHD) [1].

Two subtypes of RLS are recognised. The first, with early onset, accounts for some 25% of cases, is often familial, and is associated with a childhood history of 'growing pains' [8]. The second (idiopathic RLS) lacks a family history, and has a late onset with milder paraesthesiae or dysaesthesia, and insomnia.

Sensory symptoms include painful legs and arms, and pain at 'internal' sites. Many patients with RLS have been diagnosed with a musculoskeletal disorder, such as joint and back pains. In RLS, there is a significant association with depression and other neuropsychiatric symptoms [1,2]. Morning and daytime headaches occur frequently, and hypertension and heart problems have been reported in men.

The International Restless Leg Syndrome Study Group rating scale (the international restless legs severity scale (IRLS)) is a validated measure for the presence and severity of RLS. All four essential criteria must be present for a positive diagnosis [9]:

- An urge to move the legs, usually with uncomfortable or unpleasant sensations.
- Unpleasant sensations or urges to move beginning or worsening during rest or inactivity.
- Unpleasant sensations or urges to move, partly or totally relieved by movement such as walking, bending, stretching, etc., at least during the activity.
- Unpleasant sensations or urges to move, worse (or exclusively) in the evening or night-time.

A recent fifth criterion stipulates that the four criteria must not be solely explained by another medical or behavioural condition [10].

Augmentation may occur and is characterised by more intense symptom severity, earlier symptom occurrence and often symptom spread from the legs to the arms or other body regions.

Differential diagnosis
Burning feet syndrome:
- Peripheral neuropathy
- Erythromelalgia
  Restless legs syndrome:
- Peripheral neuropathy
- Parkinsonism
- Nocturnal leg cramps
- Peripheral vascular disease
- ADHD in children

Investigations
Exclude peripheral neuropathy. Iron stores, including ferritin and transferrin saturation.

Management
Some people with RLS have adequate symptom control with non-pharmacological measures such as massage or tepid baths. First line management options include oral iron-replacement therapy in those with evidence of reduced body-iron stores; or gabapentin [4], pregabalin and dopamine agonists such as pramipexole, ropinirole

and rotigotine (can be complicated by augmentation, an iatrogenic effect whereby symptoms worsen with time [10]). Second line therapies include intravenous iron infusion in those who are intolerant of oral iron and/or those having augmentation with intense, severe RLS symptoms, and opioids including tramadol, oxycodone and methadone [**11**]. Levodopa is efficacious in the short-term treatment of RLS [12]. In some cases, benzodiazepines (clonazepam or diazepam) can be effective [10].

Treatment ladder for burning feet and restless leg syndromes

First line
- Sleep hygiene
- Tepid baths
- Iron replacement therapy
- Gabapentin or pregabalin

Second line
- Levodopa
- Dopamine agonists

Third line
- Opioids
- Benzodiazepines

Resources

Patient resources

Restless Legs Syndrome. National Institute of Neurological Disorders and Stroke. https://www.ninds.nih.gov/health-information/disorders/restless-legs-syndrome (last accessed November 2023).

HEREDITARY NEUROPATHIES

Hereditary neuropathies encompass a wide spectrum of disorders of the PNS that recognise all types of Mendelian and mitochondrial inheritance and may manifest from early infancy to late adulthood. Causative genetic defects and altered molecular pathways are extremely heterogeneous.

Two groups of hereditary neuropathies may be distinguished.

1 The molecular defects affect the PNS selectively so that the peripheral neuropathy is the unique or main constituent; this group includes Charcot–Marie–Tooth disease (CMT) and CMT-related neuropathies.
2 The second group encompasses 'complex hereditary neuropathies' that occur in multisystem disorders affecting both the PNS and the CNS and/or other organs and tissues; in these syndromes, the peripheral neuropathy may be a key heralding feature or may represent a minor component.

Hereditary neuropathies may result from mutations in genes expressed by Schwann cells or neurons that selectively affect the

PNS or may represent a minor or major component of complex inherited diseases that also involve the CNS and/or other organs and tissues. Advances of molecular genetics and next-generation sequencing continue to identify new genes and are revolutionising the diagnostic approach. In the past, diagnostic sural nerve biopsies helped in the discovery and elucidation of major genes and molecular pathways associated to most frequent hereditary motor–sensory neuropathies. A sural nerve biopsy may prove useful in selected cases for the differential diagnosis of an acquired neuropathy when clinical examination, nerve conduction studies and molecular tests are not sufficiently informative. Skin biopsy has emerged as a minimally invasive window to the PNS, which may provide biomarkers of progression and clues to the physiopathology and molecular pathology of inherited neuropathies.

Hereditary sensory and autonomic neuropathies (HSANs)

Definition and nomenclature
The HSANs encompass several rare, inherited disorders associated with sensory dysfunction (depressed reflexes, altered pain and temperature perception) and varying degrees of autonomic dysfunction (gastro-oesophageal reflux, postural hypotension, excessive sweating) [1]. As a group, HSAN is a spectrum of diseases affecting both sexes and tending to occur in families with parental consanguinity [1,2].

The classification of HSANs was modified by Dyck into five main groups of syndromes, each with a common clinical, pathophysiological and genetic phenotype [2].

Original five types of HSAN
- HSAN type I (HSAN I): Thévenard disease
- HSAN type II (HSAN II): Riley–Day syndrome
- HSAN type III (HSAN III): familial dysautonomia
- HSAN type IV (HSAN IV)
- HSAN type V (HSAN V)

For the dermatologist, a HSAN will usually be encountered in a patient with disordered sweating accompanied by severe sensory dysfunction. Advances have been made in identifying the specific loci and genes implicated in the different types of HSANs and the resulting disease mechanisms and this complex field continues to evolve; there is an excellent regularly updated online database developed by the Neuromuscular Disease Centre, Washington University, USA [3].

Diagnosis is based on clinical findings and molecular genetic testing of the mutated gene to determine the specific HSAN. Electrophysiology and neural histopathology are also useful [4]. A skin biopsy may be useful in individual cases – liaison with a neurologist and specialised neuropathology services is needed.

Management
Management of affected individuals involves trying to control the ambient temperature to help counter problems associated with sweating dysfunction. Protective aids can be used to reduce self-mutilation injuries. When necessary, wound care and antiseptic treatment should be initiated. A greasy emollient applied regularly to the skin of neuropathic limbs may moderate callus formation.

Resources

http://www.ncbi.nlm.nih.gov/books/NBK49247/
http://www.ncbi.nlm.nih.gov/books/NBK1769/
For HSAN II, III and IV http://www.ojrd.com/content/2/1/39
(All last accessed November 2023)

Midface toddler excoriation syndrome (MiTES) due to pain insensitivity

Midface toddler excoriation syndrome (MiTES) was first reported in 2017 in three unrelated children [1]. There have been a total of 15 patients described to date [2].

Introduction and general description
Habitual scratching of the face, especially the forehead, nose, inner canthi, perinasal and perioral regions and the chin, from the first year of life results in deep, chronic self-inflicted wounds in various stages of healing, breakdown and secondary atrophic scarring with postinflammatory hyperpigmentation. Physical examination is usually otherwise normal. A mild neurological deficit has been described in one child, a high pain threshold in one, a history of seizures in another and other sensory deficits in one study of five siblings from a consanguineous Irish family. Homozygous or compound heterozygous pathogenic expansion of the *PRDM12* polyalanine tract has been found, a gene also linked to hereditary sensory and autonomic neuropathy type VIII (HSAN8) [3].

Differential diagnosis
Blistering disease, vasculitis, infections and self-mutilation due to neurometabolic disease can usually be excluded on clinical and histological grounds. A severe photodermatosis can have similar appearances. Trigeminal trophic syndrome has a unilateral distribution. Factitious disease and non-accidental injury have to be considered. HSAN8 is characterised by mutilating self-inflicted wounds of the extremities, lips and tongue, but MiTES shows little or no evidence of generalised pain insensitivity. However, the condition is probably genetically heterogeneous, and other congenital insensitivity to pain and HSAN genes such as *SCN11A* may be implicated [4].

Complications and co-morbidities
Mild neurological deficit and other sensory deficits have been described in some but not all patients.

Investigations
The diagnosis is usually made clinically. In seven out of eight cases in one study, iron deficiency anaemia and thrombocytosis

were present, although it was unclear if these were related to MiTES [3]. Additional tests include MRI of the brain, lupus serology, porphyrins, and skin biopsy for histology and microbial culture. Sensory nerve conduction was abnormal in those tested; sural nerve biopsy of two patients showed a severe loss of small, myelinated A-delta fibres, whereas large-calibre axons were unaltered. Skin biopsies of two patients showed abnormal peripheral terminals of C fibres, with complete absence of nerve fibres crossing the basement membrane to innervate the epidermis. The subepidermal neural plexus and autonomic innervation of sweat glands were also reduced but were morphologically normal. The findings were consistent with developmental defects in the sensory neurons destined to become nociceptors. Autonomic neurophysiological testing and nerve conduction studies may require a general anaesthetic in young children.

Management
Treatment is largely supportive.

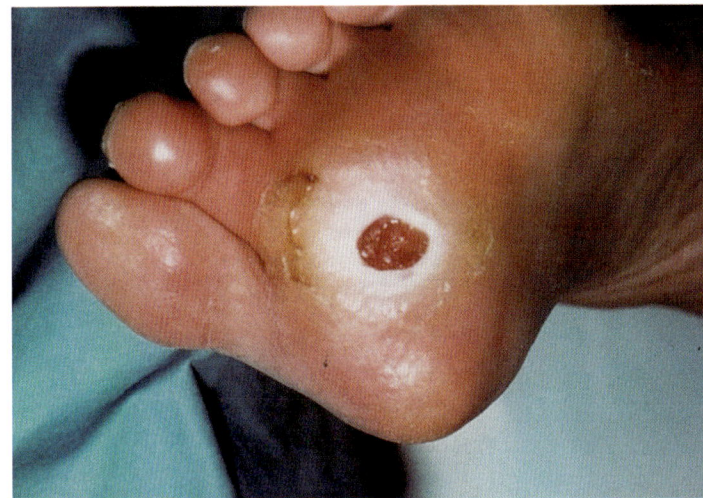

Figure 83.5 Typical neuropathic ulcers with surrounding hyperkeratosis under metatarsal heads.

Neuropathic ulcer

Definition and nomenclature
A neuropathic ulcer is a form of chronic ulceration which develops in anaesthetic skin. Characteristically, neuropathic ulcers are painless, persistent and uninflamed, appearing on areas subject to trauma or pressure although this is often unrecognised.

Introduction and general description
A neuropathic ulcer arises in an area of anaesthetic or hypoaesthetic skin and is typically painless with well-defined margins surrounding the wound. Neuropathic ulcers usually occur on weight-bearing body surfaces such as the heels and metatarsal heads.

The underlying neuropathology is commonly a distal polyneuropathy encompassing motor, sensory and autonomic components: the vast majority of neuropathic ulcers occur in patients with type II diabetes [1,2]. Other causes include peripheral nerve injury, peripheral neuropathy, renal failure, alcoholism, vitamin deficiencies, leprosy, pernicious anaemia, syringomyelia, tabes dorsalis, spinal dysraphism, spinal cord injury, and hereditary sensory and autonomic neuropathies (HSANs) [3,4].

Epidemiology
Incidence and prevalence
Of people with diabetes, 25% develop foot ulcers at some point in their lives [5]. The annual incidence of diabetic foot ulcers is ~3%, and the reported incidence in the US and UK studies is as high as 10% [6]. As the incidence of diabetes increases, so does the incidence of diabetic foot ulcers.

Pathophysiology
The major underlying factors in the development of ulcers are peripheral neuropathy and ischaemia secondary to peripheral vascular disease. In diabetic patients, hyperglycaemia leads to a complex of abnormal enzyme activity which results in a decrease in normal neuron conduction as well as nerve dysfunction and ischaemia, causing further injury to, and eventual death of, nerve cells [7].

As patients experience sensory loss, trauma to the affected site often goes unnoticed, and progressively worsens as the area is continuously subjected to repetitive pressure and shear forces.

Clinical features
Neuropathic ulcers typically occur on the foot, under the metatarsal heads or on the heel. They tend to be surrounded by thick hyperkeratosis and have a pink punched-out base that bleeds easily and is painless (Figures 83.5 and 83.6). The changes of a neuropathic foot include pes cavus and clawed toes (Figure 83.7). The foot tends to be anaesthetic, and warm with palpable pulses and dilated veins. The skin is dry and hyperkeratotic under the forefoot and heel. Primary neuropathic limbs tend to be warm, insensitive and prone to ulceration on the sole, while neuro-ischaemic limbs are usually cool, discoloured and prone to ulceration on the foot margins [2]. In diabetics, there may be a complex interplay of neuropathy and ischaemia, and when the latter is present, the foot may be cold with absent pulses, hyperkeratosis and a dark fibrotic base that does not bleed easily and is painful to touch. Continuing mechanical overload on established callus can result in fissures, increasing the risk of future ulcer formation [8].

The diagnosis is usually straightforward but arterial, venous and pressure ulcers must also be considered in the differential diagnosis. Other potential mimics of a neuropathic ulcer include pyoderma gangrenosum, amelanotic melanoma and Marjolin ulcer. In cases of clinical uncertainty, a biopsy is indicated.

When evaluating a neuropathic ulcer, it is important to screen for and assess co-morbidities which may contribute to wound evolution and/or delay wound healing. Work-up should include history including social history, smoking and alcohol use, clinical examination, baseline laboratory investigations (full blood count, urea, creatinine and electrolytes, C-reactive protein, albumin, HbA1C), nutrition evaluation and vascular assessment. On initial

PART 7: PSYCHOLOGICAL, SENSORY & NEUROLOGICAL

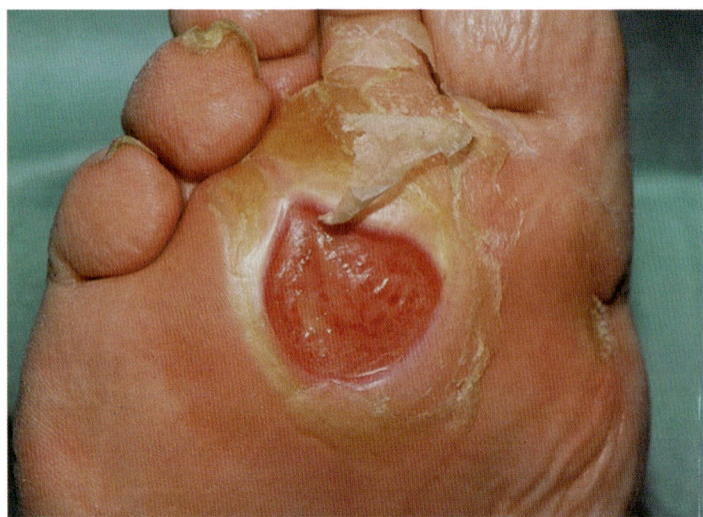

Figure 83.6 Neuropathic ulcer with hyperkeratosis removed.

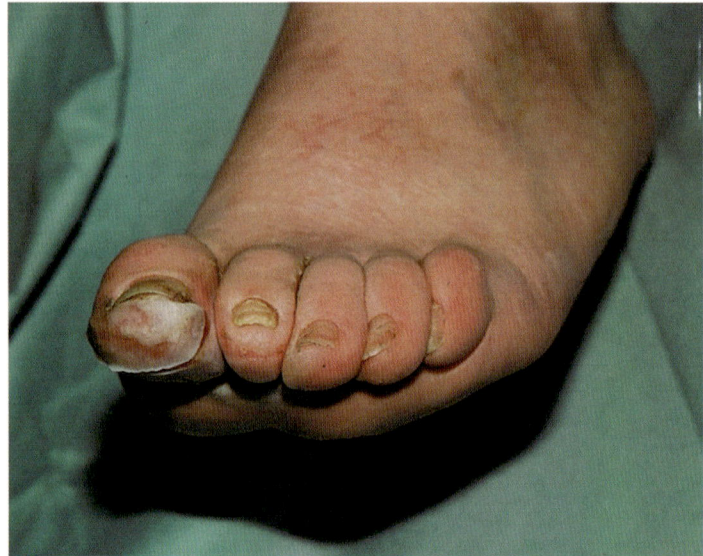

Figure 83.7 Clawing of feet occurring in neuropathic foot with painless damage to the skin on the great toe.

assessment and at follow-up, measurements and photographs of the ulcer should be taken.

Classification of severity

A well-established system is the Wagner ulcer classification (Table 83.2) to help standardise assessment, although infection and ischaemia are not considered [7].

The wound classification developed by the International Consensus of the Diabetic Foot assesses patients for ischaemia, neuropathy, linear measurement of wound diameters, depth of wound and infection [10]. The SINBAD classification (**S**ite, forefoot versus mid or hindfoot; **I**schaemia, ≥1 pedal pulse palpable versus clinical decreased pedal circulation; **N**europathy, protective sensation intact versus loss of protective sensation; **B**acterial infection, Y/N; **A**rea, < or >1 cm²; **D**epth, confined to skin/subcutis versus to muscle versus tendon or deeper tissue), is considered is a more detailed 6-point grading system and is recommended as the universal system

Table 83.2 Wagner foot ulcer classification [9].

Ulcer grade	Lesion description
0	Foot deformity or redness of skin, no erosions/ulceration
1	Superficial erosion
2	Deep ulcer involving tendon or joint capsule
3	Deep ulcer with drainage, joint sepsis or osteomyelitis
4	Local gangrene, involving forefoot or heel
5	Gangrene of foot

for clinicians to use in assessment and monitoring of neuropathic ulcers and recommended by the International Working Group on the Diabetic Foot (IWGDF) [11].

Complications and co-morbidities

A frequent complication is the presence of cellulitis or deep infection, with abscess formation or osteomyelitis. One study found that Gram-positive aerobic bacterial colonisation predominates (84%), with *Staphylococcus aureus* being the commonest organism (79%). Meticillin-resistant *Staphylococcus aureus* (MRSA) was isolated in 30% of patients, a near twofold increase over the previous 3 years [12]. Bacterial colonisation of the ulcer does not necessarily indicate infection. By contrast, infection may be present, especially in diabetics, without pyrexia. Leukocytosis, elevated erythrocyte sedimentation rate (ESR) and local signs may be less than expected. Cellulitis should alert one to the possibility of underlying osteomyelitis. Neuropathic ulcers are a leading cause of non-traumatic limb amputation in *c*.15% of individuals [13].

Investigations

In neuropathic ulcers, the reduced sensations of light touch and vibration, and sharp–blunt discrimination, can be demonstrated using a Bailey® nylon monofilament (which buckles in response to a 10 g force) (Figure 83.8), a neurothesiometer and a Neurotip®, respectively [14].

Palpable bone at the base of an ulcer on wound probing is an excellent predictor of osteomyelitis [15] (Figure 83.9). Plain X-rays may show periosteal reactions or osteolysis, and will also identify foreign bodies, tissue gas or bony abnormalities. A sinogram may be required to show communication of the sinus with a joint or a subfascial plantar abscess. A radioisotope bone scan, MRI scan or bone biopsy may help with the diagnosis [16].

Management

Neuropathic ulcers are often difficult to heal; management requires an integrated care approach from a multidisciplinary foot care team with the engagement of patients and carers, which can reduce amputations by up to 70% [17].

Prevention of ulceration is of the utmost importance. The risk of developing neuropathic ulcer can be stratified. If there is no loss of protective sensation (LOPS) or peripheral arterial disease (PAD) then ulcer risk is very low and annual assessment is indicated. In contrast, patients with a high ulcer risk have LOPS or PAD and a history of at least one foot ulcer, lower extremity amputation and end-stage renal disease merit follow-up every 1–3 months. It is important to review the residential environment for safety.

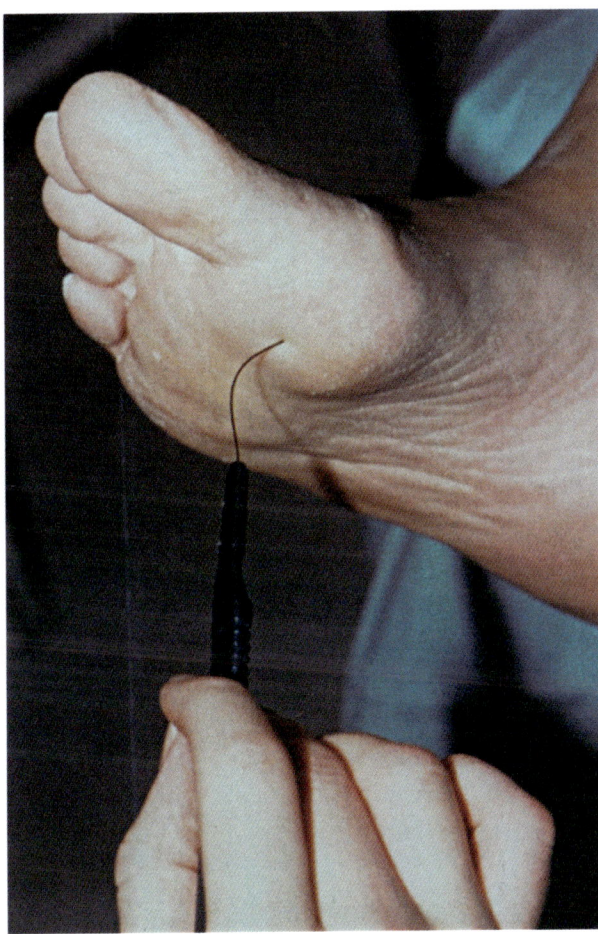

Figure 83.8 Bailey® nylon monofilament assessing sensory loss on neuropathic foot.

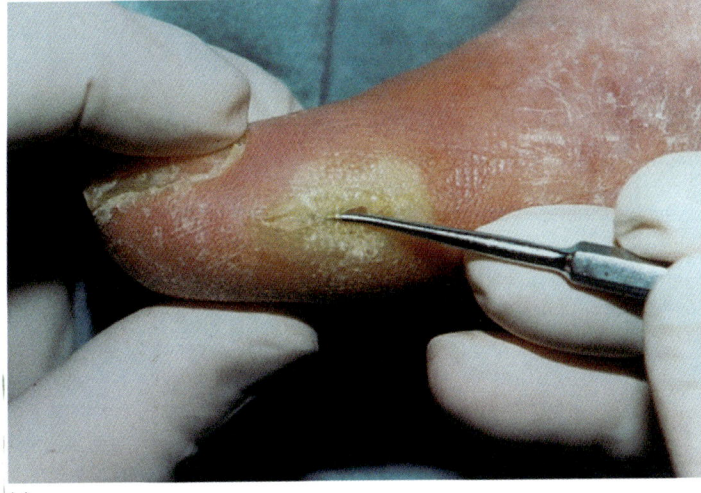

(a)

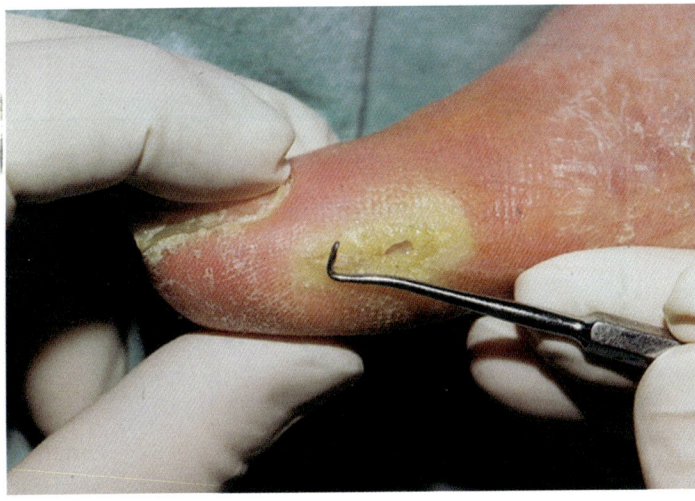

(b)

Figure 83.9 Probing a neuropathic wound: (a) probe in position, (b) with probe removed.

The patient and carers must be educated regarding the risks and the use of protective footwear. Persons at risk should receive basic foot care instruction, preferably from a podiatrist, including regular self-inspection of the feet and correct nail-cutting techniques. Shoes should accommodate deformities and be tailored to the patient's needs [18,19], with a follow-up programme to prevent further ulceration [20]. Rocker soles, custom-made insoles with metatarsal additions and a high degree of contact between the insole and foot, reduce plantar pressures in a manner that may reduce ulcer occurrence [21,22]. Urea-based products may help in managing callus [8]. Patients should be discouraged from removing callus themselves – this should be done by a podiatrist.

It is important to treat the underlying disease process: patients with reduced pulses need an ankle brachial pressure index (ABPI) test and if <0.9 this suggests peripheral arterial disease. Critical limb ischaemia should be considered for arterial revascularisation/reconstruction [23]. Diabetic control should be meticulous and the physical cause of the trauma must be addressed.

Ulcers are best treated with a combination of debridement, wound dressing and offloading of pressure. Regular local sharp debridement with scalpel, scissors and/or forceps is the gold standard.

Chronic wounds contain necrotic tissue and harbour high bacterial loads which elicit a pro-inflammatory response contributing towards poor healing [24]. Infection prevention is paramount, and dressings should maintain a moist wound bed and absorb the

exudate. Choice of dressing depends on a thorough assessment of the patient and wound [24,25].

For chronic ulcers, some novel therapeutic approaches can be considered, such as microsurgical grafts for large defects and tissue-engineered human skin, mainly as a transient method. Vacuum-assisted closure (VAC) devices improve the success of skin grafts [24]. Becaplermin, a growth factor with a proposed role in wound healing, has demonstrable efficacy [24,26]. However, there is a possible increased cancer risk with higher doses of the drug [27].

Bone marrow-derived cells may be effective in healing otherwise unresponsive wounds [28]. Hyaluronic acid dressings (Hyalofill®) are also routinely used in chronic ulcer treatment [29–31].

Studies suggest that what is removed from the foot (pressure, callus, infection and slough) is more important than what is applied to it (adjuvant treatments: hyperbaric oxygen, cytokines, growth factors, skin grafts, tissue substitute) [32]. The efficacy of hyperbaric oxygen therapy is controversial although there are studies that report a decreased amputation rate [21]. There is no evidence to support one type of skin graft over another when examining the use

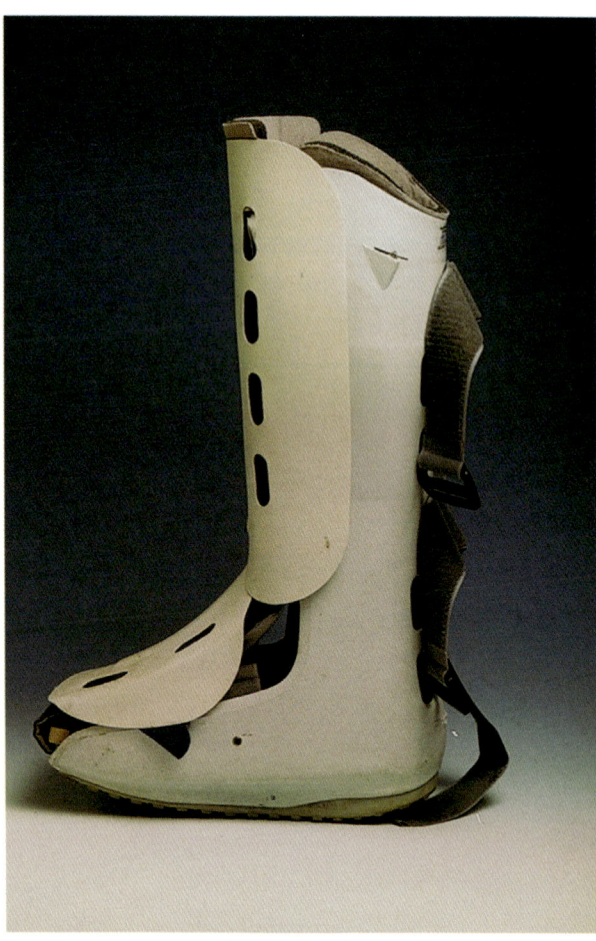

Figure 83.10 Aircast Walker® boot.

of autografts, allografts, xenografts and bioengineered or artificial skin [21].

Offloading areas of abnormal pressure on the foot is essential [33]. A contact casting (such as the Aircast Walker® foam boot; Figure 83.10), is useful for healing ulceration over metatarsal heads, but requires expert application, and is contraindicated with infected ulcers or where there is significant ischaemia [33]. A modified boot of layered adhesive foam may achieve complete removal of pressure points [34]. Plaster of Paris boots (with a rocker base) applied over weeks or months are popular in some centres [35]. Non-removable offloading devices promote better ulcer healing than removable devices, presumably because of increased patient compliance [36].

Even if healing is achieved, up to 40% of patients develop a recurrent ulcer within 1 year.

Treatment ladder for neuropathic ulcer

First line
- Basic foot care
- Proper footwear
- Control of hypertension and diabetes
- Smoking cessation

Second line
- Orthotic devices
- Electrical modalities

Third line
- Hard casting (total contact casting)
- Aircasts
- Hyperbaric oxygen therapy
- Laser therapy
- Vacuum-assisted wound closure

Resources

Wounds UK (2021) *Best Practice Statement: Care of the Person with Diabetes and Lower Limb Ulcers*. London: Wounds UK. Available to download from: 627f50978c2ed6f892ba1480f837fdba.pdf (last accessed November 2023).

Patient resources

Grennan D. Diabetic foot ulcers. *JAMA* 2019;321:114. https://jamanetwork.com/journals/jama/fullarticle/2720026 (last accessed November 2023).

Syringomyelia

Definition and nomenclature
Syringomyelia describes conditions involving abnormal fluid cavities within the spinal cord. A 'syrinx' is a fluid-filled cavity within the spinal cord parenchyma.

Synonyms and inclusions
- Hydromyelia
- Spinal cord cyst
- Morvan disease
- Syringohydromyelia

Introduction and general description
Syringomyelia is a rare disorder characterised by a longitudinal cyst in the cervical cord and/or medulla (syringobulbia) immediately anterior to the central canal which spreads, usually asymmetrically, to each side. The CNS disturbance causes dissociated sensory loss, with pain and temperature sensation being lost early in the fingers and upper limbs. The first clinical manifestation of syringomyelia is a tendency to painless burns and cuts on the hands and forearms.

Epidemiology
Incidence and prevalence
There are an estimated 8.4 cases per 100,000 population [1].

Age
Symptoms usually appear in young adults and usually progress slowly over 20–30 years. Limited self-resolution of symptoms has occurred in adults [2] and children [3,4].

Associated diseases
Chiari malformation type 1 (CM-1) is a developmental abnormality often associated with a syrinx, involving a congenital extension of the cerebellar tonsils below the foramen magnum [5].

Pathophysiology
The exact pathogenesis of syringomyelia is uncertain. The condition has several distinct cavitary patterns, which probably determine the pathogenesis and the clinical features of the condition [6]. Most lesions occur in association with type 1 Chiari syndrome. It is proposed that syrinx development, particularly in CM-1 patients, follows a differential between intracranial pressure and spinal pressure caused by a valve-like action at the foramen magnum [6]. Other causes include trauma and tumours [3].

Clinical features
History
Symptoms usually appear in young adults, and the disease generally slowly progresses over 20–30 years, although limited resolution has occurred in adults [3] and children [4,5]. An association with other abnormalities, such as a short neck and a low hairline, suggests a developmental origin. Body asymmetry or hemi-hypertrophy is known to occur in syringomyelia.

Presentation
Early involvement of pain and temperature fibres leads to a characteristic dissociated sensory loss, where pain and temperature sensation is lost early in the upper limbs, while sensory modalities carried in the posterior columns (e.g. touch, vibration and position sense) remain relatively intact. The earliest manifestation of the disease is a tendency to painless burns and cuts on the hands and forearms. Later, upper motor neuron signs in the legs may accompany weakness, wasting and loss of reflexes in the arms. Morvan syndrome, involving progressive pain loss, resultant skin ulceration, soft-tissue loss, resorption of the phalanges and muscular atrophy, occasionally occurs.

Dyshidrosis is reported in 60% of patients (either hyperhidrosis or hypohidrosis) [7]. The dyshidrosis, usually over the face and upper arms, may be spontaneous or occur on consumption of hot or seasoned food [7]. Hyperhidrosis is probably caused by stimulation of the sympathetic preganglionic neurons and, as the disease progresses, hyperreactivity is replaced by hypoactivity. Focal hyperhidrosis may be a hallmark of a relatively intact, though slightly damaged, spinal cord. Asymmetry of scalp hair can also occur, with the denervated areas having less abundant, slower-growing hair.

Complications and co-morbidities
Syringomyelia can coexist with other conditions. There is increased risk of scoliosis and a reported coexistence with Guillain–Barré syndrome. Complications include infections and decubitus ulcers.

Disease course and prognosis
The disease slowly progresses over many years. Repeated burns, and other injuries, cause the skin of the fingers to become thickened, swollen, cyanotic and keratotic. Gangrene rarely occurs, but damage to, or loss of, terminal phalanges or nails can occur.

Extension of the syrinx into the medulla may disrupt the vestibular pathways, the descending trigeminal nerve, the sympathetic and taste pathways, and the hypoglossal nerve. Patients may then experience vertigo with nystagmus, dissociated facial sensory loss, loss of taste, a wasted tongue, Horner syndrome and occasionally vocal cord paralysis or facial oedema confined to areas of sensory loss [7].

Investigations
MRI scanning of the hindbrain and upper spinal cord is best for delineation of the syrinx [3,4,5,6,7,8].

Management
A neurosurgical and orthopaedic evaluation is warranted for all patients with a syrinx. Surgical indications have been stated as progression of motor/sensory loss, scoliosis, associated pain and size of the syrinx [9].

Resources

Patient resources
Syringomyelia. National Institute of Neurological Disorders and Stroke (nih.gov); https://www.ninds.nih.gov/health-information/disorders/syringomyelia (last accessed November 2023).

Spinal dysraphism

Definition and nomenclature
Neurological disorders involving the malformation of the spinal cord due to a failure of symmetrical fusion of the embryological spinal structures are referred to as spinal dysraphisms.

Synonyms and inclusions
- Spina bifida
- Tethered cord
- Congenital dermal sinus
- Tight filum terminale
- Lipomeningomyelocele
- Split cord malformations (diastematomyelia)
- Dermal sinus tracts
- Dermoids
- Cystocoeles

Introduction and general description
Spinal cord development occurs between weeks two and six of embryonic life. Dysraphism is the failure of fusion between symmetrical embryological structures (a raphe) [1], leading to malformations of the midline dorsal structures [2]. Early embryonic defects produce spinal dysraphisms, categorised clinically into two subsets: open – exposed to the environment (e.g. spina bifida, myelomeningocoele); and closed – covered by intact skin.

Congenital dermal sinuses (CDS) are epithelium-lined tracts resulting from incomplete separation of cutaneous ectoderm from the underlying neuroectoderm. CDS may be associated with der- moid cysts and can cause complications by mass effect and by functioning as a pathway for infection [3].

Spina bifida and CDS are discussed in this section.

Epidemiology
Incidence and prevalence
For open dysraphism the incidence is around 1 : 1000 live births. The prevalence has declined worldwide over the past two decades, due to better maternal nutrition, timely folate replacement and better prenatal care with high-resolution ultrasound [4]. Spina bifida is one of the most common congenital conditions [5].

Age
From birth.

Ethnicity
In Europe, the highest incidence rates are in Ireland and Wales (5 per 1000 live births) compared with south-eastern Europe (0.1–0.6 per 1000).

In Canada and the USA, a higher incidence has been reported on the east coast, and in the USA the Hispanic population has the highest risk.

Associated diseases
Open dysraphism is associated with certain genetic disorders, including trisomy 13 or 18, congenital hemidysplasia with ichthyosiform erythroderma and limb defects (CHILD syndrome), Fraser syndrome, Waardenburg syndrome and Meckel–Gruber syndrome [6].

Pathophysiology
Predisposing factors
The cause of neural tube defects is unknown. However, genetics, folate deficiency, antiepileptic drugs (sodium valproate, carba- mazepine) and environmental conditions such as radiation can pre- dispose [6]. Folate deficiency is a major cause of open dysraphism, largely preventable by folate supplementation before conception and during early pregnancy [7].

Pathology
Dysraphisms occur at three stages of embryogenesis: primary neu- rulation, secondary neurulation and gastrulation [4].

Clinical features
Presentation
A review of 200 published cases of spinal dysraphism [8] included 102 with cutaneous abnormalities, often in combination. A derma- tologist may be the first physician to see such patients and should be aware of possible associations with underlying neurological abnor- malities. Coccygeal dimples may be unrelated to dysraphism and not require aggressive investigation, whereas lumbo-sacral dimples present a higher risk for underlying problems [9,10]. Correlation between sacral dimples and dysraphism has recently been ques- tioned [11]. Patients with congenital giant melanocytic naevi

overlying the scalp or dorsal spine can show brain abnormalities on MRI.

Many lumbo-sacral skin abnormalities have been reportedly associated with spinal dysraphism and cord tethering, includ- ing lipomas [12], port-wine stains, haemangiomas [13,14], 'faun tail' (hypertrichosis), pigmented macules, and pits or dimples. Intraspinal dermoid cysts are usually associated with either lumbar spinal dysraphism or a dermal sinus tract [15].

For occult dysraphism, midline skin abnormalities have consid- erable diagnostic value and can be divided into three groups of risk [6]:

- Group 1 (high risk): two or more lesions, subcutaneous lipoma, dermal sinus, 'queue de faune' (faun tail).
- Group 2 (low risk): atypical dimple, aplasia cutis, gluteal fold deviation.
- Group 3 (very low risk): haemangioma, port-wine stain, hypertri- chosis, fibroma pendulum, pigmentary naevus, coccygeal dimple.

Several varieties of spina bifida are described, differing in the nature and severity of the spinal defect. In the severe form, a sac protrudes through the vertebral opening and transmits an impulse on crying or coughing. In the mildest cases (spina bifida occulta) there is no such protrusion, but a defect in the vertebral lamina may be felt as a depression and is sometimes covered by a tuft of hair or a dimple (Figure 83.11). The likelihood of a midline fusion defect is increased when the cutaneous findings are associated with

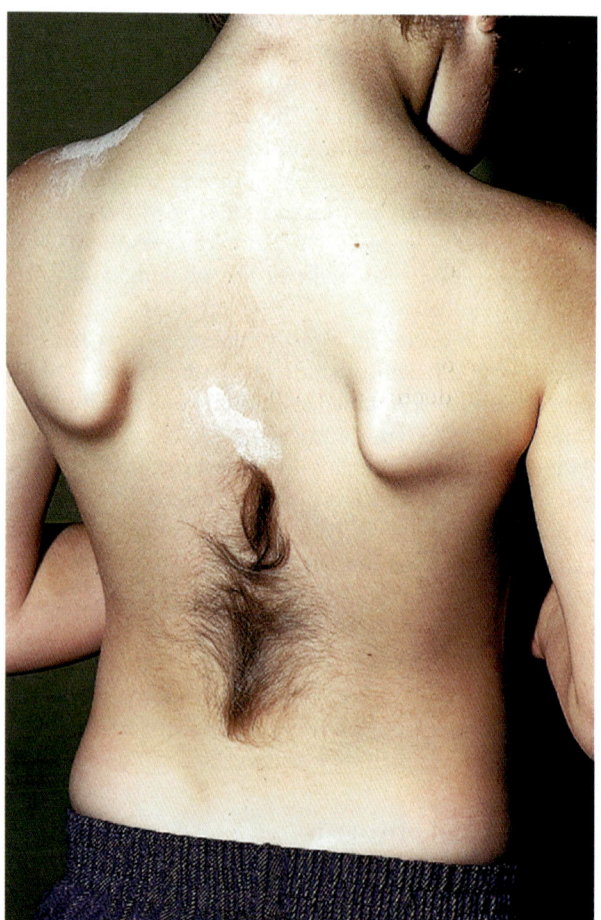

Figure 83.11 Tuft of hair in association with spina bifida.

a subcutaneous lesion such as a lipoma [12]. Spina bifida occulta may be a chance finding during routine examination.

Lesions preventing spinal cord ascent during normal growth can cause undue traction on the lower end of the cord and cauda equina. Neurological changes will then be those of a chronic cauda equina lesion. Such patients may be slow in learning to walk. Sensation may be impaired over the areas innervated by the lowest sacral segments, causing a characteristic saddle-shaped analgesic area over the buttocks and dorsa of the thighs. Trophic changes are occasionally conspicuous. In milder cases, the feet are usually cold and cyanosed. Cutaneous injuries heal slowly and tend to ulcerate, particularly on the feet and in the analgesic skin of the buttocks and thighs. The most severe neurological abnormality is a flaccid paraparesis with sphincter paralysis.

Complications and co-morbidities
Large skin defects produce complications including wound dehiscence, wound infection and cerebrospinal fluid leaks. The morbidities of wound healing and cerebrospinal fluid leaks during surgical management present significant challenges [4].

Children with spina bifida risk becoming overweight, which further reduces their mobility, increases difficulties with catheterisation and toileting, adds pressure to already vulnerable skin and increases social isolation. Urinary tract infections are a common source of morbidity among children with spina bifida [16].

People with spina bifida are prone to latex sensitivity [17] from exposure to latex products, both at the time of surgery and with indwelling catheters. They should be assessed using latex-specific serum immunoglobulin E (IgE), the radioallergosorbent test (RAST), skin prick testing with latex suspension and a latex glove usage test [17,18]. Latex-allergic patients may display urticaria, conjunctivitis, angio-oedema, rhinitis and bronchial asthma. They are at risk of anaphylaxis during health care procedures and – because of cross-sensitivity – can be allergic to fresh foods including kiwi, pear, orange, pineapple, tomato and banana.

Investigations
Estimation of α-fetoprotein in the amniotic fluid or maternal serum may successfully identify a fetus with severe CNS malformation, such as spina bifida cystica or anencephaly. Spinal ultrasound (SUS) is most helpful when supported by multiple clinical indications. It is significantly more likely to detect spinal dysraphism than imaging performed for isolated abnormalities or risk factors [11]. With antenatally diagnosed, open dysraphism caesarean section is often recommended to avoid additional trauma and infection during birth [19]. The decision to continue pregnancy or opt for termination raises many moral and ethical dilemmas for discussion with the parents.

Spinal sonography is a useful screening method in the first 4 months in newborns with a suggestive cutaneous lesion. Diagnosis is confirmed by radiography [20] which shows defective fusion of the laminae in the affected region, usually L5 and S1. Indications for ultrasound or MRI referral have recently been reviewed [9]. Because tethered spinal cord is treatable, but untreated can lead to progressive neurological degeneration, spinal MRI scanning of infants with giant melanocytic naevi involving the lumbo-sacral area is advocated [21,22,23].

Management
In open dysraphism, initial treatment is with saline gauze at 37 °C, and non-permeable dressings [6]. Management aims to provide closure of the neural tube defect and the skin without any undesirable tension within 24–48 h. Early primary closure often has an excellent outcome, although the risk of neurological sequelae varies depending on the severity of the anomalies [4].

Postnatal surgery of open spina bifida aims at covering the exposed spinal cord, preventing infection and treating hydrocephalus with a ventricular shunt. Fetal surgery with the severest form of spina bifida, myelomeningocoele, is also an option [24,25].

Due to the risk of neurological deterioration, the recommended treatment of CDS with or without a concomitant intraspinal dermoid is prompt administration of antibiotics and definitive surgical intervention [3].

Dermatoses associated with spinal cord injury

Definition
Spinal cord injury leading to a spinal cord defect results in multiple disabilities which can be complicated by skin problems.

Introduction and general description
The spinal cord may be injured directly by penetrating wounds or, more frequently, indirectly following dislocation or fracture dislocation of the vertebral column [1]. The causes of spinal cord injury are trauma, including motor vehicle accidents (36–48%), violence (5–29%), falls (17–21%) and recreational activities (7–16%).

The severity of the disability varies widely, mainly depending on the level of the injury: the worst scenario being at C1–C3, leading to ventilator dependence, limited talking ability and the need for a head- or chin-control wheelchair. As well as problems with pressure ulceration (Chapter 123), the skin of patients with spinal cord injury is prone to several inflammatory dermatoses and disorders of sweating.

Clinical features
Seborrhoea and seborrhoeic dermatitis have been reported in quadriplegic patients [2,3] with one study reporting around two-thirds developing the condition within a few weeks of injury. Nummular eczema may also occur below the level of the lesion [3], and acne on the back and buttocks may follow the onset of paralysis [3]. Changes in eccrine sweating after spinal cord injuries are complex [4]. Profuse sweating on the face, neck and upper trunk with lesions at or above T6 may occur in exaggerated response to stimuli such as bowel or bladder distension (autonomic dysreflexia). These episodes may involve facial flushing and headache. Other patients develop sweating of the face and arms after dizziness due to postural hypotension. Post-traumatic syringomyelia can lead to hyperhidrosis [5]. Dryness of the skin, particularly on the soles, is an effect of anhidrosis.

In hemiplegic stroke patients, reduction in skin temperature of the affected limb, associated with reduced limb blood flow, as well as a reduction in blood flow in the unaffected leg, have been reported.

The reduction in blood flow might contribute to tinea pedis, onychomycosis, xerosis of the extremities and reduction in hair on the lower extremities being more common in immobilised patients than in controls.

Pressure ulcers increase in severity with worsening immobility and there is a significant risk of complications, including necrotising fasciitis and Fournier's gangrene.

The concept of a localised immunocompromised area in the body has been proposed to explain subsequent immune dysregulation in an area of skin altered by preceding injury or inflammation, and can be used to explain altered neuromediator signalling as the cause of skin disease affecting the hemiplegic side [6].

Numerous case reports contrast skin changes in the plegic with the non-plegic site. Reported dermatological findings in the affected limb or below the neurological level include for example [7,8]:

- Localised fungal infections, skin thickening and nail hypertrophy [9], seborrhoea [10], crusted scabies of the legs [11], scabies burrows on the site with sensory loss [12], unilateral finger clubbing, decrease in the minimum erythema dose of ultraviolet radiation and a tendency to tan more easily.
- In contrast, localisation of skin disease on the neurologically healthy side has also been described, for example endogenous eczema, attributed to xerosis – lines on the fingernails [9] – longitudinal reddish striation, neapolitan nails, unilateral clubbing, psoriasis and scleroderma.

Bullous pemphigoid is particularly interesting in its association with various neurological conditions such as Parkinson disease, epilepsy, dementia and stroke when it may be localised to the plegic or paretic skin, or on non-neurologically affected skin [13–16].

Epitope spreading has been demonstrated in bullous pemphigoid [17]. Exposure of neural antigens during trauma or a cerebral accident could result in generation of autoantibodies and epitope spreading, explaining the limited distribution of blisters in patients with neurological diseases. Cross-antigenicity between BP180/BP230 brain and skin isoforms has been confirmed in dementia [18].

Management
Management of pressure ulcers is described in Chapter 123. Inflammatory dermatoses associated with spinal injury should be treated with appropriate topical and/or systemic therapy.

Sympathetic nerve injury

Definition
Interruption of the sympathetic innervation of the skin resulting in loss of both vasoconstrictor impulses (causing erythema) and sweating (causing anhidrosis).

Introduction and general description
Loss of sympathetic supply to the skin following nerve damage will result in vasodilation and anhidrosis.

Pathophysiology
Sympathetic nerve injury usually occurs when sympathetic axons are injured by trauma affecting major nerves. There can be dissociation of sudomotor and pilomotor activity after sympathetic ganglionectomy [1]. The areas of vasodilation generally match the areas of anhidrosis, suggesting close correspondence of sudomotor and vasoconstrictor fibres.

Clinical features
When the sympathetic supply to the skin is interrupted, loss of vasoconstrictor impulses leads to erythema with passive vasodilation. The denervated area is also anhidrotic. Affected skin may be scaly and fissured. In the denervated areas, there is no loss of cutaneous sensation, possibly due to regeneration of postganglionic cholinergic fibres. Some patients report hyperaesthesia.

When sympathetic denervation is combined with a loss of somatic sensation, as in peripheral nerve injury or severe peripheral neuropathy, neurotrophic ulcers may occur. These result from minor local trauma and are characteristically painless and slow healing. Sympathetic denervation may also slow or prevent the normal greying of the hair with ageing and may cause hyperpigmentation of the skin in the affected area.

Investigations
The affected area of skin should be physically examined for sweating, temperature, allodynia and hyperalgesia. Pupillary examination is indicated. Measurements of sweating and vasomotor responses can help determine the extent of autonomic denervation [2].

Laboratory tests include the SSR, thermoregulatory sweat test, quantitative sudomotor axon reflex test, skin wrinkling on water immersion and microneurography.

Management
Appropriate neurological/neurosurgical management of damaged nerve(s).

Complex regional pain syndrome

Definition and nomenclature
Complex regional pain syndrome (CRPS) is a rare, debilitating, painful condition affecting a limb – usually an acral site, commonly arising after injury, associated with sensory, motor, autonomic nerve problems, with abnormalities in the bone and skin of the affected limb [1].

Synonyms and inclusions

- Causalgia
- Algoneurodystrophy
- Reflex sympathetic dystrophy
- Reflex neurovascular dystrophy
- Sudeck atrophy
- Shoulder–hand syndrome

Introduction and general description
CRPS is a debilitating painful condition which usually affects a limb and is generally preceded by minor trauma to that body part.

It is considered a neurological disorder. There appears to be no relationship with the severity of injury; indeed in a few cases there is no precipitating trauma. CRPS results in neurological, cutaneous and skeletal abnormalities in the affected limb. It is described by the International Association for the Study of Pain as 'a condition that appears regionally after an injury with a variety of symptoms that often exceed the expected clinical course both in magnitude and duration, causing impairment of motor function and variable progression' [2]. CRPS is a difficult condition to treat effectively; the primary aims are to reduce pain and to preserve or restore function.

Epidemiology
Incidence and prevalence
The European incidence rate of CRPS is 26/100 000 person-years [3].

Age
It commonly occurs in the 30–50-year-old age group.

Sex
Female : male 4 : 1.

Pathophysiology
The pathogenesis is poorly understood, although abnormalities in the PNS and CNS have been described, with and without major nerve lesions. The earlier belief that the predominant problem is sympathetic dysfunction and that CRPS occurs in (stereotyped) stages is now obsolete. CRPS is not usually associated with a history of preceding psychological problems, somatisation or malingering although there is significant overlap with functional neurological disorder [4,5]. Hypotheses to explain the disorder include the release of neuropeptides from peripheral unmyelinated fibres, which causes pain and vasodilation. Other proposed pathogenetic pathways are an enhanced α-adrenergic receptor activity and upregulation of afferent nociceptors in response to norepinephrine release from sympathetic efferents. Excessive inflammation at the injury site with inflammatory cytokine release and microcirculatory dysfunction, causing tissue injury and/or immune system involvement or CNS sensitisation to thermal, mechanical and pain stimuli, may also contribute to the pathogenesis of CRPS [6].

Predisposing factors
Stroke, myocardial infarction, tuberculosis, herpes zoster and certain drugs may predispose to CRPS [6]. Dermatological conditions such as vasculitis and panniculitis may precede the condition. Excisional skin biopsies, including nail biopsies, have been reported as triggering CRPS [7].

Box 83.6 lists the reported dermatological triggers of CRPS [6].

Clinical features
Presentation
CRPS is usually preceded by physical trauma, although there is no relationship with the severity of trauma [3]. Common triggers include soft-tissue injury, fractures, orthopaedic surgery and medical illness, e.g. myocardial infarction and stroke [6]. Prolonged immobilisation of a limb is an important predisposing factor present

---

Box 83.6 Dermatological triggers of complex regional pain syndrome (CRPS)

- Acrodermatitis continua of Hallopeau
- Chronic venous ulceration
- Dupuytren contracture
- Epithelioid haemangioendothelioma
- Herpes zoster
- Human parvovirus B19
- Cutaneous surgery
- Nail biopsy
- Osteogenesis imperfecta
- Psoriatic arthritis
- Systemic lupus erythematosus
- Vasculitis
- Panniculitis

From Veldman *et al.* 1993 [1], Phelps and Wilentz 2000 [6], Royal College of Physicians 2012 [7], Harden 2001 [8], McBride and Atkins 2005 [9].

---

in almost 50% of cases [2]. CRPS can be divided into two types: in type I CRPS, also known as reflex sympathetic dystrophy (the commonest type), a major nerve lesion is absent; in type II CRPS, also known as causalgia, a peripheral nerve injury is present usually following more notable trauma [7]. CRPS usually affects one limb, but in 7% of cases can spread to others [8,9]. Onset of symptoms is usually within 1 month of the trauma or immobilisation of the limb.

The Budapest criteria have been proposed for use as an aid to clinical diagnosis (Box 83.7).

Box 83.7   Budapest clinical diagnostic criteria for chronic regional pain syndrome

1 Continuing pain, which is disproportionate to any inciting event.
2 Must report at least one symptom in three of the four following categories:
- Sensory: reports of hyperaesthesia and/or allodynia.
- Vasomotor: reports of temperature asymmetry and/or skin colour changes and/or skin colour asymmetry.
- Sudomotor/oedema: reports of oedema and/or sweating changes and/or sweating asymmetry.
- Motor/trophic: reports of decreased range of motion and/or motor dysfunction (weakness, tremor, dystonia) and/or trophic changes (hair, nail, skin).
3 Must display at least one sign at time of evaluation in two or more of the following categories:
- Sensory: evidence of hyperalgesia (to pinprick) and/or allodynia (to light touch and/or deep somatic pressure and/or joint movement).
- Vasomotor: evidence of temperature asymmetry and/or skin colour changes and/or asymmetry.
- Sudomotor/oedema: evidence of oedema and/or sweating changes and/or sweating asymmetry.
- Motor/trophic: evidence of decreased range of motion and/or motor dysfunction (weakness, tremor, dystonia) and/or trophic changes (hair, nail, skin).
4 There is no other diagnosis that better explains the signs and symptoms.

Symptoms fall into three serial worsening stages. The first begins after several days or weeks and lasts about a month, involving spontaneous burning and stinging, or tearing or shooting pain, precipitated by mechanical stimuli such as bathing, clothing on the skin or draughts [9].

Stage two occurs 1–7 months after injury and lasts 3–6 months. Symptoms relate to sympathetic hyperactivity and include cool, oedematous skin, hyperhidrosis and cyanosis, or livedo-like changes. Hair growth may increase or decrease. Nails may show decreased or increased growth or thickening, become brittle or develop striations. Pain is variable, and neuralgia may either spread or decrease. Functional limitations, e.g. limited range of movement and muscle weakness, may begin to manifest.

Stage three, starting around 8 months after injury, involves progressive tissue damage, which can become permanent. The changes may be due to vasoconstriction (resulting in skin hypoxia) or decreased motion of the skin from inactivity of underlying joints, tendons or ligaments. Usually, the skin becomes shiny, atrophic and dry; fingertips may shrink. Some patients have no trophic skin changes [10]. Deeper structures, including fascia, can thicken, resulting in contractures. If the pain is worsened by physical stimuli, the patient may protect the limb leading to trophic changes in the bone, muscle and skin (Sudeck atrophy).

Box 83.8 lists the dermatological manifestations of CRPS [6].

Box 83.8 Dermatological manifestations of complex regional pain syndrome (CRPS)

- Allodynia
- Oedema
- Erythema and warmth
- Pallor or cyanosis
- Hypopigmentation or hyperpigmentation
- Hypertrichosis or hypotrichosis
- Hypohidrosis or hyperhidrosis
- Beau lines or nail notching, leukonychia, onychodystrophy
- Petechiae
- Ulceration (may be due to external trauma)
- Dermatitis
- Erythematous papules
- Bullae
- Cutaneous atrophy
- Skin thickening and tightening

From Phelps and Wilentz 2000 [6], Montogomery and Elbuluk 2022 [11].

Differential diagnosis

The Royal College of Physicians, UK, provides an extensive list of conditions to consider in formulating a diagnosis, ranging from infections through arthritis and arthrosis, to bone, soft-tissue or neural injury [7]. A multidisciplinary approach is desirable.

Disease course and prognosis

Approximately 15% of sufferers will have unrelenting pain and physical impairment two years after the onset of CRPS, although more will suffer less ongoing pain and dysfunction [10].

Investigations

Electrodiagnostic studies (needle electromyography and nerve conduction) are normal in CRPS type I but demonstrate a peripheral nerve lesion in type II [6]. Patchy osteoporosis may be seen on some plain radiographs in CRPS II. CT or MRI scans may show atrophy or soft-tissue swelling and bone mineralisation changes. Bone scintigraphy using three-phase bone scans may usefully identify early changes. Other tests include pain relief on α_1-adrenergic blockade with intravenous phentolamine; pain exacerbation on α_2 stimulation by clonidine; and severe pain on cold stimulation. These tests help identify patients with sympathetically maintained pain (SMP). Despite having similar signs and symptoms, only some patients with CRPS type I show alleviation of the pain by selective sympathetic nervous system or α-adrenoreceptor blockade. SMP can also present in CRPS II patients, although the mechanism is probably different [7,10].

Management

Prompt diagnosis and early treatment are considered best practice to avoid secondary physical problems associated with disuse of the affected limb and the psychological consequences of living with undiagnosed chronic pain.

There is no cure for CRPS and an integrated interdisciplinary treatment approach is recommended [7,10]. Primary aims are to reduce pain, to preserve or restore function and to enable patients to manage their condition [10]. Addressing each of the four 'pillars' of care (education, pain relief, physical rehabilitation and psychological intervention) carries equal importance. However, full recovery can be elusive, even with early appropriate treatment [10]. Although there is no evidence that early physiotherapy can prevent CRPS, early diagnosis is a key prognostic factor and treatment with physiotherapy and/or occupational therapy, delivered by specifically competent therapists, is recommended to improve function and to prevent complications such as contractures, and to speed recovery [10].

Medication is indicated to minimise pain and support physical rehabilitation. Patients waiting to see a pain specialist should be seen regularly and be advised about the use of simple analgesics.

If simple medication does not reduce the pain to a mild level after 3–4 weeks, medication should be considered according to the neuropathic pain guidelines [10]. Earlier use may be appropriate. The patient should also be referred to a pain clinic for multidisciplinary pain therapy treatment, which ideally should begin within 3 months of the condition's onset [10].

The best functional advice for patients with suspected CRPS, or CRPS for which concomitant pathology has not yet been ruled out, is currently unclear. Pragmatically, encouragement of gentle limb use and active lifestyle is recommended [10].

Psychological interventions, including biofeedback, cognitive behavioural and relaxation techniques, are crucial, although often overlooked. If psychological factors (e.g. significant distress) are suspected, early referral to a psychologist specialising in pain may be advisable [7]. Treat any associated depression, anxiety or insomnia with sedative, analgesic antidepressants/anxiolytics and/or psychotherapy. If allodynia/hyperalgesia is significant, anticonvulsants and/or other sodium-channel blockers or NMDA-receptor antagonists may be used. If osteopenia, immobility and trophic changes are significant, use calcitonin or bisphosphonates. For profound vasomotor disturbance, calcium-channel blockers, sympatholytics and/or blocks may be used.

Surgery should only rarely be considered. Orthopaedic surgeons should be aware of specific treatments for chronic CRPS, such as specialist physiotherapy and occupational therapy to desensitise skin, multidisciplinary pain management programmes, sympathetic neural blockade with local anaesthetic, spinal cord stimulation to interrupt dysregulated sympathetic innervation and specialist rehabilitation programmes [7,10].

Treatment ladder for complex regional pain syndrome [2]

First line
- Mobilisation and desensitisation of affected joints by physiotherapy
- Simple analgesics
- Pain exposure physical therapy
- Psychological interventions

Second line
- Bisphosphonates
- Pain treatment ladder
- Morphine, oxycodone, tramadol, methadone, levorphanol
- If inflammation/swelling and oedema – steroids, systemic or targeted (acutely) or NSAIDs (chronically); immune modulators

Third line
Minimally invasive therapies:
- Sympathetic nerve blocks
- IV regional nerve blocks
- Somatic nerve blocks

Interventional therapies:
- Epidural and plexus catheter infusion/block(s)
- Neurostimulation (spinal cord stimulator, dorsal root gangliion)
- Intrathecal drug infusion (e.g. baclofen or clonidine)

Surgical and experimental therapies:
- Sympathectomy
- Motor cortex stimulation

Resources

Complex regional pain syndrome in adults (2nd edition). London: RCP. https://www.rcplondon.ac.uk/guidelines-policy/complex-regional-pain-syndrome-adults (last accessed November 2023).
http://guidance.nice.org.uk/CG173 (last accessed November 2023).

Horner syndrome

Definition and nomenclature

Horner syndrome follows partial or complete interruption of the sympathetic nerve pathways of the face. It is characterised by ptosis, miosis and anhidrosis.

Synonyms and inclusions
- Bernard–Horner syndrome
- Oculosympathetic palsy

Introduction and general description

Horner syndrome appears when the three-neuron sympathetic pathway is interrupted anywhere from the posteriolateral nuclei of the hypothalamus, through to the spinal cord, to the eye [1]. It is characterised by ptosis, miosis and anhidrosis.

Pathophysiology

The sympathetic fibres supplying the facial skin travel from the hypothalamus via the spinal cord, to relay at the level of the first and second thoracic segments in the lateral column of the spinal grey matter. Preganglionic fibres emerge from the first and second thoracic spinal nerves, and pass up the cervical sympathetic chain to relay in the superior cervical ganglion. From here, postganglionic fibres pass to supply the eye and the skin of a small central area of the face via the internal carotid sympathetic plexus. Other fibres pass along the external carotid artery and its branches to innervate most of the facial skin with vasomotor and sudomotor fibres.

This pathway can be interrupted centrally in the spinal cord, for example by medullary infarction, syringomyelia, multiple sclerosis or intraspinal tumours. The peripheral fibres can be damaged by aortic aneurysm, cervical lymphadenopathy, surgery, regional anaesthetic procedures or tumours. Horner syndrome may follow sympathectomy for the treatment of palmar and axillary hyper-hidrosis, and occurs in up to 40% of patients after open cervical sympathectomy, and 8% of those having transthoracic endo-scopic sympathectomy [2]. In such cases, there may be resolution of longstanding pompholyx-type hand eczema ipsilaterally, suggesting a neurological pathogenesis for endogenous pompholyx in some patients [3,4].

Clinical features

Horner syndrome is usually found in adults and only rarely in children, where it can be either congenital or acquired [1]. An irritative phase occurs rarely at the outset of Horner syndrome, charac-terised by transient unilateral hyperhidrosis and vasoconstriction. The paralytic phase involves drooping of the eyelid (ptosis) with narrowing of the palpebral fissure. The pupil is small but shows normal reflex constriction to light and accommodation. Inflam-mation of the conjunctiva is often present. Sweating is absent on the ipsilateral side of the face. There may be slight retraction of the eyeball into the orbit (enophthalmos). Bilateral cases are rare.

Sweat glands on the medial and lateral parts of the forehead are innervated separately, the former by fibres from the sympathetic plexus of the internal carotid, and the latter from the plexus surrounding the external carotid [5]. This explains the findings in Raeder syndrome, where damage involving the perivascular plexus of the internal carotid leads to anhidrosis only medially on the forehead [6].

Three cases of bilateral Horner syndrome and three cases of contralateral Horner syndrome have been reported [7–10].

Investigations

Physical examination and pupil dilatation test using hydroxyamphetamine eyedrops can confirm the diagnosis [11]. To elicit the underlying cause, X-ray, MRI and blood or urine tests might be needed.

Management

Treatment should be directed towards the underlying cause.

Gustatory hyperhidrosis

Definition and nomenclature

Gustatory hyperhidrosis describes excessive sweating occurring immediately after eating spicy or hot food. Gustatory sweating is localised to certain areas, including the scalp, upper lip, perioral region and sternum.

Synonyms and inclusions
- Frey syndrome
- Focal hyperhidrosis

Introduction and general description

Gustatory hyperhidrosis is a disorder characterised by excessive sweating on the scalp, upper lip, perioral region or sternum, immediately after eating spicy or hot food. It can occur following damage to the sympathetic cervical trunk, the vagus nerve or the auriculotemporal nerve [1].

Pathophysiology

Gustatory hyperhidrosis may complicate surgery involving the parotid gland or the temporomandibular joint. Auriculotemporal nerve injury following closed treatment for maxillomandibular joint trauma can also lead to this form of focal hyperhidrosis.

The ANS has a propensity for regrowth [2]. Damage to adjacent preganglionic parasympathetic fibres and postganglionic sympathetic fibres may result in parasympathetic fibres regrowing into the sympathetic nerves, thereby directly controlling sweat gland function. In the neck, for example, following damage to the sympathetic cervical trunk and the vagus (parasympathetic) during thyroidectomy or after trauma, such reinnervation may result in gustatory hyperhidrosis, even with bland foods [1]. A similar event may occur on the cheeks or chin following parotid or submandibular gland surgery – the auriculotemporal syndrome (Frey syndrome) [3]. Secretory sweating is now more frequently seen after endoscopic transthoracic sympathectomy [4–6]. A recent review reported a rate of gustatory hyperhidrosis of 1.1% [7].

Clinical features

Immediately following the ingestion of spicy or hot food, sweating occurs which is localised to certain areas, typically the scalp, upper lip, perioral region or sternum. Frey syndrome describes gustatory sweating and facial flushing [7], and emerges between 3 and 24 months after surgery involving the parotid or temporomandibular joint [7,8].

Investigations

Subjective symptoms should be investigated. The Minor starch iodine test and infrared thermography can be used to investigate the symptoms and confirm the diagnosis [9]. With medical thermography, images are taken after the patient has chewed a sialagogue [9,10].

Management

Topical preparations containing aluminium chloride hexahydrate can control the symptoms but may produce an irritant dermatitis. Botulinum toxin has been shown to be effective and safe in gustatory sweating [11]. The use of a 0.5% aqueous solution of glycopyrronium bromide topically has been shown to be effective, safe, well tolerated and convenient in diabetes-associated gustatory sweating [12]. Surgery can be considered in individual cases. The two surgical options are a neurectomy or the placement of a physical barrier between the parotid bed and the overlying skin – both have a risk of facial nerve injury, along with other possible surgical complications, and so should only be considered in severely symptomatic patients refractory to medical therapy [**13**].

Acknowledgements

I thank Dr David J. Eedy, Department of Dermatology, Craigavon Area Hospital, Craigavon, UK, who wrote this chapter for the 9th edition of *Rook's Textbook of Dermatology*. I would also like to thank Dr Sabine Sommers and Dr Edward Dunn who provided valuable insights on this chapter during the draft stages.

Key references

The full list of references can be found in the online version at https://www.wiley.com/rooksdermatology10e

Introduction and overview of genetic neurocutaneous disorders

1 Ruggieri M, Polizzi A, Marceca GP, Catanzaro S, Praticò AD, Di Rocco C. Introduction to phacomatoses (neurocutaneous disorders) in childhood. *Childs Nerv Syst* 2020;36:2229–68.

Cutaneous innervation

3 Zimmerman A, Bai L, Ginty DD. The gentle touch receptors of mammalian skin. *Science* 2014;346(6212):950–4.

10 Marek-Jozefowicz L, Nedoszytko B, Grochocka M et al. Molecular mechanisms of neurogenic inflammation of the skin. *Int J Mol Sci* 2023;24:5001.

Skin biopsy as an aid to diagnosis of neurological disease and neuropathies

1 Sommer C, Lauria G. Skin biopsy in the management of peripheral neuropathy. *Lancet Neurol* 2007;6:632–42.

Neuropathic pruritus and dysaesthesia

1 Kwatra SG, Kambala A, Dong X. Neuropathic pruritus. *J Allergy Clin Immunol* 2023;152:37–8.

Nerve entrapment syndromes

8 Shumway NK, Cole E, Fernandez KH. Neurocutaneous disease. *J Am Acad Dermatol* 2016;74:215–28.

Peripheral neuropathy

4 Watson JC, Dyck PJ. Peripheral neuropathy: a practical approach to diagnosis and symptom management. *Mayo Clin Proc* 2015;90:940–51.
5 Zhou L. Small fiber neuropathy. *Semin Neurol* 2019;39:570–7.

Burning feet and restless leg syndromes

11 Gossard TR, Trotti LM, Videnovic A, St Louis EK. Restless legs syndrome: contemporary diagnosis and treatment. *Neurotherapeutics* 2021;18:140–55.

Hereditary neuropathies
Midface toddler excoriation syndrome

1 Srinivas SM, Gowda VK, Owen CM *et al*. Mid-face toddler excoriation syndrome (MiTES): a new paediatric diagnosis. *Clin Exp Dermatol* 2017;42:68–71.

Neuropathic ulcer

21 Urso B, Ghias M, John A, Khachemoune A. Neuropathic ulcers: a focused review. *Int J Dermatol.* 2021;60:e383–9.
22 Ahmed S, Barwick A, Butterworth P, Nancarrow S. Footwear and insole design features that reduce neuropathic plantar forefoot ulcer risk in people with diabetes: a systematic literature review. *J Foot Ankle Res* 2020;13:30.

Syringomyelia

1 Sharma M, Coppa N, Sandhu FA. Syringomyelia: a review. *Semin Spine Surg* 2006; 18:180–4.
2 Kastrup A, Nägele T, Topka H. Spontaneous resolution of idiopathic syringomyelia. *Neurology* 2001;57:1519–20.
3 Jack CRJ, Kokmen E, Onofrio BM. Spontaneous decompression of syringomyelia: magnetic resonance imaging findings. Case report. *J Neurosurg* 1991;74:283–6.

4 Yeager BA, Lusser MA. Spontaneous resolution of idiopathic syringomyelia: MR features. *J Comput Assist Tomogr* 1992;16:323–4.
6 Williams B. Progress in syringomyelia. *Neurol Res* 1986;8:130–45.
8 Wolf M, Fürstenberg CH, Hähnel S *et al*. Spinal cord injury and syringomyelia (Rückenmarktrauma und Syringomyelie). *Radiologe* 2013;53:353–66.

Spinal dysraphism

1 Storer JS, Hawk RJ. Cutaneous signs of spinal dysraphism. In: Schachner LA, Hansen RC, eds. *Paediatric Dermatology*, Vol. 1. New York: Churchill Livingstone, 1988;275–7.
6 Zerah M, Kulkarni AV. Spinal cord malformations. In: Dulac O, Lassonde M, Sarnat HB, eds. *Handbook of Clinical Neurology*, Vol. 112. New York: Barnes & Noble, 2013;975–91.
11 McGovern M, Mulligan S, Carney O *et al*. Ultrasound investigation of sacral dimples and other stigmata of spinal dysraphism. *Arch Dis Child* 2013;98:784–6.
12 Pierre-Kahn A, Zerah M, Renier D *et al*. Congenital lumbosacral lipomas. *Child Nerv Syst* 1997;13:298–334.
13 Boyvat A, Yazar T, Ekmekci P, Gurgey E. Lumbosacral vascular malformation: a hallmark for occult spinal dysraphism. *Dermatology* 2000;201:374–6.
14 Tubbs RS, Wellons JC, Iskandar BJ, Oakes WJ. Isolated flat capillary midline lumbosacral hemangiomas as indicators of occult spinal dysraphism. *J Neurosurg* 2004;100(Suppl. Pediatrics 2):86–9.
15 Najjar MW, Kusske JA, Hasso AN. Dorsal intramedullary dermoids. *Neurosurg Rev* 2005;28:320–5.
19 Hamrick SE. Cesarean delivery and its impact on the anomalous infant. *Clin Perinatol* 2008;35:395–406.
21 Foster RD, Williams ML, Barovich AJ *et al*. Giant congenital melanocytic naevi: the significance of neurocutaneous melanosis in neurologically asymptomatic children. *Plast Reconstr Surg* 2001;107:933–41.

Dermatoses associated with spinal cord injury

1 McDonald JW, Sadowsky C. Spinal cord injury. *Lancet* 2002;359:417–25.

Horner syndrome

1 Lazar I, Cavari Y, Rosenberg E, Knyazer B. Horner's syndrome in patients admitted to the paediatric intensive care unit: epidemiology, diagnosis and clinical practice. *Anaesth Intensive Care* 2013;41:20–3.

Gustatory hyperhidrosis

13 Mantelakis A, Lafford G, Lee CW *et al*. Frey's syndrome: a review of aetiology and treatment. *Cureus* 2021;13:e20107.

CHAPTER 84

Psychodermatology

Anthony Bewley[1,2] *and Ruth E. Taylor*[3,4]

[1]Department of Dermatology, Barts Health NHS Trust, London, UK
[2]Queen Mary University, London, UK
[3]Department of Liaison Psychiatry, Barts Health NHS Trust, London, UK
[4]Queen Mary School of Medicine and Dentistry, Queen Mary University, London, UK

PART 7: PSYCHOLOGICAL, SENSORY & NEUROLOGICAL

Introduction

What is psychodermatology?

The links between the mind and the skin have long been recognised. The skin has been described as 'the mirror of the mind' and 'a window to the soul', and so it is not surprising that the interface between dermatology and psychiatry/psychology ('psychocutaneous medicine' or 'psychodermatology') has emerged as a specific subspecialty of dermatology. It encompasses diseases that involve the complex interactions between the brain, central nervous system, autonomic nervous system, cutaneous immune system and the skin [1]. Patients with psychocutaneous disease are variably managed as dermatologists struggle, in general dermatology clinics, to meet the complex needs of these patients [2,3]. Most patients with psychocutaneous disease are reluctant to attend purely psychiatric clinics. For these reasons, over the last few decades, the subspecialty of psychodermatology has emerged to address the clinical and academic needs of this group of patients.

Skin–psyche interactions may be any of the following:

1 Primarily cutaneous disorders that can be exacerbated by psychological and emotional factors, such as psoriasis and eczema.
2 Primary psychiatric disease presenting to dermatology healthcare professionals (HCPs) as a perceived dermatological disorder, for example delusional infestation, body dysmorphic disorder, dermatitis artefacta and trichotillosis.
3 Psychiatric illness or subthreshold psychological symptoms developing as a result of a skin disease, such as depression, anxiety or both, or feelings of demoralisation, helplessness and apathy.
4 Co-morbidity of a skin disease with another psychiatric disorder, for example alcoholism and obsessive compulsive disorder.

Rook's Textbook of Dermatology, Tenth Edition. Edited by Christopher Griffiths, Jonathan Barker, Tanya Bleiker, Walayat Hussain and Rosalind Simpson.
© 2024 John Wiley & Sons Ltd. Published 2024 by John Wiley & Sons Ltd.

Psychodermatology multidisciplinary teams

Although patients often present to the dermatology department, dermatologists will usually need the support of a variety of colleagues in managing patients with psychodermatological disease. For these patients, there is increasing evidence that a psychodermatology multidisciplinary team (MDT) can improve outcomes [1,2]. Specialists who make up a psychodermatology MDT (Box 84.1) require dedicated training in the management of patients with psychocutaneous disease. Such training is not always readily available, but national and international groups are now becoming pre-eminent in meeting the training needs of the psychodermatology MDT, as well as championing the clinical–academic development of the subspecialty (Box 84.2).

Box 84.1 Different specialists that may make up the psychodermatology multidisciplinary team

- Dermatologists
- Psychiatrists
- Psychologists
- Dermatology and other nursing colleagues
- Child and adolescent mental health specialists
- Paediatricians
- Geriatricians and older age psychiatrists
- Social workers
- Trichologists
- Primary care physicians
- Child and/or vulnerable adult protection teams
- Patient advocacy and support groups
- Others, e.g. physiotherapists, occupational therapists and herbalists

---

Box 84.2 National and international psychodermatology organisations

- Association of Psychoneurocutaneous Medicine of North America (APMNA): www.psychodermatology.us
- European Society for Dermatology and Psychiatry (ESDaP): www.psychodermatology.net
- Japanese Society of Psychosomatic Dermatology (JPSD): www.jpsd-ac.org/en
- Psychodermatology UK: www.psychodermatology.co.uk
- Skin Support: www.skinhealthinfo.org.uk

All last accessed June 2022.

Models of provision of psychodermatology services

There are several models of how psychodermatology services are delivered, all of which are compatible with a psychodermatology MDT. These include:

- A well-informed dermatologist who refers to a psychiatrist or psychologist when there is clinical need as a clinical adjacency.
- A dermatologist who refers to a psychiatrist or psychologist who is in a remote clinic (who will be able to support and supervise decisions taken by a dermatologist).
- A dermatologist who has a psychiatrist sitting in the clinic at the same time. Patients are seen by both specialists concurrently.
- A dermatologist who has a psychologist as a clinical adjacency (psychologists rarely sit in on clinics with dermatologists or psychiatrists).

The model where a psychiatrist and dermatologist see patients concurrently is optimal in managing disorders where there is a primary psychiatric disorder presenting via the skin and the patient lacks insight. Such patients are difficult to engage with remote psychiatric or psychological assessment.

Classification

The classification of psychodermatological disease is useful, but more complicated than it may first appear [1]. The American Psychiatric Association has published the *Diagnostic and Statistical Manual of Mental Health Disorders 5* or DSM-5 [2], the aim of which is to provide general categorisations and diagnostic criteria for psychiatric disorders. These manuals are tools for HCPs and do not represent a substitute for expert clinical opinion. The World Health Organization's *International Classification of Disease 10* or ICD-10 offers a general classification of all diseases and has a section that relates to mental health disorders. ICD-11, the next version, was adopted by the World Health Assembly in 2019 and is available to implement but has not yet fully taken over and ICD-10 remains in widespread use in mental health services [3].

Psychological co-morbidities of chronic skin disease and the 'golden rules of psychodermatology'

Psychological stress is an integral cause of skin disease either as an initiating or an exacerbating factor leading to increased disease morbidity (Chapter 15). It is therefore essential that the skin condition is treated concomitantly with the psychological co-morbidities (or the psychiatric/psychological aetiology). Part of the essential treatment of concomitant psychiatric/psychological disease is the assessment of risk both to the patients and to others (self-harm and suicidality), which should be in one's mind for every dermatology consultation. Treating the skin disease without treating the psychiatric/psychological disease makes no sense and yet a lot of training in dermatology makes little reference to the treatment of psychological disease. Empathy and compassion are needed and help develop rapport and engagement. A non-judgemental approach facilitates trust.

This leads to the 'golden rules of psychodermatology':

1 Exclude organic disease.
2 Appropriately assess and treat the dermatological disease *at the same time* as appropriately assessing and treating the psychological disease.

The following four discussions of different diseases illustrate the principle.

1 *Atopic eczema*. The complex biopsychosocial realities of living with atopic eczema are clear (see www.atopicskindisease.com for useful information; last accessed June 2022). Atopic children and adolescents show more anxiety, handle situations less well and are provoked to anger more readily. In school and college, the psychosocial issues of mixing in peer groups and making personal relationships may be blighted by feelings of stigmatisation and disfigurement. Stress makes atopic eczema worse [1]. Psychotherapies have a part to play in the holistic (skin and psychosocial) treatment plan.

2 *Psoriasis*. Psoriasis is much more than a skin disease. Functional magnetic resonance imaging (MRI) studies of patients with psoriasis show changes in the brain in response to 'disgust' images [2]. Anxiety, depression and suicidal ideation are more common than in patients with eczema, acne or alopecia [3]. Depression is particularly significant and may remain undetected but is important because patients need to be treated holistically in order to improve [4]. Many patients indicate that stress triggered the onset of the skin disease, but the latent period between a significant life stress and the onset or exacerbation of psoriasis has been difficult to assess. The response to phototherapy in highly worried individuals was almost half that of those who were deemed to have low worry and was constant for disease severity, disease duration, gender, age and skin type [5].

3 *Chronic urticaria*. Chronic spontaneous urticaria has a significant effect on quality of life. It is significantly associated with depression, dysthymia and anxiety. Psychological factors may be prominent at the onset and contribute to disease progression, and negative coping may be associated with exacerbations [6].

4 *Alopecia areata*. There has always been a strong anecdotal belief that the onset and recurrence of alopecia areata are related to stress and major life events [7]. Management of the grieving process and the psychosocial implications of living with hair loss is very much part of managing the patient's disease. Individual case reports continue to record success with individual psychotherapy and/or use of antidepressants, often selective serotonin reuptake inhibitors (SSRIs), and not always in the presence of clinical depression [7].

Stigmatisation, visible differences and coping strategies

The word *stigma* referred originally to a mark or brand on Greek slaves, distinguishing them from those who were free. The term describes the situation of an individual who is disqualified from full social acceptance. The stigmatised individual is normal until rendered abnormal by societal views. These events may occur early, for example in those afflicted by congenital skin problems, or later in individuals with an acquired visible difference. However, stigma is not just confined to alterations in the visible body. Stigmatisation may be an issue following individual behaviours and social factors such as substance abuse and unemployment. Or it may be associated with psychiatric disease. In addition, there are the population prejudices of ethnicity and religion.

Common situations where stigma may be encountered by patients include the following:

- Physical visible differences: congenital naevi (e.g. port-wine stain), acquired visible differences such as vitiligo, widespread inflammatory skin disease, surgical or post-traumatic visible differences.
- Behavioural and social factors: alcoholism and substance misuse and imprisonment.
- Psychiatric disease and learning disabilities.
- Race and religion.

Stigmatisation in later life may present a different perspective because the patient has become a physical stranger to themselves. This is most striking and obvious in those who have developed disfiguring facial scarring, but is also as valid for the patient with a late-onset dermatosis or those who suffer the odour of hidradenitis suppurativa. Patients who experience stigmatisation often refer to the guilt and shame that inhibits them from seeking help.

Stigma in psychiatry

Some people may hold a negative image of those with mental illness [1]. As with skin disease, there is a traditional stereotyping from historical attitudes towards psychiatric patients. HCPs who do not work with psychiatric patients may be inexperienced in accommodating the needs of this group. The importance of reducing the impact of stigmatisation [2] is better understood in relation to social exclusion theory, which holds that:

1 Humans possess a fundamental motive to avoid exclusion from social groupings.
2 Much social behaviour attempts to improve the chances of inclusion.
3 Negative affect (including loneliness and depression) results when a person does not or cannot achieve a desired level of social inclusion [3].

The measurement of stigma in dermatology and psychiatry has tended to rely on general measures of mental health with depression and anxiety scores, but also with psychometric measures of self-esteem such as the Rosenberg self-esteem scale. This has been used to assess stigmatisation in psoriasis and eczema as well as mental illness. Furthermore the stigma scale for mental illness [4], developed to examine discrimination, disclosure and potential positive reactions to mental illness, demonstrated that stigma scale scores were negatively correlated with global self-esteem. Interventions in dermatological stigmata are concentrated on firstly the reduction in visibility, and secondly psychological-based approaches to forestall stigmatisation.

A lot of research into stigma and dermatology is being developed, particularly through the work of the European Society for Dermatology and Psychiatry (Box 84.2). This has led to a mapping of the stigmatisation of patients with skin disease and to the better development of assessment tools [5].

Help for the stigmatised begins with information control from both the physician and family. Self-help and contact with patient advocacy groups, such as Changing Faces in the UK, can be invaluable (Box 84.3). Being part of a tolerant and informed grouping allows the expression of the normal developmental skills of the individual. Methods to change entrenched reactions within society to physical and psychological difference are more difficult to evaluate.

Box 84.3 Coping strategies suggested by Changing Faces

3-2-1-Go!

This prepares a patient with a visible difference with the following coping strategies:

- Three things to do if someone stares at you:
  - Look back and smile
  - Look back, smile and say, *'I'm sorry, do we know one another?'*
  - Ask them not to stare
- Two things to say if someone asks you what happened:
  - *'I have a skin condition but I'd rather not talk about it'*
  - *'I've had psoriasis for a few years but it's not contagious'*
- One thing to think if someone appears to turn away:
  - *'It's ok, they didn't mean any harm'*

REACHOUT

- R: reassurance – putting someone at their ease
- E: energy – creating interest in what they are saying
- A: assertiveness – taking the initiative
- C: courage – being strong and taking control
- H: humour – introducing fun or a joke
- O: over there! – distracting away from the skin condition
- U: understanding – being aware that seeing a skin condition can be difficult
- T: tenacity – try again; use a different strategy if the first does not work

From www.changingfaces.org.uk (last accessed June 2022).

Disability, quality of life and assessment in psychodermatology

Quality of life (QOL) is defined as an individual's perception of their position in life in the context of the culture and value system in which they live and in relation to their goals, expectations, standards and concerns. It is a broad-ranging concept, affected in a complex way by the person's physical heath, psychological state, level of independence and social relationships and their relationship to salient features of their environment [1]. Dermatologists increasingly understand that physical disease and QOL are intimately, but not linearly, associated. Patients with skin disease are often very clear that their condition has an impact on their lives. This impact may be huge or relatively minor. The amount of skin disease, though, does not correlate with the extent of psychosocial co-morbidity; nor does greater disease extent and longevity necessarily correlate with a lower QOL. This highlights the complexity and individuality of the illness experience which many factors contribute to – risk factors which are associated with increased difficulty in coping and resilience factors which are protective and associated with better adjustment [2,3].

Managing patients holistically means that clinicians must be able to assess how the patient is feeling and what the impact of their disease is on their QOL. Assessments may be unstructured following Socratic question principles (i.e. open-ended questions such as 'How are you feeling' or 'How are you coping at the moment', while maintaining techniques of active listening such as affirmative nodding or paraphrasing the patient's replies to questions), or may be

done using validated and reproducible tools (Box 84.4) [4]. There is a growing interest in cumulative QOL assessments (i.e. lifetime QOL).

Box 84.4 Validated tools to measure quality of life (QOL)

Dermatology-specific (but non-disease-specific) tools
- Dermatology life quality index (DLQI)
- Skindex 16 and 29

Dermatological disease-specific tools (usually validated for physical and psychosocial disease extent)
- Cardiff acne disability index
- Simplified psoriasis index
- SCORAD (eczema) score
- Vitiqol (vitiligo)
- Rosaqol (rosacea)
- HydroQOL (hyperhidrosis)

Measurements of the impact of skin disease on carers and younger patients
- Children's dermatology life quality index (CDLQI)
- Family dermatology life quality index (FDLQI)

There are some very short screening tools; for example the generalised anxiety disorder (GAD) two-question screen. If a patient answers affirmatively for either of the following questions, further assessment may be important:

Question 1 During the past 4 weeks, have you been bothered by feeling worried, tense or anxious most of the time?
Question 2 Are you frequently tense, irritable and having trouble sleeping?

These questions are used extensively in research, but are becoming increasingly important in everyday dermatology practice as they offer a standardised snapshot of patient psychosocial well-being (some research results also include scores of disease extent). There is an increasing recognition that it is not just the life of the patient affected by a skin disease, but also the lives of family, partners, carers and loved ones who are often affected by the patient's journey through treatment. Assessing the impact of disease on partners and family is crucial to the well-being of the patient. There is a growing interest in cumulative QOL scoring and meta-analyses of QOL tools.

There is also an increasing interest in QOL assessments partly driven by developments within psychodermatology, and the development of newer medicines (usually biologics) for the treatment of otherwise difficult-to-treat dermatological conditions (e.g. the use of Janus kinase (JAK) inhibitors in the treatment of nodular prurigo). These developments are leading to a greater interest in disease-specific validated and reproducible QOL tools. However, the tools must be:
- Relevant to the disease.
- Validated.
- Reproducible.
- Uniform.
- Standardised where possible.
- Translated and back translated to other languages.

It would be very useful for QOL tools to be standardised and internationally agreed, particularly so that research using QOL tools is able to use the same QOL findings between different studies [5].

DELUSIONAL BELIEFS

A true primary delusion is a false, unshakeable belief that arises from internal processes in a patient, which are not amenable to logic and are out of keeping with the person's educational and cultural background. Primary delusions can be an isolated phenomenon (a monosymptomatic hypochondriacal psychosis such as delusional infestation) or part of a broader psychosis (e.g. schizophrenia). A secondary delusion more commonly occurs with affective disorder and the delusion is secondary to the mood (e.g. a nihilistic delusion in severe depression may influence the patient into believing that their skin is rotting away). The intensity with which a delusional belief is held may be variable. Delusional infestation, for example, may arise as an overvalued idea, and this somewhat less intensely held belief may be more amenable to negotiation and reason [1].

Delusional infestation

Synonyms and inclusions
- Ekbom disease
- Delusional parasitosis
- Parasitophobia
- Monosymptomatic delusional hypochondriasis

Introduction and general description
Delusional infestation (DI) is an uncommon, but very disabling, condition where the patient is convinced that they are infested with a mite, parasite, bacteria, worm, insect, virus or animate material [1,2]. As this is a delusional disorder, the patient will hold this belief unshakeably and very often tenaciously. The patient believes wholeheartedly that they are infested even though no infesting organism or material can be found by clinicians. Although delusions are usually unshakeable and fixed, a few patients present with an overstated ideation of infestation (i.e. the patient believes that it is *possible* rather than being unshakeably *convinced* that they are infested despite all evidence to the contrary). Patients with DI will usually present to dermatologists and be extremely reticent about seeing psychiatrists; they will frequently consume large amounts of resources having often seen a wide range of HCPs while remaining unengaged with treatment [2]. Some special forms of DI exist:
- *DI as a shared delusion* (*folie à deux*, etc.). Family members, carers and friends may believe that they too are infested, or delusionally share the belief of the individual who is presenting with DI. This is common.
- *DI by proxy*. Patients complain that their child, pet or friend is infested despite all evidence to the contrary.

DI may be primary (no underlying cause is found) or secondary (to concomitant organic or psychiatric disease). Approximately half of patients presenting with DI will have secondary DI. The condition is usually a monosymptomatic delusion in that most patients hold no other delusional beliefs (as in, for example, schizophrenia). Occasionally, patients may have other delusional ideations (usually when the DI is secondary to a co-morbid psychotic disease). Most patients can 'see' the infestation but some remain uncertain whether what they see is actually the infesting organism or some other material. Patients are often isolated and have lived with their disease for a long time. Many fail to be engaged with HCPs, as the latter may try to reason that the disease is 'all in their head'. However, patients' lives can be extremely disabled by their disease and they often find themselves unemployed, in debt (e.g. some patients, in an attempt to rid their home of the infesting organisms, repeatedly buy new furniture and carpets), isolated (as loved ones may become more and more exasperated) and distraught (many patients go to great lengths to wash or clean their bodies).

The terms used prior to DI are now inappropriate as they refer to 'phobias' (DI is a delusional not a phobic disorder) and 'parasitosis' (DI patients present with a range of infesting organisms and animate material, not just parasites).

Epidemiology
Incidence and prevalence
These are unknown, but are estimated at 17 per million people per year, although this is probably an underestimate.

Age
Delusional infestation can occur at any adult age but the peak incidence is said to be in 50-year-olds. It is rare in children although shared delusions in the children of patients with DI have been reported.

Sex
The occurrence of DI is probably equally distributed in the sexes (as affected men present to clinicians much less with this disease than women do), but is reported to occur in a ratio of male : female 1 : 2.5.

Ethnicity
Delusional infestation is found in all ethnicities.

Causes
Delusional infestation may be:
- Primary (i.e. no underlying identifiable cause); this occurs in approximately 30% of all cases.
- Secondary to organic disease (Table 84.1); this occurs in approximately 60% of all cases. In many departments recreational drug usage accounts for 25–33% of all cases (Figure 84.1). Patients who have a recreational drug habit leading to their DI may not admit to using recreational drugs [3].
- Secondary to, or part of, a known psychiatric delusional disease (e.g. schizophrenia or bipolar disease) (Table 84.1); this occurs in approximately 5% of all cases.
- Iatrogenic. Some patients develop secondary organic DI as a consequence of medication, especially opiates and dopaminergic medication, commonly antiparkinsonian dopaminergics; this occurs in approximately 5% of all cases.

Table 84.1 Diseases associated with or causing delusional infestation (DI).

Primary DI	DI secondary to organic disease	DI secondary to psychiatric disease
No underlying disease	Substance abuse (Figure 84.1)	Schizophrenia
	Alcohol	Bipolar depression with psychotic symptoms
	Recreational drugs	Borderline personality disorder
	Prescribed medications, e.g. antiparkinsonian medication such as ropinirole, opioids	Anxiety disorder
	Infections	
	Tuberculosis	
	HIV	
	Endocrine disorders	
	Thyroid disease	
	Cancer	
	Tumours	
	Haematological cancer	
	Chronic or acute liver disease	
	Renal failure	
	Metabolic disease	
	Vitamin B$_{12}$ deficiency	
	Autoimmune disorders	
	Systemic lupus erythematosus	
	Multiple sclerosis	
	Brain disorders	
	Cerebrovascular disease	
	Parkinson disease	

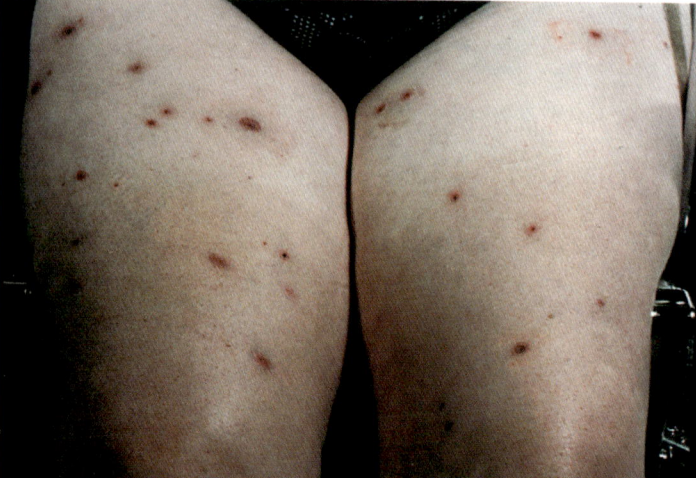

Figure 84.1 Excoriations in delusions of parasitosis in an amphetamine addict.

Pathophysiology

The pathophysiology of the DI depends on the cause. For example where there is a recreational drug habit, the brain biochemistry – for instance certain dopamine pathways – is altered; this may lead to hallucinations.

Hallucinations [4] may be:

- *Tactile.* Patients with DI, particularly secondary to certain drugs, will describe formication (sensations of crawling on the skin), itch, pain and burning sensations of the skin or the subcutaneous tissues.
- *Visual.* Many patients will see black dots and moving small material on their skin.
- *Auditory.* Some patients describe 'crackling' sensations, especially when they rub strands of hair.
- *Olfactory.* Patients may notice an unpleasant smell, although this is usually with the olfactory reference syndrome.

Many patients describe an initiating event. This can be a real insect bite, a misinterpretation of a real perception (an illusion) or a true hallucination (sensory experience in the absence of a sensory stimulus). Rather than dismissing the misinterpretation of an infestation, altered reasoning may occur (which may have a genetic and/or neurological basis), which leads the patient to believe there is a true infestation. Functional MRI in DI patients indicates that there may be abnormalities in the cortical and mid-brain areas associated with the *interpretation* of perceptions [4]. The involvement of the dopaminergic mid-brain structures and the therapeutic efficacy of antipsychotic D$_2$-dopamine antagonists may indicate dopaminergic dysfunction in DI. For patients with DI secondary to organic disease, there is often a reason why brain function may be compromised.

Predisposing factors

- There may be a genetic predisposition for patients with primary DI and DI secondary to psychiatric disease [2].
- Patients with DI may be more likely to be socially isolated (particularly those with primary DI where checks of probabilistic thinking from family and friends may not be readily available).
- There may be iatrogenic causes (particularly the use of opiates and antiparkinsonian medication).
- Recreational drug usage (although patients may not admit that they have a recreational drug habit) [3].
- Other causes of secondary DI.

Pathology

A skin biopsy is best avoided except to exclude other cutaneous differential diagnoses. Skin biopsies taken at the request of the patient to 'look for the bug' and which show no pathological evidence of an infestation are unlikely to satisfy the patient. Histology (if available) shows cutaneous excoriations or external trauma at various stages of the healing process. Other investigations are outlined here according to the clinical picture.

Clinical features

History

The diagnosis of DI is usually not difficult and is initially considered following the history alone. Patients present with a belief that they are infested by an organism or animate material. They will often describe itching, biting, burning or crawling sensations on the skin that may be localised or generalised. These sensations may be intermittent or, more often, persistent and disabling. Patients often make great effort to prove the infestation (see section on the 'specimen sign') [5].

Engagement of the patient

Although the diagnosis is usually straightforward, engaging the patient is more challenging. A negotiation around the validity of the patient's experience and attempts to question the nature of what they are experiencing may not engage and indeed may

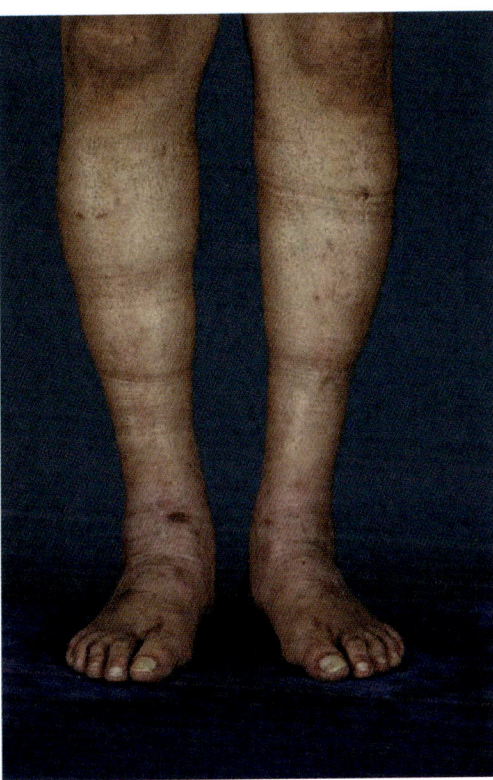

Figure 84.2 Patient with delusional infestation. The linear pressure marks on the legs are where the patient applied elastic bands to stop the 'worms' from travelling up his leg beneath the skin.

alienate them. Patients with DI are frequent 'doctor shoppers' and will react angrily or even complain to regulatory authorities if their experience is challenged (even if very sympathetically). Engagement of the patient is exceptionally important. It is crucial that HCPs carefully examine the skin of patients with suspected DI for several reasons [2]. Firstly, it is important to check for a genuine infestation. Secondly, it is important to exclude differential diagnoses and to look for clinical evidence of secondary causes of DI. It is essential for the patient to experience the clinician checking for an infestation, thereby confirming that their symptoms are being addressed. On examination, patients often have localised or generalised excoriations, erosions and sometimes ulceration. These skin changes are produced in an attempt to extricate the organism, usually with the fingernails, but occasionally nail files, scissors, needles, penknives, tweezers and nail clippers. Some patients go to much greater lengths to eradicate the perceived infestation by using surgical implements, handicraft knives and chemical corrosives (Figure 84.2). These can inflict significant damage. Occasionally there are no physical signs, but the patient will still maintain that the infestation is present and the itching/biting/stinging sensations are there.

Differential diagnosis

Differential diagnoses include:
- A genuine infestation.
- Causes of generalised pruritus (Chapter 81).
- Immunobullous disease (usually this is easily distinguished from DI by the clinical picture).
- Organic disease that leads to secondary DI.
- Part of another psychiatric disease (e.g. schizophrenia).

Complications and co-morbidities

Coexistent affective disease (anxiety, depression or both) is common in patients with DI. Assessing psychosocial co-morbidities is important. There is a considerable (but not fully charted) risk of suicide in patients with DI. Bacterial superinfection of excoriations and irritant dermatitis (e.g. from the patient's own use of cleansing agents) are common. Some patients create severe ulcers and extensive erosions from attempts to eradicate perceived organisms.

Disease course and prognosis

The crucial step in managing DI is engagement of the patient [6,7]. As with all psychodermatology disease, HCPs should treat the skin and the psychological disease concurrently (the 'golden rules'). Psychodermatology specialist centres are probably the best places to treat patients with DI, and most psychodermatologists will try to commence a treatment plan at the first appointment although this is not always possible. Treatment is usually continued for several months until the delusion has settled. Patients at this stage will tell clinicians that the infesting organisms have 'gone'. Treatment of substance abuse and co-morbid affective disease may be necessary. Treatment may be withdrawn slowly a few months after the delusion has disappeared [7,8], but recurrence of DI symptoms may occur in up to 33% of patients (especially those who have not managed to control their recreational drug and alcohol abuse). Reported adherence to medication is good once engagement of the patient is established [7], but this may be in specialist centres with extensive experience of managing patients with DI. The prognosis in these centres is favourable, with up to 75% of patients responding to treatment. Suicide is always a risk in patients with DI, and clinicians must be aware of local services to which suicidal patients can be referred urgently [9].

The prognosis is good if the patient is engaged. A proportion of patients will remit despite no medication (this is true for all delusional disease, as up to one-third of patients resolve their delusions spontaneously). A proportion of patients with DI will refuse to engage, and it is probably best if the HCPs persist with explaining the benefits of medication. For those who simply will not engage with any HCPs, an MDT approach to assess the patient's risk to themselves and others may be necessary. It is clear that patients who remain untreated with antipsychotic medication have a smaller chance of responding to any medication [10].

Some colleagues check prolactin levels to assess adherence to antipsychotic medication (prolactin levels will increase with many newer antipsychotics) [11].

Investigations, testing for recreational drugs and the 'specimen sign'

Patients with DI will usually be keen to prove their infestation. Many will bring along specimens of the organisms that they believe are infesting them (Figure 84.3). This used to be called the 'matchbox sign', but more recently clinicians have recognised that patients may have access to sophisticated equipment and may bring along hi-tech audio or computer images of material they have themselves analysed. This has been termed the 'specimen sign' [5]. It is imperative that these specimens are taken seriously and carefully reviewed by clinicians. Skin debris and specimen material may be analysed for human pathogens by microscopy in the local microbiology

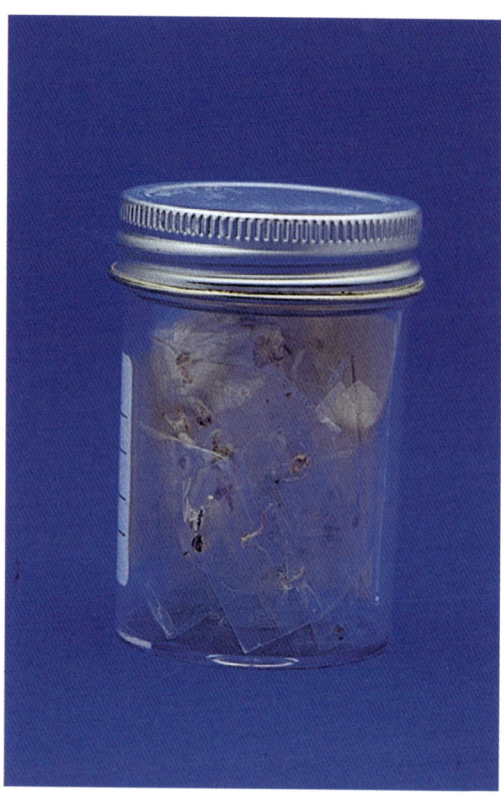

(a)

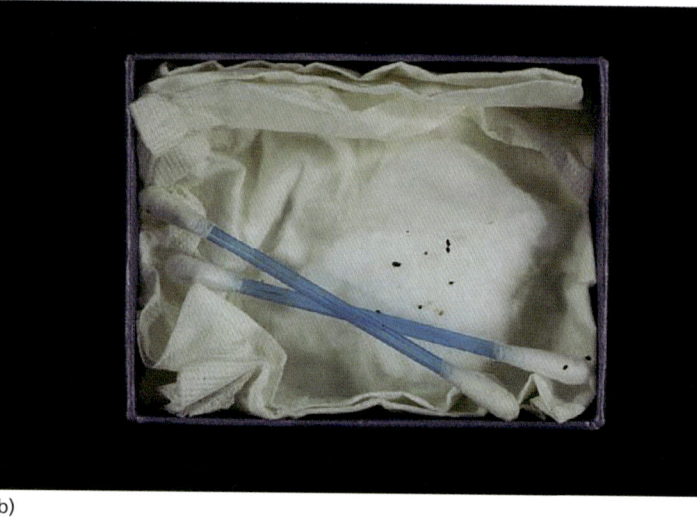

(b)

Figure 84.3 (a) Container brought in by a patient with delusional parasitosis. (b) 'Specimen sign' for delusional infestation.

laboratory. A catalogue of normal results will assist the patient in understanding that the clinician understands their experience and continues to seek and exclude a genuine infestation. Patients may repeatedly canvass clinicians to take skin biopsies to prove the infestation, and be dissatisfied with biopsies that fail to show a genuine infestation. Otherwise, investigations may be led by the clinical picture. A pruritus screen is undertaken routinely in some centres, but investigations that are informed by the clinical picture are usually acceptable. Assessment of coexistent affective disease and suicidality is imperative and careful assessment of recreational drug and alcohol usage is important.

Many psychodermatology units will now also routinely ask patients for permission to test for recreational drug usage. The techniques for this are discussed in Chapter 120. There are patients who use recreational drugs, but are embarrassed or ashamed to admit to the habit.

Some departments will take a baseline prolactin level so that objective assessments of any rise in prolactin after taking certain antipsychotics will help assess effective adherence to medication.

Finally, investigations, according to clinical picture, to exclude organic disease may be necessary.

Management
General principles of management
Engagement of the patient is crucial in the management of DI [12]. HCPs must develop a sympathetic, understanding approach to the patient. It is usually futile to try to dissuade patients of the validity of their infestation. Instead it is better to let the patient know that you understand the difficulties that they are experiencing, and that you have successfully looked after patients with similar disease. Patients with DI are often extremely debilitated by their disease. Many struggle to maintain relationships and employment and many end up considerably in debt because they have spent so much money trying to eradicate their perceived infestation from themselves and their homes.

Research in DI is difficult and very few randomised controlled clinical trials exist. Evidence tends to come from case series and is eminence based rather than evidence based. The choice of antipsychotic medication is often based on patient age, co-morbidities and lifestyle rather than any direct comparison of efficacy. Most psychodermatologists now avoid pimozide due to its cardiotoxic risks. Instead, most recommend atypical antipsychotics as the first line of treatment, together with treatment of the skin and any co-morbid affective disease (Figure 84.4).

Many patients will accept medication to help their distress even though it is not directed at the eradication of the 'parasites'. If broached in terms of using a medication that 'has helped others before' and 'getting started to help in some way' or 'to help with the sensations in the skin', psychotropic medication may be commenced in the dermatology clinic by experienced physicians [13]. Management is ideally effected with close liaison between dermatology and psychiatry. It is mandatory to refer to a psychiatrist immediately if there is any indication of risk of suicide. Adherence to medication is actually very good once the patient is engaged with medication, as is the prognosis.

In the UK the British Association of Dermatologists has recently developed and published guidelines for the management of delusional infestation [14].

First line
First line management of patients with DI includes an MDT approach and managing the skin, delusional belief and the risk of harm at the same time (Box 84.5) [15]. Antipsychotics in very low doses are the first line of pharmacological treatment. Clinicians will need to explain to patients that the use of these medications is in very low doses and not the doses usually used for the management of conditions such as schizophrenia. Clinicians may also need to engage local pharmacies as patients may leave the clinic engaged

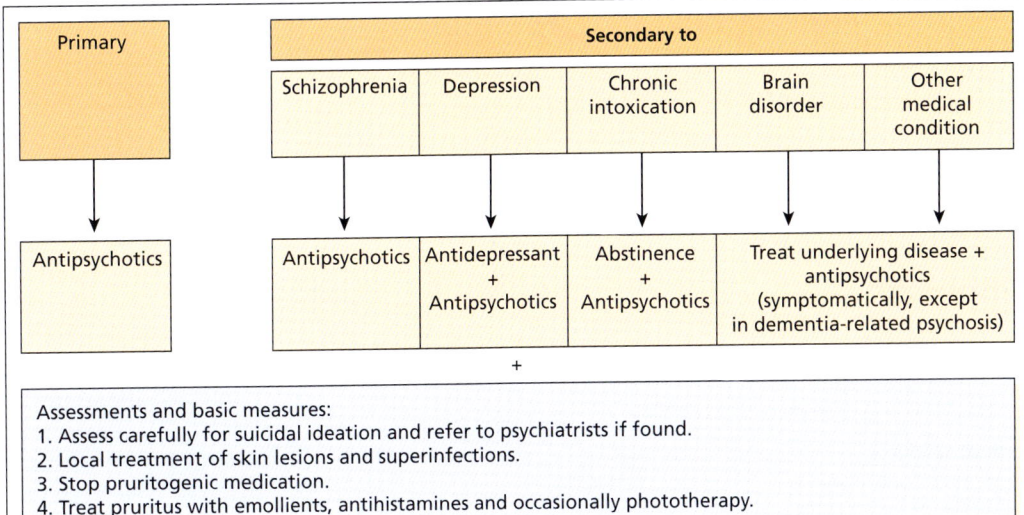

Figure 84.4 Management algorithm for delusional infestation. Reproduced from Lepping *et al.* 2014 [12] with permission of John Wiley & Sons.

and then become disengaged when other colleagues/HCPs challenge the use of antipsychotics. There is only one (fairly poor) randomised controlled clinical trial of pimozide versus placebo. However, atypical antipsychotics are probably more effective and have a better side effect profile than conventional antipsychotics [7]. The antipsychotic rispiridone is both a dopamine blocker and a serotonin antagonist and has proved of use in doses of 1–8 mg per day [8], but usually only small doses <3 mg are required. Olanzapine has a higher affinity as a serotonin blocker than a dopamine antagonist and can be effective in surprisingly small doses. The choice of the antipsychotic depends on the clinical picture and the patient's co-morbidities, which is why an MDT approach is preferred [15].

Box 84.5 Management of delusional infestation

- Engaging the patient
- Educating the patient about your understanding of how difficult the condition is for them
- Managing the patient via a multidisciplinary team (MDT) where possible [14]
- Assessing the patient for affective disease and suicidal ideation
- Assessing the patient for recreational drug usage
- Treating the skin appropriately and according to the cutaneous physical signs
- Treating the delusional belief and the skin sensations, usually with an antipsychotic in very low doses
- Considering the treatment of any affective or psychiatric disease
- Assessing the risk to others and managing that accordingly (e.g. safeguarding issues)
- Communicating with primary care colleagues
- Referring to drug and alcohol rehabilitation schemes if appropriate and agreed by the patient
- Accessing a regional/national MDT if the patient complains or is litigious or there is particular complexity
- Treating early in the course of the disease is important as the longer a patient remains untreated, the poorer the clinical outcome [10]

Treatment ladder for delusional infestation

All patients
- Topical treatment is desirable and is chosen according to clinical need, e.g. emollients, dressings
- Assessment of risk, suicidality and affective disease
- Referral to substance abuse unit if appropriate
- Topical antiseptics and/or oral antibiotics if a genuine bacterial superinfection is established

First line
- Antipsychotics (choose according to the lifestyle of the patient):
  - Risperidone (0.5–4 mg)
  - Olanzapine (2.5–10 mg)
  - Amisulpride (50–400 mg)
  - Quetiapine (25–100 mg)
  - Aripiprazole (5–15 mg)
  - Antidepressants (usually SSRIs) if depressive disorder is the underlying cause of DI

Second line
- Antidepressants (usually SSRIs) if there is coexistent affective disease

Third line
- Psychotherapy has its advocates but patients may not adhere to this line of treatment
- Phototherapy occasionally may be helpful and facilitates support from well-informed nurses

Complaints and litigation

Patients with DI can be very challenging. They may have seen a lot of HCPs and have been either dismissed or disengaged. As a consequence, HCPs managing patients with DI may be subject to complaints and litigation [16]. It is really very important that governance and regulatory bodies recognise this, as HCPs acting with all good intent may find that they become burned out, or are subject to persistent complaints from patients. There are emerging regional and national MDT support bodies in psychodermatology, so that HCPs can share their experience, expertise and well-being with colleagues managing patients with complex disease.

Resources

Clinician resources
Ahmed *et al*. 2022 [14].

Patient resources
Mind: www.mind.org.uk.
Samaritans: www.samaritans.org.
Skin Support: www.skinsupport.org.uk.
(All last accessed June 2022.)

Olfactory delusions

Synonyms and inclusions
- Delusions of smell
- Olfactory delusional syndrome
- Olfactory reference syndrome
- Bromidrosiphobia
- Cacosmia
- Phantosmia

Introduction and general description
Olfactory reference syndrome (ORS) is similar to DI in that it is a monosymptomatic delusional hypochondriasis (single symptom delusional belief which mimics a perceived illness). It is one of several unique primary psychiatric disorders that present to dermatologists. Published descriptions of ORS date back to the late 19th century and cases have been reported across the globe. The term ORS was coined by Pryse-Phillips [1] who described the condition as follows: 'The association of an "intrinsic" smell hallucination and a "contrite" reaction in the absence of a history of preceding depression' (although anxiety and depression may be a *consequence* of ORS). ORS is probably a spectrum of different disease presentations and there remains some discussion about its classification. Patients may present with a true delusional and hallucinatory illness, but some may present as part of a body dysmorphic disease (BDD) or obsessive–compulsive disorder (OCD).

Characteristically, the smell in ORS is described as being emitted from the patient – that is, intrinsic as opposed to extrinsic (the latter commonly described by patients with temporal lobe epilepsy or schizophrenia). The term 'contrite reaction' has been described in more recent literature as a 'preoccupation with body odour' where patients may become sensitive to ideas of reference (e.g. people holding/scratching noses or opening windows), have a sense of shame and excessively wash themselves and change clothing, become socially withdrawn and in some cases suffer

mild depression [2]. Hallucinations of various types occur as part of many disease processes; in ORS, however, the hallucination is olfactory only. It is accepted that persistent preoccupation with body odour may be seen in certain psychiatric illnesses or may be associated with organic brain injury and such disorders must therefore be excluded when diagnosing ORS [3,4].

Dispute has surrounded the classification of ORS [5]; this is largely due to the presence of the primary symptoms in other conditions. Most regard ORS as a delusional disorder with similarities to BDD. Since the behaviours that describe the contrite reaction are commonly seen in obsessed patients, the question has arisen as to whether or not ORS is in fact a variant of OCD. Much of the published literature is in the form of case reports, which makes this investigation more difficult; however, particular patterns have emerged and young males without any concurrent psychiatric disorder have been identified as the most frequent presenters.

Epidemiology
This is a rare condition, which is more common in young male adults (male : female 4.5 : 1) and occurs in all ethnic groups. Associated diseases include:
- Depression (especially with nihilistic symptoms).
- Other affective disease.
- Delusional infestation.
- Recreational drugs.
- Multiple sclerosis.
- Obsessive–compulsive disorders.
- Body dysmorphic disease.
- Dementia.
- Temporal lobe epilepsy.

Pathophysiology
Olfactory reference syndrome is poorly researched and the pathophysiology is not understood [6]. There are some clues, though, from case reports. People with ORS may present at the onset of dementia, and some cases are precipitated by dopaminergic medication for Parkinson disease. There are some patients who present with ORS as part of other psychiatric diseases. It has been suggested it could be seen as an anxiety-related disorder similar to post-traumatic stress disorder but with sensory olfactory symptoms [7].

ORS may be primary or secondary (as with DI). Primary ORS has no underlying cause. Secondary ORS is secondary to organic disease such as multiple sclerosis, temporal lobe epilepsy or recreational drug usage. It may also be secondary to depression, particularly that where the patient is convinced of their own worthlessness.

Clinical features
Patients will usually present with a long history of experiencing an unpleasant smell either from a specific part of the body or from all over the body [8]. The smell is almost always unpleasant and may be faecal, putrific, sweaty, metallic or acrid. Patients will usually go to great lengths to cleanse themselves of the smell and will reject any suggestion that it is not experienced by other people. Some patients have organic brain disease and others will have features of BDD, OCD or both.

Box 84.6 lists the proposed criteria for diagnosing ORS [9].

Box 84.6 Proposed criteria for diagnosing the olfactory reference syndrome (ORS)

- ORS is a preoccupation with body odour or halitosis that persists despite reassurance that it is not perceived by others
- It is seen in someone who recognises that the preoccupation is unreasonable or excessive
- It causes significant distress or impairment in function
- It is not secondary to another disorder (e.g. depression, anxiety disorders) or a consequence of substances or other organic cause
- It can be described as ORS with 'poor insight' where the person only at times recognises the preoccupation as excessive/unreasonable. However, in these cases, care must be taken not to miss a psychotic disorder

Adapted from Lochner and Stein 2003 [9].

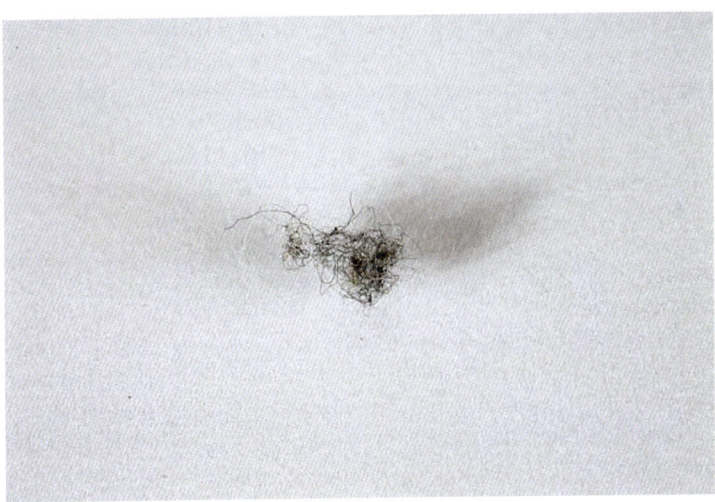

Figure 84.5 Sample of the fibres that a patient with Morgellons disease brought to clinic.

Differential diagnosis

There are a number of possible differential diagnoses:
- A genuine body odour.
- Trimethylaminuria (fish odour syndrome): the patient has a genetic amino acid metabolic syndrome caused by abnormalities of the production/function of the ezyme flavin containing mono-oxygenase 3, which leads to the build-up of trimethylamine (TMA) in body fluids. The ability to smell TMA objectively is genetic and variable. Urine analysis for TMA (usually compared with TMA oxide) is helpful in establishing the diagnosis.
- Temporal lobe epilepsy (olfactory hallucinations are common).
- Other organic brain disease: dementia, Parkinson disease, brain tumour.

Investigations

Urinalysis should be used to exclude trimethylaminuria. Clinical examination and then appropriate neurological investigations should be performed as indicated. HCPs may consider MRI of the brain and/or investigating for temporal lobe epilepsy where clinically appropriate.

Management

Management is informed by case reports and case series only [8–10]. Treatment of the underlying BDD or OCD is the prime objective for some patients; treatment of any causative neurological disease is a similar priority.

Treatment ladder for olfactory delusions

First line
- Antidepressants (usually SSRIs) together with appropriate treatment of the skin (this may be asking the patient to wash *less* often)
- Low-dose newer antipsychotics (see 'Delusional infestation' earlier in this chapter) according to the patient's clinical picture

Second line
- Atypical antipsychotics in lower doses
- Higher doses of SSRI
- Duloxetine

Third line
- Cognitive–behavioural therapy (although many believe this to be an important adjunctive first line therapy)
- Eye movement desensitisation and reprocessing (EMDR) [7]

Morgellons syndrome

Introduction and general description

The Morgellons were described by Sir Thomas Browne in 1674 in a population from Languedoc [1], one of whose characteristics was the development of a hairy back. In 2001, a biologist whose 2-year-old child developed sores on the skin discovered that the multicoloured fibres that she stated were coming from her child's lesions were undiagnosable by the many physicians she consulted. Nevertheless she chose the name Morgellons to entitle a syndrome, set up a research foundation, raised funds and generated vast media and Internet interest.

Clinical features

The phenomenon comprises:
- Sensations of crawling, stinging and biting under the skin.
- Sores that do not heal.
- Fibre-like filaments, granules and crystals that appear on or under the skin lesions (Figure 84.5).
- Joint and muscle pain and fibromyalgia.
- Debilitating fatigue.
- Cognitive dysfunction, poor concentration and memory.

Many dermatologists point to the commonalities between this constellation of symptoms and patients with DI [2]. Even so, an examination of websites shows that patients who live with Morgellons disease are certain this is not the case and that 'Morgellons disease', as yet unrecognised, really does exist. The Morgellons Foundation has suggested that Lyme disease is to blame as well as agricultural filamentous yeasts, but the US Center for Disease Control set up an independent study to evaluate the phenomenon, and has concluded that there is no objective evidence for the 'unexplained dermopathy' [3–5].

Management

Treatment responses to pimozide and risperidone have been recorded, together with treatment of the skin with topical antiseptics, systemic antibiotics and (sometimes) phototherapy.

Most dermatologists consider Morgellons to be a variant of DI and assess and manage the patients accordingly. As mentioned in the DI section, pimozide is no longer recommended due to cardiac side effects so atypical antipsychotics are favoured. The web-based connectivity of patients with Morgellons disease means that many patients actively refute that Morgellons is a delusional disease [6].

Resources

Patient resources

Skin Support: www.skinhealthinfo.org.uk.

(Both last accessed June 2022.)

OBSESSIVE AND COMPULSIVE BEHAVIOUR

Studies of obsessive–compulsive behaviour in dermatology out-patients estimate that it is present in up to 25% of patients (background prevalence in general population up to 3% of adults), but this may include some with BDD [1,2]. However, excluding this group there were still up to 15% who have other obsessive–compulsive behaviours such as [1,3]:

- Body dysmorphic disorder.
- Lichen simplex chronicus.
- Nodular prurigo.
- Skin picking disorder.
- Acné excoriée.
- Trichotillosis.
- Onychotillomania and onychophagia.
- Health anxieties.

The general principles of treatment are as follows.

1 An empathetic, supportive approach from HCPs is essential.
2 Try to find out why the patient has the 'habit'.
3 Never attempt to tell the patient that it is 'all in their head' or that they 'need to snap out of it'.
4 Psychotherapy can produce significant improvement. Cognitive–behavioural therapy (CBT) alone has helped some patients, although the management of underlying personality difficulties may require the specific skills of a psychotherapist.
5 Habit-reversal programmes may be useful. These can be accessed online or via self-help material.

6 Selective serotonin reuptake inhibitors can be helpful. Usually patients need be encouraged to start treatment with explanations that the benefit will only start to be realised after 4–6 weeks. Higher doses may be necessary but maximal recommended doses must not be exceeded.
7 The A-B-C model of habit disorders – (i) affect regulation, (ii) behavioural regulation, and (iii) cognitive control – makes use of all modalities to help patients conceptualise and manage skin picking behaviours.
8 Treatment is always based on *appropriate* treatment of the skin together with treatment of the associated psychological disease.
9 Complex disease is best managed by a psychodermatology MDT.
10 Second and third line treatments should be initiated by a psychodermatology MDT or through appropriate specialists.

Body dysmorphic disorder

Synonyms and inclusions
- Dysmorphophobia (best not used since the condition is not a 'phobia')
- Dermatological non-disease (best not used since this term is inaccurate)

Introduction and general description

Few of us believe that our skin/body is perfect and many of us tolerate our imperfections. Patients with BDD form a spectrum whereby their perception of an aspect of their appearance impacts on their lives to a greater (and sometimes very extreme) or a lesser extent. BDD is characterised by a preoccupation with a real or imagined defect (for criteria see Box 84.7) in physical appearance, or if there is a slight physical anomaly concern is out of proportion. There is a spectrum from patients with overvalued ideas to those whose beliefs are held with delusional conviction. The defect that the patient experiences may seem trivial to objective assessors, but for them it is a major focus of their consciousness [1,2].

Box 84.7 DSM-5 Definition of body dysmorphic disorder (BDD) [14]

- *Preoccupation* with one or more perceived defects or flaws in physical appearance that are *not observable or appear slight to others*
- *At some point during the course of the disorder, the individual has performed repetitive behaviours* (e.g. mirror checking, excessive grooming, skin picking, reassurance seeking) or mental acts (e.g. comparing their appearance with that of others) in response to the appearance concerns
- The preoccupation causes clinically significant distress or impairment in social, occupational or other areas of functioning
- The appearance preoccupation is not better explained by concerns with body fat or weight in an individual whose symptoms meet diagnostic criteria for an eating disorder

---

BDD is surprisingly common, occurring in 1–2% of the general population [3]. It is more common in patients seeking aesthetic and cosmetic surgery [4]. There is a high degree of co-morbidity with mood disorders, OCD and social phobia. This is a difficult group of patients to treat, one of the main obstacles being that most patients lack insight and will not accept psychiatric treatment or referral. Patients may have ideas of reference (believing that their 'defect' has been noticed by others and believing that other people's behaviour has been modified after witnessing the 'defect'). BDD is very disabling for the patient, and for those around them, since the focus on their perceived defect seems illogical but is also unshakeable. Co-morbid affective disease is common, as is suicidal ideation (up to 25% of patients will act on their suicidal ideation) [1]. Patients are therefore best seen in a joint psychodermatology clinic where possible. There are screening tools for HCPs to identify patients with BDD (especially for those patients seeking cosmetic surgery as the surgery may not address the primary BDD pathology).

Epidemiology
Age
Body dysmorphic disorder often starts in adolescence but may affect any age group. It is often linked to low self-esteem (hence the preponderance of adolescent patients). Younger patients may have a better prognosis, in that relative dissatisfaction with appearance may be a relatively normal experience in this age group and may be self-limiting. HCPs need to be more worried when patients have severe symptoms, such as social avoidance and co-morbid mood disturbances (Box 84.8).

Box 84.8 Scales and screening questions to assess body dysmorphic disorder (BDD)

Scales
- Yale–Brown obsessive–compulsive scale (Y-BOCS). There are adult and non-adult versions. This is an HCP-driven assessment that has a reliable and reproducible record
- Cosmetic procedure screening questionnaire (COPS). This is an excellent tool to screen for BDD in the cosmetic or dermatological setting [15]
- Body dysmorphic disorder questionnaire. This is an alternative screening tool for BDD [16]
- Body dysmorphic disorder symptoms scale [17]

Screening
- How much do you currently think about your skin?
- On an average day, how many hours do you spend thinking about your skin? Please add up all the time that your feature is on your mind and make your best estimate
- Do you feel your skin is ugly or very unattractive?
- How noticeable do you think your skin is?
- Does your skin currently cause you a lot of distress?
- How many times a day do you usually check your skin either in a mirror or by feeling it with your fingers?
- How often do you feel anxious about your skin in social situations? Does it lead to you avoiding social situations?
- Has your skin had an effect on dating or on an existing relationship?
- Has your skin interfered with your ability to work or study, or your role as a homemaker?

Screening section adapted from Veale *et al.* 2012 [15].

Sex
The female : male ratio is approximately 2 : 1 but this is likely to be evolving as male aesthetic concerns are now approaching those of women.

Ethnicity
This disorder occurs in all ethnic groups.

Associated diseases
The following co-morbidities may be seen:
- Chronic skin picking.
- Depression may occur in 60% with a lifetime rate of up to 80%.
- Social phobia, that is, fear of a negative impact (37%).
- Substance abuse (40%).
- Deliberate self-harm.
- Avoidant personality disorder.
- Anorexia nervosa patients very frequently have a degree of BDD.
- Suicide.

Pathophysiology [1,3,5]
Theories suggest that sufferers from BDD have self-defeating thoughts, cognitive distortions and destructive beliefs about themselves and their appearance. The development of selective processing of emotional information about body image, physical appearance and interpersonal contact may be related to anxiety disorders and social phobia. BDD patients exhibit more perfectionist thinking and maladaptive attractiveness beliefs, and it is assumed that these are aetiological rather than symptomatic. It has been suggested that childhood abusive experiences may result in body dissatisfaction, bodily shame, low self-esteem and body image distortion. Neurobiological theories relate BDD to acquired brain abnormalities and parietal lobe function. Neurochemical and psychopharmacological evidence suggests that abnormal serotonin metabolism also contributes to BDD. By contrast, social and cultural influences are assuming an increasing importance in personal bodily appearance due to the perceived concepts of beauty, and the quest for perfection, currently prominent in media-driven societies. These pressures shape the attitudes of both women and men. Women have traditionally been driven to view and treat themselves as objects while men are pushed towards an often unattainable body image, the Adonis complex of muscular perfection.

Clinical features
Patients with BDD may present with symptoms according to their gender. Women may present with a focus on the skin of the face, breasts, nose and stomach, whereas men may present with concerns about hair (usually thinning), nose, ears, genitals and body build. Facial symptoms are common, but patients with BDD may perceive 'defects' affecting any part of the body. Concerns about hair (too much, too little or hair in the 'wrong' place) are common. Some authors indicate that when patients find defects affecting the genital and (in women) breast area, HCPs may need to ask about sexual abuse. A patient's focus on their perceived defect is notoriously tenacious.

Patients will often behave in the following ways:
- Socialise poorly.
- Have a difficult relationship with mirrors (having to 'brace themselves' to look in a mirror or avoiding mirrors completely).

- Pick at their skin.
- Hide their 'defect'.
- Have very persistent and intrusive thoughts about their perceived 'defect'.
- Repeatedly seek help from different HCPs ('doctor shoppers').
- Repeatedly attend for cosmetic or aesthetic surgery.

Uncommonly, the delusional type of BDD gives rise to familial BDD where a parent imposes a delusional idea upon a child who in turn develops BDD or, even more rarely, the patient believes that their child has a bodily defect – BDD by proxy.

Prognosis

The prognosis for patients with BDD [6,7] is variable, but good, when treated by dedicated BDD teams.

Investigations

Body dysmorphic disorder is a clinical diagnosis, but objective assessments of severity and screening tools do exist:
- Assess for potential suicide risk and refer where necessary.
- Assess for any underlying abuse (physical and mental abuse in a vulnerable adult/child).
- Assess for underlying psychiatric disease (depression, anxiety or both).
- Acknowledge genuine skin disease (e.g. hair loss or skin pigmentation changes).
- Investigate skin changes appropriately (this may mean no investigations at all or may mean appropriately investigating a differential diagnosis).
- Ask about substance abuse.
- Investigate any underlying psychiatric disease appropriately.
- Consider concomitant eating disorders.

There are a number of scales (Box 83.7) and screening questions (Box 83.8) for the assessment of BDD.

Management

These treatments are in addition to the general approach to management outlined at the beginning of this section.

First line

Treatment of the skin. As always, patients with psychodermatological disease need to have their skin *and* their psychological disease treated concurrently. *Appropriate* treatment of the patient's skin will facilitate engagement of the patient – but it is appropriate treatment rather than inappropriate surgery, which may not satisfy the patient's expectations. From the outset it is important to treat the psychological disease while addressing the perceived skin disease. Often there are some skin changes (however minimal) and acknowledging these changes rather than dismissing them will facilitate patient engagement.

Education for patients and their friends and family. There are excellent patient support books and organisations (see 'Resources').

Psychopharmacological treatments. Selective serotonin reuptake inhibitors and CBT are the treatments of choice. Fluoxetine [8], fluvoxamine and citalopram are the best-studied SSRI agents, but recent evidence suggests that all SSRIs are probably effective.

Higher dosing regimens than those used for depression are usually required. Patients should receive a trial of 12–16 weeks before efficacy is assessed [9]. If one agent fails another should be substituted, as some patients idiosyncratically respond more favourably to one agent over another. Interestingly, SSRIs appear to be more effective than antipsychotic agents, despite the fact that BDD may sometimes be a delusional disorder. Only about 20% of delusional BDD patients will become free of their delusional thinking with SSRIs, however. But in delusional patients with BDD, the intrusiveness of the thoughts and distress will diminish sufficiently, such that many patients will be able to resume some social and vocational functioning. CBT may be used in conjunction with SSRIs or independently of SSRIs [10].

Talk therapies. There are various CBT techniques that can be used in the management of BDD [10,11], although there are no trials comparing the different CBT techniques in a randomised, controlled clinical setting. Supportive psychotherapy can be helpful in patients with overvalued ideas and who are not truly deluded, but it is very time consuming and emotionally demanding. Patients with BDD are often poor communicators and difficulty with interpersonal relationships may be one of the central, crucial and earliest features of this disorder. The physician undertaking supportive psychotherapy has to be patient and realise that further skilled directive intervention will eventually be needed from psychiatrists or clinical psychologists. BDD patients are often poor attendees at clinics, but the consultation may in some cases be the only opportunity that a patient has to talk to another human being, which is a reflection of the isolated life these patients often lead. The dermatologist's essential role is to recognise the problem and sympathetically steer the patient on the correct path to help. Narrative therapy addresses the sociocultural causes that may establish beliefs, in this case about the body. The change process in narrative therapy involves helping patients replace these influences by more preferred stories about their problems and lives. Single case studies have been encouraging.

CBT has been shown to be effective in the management of patients with BDD, but trials are often open labelled or uncontrolled. There are a few randomised controlled clinical trials that clearly demonstrate the benefit of CBT, although the numbers of patients in these trials is small.

Pharmacological and psychological treatment. The combination of higher-dose SSRIs and CBT (which most likely has a slightly greater benefit than supportive psychotherapy) probably has a better prognosis (chance of remission) than the use of either treatment alone [5].

Second line

Antipsychotics. The evidence that antipsychotics are beneficial for patients with BDD (even those with delusional BDD) is sporadic and solely based on case studies. It is very difficult to run controlled clinical trials with antipsychotics in patients with BDD. Although the evidence is not robust, there are some patients who will need to be treated with (usually newer atypical) antipsychotics such as risperidone, aripiprazole and others. These medications need to be initiated and monitored by specialists with extensive experience of their usage.

Dermatological surgery and BDD [12]

What is clear is that patients with BDD are much more likely to attend for cosmetic/aesthetic procedures but also much more likely to be dissatisfied with the results of the surgical intervention. It is really important that dermatologists and dermatological surgeons can identify patients with BDD early in their consultations with these patients as:

- The patients are unlikely to be satisfied with the surgical intervention.
- The patients may complain, litigate or even abuse HCPs when dissatisfied.
- Identifying the primary (psychological) problem allows HCPs to adopt a multidisciplinary approach to manage the skin (appropriately) at the same time as managing the BDD.
- Patients with BDD will often have very challenging relationships with family and friends, whose lives may in turn be disabled while trying to support their loved ones with the disorder. Treating the patient with BDD may improve the lives of family and loved ones.

Complaints and litigation

Patients with BDD can be very challenging. HCPs managing patients with BDD may be subject to complaints, abuse and litigation [13]; this may lead to burn-out and other psychological consequences for HCPs. It is therefore very important that HCPs supporting patients with BDD are supported via regional and national HCP support networks.

Resources

Patient resources

Mind: www.mind.org.uk.

OCD-UK: www.ocduk.org.

Phillips KA. *The Broken Mirror: Understanding and Treating Body Dysmorphic Disorder.* Oxford: Oxford University Press, 2005.

Skin Support: www.skinsupport.org.uk.

(All last accessed June 2022.)

Lichen simplex chronicus

Synonyms and inclusions
- Picker's nodules
- Neurodermatitis circumscripta

Introduction and general description

Lichen simplex chronicus is common and can affect various body sites including the shins, nape of neck and the genital skin (particularly the scrotal skin in men) (Chapter 81). It is also common as small 'picker's nodules' (often on the scalp, but can be anywhere on the body). Whenever the skin is chronically rubbed or excoriated, thickening of the skin in that localised area will ensue. This leads to further itch and further desire to rub/scratch or excoriate, thereby establishing the itch/scratch cycle (Figure 84.6). It is difficult to be certain which comes first, the itch or the scratch. It is likely that perceived stressors, which can be psychological or physical (e.g. an

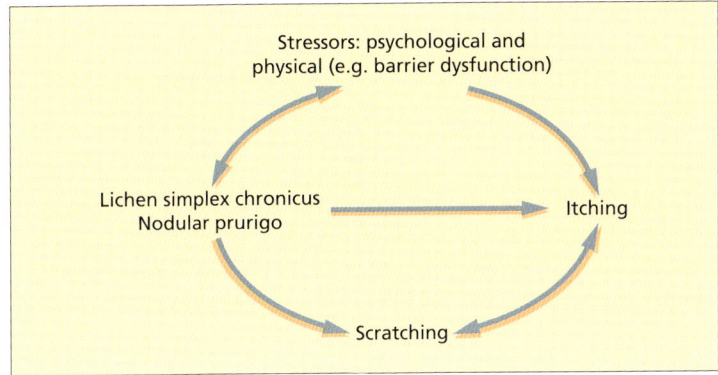

Figure 84.6 The itch/scratch cycle and nodular prurigo.

irritant or xerosis), or a combination of stressors, leads to the sensation of itch. This sensation leads to scratching and eventual habit formation. Once the scratch habit is established, thickened lichenified skin with new nerve ingrowth leads to propagation of the itch and establishment of lichen simplex chronicus or nodular prurigo.

Lichen simplex describes characteristic localised skin thickening in response to repeated rubbing and scratching. In some instances a minor initiating event, such as trauma, infection or an insect bite, precipitates episodic, insistent scratching and rubbing. Irresistible itching is the major complaint, and scratching is the chronic accompaniment. In the majority of patients, however, it is the response to anxiety, OCD or an irresistible, persistent itch [1]. Nodular prurigo is more generalised and complex (Chapter 81). Many authors believe that nodular prurigo patients fall into two categories: atopic patients (Chapter 41) and patients who are chronic skin pickers (see later in this chapter and Chapter 81).

Management

Treatment ladder for lichen simplex chronicus

First line
- Establishing skin barrier function
- Topical anti-inflammatories (usually topical corticosteroids)
- Topical corticosteroid-impregnated tapes (for picker's nodules)
- Habit reversal education and implementation

Second line
- Amitriptyline [2]
- Antihistamines
- Serotonin and norepinephrine reuptake inhibitors (SNRIs), e.g. duloxetine

Nodular prurigo

Synonyms and inclusions
- Prurigo nodularis
- Neurodermatitis
- Excoriated nodular prurigo

Epidemiology
Incidence and prevalence
Lichen simplex chronicus and nodular prurigo are common, occurring in 1–10% of the population depending on the report.

Age
Patients probably represent two populations: an early-onset atopic group with a mean age of 19 years, and a later-onset, non-atopic group with a mean age of 48 years. The earlier-onset group consists of men and women, but the older group is predominantly female.

Sex
This disease is more common in women.

Ethnicity
All ethnicities are found, although Afro-Caribbean and East and South-East Asian patients are slightly more commonly affected.

Clinical features
History and presentation
Clinical features include:
- Hyper/hypopigmented nodules.
- Hyper/hypopigmented papules.
- Patches and plaques of lichenification/cobblestoning.
- Excoriation of the above (Figure 84.7).
- There may be a few or commonly very many nodules.
- The lesions are often symmetrically distributed on the limbs but can be on any part of the body.
- Extensor surfaces are more commonly affected.
- Lesions are usually within the reach of the patient's dominant hand.
- The 'butterfly sign' of mid-back sparing is where the individual cannot reach that area of skin.
- Postinflammatory hypopigmentation and scarring are common in darker skin.
- Crusting and weeping may indicate secondary infection (usually *Staphylococcus aureus*).

Regular rubbing and pressure on the skin produces characteristic thickened, coarsely grained papules and nodules with hyperpigmentation (Figure 84.7). The classic sites of involvement are within easy reach, particularly on the nape and sides of the neck, elbows, thighs, knees and ankles. These areas may be in varying stages of evolution, from early, small, violaceous papules with surface excoriations to chronic areas that present as hyperkeratotic plaques with pigment changes, described as 'dermatological worry beads'. Affected areas are more often localised, and patches of lichen simplex chronicus affecting the vulval or scrotal skin are very common [1]. Scratching or rubbing is carried out using either the hands, back of nails or knuckles, and sometimes with the use of a convenient instrument such as a hairbrush or pen. The actions may be subconscious but more often patients engage in conscious episodes of scratching, which continue until the pruritus is relieved and is replaced by soreness and pain. The change from itch to pain is quite sudden and this abrupt cessation has been described as 'orgasm cutanée'.

Many authors categorise nodular prurigo as either atopics with nodular prurigo or non-atopics with nodular prurigo (Box 84.9).

However, there is an overlap and patients may have atopic dermatitis *and* one of the non-atopic co-morbid causes of nodular prurigo.

Box 84.9 Non-atopic causes of nodular prurigo
- Generalised causes of pruritus:
  - Renal disease
  - Liver disease
  - Haematological disease
  - Cancer
  - Psychological issues
  - Mast cell disorders
  - Urticaria-related disorders
  - Non-atopic skin disease (other inflammatory dermatoses)
  - Drugs (pharma and recreational) and alcohol
- Localised causes of pruritus:
  - Nerve root irritation (e.g. brachioradial pruritus)
  - Localised dysaesthesia (e.g. lichen simplex chronicus)
  - Picker's nodules
  - Localised inflammatory dermatoses
- Psychological distress
  - Anxiety
  - Depression
  - Anxiety and depression
  - Non-psychiatric appropriate reactive psychological distress (e.g. bereavement)
  - Others
- A combination of the above

Differential diagnosis
- Atopic skin disease.
- Other inflammatory skin diseases.
- Aetiologies in Box 84.9.
- Immunobullous disease (e.g. nodular prurigo pemphigoides).
- Genuine infestations (e.g. scabies).
- Delusional infestation.
- Cutaneous neoplasia with itching.

Complications and co-morbidities
Most authors have commented on the relationship of emotional tension to bouts of scratching [2]. Aggression and hostility related to anxiety caused by emotional disturbance may lead to itching. There is considerable evidence that habitual scratching sets up neurotransmitter changes in the brain that act as temporary 'stress busters'. Habitual scratching is often opportunistic (i.e. when the patient can get to the skin) but may become 'addictive' and so potentially out of control. The freqency of scratching episodes often increases with perceived stress.

Cutaneous complications include:
- Scarring.
- Dyspigmentaion.
- Infection (bacterial/viral).
- Cellulitis.
- Bacteraemia/septicaemia (rarely).
- Necrotising fasciitis (very rarely).
Psychological co-morbidities include:
- Anxiety.
- Depression.

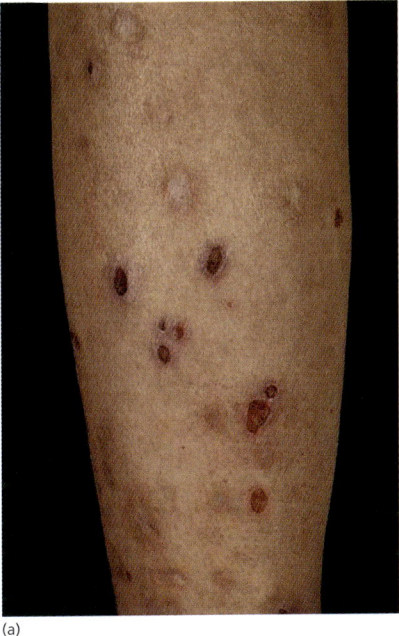
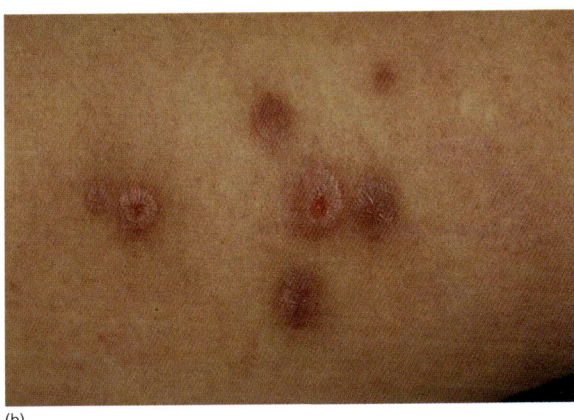
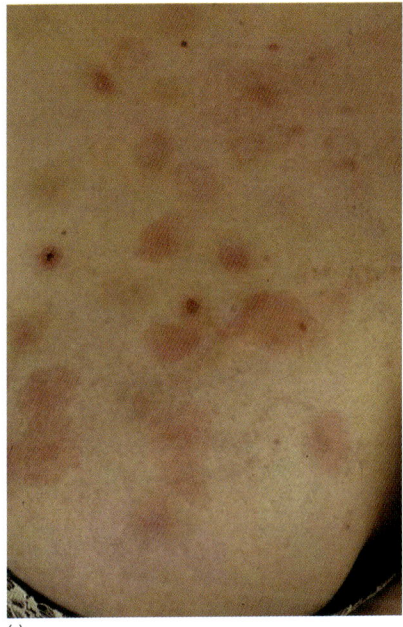

(a)   (b)   (c)

Figure 84.7 (a) Classic excoriated nodules and erosions of nodular prurigo on the shin. (b, c) Close-up of nodular prurigo.

- Anxiety and depression.
- Sleep disturbance.
- Shame/guilt.
- Coping with a visible difference.
- Body dysmorphic disease.

Management

Management of nodular prurigo involves:

1 Management of any atopic dermatitis as appropriate (Chapter 20).
2 Assessment of skin and psychological disease [3].
3 Management of the skin and the psychological disease concomitantly.

There are a number of treatments in addition to the general approach (Figure 84.8) [4–7].

Treatment ladder for nodular prurigo

Ideally after appropriate assessment, any co-morbidities should be treated with, for example, talk therapy [8] and/or psychopharmacy.

First line
Topical
- Emollients
- Topical antipruritics (menthol, laromacrogols)
- Topical anti-inflammatories (steroids, calcineurin inhibitors, tar)
- Occlusion of affected areas with cotton/viscose stretch garments or bandages
Oral
- Antihistamines
- Tricyclics (e.g. amitriptylline and doxepin)

Behavioural (crucial) [3,6]
- Habit reversal (www.atopicskindisease.com; last accessed July 2022)
- Other talk therapies

Second line
In addition to first line treatments above:
- Intralesional steroid injections
- Phototherapy/photochemotherapy [7]
- SSRIs and other antidepressants, e.g. mirtazapine, which has the benefit of being sedating
- Anticonvulsants/mood stabilisers such as pregabalin/gabapentin

Third line
- Systemic immunodulator (e.g. ciclosporin, methotrexate, azathioprine)
- Thalidomine [9]
- Serlopitant
- Naltrexone
- There is a growing interest in the management of nodular prurigo with biologic agents and JAK inhibitors. Medications such as nemolizumab [10] (anti-interleukin 31A (anti-IL-31A) monoclonal antibody), dupilumab [11] (anti-IL-4/13 monoclonal antibody), baricitinib, upadicinib and other JAK inhibitors [12,13] are being assessed by the UK National Institute for Health and Care Excellence (NICE), the European Medicines Agency (EMA) and the US Food and Drug Administration (FDA) for approval in the treatment of patients with nodular purigo. These agents are likely to be used after at least one systemic has been tried and failed, or where other systemic immunomodulators are contraindicated

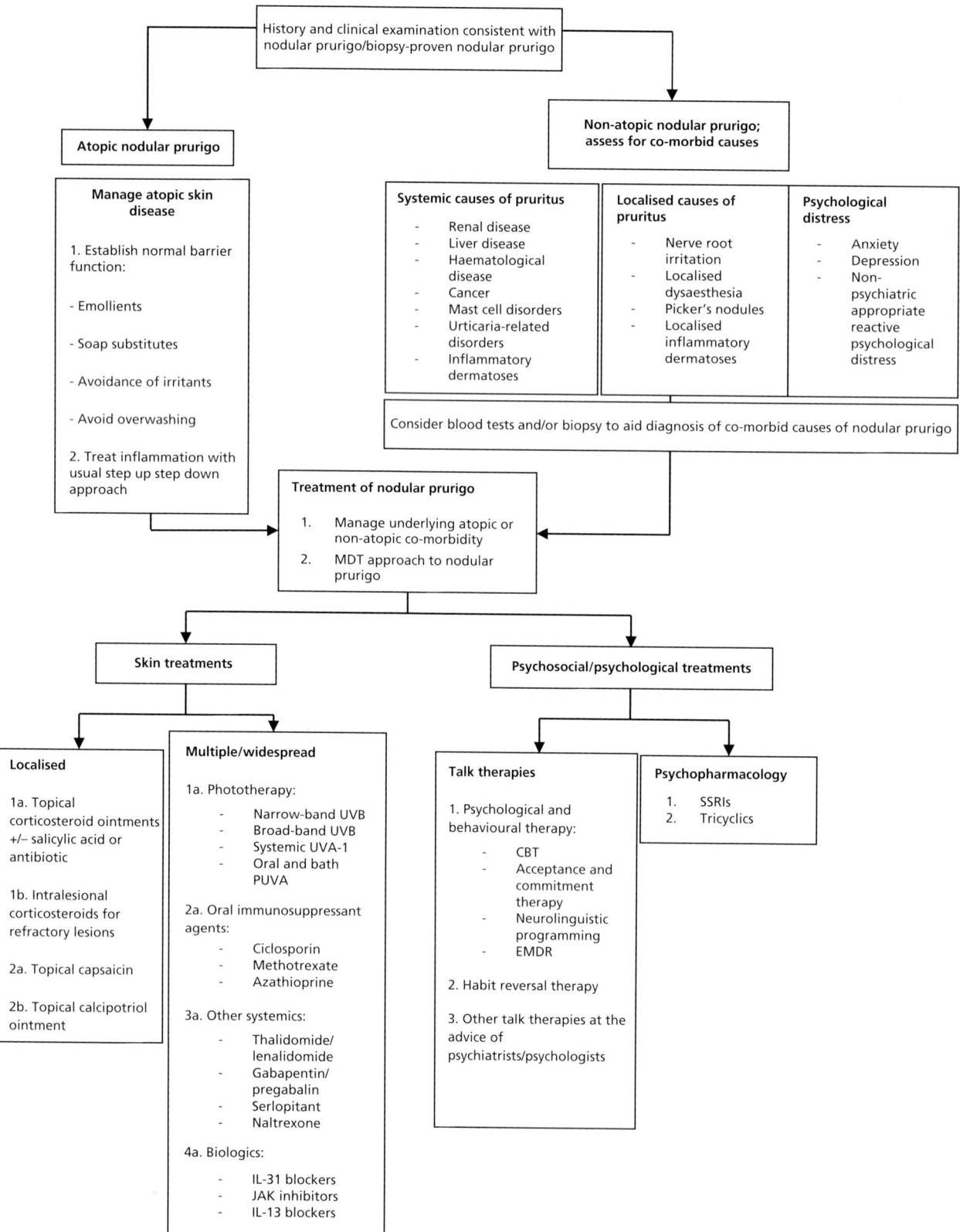

Figure 84.8 Management of nodular prurigo. CBT, cognitive–behavioural treatment; EMDR, eye movement desensitisation and reprocessing; JAK, Janus kinase; MDT, multidisciplinary team; PUVA, psoralen and ultraviolet A; SSRIs, selective serotonin reuptake inhibitors; UV, ultraviolet. Reproduced from Barlow and Bewley 2021 [12] with permission of Springer Nature.

Skin picking disorder

Synonyms and inclusions
- Psychogenic excoriations
- Neurotic excoriations
- Compulsive skin picking
- Dermatotillomania
- Psychogenic skin picking
- Pathological skin picking disease

Epidemiology

Incidence
This disorder occurs in 2% of dermatology patients, but the majority of these have pathological picking associated with atopic and other cutaneous diseases. Skin picking disease in the absence of cutaneous inflammatory disease is rarer but is still common [1].

Age
There are two peaks of occurrence: (i) in adolescence and early adult life [2,3]; and (ii) in middle-aged women. Any age can be affected, although it is rarer in younger children.

Sex
Females are more commonly affected than males.

Ethnicity
Any ethnicity can be affected.

Pathophysiology
Figure 84.9 outlines the European Society for Dermatology and Psychiatry (ESDP) algorithm for identifying and classifying skin picking disorders [4].

The medical and psychiatric causes of self-excoriating behaviour are detailed in Box 84.10.

Box 84.10 Medical and psychiatric causes of self-excoriating behaviour

Medical causes
- Urticaria
- Uraemia
- Cholestatic hepatitis
- Xerosis
- Cutaneous dysaesthesia
- Porphyria cutanea tarda
- Malignancies

Psychiatric causes
- Depression
- Anxiety
- Obsessive–compulsive disorder
- Body dysmorphic disorder
- Borderline personality disorder
- Delusions of parasitosis
- Dermatitis artefacta
- Somatoform disorders such as hypochondriasis
- Dissociative states (when patient may not recollect their behaviour)
- Malingering

Clinical features [5]
Skin picking disorder differs from true dermatitis artefacta as affected individuals admit to an urge to pick and gouge at their skin (Figure 84.10). There may be an initial reluctance to own up to the self-damage but patients are usually willing to discuss the picking as a 'response to stress'. Any area may be affected. The average duration of disease before presentation is up to 10 years. Patients spend up to 3 h per day picking, thinking about picking or resisting the urge to pick. These bouts can be ritualised to a set time and place, often the bathroom, frequently at bedtime. Although these activities are usually executed fully consciously, rarely a fugue or trance state can be apparent. Lesions may be quite deep, extending into the dermis, and are more commonly distributed within reach of the dominant hand. Older lesions show pink or red scars, some of which may be hypertrophic. Chronic lesions may also show atrophic scars, which merge and are eventually seen as linear, coalescent areas. Lesions appear at all stages of development and may number from a few to several hundred. Concealment behaviour, for example make-up and clothing, is present in 65% of chronic cases and active avoidance of social situations found in 40%. Up to a quarter of patients may increase alcohol, tobacco or recreational substance habits to counter the burden of disease.

Differential diagnosis
It is important to exclude excoriations caused by generalised pruritus, bullous disorders (such as pemphigus) and linear excoriated lesions, which may be the presenting signs of lichen planus or lupus erythematosus. Rarities such as mucinoses that cause scarring are usually distinguishable entities. Another differential is acné excoriée (see separate section).

Complications and co-morbidities
Pre-existing skin disease (e.g. atopic eczema or acne) is very common, as are psychosocial co-morbidities [6]. There may be precipitating psychological events such as divorce, bereavement, abortion or separation. Depression and/or anxiety are often found. Family members with chronic disease is also a common finding.

Cutaneous complications include:
- Cellulitis, bacteraemia and septicaemia.
- Scarring.
  Psychological co-morbidities and complications include [2–7]:
- Anxiety.
- Depression.
- Suicidal ideation.
- Other OCD spectrum disorders.
- Body image disturbance and loss of self esteem.
- BDD.
- Eating disorders.
- Substance and alcohol abuse.

Management [8–11]
1 Assess the skin disease and its extent.
2 Consider potential systemic causes of skin picking behaviour.
3 Investigate according to the clinical picture.
4 Assess for potential psychological precipitants.
5 Assess for potential safeguarding risk.
6 Commence management of the skin and psychological disease concomitantly.

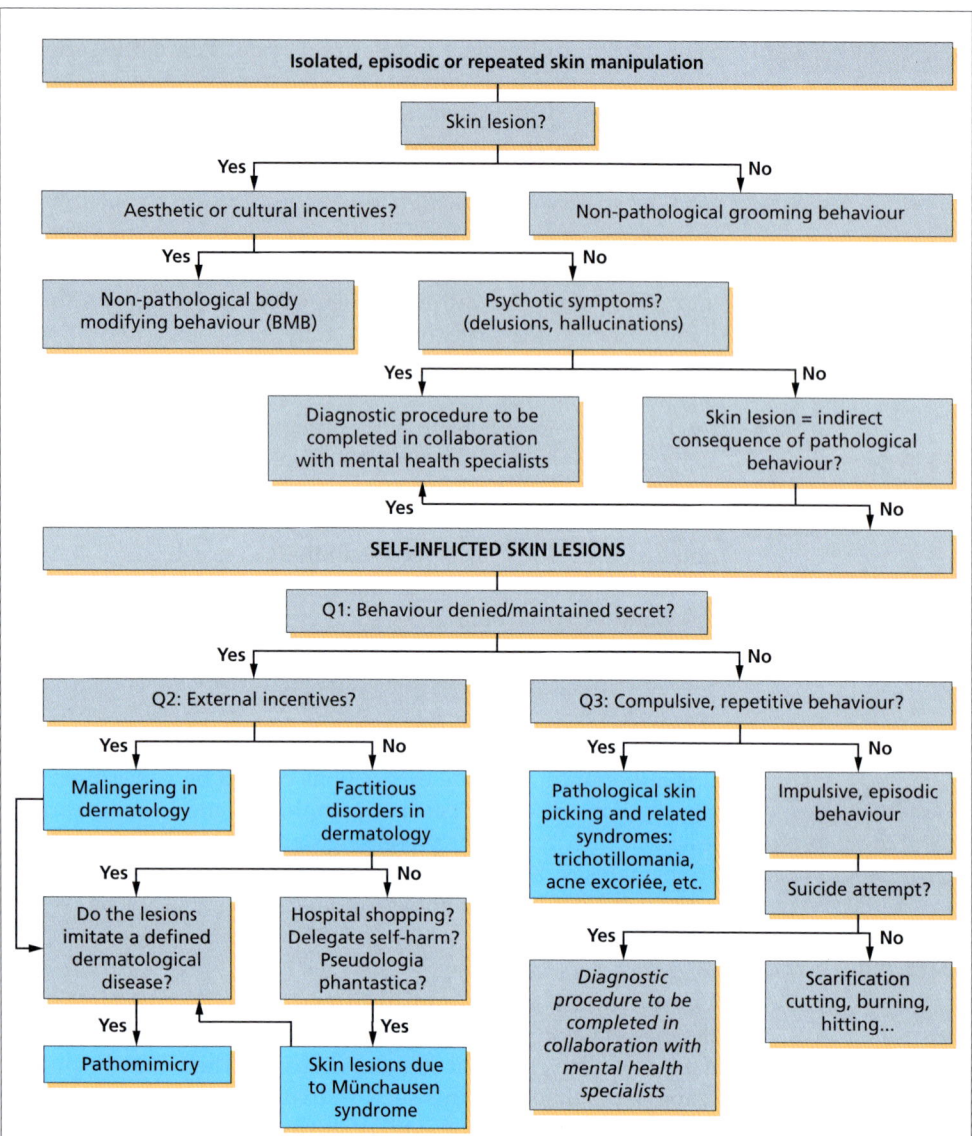

Figure 84.9 European Society for Dermatology and Psychiatry classification of skin picking. Reproduced from Gieler *et al.* 2013 [4] with permission of Acta Dermato-Venereologica.

Treatment ladder for skin picking disorder

First line
- Appropriate treatment (e.g. antibiotics if there is a clinical infection)
- Antihistamines
- Treatment of chronic pruritus

Of the picking habit and co-morbidities [12,13]
- Habit reversal (see later)
- Other talk therapies (see later)
- SSRIs, e.g. fluoxetine (usually in higher doses)
- SNRIs, e.g. duloxetine
- Tricyclics, e.g. amitriptyline

Second line
Of the skin
- Phototherapy/photochemotherapy

Of the picking habit
- Mood stabilisers (pregabalin/gabapentin)

- Other antidepressants, e.g. mirtazapine (sedating)
- Talk therapies

Third line
- Bandages and occlusion
- Intralesional steroids
- *N*-acetylcysteine
- Naltrexone
- Lamotrigine
- Topiramate [14]

Acné excoriée

Synonyms and inclusions
- Picker's acne
- Acné excoriée des jeunes filles
- Acné excoriée of Brocq

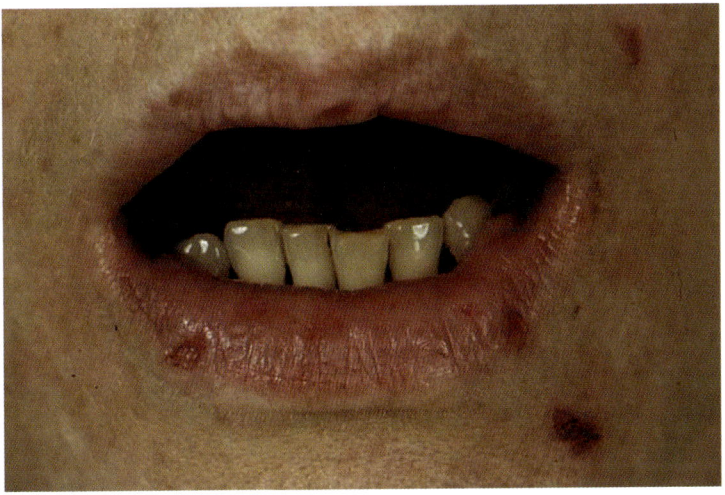

(a)

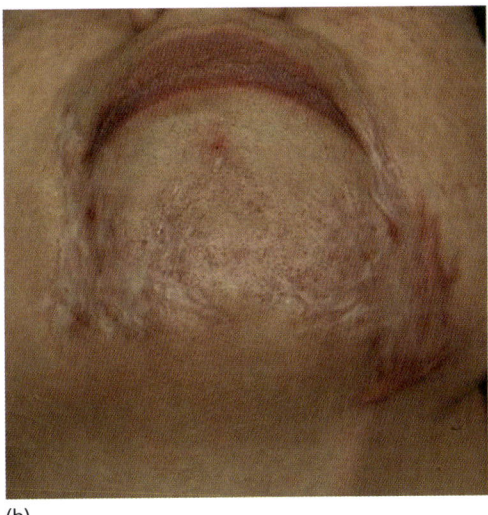

(b)

Figure 84.10 (a,b) Skin picking disorder of the face.

Introduction and general description

There are few patients with acne who can resist squeezing their spots. Brocq described acné excoriée particularly in adolescent girls under emotional stress, who picked and squeezed acne lesions repeatedly [1]. Although some patients develop these lesions after picking acne, most had no acne at all. The condition should be considered a variant of skin picking disorder with the lesions largely confined to the face (Figure 84.11) [1–3].

Epidemiology

Acné excoriée is usually seen in young (often white) women [3], with a second peak in women in their thirties.

Clinical features

The clinical lesions resemble those of chronic excoriations (Figure 86.11) [4]. They are found predominantly around the hairline, forehead, preauricular cheek and chin areas. Extension to the neck and occipital hairline is common. Chronic lesions characteristically show white, atrophic scarring with peripheral hyperpigmentation. Lesions are picked as a ritual, apparently as a response to itch

or throbbing. The lesions are excoriated until 'emptied'. There are usually some acneform lesions, at least when the disease first appears. There may be associated psychological disorders including OCD, BDD and depressive and/or anxiety disorder. Box 84.11 lists the diagnostic criteria for acné excoriée.

Box 84.11 Diagnostic criteria for acné excoriée

- Recurrent skin picking of acne that results in skin lesions
- Repeated attempts to stop the behaviour
- Symptoms cause clinically significant distress or impairment
- Symptoms are not caused by a substance misuse or medical or dermatological condition
- Symptoms are not better explained by another psychiatric disorder

---

Differential diagnosis. Differential diagnoses include the facial picking disorder (where there are no acneform lesions originating the picking habit), trigeminal trophic syndrome (Chapter 82) and dermatitis artefacta.

Management [5–9]

Treatment ladder for acné excoriée

First line

Of the acne
- Topical retinoids/antibiotics
- Systemic antibiotics

Of the habit and co-morbidities
- Habit reversal [5]
- CBT and other talk therapies [6]
- SSRIs

Second line

Of the acne
- Isotretinoin (usually in ultra-low doses, e.g. 5–10 mg/day or 20 mg once weekly; careful monitoring is necessary for all potential side effects but especially affective symptoms)
- Phototherapy

Of the habit and co-morbidities
- Other antidepressants, e.g. mirtazapine (sedating)
- Anticonvulsants/mood stabilisers, e.g. pregabalin and gabapentin [7]
- Talk therapies

Third line
- Lasers and dermabrasion are best avoided unless they are carried out together with CBT [6]
- Avoid intralesional steroids until the picking habit is under control
- Lamotrigine
- Topiramate
- Hypnosis [8]

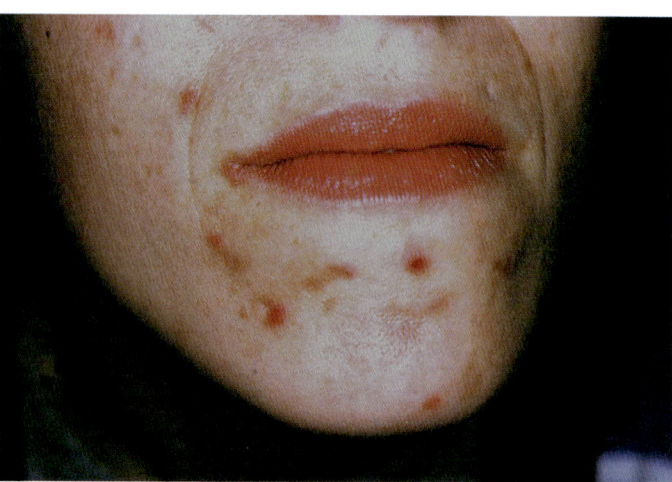

(a)

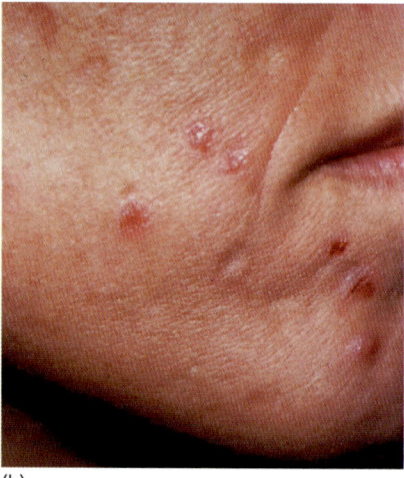

(b)

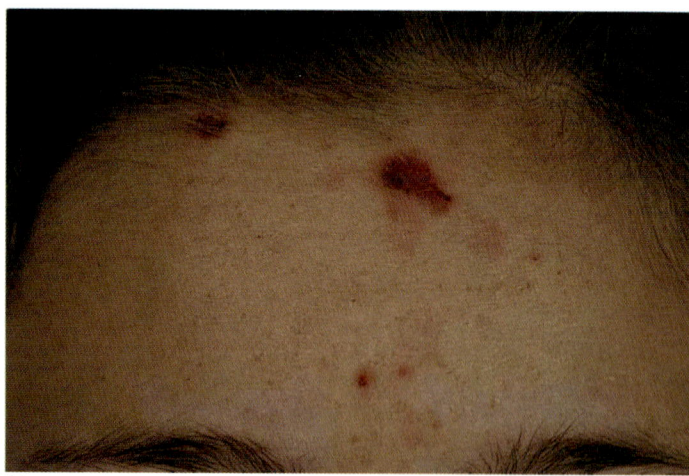

(c)

Figure 84.11 Acné excoriée. (a, b) Scarring lesions of the cheek and chin due to habitual skin interference. (c) Self-inflicted erosions on the forehead.

BODY-FOCUSED REPETITIVE BEHAVIOUR DISORDERS AND OTHER SPECIFIED OBSESSIVE–COMPULSIVE AND RELATED DISORDERS

Trichotillosis

Synonyms and inclusions
- Hair pulling disorder
- Trichotillomania

Introduction and general description

The term trichotillomania was first used by Hallopeau in 1889 and is derived from the Greek *thrix* (hair), *tillein* (pull out) and *mania* (madness). Current thinking is that the term trichotillosis is more accurate as the condition is not a 'mania' but more of an OCD spectrum disorder. Diagnostic criteria that have been cited include [1]:
- Recurrent pulling out of one's own hair resulting in hair loss.
- An increasing sense of tension immediately before pulling out the hair or when attempting to resist the behaviour.
- Pleasure, gratification or relief when pulling out the hair.
- The disturbance is not better accounted for by another mental disorder and is not due to a general medical condition (e.g. a dermatological condition).
- The disturbance provokes clinically marked distress and/or impairment in occupational, social or other important areas of functioning.

Many subdivide patients into younger and older groups and those with dissociative symptoms [2]. Patients with an earlier onset with limited progression usually have a better prognosis. Recalcitrant, obsessive and focused hair pulling is usually found in older women, and patients may deny their hair pulling. Automatic hair pulling is also found, and some patients pull their hair in a dissociative or fugue state.

Epidemiology
Incidence and prevalence

This is commoner in children and college students (rates of 0.6–3% have been reported). Overall, later and more severe trichotillosis is not common. Cosmetic hair pulling (eyebrows, etc.) is extremely common, but most do not fulfil diagnostic OCD criteria.

Age and sex

There appear to be two distinct populations: those who present in childhood, mainly between the ages of 5 and 12 years, and more chronic cases who present as adults but who started hair pulling activities in adolescence or early adult life [3]. The number of affected children may be seven times that of adults and there is evidence of a bimodal distribution with peaks in the preschool years and in adolescence [4]. Preschool children are more likely to be boys (62%), although after this older boys and male adolescents make up only 30% of the group. This early-onset group, usually aged between 2 and 10 years, show benign, self-limiting behaviour and most are probably suffering a habit disorder, perhaps as an extension of hair twirling activity and childhood stress. The adolescent group are much more likely to be female, with ratios of up to 3.5 : 1. In adults there is greater psychopathology and a distinct female preponderance, usually 4 : 1, but this is most evident in the oldest group (female : male 15 : 1).

Ethnicity
Trichotillosis is found in all ethnicities.

Associated diseases
The aetiology of trichotillosis is not fully understood, but seems to be related to the following [5]:
- Underlying anxieties.
- Depression.
- Underlying BDD.
- Psychosocial triggers.
- Family dysfunction (common).
- Other cutaneous 'habits' such as nail biting and nail pulling.
- Deliberate self-harm, 'cutting', etc.
- Eating disorders.
- Rarely substance abuse.

Familial predisposition is fairly common and successive generations of patients with trichotillosis have been described. It is always worth considering the (rarer) association with emotional or sexual abuse.

Clinical features
Most patients relate that the trichotillosis is a compulsion that is irresistible and that leads to a short-lived sense of relief or release when hair has been pulled out. But the relief usually leads rapidly to a sense of guilt and hopelessness. The habit is often hidden from the partner/close family and the hair loss is usually covered up. Patients may describe a sense of control over their body/psychosocial situation that is briefly facilitated by their hair pulling habits. Some describe pulling hair in a fugue-like state and having no control over the episodes of hair pulling.

Hair pulling and plucking are commonest from the scalp. Some patients select an apparently abnormal hair by feel or texture and extend it into an adjacent area. Most pull hair from the vertex, but temporal, occipital and frontal hair loss in children may be more obvious on the side of manual dominance. The hair loss may be minimal, commonly a solitary patch, but visible hair thinning may progress to virtual total depilation, significantly so in adult women. The hair pulling activity is usually not as a response to any skin symptoms but is either a conscious, deliberate act or more often a subconscious act, almost in some children being part of a hypnagogic (dream-like) state. Some patients may have incomplete awareness until the pattern has been established. The eyelashes, eyebrows, facial and pubic hair may also be primarily affected. Children will also pluck eyebrows and eyelashes (Figure 84.12) but adults almost exclusively pluck hair on the torso. Two-thirds of adults pulled hair from two or more sites and one-third from three areas. Involvement of a second area began after an average of 8 years. Body and pubic hair plucking, commoner in males, may become a ritualised activity done either alone or as a conjugal activity and can indicate a personality or psychotic disorder. Hair is plucked from the scalp on average two to three times per day and daily from other areas. The duration and frequency of activity are variable but adults in general

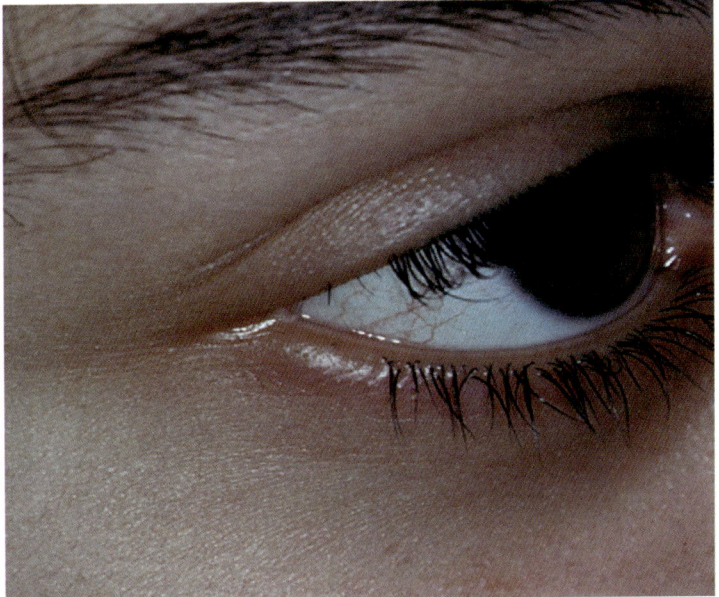

Figure 84.12 Childhood trichotillosis showing eyelash involvement with hair loss and broken-off hairs. This child also had scalp involvement.

have longer and more frequent activity. Children tend to manipulate hair at times of leisure, for example watching TV, when tired and in the evening. Adults have a more conscious, structured activity, initially seeking thicker or distorted hair and then progressing to larger areas, taking more and more time over the activity. This may become similar to a compulsion with elaboration of the rituals using instruments such as tweezers. The more frequent the plucking episodes, the greater the body image dissatisfaction and the more likely the patient will suffer depression and anxiety. There are similarities and overlap with BDD in some cases.

On examination, there are often areas of hair loss together with areas of hair regrowth (stubble and longer hairs) (Figure 84.13). This pattern may involve the eyebrows and eyelashes. There is occasionally frank scarring from where the habit has been repeated incessantly and the follicle has scarred. The patterns of plucking activity are centrifugal from a single starting point or linear, in wave-like activity. In extreme cases, the centrifugal pattern removes all hair except the most difficult to access, namely that on the occiput; this shows as a 'tonsure pattern' or 'Friar Tuck' distribution. Patients use wigs, hair weaving, false eyelashes and semipermanent use of hats and scarves to disguise the defects. Chronic folliculitis of the neck, chin, chest, pubic areas or thighs as a result of plucking activity may also be the presenting complaint.

Children may pluck the hair, or stroke or suck the hair root, before chewing and swallowing the remainder. The hair root alone may be eaten (trichorhizophagia) as a secretive activity and in a few patients the whole hair is eaten (trichophagia). Patients who eat more hair tend to swallow the longer strands and a very small percentage develop gastrointestinal bezoars.

Complications and co-morbidities
These include:
- Scarring hair loss.
- Folliculitis.

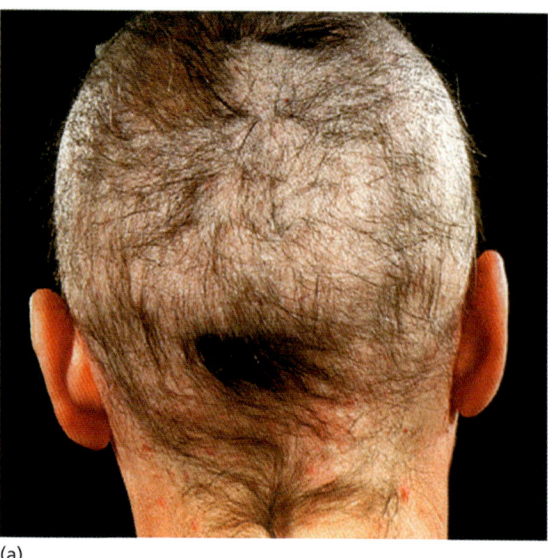
(a)

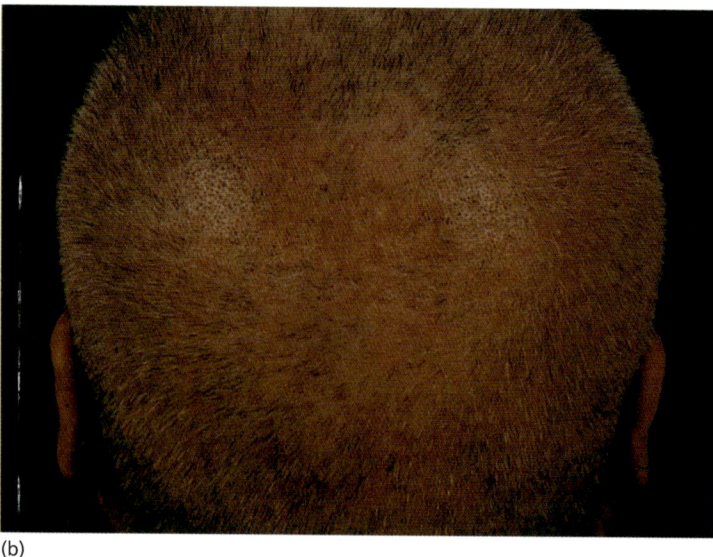
(b)

Figure 84.13 Adult trichotillosis. (a) Extensive hair loss with a preserved tuft over the occiput. (b) Patient with hairs of different lengths.

- Keloid formation.
- Trichobezoar. This name is derived from the Arabic word *badzahr*, meaning an antidote or counter-poison.It also relates to the hardened contents of the fourth stomach of the Syrian goat, much prized as a cure for many diseases. Bezoars are ball-like aggregations of vegetable or fibre-like materials in the stomach and small intestine (Figure 84.14). The true incidence of trichobezoar is unknown. It is seen almost exclusively in girls and young women. It is rare but its importance is that morbidity is high with chronicity and severe complications, which can lead to death. Longer hair is more likely to become enmeshed into a ball by the action of peristalsis, and this then becomes too large to leave the stomach via the pylorus. The larger the ball, the more likely it is that gastric atony will develop, leading to symptoms of nausea, indigestion, bloating and pain. The hair ball may eventually completely fill the stomach. Although the condition is very rare, it should be considered in children with trichotillosis who present with a combination of any of the following: abdominal pain, weight loss, nausea, vomiting, anorexia and foul breath. More common is the parental threat to their children that 'if you keep chewing your hair, eventually you'll have a hair ball in your stomach'.
- The Rapunzel syndrome [6] describes a trichobezoar with a tail that extends at least to the jejunum; sufferers are highly likely to have gastrointestinal obstructive symptoms. In a review of 27 cases, which included only one male, the mean age at presentation was 10.8 years. Most patients ingested their own long hair although cases have been recorded of bezoar by proxy where another person's hair has been eaten by the patient. In this group 37% had abdominal pain, 33% nausea and vomiting, 26% obstruction and 18.5% developed peritonitis. The hair ball can have a tail as long as 195 cm. The tail may also be broken up into numerous segments distributed throughout the small bowel. Recurrent Rapunzel syndrome has been reported [6]. Life-threatening intestinal obstruction necessitates surgical intervention.

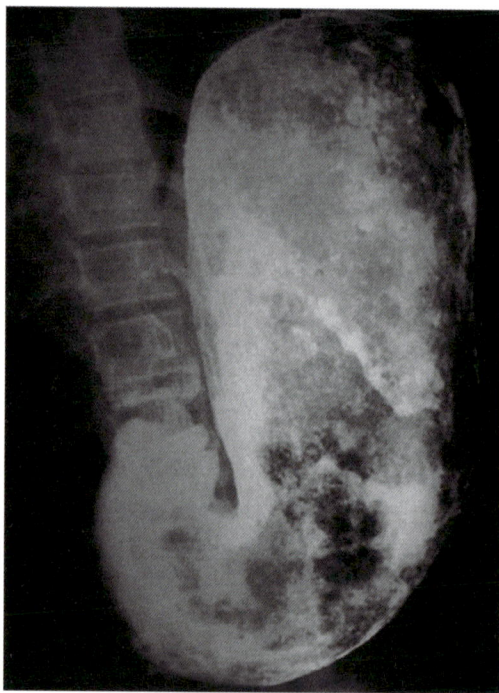

Figure 84.14 Gastric trichobezoar on barium contrast examination showing a lace-like pattern of the mass of hairs.

Investigations

The diagnosis is usually clinical [7]. Scalp biopsy is rarely necessary unless clinicians need to distinguish trichotillosis from scarring alopecia. Trichomalacia is seen as deep distortion and curling of the hair bulb. In severe damage there is intraepithelial and perifollicular damage. Trichoscopy/dermoscopy [8] has been reported as being very helpful in the presence of a corroborating history (broken hair shafts, hairs of different lengths, traumatised hair shafts, trichoptilosis (split ends), irregular coiled hairs, black dots, flame hairs and follicular hemorrhages).

Management

These treatments are in addition to the general approach to management outlined earlier in this chapter [9]:

- Try to understand *why* this pattern has developed early in the course of the condition.
- Offer cognitive–behavioural therapy early.
- Offer habit reversal technique.
- Treat the hair loss with physical measures where appropriate (weaves/appliances, etc.).
- Offer *N*-acetylcysteine.
- If *N*-acetylcysteine and behavioural treatment are ineffective, consider SSRIs, if appropriate, and other psychotropic treatment via expert advice.
- Refer to a psychodermatology clinic or a psychiatrist/mental health service.

Treament ladder for trichotillosis

First line

Of the habit
- Habit reversal [10]
- Other CBT [11]
- SSRIs usually in higher doses (especially if there is concomitant anxiety/depression) [12]
- *N*-acetylcysteine

Of the hair loss
- Hair weaves
- Hair extensions
- Treatment of any iron deficiency
- Treatment of keloid

Second line
- Mood stabilisers (e.g. gabapentin and pregabalin) [13]

Third line
- Antipsychotics (under psychodermatological supervision)
- Topiramate
- Referral to dissociative state disorder clinics

Onychotillomania and onychophagia

Introduction and general description

The compulsive habits of nail picking (onychotillomania) and nail biting (onychophagia) are common, almost a variation of normal, in children and adolescents [1]. It becomes more significant when there is damage to the nail apparatus. The aetiologies suggested include stress, imitation of family members and transference from a thumb-sucking habit. Nail biting is usually confined to the fingernails, but nail picking, especially in adults, may involve all digits. Damage to cuticles and nails causes paronychia, nail dystrophy and longitudinal nail scarring [2]. Individuals may present with anonychia and periungual ulceration imitating severe dermatoses (e.g. erosive lichen planus). In chronic cases, there is an association with trichotillosis. Compulsive biting, tearing or picking with instruments such as scissors, knives or razorblades may lead to permanent destruction.

Onychotillomania may be a feature of developmental problems in children and is a component of self-destructive behaviours in the Tourette and Prader–Willi syndromes. In adults, chronic nail biting is most commonly an isolated, self-destructive habit, which may respond to cognitive–behavioural training [3]. It is also common as a compulsive action as a part of OCD, not always at times of stress. Rarely, onychotillomania is a manifestation of a major depressive disorder that has a suicide risk. Self-induced anonychia of the toenails was produced by one man who plucked out his nails with pliers rather than suffer recurrent paronychia from previously crushed toes.

Management

Treatment ladder for onychotillomania and onychophagia

First line

Of the nails/topical/localised
- Nail lacquers
- Taping of the nails
- Gloves at night
- Emollients to the nail folds

Of the habit [4,5]
- Habit reversal treatment
- Relaxation techniques
- Meditation
- Mindfulness

Skin-related health anxieties

Synonyms and inclusions
- Cutaneous phobias

Introduction and general description

Health anxieties are irrational fears that are out of proportion with objective reality, and overwhelmingly distort everyday life. They can be regarded as *obsessional fears*. Dermatology patients may present with focused anxieties about the development of a variety of cutaneous diseases. Predominant cutaneous anxieties (or phobias) can be divided into:

1 Anxieties of contamination, e.g. dirt phobia, germ phobia, wart phobia.
2 Fear of malignancy, e.g. cancer phobia, mole phobia.
3 Others, e.g. fear of blushing, sweating.
4 Part of general health anxieties.

Dirt, infection and wart phobias [1]

These are OCDs where the patient has an overwhelming fear of contamination or infection of the skin or body. Hand washing leading to dermatitis is common, but up to 10% will admit to compulsive body washing also. The precipitating factors are fears of dirt and contamination from others who have been infected with real organisms (e.g. methicillin-resistant *Staphylococcus aureus* or MRSA) or those who might have been (e.g. those recently discharged from hospital). Situational exposure in work to dirt and waste may initiate the fear. Hand washing may occur up to 100 times per day and compulsive showering and bathing 10–20 times daily. If a patient has a recalcitrant irritant dermatitis, a sympathetic enquiry about frequent compulsive hand washing may be prudent (especially after the Covid-19 pandemic).

Mole and cancer phobias [2–5]

This is an OCD where the patient has an overwhelming fear of developing cancer and may stray into delusional intensity belief [5]. A dislike of moles and freckles may be a manifestation of BDD but for most patients who repeatedly demand mole examinations, and sometimes excision, there is an underlying cancer phobia. It occurs in response to various stimuli. For example, the patient may have had a malignant lesion removed and need constant reassurances. Or there may have been malignancy or death from melanoma in family or friends, or concern repeatedly triggered by media, medical or family pressure. It is an excessive response to disease, often related to anxiety. Patients present regularly and acutely to a screening clinic or primary care physicians. They may demand removal of some or all of their moles or even attempt self-surgery. Mole phobia by proxy is not uncommon in parents who worry about their children and their moles to such an extent that normal play activities and family holidays are curtailed because of concerns about sun exposure. Unless the primary pathology (the OCD/anxiety disorder) is addressed, the condition is likely to continue.

Other anxieties and phobias

Topical corticosteroid phobia may occur, predominantly about skin thinning and to a lesser extent stunting of growth in children [6].

Management

These treatments are in addition to the general approach to management outlined earlier in this chapter [7].

Treatment ladder for skin-related health anxieties

First line

- Reassurance about the benign nature of the condition (if it is benign)
- SSRIs, often in higher doses, have been shown to be helpful in OCD/health phobias. Mirtazepine is a sedating antidepressant that may be used if patients have sleeping disorders. Citalopram is now used to a maximum of 40 mg; at the moment fluoxetine can be used in doses up to 60 mg

- Talk therapies are essential to address the patient's anxieties and attempt to establish a more rational perspective to their disease
- Appropriate treatment of the skin may be necessary (such as treatment of irritant hand dermatitis in OCD hand washing)
- Mindfulness and relaxation techniques are proving to be very beneficial

Second and third line

- Occasionally antipsychotics may be helpful if the patient presents with delusional disease
- Mood stabilisers (e.g. lamotrigine)
- Treatment of any co-morbid affective disease
- Hypnosis

EATING DISORDERS

Eating disorders are considered primarily as psychiatric illnesses that have significant physical complications. Anorexia nervosa, bulimia nervosa and a third group called 'eating disorders not classified' are particularly common among young women and are increasing in incidence.

Anorexia nervosa and bulimia

Introduction and general description

For anorexia nervosa to be diagnosed, the following criteria must be found:
1 An inability to maintain a normal or minimum weight for age and height coupled with an intense fear of gaining weight; the body mass index (BMI) is less than 17.5 kg/m^2.
2 A distorted perception of weight, size and body configuration.
3 Amenorrhoea.
   Bulimia nervosa is defined by the following:
1 Recurrent and compulsive overeating episodes (binge eating).
2 Recurrent and inappropriate compensatory behaviour in order to avoid gaining weight; these include induced vomiting and abuse of diuretics and laxatives.
3 Binge eating and weight reduction behaviours occurring at least twice per week for 3 months.
4 Self-esteem affected by weight and body configuration.

Epidemiology
Incidence and prevalence

Anorexia nervosa now has an incidence of up to 1% and bulimia up to 5% of the general population [1]. Reviews suggest a lifetime prevalence of 2.2%, with over half the cases not detected initially in the health care system. The annual prevalence is about 0.3% for anorexia and 1% for bulimia, although this may be higher in women aged 15–24 years [2]. The incidence is 270 per 100 000 person-years in this group of younger women compared to 8 per 100 000 person-years in the group of women as a whole.

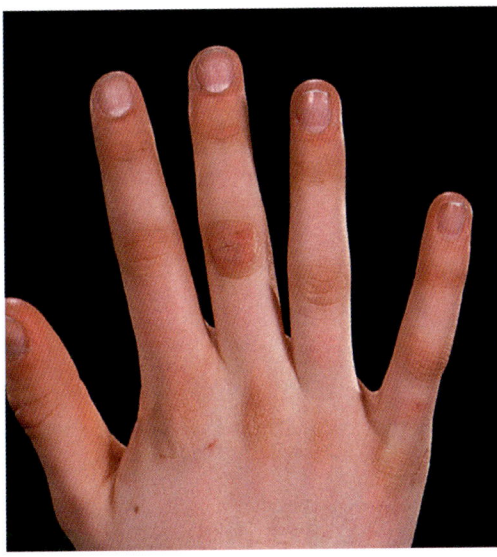

Figure 84.15 Russell sign: callosities of the knuckles from manual forced vomiting in bulimia.

Age, sex and ethnicity

Anorexia occurs earlier in life, usually in adolescence, while bulimia has its peak in the later teens and early twenties. The majority of sufferers are young women, at a ratio of female : male of 20 : 1, although there is increasing evidence that this is moving closer to 5 : 1. White races predominate in published studies. The prevalence in Afro-Caribbean and Asian women is rare. It is commoner in industrialised societies and much more frequent in those of high social class.

Clinical features
Cutaneous co-morbidities

There are a number of skin problems commonly found in sufferers of anorexia and bulimia [3]:

- Xerosis and pruritus.
- Acrocyanosis.
- Perniosis.
- Increased lanugo hairs.
- Hair loss.
- Scurvy.
- Russell sign (knuckle pads from chewing the skin overlying the knuckles) (Figure 84.15).
- Nutritional disease:
  - Pellagra
  - Dermatitis enteropathica (zinc deficiency).
  - Anaemia and hair loss secondary to iron deficiency.
- Cutaneous microvasculature:
  - Raynaud phenomenon.
  - Acrocyanosis and perniosis.
- Hair abnormalities:
  - Hypertrichosis.
  - Hair loss.

Psychodermatological co-morbidities

- Self-injurious behaviours [4].
- Trichotillosis.
- Severe onychophagia.
- Fabricated dermatitis.
- Suicide; the risk is much higher than in the normal population [5].

- Substance abuse.
- BDD [6].

Investigations

Dermatologists should suspect anorexia nervosa when presented with these suggestive signs, particularly in an underweight girl. A simple screening questionnaire is helpful for detecting eating disorders (Box 84.12) [7]. Eating disorders are largely undetected in the community.

Box 84.12 The SCOFF questionnaire for diagnosing eating disorders

- Do you make yourself **S**ick because you feel uncomfortably full?
- Do you worry you have lost **C**ontrol over how much you eat?
- Have you recently lost more than **O**ne stone (6 kg) in a 3-month period?
- Do you believe yourself to be **F**at when others say you are too thin?
- Would you say that **F**ood dominates your life?

  One point for every 'yes'; a score of ≥2 indicates a likely case of anorexia nervosa or bulimia.

Adapted from Luck *et al.* 2002 [7].

Management

Patients receptive to the suggestion of specialist care should be referred to a psychiatrist [8]. Dermatologists may be able to help with advice about treatment of skin manifestations.

Resources

Patient resources

Beat: www.beateatingdisorders.org.uk.

Mind: www.mind.org.uk.

Schmidt U, Startup H, Treasure J. *A Cognitive-Interpersonal Therapy Workbook for Treating Anorexia Nervosa: The Maudsley Model*. London: Routledge, 2019.

Virgo H, Obuaya C-C. *Hope through Recovery: A Supportive Guide to Moving Forward When in Recovery from an Eating Disorder*. London: Trigger Publishing, 2021.

(Both websites last accessed July 2022.)

PSYCHOGENIC ITCH

There is a growing interest in the research and management of itch. In the absence of organic disease, psychogenic itch is a diagnosis of exclusion, and possibly a disease entity in itself. The sensation of itch may not, according to patients, sufficiently describe the perceived sensation. Patients may describe a range of itch-pain-like sensations which are very frequently unpleasant and disabling. What patients find particularly challenging is the sense of not being in control of their bodies, and that sense of frustration is, for many, as disabling as the itch itself.

Sensations related to itch include:

- Skin pain.
- Skin burning.
- Tickling.
- Pins and needles.
- Tenderness.

Table 84.2 Proposed diagnostic criteria for psychogenic pruritus (functional itch disorder): as well as the three compulsory criteria, three out of the seven optional criteria are also required for a diagnosis.

Compulsory criteria	Optional criteria
Generalised pruritus without primary skin disease	Chronological relationship of the occurrence of pruritus with one or several life events that could have psychological repercussions
Chronic pruritus (>6 weeks)	Variations in intensity associated with stress
No somatic cause (cutaneous or systemic)	Pruritus that is worse at night
	Predominance during rest or inaction
	Associated psychological disorder
	Pruritus that could be improved by psychotropic drugs
	Pruritus that could be improved by psychological therapy

Adapted from Misery *et al.* 2007 [4] with permission of John Wiley & Sons.

Psychogenic pruritus

Classification

Pruritus can be divided in those with and those without [1] an underlying dermatosis (Box 84.13).

> #### Box 84.13   Classification of itch
>
> 1 Pruritus with associated underlying dermatosis
> 2 Pruritus with no underlying dermatosis:
>   **2a** Secondary pruritus due to underlying systemic disorder (secondary pruritus)
>   **2b** Generalised pruritus of unknown origin (GPUO)
>   Note that type 2a and 2b pruritus may have secondary cutaneous changes due to rubbing or excoriation.
>   Acute: ≤6 weeks.
>   Chronic: >6 weeks.
>
> Reproduced from Millington *et al.* 2018 [1] with permission of John Wiley & Sons.

Introduction and general description

Pruritus is a multifactorial symptom. Dermatological, neurological, iatrogenic illness and internal disease are well-recognised causes [2] (Chapter 81). The propensity for individuals to sense itch after psychological provocation by pictures of insects, rashes and watching other people scratching demonstrates the ready ability of simple measures to induce psychosomatic pruritus. Misery and colleagues have proposed diagnostic criteria for psychogenic pruritus [3,4]; there are three compulsory criteria (Table 84.2):

1 Localised or generalised pruritus *sine material*.
2 Chronic pruritus (>6 weeks).
3 Absence of a somatic cause.

Localised or generalised psychogenic itch may begin as a stress response [4]. Patterns of itching and scratching may predominantly occur during periods of relaxation or non-occupied time. Pruritic episodes may be unpredictable in onset and present with abrupt and sudden termination. The quality of itch may be unusual, described

as crawling, stinging or burning. Sites of predilection in two-thirds of subjects were the legs, arms and back. Localised itching may lead to generalised body itch within a short time. In some individuals, intense scratching can induce a feeling of pleasure which may be related to the release of opioids centrally.

The consequences of psychogenic recalcitrant itch may be [5,6]:
• Nodular prurigo.
• Anxiety.
• Depression (about 30%).
• Anxiety and depression (10% for out-patients and 20% for in-patients).
• Sleeplessness.
• Suicide.

It is recognised that recalcitrant itch (with or without underlying skin disease) is one of the main reasons why patients consider suicide [7].

Investigations

Various scales measure itch, and researchers and clinicians are attempting to standardise and validate scales. Measurements of itch include:
• The peak pruritus numerical rating scale (PP-NRS); this is the most commonly used test of pruritus in isolation of skin disease.
• The urticaria activity score over 7 days (UAS 7) (Chapter 42).
• The dermatology life quality index (DLQI); this contains a question about itch.
• The eczema area and severity score (EASI) and scoring atopic dermatitis (SCORAD); these scores have an itch factor (Chapter 41).

Management [1,8–11]

The treatment of psychogenic itch is best seen as concurrent treatment of itch sensations at the same time as treating the underlying or associated psychosocial co-morbidities.

In distressed patients with chronic pruritus, including with a likely psychogenic origin, consider psychosocial and behavioural interventions including education on how to avoid trigger factors, how to apply treatments, lifestyle interventions, relaxation techniques, cognitive restructuring and behaviour modification including habit reversal training [6]. Patient support groups can be beneficial and referral to social workers, liaison psychiatry and psychologists may be helpful in individual cases [1].

> ## Treatment ladder for psychogenic pruritus
>
> ### First line
> • Basic measures such as emollients and humectants, soap substitutes and bath additives are usually the baseline of skin treatments
> • Cooling creams such as 2% menthol in aqueous cream may provide symptomatic relief
> • Consider topical steroids and other topical anti-inflammatories if there is a co-morbid dermatitis
> • Non-sedating antihistamines
> • Sedating antihistamines may be better than non-sedating antihistamines (e.g. hydroxyzine 50–75 mg daily)
> • Behaviour-orientated therapy can be very helpful, especially habit reversal treatments [8]

Second line

- Tricyclics [1] (usually in addition to sedating antihistamines, e.g. doxepin starting at 10 mg and increasing to 125 mg/day, or amitriptyline 10–150 mg daily)
- SSRIs are next to try [10] (e.g. fluoxetine 20–40 mg/day or citalopram 20–40 mg/day)
- Phototherapy and photochemotherapy may help recalcitrant itch

Third line

- Antidepressants such as trazadone or duloxetine
- Topiramate has been reported recently as being of benefit [11]
- Serlopitant
- Naltrexone
- There is a growing interest in the management of psychogenic itch with biologic agents and JAK inhibitors. Medications such as nemolizumab [12] (anti-IL-31A monoclonal antibody), dupilumab [13] (anti-IL-4/13 monoclonal antibody), baricitinib, upadicinib and other JAK inhibitors [7,14] are being assessed by NICE, the EMA and the US FDA for approval in the treatment of patients with psychogenic pruritus. These agents are likely to be used after at least one systemic therapy has been tried and failed, or where systemic immunomodulators are contraindicated

Resources

International Society for the Study of Itch (IFSI): www.itchforum.net.

Skin Support: www.skinsupport.org.uk.

(Both last accessed July 2022.)

FACTITIOUS SKIN DISEASE

Doctors usually believe what the patient tells them. The unwritten contract of the consultation process is that the patient will relate the details of the illness as truthfully as they see it and respond to the physician's questions as openly as possible, neither deliberately hiding nor distorting the facts. The physician makes these assumptions in assessing the combination of signs and symptoms of the illness. Some patients may exaggerate or minimise symptoms. Patients may misattribute causation on the basis of experience, culture and a need to place the illness in a context. They may have mistaken beliefs because of advice from other medical or, increasingly, media- or Internet-inspired sources. These consultation behaviours are common and do not constitute a fabrication, although if persistent this conduct can compromise a clinician's objectivity.

Clinical deception refers to a spectrum of illness that lies on a continuum depending on the level of intention to deceive at the time of the act, and the motivation for the induced illness. The definition of factitious behaviour is not completely clear since the level of intention may vary, but for the dermatologist the definition by DSM-5 [1] includes:

1 Falsification of physical or psychological signs and symptoms, or induction of injury or disease, associated with identified deception.
2 The individual presents themself to others as ill, impaired or injured.
3 The deceptive behaviour is evident even in the absence of obvious external rewards.
4 The behaviour is not better explained by another mental disorder such as a delusional disorder or another psychotic disorder.

In factitious disorder imposed on another (previously factitious disorder by proxy), DSM-5 criteria are similar except criterion 2 refers to an individual presenting another person as being injured or harmed in some way.

Criterion 1 supposedly excludes disorders characterised by unintentional production of symptoms, thereby marking a distinction between factitious disorders and somatoform, conversion and dissociative disorders. Criterion 2 assumes an internal incentive which the patient may deny even to themselves, and criterion 3 excludes the intentional production of symptoms for external gain, thereby marking a distinction with malingering.

The nomenclature for dermatological lesions produced by patients, as defined above, is multifarious. Artifice is a noun meaning the use of cunning plans or devices in order to trick or deceive while an artefact is defined as man-made and artistic or decorative. A fabrication is an invention often, in certain contexts, meaning with deceitful intent, while factitious is an adjective meaning artificial or contrived. The term factitious dermatitis will be used preferentially here in keeping with the revised definition of Münchausen syndrome by proxy as factitious or induced illness (FII). Factitious falsification of information, that is, lying, is a consequence of the manufacture of skin lesions, the occult use of others (proxy disease) and disease produced for material profit or retribution. The lying may have a different quality in these cases, such that the psychosocial lies of the impulsive, immature, young girl are mainly used to avoid the shame and denigration of exposure, whereas the pathological lies (pseudologica fantastica) of the accomplished malingerer are used to embellish their performance.

There are a series of recognised factitious skin diseases characterised by the following features: firstly, the dermatoses are caused by the fully aware patient; secondly, there is a desire to hide the cause from their doctors. This definition includes dermatitis artefacta, dermatitis simulata, dermatological pathomimicry and dermatitis passivata. These syndromes are additionally distinguishable from others where there is overt secondary gain, such as Münchausen syndrome, Münchausen by proxy and malingering.

For all factitial skin disease (including dermatitis artefacta) it is crucial to make sure that organic disease is safely excluded and to try to prioritise *why* the patient is presenting with the condition rather than *how*.

Dermatitis artefacta

Introduction and general description

Dermatitis artefacta is a disorder caused entirely by the actions of the fully aware (i.e. not consciously impaired) patient on the skin,

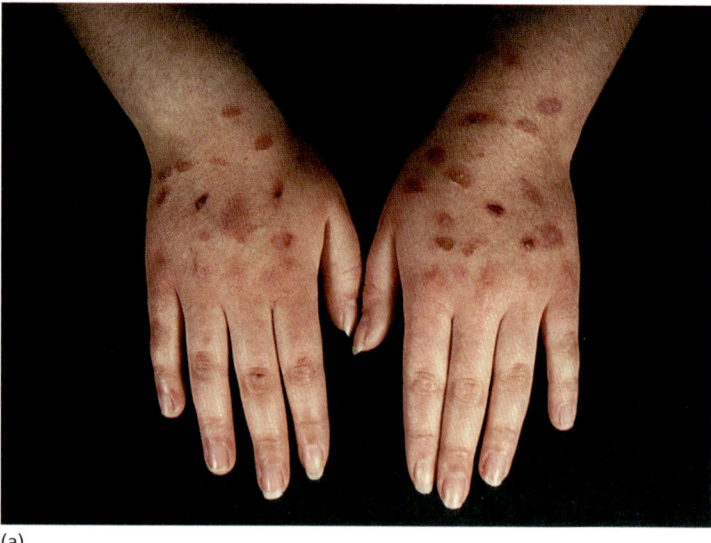

(a)

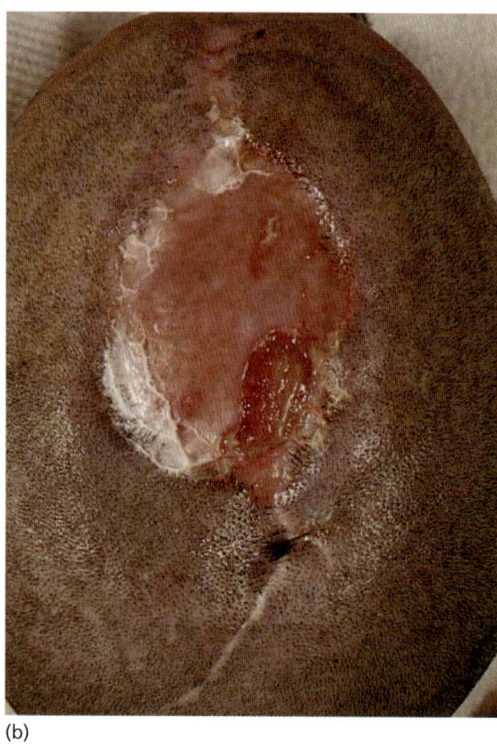

(b)

Figure 84.16 Dermatitis artefacta. (a) Symmetrical and predominantly monomorphic erosions on the dorsal hands. (b) Severe dermatitis artefacta of the scalp as a large necrotic ulcer which needed plastic surgery reconstruction.

Table 84.3 Distinguishing features from dermatitis artefacta of other self-inflicted disorders affecting the skin.

Condition	Distinguishing features from dermatitis artefacta
Self-harm	Patients deliberately cause harm, often with suicidal intent
	Intention is not to feign illness but can be a suicide attempt, a behaviour to modify emotion and cope with distress or a 'cry for help'
Self-mutilation	May be unintentional, seen in patients with severe learning disabilities/neurological patients
Skin picking disorders	Patients damage skin to relieve tension; they usually admit to this
Skin damage due to psychosis	Patients damage skin in response to hallucinations or delusions, e.g. delusional infestation
Skin damage due to body dysmorphic disorder	Damage to skin is secondary to overvalued ideas of perceived imperfection
Malingering	External motive is present, e.g. pecuniary gain
Dermatitis simulata	Individuals (usually children) apply pigments to simulate skin disease
Dermatological pathomimicry	Individuals aggravate an existing dermatosis, so that the disease looks like an exacerbation of an established skin condition with none of the bizarre physical signs
Dermatitis neglecta	Patients self-neglect and develop a build-up of keratin and debris which may mimic a primary skin disorder
Münchausen and Münchausen by proxy	With Münchausen, the patient repeatedly and deliberately acts as if they have a physical or mental illness when not really sick. Repeated acute presentations to different hospitals and different specialties is the hallmark of this extreme form of factitious disorder
	Münchausen syndrome by proxy is a mental illness and a form of abuse. The caretaker of a child, most often a mother, either makes up fake symptoms or causes real symptoms to make it look like the child is sick

Reproduced from Mohandas 2021 [1] with permission of Springer Nature.

hair, scalp, nails or mucosae (Figure 84.16) [1]. These patients hide the responsibility for their actions from their doctors. Deliberate self-harm differs from dermatitis artefacta in that patients will often own that they are 'mutilating' their skin (Table 84.3; Figure 84.17).

Epidemiology

In adults, all studies have shown a female preponderance, with the ratio of female : male varying from 20 : 1 to 4 : 1. Lesions have been found in children from the age of 8 years; prepubertal children have an equal sex ratio, which rises to 3 : 1 female predominance by the early teenage years [1]. These series confirm that the majority

of cases begin in adolescence and in adults under 30 years of age, although there is an important subgroup whose age of onset is significantly older. This latter subgroup is distinguished by being more likely to be male (male : female ratio of 2 : 1), to produce more subtle skin lesions and to have a past history of somatising illness (unexplained symptoms) such as non-epileptic attacks, abdominal pain, syncope, chronic fatigue and backache.

Pathophysiology [2]

The motivation of patients is variable. There is a distinction between disease, illness and sickness. Disease refers to primarily biological forms of pathology, illness to the subjective experience of ill health which is entirely personal, and sickness involves the *process* of being ill. People differ in the way that they perceive, assess, act or fail to act upon the symptoms that they experience. This is recognised as a personal 'illness behaviour' and shapes the role, firstly, within the family and, secondly, with professional health advisors. The psychopathology underlying the production of factitious lesions suggests that the patient *wants* the *sickness role* as the essential pathology. It is suggested that these patients have complex underlying drivers, for example self-hate and guilt, and an illness allows inappropriate regression and avoidance of adult responsibilities.

In some cultures and societies having a physical illness is acceptable, whereas having a psychiatric disease is not, therefore it is easier

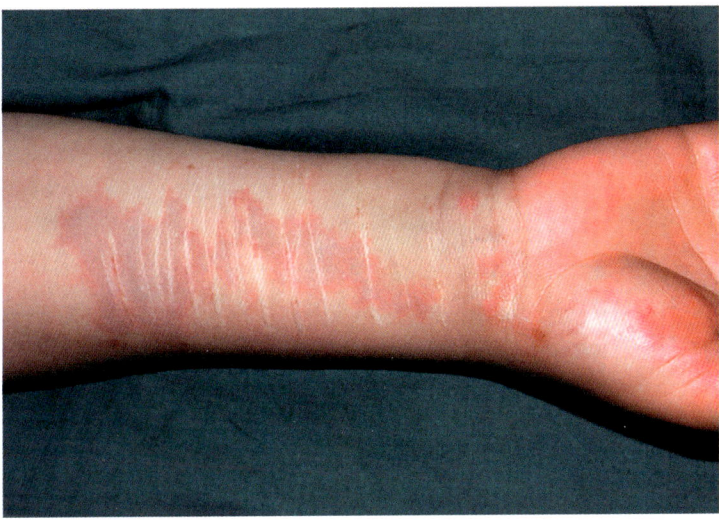

Figure 84.17 Scarring from deliberate self-cutting over a birthmark.

for a patient to mimic physical illness to adopt a sickness role when in 'emotional pain' rather than admit to psychiatric or psychological morbidity.

The precipitating life event (if there is one) may seem trivial (e.g. exam pressure from parents) or objectively be very serious (e.g. sexual or other abuse) (Box 84.14). A focus on 'why' not 'how' may be more productive in managing patients. Children and adolescents commonly show anxiety and immaturity of coping styles in response to a dysfunctional parent–child relationship, bullying, physical body changes or sexual and substance abuse. Adults may be reacting to adverse situations in an immature, impulsive manner. The more chronic patients tend to have a demonstrable personality disorder, most often borderline/emotionally unstable.

The development of dermatitis artefacta is more common in those with memorable early (and sometimes continuing) experience of illness, or in those who have a family member who is (or has been) unwell, or who is a health care professional.

Box 84.14 Psychosocial factors that may precipitate a skin disorder

Children/adolescent
- Bullying
- Family upheaval (divorce, separation)
- Emotional neglect
- Physical/sexual abuse
- Exam stress
- Bereavement
- Adoption, fostering

Adults
- See above causes for events that may have occurred in childhood
- Relationship breakdown
- Bereavement
- Financial crisis, employment
- Issues such as bullying, discrimination
- Social isolation, depression, anxiety
- Body dysmorphic disorder, personality disorders

Clinical features

The diagnosis of dermatitis artefacta can usually be suspected quite early on. The two characteristics are the physical signs and the quality, pattern and reliability of the history that accompanies them (Box 84.15) [3].

Box 84.15 Clinical clues to the diagnosis of dermatitis artefacta

- 'Hollow' history, i.e. vague/brief/lack of detail – does not seem genuine/sincere and does not add up if scrutinised
- Indifferent patient, i.e. does not seem concerned
- Lesions fully formed without precursors
- Sites of lesions may be predicted by patients
- Usually geometrical and bizarrely shaped
- Present in accessible areas, oddly distributed
- Usually present in visible areas
- Suspect historical or current abuse if on breasts or genitalia
- Poor healing/recurrent ulceration despite absence of organic pathology

---

History

The history from the patient is either incongruous or, more commonly, a 'not knowing how the skin lesions happen' (the 'hollow history'). The patient often describes the sudden appearance of complete lesions with little or no prodrome. There is no complete description of the genesis of individual skin lesions. The lesions appear or are 'discovered', often on waking. Lesions appear at an identical stage in development, in crops or groups, more often symmetrically but rarely scattered, apparently at random. There is usually a lack of disease progression on history. By contrast there is a prolonged and elaborate description of the complications and the failure to heal. Characteristically, established lesions may undergo sudden deterioration at the same time as new areas appear. Only rarely do patients use more than one method to produce lesions. It has been suggested that the patients show a 'belle indifférence' to their predicament as part of a dissociative state and that, in the presence of visible disease, they manifest a nonchalance and innocence transmitted through an enigmatic 'Mona Lisa smile' (Figure 84.18). Patients are more often passive than aggressive, even though they have a widespread disfigurement. However, considerable anger is commonplace from parents, carers, spouses or partners, who complain at the incompetence of a succession of doctors. Patients and their relatives may consume huge amounts of medical resources to seek the cause and resolution of the 'problem'. Relatives are usually convinced that the patient has a genuine disease. Official complaints to hospital management and to local or other government officials may follow.

Presentation [4,5]

The range of presentations for dermatitis artefacta is extremely wide, varying from blisters and linear tears, to huge ulcers and mutilation (Figure 84.19). Similarly, the underlying cause can vary from what would seem fairly trivial to an enormous psychological blow. For all age groups, the commonest site of involvement is the face, particularly the cheeks, representing over half the presentations in children (Box 84.16). The dorsa of the hands rather than the palms are

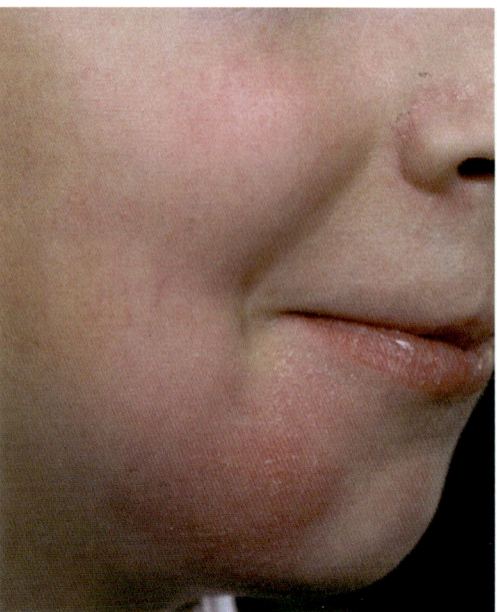

Figure 84.18 Factitious disease of skin on the chin and the 'Mona Lisa smile'.

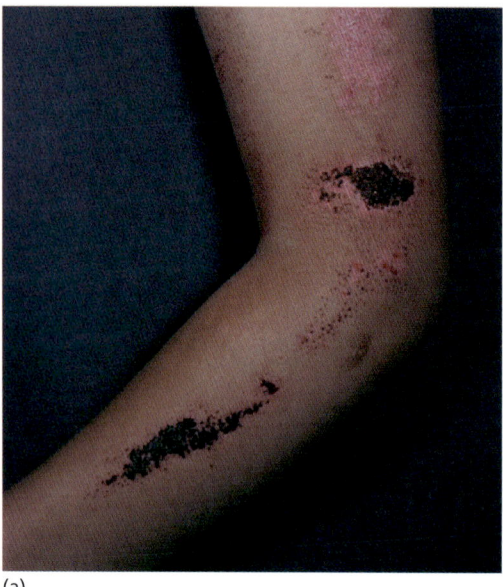

(a)

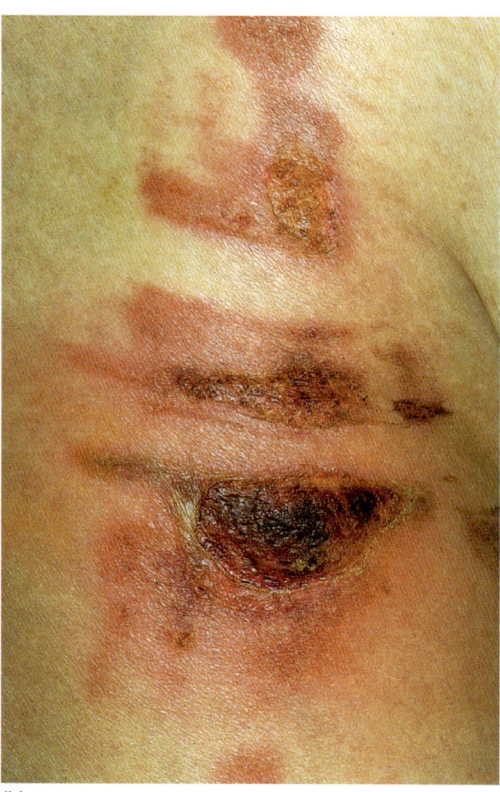

(b)

Figure 84.19 Dermatitis artefacta. (a) Crude, linear, angulated and destructive factitious dermatitis. (b) Note the straight edges and sharp angulation of some of the lesions.

the next commonest site, then the forearms, most frequently of the non-dominant limb. There is a particular covert pattern on covered skin where the clothes hide significant mutilation of the breasts, abdominal areas and sometimes the genitalia. These areas of damage in young girls should prompt inquiry about sexual abuse. Involvement of the back, axillae and external ear is uncommon.

> **Box 84.16 Common sites of artefactual skin lesions**
>
> - Head and neck – scalp, face
> - Lower limbs – shins, thighs
> - Upper limbs – forearms, wrists, upper arms
> - Torso – chest, breasts, abdomen, shoulders
> - Genitalia

Cutaneous lesions have been produced by every known means of damaging the skin and are therefore polymorphic, bizarre and mimic any of the known inflammatory reactions in the skin. Factitial dermatitis should enter the differential diagnosis of every chronic, puzzling and recurrent dermatosis. The lesions are usually linear, angulated or assume patterns that do not conform to recognised skin disease morphology, and are often the result of thermal, chemical or instrumental injury (Figure 84.20). Commonly, circular erosions or blisters of a uniform size can be manufactured (e.g. by cigarette burns or cryodamage from a closely applied pressurised aerosol such as an antiperspirant or asthma inhaler). Perfume may remain detectable in the lesions for some days. Less commonly, dermal lesions from blunt trauma presenting as odd haemorrhages or dramatic dermal indurations and necrosis are found from foreign body injections of milk, cosmetic oil or industrial grease [6]. These are found more often in the breasts, thighs or penis, the latter as covert body augmentation.

Excoriations may be made with nail files, sanding boards, cheese graters or wire brushes to produce raw, crusty, linear or arciform lesions with characteristic geometrical edges. Urticarial lesions are initially produced by chemical damage and progress subsequently to blistering, crusting and scarring (Figure 84.21). Characteristically, these areas may show the 'drip sign', where corrosive liquids have been uncontrolled and allowed to run over the skin (Figure 84.22). Bleaches, soaps and household cleaners are most commonly employed by women; industrial acids and automotive fluids by men. These chemicals may produce a persistent, detectable smell on the skin.

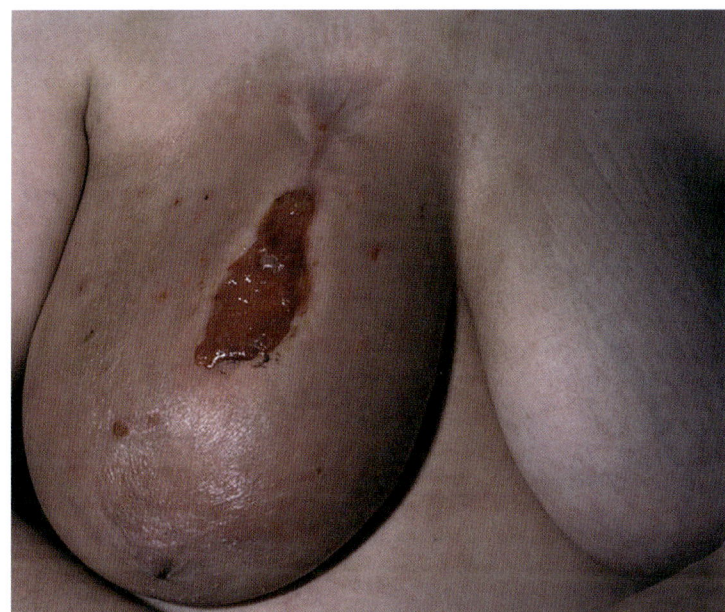

Figure 84.20 Dermatitis artefacta. Persistent ulceration of the breast from covert injections of milk and talcum powder.

Clinical variants

Factitious cheilitis. Factitious cheilitis (also known as *le tic des levres*), or the production of artefactual lesions of the lips, is not common. It is most frequently seen in girls and young women but the incidence is equal in male and female older patients. Simulation of cheilitis has been produced by applying a crust of paper, glue or colourant. Reactions of the lips are limited and appear in particular as persistent inflammation with crusting and variable haemorrhage. The crusts may be very thick with a succession of layers of congealed haemorrhagic exudates resembling a carapace or oyster shell. The haemorrhage can also be impressive, with coagulated blood and serum extruding over the lips. This is caused by picking, biting, rubbing and licking. Occasionally patients may develop crusting of the lips when they become concerned about their lips and refuse to clean them. Removal of the crusts leaves a relatively normal lip although with time there is some superficial erosion. Differential diagnosis includes contact dermatitis, actinic damage, chronic lip licking habit and causes of granulomatous cheilitis.

Factitious nail disease. Traumatic and chemical damage to both the nail and nail fold have been seen in children and adults. The paediatric cases show chronic paronychia caused by the insertion of nails, pins or splinters. Soldiers avoiding duty have habitually used caustics to damage their fingers. The characteristic lesions show purpura and haemorrhage around the nail fold but also subungual haemorrhage and pustules. A significant sign is repeated traumatic nail loss occurring singly or multiply on one hand only.

Hair artefact. A distinctive pattern of hair loss may occur after cutting or shaving. It differs from the plucked appearance of trichotillosis, with obvious gross changes such as rough, cropped areas of hair loss or unnatural, patterned or shaved alopecia of the scalp or eyebrows.

Witchcraft syndrome. Artefact dermatitis can be provoked on an unknowing and unsuspecting victim by proxy [7,8]. For example, as an act of revenge, a hairdresser applied benzyl ether to a customer's skin. This induced hyperaemia with some oedema within 10 minutes but not on the perpetrator since absorption of the agent is very low on the palm of the hand; thus she could easily apply it to the customer's skin without harm to herself.

Dermatitis artefacta with artefact of patch tests. Bullous dermatitis artefacta in a female veterinary assistant healed with occlusive dressings. New bullae on the other arm prompted the parents to demand 'allergy' tests. Ten patch tests to yellow petrolatum were applied to the back, which provoked a non-inflammatory bulla on one of the sites 2 days later [9]. In another case the patch test reaction was mimicked by scarification in an attempt to claim compensation [10].

Constriction artefact. Oedema of limbs from constricting bands has been described (Secretan syndrome). It is characteristic that one digit, usually a toe, will be constricted at a time while the others are unaffected. A repeated series of single, different ischaemic toes, while all the others are healthy, should raise suspicion of external banding. Embolic disease can be excluded by vascular scan.

Purpura artefact. Purpura and bruising are seen after suction, friction or blunt trauma. Children produce purpura on the chin by sucking on cups and on limbs by direct mouth suction or with the use of a toy or tool. Shearing stress also produces purpura, tending to present as linear limb lesions. Extensive bruising and bleeding in a child mean that factitious and induced illness (see 'Fabricated and induced illness' later in this chapter) should be excluded, caused not only by trauma but also drug-induced by anticoagulants.

Dermal artefact. Dermal skin lesions may take the form of panniculitis-type lesions and boggy, fluctuant swellings. Careful examination of an acute lesion may reveal the presence of a needle track where milk, air, faeces, urine, cooking oil, silicone, grease or engine oil has been injected. Access to needles and syringes may be via medical or paramedical family and friends.

Postsurgical artefact. There is a group of patients who present with a non-healing, postsurgical wound (Figure 84.23). This may follow a small operation after minor skin trauma, breast biopsy or instrumentation such as a laparoscopy. Wounds 'burst' after the sutures are removed, become recurrently infected and real organisms such as MRSA appear. Unfortunately, further 'wound repairs' exacerbate and legitimise the continuing wound. It is not unusual to see patients who have had up to eight operative revisions before a further referral is made to a dermatologist.

Differential diagnosis

The differential dermatological diagnoses for dermatitis artefacta include:

- Autoimmune bullous disease (bullous pemphigoid, cicatricial pemphigoid, linear IgA disease).
- Porphyria cutanea tarda.
- Pyoderma gangrenosum.
- Vasculitis.
- Connective tissue disorder.
- Cutaneous lymphoma.
- Folliculitis (bacterial/fungal).

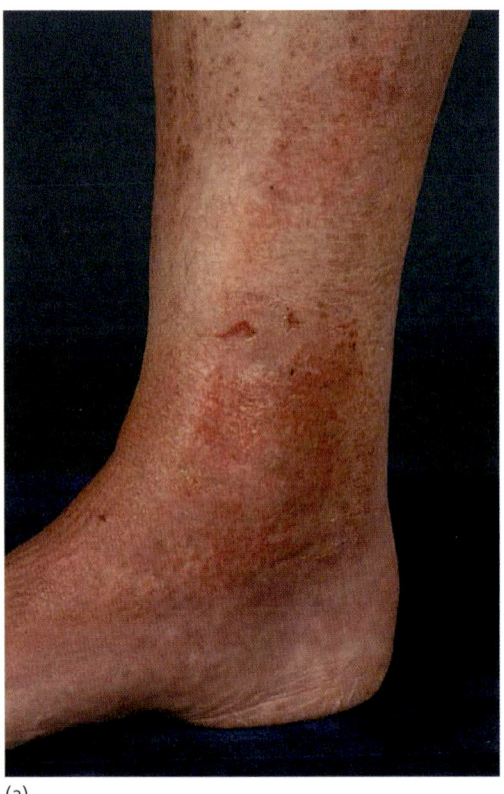

(a)

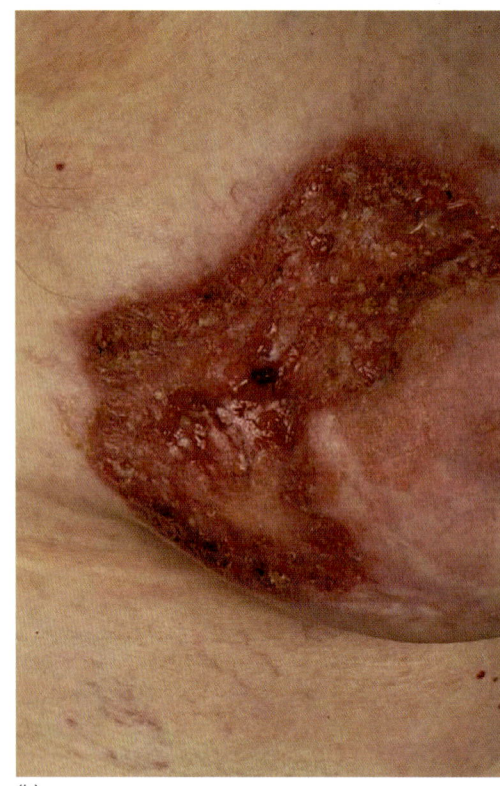

(b)

Figure 84.21 Dermatitis artefacta of (a) the ankle and (b) left breast (different patients).

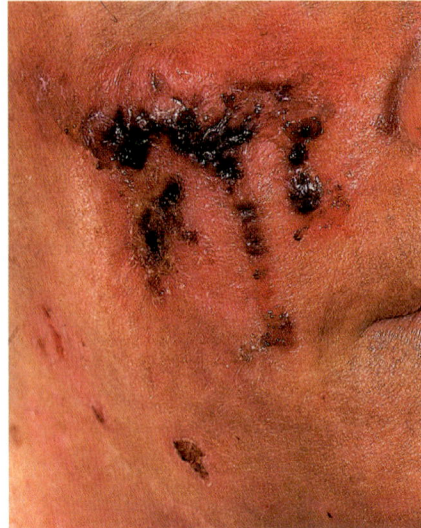

Figure 84.22 Dermatitis artefacta showing the drip sign.

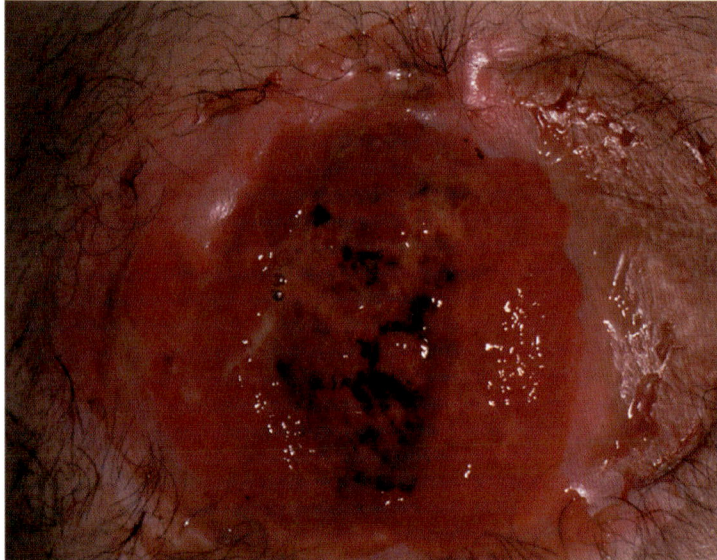

Figure 84.23 Non-healing wound after surgery with characteristic central 'interference haemorrhage'.

- Granulomatous infection (mycobacterial, deep fungal).
- Folliculitis decalvans.
- Arthropod bites.
- Dermatitis herpetiformis.
- Pinch purpura secondary to systemic amyloidosis.

Complications and co-morbidities

Twenty per cent of patients have a somatisation disorder and hypochondriasis. These are co-morbid with anxiety, depression and substance abuse. Borderline/emotionally unstable personality disorder is a factor for chronicity in both sexes. Dissociative states, where there is dissociation between the act of self-damage and the awareness of performing the action, is debated at length based on the premise that the patient may be performing the act without awareness for unconscious reasons.

Complications of dermatitis artefacta include:
- Pigmentation disturbances.
- Scarring.
- Cutaneous infection.
- Osteomyelitis.

- Fistulae.
- Severe infection such as cerebral abscess.

Investigations [11]

The diagnosis is not difficult to make and is usually considered quite early on in the patient's journey. Nevertheless, it is essential to exclude organic disease (see the 'golden rules of psychodermatology' earlier in this chapter). Any skin biopsies must be carefully assessed with very close clinicopathological correlation to avoid under- and overdiagnosis. For this and a range of other reasons, it is essential that dermatitis artefacta is managed in a psychodermatology MDT setting. A skin biopsy is not necessary in the majority of cases but can provide essential supportive information to help to exclude organic disease. Similarly, if a skin biopsy shows minor inflammatory features and the clinicopathological correlation suggests dermatitis artefacta, then it is important to consider the diagnosis as a likely cause of the presenting disease.

Histological appearances can include an epidermis damaged by friction or chemicals with a vacuolar dermatitis and lymphocytes around degenerating keratinocytes. Superficial acute and dramatic epidermal necrosis from physical and chemical damage is characteristic of crude damage to the skin. Subepidermal blistering can be produced by thermal and cryodamage. In contrast, the subjacent deeper dermal tissues can appear spared. Some chemicals, for example toothpaste, can induce unusual inflammatory dermal appearances suggestive of cutaneous lymphoma (pseudolymphoma). Injections into subcutaneous tissues can also produce deeper lesions that show as vasculitis or an odd panniculitis. Ink shows as pigment with limited inflammation, and talc excites a macrophage reaction with giant cells. Injected oils and greases produce deep continuing panniculitis.

Special stains can reveal silver from silver nitrate caustic damage. Examination under polarised light can identify foreign material and further refinement can be found with energy-dispersive X-ray analysis and infrared spectrometry. Unlike disease states, the histopathology of factitious disease may vary with time and it has been shown that serial biopsies may be diagnostically helpful because differing patterns of change may be present on each occasion. Occasionally, patients will completely bury needles into their skin to produce recurrent abscesses. A plain X-ray will visualise these. Some patients have inserted hundreds of needles throughout the skin; if one is identified, then other body areas should also be X-rayed. Wooden skewers may also be inserted; these are best seen via MRI scan.

There are psychometric tests that can be used for the assessment of factitial disorders, but these are essentially research tools.

Management [11–13]

The management of dermatitis artefacta is not an interrogation. There are three therapeutic aims:

1 Treat the skin appropriately. The skin damage may be extensive, disfiguring and infected, with the potential for scarring and dyspigmentation. The process of tissue repair may take time but this allows the opportunity for patient–clinician relationship building. It is important that the physician has a helpful, non-aggressive, sympathetic approach. Very occasionally, occlusive bandaging will allow lesions to heal (except for those of the most determined patients). Establishing a trusting relationship with the patient is crucial.

2 Time should be taken to identify the nature and extent of the psychological problem. The dilemma has always been whether patients should be confronted or not. Generally, most psychodermatologists advocate not confronting the patient unless there are specific benefits (secondary gain, fugue states, etc.). The doctor must avoid personalising the episode and needs to consider the approach that is most likely to change the patient's behaviour. The patient's psychological problems should be approached in a non-intrusive manner, allowing the patient freedom to express their difficulties in a confidential environment. Children usually respond well to this approach, particularly if a cause of psychosocial pressure is identifiable. Any concerns about abuse should be addressed with child protection teams immediately, and concerns about significant psychiatric disease warrant an urgent referral to psychiatric services. Patients will often be engaged with psychological assessment if the clinician acknowledges how difficult and stressful the skin disorder must be and then goes on to explore mood anxiety, impact on life and other psychosocial stressors via this approach. This may be more successful than a direct approach to suggesting the disorder is stress related.

3 Clinicians need to address *why* the patient is presenting with dermatitis artefacta. Usually a cause for the dermatitis artefacta will be revealed as soon as the patient feels safe with the clinician and the environment. This can be very quickly after presentation or may take a long time. The reasons why a patient presents with dermatitis artefacta are very variable and may be relatively easily addressed (e.g. parental pressure to succeed at examinations) or may be difficult to address (e.g. sexual and physical abuse). Concomitant affective disease may need to be treated at the same time.

Adult patients may respond to a non-confrontational 'narrow escape', 'quasi-confession', 'recovery', 'face saving' or 'escape with honour' strategy. This mechanism works by suggesting that the patient does some 'personal homework' to find a solution to their illness by offering a rationale for recovery. The patient may claim that an alternative medicine such as hypnosis, homeopathy or fringe methods such as manipulation and aromatherapy has 'cured' them. It is important to follow up the patient to establish that psychological and social factors were intrinsic to the remission.

One additional technique is the double-bind strategy where the physician explains that the treatment carries an expectation for recovery. If this does not occur then they will be forced to conclude that failure to improve constituted conclusive evidence that the problem is psychological or factitious. A study of behavioural interventions of this type in acute and chronic non-organic (conversion/factitious) motor disorders showed that this produced positive resolution in chronic cases resistant to more passive techniques. This strategy worked particularly well where members of the family were angry or sceptical about the nature of the symptoms.

The prognosis is that of the primary psychological disorder. Acute stress reaction can be addressed in a series of short consultations at the time when the dressings are changed. Approximately one-third to one-half of patients continue to develop chronic lesions. Such patients may have a personality disorder (commonly borderline/emotionally unstable) and need psychiatric assessment.

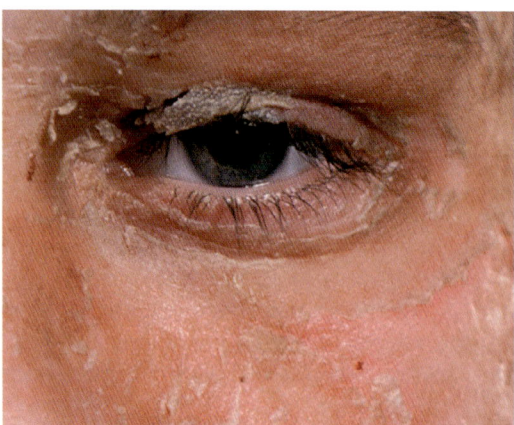

Figure 84.24 Dermatitis simulata. Glue applied to look like herpes zoster.

Unfortunately, this is frequently unacceptable to the patient who may fail to attend the clinic or ask to be referred elsewhere.

Dermatitis simulata

Apparent skin disease can be represented by patients who are ingenious enough to use external disguise to simulate disease (Figure 84.24). These patients do not significantly damage their skin. Make-up has been used to paint on a rash or simulate a birthmark. This is most common in children. Glue and crystallised sugar can produce a coagulum to simulate a desquamating rash or chronic cheilitis, drugs to induce skin discoloration and topical printing dyes to produce discoloured sweat. These discolorations can be removed by aqueous or alcohol swabs and analysed if necessary. Sugar crusts dissolve easily in water, keratin ones do not. Red make-up has been used to simulate a port-wine stain on the face. These deceptions may be clever enough to confuse attending doctors for months.

Dermatological pathomimicry

Some patients may intentionally aggravate an existing dermatosis using the explanation of its genesis given by their dermatologist. It is distinguishable from dermatitits artefacta because the disease looks like an exacerbation of an established skin disease with none of the bizarre physical signs typical of mechanical, chemical or thermal interference. It should also be differentiated from self-inflicted, delayed healing of surgical and traumatic wounds, which is achieved by external damage. A clinical suspicion should arise when patients suffer unexplained exacerbations of disease or are particularly unresponsive to adequate supervised therapy. More direct confrontational discussion without recrimination may prove useful.

Dermatitis passivata

Synonyms and inclusions
• Terre firme forme
• Dermatitis neglecta

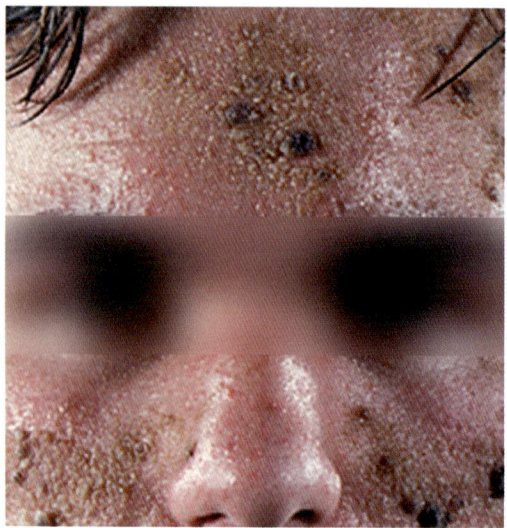

Figure 84.25 Dermatitis passivata in a younger patient.

The cessation of normal skin cleansing will produce an accumulation of keratinous crusts (Figure 84.25). This is commonly seen in geriatric or demented patients who suffer from self-neglect. The lesions are the result of self-neglect and comprise cumulative accretions of keratin and dirty debris that form a thick carapace with time. Younger patients may present with purposefully uncleaned areas of skin (terra firme forme) as a way of mimicking what they may consider to be skin disease. These patients (as opposed to the elderly self-neglect patients) usually seek help to diagnose and manage their skin 'disease'.

Malingering

Asher defined malingering as the imitation, production or encouragement of illness for a deliberate end [1]. The American Psychiatric Association DSM-5 definition states that the 'essential feature of malingering is the intentional production of false or grossly exaggerated physical or psychological symptoms, motivated by external incentives such as avoiding military duty, avoiding work, seeking financial compensation, evading criminal prosecution, or obtaining drugs'.

Malingering may be co-morbid with conversion disorders [2], personality disorders [3] and other factitial behaviour. However, it usually differs from most factitial disease in being short term and opportunistic. Other illness falsification tends to be chronic and persistent. Fear, desire and escape are the three main motives for producing false or grossly exaggerated physical or psychological symptoms [4]. Soldiers feigning disease and disability hope to avoid duty, suspend transfer or be discharged from the service [5]. Workers can prolong sick leave, delay corporate change of job or seek to obtain early retirement with an apparently extended illness. Some patients may seek compensation for a contrived illness, for example alleged burns, or aggravate and continue an existing disease, for example industrial dermatitis, out of a sense of grievance or retribution. Prolonged legal cases of supposed medical negligence are common in those with manufactured illness whose dissatisfaction with their doctors, or the care they have been given, may lead to a financial settlement as a reward [6]. Chronic, non-healing, post-operative scars are manipulated with instruments, or even faecal injection, to maintain sepsis. Hand dermatitis, both irritant and allergic contact, may be perpetuated to seek higher compensation awards.

Treatment depends on the underlying psychiatric illness, if significant psychopathology can be found, but the opportunist response in patients with an underlying personality disorder is poor [7].

Pseudologia fantastica and Münchausen syndrome

Asher used the term Münchausen syndrome to describe notorious hospital hoppers who present with a dramatic and untruthful story of illness [1]. This is a chronic, severe and dramatic subtype of factitious disease. The essential elements are the recurrent nature of the illness, and the frequency and similarity of the repetitive pattern of the complaint in different hospitals (peregrination). The simulated illnesses may be esoteric and rare, with the patient often presenting a dossier to the doctors. While dermatological complaints are uncommon in Münchausen syndrome, simulated porphyria and connective tissue disease, for example, may present to the dermatologist. The last element in the syndrome is pseudologia fantastica (pathological lying) [2,3]. This describes the telling of lies about past social history and connections, exploits, wealth and invention of an alias. The patients are usually male, over 30 years of age and travel widely from hospital to hospital. They complain of abdominal pain, haemorrhage or some neurological incapacity; skin lesions are rare. The commonest signs are non-healing wounds, widespread blistering or multiple excoriations associated with other somatic complaints. Serious consequences such as septicaemia and paraplegia have occurred from induced cutaneous ulceration. Characteristically, patients take their own discharge if they sense their deception has been discovered.

The Internet provides access to those interested in health and medicine and is a rich resource for some patients [4]. In the way that the Internet offers 'virtual support groups', these individuals may offer 'virtual' factitious disorders. Cases have been reported showing the facility with which they can attract attention, mobilise sympathy and control others.

Fabricated and induced illness

Synonyms and inclusions
- Münchausen syndrome by proxy
- Meadow syndrome

In 1977, Meadow had the clinical acuity and personal courage to describe the syndrome of Münchausen by proxy where the illness in a child is fabricated by the parent, usually the mother, or someone *in loco parentis* [1]. This phenomenon has been redefined as fabricated and induced illness [2]. Other carers may be involved and may include health professionals [3].

Doctors and others may not only fail to understand the origins of a child's symptoms but also institute further harm by inappropriate investigations, treatment and surgery. The guidelines for identifying cases mirror many of those discussed for dermatitis artefacta. The history is 'hollow' with a lack of detail. Most parents and carers can give a clear account of an accident. Risk factors include single parent, previous abuse, frequent visits to the GP or accident and emergency departments, poverty, overcrowding and young parents [4]. The victims have a persistent or recurrent illness that cannot be readily explained. The previous diagnoses remain descriptive and not stringent. Symptoms do not respond and laboratory tests are incongruous. The reported symptoms are inconsistent with the presenting health and the symptoms fail to appear in the absence of a certain parent (usually the mother) [5]. The perpetrator is reluctant to leave the child even for a few minutes, but remains oddly impassive even in an emergency. They refuse treatments and hospital admission and may become hostile and abusive. Characteristically, these carers attempt to make close relationships with some medical staff, usually nurses, with a blurring of the professional–parent objective relationship. There may be fabrication of family details and a disturbed marital and social structure. Rarely, parents exhibit the syndrome themselves and produce proxy lesions on the child.

The victims are usually infants or toddlers with a mean age at diagnosis of 40 months. The mean delay between presentation and diagnosis is approximately 15 months. The most common presentations in a literature review [6] were bleeding and bruising (44%), central nervous system depression (19%), apnoea (15%), diarrhoea (11%), vomiting (10%), fever (10%) and rash (9%). Skin lesions are among the five commonest signs. Bruises in children are common on the lower legs and arms. Bruises at certain sites should raise concern – these sites are the face and head of a child less than 1 year old, the sides of the face and ears, black eyes and bruising on the buttocks/lower back and outer thighs. These are the 'punishment' sites [7]. The pattern of bruising may show fingertip marks, striate finger stripe effects from slapping or pinch marks as opposing crescent-shaped lesions. Kicks to the lower body show as irregular, large, deep bruises. Belt and strap damage appears on the trunk as parallel curved marks. The other skin lesions are usually crude forms of factitious dermatitis produced by thermal burns or caustic corrosives on the skin [8].

A large review of countries outside the English-speaking industrialised populations produced similar results [9]. The long-term consequences of childhood victimisation might contribute to the development of factitious disease in adult life. Elements of the child victim experience, including feelings of powerlessness, lack of control and disappointment in the physician, are the suggested dynamics for the development of independent illness falsification. A full discussion of the issues in these cases with paediatric services is essential.

Fabricated and induced illness is occasionally seen in the elderly, special needs or other vulnerable adults perpetrated by relatives, nurses and care home personnel [10].

Medicolegal issues in suspected factitious skin diseases by proxy

The most important action for the physician who suspects factitious disease by proxy is to share the suspicion with colleagues at a very early stage [1] and involve child or adult protection services as appropriate. Case conference discussion and involvement of the institution's management and legal services after these group discussions help to avoid isolation and persecution of the physician. Structures will differ according to health providers in each country but the solitary physician may find support disappointing if an acrimonious dispute arises and legal action has been taken.

DELIBERATE SELF-HARM

Synonyms and inclusions
- Self-injury
- Self-mutilation

Self-mutilation of the skin may present with a wide range of lesions. Cutting and scratching are frequent, but other methods, such as grazing, burning with fire or chemicals, or the insertion of foreign bodies under the skin, are also seen [1]. The damage can be to a wide range of body parts, including the face and genitals. Cases of self-harm may present to accident and emergency departments with acute damage in need of treatment, or to the clinic with chronic lesions or scarring [2].

The relationship between such self-harming behaviours and suicide is complex and varies widely among cases. Authors have made a distinction between repetitive cases of self-mutilation that occur in the context of suicidal ideation, or ambivalence towards suicide, and those cases that clearly occur outside the context of suicidal ideation [3]. It should be noted, however, that there is a potential for overlap between the two, due to the difficulty in measuring or categorising 'intent' and because there are cases of repetitive self-harm, apparently without suicidal intent, progressing to completed suicide [4].

Deliberate self-harm with suicidal ideation

Self-mutilating behaviour is often grouped with other behaviours, such as self-poisoning, attempted hanging or jumping from heights, as 'parasuicide' or 'deliberate self-harm' [1]. The patient describes suicidal ideation, or ambivalence about continuing to live, at the mental state examination. The most frequent lesions are caused by self-cutting, often to the wrists. Burns and ligature marks, and their scars, may also be seen. The predisposing and precipitating factors for this behaviour are numerous. The act may be in response to the symptoms of an underlying psychiatric illness, such as depression, substance misuse or schizophrenia. Vulnerable individuals may respond with parasuicidal behaviour to social or interpersonal stressors. Often a combination of psychiatric and social factors is elicited from the history. Patients often present to accident and emergency departments with acute lesions; in many areas, psychiatric screening of such cases by specialist services is standard. The rate of repeated self-harm in the year following a self-harm presentation to an emergency department is high. The

rate of completed suicide in the year following such a presentation with self-harm is 37 times higher than in the general population. The risk is particularly high after violent self-harm (e.g. the use of firearms) [2].

Some patients, however, commit these acts and do not present for emergency medical treatment. Patients may present with chronic lesions or scarring when this behaviour has become a frequent response to stressors, and such stressors are chronic, such as untreated illness or continuing social problems. Referral for treatment of underlying psychiatric illnesses is indicated where one is present. The evidence for psychosocial interventions after deliberate self-harm is limited but there is some evidence CBT reduces repetition, and a brief intervention and follow-up contact reduce the subsequent rate of completed suicide [3].

Deliberate self-harm without suicidal intent

Introduction and general description

A number of authors have made the case for a distinct syndrome of self-injurious behaviour, or self-mutilation, occurring outside the context of conscious suicidal ideation. Further classification into categories is based on the degree of tissue damage and the rate and pattern of the destructive behaviour [1]:
- Major.
- Stereotypic.
- Superficial/moderate.

Epidemiology
Age
The onset is typically in early life, below the age of 30 years. The mean duration of the syndrome is 12 years.

Sex
An increased prevalence in women is reported.

Pathophysiology
Predisposing factors
Recent work has demonstrated a potential genetic link [2]. Deliberate self-harm has been associated with numerous other psychiatric conditions. Personality disorders, especially borderline/emotionally unstable type [3], are found in many studies and reviews. There is an association with childhood trauma, including abuse. Eating disorders, depressive and bipolar affective disorders, anxiety disorders, somatoform disorders, OCD, substance misuse disorders and schizophrenia have also been described in association with self-harm. Another major group of patients who self-mutilate is found in those with learning disability.

Psychological symptoms described by repetitive self-mutilators include dysphoria, anxiety, depersonalisation and aggression. The patient may experience and describe a strong compulsion to self-harm, similar to compulsion in OCD. The act of self-mutilation may provide relief from the unpleasant emotions or compulsion to self-mutilate, and may also induce feelings of self-control, power or euphoria. Relief may last from several hours to several weeks. In addition, a marked reduction in pain sensation, or increase in pain tolerance, is described in self-mutilators, although this is not uniform. The act is usually performed in private.

Reviews of biological correlates of self-injurious behaviour have suggested changes in opiate, dopaminergic and serotonin systems [4]. One study found reduced imipramine-binding sites in platelets, a marker for serotinergic dysfunction, associated with self-harm. Other proposed biological mechanisms are reinforcement of self-mutilating behaviour due to dysregulations of the dopamine system. A recent study of neuropsychological correlates of self-injurious behaviour in borderline/emotionally unstable personality disorder found impaired executive function and disinhibitory processes [5].

Management [6]

Treatment should include appropriate referral where the disease is associated with another psychiatric diagnosis. There are no clear guidelines for pharmacological treatment of self-mutilation syndrome itself, and a lack of randomised trials. Indeed some authors do not believe there are any general recommendations for the use of psychotropic medication. Where suggestions have been made, SSRIs have been used, in line with the serotonergic hypofunction hypothesis. Dopamine antagonists and opiate antagonists have also been suggested. Mood stabilisers, β-blockers and analgesics have all been used.

Psychological approaches to treatment are varied. Behavioural and psychodynamic techniques are used in group and individual settings. Dialectical behaviour therapy has been described as successful, but access to this therapy varies regionally. Authors make the point that therapy can be long term, difficult and, in serious cases, involve periods of in-patient care.

Patients presenting with self-harm are a heterogeneous group, and likely to have complex problems in any of the biological, psychological and social domains. An understanding of the aetiological factors behind an individual's presentation is a key first step to deciding upon a programme of treatment. This may include pharmacological strategies, but there is as yet no clear core medication recommendation for these cases, and treatment is often complex and specialised.

OTHER PSYCHODERMATOLOGY AND PSYCHOCUTANEOUS CONSIDERATIONS

Cutaneous disease and alcohol misuse

Alcohol may have an effect on the skin either directly (toxicity) or indirectly (via mast cells and the peripheral and central nervous system) [1,2]. The effect of alcohol on the liver may also lead to skin disease (porphyria cutanea tarda). Alcohol dependence and alcohol abuse are on the increase. They rank among the three commonest psychiatric disorders in the community. The prevalence of alcohol abuse and dependence in the USA is 4.65% and 3.8%, respectively,

according to the American Psychiatric Association [3]. There are significant medical and economic consequences because of differing effects of alcohol on metabolism, health, treatment behaviour and motivation.

Alcohol abuse can be missed as a diagnosis by experienced physicians even though the problem is common. Mechanisms for screening and brief interventions are well established and show robust stringency [4]. The four-question CAGE questionnaire (Box 84.17) used as part of a general health enquiry is a consistent indicator of alcohol problems [5]. A two-question screen consisting of, firstly, an enquiry about past alcohol problems and, secondly, significant drinking within the last 24 h is also a sensitive index. The combined sensitivity of these tests shows a 90% accuracy.

Box 84.17 The CAGE questionnaire

- Have you ever felt you should **C**ut down on your drinking?
- Have people **A**nnoyed you by criticising your drinking?
- Have you ever felt bad or **G**uilty about your drinking?
- Have you ever had a drink first thing in the morning to steady your nerves or get rid of a hangover (**E**ye opener)?

  Item responses are scored 0 or 1 with a score over 2 being clinically significant.

Up to 15% of admissions to hospital are directly or partially related to alcohol intake. Alcohol abuse is also co-morbid with psychiatric disorders such as depression, OCD and anxiety states. The cutaneous manifestations of alcohol abuse include diseases that may be exacerbated or caused by the alcohol (Box 84.18) [6,7].

Box 84.18 Skin diseases related to alcohol abuse

Diseases that may be exacerbated by alcohol

- Psoriasis
- Rosacea
- Atopic and other eczemas (especially seborrhoeic dermatitis)
- Pruritus (most causes)
- Chronic spontaneous urticaria
- Other inflammatory skin disease
- Nodular prurigo
- Skin disease associated with metabolic disease (e.g. skin manifestations of diabetes and thyroid dysfunction)

Diseases that may be caused by alcohol

- Porphyria cutanea tarda
- Delusional infestation
- Chronic skin picking disorder

Adapted from Rao 2004 [6] and Kostovic and Lipozecik 2004 [7].

The psychosocial effects of chronic and disfiguring skin disease often produce feelings of stigma and rejection. Recreational substances such as alcohol are commonly used by affected patients as a negative coping mechanism [8]. Most itchy skin diseases are at least exacerbated by alcohol abuse. Seborrhoeic dermatitis is twice as common with alcohol abuse and this may be related to immunosuppression and the effect on cutaneous microflora.

Studies have suggested that female as well as male psoriatics showed an excess rate of alcoholism [9]. Also, while alcohol abuse was not a factor in the onset of psoriasis, it became significant in women after the disease was present. Up to 30% of patients with psoriasis thought they had difficulties with alcohol and 13% a current drinking problem. Furthermore, a daily intake of alcohol of more than 80 g was associated with poor treatment responsiveness in patients with psoriasis. It also appears that the changed character and distribution of psoriasis make it more difficult to treat. In studies of patients with psoriasis, alcohol abuse was not marked by elevated liver enzymes [10]. Alcohol abstinence helped to induce remission, and relapse was induced by re-consumption. The effects of alcohol on immune function and skin vasculature are thought to precipitate exacerbations of rosacea and postadolescent acne.

Genuine infestations of the skin (scabies and pediculosis) and superficial skin infections (usually related to *Staphylococcus aureus*) were found more frequently in alcoholic vagrants than in non-alcoholics and those with other psychiatric disorders. This also suggests that more specific alcohol-related immune factors may be active.

Depression in dermatological patients

The concept of depression is frequently used to mean disillusion, disenchantment, helplessness, frustration or mental fatigue. True depressive illness is an important but frequently missed diagnosis for non-psychiatrists. Up to one-third of medically ill patients have depressive symptoms and depression has a greater impact on mean health scores than angina, asthma or diabetes and more so when combined with chronic physical illness [1]. This is also true for dermatology. A study of the UK General Practice Research Database involving more than 900 000 patients found that patients with psoriasis were 37% more likely to have a diagnosis of depression than matched controls, and that this increased with the severity of the psoriasis [2]. Depression, and to a lesser extent all forms of substance abuse, were the most overlooked diagnoses by dermatologists in 500 unselected dermatology patients examined by Musalek [3]. Screening for depressive diseases in patients with skin disease showed a prevalence of major depressive disorder in 8.4% and dysthymic disorder in 6.3%. Clinicians may underestimate the importance of depression believing that it is an almost inevitable reaction to a severe chronic skin condition. However, the importance of a mood disorder in skin disease is that it may increase distress, cause loss of function and reduce treatment adherence (Chapter 15).

Depression may affect the skin in several ways:
• Skin disease may lead to a loss of self-esteem and thus to depression.
• Depression may be a co-morbidity of skin disease.
• Depression may lead to skin disease.
• Medication for depression may lead to skin disease (e.g. lithium and psoriasis).

Clinicians need to be able to make a clear distinction between appropriate sadness in response to life events and a clinical depression. This is not to say that appropriate sadness should be dismissed or not addressed (for example, by suggesting opportunities for bereavement counselling or other support where suitable). There are three main types of mood disorder:
• Major depressive disorder.
• Dysthymia.
• Bipolar disorder.

Major depressive disorder. DSM-5 criteria for major depressive disorders are the duration of 2 weeks or longer of one of the following:
1 Depressed mood most of the day, nearly every day.
2 Diminished pleasure or interest in the activities of the day (anhedonia).
 Plus three or more of the following:
3 More than 5% weight loss in a month or persistent increase or decrease in appetite.
4 Insomnia or hypersomnia most days.
5 Psychomotor retardation or agitation.
6 Fatigue or loss of energy.
7 Feelings of worthlessness or inappropriate guilt (which may be delusional).
8 Reduced concentration or indecisiveness.
9 Suicidal ideas.

Dysthymia. This is a chronic state of depression that may not be severe enough to meet the criteria for major depression. A depressed mood must be present for most of the day on most days for at least 2 years. The patient must not have gone more than 2 months without experiencing at least two of the following symptoms:
1 Poor appetite or overeating.
2 Insomnia or hypersomnia.
3 Low self-esteem.
4 Poor concentration.
5 Feelings of hopelessness.

Bipolar disorder. This is defined by episodes of low mood as well as those of elevated mood. Manic episodes occur in type 1, while in type 2 milder hypomanic episodes occur.
 DSM-5 mania is defined by the duration of 1 week (or any duration requiring hospitalisation) of three (or four if mood is only irritable) of the following:
1 Inflated self-esteem/grandiosity.
2 Reduced need for sleep.
3 Being more talkative.
4 Subjective experience of racing thoughts or flight of ideas.
5 Increased goal-directed activity or agitation.
6 Increased distractability.
7 Increased risk-taking in pursuit of pleasure.
 DSM-5 hypomania is defined by the duration of 4 days or longer of three (or four if mood is only irritable) of the symptoms of mania above plus all three of the following:
1 Definite uncharacteristic changes in behaviour.
2 Disturbance of mood observable by others.
3 Episode not severe enough to disturb function markedly, hospitalisation is not required, and no psychotic features.

Assessment of mood disorders

This is undertaken by careful history taking and mental state examination. There are several depression screening questions that dermatology HCPs can ask patients. It is important to be mindful of the privacy of the interview situation, and reassurance of the patient about confidentiality of record keeping in order to optimise the assessment of depressive and other mental health symptoms.

Patients with chronic forms of depression are at risk of subsequent major depression, considerable social disability and unhealthy lifestyle choices such as poor diet, alcohol abuse and smoking. Depression in the elderly may be more manifested by irritability, self-neglect, somatic complaints or forgetfulness than conventional symptoms. In children, depression may be insidious and present as disruptive behaviour, irritability, truancy or somatic complaints [4]. In patients with physical illness, somatic symptoms of depression such as poor sleep, poor appetite and weight loss are less useful in assessing depression than cognitive symptoms such as guilt, negative thoughts and hopelessness. Non-dermatological symptoms such as burning sensations, failure to cope with dermatology treatment regimens, negative feelings about body image or failure to resume usual function after recovery from a skin condition can also be indicators of depressive disorder.

A number of robust questionnaires [5] have been developed and validated to screen for depression. These can be either administered by the physician (e.g. the Beck depression inventory (BDI) or the hospital anxiety and depression (HAD) scale) or self-reported. One- and two-question screening tools have the merit of speed but a high false positivity. The patient health questionnaire 9 (PHQ 9) for depression appears well validated as a diagnostic and treatment outcome measure [6].

Suicide in dermatological patients

The mistake that is often made by non-dermatology HCPs is that skin disease does not carry a mortality risk. Suicidal behaviour refers to a range of self-destructive behaviours ranging from non-lethal acts, which have been called suicidal gestures, attempted suicide, parasuicide and more recently self-injury, to a lethal action in which a patient dies, defined as a completed suicide. The rates of completed suicide in the UK are 11 per 100 000 [1]. Rates are higher in men than women and highest in men aged 45–49 years [1]. The rate is rising in young people, particularly in those with behavioural disturbance, substance misuse (25%) and persistent psychosocial difficulties [1]. Psychiatric disorders are the main risk factors for suicide, but numerous studies have also identified physical illness as an important contributory factor. Chronic illness is a risk factor in suicidal ideation and 50% of patients who attempt suicide have a physical illness, especially chronic debility and pain [2]. Not surprisingly, disfiguring chronic dermatoses have been shown to put patients at risk. In a study of 217 patients with psoriasis [3], 10% of patients reported a death wish and 6% reported active suicidal ideation at the time of the study. In another group, 2.5% of out-patients and 7.2% of in-patients with psoriasis expressed suicidal ideas. The severity of the psoriasis was reflected in the frequency of suicidal ideation and the level of measurable clinical depression. Facial acne was also associated with significant risk (5.6%) of suicidal ideation [4], which

is also higher than the levels reported in general medical patients. Suicidal ideation was found in 7 of 11 patients with Darier disease related to the disfigurement, intractability, social exclusion and smell of the dermatosis [5].

Unfortunately, some dermatological patients become so unhappy that they intentionally end their life. A group of 16 patients – 7 males and 9 females – who died by suicide after presenting with dermatological problems to two dermatologists working in the same skin department has been described [6]. The majority of these patients had either body image disorders (BDD) or a chronic, potentially disfiguring skin disorder. It is important to recognise that patients with BDD, and particularly females with facial complaints, may be extremely depressed and at risk of suicide. Even more strikingly, BDD in children and adolescents carries a much larger risk: 67% had experienced suicidal ideation and 21% had attempted suicide [7]. Acne scarring can have just as profound an effect, or even a more profound effect, on body image, self-esteem and confidence as inflammatory acne. The positive therapeutic role of isotretinoin in the management of moderate to severe acne has been described for many years [8], and this may need to be borne in mind when considering the more recently reported association of suicidal ideation in patients treated with isotretinoin as discussed here. Controversy remains over the relationship between isotretinoin and suicidal thoughts, so it is important for the prescriber to make patients and their families aware of this risk, monitor suicidal ideas and refer high-risk patients to the mental health services.

Assessment of risk

Dermatologists are not always accustomed to asking patients about their intentions to self-harm. However when a depressed patient has confided their distress, it is essential that they should be asked about suicidal thoughts. Dermatology HCPs, like all HCPs, have a duty to assess suicidal risk and to make sure that their patients are safe. Dermatologists should be aware of the risk factors for suicide (Box 84.19).

Box 84.19 Risk factors for suicide

- Male
- Older age
- Prior suicide attempts especially with violent methods
- Suicide plans
- Ruminations about suicide
- Depression or anxiety disorder
- Psychotic symptoms
- Unstable mood states, for example as in emotionally unstable personality disorder or in bipolar illness
- Family history of suicide or suicide in close other
- Hopelessness
- Substance misuse
- Social isolation
- Unemployment
- Physical illness, especially those that are chronic, painful and debilitating
- Recent substantial loss, for example bereavement, job loss, relationship loss or recent health deterioration
- Impaired insight or impulsivity

Dermatologists must explore suicidal thoughts. There is no evidence that this increases the risk of sucide. It is appropriate to ask 'How difficult have things become? Do you wonder whether you can go on?', gradually pressing on to 'Have you ever thought you can't go on, or even don't want to go on?', ask about passive suicidal ideas, 'Have you ever wished you could not wake up in the morning?', and eventually 'Have you ever thought about harming yourself, or even ending your life?' It is important not to try and persuade the patient out of their suicidality by false reassurances but to assess whether they have suicidal thoughts, have an intention to act, have plans and have the means to implement the plan. Asking about protective factors is useful and it is important to ask whether the patient feels safe and knows who to contact if they feel unsafe and in danger of acting on these feelings. Record the interview and seek permission to call a psychiatrist for advice and referral.

Dermatology HCPs need to act on expressions of suicidal ideation from patients by assessing if the patient is at risk of harming themselves or those around them; and if sufficiently worried, then an immediate referral to the local acute mental health team is crucial. The acute mental health team will assess the risk and consider admission or crisis home treatment where the risk is high. Rarely, where a patient is considered to be at high risk but is declining admission, they may be assessed and admitted using the legal powers in the UK Mental Health Act 1983, amended by the Mental Health Act 2007. Other countries often have similar legislation to cover capacity and self-harm.

Isotretinoin and mood changes

Following the introduction of oral isotretinoin for the systemic treatment of acne in 1982 there has been some controversy over the relationship of this treatment to the apparent development of depression and suicidality (Chapter 88). Shortly after the introduction of oral isotretinoin there were isolated case reports of mood change and depression. Large doses of vitamin A have well-recognised toxic effects including fatigue, confusion, headache and diplopia. Reported psychological effects include aggression, personality changes, poor concentration, tearfulness, depression, ruminations of guilt and psychosis. These neuropsychological adverse effects have been suggested as a general model for retinoid side effects. The relationship between the drug and depressive illness was made more acute by reports of suicide in isolated rare cases. Some case reports have described depression developing during treatment, some with resolution during the discontinuation of the drug – so-called positive dechallenge – and a few with the recurrence of symptoms on rechallenging with the drug. In addition, there have been descriptions of an increase in frequency and/or severity with increased dosage, simulating a dose–response relationship.

A recent study reported a rise in the risk of attempted suicide in patients both on treatment and after treatment with isotretinoin (standardised incidence ratio 1.78 (95%CI 1.04–2.85)) [9]. However, the risk of attempted suicide had been increasing before the treatment was started, so it could not be established whether the increased risk during and after treatment was because of the isotretinoin. A systematic literature search for studies reporting primary data on depression and suicidal behaviour in patients treated with isotretinoin for acne could only analyse 9 studies that met the inclusion criteria out of 214 studies examined [10]. Rates of depression varied from 1% to 11%. A period prevalence of 11% was found in a 4-month treatment period in one study and a monthly prevalence of 4% in another [10]. These rates are similar to those seen in the 12-month prevalence rates of 10% in the USA, 6% in Canada and 9% in Europe [11]. Although studies have found an association between isotretinoin treatment and depression [12,13], more recent studies have found an effect of isotretinoin reducing depression, possibly through the positive psychological benefit of improved acne [14–18]. A recent analysis of US FDA databases [19] found a completed suicide rate in patients on isotretinoin lower than that in the general US population. Therefore, although there is evidence of an association there is also evidence that treatment of acne with isotretinoin can be positive for mood and that delays in adequate treatment may result in harm to mental health.

There still remains enough doubt about the validity of a relationship between isotretinoin and mood changes to advise that clinicians need specifically to enquire about depression at each out-patient visit. Most national dermatology associations have produced guidelines to assess this risk of mood change in patients on isotretinoin. Most dermatologists will now routinely ask about mood change at each clinic visit and if indicated use a depression inventory, for example the BDI or the HAD scale. Positive scores (BDI >10) should prompt withdrawal of the drug and referral to the psychiatry team. Similarly, regular assessments for suicide before, during and after treatment should be routine for patients with acne and psychosocial co-morbidities, especially those for whom isotretinoin is prescribed. In the UK the Medicines and Health Care Products Regulatory Agency (MHRA) is in the process of reviewing the guidelines for the use of isotretinoin.

Psychiatric therapies in dermatology

Psychiatric treatments are traditionally divided into physical and psychological. Physical treatments now most often refer to medication, but also include some other less frequently used modalities, such as electroconvulsive therapy, light box treatment and even psychosurgery. Psychological treatments cover a wide range of interventions, including anxiety management techniques, cognitive–behavioural therapies and psychoanalytical therapies. The treatment of psychiatric conditions also often involves social interventions, such as attention to housing, occupational or educational interventions and arranging appropriate access to benefits or resources. The synthesis of the three approaches is often termed the biopsychosocial approach.

Several dermatologists are beginning to become increasingly familiar with psychopharmacological interventions and also recommending talk therapies. The rise of psychodermatology as a subspecialty has seen more dermatologists experienced and trained in basic psychiatric and psychological interventions (albeit under the supervision of trained psychiatrists and psychologists). Useful guidance in this may be found in the UK NICE recommendations published for psychiatric interventions that cover primary care and secondary care. Guidelines have been produced for anxiety, bipolar affective disorder, dementia, depression (both in adults and children and in adults with chronic physical health problems), drug misuse, eating disorders, OCD (which contains specific guidelines for BDD), post-traumatic stress disorder, pre- and postnatal mental health disorders, schizophrenia and self-harm [1–8]. A useful publication is the NICE pathway on common mental health disorders [9], which is a 'one-stop shop' for advice; this brings together all the NICE recommendations for non-psychotic mental health conditions. There is also a growing literature in psychodermatology that is written by dermatologists, psychiatrists and psychologists who work in psychodermatology clinics and which offers clear guidance for the psychopharmacological and psychological management of psychodermatological disease [10,11].

Drug therapies (medications)
Antidepressants
Antidepressants are widely used, not only for the management of depression but also for anxiety and panic disorder, OCD and BDD, post-traumatic stress disorder, bulimia nervosa and pain. They are also occasionally used cautiously in depression in the context of bipolar affective disorder, but as there is a risk of triggering a manic episode they should only be prescribed in such patients by a mental health specialist. The introduction of antidepressants with a better safety profile in overdosage than the old tricyclics has led to an increase in their prescription in recent years. Arguments have been made that there is now overprescription, and there are concerns that SSRIs may be associated with suicide, particularly in adolescents [12]. These concerns have been contested but guidelines for treatment now reflect an increased caution in the prescribing of antidepressants. Fluoxetine is the only antidepressant that has been shown in clinical trials to be effective for treating depression and anxiety in children but, as with other SSRIs, it is associated with a small risk of suicidal thoughts and self-harm behaviours. It should only be prescribed by specialists in child and adolescent mental health and is never used as first line treatment in children.

General considerations in antidepressant prescribing
Before starting an antidepressant it is important to ensure that the patient understands the rationale for their use and has information about what to expect. Emphasise to the patient that depression is an illness which is treatable. Explain that antidepressants work by increasing the levels of certain brain chemicals and that this takes a while so there will be no immediate therapeutic effect. Antidepressant effects can be evident at 1 week, and by 2–3 weeks at therapeutic dose an effect is often seen. If there is minimal effect, consider increasing the dose after 3–4 weeks, but if there is no response at all after 3–4 weeks on the maximum dose the patient will tolerate, consider changing to another agent from a different antidepressant group. Side effects, however, can be more immediate, for example the sedative and appetite-increasing side effect of mirtazapine. Explain what side effects to expect and whether these will settle. For example, SSRIs often have an immediate effect of causing nausea and sometimes increased anxiety but this usually settles in a few days. Patients are often concerned that antidepressants are addictive. Explain that they are not but they can have a discontinuation syndrome in which if the antidepressant is stopped suddenly the patient may experience flu-like symptoms and odd electric shock sensations. These symptoms disappear on restarting the antidepressant, which should then be withdrawn gradually. Antidepressants with a shorter half-life, for example paroxetine, are

particularly prone to having a discontinuation syndrome, whereas fluoxetine with its long half-life is much less likely to manifest this problem. After starting an antidepressant the patient should be monitored carefully for suicidal ideation; this is especially important for patients under the age of 25 where the risk of this effect is greater.

A review after 1 week may be important for those considered to be at high risk of self-harm, or those under 25 years of age, while a review after 2–6 weeks is suitable for others. Antidepressants should be continued for 6–9 months past the remission of symptoms as this helps reduce the risk of relapse. The Maudsley prescribing guidelines, published in the UK, provide an up-to-date and comprehensive reference for psychotropic prescribing [13]. The Royal College of Psychiatrists in the UK has produced useful patient information leaflets on antidepressants and the antidepressant discontinuation syndrome.

Selective serotonin reuptake inhibitors
Selective serotonin reuptake inhibitors are now recommended for first choice use in depression and OCD, specifically for BDD and anxiety disorders, due to their relatively low side effect profile and lower toxicity in overdosage when compared with the older tricyclic antidepressants (Table 84.4). They are usually very well tolerated. The most common side effects are nausea, dyspepsia and gastrointestinal upset, headache, agitation and anxiety, sweating, rashes, insomnia and sexual dysfunction. Rarely, SSRIs may lead initially to an exacerbation of anxiety; in the under 18 years age group, the association with agitation leading to increased suicidal behaviour and hostility has led to the recommendation that SSRIs should only be prescribed by child and adolescent mental health specialists. Hyponatraemia and increased risk of bleeding due to an effect on platelets can rarely occur. There is increasing concern about the propensity for some psychotropics to prolong the QT interval, thus increasing the risk of fatal arrhythmias. SSRIs are generally regarded as having low cardiotoxicity but recent studies have indicated that of this group citalopram and escitalopram can prolong the QT interval. Citalopram should not now be used in daily doses above 40 mg. Caution should be exercised and the prescriber should avoid combination with other drugs known to cause a prolonged QT interval.

Other newer antidepressants
The serotonin and norepinephrine reuptake inhibitors (SNRIs) act on both serotonin and norepinephrine (e.g. venlafaxine and duloxetine). They tend to be used as second line agents. Generally they are less well tolerated than SSRIs but are better than the old tricyclic agents. They have similar side effects to the SSRIs in terms of gastrointestinal side effects and increased anxiety, but generally have fewer sexual side effects (Table 84.5). They can be alerting, which may worsen insomnia. Mirtazapine belongs to the class called noradrenergic and specific serotonergic antidepressants (NaSSAs). It has minimal sexual side effects but is sedative and causes increased appetite and weight gain. These side effects can be helpful in patients with insomnia and loss of appetite, but it is important to warn normal-weight patients of the propensity to gain weight and it is best avoided in overweight patients.

Tricyclic antidepressants
Tricyclic antidepressants are no longer recommended for first line use in depression. They are still useful when sedation is required,

Table 84.4 Use of selective serotonin reuptake inhibitor (SSRI) antidepressants in depression.

Name	Dose (adult <65 years)	Indications [27,28]	Notes
Citalopram	10–40 mg/day	Depression Panic disorder	Recommended as good choice in hepatic impairment [30] Few drug interactions Prolongs QT interval
Escitalopram	5–20 mg/day	Depression Panic disorder Social anxiety disorder Generalised anxiety disorder	Isomer of citalopram Few side effects and tends to be well tolerated Few drug interactions Prolongs QT interval
Fluoxetine	20–60 mg/day	Depression OCD BDD Bulimia nervosa	Long half-life, useful in patients with poor adherence who may miss doses Does not cause discontinuation syndrome if abruptly stopped SSRI with most experience of use in pregnancy Sedative, so give at night
Fluvoxamine	50–300 mg/day	Depression OCD	Split dosing if above 150 mg/day
Paroxetine	10–60 mg/day	Depression OCD Panic disorder PTSD Social anxiety disorder Generalised anxiety disorder	Marked withdrawal syndrome Associated with extrapyramidal side effects Recommended as good choice in liver impairment [29] Recommended as good choice in breastfeeding [30]
Sertraline	50–200 mg/day	Depression OCD Panic disorder	Recommended as good choice in hepatic impairment [30] Few side effects and drug interactions

BDD, body dysmorphic disorder; OCD, obsessive–compulsive disorder; PTSD, post-traumatic stress disorder.

Table 84.5 Use of noradrenergic and specific serotonergic antidepressants (NaSSAs) and serotonin and norepinephrine reuptake inhibitors (SNRIs) in depression.

Name	Dose (adult <65 years)	Indications	Notes
Duloxetine	30–120 mg/day	Depression Generalised anxiety disorder (Also diabetic neuropathy and stress incontinence)	SNRI Often used by pain clinics as there is some evidence it is helpful in neuropathic pain
Mirtazapine	15–45 mg/day	Depression	NaSSA Relatively free of anticholinergic and sexual side effects Appetite increase and weight gain Sedating, often used if sleep is poor
Reboxetine	8–12 mg/day	Depression	Not sedating Sexual side effects can occur Split dosing
Venlafaxine	37.5–225 mg/day	Depression Generalised anxiety disorder	SNRI Tends to be used as second line Split dosing, or up to 225 mg/day can be given as a modified-release form Blood pressure should be monitored at higher doses

as this can provide some immediate relief from the insomnia of depressive states and aid concordance (Table 84.6). In lower doses tricyclics are commonly used by dermatologists for pruritus and urticaria (as patients may find both the antipruritic and sedative effects useful), and for dysaesthesias and atypical pain syndromes (e.g. burning mouth syndrome). Side effects include dry mouth, blurred vision, constipation, sedation, urinary retention, open-angle glaucoma and postural hypotension. Cardiotoxicity, including heart block, is recognised in larger doses and overdoses. Prolongation of the QT interval is caused by most tricyclics and amitriptyline in particular can cause marked QT prolongation, so caution needs to be exercised in the use of high doses or if there is a potential combination with other drugs that prolong the QT interval. Do not prescribe in patients where there is a risk of overdose as they are lethal in overdose. Reduction of the seizure threshold is greater than with the SSRIs so they should be avoided in epilepsy.

Switching antidepressant drugs
The need to switch between antidepressant drugs is common, not only because response rates to the first drug are around 50% [14] but also due to the intolerance of side effects or troublesome interactions. When switching from drug to drug it is necessary to consider both the potential for withdrawal reactions from the first drug, and also the possibility of interactions between the old and new agents. It has been recommended that if antidepressants have been taken continuously for 6 weeks or more they should not be stopped

Table 84.6 Use of tricyclic antidepressants (TCAs) in depression.

Name	Dose (adult <65 years)	Indications [31]	Notes
Amitriptyline	10–200 mg/day	Depression Neuropathic pain	Noted cardiotoxicity
Clomipramine	10–250 mg/day	Depression Phobic states Obsessional states	Cardiotoxic
Dosulepin	75–225 mg/day	Depression	Cardiotoxic Previous name dothiepin
Imipramine	75–300 mg/day	Depression	Cardiotoxic Less sedating Split dose twice daily above 150 mg/day
Lofepramine	140–210 mg/day	Depression	Less cardiotoxicity than other TCAs Split dose twice daily Less toxic in overdose Occasionally hepatotoxic
Nortriptyline	10–150 mg/day	Depression Neuropathic pain	Cardiotoxic Plasma level monitoring often available
Trimipramine	50–300 mg/day	Depression	Regarded as most sedating

abruptly unless a serious adverse event has occurred (e.g. arrhythmia). They should be withdrawn gradually and doses of new drugs are cross-tapered upwards if possible. Interactions described on switching include the serotonin syndrome, cholinergic rebound, elevated levels of drugs due to pharmacokinetic interactions and excessive side effects due to pharmacodynamic interactions. Certain drugs are particularly troublesome in switches, such as monoamineoxidase inhibitors (MAOIs) (due to their mechanism of action) and fluoxetine (due to a long half-life). A good rule of thumb is to wait 2 weeks after withdrawing an antidepressant before starting an MAOI and 2 weeks after stopping the MAOI before starting another agent, but due to its long half-life this should be extended to 6 weeks for fluoxetine. Read the manufacturer's prescribing guidelines; MAOIs are best left to mental health specialists.

Antipsychotics

Increasingly, some dermatologists (with appropriate training and experience) are in a position to prescribe antipsychotics. Dermatologists are most likely to consider prescribing antipsychotics in DI or in other delusional disorders. In these conditions, particularly where there are somatic delusions and no insight, it is unlikely that the patient will accept referral to psychiatry and therefore prescription by the dermatologist is the only possibility of attempting a pharmacological intervention. There is no robust evidence from randomised controlled trials for the treatment of DI or other delusional disorders [15]. However, as mentioned in the section on DI, there is case series evidence that antipsychotics help [16] and a review by Manschrek and Khan [17] suggested antipsychotics are effective in delusional disorders.

Second and subsequent generation antipsychotics

For most dermatology-related psychotic conditions, the agents of choice are the second and subsequent generation antipsychotic drugs as they have a lower incidence of extrapyramidal and cardiotoxic side effects (Table 84.7). Some second and subsequent generation antipsychotics may be associated with drowsiness, weight gain, metabolic syndrome (abnormal glucose tolerance and

lipid metabolism) and hyperprolactinaemia. Olanzapine has been particularly problematic in causing the metabolic syndrome. Some are still associated with prolongation of the QT interval and possible cardiotoxicity, although this is less common than in the first generation antipsychotics. Rarely, there is an association with impaired glucose tolerance. Clozapine, in particular, is reserved for psychiatrist only use due to its association with severe agranulocytosis which requires close monitoring of the full blood count.

First generation antipsychotics

A wide number of first generation antipsychotics are still available, although these are unlikely to be prescribed by a dermatologist. Chlorpromazine, the first of the antipsychotics, is still available. Haloperidol has a wide range of uses, not only in psychoses, but also in tic disorders, hiccup and nausea. Some dermatologists have used it in the early part of their medical career to treat delirium in elderly in-patients. Sulpiride is very similar in structure to amisulpiride, and is less expensive. Many antipsychotics prolong the QT interval and this is particularly a problem with haloperidol and pimozide.

Second generation antipsychotics

The newer antipsychotics, amisulpiride, olanzapine and quetiapine, have been found to have minimal effect on the QT interval, and aripiprazole has no effect on the QT interval. Some dermatologists may still be familiar with pimozide for the management of DI but it has been associated with sudden death syndrome and so should be avoided in favour of newer, safer agents. Antipsychotics should be used with caution in patients with cardiac disease, and a pretreatment electrocardiogram (ECG) with subsequent ECG monitoring should be completed. It is important to be aware of the risk of weight gain and metabolic syndrome particularly with quetiapine and olanzapine. Glucose tolerance and weight should be monitored at baseline and follow-up. Many antipsychotics cause raised prolactin, where this results in symptoms (e.g. galactorrhoea) they may need to be stopped and changed to an alternative. Baseline and follow-up prolactin can for some agents be used to give an indication about whether the patient is taking the medication. In elderly

Table 84.7 Use of second generation antipsychotics (SGAs) in delusional infestation (DI).

Drug	Dose[a]	Side effects (rated in ascending order: some/low, moderate, high/large)	Notes
Amisulpride	200–400 mg	Not sedating No/minimal weight gain Moderate increase prolactin level Low risk of EPSE Some QT prolongation	Suggest dose splitting Renally excreted Consider dose reduction if GFR is reduced Does not usually affect liver function
Aripiprazole	5–15 mg	Some sedation Not clearly associated with weight gain or dyslipidaemia Unlike other SGAs, this drug decreases prolactin level Some EPSE No QT prolongation	Increased risk of cardiovascular events in patients with dementia
Olanzapine	2.5–10 mg	Highly sedating Large weight gain, risk of metabolic syndrome, risk of dyslipidaemias Usually no increased prolactin (<20 mg) Some anticholinergic effects Low risk of EPSE Some QT prolongation	Increased risk of cardiovascular events in patients with dementia
Quetiapine	50–300 mg	Moderately sedating Moderate weight gain Usually no/minimal increased prolactin Some anticholinergic effects Low risk of EPSE; common choice in patients with Parkinson disease Some QT prolongation	Increased risk of cardiovascular events in patients with dementia but there is a suggestion that this effect is less than with other SGAs
Risperidone	0.5–3 mg	Some sedation Some weight gain Moderate increase in prolactin level Some anticholinergic effects Moderate risk of EPSE Some QT prolongation	Increased risk of cardiovascular events in patients with dementia

[a] Note that the doses given are the ranges which are usually used in DI where patients often respond to much lower doses than those used in schizophrenia. Please refer to the *British National Formulary* for the maximum licensed doses in schizophrenia.
EPSE, extrapyramidal side effects; GFR, glomerular filtration rate.

patients with dementia there is an association beween antipsychotic use and increased risk of stroke and transient ischaemic attack. There is a suggestion that quetiapine and aripiprazole have a lower risk of cerebrovascular accident but this is not a consistent finding. These risks should be considered before prescribing in the elderly, and a risk–benefit assessment undertaken together with appropriate monitoring. When antipsychotics are prescribed in patients with dementia very low doses should be used.

Although there are no randomised controlled trials of the use of second generation antipsychotics, there are accumulating data in the literature about their use. A systematic review found that response rates for second generation antipsychotics are about 75% [16]. The most widely used for DI are probably risperidone and olanzapine, but amisulpiride has also been recommended. DI often responds to lower doses than those used in schizophrenia (e.g. risperidone 0.5–3 mg daily, olanzapine 2.5–10 mg daily, amisulpiride 200–400 mg daily, aripiprazole 5 mg daily).

Any prescribing of antipsychotics should be done with appropriate monitoring according to national guidelines. It may be appropriate to negotiate with the primary care physician about such monitoring, which can be done in primary care.

Anxiolytics

The benzodiazepine anxiolytics can appear initially very effective in alleviating anxiety symptoms and states, but problems with tolerance and dependence rapidly develop, and they are frequently misused. They should be avoided, but if needed use should be limited to the short term (2 weeks). Buspirone has low dependence potential and is rarely misused, and is licensed for short-term use in anxiety. β-Blockers are used for autonomic anxiety symptoms but do not affect psychic symptoms or muscle tension. Many of the SSRIs and some other antidepressants are licensed for use in anxiety disorders (see Tables 84.4, 84.5 and 84.6) and are effective anxiolytics.

Mood stabilisers

Mood stabilisers are usually used in dermatology for dysaesthesias and postherpetic neuralgia, or are encountered when other specialists have initiated them. Many anticonvulsants are used as mood stabilisers. Pregabalin and gabapentin are the commonest medications to be commenced by dermatologists. These drugs are often started at lower doses and then titrated upwards according to clinical benefit. Some patients experience sedation and/or weight gain. There is increasing awareness of the abuse potential of pregabalin and gabapentin and in the UK NICE guidelines take account of this. Valproate in various forms is used for different reasons in dermatology (including dysaesthesias and postherpetic neuralgia). Modified-release forms of valproate are frequently used off licence for prophylaxis of bipolar disorders. Carbamazepine is licensed for the prophylaxis of bipolar disorder, and is also used in augmentation strategies for refractory depression. Other antiepileptic drugs have been used off licence for treatment and for prophylaxis. The use of lamotrigine has become widespread, and topiramate and gabapentin have also been used. Lithium is the oldest of the mood stabilisers, but is still widely used and is effective in acute mania, prophylaxis of bipolar disorder and augmentation of treatment in refractory depression. It has a narrow therapeutic index and a wide array of side effects, especially on the kidneys and thyroid, and requires careful monitoring through blood tests. It is also known for causing exacerbations of psoriasis. Lithium and anticonvulsants are known teratogens and should be avoided in women of childbearing age. They should only be used in this group with appropriate consideration of the risks and counselling about potential hazards if the patient becomes pregnant.

Psychological therapies

The use of psychotherapies in disorders that combine somatic and psychological factors is widespread, but there is often confusion about how these conditions are defined, and the evidence base is incomplete [18]. An example of the difficulties in this area is given by a Cochrane review of conversion disorder [19] in which all but 3 of only 43 identified references were excluded on grounds of quality. There is more evidence for specific therapies in certain psychiatric illnesses, and recommendations for the use of therapies have been included in clinical guidelines [1–9].

The therapeutic relationship

The relationship between the clinician and patient has a potentially powerful therapeutic (or sometimes counter-therapeutic) effect, even before formal psychological techniques are considered. The effect of an empathic approach can be very powerful in those cases presenting with emotional distress related to dermatological problems. Although efforts are constantly made to reduce stigma, some patients may feel stigmatised by both their skin and psychiatric symptoms. The opportunity to express their anxieties and fears may provide significant relief. It may be necessary for the clinician to question gently any defensive explanations that a patient uses for their symptoms. The effect of touch during examination has been described as relieving the anxiety of patients who feel stigmatised by their skin lesions. The effect of actively listening within a therapeutic relationship allows patients to address their own problems, and is the basis of client-centred counselling, described by Rogers [20]. Of course, the dermatologist will need to give clinical advice, but a confident, authoritative rather than authoritarian approach, where the clinician offers explanation and clinical advice when indicated, but is able to tolerate this advice initially being partially taken or prevaricated on, will aid sustained engagement.

It should also be noted that a small, but significantly morbid, population of patients can experience a marked negative effect through the therapeutic relationship. With such patients, who usually have severe neurotic or personality pathologies, the clinician can feel pressed into making unusual decisions, ordering unusual investigations and going to extreme lengths to manage the patient's anxiety, anger or demands. It is not unusual for such patients to initially present with the impression that the clinician is 'the best they have seen' or 'the only one who has understood' – a relationship

that can rapidly change to one of dissatisfaction, complaint or litigation. In such patients, although presenting as seeking a 'cure', there may be an unspoken or unconscious need to remain in the sick role, and the clinician has an apparently impossible task. It is important for the clinician to recognise when such dynamics are potentially distorting practice, and seek appropriate advice if severe anxiety or personality disorder is suspected.

Cognitive–behavioural therapy

Increasingly, CBT has become the first line psychological therapy in depression and anxiety disorders, including BDD [1–8]. Randomised trials have found efficacy of CBT in BDD [21] and it is recommended in UK national guidelines for the treatment of BDD [4].

The theory of CBT is that the patient automatically responds to certain situations and stimuli with ingrained negative thoughts. These thoughts in turn lead to negative emotions such as fear or depression, and behavioural consequences such as avoidance or rituals. Treatment in CBT is based around the process of sympathetically challenging these negative automatic thoughts and exploring alternative responses that may not lead to behavioural and emotional pathology. The therapeutic process may include exposure and response prevention, wherein the patient is exposed to a troubling thought or stimulus (often, initially, in imagination or abstract) and encouraged to explore alternative thoughts and responses to their ingrained pathological reaction. Often, adjunctive relaxation and anxiety management techniques are an integral part of the therapy. CBT techniques are widely used and have been published in 'self-help' formats, for example *Overcoming Depression and Low Mood* [22]. The clinician can incorporate CBT principles and techniques in their clinical practice. Computer packages have been developed to deliver CBT, although guidelines state the evidence is better in depression and anxiety than in OCD [23].

Formal CBT treatment, when provided by a trained therapist, can consist of 6–20 or more hour-long sessions, depending on the severity of the case, complexity, co-morbidities and response. The main concern for many health care providers is insufficient therapist hours to meet demand, resulting in lengthy waiting lists. The therapy can be provided in group as well as individual settings. In the UK, the provision of psychological therapies has been enhanced through the Improving Access to Psychological Therapies (IAPT) programme. This is a government-funded initiative to increase the provision of psychotherapy and has mostly provided increased access to CBT delivered by psychologists. Further information and a list of services are provided via the IAPT website on the NHS England website (www.england.nhs.uk; last accessed July 2022). Although usually effective, CBT is not suitable for all cases and alternate modalities of therapy still need to be considered.

Habit reversal therapy

Habit reversal is a treatment based on principles of behavior modification, originally developed for undesirable habits such as nail biting. It has been adapted to treat habitual and circumstance-driven scratching behaviour in atopic eczema. Behaviour modification changes a negative behaviour and develops or strengthens a new behaviour which is then maintained over time. The aim of habit reversal in atopic eczema is to reduce scratching and the related skin damage, allowing skin to heal. This technique has been developed both as an individual therapy and in group work, and there is ongoing work to produce self-help and computer-assisted versions. Studies have demonstrated that those who received topical steroid and emollient treatment in addition to habit reversal therapy had greater improvement in skin and scratching compared with those who only got habit reversal [24,25]. This approach of steroid and emollients alongside habit reversal has been called the combined approach [26] and a manual and website have been produced to assist patients and clinicians (www.atopicskindisease.com; last accessed July 2022). Scratching behaviour can become habitual or it can be driven by emotional distress. Habit reversal has greater success in habitual scratching, with 80% of patients who complete the treatment course improved. Emotional scratching requires further psychological evaluation and other treatment modalities, for example stress management techniques, alongside the habit reversal [27]. The combined treatment of habit reversal plus steroids can be delivered by a variety of health care professionals and often dermatology nurse specialists are ideally placed to be trained in and deliver this treatment. It is a simple, relatively brief intervention effective in suitable motivated patients.

Interpersonal psychotherapy and interpersonal counselling

These forms of therapy are based on the work of Klerman and associates [28]. The focus of interpersonal psychotherapy (IPT) is on the relationships of the patient and how they affect mood states. Problems in relationships are categorised as one of dispute, change in role, grief or deficit. The therapist then assists the patient in working through the problems using techniques such as role play and analysis of communications within relationships. Like CBT, the therapy takes place over a number of hour-long sessions, usually 12–16 sessions.

Interpersonal counselling (IPC) is a modification of IPT, of a simpler form that can be integrated into the work of health professionals. It was designed for primary care, but can be used in other health settings. IPT has been shown to be effective, and equivalent to the use of CBT in depression and eating disorders. Unlike CBT, it has not yet been shown to be effective in OCD or BDD. It has been suggested that IPT be offered as an alternative to CBT for patients who prefer this approach. However, provision, especially outside the USA, is often limited by a shortage of trained practitioners.

Dynamic psychotherapies and psychoanalysis

There is not scope here to describe the range of these psychotherapies. Some awareness of, or even familiarity with, the concepts first described by Freud are common in western and European cultures. There are numerous therapists and theorists who have written on the subject. Psychodynamic concepts such as transference, counter-transference, projection and identification can help the clinical interview, and good descriptions can be found for the interested in textbooks such as *Introduction to Psychotherapy* [29].

Short-term forms of dynamic therapies (defined as fewer than 40 sessions) have been shown to have efficacy in a wide range of common mental health disorders [30]. Many forms of dynamic therapies and psychoanalytic therapy are long lasting and intensive, with three or more sessions weekly. Due to the complexity of the longer forms of therapy, especially around conducting

controlled studies and defining outcomes, there are difficulties with an evidence-based approach to demonstrating efficacy [31]. While this is acknowledged by practitioners writing in this field, the point is often made that these forms of therapy are complex, and used in complicated conditions where the 'drug paradigm' or 'single intervention for single condition' approach may not be strictly relevant.

Varieties of psychiatric syndromes presenting to the dermatologist, either as part of or alongside a cutaneous presentation, can be effectively treated by clinicians familiar with the stratagems used in primary care. Although specialist knowledge and training are required to deliver formal psychotherapy, techniques from psychotherapy – especially empathy, a non-judgemental approach, understanding, patience and reflection – can be used to augment safe prescribing where indicated. Specialist referral should be arranged when symptoms are severe or specialist drugs or therapies needed.

Alternative therapies

There has been a long tradition of the use of complementary therapies in dermatology, but especially for those diseases where there is a psychological component. Most reports of therapy are anecdotal, often single cases with no randomised controlled trials. Therapies with a neurogenic basis are claimed to work through neuroimmune mechanisms although no hard evidence is available. Acupuncture, biofeedback and hypnosis in skin disease are summarised by Shenefelt [32] and Freid [33]. The mechanisms of action may be related to the beneficial effects of supportive psychotherapy and relaxation rather than any specific therapeutic component measurable for each treatment type. Hypnotherapy has been the most frequently studied in western literature. Despite the lack of trials, there are strong advocates for the use of hypnosis as an adjunct to control itch [34] and pain [35]. Hypnotherapy for warts in children showed a 53% success at 3 months compared with none in the control group [36]. The practicality and cost were not assessed.

Alternative herbal medications are used both topically and systemically. In an evidence-based review of the literature [37] there was no compelling evidence for the efficacy of diet, herbal medicines or dietary supplements in atopic eczema. The authors suggested promising data for treatments with a psychological component such as hypnosis, autogenic training and biofeedback. For chronic venous insufficiency, oral horse chestnut seed extract appeared to have a real effect as opposed to topical aloe vera gel or tea tree oil. Two fuller reviews of phytopharmaceutical agents explored not only the therapeutic uses of herbs but also the toxic and allergic skin reactions [38,39].

Key references

The full list of references can be found in the online version at https://www.wiley.com/rooksdermatology10e

Introduction
What is psychodermatology?
  2 Poot FR, Sampogna F, Onnis L. Basic knowledge in psychodermatology. *J Eur Acad Dermatol Venereol* 2007;21:227–34.
  3 Poot F. Doctor-patient relations in dermatology: obligations and rights for a mutual satisfaction. *Eur Acad Dermatol Venereol* 2009;23:1233–9.

Psychodermatology multidisciplinary teams

2 Bewley A, Affleck A, Bundy C, Higgins E, McBride S. Psychodermatology services guidance: the report of the British Association of Dermatologists' Psychodermatology Working Party. *Br J Dermatol* 2013;168:1149–50.

Delusional beliefs
Delusional infestation

4 Eccles JA, Garfinkel SN, Harrison NA *et al*. Sensations of skin infestation linked to abnormal frontolimbic brain reactivity and differences in self-representation. *Neuropsychologia* 2015;77:90–6.

5 Freudenmann RW, Lepping P, Huber M *et al*. Delusional infestation and the specimen sign: a European multicentre study in 148 consecutive cases. *Br J Dermatol* 2012;167:247–51.

Olfactory delusions

1 Pryse-Phillips W. An olfactory reference syndrome. *Acta Psychiatr Scand* 1971;47:484–509.

CHAPTER 85

Acquired Disorders of Epidermal Keratinisation

Matthew J. Scorer and Graham A. Johnston

Leicester Royal Infirmary, University Hospitals of Leicester NHS Trust, Leicester, UK

Acquired ichthyosis

Definition and nomenclature

Acquired ichthyosis is a condition that arises in adulthood but is clinically and histopathologically similar to hereditary ichthyosis vulgaris. It is rare, and should raise the suspicion of an associated internal disease, particularly malignancy, endocrinopathy, infections, autoimmunity or an adverse drug reaction [1].

Synonyms and inclusions

* Ichthyosis acquisita

Introduction and general description

Acquired ichthyosis usually arises in adult life and clinically resembles hereditary ichthyosis. It is not, however, inherited and may be associated with a systemic disorder.

Epidemiology

Incidence and prevalence

Acquired ichthyosis is a rare condition. There are no available data on prevalence.

Age

Acquired ichthyosis occurs mainly in adulthood but acquired ichthyosis in children with systemic disease has been reported [2].

Associated diseases

See Box 85.1 for diseases that are associated with acquired ichthyosis [3–25].

Box 85.1 Disorders that have been associated with acquired ichthyosis

* Neoplasia: particularly Hodgkin disease, mycosis fungoides, primary cutaneous CD30+ lymphoproliferative disorders, multiple myeloma, Kaposi and other sarcomas, and carcinomas (lung, breast, ovary, cervix; Chapter 148) [3–8]
* Medications: statins, nicotinic acid, cimetidine, clofazimine [9], acitretin [10] and tyrosine kinase inhibitors [11]
* Endocrinopathies: diabetes [12], thyroid disease [2], hyperparathyroidism [13] and hypopituitarism [14]
* Infections: leprosy, tuberculosis, HIV [15] and HTLV-1 infection [16]
* Autoimmune conditions: dermatomyositis, systemic lupus erythematosus and scleroderma/lupus overlap syndrome [17–19]
* Chronic metabolic disease: including malnutrition [20], vitamin A deficiency [21], malabsorption syndromes [22], essential fatty acid deficiency [23] and pancreatic insufficiency (Shwachman syndrome) [24]
* Anorexia nervosa
* Miscellaneous: bone marrow transplantation and chronic renal failure [25] and consumption of kava

HIV, human immunodeficiency virus; HTLV-1, human T-cell leukaemia virus 1.

Pathophysiology

The pathogenesis of acquired ichthyosis is not fully understood and it differs according to the entity with which it is associated.

In cases associated with diabetes, it is hypothesised that the changes in the skin are due to structural abnormalities in proteins resulting from non-enzymatic glycosylation [26,27]. However,

Rook's Textbook of Dermatology, Tenth Edition. Edited by Christopher Griffiths, Jonathan Barker, Tanya Bleiker, Walayat Hussain and Rosalind Simpson.

© 2024 John Wiley & Sons Ltd. Published 2024 by John Wiley & Sons Ltd.

PART 8: SPECIFIC CUTANEOUS STRUCTURES

well-controlled diabetics can also show ichthyotic changes, and for these an abnormal host immune response has been proposed, probably against components of the granular cell layer [12]. The same hypothesis has also been advanced to explain acquired ichthyosis associated with autoimmune disorders [19], whereas those cases associated with tumours seem to be due to secretion by neoplastic cells of transforming growth factor α (TGF-α), which may exert a mitogenic action on keratinocytes [28].

Pathology
Histologically, the epidermis shows compact hyperkeratosis with a thinned or absent granular cell layer.

Environmental factors
Living in a hot and humid climate may hide the clinical manifestations of filaggrin deficiency [29]. Severe xerosis mimicking acquired ichthyosis can be observed in atopic individuals who immigrate from very humid atmospheres such as South-East Asia to Europe. In their home country xerosis is not evident, but the low humidity in Europe may precipitate an ichthyotic change in the skin.

Clinical features
History
The onset of acquired ichthyosis is typically sudden with initial involvement of the lower limbs after which it may generalise.

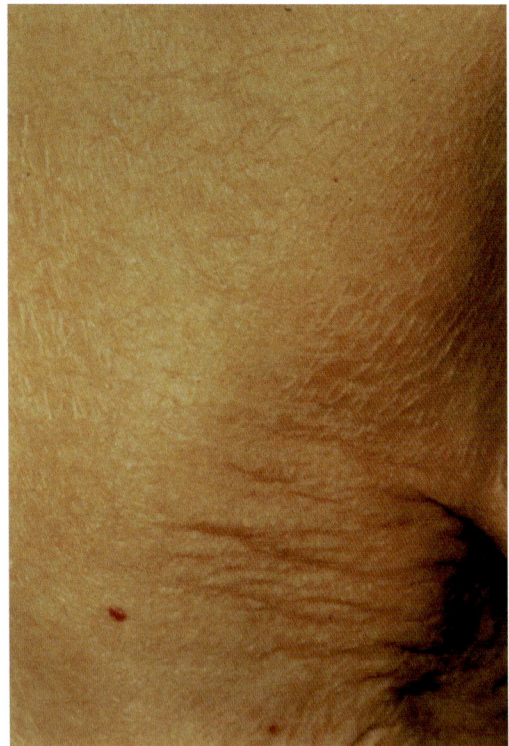

Figure 85.1 Acquired ichthyosis secondary to lymphoma.

Presentation
Symmetrical, dark, thick scaling appears on the legs in a pattern likened to the skin of lizards. The arms and trunk can also be involved, especially the back (Figures 85.1 and 85.2), but flexures are spared, due to the higher humidity in these areas. The face is unaffected in most cases, probably due to the size and number of its sebaceous glands, but the scalp shows abundant fine scales. Pruritus can be pronounced. There may be palmoplantar hyperkeratosis, with fissures that can become infected [1].

Differential diagnosis
The differential diagnosis includes:
- Xerosis cutis.
- Asteatotic eczema.
- Atopic eczema.
- Drug eruptions.
- Hereditary ichthyoses.
- Icthyosiform sarcoidosis [30].

Disease course and prognosis
Acquired ichthyosis may improve with successful treatment of the underlying disease or cessation of the responsible drug.

Investigations
The diagnosis of acquired ichthyosis is made clinically and confirmatory tests are unnecessary. Once the diagnosis has been made, a careful search for an underlying cause should be undertaken, with a full history, clinical examination, a detailed drug history and appropriate investigations to identify potential causes.

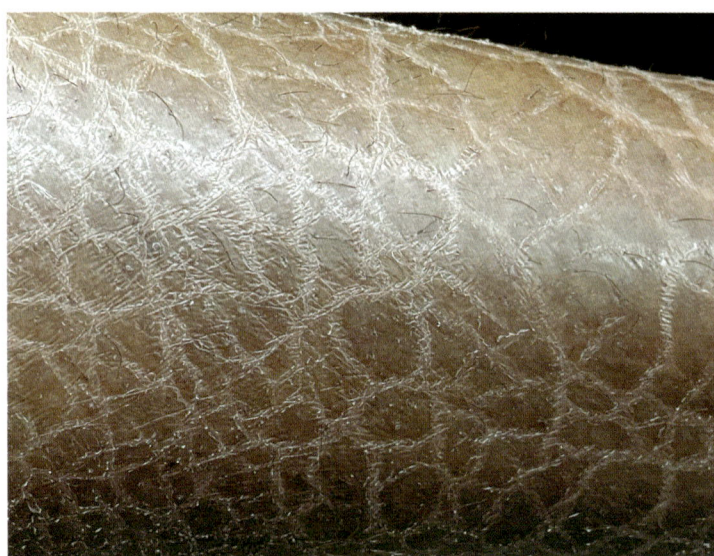

Figure 85.2 Acquired icthyiosis in a female with hypothyroidism. Courtesy of Dr Shyam Verma, Vadodara, India.

Management
The primary aim in the management of acquired ichthyosis is to identify the underlying cause of the disorder. Its treatment can lead to improvement of the dermatosis.

Treatment of the acquired ichthyosis is symptomatic and involves the use of retinoids and keratolytic agents.

Treatment ladder for acquired ichthyosis

First line
- Topical retinoids, particularly tretinoin and tazarotene, reduce the cohesiveness of keratinocytes [31]

Second line
- Beta-hydroxyacids (salicylic acid) help to disaggregate the corneocytes

Third line
- Alpha-hydroxyacids (lactic or glycolic acids) produce loosening and desquamation of corneocytes, when applied twice daily
- Urea 10–20% cream is an excellent humectant
- Propylene glycol as a 20% preparation in aqueous cream hydrates the stratum corneum

Acanthosis nigricans

Definition
Acanthosis nigricans (AN) manifests as asymptomatic and symmetrical darkening affecting the skin of intertriginous areas, in particular the axillae, groins, submammary folds and neck. The skin is thickened with a velvety texture, and may be studded by skin tags. It is particularly associated with obesity and insulin resistance.

Introduction and general description
Acanthosis nigricans may present as an isolated skin condition but may be associated with a large range of conditions ranging from obesity to endocrinopathies to internal neoplasms.

Epidemiology
Incidence and prevalence
Benign AN is very common, and affects up to 20% of adults and 7% of children; this increases threefold if only overweight children are considered [1,2,3]. Malignant AN is rare.

Age
Acanthosis nigricans can occur at any age. The benign form is most common in adults but may be present at birth and is not uncommon in obese children. The malignant form, which is rare, usually arises in older age groups but has been observed in children with Wilms tumours and osteogenic sarcomas [3].

Sex
It has an equal sex ratio.

Ethnicity
Acanthosis nigricans is more common in patients with skin of colour. In one epidemiological study AN was observed in 1% of white, 5.5% of Latino and 13.3% of African American populations [4].

Associated diseases
Insulin resistance is the most common association with AN (previously called pseudo-AN) [5], which can regress with treatment of the insulin resistance including low-carbohydrate diet and exercise, resulting in weight loss.

Many syndromes (Box 85.2) have been associated with AN; they usually involve the endocrine system or accompany autoimmune disorders.

Box 85.2 Disorders associated with acanthosis nigricans

- Acromegaly and gigantism
- Alström telangiectasia
- Bartter syndrome
- Beare–Stevenson syndrome
- Benign encephalopathy
- Bloom syndrome
- Capozucca syndrome
- Chondrodystrophy with dwarfism
- Costello syndrome
- Crouzon syndrome [28,29]
- Dermatomyositis
- Diabetes
- Familial pineal body hypertrophy
- Gigantism
- HAIR-AN syndrome
- Hashimoto thyroiditis
- Hirschowitz syndrome
- Laurence–Moon–Bardet syndrome
- Lawrence–Seip syndrome
- Lipoatrophic diabetes
- Lupoid hepatitis
- Lupus erythematosus
- Motor tract degeneration
- Phenylketonuria
- Polycystic ovary syndrome
- Prader–Willi syndrome
- Primary hypogonadism
- Pseudoacromegaly
- Pyramidal tract degeneration
- Rud syndrome
- SADDAN syndrome
- Systemic sclerosis
- Thanatophoric dwarfism
- Werner syndrome
- Wilson syndrome

HAIR-AN, hyperandrogenism, insulin resistance and acanthosis nigricans; SADDAN, severe achondroplasia with developmental delay and acanthosis nigricans.

Malignant AN (described in more detail in Chapter 148) has been associated with an extensive range of solid tumours, but over 90% have been seen in patients with gastrointestinal cancer, of which two-thirds are gastric [6–8]. Other tumours associated with AN are listed in Box 85.3. Malignant AN may be accompanied by other cutaneous paraneoplastic phenomena, particularly florid cutaneous papillomatosis in which there is a rapid development of numerous warty papules on the trunk and the extremities that are clinically indistinguishable from viral warts (Chapter 148).

> ### Box 85.3 Internal malignancies associated with acanthosis nigricans
>
> - Bladder adenocarcinoma
> - Breast adenocarcinoma
> - Cervical squamous cell carcinoma
> - Gall bladder and bile duct adenocarcinoma
> - Gastric adenocarcinoma
> - Hodgkin disease
> - Lung adenocarcinoma and squamous cell carcinoma
> - Osteogenic sarcoma and Wilms tumour (in children)
> - Ovarian adenocarcinoma
> - Pancreatic adenocarcinoma
> - Prostatic adenocarcinoma
> - Renal cell carcinoma
> - Testicular carcinoma
> - Thyroid adenocarcinoma

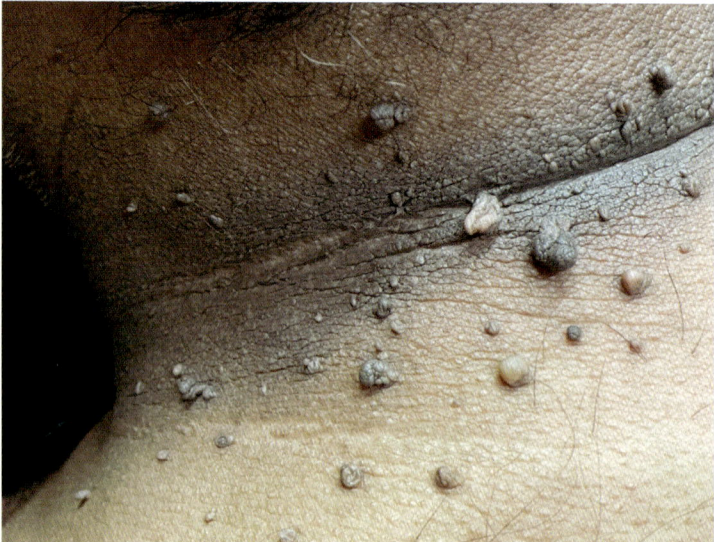

Figure 85.3 Acanthosis nigricans affecting the neck with associated skin tags. Courtesy of Dr Shyam Verma, Vadodara, India.

Pathophysiology

The most common associations reported with benign AN are insulin resistance [1,9–11] and obesity [2,12]. There is increasing evidence that obesity is a consequence of insulin resistance in the presence of a high-carbohydrate diet [13], therefore insulin resistance may be the common causative factor rather than obesity being a direct cause of AN. Insulin-derived growth factor (IGF-1) receptors are overexpressed in patients with hyperinsulinaemia and insulin resistance [14]. IGF-1 can stimulate the proliferation of keratinocytes and dermal fibroblasts. Epidermal growth factor receptors and fibroblast growth factor receptors (FGFRs) are also implicated. In Beare–Stevenson syndrome, activating mutations of FGFR2 have been identified, and activating mutations of FGFR3 are associated with thanatophoric dysplasia and the rare severe achondroplasia with developmental delay and acanthosis nigricans (SADDAN syndrome). Crouzon syndrome is associated with both [15]. FGFR3 mutations have been identified in the familial form of AN [16].

Some drugs may contribute to AN development: FGFR activation can be produced by certain medications used in stem cell transplantation, such as palifermin [17], and insulin can provoke the development of AN at injection sites by activation of IGF receptors.

In malignant AN, tumour-derived growth factors are produced, especially TGF-α, which binds to epidermal growth factor receptors. The levels of TGF-α decrease with tumour debulking, which may be followed by regression of the paraneoplastic phenomena [18].

Predisposing factors

Acanthosis nigricans is associated with a number of benign and malignant conditions with a common pathway of keratinocyte and fibroblast proliferation. Perspiration and/or friction are mechanical contributing factors which may be important in determining the characteristic distribution of AN in flexural areas.

Pathology

Despite its name, AN shows no or minimal acanthosis or hyper-pigmentation microscopically. Histology shows hyperkeratosis and papillomatosis with finger-like upward projections of dermal papillae. Pigmentation is due to the hyperkeratosis; there is no increase in melanocyte numbers or in melanin production. Pseudo-horn cysts may be present. In mucosal lesions, parakeratosis may be observed [3].

Genetics

The familial form of AN is inherited in an autosomal dominant fashion and *FGFR3* mutations have been identified [16].

Clinical features

History

Acanthosis nigricans usually starts as asymptomatic darkening of the skin of the dorsae of the knuckles, neck, axillae and groins. With time, the patches become thicker and may develop skin tags in the affected areas (Figure 85.3). Pruritus is not common. Pigmentation under the eyes may result.

Presentation

It presents as symmetrical, velvety, dark patches which are most commonly seen in the axillae, groins and on the back and sides of the neck (Figure 85.4). The back of the neck is the most common site in children. Skin tags (acrochordons) may be present in affected areas. AN may become widespread with delicate velvety furrowing of mucosal surfaces and involvement of the eyelids and conjunctivae. Associated nail changes include leukonychia and subungual hyperkeratosis.

Clinical variants

A familial syndrome, HAIR-AN, manifests as hyperandrogenism, insulin resistance and acanthosis nigricans. It typically presents in girls with polycystic ovaries, hirsutism and clitoral hypertrophy,

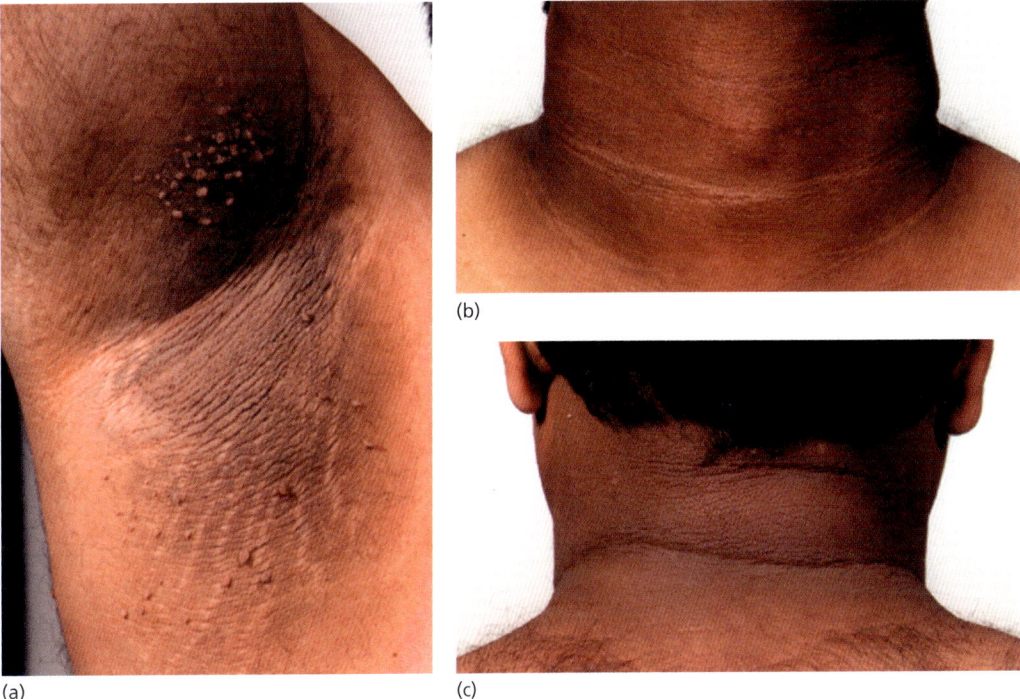

(a)

(b)

(c)

Figure 85.4 (a–c) Typical acanthosis nigricans in an obese 41-year-old man of South Asian descent with type 2 diabetes. Note the associated striae and skin tags in the axilla (a), and darkening and velvety thickening of the skin around the root and nape of the neck (b, c).

and frequently with high plasma testosterone levels. This condition, which is also known as type A insulin resistance syndrome, is described in more detail in Chapters 88 and 150.

Type B insulin resistance syndrome is characterised by the association of AN with diabetes and hyperandrogenism, or with an autoimmune disease (including systemic lupus erythematosus, systemic sclerosis, Hashimoto thyroiditis and Sjögren syndrome).

Familial AN is rare and transmitted as an autosomal dominant trait with variable penetrance. It manifests early in life and tends to stabilise in the teenage years. In some patients, it can improve with age.

Drug-induced AN has been associated with many different medications, particularly hormones, insulin, systemic corticosteroids, testosterone and exogenous oestrogens, including oral contraceptives [19,20]. One of the most common associations is with nicotinic acid. The dermatosis tends to resolve after discontinuation of the offending agent.

Generalised AN is very rare, and seen only in children. There is generalised hyperpigmentation and velvety thickening of the skin, and extensive investigation fails to show any associated systemic abnormality [21–23].

Acral AN is more common in skin phototypes 5 and 6. It is not associated with systemic disease, and manifests as a velvety thickening and hyperpigmentation of the skin on the dorsa of the hands and feet, especially the knuckles [24].

Unilateral AN (or naevoid AN) is very rare, and is assumed to arise from a somatic mutation during embryogenesis. It can appear in infancy, but cases have been reported with onset in childhood or adulthood. Clinically, it appears as a pigmented plaque, solitary or along a line of Blaschko, and resembles an epidermal naevus. Histopathologically, the typical changes of AN are seen. It has been described on the face and scalp, chest and abdomen, back and thighs [25].

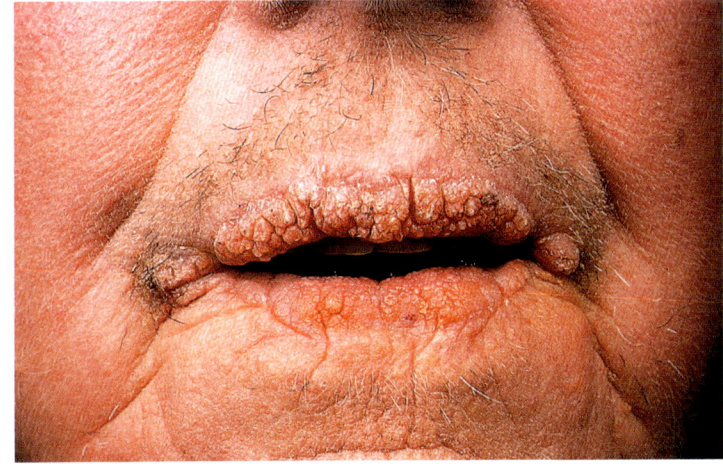

Figure 85.5 Malignant acanthosis nigricans: rugose hypertrophy leading to warty thickening of the oral margins in a patient with carcinoma of the breast.

Malignant or paraneoplastic AN (Figure 85.5) can be associated with a wide range of solid tumours (see earlier and Box 85.3).

Differential diagnosis
The major differential diagnoses are:
- Addison disease.
- Pellagra.
- Haemochromatosis.

Disease course and prognosis
Benign AN is not associated with systemic disease but is chronic and may become a significant cosmetic problem. However, all AN patients should be investigated to rule out insulin resistance.

AN associated with metabolic abnormalities and insulin resistance may improve with treatment of the underlying condition.

PART 8: SPECIFIC CUTANEOUS STRUCTURES

AN associated with obesity may improve with dietary restriction and weight loss.

The prognosis of patients with malignant AN is poor, with an average survival of only 2 years from diagnosis due to the frequently advanced stage of malignancy at diagnosis.

Investigations

Patients should be screened for underlying endocrinopathy and malignancy. Insulin sensitivity can be assessed by a calculation utilising fasting glucose and insulin called HOMA-IR (homeostatic model assessment for insulin resistance), with an elevated result indicating insulin resistance [26].

Management

Management of AN is the management of the underlying condition, usually insulin resistance. In familial AN or AN not associated with an underlying condition, treatment is aimed at improving the cosmetic appearance of the condition.

General measures

Refer to a dietician for guidance about low-carbohydrate diets and exercise regimes. Metformin is often needed in individuals who also have obesity.

Other than addressing underlying insulin resistance, therapies aim to improve the cosmetic appearance by modifying keratinisation [27].

> **Treatment ladder for acanthosis nigricans**
>
> **First line**
> - Topical retinoids – may reduce the hyperkeratosis
>
> **Second line**
> - Topical α-hydroxyacids and keratolytics such as salicylic acid may improve appearance by reducing hyperkeratosis
> - Topical vitamin D analogues
>
> **Third line**
> - In extensive cases, oral isotretinoin and acitretin have been reported to improve the skin [27]

Confluent and reticulated papillomatosis

Definition and nomenclature

Confluent and reticulated papillomatosis (CARP) is an uncommon disorder of epidermal keratinisation characterised by the development of hyperkeratotic papules which coalesce into confluent and, in places, reticulated plaques on truncal skin. An abnormal reaction to commensal microorganisms has been postulated to play an aetiological role.

> **Synonyms and inclusions**
> - Papillomatose pigmentée innominée
> - Papillomatose pigmentée confluente et réticulée
> - Gougerot–Carteaud syndrome

Introduction and general description

Gougerot and Carteaud first described this entity in 1927 [1]. While it had been considered to be a specific form of AN [2], diagnostic criteria have been established and it is now considered a specific form of cutaneous papillomatosis [3,4].

Epidemiology
Incidence and prevalence

This is a rare disease and there are no data on prevalence.

Age

It is predominantly a disease of young adults. In one series of patients, the mean age at onset was 19 years [2].

Sex

It is likely that the sex incidence is equal but different reports have shown a predominance of women in white populations but a predominance of men in Japan. A study from the USA [4] and one from Lebanon [5] show equal sex incidence.

Ethnicity

Confluent and reticulated papillomatosis has been reported in multiple ethnic groups with no clear predilection.

Pathophysiology

The pathogenesis of CARP is poorly understood. It is thought that an abnormal host reaction to *Malassezia* organisms may be relevant in some patients [6,7] and it has also been suggested that actinomycete bacteria may play a role [8]. These hypotheses are discussed in more detail later. However, the anti-inflammatory properties of the antibiotics used in treatment might be the true reason for the response.

Abnormal keratinocyte differentiation has been found on transmission electron microscopy and by immunohistochemical studies, which show an increased expression of involucrin, keratin 16 and Ki-67 [9]. These changes might explain the clustering of the condition in some families [10,11]. The number of Odland bodies is increased and this is associated with a higher turnover of epidermal keratinocytes, as seen in psoriasis [12]. The role of metabolic abnormalities in the development of CARP is gaining support [2]. CARP has been associated with obesity and insulin resistance [13], as well as thyroid dysfunction and Cushing disease [14].

Pathology

There is hyperkeratosis and papillomatosis, with a decrease in the thickness or disappearance of the granular cell layer. There may be increased melanin in the basal cell layer and in the stratum corneum, and this is reflected in the colour of the plaques. The dermis shows at most a mild, non-specific inflammatory infiltrate [15].

Fungal stains frequently show *Malassezia* yeasts on the surface of the epidermis.

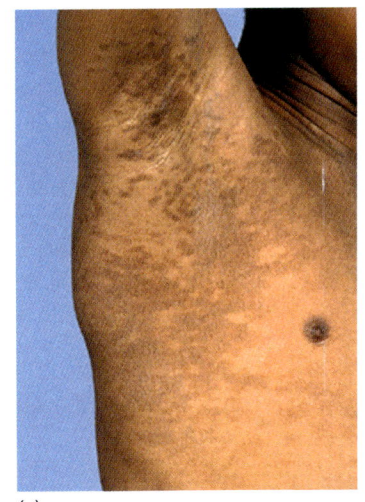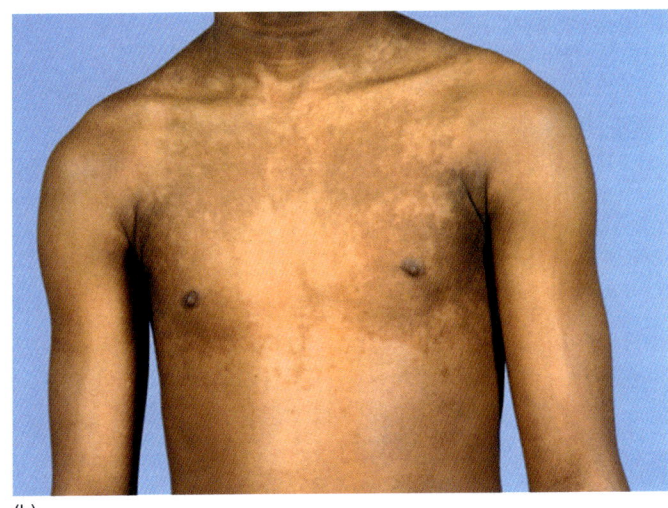

Figure 85.6 (a, b) Confluent and reticulate papillomatosis: an asymptomatic rash appeared 6 months earlier around the neck of this of 12-year-old boy before spreading to the axillae and upper torso. There was no response to antifungal medication.

(a)   (b)

Causative organisms

A number of reports have demonstrated the presence of *Malassezia* organisms in CARP. This has led to speculation that CARP is due to an abnormal host reaction to *Malassezia*. Several studies have shown, however, that only about one-half of patients with CARP have significant yeast populations on affected skin [2,6,7]. Although some patients with CARP respond to topical imidazoles and other antifungal agents, half of cases fail to respond [5–7] and in those cases only a few spores can be retrieved from the skin surface.

Some patients with CARP appear to respond to tetracycline and macrolide antibiotics, which has led to the suggestion that skin bacteria may be responsible for this disease. In 2005, a previously unknown actinomycete bacterium of the genus *Dietzia* was isolated from the skin of a patient with CARP. Sensitivity studies showed sensitivity to tetracycline and erythromycin and the patient cleared with tetracycline. The organism, which has subsequently been named *Dietzia papillomatosis*, has been implicated in a case of septicaemia but, to date, there have been no further reports linking it with CARP [8]. It has been suggested, however, that the response to antibiotics may be due to their anti-inflammatory rather than their antibacterial properties.

Genetics

Although familial forms of CARP have been reported [10,11], they are too rare to postulate a genetic inheritance.

Clinical features

History

The patient is usually a young, postpubertal individual. Plaques of CARP are located mainly on the trunk, especially on the presternal, interscapular and epigastric areas. They are generally asymptomatic.

Presentation

Patients first notice pigmented, 1–2 mm diameter hyperkeratotic papules on the trunk. These coalesce to form greyish blue plaques which are confluent at the centre but become reticular towards the periphery of the plaques (Figure 85.6). Over weeks or months, the plaques spread to involve the lower abdomen and pubic areas [2]. The face and limbs may be affected. Localised forms affecting only the face or pubic area have been reported [16,17]. Mucous membranes are not involved. A number of different patterns of skin involvement have been described [18].

Differential diagnosis

The most common differential diagnoses proposed in cases of CARP include:
- Acanthosis nigricans.
- Prurigo pigmentosa.
- Macular amyloid.
- Darier disease.
- Epidermal naevus.
- Plane warts.
- Pityriasis versicolor.
- Dermatitis neglecta (inadequate frictional cleansing).

Disease course and prognosis

It is a chronic disease with remissions and exacerbations. If CARP responds to treatment, it may relapse when treatment is withdrawn although persistent remission after tetracyclines is reported [19].

Management

It is a chronic disease and is purely cosmetic, so no treatment is an option if the condition does not bother the patient. Spontaneous improvement has been reported [20,21]. In overweight patients, weight reduction may result in improvement. In some women, CARP may improve during pregnancy or with the use of the oral contraceptive.

Treatment ladder for confluent and reticulated papillomatosis

First line
- A wide range of oral antibiotics have been found to be effective in CARP: the most effective appears to be minocycline [4,22,23]; azithromycin is an alternative [24]

- Topical mupirocin ointment has been of benefit in some cases [25]

Second line
- Topical and systemic antifungal agents, including selenium sulphide shampoo, have been used with success in some patients [2,26] but the results have been very variable
- Topical retinoids and vitamin D analogues have been used with mixed results [27–29]

Third line
- Both high- and low-dose isotretinoin have been used in the treatment of CARP with varying results [30,31]

Pityriasis rotunda

Definition and nomenclature
Pityriasis rotunda (PR) is a dermatosis of unknown cause that presents as perfectly round, slightly red or hyperpigmented plaques, with fine scaling, usually located on the trunk or buttocks, arms and legs [1].

Synonyms and inclusions
- Pityriasis circinata
- Acquired pseudo-ichthyosis

Introduction and general description
Pityriasis rotunda is a rare condition with very few reports in the literature. The most common form of PR is type 1 PR, which is typically seen in older individuals from Asian or African origin. Type 1 is usually associated with underlying systemic disease or malignancy [2] and may resolve with treatment of the underlying condition [2,3]. Type 2 PR is sometimes familial and presents in younger white patients; it is not associated with underlying disease.

Epidemiology
Incidence and prevalence
This disease is rare, with most reports coming from South Africa, Sardinia or Japan.

Age
Type 1 PR is usually seen in patients in their 60s. Type 2 PR is usually seen in younger patients with a large case series from Jordan reporting a younger cohort with a mean age of 19 (range 9–38 years) [4].

Sex
Pityriasis rotunda has an equal sex incidence.

Ethnicity
Most case reports of PR have come from South Africa in black populations and the few reports from the UK have been in patients of African descent [5]. Type 1 disease is also seen in East Asian patients,

with most reports from Japan; it is rare in white populations [6]. Familial type 2 PR has been reported principally from Sardinia.

Associated diseases
Type 1 PR has been associated with hepatocellular carcinoma. In a series of 10 black patients from South Africa with PR, 70% were associated with hepatocellular carcinoma [7]. In a further study from South Africa examining hepatocellular carcinoma, 15.9% of 63 patients had PR [8]. In the South African black population, PR has been associated with a number of systemic diseases (Box 85.4).

Box 85.4 Diseases associated with pityriasis rotunda

- Hepatocellular carcinoma
- Chronic myeloid leukaemia
- Squamous cell carcinoma of the hard palate
- Tuberculosis
- Liver disease
- Cardiac disease
- Nutritional disease
- Other malignancies
- Pulmonary disease
- Chronic renal failure
- Osteitis
- Chronic diarrhoea
- Systemic sclerosis

In Asian populations, PR is associated with underlying malignancy but not specifically with hepatocellular carcinoma [9].

Pathophysiology
The aetiopathogenesis of PR is unknown. Histologically, it shares some characteristics with ichthyosis vulgaris and some authors feel it is a variant of this disease [10]. In South African patients it has been associated with malnutrition, but this is not generally accepted as a cause of the disease. Diminished expression of loricrin and filaggrin has been demonstrated [11].

Pathology
Histological changes are restricted to the epidermis with hyperkeratosis and loss of the granular cell layer.

Genetics
Type 2 PR is inherited as an autosomal dominant trait [12].

Clinical features
History
It is an asymptomatic condition and is often diagnosed incidentally in patients being investigated for other disease.

Presentation
The disease presents as asymptomatic, thin, finely scaling plaques ranging from 0.5 to more than 20 cm in diameter located on the trunk, buttocks, arms and legs. The plaques, ranging in number from a few to more than 100, are sharply demarcated and can coalesce,

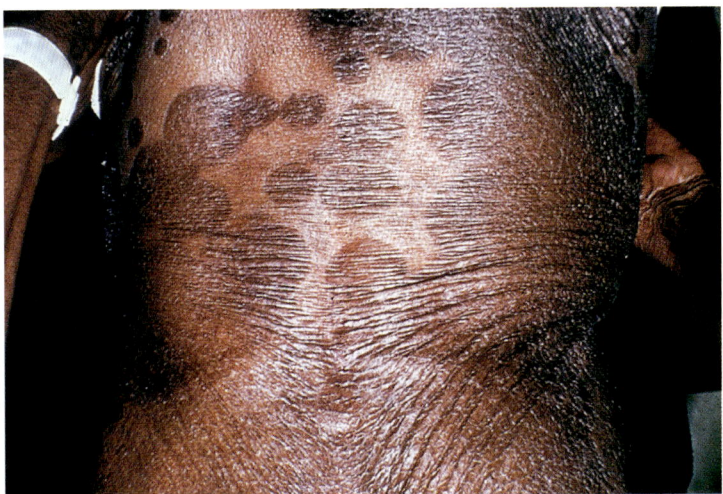

Figure 85.7 Pityriasis rotunda.

forming polycyclic plaques. They are pink in lightly pigmented skin to dark brown in skin of phototypes 5 and 6 (Figure 85.7).

Clinical variants
Types 1 and 2 PR are sporadic and familial, respectively.

Differential diagnosis
The differential diagnosis includes postinflammatory hyperpigmentation following fixed drug eruption, erythrasma, tinea corporis, pityriasis versicolor and psoriasis.

Disease course and prognosis
In type 1 PR associated with an underlying disease, treatment of the disease may result in resolution of the PR. Once type 2 PR develops, it is usually lifelong.

Investigations
A skin biopsy can be helpful to exclude other conditions, as the diagnosis of PR is one of exclusion. Skin scraping and mycological examination will exclude dermatophytosis and pityriasis versicolor. Examination with a Wood lamp can exclude erythrasma in flexural lesions.

Management
Lesions of PR are notoriously resistant to therapy, but some improvement has been reported with topical treatment.

Treatment ladder of pityriasis rotunda

First line
- Topical retinoids, such as tretinoin, isotretinoin or tazarotene

Second line
- Topical 10% lactic acid

Third line
- 5% salicylic acid ointment

Keratosis pilaris

Definition and nomenclature
Keratosis pilaris (KP) is an inherited abnormality of keratinisation affecting the follicular orifices with varying degrees of keratotic follicular plugging, perifollicular redness and follicular atrophy.

Synonyms and inclusions
- Follicular keratosis
- Lichen pilaris

Introduction and general description
Keratosis pilaris is a common skin condition, characterised by follicular keratotic papules and perifollicular redness or hyperpigmentation [1,2]. Because up to half of the population present with the condition to some degree, it can be considered a variant of normal rather than a disease.

Epidemiology
Incidence and prevalence
It is a very common condition affecting 50–80% of adolescents and about 40% of adults.

Age
Keratosis pilaris often presents in the first decade of life and may worsen around puberty. In some patients the disorder improves with age, but any age group can be affected from childhood to old age.

Sex
Females appear to be more frequently affected than males.

Ethnicity
It is not more prevalent in any racial group.

Associated diseases
Keratosis pilaris may be associated with ichthyosis vulgaris and atopic eczema [3]. These conditions are, however, all common and the association may be coincidental. Some other reported associations are listed in Box 85.5 [4–17]. More recently, patients with *BRAF*-positive tumours treated with vemurafenib and sorafenib can develop KP as a side effect [17].

Pathophysiology
A plug of excess keratin is formed, possibly due to a defect of corneocyte adhesion at the follicular orifice, which impedes the hair from emerging. The hair can become ingrown and result in an inflammatory response [18].

Pathology
Histology of KP shows hyperkeratosis, hypergranulosis and plugging of hair follicles. In the dermis, there is a mild perivascular lymphocytic infiltrate in the upper dermis.

Box 85.5 Disorders with which keratosis pilaris and follicular hyperkeratoses have been associated

- Ichthyosis vulgaris [3]
- Atopic eczema [3]
- Obesity [4]
- Insulin-dependent diabetes (seen in types 1 and 2) [4]
- Noonan syndrome [5]
- Cardio-facio-cutaneous syndrome [6]
- Prolidase deficiency [7]
- Down syndrome [8]
- Fairbanks syndrome [9]
- Olmsted syndrome [10]
- Renal failure and hypervitaminosis A [11]
- Monilethrix [12]
- Pachyonychia congenita [13]
- Ectodermal dysplasias [14]
- Systemic corticosteroid therapy [15]
- Lithium [16]
- Vemurafenib and sorafenib [17]

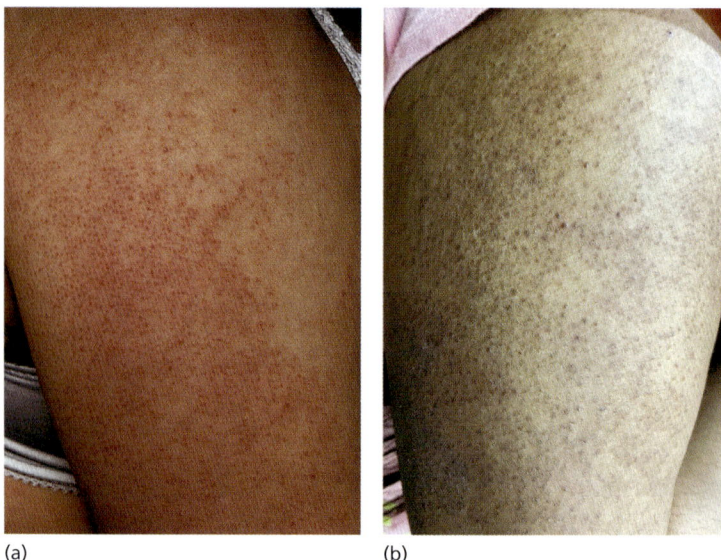

(a)   (b)

Figure 85.8 (a, b) Keratosis pilaris on the extensor aspect of the upper arm.

Genetics

It is inherited as an autosomal dominant trait with variable penetrance [18]. Reports have identified a partial monosomy in the short arm of chromosome 18 in patients with severe forms of KP and ulerythema ophryogenes [19].

Environmental factors

Keratosis pilaris may show seasonal variation, improving in the summer [20].

Clinical features

History

It generally starts in children, most commonly on the extensor surfaces of the upper arms, and can worsen around puberty.

Presentation

There are small, keratotic papules on the extensor aspects of the limbs, particularly the arms (Figure 85.8) and thighs [20]. The buttocks and the lumbar areas are also frequently affected. These areas acquire a 'goose-bump' appearance and rough texture. Lesions can become pustular with superficial pustules developing in affected follicles, precipitated by rubbing on clothing. On the buttock, deeper inflammatory lesions and nodules may develop.

Clinical variants

Erythromelanosis follicularis faciei et colli (EFFC). EFFC is a condition that has been described as a subtype of KP seen in India and other countries in Asia. It manifests as follicular hyperkeratosis accompanied by redness and hyperpigmentation, and affects, as the name indicates, the face, particularly the cheeks and neck (Figure 85.9) [21–23].

Keratosis pilaris rubra faciei. This is a common variant with prominent facial redness, but without the hyperpigmentation or atrophy

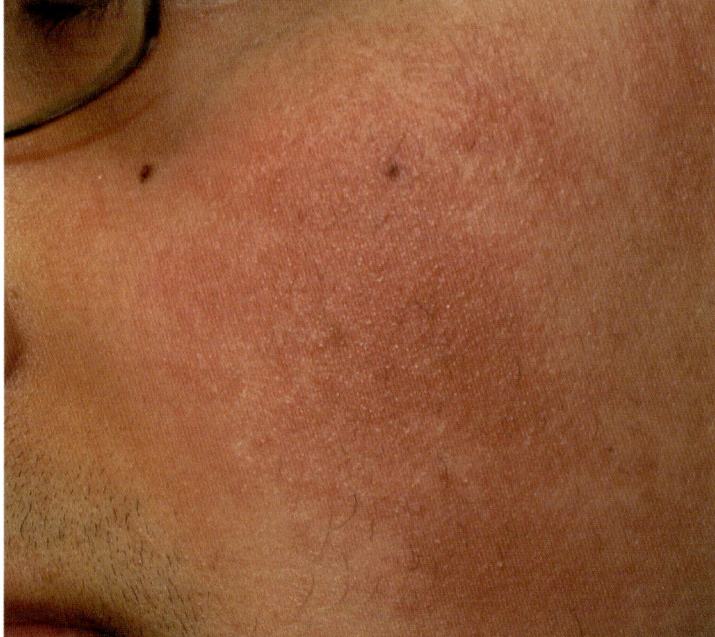

Figure 85.9 Erythromelanosis follicularis faciei et colli in a young Asian man.

associated with other variants [24]. It affects up to 25% of patients with KP [25]. The clinical presentation overlaps with EFFC and may represent a spectrum with differing degrees of pigmentation.

Keratosis pilaris atrophicans. This is a more inflammatory form of KP which results in follicular fibrosis and atrophy progressing to scarring alopecia. Three variants have been recognised:
1 *Keratosis pilaris atrophicans faciei*, also called ulerythema ophryogenes [26] or keratosis rubra pilaris faciei atrophicans, affects the cheeks and lateral eyebrows (Figure 85.10). There is fixed redness, follicular plugging, pitted scarring and hair loss. It may be associated with common KP and may be inherited as an autosomal dominant trait [27].

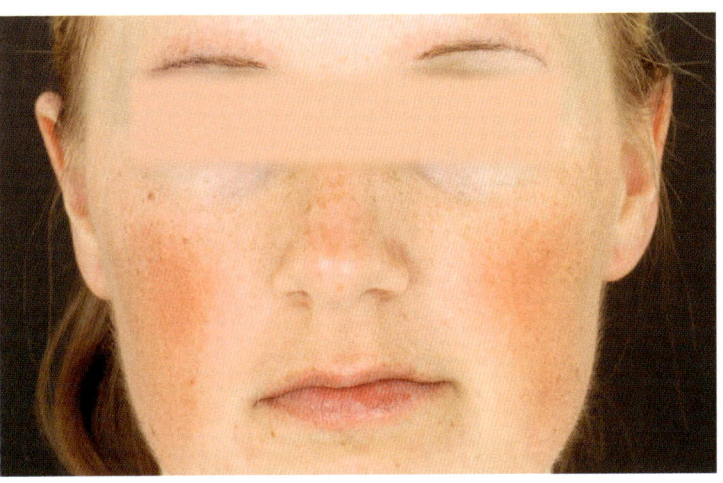

(a)

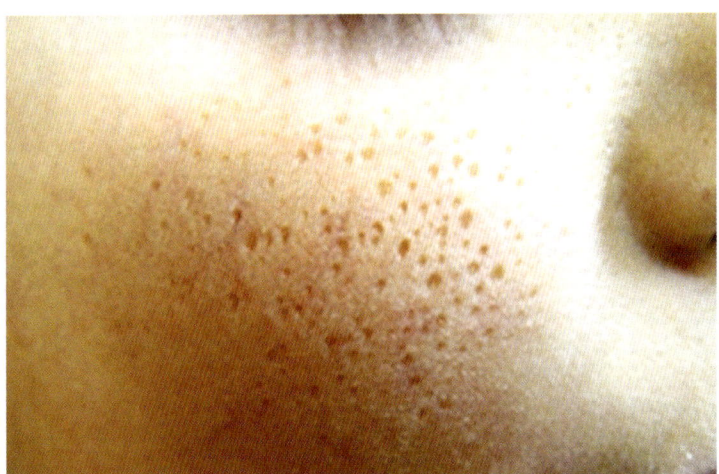

Figure 85.11 Atrophoderma vermiculatum on the cheek of a 10-year-old boy. Reproduced from Apalla *et al.* 2009 [33] with permission of Specjalisci Dermatolodzy.

If follicular lesions become inflamed KP may be confused with the following:
- Acne.
- Folliculitis.

KP atrophicans faciei may be confused with rosacea.

Disease course and prognosis

In the majority of patients, KP is a mild cosmetic disorder which improves with age. Hypopigmentation, hyperpigmentation and scarring may occur. The condition may cause embarrassment and loss of self-esteem in teenage patients and affect their quality of life.

Investigations

Keratosis pilaris is a clinical diagnosis for which no tests are normally required.

Management

Keratosis pilaris is principally a cosmetic problem and many people do not know they have it. If it does not bother the patient, treatment is unnecessary. However, if the condition is affecting the patient psychologically then treatment and reassurance are necessary. Topical lactic acids and retinoids can smoothen the keratotic papules but the redness or pigmentation requires topical steroids and sometimes laser therapies.

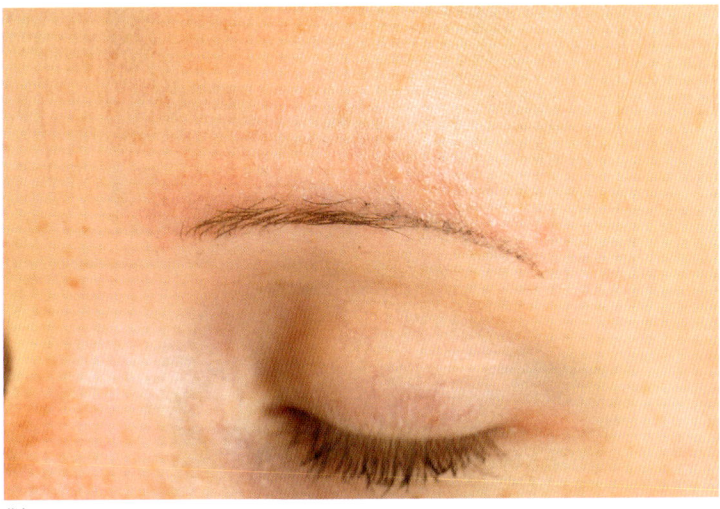

(b)

Figure 85.10 Keratosis pilaris atrophicans faciei (ulerythema ophryogenes). (a) Note the well-defined symmetrical redness on the cheeks and above sparse residual eyebrow hairs. (b) The complete loss of hair from the lateral half of the eyebrows has been disguised by pencilling.

2 *Keratosis follicularis spinulosa decalvans* has its onset in infancy, and affects the cheeks and nose [28]: follicular plugging results in follicular atrophy. The scalp may also be involved, resulting in scarring alopecia. It can be associated with palmoplantar hyperkeratosis.

3 *Atrophoderma vermiculatum* manifests in late childhood, and affects the cheeks and preauricular skin. The follicular plugging evolves towards reticulated atrophy of the skin (Figure 85.11) [29].

Differential diagnosis

Keratosis pilaris may be confused with a large number of dermatoses including the following:
- Darier disease.
- Pityriasis rubra pilaris.
- Atopic eczema.
- Lichen nitidus.
- Eruptive vellous hair cysts.

Treatment ladder for keratosis pilaris

First line
- Keratolytics, particularly salicylic acid
- Lactic and glycolic acid preparations also reduce roughness of the skin
- Treatment may need to be continued for many years

Second line
- Topical retinoids may reduce hyperkeratosis and can be very successful when combined with 10% urea-containing moisturisers

- Topical retinoids are particularly useful for KP atrophicans faciei [30]

Third line
- In severe KP, oral isotretinoin has been successfully used but relapse occurs on cessation [31]

Fourth line
- Pulsed dye laser and intense pulsed light can be effective for fixed redness in KP rubra faciei and KP atrophicans
- Q-switched neodymium:yttrium-aluminium-garnet (Nd:YAG) laser can be effective in reducing roughness as well as redness in refractory KP [32]

Lichen spinulosus

Definition and nomenclature
Lichen spinulosus (LS) is a rare idiopathic condition, characterised by the appearance of hyperkeratotic follicular papules arranged into large plaques [1–3].

Synonyms and inclusions
- Keratosis spinulosa

Introduction and general description
Lichen spinulosus is an acute eruption of grouped keratotic papules which form into plaques. They appear suddenly and are distributed symmetrically on the extensor surfaces of the limbs or on the trunk and neck [1,2,3]. They are coarse to the touch and typically measure 2–5 cm in diameter.

Epidemiology
Incidence and prevalence
Lichen spinulosus is a rare disorder. From the first description in 1908 [4], few reports of the disease appeared in the literature until 1990, when Friedman described 35 patients in a survey of 7435 patients attending a dermatology clinic in the Philippines, accounting for 0.5% of patients surveyed [3].

Age
Lichen spinulosus is a disease of children and young adults with a reported age of onset ranging from 6 to 26 years (average 16 years) [3].

Sex
Case reports suggest an equal distribution of LS in males and females.

Ethnicity
There is no predilection of LS in any ethnic group.

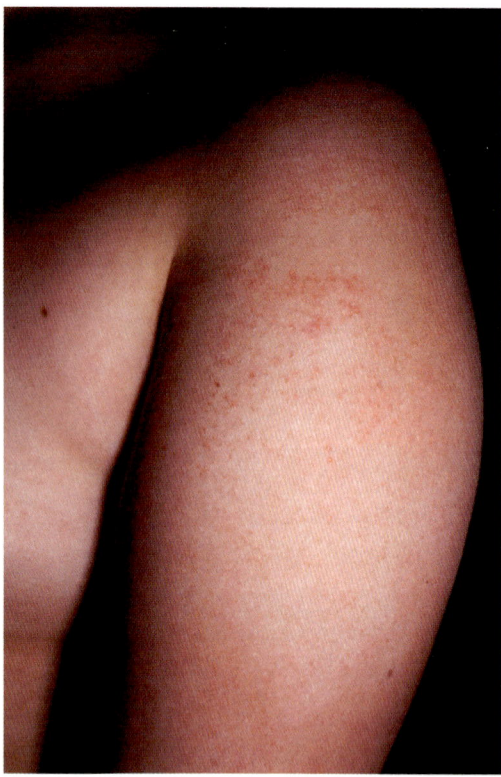

Figure 85.12 Lichen spinulosus present for 18 months as an asymptomatic eruption on the back, shoulder and upper arm of an 8-year-old girl.

Associated diseases
Lichen spinulosus is not usually associated with any underlying systemic disease. There have been case reports of LS in human immunodeficiency virus (HIV) infection, Crohn disease, Hodgkin disease and syphilis [5–7]. Lichen spinulosus has been associated with certain drugs including thallium, gold and diphtheria toxin.

Pathophysiology
The cause of LS is unknown. Some authors feel that it is a variant of KP: the conditions share the same features on histology.

Pathology
Hair follicles are dilated by a thick keratinous plug, and surrounded by a mild to moderate chronic inflammatory infiltrate.

Clinical features
History
Lichen spinulosus generally erupts acutely and is asymptomatic.

Presentation
Individual papules are follicular, measuring 2–3 mm in diameter and raised 1 mm above the surface of the skin with a pointed keratotic spine. Papules coalesce into plaques ranging from 2 to 5 cm in diameter. The patches are symmetrical and distributed on the trunk (Figure 85.12), buttocks, neck, knees and elbows. The face, hands and feet are usually spared. Plaques erupt in crops, grow rapidly and then remain stationary.

Clinical variants
Spinulosis of the face, presenting with tiny keratotic spicules on the cheeks, may be a variant of lichen spinulosus.

Differential diagnosis
All other causes of follicular papules should be considered in the differential diagnosis, including KP, lichen nitidus, phrynoderma and pityriasis rubra pilaris.

Disease course and prognosis
Lichen spinulosus is a chronic but purely cosmetic disease. It can persist for many years, but in most patients it resolves spontaneously within 1–2 years.

Investigations
Diagnosis of LS is made clinically and can be supported by histology. Investigation for immunosuppression including HIV should be considered in severe cases.

Management
Management of LS is aimed at improving the cosmetic appearance. The mainstays of treatment are topical retinoids and keratolytics [8].

Treatment ladder for lichen spinulosus

First line
- Topical keratolyic agents including lactic acid, salicylic acid and urea can be used

Second line
- Topical retinoids [9]

Third line
- Successful use of topical tacalcitol in two children with an atypical presentation of submental LS has been reported [10]

Keratosis circumscripta

Definition
Keratosis circumscripta (KC) is a rare condition characterised by circumscribed areas of follicular hyperkeratosis

Introduction and general description
Keratosis circumscripta was first described by Shrank in 1966 in 10 members of the Yoruba tribe in Nigeria [1]. It is rare and there remains controversy over its status as an individual dermatosis. In one report and review of the literature, the authors suggested that KC was in fact a form of psoriasis modified by environmental factors [2]. It has also been suggested that it is the same as type IV circumscribed juvenile-onset pityriasis rubra pilaris (Chapter 36). Shrank's findings were, however, supported by a report of 10 patients from Kenya [3] and other authors have supported its recognition as an individual entity [4,5].

Epidemiology
Incidence and prevalence
Keratosis circumscripta is rare.

Age
Keratosis circumscripta first develops in childhood and is persistent thereafter.

Ethnicity
It was first described in an African tribe and is more common in patients with phototype 6 skin.

Pathophysiology
The aetiopathogenesis of KC is unknown.

Pathology
Histology shows follicular plugging and moderate hyperkeratosis (Figure 85.13a). There is no involvement of the dermis.

Genetics
The condition appears to be sporadic but clustering of cases within a particular ethnic group would support a genetic predisposition.

Clinical features
History
Keratosis circumscripta normally starts at the age to 3–5 years with lesions developing quickly over a period of 2–3 weeks.

Presentation
The lesions of KC are well-defined areas of diffuse and follicular hyperkeratosis affecting the extensor surfaces of the arms and legs (Figure 85.13b) and the trunk. In his original report, Shrank described elbow and knee involvement in all his patients and 4–5 cm round discs of follicular hyperkeratosis on each hip. The dorsa of the hands and feet were occasionally involved but the palms and soles were rarely affected. Lesions may become thickened and hyperpigmented or violaceous in colour.

Differential diagnosis
A number of dermatoses can be confused with KC but can be clinically differentiated from this disease. These include the following:
- Type IV circumscribed juvenile pityriasis rubra pilaris (Chapter 36).
- Lichen spinulosus.
- Psoriasis (Chapter 35).

Disease course and prognosis
Once established, the condition persists. Patients tend not to develop new lesions but existing lesions may slowly increase in size and become more keratotic.

Management
KC is poorly responsive to treatment and generally does not improve with topical corticosteroids, topical retinoids or conventional keratolytics. The appearance of KC was improved in one patient using 40% urea in white soft paraffin [3].

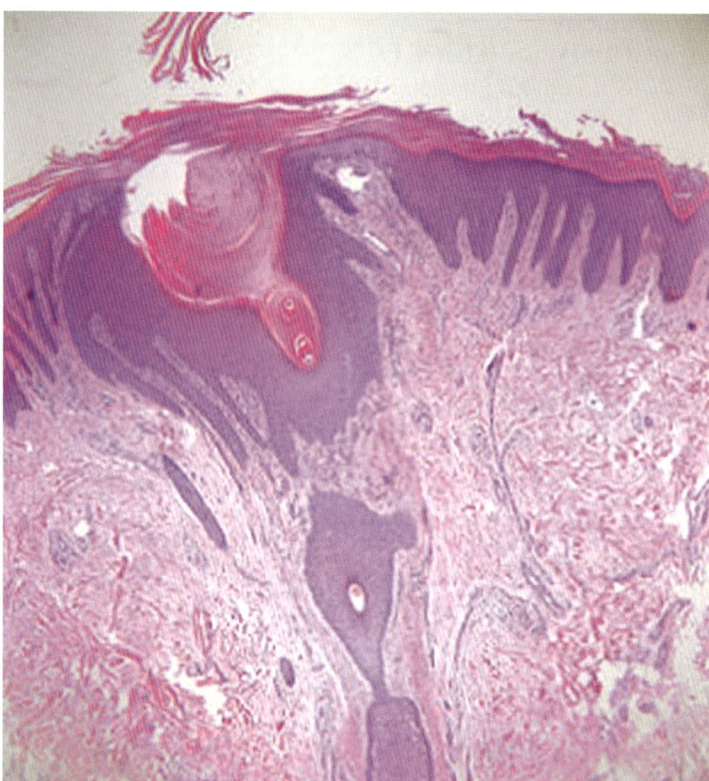

(a)

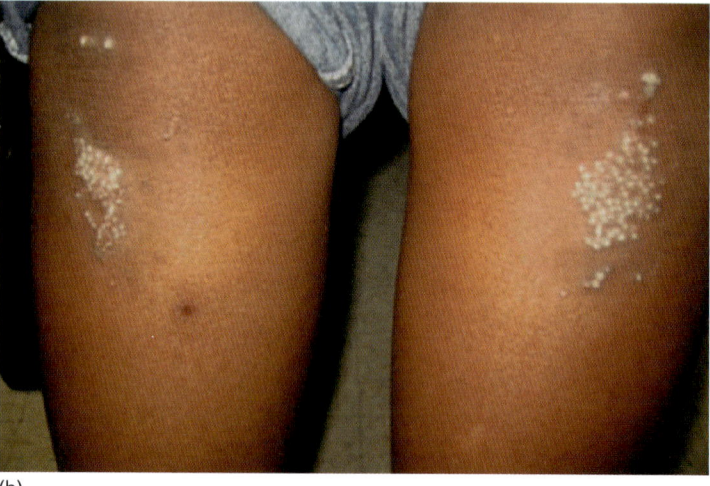

(b)

Figure 85.13 Keratosis circumscripta. (a) Psoriasiform dermatitis with prominent follicular plugging but without neutrophils. (b) Coalescing hyperkeratotic papules on the thighs of a 10-year-old African American girl. Reproduced from Shams *et al.* 2011 [5] with permission of John Wiley & Sons.

Phrynoderma

Definition

Phrynoderma, which literally means toad skin, is one of the cutaneous manifestations of vitamin A deficiency and may also be associated with other nutritional deficiencies. It manifests as follicular hyperkeratosis. It is described in more detail in Chapter 61.

Introduction and general description

Phrynoderma was first described by Nicholls in 1933 in African labourers and was recognised as a manifestation of vitamin A deficiency [1]. It is usually seen in children living in economically deprived countries.

Epidemiology

Incidence and prevalence

Phrynoderma is more common in countries where malnutrition is prevalent, but can also be seen in Europe in individuals with liver cirrhosis, malabsorption syndromes or anorexia nervosa and in those who abuse alcohol or are homeless [2]. In economically deprived countries, it is seen in <5% of children and adolescents [3]. Recently, it has been recognised as a complication of bariatric surgery [4,5].

Age

Phrynoderma is commonest in children between the ages of 5 and 15 years in economically deprived countries.

Sex

Sexes are equally affected.

Ethnicity

No data are available.

Associated diseases

These include:
• Liver cirrhosis.
• Malabsorption syndromes.
• Anorexia nervosa.
• Alcohol abuse.
• Nutritional deficiency following bariatric surgery.

Pathophysiology

Phrynoderma was initially thought to be due purely to vitamin A deficiency. Vitamin A is essential for normal cellular growth and division, and maintenance of the immune response. Lack of this vitamin results in abnormal epidermal keratinisation as well as immunosuppression [6–8]. Phrynoderma has now been described in patients with normal vitamin A levels and has been associated with other nutritional deficiencies including B complex, riboflavin, vitamin C, vitamin E, essential fatty acids and malnutrition [1].

Pathology

Follicles are dilated with compact keratin and patchy parakeratosis with no dermal reaction.

Clinical features

History

Phrynoderma starts gradually with mostly non-pruritic lesions on the elbows (Figure 85.14).

Presentation

Phrynoderma manifests as groups of papules, each one around 3–4 mm in diameter, with a central keratotic plug [9,10,11]. The papules

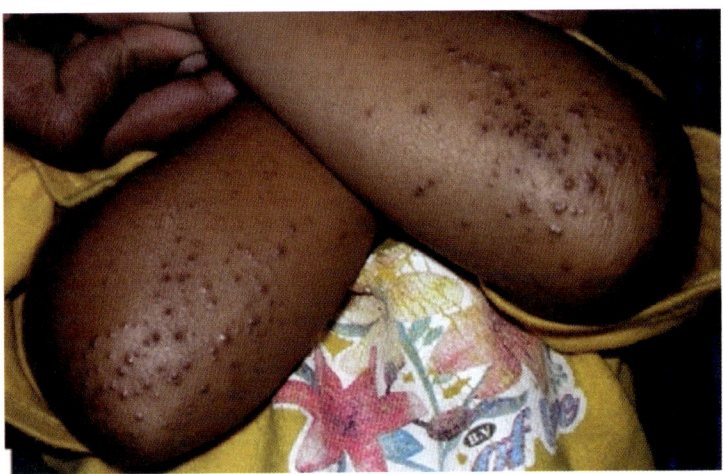

Figure 85.14 Phrynoderma: keratotic papules with intrafollicular plugging on extensor surfaces of the forearms of a 3-year-old Indian girl presenting with night blindness. Both conditions responded within 1 month to vitamin A supplementation. Reproduced from Murthy and Prabhakaran 2010 [14] with permission of Wolters Kluwer.

have a follicular distribution and give the skin a rough texture. The elbows and knees are the most commonly affected areas but the buttocks and extensor surfaces of the limbs may be affected. In generalised disease, the trunk and face may be affected. Papules are skin coloured or hyperpigmented. The condition is usually associated with ocular signs, such as night blindness, conjunctival xerosis and ulcerations [12].

Differential diagnosis

The differential diagnosis of phrynoderma includes:

- Keratosis pilaris.
- Lichen nitidus.
- Lichen spinulosus.
- Multiple minute digitate keratoses.
- Perforating dermatoses.
- Pityriasis rubra pilaris.

Complications and co-morbidities

Ocular involvement including conjunctival xerosis, triangular, dry, white, foamy conjunctival lesions (Bitot spots) and blindness may be associated with phrynoderma.

Investigations

All patients with phrynoderma should have their vitamin A levels measured. Serum vitamin A levels lower than 35 µmol/dL indicate hypovitaminosis. In some patients with nutritional deficiency, there will be concomitant hypoproteinaemia. In this circumstance, values of vitamin A can appear reduced despite adequate vitamin A stores.

Management

Treatment involves the correction of poor diet and administration of a multivitamin preparation containing vitamin A, since poor diet often results in other concurrent deficiencies. Oral administration is preferred over parenteral therapy. The dosage in children aged 8 years or above and adults is 100 000 units daily for 3 days, followed by 50 000 units daily for 2 weeks, and then 10 000 units daily for 2 months, until liver storage is adequate [13].

Treatment ladder for phrynoderma

First line
- Improved nutrition, vitamin supplementation and management of underlying disease

---

Trichodysplasia spinulosa

Definition and nomenclature

Trichodysplasia spinulosa is a rare and disfiguring condition caused by infection of the hair inner root sheath by a polyomavirus in immunocompromised patients.

Synonyms and inclusions
- Polyomavirus-associated trichodysplasia
- Trichodysplasia of immunosuppression

Introduction and general description

This is a rare condition seen in immunocompromised patients. It was first named trichodysplasia spinulosa in 1999 [1], although earlier reports of a lichen spinulosus-like eruption associated with HIV infection are likely the same disorder [2]. It is due to a novel polyomavirus that appears to infect keratinocytes of the inner root sheath of the hair follicle. Polyomaviruses are small, non-enveloped DNA viruses, which are widespread in nature where they cause benign skin tumors (papillomas or warts) in birds and can affect 80% of humans.

Epidemiology

Incidence and prevalence

Trichodysplasia spinulosa is rare with only a small number of reported cases in the world literature.

Age

Trichodysplasia spinulosa has been reported in immunosuppressed patients of all age groups [3].

Ethnicity

All ethnic groups can be affected.

Associated diseases

Most patients with trichodysplasia spinulosa are immunosuppressed following organ transplantation [4]. The disease has been reported in a patient with lymphocytic leukaemia [5]. There have been rare reports of trichodysplasia spinulosa associated with systemic lupus erythematosus [6].

Pathophysiology

Predisposing factors

The trichodysplasia spinulosa polyomavirus (TSPyV) is an opportunistic virus: immunosuppression, whether caused by disease or medication, is a prerequisite for the development of trichodysplasia spinulosa.

Pathology

In affected areas, the hair follicles show abnormal maturation with dilatation of the follicular infundibulum, which is plugged by cornified eosinophilic keratinocytes containing large trichohyalin granules (Chapter 87). Electromicroscopy shows 28 nm intracellular viral particles consistent with polyomavirus. Immunofluorescence studies using antibodies to trichohyalin and TSPyV VP1 protein have shown that the virus is restricted to the nuclei of inner root sheath cells [7]. However, virus has been identified using molecular techniques in a renal allograft [8], urine [9,10] and the respiratory tract [11].

Causative organisms

Trichodysplasia spinulosa is caused by TSPyV. TSPyV is a group I double-stranded DNA virus of the family Polyomaviridae and genus *Orthopolyomavirus* and is related to the Merkel cell polyomavirus. A study in the Netherlands [12] has shown that the virus is common in the general population with a seroprevalence of 70%; it only becomes symptomatic if a carrier is immunocompromised. In contrast to Merkel cell polyomavirus, TSPyV causes dysplasia rather than neoplasia.

Clinical features

History

Patients report the eruption of spiny papules, typically on the central face and eyebrows but sometimes becoming generalised. The condition is usually asymptomatic but may be mildly pruritic.

Presentation

Shiny follicular papules with central spiny keratotic spikes are seen on the facial skin (Figure 85.15). The condition progresses rapidly with multiple disfiguring lesions. Alopecia of the eyebrows and scalp may occur.

Differential diagnosis

Trichodysplasia spinulosa is a very distinctive disease but in the early stages may be confused with other follicular keratotic dermatoses, including the following:

- Keratosis pilaris.
- Lichen nitidus.
- Follicular mucinosis.

Complications and co-morbidities

All patients are immunocompromised.

Disease course and prognosis

Trichodysplasia spinulosa progresses unless specifically treated or unless immunosuppression is withdrawn. There have been no long-term reports of this disease so long-term prognosis is speculative.

Investigations

Skin biopsy shows characteristic changes in the hair follicle. The virus can be identified using molecular or immunofluorescence techniques.

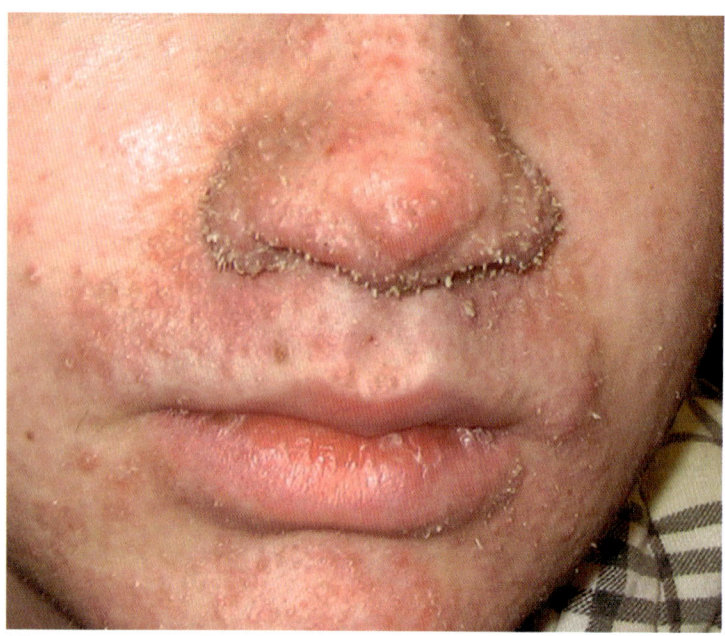

(a)

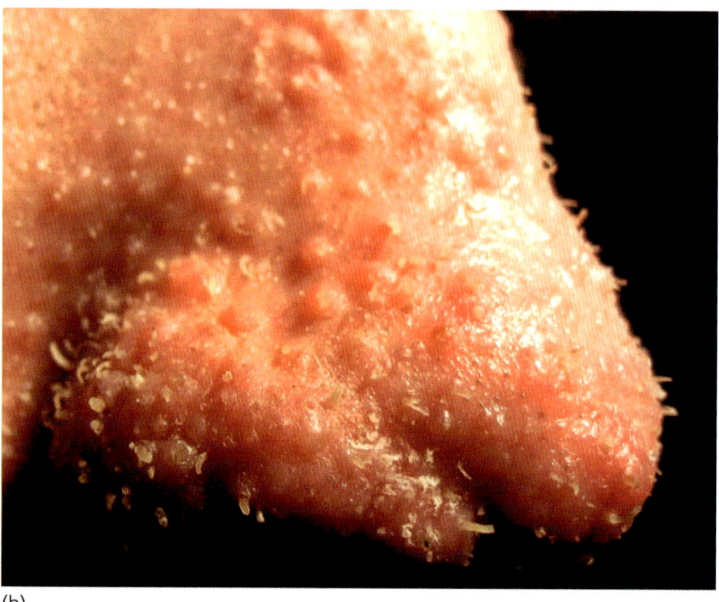

(b)

Figure 85.15 (a, b) Trichodysplasia spinulosa: multiple keratotic spicules on the nose of a heart transplant recipient. Reproduced from van der Meiden *et al.* [18] with permission of Public Library of Science (PLOS).

Management

Trichodysplasia spinulosa is a persistent disease. In organ transplant recipients, reduction of immunosuppression has resulted in some improvement. Antiviral treatment has been successful in some patients [13,14] and one patient responded to surgery followed by topical tazarotene [15]. Firm guidance on management cannot be given due to the paucity of reports but topical or oral antiviral therapy would appear to be the treatment of choice.

Treatment ladder for trichodysplasia spinulosa

First line
- Reduction of immunosuppression if feasible
- Topical cidofovir 3% (if available) **[16]**
- Oral valganciclovir: successful response has been reported in four patients

Second line
- Topical tazarotene: one patient improved with topical tazarotene after skin lesions were shaved off under local anaesthesia [15]

Third line
- One patient treated with a topical compound of aciclovir, 2-deoxy-D-glucose and epigallocatechin (green tea extract) showed improvement [17]

Flegel disease

Definition and nomenclature
Flegel disease (FD) is a rare dermatosis, first described by Flegel in 1958 [1]. It is characterised by the presence of flat keratotic papules on the lower legs and dorsa of the feet. It is a disease of the older adult, but it can be seen occasionally in younger persons.

Synonyms and inclusions
- Hyperkeratosis lenticularis perstans

Introduction and general description
Flegel disease is a rare dermatosis characterised by flat keratotic papules on the lower legs and dorsa of the feet. It is more commonly found in older adults, but can appear occasionally in younger people. Each papule measures 1–5 mm in diameter and is topped by a horny keratotic scale, the removal of which causes bleeding.

Epidemiology
Incidence and prevalence
It is a rare disease and there are no prevalence data in the literature.

Age
Flegel disease is most commonly seen in mid to late adult life but cases in children have been reported [2].

Ethnicity
It is seen in all racial groups but appears to be more common in white populations.

Associated diseases
A number of reports have suggested an association between endocrinopathies and FD [3], particularly diabetes.

Pathophysiology
The cause of FD is unknown. A number of hypotheses have been put forward. Some authors have suggested that ultraviolet (UV) light may play a role [4]. Electron microscopic studies have demonstrated a lack or paucity of Odland bodies in the stratum granulosum. Odland bodies contain proteases and regulate desquamation of keratinocytes suggesting a possible mechanism for localised hyperkeratosis [5,6]. Immunological studies have shown that the dermal infiltrate in FD is predominantly T cells and that these cells are activated, suggesting that the disease could be the result of a cell-mediated immune response to keratinocytes [7].

Pathology
Microscopic examination of a well-developed papule shows characteristic histological features. The stratum corneum is markedly thickened, eosinophilic and compact, and the underlying stratum spinosum is compressed. Patchy parakeratosis may be present. The intervening granular layer is thinned or absent. The surrounding epidermis can show papillomatosis. There is a lymphocytic dermal infiltrate in a band-like distribution beneath the affected epidermis [5].

Genetics
Both a familial and a non-familial variant have been recognised. At least in some cases, the disease is inherited as an autosomal dominant trait [8].

Environmental factors
Some authors suggest that exposure to the sun may be involved in the pathogenesis of FD.

Clinical features
History
Small keratotic papules develop on the lower legs in middle-aged to elderly patients and slowly spread up the legs (Figure 85.16). The lesions are asymptomatic.

Presentation
The lesions of FD are red-brown non-follicular keratotic papules measuring 1–5 mm in diameter. Rarely, the disease may affect the outer ear lobes, arms, palms, soles and oral mucosa [9]. If the scale is removed, the site is red and may have bleeding points. Involvement of the trunk is unusual but a generalised form of FD has been described [10].

Differential diagnosis
Diseases with localised areas of hyperkeratosis are considered in the differential diagnosis, as listed in Box 85.6.

Box 85.6 Differential diagnosis of Flegel disease

- Acquired reactive perforating dermatosis (Kyrle disease)
- Actinic keratosis
- Arsenical keratosis
- Darier disease
- Porokeratosis
- Stucco keratosis

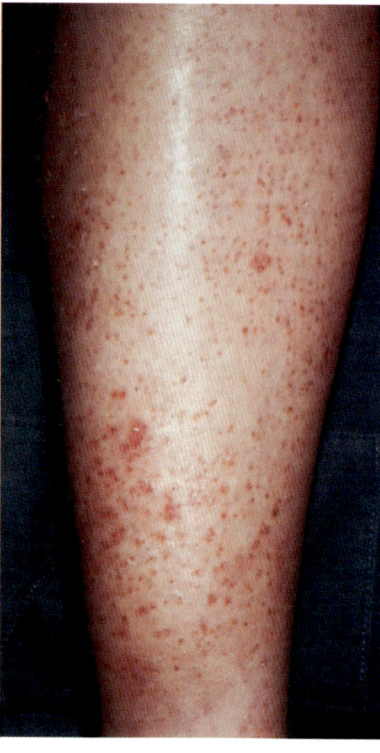

Figure 85.16 Flegel disease: multiple, tiny, thorn-like keratotic papules on the skin of the lower leg.

Investigations
Skin biopsy will show the characteristic changes and will confirm a clinical diagnosis.

Management
Flegel disease is difficult to treat and medical treatment needs to continue for prolonged periods.

First line
The most consistent treatment results have been achieved with 5% fluorouracil, which needs to be continued for several months [11,12,**13**], dermabrasion and local excision [14].

Second line
Various systemic retinoids have been used with variable responses. Lesions tend to reform on cessation of treatment [15].

Third line
Treatment with topical vitamin D analogues has been reported with variable and inconsistent results [16,17]. Topical retinoids and keratolytics have been used with disappointing results [12].

Multiple minute digitate keratoses

Definition and nomenclature
The term multiple minute digitate keratoses (MMDK) describes a rare, clinically distinctive but aetiologically heterogeneous disorder of epidermal keratinisation occurring in adults.

Synonyms and inclusions
- Multiple minute digitate hyperkeratoses
- Spiny hyperkeratosis
- Digitate keratoses
- Disseminated spiked hyperkeratosis
- Familial disseminated filiform hyperkeratosis
- Filiform keratoses
- Minute aggregated keratoses

Introduction and general description
Multiple minute digitate hyperkeratoses is a term introduced by Goldstein in 1967 [1] and more fully characterised by Ramselaar and Toonstra in 1999 [2] as a rare disorder of keratinisation in which multiple, tiny, spiky cutaneous keratoses appear in adult life. The more appropriate label MMDK is preferred to define this disorder [3].

Epidemiology
Incidence and prevalence
This is a rare disorder.

Age
The genetic form generally presents between the ages of 20 and 30 years. MMDK associated with malignancy or other systemic disease presents later in life, typically in the sixth decade of life [4].

Sex
There is a slight male preponderance [1].

Ethnicity
No racial predilection has been identified.

Associated diseases
Postinflammatory/reactive cases of MMDK may be associated with solar damage, radiotherapy or the use of drugs including acitretin, simvastatin and ciclosporin [5].
Sporadic cases of MMDK may be associated with systemic disease or may be paraneoplastic [1,6–8].

Pathophysiology
Three forms of MMDK have been proposed, although these divisions may not represent distinct disorders.
The genetic form appears to be inherited as an autosomal dominant trait and the disease becomes clinically apparent in the second and third decades of life.
MMDK has been associated with various drugs as well as following radiotherapy or chronic sun exposure.
Sporadic MMDK may be a paraneoplastic phenomenon but due to its rarity it is difficult to determine whether the associations with underlying neoplasms which have been noted are simply coincidental [6].

Pathology
Histologically, MMDK shows discrete columns of compact hyperkeratosis arising from an acanthotic interfollicular epidermis (Figure 85.17a). The granular cell layer is intact. The dermis is uninvolved. Under the electron microscope, keratohyalin bodies

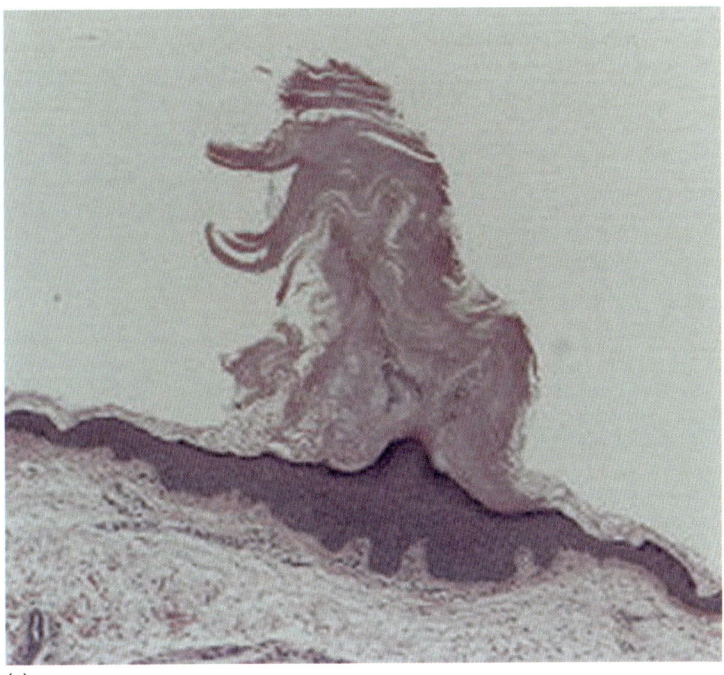

(a)

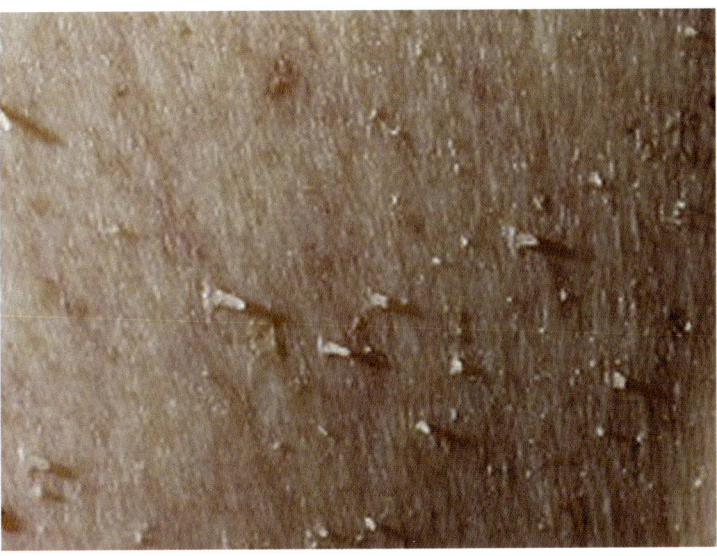

(b)

Figure 85.17 Multiple minute digitate keratoses. (a) Photomicrograph of a hyperkeratotic spicule. (b) Close-up view of spicules on the back. From Caccetta *et al.* 2012 [10] © 2010 American Academy of Dermatology, Inc. Published by Mosby, Inc. All rights reserved.

are smaller than normal but Odland bodies are present. The pattern of keratin is otherwise normal [9].

Genetics
The early-onset familial form is inherited in an autosomal dominant fashion.

Clinical features
History
Patients report the sudden appearance of asymptomatic tiny spiny keratoses on the skin.

Presentation
The keratoses are typically located on the trunk and proximal limbs and may number in the hundreds (Figure 85.17b). They are tiny flesh-coloured spikes that measure up to 2 mm in length and are non-follicular. Case reports have described patients with lesions restricted to the palms and soles [7,8].

Differential diagnosis
Other digitate keratoses should be considered including lichen spinulosus, phrynoderma, multiple filiform viral warts, trichodysplasia spinulosa and arsenical keratoses [10].

Investigations
In sporadic cases of MMDK, investigations for age-related underlying malignancy should be performed.

Management
There is no evidence for the treatment of MMDK. Reports have shown response to a number of treatments.

Treatment ladder for multiple minute digitate keratoses

First line
- Keratolytic agents, particularly salicylic acid and lactic acid, with emollients

Second line
- Topical retinoids in combination with emollients and urea-containing moisturisers

Third line
- Topical 5-fluorouracil

Porokeratoses

Definition and nomenclature
A porokeratosis is a clonal expansion of keratinocytes which differentiate abnormally but are not truly neoplastic. All forms of porokeratosis show a thin column of parakeratosis, the cornoid lamella, representing the active border. Squamous cell carcinomas may develop within lesions.

Synonyms and inclusions
- Porokeratosis of Mibelli
- Disseminated superficial actinic porokeratosis (DSAP)
- Linear porokeratosis
- Punctate porokeratosis
- Disseminated actinic porokeratosis
- Disseminated palmoplantar porokeratosis

Introduction and general description

A porokeratosis is a clonal expansion of keratinocytes which differentiate abnormally but are not hyperproliferative. Porokeratoses may present as single or multiple lesions and may be localised or disseminated. All forms show a thin column of parakeratosis, the cornoid lamella, representing the active border [1,2].

Mibelli described the classic form which bears his name in 1893. This was followed by descriptions of superficial and disseminated forms of porokeratosis by Respighi in 1893, linear porokeratosis in 1918, disseminated superficial actinic porokeratosis (DSAP) by Chernosky in 1966, disseminated palmoplantar porokeratosis by Guss in 1971 and punctate porokeratosis by Rahbari in 1977.

A working clinical classification of porokeratoses is shown in Box 85.7 [1,2]. Lesions start as papules or plaques that develop into annular lesions with a thin, often thread-like elevated rim. Diagnosis is confirmed by finding the pathognomonic cornoid lamella on histological examination (Figure 85.18). It is likely that the different variants are related, as more than one type of porokeratosis has been reported in the same patient [3] and different types have been reported in different members of the same family [4]. Malignant change with development of squamous cell carcinoma may occur.

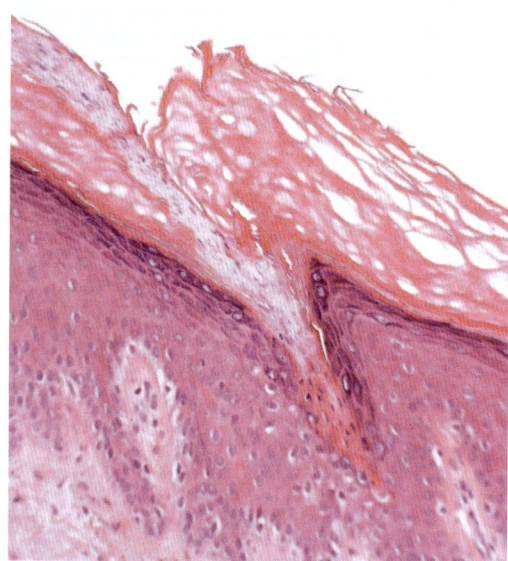

Figure 85.18 Cornoid lamella forming the edge of a porokeratosis: a column of parakeratotic keratinocytes can be seen arising from invagination of the underlying epidermis.

Box 85.7 Clinical classification of porokeratoses

Localised forms
- Porokeratosis of Mibelli
- Linear porokeratosis
- Punctate palmoplantar porokeratosis
- Genital porokeratosis
- Porokeratosis ptychotropica

Disseminated forms
- Disseminated superficial actinic porokeratosis
- Disseminated superficial porokeratosis
- Systematised linear porokeratosis
- Disseminated palmoplantar porokeratosis

Adapted from Sertznig *et al.* 2012 [1] and Ferreira *et al.* 2013 [2].

Epidemiology

Incidence and prevalence

Porokeratosis is listed as a rare disease and classified as such by Orphanet and the Office of Rare Diseases (ORD) of the National Institutes of Health. DSAP is the most common form [5].

Age

Classic porokeratosis of Mibelli and linear porokeratosis typically appear during infancy or childhood. Punctate palmoplantar porokeratosis and disseminated palmoplantar porokeratosis usually appear in adolescence, while DSAP generally first manifests in adult life.

Sex

Porokeratosis of Mibelli, genital porokeratosis and punctate porokeratosis are more common in males, whereas DSAP is more common in women. Linear porokeratosis has an equal sex ratio.

Ethnicity

All forms of porokeratosis are seen predominantly in pale, fair-skinned ethnic groups.

Associated diseases

These include:
- HIV infection [6].
- Crohn disease [7].
- Diabetes [8].
- Liver disease [9].
- Chronic renal failure [10].
- Haematological and solid tumours [11].

Pathophysiology

Porokeratosis represents a clonal expansion of keratinocytes [12] that show abnormal differentiation but are not hyperproliferative [13]. The cornoid lamella, which is the hallmark of porokeratosis, is composed of parakeratotic keratinocytes which result from either faulty maturation or an acceleration of epidermopoiesis. It has been shown that there is reduced keratinocyte loricrin and filaggrin expression and abnormal premature keratinocyte apoptosis underlying the cornoid lamella, indicating dysregulation of terminal differentiation [1]. Furthermore, abnormal DNA ploidy in keratinocytes has been demonstrated [14]. In DSAP mutations in the *SART3* (Squamous Cell Carcinoma Antigen Recognized by T-cells) and *MVK* (MeValonate Kinase) genes have been found [5]: *MVK* has a role in keratinocyte differentiation and may protect keratinocytes from apoptosis in response to damage from UV radiation [15].

Predisposing factors

Drug-induced immunosuppression in various diseases including organ transplantation may predispose to porokeratosis [16]. Natural or therapeutic exposure to UV radiation is a recognised trigger factor for DSAP and porokeratosis of Mibelli.

Pathology

Identification of the cornoid lamella is essential for the diagnosis of porokeratosis. As this represents the peripheral thread-like border of the lesion it is essential that biopsy includes this border. Histologically, the cornoid lamella is a thin column of tightly packed parakeratotic keratinocytes within a keratin-filled invagination of the epidermis through the stratum corneum (Figure 87.18) [1]. The underlying stratum granulosum may be absent or attenuated but is normal in other parts of the lesion. There is a perivascular or lichenoid lymphocytic infiltrate. Amyloid deposits have been reported in DSAP and in the intertriginous portion of perianal porokeratosis (porokeratosis ptychotropica). The central portion of a porokeratosis may show epidermal atrophy and areas of liquefaction degeneration.

Genetics

All forms of porokeratosis have been reported to have familial clusters with autosomal dominant patterns of inheritance but with variable penetrance. A number of very different chromosomal loci have been identified in DSAP, including 12q23.2-24.1, 1p31.3-p31, 16q24.1-24.3 and 18p11.3 [17]. Linear porokeratosis follows the lines of Blaschko and may be systematised, indicating genetic mosaicism.

Environmental factors

Exposure to UV radiation is a factor in the induction of superficial actinic porokeratosis and porokeratosis of Mibelli.

Clinical features

History

Porokeratoses present with single or multiple papules or plaques that develop into annular lesions with a thin raised border. They are usually asymptomatic but may be pruritic and, if verrucous, may cause discomfort from pressure.

Clinical variants of localised forms

Porokeratosis of Mibelli. This starts as a single or small group of keratotic papules which may be pigmented. These gradually grow over years to form one or more irregular plaques with a thin, keratotic and well-demarcated border. The central area may be atrophic, either hyper- or hypopigmented, hairless and anhidrotic (Figure 85.19). Lesions are generally distributed on the extremities but can occur anywhere on the body. Occasionally, giant and verrucous forms of the disease may occur [18].

Linear porokeratosis. This generally occurs in infancy as unilateral streaks or plaques of reddish brown papules along limbs or the side of the trunk, head or neck following Blaschko lines, indicating underlying somatic mosaicism (Figure 85.20). There is a higher risk of malignant change in linear porokeratosis than in other forms of porokeratosis [19].

Punctate palmoplantar porokeratosis. This is a rare type of porokeratosis in which seed-like punctate keratoses form on the palms and soles during adulthood [1].

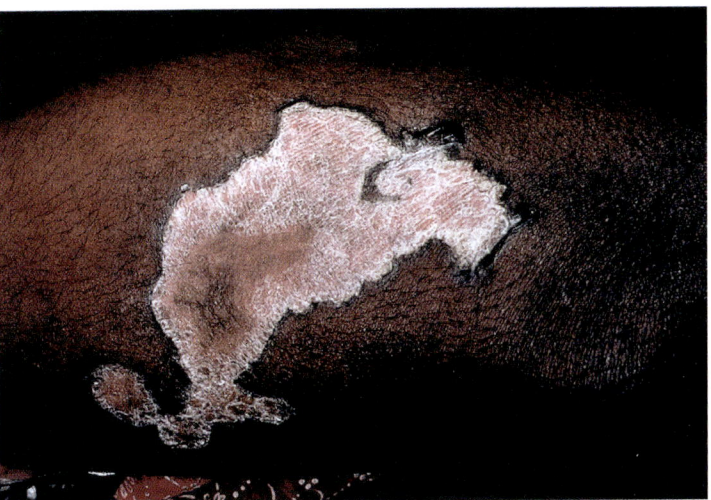

Figure 85.19 Porokeratosis of Mibelli.

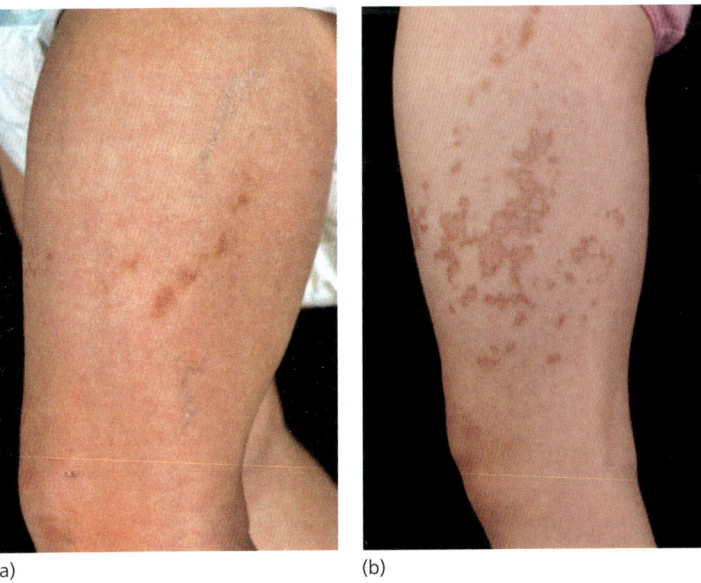

(a)　　　　　　　　　　　　(b)

Figure 85.20 (a, b) Linear porokeratosis: irregular linear and polygonal 'Chinese character' plaques developing in a blaschkoid distribution on the thigh, showing progression from 23 months to 5 years of age.

Genital porokeratosis. Genital porokeratosis is a rare localised type which it is important to be aware of as it is frequently misdiagnosed clinically. It occurs almost exclusively in men, more often affecting the scrotum than the penis (Figure 85.21) [20]. Vulval porokeratosis is much rarer [21].

Ptychotropic porokeratosis. Ptychotropic porokeratosis (affecting the natal cleft and buttocks) [22] is another very rare type which may be very inflammatory and thus elude diagnosis until appropriate biopsies have been taken (Figure 85.22).

Clinical variants of disseminated forms

Disseminated superficial actinic porokeratosis. DSAP is the most common form of porokeratosis [1,5], representing more than half of all cases. The condition is often overlooked as the lesions may be quite inconspicuous to the casual observer. Multiple flesh-coloured,

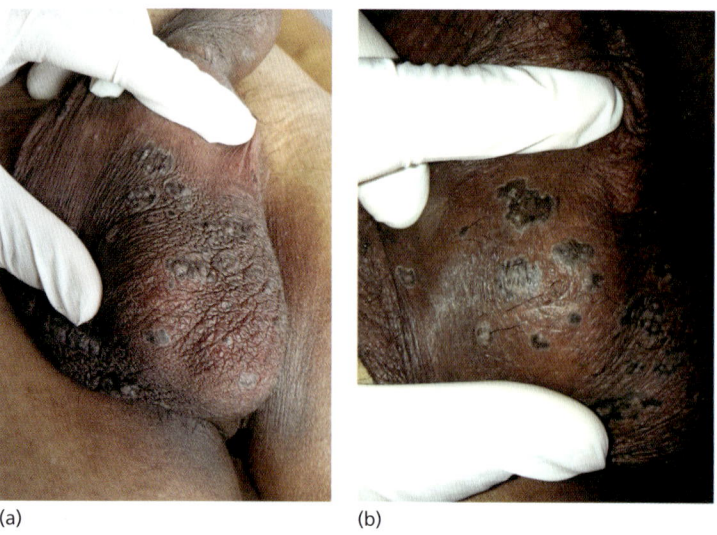

(a)   (b)

Figure 85.21 (a, b) Genital porokeratosis: multiple lesions limited to the scrotum. Reproduced from Joshi and Minni 2018 [34] with permission of Dove Medical Press Limited, CC BY-NC 3.0.

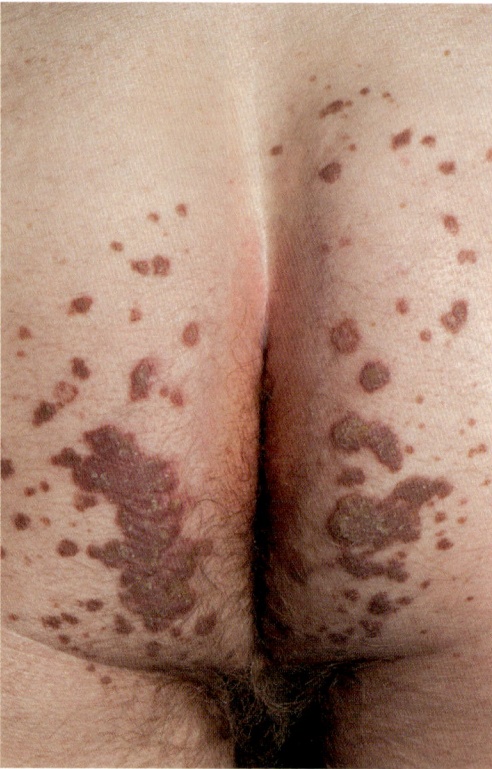

Figure 85.22 Ptychotropic porokeratosis. Courtesy of Dr P. Laws.

pink or reddish brown, finely scaling macules with a thin but well-defined raised border start to appear in early adult life, predominantly on the lower legs and arms (Figure 85.23). The palms and soles are not affected. The lesions are generally small, <1 cm diameter, and usually asymptomatic. Patients will often give a history of worsening of the condition following sun exposure.

Disseminated superficial porokeratosis. This is not necessarily related to sun exposure and will present in both sun-exposed

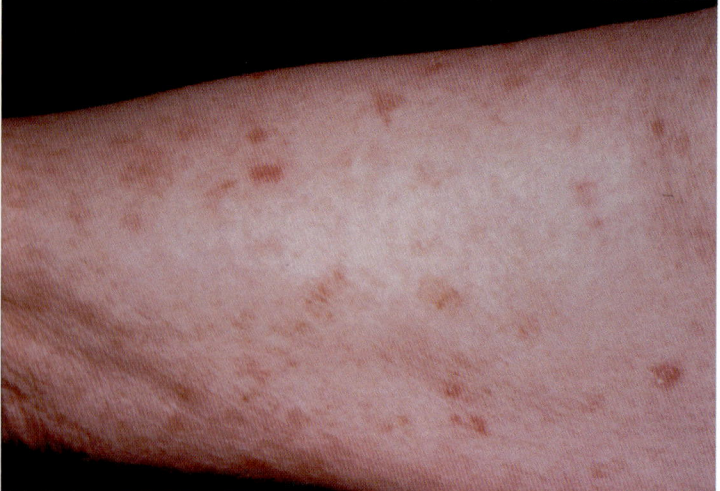

Figure 85.23 Disseminated superficial actinic porokeratosis: view of the upper arm.

and sun-protected sites, including sometimes the oral mucosa and genitalia. It may be associated with immunodeficiency (e.g. organ transplantation, malignancy, HIV infection) or may develop sporadically during childhood [1].

Systematised linear porokeratosis. This is a disseminated variant of linear porokeratosis that may be unilateral or generalised and follows the lines of Blaschko [1,23].

Disseminated palmoplantar porokeratosis. Disseminated palmoplantar porokeratosis (porokeratosis palmaris et plantaris disseminata) is a rare generalised form of punctate palmoplantar porokeratosis in which palmoplantar lesions, which first appear in the third decade of life, are succeeded by multiple, widely disseminated, wart-like keratoses in both sun-exposed and sun-protected areas including the oral mucosa and genitalia and often following Blaschko lines [1,24].

CDAGS syndrome. CDAGS syndrome is a rare autosomal recessive disorder defined as *c*raniostenosis, *d*elayed closure of the fontanelles, cranial defects or deafness, *a*nal anomalies, *g*enitourinary abnormalities and *s*kin eruption, which is often porokeratosis [25].

Differential diagnosis
The differential diagnoses of porokeratosis of Mibelli and disseminated palmoplantar porokeratosis include psoriasis, Bowen disease and actinic keratoses. Disseminated superficial actinic porokeratosis may be confused with actinic keratosis or stucco keratoses. The differential diagnosis of linear porokeratosis includes linear verrucous epidermal naevus, lichen striatus and incontinentia pigmenti. Punctate palmoplantar porokeratosis may be mistaken for viral warts.

Complications and co-morbidities
Cutaneous malignancies, particularly squamous cell carcinoma, may occur. The rate of malignant transformation varies between subtypes, with the highest rate (19%) in linear porokeratosis and the lowest in DSAP (3%) [26]. The necessary role of UV radiation in

the pathogenesis of DSAP and the frequent concurrence of actinic keratosis make the latter relationship uncertain.

Disease course and prognosis

All forms of porokeratosis are chronic with no tendency for spontaneous resolution.

Investigations

Patients presenting with sudden onset of porokeratosis should be investigated for causes of immunosuppression including HIV and haematological malignancies.

Management

In many patients, regular monitoring for evolving skin cancer may be all that is needed. In patients with immunosuppression or in linear porokeratosis where the malignancy rate is increased, or in those requesting treatment, there are principally two approaches:
1 Target the underlying abnormal clone of cells using the same approach that is used for actinic keratosis.
2 Target the abnormal keratinisation with topical or systemic retinoids.

First line

Cryotherapy, 5-fluorouracil [27], imiquimod [28], curettage and cautery, photodynamic therapy, laser modalities [29], topical diclofenac [30] and topical vitamin D analogues such as calcipotriol [31] have all been used to treat porokeratosis with varying degrees of success.

Topical cholesterol/lovastatin has been reported as an effective and well-tolerated therapy in five patients with various porokeratoses [32].

Second line

Oral retinoids including isotretinoin and acitretin have been advocated in patients with porokeratosis who are immunosuppressed or have the linear form of the disease in order to reduce the risk of malignant change [33].

Transient acantholytic dermatosis

Definition and nomenclature

Transient acantholytic dermatosis (TAD) is a relatively common transient or persistent monomorphous, papulovesicular eruption mainly affecting the trunk. It may be pruritic or asymptomatic and was first described by Grover in 1970 [1].

Synonyms and inclusions
- Grover disease
- Papular acantholytic dermatosis

Introduction and general description

The term TAD is possibly misleading [2], for although it is self-limiting in some patients, it may be very persistent in others.

The physician needs a high index of suspicion to diagnose this disease as clinically it resembles a number of inflammatory dermatoses and histologically is similar to several other dermatoses.

Epidemiology

It is a relatively common inflammatory dermatosis but there are no incidence data available. In a Swiss study [2], only 24 cases of TAD were found among 30 000 biopsies taken. Similarly, studies of incidence in hospital referrals in the USA and France have shown an incidence of about 0.1% [3].

Age

It is a disease of older patients with a mean age at diagnosis of 59 years, but may manifest throughout adult life [4].

Sex

The disease has a male predominance with a male to female ratio of 3.95 : 1 [4].

Ethnicity

Transient acantholytic dermatosis is commonest in white populations.

Associated diseases

It may be seen in conjunction with a number of other inflammatory dermatoses including psoriasis, asteatotic eczema, contact allergic dermatitis and contact irritant dermatitis. In one study, 11% of patients with TAD were found to have a concurrent inflammatory dermatosis [5].

TAD may also be associated with malignant disease including skin cancer and haematological malignancies [5].

Pathophysiology

The cause of TAD is unknown. A recent study has demonstrated autoantibodies against a number of proteins involved in keratinocyte development, activation, growth, adhesion and motility using proteomic microarrays to analyse immunoglobulin A (IgA) and IgG autoantibodies [6]. It is still unclear whether these autoantibodies are causative or are a reaction to the damage to keratinocytes seen in this disease.

Predisposing factors

Transient acantholytic dermatosis has been associated with exposure to natural UV radiation, heat and sweating, which has led to the hypothesis that the eccrine sweat glands are aetiologically involved. The disease has not, however, been associated with artificial UV exposure and in some reports is more common in the winter [7]. A number of case series have reported the association of TAD with hospitalised and bedridden patients [8]. TAD occurs commonly in patients receiving long-term BRAF (B-rapidly accelerated fibrosarcoma protein) inhibitor therapy for metastatic melanoma [9].

Recently, Grover-like eruptions have been described as one of the papulovesicular presentations associated with SARS-CoV-2 infection [10].

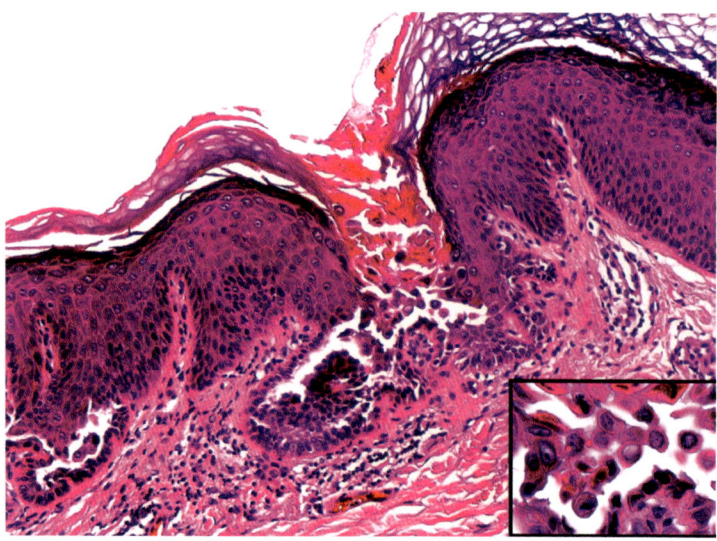

Figure 85.24 Transient acantholytic dermatosis: histopathological image of a papule demonstrating intraepidermal clefting and acantholytic cells (inset). Courtesy of Professor Luis Requena.

Table 85.1 Histological patterns in transient acantholytic dermatosis.

Pattern	Features
Darier-like	Suprabasal acantholysis with scattered dyskeratosis and apoptotic cells (corps ronds and grains) throughout the epidermis
Hailey–Hailey-like	Acantholyisis throughout the stratum spinosum with more hyperplastic epidermis and no significant dyskeratosis
Pemphigus vulgaris-like	Suprabasal acantholyisis, often with large numbers of eosinophils present
Spongiotic	Epidermal oedema causing separation of keratinocytes and prominent desmosomes
Pemphigus foliaceus-like	Superficial clefting in the superficial epidermis

Adated from Streit *et al.* 2000 [2].

Pathology

The primary histological feature of TAD is the presence of small foci of acantholysis with dyskeratosis, intraepidermal clefting and sometimes vesicle formation (Figure 85.24). Five patterns of acantholysis have been described, present either singly or in combination. The incidences of these patterns observed in the three largest studies on TAD are pemphigus vulgaris-like (47%), Darier-like (18%), spongiotic (9%), pemphigus foliaceus-like (9%) and Hailey–Hailey-like (8%) (Table 85.1) [2].

Within the dermis, there is usually a sparse lymphohistiocytic, perivascular infiltrate. Lichenoid change with basal vacuolisation has been reported; eosinophils and neutrophils may be present [11].

Environmental factors

Transient acantholytic dermatosis is reported to be more common in the winter but may be exacerbated by UV exposure and sweating.

Clinical features

History

Patients usually give a history of the sudden onset of itchy papules on the trunk.

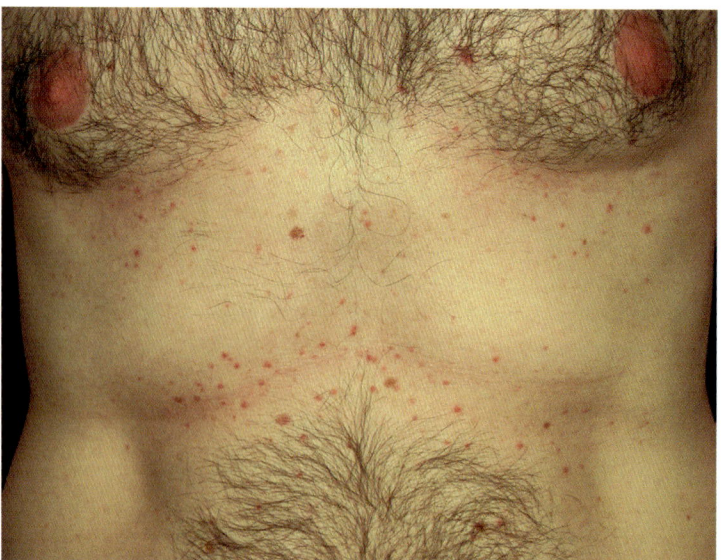

Figure 85.25 Transient acantholytic dermatosis: typical appearance on the abdomen. Courtesy of Professor Luis Requena.

Presentation

The normal presentation is of a papulovesicular red eruption on the trunk of a middle-aged or elderly white male. It starts with small papules and vesicles that quickly crust and develop keratotic erosions (Figure 85.25). The eruption is usually very itchy and the patient presents with multiple excoriations, although in some patients there is no pruritus. In others, the distribution extends to cover the proximal limbs. In many patients, it may live up to its name and be transient, lasting 2–4 weeks; in some it may, however, persist for months or years or follow a chronic relapsing course.

Some authors use the term 'persistent and recurrent acantholytic dermatosis' to encompass those cases that do not rapidly resolve.

Differential diagnosis

Transient acantholytic dermatosis has very characteristic clinical features and usually presents little problem in diagnosis. It may be confused with folliculitis, papular urticaria, scabies and herpes zoster. Galli–Galli disease, a rare acantholytic variant of Dowling–Degos disease, occurs in a similar age group and may clinically resemble TAD but is usually more widespread, affecting the hands and groins. The reticulate pattern seen in Dowling–Degos disease may be present [12].

Complications and co-morbidities

It has been shown to be associated with skin cancer and in one study 8% of patients had a haematological malignancy [3].

Disease course and prognosis

Transient acantholytic dermatosis may resolve spontaneously after weeks or months or persist for years. There are no clinical or histological prognostic signs in this disease.

Investigations

Skin biopsy will confirm the clinical diagnosis. In view of the raised incidence of haematological malignancies seen in this disease, haematological work-up is advised.

Management

Patients should be advised to avoid sunlight exposure, strenuous exercise and heat, all of which may exacerbate the disease.

First line

In many patients, the disease resolves spontaneously after a few weeks and all that is needed is a potent topical corticosteroid for symptomatic relief. Topical vitamin D analogues and calcineurin inhibitors have been used. Systemic antihistamines can be used to control pruritus.

Second line

In more severe cases, short courses of systemic corticosteroids have been shown to give sustained improvement but rebound may occur. Systemic retinoids [13], phototherapy [14] and methotrexate have been used in more severe and refractory cases.

Third line

Recent case reports have claimed benefit from etanercept [15] and, in one patient with recalcitrant TAD, from photodynamic therapy [16].

Keratolysis exfoliativa

Definition and nomenclature

Keratolysis exfoliativa is a common disease of young adults in which discrete areas of superficial skin peeling occur on the palms, starting as air-filled blisters and leading to a circinate or irregular annular pattern of scaling. This may be associated with localised hyperhidrosis.

Synonyms and inclusions

- Exfoliative keratolysis
- Dyshidrosis lamellosa sicca
- Focal palmar peeling
- Recurrent focal palmar peeling
- Desquamation en aires

Introduction and general description

Keratolysis exfoliativa represents an acquired form of non inflammatory skin peeling. The condition was first described by Wende in 1919 [1].

Epidemiology
Incidence and prevalence

Keratolysis exfoliativa is a common condition but there are no epidemiological data available on it.

Age

Keratolysis exfoliativa typically affects young adults.

Sex

No sex predilection has been described.

Ethnicity

There are no data.

Associated diseases

Keratolysis exfoliativa may be associated with local hyperhidrosis.

Pathophysiology

The cause is unknown but a recent study suggests that premature corneodesmolysis is the main pathological mechanism [2]. This study showed no association with atopy and filaggrin mutations were not found.

Pathology

Histology and electron microscopy show cleavage and partially degraded corneodesmosomes within the stratum corneum [2]. There is no inflammatory infiltrate.

Environmental factors

Keratolysis exfoliativa often presents in the summer with warmer weather. It can be aggravated by detergents, solvents and irritants.

Clinical features
History

Keratolysis exfoliativa starts as a sudden onset of discrete scaling on the palms of the hands (Figures 85.26 and 85.27).

Presentation

Keratolysis exfoliativa presents initially as small, superficial blister-like, air-filled pockets on the palms and palmar aspects of the fingers or occasionally the feet. These are formed as the result of focal separation of superficial layers of corneocytes from the stratum corneum. The roofs of the pockets rupture centrally as they expand centrifugally, leaving a ragged rim of residual scale surrounding an irregular superficial dry erosion. There is no irritation and vesicles are not present. Peeled areas of skin lack normal barrier function and may become dry and fissured, particularly on the fingertips.

Differential diagnosis

Keratolysis exfoliativa is a very distinctive disorder but may be confused with pompholyx, psoriasis, tinea manuum, epidermolysis bullosa simplex or acral skin peeling syndrome (Chapter 63).

Complications and co-morbidities

Keratolysis exfoliativa may be associated with local hyperhidrosis.

Disease course and prognosis

Keratolysis exfoliativa is generally self-limiting but may recur each summer.

Investigations

No investigations are needed.

Management

Keratolysis exfoliativa is usually a self-limiting condition and treatment may not be needed. Patients should be advised to avoid contact with detergents and other irritants.

PART 8: SPECIFIC CUTANEOUS STRUCTURES

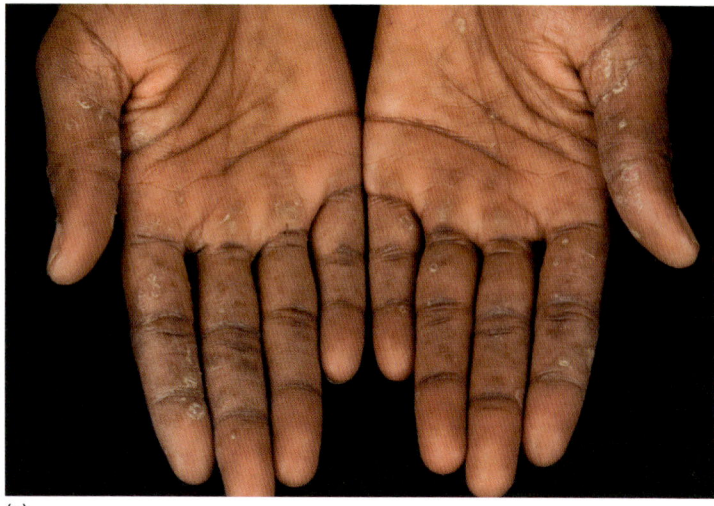

(a)

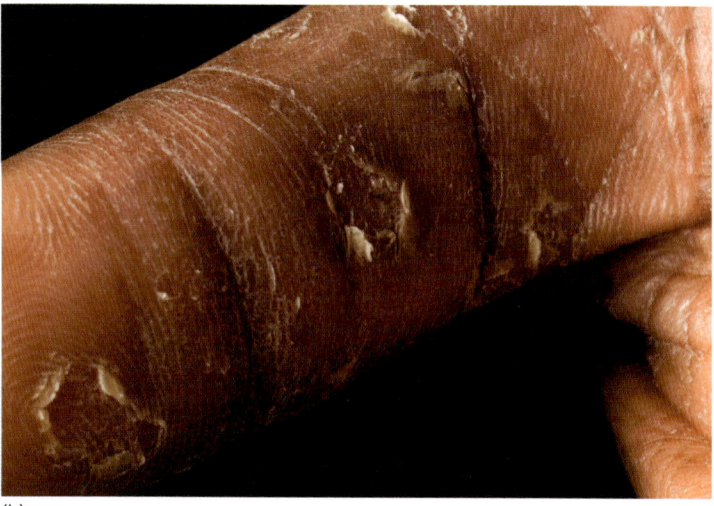

(b)

Figure 85.26 Keratolysis exfoliativa: (a) view of the palms with (b) close-up of the right index finger.

First line

Emollients and moisturisers, particularly those containing urea or salicylic acid, may be useful. Topical steroids may exacerbate the condition by further drying the skin.

Xerosis cutis and asteatosis

Definition and nomenclature

Xerosis cutis (dry skin) and asteatosis (lacking in fat) are alternative terms used to describe an acquired abnormality of the skin that has lost its normal soft smooth surface and feels dry and rough to the touch.

Synonyms and inclusions

- Xeroderma
- Winter itch
- Dry skin

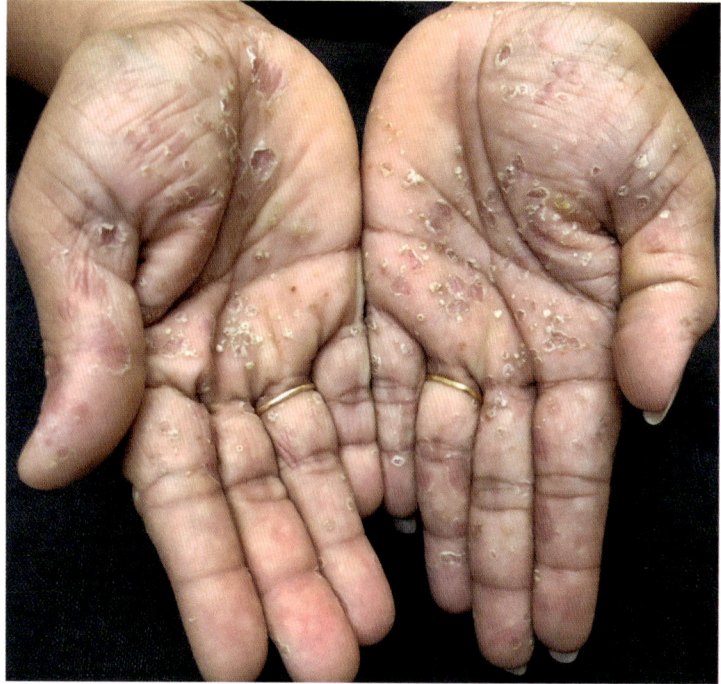

Figure 85.27 Keratolysis exfoliativa affecting the palmar surface of the hands in a female patient. Courtesy of Dr Shyam Verma, Vadodara, India.

Introduction and general description

Xerosis cutis is very common and almost physiological in old age. Xerosis cutis and asteatosis may be the result of a range of endogenous and exogenous factors, especially ageing and low ambient humidity, and are associated with impaired epidermal barrier function. Xerosis cutis may be accompanied by pruritus (winter itch) and predisposes to eczematous inflammation (asteatotic eczema or eczéma craquelé). The condition is associated with an impaired barrier function of the stratum corneum, as reflected by increased transepidermal water loss (TEWL) and reduced water content. Xerosis is generally assessed by clinical examination [1].

Xerosis is also a common component of eczematous skin diseases, for example atopic eczema, where it is present in up to 90% of cases. This is discussed in detail in Chapter 41.

Epidemiology
Incidence and prevalence

Xerosis cutis is very common and almost universal in old age.

Age

It generally first manifests in the seventh decade of life and progresses with age.

Sex

It appears to be slightly more common in men.

Ethnicity

Xerosis cutis is universal in older age groups. In children, it is said to be more prevalent in sub-Saharan Africa, possibly due to high local temperatures. TEWL has been shown to be higher in phototype 6 skin compared with other skin types [2].

Associated diseases

It may be observed in association with marasmus, malnutrition, diabetes, renal failure and renal dialysis.

Pathophysiology

Xerosis cutis was initially thought to be due to reduced sebum production with age. The major factors in the development of dry skin, however, appear to be changes in stratum corneum function and lipids [3]. There is a deficiency of all stratum corneum lipids as well as premature expression of involucrin and persistence of corneodesmosomes [4–7]. Loricrin expression does not appear to be changed [5]. Dry skin also shows decreases in keratin 1 and 10 and an increase of keratin 5 and 14. In women, oestrogen substitution ameliorates dry skin, indicating a role for sex hormones [8].

Predisposing factors

It is more common in winter where humidity is low, and central heating tends to aggravate the condition. Damage to the stratum corneum by excessive contact with soap or detergents or from frequent and prolonged bathing have each been proposed as additional exacerbating factors, although one study found no difference in bathing habits between patients with widespread asteatotic eczema and controls [9]. Lack of oestrogen is thought to be a contributory factor in postmenopausal women [8].

Pathology

There are no histological abnormalities apart from a slight irregularity in the stratum corneum.

Environmental factors

Low humidity in the winter and the drying effects of central heating exacerbate xerosis cutis. The generally dry atmosphere in hospital wards increases the risk in frail elderly patients confined to hospital for prolonged periods. Targeted anticancer therapies may induce xerosis [10].

Clinical features

History

Dryness and scaliness of the skin is generally the first manifestation of the condition, followed by itching.

Presentation

Xerosis cutis most often affects the shins and may not affect any other area of the skin. It may become widespread but spares the face, neck, palms and soles. In elderly, immobile, hospitalised patients, it will frequently affect the abdomen and, in women, the anterior surfaces of the breasts, but spares the back and the undersurfaces of the breasts.

Affected skin looks dull, dry and covered with fine scale which sheds readily. The surface may become crazed with criss-cross superficial cracks in the stratum corneum giving the skin a 'crazy-paving' look (Figures 85.28 and 85.29).

Clinical variants

Asteatotic eczema (eczéma craquelé). Xerosis cutis may progress to an eczematous inflammation in which the fissures in the skin

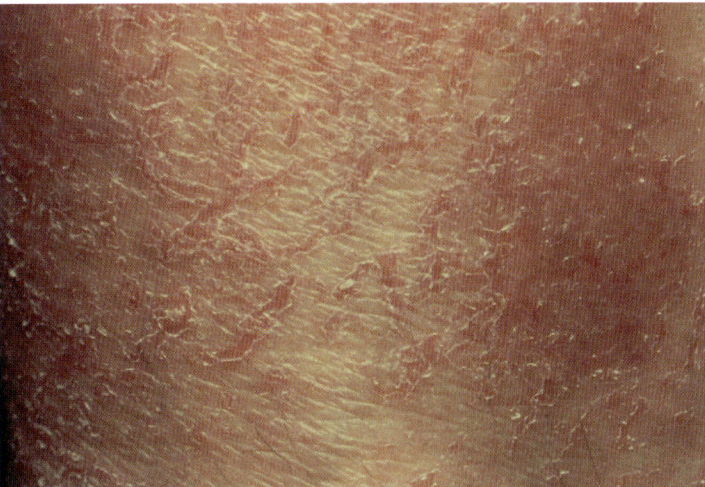

Figure 85.28 Xerosis cutis: scaling is present, with a degree of redness. When a higher degree of redness and pruritus is present, the diagnosis may be considered to be asteatotic eczema, which is a clinical variant on the same disease spectrum.

Figure 85.29 Xerosis cutis affecting the flank of a patient with dark skin. Courtesy of Dr Shyam Verma, Vadodara, India.

surface become red, inflamed and itchy (Figure 85.30). Asteatotic eczema may sometimes be seen after episodes of acute distension of the skin, usually due to acute oedema (see Figure 85.32).

Differential diagnosis

Dry scaly skin is a component of many inflammatory skin diseases. These include atopic eczema (Chapter 41), hereditary ichthyosis (Chapter 63) and acquired ichthyosis (see earlier in this chapter). Apart from the latter, these generally manifest at an early age.

Disease course and prognosis

Xerosis cutis is often seasonal, being worse or occurring only in the winter; it tends to worsen and become more persistent with age.

Management

Basic skin care in the treatment of xerosis cutis is intended to improve skin hydration, compensate the lack in barrier lipids and improve the skin's barrier function [11].

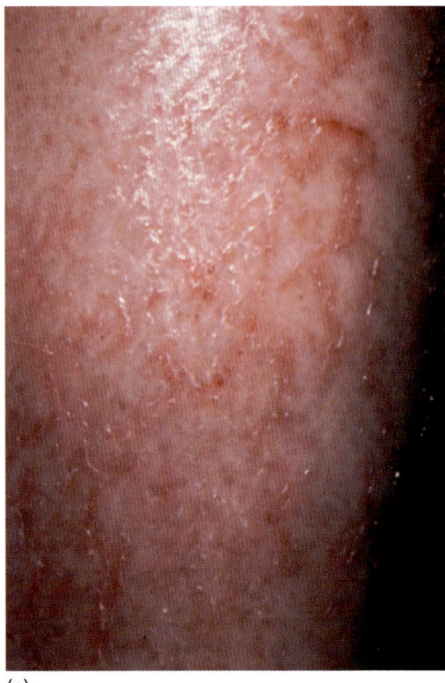

(a)

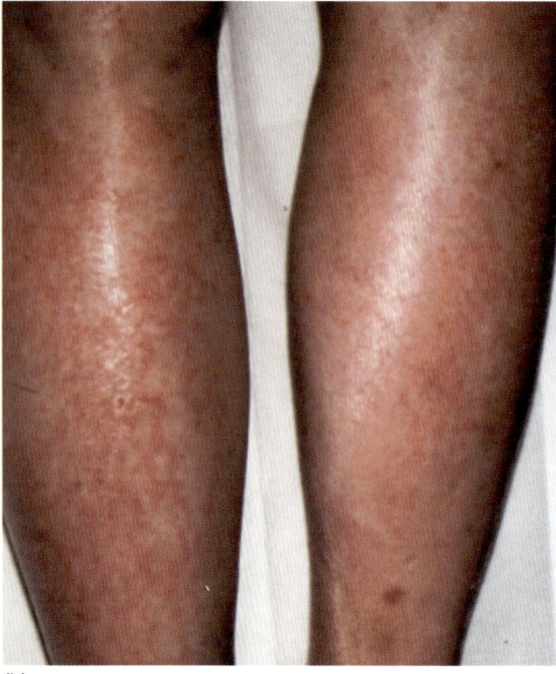

(b)

Figure 85.30 (a, b) Asteatotic eczema: deeper redness and rhagades (linear cracks) signify a more inflammatory process than typical xerosis cutis.

Precipitating factors should be removed. Patients should be instructed to avoid applying any irritants to the skin. Limiting luke-warm baths to a maximum of 5 minutes and avoiding hot showers and baths is recommended [11]. Simple measures to increase the humidity of centrally heated rooms (e.g. placing a bowl of water close to radiators) may alleviate environmental factors.

First line
Emollients and moisturisers are the treatment of choice and usually result in rapid improvement when compliance is good. Emollients with hydrophilic ingredients such as urea, alongside physiological lipids such as ceramides to replenish the skin barrier, are the most effective [11].

Second line
If asteatotic eczema develops, anti-inflammatory treatment with a mild corticosteroid ointment may be necessary but long-term topical corticosteroids should be avoided, as these may further damage the skin barrier. Topical tacrolimus and pimecrolimus have also been advocated for the treatment of asteatotic eczema [12,13].

Acute epidermal distension and acute oedema blisters

Definition and nomenclature
There are certain situations where the epidermis is unable to with-stand forces that would normally not affect its integrity. Acute distension of uninflamed skin in the absence of disordered epi-dermal integrity may at times result in epidermal separation or disruption. Most commonly, this is due to acute dependent oedema,

as from acute congestive heart failure, and results in large bullae which may be mistaken for bullous pemphigoid. Alternatively, the distension may result in disruption of epidermal cohesion manifesting as asteatotic eczema.

Synonyms and inclusions
- Acute oedema blisters
- Eczéma craquelé due to acute cutaneous distension
- Fracture blisters

Introduction and general description
Subepidermal blistering is a well-recognised component of many skin disorders in which there are hereditary or acquired abnor-malities affecting the normal adhesion of the epidermis to the

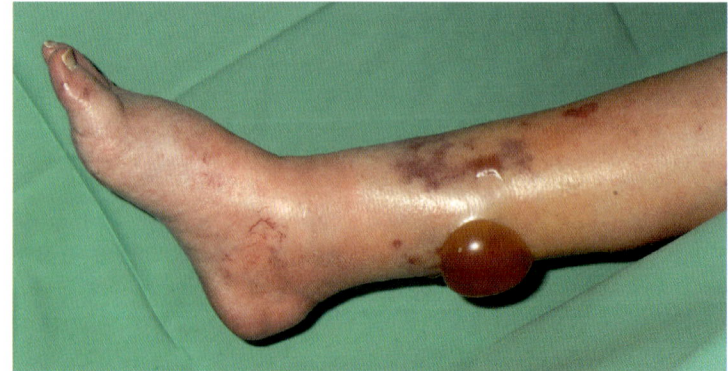

Figure 85.31 Acute oedema blisters in an elderly female: acute swelling of the lower limbs after withdrawal of diuretic therapy given for congestive heart failure (complicated by cellulitis which responded rapidly to antibiotics but left residual purpura).

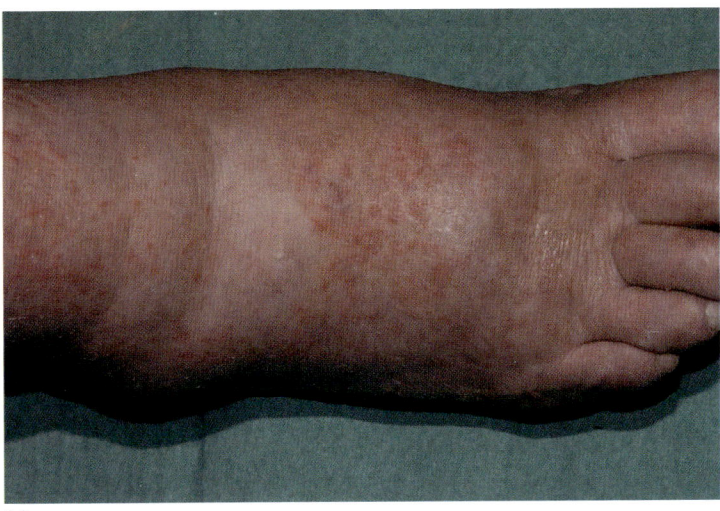

(a)

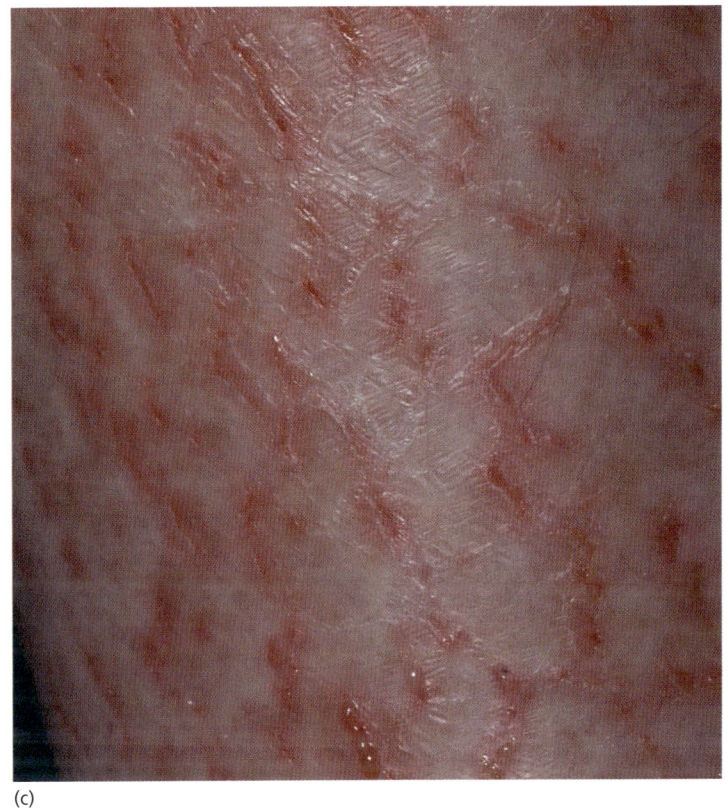

(c)

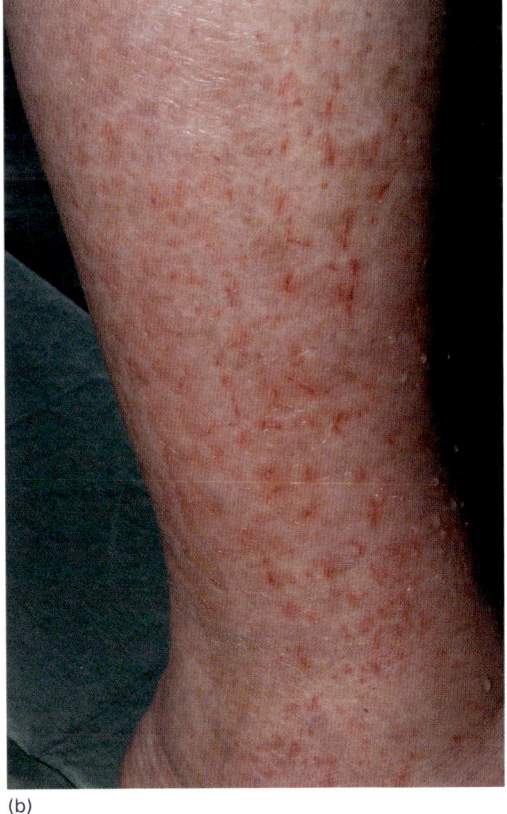

(b)

Figure 85.32 (a–c) Asteatotic eczema following acute onset of oedema due to congestive heart failure.

dermis. It is also a normal reaction to excessive thermal or frictional trauma.

Bullae may also occur in otherwise normal skin as a consequence of the rapid onset of oedema. The speed of development of such acute oedema appears to be a more important risk factor than the degree of oedema. The blisters respond rapidly to reduction of the oedema [1]. It has been described after attacks of angioedema as well as in the elderly following the sudden onset or exacerbation of oedema, such as after acute congestive heart failure [1,2–4].

Epidemiology
Incidence and prevalence
It has been only reported in case series, and no structured studies are available.

Age
It may appear in any person who develops oedema acutely, and the elderly appear to be more susceptible [2].

Pathophysiology

Little is known about the pathophysiology of this disease. Ultrasound studies of acute oedema suggest that fluids accumulate more superficially in the dermis than following lymphoedema or chronic venous stasis [5,6], which may sometimes be a contributory factor.

Pathology

Biopsies have shown marked epidermal spongiosis and a slight lymphohistiocytic inflammatory infiltrate. Direct immunofluorescence was negative [2].

Clinical features

History

There is an acute onset of oedema without itching.

Presentation

Tense, unilocular, non-pruritic bullae appear in areas of acute oedema (Figure 85.31).

Clinical variants

Acute cutaneous distension may alternatively result in disruption of the epidermis as seen in asteatotic eczema with crazing and fissuring of the epidermis and leakage of oedema fluid to the surface (Figure 85.32) [1,7,8].

A combination of shearing stress on the dermal–epidermal junction plus resultant soft-tissue oedema can cause tense bullae overlying the site of fractures, known as fracture blisters [9].

Differential diagnosis

In the elderly population, autoimmune bullous diseases, particularly bullous pemphigoid, are an important differential diagnosis. The close temporal association with acute oedema, the absence of itching and the lack of spread to other areas of the body form important clues to the diagnosis.

Diabetic bullae (Chapter 62) may resemble acute oedema blisters but are generally not so tense and they are not associated with acute oedema (Figure 85.33).

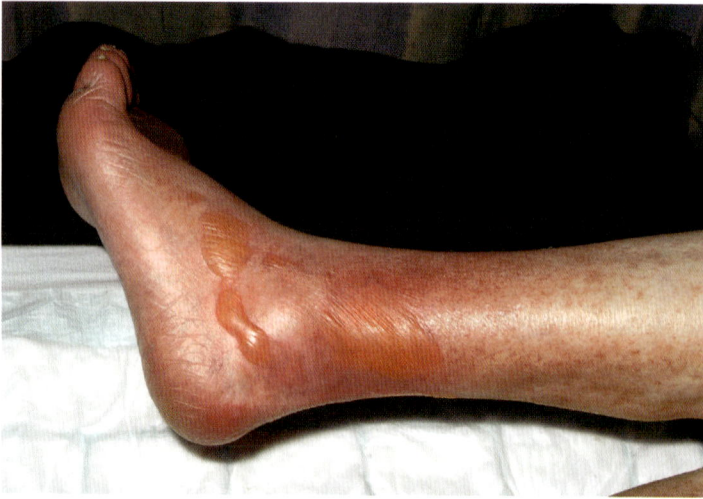

Figure 85.33 Diabetic bullae: recent development of extensive large bullae on the lower legs and feet in the absence of inflammation or oedema in a patient with longstanding diabetes: the bullae are less tense but more irregular in shape and there is no oedema.

Disease course and prognosis

The lesions resolve rapidly as the oedema resolves, leaving no scars.

Investigations

This is a clinically defined disease without known pathognomonic tests. In some cases, the attending dermatologist may wish to rule out autoimmune bullous disorders through direct immunofluorescence or identification of circulating antibodies.

Management

First line

Oedema should be reduced through the appropriate management of the underlying disease. Aseptic puncture of individual lesions can be done to reduce the risk of ulceration.

Key references

The full list of references can be found in the online version at https://www.wiley.com/rooksdermatology10e

Acquired ichthyosis

 1 Patel N, Spencer LA, English JC, III et al. Acquired ichthyosis. *J Am Acad Dermatol* 2006;55:647–56.

Acanthosis nigricans

 1 Brickman WJ, Binns HJ, Jovanovic BD, Kolesky S, Mancini AJ, Metzger BE. Acanthosis nigricans: a common finding in overweight youth. *Pediatr Dermatol* 2007;24:601–6.

Confluent and reticulated papillomatosis

 2 Scheinfeld N. Confluent and reticulated papillomatosis: a review of the literature. *Am J Clin Dermatol* 2006;7:305–13.

Pityriasis rotunda

 2 Findlay GH. Pityriasis rotunda in South African Bantu. *Br J Dermatol* 1965;77:63–4.

Keratosis pilaris

32 Maghfour J, Ly S, Haidari W et al. Treatment of keratosis pilaris and its variants: a systematic review. *J Dermatolog Treat* 2022;33:1231–42.

Lichen spinulosus

 3 Friedman SJ. Lichen spinulosus. Clinicopathologic review of thirty-five cases. *J Am Acad Dermatol* 1990;22:261–4.

Keratosis circumscripta

 5 Shams M, Blalock TW, Davis LS. Keratosis circumscripta: a unique case and review of the literature. *Int J Dermatol* 2011;50:1259–61.

Phrynoderma

 9 Ragunatha S, Kumar VJ, Murugesh SB. A clinical study of 125 patients with phrynoderma. *Indian J Dermatol* 2011;56:389–92.

Trichodysplasia spinulosa

16 Curman P, Näsman A, Brauner H. Trichodysplasia spinulosa: a comprehensive review of the disease and its treatment. *J Eur Acad Dermatol Venereol* 2021;35:1067–76.

Flegel disease

13 Pearson LH, Smith JG, Jr, Chalker DK. Hyperkeratosis lenticularis perstans (Flegel's disease). Case report and literature review. *J Am Acad Dermatol* 1987;16:190–5.

Multiple minute digitate keratoses

10 Caccetta TP, Dessauvagie B, McCallum D, Kumarasinghe SP. Multiple minute digitate hyperkeratosis: a proposed algorithm for the digitate keratoses. *J Am Acad Dermatol* 2012;67:e49–55.

Porokeratoses

26 Sasson M, Krain AD. Porokeratosis and cutaneous malignancy. A review. *Dermatol Surg* 1996;22:339–42.

32 Atzmony L, Young HL, Hamilton C *et al.* Topical cholesterol/lovastatin for the treatment of porokeratosis: a pathogenesis-directed therapy. *J Am Acad Dermatol* 2020;82:123–31.

Transient acantholytic dermatosis

9 Anforth R, Carlos G, Clements A *et al.* Cutaneous adverse events in patients treated with BRAF inhibitor-based therapies for metastatic melanoma for longer than 52 weeks. *Br J Dermatol* 2015;172:239–43.

Keratolysis exfoliativa

2 Chang YY, van der Velden J, van der Wier G *et al.* Keratolysis exfoliativa (dyshidrosis lamellose sicca): a distinct peeling entity. *Br J Dermatol* 2012;167:1076–84.

Xerosis cutis and asteatosis

1 Berry N, Charmeil C, Goujon C *et al.* A clinical, biometrological and ultrastructural study of xerotic skin. *Int J Cosmet Sci* 1999;21:241–52.

Acute epidermal distension and acute oedema blisters

1 Cox NH, Chalmers RJG, Bhushan M. The acute edema/cutaneous distension syndrome. *Arch Dermatol* 2003;139:224–5.

Index

Note: Page numbers in *italics* refer to figures and those in **bold** refer to tables and boxes, where they fall outside the main text range. References are to pages within chapters, thus 58.10 is page 10 of Chapter 58.